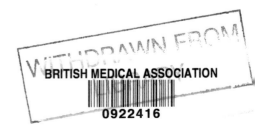

Principles and Practice of Surgical Oncology

Multidisciplinary Approach to
Difficult Problems

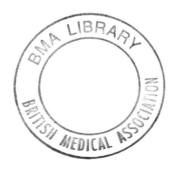

Principles and Practice of Surgical Oncology

Multidisciplinary Approach to Difficult Problems

Editors:

Howard Silberman, MD

Professor of Surgery
Keck School of Medicine
University of Southern California
Los Angeles, California

Allan W. Silberman, MD, PhD

Robert J. and Suzanne Gottlieb Endowed Chair in Surgical Oncology
Samuel Oschin Comprehensive Cancer Institute
Cedars-Sinai Medical Center
Los Angeles, California

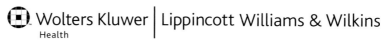

Wolters Kluwer | Lippincott Williams & Wilkins
Health

Philadelphia · Baltimore · New York · London
Buenos Aires · Hong Kong · Sydney · Tokyo

Senior Executive Editor: Jonathan W. Pine, Jr.
Senior Product Managers: Joyce Murphy, Emilie Moyer
Vendor Manager: Alicia Jackson
Senior Manufacturing Manager: Benjamin Rivera
Senior Marketing Manager: Angela Panetta
Cover Designer: Joseph DePinho
Production Service: Aptara Corp.

Printed in China

Library of Congress Cataloging-in-Publication Data

Principles and practice of surgical oncology : multidisciplinary approach to difficult problems / editors, Howard Silberman, Allan W. Silberman.
    p. ; cm.
   Includes bibliographical references and index.
   ISBN-13: 978-0-7817-6546-6 (hardback : alk. paper)
   ISBN 0-7817-6546-3 (hardback : alk. paper) (invalid) 0-7817-6546-6
1. Cancer—Surgery.   I. Silberman, Howard.   II. Silberman, Allan W.
   [DNLM: 1. Neoplasms—surgery.   2. Combined Modality Therapy.
QZ 268 P9564 2010]
   RD651.P85   2010
   616.99′4059—dc22   2009022111

Care has been taken to confirm the accuracy of the information presented and to describe generally accepted practices. However, the authors, editors, and publisher are not responsible for errors or omissions or for any consequences from application of the information in this book and make no warranty, expressed or implied, with respect to the currency, completeness, or accuracy of the contents of the publication. Application of the information in a particular situation remains the professional responsibility of the practitioner.

The authors, editors, and publisher have exerted every effort to ensure that drug selection and dosage set forth in this text are in accordance with current recommendations and practice at the time of publication. However, in view of ongoing research, changes in government regulations, and the constant flow of information relating to drug therapy and drug reactions, the reader is urged to check the package insert for each drug for any change in indications and dosage and for added warnings and precautions. This is particularly important when the recommended agent is a new or infrequently employed drug.

Some drugs and medical devices presented in the publication have Food and Drug Administration (FDA) clearance for limited use in restricted research settings. It is the responsibility of the health care provider to ascertain the FDA status of each drug or device planned for use in their clinical practice.

To purchase additional copies of this book, call our customer service department at (800) 638-3030 or fax orders to (301) 223-2320. International customers should call (301) 223-2300.

Visit Lippincott Williams & Wilkins on the Internet: at LWW.com. Lippincott Williams & Wilkins customer service representatives are available from 8:30 am to 6 pm, EST.

10 9 8 7 6 5 4 3 2 1

In memory of
Mom and Dad and Auntie
In honor of
Kathy and Samantha

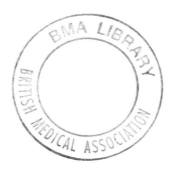

Preface

The management of solid tumors has undergone dramatic evolution in the last century. The earlier approach to cure called for increasingly more radical surgical extirpation in accordance with the Halstedian concept that cancer spreads primarily by contiguous extension throughout the body. Advances in cancer biology, pathology, and imaging sciences have led to more limited, conservative surgery with perioperative adjunctive therapies designed to address micrometastatic deposits that are now known to frequently exist at even the earliest stages of clinically evident disease. Such occult systemic disease undoubtedly explains the treatment failures commonly observed after apparently successful surgical resection alone.

Thus, to provide optimal oncologic care in the 21st century, the surgeon must not only be technically adroit but must also be well versed in the biology of cancer and have a thorough understanding of the range of therapies that other oncologic disciplines can offer patients in order to enhance outcome. The advantages of a multidisciplinary approach in the evaluation and treatment of patients with solid tumors has become increasingly clear over the last two decades. It is our view that neoadjuvant and/or adjuvant therapy is worthy of consideration in many, even the majority, of our patients at the present time, and we expect that adjunctive treatments will be an essential component of therapy in virtually all patients with solid tumors as research yields effective new therapies, including more potent pharmacologic and biologic agents, and advances in other treatment modalities, such as radiation therapy, cryosurgery, and radiofrequency ablation.

We present a multidisciplinary analysis of the common solid malignancies, highlighting the controversial issues in clinical judgment surrounding each problem. We include 59 chapters, contributed by authorities representing the whole spectrum of disciplines contributing to the evaluation and management of patients with cancer. Nonsurgical topics include genetics and cancer pathogenesis; nutritional support of the cancer patient; targeted therapy; imaging techniques, including detailed discussions of breast-imaging techniques; an overview of radiation therapy; cancer and pregnancy; and pain management. Surgical topics include the surgical approach to metastatic melanoma; bone tumors; tumors of the spleen; laparoscopic versus open colon surgery; pelvic exenteration; neuroendocrine tumors; gastrointestinal stromal tumors; small bowel tumors; tumors arising in inflammatory bowel disease; primary vascular tumors; thyroid cancer; surgical and adjuvant treatment of lung cancer; surgical and adjuvant therapy of urologic cancers; ovarian cancer; and biliary cancers. The inclusion of these chapters broadens the scope from general surgical oncology to cover related subspecialties such as, thoracic, vascular, orthopaedic, urologic, head and neck, and gynecologic oncology.

Clinical judgments that must be rendered prior to the availability of conclusive scientific evidence often differ among even the most experienced physicians. We believe that other viewpoints are often necessary to highlight and emphasize the problem in order to understand such controversial issues. Thus, each of our primary chapters is followed by a commentary written by other experts in the field and offers a contrasting opinion or discusses a tangential issue that may not have been presented by the primary authors.

Finally, we wish to express our gratitude to Jonathan W. Pine Jr., Senior Executive Editor at Lippincott Williams & Wilkins, who, after favorably evaluating our proposal to update and expand our original volume, provided us the much-appreciated opportunity to prepare this work. In addition, we must acknowledge the assistance of our editors, Anne Jacobs, Joyce Murphy, and Emilie Moyer at Lippincott, and Larry Fox at Aptara Corp., whose extraordinary attention to the details of organizing and reviewing the various materials comprising the book greatly improved the quality of the final product.

Allan W. Silberman
Howard Silberman
Los Angeles, California

Contents

Contributors

Elke R. Ahlmann, MD
Department of Orthopaedics
Division of Oncology
Los Angeles County-University of Southern
California Medical Center
Los Angeles, California

Randa Alsabeh, MD
Associate Clinical Professor
David Geffen School of Medicine
University of California, Los Angeles
Director, Immunopathology Laboratory
Co-Director Special Testing
Cedars-Sinai Medical Center
Los Angeles, California

Farin F. Amersi, MD, FACS
Attending Surgical Oncologist
Samuel Oschin Comprehensive Cancer Institute
Associate Director, Surgery Residency Program
Department of Surgery
Cedars-Sinai Medical Center
Los Angeles, California

Benjamin O. Anderson, MD
Professor of Surgery
Director, Breast Health Center
University of Washington
Seattle Cancer Care Alliance
Seattle, Washington

Pramila Rani Anné, MD
Instructor
Department of Radiation Oncology
Kimmel Cancer Center
Jefferson Medical College
Philadelphia, Pennsylvania

Karen Antman, MD
Provost, Boston University Medical Campus
Dean and Professor of Medicine
Boston University School of Medicine
Boston, Massachusetts

Bach Ardalan, MD
Professor of Medicine and Cellular Pharmacology
Sylvester Comprehensive Cancer Center
University of Miami
Miami, Florida

M. William Audeh, MD
Associate Clinical Professor of Medicine
David Geffen School of Medicine
University of California, Los Angeles
Los Angeles, California
Medical Oncologist
Department of Medicine
Cedars-Sinai Medical Center
Los Angeles, California

Glenn T. Ault, MD
Assistant Professor of Surgery
Division of Colorectal Surgery
Keck School of Medicine
University of Southern California
Los Angeles, California

Laurence H. Baker, DO
Executive Director
Sarcoma Alliance for Research Through Collaboration (SARC)
Professor of Medicine and Pharmacology
University of Michigan
Ann Arbor, Michigan

Marija Balic, MD
Department of Pathology
Kenneth Norris Comprehensive Cancer Center
Keck School of Medicine
University of Southern California
Los Angeles, California

Charles M. Balch, MD
Professor of Surgery, Oncology, and Dermatology
Johns Hopkins Medical Center
Baltimore, Maryland

Robert W. Beart, Jr., MD
Professor of Surgery
Division of Colorectal Surgery
Keck School of Medicine
University of Southern California
Los Angeles, California

Chandra P. Belani, MD
Miriam Beckner Professor of Medicine
Penn State Milton S. Hershey Medical Center
Deputy Director
Penn State Cancer Institute
Hershey, Pennsylvania

George Berci, MD, FACS, FRCS, ED (Hon)
Senior Director, Minimally Invasive Surgery Research
Department of Surgery
Cedars-Sinai Medical Center
Los Angeles, California

J. Sybil Biermann, MD
Associate Professor of Orthopaedic Surgery
University of Michigan
Ann Arbor, Michigan
Director, Musculoskeletal Oncology
Medical Director, Sarcoma Clinic
Ann Arbor, Michigan

Leslie H. Blumgart, MD, FACS, FRCS
Enid A. Haupt Chair in Surgery
Attending Surgeon
Department of Surgery
Memorial Sloan Kettering Cancer Center
New York, New York

Michael L. Blute, MD
Professor and Chair
Department of Urology
Mayo Medical School and Mayo Clinic
Rochester, Minnesota

William D. Boswell, MD
Professor of Clinical Radiology
Chief, Department of Radiology
Kenneth Norris Comprehensive Cancer Center
Keck School of Medicine
University of Southern California
Los Angeles, California

Leslie Botnick, MD
Chief Medical Officer
Vantage Oncology, Inc.
Manhattan Beach, California

Glenn D. Braunstein, MD
Chairman, Department of Medicine
The James R. Klinenberg Chair in Medicine
Cedars-Sinai Medical Center
Professor of Medicine
The David Geffen School of Medicine
University of California, Los Angeles
Los Angeles, California

Murray F. Brennan, MD, FACS
Professor of Surgery
Weill Medical College of Cornell University
Benno C. Schmidt Chair in Clinical Oncology
Department of Surgery
Memorial Sloan-Kettering Cancer Center
New York, New York

Earl Brien, MD
Director, Musculoskeletal Tumor Service
Cedars-Sinai Medical Center
Los Angeles, California

Thomas A. Buchholz, MD
Professor and Chairman
Department of Radiation Oncology
The University of Texas, MD Anderson
    Cancer Center
Houston, Texas

Ronald W. Busuttil, MD, PhD
Professor of Surgery
David Geffen School of Medicine
University of California at Los Angeles
Los Angeles, California
Chairman
Department of Surgery
Ronald Reagan-University of California at Los Angeles
    Medical Center
Los Angeles, California

John A. Butler, MD
Professor of Surgery
Chief
Division of Surgical Oncology
University of California, Irvine Medical Center
Orange, California

Blake Cady, MD
Professor of Surgery
Brown Medical School
Interim Director, Comprehensive Breast Center
Rhode Island Hospital
Providence, Rhode Island

Kristine E. Calhoun, MD
Assistant Professor of Surgery
Section of Surgical Oncology
Department of Surgery
University of Washington
Seattle, Washington

Ilana Cass, MD
Division of Gynecologic Oncology
Department Obstetrics and Gynecology
Cedars-Sinai Medical Center
Associate Professor of Obstetrics and Gynecology
David Geffen School of Medicine
University of California, Los Angeles
Los Angeles, California

Bruce A. Chabner, MD
Clinical Director, MGH Cancer Center
Massachusetts General Hospital
Professor of Medicine
Harvard Medical School
Boston, Massachusetts

Parakrama Chandrasoma, MD
Professor of Pathology
Keck School of Medicine
Chief of Anatomic Pathology
Los Angeles County-University of Southern California
    Medical Center
Los Angeles, California

Antony J. Charles, MD
Mayo Clinic
Jacksonville, Florida

H. H. Tony Chen, DDS, PhD
Professor of Epidemiology and Statistics
Graduate Institue of Epidemiology
College of Public health
National Taiwan University
Taipei, Taiwan

Sherry Yueh-Hsia Chiu, PhD
Graduate Institute of Epidemiology
College of Public Health
National Taiwan University
Taipei, Taiwan

Michael A. Choti, MD, MBA, FACS
Jacob C. Handelsman Professor of Surgery
Johns Hopkins School of Medicine
Baltimore, Maryland

Toni K. Choueiri, MD
Department of Solid Tumor Oncology
Cleveland Clinic Taussig Cancer Center
Cleveland, Ohio

Gregory M. Chronowski, MD
Assistant Professor
Department of Radiation Oncology
The University of Texas, MD Anderson Cancer Center
Houston, Texas

Cathie T. Chung, MD, PhD
Staff Physician
Medical Oncology and Therapeutics Research
City of Hope National Medical Center
Duarte, California

Mary E. Cianfrocca, DO
Assistant Professor of Medicine
Division of Hematology/Oncology
Feinberg School of Medicine
Northwestern University
Chicago, Illinois

Orlo H. Clark, MD
Professor and Vice Chair
Department of Surgery, University California,
    San Francisco,
Comprehensive Cancer Center at Mount Zion,
    Medical Center
San Francisco, California

Steven D. Colquhoun, MD
Associate Professor
Department of Surgery
University of California, Los Angeles
Director of Liver Transplant Program
Department of Surgery
Cedars-Sinai Medical Center
Los Angeles, California

David V. Cossman, MD
Attending Surgeon
Medical Director, Cedars-Sinai Vascular Laboratory
Co-Director of Vascular Trauma
Division of Vascular Surgery
Cedars-Sinai Medical Center
Los Angeles, California

Richard J. Cote, MD, FRCPath
Professor and Chair
Department of Pathology
Leonard M. Miller School of Medicine
University of Miami
Miami, Florida

Peter F. Crookes, MD
Associate Professor of Surgery
Keck School of Medicine
University of Southern California
Los Angeles, California

Jason Cundiff, MD
Department of Surgery
Louisiana State University Health Sciences Center
New Orleans, Louisiana

Walter J. Curran, Jr., MD
Professor and Chair
Department of Radiation Oncology
Emory School of Medicine
Chief Medical Officer
Emory Winship Cancer Institute
Atlanta, Georgia

John M. Daly, MD
Harry C. Donahoo Professor of Surgery and Dean
Temple University School of Medicine
Philadelphia, Pennsylvania

Michael D'Angelica, MD
Assistant Professor of Surgery
Weil Medical College of Cornell University
Assistant Attending Surgeon
Memorial Sloan Kettering Cancer Center
New York, New York

Peter B. Dean, MD
Professor of Radiology
University of Turku
Director of Breast Imaging
Turku University Hospital
Turku, Finland

Robert W. Decker, MD
Tower Hematology Oncology Medical Group
Beverly Hills, California

Wendy DeMartini, MD
Assistant Professor of Radiology
Section of Breast Imaging
University of Washington
Seattle, Washington

John F. DiPersio, MD, PhD
Professor of Medicine
Washington University in St. Louis
St. Louis, Missouri
Chairman of Oncology
Division of Oncology
Department of Medicine
Barnes-Jewish Hospital
St. Louis, Missouri

John H. Donohue, MD
Professor of Surgery
Mayo Medical School
Division of Gastroenterologic and General Surgery
Mayo Clinic and Mayo Foundation
Rochester, Minnesota

Vinay A. Duddalwar, MD, FRCR
Assistant Professor of Radiology
Keck School of Medicine
University of Southern California
Section Chief, Abdominal Imaging
Department of Radiology
Norris Cancer Center
University of Southern California
Los Angeles, California

Stanley J. Dudrick, MD, FACS
Professor of Surgery
Department of Surgery
Yale School of Medicine
New Haven, Connecticut
Chairman Emeritus
Department of Surgery
Saint Mary's Hospital
Waterbury, Connecticut

John P. Duffy, MD
Clinical Instructor
Department of Surgery
Division of Liver and Pancreas Transplantation
David Geffen School of Medicine
University of California at Los Angeles
Los Angeles, California

Stephen W. Duffy, MSc
Cancer Research UK Centre for Epidemiology, Mathematics,
    and Statistics
Wolfson Institute for Preventive Medicine
Charter House Square, London
United Kingdom

James S. Economou, MD, PhD
Beaumont Professor of Surgery
Chief, Division of Surgical Oncology
Professor of Microbiology, Immunology, and Molecular Genetics
Professor of Molecular and Medical Pharmacology
Director, Human Gene Medicine Program
Deputy Director, Jonsson Comprehensive Cancer Center
David Geffen School of Medicine
University of California at Los Angeles
Los Angeles, California

Frederick R. Eilber, MD
Professor of Surgery
Division of Surgical Oncology
University of California, Los Angeles
Los Angeles, California

Fritz C. Eilber, MD
Assistant Professor of Surgery
Division of Surgical Oncology
University of California, Los Angeles
Los Angeles, California

Anthony B. Elkhouiery, MD
Assistant Professor of Medicine
University of Southern California
Keck School of Medicine
Norris Comprehensive Cancer Center
Los Angeles, California

Richard Essner, MD
Assistant Director, Surgical Oncology
Director, Molecular Therapeutics
John Wayne Cancer Institute
Santa Monica, California

David A. Etzioni, MD, MPH
Assistant Professor of Surgery
Division of Colorectal Surgery
Keck School of Medicine
University of Southern California
Los Angeles, California

Laurie L. Fajardo, MD, MBA
Professor
Department of Radiology
University of Iowa Hospital
Chair
Department of Radiology
University of Iowa Hospitals & Clinics
Iowa City, Iowa

Yuri Falkinstein, MD
Department of Orthopaedics
Los Angeles County-University of Southern
    California Medical Center
Los Angeles, California

Daniel L. Farkas, PhD
Director, Minimally Invasive Surgical Technologies Institute
Vice Chairman for Research
Department of Surgery
Cedars-Sinai Medical Center
Los Angeles, California

Jeffrey M. Farma, MD
Department of Surgery
Temple University School of Medicine
Philadelphia, Pennsylvania

Robert A. Figlin, MD
Professor and Chair, Medical Oncology and
    Therapeutics Research
City of Hope National Medical Center and Beckman Research
    Institute
Associate Director for Clinical Research
City of Hope Comprehensive Cancer Center
Duarte, California

Phillip R. Fleshner, MD
Director, Colorectal Residency Program
Cedars-Sinai Medical Center
Clinical Professor of Surgery
School of Medicine
University of California
Los Angeles, California

Yuman Fong, MD
Professor of Surgery
Weill Cornell Medical Center
Murray F. Brennan Chair in Surgery
Department of Surgery
Memorial Sloan-Kettering Cancer Center
New York, New York

Charles A. Forscher, MD
Medical Director, Sarcoma Service
Samuel Oschin Comprehensive Cancer Institute
Cedars-Sinai Medical Center
Los Angeles, California

Kevin R. Fox, MD
MacDonald Professor of Medicine
Medical Director, Rena Rowan Breast Center
Abramson Cancer Center
University of Pennsylvania
Philadelphia, Pennsylvania

Julie A. Freischlag, MD
William Stewart Halsted Professor of Surgery
Chair, Department of Surgery
Johns Hopkins University School of Medicine
Baltimore, MD

Marc L. Friedman, MD
Director, Vascular/Interventional Radiology
Cedars-Sinai Medical Center
Los Angeles, California

David J. Gallagher, MD
Memorial Sloan-Kettering Cancer Center
New York, New York

Hans Gelderblom, MD, PhD
Department of Clinical Oncology
Leiden University Medical Center
Leiden, The Netherlands

Bruce L. Gewertz, MD
Surgeon-in-Chief
H and S Nichols Endowed Chair in Surgery
Chairman, Department of Surgery
Vice-President for Interventional Services
Cedars-Sinai Medical Center
Los Angeles, California

Mark A. Gittleman, MD
Director
Breast Cancer Specialists
Allentown, Pennsylvania

Armando E. Giuliano, MD
Chief of Science and Medicine
Director, Breast Surgical Oncology
Director, Joyce Eisenberg Keefer Breast Center
John Wayne Cancer Institute
Santa Monica, California

David M. Goldenberg, ScD, MD
President
Center for Molecular Medicine and Immunology
Garden State Cancer Center
Belleville, New Jersey

Leo A. Gordon, MD
Outpatient Cancer Center
Samuel Oschin Comprehensive Cancer Institute
Cedars-Sinai Medical Center
Los Angeles, California

Ora Karp Gordon, MD, MS
Associate Professor
David Geffen School of Medicine
University of California, Los Angeles
Los Angeles, California
Director
GenRISK Adult Program
Medical Genetics
Cedars-Sinai Medical Center
Los Angeles, California

William J. Gradishar, MD
Professor of Medicine
Director of Breast Oncology
Lynn Sage Breast Cancer Program
Robert H. Lurie Comprehensive Cancer Center
Feinberg School of Medicine
Northwestern University
Chicago, Illinois

Frederick L. Greene, MD
Chairman, Department of General Surgery
Department of Surgery
Carolinas Medical Center
Charlotte, North Carolina

Gauree Gupta, MD
Department of Internal Medicine
Cedars-Sinai Medical Center
Los Angeles, California

Alan W. Hackford, MD
Associate Professor of Colorectal Surgery
Tufts University School of Medicine
Chief, Department of Colorectal Surgery
Caritas St. Elizabeth's Medical Center
Boston, Massachusetts

Masanobu Hagiike, MD, PhD
Postgraduate Research Fellow
Department of Surgery
Cedars-Sinai Medical Center
Los Angeles, California

Omid Hamid, MD
Instructor, Division of Medical Oncology
Department of Medicine
Keck School of Medicine
University of Southern California
The Angeles Clinic and Research Institute
Los Angeles, California

Heitham T. Hassoun, MD
Assistant Professor of Surgery
Endovascular and Vascular Surgery
Johns Hopkins University School of Medicine
Baltimore, Maryland

Debra Hawes, MD
Department of Pathology
Kenneth Norris Comprehensive Cancer Center
Keck School of Medicine
University of Southern California
Los Angeles, California

Dennis R. Holmes, MD
Assistant Professor of Clinical Surgery
Harold E. and Henrietta C. Lee Breast Center
Kenneth Norris Comprehensive Cancer Center
Keck School of Medicine
University of Southern California
Los Angeles, California

David S. B. Hoon, MSc, PhD
Full Member, Director
Department of Molecular Oncology
John Wayne Cancer Institute at St. John's Health Center
Santa Monica, California

Mustafa Hussain, MD
Department of Surgery
New York University
New York, New York

James F. Huth, MD
Professor of Surgery
Occidental Chemical Chair in Cancer Research
University of Texas Southwestern School of Medicine
Dallas, Texas

Nola Hylton, PhD
Professor in Residence
Department of Radiology
University of California, San Francisco
San Francisco, California

Syma Iqbal, MD
Assistant Professor of Medicine
Division of Medical Oncology
Kenneth Norris Jr. Comprehensive Cancer Center
Keck School of Medicine
University of Southern California
Los Angeles, California

Yuichiro Ito, MD
Research Fellow
Minimally Invasive Surgery
Cedars-Sinai Medical Center
Los Angeles, California

Nicolas Jabbour, MD
Medical Director
Nazih Zuhdi Transplant Institute
INTEGRIS Baptist Medical Center
Oklahoma City, Oklahoma

Lisa K. Jacobs, MD
Assistant Professor of Surgery
Johns Hopkins Medical Center
Baltimore, Maryland

Hossein Jadvar, MD, PhD, MPH, MBA
Associate Professor of Radiology and Biomedical Engineering
Department of Radiology
Keck School of Medicine
University of Southern California
Los Angeles, California
Director of Radiology Research
Department of Radiology
University of Southern California Medical Center
Los Angeles, California
Visiting Associate in Bioengineering
California Institute of Technology
Pasadena, California

Ajay Jain, MD
Department of Surgery
Johns Hopkins University School of Medicine
Baltimore, Maryland

Larry R. Kaiser, MD
President
University of Texas Health Science Center
Houston, Texas
Formerly, The John Rhea Barton Professor and Chairman
Department of Surgery
University of Pennsylvania Surgeon-in-Chief
University of Pennsylvania Health System
Philadelphia, Pennsylvania

John J. Kavanagh, Jr., MD
Professor of Medicine
Chair, International Oncology Program
Chulalongkorn University
Bangkok, Thailand
Formerly Professor of Medicine
Department of Gynecologic Medical Oncology
The University of Texas MD Anderson Cancer Center
Houston, Texas

Nancy E. Kemeny, MD
Professor of Medicine
Weill Medical College of Cornell University
Attending Physician
Gastrointestinal Oncology Service
Memorial Sloan-Kettering Cancer Center
New York, New York

Andrew S. Klein, MD, MBA
Professor of Surgery
David Geffen School of Medicine
University of California, Los Angeles
Los Angeles, California
Director
Comprehensive Transplant Center
Cedars-Sinai Medical Center
Los Angeles, California

David A. Kooby, MD
Assistant Professor of Surgery
Emory University School of Medicine
Atlanta, Georgia

Olga Kozyreva, MD
Department of Medicine
Tufts University
Boston, Massachusetts

S. Ram Kumar, MD, PhD
Division of Cardiothoracic Surgery
Department of Surgery
Keck School of Medicine
University of Southern California
Los Angeles, California

David Krag, MD
SD Ireland Professor of Surgical Oncology
University of Vermont
College of Medicine
Burlington, Vermont

David I. Kuperman, MD
Instructor
Division of Oncology
Department of Medicine
Washington University in St. Louis
Staff Physician
Division of Oncology
Department of Medicine
Barnes-Jewish Hospital
St. Louis, Missouri

John C. Kucharczuk, MD
Assistant Professor of Surgery
University of Pennsylvania School of Medicine
Philadelphia, Pennsylvania

Karen T. Lane, MD
Assistant Professor
Department of Surgery
University of California, Irvine
Clinical Director, Breast Health Center
University of California, Irvine Medical Center
Orange, California

Julie R. Lange, MD
Assistant Professor of Surgery, Oncology, and Dermatology
Johns Hopkins Medical Center
Baltimore, Maryland

Linda Hovanessian Larsen, MD
Associate Professor of Clinical Radiology
Keck School of Medicine
University of Southern California
Los Angeles, California

James A. Lee, MD
Professor and Vice Chair
Department of Surgery, University California, San Francisco
Comprehensive Cancer Center at Mount Zion,
    Medical Center
San Francisco, California

Sarah J. Lee, MD
Clinical Fellow
Minimally Invasive Surgery
Cedars-Sinai Medical Center
Los Angeles, California

Alan T. Lefor, MD, MPH
Professor
Department of Surgery
Jichi Medical University
Tochigi, Japan
Director, Division of Surgical Oncology
Director, Surgical Education and Academic Affairs
Department of Surgery
Cedars-Sinai Medical Center
Los Angeles, California

Constance D. Lehman, MD, PhD
Professor of Radiology
Director, Section of Breast Imaging
University of Washington
Director, Breast Imaging
Seattle Cancer Care Alliance
Seattle, Washington

Cynthia Gail Leichman, MD
Director, Clinical Research
Desert Regional Medical Cancer
Aptium Oncology Inc.
Palms Springs, California

Lawrence Leichman, MD
Director, Gastrointestinal Oncology Program
Aptium Oncology Inc.
Palm Springs, California

Heinz-Josef Lenz, MD
Professor of Medicine and Preventive Medicine
Division of Medical Oncology
Kenneth Norris Comprehensive Cancer Center
Keck School of Medicine
University of Southern California
Los Angeles, California

Angela D. Levy, MD
Division of Abdominal Imaging
Department of Radiology
Georgetown University Hospital
Washington, DC
Formerly, Associate Professor of Radiology
Department of Radiology
Uniformed Services University of the Health Sciences
Bethesda, Maryland

Bernard S. Lewinsky, MD
Director
West Hills Radiation Therapy Center
Vantage Oncology, Inc.
West Hills, California

Michael Lill, MB, BS
Clinical Professor of Medicine
David Geffen School of Medicine
University of California, Los Angeles
Director, Blood and Marrow Transplant Program
Medical Director, Outpatient Cancer Center
Samuel Oschin Comprehensive Cancer Institute
Cedars-Sinai Medical Center
Los Angeles, California

Keith D. Lillemoe, MD
Jay L. Grosfeld Professor and Chair
Department of Surgery
Indiana University
Indianapolis, Indiana

Stephen W. Lim, MD
Associate Clinical Professor of Medicine
David Geffen School of Medicine
University of California, Los Angeles
Associate Director, Blood and Marrow Transplant Program
Samuel Oschin Comprehensive Cancer Institute
Cedars-Sinai Medical Center
Los Angeles, California

Alan S. Livingstone, MD
Professor and Chairman
DeWitt Daughtry Family Department of Surgery
Leonard M. Miller School of Medicine
University of Miami
Miami, Florida

Simon K. Lo, MD
Director of Endoscopy
Cedars-Sinai Medical Center
Clinical Professor of Medicine
David Geffen School of Medicine
University of California, Los Angeles
Los Angeles, California

Marvin J. Lopez, MD
Professor of Surgery
Tufts University School of Medicine
Chief, General and Oncologic Surgery
Caritas St. Elizabeth's Medical Center
Boston, Massachusetts

Ann C. Lowry, MD
Adjunct Professor of Surgery
Division of Colon and Rectal Surgery
Department of Surgery
University of Minnesota Medical School
Minneapolis, Minnesota

John Lyons, MD
Department of Surgery
Louisiana State University Health Sciences Center
New Orleans, Louisiana

Helen Mabry, MD
Assistant Director, Breast Surgical Oncology
Assistant Director, Joyce Eisenberg Keefer
    Breast Center
John Wayne Cancer Institute
Santa Monica, California

John S. Macdonald, MD
Lynn Wood Neag Distinguished Professor of Gastrointestinal
 Oncology
New York Medical College
Saint Vincent's Cancer Center
New York, New York
Chief Medical Officer
Aptium Oncology, Inc.
Los Angeles, California

Shishir K. Maithel, MD
Department of Surgery
Memorial Sloan-Kettering Cancer Center
New York, New York

Gary N. Mann, MD
Associate Professor of Surgery
University of Washington
Seattle, Washington

Christian Marth, MD, PhD
Department of Obstetrics and Gynecology
Innsbruck Medical University
Innsbruck, Austria

Lea Matsuoka, MD
Keck School of Medicine
University of Southern California University Hospital
Division of Hepatobiliary/Pancreatic Surgery and Abdominal
 Transplant Surgery
Los Angeles, California

Philomena McAndrew, MD
Tower Hematology Oncology Medical Group
Cedars-Sinai Medical Center
Beverly Hills, California

Robert J. McKenna, Jr., MD
Department of Surgery
Cedars-Sinai Medical Center
Los Angeles, California

James M. McLoughlin, MD
Department of Surgery
H. Lee Moffitt Cancer Center and Research Institute
Tampa, Florida

Lawrence R. Menendez, MD
Professor of Clinical Orthopaedics
Chief, Division of Orthopaedic Oncology
Keck School of Medicine
University of Southern California
Los Angeles, California

Steven G. Meranze, MD
Professor of Radiology
Vanderbilt University Medical Center
Nashville, Tennessee

Robert D. Moore, MD
Department of Surgery
University of Massachusetts Medical School
Worcester, Massachusetts

Leon Morgenstern, MD
Emeritus, Professor of Surgery
David Geffen School of Medicine
University of California, Los Angeles
Emeritus, Director of Surgery
Cedars-Sinai Medical Center
Los Angeles, California

Lilah F. Morris, MD
Division of Surgical Oncology
Department of Surgery
David Geffen School of Medicine
University of California at Los Angeles
Los Angeles, California

Monica Morrow, MD
Chief, Breast Surgery Service
Anne Burnett Windfohr Chair of Clinical Oncology
Memorial Sloan-Kettering Cancer Center
New York, New York

Franco M. Muggia, MD
Anne Murnick Cogan and David H. Cogan
 Professor of Oncology
New York University Clinical Cancer Center
New York, New York

Attila Nakeeb, MD
Department of Surgery
Indiana University
Indianapolis, Indiana

Ronald B. Natale, MD
Senior Research Advisor and National Director
Lung Cancer Research Program
Aptium Oncology, Inc.
Attending Physician
Cedars-Sinai Outpatient Cancer Center
Samuel Oschin Comprehensive Cancer Institute
Cedars-Sinai Medical Center
Los Angeles, California

A. Munro Neville, MD, DSc
Ludwig Institute for Cancer Research
London, England

Elliot Newman, MD
Associate Professor of Surgery
New York University
New York, New York

Ankesh Nigam, MD
Associate Professor
Chief of Surgical Oncology
Department of Surgery
Albany Medical College
Albany, New York

Johannes W. R. Nortier, MD, PhD
Professor
Department of Clinical Oncology
Leiden University Medical Center
Leiden, The Netherlands

Theodore X. O'Connell, MD, FACS
Clinical Professor of Surgical Oncology
David Geffen School of Medicine
University of California, Los Angeles
Chief of Surgery
Kaiser Permanente Los Angeles Medical Center
Los Angeles, California

James R. Ouellette, DO
Assistant Professor of Surgery
Division of Surgical Oncology
Wright State University
Kettering Memorial Hospital
Dayton, Ohio

J. Alexander Palesty, MD
Assistant Professor
Department of Surgery
University of Connecticut
Farmington, Connecticut
Associate Program Director
Department of Surgery
Saint Mary's Hospital
Waterbury, Connecticut

Yuri Parisky, MD
Director, Medical Imaging Center
Mammoth Hospital
Mammoth Lakes, California

David J. Park, MD
Virginia K. Crosson Cancer Center
St. Jude Heritage Medical Group
Fullerton, California

Janelle L. Park, MD
Assistant Professor
Radiation Oncology
Mount Sinai School of Medicine
New York, New York
Practice Chief, Radiation Therapy
James J. Peters Veterans Administration
    Medical Center
Bronx, New York

Jeong Mi Park, MD
Professor and Director
Division of Breast Imaging and Intervention
Director of Breast Imaging Fellowship
Department of Radiology
University of Iowa
Iowa City, Iowa

Edith A. Perez, MD
Professor of Medicine
Director
Breast Cancer Program
Mayo Clinic
Jacksonville, Florida

Edward H. Phillips, MD
Vice-Chairman, Department of Surgery
Director, Division of General Surgery
Director, Center for Minimally Invasive & Weight Loss Surgery
Director, Saul & Joyce Brandman Breast Center
Chair Holder of the Karl Storz Chair in Minimally Invasive Surgery
Cedars-Sinai Medical Center
Los Angeles, California

Elisa R. Port, MD
The Breast Service
Department of Surgery
Memorial Sloan-Kettering Cancer Center
Assistant Professor of Surgery
Weill Medical College of Cornell University
New York, New York

Mitchell C. Posner, MD
Thomas D. Jones Professor of Surgery
Chief, Section of General Surgery and
    Surgical Oncology
Vice Chair, Department of Surgery
The University of Chicago Medical Center
Chicago, Illinois

David I. Quinn, MBBS, PhD
Assistant Professor of Medicine
Director, Clinical Investigation Support Office
University of Southern California
Keck School of Medicine
Norris Comprehensive Cancer Center
Los Angeles, California

Derek Raghavan, MD, PhD
M. Frank & Margaret Domiter Rudy Distinguished Chair
    and Director, Taussig Cancer Institute
Cleveland Clinic
Cleveland, Ohio

Chandrajit P. Raut, MD, MSc
Instructor of Surgery
Harvard Medical School
Division of Surgical Oncology
Brigham and Women's Hospital
Center for Sarcoma and Bone Oncology
Dana-Farber Cancer Institute
Boston, Massachusetts

Polina Reyblat, MD
Department of Urology
Keck School of Medicine
University of Southern California
Los Angeles, California

Dror Robinson, MD, PhD
Sackler School of Medicine
Tel Aviv University
Tel Aviv, Israel
Rabin Medical Center
Petah Tikwa, Israel

Christopher M. Rose, MD
Radiation Oncology
Keck School of Medicine
University of Southern California
Los Angeles, California
Technical Director
Valley Radiotherapy Associates
Manhattan Beach, California

Peter J. Rosen, MD
Professor Emeritus
School of Medicine
University of California, Los Angeles
Los Angeles, California
Medical Director
Tower Cancer Research Foundation
Beverly Hills, California

Daniel F. Roses, MD
Jules Leonard Whitehill Professor of Surgery and
    Oncology
Division of Oncology
Department of Surgery
New York University School of Medicine
Senior Attending Surgeon
New York University Medical Center
New York, New York

Howard L. Rosner, MD
Medical Director
The Pain Center
Cedars-Sinai Medical Center
Los Angeles, California

Vivek Roy, MD
Associate Professor of Medicine
Mayo Clinic
Jacksonville, Florida

Mary K. Russell, MS, RD, LDN, CNSD
Assistant Director, Nutrition Services
Adult Lung Transplant Dietician
University of Chicago Hospitals
Chicago, Illinois

Michael S. Sabel, MD
Associate Professor of Surgery
Division of Surgical Oncology
University of Michigan Comprehensive Cancer Center
Ann Arbor, Michigan

Gregory P. Sarna, MD
Clinical Professor of Medicine
David Geffen School of Medicine
University of California, Los Angeles
Research Director, Outpatient Cancer Center
Samuel Oschin Comprehensive Cancer Institute
Cedars-Sinai Medical Center
Los Angeles, California

Thomas Schnelldorfer, MD
GI Surgical Scholar
Division of Gastroenterologic and General Surgery
Mayo Clinic and Mayo Foundation
Rochester, Minnesota

Lawrence H. Schwartz, MD
Professor of Radiology
Weill Medical College of Cornell University
Vice Chair for Technology Development
Director, Magnetic Resonance Imaging
Department of Radiology
Memorial Sloan-Kettering Cancer Center
New York, New York

Rick Selby, MD
Keck School of Medicine and University of Southern California
    University Hospital Division of Hepatobiliary/Pancreatic
    Surgery and Abdominal Transplant Surgery
Los Angeles, California

Jatin P. Shah, MD, PhD (Hon)
Professor of Surgery
Elliot W. Strong Chair in Head and Neck Oncology
Chief, Head and Neck Service
Memorial Sloan-Kettering Cancer Center
New York, New York

Robert M. Sharkey, PhD
Director of Clinical Research Administration
Center for Molecular Medicine and Immunology
Garden State Cancer Center
Belleville, New Jersey

Pulin A. Sheth, MD
Director of Breast Imaging
H. Lee Breast Center, USC Norris Cancer Hospital
Assistant Professor of Clinical Radiology
Keck School of Medicine
University of Southern California
Los Angeles, California

Karen S. Sibert, MD
Attending Anesthesiologist
Department of Anesthesiology
Cedars-Sinai Medical Center
Los Angeles, California

Allan W. Silberman, MD, PhD
Robert J. and Suzanne Gottlieb Endowed Chair in Surgical
    Oncology
Samuel Oschin Comprehensive Cancer Institute
Cedars-Sinai Medical Center
Los Angeles, California

Howard Silberman, MD
Professor of Surgery
Keck School of Medicine
University of Southern California
Los Angeles, California

Melvin J. Silverstein, MD
Clinical Professor of Surgery
Keck School of Medicine
University of Southern California
Los Angeles, California
Medical Director
Hoag Breast Care Center
Hoag Memorial Hospital Presbyterian
Newport Beach, California

Gagandeep Singh, MD
Director, Liver and Pancreas Center
Gastrointestinal Surgical Oncology
John Wayne Cancer Institute
Santa Monica, California

Donald G. Skinner, MD (Retired)
Professor of Urology
Chairman, Department of Urology
Hanson-White Chair in Medical Research
Keck School of Medicine
University of Southern California
Los Angeles, California

Andrew S. Sloan, MD
Assistant Professor of Surgery
Department of Interdisciplinary Oncology
College of Medicine
University of South Florida
Division of Neurooncology
H. Lee Moffitt Cancer Center and Research Institute
Tampa, Florida

Brian R. Smith, MD
Department of Surgery
Harbor University of California, Los Angeles Medical Center
Torrance, California

Vernon K. Sondak, MD
Professor of Surgery
Departments of Interdisciplinary Oncology and Surgery
College of Medicine
University of South Florida
Chief, Division of Cutaneous Oncology
H. Lee Moffitt Cancer Center and Research Institute
Tampa, Florida

Seth A. Spector, MD
Assistant Professor of Surgery
DeWitt Daughtry Family Department of Surgery
Leonard M. Miller School of Medicine
University of Miami
Miami, Florida

Bruce E. Stabile, MD
Professor of Surgery
School of Medicine
University of California, Los Angeles
Los Angeles, California
Chairman
Department of Surgery
Harbor University of California, Los Angeles
     Medical Center
Torrance, California

Steven C. Stain, MD
Neil Lempert Professor and Chair
Department of Surgery
Albany Medical College
Albany, New York

Valerie L. Staradub, MD
Visiting Assistant Professor of Surgery
Harvard Medical School
Boston, Massachusetts

Ezra Steiger, MD
Professor of Surgery
Cleveland Clinic Lerner College of Medicine
Case Western Reserve University
Consultant
Digestive Disease Center
Cleveland Clinic
Cleveland, Ohio

John P. Stein, MD
Associate Professor of Urology
Norris Comprehensive Cancer Center
Keck School of Medicine
University of Southern California
Los Angeles, California

LeAnn S. Stokes, MD
Assistant Professor of Radiology
Vanderbilt-Ingram Cancer Center
Vanderbilt University Medical Center
Nashville, Tennessee

Oscar E. Streeter, Jr., MD
Professor and Chair
Department of Radiation Oncology
Howard University College of Medicine
Washington, DC

Paul H. Sugarbaker, MD
The Washington Cancer Institute
Washington Hospital Center
Washington, DC

László Tabár, MD
Professor of Radiology
University of Uppsala School of Medicine
Uppsala, Sweden

Hiroomi Tada, MD, PhD
Assistant Professor of Surgery
Temple University School of Medicine
Philadelphia, Pennsylvania

Snehal G. Thakkar, MD
Department of Solid Tumor Oncology
Cleveland Clinic Taussig Cancer Center
Cleveland, Ohio

R. Houston Thompson, MD
Department of Urology
Mayo Medical School and Mayo Clinic
Rochester, Minnesota

Przemyslaw Twardowski, MD
Assistant Professor, Medical Oncology and Therapeutics
     Research
City of Hope Comprehensive Cancer Center
Director, Medical Oncology Prostate Program
City of Hope Comprehensive Cancer Center
Duarte, California

Thomas A. Ullman, MD
Assistant Professor of Medicine
The Dr. Henry D. Janowitz Division of Gastroenterology
The Mount Sinai School of Medicine
New York, New York

Cornelis J. H. van de Velde, MD, PhD
Professor of Surgery
Leiden University Medical Center
Leiden, The Netherlands

Anneke Q. van Hoesel, MD
Postdoctoral Research Fellow
Department of Molecular Oncology
John Wayne Cancer Institute at St. John's Health Center
Santa Monica, California

Liselot B. J. van Iersel, MD
Department of Clinical Oncology
Leiden University Medical Center
Leiden, The Netherlands

Kimberly A. Varker, MD
Division of Surgical Oncology
The Ohio State University Comprehensive Cancer Center
Columbus, Ohio

Harold J. Wanebo, MD
Landmark Medical Center
Adjunct Professor of Surgery
Brown University School of Medicine
Providence, Rhode Island
Professor of Surgery
Boston University School of Medicine
Boston, Massachusetts

Hanlin L. Wang, MD, PhD
Director of Gastrointestinal Pathology
Department of Pathology and Laboratory Medicine
Cedars-Sinai Medical Center
Los Angeles, California

Alan D. Waxman, MD
Clinical Professor of Radiology
School of Medicine
University of Southern California
Co-Chairman, Department of Imaging
Director, Nuclear Medicine
S. Mark Taper Imaging Department
Cedars-Sinai Medical Center
Los Angeles, California

Jeffrey S. Weber, MD, PhD
Professor of Internal Medicine and Oncologic Sciences
College of Medicine
University of South Florida
Director
Donald A. Adam Comprehensive Melanoma Research Center
H. Lee Moffitt Cancer Center and Research Institute
Tampa, Florida

Edward M. Wolin, MD
Attending Physician (Medical Oncology)
Cedars-Sinai Outpatient Cancer Center
Samuel Oschin Comprehensive Cancer Institute
Cedars-Sinai Medical Center
Los Angeles, California

Eugene A. Woltering, MD
The James D. Rives Professor of Surgery and Neurosciences
Chief, Sections of Surgical Oncology and Endocrine Surgery
Director of Surgical Research
Department of Surgery
Louisiana State University Health Sciences Center
New Orleans, Louisiana

Linda L. Wong, MD
Professor of Surgery
Vice-chairman for Clinical Research
Department of Surgery
John A. Burns School of Medicine
University of Hawaii
Transplant Institute
Hawaii Medical Center–East
Honolulu, Hawaii

Amy Ming-Fang Yen, PhD
Graduate Institute of Epidemiology
College of Public Health
National Taiwan University
Taipei, Taiwan

Jonathan S. Zager, MD
Assistant Professor of Surgery
Department of Interdisciplinary Oncology
College of Medicine
University of South Florida
Division of Cutaneous Oncology
H. Lee Moffitt Cancer Center and Research Institute
Tampa, Florida

Robert P. Zimmermann, MD
Valley Radiotherapy Associates
Western Tumor Medical Group, Inc.
Sherman Oaks, California

Nicholas J. Zyromski, MD
Department of Surgery
Indiana University
Indianapolis, Indiana

Contributors by Specialty

SURGERY

Elke R. Ahlmann, MD	Orthopedic Oncology
Farin F. Amersi, MD, FACS	Surgical Oncology
Glenn T. Ault, MD	Colorectal Surgery
Benjamin O. Anderson, MD	Surgical Oncology
Charles M. Balch, MD	Surgical Oncology
Robert W. Beart, Jr., MD	Colorectal Surgery
George Berci, MD, FACS, FRCS, ED (Hon)	General Surgery/Laparoscopy
J. Sybil Biermann, MD	Orthopedic Oncology
Leslie H. Blumgart, MD, FACS, FRCS	Surgical Oncology/Hepato-Biliary
Michael L. Blute, MD	Urology
Murray F. Brennan, MD, FACS	Surgical Oncology
Earl Brien, MD	Orthopedic Oncology
Ronald W. Busuttil, MD, PhD	Transplant Surgery
John A. Butler, MD	Surgical Oncology
Blake Cady, MD	Surgical Oncology
Kristine E. Calhoun, MD	Surgical Oncology
Ilana Cass, MD	Gynecologic Oncology
Michael A. Choti, MD, MBA, FACS	Surgical Oncology
Orlo H. Clark, MD	General Surgery/Endocrine
Steven D. Colquhoun, MD	Transplant Surgery
David V. Cossman, MD	Vascular Surgery
Peter F. Crookes, MD	General Surgery
Jason Cundiff, MD	General Surgery
Michael D'Angelica, MD	Surgical Oncology
John M. Daly, MD	Surgical Oncology
John H. Donohue, MD	Surgical Oncology
Stanley J. Dudrick, MD, FACS	Surgical Oncology
John P. Duffy, MD	Transplant Surgery
James S. Economou, MD, PhD	Surgical Oncology
Frederick R. Eilber, MD	Surgical Oncology
Fritz C. Eilber, MD	Surgical Oncology
Richard Essner, MD	Surgical Oncology
David A. Etzioni, MD	Colorectal Surgery
Yuri Falkinstein, MD	Orthopedic Oncology
Jeffrey M. Farma, MD	Surgical Oncology
Phillip R. Fleshner, MD	Colorectal Surgery
Yuman Fong, MD	Surgical Oncology
Julie A. Freischlag, MD	Vascular Surgery
Bruce L. Gewertz, MD	Vascular Surgery
Mark A. Gittleman, MD	Surgical Oncology
Armando E. Giuliano, MD	Surgical Oncology
Leo A. Gordon, MD	General Surgery
Frederick L. Greene, MD	Surgical Oncology
Alan W. Hackford, MD	Colorectal Surgery
Masanobu Hagiike, MD, PhD	Research Fellow/Laparoscopy
Heitham T. Hassoun, MD	Vascular Surgery
Dennis R. Holmes, MD	Surgical Oncology
Mustafa Hussain, MD	General Surgery
James F. Huth, MD	Surgical Oncology
Yuichiro Ito, MD	Research Fellow/Laparoscopy

Nicolas Jabbour, MD	Transplant Surgery
Lisa K. Jacobs, MD	Surgical Oncology
Ajay Jain, MD	Vascular Surgery
Larry R. Kaiser, MD	Thoracic Oncology
Andrew S. Klein, MD, MBA	Transplant Surgery
David A. Kooby, MD	Surgical Oncology
David Krag, MD	Surgical Oncology
John C. Kucharczuk, MD	Thoracic Oncology
S. Ram Kumar, MD, PhD	General Surgery
Karen T. Lane, MD	Surgical Oncology
Julie R. Lange, MD	Surgical Oncology
James A. Lee, MD	General Surgery/Endocrine
Sarah J. Lee, MD	General Surgery/ Laparoscopy
Alan T. Lefor, MD, MPH	Surgical Oncology
Keith D. Lillemoe, MD	General Surgery
Alan S. Livingstone, MD	Surgical Oncology
Marvin J. Lopez, MD	Surgical Oncology
Ann C. Lowry, MD	Colorectal Surgery
John Lyons, MD	General Surgery
Helen Mabry, MD	Surgical Oncology
Shishir K. Maithel, MD	Surgical Oncology
Gary N. Mann, MD	Surgical Oncology
Christian Marth, MD, PhD	Gynecologic Oncology
Lea Matsuoka, MD	Transplant Surgery
Robert J. McKenna, Jr., MD	Thoracic Oncology
James M. McLoughlin, MD	Surgical Oncology
Lawrence R. Menendez, MD	Orthopedic Oncology
Robert D. Moore, MD	Colorectal Surgery
Leon Morgenstern, MD	General Surgery
Lilah F. Morris, MD	Surgical Oncology
Monica Morrow, MD	Surgical Oncology
Attila Nakeeb, MD	General Surgery
Elliot Newman, MD	Surgical Oncology
Ankesh Nigam, MD	Surgical Oncology
Theodore X. O'Connell, MD, FACS	Surgical Oncology
James R. Ouellette, DO	Surgical Oncology
J. Alexander Palesty, MD	Surgical Oncology
Edward H. Phillips, MD	General Surgery/Laparoscopy
Elisa R. Port, MD	Surgical Oncology
Mitchell C. Posner, MD	Surgical Oncology
Chandrajit P. Raut, MD, MSc	Surgical Oncology
Polina Reyblat, MD	Urology
Dror Robinson, MD, PhD	Orthopedic Oncology
Daniel F. Roses, MD	Surgical Oncology
Mary K. Russell, MS, RD, LDN, CNSD	Nutrition
Michael S. Sabel, MD	Surgical Oncology
Thomas Schnelldorfer, MD	General Surgery
Rick Selby, MD	Transplant Surgery
Jatin P. Shah, MD, PhD (Hon)	Surgical Oncology/ENT
Allan W. Silberman, MD, PhD	Surgical Oncology
Howard Silberman, MD	Surgical Oncology
Melvin J. Silverstein, MD	Surgical Oncology
Gagandeep Singh, MD	Surgical Oncology/Hepato-Biliary
Donald G. Skinner, MD (Retired)	Urology
Andrew S. Sloan, MD	Surgical Oncology
Brian R. Smith, MD	General Surgery
Vernon K. Sondak, MD	Surgical Oncology
Seth A. Spector, MD	Surgical Oncology
Bruce E. Stabile, MD	General Surgery

Steven C. Stain, MD	General Surgery/Hepato-Biliary
Valerie L. Staradub, MD	Surgical Oncology
Ezra Steiger, MD	General Surgery
John P. Stein, MD	Urology (Deceased)
Paul H. Sugarbaker, MD	Surgical Oncology
Hiroomi Tada, MD, PhD	General Surgery
R. Houston Thompson, MD	Urology
Cornelis J. H. van de Velde, MD, PhD	General Surgery
Kimberly A. Varker, MD	Surgical Oncology
Harold J. Wanebo, MD	Surgical Oncology
Eugene A. Woltering, MD	Surgical Oncology
Linda L. Wong, MD	Transplant Surgery
Jonathan S. Zager, MD	Surgical Oncology
Nicholas J. Zyromski, MD	General Surgery

MEDICAL ONCOLOGY/HEMATOLOGY

Karen Antman, MD
Bach Ardalan, MD
M. William Audeh, MD
Laurence H. Baker, DO
Chandra P. Belani, MD
Bruce A. Chabner, MD
Antony J. Charles, MD
Toni K. Choueiri, MD
Cathie T. Chung, MD, PhD
Mary E. Cianfrocca, DO
Robert W. Decker, MD
John F. DiPersio, MD, PhD
Anthony B. Elkhouiery, MD
Robert A. Figlin, MD
Charles A. Forscher, MD
Kevin R. Fox, MD
David J. Gallagher, MD
Hans Gelderblom, MD, PhD
William J. Gradishar, MD
Omid Hamid, MD
Syma Iqbal, MD
John J. Kavanagh, Jr., MD
Nancy E. Kemeny, MD
Olga Kozyreva, MD

David I. Kuperman, MD
Cynthia Gail Leichman, MD
Lawrence Leichman, MD
Heinz-Josef Lenz, MD
Michael Lill, MB, BS
Stephen W. Lim, MD
John S. Macdonald, MD
Philomena McAndrew, MD
Franco M. Muggia, MD
Ronald B. Natale, MD
Johannes W. R. Nortier, MD, PhD
David J. Park, MD
Edith A. Perez, MD
David I. Quinn, MBBS, PhD
Derek Raghavan, MD, PhD
Peter J. Rosen, MD
Vivek Roy, MD
Gregory P. Sarna, MD
Snehal G. Thakkar, MD
Przemyslaw Twardowski, MD
Liselot B. J. van Iersel, MD
Jeffrey S. Weber, MD, PhD
Edward M. Wolin, MD

MOLECULAR BIOLOGY/IMMUNOLOGY/GENETICS

Daniel L. Farkas, PhD
David M. Goldenberg, ScD, MD
Ora Karp Gordon, MD, MS

David S. B. Hoon, MSc, PhD
Robert M. Sharkey, PhD
Anneke Q. van Hoesel, MD

INTERNAL MEDICINE

Glenn D. Braunstein, MD	Endocrinology
Gauree Gupta, MD	Gastroenterology
Simon K. Lo, MD	Gastroenterology
Thomas A. Ullman, MD	Gastroenterology

ANESTHESIOLOGY/PAIN MANAGEMENT

Howard L. Rosner, MD
Karen S. Sibert, MD

PATHOLOGY

Randa Alsabeh, MD

Marija Balic, MD

Parakrama Chandrasoma, MD

Richard J. Cote, MD, FRCPath

Debra Hawes, MD

A. Munro Neville, MD, DSc

Hanlin L. Wang, MD, PhD

IMAGING

William D. Boswell, MD

Peter B. Dean, MD

Wendy DeMartini, MD

Vinay A. Duddalwar, MD, FRCR

Laurie L. Fajardo, MD, MBA

Marc L. Friedman, MD

Nola Hylton, PhD

Hossein Jadvar, MD, PhD, MPH, MBA

Constance D. Lehman, MD, PhD

Linda Hovanessian Larsen, MD

Angela D. Levy, MD

Steven G. Meranze, MD

Yuri Parisky, MD

Jeong Mi Park, MD

Lawrence H. Schwartz, MD

Pulin A. Sheth, MD

LeAnn S. Stokes, MD

László Tabár, MD

Alan D. Waxman, MD

RADIATION ONCOLOGY

Pramila Rani Anné, MD

Leslie Botnick, MD

Thomas A. Buchholz, MD

Gregory M. Chronowski, MD

Walter J. Curran, Jr., MD

Bernard S. Lewinsky, MD

Janelle L. Park, MD

Christopher M. Rose, MD

Oscar E. Streeter, Jr., MD

Robert P. Zimmermann, MD

EPIDEMIOLOGY

H. H. Tony Chen, DDS, PhD

Sherry Yueh-Hsia Chiu, PhD

Stephen W. Duffy, MSc

Amy Ming-Fang Yen, PhD

Drs. Howard and Allan Silberman have compiled a textbook on surgical oncology that is both comprehensive in subject and rich in content. Indeed, this outstanding book covers the universe of cognitive knowledge that defines our specialty. In addition, definitive chapters have been written by a broad array of distinguished authors, and each chapter is supplemented by a commentary by yet another expert that brings a balanced perspective and context to the reader.

This book is an important resource because the specialty of surgical oncology exists as a distinctive body of knowledge that uniquely defines it as a surgical specialty. As described in various chapters, the surgical oncologist brings a body of knowledge that extends to all facets of cancer, including prevention, diagnosis, treatment, rehabilitation, and surveillance. Although surgical treatment is the centerpiece of our subspecialty, what differentiates surgical oncology is the oncology expertise needed to manage and coordinate all aspects of cancer management in a multidisciplinary fashion. Thus, surgical oncology is both a technical and a cognitive specialty involving a chronic disease process that encompasses all organ systems and, therefore, involves many physiologic and biologic processes. Surgical oncologists must also be knowledgeable about basic science, especially as it relates to molecular and cellular processes, as well as have a firm background in immunology, as summarized in the first section of this textbook.

The surgical component of our specialty comprises the judgment and experience to safely and adeptly perform cancer operations with the goals of cure, local disease control, staging, or a combination thereof. Usually this involves an *en bloc* resection of the primary tumor and any regional extensions in order to minimize the probability of tumor recurrence, prevent further spread, and reduce or eliminate the tumor burden. On the other hand, he or she must have the judgment to know when to apply more conservative surgery where appropriate and safe, especially when it preserves a function, reduces morbidity, or is less disfiguring than more radical surgery. The surgeon must also know how to perform palliative operations to resect tumors that threaten bodily functions, relieve existing symptoms, reduce tumor burden, and enhance the capabilities of other modalities to eradicate the cancer. All these facets of surgical management are covered in this book.

In addition to being an excellent surgeon, the surgical oncologist brings the perspective of a cancer specialist to the realm of decision-making and multidisciplinary treatment planning for the surgical patient. This is a defining part of the specialty—to participate in coordinating multidisciplinary cancer care and counseling patients about the appropriate combinations and sequences of cancer treatment options for their stage of disease. Thus, the surgical oncologist has a pivotal role in therapy planning and management. To do this, the surgeon must fully understand the indications, risks, and benefits of using adjuvant chemotherapy, hormone therapy, and radiotherapy, especially when there is demonstrable benefit from prospective clinical trials. Because systemic drugs and biologics are now so effective, there is an increasing role for surgery as a component of managing stage IV disease. This textbook provides up-to-date chapters on each of these subjects.

The role of the surgical oncologist will increase substantially during the next decade and research advances in cancer management (many made by surgeons) will require an expanding cadre of surgical specialists to fulfill the functions described in this book. It is uncommon today and will be rare in the future for a cancer patient not to be treated in a multidisciplinary environment; therefore, all surgeons must be trained and equipped to participate meaningfully in this rapidly evolving oncology field. Powerful new molecular and genetic tools and radiological techniques will allow us to understand this complex and diverse disease at a much more fundamental level in the near future. This, in turn, will lead to more precise staging of patients and allow us to precisely apply a combination and sequence of treatments calibrated to the biological aggressiveness of the cancer and designed to eradicate the disease and restore our patients to health. This textbook can be a primary resource to educate all surgeons caring for cancer patients to better know how to bring both innovative therapies and optimal cancer management for their patients.

Charles M. Balch, MD, FACS
Professor of Surgery, Oncology, and Dermatology
Johns Hopkins Medical Institutions
Baltimore, Maryland

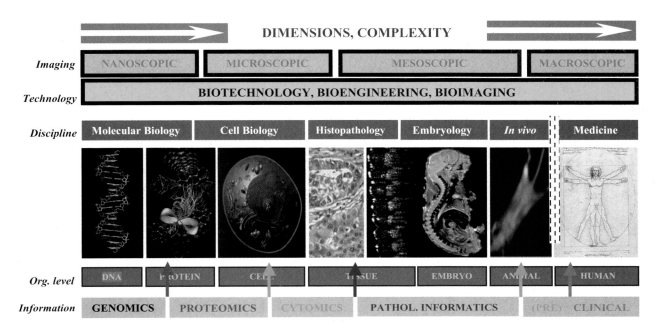

Color Plate 1C.1

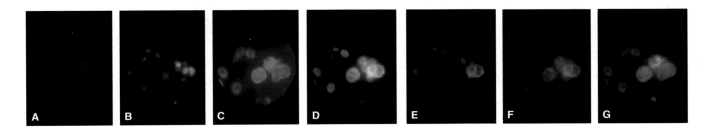

Color Plate 1C.2

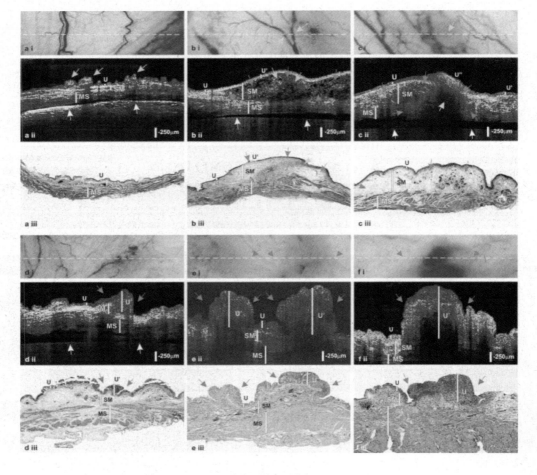

Color Plate 1C.4

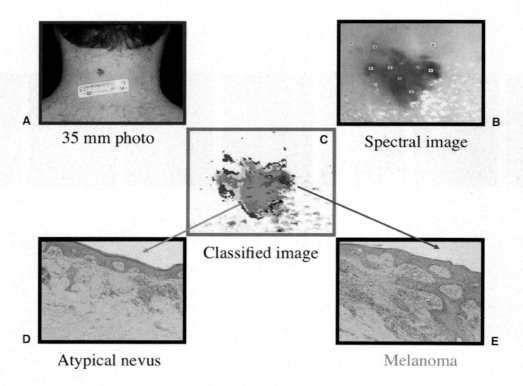

A — 35 mm photo

B — Spectral image

C — Classified image

D — Atypical nevus

E — Melanoma

Color Plate 1C.5

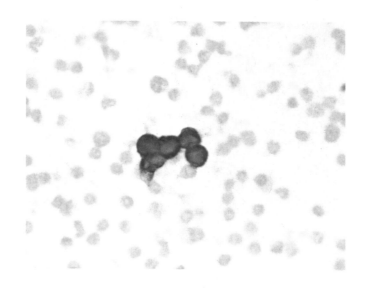

Color Plate 4.1

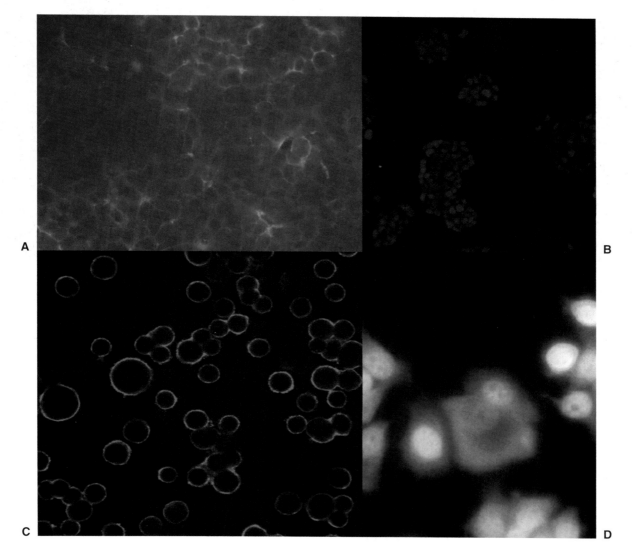

Color Plate 4.3

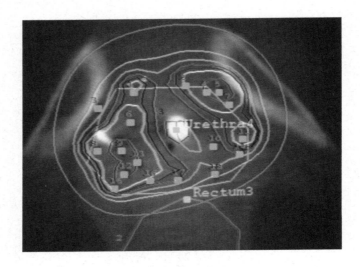

Color Plate 12.3

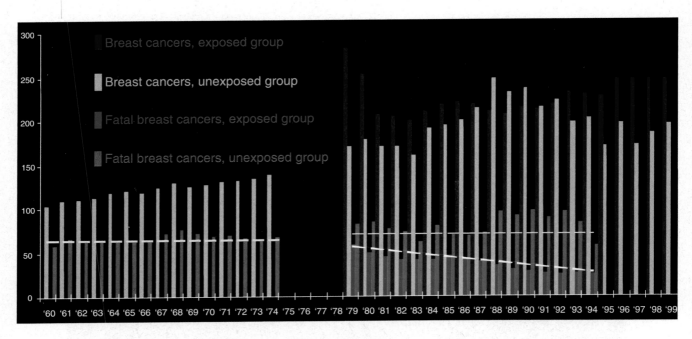

Breast cancers, exposed group

Breast cancers, unexposed group

Fatal breast cancers, exposed group

Fatal breast cancers, unexposed group

'60 '61 '62 '63 '64 '65 '66 '67 '68 '69 '70 '71 '72 '73 '74 '75 '76 '77 '78 '79 '80 '81 '82 '83 '84 '85 '86 '87 '88 '89 '90 '91 '92 '93 '94 '95 '96 '97 '98 '99

Color Plate 16A.1

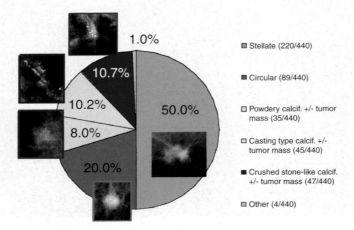

1.0%

10.7%

10.2%

8.0%

50.0%

20.0%

■ Stellate (220/440)

■ Circular (89/440)

□ Powdery calcif. +/- tumor mass (35/440)

□ Casting type calcif. +/- tumor mass (45/440)

■ Crushed stone-like calcif. +/- tumor mass (47/440)

□ Other (4/440)

Color Plate 16A.8.1

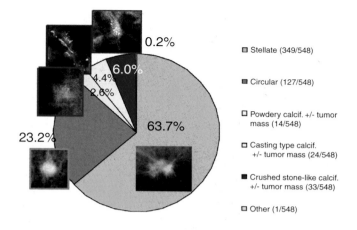

Stellate (349/548)

Circular (127/548)

Powdery calcif. +/- tumor mass (14/548)

Casting type calcif. +/- tumor mass (24/548)

Crushed stone-like calcif. +/- tumor mass (33/548)

Other (1/548)

0.2%
6.0%
4.4%
2.6%
63.7%
23.2%

Color Plate 16A.8.2

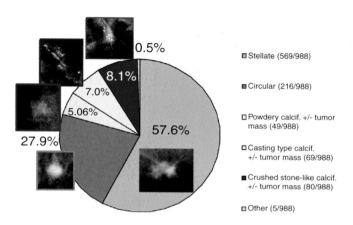

Stellate (569/988)

Circular (216/988)

Powdery calcif. +/- tumor mass (49/988)

Casting type calcif. +/- tumor mass (69/988)

Crushed stone-like calcif. +/- tumor mass (80/988)

Other (5/988)

0.5%
8.1%
7.0%
5.06%
57.6%
27.9%

Color Plate 16A.8.3

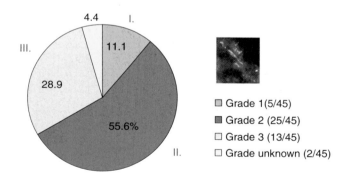

4.4
I.
III.
11.1
28.9
55.6%
II.

☐ Grade 1(5/45)
☐ Grade 2 (25/45)
☐ Grade 3 (13/45)
☐ Grade unknown (2/45)

Color Plate 16A.12.1

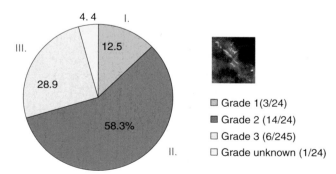

4. 4
I.
III.
12.5
28.9
58.3%
II.

☐ Grade 1(3/24)
☐ Grade 2 (14/24)
☐ Grade 3 (6/245)
☐ Grade unknown (1/24)

Color Plate 16A.12.2

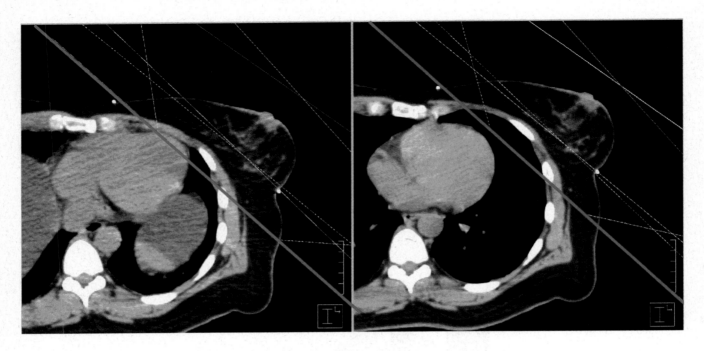

Color Plate 19C.1

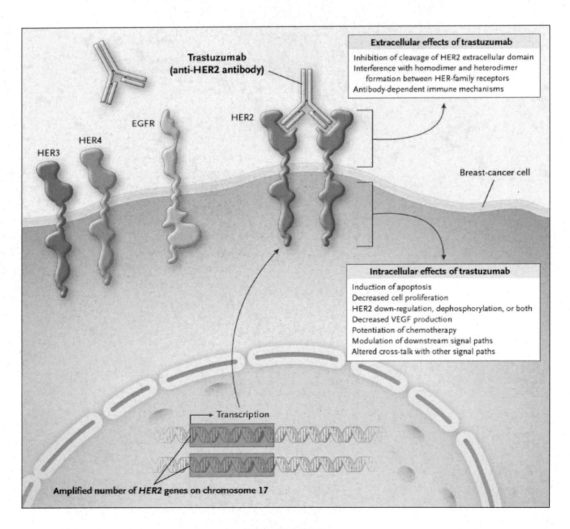

Color Plate 20.4

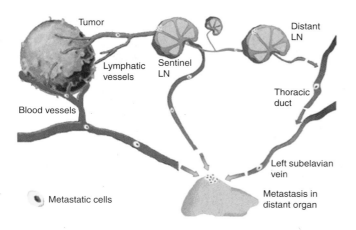

Color Plate 21.1

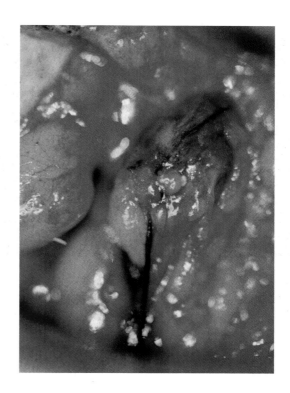

Color Plate 22.2

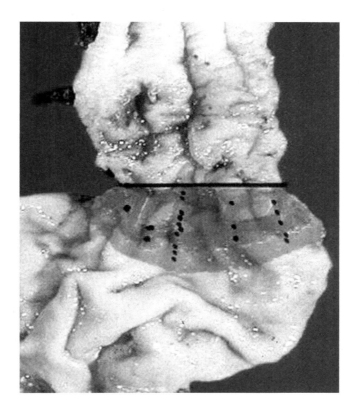

Color Plate 30.3

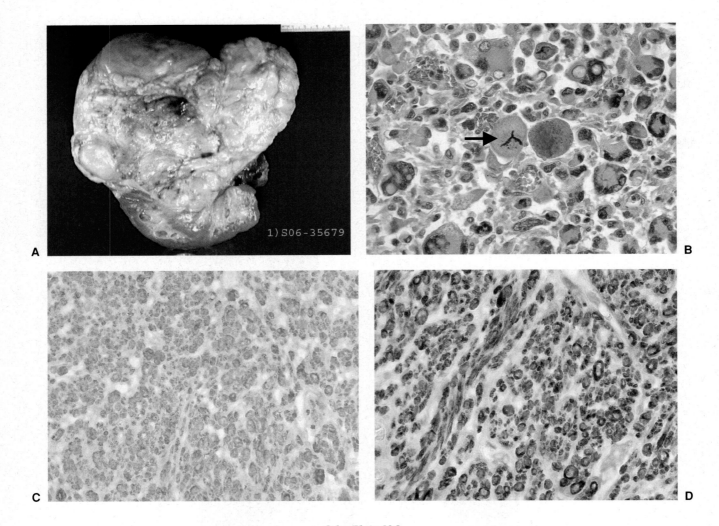

Color Plate 49.2

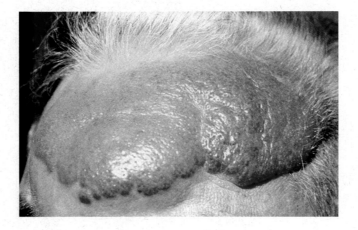

Color Plate 49.5

Principles of Molecular Biology for Cancer Surgeons

S. Ram Kumar

Recent advances in the techniques and understanding of molecular biology have significantly furthered our grasp of the pathophysiology of cancer. It is commonplace knowledge today that Cancer Results from genetic mutations resulting in survival and metastatic advantage to tumor cells. Several components in these complex molecular pathways and the downstream signaling events orchestrated by them are now beginning to be better understood. Such an explosion in knowledge has added a new dimension to the armamentarium of the cancer therapist, and biological therapy heralds the next wave of cancer treatment. Several agents—some already in the clinic and others in the pipeline—have brought to fruition the cherished goal of disease-focused therapy with minimal side effects. In the not-so-far future, translation of molecular biologic principles from the bench to bedside will provide targeted therapy aimed at patient-specific genetic derangements that reverse the survival advantage acquired by cancer cells at the molecular level. This chapter is an overview of some of the principles of cancer pathogenesis, disease-specific mutations, and their potential clinical applications.

MOLECULAR MECHANISMS GOVERNING NORMAL CELLULAR PROLIFERATION AND TURNOVER

In order to understand the biology of cancer, it is necessary to first understand the biology of normal cellular processes. The normal cell undergoes a tightly regulated cycle of growth and division called the *cell cycle*. Control of cellular proliferation involves a cascade of events, including those regulated by oncogenes and tumor suppressor genes, connecting extracellular signals to intracellular responses. Cell density is maintained via a maintenance pathway called *apoptosis* that programs death of senescent or abnormal cells. Angiogenesis provides nutrients to the growing mass of cells and renders them capable of continued independent growth. The interaction between growing cells and their microenvironment allows seeding and growth and facilitates migration and selective homing of cells in their appropriate growth niche.

Cell Cycle and Its Regulation

Replicating somatic cells progress through a defined process prior to cell division: an initial growth phase in the absence of

DNA replication (G1), a period of DNA replication (S), a growth phase following DNA synthesis (G2), and, finally, mitosis (M). At the completion of mitosis, daughter cells can continue to divide by entering G1 phase or remain growth-arrested, entering the so-called G0 phase (Figure 1.1). The cell cycle is largely regulated by a special class of protein kinases called *cyclin-dependent kinases* (CDKs). These kinases are active only when complexed with unstable regulatory elements, called *cyclins,* that fluctuate in abundance during the cell cycle (1). Tight control of the cell cycle is achieved by regulating the cyclins and CDKs at various levels. Cyclin levels are maintained by transcriptional regulation of their synthesis and periodic destruction of formed proteins via proteolysis. CDK function is regulated by binding to specific CDK inhibitors such as pI5, pI6, p2I, p27, or other proteins such as sic1, an S-phase CDK inhibitor. Finally, cyclin-CDK complexes are subject to both activating and inactivating phosphorylations.

Each step in the cell cycle is tightly regulated, and progression depends on the completion of events in the previous step (2). At the completion of mitosis, most cells enter a resting state, the G0 phase. When the cell receives signals to proliferate (e.g., growth factors, nutritional signals) cyclin D is produced, which complexes with and activates CDK4 and CDK6. Progression through G1 is regulated by cyclin D in complex with CDK4 or CDK6. These active kinases phosphorylate and inactivate *pRB*, the gene product of the retinoblastoma tumor suppressor gene. Inactivation of *pRB* leads to the activation of E2F, a transcription factor, which then activates transcription of many genes that are required for DNA synthesis and chromosome duplication. Further, accumulation of the G1 CDKs leads to the activation of the S-phase CDKs and the inactivation of the anaphase-promoting complex (An-PC) that regulates the completion of mitosis. The inactivation of An-PC allows M-phase CDKs to accumulate. Finally, proteins synthesized during G1 allow assembly of prereplication complexes at DNA origins of replication, rendering the DNA competent for replication. Cells now enter the S phase of the cell cycle and progression through this phase is regulated by cyclin E or cyclin A in complex with CDK2. Active CDK2 triggers replication of DNA from origins assembled with complete prereplication complexes, and inhibits the formation of new prereplication complexes. DNA synthesis thus occurs during S-phase and chromosome duplication ensues. Cells then enter the G2 growth phase and activation of CDK1 by complexing with cyclin A or B in late G2 is required for progression into mitosis. Active CDK1 and M-phase CDKs

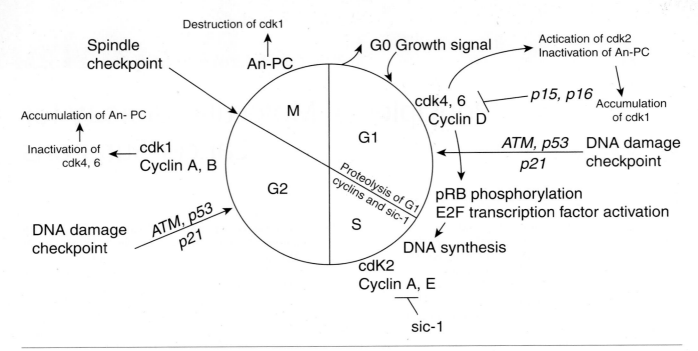

Figure 1.1 Cell-cycle control. Cells rest in G0 unless stimulated by a growth signal, at which time they enter G1 growth phase via activation of cyclin D. Cyclin D, in turn, activates the G1 cyclin-dependent kinases (CDKs), CDK4 and CDK6. Inhibitors of the G1 CDKs include *p15*, *p16*, and *p21*. G1 CDKs activate the S-phase CDK, CDK2, and inactivate the anaphase promoting complex (An-PC), allowing accumulation of CDK1. *ATM*, *p53*, and *p21* mediate the DNA damage checkpoint in G1 and G2. If this checkpoint is successfully negotiated, the G1 CDKs phosphorylate the retinoblastoma protein (pRB), leading to activation of the E2F transcription factor and induction of the proteins required for DNA synthesis. At the G1/S interface, the G1 cyclins and sic-1, an inhibitor of S-phase CDKs, are inactivated, allowing progression of S phase. After DNA synthesis and chromosome duplication are complete, the cell enters another growth phase, G2, during which the mitotic CDK, CDK1, is activated, leading to inactivation of the G1 CDKs, and allowing accumulation of An-PC. At the G2/M interface, the spindle checkpoint ensures proper spindle formation and segregation of the chromosomes before mitosis begins. Completion of mitosis is mediated by An-PC. Accumulation of An-PC leads to inactivation of mitotic CDKs. At the completion of mitosis, the cells enter the resting stage, G0, unless stimulated by further growth signals.

induce chromosome alignment and spindle formation, as well as the inactivation of G1 cyclins. Once the spindle forms and the chromosomes are correctly aligned, the An-PC is formed. An-PC causes segregation of the sister chromatids and the completion of mitosis. An-PC also triggers the proteolysis of mitotic CDKs and the accumulation of G1 cyclins. This prevents continued cell division and allows for directing daughter cells to growth arrest or further proliferation.

There are two known checkpoints that ensure that the processes of DNA replication and cell division are completed with the necessary fidelity to ensure production of two identical daughter cells (3). The first checkpoint is the DNA damage checkpoint. This is a mechanism that detects DNA damage and generates a signal that arrests cells in G1, slows down S phase, or arrests cells in G2, and induces transcription of DNA repair genes. In this way, damaged DNA is repaired before a round of cell division is allowed to proceed. If cells are not able to repair the DNA damage, they are then subject to apoptosis (vide infra). The signal that activates this pathway is DNA damage. The sensor is thought to be a protein encoded by the *RAD9* gene, which activates the ataxia-telangiectasia mutated (*ATM*) gene, a member of the phosphinositide kinase superfamily. ATM then activates

the *TP53* tumor suppressor gene, which in turn activates the p21 CDK inhibitor, thereby blocking cell cycle progression, and activates the DNA repair genes or triggers apoptosis. The second checkpoint is the spindle assembly checkpoint. This checkpoint is a mechanism that assures proper segregation of chromosomes at mitosis. Proper segregation requires assembly of a bipolar spindle, attachment of kinetochores of the sister chromatids to fibers from opposite poles of the spindle, and arrival of the chromosomes at the metaphase plate. If these events do not occur properly, anaphase is prevented. This mechanism ensures that each daughter cell receives a single copy of each chromosome at anaphase.

In summary, it is clear that the cell cycle is tightly regulated in normal cells so that each step must be completed before subsequent steps are initiated. Entry into a subsequent step removes the proteins that drove the previous step in the absence of signals for their continued production. DNA can be replicated only once per cell cycle. Chromosomes can segregate only after they have correctly aligned. Checkpoints are in place to ensure that each daughter cell is an accurate copy of the parental cell. In cancer cells, these regulatory processes become altered. Oncogenic processes primarily target regulators of G1 phase. Cells respond to extracellular signals during the G1 phase either by advancing toward division or by withdrawing from the cell cycle and entering the G0 phase (4).

Regulation of Cell Proliferation

Most somatic cells reside in G0 phase until they receive a signal to proliferate, at which time they re-enter the G1 phase. Proliferation signals include exposure to growth factors, electrolyte imbalances, and loss of contact inhibition. These signals originate in the extracellular domain and are transduced through complex networks of molecules to nuclear signals that alter gene expression, leading to cell growth and proliferation. The signal transduction pathways are voluminous, intricate, and complex, and their complete description is beyond the scope of this chapter, but a generalized schematic is provided as an overview of the process.

The cell membrane is a fluid structure with protein channels and receptors embedded in it. For the most part, these receptors are ligand-specific, binding ligand with their extracellular domain and initiating signals with their intracellular domain. The signal is then carried to the nucleus through a series of second messenger molecules that typically act to alter the phosphorylation state of other molecules, resulting in activation of other messengers. The ultimate result is the activation of transcription factors, which turn on the expression of the "immediate-early response genes," which are required for cell proliferation. These genes, in turn, activate other genes and processes, ultimately leading to cell growth, DNA synthesis, and cell division (5) (Figure 1.2).

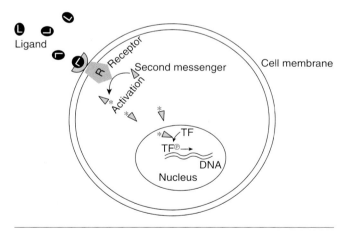

Figure 1.2 A simplified illustration of the control of cellular proliferation. Proliferation is initiated when a growth signal, or ligand (L), binds to its receptor (R) on the cell membrane. Ligand-receptor binding leads to activation (*) of a second messenger system. The activated second messenger carries the signal to the nucleus (sometimes through other mediators), where the signal is translated into the activation of transcription factors (TF), typically through phosphorylation. These transcription factors can then bind DNA, leading to expression of genes required for proliferation.

Apoptosis

Apoptosis, or programmed cell death, is a fundamental mechanism that maintains a check on cell population density and prevents the proliferation of genotypically or phenotypically abnormal cells. It is derived from the Greek word for "falling off" and is one of the most intensely researched aspects in cancer today. It is now known that complex molecular mechanisms exist to put into motion apoptotic signaling that ultimately result in the activation of enzymes called *caspases* that induce cell death (6,7). There are two fundamental mechanisms by which apoptosis can be induced in cells.

The extrinsic apoptotic pathway originates in the cell membrane (8). Proteins expressed on the membrane of cancer cells differ substantially from those on normal cells. The human body contains several circulating policing molecules that recognize these abnormal proteins and induce cell death. A cardinal example of this process is the tumor necrosis factor-α–related apoptosis-inducing ligand or TRAIL. TRAIL is a circulating protein endogenously produced by several cells in the human body. TRAIL binds to death receptors expressed on cell membranes and induces the formation of death-inducing signaling complex (DISC) of a variety of proteins on the inside of these cells. The fundamental outcome of the formation of DISC is the activation of pro-caspase 8, an inactive protein, to caspase 8. Caspase 8 is a potent inducer of apoptosis. It activates a series of intracellular proteins including caspases 7 and 9, ultimately resulting in the induction of caspase 3. Normal cells evade TRAIL-induced cell death by several mechanisms, the most remarkable of which is the expression of the so-called decoy receptors. These receptors resemble death receptors in their extracellular domain, but lack the intracellular domain that is capable of assembling DISC. Hence, they serve to sequester TRAIL from binding to and activating the death receptors, while themselves incapable of inducing apoptosis. The hallmark of the extrinsic apoptotic pathway is that it recognizes phenotypically abnormal cells with differential protein expression at the cell surface. T-cell turnover in the body—in particular, the destruction of T cells after their function in fighting infection is served—is a TRAIL-dependent mechanism. Cancer cells frequently do not express decoy receptors or express dysfunctional decoy receptors, making them susceptible to circulating TRAIL.

Intrinsic apoptotic pathway, on the other hand, originates in the mitochondria (9). Several factors—extracellular, such as radiation and hypoxia, and intracellular, such as DNA mutations—result in DNA damage. In response to DNA damage, the mitochondrial membrane secretes proteins that cleave pro-caspase 9 to the active caspase 9. Caspase 9 then activates a series of downstream enzymes that ultimately result in activation of caspase 3 and apoptosis. During cell cycle progression, the identification of DNA mutations sets in motion DNA repair machinery (vide supra). When complete repair is not feasible, the protein p53, among others, induces the intrinsic apoptotic pathway. Although there is some overlap between the two pathways, intrinsic pathway does not use caspase 8 and generally responds to genotypic alterations in cells.

Regardless of the stimulus, activation of caspase 3 leads to the activation of several proteases and endonucleases. Endonucleases induce the classic internucleosomal DNA fragmentation producing a series of 180 to 200 base pair long nucleosomes (DNA laddering) and chromatin condensation. Proteases disrupt cellular cytoskeleton and induce cell shrinkage and intracellular protein cross-linking. Cells then undergo surface blebbing and fragmentation into a number of membrane-bound apoptotic bodies. These apoptotic bodies express specific proteins that signal macrophage-induced phagocytosis. Such a complex process resulting in cell death is testimony to the central importance of apoptosis as a regulatory pathway in maintaining cellular homeostasis, and deregulation of apoptosis is a central event in virtually all cancers.

Angiogenesis and Its Regulation

When cells multiply, they depend on surrounding cells and existing blood vessels for nutrition. Once a critical mass of cells is reached, existing blood vessels are no longer adequate to support this growing mass of cells. Subsequent cellular proliferation is critically dependent on establishing new blood supply to the cells, a process loosely termed *angiogenesis*. Formation of blood vessels is a tightly regulated process that happens routinely during embryonic growth and at sites of neovascularization in the adult, such as in the ovary in reproductive women, during inflammation and wound healing (10). In the embryo, mesodermal precursor cells are directed to form hemangioblasts that provide the cellular source for hematopoietic stem cells and vascular stem cells or angioblasts. The vascular stem cells, or angioblasts, are organized into blood vessels de novo by a process termed *vasculogenesis* that is critically dependent in a dose-dependent fashion on vascular endothelial growth factor (VEGF) (11). Once a niche of blood vessels is formed, these divide to form additional blood vessels through angiogenesis. These processes lead to a juvenile angiomatous capillary-like network of blood vessels. Subsequent pruning of the juvenile vascular plexus calls into action a slew of vessel maturation proteins, many of which are only now being identified and characterized. Vessel maturation proteins induce arterial and venous distinction, leading to blood vessel hierarchy and pericyte or smooth muscle cell coverage of endothelial cells, through a process termed *arteriogenesis*. Mature vessels then integrate into the primary circulation, establishing new blood supply to the target site.

Although the role of VEGF in angiogenesis has been well established, the role played by vessel maturation proteins has only recently come to the fore (12). The vessel maturation protein EphB4, a member of the largest family of receptor tyrosine kinases called *Ephs*, and its cognate ligand ephrinB2, are mutually exclusively expressed by endothelial cells. Expression of these proteins directs arterial (ephrinB2) and venous (EphB4) lineage of endothelial cells even before the onset of circulation, indicating that endothelial cells are genetically programmed to generate arteries or veins. In addition, the interaction between these proteins at the capillary junctions of venules and arterioles is critically required for blood vessel maturation. When either protein is lost, vessel development is arrested at the capillary stage, resulting in embryonic lethality (13) and impaired angiogenesis at sites of neovascularization in the adult (14). An additional family of receptor tyrosine kinases, called *Tie receptors*, also plays an important role in blood vessel maturation.

The Tie-2 receptor is exclusively expressed by endothelial cells and has two natural ligands, angiopoietin-1 (Ang-1) and Ang-2. Ang-1 induces the generation of leakage-resistant blood vessels (15) by increasing pericyte deposition; such mature vessels rest in a dormant nonproliferative state. The naturally occurring antagonist to Ang-1 is Ang-2, which competitively inhibits Ang-1 binding to Tie-2. Ang-2 induces breakdown of pericytes, exposing endothelial cells to surrounding matrix proteins. In the absence of stimuli for blood vessel proliferation, these blood vessels lacking pericyte coat are destroyed; to the contrary, when angiogenic factors are present, angiogenesis ensues.

A third and more interesting family of proteins belong to the Notch-Delta superfamily. In particular, the Deltalike ligand-4 (Dll-4) is exclusively expressed by arterial endothelial cells and can suppress venous fate of endothelial cells. Dll-4 is required in a dosage-sensitive manner for arterial patterning and normal arterial and venous development (16). Dll-4 expression arrests blood vessel proliferation, and directs their functional maturation and integration into the primary circulation (17).

It is hence clear that blood vessel formation and maturation is a complex process. Although initiated by well-known angiogenic molecules like VEGF and fibroblast growth factor (FGF), several additional proteins play a key role in the maturation of juvenile vessels, their pruning and integration into primary circulation. These proteins also determine the artery-vein fate of endothelial cells, the extent of pericyte coat on nascent vasculature, and, finally, the ability of these cells to continue to generate additional vessels. This maturity in our understanding of blood vessel formation has allowed refining the strategies aimed at inhibiting tumor angiogenesis, and cancer therapy has moved from the first-generation, generic, and poorly functional antiangiogenic molecules like angiostatin, to the more modern and targeted VEGF antagonist, Avastin. Continued research with other molecules that regulate angiogenesis will soon bring to the fray more potent and less toxic angiogenesis inhibitors.

MOLECULAR DERANGMENTS IN CANCER

Molecular Changes That Deregulate Normal Cellular Proliferation

Cancer results from complex changes in the tightly regulated molecular pathways that control cell proliferation and differentiation. Several naturally occurring processes serve to check and correct these derangements before they result in uncoordinated cell proliferation and tumorigenicity. The first clear description of the so-called two-hit theory of carcinogenesis in the colon recognizes the requirement of multiple complementary changes to evade cellular checkpoints and cause cancer. These changes can be induced by many different cellular processes, some of which will be considered here.

Genetic abnormalities that induce cancer can occur sporadically, as seen in a majority of cancers, or be inherited, such as *BRCA-1* mutations associated with breast cancer or *ret* proto-oncogene mutations in multiple endocrine neoplasia type 2 syndrome. At the most simplistic level, mutations in genes can cause the amplification of loci coding for oncogenic proteins, such as

HER-2/neu amplification in a proportion of breast cancers (18), or result in the deletion of loci coding for tumor suppressor genes, such as loss of *VHL* gene in von Hippel-Lindau syndrome (19). Such mutations result in quantitatively altered protein expression. Alternatively, mutations can result in qualitatively altered proteins that are overactive or unable to perform their intended function. Mutations in the ras protein reduce its GTPase activity and mutant ras remains in the active GTP-bound form, inducing cell proliferation. Mutations in p53 DNA result in an abnormal protein that is less easily degraded, but functionless. *APC* mutations in colon cancer introduce a premature stop codon in the gene, leading to the formation of a truncated protein incapable of inducing β-catenin degradation.

A third type of DNA mutation frequently observed in cancer is chromosomal translocation. One form of DNA translocation causes generation of a new hybrid protein with oncogenic activity, best exemplified by the Philadelphia chromosome in chronic myeloid leukemia. A reciprocal translocation results in transfer of the c-*abl* proto-oncogene from chromosome 9 to the breakpoint cluster region in chromosome 22. The resultant hybrid c-*abl*-*bcr* gene codes a chimeric protein that induces uncontrolled leukocyte proliferation. Alternatively, chromosomal translocation can transfer genes from regions wherein their expression is tightly controlled to regions where they can be constitutively expressed. Translocation of the c-*myc* gene from its location on chromosome 8 to chromosome 14 in Burkitt lymphoma is an example of this type of DNA mutation.

Viral infection has been implicated in several epithelial cancers, including nasopharyngeal carcinoma (Epstein-Barr virus) and cervical carcinoma (human papillomavirus [HPV]) and following human immunodeficiency virus infection, such as lymphoma and Kaposi sarcoma. Although the exact mechanism of viral oncogenesis is not known, several DNA mutations have been implicated in these tumors. In cervical cancers, for example, infection with HPV16 or HPV18 strains results in integration of the HPV DNA into the host genome. In particular, the open reading frames of oncogenes E6 and E7 integrate at sites in the host genome wherein their transcription is regulated by constitutively activating promoters. The resultant overexpression of these oncogenic proteins induces uncontrolled cell proliferation and cancer. In addition, such integration may also disrupt expression of genes near the site of integration, thereby silencing some tumor suppressor genes.

Curiously, in some forms of carcinogenesis, structurally normal and functionally competent proteins can assume altered functions, through as yet unknown mechanisms. The canonical Wnt/β-catenin signaling pathway is an excellent example of this alteration in protein function. Under normal conditions, Wnt signaling via β-catenin leads to the formation of a transcriptional activation complex composed of different proteins in the nucleus. These complexes can include the transcriptional coactivator CREB-binding protein (CBP) or its homolog p300. The CBP-containing complex induces proteins that maintain the cell in an immature, proliferative, dedifferentiated state, whereas the p300-containing complex drives cellular maturation and differentiation (20). It has been proposed that aberrant regulation of the balance between these two related transcriptional programs underlies the differential gene regulation observed in cancer. Nuclear accumulation of β-catenin in cancer is believed to pref-erentially use the CBP-containing transcriptional complex over p300. This favors continued cellular proliferation and maintenance of cells in the poorly differentiated state.

In the absence of overt DNA mutations, histone modifications and changes in chromatin structure can alter the ability of the nuclear transcriptional machinery to access genes for transcription. Epigenetic changes refer to such reversible phenotypic changes in cells that can be inherited and the field of cancer epigenetics is evolving rapidly on several fronts (21). One of the best-studied epigenetic alterations in cancer is DNA methylation. In general, promoter regions of genes contain recurrent CG bases, called *CpG islands*. Methylation of the cytosine residues is a reversible event that significantly impairs the ability of transcriptional activators to bind to gene promoters to induce transcription. Whereas there is global hypomethylation in cancer, promoter regions of tumor suppressor genes are consistently hypermethylated, and, thereby, expression of these genes is silenced.

Activation of Oncogenes

Many genetic alterations occur in tumor cells as a result of cellular transformation rather than as a cause of it. Therefore, by strict definition, an oncogene is a gene that, when introduced in a cell, causes transformation and/or tumor formation. The first oncogene was described in the mid-1970s as a gene carried by the Rous sarcoma virus, an animal RNA tumor virus. Stehelin et al. (22) showed in 1976 that the transforming gene was derived from a normal cellular gene named *src*. Infection by the virus led to overexpression and activation of *src*, resulting in transformation of infected cells and tumor formation. Over the next decade, many other viral oncogenes were identified, along with their cellular homologues. Subsequently, it has been shown that these cellular oncogenes are activated by mutations or genetic rearrangements in many human tumors (23).

In general, cellular oncogenes are genes involved in cell proliferation and can be classified into several groups (24) (Table 1.1). The first group of oncogenes encodes growth factors. When aberrantly expressed, these oncogene products will stimulate cell growth through the normal mechanisms of the parent growth factor. Examples include the *sis* oncogene (platelet-derived growth factor), *int-l* (unknown growth factor), *int-2* (FGF-related), and *hst* (also FGF-related). The second group of oncogenes encodes proteins that resemble growth factor receptors. Whereas wild type growth factor receptors are activated only on specific ligand binding, oncogene products are constitutively active forms of these receptors, which signal continuously, regardless of presence of the ligand. Oncogenes in the third group encode members of the signal transduction pathways within the cell. Normally, members of these pathways require activation by the previous step in the pathway. However, when overexpressed or aberrantly expressed, these oncogene products are constantly active and induce cell proliferation. The final group is the nuclear transcription factors. These genes are normally regulated by the signal transduction pathways and regulate expression of proliferation-associated genes. When aberrantly expressed they lead to unbridled proliferation. Oncogenes, then, are positive regulators of proliferation and gain of function of oncogenes leads to tumor formation.

Table 1.1

Oncogenes

Growth Factor Type	Receptor Type	Signal Transducer Type	Transcription Factor Type
hst (fibroblast growth factor related)	c-erb B2 (HER-2/neu) (receptor like)	abl (cytoplasmic/nuclear protein tyrosine kinase)	ets (sequene-specific DNA-binding protein)
int-1 (?)	erb-B (truncated epidermal growth factor)	fgr (membrane-associated protein tyrosine kinase)	fos (component of AP-1 transcription factor)
int-2 (fibroblast growth factor related)	fms (mutant CSF-1 receptor)	fps/fcs (cytoplasmic protein tyrosine kinase)	jun (sequene-specific DNA-binding protein)
sis (platelet-derived growth factor β-chain)	kit (truncated stem cell receptor-like protein)	fgr (membrane-associated protein tyrosine kinase)	myb (sequene-specific DNA-binding protein)
	met (soluble truncated receptor-like protein)	lck (membrane-associated protein tyrosine kinase)	L-myc (sequene-specific DNA-binding protein)
	ret (truncated receptor-like protein)	src (membrane-associated protein tyrosine kinase)	N-myc (sequene-specific DNA-binding protein)
	ros (receptor-like protein)	yes (membrane-associated protein tyrosine kinase)	myc (sequene-specific DNA-binding protein)
	trk (soluble truncated receptor-like protein)	H-ras (membrane-associated G-protein)	erbA (dominant negative mutant of thyroxine receptor)
		K-ras (membrane-associated G-protein)	rel (dominant negative mutant of NF-B-related protein)
		N-ras (membrane-associated G-protein)	evi-1 (transcription factor?)
		gip (mutant-activated form of Gi)	ski (transcription factor?)
		gsp (mutant-activated form of Gs)	vuv (transcription factor?)
		B-raf (protein-serine kinase)	
		cot (protein-serine kinase)	
		pim-1 (protein-serine kinase)	
		raf/mil (protein-serine kinase)	
		mos (cytostatic factor)	
		crk (SH2/SH3-containing protein)	

Inhibition of Tumor Suppressor Genes

The first experimental evidence for tumor suppressor genes came nearly 30 years ago, when tumor cells were fused with normal cells and the resulting hybrid cells were found to have lost the potential to form tumors (25–27). It was noted that the tumorigenic potential was regained if specific chromosomes derived from the normal parental cell were subsequently lost from the hybrid cell. Further, these same specific normal chromosomes were able to suppress the tumorigenic phenotype when introduced into tumor cells, and therefore were identified as carrying "tumor suppressing" genes. Unlike oncogenes, a tumor suppressor gene is a gene whose loss of function confers a malignant phenotype. It acts in a recessive fashion in that both copies of the gene must be inactivated for the effect to be seen, through mutation, deletion, loss of heterozygosity, or transcriptional silencing. Finally, returning a functional allele to a cell lacking a tumor suppressor gene would reverse the tumorigenic phenotype (27).

The first tumor suppressor genes were identified through the study of human familial cancer syndromes. Chromosomal analysis of disease carriers reveals areas of consistent chromosomal loss or abnormality, identifying potential tumor suppressor genes. As more and more detailed genetic linkage analyses are undertaken, the specific gene can be identified (28). In this manner, the first tumor suppressor gene, the retinoblastoma gene (Rb), was identified and cloned in 1987 (29). Subsequently, many other tumor suppressor genes have been identified and their functions are beginning to be elucidated (Table 1.2). In general, the function of tumor suppressor gene products is to control cellular proliferation. Although the exact mechanism of action of many of the tumor suppressor genes is not understood, the molecular pathways regulated by the Rb and TP53 genes provide valuable prototypes.

The Retinoblastoma Pathway

The retinoblastoma gene encodes a 105-kilodalton protein, pRb, which is unphosphorylated in the G0/G1 phase of the cell cycle. The unphosphorylated form is capable of binding to and inhibiting the activity of the E2F transcription factor. E2F is required for transcription of genes required for proliferation, DNA synthesis, and replication; therefore, when E2F is sequestered by pRb, the cell is unable to proliferate. In late G1, pRb is phosphorylated by CDK4 or CDK6, releasing E2F, thereby allowing transcriptional activation of cell cycle-promoting genes. The CDK inhibitor p16/ink-4α inhibits phosphorylation of pRb by CDK4 and CDK6 and therefore maintains G1 arrest (30,31). Mutant pRb is incapable of binding E2F and, hence, unable to restrict cellular proliferation.

The *TP53* Pathway

Alterations in *TP53* are the most common genetic changes documented in human malignancies, with over half of all cancers carrying such mutations. *TP53* is a tumor suppressor gene that is induced in the presence of DNA damage and encodes the protein, p53. p53 acts as a transcription factor and activates other genes that in turn transcriptionally regulate proteins required for G1 arrest and DNA repair. p53 can also act to trigger apoptosis in the face of DNA damage. Thus, up-regulation of p53 leads to G1 arrest, allowing the cell adequate time for DNA repair. If DNA repair fails, p53 eliminates these abnormal cells by inducing programmed cell death (31). The end result is that mutations are prevented from accumulating and the fidelity of the genome is preserved through successive rounds of the cell cycle. The oncogene *mdm2*, overexpressed in 30% to 40% of sarcomas, encodes a protein that binds to and degrades *p53*, inhibiting its effects. The *p19/ARF* tumor suppresser gene encodes a protein that specifically binds to the mdm2 protein and leads to its degradation, blocking the inhibition of *p53* (32,33).

Angiogenic Switch

Angiogenesis represents a sentinel event in cancer progression. Whereas an initial mass of cancer cells can survive using nutrition from existing blood vessels and surrounding tissues, continued tumor growth critically depends on the ability to induce blood vessel formation to exclusively supply the tumor. The theory of "angiogenic switch" that was popularized by Judah Folkman (34) argues that several nests of tumor cells can be identified in patients with no overt malignancy. The ability of these tumor nests to progress into clinically significant cancer depends on their ability to induce angiogenesis. Tumor cells can induce angiogenesis in a variety of ways. Tumor cells can produce soluble angiogenic factors themselves, such as Kaposi sarcoma cells producing VEGF, which binds to its cognate receptors on endothelial cells to induce angiogenesis (35). Alternatively, tumor cells may express proteins on their surface that can interact with other proteins expressed on endothelial cells and thereby induce angiogenesis. The EphB4 vessel maturation protein is expressed by a variety of epithelial cancers and is capable of signaling via ephrinB2 expressed on host endothelial cells to stimulate angiogenesis (36). Some tumors cause the release of angiogenic factors from the extracellular matrix or from host cells, such as macrophages or other inflammatory cells. Lastly, some signals initiated in tumor cells can down-regulate local expression of inhibitors of angiogenesis. For example, loss of function of the tumor suppressor gene *TP53* leads to down-regulation of thrombospondin, a potent inhibitor of angiogenesis.

Regardless of the mechanism, the end result is an increase in the local concentration of angiogenic factors relative to the concentration of angiogenic inhibitors. The angiogenic factors, then, induce the expression and secretion of enzymes by tumor cells, endothelial cells, and stromal cells that break down the extracellular matrix and vascular basement membrane. Breakdown of the extracellular matrix allows migration of both tumor cells and endothelial cells. In addition, angiogenic factors provide a chemotactic signal for the endothelial cells, promoting migration, proliferation, lumen formation, and finally vessel maturation (10) (Figure 1.3). Immature capillaries have a fragmented basement membrane and are leaky, making them more penetrable to tumor cells, thus facilitating metastasis as well (37).

Cell-Matrix Interaction and Metastatic Potential

The growth of tumor cells within an environment represents a dynamic process and calls for continuous interaction between the tumor cells and the surrounding matrix and host cells. Tumor cells have a highly evolved mechanism of interacting with

Table 1.2

Tumor Suppressor Genes

Gene	Proposed Function	Associated Cancer or Disorder	Syndrome
APC	Regulation of β-catenin, signal transduction	Colon cancer, colon polyps, gastric and duodenal tumors, desmoid tumors (Gardner's syndrome)	Familial polyposis coli
ATM	DNA repair, induction of TP53	Lymphoma, cerebellar ataxia, immunodeficiency, breast cancer in heterozygotes	Ataxia-telangiaectasia
BLM	? DNA helicase	Solid tumors, immunodeficiency, small stature	Bloom's syndrome
BRCA1	Interact with RAD51, repair of double-stranded DNA breaks	Breast cancer, ovarian cancer	Familial breast cancer 1
BRCA2	? Interact with RAD51, repair of double-stranded DNA breaks?	Breast cancer, male breast cancer, pancreatic cancer?, others	Familial breast cancer 2
CDK4	Cyclin-dependent kinase	Melanoma	Familial melanoma
?DCC	Cell surface receptor similar to NCAM	Colon cancer	?
E-cadherin	Intracellular signaling	Gastric cancer	?
EXT1, EXT2, EXT3	?	Exostoses, chondrosarcoma	Multiple exostoses
FACC	? DNA repair	Acute myelogenous leukemia, pancytopenia, skeletal abnormalities	Fanconi's anemia
MEN1	?	Pancreatic islet cell tumors	Multiple endocrine neoplasia type 1
MET	Receptor for HGF	Renal cancers, ?others	Hereditary papillary renal cancer
MLH1, MSH1, PMS1, PMS2	DNA mismatch repair	Colon cancer, endometrial, ovarian, hepatobiliary, genitourinary	Hereditary non-polyposis colorectal cancer
NF1	GTPase-activating protein for p21 ras proteins	Neurofibromas, neurofibromosarcoma, brain tumors	Neurofibromatosis type 1
NF2	Links membrane proteins to cytoskeleton	Acoustic neuromas, meningiomas, gliomas, ependymomas	Neurofibromatosis type 2
P15	Cyclin-dependent kinase inhibitor	Hematologic malignancies	?
P16/INK-4A	Cyclin-dependent kinase inhibitor	Melanoma, pancreatic cancer, other	Familial melanoma
P19ARF	Binds and degrades mdm2	?	?
P57/K1P2	Cell-cycle regulator	Wilms' tumor	Wiedmann–Beckwith syndrome
PTCH	Receptor for hedgehog signaling molecule	Basal cell carcinoma	Nevoid basal cell carcinoma syndrome
PTEN	Phosphatase with similarity to tensin	Breast cancer, follicular thyroid cancer, intestinal hamartomas, skin lesions	Cowden's disease
RB1	Cell-cycle and transcriptional regulator through E2F binding	Retinoblastoma, osteosarcoma, small-cell lung cancer, many others	Familial retinoblastoma
RET	Receptor tyrosine kinase for GDNF	Medullary thyroid cancer, pheochromocytoma, parathyroid hyperplasia, mucosal hamartomas	Multiple endocrine neoplasia type 2, familial medullary thyroid cancer
TP53	Transcription factor, response to stress and DNA damage, apoptosis	Sarcomas, breast cancers, brain tumors, leukemia, many others	Li–Fraumeni syndrome
VHL	Regulates transcriptional elongation by RNA polymerase III	Renal cell carcinoma, pheochromocytoma, retinal angiomas, hemangioblastomas	Von Hippel–Lindau syndrome
WT1	Transcriptional repressor	Wilms' tumor	Wilms' tumor
XPA, XPB, XPD	DNA repair helicases, nucleotide excision repair	Skin cancer, pigmentation abnormalities, hypogonadism	Xeroderma pigmentosum

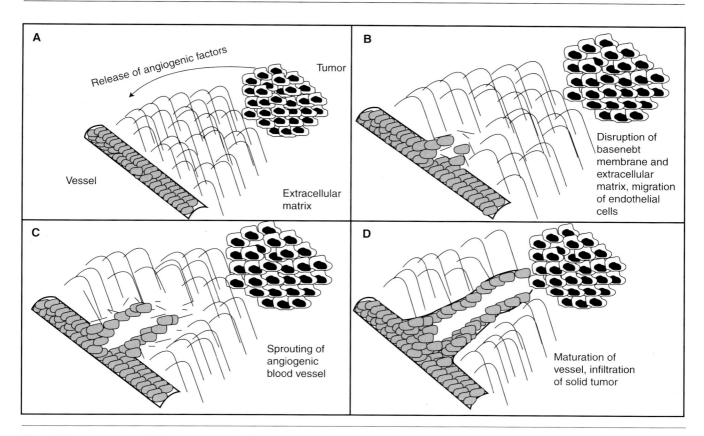

Figure 1.3 Angiogenesis. (**A**) Tumor-associated angiogenesis begins when tumor cells, or the surrounding stroma, release angiogenic factors. (**B**) The angiogenic factors induce collagenase and matrix metalloproteinases that lead to the digestion of the vascular basement membrane and the extracellular matrix. The angiogenic factors also provide a chemotactic signal for vascular endothelial cells, leading to endothelial migration. (**C**) Further extracellular matrix destruction and cell migration culminate in the sprouting of angiogenic vessels. (**D**) Finally, the angiogenic vessels infiltrate the solid tumor and mature.

their microenvironment, and some of the complexity and benefit of such interactions, such as angiogenesis, has already been alluded to. Tumor cells need to anchor to the surrounding matrix to establish intercellular trafficking and promote growth, while metastasis calls for displacement of tumor cells from their primary site. In line with this altered functional requirement, cancer cells are known to variably express adhesion molecules, such as laminin and integrin, depending on the stage of their growth. The proclivity that tumors have for specific organs as metastatic targets ("seed and soil" theory) is almost certainly orchestrated by molecular alterations, the exact nature of which is poorly understood.

Tumor cells harvested from metastatic deposits frequently have a very different genetic signature from a majority of the cells at the primary tumor site. Exactly when tumors acquire this metastatic advantage is not known. It has been proposed that extensive genomic instability seen in cancers generates a heterogenous polyclonal pool of tumor cells and, over time, cells with metastatic advantage are naturally selected. Indeed, molecular derangements in this subset of cells facilitates tumor cell invasion, embolization, survival in the circulation, arrest in a distant capillary bed, and extravasation into and multiplication within the organ parenchyma (38). It is possible that some molecular derangements have overlapping functions inducing

primary tumor growth and metastases. One example of such a multifunctional protein is the vessel maturation protein EphB4. EphB4 is overexpressed in a variety of epithelial cancers and provides direct survival advantage to tumor cells by inhibiting apoptosis. Furthermore, tumor cell-expressed EphB4 can promote angiogenesis by signaling via endothelial cell ephrinB2. In addition, EphB4 increases the levels of collagenases, in particular MMP-9 and MMP-2, and other proteases in tumor cells, which allows for tumor cells to invade the surrounding basement membrane and migrate to distant targets (39). Consistent with this idea, cells isolated from metastatic deposits form more aggressive tumors (40), and metastases themselves have the molecular advantage to metastasize. Alternatively, when tumor cells gain survival advantage because of genetic alterations that are not capable of inducing metastases, even tumors that are locally aggressive do not metastasize.

Some Tumor-Specific Abnormalities and Tumor Markers

Breast Cancer

Biologic therapy aimed at tumor-specific molecular abnormalities first saw the light in the solid-organ malignancy realm for the management of breast cancer. Overexpression of HER2/neu is observed in about 30% breast cancers (18) and is associated with a poorer clinical outcome, particularly in node-positive breast cancer patients. In addition, HER-2/neu expression is associated with relative resistance to cyclophosphamide therapy (41) and hormonal therapy (42). More importantly, the discovery of Herceptin, a monoclonal antibody directed against human HER-2/neu receptor, has dramatically advanced our ability to treat breast cancer. Treatment of metastatic breast cancers that overexpress HER-2/neu with Herceptin improves outcome even when used as a single agent (43) and also increases the clinical benefit of first-line chemotherapy (44).

Inherited predisposition to breast cancer is mediated by mutations in the *BRCA-1* and *BRCA-2* genes, which serve as potent tumor suppressors in normal population. Expression of the hormone receptors, estrogen receptor, and progesterone receptor, by breast cancer cells predicts response to hormonal therapy and has prognostic significance (45). Numerous other tumor markers for breast cancer have been described. These include expression of the DF3 antigen, a high-molecular-weight mucin, and of the estrogen-related protein pS-2. Both markers are associated with a favorable clinical outcome (46,47). Other studies have implicated that overexpression of certain enzymes, such as cathepsin D or urokinase plasminogen activator, or an adhesion molecule such as the laminin receptor, may be associated with development of metastases (48–50). However, these markers are not widely used clinically.

Another potential use of biologic markers is to follow patients once the primary tumor has been removed. Of the many markers described, carcinoembryonic antigen (CEA), carbohydrate antigen (CA) 27–29, and CA15-3 have been shown to become elevated prior to the development of symptoms or the detection of metastatic disease by physical examination or radiographic findings (51–54). In general, approximately 40% to 50% of patients who develop metastases have a preceding rise in either CEA, CA 27–29 or CA15-3 levels, with lead times ranging from 3 to 18 months. However, the clinical utility of tumor markers in predicting relapse has not been proven, and the treatment of asymptomatic patients has not been shown to improve palliation (55,56).

Colorectal Cancer

Several oncogenes and tumor suppressor genes have been described in colon cancer. The canonical Wnt/β-catenin pathway is mutated in most colon cancers, leading to decreased β-catenin degradation and its consequent nuclear accumulation. Adenomatous polyposis coli (*APC*) protein inhibits β-catenin dephoshorylation and directs it toward degradation, serving as a tumor suppressor. Inactivating *APC* mutations are observed in over 80% of sporadic colon cancers, and inherited *APC* mutation leads to familial adenomatous polyposis and a near-certain incidence of colorectal malignancy by the age of 40. Inability of duplicating cells to correct DNA mismatch because of an inherited mismatch repair gene mutation also leads to colonic polyposis and right-sided colon cancers at an early age (Lynch syndrome). Other tumor suppressors with mutations in colorectal cancers include *p53* and deleted in colon cancer (*DCC*) genes.

There is no tumor marker available for screening for colon cancer. CEA has been shown to be ineffective for screening, even in high-risk patients such as those with ulcerative colitis, adenomatous familial polyposis, or hereditary nonpolyposis colon cancer syndrome (57). CEA has been shown to be elevated in 65% of patients with stage D colon cancer, but significant elevations are less common among patients with potentially curable disease (58,59). Preoperative CEA levels have been shown to have a prognostic value independent of tumor stage (60). Elevated preoperative CEA levels should return to normal following resection; failure to do so is associated with a high risk of recurrence (61). Some patients continue to maintain a marginally elevated level despite no evidence of recurrent disease; thus, although highly predictive of relapse, an elevated postoperative CEA is not absolute (62). Several studies have evaluated the utility of CEA monitoring in postoperative patients. Approximately half of patients who might benefit from a second resection are identified by routine CEA testing (62).

Lung Cancer

Serum tumor markers play a less concrete role in lung cancer than in other solid malignancies, and the currently defined markers are not suitable for screening asymptomatic patients. The most promising molecular target for therapy in lung cancer is the epidermal growth factor receptor (EGFR). Several EGFR activating mutations have been described in lung cancer, and small-molecule inhibitors such as erlotinib and gefitinib have been developed for the treatment of advanced non-small cell lung cancer (NSCLC). In particular, mutations in exons 18 through 21 of the *EGFR* gene render NSCLC responsive to gefitinib (63). Cytokeratin 19 fragment 21-1 (CYFRA 21-1) is another useful tumor marker in NSCLC (64). Elevated pretreatment levels predict shorter survival (65,66). In addition, serum levels drop to the normal range after curative resection, and rise in levels may be used to monitor recurrence (67,68). CYFRA 21-1 levels also correlate with clinical response to chemotherapy in patients with inoperable squamous cell cancer (69). A few studies have evaluated the prognostic value of CEA in resectable early-stage NSCLC. Elevated preoperative CEA levels correlates with a higher likelihood of recurrence (70). CA 125 may also be a useful marker for predicting stage, respectability, and survival in NSCLC patients (71,72). For squamous cell cancer in particular, the squamous cell carcinoma antigen level should drop to baseline after curative resection, and a subsequent rise in levels indicates tumor relapse (73). The squamous cell carcinoma antigen level is not affected by smoking, and thus eliminates the interference that is seen with CEA.

For small cell lung cancer (SCLC), the best tumor marker available is neuron-specific enolase (NSE). NSE can be used to differentiate between SCLC and lymphoma, both Hodgkin and non-Hodgkin (74). NSE levels may be useful to monitor patients for SCLC recurrence, but they have not been shown to differentiate between a complete and partial remission (75). CEA has also been used as a marker for SCLC; however, it is not specific, as it may be elevated in benign pulmonary conditions such as chronic obstructive pulmonary disease and tuberculosis. CEA has been shown to be more elevated in SCLC patients with more extensive disease than those with limited tumor involvement, and a fall in CEA predicts response to chemotherapy (76). In addition, survival is significantly shorter for patients with marked CEA elevations (77).

Pancreatic Cancer

Oncogenic activation of the *K-ras* gene occurs in over 90% of pancreatic ductal adenocarcinoma early in the carcinoma progression sequence. *K-ras* mutations induce transformation in pancreatic duct epithelial cells by activating a variety of molecular pathways that induce cell proliferation (78). CA 19-9 has been the main tumor marker for pancreatic cancer, although it is not specific. High CA 19-9 levels can differentiate pancreatic cancer from chronic pancreatitis, but not from other hepatobiliary malignancies, or cholangitis (79). Serum CA 19-9 levels correlate with extent of disease (80,81); failure to normalize values following resection is a poor prognostic indicator. Similarly, a subsequent rise in the marker following normalization indicates recurrence; in fact, the level may rise prior to clinical presentation (62). There has not been a clear delineation between CA 19-9 levels and response to chemotherapy, in part because of limitations of the currently available treatments for the disease. CEA may be associated with pancreatic cancer in 20% to 40% of patients, but is much less specific and sensitive than CA 19-9 (81). Some authors have found that a low CEA level is associated with a better prognosis (82).

Gastric Cancer

CA 72-4 is found in a variety of human malignancies of epithelial origin including NSCLC, breast, ovarian, pancreatic, esophageal, and gastric cancers. It is rarely expressed in benign lesions, and only appears in normal adult human tissue in the secretory endometrium. In gastric cancer, CA 72-4 levels correlate with the presence of nodal or serosal involvement (83). Because levels of CA 72-4 drop following curative resection, a subsequent rise is useful as a marker of recurrence, or a persistent elevation as an indication of incomplete resection. CEA has also been used to monitor patients with gastric cancer, but it has a low sensitivity, and thus is not advocated as a first-choice tumor marker (84,85). The serum CEA level appears to correlate with the tumor stage, and falls to normal levels following curative resection. Whereas approximately 40% to 60% of all gastric cancers express CEA, only 10% to 20% of patients with stage I and II disease have an elevated CEA level, compared with 30% of stage III disease (62,86). Although an elevated CEA level is a predictor of unresectable disease, a normal level does not reliably predict curability. Alpha-fetoprotein (AFP) may also be elevated in 30% of gastric cancers and in as many as 40% of patients with liver metastases (87). The elevations in CEA and AFP are nonoverlapping in gastric cancer. CA 19-9 has also been shown to be elevated in gastric cancer.

Ovarian Cancer

Estrogen and progesterone play an important role in the turnover of ovarian epithelial cells and, similar to their role in breast cancer, the expression of estrogen receptor and progesterone receptor has therapeutic and prognostic significance in ovarian cancer. Serum CA-125 levels are elevated in 80% to 90% of women with epithelial ovarian cancer. The expression is highest in serous, mixed, and unclassified adenocarcinomas and lowest in mucinous types (98). CA-125 does not have a high enough sensitivity to be used for screening, as up to 50% of patients with early disease will have a normal level, as well as a low specificity, with benign conditions such as pelvic inflammatory disease producing elevations (88). It may be used to differentiate between benign and malignant disease in women presenting with a pelvic mass, with a sensitivity of 78% and a specificity of 93% (88). The degree of elevation appears to relate to extent of disease (89). It appears that CA-125 levels preoperatively do not have independent prognostic significance (88,90). However, the presence of a persistently elevated level postoperatively might reflect the presence of residual or recurrent disease, and has been used as an indicator for a second-look operation. Some reports indicate that a change in CA-125 level during chemotherapy induction is associated with improved survival (91).

Prostate Cancer

Prostate epithelial cell turnover is regulated by androgens, and these cells maintain their androgen-dependence even in the transformed state. Androgen ablation is an effective strategy for the treatment of prostate adenocarcinoma; in particular, metastatic disease. Unfortunately, androgen ablation eventually results in the emergence of a hormone-refractory stage, complicating treatment options. *PTEN* is a tumor suppressor gene that plays a central role in prostate cancer. The *PTEN* gene product is a lipid phosphatase that negatively regulates the phosphatidylinositol 3′-kinase-AKT pathway, which induces cell proliferation and has antiapoptotic effects. Loss of *PTEN* expression, therefore, leads to inappropriate activation of AKT and correlates with increasing Gleason score and advanced grade prostate cancer (92). *NKX3.1* is a homeobox gene expressed specifically in prostatic epithelium and has been implicated in prostate cancer initiation. It is located on chromosome 8p21, which undergoes allelic deletion in a majority of prostate cancers (93).

The prostate-specific antigen (PSA) has greatly improved our ability to diagnose prostate cancer, and there is growing evidence that PSA-diagnosed tumors are more likely to be organ-confined and thus curable (94). PSA is produced by both normal and malignant prostate tissue, and is thus prostate-specific, although not prostate cancer-specific. The elevation in PSA in benign prostatic hypertrophy is usually mild, in contrast to the more striking elevations seen in prostatitis (95). PSA appears to predict success of radiotherapy as primary treatment (96,97). In addition, PSA levels rapidly decline following radical prostatectomy, and thus can be used as a marker for either incomplete resection or recurrence.

Hepatocellular Cancer

AFP is the major tumor marker associated with hepatocellular carcinoma, and may even be used for screening in high-risk population. Approximately 20% to 35% of tumors are not associated with an elevated AFP level (98,99). In general, the degree of AFP elevation relates to tumor size. Currently, a screening combination of ultrasound and AFP determination is recommended for patients with hepatitis B or C and cirrhosis or chronic active hepatitis (100). The level of AFP will fall following resection or chemoembolization, and a subsequent rise indicates recurrence (101).

CLINICAL APPLICATIONS OF MOLECULAR BIOLOGY IN CANCER MANAGEMENT

Therapy for Cancer

The cherished goal of a better understanding of the molecular biology of cancer is to provide better therapeutic options: more potent, highly targeted and less toxic. Biological therapy aims at reversing molecular derangements specific to the cancer at hand. Although some forms of therapy may generically target any cancer, such as antiangiogenic therapy, others will be used exclusively for a subset of cancers, such as Herceptin for HER2/neu overexpressing breast cancers. There are a variety of molecules that may be used for biologic therapy, of which proteins are the most extensively studied. Herceptin and Avastin are antibodies that target HER2/neu and VEGF, respectively. In other instances, proteins that compete with natural ligand for binding with growth-promoting receptors can be used to inhibit receptor function. For example, the soluble extracellular domain of EphB4 (sEphB4) competes for ephrinB2 binding and inhibits EphB4 stimulation and angiogenesis in murine models of human cancers (14). Alternatively, proteins that alter structure or sequester critical parts of oncogenic proteins can inhibit their function. For example, the EGFR family of receptors needs to form dimers for signaling. Inhibiting dimerization by binding to cysteine-rich domains that mediate receptor-receptor interaction inhibits EGFR signaling even in the presence of ligands.

A second class of molecules with application in cancer therapy is RNA. Protein synthesis in dividing cells requires translation of message from a single-stranded mRNA in cytoplasm. A multistranded cytoplasmic mRNA is considered abnormal by the cell and is appropriately degraded. Introduction of single-strand antisense nucleotides with sequence complementary to a portion of the mRNA of the overexpressed oncogenic protein will lead to the formation of a double-stranded piece of mRNA in the cytoplasm and its subsequent degradation without the production of the oncogenic protein. VEGF antisense is a good example of a single-strand oligonucleotide that targets VEGF and inhibits angiogenesis in tumors (102). Double-stranded small interfering RNA (siRNA) are 22 base pair-long double strands of RNA with sequence complementary to a portion of the mRNA of interest. These molecules are more potent than antisense nucleotides and are also highly specific. Similar to antisense oligonulceotides, siRNA also bind to target mRNA and generate RNA-induced silencing complexes that degrade the mRNA of interest (103). Antioncogene ribozymes are RNA molecules with catalytic activity, like protein enzymes that are able to bind and cleave specific target RNA sequences, preventing translation of the gene into a protein product. Anti-*ras* ribozymes have been designed to cleave the H-*ras* mRNA in human bladder carcinoma cells and result in growth suppression.

The third class of molecules for therapy in cancer includes DNA. Introduction of a gene that codes for a missing tumor suppressor gene will replace the molecular deficiency at source. Replenishing the thymidylate synthase DNA will produce the appropriate protein to restore colon cancer sensitivity to fluorouracil, for example. Transfer of normal *Rb* gene into retinoblastoma or osteosarcoma cells with inactivated *Rb* genes inhibits cell

growth and tumorigenicity in nude mice (104). Replacement of the wild type *TP53* gene by viral vectors has been shown to inhibit tumor growth in human lung cancer, head and neck cancer, and prostate cancer (105–107).

Lastly, several small molecules have been designed to specifically inhibit the function of oncogene products. Kinase inhibitors of EGFR such as imatinib are examples of such molecules. Small molecule targets include tyrosine kinases, phosphatases, acetylases, and a variety of other molecules that play an important role in intracellular signal transduction.

The delivery of biological agents to tissues of interest can be a particular challenge. Proteins and small molecules can be efficiently delivered by traditional parenteral and enteral routes with good bioavailability. However, nucleotide delivery, both RNA and DNA, poses a major hurdle. The best vector for nucleotide transfer would be safe to the host, easily produced in high quantities, efficient at transferring the molecule of interest, and result in long-lasting effects. The earliest vehicles for gene delivery were viral vectors, because a natural part of the viral life cycle is to infect host cells and transfer their genetic material. Several types of viral vectors have been used for gene delivery with mixed success and variable adverse effects. Replication-incompetent retroviruses, adenoviruses, adeno-associated viruses, and herpes simplex viruses are some the viral vectors that have been studied so far. These viral-dependent approaches probably remain the most efficient methods of gene delivery. However, issues of safety and possible host inflammatory responses led to the development of other nonviral strategies.

Liposomes have been engineered for gene delivery by mixing positively charged lipids with negatively charged DNA. Synthetic liposomes tend to be better absorbed by rapidly proliferating cells and vascular endothelial cells, leading to nonspecific fusion of the liposome with the cell membrane and release of the DNA into the cytoplasm (108). Gene transfer efficiency can be quite variable with the various compositions of liposomes under investigation, although up to 90% gene transfer has been reported (109). To improve the efficacy of liposome entry into the target cell, liposomes have been complexed with viral proteins as well as target cell-specific antibodies to create "virosomes" and "immunoliposomes" (109,110). The clinical applicability of liposome-mediated gene transfer is still limited by the transient nature of gene expression.

Nucleotide delivery can also be achieved by simple injection into target tissue. The exact mechanism of incorporation of the DNA into cells is not fully understood but appears to involve endocytic or electrical processes resulting in internalization of the DNA (111). Specific tissues seem to be more capable of expressing directly injected DNA such as muscle, subcutaneous tissue, liver, and thyroid follicular cells (112–114). A recently developed device, the Accell gene gun (Accell, GENIVA, Middleton, NI), is able to deliver DNA, coated with gold particles, at high velocities with a burst of helium gas into the target tissue. Alternatively, electrical current can be used to transiently generate pores in cell membranes through which nucleotides of interest can enter cells, a process termed *electroporation*. Hydroporation involves injecting large volumes of liquid into cells, causing them to swell, resulting in stretching of the cell membrane and leakiness through pores that form portals of entry for foreign nucleotides. A variation of direct gene injection uses engineered skeletal muscle cells to express the gene of interest. Skeletal myoblasts are harvested and gene of interest introduced into them ex vivo. When the genetically engineered myoblasts are injected into the host skeletal muscle, they are able to produce and secrete the foreign protein locally as well as systemically.

Biological therapy for cancer is a multifaceted approach that targets several molecular events that are aberrant in cancer. A brief overview of some of the techniques that hold promise follows.

Oncogene and Tumor Suppressor Homeostasis

In its simplest form, biological therapy re-establishes the balance between oncogenes and tumor suppressor genes. Ablation of the function of an oncogene or enhancing the function of tumor suppressor genes restores the normal mechanisms for growth control and differentiation. Tumor suppressors can be replenished by reintroducing deleted genes, or by demethylating tumor suppressor gene promoter regions. Oncogene synthesis can be inhibited by antisense RNA or siRNA. Synthesized proteins can be degraded using antibodies that induce membrane receptor endocytosis. Small molecules and dominant negative proteins can inhibit oncogene-induced signaling. Gleevac, Herceptin, and imatinib are agents currently in clinical use that inhibit oncogenic function to treat cancer.

Antiangiogenic Therapy

There are three main strategies on which antiangiogenic therapies are based (115). First, because antiangiogenic therapy targets sites of neovascularization only, tumor vasculature is selectively targeted, and the more dormant developed vasculature is spared. Endothelial cells engaged in active tumor angiogenesis have a much more rapid turnover than do normal adult endothelial cells and, hence, undergo little genetic mutation compared with cancer cells, reducing the risk of developing drug resistance (116). Second, endothelial cells release growth factors in a paracrine manner that have direct influence on tumor growth. Two such examples are insulin-like growth factors 1 and 2 and basic fibroblast growth factor, which have been shown to promote tumor cell growth and migration (117). Therefore, through inhibiting endothelial proliferation, it may be possible to inhibit tumor cell growth.

Finally, through preventing peripheral capillary formation, it may be possible to prevent spread of tumor cells to distant sites via the leaky neovasculature. Avastin, a VEGF antibody, is a potent antiangiogenic molecule currently in clinical use for the treatment of several solid-organ tumors, including colon cancer and lung cancer. The extent of response seen to anti-VEGF therapy will depend on the extent the tumor relies on VEGF for its survival and the magnitude of VEGF induction by tumor cells.

Immunotherapy

Three main strategies have been proposed using gene therapy techniques to stimulate the immune response to treat tumors: enhancement of the immunogenicity of the tumor, blocking mechanisms by which tumor cells evade immunologic destruction, and increasing antitumor activity of immune cells. Tumor cells are poor immunogens, although they express several tumor-associated antigens. Attempts have been made to immunize patients with cancer-specific antigens such as CEA to invoke an antitumor response in the host (118–120). A plasmid carrying the human CEA cDNA was shown to elicit humoral and cellular immune responses that were CEA-specific in vivo. In addition, the plasmid was able to function as a vaccine and protect against syngeneic colon carcinoma cells that expressed CEA (119). Alternatively, because all tumors contain necrotic areas, immunizing the host with necrosis-specific proteins is another way to induce tumor immunogenicity.

Genes encoding accessory proteins in the immune response have been incorporated in tumor vaccines. The B7 family of molecules is expressed on the surface of antigen-presenting cells and is required as a costimulation factor to activate T lymphocytes by interaction with the CD28 and CTLA-4 molecules on the lymphocytes. When the *B7* gene was transfected into tumor cells in animals, tumor regression was observed and subsequent injections of tumor cells were rejected (121,122). In a human clinical trial for melanoma, liposomes containing the *HLA-B7* gene were directly injected into subcutaneous melanoma nodules. In four of five patients, the injected nodules regressed. In one patient, the regression was seen in the injected nodule as well as distant metastases (123). Another strategy to boost host immunity is to inhibit the regulatory T cells that specifically blunt host immune responses in general.

Other methods to induce immunity against tumors include forcing tumor cells to secrete cytokines that can sensitize cytotoxic T cells to attack them. Alternatively, tumor-infiltrating lymphocytes can be isolated and stimulated in vitro. When reinjected into the subject, these cells target the tumor and elicit a local cytokine response and initiating T-cell–mediated tumor cell death.

Restoring Response to Chemotherapy

As previously discussed, expression of certain proteins or deletion of specific molecules portends poor response to chemotherapy. Restoring the deleted gene product or inhibiting overexpressed molecule can restore tumor cell sensitivity to traditional chemotherapy. When human NSCLC cells with a deletion of *TP53* are engineered to express wild type *TP53* gene product, their sensitivity to cisplatin is significantly increased (124).

Utility of Suicide Genes

A gene encoding an enzyme is transferred into tumor cells and this enzyme activates a nontoxic prodrug to produce a toxic agent, resulting in death of the tumor cell. In the best-known system, the herpes simplex virus thymidine kinase (*HSV-tk*) gene is transduced into tumor cells. When the tumor cell is exposed to the prodrug ganciclovir, thymidine kinase phosphorylates the molecule, producing an intermediate that interferes with DNA synthesis and leads to cell death (125). Theoretically, cytotoxic effects could be directed specifically to tumor cells transferred with the *HSV-tk* gene without systemic toxicity. Other investigators have transduced the gene encoding cytosine deaminase into tumor cells, allowing the metabolism of the nontoxic prodrug 5-fluorocytosine to the toxic metabolite 5-fluorouracil (126). In the first clinical trial using suicide gene therapy, a positive response was seen in five of the eight patients with glioblastoma multiforme treated with a retroviral*HSV-tk* vector (127). The delivery of the *HSV-tk* gene, and thus cell killing, can be targeted to specific tumor cells by the use of tumor-specific promoters. For instance, when the CEA promoter was linked to the *HSV-tk* gene in a plasmid and transfected into lung cancer cells, only CEA-positive cells were killed in response to ganciclovir treatment. Similarly, viral vectors containing the AFP promoter have been effective against hepatocellular carcinomas and the HER2/neu promoter for pancreatic and breast cancers (128,129).

Toxins

Naked cytotoxins have systemic side effects and do not achieve desired tumor-specific levels to effect efficient tumor killing. It is known that several receptors endocytose ligands as part of their signaling mechanism. Using this concept, ligands of receptors overexpressed on cancer cells can be linked to toxins and delivered systemically. Receptor-ligand interaction occurring at the receptor-rich tumor cell surface leads to ligand endocytosis and, consequently, toxin intake by cancer cells and their targeted killing. Interleukin-2-toxin is an example of this strategy applied in the treatment of chemorefractory T-cell leukemias (130).

Cancer Screening and Diagnosis

Molecular diagnostic techniques are constantly being improved. With better understanding of genomics, transcriptomics, and proteomics, our ability to detect molecular changes in small tissue samples with exceeding accuracy continues to evolve. Already, the detection of *BRCA-1* mutations and *APC* deletions in first-degree relatives of patients with documented disease is a clinical reality. This allows us to detect patients at risk for known diseases and allows for aggressive screening by conventional techniques and possibly prophylactic intervention. In the future, it is likely that we will develop pharmacologic or biologic therapy to reverse this derangement or slow its progression. Refining assays for screening and diagnosis, while greatly improving our diagnostic capability, can reduce patient discomfort as well. Consider, for example, an ex-smoker who is at risk for squamous cell carcinoma of the mouth. Amplifying millions of times the small amount of RNA extracted from the few cells secreted into the patient's saliva will allow us to identify genetic mutations and early buccal cancer.

Molecular derangements also afford diagnostic capabilities using generic or patient-specific abnormalities. For example, $\alpha v \beta 5$ integrin is specifically expressed at sites of active angiogenesis. Scans aimed at targeting proteins that specifically detect this integrin can be generically used to detect angiogenesis and, consequently, small foci of cancer growth early, regardless of the cancer type. Alternatively, analysis of primary tumor samples will delineate overexpressed or mutated proteins and a patient-specific molecular signature unique to that cancer can be identified. This allows us immense capability to diagnose disease in other parts of the body through both invasive and noninvasive methods. Staining for this protein in biopsy specimens will allow far greater accuracy in detecting cancer spread compared with traditional hematoxylin and eosin staining. Antibodies generated against this protein can be applied in whole-body scans to identify even a few systemic cancer cells.

Cancer Prognosis and Follow-Up

Specific molecular abnormalities are known to portend poor prognosis. We have already seen the prognostic benefit of evaluating hormone receptors in breast cancer, or monitoring the response to therapeutic intervention by measuring levels of tumor-specific antigens. In addition, certain molecular signatures predict poor response to chemotherapy, such as HER2/neu expression in breast cancer and cyclophosphamide therapy, thymidylate synthase deficiency in colon cancer and fluorouracil therapy, and EphB4 expression in ovarian cancer and conventional chemotherapy (131). In one study, Lloyd et al. (132) showed that presence of EphB4 mRNA in peritoneal fluid of colon cancer patients at the time of resection of primary disease predicts recurrence and poor survival. Thus, a keen knowledge of the molecular derangements in cancer and their biological outcome helps predict the behavior of the tumor, the likelihood it will respond to other forms of therapy, and overall recurrence and outcome.

Follow-up regimen can be tailored to the molecular nature of the patient's disease. The duration and extent of follow-up will be dictated by the predicted aggressiveness of the disease. Agents that target molecular changes in the tumor will allow more sophisticated methods to identify early sites of recurrence, and sensitive diagnostic tools will use small quantities of easily accessible tissue to monitor disease remission.

CONCLUSION

Advances in the techniques and our grasp of molecular biology have opened the door to a new paradigm in cancer screening, diagnosis, and management. The slow but steady unraveling of the complex signaling pathways that are deranged in cancer is allowing more varied, more targeted, and more potent therapeutic options to traditionally difficult methods to manage cancers. Several roadblocks in our comprehension of cancer biology and the delivery of active molecules continue to retard progress in the field. A multidisciplinary approach to cancer therapy guided by translational application of basic science strategies is certain to bring to reality many possibilities that are now considered theoretical. All these tremendous improvements will make cancer a curable disease, most likely in the not-so-distant future.

ACKNOWLEDGMENTS

The authors acknowledge the contributions of Rosa F. Hwang, Nicole Baril, Megan McGarvey, Mimi H. Chiang, Silvia C. Formenti, and Kristin Skinner, who contributed the chapter on molecular biology in the first edition of this book. The present authors have used portions of that chapter in the current work.

REFERENCES

1. Nasmyth K. Viewpoint: putting the cell cycle in order. *Science.* 1996;274:1643–1646.
2. Edgar BA, Lehner CF. developmental control of cell cycle regulators: a fly's perspective. *Science.* 1996;274:1646–1652.

3. Elledge SJ. Cell cycle checkpoints: preventing an identity crisis. *Science.* 1996;274:1664–1672.

4. Scherr CJ. Cancer cell cycles. *Science.* 1996;274:1672–1677.

5. Hunter T. Oncoprotein networks. *Cell.* 1998;88:333–346.

6. Steller H. Mechanisms and genes of cellular suicide. *Science.* 1995;267:1445–1449.

7. Peter ME, Budd RC, Desbarats J, et al. The CD95 receptor: apoptosis revisited. *Cell.* 2007;129:447–450.

8. Ashkenazi A, Dixit VM. Death receptors: signaling and modulation. *Science.* 1998;281:1305–1308.

9. Nicholson DW, Thornberry NA. Apoptosis. Life and death decisions. *Science.* 2003;299:214–215.

10. Risau W. Mechanisms of angiogenesis. *Nature.* 1997;386:671–674.

11. Ferrara N, Carver-Moore K, Chen H, et al. Heterozygous embryonic lethality induced by targeted inactivation of the VEGF gene. *Nature.* 1996; 380:439–442.

12. Yancopoulos GD, Davis S, Gale NW, et al. Vascular-specific growth factors and blood vessel formation. *Nature.* 2000;407:242–248.

13. Gerety SS, Wang HU, Chen ZF, Anderson D. Symmetrical mutant phenotypes of the receptor EphB4 and its specific transmembrane ligand ephrin-B2 in cardiovascular development. *Mol Cell.* 1999;4:403–414.

14. Kertesz N, Krasnoperov V, Reddy R, et al. The soluble extracellular domain of EphB4 (sEphB4) antagonizes EphB4-EphrinB2 interaction, modulates angiogenesis, and inhibits tumor growth. *Blood.* 2006;107:2330–2338.

15. Thurston G, Suri C, Smith K, et al. Leakage-resistant blood vessels in mice transgenically overexpressing angiopoietin-1. *Science.* 1999;286:2511–2514.

16. Duarte A, Hirashima M, Benedito R, et al. Dosage-sensitive requirement for mouse Dll4 in artery development. Genes Dev 2004;18:2474–2478.

17. Scehnet JS, Jiang W, Kumar SR, et al. Inhibition of Dll4-mediated signaling induces proliferation of immature vessels and results in poor tissue perfusion. *Blood.* 2007;109:4753–4760.

18. Slamon D, Clark G, Wong S, et al. Human breast cancer: Correlation of relapse and survival with amplification of the HER-2/neu oncogene. *Science.* 1987;235:177–182.

19. Pluda J. Tumor-associated angiogenesis: mechanisms, clinical implications, and therapeutic strategies. *Semin Oncol.* 1997;24:203–218.

20. McMillan M, Kahn M. Investigating Wnt signaling: a chemogenomic safari. Drug Discov. *Today*. 2005;10:1467–1474.

21. Laird PW. Cancer epigenetics. *Hum Mol Genet.* 2005;14:R65–R76.

22. Stehelin D, Varmus HE, Bishop JM, Vogy PK. DNA related to the transforming gene9S) of avian sacroma virus is present in normal avian DNA. *Nature.* 1976;260:170–173.

23. Weinberg RA. Oncogenes and tumor suppressor genes. *CA: A Cancer Journal for Clinicians* 1994;44:160–170.

24. Yamamoto T. Molecular basis of cancer: oncogenes and tumor suppressor genes. *Microbiol Immunol.* 1993;37:11–22.

25. Weinberg RA. Tumor suppressor genes. *Science.* 1991;254:1138–1145.

26. Marshall C. Tumor suppressor genes. *Cell.* 1991;64:313–328.

27. Levine J. The tumor suppressor genes. *Annu Rev Biochem.* 1993;62:623–651.

28. Fearon ER. Human cancer syndromes: clues to the origin and nature of cancer. *Science.* 1997;278:1043–1050.

29. Lee W-H, Bookstein R, Hong F, et al. Human retinoblastoma susceptibility gene: cloning, identification, and sequence. *Science.* 1987;235:1394–1399.

30. Sager R. Tumor suppressor genes in the cell cycle. *Curr Opin Cell Biol.* 1992;4:155–160.

31. Hoppe-Seyler F, Butz K. Tumor suppressor genes in molecular medicine. *Clin Investig.* 1994;72:619–630.

32. Zhang Y, Xiong Y, Yarbrough W. ARF promotes MDM2 degradiation and stabilizes p53: ARF-INK4a locus deletion impairs both the Rb and p53 tumor suppression pathways. *Cell.* 1998;92:725–734.

33. Pomerantz J, Schrerer-Agus N, Liegeois N, et al. The Ink4a Tumor suppressor gene product, p 19Arf, interacts with MDM2 and neutralizes MDM2's inhibition of p53. *Cell.* 1998;92:713–723.

34. Folkman J. Tumor angiogenesis: therapeutic implications. *N Engl J Med.* 1971;285:1182–1186.

35. Masood R, Cai J, Zheng T, Smith DL, et al. Vascular endothelial growth factor (VEGF) is an autocrine growth factor for VEGF receptor-positive human tumors. *Blood.* 2001;98:1904–1913.

36. Noren NK, Lu M, Freeman AL, et al. Interplay between EphB4 on tumor cells and vascular ephrin-B2 regulates tumor growth. *Proc Natl Acad Sci U S A.* 2004;101:5583–5588.

37. Gastl G, Hermann T, Steurer M, et al. Angiogenesis as a target for tumor treatment. *Oncology.* 1997;54:177–184.

38. Fidler IJ. The pathogenesis of cancer metastasis: the 'seed and soil' hypothesis revisited. *Nat Rev Cancer.*2003;3:453–458.

39. Kumar SR, Singh J, Xia G, et al.Receptor tyrosine kinase EphB4 is a survival factor in breast cancer. *Am J Pathol.* 2006;169:279–293.

40. Minn AJ, Gupta GP, Siegel PM, et al. Genes that mediate breast cancer metastasis to lung. *Nature.* 2005;436:518–524.

41. Gusterson B, Gelber R, Goldhirsch A, et al. Prognostic importance of c-erbB-2 expression in breast cancer. *J Clin Oncol.* 1992;10:1049–1056.

42. Wright C, Nicholson S, Angus B, et al. Relationship between c-erbB-2 protein product expression and response to endocrine therapy in advanced breast cancer. *Br J Cancer.* 1992;65:118–121.

43. Vogel CL, Cobleigh MA, Tripathy D, et al. Efficacy and safety of trastuzumab as a single agent in first-line treatment of HER2-overexpressing metastatic breast cancer. *J Clin Oncol.* 2002;2:719–726.

44. Slamon DJ, Leyland-Jones B, Shak S, et al. Use of chemotherapy plus a monoclonal antibody against HER2 for metastatic breast cancer that overexpresses HER2. *N Engl J Med.* 2001;344:783–792.

45. Osborne C. *Receptors.* Philadelphia: Lippincott; 1991.

46. Foekins J, Rio M, Sequin P, et al. Prediction of relapse and survival in breast cancer patients by pS2 protein status. *Cancer Res.* 1990;50:3832–3837.

47. Hayes D, Mesa-Tejada R, Papsidero L, et al. Prediction of prognosis in primary breast cancer by detection of a high molecular weight mucin-like antigen using monoclonal antibodies DF3, F36/22 and CUI8: A cancer and Leukemia Group B study. *J Clin Oncol.* 1991;9:1–10.

48. Duffy M, O'Grady P, Devaney D, et al. Tissue plasminogen activator, a new prognostic marker in breast cancer. *Cancer Res.* 1988;48:1348–1349.

49. Marques L, Franco E, TorIoni H, et al. Independent prognostic value of laminin receptor expression in breast cancer survival. *Cancer Res.* 1990;50:1479–1483.

50. Tandon A, Clark G, Chamness G, et al. Cathepsin D and prognosis n breast cancer. *N Engl J Med.* 1990;322:297–302.

51. Colomer R, Ruibal A, Genoballa J, et al. Circulating CA15-3 levels in the post surgical follow-up of breast cancer patients and in nonmalignant diseases. Breast *Cancer Res.* Treat 1989;13:123–133.

52. Kallioniemi 0, Oksa H, Aaran R, et al. Serum CA15-3 assay in the diagnosis and follow-up of breast cancer. *Br J Cancer.* 1988;58:213–215.

53. Safi F, Lohler 1, Rottinger, et al. Comparison of CA 15-3 and CEA in diagnosis and monitoring of breast cancer. *Int J Biol Markers.* 1989;4:207–214.

54. Chan D, Beveridge R, Muss H, et al. Use of truquant BR radioimmunoassay for early detection of breast cancer recurrence in patients with stage II and III disease. *J Clin Oncol.*1997;15:2322–2328.

55. Stierer M, Rosen H. Influence of early diagnosis on prognosis of recurrent breast cancer. *Cancer.* 1989;64:1128–1131.

56. Hayes D, Kaplan W. Evaluation of patients following primary therapy. Philadelphia: JB Lippincott, 1991.

57. Fletcher R. Carcinoembryonic antigen. *Ann Intern Med.* 1986;104:66–73.

58. Goslin R, Steele G, Mcintyre J, et al. The use of preoperative plasma CEA levels for the stratification of patients after curative resection of colorectal cancers. *Ann Surg.* 1980;192:747–751.

59. Wolmark N, Fisher B, Wieand S, et al. The prognostic significance of pre-operative carcinoembryonic antigen levels in colorectal cancer. *Ann Surg.* 1984;199:375–382.

60. Moertel C, O'Fallon J, Go V, et al. The preoperative carcinoembryonic antigen test in the diagnosis, staging and prognosis of colorectal cancer. *Cancer.* 1986;58:603–610.

61. Wanebo H, Stearns M, Schwartz M. Use of CEA as an indicator of early recurrence and as a guide to a selected second-look procedure in patients with colorectal cancer. *Ann Surg.*ery 1978;188:481–493.

62. Steele G, Ellenberg D, Ramming K, et al. CEA monitoring among patients in multi-institutional adjuvant GI therapy protocols. *Ann Surg.* 1982;196:162–169.

63. Lynch TJ, Bell DW, Sordella R, et al. Activating mutations in the epidermal growth factor receptor underlying responsiveness of non-small-cell lung cancer to gefitinib. *N Engl J Med.* 2004;350:2129–2139.

64. Steiber P, Dienemann H, Hasholzener U, et al. Comparison of CYFRA 21-1, TPA and TPS in lung cancer, urinary bladder cancer and benign disease. *Int J Biol Markers.* 1994;9:82–88.

65. Ebert W, Bodenmuller H, Holzel W. CYFRA 21-1—Medical decision making and analytical standardization and requirements. *Scand J Clin Lab Invest.* 1995;55(SuppI221):72–80.

66. Pujol J-L, Grenier J, Daures J-P, et al. Serum fragment of cytokeratin subunit 19 measured by CYFRA 21-1. Immunoradiometric assay as a marker of lung cancer. *Cancer Res.* 1993;53:61–66.

67. Ebert W, Muley T, Drings P. Does the assessment of serum markers in patients with lung cancer aid in the clinical decision making process? *Anticancer Res.* 1996;16:2161–2168.

68. Ebert W, Dienemann H, Fateh-Moghadam A, et al. Cytokeratin 19 FRAGMENT (CYFRA 21-1) compared with carcinoembryonic antigen, squamous cell carcinoma antigen and neuron-specific enolase in lung cancer: results of an international multicentre study. *Eur J Clin Chem Clin Biochem.* 1994;32:189–199.

69. Van der gaast A, Schoenmakers C, Kok T, et al. Evaluation of a new tumor marker in patients with non-small cell lung cancer: CYFRA 21-1. *Br J Cancer.* 1994;69:525–528.

70. Gail M, Eagan R, Feld R, et al. Prognostic factors in patients with resected stage I NSCLC: A report from the Lung Center Study Group. *Cancer.* 1984;54:1802–1813.

71. Diez M, Cerdan F, Ortega M, et al. Evaluation of serum CA-125 as a tumor marker in non-small cell lung cancer. *Cancer.* 1991;67:150–154.

72. Kimura Y, Fujii T, Hamamoto K, et al. Serum CA-125 is a good prognostic indicator in lung cancer. *Br J Cancer.* 1990;62:676–678.

73. Ebert W, Leichweis B, Bulzebruck I, Drings P. The role of Imx SCC assays in the detection and prognosis of primary squamous carcinoma of the lung. *Diagn Oncol.*1992;2:203–210.

74. Hansen M. Serum tumor markers in lung cancer. Comments and critique. *Eur J Cancer.* 1993;29A:483–484.

75. Cooper E, Splinter T, Brown D, et al. Evaluation of radioimmunoassay for neuro-specific enolase in small cell lung cancer. *Br J Cancer.* 1985;52:333–338.

76. Sculier J, Field R, Evans W, et al. Carcinoembryonic antigen: a useful prognostic marker in small cell lung cancer. *J Clin Oncol.* 1985;3:1349–1354.

77. Laberge F, Fritsche H, Umsawasdi T, et al. Use of carcinoemryonic antigen in small cell lung cancer. *Cancer.* 1987;59:2047–2052.

78. Qian J, Niu J, Li M, et al. In vitro modeling of human pancreatic duct epithelial cell transformation defines gene expression changes induced by K-ras oncogenic activation in pancreatic carcinogenesis. *Cancer Res.* 2005;65:5045–5053.

79. Gullo L. CA 19-9: The Italian experience. *Pancreas.* 1994;9:717–719.

80. Glenn J, Steinberg W, Kurtzman S, et al. Evaluation of the utility of radioimmunoassay for serum CA 19-9 levels in patients before and after the treatment of carcinoma of the pancreas. *J Clin Oncol.*1988;6:462–468.

81. Pleskow D, Berger H, Gyves J, et al. Evaluation of serologic marker, CA 19-9, in the diagnosis of pancreatic cancer. *Ann Intern Med.* 1989;110:704–709.

82. Yasue M, Sakamoto J, Teramukai S, et al. Prognostic values of pre-operative CEA and CA 19-9 levels in pancreatic cancer. *Pancreas.* 1994;9:735–740.

83. Byrne DJ, Browning MC, Cuschieri A. Ca72-4: a new tumour marker for gastric cancer. *Br J Surg.* 1990;77:1010–1013.

84. Koga T, Kano T, Souda K, et al. The clinical usefulness of preoperative CEA determination in gastric cancer. *Jap J Surg* 1987;17:342–347.

85. Hamazoe R, Maeta M, Matsui T, et al. CA 72-4 compared with carcinoembryonic antigen as a tumor marker for gastric cancer. *Eur J Cancer.* 1992;28A:1351–1354.

86. Maehara Y, Sugimachi K, Akagi M, et al. Serum carcinoembryonic antigen level increases correlate with tumor prgression in patients with differentiated gastric carcinoma following noncurative resection. *Cancer Res.* 1990;50:3952–3955.

87. Ravry M, McIntire R, Moertel C, et al. Brief communication: Carcinoembryonic antigen and alpha fetoprotein in the diagnosis of gastric and colonic cancer: A comparative clinical evaluation. *J Natl Cancer Inst.* 1974;52:1019–1024.

88. Ozols R. Gynecologic Oncology. Norwell: Kluwer, 1998.

89. Makar A, Kristensen G, Kaern J, et al. Prognostic value of pre- and postoperative serum CA-125 levels in ovarian cancer: New aspects and multivariate analysis. *Obstet Gynecol.* 1992;79:1002–1010.

90. Makar AP, Kristensen GB, Kaern J, et al. Prognostic value of pre- and postoperative serum CA 125 levels in ovarian cancer: New aspects and multivariate analysis. *Obstet Gynecol.* 1992;79:1002–1010.

91. Rustin G, Gennings J, Nelstrop A. Use of CA-125 levels to predict survival of patients with ovarian cancer. *J Clin Oncol.*1989;7:1667–1671.

92. McMenamin M E, Soung P, Perera S, et al. Loss of PTEN expression in paraffin-embedded primary prostate cancer correlates with high Gleason score and advanced stage. *Cancer Res.* 1999;59:4291–4296.

93. Dong JT. Chromosomal deletions and tumor suppressor genes in prostate cancer. *Cancer Metastasis Rev.* 2001;20:173–193.

94. Catalona W, Smith D, Ratliff T, et al. Detection of organ confined prostate cancer is increased through prostate-specific antigen-bsed screening. *JAMA.* 1993;270:948–954.

95. Neal D, Clejan S, Sarma D, Moon T. Prostate specific antigen and prostatitis. Effect of prostatitis on serum PSA in the human and non-human primate. *Prostate.* 1992;20:105–111.

96. Zagars G. Prostate-specific antigen as a prognostic factor for prostate cancer treated by external beam radiotherapy. *Int J Radiat Oncol Biol Phys.* 1992;23:47–53.

97. Pisansky T, Cha S, Earle J, et al. Prostate-specific antigen as a pre-therapy prognostic factor in patients treatment with radiation therapy for clinically localized prostate cancer. *J Clin Oncol.* 1993;11:2158–2166.

98. Taketa K. Alpha-fetoprotein: Reevaluation in hepatology. *Hepatology* 1990;12:1420–1432.

99. Tsukuma H, Hiyama T, Tanaka S, et al. Risk factors for hepatocellular carcinoma among patients with chronic liver disease. *N Engl J Med.* 1993;328:1797–1801.

100. Di Biscegile AM, Rustgi VK, Hoffnagle JH, et al. Hepatocellular carcinoma. *Ann Intern Med.* 1988;108:390–401.

101. Posner MR, Mayer RJ. The use of serologic tumor markers in gastrointestinal malignancies. *Hematol Oncol Clin North Am.* 1994;8:533–553.

102. Levine A M, Tulpule A, Quinn DI, etal. Phase I study of antisense oligonucleotide against vascular endothelial growth factor: decrease in plasma vascular endothelial growth factor with potential clinical efficacy. *J Clin Oncol.* 2006;24:1712–1719.

103. Shuey DJ, McCallus DE, Giordano T. RNAi: gene-silencing in therapeutic intervention. *Drug Discov Today.* 2002;7:1040–1046.

104. Huang H, Yee J, Shew J, et al. Suppression of the neoplastic phenotype by replacement of the RB gene in human cancer cells. *Science.* 1988;242:1563–1566.

105. Cai D, Mukhopadhyay T, Liu Y, et al. A stable expression of the wild-type p53 gene in human lung cancer cells after retrovirus-mediated gene transfer. *Hum Gene Ther.* 1993;4:617–624.

106. Liu T, Zhang W, Taylor D, et al. Growth suppression of human head and neck cancer cells by the introduction of a wild-type p53 gene via a recombinant adenovirus. *Cancer Res.* 1994;54:3662–3667.

107. Eastman J, Hall S, Sehgal I, et al. In vivo gene therapy with p53 or p21 adenovirus for prostate cancer. *Cancer Res.* 1995;55:5151–5155.

108. Felger P, Tsai Y, Sukhu L, et al. Improved cationic lipid formulations for in vivo gene therapy. *Ann NY Acad Sci.* 1995;772:126–139.

109. Ledley F. Non-viral gene therapy: the promise of genes as pharmaceutical products. *Hum Gene Ther.* 1995;6:1129–1144.

110. Trubetskoy V S, Torchilin VP, Kennel S, Huang L. Cationic liposomes enhance targeted delivery and expression of exogenous DNA mediated by N-terminal modified poly (L-lysine)-antibody conjugate in mouse lung endothelial cells. *Biochim Biophys Acta.* 1992;1131:311–333.

111. Manthorpe M, Cornefert-Jensen F, Hartikka J, et al. Gene therapy by intramuscular injection of plasmid DNA: studies on firefly luciferase gene expression in mice. *Hum Gene Ther.* 1993;4:419–431.

112. Raz E, Carson D, Parker S, et al. Intradermal gene immunization: the possible role of DNA uptake in the induction of cellular immunity to viruses. *Proc Natl Acad Sci U S A.* 1994;91:9519–9523.

113. Hickman M A, Malone R W, Lehmann-Bruinsma K, et al. Gene expression following direct injection of DNA into liver. *Hum Gene Ther.* 1994;5:1477–1483.

114. Sikes M, O'Malley BJ, Finegold M, Ledley F. In vivo gene transfer into rabbit thyroid follicular cells by direct DNA injection. *Hum Gene Ther.* 1994;5:837–844.

115. Twardowski P, Gradishar WJ. Clinical trials of anti-angiogenic agents. *Curr Opin Oncol.* 1997;9:584–589.

116. Boehm T, Folkman J, Browder T, O'Reilly MS. Antiangiogenic therapy of experimental cancer does not induce acquired drug resistance. *Nature.* 1997;390:404–407.

117. Pluda JM. Tumor-associated angiogenesis: mechanisms, clinical implications, and therapeutic strategies. *Semin Oncol.* 1997;24:203–218.

118. Zweibel J, Su N, MacPherson A, et al. The gene therapy of cancer: transgenic immunotherapy. *Sem Hematol.* 1993;30:119–129.

119. Conry R, LoBuglio A, Loechel F, et al. A carcinoembryonic antigen polynucleotide vaccine has in vivo antitumor activity. *Gene Ther.* 1995;2:59–65.

120. Pardoll D. Immunotheraphy with cytokine gene-transduced tumor cells: the next wave in gene therapy for cancer. *Curr Opin Oncol.*1992;4:1124–1129.

121. LaMotte R, Rubin M, Barr E, et al. Therapeutic effectiveness of the immunity elicited by P815 tumor cells engineered to express the B7-2 co stimulatory molecule. *Cancer Immunol Immunother.* 1996;42:161–169.

122. Dunussi-Joannopoulos K, Weinstein H, Nickerson P, al e. Irradiated B7-1 transduced primary acute myelogenous leukemia (AML) cells can be used as therapeutic vaccines in murine AML. *Blood.* 1996;87:2938–2946.

123. Nabel G, Nabel E, Yang Z, et al. Direct gene transfer with DNA liposome complexes in melanoma: expression, biologic activity and lack of toxicity in humans. *Proc Natl Acad Sci U S A.* 1993;90:11307–11311.

124. Fujiwara T, Grimm E, Mukhopadhyay T, et al. Induction of chemosensitivity in human lung cancer cells in vivo by adenovirus-mediated transfer of the wild-type p53 gene. *Cancer Res.* 1994;54:2287–2291.

125. Moolten F. Tumor Chemosensitivity conferred by inserted herpes thymidine kinase genes: paradigm for a prospective cancer control strategy. *Cancer Res.* 1986;46:5276–5281.

126. Mullen C, Kilstrup M, Blaese R. Transfer of the bacterial gene for cytosine deaminase to mammalian cells confers lethal sensitivity to 5-fluorocytosine: a negative selection system. *Proc Natl Acad Sci U S A.* 1992;89:33–37.

127. Ram Z, Culver K W, Walbridge S, et al. Toxicity studies of retroviral-mediated gene transfer for the treatment of brain tumors. *Neurosurgery.* 1993;79:400–407.

128. Walther W, Stein U. Cell type specific and inducible promoters for vectors in gene therapy as an approach for cell targeting. *J Mol Med.* 1996;74:379–392.

129. Sikora K, Harris J, Hurst H, et al. Therapeutic strategies using c-erb B-2 promoter-controlled drug activation. *Ann NY Acad Sci.* 1994;716:115–124.

130. Frankel AE, Fleming DR, Hall PD, et al. A phase II study of DT fusion protein denileukin diftitox in patients with fludarabine-refractory chronic lymphocytic leukemia. *Clin Cancer Res.* 2003;9:3555–3561.

131. Wu Q, Suo Z, Kristensen GB, Baekelandt M, Nesland JM. The prognostic impact of EphB2/B4 expression on patients with advanced ovarian carcinoma. *Gynecol Oncol.* 2006;102:15–21.

132. Lloyd JM, McIver CM, Stephenson SA, et al. Identification of early-stage colorectal cancer patients at risk of relapse post-resection by immunobead reverse transcription-PCR analysis of peritoneal lavage fluid for malignant cells. *Clin Cancer Res.* 2006;12:417–423.

COMMENTARY
Daniel L. Farkas

The principles and potential application of multispectral and multimode molecular imaging are reviewed in this commentary to complement the comprehensive chapter on molecular biology by Dr. Kumar.

EMERGENCE OF AND NEED FOR MOLECULAR IMAGING

Advances in medicine and surgery depend strongly on our understanding of the human body's anatomy and physiology, and of its biological underpinnings. What we do with this knowledge and how useful we can make it in healing patients depends not only on the skills of the physicians and surgeons but also on the technologies available to them.

There is no discipline that brings these two critical components of health care together better and with more promise than biomedical imaging. The field has experienced explosive growth recently, as anatomic imaging is supplemented with dynamic, high-specificity methods providing access to molecular mechanisms of relevant processes (senescence, apoptosis, immune response, angiogenesis, metastasis). Most advanced imaging is no longer only topological in nature, as most currently established imaging methods, but also provides molecular specificity, usually by labeling with appropriate biomarkers. Even more exciting, optical molecular imaging has the potential of additionally delivering *microscopic* resolution in vivo, thus performing a role previously reserved for the gold standard in surgical decision making, pathology.

Cancer detection and treatment are particularly important and appropriate application areas for such *molecular imaging*, and are being pursued vigorously. The potential is thus created for earlier detection of disease, individualized care, detailed monitoring of treatments, and new avenues for drug development. In order for such plans to succeed in the surgical management of cancer, we must design, implement, and deploy the kind of *translational* molecular imaging that (a) incorporates newly emerging molecular-biological information, both genomic and epigenomic; (b) takes advantage of major developing technology trends, including many outside the field of medicine; and (c) is deployable in the setting of the operating room (see Figure 1C.1 for a schematic plan).

We briefly review the potential of optical (1) molecular imaging for cancer detection and treatment, with emphasis on spectral and multimode approaches (2–4). Excellent reviews are available for the broader field of molecular imaging (5,6).

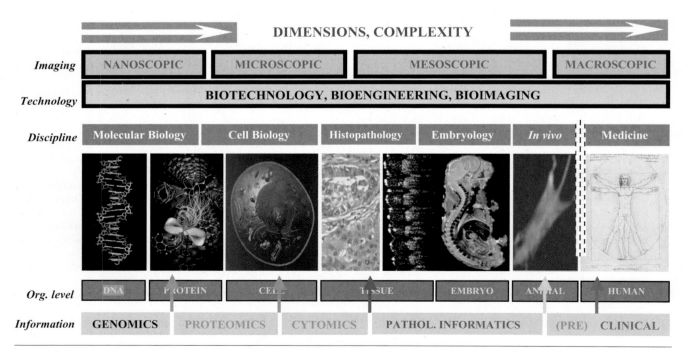

Figure 1C.1 Translational research from molecules to humans, highlighting challenges and central role of bioimaging. Pharma and biotech are focusing on protein-level solutions (*green arrow*), our best imaging is at the cellular level (*orange arrow*), and most of the advanced optical imaging stops at the preclinical level (*turquoise arrow*). Most diagnosis and clinical decision making is based on pathology (*blue arrow*), while clearly the need and resources peak at the clinical level (*red arrow*). We should aim to superimpose all these arrows toward the clinical end, overcoming the translational brick wall. (Modified from Farkas DL. Invention and commercialization in optical bioimaging. *Nature Biotechnol.* 2003;21:1269–1271.) (See color plates.)

CANCER DETECTION AND DIAGNOSIS

The importance—human, financial, scientific—of cancer research and treatment, and the inherent difficulty of the challenges they face, make it very important to try designing *strategic* approaches. To achieve this, we have to extract as much useful information as possible from in vitro models, ex vivo (biopsy) specimens, from in vivo animal models, and from surgical intervention. Imaging at these different levels of organization, of varying levels of complexity, and regulatory hurdles, requires different technologies; ideally, these should be complementary, or even synergetic in providing solutions for better patient outcomes. The excitement around molecular imaging arises from its potential to detect early derangements and predisease states, before structural modifications associated with cancer progression have occurred, thus yielding better treatment results.

Quantitative Premolecular Imaging: Spectral Pathology

Most of the derangements to the molecular machinery of the cell that yield disease states are assessed at the tissue level by histopathology. Decisions in surgical oncology, more so than in almost any other field, are made based on the input of the pathologists. The most commonly used stain in histopathology, hematoxylin and eosin (H&E), is somewhat nonspecific and has yet to be standardized, but provides morphologic cues. Molecular specificity is present in immunohistochemistry and immunofluorescence, but these techniques are far from perfect because the biological material needs to be extracted from the patient (usually by biopsy or complete removal) and laboriously processed and stained. In addition, the result is based on subjective evaluation rather than, for example, advanced digital imaging.

We have introduced spectral imaging methods (acquisition and analysis) derived from satellite reconnaissance, to cyto- and histopathology (3,7), and achieved highly reproducible segmentation of the digital tissue images, based on spectral signature, followed by easy quantitation. In immunofluorescence, several markers, neatly separated spectrally, could be studied simultaneously, yielding a more complete picture.

Intracellular Proteomics: Imaging of Molecular Topology and Expression Levels

Any tissue specimen obtained from a patient contains potentially a very large amount of specific information. The cell, as the basic unit of life, is also the locus of the derangements that ultimately cause cancer, and should be the focus of studies aiming to understand mechanisms. Tumors arise as the result of the gradual accumulation of genetic changes in single cells, and identifying which genes encoded within the human genome can contribute to the development of cancer remains a challenge and a high priority in cancer research. Describing, evaluating, and quantifying the molecular alterations that distinguish any particular cancer cell from a normal one can predict the behavior of that cancer cell, as well as the responsiveness to treatment of that particular tumor in an individual. Understanding the profile of molecular changes in any particular cancer allows correlating its resulting phenotype with molecular events and should yield new targets and strategies for therapy.

Recent discoveries indicate that alterations in many of the cellular processes, pathways, or networks may contribute to the onset of cancer and could be used for therapeutic intervention. Therefore, it is important to put in place technologies that can detect molecular changes *within the cell*, without preconceived ideas about which information will be most valuable to monitor or what technologies will have the greatest impact. It is currently possible to study very specific changes in the expression and function of genes and gene products at the DNA, RNA, or protein level. However, many existing technologies do not adequately address specific issues such as restrictions on the number of components studied in an experiment, limited cell number, sample heterogeneity, variability of specimen types, and cost-effectiveness. Innovation-yielding novel technologies to study tumor specimens are needed. Recent advances in molecular genetics have made it possible to perform multiple correlated measurements on the cells of individual tumors, to use such measurements to identify specific molecular subtypes of cancer, and to develop tumor subtype-specific combinations of targeted therapeutic agents.

Development and translation of new in vitro technologies for the multiplexed analysis of molecular species in clinical specimens require a multidisciplinary approach. Progress in the application of prognostic factors in cancer will ultimately depend on the intelligent use of such factors *in combination*. The most robust combinations of such predictive factors are likely to be those based on relationships between tumor biology at the molecular level and clinical aggressiveness. A *systematic hypothesis-testing* approach for developing such combinations is both desirable and feasible, and has been greatly facilitated by several recent developments. First, it has become increasingly apparent that there are specific patterns of molecular abnormalities that occur in individual tumors that are recapitulated in tumors from different patients (8,9), and that these patterns are of clinical prognostic value. These patterns provide useful starting points for the conceptual formulation of hypotheses regarding derangements in intracellular molecular network behavior and their effects on tumor aggressiveness. However, there are special difficulties in actually testing these hypotheses in studies on clinical samples, because the material available for study is limited in quantity, because there is extensive clonal heterogeneity within clinical tumor samples, and because of the limited degree to which fresh clinical material can be manipulated experimentally. Recent advances in laser scanning cytometry, a newly emerging technology that is especially well suited for the analysis of tumor cells in clinical samples, have some, but certainly not all, of these difficulties (8–10).

Lung cancer continues to be the most common cause of cancer-related mortality in the United States and worldwide (11,12). The lung cancer survival rate has remained about 12% to 15% throughout the past 3 decades, despite innovations in diagnostic testing, surgical technique, and development of new chemotherapeutic agents. A fuller understanding of etiology and pathology of lung cancer requires the elucidation of molecular mechanisms, which would in return lead to more effective therapeutic intervention for improved clinical outcomes. It is clear that the molecular mechanisms involved are extremely complex. Duplication, cross-talk, and redundancy of molecules and pathways contribute to this complexity, which far exceeds initial

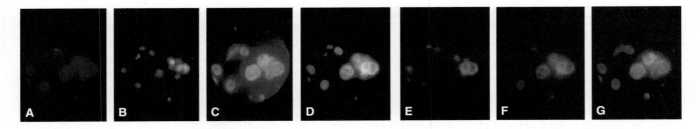

Figure 1C.2 Seven-color intracellular *imaging* "proteomics" in human breast cancer cells. Cells labeled simultaneously with seven different probes (*left to right*): (**A**) the nucleus labeled with DAPI; (**B**) *Her-2/neu* labeled with FITC; (**C**) vascular endothelial growth factor (VEGF) labeled with Cy3; (**D**) cyclin D1 labeled with Cy3.5; (**E**) ras labeled with Cy5; (**F**) c-myc labeled with Cy5.5; (**G**) *p53* labeled with Cy7. These images were acquired using four separate microscopy filter sets: a DAPI set, a FITC set, a Cy3 set, and a combined Cy5-Cy7 set. The acousto-optical tunable filter spectral imaging module was used to distinguish between the two dyes contained within the Cy3 filter set (Cy3 and Cy3.5) and between the three dyes contained within the Cy5-Cy7 filter set (Cy5, Cy5.5, and Cy7). (See color plates.)

assumptions based on molecular amplification cascades within single pathways (13). Despite more than 400 publicly available lung cancer expression profiles generated with different methods, the results so far have raised as many questions as answers. Many studies have clearly demonstrated correlations between expression profile and clinical outcome, but most of the gene sets that have been identified have little overlap with each other (14). Recently, microarrays have been used for lung tumor expression analysis (15–17). All data sets recapitulate the morphologic classification, but all of the identified groups selected quite different sets of genes that influenced patient survival.

As gene products exert their function in a timely and spatially defined manner within a specific molecular and cellular environment, knowledge of qualitative, in relation to quantitative, gene expression profiles is central to the understanding of the role and activity of gene products in complex biological processes. We developed new imaging technologies (2–4) for replacement of laser scanning microscopy with a more powerful approach, allowing simultaneous imaging and quantitation of a large number of molecular species within the same cell. We have imaged 6 to 10 cancer-relevant proteins (including p53, HER2/neu, c-myc, ras, p21, cyclin D) in breast and lung cancer specimens from patients (Figure 1C.2). It is based on multispectral imaging (3), which in our definition consists in using several spectral methods for imaging, simultaneously. It enables the optical probing and discrimination of intra- and extracellular molecules within tissues and provides a quantitative, dynamic picture of in situ and in vivo molecular interactions. Therefore, multispectral imaging has major advantages in clinicopathologic diagnosis and prognosis, and in therapy design and validation. The output is a digital, segmented, quantitated, and partially interpreted image of a fixed cell or tissue (on a microscopic slide). While in vitro gene expression and proteomic analysis provide only crude quantitative information of bulk tumor tissue, spectral imaging can generate quantitative biomarker information on a per-cell basis, and thus insights into complex interactions within the cellular pathways. This single-cell focus and subcellular resolution information is also extremely valuable in the assessment of the heterogeneous tumor composition in breast cancer as well as lung carcinoma. Because multispectral imaging is amenable to automation and electronic data transfer and

storage, it offers great improvement in time and cost reduction in the clinicopathologic routine to classify cancer disease processes through the analysis of a defined cluster of prognostic markers. Additionally, the effort in imaging a large number of intracellular components simultaneously is well spent: one six-color panel contains as much information as 30 four-color panels (the limit of current laser scanning cytometry), and one seven-color panel contains as much information as 210 four-color panels.

Our spectral selection devices of choice in achieving the spectral imaging performance needed are acousto-optical tunable filters (3,4). Because the cells are studied in vitro, a large number of dyes and other markers (such as quantum dots; see later discussion) can be used, potentially raising the number of components that can be simultaneously imaged to a record 18 to 20.

In an elegant recent study, Kumar et al. (18) investigated complex intracellular signaling networks and modeled cell migration, proliferation, and differentiation as they pertain to understanding cancerization. Their argument was as follows: cells in the human body react to external cues, and many diseases, such as cancer, occur when these decision-making processes are disturbed. They studied *HER2*, a receptor overexpressed in 30% of breast cancers and associated with a worse prognosis. Their model was able to identify a small subset of phosphorylation events that were predictive of changes in cellular behavior with *HER2* overexpression; this in turn suggested critical elements of cellular network architecture (probably no more than six to nine per cell), leading to potential biomarkers and targets for therapy in *HER2* overexpressing cancers. We believe that multiplexed intracellular imaging as previously outlined could greatly facilitate the quantitative monitoring of such targets and their behavior, including response to treatments.

Preclinical Molecular Imaging of Cancer in Small Animals

Antibody-Based Molecular Imaging *in vivo*

Tumor localization using fluorescence has been made practical by current improvements in tumor targeting molecules, by the development of convenient near-infrared emitting fluorochromes, and by the availability of digital cameras having high sensitivity in this spectral region. Recent studies in animals have demonstrated that fluorochrome labeling of monoclonal antibodies confers adequate sensitivity and improved resolution. Simultaneous localization of multiple reagents is made possible by labeling with several different near-infrared emitting fluorochromes; thus, background subtraction and differential labeling of multiple tumor-associated components can be performed. Difficulties in using the fluorochrome labels are mainly related to light scattering and absorption in tissues, but detection of small tumors at depths of several millimeters is feasible. The major medical use of this new technology is likely to be endoscopic location of tumors. Scientific uses include studies of tumor metastasis, uptake and distribution of drugs and tumor-targeting molecules by tumors, and migration patterns of near-infrared labeled cells in vivo.

One of the promising areas of research is tumor visualization in vivo using fluorochrome-conjugated monoclonal antibodies. Relatively new cyanine conjugates that fluoresce in the near-infrared offer improved resolution and high sensitivity for in situ studies of tumor growth and metastasis in animal models (19).

Fluorochrome labeling for tumor detection seemed unlikely to be useful until the last decade. However, near-infrared emitting fluorochromes have been developed that have high quantum yields, are easily conjugated to antibodies or other tumor-targeting agents, are visible through millimeter thicknesses of tissue, and have the needed stability for labeling in vivo (20–24). These fluorochromes are now commercially available. Moreover, high-resolution cooled charge-coupled device cameras that have adequate sensitivity in the near-infrared are now both available and affordable. Improved targeting agents—including second- and third-generation antibodies and antibody fragments, peptides selected from combinatorial libraries, and ligands for receptors that are altered, overexpressed, or selectively accessible in tumors—are emerging almost daily.

Many studies have demonstrated tumor location using monoclonal antibodies and derived reagents in both animal models and humans, but despite occasional successes, these antibodies have not yet found general use in either tumor location or therapy. The major limitation is pharmacokinetic. In humans, a long time is required for a significant fraction of circulating blood to access a small tumor, while the circulating half-life of antibodies is much shorter. Thus the majority of the antibody will be cleared before it has accessed the tumor (26). It is therefore difficult to attain high concentrations of conjugated monoclonal(s) in human tumors while maintaining acceptably low exposure of patients to conjugated radioisotopes or drugs. It is mainly for this reason that the high levels of antibody targeting and successful therapies seen in small animal models have not been matched in clinical practice. Moreover, antigenic heterogeneity within and between tumors, poor or variable access to antigens, low diffusion rates of macromolecules, poor vascularization, high internal tumor pressure, and a putative "binding site barrier" have all been identified as contributors to poor antibody binding in vivo (27,28). The problem shows itself most dramatically in tumor visualization: large amounts of input label, long exposure times, and high sensitivity are required to attain acceptable tumor visualization. Long clearance times are

required to see small tumors. Therefore, labels detectable at very low levels of targeting are highly desirable. Solutions to the problems indicated here have been actively pursued for the past 3 decades. The requirements are different for therapy and visualization. For therapeutic purposes, the important factors are high tumor uptake while minimizing damage to normal tissues and increasing the selective toxicity of conjugates to maximize killing of tumor cells by the conjugates that do reach the tumor. For imaging, however, it is necessary to reduce the background in normal tissues and in the circulation while maintaining good tumor targeting; also, targeting must be accomplished within a fairly short time for the technique to be practical.

The search for better targets in tumors is continuing. The overwhelming majority of antibodies now in use were selected in vitro for higher binding to tumor tissue or tumor cell lines than to normal tissues or normal cells. Reintgen et al. (29) and Ballou et al. (30) observed that specificity in vitro did not predict targetability in vivo. Both groups found that some antigens in tumors were selectively targeted in vivo, even though normal tissues had equal or even higher concentrations of the antigens. Mann et al. (31) demonstrated the contrary: even highly specific antigens were not necessarily targeted. Thus, in vitro specificity does not predict in vivo targetability (32).

Selection for targeting in vivo, rather than for tumor specificity in vitro, has only recently begun (19,25). In another approach to selection in vivo, phages that express random peptides were injected into normal animals, and organ-targeting phages were selected by removing organs of interest, amplifying the phage absorbed by the organ, and reselecting. Three cycles of selection yielded phage clones that had improved targeting to the organs used for selection. Synthetic peptides having sequences derived from the selected phage were shown to block phage uptake specifically. It seems likely that this approach can be used to select tumor-targeting sequences (33). We expect that combinatorial libraries other than antibodies and peptides will be used for selection in vivo.

Fluorochrome-Labeled Antibody Targeting

Fluorochrome molecules can undergo many cycles of excitation and emission, yielding many photons, rather than giving rise to a single signal, as does radioactive decay. Light can be focused by lenses, allowing both a wide field for collection of photons and good resolution. Red or near-infrared excitation light is used, not ionizing radiation. Differential targeting can be easily accomplished by using two or more separate fluorochromes, emitting at different wavelengths, as in differential isotope labeling.

A first step in fluorochrome labeling in vivo was accomplished by Jain, whose group used fluorescein-conjugated monoclonal antibodies to study the details of antibody uptake in xenografted tumors implanted in rabbit ears, then in nude mice (34). Fluorescein has the advantage of being readily visible to the naked eye; however, a significant background of tissue fluorescence occurs at the wavelengths used for fluorescein excitation and emission. Another problem with fluorescein is that its emission is sensitive to pH; emission is best above pH 8 and decreases sharply below pH 6. Thus, we would expect less than optimal fluorescence at blood pH, and intracellular fluorescein derivatives in acidic endosomes would be still less fluorescent.

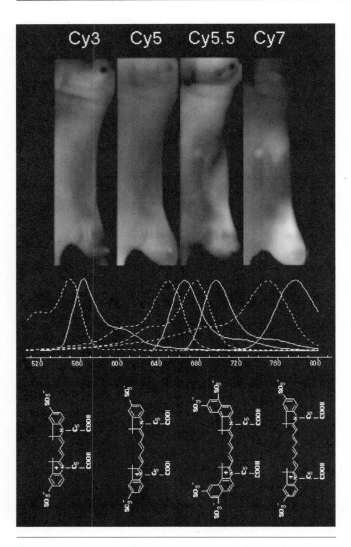

Figure 1C.3 In vivo imaging of fluorescently targeted tumors: importance of wavelength. Tumors induced in a nude mouse were targeted with antibody, labeled with an equimolar mixture of Cy3, Cy5, Cy5.5, and Cy7. As the number of carbon atoms in the chains increases (*bottom*), so does the wavelength (excitation and emission) of the fluorophore (*middle*). Because the images (*top*) are of the same mouse, at the same time (but in different wavelength channels), one can see that the tumors (including a necrotic area) are better visualized the longer the wavelength. Cy7 yields by far the best "transparency" because of lowered scattering. (Modified from Hoffman RM. Green fluorescent protein imaging of tumour growth, metastasis, and angiogenesis in mouse models. *Lancet Oncol.* 2002;3:546–556.)

Better fluorochromes are now available. Researchers at Carnegie Mellon University have synthesized a series of blue to far-red and near-infrared emitting fluorescent dyes, among them cyanine (Cy)2, Cy3, Cy5, Cy5.5, and Cy7 (see Figure 1C.3 for structures). These fluorochromes are tailored for high quantum yield, good chemical stability, and ease of conjugation to various carriers (22,23) and are now commercially available from GE Healthcare (formerly Amersham). For Cy5, Cy5.5, and Cy7, both excitation and emission are at wavelengths at which blood

has relatively low absorbance. Fluorescence is insensitive to pH in the range from pH 4 to 9, and self-quench is low. Moreover, both scattering and background due to intrinsic tissue fluorescence are reduced by working at longer wavelengths, and the fluorochromes have high resistance to photobleaching. At high substitution levels, Cy5-antibody conjugates retain their brightness, in contrast to the quenching observed at high levels of fluorescein or rhodamine conjugation. The result is high sensitivity and a signal-to-noise ratio far superior to that of fluorescein, as assessed by fluorescence microscopy. The fluorochromes are stable in vivo in circulation. Erythrocytes surface-labeled using Cy3 and Cy5 were found to have a half-life of 40 days in rabbits with no diminution of fluorescence per cell. Because the fluorochromes have a convenient range of excitation and emission maxima, it is possible to visualize several fluorochromes in a given experiment by using multiple filters and image processing to remove spurious signals from spectral overlap. Thus, background subtraction using a differentially labeled nontargeting antibody is possible (24,25). Alternatively, multiple targeting reagents can be followed in a single experiment. Recent adaptation of acousto-optic tunable filter technology to deliver good-quality, high-resolution images makes visualization of multiple fluorochromes much more practical, as bandpass can be tailored to the needs of the individual experiment, and there is no need to use several different filters (2,3). Because of the poor sensitivity of the human eye in the far-red and near-infrared, the fluorochromes must be visualized using a camera. This is not a disadvantage, because electronic cameras have spectral sensitivity peaking in the near-infrared.

We have performed studies aimed at determining which of the currently available cyanine fluorochromes is most useful for in vivo tumor location. Direct comparison of four commercially available cyanine fluorochromes conjugated to monoclonal antibodies showed that Cy7 and Cy5.5 were superior to the shorter wavelength dyes (Cy2, Cy3, and Cy5) for in vivo visualization of two different mouse model tumors (25).

Scattering and absorption are the two key factors that diminish light flux significantly. In a homogenous, isotropic medium, Rayleigh scattering diminishes with the fourth power of wavelength; thus, visualization in the infrared should be appreciably better than in visible light. In biological tissues, this simple wavelength dependence holds only qualitatively. We have taken a different approach to quantitate light penetration in biological tissues. We investigated the effects of tissue thickness on detectability and resolution by using multiple views of living animals labeled using fluorescent probes. Back-projection was used to reconstruct tomographic images of the fluorescence emission. Thus, we may view fluorescent structures in living mice to judge how well light penetrates at successively longer wavelengths. This approach provides a good method for assessing depth and resolution in a realistic in vivo model (34).

Studies of tumor models in animals are simplified by using cyanine fluorochrome labeling. No radioisotopes are needed, so associated problems of radiation and disposal of radioactive tissue are avoided. Resolution is far better than that offered by conventional gamma cameras; in addition, superficial tumors and growth and patterns of metastasis are easily investigated using fluorochromes (19). Current results from targeting studies in vivo show that cyanine fluorochrome labels are a promising tool. The desirability of noninvasive, high-resolution imaging in living organisms, coupled with significant advances in component technologies, fluorophore synthesis, antibody purification, detectors, and digital image processing, makes this an exciting and fast-evolving field. Major recent advances are based on better fluorescent antibody targeting, differential detection, and improved probes and optical design (6).

Fluorescent Proteins

Today's molecular fluorescence imaging in animal models is dominated by the use of fluorescent proteins (the first of which, green fluorescent protein, was introduced a little over a decade ago). The combination of very high specificity, high fluorescence levels, and choice of wavelengths is quite powerful (36), and has made this one of the most successful areas of optical imaging in vivo. However, it is unlikely that this method will be used in human trials because of regulatory issues.

Fluorescent Nanoparticles

These very bright, nonbleaching particles of controllable emission wavelength (via size and composition variation) were also introduced into the field of biological imaging about a decade ago (33,37), and have enjoyed fast progress in both technologies and applications, including cancer research (38). Quantum dots are the best-known example, widely available commercially. Because of their composition, they are also unlikely to be used in the clinic, but have become excellent tools for in vitro and animal studies.

Three-Dimensional Optical Tomography

With instrumentation and probes steadily improving, it has become more feasible to conduct studies in small animals in three dimensions, using sophisticated image acquisition and processing schemes. It is a promising field, helped by theoretical knowledge from other three-dimensional bioimaging fields, and was recently reviewed (39).

Bioluminescence Imaging

Another highly useful and popular method, developed in the mid-1990s at Stanford University, bioluminescence imaging of small animals is able to monitor live gene expression patterns and other cancer-relevant variables in small animals, with high specificity. The field has received wide acceptance in preclinical studies because of the commercial availability of the instruments needed, and has been reviewed mostly by the technology's developers (40).

Multimode Optical Imaging for Tumor Detection and Treatment

Small animal imaging has become widely used as a noninvasive monitoring tool as it allows the detection of both primary and metastatic tumors, as well as monitoring of specific effects of pharmacologic interventions (41–43). In the past it was necessary to sacrifice the animals in order to detect tumors or monitor tissues and drug molecules inside them. The excised tissues are dead; thus, the normal physiology such as blood flow, cell-cell interactions, and metabolic activity is suspended or even degraded, making impossible the continuous monitoring of

biochemical, genetic, and pharmacologic processes in vivo and in the same animal, repeatedly. Thus, better methods to track tumor development and to monitor tissues and molecules within living animals were needed, and optical small animal imaging has been developed as a useful alternative (44–45).

Currently, many noninvasive technologies such as ultrasound, computerized tomography, magnetic resonance imaging (MRI), positron emission tomography, single-photon emission computed tomography, and optical imaging are available for small animal imaging. Interestingly, they were originally developed for medical applications, but have been redesigned for small animal imaging. Ultrasound, computerized tomography, and MRI are capable of resolving the anatomy and physiology through the energy-tissue interaction, whereas positron emission tomography and single-photon emission computed tomography require reporter probes or contrast agents in order to monitor metabolism of organisms (42). Various optical imaging technologies ranging from simple two-dimensional imaging to sophisticated devices for three-dimensional tomography of internal organs and tissues have been developed for small animals (3,19,34,39,40,44). These methods have several advantages over nonoptical methods: they allow simultaneous monitoring of multiple targets or molecular pathways, and are cheaper, simpler, and less harmful.

In particular, whole-body in vivo imaging techniques using fluorescence and luminescence markers have been used for the monitoring of primary and metastatic tumor growth, angiogenesis, gene expression, infection, and stem cell and other cell tracking in intact animals. A number of companies have developed optical imaging systems for small animal imaging. However, although the commercial systems perform well for the tasks they have been designed, they are expensive (for performing a single task) and do not have advanced capabilities such as the use of multiple excitation sources, or multiple optical detection methods. These limitations, and the need for more versatile, advanced in vivo imaging, prompted us to develop a new multimode optical imaging system that can resolve less than 1 mm size objects below the small animal surface, detect light at single photon level, distinguish multiple targets, provide quantification of marker (fluorochrome) biodistribution, and allow simple switching between multiple imaging modes and various illumination sources, including advanced lasers for applications such as nonlinear imaging.

Our first-generation multimode system included the following imaging modes: bioluminescence, fluorescence, fluorescence lifetime, hyperspectral, and transillumination (47). Cancer-related applications of this system included (a) observing and quantitating drug nanoconjugate carrier accumulation within cancerous tumor and several organs in real-time, in mice; (b) examining the extent and topology of targeted drug delivery into specific organs and the tumor by hyperspectral imaging and spectral unmixing analysis; (c) detecting adenosine triphosphate and enzymatic activity in engineered nude mice by bioluminescence imaging; (d) resolving the targets of interest in nude mice using fluorescence lifetime imaging; and (e) resolving small objects inside thick tissues using transillumination imaging. A more recent version added scanned fluorescence lifetime imaging and full-field two-photon excitation imaging for chemotherapy assessment (48).

THE FUTURE OF MOLECULAR IMAGING: OPTIMIZED TREATMENTS

In Vivo Imaging Requiring no Contrast Agents

Spectral imaging has recently been introduced in the biomedical field as a noninvasive, quantitative means of studying biological tissues (49). Many potential applications have been demonstrated (in vitro and, to a lesser degree, in vivo) with the use of stains or dyes. Translation to the clinical environment has been largely lagging because of safety considerations and regulatory limitations preventing use of contrast agents in humans.

To avoid this trap, we designed experiments to show the feasibility of high-resolution imaging of cancer without the use of contrast agents, thus completing the continuum of translational research (Figure 1C.1) to in vivo imaging that will be directly applicable in the clinical environment.

Optical Coherence Tomography

This elegant imaging method, optical coherence tomography (OCT), invented at the Massachusetts Institute of Technology, uses coherence properties of light to detect the photons of interest for imaging from a background that could be six to seven orders of magnitude higher. Similar in concept to ultrasound imaging, it allows better penetration into tissue (2 to 3 mm) than conventional optical imaging, and has reached the speed (approximately video rate) and spatial resolution that allow it to produce highly useful images of cells, in vivo, with no contrast agents, in real-time (50).

We developed a high-fidelity OCT system with high-resolution and superior dynamic range. We examined its utility in imaging urinary bladders and systematically studied the morphologic alternations associated with diseases of the bladder, including urothelial tumors in an animal (porcine) model closely approximating the human situation. The method, incorporating and comparing OCT with cystoscopy (by surface imaging) and excisional biopsy (by histologic evaluation), allowed evaluation of the potential of OCT for the noninvasive diagnosis of transitional cell cancers.

Bladder cancer is the fifth most common cancer in the United States. If detected and excised prior to invasion or metastasis, bladder carcinoma is curable. However, none of the current detection methods (e.g., urine cytology, intravenous pyelogram, MRI and ultrasound), provide sufficient sensitivity or specificity in predicting either the prognosis or stage of early bladder cancer because of resolution limitations or technical imperfections of these methods. In a methyl-nitroso-urea instillation-induced cancerization model, experiments using the OCT system showed that the micromorphology of porcine bladder such as the urothelium, submucosa, and muscle is identified by OCT and well correlated with the histologic evaluations (51). OCT detected edema, inflammatory infiltrates, and submucosal blood congestion as well as the abnormal growth of urothelium (e.g., papillary hyperplasia and carcinomas). By contrast, surface imaging, which resembles cystoscopy, provided far less sensitivity and resolution than OCT. Histologic evaluation showed obvious changes in tissue during cancerization but, compared with OCT, also demonstrated additional changes that were due to

tissue preparation for histopathology. This was the first OCT study of any tumor documented in a systematic fashion. This showed the potential of OCT for the noninvasive diagnosis of both bladder inflammatory lesions and early urothelial abnormalities by imaging characterization of the increases in urothelial thickening and backscattering (Figure 1C.4).

Fresh *Ex Vivo* Imaging with no Contrast Agents

With proper experimental planning, light originating in a sample (including a living body) is both target-specific and content-rich. Semantic optical imaging is thus enabled, allowing attribution of instant significance to a signal. The often-used (but sometimes misused) term *optical biopsy* captures this exciting concept, in the sense that an entity or feature of interest could be detected, located, and quantitated within the body, noninvasively, with diagnostic power approximating that of a traditional biopsy. We have come to believe that a major obstacle in moving optical imaging diagnostic technologies from the laboratory to the bedside is that the heavy use of contrast agents in research cannot be duplicated in humans. Although imparting higher specificity and signal-to-noise ratio to imaging, agents routinely used in live cell, fixed tissue, and animal experiments are not approved by the Food and Drug Administration, and thus not transferable for use in humans. This is not likely to change soon, and underscores the need to concentrate on optical imaging requiring no extrinsic contrast agents. We aimed to test these methods on unstained cancer specimens, ex vivo and in vivo.

A key issue in comparing an in vivo test with the gold standard is that the chemical processes applied by the pathologist to the specimen distinctly alter it. Often, when the processing is complete, the specimen has been deformed and toxic contrast agents have been added. We chose to address this issue through the use of odd-even slicing of the sample. This involves having the pathologist prepare the embedded sample and then slice it using the microkeratome. Then, the rest of the traditional H&E staining procedure is completed using only the odd-numbered slices. The even-number slices are instead placed on microscopy slides for *unstained* spectral imaging, with the paraffin removed from the slide. The unstained (even) slides were then imaged using reflected light, and we compared spectral imaging on unstained slides (even) to their corresponding stained slide (odd) that exhibits the same topology to verify our results against the gold standard, as defined by the pathologist. We settled on the use of ink as a fiducial marker. The remainder of this experiment had two phases:

For the first phase, nine pairs of stained-unstained slides were obtained and classified. From these preliminary results, we were able to segment regions of breast cancer from regions of normal tissue using the minimum squared error classification scheme. The segmentation results of the stained slide are very similar to the results of the corresponding unstained slides of breast cancer.

For the second phase, we progressed to imaging fresh unstained ex vivo specimens, the images from which the library was defined with separate images of normal breast tissue, normal breast tissue stained with ink, and pure breast cancer from a 10-day old tumor. A total of 22 animals were induced with cancer, and more than 2,000 images were taken. We experimented

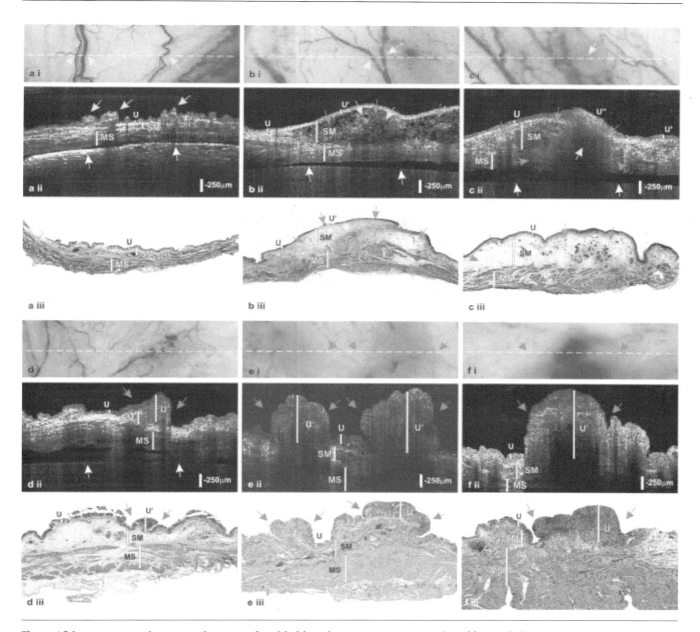

Figure 1C.4 Ex vivo two-dimensional images of rat bladders during tumorigensis induced by methyl-nitroso-urea (MNU) installation. At each time point, Panels i, ii, iii (*top to bottom*) are surface red/green/blue (RGB), optical coherence tomography (OCT), and hematoxylin and eosin stained histology, respectively. Image size: X/4.2 mm, Z/1.9 mm. For normal control (group a), the low scattering U and the underlying high scattering SM and MS layers are identified and indicated by white bars. *Yellow and white arrows* point to superficial blood vessels and the supporting silicon pad, respectively. At 24 hours after MNU instillation (group b), acute chemical cystitis involving inflammatory infiltrate with SM fluid buildup is identified by OCT and evidenced by histology, whereas surface imaging fails to provide any specific feature. The whole mount bladder wall is thickened. At 48 hours (group c), continued damage to the bladder involving inflammatory infiltrate with SM vasodilation or blood congestion within the SM blood vessels (e.g., severe edema) is identified by OCT and evidenced by histology. *Blue arrows* point to the SM inflammatory lesion, *yellow arrows* point to blood congestion. U″ shows the completely denuded urothelium following MNU installation. At 20 weeks (group d), in addition to inflammatory infiltrate, chronic damage (e.g., early papillary hyperplasia) is identified by OCT as thickened urothelium and evidenced by histology. *Blue arrows* point to the thickened urothelium (U′). The underlying bladder wall (e.g., SM and MS) are still visible. At 30 weeks (group e), more severe damage is identified by OCT as indicated by *blue arrows* and evidenced by histology. At 40 weeks, thickened urothelium and increased vascularization are identified by OCT and evidenced by histology. High-magnification histology provides subcellular evidence of the growth of an incipient papillary carcinoma. (Modified from Pan Y, Lavelle JP, Meyers S, et al. High fidelity optical coherence tomography of tumorigenesis in rat bladders induced by N-Methyl-N-NitrosoUrea (MNU) instillation. *Med Physics.* 2001;28:2432–2440.) (See color plates.)

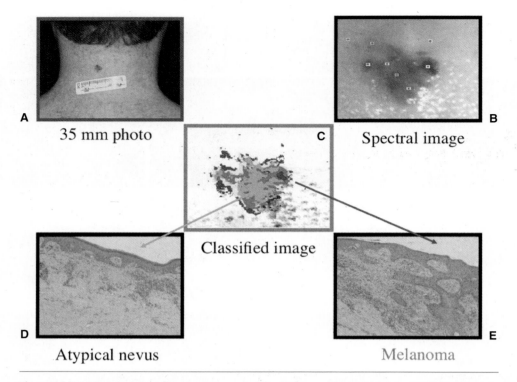

Figure 1C.5 Melanoma detection in patients, by in vivo spectral imaging. Macroscopic spectral imaging analysis of an RGP melanoma arising in an atypical nevus. (**A**) represents 35-mm photographs of the melanocytic lesion. (**B**) A red/green/blue (RGB) image was derived from the spectral cube of the melanocytic lesion. The pixels in the RGB image were used to select spectra for classification. (**C**) In the spectral image, the area pseudocolored green represents the spectrally segregated region of the atypical nevus. The areas pseudocolored red and blue display the spectrally segregated regions containing the RGP melanoma. The areas pseudocolored yellow correspond to heavily pigmented regions in the atypical nevus. The hematoxylin and eosin-counterstained tissue sections, shown in panels (**D**) and (**E**), depict the histology of the atypical nevus (**D**) and the RGP melanoma (**E**). See reference 2 for more details. (See color plates.)

with various classification schemes and normalization techniques, and ultimately arrived at using a normalized dimensional analysis with Mahalanobis distance. We calculated the sensitivity, specificity, positive predictive value, and negative predictive value using generally accepted clinical calculations to be 96%, 92%, 95%, 95%, respectively. Our results demonstrate that spectral imaging and classification has the potential to detect cancer regions within fresh *unstained* breast tissue (52,53). We plan to pursue this approach for in vivo imaging, as the results summarized here illustrate *our ability to achieve quality pathologic assessment of unstained tissue.* The approach likely to yield the best results (including margin assessment during cancer surgery) will require combining spectral imaging with one or more other optical methods, similar to the multimode studies described here for animal models.

In vivo Imaging in Patients, with no Contrast Agents: Melanoma Detection

If a cancer-related lesion, such as an atypical melanocytic nevus, has a contrast-providing feature of its own (pigmentation), early detection could be aided, provided that a sensitive, reproducible,

and quantitative link can be established. We have achieved this in spectral imaging studies (2) (Figure 1C.5). A more careful study with larger number of patients is required, but the potential for increased accuracy and earlier detection using a fast, noninvasive method is significant and exciting.

Surgical Management: Image-Guided Therapy

The greatest impact of the optical molecular imaging methods reviewed here may be in the setting of minimally invasive surgery for guidance of intervention. Endoscopic implementation of the multimode imaging concept combining several ways of assessing the surgical field may lead to an optical biopsy or guiding an actual biopsy, tumor excision, or tumor margin evaluation.

Advanced Multimode and Multimodality Imaging

Currently at least six optical methods are potentially available for discriminating normal from abnormal tissue with high spatiotemporal imaging resolution, without using contrast agents. These include spectral reflectance, autofluorescence,

fluorescence lifetime, Raman, Stokes shift, and elastic (Mie) scattering imaging. Each method has potential advantages and disadvantages as a stand-alone technique, and several such methods have already been verified to be useful adjuncts to surgery. The effort to test each of these individual methods against each other would be quite significant, and result in delays in the development of clinically meaningful tools. However, the capacity to *combine* these methods in a single platform and subsequently analyze the potentially additive and even synergistic information gained by multimode imaging presents a unique opportunity for the advancement of this field. The use of a recently developed and commercially available supercontinuum laser light source to enable and deploy all such imaging methods in a single platform may prove important in advancing this agenda. The result should be a hyperreality (interpreted) image available to the surgeon in real time. Once the size, shape, orientation, and location of the lesion (e.g., tumor, lymph node) are assessed by digital imaging, it becomes easy to "paint a target" for intervention such as robotic excision or laser ablation.

Molecular Imaging in the Operating Room of the Future

Until major new approaches (such as gene or cellular therapies) open unforeseen possibilities in treatment, our brightest hope for better outcomes in cancer treatment is a thorough retuning (or maybe even re-thinking) of our current approaches that show success: early detection, improved surgery, and individualized postoperative therapies. For all these, the critically important step appears to be the ability to discriminate abnormal from normal tissue (preferably quantitatively, and during surgical intervention). Up until now, this task has been delegated to pathologists, who make this important decision "off-line" (hence, slowly), and without sophisticated tools. Not surprisingly, results are far from spectacular.

We believe that the time has come for the equivalent of real-time, quantitative intrasurgical pathology, based on a combination of advanced optical methods. The intervention thus enabled is image-guided in a manner that is of much higher spatiotemporal resolution and specificity than current practice; it should therefore also be appealing for robotic and other automated implementations. Although based on established methods (excision, laser ablation, photodynamic therapy), the resulting surgical procedures should also be new, at least in precision and speed.

In order for the high-tech scenario presented here to become realistic, one has to go beyond developing the needed technologies (54): one has to ensure that these are compatible with, and thus deployable into, the operating room of the future. Even the most advanced, fully integrated operating rooms are rather monolithic in concept and implementation today, and we (and others) are working on new versions, with more flexibility. What is needed is an all-digital, networking-based versatility, so that advanced new instruments could be brought into this environment seamlessly.

Ultimately, will molecular imaging be able to provide the much-needed closer link—spatially and temporally—between cancer detection and treatment, thus improving both? As always, what happens is governed by a mixture of what is available (tech-

nologically), what is acceptable (performance and compatibility-wise), what is allowable (regulation-wise) and what is affordable (economically). The noninvasive, intuitive nature, high resolution, and relatively low cost of optical molecular imaging strongly recommend it, but in the meantime we have to keep in mind the words of Jorge Louis Borges: *Nothing is built on stone; all is built on sand, but we must build as if the sand were stone.*

ACKNOWLEDGMENT

This work was supported in part by the U.S. Navy Bureau of Medicine and Surgery.

REFERENCES

1. Farkas DL. Invention and commercialization in optical bioimaging. *Nature Biotechnol.* 2003;21:1269–1271.
2. Farkas DL, Becker D. Applications of spectral imaging: detection and analysis of human melanoma and its precursors. *Pigment Cell Res.* 2001;14:2–8.
3. Burton K, Jeong J, Wachsmann-Hogiu S, et al. Spectral optical imaging in biology and medicine. In: Fujimoto J, Farkas DL, eds. *Biology and Medicine in Biomedical Optical Imaging* Oxford University Press; 2009, pp. 29–72.
4. Wachsmann-Hogiu S, Farkas DL. Nonlinear multispectral imaging microscopy: Concepts, instrumentation and applications. In: *Handbook of Biomedical Nonlinear Optical Microscopy.* Oxford University Press; 2008;461–483.
5. Weissleder R. Scaling down imaging: molecular mapping of cancer in mice. *Nature Rev Cancer.* 2002;2:11–18.
6. Weissleder R. Molecular imaging in cancer. *Science.* 2006;312:1168–1171.
7. Levenson RM, Balestreire EM, Farkas DL. Spectral imaging: prospects for pathology. In: Kohen E, ed. *Applications of Optical Engineering to the Study of Cellular Pathology.* 1999;133–149.
8. Pollice AA, Smith CA, Brown,, K, et al. Multiparameter analysis of human epithelial tumor cell lines by laser scanning cytometry. *Cytometry.* 2000;42:347–356.
9. Smith CA, Pollice A, Emlet D, et al. A simple correction for cell autofluorescence for multiparameter cell-based analysis of human solid tumors. Multiparameter analysis of human epithelial tumor cell lines by laser scanning cytometry. *Cytometry B Clin Cytom.* 2006;70:91–103.
10. Shackney S, Emlet DR, Pollice A, et al. Guidelines for improving the reproducibility of quantitative multiparameter immunofluorescence measurements by laser scanning cytometry on fixed cell suspensions from human solid tumors. *Cytometry B Clin Cytom.* 2006;70:10–19.
11. Virtanen C, Ishikawa Y, Honjoh D, et al. Integrated classification of lung tumors and cell lines by expression profiling. *Proc Natl Acad Sci U S A.* 2002;99:12357–12362.
12. Stellman SD, Muscat JE, Thompson S, et al. Risk of squamous cell carcinoma and adenocarcinoma of the lung in relation to lifetime filter cigarette smoking. *Cancer.* 1997;80:382–388.
13. Bhattacharjee A, Richards WG, Staunton J, et al. Classification of human lung carcinomas by mRNA expression profiling reveals distinct adenocarcinoma subclasses. *Proc Natl Acad Sci U S A.* 2001;98:13790–13795.
14. Beer DG, Kardia SL, Huang CC, et al. Gene-expression profiles predict survival of patients with lung adenocarcinoma. *Nat Med.* 2002;8:816–824.
15. Wigle DA, Jurisica I, Radulovich N, et al. Molecular profiling of non-small cell lung cancer and correlation with disease-free survival. *Cancer Res.* 2002;62:3005–3008.

16. Garber ME, Troyanskaya OG, Schluens K, et al. Diversity of gene expression in adenocarcinoma of the lung. *Proc Natl Acad Sci U S A.* 2001;98:13784–13789.

17. Aljada IS, Ramnath N, Donohue K, et al. Upregulation of the tissue inhibitor of metalloproteinase-1 protein is associated with progression of human non-small-cell lung cancer. *J Clin Oncol.* 2004;22:3218–3229.

18. Kumar N, Wolf-Yadlin A, White FM, et al. Modeling HER2 Effects on cell behavior from mass spectrometry phosphotyrosine data. *PLoS Computational Biology.* 2007;3:35–48.

19. Ballou BT, Fisher GW, Hakala T, et al. Tumor visualization using fluorochrome-labeled antibodies. *Biotechnology Progress.* 1997;13:649–658.

20. Ballou B, Fisher G, Waggoner AS, et al. Tumor labeling *in vivo* using Cy5-monoclonal antibody. *Proc Am Assoc Cancer Res.* 1994;35: 504.

21. Folli S, Westerman P, Braichotte D, et al. Antibody-indocyanine conjugates for immunophotodetection of human squamous cell carcinoma in nude mice. *Cancer Res.* 1994;54:2643–2649.

22. Mujumdar RB, Ernst LA, Mujumdar SR, et al.Cyanine labeling reagents: sulfoindocyanine succinimidyl esters. *Bioconjugate Chem.* 1993;4:105–111.

23. Mujumdar SR, Mujumdar RB, Grant CM, et al.Cyanine labeling reagents: sulfobenzindocyanine succimimidyl esters. *Bioconjugate Chem.* 1996;7:356–362.

24. Ballou B, Fisher GW, Waggoner AS, et al. Tumor labeling *in vivo* using cyanine-conjugated monoclonal antibodies. *Cancer Immunol Immunother.* 1995;41:257–263.

25. Ballou BT, Fisher GW, Hakala TR, et al. Fluorochromes for tumor imaging *in vivo, Cancer Detection and Prevention,* 1998; 22: 251–257.

26. Weinstein JN, Eger RR, Covell DG, et al. The pharmacology of monoclonal antibodies. *Ann NY Acad Sci.* 1987;507:199–210.

27. Weinstein JN, van Osdol W. Early intervention in cancer using monoclonal antibodies and other biological ligands: micropharmacology and the "binding site barrier." *Cancer Res.* 1992;52:2747s–2751s.

28. Buchsbaum DJ. Experimental approaches to increase radiolabeled antibody localization in tumors. *Cancer Res.* 1995;55:5729s–5732s.

29. Reintgen DS, Shimizu K, Coleman E, et al. Immunodiagnosis of tumors in vivo using radiolabeled monoclonal antibody A2B5. *J Surg Oncol.* 1983;23:205–211.

30. Ballou B, Jaffe R, Taylor RJ, et al.Tumor radioimmunolocation: differential antibody retention by antigenic normal tissue and tumor. *J Immunol.* 1984;132:2111–2116.

31. Mann BD, Cohen MB, Saxton RE, et al. Imaging of human tumor xenografts in nude mice with radiolabeled monoclonal antibodies. *Cancer.* 1984;54:1318–1327.

32. McCready DR, Balch CM, Fidler IJ, et al. Lack of comparability between binding of monoclonal antibodies to melanoma cells in vitro and localization in vivo. *J Natl Cancer Inst.* 1989;81:682–687.

33. Pasqualini R, Ruoslahti E. Organ targeting in vivo using phage display peptide libraries. *Nature.* 1996;380:364–366.

34. Farkas DL, Ballou B, Du C, et al. Optical image acquisition, analysis and processing for biomedical applications. *Springer Lecture Notes in Computer Science.* 1997;1311:663–671.

35. Hoffman RM. Green fluorescent protein imaging of tumour growth, metastasis, and angiogenesis in mouse models. *Lancet Oncol.* 2002;3:546–556.

36. Alivisatos AP. Semiconductor clusters, nanocrystals, and QDs. *Science.* 1996;271:933–937.

37. Bruchez M Jr, Moronne M, Gin P, et al. Semiconductor nanocrystals as fluorescent biological labels. *Science.* 1998;281:2013–2015.

38. Nie S, Xing Y, Kim GJ, et al. Nanotechnology applications in cancer. *Annu Rev Biomed Eng.* 2007;9:257–288.

39. Ntziachristos V. Illuminating disease with fluorescence molecular tomography. Biomedical Imaging: Nano to Macro. Proceedings of the 3rd IEEE International Symposium. 2006;375–377.

40. Contag CH, Bachmann MH. Advances in *in vivo* bioluminescence imaging of gene expression. *Annu Rev Biomed Eng.* 2002;4:235–260.

41. Graves EE, Ripoll J, Weissleder R, et al. A submillimeter resolution fluorescence molecular imaging system for small animal imaging. *Med Physics.* 2003;30:901–911.

42. Koo V, Hamilton PW, Williamson K. Non-invasive in vivo imaging in small animal research. *Cellular Oncol.* 2006;28:127–139.

43. Rice BW, Cable MD, Nelson MB. In vivo imaging of light-emitting probes. *J Biomed Optics.* 2001;6:432–440.

44. Zacharakis G, Kambara H, Shih H, et al. Volumetric tomography of fluorescent proteins through small animals in vivo. *Proc Natl Acad Sci U S A.* 2005;102:18252–18257.

45. Bouvet M, Wang JW, Nardin SR, et al. Real-time optical imaging of primary tumor growth and multiple metastatic events in a pancreatic cancer orthotopic model. *Cancer Res.* 2002;62:1534–1540.

46. Yamauchi K, Yang M, Jiang P, et al. Real-time in vivo dual-color imaging of intracapillary cancer cell and nucleus deformation and migration. *Cancer Res.* 2005;65:4246–4252.

47. Hwang JY, Moffatt-Blue C, Equils O, et al. Multimode optical imaging of small animals: development and applications. *Prog Biomed Optics Imaging.* 2007;8:1–10.

48. Hwang JY, Agadjanian H, Medina-Kauwe LK, et al. Large field of view scanning fluorescence lifetime imaging system for multi-mode optical imaging of small animals. *Prog Biomed Optics and Imaging.* 2008; in press.

49. Farkas DL. Spectral microscopy for quantitative cell and tissue imaging.In: Periasamy A, ed. *Methods in Cellular Imaging.* Oxford University Press; 2001;345–361.

50. Boppart SA, Bouma BE, Pitris C, et al. In vivo cellular optical coherence tomography imaging. *Nat Med.* 1998;4:861–865.

51. Pan Y, Lavelle JP, Meyers S, et al. High fidelity optical coherence tomography of tumorigenesis in rat bladders induced by N-Methyl-N-NitrosoUrea (MNU) instillation. *Med Physics.* 2001;28:2432–2440.

52. Chung A, Wachsmann-Hogiu S, Zhao T, et al. Advanced optical imaging requiring no contrast agents: a new armamentarium for medicine and surgery. *Curr Surg.* 2005;62:365–370.

53. Chung A, Karlan S, Lindsley E, et al. In vivo cytometry: a spectrum of possibilities. *Cytometry A.* 2006;69:142–146.

54. Farkas DL, Demetriou AA. New surgery for better outcomes: factors shaping it, and the need for high technology. *Global Surg.* 2003;21–25.

2

Genetic and Environmental Factors in Cancer Pathogenesis

M. William Audeh

"...in Biology, nothing makes sense except in the light of Evolution."

Theodosus Dobzhansky (1)

"Evolutionary Biology is the foundation for all Biology, and Biology is the foundation for all Medicine."

Nesse and Williams (2)

Carcinogenesis, the process by which cancer develops, and invasive cancer, the ultimate outcome of this process, are best understood as biological entities that operate within the laws of biology. The biology of all living things, when viewed through the prism of evolution, is essentially the means by which organisms survive, thrive, and reproduce within their environment, through the action of natural selection. The acquisition of genetic variation, which enhances survival in a particular environment and allows for successful reproduction, is the cornerstone of evolutionary biology, whether considering populations of organisms, such as species, or populations of cells, such as the clonal development of malignancy. Evolutionary biology, therefore, provides an informative framework with which to understand the factors that drive carcinogenesis and the behavior of established cancers—the factors that enhance genetic diversity, impose selective pressures on survival, and allow reproduction of the malignant cell. As with all living organisms, these factors are determined by the interaction between the genetic structure of the organism, its genome, and the environment.

The burden of cancer in the human population may also be examined and understood through evolutionary biology. The potential for the development of cancer may be a risk inherent in human biology, a risk that does not appear to have arisen as a significant threat to human health until modern times. Although cancer has always plagued mankind, having been found even in the mummified remains of ancient Egyptians (3), and named "carkinos" by the ancient Greeks (4), it is primarily in modern times that cancer appears to have become epidemic, particularly in the Western world. One in three individuals in the Western world will develop cancer in their lifetime, and one in five will die from cancer (5). As cancer is essentially a disease of genetic dysregulation of growth, it may be considered the most common "genetic" disease afflicting the human species. Why has this genetic disease reached epidemic proportions? The answer would seem to come from the study of the human genome, and the genes themselves, particularly those found to predispose to cancer development, as well as the environment in which the human genome operates.

If the human genome appears to possess an increased susceptibility to the development of malignancy in the current environment, it may be as a consequence of rapid change: the human genome developed in an environment very different from that in which we live today. Life in the modern environment entails increased exposure to DNA-damaging chemicals and physical factors, and growth-promoting substances, as well as changes in diet and lifestyle, all of which have occurred recently in human history, in an instant of evolutionary time. Therefore it is likely that cancer is the result of the human genome being maladapted to the current environment. All human beings may then be considered to carry some level of genetic predisposition to cancer, by virtue of possessing a human genome and living in the current environment. However, the genetic variation that exists between populations and between individuals, and that is being uncovered through the mapping of the human genome (6), produces varying responses to the environment, and in turn, a varying likelihood of developing cancer.

Medicine has traditionally focused on intervention only at the final stage of the long process of carcinogenesis, the invasive or metastatic cancer, with arguably little therapeutic success. However, the growing understanding of the genetic and environmental factors involved in carcinogenesis provides the ability to identify individuals at increased risk for cancer, and those environmental factors that alter their risk. Understanding how cancer "evolves" allows attention to ultimately be turned toward the prevention of cancer.

CARCINOGENESIS: THE EVOLUTION OF CANCER

Cancer develops in a long, multistep process in a population of cells, through the sequential acquisition of primarily somatic mutations in critical genes, which under selective pressures for survival ultimately leads to the evolution of a malignant, autonomously growing clone of cells (7). The principles of Darwinian evolution, when applied to this process, predict that genetic variation, in the form of mutations that enhance survival, will be selected and retained in a population of cells, and that those mutations that overcome common obstacles of growth controls and cell death in the cellular environment will be a common feature of all cancers. The process of carcinogenesis will therefore be facilitated by those genetic and environmental factors that enable the acquisition of genetic variation and promote growth. Such a survival strategy is phylogenetically ancient, having first developed in the most successful and ubiquitous of all life forms, bacteria (8). Increased genetic variation, in response to environmental selective pressures, is generated in bacterial populations by a rise in the rate of endogenous mutations, or hypermutability, accomplished by a variety of means. These include the induction of diminished fidelity of replication through the use of error-prone DNA polymerases, increased chromosomal instability, and diminished DNA mismatch repair. Adaptive hypermutability via diminished DNA mismatch repair is accomplished in bacteria by the horizontal transfer of defective mismatch repair genes, and is considered a hallmark of adaptive evolution (9).

The inducible hypermutability of bacteria directly parallels the observation of a "mutator phenotype" in human malignancy, as both provide the mechanism by which genetic diversity may be generated and evolutionary adaptation accelerated (10). The "universal" selective pressures that drive the clonal evolution of solid tumors have been identified as the hallmarks of cancer (see later discussion), and very likely account for nearly all of the recurring genetic changes that appear essential for cancer development. Inherited (germ line) mutations or polymorphisms that aid in the acquisition of these critical mutations will be associated with an increased risk of cancer, as is the case, for example, with mutations in the *BRCA* genes that increase the mutation rate, and polymorphisms in carcinogen-metabolizing genes, which may permit increased DNA damage. The stepwise acquisition of additional somatic mutations may then occur through interactions with environmental, dietary, or lifestyle factors, which also enhance DNA damage and proliferation, or simply due to the underlying genetic instability in neoplasia (11). Opportunities exist for intervention during the long process of carcinogenesis, a strategy that would be aided by the identification of individuals with any form of underlying genetic predisposition to accelerated carcinogenesis.

Genetic Instability, Cell Division, and Carcinogenesis

Genetic instability is a feature of all cancers. There is general agreement that genetic instability is a necessary and early step facilitating carcinogenesis, rather than an epiphenomenon of dysregulated and rapid growth (12). It is clear, however, that simple genetic instability and mutation are not sufficient to produce cancer; the mutations that promote carcinogenesis must also provide a survival advantage to the mutated cells, as most mutations are likely to be deleterious to cell survival (13,14). It is during the process of cell division and replication of the DNA that the genetic material is most susceptible to mutation. Errors in copying or damage to the DNA molecule must be detected and repaired during the window of cellular time between DNA replication and completion of the cell cycle, otherwise, the mutated DNA will be passed on to subsequent generations of cells. It follows, then, that with every cell division, the integrity of the DNA is placed at risk. It is well known in animal models of cancer that if the application of a chemical insult that damages DNA is coupled with a drive to proliferate, the process of carcinogenesis is facilitated (15). In the human body, there are 10^{13} cells, and in the lifetime of an individual, 10^{17} cell divisions from conception

to death, an enormous number of opportunities for the acquisition of mutation during replication (16). Fortunately, there are many genes involved in the protection of the integrity of the genetic information: those that detect and repair DNA damage and copying errors, and those that respond to environmental insults that may threaten the integrity of DNA. It is these genes that form the first line of defense against carcinogenesis, and are also frequently associated with predisposition to cancer when mutated or malfunctioning. Genetic analysis of premalignant precursor lesions such as hyperplasia has confirmed that the earliest abnormality, prior to the appearance of genetic instability, is activation of DNA damage checkpoints, usually in response to double-strand breaks (17,18). Critical detectors of DNA damage such as *p53*, *ATM*, and *CHk2* appear to be activated as one of the earliest steps in hyperplasia, indicating that DNA damage, either due to endogenous or exogenous factors, is indeed an initial step in carcinogenesis. The natural result of this DNA damage response should be cell cycle arrest and repair, or cell death (apoptosis) if repair cannot be accomplished. However, such controls provide a selective pressure for the emergence of escape from repair (i.e., the avoidance of cell death despite genetic instability), allowing the DNA damage to become fixed in the genome, and proceeding along the course of carcinogenesis. The clinical observation of a high risk of cancer development in individuals with inherited defects in DNA repair supports this view (19). In addition, nearly all environmental factors associated with carcinogenesis also either directly increase the likelihood of DNA damage, or increase the drive for cells to divide and enter the cell cycle, thus indirectly placing genomic integrity at risk. Table 2.1A,B summarizes the genetic and environmental factors associated with carcinogenesis.

The Selective Pressures of Carcinogenesis: The Hallmarks of Cancer

During the evolution of the cells of a tissue from normal cellular function to invasive cancer, the phenotype of malignancy, an enormous amount of change has occurred at the genetic level. It is estimated, for example, that a colonic adenoma will have over 11,000 genetic alterations (20) relative to normal colonic epithelium. If among these thousands of mutations are those that confer a survival advantage, the combination of genetic variability and selective advantage will promote the development of cancer. In order for cancer to evolve, a cell and its progeny must acquire mutations that overcome the selective pressures opposing the development of cancer. There are universal obstacles to cancer development that all cells must overcome to progress through carcinogenesis, and the capabilities that all cells must acquire to overcome these obstacles have been dubbed the *hallmarks of cancer* (10) and are summarized in Table 2.2.

The hallmarks of cancer are the phenotype of malignancy, and acquiring them would appear to be the "Holy Grail" of carcinogenesis. The primary factor that facilitates the acquisition of mutations in these critical genetic pathways is genetic instability. Not surprisingly, many of the genes associated with human cancer predisposition syndromes are involved in the maintenance of genetic stability and DNA repair. Germ line mutations or polymorphic variants that enhance genetic instability and increase the mutation rate will accelerate the acquisition of the hallmarks

Table 2.1A

Inherited Genetic Factors that Drive Carcinogenesis

Genes	Direct Effect	Carcinogenic Effect
Mutated		
BRCA1 and BRCA2	Defective DNA repair	Increased mutation rate
Mismatch repair genes (MLH1, MSH2, MSH6)	Defective mismatch repair	Increased mutation rate
APC	Increased stem cell population	Increased proliferating cells susceptible to mutation
RET	Increased cellular proliferation	Increased proliferating cells susceptible to mutation
Polymorphic		
Cytochrome P-450 system	Enhanced carcinogen activation	Increased mutation rate
Glutathione S-transferases	Diminished excretion of carcinogens	Increased mutation rate
MTHFR	Diminished folate levels	Increased mutation rate
Estrogen metabolizing enzymes	Increased estrogen levels	Increased cellular proliferation

of cancer. Key genes such as *p53, BRCA 1,* and *MLH1* not only participate in DNA repair, but also in the signaling system that identifies that a cell has sustained too much DNA damage to be repaired and should undergo apoptosis. These genes, when mutated, are highly penetrant "cancer predisposition" genes producing early-onset cancer, because they not only accelerate the mutation rate, but also provide at least one of the necessary hallmarks of cancer by allowing the escape from the programmed cell death response to DNA damage. Other cancer predisposition genes such as *APC* and *RET* also provide the hallmarks of cancer by increasing growth rates and decreasing apoptosis in the colonic epithelium and thyroid gland, respectively. Genetic predisposition to cancer may therefore be viewed as any inherited gene or set of genes that facilitates the acquisition of mutations that overcome the selective pressures of carcinogenesis

and achieve the functional hallmarks of cancer, the phenotype of malignancy.

GENOMIC MEDICINE AND CANCER

The year 2003 marked the 50th anniversary of the discovery of the structure of DNA, the Watson-Crick double-helix whose form elegantly suggested its function, and the mechanism by which genetic information is stored, replicated, damaged and repaired in all living things. Medical science entered the era of "genomic medicine" with the publication of the draft sequence of the human genome in 2001 (21), and it is clear that human genetic information, in the form of DNA (the genome), transcribed RNA (the transcriptome), and translated proteins

Table 2.1B

Environmental Factors that Drive Carcinogenesis

Environmental Factors	Direct Effect	Carcinogenic Effect
Exposures		
Hydrocarbon pollutants (aromatic hydrocarbons)	DNA damage	Increased mutation rate
Polychlorinated biphenyls (PCBs)	Estrogen mimic	Increased proliferation in hormone-responsive tissues
Cigarette smoke (aromatic hydrocarbons, nitrosamines)	DNA damage Tissue damage and inflammation	Increased mutation rate Increased cell proliferation
Diet		
Low fruit and vegetable intake	Decreased antioxidant levels	Increased mutation rate
Saturated fat	Increased oxidant damage	Increased mutation rate
Folate deficiency	Diminished DNA repair	Increased mutation rate
Infectious agents (see Table 2.3)	Tissue damage and inflammation Increased proliferation	Increased mutation rate Increased cell proliferation

Table 2.2

Hallmarks of Cancer: The Phenotype of Malignancy

Phenotype	Carcinogenic Effect
Self-sufficiency in growth signals	Increased cell proliferation Susceptibility to mutation
Insensitivity to antigrowth signals	Increased cell proliferation Susceptibility to mutation
Evading apoptosis	Decreased cell death relative to cell proliferation
Limitless replicative potential	Cell proliferation not limited by chromosomal instability and cell death
Sustained angiogenesis	Increased nutritional support for cell proliferation
Tissue invasion and metastasis	Expanded environment and access to growth factors for cell proliferation
Genetic instability	Increased mutation rate

Data from Hanahan D, Weinberg R. The Hallmarks of Cancer. *Cell.* 2000;100:57–70, with permission.

(the proteome), is essential to our understanding of cancer and carcinogenesis. The mapping of the human genome has provided a finite catalogue of the body of human genes, human "anatomy" at the molecular level, in addition to providing an understanding of the structure and organization of the genomic information (6,16). The insights gained from genomic medicine have facilitated the understanding of the susceptibility of the human genome to carcinogenesis, as well as the identification of specific genes associated with cancer risk.

The Human Genome and Carcinogenesis: Predisposition to Genetic Instability?

The human genome is by its very structure predisposed to mutational change and therefore innately susceptible to cancer development (22). The capacity to change, to generate genetic diversity by point mutation or recombination, is essential for the survival of any species, particularly when faced with environmental selective pressures. A key to this mutational trait may be found in the vast biological difference between the human species and our nearest genetic relative, the chimpanzee, a difference that has arisen within a relatively short period of time in evolutionary terms. Of the 22,000 to 30,000 genes currently believed to comprise the human genome, fully 98.8% of the genetic sequence of these genes are identical to that of the chimpanzee (23). However, dramatic change has occurred in the arrangement of these genes, the architecture of the human genome, which explains the wide biological gulf between humans and our nearest genetic relatives. Despite being identical in sequence, the organization of these 98.8% of genes has nevertheless changed, with resulting changes in regulatory control and gene expression; many genes have been shuffled to different locations in the genome, and in some cases lost or duplicated, such that genes are

expressed in different combinations, at different times, and to a differing extent in the human genome. Gene expression and regulation has changed because of recombination events, mediated by the presence of "hot spots" that are predisposed to breakage and reconnection (24,25). Such hot spots are actually part of the innate structure of the human genome, which contains a high density of GC-regions, and of short, repeating DNA sequences (25), both of which are prone to recombination events. The insertion—relatively recently in primate history—of highly homologous low-copy repeat and *Alu* elements throughout the genome, some between genes and some within coding regions, allows for recombination of nonhomologous chromosomal segments, reshuffling of genes, and changes in gene expression (see later discussion). Although this mutable quality of our genomic architecture may have fostered the rapid evolutionary change that makes us human, it has also predisposed our chromosomes to somatic mutations that promote malignant transformation. Indeed, many oncogenic chromosomal translocations occur between these recombination hot spots.

Significant genetic variation exists within the human population—approximately one in every 1,000 bases varies between individuals and is referred to as a *single nucleotide polymorphism* (21). However, many general features are present in all individuals (26). Only 1% to 2% of the human genomic DNA contains genes encoding proteins; over half of the genome is made up of repetitive sequences that do not contain genes. In fact, of all the DNA in the genome, the majority, over 45%, is made up of the repeated sequences previously described, which have been inserted into the genome during the course of mammalian, primate, and human evolution (27–29). The small fraction of the genome that encodes proteins, and varies between individuals, is the source of the most significant genetic predisposition to cancer: the individual genes involved in cancer development.

Human Genes That Predispose to Cancer

Cancer is a disease caused by the loss of integrity of the genetic information contained in the genome, and as such, cancer must be viewed as a truly "genetic" disease. Genetic diseases are those that are observed to be the result of heritable factors, most easily recognized in medical terms by a "positive" family history, the presence of the same disease in genetically related individuals. Cancer has long been known to "run in families," yet the majority of individuals developing cancer do not have a significant family history of cancer. This paradox may be explained by the fact that only a small proportion of cancer is attributable to single genes with a clear pattern of mendelian inheritance. The majority of human cancer is more appropriately understood as the phenotype of a "complex genetic trait," which develops as a result of the interaction of common polymorphic genes with the environment, and with other genes (30).

There are approximately 1,200 human genes (only 4% to 5% of all genes) that have been identified thus far as causing "mendelian" disease, or diseases attributable to single genes with identifiable patterns of inheritance (31). Of these, over 200 are thought to be associated with predisposition to cancer (32), and only 31 loci have been associated with clinically recognizable cancer-predisposition syndromes (19). Human disease genes may be grouped into specific functional categories, with the majority of adult-onset genetic diseases due to mutations in genes encoding enzymes, or modulators of protein function (33). Nearly all inherited genes predisposing to cancer fall into these categories. The majority of these disease-related genes have been identified since 1989, through the study of affected families, using the approach of locating the position of the single gene associated with disease by linkage analysis and then cloning the DNA sequence, a technique known as *positional cloning*. The major known cancer-predisposing genes, such as *BRCA1* and *BRCA2* associated with breast and ovarian cancers, and the *APC* gene associated with familial adenomatous polyposis (FAP), were discovered with this technique.

Positional cloning has the advantage of not requiring knowledge of the function of a gene, nor the mechanism by which malfunction of the gene contributes to disease. However, this method of identifying cancer-causing genes may only succeed when two important criteria are met: first, that the gene produces a positive family history of cancer, and second, that the cancer "phenotype" caused by the gene be accurately identified. The enormous phenotypic heterogeneity of cancer creates a significant challenge to this approach to gene discovery. Cancer is actually over 100 different diseases (16), each with multiple subtypes that differ substantially in their biological and clinical behavior. In the case of *BRCA1*, for example, the gene could not be located and identified simply by studying large families with breast cancer, but only after study was restricted to families with *early-onset* breast cancer, further refining the cancer phenotype associated with the gene (34).

Genes That Predispose to Carcinogenesis: Malfunction Versus Maladaptation

It is likely that the single-gene disorders associated with cancer predisposition represent the most readily apparent causes of inherited disposition to cancer: those genes with the highest penetrance, but which overall are quite rare in the human population and account for only a small proportion of the total burden of human cancer. The inherited mutations that lead to a frank *malfunction* of genes, such as those that inactivate powerful cancer-predisposing genes such as *BRCA1* and *BRCA2*, or *MSH2, MLH1,* and *APC*, account for no more than 5% to 15% of all breast and colorectal cancer patients, respectively. The remaining 85% to 95% of the cancer burden must be attributed, from the genetic perspective, to the action of far more common, but less powerful (i.e., low penetrance) genes. Common genes, with high gene frequency in a particular population, occur as a result of positive selection, population bottlenecks, or genetic drift (35). Common genes are common, therefore, by being either adaptive to a past environment or neutral in their adaptive benefit. Common genes, by definition, cannot be significantly malfunctioning in a manner detrimental to health or they would not have become common in human populations. Rather, common genes with minor functional differences between individuals (polymorphisms) are much more likely to be functioning adequately, but may contribute to the development of cancer when present in a particular environment, or in combination with certain other low penetrance genes. Genes that function appropriately but produce disease in a certain environment would be considered *maladapted* to that environment, rather than malfunctioning (36).

Many, if not all, common human diseases are very likely the consequence of the human genome being maladapted to our modern environment, which includes diet, mode of living, or lifestyle. The high incidence of cancer, as well as cardiovascular disease, hypertension, diabetes mellitus, and obesity may reflect the fact that our genetic construction is poorly adapted to the dietary and lifestyle changes (37), as well as new environmental exposures that have occurred since the human species originally evolved (2). Some have argued that cancer, which increases in incidence with age, is simply the result of increasing human longevity, that the human body is maladapted, not to the environment but to maintaining health beyond the reproductive years, because this would not be evolutionarily advantageous (38). However, the enormous number of individuals developing cancer before and during reproductive age argues against cancer as simply being an inevitable result of aging, and suggests a more complex process of deleterious gene-environment interactions. Studies indicating the major effect of environmental and dietary factors on cancer incidence, and the variation of cancer incidence around the world, also support the importance of gene-environment interactions (39).

The evidence would suggest that many inherited genes confer a genetic predisposition to cancer; a few due to frank malfunction of critical genes relevant to carcinogenesis, and the majority due to the effects of common genes that are maladapted to the modern environment and vary within and between populations. Common low-penetrance genes with relevance to carcinogenesis include metabolic polymorphisms responsible for responding to and detoxifying environmental chemicals (40), and polymorphic genes involved in DNA replication (41) and DNA damage repair (42). These polymorphisms with relevance to cancer development are widespread throughout the world, although their distribution varies greatly from one population to another. It is estimated that such common variants are phylogenetically ancient, having appeared within the human genome well over 10,000 years ago in most cases, as opposed to mutations in mendelian cancer genes such as *BRCA1*, which are estimated to be of more recent origin (2000 years or less) (19).

HUMAN GENETIC VARIATION AND ADAPTATION TO THE ENVIRONMENT: FORCES THAT SHAPED THE HUMAN GENOME

In order to understand the diseases caused by the maladaptation of human genes to the environment, it is necessary to understand the original adaptive forces that formed the human genome and produced the patterns of genetic variation observed in human populations. The human genome has significant amounts of variation in gene sequence, some of which is of no biological significance, but much of which reflects the action of natural selection in the past (26). Natural selection occurs over long spans of evolutionary time, in response to selective pressures from the surrounding environment. The modern human genome has been shaped and formed by the effects of prior darwinian natural selection and historical migrations of human populations (causing genetic drift and founder effects in isolated populations). During the course of history of the human species, it is clear that the majority of human existence (the several million years since the emergence and separation of the hominid line from that of the great apes) has been spent in the environment of prehistoric Africa, eating the diet and living the lifestyle of a hunter-gatherer. It is this long period of evolution that has been the primary shaper of our genome (43).

Important forces of natural selection in the genetic history of the human population have been infectious disease, climate, and diet (35). The genetic "signature" of ancient natural selection is still present in the human genome of today, in the form of polymorphic genes such as hemoglobin S, *G6PD*, factor V Leiden, and *HCE* (hemochromatosis), which may have provided a survival advantage for heterozygotes in certain populations in the past, but which today cause disease when two copies of the abnormal gene are inherited in homozygotes (44).

With a genome adapted primarily to the environment of Paleolithic Africa, the human species then spread rapidly throughout all the other environments of the world. There is strong evidence for the belief that all humans living today are descended from small populations of *Homo sapiens* that left the ancestral home of East Africa and populated the world at various times between 80,000 and 160,000 years ago (45). The initial ancient expansions of these groups, into Asia, the Middle East, and Europe were followed by the much more recent radiation of human populations into the new environments of the South Pacific and North and South America, all within the past 10,000 to 20,000 years (46,47).

In addition to the geographic variation in climate and environment that human populations encountered, the advent of agriculture and domestication of food animals beginning approximately 10,000 years ago served to further distance human populations from the hunter-gatherer diet, environment, and lifestyle in which humans had evolved.

The branches of the human family tree that developed in different geographic regions of the world provide the basis of the genetic variation observed between ethnic groups today. As the study of the genetic basis of cancer progresses beyond high-penetrance mendelian genetics limited primarily to families and extends to the search for common low-penetrance genes whose frequencies vary between ethnic groups and may contribute to cancer risk, it will become important to identify to which branch of the tree an individual belongs. This will likely be based on determining genetic identity through whole-genome analysis, rather than the archaic physical definitions of race (48,49), although the genetic background of an individual may be predicted in some cases by continent of origin (50) or by using haplotype structure, large blocks of DNA sequence that may categorize human lineage more accurately (49).

Genetic Maladaptation to the Environment and Carcinogenesis

In biological time, this period "out of Africa" has been extremely short; long enough to allow for minor genetic variations in traits

such as skin color as a gradual adaptation to differing climates, but not long enough to adapt to the extreme changes in diet, environment, and lifestyle of the past few thousand years. These changes have occurred far too quickly for human evolution to have produced any genetic adaptation to this new world, and the result instead has been genetic maladaptation, a component of the human genetic predisposition to cancer.

A well-known example of genetic maladaptation to the environment leading to an increased risk of cancer has been observed in Australia in the past century (51). Individuals from populations that had evolved for hundreds of generations in the colder northern latitudes, having lost genes for pigmentation as the result of adaptation to diminished exposure to solar radiation, emigrated approximately 300 year ago from the northern hemisphere, the British Isles, to the southern hemisphere, Australia. There they encountered high levels of solar radiation to which they were genetically maladapted because of lack of pigmentation. The result has been an increased susceptibility to superficial DNA damage in the skin and a significant incidence of skin cancer, particularly melanoma. Rates of melanoma are higher in Australia than anywhere in the world, although this increased incidence is only observed in the nonindigenous, or maladapted, population. Importantly, the genetic basis for the particularly high risk of melanoma has been attributed to inheritance of mutations or polymorphisms in a number of specific genes, including those involving pigmentation (*MICR* [52]), cell cycle control (*CDK2NA* [53]), and DNA damage repair (54).

ENVIRONMENTAL CHANGE AND CANCER RISK

A number of significant changes in environment, diet, and lifestyle have occurred in recent history, outpacing the adaptive change in the human genome and rendering large numbers of individuals genetically predisposed to cancer. Changes in the environment have been attributed to the enormous volume of synthetic substances with carcinogenic potential that have been manufactured in the past century and released into the air, water, and soil, often finding their way into dietary constituents (4). Significant changes of historically recent origin also include dietary changes associated with the Western diet such as reduced fruit and vegetables and increased fat and overall caloric intake, relative to the Paleolithic diet. Lifestyle factors have also contributed to the increased risk of cancer, including genotoxic exposures from cigarette smoking and other sources of combustion of organic materials, decreased physical activity, and the sedentary lifestyle, as well as changes in reproductive patterns in women. Women living in developed countries have prolonged and increased levels of estrogen exposure, a risk factor for breast and endometrial cancer (55). Increased estrogen exposure results from factors such as delay or avoidance of pregnancy, the use of hormone-replacement therapy, and possibly exposures to environmental estrogens such as polychlorinated biphenyl (56). The effect of such changes may be accentuated by the underlying genetics of hormone metabolism, which differs widely between individuals, and may add to the already increased levels of estrogen through the variable activity of polymorphic genes such as *CYP17, COMT, 17βHD*, and the estrogen receptor itself (57,58).

The environment to which our genome is adapted bears little resemblance to the current environment we encounter, particularly in the Western world. The genes that have evolved to respond to the minor and manageable genotoxic stresses of the ancient environment are maladapted to handle the array of carcinogens in today's world and the dietary deficiencies and excesses that characterize the Western diet. The genetic variation in environmental response genes controlling xenobiotic metabolism and DNA repair within human populations is likely to explain much of the difference in susceptibility to cancer between individuals in whom there is no family history or mendelian cancer gene identified. Although traditional cancer epidemiology has succeeded in identifying many of the environmental and lifestyle factors associated with an increased risk of cancer risk, the field is only now beginning to acknowledge the importance of genetic predisposition and the key role of gene-environment interactions in carcinogenesis (59).

Genomic Cancer Epidemiology

Consideration of the involvement of genetic factors in cancer has traditionally been limited to mendelian cancer syndromes, with cancers being classified as " hereditary," "familial," or "sporadic," on the basis of whether a positive family history is present and whether the pattern of inheritance is compatible with a single disease-causing gene (60). *Hereditary cancer* therefore applies to cancer caused by mendelian cancer genes such as *BRCA1* and *APC*, while *familial cancer* is applied to cancers that run in

families but for which a single gene has not clearly been identified and the pattern of inheritance is unpredictable. *Sporadic cancer* is the term that has been applied to all other cancers: the majority of cancer in which no familial or inherited pattern has been observed. It is therefore assumed by some that sporadic cancer has no genetic basis, and this misconception has contributed to the belief that most cancers are caused solely by environmental exposures. The current understanding of the biological basis of carcinogenesis does not support such distinctions, and it is more appropriate to think of the risk of cancer development as a continuum of the relative contribution of genes of variable penetrance, environmental exposures, and the interaction between the two. As shown in Figure 2.1, cancer may also develop in the rare extremes of this spectrum.

For example, the inheritance of rare malfunctioning genes such as mutated *APC*, with 100% penetrance, will lead to colorectal cancer with 100% frequency, regardless of environment. The other extreme, rare environmental exposures with such potent carcinogenicity that cancer will develop in 100% of those exposed, may occur, for example, with profound, catastrophic radiation exposure. Most cancers developing in the human population, however, fall somewhere between these extremes, representing the interaction between genes and environment. Even highly penetrant inherited mutations, such as those associated with hereditary nonpolyposis colorectal cancer (HNPCC) or *BRCA1* and *BRCA2*, do not produce cancer in all carriers (with penetrance estimates ranging from 33% to 87% for *BRCA*), and are therefore modified by environment, lifestyle, diet, and other

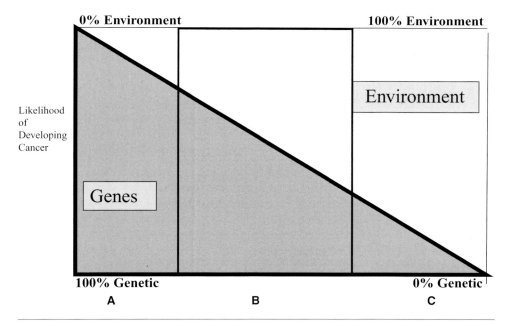

Figure 2.1 Carcinogenesis occurs as the result of interactions between genes and environment, and rarely occurs as the result of entirely one or the other. **Panel A** represents the rare occurrence of a highly penetrant inherited gene mutation, such as in the adenomatous polyposis coli (*APC*) gene, which confers a 100% likelihood of cancer of the colon, regardless of environment. **Panel B** represents the vast majority of cancers, in which carcinogenesis is driven by gene/environment interaction, is represented. **Panel C** represents the rare occurrence of an overwhelmingly carcinogenic exposure, such a radiation accidents, will lead to cancer in exposed individuals regardless of genetic background.

genes (41,61). Less penetrant genes such as those involved in carcinogen metabolism and DNA damage repair may contribute to the risk of cancer through their maladaptive interaction with the modern environment, and represent the basis for most of those cancers formerly considered sporadic. Because these low-penetrance genes are nevertheless inherited germ line genes, some contribution of inherited genetic background to the risk of cancer would appear to be present in virtually every individual diagnosed with cancer, regardless of family history.

Gene-Environment Interactions As the Cause of Most Cancers

The role of environmental exposures in cancer causation has been the subject of considerable public concern and scientific debate (62). It is generally assumed by the public that cancer is primarily a consequence of chemical or radiation exposure, perhaps as a result of the well-known association between cigarette smoking and lung cancer, as well as celebrated cases of insidious industrial pollution associated with geographic increases in cancer incidence, or "cancer clusters" (63,64). Indeed, the notion of environmental exposure as the sole cause of cancer is so firmly accepted by the lay public and some cancer activists that when studies seeking to detect assumed cancer-exposure associations produce negative results (e.g., pesticide exposure and breast cancer in Long Island, New York [65]), they are often met with skepticism and anger (66). Such misconceptions ignore the central fact of cancer causation: an individual's genetic background acts as a "filter" for the effects of environmental exposures (67) and is therefore the key to understanding the process of carcinogenesis and designing effective strategies for cancer prevention (68–70).

THE RELATIVE CONTRIBUTION OF GENETIC AND ENVIRONMENTAL FACTORS TO CARCINOGENESIS

The relative contribution of genetics and environment, of "nature versus nurture," in carcinogenesis has been debated for many years (68), although it is apparent that any analysis that attempts to separate genes from environment risks ignorance of the true process of carcinogenesis. A recent attempt to define the contribution of genetic susceptibility to cancer "versus" environment involved the study of cancer incidence among twins in Scandinavia (71). The value of twin studies in cancer epidemiology is based on the assumption that genetic susceptibility to disease will be manifest as a difference in disease incidence between monozygotic (genetically identical) and dizygotic (genetically separate) twins, while environmental factors will affect both types of twins equally (70). The study analyzed over 10,000 cancers in near 45,000 pairs of twins from the Swedish, Danish, and Finnish twin registries, comparing cancer incidence between identical and fraternal twins and unrelated controls. The study has been criticized for addressing only a few major cancers and lacking data on exposures or screening practices. Nevertheless, the study found significant differences between monozygotic and dizygotic twins in the incidence of several cancers, and suggested that at least 26% to 42% of common cancers such as breast and prostate might be attributable to genetic susceptibility.

CANCER EPIDEMIOLOGY: ENVIRONMENTAL FACTORS IN CARCINOGENESIS

Epidemiologic studies have identified a number of environmental factors associated with increased or decreased risk of cancer, including diet, infection, solar radiation exposure, and industrial and synthetic chemical exposures (72). Greatest attention, perhaps for reasons previously mentioned, has been paid to chemical exposures and methods by which carcinogenic chemicals may be identified, and their potency as carcinogens quantified (73). Focus has also been paid to "natural" carcinogens present in the diet and dietary deficiencies in micronutrients such as folate, encountered in the modern diet and known to increase the likelihood of DNA damage (74). The common thread connecting these factors derives from the understanding of the process of carcinogenesis and the dependence of this process on DNA damage and cellular proliferation—nearly all identified synthetic and natural chemical carcinogens appear to be capable of inducing either DNA damage or cellular proliferation, or both, and are therefore plausible contributors to cancer risk (75). It is likely that both synthetic carcinogens and dietary factors play important and complementary roles in carcinogenesis.

A number of public and private agencies conduct assays for carcinogenicity and attempt to classify substances accordingly. The current list of known or suspected carcinogens, released by the National Institute of Environmental Health Sciences in 2003, includes 228 substances, many of which are from identifiable industrial sources, while others are ubiquitous and unavoidable for most individuals in Western societies (76). In addition to well-known cancer-causing chemicals such as benzene, the current list includes steroidal estrogens used in hormone-replacement therapy; methyleugenol, a naturally occurring substance in herbs, oils, and spices, used in synthetic flavoring and sunscreen; and IQ (2-amino-3-methylimidazo (4,5-f)-quinoline), a common dietary chemical produced when various meats and fish are grilled at high temperatures.

Diet and Carcinogenesis

Diet and dietary constituents are perhaps the most important controllable "exposures" for any individual, and while these factors represent a minority of identified carcinogens in the National Institute of Environmental Health Sciences report of carcinogens, carcinogenic substances are certainly present in dietary sources. Of the many chemicals in the human diet, nitrosamines, polycyclic aromatic hydrocarbons, and fungal contaminants (mycotoxins) such as aflatoxin directly damage DNA and are unequivocal carcinogens (77), while controversy continues regarding the contribution of more general elements such as saturated fats (78) and other potential "indirect" carcinogens. Dietary exposures produce extraordinarily complex biological responses because of the presence or absence of protective (e.g., folate, antioxidants) and harmful factors (e.g., nitrosamines and oxidizing fats) and total energy intake (79), which itself may be a proxy for exposure to free radicals generated by oxidative metabolism (see later discussion). Genetic factors such as variation in metabolic enzymes and DNA damage repair (low-penetrance genes) will influence the effects of dietary constituents on cancer development, and dietary constituents in turn are likely to be modifiers of the effects of high-penetrance genes predisposing to cancer (80). For example, dietary oxidant load may enhance the carcinogenic effects of defective mismatch repair genes in hereditary nonpolyposis colon cancer (81), while intake of plant phenolics such as curcumin may reduce the effects of a mutated *APC* gene in familial adenomatous polyposis (82).

Environmental Exposures and Carcinogenesis

The ubiquitous nature of the known carcinogens present in the current environment, either due to industrial activity or as a result of common practices in everyday life, suggests that millions of individuals are regularly exposed to these substances and only a minority of those exposed will actually develop cancer. If this is so, then clearly exposure alone is insufficient to determine whether cancer will develop in a given individual. Environmental causes of cancer cannot be accurately considered without knowledge of the genetic susceptibility of the exposed individuals. However, most epidemiologic studies have traditionally been limited to the careful cataloguing of exposures and have historically had mixed and often uninterpretable results because of the absence of any data on the genetic predisposition of the subjects being studied (83,84). The likelihood that exposure to environmental carcinogens will lead to cancer depends in large part on the manner in which these substances are handled by the human body; such exogenous factors, whatever their source, are known to be affected by heritable factors, "environmental response genes," which vary widely between individuals and determine such diverse functions as metabolism of carcinogens (e.g., cytochrome P-450 genes, glutathione S-transferase [GST]) and detection and repair of DNA damage (e.g., *ATM, BRCA*) (84).

These genes will therefore determine whether an environmental carcinogen is effectively detoxified and excreted or allowed to inflict DNA damage, and whether or not that damage will be detected and repaired before being passed on to daughter cells. Genetic predisposition to cancer may therefore be manifest as a sensitivity to environmental carcinogens, an inherited "trait" that will not necessarily be identified as a family history of cancer owing to the variation in exposure histories from generation to generation.

ENDOGENOUS VERSUS EXOGENOUS FACTORS

DNA damage is arguably the most important of factors promoting the development of cancer, and it is well known that a major source of DNA damage comes from endogenous sources such as oxidative metabolism and chronic inflammation. Oxidative metabolism produces free radicals, highly reactive oxygen species that readily react with and alter macromolecules within the cell, principally DNA, as well as proteins and lipids (85). Oxidative DNA damage is a biologically ancient threat to genetic integrity, as evidenced by the nearly universal presence in all bacteria and eukaryotic cells of extensive DNA repair systems designed to identify and replace oxidized bases (86). The base excision repair (BER) system is present from *Escherichia coli* to human cells, and the activity of any component of the BER system will greatly affect the overall mutation rate. Recently, a polymorphic variant of the human BER enzyme, XRCC1 (R194W), was found to be associated with a reduced risk of breast, lung, and bladder cancer, while another polymorphic BER enzyme, OGG1, produced an increased risk of various cancers associated with the common variant S326C (42).

INFECTIOUS AGENTS AND CARCINOGENESIS

A variety of infectious agents have been associated with an increased risk of malignancy (Table 2.3). Human genetic variation in immune response also affects the natural history of infection

Table 2.3

Infectious Agents and Carcinogenesis

Agent	Affected Tissue/Cells	Carcinogenic Effect
Hepatitis B	Hepatocytes	Chronic inflammation: DNA damage Cell proliferation
Epstein-Barr virus	B-Lymphocytes	Increased
Human papillomavirus	Cervical epithelium	Chronic inflammation: DNA damage Cell proliferation Increased cell proliferation driven by virus
Helicobacter pylori	Gastric epithelium	Chronic Inflammation: DNA damage Cell proliferation
Helicobacter pylori	MALT B-Lymphocytes	Increased cell proliferation driven by antigenic stimulation

MALT, mucosa-associated lymphoid tissue.

with these agents and contributes to variability in cancer risk across ethnic groups. In most cases, these organisms are those that have co-evolved with the human species, and therefore have a lengthy evolutionary history of genetic adaptations to the human host (35,87,88). Such adaptations result in escape from eradication by the host immune system, the ability to produce chronic and persistent infection or colonization, and, in the case of viruses, to use human cellular proliferative pathways to replicate the viral genome. Infectious organisms that have co-evolved with the human species are characterized by high prevalence rates of colonization and/or infection in the population, the most important examples being viral (e.g., human papillomavirus [HPV], hepatitis B, Epstein-Barr virus) and bacterial (*Helicobacter pylori*). While few if any of these organisms are able to directly transform human cells and produce outright malignancy in the manner of oncogenic tumor viruses in animal models (16), the chronic inflammatory response induced by the presence of the organism or the chronic proliferative drive in the infected tissue, or both, lead to the acquisition of somatic mutations and selection for malignant clones (87).

HPV is the principle cause of human cervical cancer, with the greatest risk of cancer arising from chronic infection, particularly with subtypes 16 and 18. HPV is carried by every branch of the human family tree, and evidence of infection is found in all ethnic groups tested around the world (88). Numerous variants of the oncogenic subtypes 16 and 18 of HPV have evolved, adapted specifically to a particular human ethnic group, thus allowing for greater likelihood of chronic infection by that subtype in that ethnic group (89). As a result, HPV 16 or 18 variants adapted to caucasians, for example, are less easily cleared by the immune system of caucasian hosts and more likely to cause cervical cancer in whites from chronic infection. The recent development of a nontherapeutic vaccine directed against HPV may eradicate this ancient "passenger" from the human population, and is thus expected to reduce the incidence of cervical cancer (88). The HPV vaccine, by artificially generating an immune response, is attempting to circumvent millions of years of adaptation of HPV to its human host.

Helicobacter pylori colonization of the gastric epithelium has been highly associated with risk of mucosa-associated lymphoid tissue lymphoma and gastric carcinoma. The mechanism of association of infection with risk of mucosa-associated lymphoid tissue lymphoma may be chronic antigenic stimulation and proliferation. For carcinoma in the gastric epithelium, this mechanism is chronic inflammation in response to the bacterium, local production of oxidative free radicals by the human cellular immune response, and the resulting oxidative DNA damage to the nearby epithelial cells as "innocent bystanders" (90). Interestingly, *H. pylori* does not colonize premalignant lesions, and therefore evidence of infection may diminish by the time frank malignancy has developed. The association of infection with the risk of gastric cancer is limited to noncardia gastric cancer, while the presence of *H. pylori* may be protective against cancer of the gastric cardia or cancer of the gastroesophageal junction. The eradication of *H. pylori* by recently introduced medical therapy appears to be associated with an increased risk of gastric cardia cancer, despite reducing the risk of gastric noncardia cancer (91). This finding may help to explain the changing rates and distributions of these cancers in Western countries over the past century. A possible mechanism to explain this observation is that chronic colonization with *H. pylori* leads to gastric atrophy and diminished acid secretion and reflux, thereby reducing a causative factor in gastric cardia cancer. Another hypothesis may be that the eradication of a long-term commensal or passenger organism in the human body leads to alteration of the ecology of the upper digestive tract in a manner that promotes carcinogenesis in some tissues (90,91). If eradication of a phylogenetically ancient passenger organism from the human body poses potential harmful consequences, the introduction of the HPV vaccine may, despite diminishing virally associated cervical cancer, produce other, undesirable consequences.

GENETIC FACTORS AFFECTING CARCINOGENESIS: MAINTENANCE OF GENETIC INTEGRITY BY DNA REPAIR SYSTEMS

Over 130 genes involved in DNA repair have been identified in the human genome (92). In addition to DNA repair in response to damage, a number of genes maintain genetic integrity through DNA replication by detecting and correcting copying errors (93). Four major repair systems exist in the human genome for the purpose of repairing specific lesions: *base excision repair* (BER) for repair of oxidative damage, *nucleotide excisions repair* for bulky adducts such as carcinogens that bind to DNA, *mismatch repair* for repair of replication mismatch, and *recombinational repair* for the repair of double-strand breaks (Table 2.4). These repair systems contain genes that are polymorphic between individuals and populations, and are inherited genes conferring differing levels of DNA repair capacity. These differences in DNA repair capacity become biologically and clinically important in the presence of DNA damaging agents, particularly those that arise from exogenous sources such as polycyclic aromatic hydrocarbons and nitrosamines, bulky adducts that bind to DNA and disrupt its structure (42). Over 30 studies have evaluated genetic predisposition to cancer associated with polymorphisms in DNA repair genes. Although associations with single genes have been seen, most studies have been of insufficient sample size to be anything more than suggestive of an association. However, DNA repair genes that are inherited in a frankly malfunctioning form are the cause of well-known but rare cancer syndromes. Defects in any of a number of nucleotide excisions repair enzymes will cause xeroderma pigmentosum, a rare condition with high rates of cutaneous and visceral cancers. Defects in the DNA damage-signaling molecule, ATM, produce ataxia telangiectasia, a rare condition characterized by a high risk of lymphoid malignancy and neurologic abnormalities. Defects in double-strand break repair and in mismatch repair are the basis of the cancer syndromes associated with *BRCA1* and *BRCA2*, and the HNPCC genes *MLH1* and *MSH2*, and will be described separately.

Environmental Response Genes and Cancer

Enzyme systems have evolved to detoxify and remove non-nutritive chemicals that enter the body from the environment. The goal of this process is to render such chemicals water-soluble, so that they may be excreted in the urine, or fat-soluble, so they may be excreted via the biliary system. The phase I

Table 2.4

DNA Repair Systems

Repair System	Repair Enzymes	Type of Damage	Causes of Damage
Recombinational	*BRCA1,2* *ATM*	Double-strand breaks	DNA-binding chemicals (alkylating agents) X-radiation
Nucleotide excision	Xeroderma pigmentosum genes (XP)	Nucleotide chemical modification	DNA-binding chemicals (bulky adducts) Ultraviolet radiation
Base excision	*XRCC1* *OGG, MYH*	Single-strand breaks	Oxidative damage Radiation
Mismatch	*MLH1* *MSH2, 6*	Mispairing of bases	Replication error Slippage of replication in repeating sequences

Data from Wood RD, Mitchell M, Sgouros J, et al. Human DNA repair genes. *Science.* 2001;291:1284–1289.

enzyme system, an example of which is the cytochrome P-450 system, or CYP, is highly polymorphic and variable between individuals and ethnic groups (40). These systems evolved in an ancient environment that did not contain any of the man-made carcinogens to which we are now exposed every day. The function of the CYP enzymes is to render a compound chemically able to be made soluble or conjugated to another molecule that will carry it out of the body. The paradox is that this action of the phase I enzymes will actually "activate" a number of carcinogens, making them more highly reactive with DNA, before the phase II enzymes are able to step in and conjugate the compound to an inactivating moiety such as glutathione. Polymorphic variants of CYP genes encode proteins that are increased in their activation function and confer a small but significant increased risk of cancer with certain environmental exposures.

Phase II enzymes, an example of which is the GST system, function to conjugate compounds with inactivating moieties such as glutathione, which also acts as an antioxidant to absorb oxygen-free radicals in the cell. The GST system is highly polymorphic within human populations, and some GSTs are actually absent from certain populations. For example, GST-M is absent in 50% of all caucasians. Absence or inactivity of the GST enzymes would be expected to increase cancer risk by delaying the excretion of DNA-damaging carcinogens, and epidemiology studies have confirmed this for the most part, although the increased relative risk has been no more than 1.5 to 2 for any single gene. Studies that have combined CYP and GST polymorphisms have found marked differences in cancer risk, ranging from 40- to 100-fold differences, although the confidence intervals for such studies are large, owing to small sample sizes.

MENDELIAN CANCER GENES

DNA Damage Repair-Associated Genes and Common Cancers

BRCA1 and *BRCA2* and Breast Cancer

BRCA1 and *BRCA2* genes encode large proteins with complex functions in the maintenance of chromosomal stability, most important of which is detection and repair of DNA double-strand breaks (94). *BRCA1* and *BRCA2* also activate checkpoints within the cell cycle that determine whether a cell will proceed through the cycle, stop for repairs, or undergo apoptosis. Inherited mutations in *BRCA1* and *BRCA2* will therefore lead to an increased mutation rate and accelerate the process of carcinogenesis. As a result, the average age of onset of breast cancer in *BRCA1* and *BRCA2* mutation carriers is 20 years younger than the average age of onset of breast cancer in the general population.

BRCA1 and *BRCA2* mutations confer a lifetime risk of breast cancer of between 33% and 85%, depending on genetic background and other modifying factors. A number of modifying factors have been observed to affect the likelihood of cancer development in carriers of *BRCA* mutations, including environmental exposures to carcinogens, reproductive history, and other modifying genes involved in estrogen and androgen metabolism (61) and transcription factors (34). Germ line mutations in *BRCA* predispose primarily to breast and ovarian cancer, although a growing number of other cancers are now known to be associated with these genes, including colon, liver, pancreatic, uterine, and cervical cancers in female carriers of *BRCA1* mutations (95), and melanoma, pancreatic and laryngeal cancer, among others, in *BRCA2* carriers. The risk of prostate cancer is also elevated in male carriers of *BRCA1* and *BRCA2*. These genes account for a large proportion of families with numerous family members affected by breast or ovarian cancer, although there are clearly other genes that contribute to familial patterns of inheritance (96), as shown by the differing patterns of gene expression in these non-*BRCA* familial tumors.

Hundreds of different *BRCA1* and *BRCA2* mutations have been found in families with breast and ovarian cancer, although certain recurring mutations have been detected in individuals who are genetically related by virtue of belonging to an ethnically or geographically defined group. Examples are individuals of Ashkenazi Jewish descent, French Canadian descent, or from the population of Iceland. Such genetic "founder effects" are likely be detected in other groups as well. As the number of individuals and families tested grows around the world, the possibility of uncovering more "group-specific" mutations or polymorphisms will also increase and will assist with the identification of high-risk individuals.

Cancers that develop in *BRCA1* carriers are generally of higher grade than cancers in *BRCA2* carriers, and are more likely to be estrogen receptor-negative, perhaps reflecting a different pathogenesis or an acceleration of carcinogenesis that limits estrogen dependence to a brief and early phase of the process. There is evidence that cancers arising from *BRCA* mutations will respond differently to DNA-damaging cancer therapy because of their innate difference in the DNA damage response (97). The recognition of a genetically defined subset of breast cancer may eventually require a cancer therapy tailored to the specific nature of the genetic defect in these cancers.

Opportunities for Cancer Prevention in *BRCA1* and *BRCA2* Mutation Carriers.

Three approaches to cancer prevention exist for individuals with genetic predisposition to cancer: screening for premalignant lesions (screening for malignant lesions is not technically "prevention" but early detection), surgical removal of the tissue at risk, or biological alteration of the tissue at risk to inhibit carcinogenesis. For BRCA-related breast cancer, effective preventive screening remains to be defined (60). Mastectomy clearly reduces the likelihood of cancer development by as much as 90% to 95%, although microscopic rests of breast cells may remain even after surgery. Biological interventions such as reduction of estrogen effect by oophorectomy or medication (e.g., tamoxifen) have shown similar results, with a reduction in risk of approximately 50%. The National Surgical Adjuvant Breast and Bowel Project (NSABP)-P1 trial results suggested that estrogen blockade strategy may be ineffective in inhibiting breast carcinogenesis in BRCA1 carriers, although the results did not approach statistical significance. In view of the fact that estrogen is an important growth factor for the breast epithelium, it is likely that BRCA1 tumors do proceed through a period of estrogen dependence, but accelerated carcinogenesis may render this a brief and early step. Therefore, estrogen deprivation may be effective in preventing BRCA1-associated breast cancers, but only if applied early. Other molecularly targeted approaches using differentiating agents such as retinoids or epidermal growth factor inhibitors (preventing acquisition of the first hallmark of cancer) have entered clinical trials in BRCA1 carriers and offer great hope for an effective alternative to surgery or estrogen deprivation (98,99).

Mismatch Repair Genes and Colorectal Cancer

HNPCC, also known as the *Lynch syndrome*, is due to inherited germ line mutations in DNA mismatch repair genes, primarily *MLH1* and *MSH2* (100). However, there are over 20 genes involved in this system and it is likely that additional genes associated with cancer risk will be uncovered (101). These genes are involved in detection and repair of mismatches or slippage that occurs during DNA replication in areas that are prone to such errors, the repetitive sequences known as *microsatellites*. The genetic signature of defective mismatch repair proficiency is extreme variation in the length of microsatellite sequences due to the insertions and deletions that result from mismatches, microsatellite instability (MSI). In addition, there is evidence that

these genes also function in triggering the apoptosis response to irreparable DNA damage caused by oxidative stress, as the oxidized DNA base may resemble an area of mismatch (102). Therefore, the absence or malfunction of these genes will lead to genetic instability and an increased mutation rate within repetitive DNA sequences. Although most of these sequences occur in noncoding DNA, there are repeat sequences within the coding region of multiple genes know to be critical to the process of carcinogenesis, genes that participate in producing the hallmarks of cancer. Genes such as transforming growth factor-beta receptor type II, a growth-controlling gene, and *MSH2* itself, possess microsatellites within coding regions, leading to mutation of these genes and accelerated carcinogenesis.

Individuals with germ line mutations in mismatch repair genes have an 80% likelihood of developing colorectal cancer, as well as elevated risks of uterine, ovarian, genitourinary, upper gastrointestinal, hepatobiliary, and central nervous system tumors. Interestingly, the phenotype of HNPCC (i.e., the pattern of cancers developing in affected individuals) varies between populations, with an excess of gastric and pancreatic cancer being evident in Japanese and Korean patients, reflecting the modifying effects of environment, genetic background, or both (103).

Additional examples of modifying genes comes from the observation that two polymorphisms may affect the cancer risk in these individuals. The first, in a gene controlling DNA methylation, DNA methyltransferase 3b, may alter the age of onset of colorectal cancer in individuals with HNPCC (101). The polymorphic variant, a C-to-T transition in the promoter region, leads to increased gene expression, suggesting an increase in the potential for hypermethylation, an epigenetic event that may silence tumor suppressor genes and promote carcinogenesis. The second polymorphism, the common C677T variant found in methylenetetrahydrofolate reductase (MTHFR) confers a lower activity to this enzyme, resulting in a lower level of serum folate when diet is not supplemented with folate. Low folate levels are associated with diminished capacity for DNA repair, as folate is critical for the production of nucleotides. Individuals with this variant appear to have an increased risk of MSI-positive colorectal cancer, suggesting a synergistic interaction between mismatch repair, folate metabolism, and diet.

Although germ line mutations in mismatch repair genes are the basis of HNPCC, somatic mutations that delete or inactivate mismatch repair genes are a frequent occurrence in colorectal cancer and adenomas, with MSI being detected in 15% to 20% of all patients. The remainder of colorectal cancers display marked chromosomal instability and are presumed to develop through a different path of genetic changes that do not necessarily involve mismatch repair defects (20). Although the somatic mutations in mismatch repair genes that lead to MSI are thought to be stochastic events that produce a survival advantage in the process of neoplasia, they occur by a variety of means, including point mutation, loss of heterozygosity, and most frequently, methylation of the *MLH1* promoter, with silencing of gene expression. The factors leading to abnormal methylation are unknown, but may be related to diet and carcinogen exposure. Recent evidence suggests that the tendency to develop *MLH1* promoter hypermethylation may itself be an inherited trait (104). First-degree relatives of individuals affected by colorectal cancer (but without FAP or HNPCC) are known to have a doubled risk of developing colorectal neoplasia, although the basis for this familial risk has yet to be identified. However, adenomatous polyps developing in individuals with a single first-degree relative with colorectal cancer appear to be far more likely to possess MSI than polyps from individuals without a family history (29.6% vs. 9.3%, $p < 0.02$). The majority of these MSI-positive polyps displayed methylation of the *MLH1* promoter. The genetic basis for this inherited predisposition to promoter hypermethylation is unknown and may be related to enzymes such as DNA methyltransferase, and indicate another form of genetic predisposition to cancer.

The importance of genetic instability in the development of colorectal cancer is also illustrated by the identification of two additional types of genetic predisposition to colorectal cancer. Individuals who carry a single defective copy of the *BLM* gene, RecQ DNA helicase, have an increased risk of colorectal cancer. This gene is normally involved in maintaining the stability of chromosomes during replication, and when homozygous, is the basis for the cancer-prone Bloom syndrome. Also, germ line mutations in the BER gene *MYH* have been recently associated with the inheritance of multiple colorectal adenomas and an increased risk of colorectal cancer (105).

Opportunities for Prevention of Colorectal Cancer

Screening is an effective method of cancer prevention for colorectal cancer because of the ability to detect and remove the premalignant lesion, the adenomatous polyp. Screening in HNPCC has been proven to save lives and reduce cancer incidence (106). Total colectomy may be an unnecessarily aggressive intervention in view of the efficacy of screening. Chemoprevention for colorectal cancer in general has been evaluated with a variety of compounds, although specific interventions for HNPCC have not been well studied. Cyclooxygenase (COX)-2 inhibitors have been effective in reducing polyp formation in *APC* gene carriers (see later discussion), but this may represent a different path of carcinogenesis and may or not be effective in HNPCC or other genetic instability syndromes.

Interestingly, the use of a less specific COX inhibitor, aspirin, has been observed to reduce the risk of adenomatous polyps to a small degree. Two recent studies showed a reduction of 5.2% in adenomas in at-risk individuals identified by prior history of adenomas and 10% reduction in adenomas in at-risk individuals identified by a history of colorectal cancer, with the use of low doses of aspirin (107,108). The differences between the responses of these two at-risk populations to this chemoprevention agent may derive from the variation in the biological basis of their risk, the adenoma population being more heterogeneous in "genotype" than the colorectal cancer population. It is also likely that the reduction in adenoma incidence related to chemoprevention with aspirin is greatest in, or limited to, a specific, genetically defined subset, admixed within the study population. Such a genetic subset may be those individuals with a polymorphic variant of the ornithine decarboxylase gene (ODC), an enzyme important in polyamine synthesis, a pathway whose activity is associated with colorectal cancer (109). Individuals in the adenoma prevention trial with the polymorphic ODC "A" allele (which confers lower levels of the enzyme) appeared to benefit most profoundly from aspirin chemoprevention, with a 25% reduction in adenoma formation. Importantly, the population frequency of this aspirin-sensitive allele varies by ethnicity, with only 25% of caucasians carrying this allele, as opposed to 35% of African Americans and 63% of Asian Americans. Such findings suggest that chemoprevention, as well as cancer risk, will be affected by the genetic background of the individual.

High-Penetrance Cancer Syndromes Not Associated with DNA Repair Defects

APC: Loss of Function, Increased Stem Cell Number, and Familial Adenomatous Polyposis

The *APC* gene is the basis for FAP, a syndrome accounting for less than 1% of all colorectal cancer and manifest by the phenotype of innumerable colonic polyps, and a 100% penetrance for colon cancer (110). Unlike the other examples of genetic predisposition to colorectal cancer previously described, the function of the *APC* gene does not significantly affect genetic stability. The *APC* gene is a member of the Wnt signaling pathway, a critical pathway that regulates developmental programs during embryogenesis, and maintenance of renewable tissues after development (111). During embryogenesis, the *APC* gene appears essential for determining the fate of epithelial cells in organs that require epithelial-mesenchymal interactions for their development. In the normal colonic epithelium, the primary function of *APC* is to regulate the number and fate of proliferating stem cells within the colonic crypts. Germ line mutations that disrupt this vital function lead to large numbers of stem cells continuing to divide, rather than undergoing terminal differentiation and apoptosis. The result is the hyperplastic, polypoid epithelium, with vast numbers of proliferating cells exposed to the mutagenic environment of the intestinal tract, raising the likelihood of the eventual appearance of a malignant clone to 100%. Interestingly, a polymorphism of this gene, I1307K, which retains function but renders the gene more susceptible to somatic inactivation, has been identified in the Ashkenazi population and may double the risk of colorectal cancer (100). As previously described, it is the colon cancers resulting from *APC* mutations that may benefit most from chemoprevention with COX-2 inhibitors.

RET Gain of Function, Growth Promotion, and Familial Thyroid Cancer

The *RET* gene encodes a receptor tyrosine kinase that activates growth on the binding of ligand (32). Germ line mutations in this gene, in certain exons, will produce a constitutively activated protein that promotes growth signals in the absence of ligand binding. This inherited gene is associated with familial endocrine malignancies, such as multiple endocrine neoplasia type 2 (MEN2) syndrome, which is characterized by the triad of medullary thyroid cancer (MTC), pheochromocytoma, and hyperparathyroidism. Although familial MTC has nearly always been associated with MEN2 and germ line mutations in *RET*, nonfamilial MTC was assumed to be sporadic until recently (112). A subset of sporadic MTC was found to be associated with an ancient, low-penetrance founder locus, suggesting a polymorphic variant predisposing to isolated MTC. Until very recently, prevention of cancer in individuals with an inherited mutation in *RET* has been limited to surgical excision of the tissue at risk. The advent of molecularly targeted cancer therapy has led to the development of compounds that inhibit the activity of mutated, hyperactive tyrosine kinases such as *RET* (113) and may offer a form of chemoprevention in the future.

GENETIC AND ENVIRONMENTAL FACTORS IN CARCINOGENESIS: SEEKING CANCER PREVENTION THROUGH GENOMIC MEDICINE

Carcinogenesis is an evolutionary process requiring the interaction of genetic and environmental factors. The current burden of cancer in the human population is partly due to the unique susceptibility of the human genome to mutational change and to the numerous environmental factors, including diet and lifestyle, which reveal this susceptibility by increasing the opportunities for sustained mutational change that drives carcinogenesis. Even though all humans are at risk for developing cancer, certain individuals and groups of individuals, by virtue of the genetic variation they possess, may be more or less susceptible to carcinogenesis. The ideal outcome of the application of genomic medicine to the problem of human cancer will be the reduction in cancer incidence resulting from the identification of genetically predisposed individuals, and the use of molecularly targeted therapies and other prevention strategies to interfere with the process of carcinogenesis to which they are most susceptible. Genome-wide analysis may soon be capable of identifying not only genomic patterns associated with varying levels of cancer risk, but also the environmental susceptibilities that result from these genomic patterns. It is hoped that the growing understanding of the genetic and environmental factors involved in carcinogenesis will allow the emphasis of cancer medicine to shift from the therapy of established cancer to the prevention of carcinogenesis.

REFERENCES

1. Dobzhansky T. *Genetics of the Evolutionary Process*. New York: Columbia University Press; 1970.
2. Nesse R, Williams G. *Why We Get Sick: The New Science of Darwinian Medicine*. New York: Random House; 1994.
3. Filer J. *Disease* (Egyptian Bookshelf series). Austin, TX: University of Texas Press; 1995.
4. Nicolopoulou-Stamati P, Hens L, Howard CV, Van Larebeke N, eds. *Cancer as an Environmental Disease*. Environmental Science and Technology Library. Kluwer Academic Publishers: Dordrecht, the Netherlands; 2004.
5. Futreal PA, Kasprzyk A, Birney E, et al. Cancer and genomics. *Nature*. 2001;409:850–852.
6. Collins F, Guttmacher A. Genetics moves into the medical mainstream. *JAMA*. 2001;286:2322–2324.
7. Nowell P. The clonal evolution of tumor cell populations. *Science*. 1976;194:23–28.
8. Hoffmann AA, Parsons PA. *Evolutionary Genetics and Environmental Stress*. New York: Oxford University Press; 1993.
9. Denamur E, Lecointre G, Darlu P, et al, Evolutionary Implications of the Frequent Horizontal Transfer of Mismatch Repair Genes. *Cell*. 2000;103:711–721.
10. Hanahan D, Weinberg R. The Hallmarks of Cancer. *Cell*. 2000; 100:57–70.
11. Loeb LA. A Mutator Phenotype in Cancer. *Cancer Res*. 2001;61(8): 3230–3239.
12. Loeb LA, Loeb KR, Anderson JP. Multiple mutations and cancer. *PNAS*. 2003;100(3):776–781.
13. Steen HB. The origin of oncogenic mutations: where is the primary damage? *Carcinogenesis*. 2000;21(10):1773–1776.
14. Strauss BS. Hypermutability in Carcinogenesis. *Genetics*, 1998;148(4):1619–1626.
15. Breivik J. Don't stop for repairs in a war zone: Darwinian evolution unites genes and environment in cancer development. *PNAS*. 2001;98(10):5379–5381.
16. Weinberg R. *The biology of cancer*. New York: Garland Science; 2006.
17. Bartkova J. DNA damage response as a candidate anti-cancer barrier in early human tumorigenesis. 2005;434(7035):864–870.
18. Gorgoulis VG. Activation of the DNA damage checkpoint and genomic instability in human precancerous lesions. 2005;434(7035):907–913.
19. Frank SA. Genetic Predisposition to Cancer—Insights from Population Genetics. *Nature Reviews Genetics Nat Rev Genet*. 2004;5(10):764–772.
20. Boland CR, Ricciardiello L. How many mutations does it take to make a tumor? *PNAS*. 1999;96(26):14675–14677.
21. Consortium IHGS. Initial sequencing and analysis of the human genome. *Nature*. 2001;409:860–921.
22. Shaw CJ, Lupski JR. Implications of human genome architecture for rearrangement-based disorders: the genomic basis of disease10.1093/hmg/ddh073. *Hum Mol Genet*. 2004:ddh073.
23. Navarro A. Barton NH. Chromosomal speciation and molecular divergence—accelerated evolution in rearranged chromosomes10.1126/science.1080600. *Science*. 2003;300(5617):321–324.
24. Sanjuan R, Elena SF. Epistasis correlates to genomic complexity 10.1073/pnas.0604543103. *PNAS*. 2006;103(39):14402–14405.
25. Spencer CCA. The influence of recombination on human genetic diversity. *PLoS Genetics*. 2006;2(9):e148.
26. Baltimore D. Our genome unveiled. *Nature*. 2001;409:814–816.
27. Lupski JR. Genomic disorders: recombination-based disease resulting from genome architecture. *Am J Hum Genet*. 2003;72:246–252.
28. Haig H Kazazian Jr. LINE drive: Retroposition and genome instability. *Cell*. 2002;110:277–280.
29. Inoue K, Lupski JR. Molecular mechanisms for genomic disorders. *Annu Rev Genom Hum Genet*. 2002;3(1):199–242.
30. Balmain A. Cancer as a complex genetic trait: tumor susceptibility in humans and mouse models. *Cell*. 2002;108:145–152.
31. Botstein D, Risch N. Discovering genotypes underlying human phenotypes: past successes for mendelian disease, future approaches for complex disease. *Nature Genetics—Supplement*. 2003;33:228–237.
32. Mulvihill J. *Catalog of Human Cancer Genes: McKusick's Mendelian Inheritance in Man for Clinical and Research Oncologists*. Baltimore: The Johns Hopkins University Press; 1999.
33. Jimenez-Sanchez G, Childs B, Valle D, et al. Human disease genes. *Nature*. 2001;409:853–855.
34. Rebbeck TR. Modification of BRCA1- and BRCA2-associated breast cancer risk by AIB1 genotype and reproductive history. *Cancer Res*. 2001;61(14):5420–5424.
35. Jobling MA, Hurles ME, Tyler-Smith C, et al. *Human Evolutionary Genetics: Origins, Peoples and Disease*. New York: Garland Publishing; 2004.
36. Greaves M. Cancer causation: the Darwinian downside of past success? *Lancet Oncology*. 2003;3:244–251.

37. Simopoulos AP, Nestel PJ., eds. Genetic variation and dietary response. *World Review of Nutrition and Dietetics.* Vol. 80. Karger: Basel; 1997.

38. McKeown T. *The Origins of Human Disease.* Blackwell Publishers: Cambridge; 1988:140–142.

39. Fraser GE. Diet and the risk of cancer. In *Diet, Life Expectancy and Chronic Disease.* Oxford University Press: New York; 2003:85–108.

40. Pelkonen O, Raunio H, Lang M, et al. Xenobiotic-metabolizing enzymes and cancer risk. In: Vineis P, ed. *Metabolic Polymorphisms and Susceptibility to Cancer.* IARC: Lyon; 1999:77–88.

41. Sharp L, Julian L. Methylenetetrahydrofolate reductase gene (MTHFR), folate, and colorectal neoplasia. In: Khoury MJ, Little J, Burke W., ed. *Human Genome Epidemiology.* New York: Oxford University Press; 2004:333–364.

42. Goode EL, Ulrich CM, Potter JD, et al. Polymorphisms in DNA repair genes and associations with cancer risk. *Cancer Epidemiol Biomarkers Prev.* 2002;11(12):1513–1530.

43. Paabo S. The mosaic that is our genome. *Nature.* 2003;421:409–412.

44. Bamshad M, Wooding S. Signatures of natural selection in the human genome. *Nat Rev Gen.* 2003;4:99–111.

45. Cavalli-Sforza LL, Menozzi P, Piazza A, et al. *The History and Geography of Human Genes.* Princeton: Princeton University Press; 1994.

46. Cavalli-Sforza LL, Feldman MW. The application of molecular genetic approaches to the study of human evolution. *Nat Gen.* 2003;33:266–275.

47. Goldstein DB, Chikhi L. Human migrations and population structure: what we know and why it matters. *Annu Rev Genom Hum Genet.* 2002;3(1):129–152.

48. Rosenberg NA. Genetic structure of human populations. *Science.* 2002;298(5602):2381–2385.

49. Foster MW, Sharp RR. Beyond race: towards a whole-genome perspective on human populations and genetic variation. *Nat Rev Genet.* 2004;5(10):790–796.

50. Bamshad MJ, Wooding S, Watkins WS, et al. Human population genetic structure and inference of group membership. *Am J Hum Genet.* 2003;72:578–589.

51. Jablonski N, Chambers G. Skin deep: human skin color. *Scientific American.* 2002 October;74–83.

52. Sturm R. Skin colour and skin cancer—MICR, the genetic link. *Melanoma Research.* 2002;12:405–416.

53. Bishop DT. Geographical variation in the penetrance of CDKN2A mutations for melanoma. *JNCI Cancer Spectrum.* 2002;94(12):894–903.

54. Wei Q. Repair of UV light-induced DNA damage and risk of cutaneous malignant melanoma. *JNCI Cancer Spectrum.* 2003;95(4):308–315.

55. Audeh MW. Commentary: risk factors for breast cancer: The biological perspective. In Silberman A, ed. *Surgical Oncology: Multidisciplinary Approach to Difficlut Problems.* Arnold: London; 2002:261–267.

56. Shields PG. Understanding population and individual risk assessment: the case of polychlorinated biphenyls 10.1158/1055-9965. EPI-06-0222. *Cancer Epidemiol Biomarkers Prev.* 2006; 15(5):830–839.

57. Henderson B, Ponder B, Ross RK, et al. *Hormones, Genes, and Cancer.* New York: Oxford University Press; 2003.

58. Ambrosone C. CYP17 genetic polymorphism, breast cancer, and breast cancer risk factors. *Breast Cancer Res.* 2003;5(2): R45–R51.

59. Perera F. Molecular Epidemiology: on the path to prevention? *JNCI Cancer Spectrum.* 2000;19:602–612.

60. ASCO. *ASCO Comprehensive Review of Clinical Cancer Genetics.* in *2002 ASCO Annual Meeting.* FL: Orlando; 2002.

61. Narod S. Modifiers of risk of hereditary breast and ovarian cancer. *Nat Rev Cancer.* 2002;2(2):113–123.

62. Chakravarti A, Little P. Nature, nurture, and human disease. *Nature.* 2003;421:412–414.

63. Harr J. *A Civil Action.* New York: Vintage/Random House; 1996.

64. Gibbs LM. *Love Canal: the story continues.* Stony Creek, CT: New Society Publishers; 1998.

65. Gammon MD. Environmental toxins and breast cancer on long island. ii. organochlorine compound levels in blood. *Cancer Epidemiol Biomarkers Prev.* 2002;11(8):686–697.

66. Twombly R. Long Island study finds no link between pollutants and breast cancer. *JNCI Cancer Spectrum.* 2002;94(18):1348–1351.

67. Olden K, Wilson S. Environmental health and genomics: visions and implications. *Na Rev Genetics.* 2000;1:149–153.

68. Hoover RN. Cancer—Nature, nurture, or both. *N Engl J Med.* 2000;343(2):135–136.

69. Safe SH. Interactions between hormones and chemicals in breast cancer. *Annu Rev Pharmacol Toxicol.* 1998;38(1):121–158.

70. Risch N. The genetic epidemiology of cancer: interpreting family and twin studies and their implications for molecular genetic approaches. *Cancer Epidemiol Biomarkers Prev.* 2001;10(7):733–741.

71. Lichtenstein P. Environmental and heritable factors in the causation of cancer—analyses of cohorts of twins from Sweden, Denmark, and Finland. *N Engl J Med.* 2000;343(2):78–85.

72. Ames BN, Gold L. Willett W, et al. The causes and prevention of cancer. *PNAS.* 1995;92:5258–5265.

73. Ames BN, Gold L. Pollution, pesticides, and cancer misconceptions. *FASEB J.* 1997;11:1041–1052.

74. Blount BC. Folate deficiency causes uracil misincorporation into human DNA and chromosome breakage: Implications for cancer and neuronal damage. *PNAS.* 1997;94(7):3290–3295.

75. Tomatis L. Alleged misconceptions' distort perceptions of environmental cancer risks. *FASEB J.* 2001;15(1):195–203.

76. Twombly R. New carcinogen list includes estrogen, UV radiation. *JNCI Cancer Spectrum.* 2003;95(3):185–186.

77. Sugimura T. Food and cancer. *Toxicology.* 2002;181–182:17–21.

78. Kushi L, Giovannucci E. Dietary fat and cancer. *Am J Med.* 2002;113;Suppl 9B:63S–70S.

79. Weisburger J. Lifestyle, health and disease prevention: the underlying mechanisms. *Eur J Cancer Prev.* 2002;11 Suppl 2:S1–7.

80. Choi SW, Friso S, ed. *Nutrient-Gene Interactions in Cancer.* Taylor and Francis: Boca Raton; 2006.

81. Bruce WR, Giacca A, Medline A, et al. Possible mechanisms relating diet and risk of colon cancer. *Cancer Epidemiol Biomarkers Prev.* 2000;9(12):1271–1279.

82. Mahmoud NN. Plant phenolics decrease intestinal tumors in an animal model of familial adenomatous polyposis. *Carcinogenesis.* 2000;21(5):921–927.

83. Tarasuk VS, Brooker AS. Interpreting epidemiologic studies of diet-disease relationships. *J Nutr.* 1997;127(9):1847–1852.

84. Peltonen L, McKusick VA. Genomics and medicine: dissecting human disease in the postgenomic era. *Science.* 2001;291(5507): 1224–1229.

85. Wallace S. Oxidative damage to DNA and its repair. In: Scandalios JG., ed. *Oxidative Stress and the Molecular biology of Antioxidant defenses.* Plainview, NY: Cold Spring Harbor Laboratory Press; 1997:49–91.

86. Marnett LJ, Riggins JN, West JD, et al. Endogenous generation of reactive oxidants and electrophiles and their reactions with DNA and protein. *J Clin Invest.* 2003;111(5):583–593.

87. Coussens LM, Werb Z. Inflammation and cancer. *Nature*. 2002;420:860–867.

88. Burk RD, DeSalle R. The tango and tangle of human papillomavirus and the human genome 10.1093/jnci/djj322. *J Natl Cancer Inst*. 2006;98(15):1026–1027.

89. Xi LF. Human Papillomavirus Type 16 and 18 variants: race-related distribution and persistence 10.1093/jnci/djj297. *J Natl Cancer Inst*. 2006;98(15):1045–1052.

90. Nyren O, Blot WJ. Helicobacter pylori infection: mainly foe but also friend? 10.1093/jnci/djj422. *J Natl Cancer Inst*. 2006;98(20):1432–1434.

91. Kamangar F. Opposing risks of gastric cardia and noncardia gastric adenocarcinomas associated with helicobacter pylori seropositivity 10.1093/jnci/djj393. *J Natl Cancer Inst*. 2006;98(20):1445–1452.

92. Wood RD. Human DNA repair genes. *Science*. 2001;291(5507):1284–1289.

93. Kunkel TA, Bebenek K. DNA replication fidelity. *Annu Rev Biochem*. 2000;69(1):497–529.

94. Venkitaraman A. Cancer susceptibility and the functions of BRCA1 and BRCA2. *Cell*. 2002;108(171–182).

95. Thompson D, Easton DF, and the Breast Cancer Linkage Consortium. Cancer incidence in BRCA1 mutation carriers. *JNCI Cancer Spectrum*. 2002;94(18):1358–1365.

96. Hedenfalk I. Molecular classification of familial non-BRCA1/BRCA2 breast cancer. *PNAS*. 2003;100(5):2532–2537.

97. Farmer H. Targeting the DNA repair defect in BRCA mutant cells as a therapeutic strategy. *Nature*. 2005;434(7035):917–921.

98. Wu K. The retinoid X receptor-selective retinoid, LGD1069, prevents the development of estrogen receptor-negative mammary tumors in transgenic mice. *Cancer Res*. 2002;62(22):6376–6380.

99. Suh N. Prevention and treatment of experimental breast cancer with the combination of a new selective estrogen receptor modulator, arzoxifene, and a new rexinoid, LG 100268. *Clin Cancer Res*. 2002;8(10):3270–3275.

100. Lynch HT, de la Chapelle A. Hereditary colorectal cancer. *N Engl J Med*. 2003;348(10):919–932.

101. Jones JS. DNMT3b polymorphism and hereditary nonpolyposis colorectal cancer age of onset 10.1158/1055-9965.EPI-05-0644. *Cancer Epidemiol Biomarkers Prev*. 2006;15(5):886–891.

102. Hardman RA, Afshari CA, Barrett JC, et al. Involvement of mammalian MLH1 in the apoptotic response to peroxide-induced oxidative stress. *Cancer Res*. 2001;61(4):1392–1397.

103. Park J. Gene-environment interaction in hereditary non-polyposis colorectal cancer with implications for diagnosis and genetic testing. *Int J Cancer*. 1999;82:516–519.

104. Ricciardiello L. Frequent loss of hMLH1 by promoter hypermethylation leads to microsatellite instability in adenomatous polyps of patients with a single first-degree member affected by colon cancer. *Cancer Res*. 2003;63(4):787–792.

105. Sieber OM. Multiple colorectal adenomas, classic adenomatous polyposis, and germ-line mutations in MYH. *N Engl J Med*. 2003;348(9):791–799.

106. de la Chapelle A. Inherited human diseases: victories, challenges, disappointments. *Am. J Hum Genet*. 2003;72:236–240.

107. Baron JA. A randomized trial of aspirin to prevent colorectal adenomas. *N Engl J Med*. 2003;348(10):891–899.

108. Sandler RS. A randomized trial of aspirin to prevent colorectal adenomas in patients with previous colorectal cancer. *N Engl J Med*. 2003;348(10):883–890.

109. Barry ELR. Ornithine decarboxylase polymorphism modification of response to aspirin treatment for colorectal adenoma prevention 10.1093/jnci/djj398. *J Natl Cancer Inst*. 2006;98(20):1494–1500.

110. Fearnhead NS, Britton MP, Bodmer WF, et al. The ABC of APC. *Hum Mol Genet*. 2001;10(7):721–733.

111. Kuraguchi M. Adenomatous polyposis coli (APC) is required for normal development of skin and thymus. *PLoS Genetics*. 2006;2(9):e146.

112. Borrego S. A Founding locus within the RET proto-oncogene may account for a large proportion of apparently sporadic Hirschsprung disease and a subset of cases of sporadic medullary thyroid cancer. *Am J Hum Genet*. 2003;72:88–100.

113. Milano A, Chiofalo MG, Basile M, et al. New molecular targeted therapies in thyroid cancer. *Anticancer Drugs*. 2006;8:869–879.

COMMENTARY
Ora Karp Gordon

Dr. Audeh has provided a broad and comprehensive discussion of the genetic and environmental factors in the pathogenesis of malignant disease. In this *Commentary*-I summarize the current state of our knowledge of hereditary breast cancer.

ONCOGENETICS OF BREAST CANCER: CLINICAL IMPLICATIONS

Breast cancer is the most common cancer in women, with lifetime estimates up to 1 in 8 (1). A subset of women affected with breast cancer has clear hereditary susceptibility, usually presenting as an autosomal dominant pattern of inheritance. Overall, it is estimated that 5% to 10% of breast cancers are due to highly penetrant single-gene mutations (2), but over 20% of women diagnosed with breast cancer have some family history (3). The discovery of several genes responsible for hereditary cancer syndromes have allowed for significant advances in prevention, early detection, and targeted therapeutics for breast cancer and other malignancies. Although identification of these mutations is of critical importance to clinical care, it is equally important to recognize the limitations of genetic testing, particularly for the best-known *BRCA* genes, and the role of genetic testing in risk prediction at large.

High-Penetrant Breast Cancer Susceptibility Genes

The best described and most widely clinically available genetic testing is for the *BRCA* genes, *BRCA1* and *BRCA2*. The *BRCA* genes were identified in the 1990s via linkage studies of very highly penetrant breast, and breast/ovary families. Although the protein products of both genes are involved in DNA repair, the cancers associated with mutations in either gene have distinct and unique features. *BRCA1* mutations are associated with early age of onset (average, 2 decades earlier than sporadic cancer) and high-grade and highly proliferative tumors with a "basal phenotype." This is characterized molecularly by estrogen and progesterone negativity, and lack of HER2/eu overexpression, as well as cytokeratin 5,14 positive staining (4). *BRCA1* mutations are also associated with a high risk of ovarian cancer.

BRCA2 mutations result in cancers more typical of post-menopausal sporadic breast cancers both in terms of age on onset as well as hormonal and molecular characteristics. *BRCA2* mutations are in general associated with lower risk of ovarian cancer than *BRCA1* mutations; however, confer risk of male breast cancer, pancreatic, laryngeal carcinoma, and melanoma (5). Pancreatic cancer has recently been associated with *BRCA1* as well although there are no specific risk levels or screening recommended at present (6). Some earlier associations have been largely discounted, such as the colon cancer risk (7). Clearly there is an increase in cancer incidence overall in *BRCA* families, which is likely due to combined environmental and modifying genetic effects (8).

Genotype-Phenotype Correlation

There has been much debate in the literature regarding the "true" risk of cancer in hereditary breast ovary syndrome and carriers of deleterious *BRCA* mutations. Cancer risk estimates vary broadly in the literature, from 55% to 85% lifetime risk for breast cancer, depending on the study design and mode of ascertainment of cases. The original studies from the Breast Cancer Linkage consortium (which led to the discovery to the *BRCA* genes) estimated the breast cancer risk at 85% to 87% lifetime and the ovarian cancer risk at 27% to 50%, with a contralateral breast cancer risk of 60% (9,10). More recently, the contralateral breast cancer risk among *BRCA* carriers was estimated at 30% within 10 years of first diagnosis without other interventions such as estrogen depletion (11). These risk estimations have been criticized as overestimations of risk for all *BRCA* carriers as the data were generated from the most penetrant, highest risk families (12). Cancer risk estimates among unselected population-based *BRCA* testing, typically for a few specific mutations to age 70, have been lower, 28% to 60% (13–15).

A meta-analysis that combined data from 22 studies of *BRCA* carriers estimated the penetrance of breast cancer to be 65% lifetime for *BRCA1* and 45% for *BRCA2*. The ovarian cancer risk was 39% for *BRCA1* and 11% for *BRCA2*, but there was variation in risk by age of diagnosis of the index case, consistent with other genetic or modifying affects (16). More recently, a meta-analysis of 10 studies estimated breast cancer risk at 57% for *BRCA1* and 49% for *BRCA2* mutation carriers, and ovarian cancer risk of 40% for *BRCA1* and 18% for *BRCA2* mutation carriers (17). In the New York Breast Cancer Study, 1,000 incident cases of breast cancer in Ashkenazi Jewish women were screening for one of the three founder mutations regardless of age of onset or family history; 10.8% of women were found to carry a deleterious mutation. Seven hundred family members then underwent genetic testing, and cancer risk estimates were derived from that data. They demonstrated that, as expected for an autosomal dominant condition, half of the mutations were paternally inherited, thus reducing the apparent penetrance because male carriers of *BRCA* mutations have much lower cancer risks. Lifetime risk for breast cancer was 81% for *BRCA1* and 84% for *BRCA2*, and 54% and 27% risk of ovarian cancer in *BRCA1* and *BRCA2*, respectively (18) (Table 2C.1). Thus the question remains: how much of the variability in cancer estimates is due to study ascertainment issues and how much may be due to differences in environmental or modifier gene effects in the higher cancer-expressing kindreds?

In certain cancer predisposition genes, the risk of malignancy or other associated clinical findings are specific to the location of the mutation within the gene. This is true for *APC* mutations that lead to familial adenomatous polyposis syndrome and the *RET* gene (a proto-oncogene that leads to multiple endocrine neoplasia type 2), where the location of a specific mutation within the gene can be used to predict clinical outcome and disease risk (19,20). For the *BRCA* genes this is not as well correlated. There is a region within *BRCA2* known as the *ovarian cancer cluster region* between nucleotide number 3035 and 6629. Mutations within this region are associated with elevated risk of ovarian cancer and lower breast cancer risk. The 999del5 Icelandic founder associated with a higher risk of prostate cancer (21). This positional effect has not been seen with *BRCA1*.

A number of studies have interrogated candidate genes as modifiers of risk for either type or likelihood of cancer in *BRCA*

Table 2C.1

Lifetime Accumulative Risk (%) for Breast and Ovarian Cancer in Ashkenazi Jewish Women with *BRCA1* Founder Mutations

Risk By Age	Breast Cancer		Ovarian Cancer	
	BRCA1	*BRCA2*	*BRCA1*	*BRCA2*
30	3	0	—	0
40	21	17	3	2
50	39	34	21	2
60	58	48	40	6
70	69	74	46	12
80	81	85	54	23

Adapted from King MC, Marks JH, Mandel JB, *New York Breast Cancer Study Group*. Breast and ovarian cancer risks due to inherited mutations in *BRCA1* and *BRCA2*. *Science*. 2003;302;643–646.

carriers including *CHEK2, TGFB, FANC*, and *RAD51*. Although individually each seems to confer modest risk for breast or other cancers, none clearly distinguish risk among *BRCA* carriers (22). Further complicating issues of penetrance are "phenocopies," which is when an individual with a particular disorder does not carry a mutation found in other affected members of the family. Excess of breast cancer has been previously reported in *BRCA* families (12). Recently a study from a British hereditary breast/ovary registry demonstrated an excess of breast cancer in relatives of *BRCA* carriers who themselves have tested negative for a mutation. In this series, 12% of first-degree relatives with breast cancer of index cases from *BRCA* families tested negative for a mutation, giving a standardized index ratio of 3.2, suggesting significant modifier gene effect among high-risk families (24). These data, however, have been criticized as not all individuals within the families actually underwent testing. In a study by Gronwald et al. (24), genetic testing was offered to 261 sisters of 188 mutation-positive cases. One of 72 mutation-negative sisters was diagnosed with breast cancer. Of the 17 sisters diagnosed with breast cancer, only one was a phenocopy, thus not supporting the previous findings.

Modifiable risk factors have been associated with cancer expression. The most profound is probably the use of oral contraceptive pills on ovarian cancer (26), with up to 60% reduction in risk with 5 years of use, and the effect of oophorectomy on reducing the risk of breast cancer by 50% if completed by age 40 (27,28). Salpingo oophorectomy also reduces the risk of ovarian cancer by 90% or more, but does not eliminate the risk of primary peritoneal carcinoma in *BRCA1* carriers. Normal weight and physical activity at age 18 delayed the age of onset of breast cancer in *BRCA* carriers (18). Tamoxifen use in carrier women previously affected with breast cancer substantially reduced the risk of contralateral breast cancer, as did oophorectomy, with a synergistic combined use affect seen, even for *BRCA1* carriers (11).

The prevalence of *BRCA* mutations varies among ethnic populations, and estimations of the frequency of mutations are influenced by mode of ascertainment and study method. Unlike other cancer predisposition genes, where new or de novo mutations are frequent, overwhelmingly, *BRCA* mutations are stable, resulting from an ancestral mutation that is passed on through many generations (14). There are a few case reports in the literature that have proven a de novo *BRCA* mutation by paternity testing and haplotype analysis (17). Because of population genetic effects—genetic drift, population isolates—certain recurrent mutations have become fairly frequent (14,18). Examples include Eastern European Ashkenazi Jewish, French Canadian, and Icelandic founder mutations where the population prevalence of *BRCA* mutations can be as high as 1 in 40 (19), and the prevalence of mutations among incident cases of Ashkenazi Jewish women with ovarian cancer is over 30% (32). Common recurrent mutations have also been described in Polish and Filipino populations (33). In low-frequency groups, the estimated prevalence of a mutations may be a little as 1 in 500 (34).

Thus the a priori likelihood of a *BRCA* mutation is influenced by these ethnic variations and has clinical implications regarding testing. For example, individuals from high-risk, high-prevalent ethnic groups could undergo more limited genetic testing for those common mutations, rather than comprehensive full gene sequencing. Additionally, there has been significant research of hereditary breast ovary families wherein no mutation has been detected. Since the discovery of the *BRCA* genes, several genomic rearrangements, duplications, and deletions, common founder mutations in certain ethnic groups such as the Dutch and British Isles descendents have been discovered (34–36) and five common rearrangements in *BRCA1* were added to the patented commercial BRCA test in the United States and Europe in late 2002 (37). Multiplex ligation-dependent probe amplification identifies up to 6% of mutations missed by direct sequence analysis (38). In a study of high-risk families (defined as four or more breast or ovarian cancer cases), 12% were found to carry previously undetected *BRCA* mutations, 5% *CHEK2* mutations, and 1% *TP53* mutations (39).

Predictive Value of *BRCA* Testing

Numerous guidelines for testing have been established over the past few years. None are completely comprehensive, and as information evolves indications for testing have broadened substantially. Generally accepted insurance indications for *BRCA* testing are summarized in Table 2C.2 but are not meant to be all-inclusive. Insurance coverage in the United States varies considerably by policy and location, but serves as a reference point for genetic testing coverage. As previously described, studies have found the molecular pattern referred to as "basal" to be strongly predictive of an underlying *BRCA* germ line mutation, even without a very early age of onset or family history (40), and thus may become an independent indication for genetic testing even when other criteria are not met.

Various models have been developed to aid in the clinical estimation that any one individual will harbor a *BRCA* mutation. The BRCApro (41) model is a widely available online tool that estimates the likelihood of a *BRCA1* or *BRCA2* mutation, but tends to overestimate the probability of a mutation in Ashkenazi Jewish individuals and underestimate the probability in families with breast cancer only. Tyrer-Cusick is a breast cancer risk prediction model developed in England that has been shown to have higher discriminatory accuracy in predicting likelihood of breast cancer as it incorporates reproductive risk information and family history information, but it does not predict risk of a *BRCA* mutation (42). However, an easy-to-use electronic format has not been made available, thus limiting the clinical utility of this model for now. Myriad Genetic Laboratory in Salt Lake City, UT, provides both online and handheld table of *BRCA* probabilities (43). These data are constructed from clinical history information provided on the test requisition forms and are therefore limited by the extent and accuracy that personal and family history information is completed by the ordering clinician.

What began as best-practice expert recommendations now, for the most part, has proven evidenced-based efficacy. The National Comprehensive Cancer Network guidelines and National Institute of Health and Clinical Excellence (United Kingdom) provide a comprehensive summary of screening guidelines for hereditary breast cancer, the most significant of which is the addition of regular breast magnetic resonance imaging for *BRCA* carriers beginning at age 25. Surgical risk reduction has the

Table 2C.2
Sample Insurance Criteria for *BRCA* Testing

Women with a personal history of breast cancer and any of the following:

1. Breast cancer is diagnosed at age 40 years or younger, with or without family history; *or*
2. Breast cancer is diagnosed at age 50 years or younger, with at least one close blood relative with breast cancer at age 50 years or younger; *or*
3. Breast cancer is diagnosed at age 50 years or younger, with at least one close blood relative with ovarian cancer; *or*
4. Breast cancer is diagnosed at any age, with at least two close blood relatives with ovarian cancer at any age; *or*
5. Two breast primaries with at least one close blood relative with breast cancer at age 50 years or younger; *or*
6. Two breast primaries with at least one close blood relative with ovarian cancer; *or*
7. Breast cancer is diagnosed at any age, with at least two close blood relatives with breast cancer, especially if at least one woman is diagnosed before age 50 years or has two breast primaries; *or*
8. Close male blood relative with breast cancer; *or*
9. Personal history of ovarian cancer; *or*
10. If of certain ethnic descent associated with deleterious mutations (for example, founder populations of Ashkenazi Jewish, Icelandic, Swedish, Hungarian, or other) or history of breast and/or ovarian cancer in close blood relative, no additional family history required

Women with a personal history of ovarian cancer and any of the following:

11. Personal history of breast cancer; *or*
12. At least one close blood relative with ovarian cancer; *or*
13. At least one close female blood relative with breast cancer diagnosed at age 50 years or younger or two breast primary cancers
14. At least two close blood relatives with breast cancer; *or*
15. At least one close male blood relative with breast cancer; *or*
16. If of Ashkenazi Jewish descent, no additional family history is required

Medicare criteria for BRCA testing:

1. Clinically affected individuals (invasive breast cancer or ovarian cancer at any age) meeting at least one of the following criteria:
   - One or more first-degree relatives (mother, father, sister, daughter) or second-degree relative (aunt, uncle, grandmother, niece, granddaughter) with invasive breast cancer diagnosed before age 50 years, *or*
   - One or more first- or second-degree relatives with ovarian cancer, *or*
   - One or more first- or second-degree relatives with male breast cancer.
2. Individuals with a personal history of at least one of the following (no family history required):
   - Invasive breast cancer before age 50 years, *or*
   - Ovarian cancer at any age, *or*
   - Both invasive breast cancer and ovarian cancer at any age, *or*
   - Male breast cancer at any age
3. Clinically unaffected patients with a family member with a known *BRCA1* or *BRCA2* mutation
4. Individuals of Ashkenazi (Eastern European) Jewish ancestry with invasive breast cancer at any age, or meeting any of the above-listed (1–3) criteria

Adapted from Aetna clinical criteria for *BRCA* testing, July 2006, and Center for Medicare Services www.mydriadtests

greatest efficacy for both breast and ovarian cancer, but does not completely eliminate risk and is associated with substantial potential morbidity (44,45).

RARE HEREDITARY BREAST CANCER SYNDROMES

There are several well-described genetic syndromes that predispose to breast and other cancers that should always be considered in the evaluation of the breast cancer patient. Li-Fraumeni syndrome is a hereditary cancer syndrome first described in the 1960s that in over 70% of cases is due to mutations in the *TP53* gene, and thought to account for about 1% of hereditary breast cancer. The classic triad is of early-onset breast cancer, soft tissue sarcoma, and adrenal cortical carcinoma. The original diagnostic criteria was for a very early-onset cancer syndrome: a proband with a sarcoma age less than 45, plus a first-degree relative with any cancer age less than 45, and other first- or second-degree relative with the same (46,47). Since then, a Li-Fraumeni-like syndrome with more broadly inclusive criteria has emerged as mutations have been found in families not meeting the original criteria (35). However, sarcoma—particularly childhood osteosarcoma or rhabdomyosarcoma—and childhood adrenocortical carcinoma are the strongest predictor of a *TP53* mutation, with 80% of unselected adrenocortical carcinoma patients having germ line *TP53* mutations (46). The breast cancer risk in Li-Fraumeni may be as high as 56% by age 45 (47) and has been identified in a series of unselected women with breast cancer under the age of 30 with a frequency of 4%, half of which were de novo mutations (48).

Cowden syndrome is a hamartomatous cancer predisposition syndrome due to mutations in the *PTEN* gene. Cowden syndrome is unique in that it has pathognomic clinical features including hamartomas of the colon, trichellemoma of the skin, and a cerebellar malformation that causes Lermitte-Duclos disease and megencephaly, which results in macrocephaly. Cowden syndrome is associated with risk of breast, thyroid, and endometrial cancer as well as a variety of benign tumors such as multinodular goiter, lipomas, and papillomas (52). *PTEN* mutations are frequently found in somatic breast cancers, and some series have found up to 5% of breast cancers under age 40 associated with a germ line *PTEN* mutation, although in general *PTEN* mutations are thought to be a rare etiology of breast cancer (53).

As noted previously, pedigrees consistent with hereditary breast ovary syndrome (multiple affected individuals within successive generations, and at least one with ovarian or breast and ovarian cancer) greatly increases the probability of an underlying *BRCA* mutation, and account for 90% of the genetic risk in hereditary ovarian cancer. Yet *BRCA* mutations account for only about half of site-specific breast cancer (e.g., families affected with breast cancer only), demonstrating the much broader genetic heterogeneity for breast cancer. In these families, a negative *BRCA* test can provide substantial clinical reassurance that there is no increased susceptibility to ovarian cancer (54), but much less information regarding the risk of breast cancer or a second primary breast cancer. Contralateral breast cancer risk is as high as 27.3% in affected individuals who have a family history consistent with hereditary breast cancer, but are *BRCA*-negative (55). Investigations to identify another *BRCA* locus, "*BRCA3*," have for the most part not been successful (8), and this has led to a change in approach to investigating the role of more common lower penetrant genetic effects, individually and in combination to explain the clustering of breast cancer within families.

Moderate Penetrant Genes

CHEK2 is a serine threonine kinase, which is activated in response to ionizing radiation and other agents that induce double-strand breaks. Ataxia telangiectasia mutated protein activation phosphorylates a variety of substrates including *BRCA1* and *CHEK2* (56). On activation, *CHEK2* acquires the ability to carry out the following: (a) regulate the S phase cell cycle checkpoint, (b) modulate P53 activity by direct phosphorylation, (c) activate P53-independent damage response pathways, (d) phosphorylate *BRCA1*.

Because of its integral role in the P53 pathway, *CHEK2* was initially considered a candidate gene for Li-Fraumeni and Li-Fraumeni-like syndrome (57). A common variant in *CHEK2*, 1100delC, is predicted to result in a truncated version of the protein. This variant is found with a frequency of approximately 1.4% in whites of northern European descent (58), and has been associated with an increased risk for breast cancer. Although

literature is conflicting on the effect of *CHEK2* on breast cancer risk, an international pooled consortium supported a twofold increased risk among carriers of the variant than controls (59). Since then there have been several studies implicating *CHEK2* as a significant risk for contralateral breast cancer and possibly as a susceptibility to the effects of ionizing radiation such as chest x-ray (60).

Low-Penetrant Genes and Breast Cancer

The modern era of breast cancer risk assessment began with the identification of the highly penetrant *BRCA1* and *BRCA2* genes as well as the other rare high-penetrant genes such as *TP53* and *PTEN*. However, the majority of breast cancer cases occur sporadically or in familial clusters not consistent with a mendelian pattern of inheritance. Studies investigating lower risk genes such as *CHEK2* do not account for enough risk to be solely responsible for the breast cancer in the majority of cases. Thus it is likely that a predisposition to breast cancer is associated with common but weakly penetrant genetic variants in multiple genes (61–62). Single nucleotide polymorphisms (SNPs) have been associated with breast cancer risk in a variety of genes including those involved in the steroid hormone pathway, including *COMT* (49), *CYP17*, and *UGT* transferase family (65). Although much research has focused on the endogenous estrogen state of women on breast cancer risk (66–67) and some predictive models for breast cancer susceptibility from multiple SNPs have emerged (52), these SNPs have not been investigated in relationship to the effect based on age or menopausal status of the woman because of the complexity of analysis or sample size.

Data are now emerging on the age-specific association of various SNPs on breast cancer risk (69). These studies investigated age-specific cohorts defined as young (less than 44 years), middle (44 to 54 years), and old age (55 to 69 years) correlating with pre-, peri-, and postmenopausal status. Multiple genes demonstrated a significant association with breast cancer, but with genotypes for *CYP11B2* and *UGT1A7*, risk associations reversed between young and old groups, such that increased risk in the young group was associated with protective effect in the old group and vice versa. Other genes only demonstrated association in one age group. This demonstrates the nonlinear association between various genetic and environmental affects (e.g., hormonal status) and breast cancer risk (70,71). Application of this type of data into models for breast cancer prediction are currently under investigation and hold promise for the future of genetic risk prediction with a much broader clinical application.

CONCLUSIONS

The advances in the molecular basis of inherited breast cancer have been substantial, yet most breast cancer is not explained by these single gene effects. Thus the future of the genetic basis of susceptibility to cancer will likely require novel analysis of combinations of polymorphisms and epistatic genetic mechanisms. It is critical for the clinician attending to the care and prevention of patients and those at risk for breast cancer to recognize the contribution of known hereditary factors, as well as the limitations of current clinical tests in the interpretation of risk. This applies to both known single gene effects such as *BRCA*, *TP53*,

PTEN, STK11, and *CHEK2* as well as the emerging combined effects of lower penetrant genes. Management recommendations therefore can never be based on a single genetic test alone, but must be interpreted within the context of that patient's personal and family history, as well as the predictive power of the genetic test itself.

REFERENCES

1. Althuis M, Dozier JM, Anderson WF, et al. Global trends in breast cancer incidence and mortality 1973-1997. *Int J Epidemiol.* 2005;34:405–412.
2. The Breast Cancer Linkage Consortium. Cancer risks in BRCA2 mutation carriers. *J Natl Cancer Inst.* 1999;91:1310–1316.
3. Amir E, Evans DG, Shenton A, et al. Evaluation of breast cancer risk assessment packages in the family history evaluation and screening programme. *J Med Genet.* 2003;40:807–814.
4. Lakhani SR, Van De Vijver MJ, Jacquemier J, et al. The pathology of familial breast cancer: Predictive value of immunohistochemical markers estrogen receptor, progesterone receptor, HER-2, and p53 in patients with mutations in BRCA1 and BRCA2. *J Clin Oncol.* 2002;20:2310–2318.
5. Loman, et al. Cancer incidence in relatives of a population-based set of cases of early-onset breast cancer with a known BRCA1 and BRCA2 mutation status. *Breast Cancer Res.* 2003;5:175–186.
6. Greer J, Whitcomb D. Role of BRCA1 and BRCA2 mutations in pancreatic cancer. *Gut.* 2007;56:601–605.
7. Kirchhoff T, Satagopan JM, Kauff ND, et al. Frequency of BRCA1 and BRCA2 mutations in unselected Ashkenazi Jewish patients with colorectal cancer. *J Natl Cancer Inst.* 2004;96:68–70.
8. Antoniou AC, Pharoah PD, McMullan G, et al. Evidence for further breast cancer susceptibility genes in addition to BRCA1 and BRCA2 in a population-based study. *Genet Epidemiol.* 2001;21:1–18.
9. Ford D, Easton DF, Bishop DT, et al. Risks of cancer in BRCA1-mutation carriers. Breast Cancer Linkage Consortium. *Lancet.* 1994;343:692–695.
10. Ford D, Easton DF, Stratton M, et al. Genetic heterogenity and penetrance analysis of the BRCA1 and BRCA2 genes in breast cancer families. *Am J Hum Genet.* 1998;62:676–689.
11. Metcalfe K, Lynch HT, Ghadirian P, et al. Contralateral breast cancer in BRCA1 and BRCA2 mutation carriers. *J Clin Oncol.* 2004; 22:2328–2335.
12. Begg CB. On the use of familial aggregation in population-based case probands for calculating penetrance. *J Natl Cancer Inst.* 2002. 94: p. 1221–1226.
13. Struewing JP, Hartge P, Wacholder S, et al. The risk of cancer associated with specific mutations of BRCA1 and BRCA2 among Ashkenazi Jews. *N Engl J Med.* 1997;336:1401–1408.
14. Warner E, Foulkes W, Goodwin P, et al. Prevalence and penetrance of BRCA1 and BRCA2 gene mutations in unselected Ashkenazi Jewish women with breast cancer. *J Natl Cancer Inst.* 1999;91:1241–1247.
15. Hopper JL, Southey MC, Dite GS, et al. Population-based estimate of the average age-specific cumulative risk of breast cancer for a defined set of protein-truncating mutations in BRCA1 and BRCA2. Australian Breast Cancer Family Study. *Cancer Epidemiol Biomarkers Prev.* 1999;8:741–747.
16. Antoniou AC, Pharoah PD, Narod S, et al. Breast and ovarian cancer risks to carriers of the BRCA1 5382insC and 185delAG and BRCA2 6174delT mutations: a combined analysis of 22 population based studies. *J Med Genet.* 2005;42:602–603.
17. Chen S, Parmigiani G. Meta-analysis of BRCA1 and BRCA2 penetrance. *J Clin Oncol.* 2007;25:1329–1333.
18. King MC, Marks JL, Mandel JB, New York Breast Cancer Study Group. Breast and ovarian cancer risks due to inherited mutations in BRCA1 and BRCA2. *Science.* 2003;302:643–646.
19. Knudsen A. Attenuated familial adenomatous polyposis (AFAP).A review of the literature. *Familial Cancer.* 2003;2:43–55.
20. Koch C. Molecular pathogenesis of MEN2-associated tumors. *Familial Cancer.* 2005;4:3–7.
21. Thompson D, Easton D. Variation in cancer risks by mutation position, in BRCA2 mutation carriers. *Am J Hum Genet.* 2001;68:410–419.
22. Kadouri L, Kote-Jarai Z, Hubert A, et al. A single-nucleotide polymorphism in the RAD51 gene modifies breast cancer risk in BRCA2 carriers, but not in BRCA1 carriers or noncarriers. *Br J Cancer.* 2004;90:2002–2005.
23. Smith A, et al. Phenocopies in BRCA1 and BRCA2 families: evidence for modifier genes and implications for screening. *J Med Genet.* 2006;0:1–6.
24. Gronwald J, Cybulski C, Lubinski J, et al. Phenocopies in breast cancer 1 (BRCA1) families: implications for genetic counselling. *J Med Genet.* 2007;44:e76.
25. Narod SA. Modifiers of risk of hereditary breast cancer. *Oncogene.* 2006;25:5832–5836.
26. Eisen A, Lubinski J, Klijn J, et al. Breast cancer risk following bilateral oophorectomy in BRCA1 and BRCA2 mutation carriers: an international case-control study. *J Clin Oncol.* 2005;23:7491–7496.
27. Kramer JL, Velazquez IA, Chen BE, et al. Prophylactic oophorectomy reduces breast cancer penetrance during prospective, long-term follow-up of BRCA1 mutation carriers. *J Clin Oncol.* 2005;23: 8629–8635.
28. Kaufman DJ, Beaty TH, Struewing JP. Segregation analysis of 231 Ashkenazi Jewish families for evidence of additional breast cancer susceptibility genes. *Cancer Epidemiol Biomarkers Prev.* 2003;12:1045–1052.
29. Shaag A, Walsh T, Renbaum P, et al. Functional and genomic approaches reveal an ancient CHEK2 allele associated with breast cancer in the Ashkenazi Jewish population. *Hum Mol Genet.* 2005;14: 555–563.
30. Moslehi R, Chu W, Karlan B, et al. BRCA and BRCA2 mutation analysis of 208 Ashkenazi Jewish women with ovarian cancer. *Am J Hum Genet.* 2000;66:1259–1272.
31. De Leon Matsuda ML, Liede A, Kwan E, et al. BRCA1 and BRCA2 mutations among breast cancer patients from the Philippines. *Int J Cancer.* 2002;98:596–603.
32. Eccles DM, Englefield P, Soulby MA, et al. BRCA1 mutations in Southern England. *Br J Cancer.* 1998;77:2199–2203.
33. Woodward AM, Davis TA, Silva AG, et al. Large genomic rearrangements of both BRCA2 and BRCA1 are a feature of the inherited breast/ovarian cancer phenotype in selected families. *J Med Genet.* 2005;42:e31.
34. Mazoyer S. Genomic rearrangements in the BRCA1 and BRCA2 genes. *Hum Mutat.* 2005;25:415–422.
35. Hendrickson BC, Judkins T, Ward BD, et al. Prevalence of five previously reported and recurrent BRCA1 genetic rearrangement mutations in 20,000 patients from hereditary breast/ovarian cancer families. *Genes Chromosomes Cancer.* 2005;43:309–313.
36. Evans DG, Bulman M, Young K, et al. Sensitivity for BRCA1/2 mutation testing in 466 breast/ovarian cancer families. *J Med Genet.* 2003;40:e107.
37. Lakhani SR, Reis-Filho JS, Fulford L, et al. Prediction of BRCA1 status in patients with breast cancer using estrogen receptor and basal phenotype. *Clin Cancer Res.* 2005;11:5175–5180.
38. Marroni F, Aretini P, D'Andrea E, et al. Evaluation of widely used models for predicting BRCA1 and BRCA2 mutations. *J Med Genet.* 2004; 41:278–285.

39. E Amir, et al. Evaluation of breast cancer risk assessment packages in the family history evaluation and screening programme. *J Med Genet*. 2003;40:807–814.

40. Http/: www.Myriad.com/prevtables. Accessed October 9, 2009.

41. Metcalfe. Time to reconsider subcutaneous mastectomy for breast cancer prevention? *Lancet Oncol*. 2005;6:431–434.

42. Robson M, Offit K. Clinical practice. Management of an inherited predisposition to breast cancer. *N Engl J Med*. 2007;357:154–162.

43. Li FP, Fraumeni JF. Soft tissue sarcomas, breast cancer and other neoplasms. A familial syndrome? *Ann Intern Med*. 1969;71:747–752.

44. Li FP, Fraumeni JF Jr, Mulvihill JJ, et al. A cancer family syndrome in twenty-four kindreds. *Cancer Res*. 1988;48:5358–5362.

45. Evans DGR, Birch JM, Thorneycroft M, et al. Low rate of TP53 germline mutations in breast cancer/sarcoma families not fulfilling classical criteria for Li-Fraumeni syndrome. *J Med Genet*. 2002;39:941–944.

46. Varley JM McGown G, Thorncroft M, et al. Are there low-penetrance TP53 alleles? Evidence from childhood adrenocortical tumors. *Am J Hum Genet*. 1999;65:995–1006.

47. Nichols KE, Malkin D, Garber JE, et al. Germ-line p53 mutations predispose to a wide spectrum of early-onset cancers. *Cancer Epidemiol Biomarkers Prev*. 2001;10: p. 83–87

48. Chompret A, Brugières L, Ronsin M, et al. P53 germline mutations in childhood cancers and cancer risk for carrier individuals. *Br J Cancer*. 2000;82:1932–1937.

49. Lynch ED, Ostermeyer EA, Lee MK, et al. Inherited mutations in PTEN that are associated with breast cancer, Cowden disease and juvenile polyposis. *Am J Hum Genet*. 1997;61:1254–1260.

50. FitzGerald MG, Marsh DJ, Wahrer D, et al. Germline mutation in PTEN are an infrequent cause of genetic predisposition to breast cancer. *Oncogene*. 1998;17:727–731.

51. Walsh et al. Risk of ovarian cancer in BRCA1 and BRCA2 mutation-negative hereditary breast cancer families. *J Natl Cancer Inst*. 2005;97:1382–1384.

52. Shahedi K, Emanuelsson M, Wiklund F, et al. High risk of contralateral breast carcinoma in women with hereditary/familial non-BRCA1/BRCA2 breast carcinoma. *Cancer.*2006;106:1237–1242.

53. Bernstein JL, Teraoka SN, John EM, et al. The CHEK2*1100delC allelic variant and risk of breast cancer: screening results from the Breast Cancer Family Registry. *Cancer Epidemiol Biomarkers Prev*. 2006;15:348–352.

54. Cybulski C, Górski B, Huzarski T, et al. CHEK2 Is a multiorgan cancer susceptibility gene. *Am J Hum Genet*. 2004;75:1131–1135.

55. Meijers-Heijboer H, van den Ouweland A, Klijn J, et al. Low penetrance susceptibility to breast cancer due to CHEK2*1100delC in noncarriers of BRCA1 or BRCA2 mutations. *Nat Gen*. 2002;31: 55–59.

56. CHEK2 Breast Cancer Case-Control Consortium. CHEK2*1100 delC and susceptibility to breast cancer: a collaborative analysis involving 10,860 breast cancer cases and 9,065 controls from 10 studies. *Am J Hum Genet*. 2004;74:1175–1182.

57. Johnson N, Fletcher O, Naceur-Lombardelli C, et al. Interaction between CHEK2*1100delC and other low-penetrance breast cancer susceptibility genes: a familial study. *Lancet*. 2005;366:1554–1557.

58. Ponder BA, Antoniou A, Dunning A, et al. Polygenic inherited predisposition to breast cancer. *Cold Spring Harb Symp Quant Biol*. 2005;70:35–41.

59. Pharoah PD, Antoniou A, Bobrow M, et al. Polygenic susceptibility to breast cancer and implications for prevention. *Nature Genet*. 2002;31:33–36.

60. Ioannidis JP, Ntzani EE, Trikalinos TA, et al. Replication validity of genetic association studies. *Nature Genet*. 2001;29:306–309.

61. Wedrén S, Rudqvist TR, Granath F, et al. Catechol-O-methyltransferase gene polymorphism and post-menopausal breast cancer risk. *Carcinogenesis*. 2003;24:681–687.

62. Van der Logt EM, Bergevoet SM, Roelofs HM, et al. Genetic polymorphisms in UDP-glucuronosyltransferases and glutathione S-transferases and colorectal cancer risk. *Carcinogenesis*. 2004;25: 2407–2415.

63. Thompson P, Ambrosone C. *Chapter 7:* Molecular epidemiology of genetic polymorphisms in estrogen metabolizing enzymes in human breast ancer. *J Natl Cancer Inst Monog*. 2000;27:125–134.

64. Kristensen V, Børresen-Dale AL. Molecular epidemiology of breast cancer: genetic variation in steroid hormone metabolism. *Mutant Res*. 2000;462:323–323.

65. Listgarten J, Damaraju S, Poulin B. Predictive models for breast cancer susceptibility from multiple single nucleotide polymorphisms. *Clin Cancer Res*. 2004;10:2725–2737.

66. Anderson et al. Estimating age specific breast cancer risks: a descriptive tool to identify age interactions. *Cancer Causes Controls*. 2007; Jan 9 {epub}.

67. Aston CE, Ralph DA, Lalo DP, et al. Oligogenic combinations associated with breast cancer risk. *Hum Genet*. 2005;116:208–221.

68. Ralph D, Zhao LP, Aston CE, et al. Age-specific association of steroid hormone pathway gene polymorphisms with breast cancer risk. *Cancer*. 2007;109:1940–1948.

WEB SITES FOR ADDITIONAL INFORMATION

BRCApro: http://astor.som.jhmi.edu/BayesMendel/brcapro.html

Medicare Criteria for BRCA testing: http://www.cms.hhs.gov/Coverage GenInfo/

National Comprehensive Cancer Network (Breast cancer screening and diagnosis guidelines): http://www. nccn.org

National Institute of Health and Clinical Excellence (familial breast cancer guidelines): http://www.guidance.nice.org.uk/cg41

3

Specialized Nutritional Support for Cancer Patients

Mary K. Russell and Ezra Steiger

Malnutrition is a frequent accompaniment of malignant disease, and when it occurs, prognosis is adversely affected. Consequently, the recognition of malnutrition, its prevention, and its treatment are important considerations in the management of patients with cancer. In this chapter, we consider the pathogenesis of malnutrition in malignant disease (the *cancer-cachexia syndrome*), assessment of nutritional status of cancer patients, the impact of malnutrition on morbidity and mortality, the special techniques available for providing required nutrients for patients in whom oral nutrition has proved inadequate or ineffective, and the applicability of such specialized nutritional support in cancer patients receiving antitumor therapy, including surgery, chemotherapy, and radiation.

PATHOGENESIS OF THE CANCER-CACHEXIA SYNDROME

The malnutrition occurring in patients with malignant disease is associated with a series of physical and biochemical features that constitute the syndrome of *cancer-cachexia*. Forty percent to 80% of patients with cancer develop some degree of clinical malnutrition (1–5). Although anorexia is present in more than half of patients with cancer at diagnosis (6,7), cachexia often precedes a reduction in food intake (8), and affects more than 50% of untreated cancer patients. This syndrome may be responsible for the deaths of 10% to 22% of patients with cancer, with the frequency and severity of malnutrition dependent on tumor type (8,9). The anorexia-cachexia syndrome may be present at time of death in as a many as 80% of cancer patients (10).

The cachexia syndrome is characterized by a mixture of metabolic abnormalities that lead to progressive weight loss as a result of reduced nutrient intake and absorption, accelerated depletion of skeletal muscle and adipose tissue stores (5,8,9), and impaired ability of the host to effectively use provided nutrients, so that weight loss may not respond well even to adequate nutritional intake (11–13). The abnormalities of cancer cachexia, in addition to anorexia, may include early satiety, progressive asthenia, inappropriate increases in energy expenditure, defects in carbohydrate, protein, and lipid metabolism, anemia, and muscle protein loss and atrophy (8,9,11,14,15). These complications result in a greater risk for organ dysfunction and death (5,11,15).

The etiology of the metabolic abnormalities observed in cancer cachexia is poorly understood, although a number of factors are thought to contribute (5,11,14,16,17). These factors, many similar to those seen during the inflammatory processes of injury and sepsis, include the following:

- Altered metabolism of carbohydrate (including increased Cori cycle activity, hepatic gluconeogenesis, glucose turnover, and insulin resistance), lipid (including increased adipose tissue lipolysis, increased hepatic lipogenesis, hyperlipidemia), and protein (tumor-directed proteolysis, increased whole-body protein turnover, decreased muscle amino acid uptake)
- Tumor cell lactate production
- Tumor-induced secretion of host mediators, including various glycoproteins (*proteolysis-inducing factor* and *lipid-mobilizing factor*); proinflammatory cytokines (*interleukin-1*, *interleukin 6*, and *tumor necrosis factor-α*); and neuropeptides (*neuropeptide Y* and *corticotrophin-releasing factor*), which produce a chronic inflammatory state with adverse effects on nutrient metabolism and appetite (3,18,19)
- Altered metabolism of peripheral hormones (such as leptin and ghrelin) and neuropeptides (melanocortin, neuropeptide Y), which regulate appetite
- Altered intestinal secretory metabolism and gastrointestinal tract abnormalities associated with infection
- Learned food aversion
- Nutritional consequences of antitumor therapy (chemotherapy, surgery, radiation)

Although decreased energy and protein intake plays a significant role in the development of cachexia, weight loss and tissue wasting have been observed even in patients with presumably adequate intake for their body weight (5,7). A hypermetabolic state may contribute to this finding in some, but not all, cancer patients. In a study of 200 malnourished patients conducted by Knox and colleagues (20), 41% had normal resting energy expenditure (REE), 33% had decreased REE, and 26% had increased REE. Bosaeus et al. (13) measured REE in 295 adults with advanced solid tumors, primarily colorectal, biliary, pancreatic, and upper gastrointestinal. Hypermetabolism was noted in 48.5% of these patients; 50% of the patients were normometabolic. Patients with a >10% weight loss had a higher REE than did weight-stable patients, but absolute energy intake did not differ between the two groups. The authors postulated a failure of feedback regulation between energy expenditure and dietary intake, contributing to the weight loss (5,13).

It is clear that reduced food intake alone is not responsible for the array of alterations seen in cachexia. Thus, attempts to improve food intake via nutrition and supplementation nutrition (oral, enteral, or parenteral) may not consistently prevent loss of lean body mass (3,8). Weight gain associated with the administration of parenteral nutrition (PN) often may be the result of increased fluid volume and an increase in fat stores, rather than increased protein mass (18,21).

EFFECT OF MALIGNANCY ON NUTRIENT METABOLISM, INTAKE, AND ABSORPTION

Carbohydrate Metabolism

In the presence of cancer cachexia, as opposed to "simple" starvation such as that seen in anorexia nervosa, glucose production via gluconeogenesis is maintained. Ketone bodies are not used preferentially to spare protein catabolism and lean body mass, leading to muscle wasting and early lean body mass depletion (21). In a study of glucose turnover, normal volunteers and patients with early colon cancer were compared with patients with advanced esophageal, stomach, and pancreatic cancer. Basal rates of glucose turnover were significantly higher in the advanced cancer group than in either of the other two groups (22). Glucose infusion only partially suppressed glucose production in the persons with early and advanced cancer; in the healthy volunteers glucose production was suppressed by 94% (22). Early research had suggested that increased Cori cycle activity, with anaerobic glycolysis by tumor cells with release of lactate, might be responsible for the altered glucose metabolism (3,23). A later study, however, suggested that the Cori cycle may play only a small role in altered glucose metabolism (24), but other futile cycles have been identified (3).

Protein Metabolism

In simple starvation, lean body mass is relatively preserved as protein catabolism gradually slows in response to reduced intake (3). In cancer, rates of whole-body protein turnover and the synthesis and catabolism of protein increase with the amount of weight loss and with stage of the disease (25,26). The protein turnover results from increased muscle protein degradation and increased hepatic protein synthesis and is not reversed by administration of PN (3,27). Patients with cancer have reduced lean body muscle mass, with a relatively larger percent of non-muscle lean mass. Currently, research is underway with pentoxifylline and eicosapentaenoic acid, agents that have been shown in animal models to attenuate muscle loss via the ubiquitin-proteasome pathway (28,29).

Lipid Metabolism

Patients with cancer have depleted adipose and lipid stores, likely related to an imbalance between lipolysis and lipogenesis (30). The mechanism for deceased lipogenesis is not well understood. Proposed causes for increased lipolysis include release of lipolytic factors by the tumor, the stress response, and decreased food intake (3).

Changes in Intake and Absorption

Changes in taste and appetite, gastrointestinal symptoms (abdominal fullness, early satiety, intestinal dysmotility, malab-sorption, diarrhea, constipation), and depression are common in cancer patients (31,32). Anorexia and food aversion may be induced or aggravated by intensive chemotherapy. Small bowel bacterial overgrowth (3) and exocrine pancreatic insufficiency (33) may cause malabsorption in patients with strictures or blind loops, and after pancreatic resections, respectively. Fistulas resulting from tumor invasion or from surgery or radiation therapy may also cause malabsorption with significant loss of fluid and electrolytes (3). Protein-losing enteropathies, such as those associated with melanoma or gastric cancer, result in hypoalbuminemia and hypoglobulinemia (3). The component of malnutrition based on these kinds of abnormalities may well respond to specialized nutritional support with enteral or PN (34).

CLINICAL CONSEQUENCES OF THE CANCER-CACHEXIA SYNDROME

The adverse effects of malnutrition in cancer patients include impaired wound healing, compromised immune function, anastomotic leaks, wound dehiscence, endocrine abnormalities, and fluid and electrolyte imbalances (3,4). Weight loss is an independent predictor of response to therapy, quality of life, and decrease in survival (35), and, according to Alexandre et al. (36), malnutrition increases the risk of chemotherapy-induced hematologic toxicities such as neutropenic fever and severe thrombocytopenia. In a Veterans Administration study, malnourished patients who underwent a major operation were at greater risk for postoperative morbidity and mortality than were well-nourished patients (37). In patients with recurrent head and neck cancer, weight loss was found to be a better predictor of mortality than the stage of the disease (38).

PHARMACOLOGIC TREATMENT OF CANCER CACHEXIA

Use of pharmacologic agents, including appetite stimulants, anticytokine agents, anabolic agents, metabolic inhibitors, and anti-inflammatory agents, has been proposed to help manage cancer anorexia and cachexia (5,39). The first-line orexigenic agents are dexamethasone, methylprednisolone, prednisolone, medroxyprogesterone, and megestrol acetate (5,39). Other agents, such as dronabinol, cyproheptadine, thalidomide, and melatonin, may be secondary options if first-line treatment fails. Effects of these agents on appetite are controversial, and some of these compounds have been recommended for investigational use only (5).

According to Mattox (5), the properties of an ideal orexigenic agent include sustained positive effects on appetite, minimal adverse effects, minimal or no negative effects on tumor treatment, positive effects on quality of life, and a positive association between use and maintenance or repletion of body cell mass. Two meta-analyses of megestrol acetate, the progestational agent most frequently investigated as an orexigenic agent in controlled trials of cancer patients, concluded that patients who received megestrol acetate were more than twice as likely as patients who received placebo to gain weight and exhibit improved appetite (40,41). However, several important points should be considered in interpreting these results (5). The patients studied had a variety of malignancies, may or may not have had cancer treatment, tended to be older than 60, and the attrition rate in the studies exceeded 30% to 50% (40,41). The amount of weight gained was often small; some patients gained no weight; and weight gain in some patients was found to be fat rather than lean tissue. The recommended dose of megestrol acetate to maximize benefit and minimize side effects and its cost is unknown; an initial dose of 400 mg/day, with titration to maximum of 800 mg/day has been suggested by several authors (5,40,41).

A randomized controlled trial of fluoxymesterone, dexamethasone, and megestrol acetate found that the latter two agents had similar effect on appetite and weight gain (an average 2 to 2.5 kg over 7 to 9 weeks of treatment) (42). Patients in the fluoxymesterone group gained an average 1.77 kg. Many patients in all groups continued to lose weight even with intervention, and all agents caused toxicities to varying degrees. The authors used cost and toxicity data as the basis for their recommendation to use corticosteroids for short-term (days to weeks) appetite stimulation and megestrol acetate for stimulation over weeks to months (42). Mattox (5), however, states that adverse effects, such as muscle wasting and immunosuppression, outweigh the benefits of corticosteroid use for appetite stimulation, except possibly in terminal patients with poor performance status (5).

Because of inconsistent evidence of positive outcomes in cancer patients, routine use of the dronabinol, a cannabinoid-based compound, as an appetite stimulant in cancer patients is not recommended (39). Cyproheptadine has not been well studied in cancer patients (5), and sedation is a frequent side effect of use. This drug also is not recommended as an appetite stimulant (39). Thalidomide, an immune-modulating agent that has been shown to reduce tumor necrosis factor-α activity, and melatonin, an endogenous hormone that may have antitumor and anti–tumor necrosis factor-α activity, may have positive effects on weight gain in cancer patients, but further study is required (5). Unfortunately, current data suggest that no single agent successfully treats unintentional weight loss in patients with cancer, and expectations for effective pharmacologic management may be unrealistic (5,43).

ASSESSMENT OF NUTRITIONAL STATUS

Screening Tools

Several nutrition assessment tools have been developed specifically for use in patients with cancer (4). They include the following:

- Subjective Global Assessment (SGA) of Detsky et al. (44) from Toronto General Hospital. This method of nutritional assessment is based on specific features of history and physical examination that lead to score of A, *well-nourished*; B, *moderately malnourished*; or C, *severely malnourished*. According to the authors, this clinical method of assessment, after appropriate training, correlates well with assessment protocols employing objective anthropometric measurements and laboratory tests. In addition, the authors reported that with SGA, infections

following gastrointestinal surgery were predicted to a degree that was equal to or better than with objective measurements. Four features in the history are elicited. The first is weight loss in the previous 6 months. Weight loss of <5%, 5% to 10%, or >10% was considered as a "small" loss, "potentially significant" loss, and "definitely significant" loss, respectively. Weight gain in the 2 weeks prior to assessment was interpreted as diminishing the significance of the weight loss. The second feature of the history assesses the patient's dietary intake as normal or abnormal, with attention the severity of reduced intake. The third feature is an assessment of significant gastrointestinal symptoms, including anorexia, vomiting, and diarrhea. The final historical feature is the patient's functional capacity or energy level, ranging from bedridden to full capacity. The five relevant findings on physical examination, rated normal, mild, moderate, or severe, include loss of subcutaneous fat, muscle wasting, ankle edema, sacral edema, and ascites.

- Modified Patient-Generated Subjective Global Assessment of Ottery (45) and colleagues at the Fox Chase Cancer Center. This tool is completed in part by the patient or caregiver (weight history, food intake, symptoms) and in part by the clinician (disease state, metabolic demands, physical findings). A three-level rating similar to that of the SGA is then derived. This method is intended to help diagnose nutritional problems or deficits at baseline or very early in the clinical course (4). In one author's experience, use of this tool has markedly improved the referral of at-risk head and neck cancer patients to the radiation oncology clinic dietitian and anecdotally resulted in reduction of weight loss and better quality of life. A formal study is in progress.
- Oncology Screening Tool from the Memorial Sloan-Kettering Cancer Center (4). This tool is used by a qualified clinician to assess presence of weight loss and physical symptoms associated with poor oral intake. Based on diagnosis, complications, treatment, and weight status, patients are classified as at low or moderate to high risk, and appropriate intervention and follow-up is established.

Other general screening tools for use with individuals with cancer are available in publications from the American Society for Parenteral and Enteral Nutrition (www.nutritioncare.org) and the American Dietetic Association (www.eatright.org).

Assessing Response to Nutrition Therapy

Parameters used to assess the response of a patient with cancer to nutrition therapy include improvements in the one or more of the components of the SGA (e.g., body weight, gastrointestinal symptoms, ability to perform daily activities, muscle wasting, and presence of edema) and improved sense of well-being and quality of life. Serum levels of hepatic transport proteins (e.g., albumin, prealbumin, transferrin), also known as *negative acute-phase proteins*, will remain depressed as long as a significant inflammatory process continues. Levels of these proteins are most useful as prognostic indicators for morbidity and mortality, and prealbumin and transferrin may be of value in following nutrition support of the nonseptic, stable patient.

NUTRITIONAL SUPPORT

Oral Nutrition

When anatomically and physiologically feasible, the oral route is the preferable method of providing all required nutrients. The registered dietitian is extremely helpful in achieving this goal by designing oral diets that take into account specific problems encountered in cancer patients, such as taste fatigue, altered perceptions of sweetness, lactase deficiency, stomatitis, gastrointestinal intolerance of various food stuffs, and early satiety. Although oral intake is the most acceptable method of feeding to cancer patients and to their family members, the disease and its treatment may limit a patient's ability to consume a "regular" diet. Regimens with the fewest number of dietary modifications are most likely to be acceptable to the patient. Restrictions in sodium, fat, fluid, and carbohydrate content of the diet and texture modifications should be made judiciously and only if absolutely necessary. Patients and families must understand that dietary restrictions once deemed immutable, such as low cholesterol, have little or no place when the diagnosis of most concern is cancer (4). Small, frequent feedings of calorically dense foods, altered in texture and temperature as needed depending on the nutritional issues addressed, are accepted best. Imagination and individual tailoring of food to the patient's needs can positively affect intake and potentially avoid the need for more complex methods of nutritional support (4). Unfortunately, many acute care facilities adhere to rigorous meal schedules that do not easily allow patients to eat what they desire when they feel hungry. The "room service" method of food service, while expensive in terms of labor and food cost, can appreciably affect patient satisfaction with food, and potentially result in greater intake. Oral supplements are available in a variety of caloric densities and flavors. Many are both lactose-free and ready to serve. Others must be mixed, often with milk, prior to consumption. Taste fatigue, altered perceptions of sweetness, lactase deficiency, gastrointestinal intolerance, and early satiety may interfere with patient acceptance. Thus, it is vital to frequently monitor the patient's acceptance of any supplement.

Enteral and Parenteral Nutrition

If oral nutrition is inadequate in volume or composition to meet nutritional needs, or is contraindicated as a consequence of the disease or its treatment, specialized nutritional support with enteral nutrition or PN may be indicated. Such therapy should be directed to a specific measure or outcome, such as increase in body weight, meeting specific nutrient requirements, or improving the outcome of a surgical procedure (4). The decision to prescribe enteral nutrition or PN in patients depends on several factors, including the functional status of the gastrointestinal tract, the type and location of the tumor, the extent and duration of therapy, the availability of antitumor therapy, and the wishes of the patient and family.

Rationale for Specialized Nutritional Intervention in Patients with Cancer

With the development of safe parenterally administered nutrient solutions and, subsequently, enteral feeding products, innumerable clinical trials employing specialized interventions, parenteral or enteral nutrition, have been conducted in patients with malignant disease to answer the following questions:

1. Can specialized nutritional intervention allow patients to receive aggressive antitumor therapy when the inherent toxicity of such therapy would otherwise preclude treatment because of severe malnutrition?
2. Can specialized nutritional intervention reduce the morbidity of antitumor therapy that may be aggravated by malnutrition?
3. Can specialized nutritional intervention improve tumor response to specific cancer treatment independent of the pretreatment nutritional status?
4. Can specialized nutritional intervention improve quality of life sufficiently to ethically justify its use in patients with end-stage disease no longer amenable to specific antitumor therapy?

Parenteral and Enteral Nutrition as an Adjunct to Surgery

Many studies have been conducted to assess the benefit of parenteral and enteral nutrition in patients undergoing oncologic surgery (46). Smale and associates (47) analyzed the postoperative course of a series of patients who had undergone a major intra-abdominal, intrathoracic, or head and neck operation for palliation or cure of malignancy after receiving 6 or more days of total PN providing over 35 kcal/kg/day. The preoperative PN did not alter morbidity or mortality in the patients deemed well nourished. In contrast, however, among the poorly nourished patients, the preoperative nutritional support was associated with a 2.1-fold reduction in all postoperative complications ($p < 0.001$), a 2.9-fold reduction in major sepsis ($p < 0.005$), and a 2.7-fold reduction in mortality ($p < 0.025$). Brennan et al. (48) randomized patients undergoing resection for pancreatic cancer *regardless of their nutritional status* to either a postoperative regimen of adjuvant PN or routine dextrose-salt intravenous fluid. They found no benefit to the routine use of postoperative PN, and, in fact, noted that patients who received PN had a significant increase in postoperative infectious complications. Assessing the worth of PN in this study is confounded because malnutrition was not an eligibility criterion. In fact, the mean preoperative body weight loss in the total parenteral (TPN) group was only 5.8% and the mean albumin level was 3.1 g/dL.

The principle that perioperative PN should be restricted to patients with significant malnutrition is further supported by the findings of the Veterans Affairs Total Parenteral Nutrition Cooperative Study Group (37). In this trial 395 malnourished patients who required laparotomy or noncardiac thoracotomy, many for gastrointestinal or lung cancer, were randomly assigned to receive either PN for 7 to 15 days before surgery and 3 days afterward (the PN group) or no perioperative PN (the control group). The patients were monitored for complications for 90 days after surgery. The rates of major complications during the first 30 days after surgery in the two groups were similar (PN group, 25.5%; control group, 24.6%), as were the overall 90-day mortality rates (13.4% and 10.5%, respectively). There were more infectious complications in the PN group than in the controls (14.1% vs. 6.4%; $p = 0.01$; relative risk, 2.20; 95% confidence interval, 1.19–4.05), but slightly more noninfectious complications in the control group (16.7% vs. 22.2%; $p = 0.20$; relative risk, 0.75; 95% confidence interval, 0.50–1.13). The increased rate of infections was confined to patients categorized as either borderline or mildly malnourished, according to SGA or an objective nutritional assessment, and these patients had no demonstrable benefit from PN. In contrast, severely malnourished patients who received PN had significantly fewer noninfectious complications than controls (5% vs. 43%; $p = 0.03$; relative risk, 0.12; 95% confidence interval, 0.02–0.91), with no concomitant increase in infectious complications. The authors concluded that the use of preoperative PN should be limited to patients who are severely malnourished unless there are other specific indications.

More recently, 13 randomized trials that had been conducted to assess the value of perioperative TPN were reviewed at a conference sponsored by the National Institutes of Health, American Society for Parenteral and Enteral Nutrition, and the American Society of Clinical Nutrition (49). In a consensus statement published in 1997, the following conclusions were reached:

1. PN given to malnourished patients with gastrointestinal cancer for 7 to 10 days before surgery decreases postoperative complications by approximately 10%.
2. Routine use of postoperative PN in malnourished general surgical patients who do not receive preoperative PN increases postoperative complications by approximately 10%.
3. To avoid the adverse effects of starvation because of inability to eat for a prolonged period postoperatively, PN should be considered 5 to 10 days after operation for patients still unable to eat or tolerate enteral feedings.

In the absence of specific contraindications, such as short bowel syndrome, intestinal obstruction, and gastrointestinal intolerance, enteral nutrition appears to be well tolerated by patients with a variety of cancers. Several reports indicate that among surgical patients with tumors affecting the alimentary tract, early postoperative enteral feedings, prior to the anticipated resumption of an adequate oral diet, is associated with decreased cost, decreased length of hospital stay, reduction in infectious and wound complications, improvement in weight, and decreased treatment interruptions (50–52). In a randomized study of early postoperative enteral nutrition conducted by Farreras and associates (53), 66 patients undergoing operation for gastric cancer were fed within 12 to 18 hours of surgery with an "immune-supplemented" formula containing arginine, omega-3 fatty acids, and RNA, or an isocaloric isonitrogenous control diet. Patients who received the specialized formula had significantly fewer wound healing complications (0% vs. 26.7%; $p = 0.005$).

In contrast, several studies fail to confirm any benefit associated with routine postoperative enteral feedings, including immune-supplemented preparations, compared with standard intravenous hydration (54–57). In fact, Watters and associates (57) observed an impairment of respiratory mechanics among a series of well-nourished patients receiving postoperative enteral feedings.

Significant salutary effects, however, have been reported in trials studying perioperative enteral nutrition limited to patients with significant malnutrition. Braga and colleagues (58) conducted a prospective randomized controlled trial of perioperative enteral nutrition in which 196 patients malnourished patients (weight loss $\geq$10%) who were candidates for major elective surgery for malignancy of the gastrointestinal tract were assigned to one of three groups; Group 1, the control group, received postoperative feedings with a standard oral liquid diet within 12 hours of surgery. Group 2, the preoperative group, received 1 L/day for 7 days of an oral liquid diet enriched with arginine, omega-3 fatty acids, and RNA ("immunonutrition"). Postoperatively, patients in this group received the standard oral liquid diet. Group 3, the perioperative group, received the enriched diet preoperatively and postoperatively. Results showed that the total number of patients with complications overall was 24 in the control group, 14 in the preoperative group, and 9 in the perioperative group ($p = 0.02$, control group vs. perioperative group). However, the incidence of infection was not significantly different among the three groups. Postoperative length of stay was significantly shorter in the preoperative (13.2 days) and perioperative (12.0 days) groups than in the control group (15.3 days) ($p = .01$ and $p = .001$, respectively, vs. the control group). The authors concluded that perioperative immunonutrition seems to be the best approach to support malnourished patients with cancer.

In contrast to patients in whom early postoperative resumption of oral intake is anticipated within 7 to 14 days and for whom the benefits of enteral or parenteral feedings are uncertain, patients with treatable tumors or with conditions secondary to aggressive antitumor therapy that preclude oral intake for prolonged periods or indefinitely, should receive some form of specialized nutritional support (59,60).

Parenteral and Enteral Nutrition as an Adjunct to Chemotherapy and Radiotherapy

PN for patients receiving chemotherapy with or without radiation can result in increased body weight and fat mass, improved hydration, and correction of vitamin and mineral deficiencies (3). However, the primary concerns for clinicians include the effect of PN on morbidity and mortality, the ability of PN to improve nutritional status sufficiently to allow more intense antineoplastic therapy, and any adjuvant impact of PN on the efficacy of the antitumor treatment (3). Klein et al. (61) pooled data from 28 prospective, randomized, controlled clinical trials evaluating the use of TPN in cancer patients No statistically significant benefit could be demonstrated in survival, treatment tolerance, treatment toxicity, or tumor response in patents receiving chemotherapy or radiotherapy. Moreover, in their analysis of the data, McGeer and associates (62) concluded that PN was associated with higher infection rates, decreased overall survival, and poorer tumor responses in patients receiving chemotherapy. However, the applicability of these conclusions in determining the indications for PN in malnourished patients requiring chemotherapy or radiotherapy is uncertain because many of the original investigations were of poor quality and often excluded the key population of interest, the severely malnourished patient unable to tolerate oral or enteral feedings. In fact, most of the patients in the published series were not severely malnourished and were able to tolerate oral or tube feedings (60,63,64).

Consequently, current guidelines published by the American Society of Parenteral and Enteral Nutrition again call for the administration of PN to this group of malnourished cancer patients who are receiving active treatment and have conditions that have precluded or are expected to preclude enteral intake for 7 to 14 days (59,60).

Enteral nutrition is a particularly useful adjunct in patients with malignancies of the head and neck requiring radiotherapy alone or combined with surgery and chemotherapy. Approximately 40% of these patients present with weight loss because of their cancer, and their nutritional reserve can be further compromised as the result of treatment. Thus, taste changes, xerostomia, mucositis, odynophagia, dysphagia, and anorexia are to be expected, and all are conditions that can limit oral intake during treatment and even for prolonged periods after treatment is completed (65). Enteral nutrition using a feeding tube, such as a percutaneous endoscopic gastrostomy tube, inserted prophylactically prior to the commencement of radiotherapy has been associated with decreased weight loss, reduced number of hospitalizations for mucositis and dehydration, a reduced rate of treatment interruptions, and a higher rate of compliance with and completion of therapy (52,60,65–67).

Specialized Nutritional Support in Patients with Advanced Cancer

The indications for parenteral or enteral nutrition are controversial in patients unable to eat and who have advanced malignant disease for which there is no remaining specific antitumor treatment available. The decision to treat or withhold nutrition therapy sometimes raises difficult moral, ethical, and even legal issues (46). In most patients with widely metastatic disease and a poor prognosis, nutritional support offers limited benefit (3). A study of terminally ill cancer patients in a long-term care facility suggested that most patients experienced neither hunger nor thirst, and when it occurred, a small amount of food alleviated the symptoms (68).

Hoda et al. (69) reviewed the records of 52 patients with incurable cancer who received TPN at home. Median survival was 5 months from the initiation of PN; however, 16 patients survived >1 year with little PN-related morbidity. Thus, these authors and others (70–73) have suggested that palliative specialized nutritional support occasionally is indicated in a small subset of terminally ill patients in whom it may be possible to improve nutritional status, increase survival, or improve quality of life. Such nutritional support is generally restricted to those with a predicted survival exceeding 3 months, those with a good performance status, such as a Karnofsky score >50, and those with relatively indolent disease progression. Candidates may also include those with an inoperable malignant bowel obstruction or those with minimal symptoms from disease involving major organs, such as the brain, liver, or lungs (60,74–76). Other relevant issues bearing on the decision to treat have been discussed by Glick (77) and Fuhrman and Hermann (73). Glick (77) discusses the use of advanced health care directives regarding artificial nutrition and hydration, and stresses the need to assure that the patient and his or her family understand the intricacies of the treatment, especially if it is to be administered at home. The decision to provide nutritional support also must take into consideration the realistic therapeutic goals, the patient's perception of the benefits compared to the burdens of the therapy, and what constitutes quality of life (73).

Nutritional Support and Tumor Growth

Accelerated tumor growth induced by provision of energy and essential nutrients, as well as the influence of hormones and growth factors that may be stimulated in response to nutritional support, is a theoretical consideration that, if demonstrated, could well have important clinical implications. In fact, experimental studies in tumor-bearing animals indicate that nutritional repletion with PN increases tumor growth, often out of proportion to the nutritional benefit to the host (3,46). Despite these findings in animal tumor models, no clinically significant tumor growth has been documented in human cancer patients receiving nutritional support (3,46).

Refeeding Syndrome

The rapid induction of the anabolic state in severely malnourished, cachectic patients using standard nutrient solutions has been associated with a variety of adverse effects constituting the "refeeding syndrome" (46,78–85). Cardiac decompensation, the most serious feature of the refeeding syndrome, may be due to overhydration and salt retention in the face of starvation-induced low cardiac reserve. Hypophosphatemia consequent to rapid refeeding is another important contributing factor to cardiac failure as well as to acute respiratory failure. Rapid nutritional repletion also is implicated in deficits of the other major intracellular ions, magnesium, and potassium, as well as acute deficiencies of vitamin A, thiamine, and zinc (46).

To avoid manifestations of the refeeding syndrome in severely malnourished patients, nutritional support should be introduced very gradually, providing approximately only 25% to 50% of the calculated energy goal on the first day with graded increases over the next 3 to 5 days (79–81). Serum electrolyte levels (particularly phosphorus, potassium, and magnesium) should be measured and corrected to normal before nutritional support is begun (79) and closely monitored thereafter as caloric intake is increased. Fluid and sodium may need to be restricted initially to avoid cardiac decompensation (82). Weight gain exceeding 1 kg/week would likely be attributable to fluid retention and should be avoided (82). Supplemental vitamins, especially thiamine, also may be advisable (46).

SUMMARY AND CURRENT RECOMMENDATIONS

Although specialized nutritional support does not directly contribute to the effectiveness of antitumor therapy and, therefore, should not be *routinely* prescribed, its use as an important supportive adjunctive modality has substantial benefits under a variety of specific circumstances. Malnourished patients requiring surgery experience a reduction in postoperative morbidity if they receive a period of preoperative nutritional repletion, usually with PN. Nutritional support is also recommended for other patients receiving active cancer therapy when conditions resulting from the disease or the therapy itself have prevented, or by clinical experience is expected to prevent, adequate oral consumption for periods exceeding 7 to 14 days. Occasionally, patients with advanced cancer who are no longer candidates for antitumor therapy and who unable to eat experience an improvement in well-being and even a modest increase in survival when nutritional supplements are provided by feeding tube or by vein, preferably in the home setting. Candidates for such support are generally those with relatively indolent disease, a good performance status, and anticipated survival of at least 3 months.

REFERENCES

1. Kern KA, Norton JA. Cancer cachexia. *J Parenter Enteral Nutr.* 1988;12:286–298.
2. Ollenschlager G, Veill B, Thomas W, et al. Tumor anorexia: causes, assessment, treatment. *Recent Results Cancer Res* 1991;121:249–259.
3. Schattner M, Shike M. Nutrition support of the patient with cancer. In: Shils ME, Shike M, et al., eds. *Modern Nutrition in Health and Disease.* 10th ed. Baltimore: Lippincott Williams & Wilkins; 2006:1290–1313.
4. Bloch AS. Cancer. In: Matarese LE, Gottschlich MM, eds. *Contemporary Nutrition Support Practice: A Clinical Guide.* 2nd ed. Philadelphia: WB Saunders Company; 2003:484–508.
5. Mattox TW. Treatment of unintentional weight loss in patients with cancer. *Nutr Clin Prac.* 2005;12:400–410.
6. Lorite MJ, Cariuk P, Tisdale MJ. Induction of muscle protein degradation by a tumour factor. *Br J Cancer.* 1997;76:1035–1040.
7. Costa G. Weight loss and cachexia in lung cancer. *Nutr Cancer.* 1980;2:98–103.
8. Delano M, Moldawer L. The origins of cachexia in acute and chronic inflammatory diseases. *Nutr Clin Prac.* 2006;21:68–81.
9. Warren S. The immediate cause of death in cancer. *Am J Med Sci.* 1932;184:610–613.
10. Nelson KA. The cancer anorexia-cachexia syndrome. *Semon Oncol.* 2000;27:64–68.
11. Palesty JA, Dudrick SJ. What we have learned about cachexia in gastrointestinal cancer. *Dig Dis.* 2003;21:198–213.
12. Bosaeus I, Daneryd P, Svanberg E, et al. Dietary intake and resting energy expenditure in relation to weight loss in unselected cancer patients. *Int J Cancer.* 2001;93:380–383.
13. Bosaeus I, Daneryd P, Lundholhm K. Dietary intake, resting energy expenditure, weight loss and survival in cancer patients. *J Nutr.* 2002;132(Suppl 11):3465S–3466S.
14. Argiles JM, Alvare B, Lopez-Soriano FJ. The metabolic basis of cancer cachexia. *Med Res Rev.* 1997;17:477–498.
15. Dahele M, Fearon KHC. Research methodology: cancer cachexia syndrome. *Palliat Med.* 2004;18:409–417.
16. Douglas RC, Shaw JHF. Metabolic effects of cancer. *Br J Surg.* 1009;77:246–254.
17. Tisdale MJ. Cancer cachexia: metabolic alterations and clinical manifestations. *Nutrition.* 1997;13:1–7.
18. Ramos EJB, Suzuki S, Marks D, et al. Cancer anorexia-cachexia syndrome: cytokines and neuropeptides. *Curr Opin Clin Nutr Metab Care.* 2004;7:427–434.
19. Tisdale MJ. Pathogenesis of cancer cachexia. *J Support Oncol.* 2003;1:159–168.
20. Knox LS, Crosby LO, Feurer ID, et al. Energy expenditure in malnourished cancer patients. *Ann Surg.* 1983;197:152–162.
21. Evans WK, Makuch R, Clamon GH, et al. Limited impact of PN on nutritional status during treatment for small cell lung cancer. *Cancer Res.* 1985;45:3347–3353.
22. Shaw JH, Wolfe RR. Glucose and urea kinetics in patients with early and advanced gastrointestinal cancer: the response to glucose infusion, parenteral feeding, and surgical resection. *Surgery.* 1987;101:181–191.
23. Holruyde CP, Gabuxda TG, Putnam RC, et al. Altered glucose metabolism in metastatic carcinoma. *Cancer Res.* 1975;35:3710–3714.
24. Cersosimo E, Pisters PW, Pesola G, et al. The effect of graded doses of insulin on peripheral glucose uptake and lactate release in cancer cachexia. *Surgery.* 1991;109:450–467.
25. Eden E, Ekman L, Bennegard K, et al. Whole-body tyrosine flux in relation to energy expenditure in weight-losing cancer patients. *Metabolism.* 1984;33:1020–1027.
26. Smith KL, Tisdale MJ. Mechanism of muscle protein degradation in cancer cachexia. *Br J Cancer.* 1993;68:314–318.
27. Norton JA, Stien TP, Brennan MF. Whole body protein synthesis and turnover in normal man and malnourished patients with and without known cancer. *Ann Surg.* 1981;194:123–128.
28. Combaret L, Ralliere C, Taillandier D, et al. Manipulation of the ubiquitin-proteasome pathway in cachexia: pentoxifylline suppresses the activation of 20S and 26S proteasomes in muscles from tumor-bearing rats. *Mol Biol Rep.* 1999;1–2:95–101.
29. Whitehouse AS, Smith HJ, Drake JL, et al. Mechanism of attenuation of skeletal muscle protein catabolism in cancer cachexia by eicosapentaenoic acid. *Cancer Res.* 2001;61:3604–3609.
30. Nitenberg G, Raynard B. Nutritional support of the cancer patient: issues and dilemmas. *Crit Rev Oncol Hematol.* 2000;34:137–168.
31. Grosvenor M, Bulcavage L, Chlebowski RT. Symptoms potentially influencing weight loss in a cancer population: correlations with primary site, nutritional status, and chemotherapy administration. *Cancer.* 1989;63:330–334.
32. Komurcu S, Nelson KA, Walsh D, et al. Gastrointestinal symptoms among inpatients with advanced cancer. *Am J Hosp Palliat Care.* 2002;19:351–355.
33. Gnaneh P, Neoptolemos JB. Exocrine pancreatic function following pancreatectomy. *Ann NY Acad Sci.* 1999;880:308–318.
34. Makhdoom ZA, Komar MJ, Still CD. Nutrition and enterocutaneous fistulas. *J Clin Gastrolenterol.* 2000;31:195–204.
35. Persson C, Gilmelius B. The relevance of weight loss for survival and quality of life in patients with advanced gastrointestinal cancer treated with palliative chemotherapy. *Anticancer Res.* 2002;22:3661–3668.
36. Alexandre J, Gross-Goupil M, Falissard B, et al. Evaluation of the nutritional and inflammatory status in cancer patients for the risk assessment of severe haematological toxicity following chemotherapy. *Ann Oncol.* 2003;14:36–41.
37. The Veterans Affairs Total Parenteral Nutrition Cooperative Study Group. Peroperative total parenteral nutrition in surgical patients. *N Engl J Med.* 1991;325:525–532.
38. Nguyen TV, Yueh B. Weight loss predicts mortality after recurrent oral cavity and oropharyngeal carcinomas. *Cancer.* 2002;95:553–562.
39. Desport JC, Gory-Delabaere G, Blanc-Vincent MP, et al. Standards, options, and recommendations for the use of appetite stimulants in oncology (2000). *Br J Cancer* 2003;89(Suppl 1):S98–S100.
40. Maltoni M, Nanni O, Scarpi E, et al. High-dose progestins form the treatment of cancer anorexia-cachexia syndrome: a systematic review of randomized clinical trials. *Ann Oncol.* 2001;12:289–300.
41. Lopez AP, Roque I, Figuls M, et al. Systematic review of megastrol acetate in the treatment of anorexia-cachexia syndrome. *J Pain Symptom Manage.* 2004;27:360–369.
42. Loprinzi CL, Kugler SJ, Sloan JA, et al. Randomized comparison of megestrol acetate versus dexamethasome versus fluoxymesterone

for the treatment of cancer anorexia/cachexia. *J Clin Oncol.* 1999;17: 3299–3306.

43. Mattox TW. Intravenous hyperalimentation and cancer: a historical perspective. *Nutr Clin Prac.* 2002;17:249–252.

44. Detsky AS, McLaughlin JR, Baker JP, et al. What is subjective global assessment of nutritional status? *JPEN J Parenter Enteral Nutr.* 1987;11:8–13.

45. Ottery FD. Cancer cachexia prevention, early diagnosis, and practice. *Cancer Pract.* 1994;2:123–131.

46. Silberman H. Nutrition therapy: clinical applications: cancer. In: Silberman H, ed. *Parenteral and Enteral Nutrition.* 2nd ed. Norwalk, CT: Appleton and Lange; 1989:395–407.

47. Smale BF, Mullen JE, Buzby GP, et al. The efficacy of nutritional assessment and support in cancer surgery. *Cancer.* 1981;47: 2375–2381.

48. Brennan MF, Pisters PWT, Posner M, et al. A prospective randomized trial of total parenteral nutrition after major pancreatic resection for malignancy. *Ann Surg.* 1994;220:436–441.

49. Klein S, Kinney J, Jeejeebhoy MB, et al. Nutrition support in clinical practice: review of published data and recommendations for future research directions. *JPEN J Parenter Enteral Nutr.* 1997;21:133–150.

50. Braga M, Gianotti L, Gentilimi O, et al. Feeding the gut early after digestive surgery: results of a nine-year experience. *Clin Nutr.* 2002;21:59–65.

51. Daly JM, Weintraub FN, Shou J, et al. Enteral nutrition during multimodal therapy in upper gastrointestinal tract cancer patients. *Ann Surg.* 1995;221:327–338.

52. Beer K, Krause K, Zuercher T, et al. Early percutaneous endoscopic gastrostomy insertion maintains nutritional state in patients with aerodigestive tract cancer. *Nutr Cancer.* 2005;52:29–34.

53. Farreras N, Artigas V, Cardona D, et al. Effect of early postoperative enteral nutrition on wound healing in patients undergoing surgery for gastric cancer. *Clin Nutr.* 2005;24:55–65.

54. Heslin MJ, Latkany L, Leung D, et al. A prospective, randomized trial of early enteral feeding after resection of upper gastrointestinal malignancy. *Ann Surg.* 1997;227:567–577.

55. Page RD, Oo AY, Russell GN, et al. Intravenous hydration versus naso-jejunal enteral feeding after esophagectomy: a randomised study. *Eur J Cardiothoraic Surg.* 2002;22:666–672.

56. Lobo DN, Williams RN, Welch NT, et al. Early postoperative jejunostomy feeding with an immune modulating diet in patients undergoing resectional surgery for upper gastointestinal cancer: a prospective, randomized, controlled, double-blind study. *Clin Nutr.* 2006;25: 716–726.

57. Watters JM, Kirkpatrick SM, Norris SB, et al. Immediate postoperative enteral feeding results in impaired respiratory mechanics and decreased mobility. *Ann Surg.* 1997;226: 369–377.

58. Braga M, Gianotti L, Nespoli L, et al. Nutritional approach in malnourished surgical patients. *Arch Surg.* 2002;137:174–180.

59. A.S.P.E.N. Board of Directors and the Clinical Guidelines Task Force. Guidelines for use of parenteral and enteral nutrition in adult and pediatric patients. *JPEN J Parenter Enteral Nutr.* 2002;26:1SA–138SA.

60. Roberts S, Mattox T. Cancer. In: Gottschlich MM, ed. *The A.S.P.E.N. Nutrition Support Core Curriculum: A Case- Based Approach—The Adult Patient.* Silver Spring, MD: The American Society for Parenteral and Enteral Nutrition; 2007:649–675.

61. Klein S, Simes J, Blackburn GL. Total parenteral nutrition and cancer clinical trials. *Cancer.* 1986;58: 1378–1386.

62. McGeer AJ, Detsky AS, O'Rourke KD. Parenteral nutrition in cancer patients undergoing chemotherapy: a meta-analysis. *Nutrition.* 1990;6:233–240.

63. Zaloga G. Parenteral nutrition in adults with functioning gastrointestinal tracts: assessment of outcomes. *Lancet.* 2006;367:1101–1111.

64. American College of Physicians. Parenteral nutrition in patients receiving cancer chemotherapy. *Ann Intern Med.* 1989;110:734–736.

65. Scolapio JS, Spangler PR, Romano MM. Prophylactic placement of gastrostomy feeding tubes before radiotherapy in patients with head and neck cancer: Is it worthwhile? *J Clin Gastroenterol.* 2001;33: 215–217.

66. Bahl M, Siu LL, Pond GR, et al. Tolerability of the Intergroup 0099 (INT 0099) regimen in locally advanced nasopharyngeal cancer with a focus on patients' nutritional status. *Int J Radiation Oncology Biol Phys.* 2004;60: 1127–1136.

67. Raykher A, Russo L, Schattner M, et al. Enteral nutrition support of head and neck cancer patients. *Nutr Clin Prac.* 2007;22: 68–73.

68. McCann RM, Hall WJ, Groth-Junker A. Comfort care for terminally ill patients. The appropriate use of nutrition and hydration. *JAMA.* 1994;272:1263–1266.

69. Hoda D, Jatol A, Lopinzi C, et al. Should patients with advanced, incurable cancers ever be sent home with total parenteral nutrition? A single insititution's 20-year experience. *Cancer.* 2005;103:863–868.

70. August DA, Thorn D, Fischer RL, et al. Home parenteral nutrition for patients with inoperable malignant bowel obstruction. *JPEN J Parenter Enteral Nutr.* 1991;15:323–327.

71. Ripamonti C, Twycross R, Baines M, et al. Clinical practice recommendations for the management of bowel obstruction in patients with end stage cancer. *Support Care Cancer.* 2001;9:223–233.

72. Whitworth MK, Whitfield A, Holm S, et al. Doctor, does this mean I'm going to starve to death? *J Clin Oncol.* 2004;22:199–201.

73. Fuhrman MP, Hermann VM. Bridging the continuum: nutrition support in palliative and hospice care. *Nutr Clin Prac.* 2006;21:134–141.

74. Bachmann P, Marti-Massoud C, Blanc-Vincent MP, et al. Summary version of the standards, options and recommendations for palliative or terminal nutrition in adults with progressive cancer (2001). *Br J Cancer.* 2003;89(Suppl 1):S107–S110.

75. Mirhosseini N, Faisinger RI, Baracos V. Parenteral nutrition in advanced cancer : indications and clinical prctice guidelines. *J Palliative Med.* 2005;8:914–918.

76. Bozzetti F, Cozzaglio E, Biganzoli E, et al. Quality of life and length of survival in advanced cancer patients on home parenteral nutrition. *Clin Nutr.* 2002;21:281–288.

77. Glick MR. The use of advance care planning to guide decisions about artificial nutrition and hydration. *Nutr Clin Prac.* 2006;21:126–133.

78. Weinsier RL, Krumdieck CL. Death resulting from overzealous total parenteral nutrition: the refeeding syndrome revisited. *Am J Clin Nutr.* 1980;34:393–399.

79. Kraft MD, Btaiche IF, Sacks GS. Review of the refeeding syndrome. *Nutr Clin Prac.* 2005;20:625–633.

80. Solomon SM, Kirby DF. The refeeding syndrome: a review. *JPEN J Parenter Enteral Nutr.* 1990;14:90–97.

81. Brooks MJ, Melnik G. The refeeding syndrome: an approach to understanding its complications. *Pharmacotherapy.* 1995;15:713–726.

82. Apovian CM, McMahon MM, Bistrian BR. Guidelines for refeeding the marasmic patient. *Crit Care Med.* 1990;18:1030–1033.

83. Klein CJ, Stanek GS, Wiles CE. Overfeeding macronutrients to critically ill adults: metabolic complications. *J Am Diet Assoc.* 1998;98:795–806.

84. Crook MA, Hally V, Panteli JV. The importance of the refeeding syndrome. *Nutrition.* 2001;17:632–637.

85. Flesher M, Archer K, Leslie B, et al. Assessing the metabolic and clinical consequences of early enteral feeding in the malnourished patient. *JPEN J Parenter Enteral Nutr.* 2005;29:108–117.

COMMENTARY
Stanley J. Dudrick and J. Alexander Palesty

Having been asked by Dr. Howard Silberman to contribute this commentary to the outstanding textbook that he and his brother, Dr. Allan Silberman, have conceived and edited, the senior author of this commentary is most honored, privileged, and delighted to accept the gracious invitation for several reasons. Foremost, is the opportunity to participate in the production of the second edition of this useful and unique educational volume by a distinguished surgeon, investigator, and educator, whose continuous and cherished friendship dates back to our association during residency training in surgery at the Hospital of the University of Pennsylvania more than 40 years ago. Additionally, but no less exciting and gratifying, is the opportunity to learn from, add to, modulate, and emphasize the knowledge, experience, wisdom, and philosophy of Dr. Ezra Steiger (who was in the same intern group as Dr. Silberman), who was my first surgical intern when I was Chief of Surgery of the University of Pennsylvania Service at the Veterans Administration Hospital in Philadelphia; who was an invaluable, dedicated, indefatigable, and innovative member of our nutritional and metabolic research team in the Harrison Department of Surgical Research at the University of Pennsylvania; who inserted a subclavian vein feeding catheter into my seriously ill father and supervised his total parenteral nutrition therapy perfectly in the days of its clinical infancy; who has subsequently had a distinguished career in surgical nutrition and metabolism; and who has also been a most cherished and treasured collaborator, advocate, and friend throughout our more than 40-year association with each other. Additionally, it is an especially gratifying bit of luck to be able to work together on this commentary with a highly esteemed and treasured former outstanding student and surgical resident, and currently a most valued colleague and coworker continuously for more than 12 years, Dr. J. Alexander Palesty, Chief of Surgical Oncology and Assistant Program Director in Surgery at Saint Mary's Hospital in Waterbury, and Assistant Professor of Surgery at the University of Connecticut School of Medicine. Finally, it is always a pleasurable and satisfying experience to participate in a relevant and significant endeavor with relatively newly acquired, able, accomplished, and eminent collaborators such as Dr. Allan Silberman and Mary K. Russell in this important undertaking.

No data have been published in the literature to document that the successful and/or optimal treatment of any pathophysiologic process can more likely be achieved in a malnourished patient than in a comparable, well-nourished patient with the same condition and collateral factors. Russell and Steiger emphasize that malnutrition is a frequent accompaniment of malignant disease; that when it occurs, prognosis is adversely affected; and consequently, that the recognition of malnutrition, its prevention, and its treatment are important considerations in the management of patients with cancer. Accordingly, if a patient is expected to respond optimally to one or more forms of oncologic therapy, the patient should simultaneously be in the best possible nutritional and metabolic condition to withstand the rigors and challenges of both the therapy and the disease. Nutrient substrates are required by the human body in sufficient quality and quantity, not only to satisfy basal metabolic requirements, but to support a state of nutritional equilibrium and positive nitrogen balance under a wide variety of conditions associated with catabolism. Furthermore, nutrient requirements have been shown to be significantly increased by major trauma, major burns, sepsis, various metabolic disorders, in addition to many forms and stages of malignant diseases.

Often, when the initial diagnosis of a malignancy is made, patients are adequately nourished. However, the various forms of effective antineoplastic therapy commonly result in severe associated nutritional defects, including weight loss, protein malnutrition, weakness, and inanition. On the other hand, in patients with specific malignant disorders such as leukemia, lymphoma, and oat cell carcinoma of the lung, significant loss of body mass can be the initial clinical sign of the problem. In such patients, tumor burden or bulk can achieve rather large proportions before symptoms and other signs become manifest, and the weight loss may in part reflect the increased nutritional and metabolic demands imposed on the host by the progressive tumor growth. Conversely, breast cancer, melanoma, most soft-tissue sarcomas, and the majority of gastrointestinal neoplasms produce relatively early signs and symptoms, including bleeding or a palpable mass, even while the tumor mass is relatively small and before any weight loss secondary to the increased metabolic demands imposed by the tumor can be identified or appreciated. Additionally, some specific neoplasms of the alimentary tract, especially those of the oropharynx and esophagus, compound the weight loss induced by the increased tumor cell metabolism by causing voluntarily reduced oral intake secondary to dysphagia or luminal mass obstruction. Moreover, malnutrition secondary to malabsorption can accompany neoplasms such as lymphoma of the small bowel and hormone-secreting tumors, such as islet cell carcinoma of the pancreas. Nonetheless, the malnutrition we have observed in patients with malignant disorders is usually iatrogenic as a result of oncologic therapy, except in those patients who have neglected their symptoms for several weeks or months and have become cachectic secondary to diminished oral intake and increased tumor mass before seeking professional medical help (1).

Cancer cachexia was first reported as a commonly occurring syndrome more than 70 years ago when an autopsy series of 500 cancer patients documented that the immediate cause of death in cancer patients was inanition in 114 (22%) of the patients, and that up to two thirds of this group of patients exhibited some degree of cachexia (2). Russell and Steiger point out that the frequency and severity of malnutrition often depends on tumor type. In 3,047 patients enrolled in Eastern Cooperative Oncology Group (ECOG) chemotherapy protocols, and who were all assessed for weight loss before initiating chemotherapy, survival was significantly lower in the patients who demonstrated weight loss when compared with those who had not lost weight prior to starting chemotherapy (3,4). Patients with breast cancer or sarcomas had the lowest frequency of weight loss (31% to 40%), patients with colon cancer had an intermediate frequency of weight loss (48% to 61%), and patients with pancreatic or gastric cancer had the highest frequency of weight loss (83% to

87%), with about one third of these patients having presented initially with >10% weight loss (3,4). In another prospective study of 280 cancer patients, malnutrition was related predominantly to tumor type and site, with esophageal and gastric cancer patients demonstrating significantly higher degrees of malnutrition compared with the patients with other sites and types of cancer. Moreover, as expected, malnutrition was shown to increase in severity as the malignant process progressed (5). In yet another study of 365 patients with gastrointestinal cancer, virtually 50% were shown to be malnourished. The incidence of malnutrition was related to the site of the disease, and the stage of the disease was identified as a reliable predictor of weight loss, with over 50% of patients with stage III malignancies manifesting malnutrition (6).

Russell and Steiger have appropriately emphasized that the anorexia-cachexia syndrome may be present at the time of death in as many as 80% of cancer patients. They also point out the other factors and accompanying complications of cancer cachexia that result in a greater risk for organ dysfunction and death. Finally, the cachectic patient with cancer exhibits a much narrower safe therapeutic margin for tolerating chemotherapy than does the well-nourished host in the early stages of metastatic disease, and malnutrition often eliminates such patients as candidates for adequate oncologic treatment. This was documented clearly by Copeland et al. (7) more than 30 years ago in a group of 58 nutritionally depleted patients with cancer who had been denied adequate antitumor therapy because of the fear of complications related to malnutrition and inanition. Following an average of 3 to 4 weeks of nutritional rehabilitation therapy, primarily in the form of total parenteral nutrition, 52 patients gained an average of 6.8 pounds, whereas 6 patients lost an average of 7 pounds. The patients then received chemotherapeutic regimens in accordance with established protocols at that time for their tumor types and stages, and a 36% response rate was obtained in these 58 nutritionally depleted patients who otherwise would have been denied an adequate course of antineoplastic therapy. A 50% reduction in measurable tumor metastases occurred in 21 of the patients, and a 25% reduction occurred in another 3 patients. The conclusion of this study was that intravenous hyperalimentation, as total parenteral nutrition was known at that time, can be a valuable adjunct to cancer chemotherapy by improving the nutritional status, increasing the total deliverable dose of anticancer agent per unit of time, and reducing the incidence and severity of the toxic gastrointestinal side effects without adversely stimulating malignant cell growth or producing septic complications (7).

When the alimentary tract cannot be used effectively for feeding cancer patients, parenteral nutrition can be life saving. Moreover, patients who are poor candidates or noncandidates for any antineoplastic therapy because of their debility or cachexia can be converted to reasonable candidates following a course of supplemental or total parenteral nutrition (8). The morbidity and mortality of cancer patients can be significantly reduced without stimulating tumor growth when applied conscientiously according to the established principles and techniques and when integrated with specific effective antitumor therapy (8). The most natural and practical method of nutrient administration is by mouth, and the next most feasible method of nutrient delivery is via nasogastric or nasoduodenal feeding tubes. However, min-

imally invasive operative insertion of a gastrostomy or jejunostomy tube may be necessary for long-term nutritional maintenance in some patients. Unfortunately, optimal nutritional rehabilitation via the alimentary tract can sometimes require an inordinate amount of time, and specific antineoplastic therapy cannot always be deferred until protein and energy stores have been replenished adequately and in a timely manner by this route alone (1).

Russell and Steiger outline and discuss briefly the etiology of the metabolic abnormalities observed in cancer cachexia and also affirm that a unified cause of this vexing problem has yet to be defined. Many questions remain unanswered: why is it that the metabolism of carbohydrates, fats, and proteins are altered in tumor cells? Clearly, the metabolic changes appear to place the tumor cells in a position of predominance over the nontumor cells. This is obvious from the inevitable outcomes in untreated cancer patients. What is the fundamental difference in the metabolism of malignant cells from that of normal cells? Can it possibly be a "mass" effect or the result of a large tumor burden? If so, the deranged metabolism should respond to excision or debulking of the tumor, but does it? This certainly does not occur uniformly or obviously.

Additional questions include: why do malignant cells appear to inherently induce the secretion of a large number and variety of host mediators that ultimately produce a chronic inflammatory state with adverse effects on nutrient metabolism and appetite? Normal host cells either do not act the same under normal conditions or do so to a much lesser degree. Does the inflammatory response associated with neoplasia indicate that tumor cells are recognized as foreign bodies or "invaders?" Does the tumor-induced inflammatory response have any measurable beneficial effect in containing, controlling, or destroying the neoplasm? If not, the inflammatory reaction appears to be "hysterical" or futile. How and why is it that the tumor cells multiply and function apparently autonomously from the rest of the host's body cell mass?

The altered metabolism of peripheral hormones that regulate appetite indicates a de facto difference in the processing of the usual nutrients ingested by a patient with cancer from that while the host is cancer-free. This strongly intimates a different metabolism of "normal diet" and suggests that special diets specifically tailored from individual nutrient components may help the patient by placing the cancer cell at a relative disadvantage compared with the normal cells, rather than vice versa, which appears to be the rule. Investigations in this critically important area are long overdue. Clinicians and investigators have preferred to attempt to develop "magic bullet" surgical operations, radiotherapy, chemotherapy, immunotherapy, and targeted therapy, various combinations of these, and other directed therapies. Preferably, they should be attempting to identify clearly the differences in the cell biology of the various neoplastic cells from the normal cells from which they originate in order to take advantage of such differences to treat or help to treat the patient specifically, prudently, rationally, scientifically, and effectively. The learned food aversion, which Russell and Steiger appropriately mention, likely occurs as a result of "bad experience" with some forms of foods that the patients formerly had enjoyed in their normal diet prior to development of their cancers. What is it about the foods they avert that causes the patient to reject them? A study of the most highly avoided foods and the composition of those foods might possibly point the way toward formulating a diet that is not as adverse and that might actually nourish the normal body cell mass better than the tumor cell mass is nourished, thus placing the malignant cells at a disadvantage.

Another area that requires more intensive study is the hypermetabolic state that occurs in some, but not all, cancer patients. Why is it that only one fourth of cancer patients are hypermetabolic at rest, while one-third are actually hypometabolic and two-fifths have normal resting energy expenditure? In the opinion of the senior author of this commentary, all too often, the metabolic data reported in cancer patients have been selective and used to the advantage of the theories of the proponents rather than used to the advantage of the patient. Another enigmatic attitude among a rather disturbingly large number of clinicians and clinical investigators is that initial weight gain in cachectic patients often may result from increased fluid volume and an increase in fat stores rather than an early increase in protein mass. Why should this surprise them, when the body water compartment that comprises 60% of total body weight and the body fat compartment that comprises between 15% and 25% or more of total body weight are the first areas to be depleted? Restoring body protein mass to normal may actually be a second or third priority and may take a longer period of time to restore, but might occur with persistent provision of a high-protein diet and specific tailoring of the amino acid formulation of the dietary nitrogen or protein provided.

Contradictions and inconsistencies in the results of studies of carbohydrate metabolism in cancer patients may be related to the facts that many malignant cell types exist, that all cancers are not the same, and that the extent of all cancers in all patients is not identical. Moreover, the biology of the disease, differing tumor actions, and the variety of antineoplastic agents and techniques used in treating the many different malignancies, the variations and collateral factors and comorbidities, and so forth, are some of the multiple complicating factors that have effects on the metabolism of carbohydrates. Thus, it is difficult to standardize carbohydrate metabolism globally in cancer patients, and accordingly, it is difficult to obtain definitive or conclusive data. As an analogy, two other conditions that are difficult to standardize in studying the metabolism of critically ill patients are major trauma and sepsis, most simply because it is virtually impossible to have identical types and extents of trauma and sepsis in nearly identical patients, much less in those having additional identical collateral factors, such as age, gender, and comorbidities.

The differences in protein metabolism with simple starvation and in patients with cancer imply the relative autonomy of the cancer cells compared with normal cells. The etiology of this "difference" is essential to identify, define, and then to neutralize, diminish, or reverse if success in treating the cancer patient comprehensively is to be achieved. Certainly, the basic cell biologists have not been able to elucidate the answers to date. Perhaps research in the area of genomics will be more successful in identifying "the cause" of the differences in protein metabolism among normal and neoplastic cells. It is well known that the current forms of parenteral nutrition have not been successful in decreasing protein turnover, decreasing muscle protein degradation, or altering hepatic protein synthesis favorably. The therapeutic nihilists among us, therefore, condemn and advise against the use of parenteral nutrition support in the management of cancer patients. They do not seem to give consideration to the fact that the current parenteral nutrition formulations were designed to correct malnutrition secondary to periods of starvation rather than for the specific therapy of the special forms of malnutrition and anorexia-cachexia that occur in patients with malignant disorders, severe trauma, sepsis, and other complex pathophysiologies. Successful nutritional rehabilitation, whether by the enteral or the parenteral route, will require special formulations of the components, tailored to the individual patients, their cancer cell types, the stages of their disease, and their extent of malnutrition, similar to the way cytotoxic drugs and regimens have been designed for specific cancer types. A new hybrid of clinician scientist must be developed and trained to incorporate the best knowledge, skills, and motivations of basic scientists (including molecular biologists, immunologists, and geneticists) with those of medical oncologists, radiotherapists, pharmacologists, and surgeons, if optimal therapeutic results are to be achieved in the management of cancer patients. It is time for the profession to stop seeking the "silver bullet" or "holy grail" and to design collaborative studies that are comprehensive in all aspects of the management of the cancer patient. Nutritional support must be an essential component of optimal treatment of the cancer patient, regardless of the specific other components of the antineoplastic protocol.

Regarding lipid metabolism in the cancer patients, why is it that we know that increased lipolysis occurs with virtually all cancers, but we still have not identified, defined, or classified the contributions of the various potential causes of the increased lipolysis? This simply must be accomplished before rational attempts at its prevention, reversal, or correction are attempted. Too much time and effort have been spent on relatively fruitless generalizations and observational investigations rather than directing efforts and resources toward specific answers to specific questions. In their summation of the causes of changes in intake and absorption of cancer patients, Russell and Steiger succinctly point out the wide variety of causes for these adverse situations, and they essentially mandate that cancer patients require the services of a special nutritional support team that can provide specific, individually tailored, and formulated nutritional support, comprehensively and integrated with the total antineoplastic care of the patient. We agree that this is absolutely key to the successful optimal management of the cancer patient. We also strongly agree that it is of utmost importance to attempt to achieve a state of anabolism in cancer patients if at all possible prior to any and all forms of antineoplastic therapy in order to maximize positive outcomes and to minimize morbidity.

To carry our point of view a step further, anorexia may be regarded virtually as a marker for failure of effective antineoplastic therapy, and rather than further compounding the patient's system with pharmacologic agents to overcome the anorexia, it would seem prudent to us that it would be best to feed the patients enterally and/or parenterally with specifically tailored diets while using an effective anticancer therapy. Thus, the diminished appetite either will not matter in the ultimate outcome of the patient or will return to or toward normal spontaneously with the eradication or diminution of the tumor as a result of the success of optimal neoplastic therapy and specialized nutritional support. Regarding further the pharmacologic treatment of cancer cachexia, we have had no positive or useful experience with megestrol acetate in alleviating cancer anorexia-cachexia. Moreover, all agents used for this purpose to date have shown toxicities to various degrees in cancer patients. Also, there has been much individual variation in the response to pharmacologic agents and, as an analogy, this should not be unexpected, considering the great variations in the effectiveness of the myriad approaches and responses to the promotion of weight loss in obese patients. Again, there is no magic bullet. Finally, we would like to emphasize our concurrence with the strong statement by Russell and Steiger that the adverse effects, such as muscle wasting and immunosuppression outweigh the benefits of corticosteroid use for appetite stimulation, except possibly in terminal patients with poor performance status; that unfortunately, current data suggest that no single agent successfully treats unintentional weight loss in patients with cancer; and that expectations for effective pharmacologic management of cancer anorexia-cachexia may be unrealistic (9,10).

In their section on nutritional assessment, Russell and Steiger essentially demonstrate that there is more than one way to assess nutritional status, just as there is more than one way to treat cancer patients. Accordingly, practitioners should use whatever means of nutritional assessment seem to work consistently for them and their patients. The more experienced practitioners often evaluate the nutritional status of their patients intuitively "by the seat of their pants," whereas formal nutritional status protocols are more useful for the novice or for physicians or surgeons engaged in clinical research protocols. The senior author of this commentary has been engaged in nutritional support for more than 45 years, even before formal nutritional assessment became a clinical entity; thus, a four-point assessment of nutritional status was devised de novo. We have defined and graded the extent of malnutrition in accordance with the following minimal criteria: (a) an unintentional or unexplainable recent loss of 10% or more of usual body weight; (b) a serum albumin concentration <3.5 g/dL or a serum total protein concentration <5.5 g/dL; (c) a peripheral lymphocyte count <20% or a total lymphocyte count <1,200/mm^3; and (d) impaired immunocompetence manifested originally by delayed cutaneous hypersensitivity, but more recently by sophisticated blood tests of immunocompetence, which are more reliable and better tolerated by the patients than reactive skin tests. If any of these criteria are evident, the patient is graded as mildly malnourished; if any two are present, the patient is considered moderately malnourished; if any three are manifested, the patient is deemed moderately to severely malnourished; and if all four of the criteria are met, the patient is classified as severely malnourished. This definition and classification of malnutrition has served the purposes of our nutritional support teams very well for the past 40 years, and we continue to use it as a fundamental index of nutritional assessment to this day. More recently, the serum prealbumin level has been added as an important and dynamic indicator of protein nutritional status and as a highly responsive marker for the effectiveness of the provision of adequate amounts of high-quality protein or amino acids in addition to the other essential components for protein synthesis, that is, calories, vitamins, minerals, trace elements, and essential fatty acids.

The nutritional support section is excellent, erudite, and reflects the wisdom of the authors. The fundamental philosophy of our team is that food must be considered therapeutic by the patient as if it were "a medicine," and taken conscientiously and precisely as directed, just as if it were a specifically determined chemotherapy or programmed radiotherapy regimen. It is strongly and repeatedly emphasized to the patients that their diets are equally important to their specific antineoplastic treatment modalities and should be consumed as completely as possible, regardless whether it is enjoyable, satisfying, or providing pleasant gustatory sensations. The nutritional support team must not only calculate the optimal requirements and formulate an optimal nutritional regimen, but must then exercise relentless, conscientious surveillance of the patient's nutrient intake. Essentially, the nutritional support team and other caregivers must be highly motivated and capable about optimally nourishing the cancer patient. In the enteral and parenteral nutrition section, which is very succinct and well presented, we would add to the goals presented, additional functional goals that are also desirable, including increasing strength, ambulation, exercise, participation and improvement in activities of daily living, which would likely promote a feeling of well-being and comfort.

We are in complete agreement with the authors regarding their rationale for specialized nutritional intervention in patients with cancer and appreciate their Socratic approach to this aspect of their chapter. The questions posed are essential to answer in a positive, constructive manner if optimal therapy is to be achieved. This cannot possibly be overemphasized.

In their section on parenteral and enteral nutrition as an adjunct to surgery, Russell and Steiger expound wisely and fairly with representative data from the literature relating both to some positive and negative aspects of these forms of nutritional support in cancer patients. Because we have had a longer experience, and perhaps even a broader experience, with the use of parenteral and enteral nutrition in the management of cancer patients than anyone in the world, we welcome the opportunity to comment on some of our personal principles, practices, and attitudes in this important matter. Historically, when the senior author was a resident in surgery, a cadre of more than three dozen patients with advanced stages of various cancers was studied at the Hospital of the University of Pennsylvania, using an early and rudimentary parenteral technique of providing nutrition to these cachectic patients who could not support themselves nutritionally and metabolically by mouth. They were nourished with peripheral intravenous feedings providing up to 5 L of a 10% to 15% solution daily, which could provide as much as 100 g of protein in the form of fibrin hydrolysate and 2,000 calories, plus the available vitamins and minerals that could be given intravenously at that time, and using intravenous chlorothiazide as a diuretic to help excrete the "excess water" required to provide the nutrients intravenously. In this seminal pilot study, the fundamental goals were to study the feasibility and safety of providing nutrients intravenously to cancer patients who were unable to be nourished adequately by the alimentary tract. Tumor types were not standardized, and therapeutic options were rudimentary at that time. Furthermore, it had been determined by the primary physician or surgeon that each of the patients studied had received maximum available therapeutic benefit, were "preterminal," and were destined to die in the hospital during that admission. It was impressive that virtually all of the patients tolerated the therapy without infection or sepsis. Two of the patients exhibited mild fluid overload that responded promptly to adjustments in their regimen. All of the patients improved in their feeling of well-being, strength, activities of daily living, and attitude. Their quality of life improved so obviously, not only to their caregivers and investigators but to the patients themselves, such that several of the patients thought that the nutritional regimen might actually be promoting antineoplastic therapeutic results. Indeed, some of them, and their families, had to be cautioned against that optimistic conjecture, lest the inevitable fatal outcome that might be delayed somewhat by the nutritional support, be misunderstood, disappointing, or even devastating (11). Subsequently, patients at the Philadelphia Veterans Administration Hospital, and a series of patients at the MD Anderson Hospital and Tumor Institute in Houston, who had significant malnutrition (30- to 40-pound weight loss) secondary to esophageal cancer, had better operative outcomes than would have been expected or that were obtained in patients who did not have nutritional support in the form of parenteral nutrition perioperatively (12).

A major difficulty during the early development and application of total parenteral nutrition to the management of cancer patients appears to have been, and continues to be, an inherent resistance among medical oncologists to add or include this important modality in their various protocols. Their usual rationalization is that adding nutritional support to their patient management would introduce a confounding factor to their original protocols. The time is long overdue to overcome this negative attitude and to carry out prospective, controlled studies in comparable cancer patients to measure the effects of malnutrition and its correction or amelioration in cancer patients when the nutritional support regimen is tailored, formulated, conducted, and/or supervised by a competent nutritional support team. In the opinion of the senior author of this commentary, virtually none of the studies reported in the literature during the past decade or more satisfy these criteria and are thereby fundamentally flawed. Until this unacceptable situation is corrected, the optimal nutritional support of cancer patients will be compromised and will not reach its full adjunctive therapeutic potential.

As documented by Russell and Steiger, one of the studies most frequently quoted in this area provided 35 kcal/kg/day to all of the cancer patients. Perhaps the results would have been better if the caloric ration had been increased up to 45 kcal/kg/day in patients who required and tolerated this caloric level, together with a concomitant increase in amino acid nitrogen (13). It has seemed to be prudent in our experience to maximize parenteral nutritional support rather than simply following "boiler plate" recommendations, as if every patient were exactly the same. A malnourished or cachectic cancer patient is obviously the same person as he or she was when in optimal nutritional condition and health, but the body cell mass does not act, react, or respond in the same manner under both sets of circumstances. More simply stated, the patients with cancer are not the same nutritionally or metabolically as they had been when they were cancer-free, and this must be taken into consideration in carrying out their treatment. Optimal results cannot possibly be obtained uniformly with any therapeutic endeavor in a malnourished or cachectic patient. Their systems require adequate

nutrient substrates at all times to function at their maximum potential. Because infection associated with parenteral nutrition has been the single most important impediment to its optimal application in critically ill patients and in cancer patients, and has been obviously related primarily to catheter and other related administrative aspects of the technique, it is of paramount importance that dedicated and competent nutritional support teams are actively and conscientiously engaged in the comprehensive management of the cancer patient daily.

It is well known that patients who are relatively well nourished, or only mildly malnourished, are not likely to exhibit benefits that are readily measurable clinically following specialized nutritional support. However, patients with moderate-to-severe malnutrition are likely to respond more favorably to other therapeutic modalities when they receive adequate nutritional support enterally and/or parenterally. The techniques used for providing optimal specialized nutritional support, however, must be applied just as conscientiously and competently as, for example, the management of blood sugar levels in critically ill patients, especially postoperatively, in intensive care situations. A fundamental problem with providing nutritional support is that caregivers, especially physicians and surgeons, have become virtually too familiar and comfortable with the existence of the technology without mastering the essential principles and practices mandatorily associated with the desired optimal outcomes. In some quarters, total parenteral nutrition is still considered for use primarily as a "last-ditch effort" rather than having been applied earlier and more rationally in the clinical course. Inevitably, the conclusion drawn from this predictably suboptimal experience is that, "the TPN doesn't work." Total parenteral nutrition is not "holy water" and should be used prudently and judiciously when indicated for patients who are significantly malnourished and who cannot otherwise obtain adequate nutrition in a timely manner.

Finally, the composition of total parenteral nutrition is so variable in different institutions that it is difficult or impossible to derive meaningful data from meta-analysis, which has been used so frequently to discredit its use. In the opinion of the senior author of this commentary, the meta-analysis of nutritional support using parenteral and enteral techniques has been flawed and has propagated more misinformation than useful information. Moreover, meta-analysis is to science what alchemy is to chemistry; it is really pseudoscience rather than real science. In the frequently quoted study by Brennan et al. (14), the data are flawed by the facts that patients were included in the study and randomized without regard to their nutritional status; all of the patients received the same parenteral nutrition regimen providing 2,000 calories, an inordinately high fat content approaching 60% of total calories, and inadequate protein; the total parenteral nutrition was administered autonomously by the "medical TPN team," and the composition and ratios of the components of the parenteral diet would certainly not be considered a healthy diet if given by mouth or enterally. This study has resulted in a widespread attitude among oncologic surgeons that parenteral nutritional support is not only unnecessary as an adjunct to the management of all patients with pancreatic malignancies, but that its use may actually be contraindicated. This is not only an invalid, but a dangerous attitude, as there are patients at various stages of pancreatic cancer and its treatment who clearly can benefit from parenteral nutritional support when enteral or oral nutritional support cannot be provided adequately or at all.

The consensus statement published in 1997 by the American Society for Parenteral and Enteral Nutrition and included in this section represents the best published principles in this area to date (15). Our primary modification of the statement is that we believe that parenteral nutrition should be either strongly considered or mandated 5 to 10 days after operation for patients still unable to eat or tolerate enteral feedings rather than merely "considered," which to us is a bit too "soft, weak, or polite." Too often, clinicians tend to put off or delay the initiation of specialized nutritional support postoperatively "to see how the patient feels tomorrow" in the hope that the patient will then begin to ingest adequate nutrients. However, the tomorrows often become successive, so that by the time the specialized nutritional support technologies are initiated or fully undertaken, the nutritional status of the patient has deteriorated to a rather severe state, which can either be difficult or impossible to overcome nutritionally. To emphasize this common error in clinical judgment, we reinforce the teaching of prudent application of specialized nutritional support postoperatively to our students and residents by relating to them the anecdote of the local pub, which has a sign behind the bar that states, "free beer tomorrow." The obvious "catch" is that if one returns tomorrow for the free beer advertised by the sign, the bartender will point out that the sign still says, "free beer tomorrow." Obviously, the tomorrow never becomes today, and the beer never becomes free. Unfortunately, in the clinical situation, the patient pays the price for this conundrum.

The concluding four paragraphs in this important section by Russell and Steiger provide excellent data, experience, and principles that are encouraging to those of us who believe strongly in the importance of feeding all patients optimally, under all conditions, at all times.

In the section of their chapter on parenteral and enteral nutrition as an adjunct to chemotherapy and radiotherapy, they dutifully outline the goals and point out the flaws in studies of the impact of parenteral nutritional support on the efficacy of antitumor treatment. It is important in such studies that not all patients with cancer who are receiving chemotherapy and/or radiation therapy are "lumped" together. The subgroups of severely malnourished patients must be treated differently nutritionally no matter what their primary pathophysiologic process is, but this especially is relevant to cancer patients. The final sentence in the section emphasizing the importance of prophylactic enteral nutrition support prior to the commencement of radiotherapy is absolutely key to the achievement of optimal results.

Our philosophy is essentially in agreement with Russell and Steiger regarding specialized nutritional support in patients with advanced cancer. Indeed, the senior editor of this textbook had contributed to this important area almost 20 years ago in his tome entitled, *Parenteral and Enteral Nutrition* (16). This is an area that had been particularly difficult for clinicians who care for cancer patients. The decision is not obvious and requires a great deal of experience, judgment, wisdom, courage, self-confidence, and angst on the part of the surgeon. Patients present with a wide variety of situations even when their diagnosis is the same; collateral factors and comorbidities are also very important obvious modifiers in decision making. Economical,

practical, and humane issues must be considered in addition to the moral, ethical, and legal issues, notwithstanding the personal preferences or wishes of the patient, especially regarding quality of life, comfort, and feeling of well-being. A problem with morals and ethics is that they are not well defined, are not uniformly held or accepted, are not standardized, and are certainly not scientific. Indeed, medical ethics have become so significantly complex that it is often helpful or advisable to seek the services of a medical ethics committee in decision making. Furthermore, medical ethics is actually evolving into a specialty area of academic and professional pursuit and development, and is likely to become a more integral force in the future practice of medicine.

On a personal note, we adhere to the philosophy that whenever it is obvious that everything that can be done for the benefit of the patient has been done and that the patient is nonetheless deteriorating toward an inevitable, imminent, but comfortable demise, we shift much of our primary attention and consideration from the patient to the patient's family and other significant survivors in order to minimize or alleviate their inevitable guilt associated with the impending or real loss of their loved one. Accordingly, meaningful communication and consideration of the beliefs, wishes, and opinions of the survivors becomes foremost. The survivors also must be reassured that nothing else can be, nor could have been, done by them, nor by the caregivers, to save the patient's life. From a practical standpoint, their survivors virtually all become our patients, and if they are not treated in a most considerate and judicious manner, they may well become victims of guilt for prolonged times, or even for the rest of their lives. This is a high price to pay, especially for the inexorable death of a terminally ill elderly patient with widespread cancer. Finally, the primary physician or surgeon making these difficult decisions must also do so in such a manner as to relieve his or her own guilt, together with the guilt of fellow caregivers who all are adversely affected by their individual and collective failure to save the patient. These are powerful human instincts that require great strength and effort in order to maintain perspective, self-confidence, and peace of mind.

Russell and Steiger and others have suggested that palliative specialized nutritional support occasionally is indicated in a small subset of terminally ill patients in whom it may be possible to improve nutritional status, increase survival, or improve quality of life despite the fact that the ultimate outcome will be the same (17–20). We strongly support that philosophy, having been influenced by countless patients in this situation throughout the past 4 to 5 decades. Subjective input influencing this philosophy is derived in part from the fact that the senior author has never cared for a fellow physician or a fellow physician's family member who has opted for starvation as the modus exodus rather than succumbing secondary to the other collateral causes of death in cancer patients, such as massive hemorrhage, sepsis, or organ failure. Furthermore, tumor biology is often so variable in individual patients that a process that might predictably lead to death within a year or less in one patient may be extended to 5 years or more in another patient. A current patient of the two commentators is a 78-year-old woman with metastatic carcinoid of the small bowel who underwent a major debulking procedure and a subsequent intestinal bypass of the residual recurrent tumor that could not be resected more than 5 years ago. Following perioperative nutritional support, she was then encouraged to follow her wishes to spend her putative last months in her beloved Florida condominium. This all occurred after she and her family had been advised by her primary physician and oncologists to go home and prepare for her death because nothing else could be done for her. She and her family are most grateful for the quantity and quality of life she has experienced during these more than 5 years, including five winters in Florida and five summers in New England. At the time of this writing, she is in an extended care facility where she is being maintained comfortably with modified nutritional, fluid, and electrolyte support as her now greatly increased tumor burden threatens imminently to overwhelm her. She and her family are most grateful for the years she has lived and the lifestyle she has enjoyed as a result of the surgical and nutritional care we have provided to her. Although the family is grieving her inevitable loss, they appreciate what has been done to keep her alive and functioning for 5 years longer than they originally anticipated. There is no way to design or report a controlled series of patients treated in this manner, indicating that comprehensive management of cancer patients is not exclusively the domain of science, but also of the more ancient art of the practice of medicine.

In the section on nutritional support and tumor growth, the authors of the chapter admit that this is a theoretical consideration that has garnered consideration and support from some animal studies. However, it is important to emphasize that no clinically significant increases in the rate of tumor growth has been documented in human cancer patients receiving nutritional support, especially when simultaneously being treated by effective antineoplastic therapy (16,21). This has certainly been our experience throughout the past half century. The cancer cells appear to be functioning, multiplying, and obtaining nourishment from the host maximally regardless of the host's nutritional intake and status, which is consistent with the autonomous and parasitic nature of malignant neoplasia.

Regarding the refeeding syndrome, both commentators believe that nutritional emergencies virtually do not exist. Therefore, in the treatment of a malnourished patient who obviously requires nutritional rehabilitation, the process must be undertaken rationally and judiciously, and applied in a manner in which the patient can effectively use all of the nutrients efficiently without having his or her metabolic capabilities overwhelmed by excessive provision of biochemically active nutrient substrates and large volumes of water. We agree whole-heartedly with the principles put forth by the authors of the chapter. The commentators have published previously on this subject and employ the "Goldilocks" analogy in providing nutritional support to severely malnourished patients in order to prevent the refeeding syndrome, that is, "too little, too much, or just right" when providing nutrients (22). The refeeding syndrome is completely avoidable and should neither occur nor be tolerated in this day and age. Patients should always be fed "just right."

In drawing this commentary to a close, we congratulate the authors on their outstanding contribution to this textbook and to the profession. Especially noteworthy are their summary and current recommendations, which outline and emphasize the essentials of this complex yet important area of endeavor, and with which we are in complete agreement. Neither our knowledge nor our care of cancer patients with significant malnutrition is comprehensive nor ideal at this time, and we must continue to strive for ultimate excellence in providing optimal nutritional support to cancer patients. Space limitations have not allowed either the chapter authors or commentators to address the recent issues in the literature concerning the questions raised regarding the possibility that antioxidants and other nutrients might interfere with chemotherapy or radiation therapy and can actually increase morbidity and decrease survival. In a recent review of this important subject, it has been reported that since the 1970s, 280 peer-reviewed in vitro and in vivo studies, including 50 human studies involving 8,521 patients, 5,081 of whom where given nutrients, have consistently shown that the nutrients do not interfere with the therapeutic modalities for cancer. Furthermore, nonprescription antioxidants and other nutrients actually enhance the killing of therapeutic modalities for cancer, decrease their side effects, and protect normal tissue. In 15 human studies, 3,738 patients who took nonprescription antioxidants and other nutrients actually had increased survival compared with the others in the group (23). It is obvious that the importance of individual nutrients as adjuncts to specific antineoplastic therapy must be undertaken to define their efficacy and role in comprehensive cancer patient management.

Another reality of clinical practice is that patients often combine prescription medications with herbal and dietary substances on their own in an attempt at times to make up for what they perceive are deficiencies or inadequacies in conventional medical knowledge or treatment of their malignances. The use of herbal and dietary substances in the United States has increased substantially during the last decade, the percentage of patients using herbal remedies having increased from 2.5% in 1990 to 18.8% in 2002 (24–26). It is estimated that 18% to 22% of patients use herbal medicines today, and approximately 16% of patients combine herbal medicines with their prescription medications (24,27–29). Although herbal medicines have been associated with a variety of adverse herb-drug interactions, the actual incidence of such adverse interactions in patients using multiple herbal and prescription medications has not been measured (24,30,31). These are important considerations for those of us who manage cancer patients with malnutrition, and it is imperative that we attempt to help define this area further. The published data are a testament to that fact that patients and families who do not think that the members of the medical profession are doing all they can to manage both the malnutrition and the neoplasm of the patients are increasingly taking matters into their own hands and seeking whatever other forms of therapy might be available to them.

We conclude this commentary by emphasizing again that there is more to the nutritional support of the cancer patient than the current science and clinical practice mandate or justify. The emotional and psychological support of the patient and significant others, and the social aspects of food intake and "breaking bread" with family and friends cannot be denied. These needs do exist, and we eventually must address and do something about them rather than ignore them, as is all too often done. Finally, when we have exhausted all reasonable, rational, or justifiable antineoplastic, or even nutritional, therapy provided for the patient with an inexorably lethal cancer, it is of utmost importance that we never abandon the patient or the family, and at the very least, continue to support them, bond with them, relieve their guilt, and above all, reinforce their faith in the humane and human core values by "being there" for them and providing a feeling of comfort and hope that cannot otherwise be accomplished. The frontiers for specialized nutritional support of cancer patients await our exploration, discovery, and judicious clinical application.

REFERENCES

1. Dudrick SJ, MacFadyen BV Jr, Souchon EA, et al. Parenteral nutrition techniques in cancer patients. *Cancer Res.* 1977;37(7 Pt 2): 2440–2450.
2. Warren S. The immediate causes of death and cancer. *Am J Med Sci.* 1932;184:610–615.
3. Dewys WD, Begg C, Lavin PT, et al. Prognostic effect of weight loss prior to chemotherapy in cancer patients. Eastern Cooperative Oncology Group. *Am J Med.* 1980;69:491–497.
4. Harrison LE, Fong FY. Enteral nutrition in the cancer patient. In: Rombeau JL, ed. *Clinical Nutrition Enteral and Tube Feeding.* Philadelphia: Saunders; 1997:300–323.
5. Bozzetti F, Migliavacca S, Scotti A, et al. Impact of cancer, type, site, stage and treatment on the nutritional status of patients. *Ann Surg.* 1982;196:170–179.
6. Meguid MM, Meguid V. Preoperative identification of the surgical cancer patient in need of postoperative supportive total parenteral nutrition. *Cancer.* 1985;55(1 Suppl):258–262.
7. Copeland EM 3rd, MacFadyen BV Jr, Lanzotti VJ, et al. Intravenous hyperalimentation as an adjunct to cancer chemotherapy. *Am J Surg.* 1975;129:167–173.
8. Palesty JA, Dudrick SJ. What we have learned about cachexia in gastrointestinal cancer. *Dig Dis.* 2003;21:198–213.
9. Mattox TW. Treatment of unintentional weight loss in patients with cancer. *Nutr Clin Pract.* 2005;20:400–410.
10. Mattox TW. Intravenous hyperalimentation and cancer: a historical perspective. 1986. *Nutr Clin Pract.* 2002;17:249–251.
11. Dudrick SJ. Early developments and clinical applications of total parenteral nutrition. *JPEN J Parenter Enteral Nutr.* 2003;27:291–299.
12. Daly JM, Massar E, Giacco G, et al. Parenteral nutrition in esophageal cancer patients. *Ann Surg.* 1982;196:203–208.
13. Smale BF, Mullen JL, Buzby GP, et al. The efficacy of nutritional assessment and support in cancer surgery. *Cancer.* 1981;47:2375–2381.
14. Brennan MF, Pisters PW, Posner M, et al. A prospective randomized trial of total parenteral nutrition after major pancreatic resection for malignancy. *Ann Surg.* 1994;220:436–444.
15. Klein S, Kinney J, Jeejeebhoy K, et al. Nutrition support in clinical practice: review of published data and recommendations for future research directions. National Institutes of Health, American Society for Parenteral and Enteral Nutrition, and American Society for Clinical Nutrition. *JPEN J Parenter Enteral Nutr,* 1997;21:133–156.
16. Silberman H. Nutritional therapy: clinical applications: cancer. In: Silberman H, ed. *Parenteral and Enteral Nutrition.* 2nd ed. Norwalk, CT: Appleton and Lange;1989:395–407.
17. August DA, Thorn D, Fisher RL, et al. Home parenteral nutrition for patients with inoperable malignant bowel obstruction. *JPEN J Parenter Enteral Nutr.* 1991;15:323–327.
18. Fuhrman MP, Herrmann VM. Bridging the continuum: nutrition support in palliative and hospice care. *Nutr Clin Pract.* 2006;21: 134–141.
19. Ripamonti C, Twycross R, Baines M, et al. Clinical-practice recommendations for the management of bowel obstruction in patients with end-stage cancer. *Support Care Cancer.* 2001;9:223–233.
20. Whitworth MK, Whitfield A, Holm S, et al. Doctor, does this mean I'm going to starve to death? *J Clin Oncol.* 2004;22:199–201.
21. Schattner M, Shike M. Nutrition support of the patient with cancer. In: Shils ME, Shike M, Ross AC, Caballero B, Cousins RJ, eds. *Modern Nutrition in Health and Disease*, Baltimore: Lippincott Williams & Wilkins; 2006:1290–1313.
22. Palesty JA, Dudrick SJ. The goldilocks paradigm of starvation and refeeding. *Nutr Clin Pract.* 2006;21:147–154.
23. Simone CB 2nd, Simone NL, Simone V, et al. Antioxidants and other nutrients do not interfere with chemotherapy or radiation therapy and can increase kill and increase survival, Part 2. *Altern Ther Health Med.* 2007;13:40–47.
24. Bush TM, Rayburn KS, Holloway SW, et al. Adverse interactions between herbal and dietary substances and prescription medications: a clinical survey. *Altern Ther Health Med.* 2007;13:30–35.
25. Eisenberg DM, Kessler RC, Foster C, et al. Unconventional medicine in the United States. Prevalence, costs, and patterns of use. *N Engl J Med.* 1993;328:246–252.
26. Kelly JP, Kaufman DW, Kelley K, et al. Recent trends in use of herbal and other natural products. *Arch Intern Med.* 2005;165:281–286.
27. Kaufman DW, Kelly JP, Rosenberg L, et al. Recent patterns of medication use in the ambulatory adult population of the United States: the Slone survey. *JAMA.* 2002;287:337–344.
28. Rao JK, Mihaliak K, Kroenke K, et al. Use of complementary therapies for arthritis among patients of rheumatologists. *Ann Intern Med.* 1999;131:409–416.
29. Rhee SM, Garg VK, Hershey CO. Use of complementary and alternative medicines by ambulatory patients. *Arch Intern Med.* 2004;164:1004–1009.
30. Ernst E. Harmless herbs? A review of the recent literature. *Am J Med.* 1998;104:170–178.
31. Fugh-Berman A. Herb-drug interactions. *Lancet.* 2000;355:134–138.

4

Occult Metastases: Detection and Prognostic and Therapeutic Implications

Marija Balic, Debra Hawes, A. Munro Neville, and Richard J. Cote

The goal of diagnostic surgical oncology is to diagnose and stage tumors. Using these pathologic criteria in conjunction with clinical parameters, pathologist and clinician attempt to determine the appropriate treatment of a patient and predict the outcome.

One and possibly the most important factor in predicting clinical outcome is the extent of disease. It must be established whether the lesion is truly localized (T) or has spread to regional nodes (N) or distant metastatic sites (M) (1). However, a proportion of patients with no evidence of systemic dissemination after primary therapy will develop recurrent disease. Small numbers of tumor cells disseminated from the primary tumor cannot be readily detected and conventional pathologic TNM tumor staging methods (careful pathologic, clinical, biochemical, and radiologic evaluation) do not take the presence of such occult tumor cells into account. Such occult metastases have also been described in literature as micrometastases, disseminated tumor cells, minimal residual cancer, or minimal residual disease or, when circulating in blood, as circulating tumor cells.

The success of adjuvant therapy is assumed to stem from its ability to eradicate or render quiescent occult tumor cells. Methods for the detection of these cells in patients with the earliest stage of cancer (i.e., prior to detection of metastases by any other clinical or pathologic analysis) have received a great deal of attention. This chapter focuses on the detection and significance of occult tumor cells in the bone marrow, peripheral blood, and lymph nodes of patients with various types of tumors, as well as its therapeutic implications.

Detection of occult disease, irrespective of the method, carries valuable clinical data and should be given consideration for inclusion in a modified TNM classification and in designing therapy particularly for breast cancer at this time.

METHODS USED FOR DETECTION OF OCCULT TUMOR CELLS

Sample Collection

Bone Marrow and Peripheral Blood

Bone marrow is a frequent site of distant metastasis in a variety of cancers, such as carcinoma of the breast and prostate. Epithelial cancer cells detected in the bone marrow do not necessarily have the potential to form metastatic lesions at the sample site; rather, they may merely be cells in transit. In this regard, we have found that extrinsic cells could be identified in the bone marrow of patients with metastatic disease, even when aspirates were taken from sites distant from the areas of clinically detectable tumor involvement (2). Moreover, even in tumors that do not usually metastasize to the bone marrow, such as colon cancer, disseminated tumor cells can be detected in the bone marrow aspirates in patients with early-stage disease (3). Bone marrow aspirates collected at the time of surgery are analyzed for presence of epithelial cells. Several authors have suggested that the yield of positive cells improves when aspirates from multiple sites are obtained (4,5). The general practice is that while the patient is under general anesthesia, bone marrow samples are obtained from each upper iliac crest by needle aspiration during primary surgery (6).

Because of the difficulty in obtaining bone marrow, peripheral blood would clearly be a more convenient sample site for studies to detect disseminated tumor cells; however, the yield of disseminated tumor cells from peripheral blood is known to be lower than that in the bone marrow (5,7). A possible reason for this is that the bone marrow vasculature consists of a unique sinusoidal system that may simply act as a filter that traps or concentrates malignant cells. Therefore, with currently available techniques bone marrow still offers the maximum opportunity to detect cancer cells that have been released into the blood, and the majority of studies to detect disseminated tumor cells in the systemic circulation have investigated bone marrow as a site of spread.

One of the reasons for the lower rate of detection of circulating tumor cells in blood could be the limitations of the current methods. Because of the advantages of using peripheral blood, technical advances to increase the yield of circulating tumor cells have received more attention in recent years.

Lymph Nodes

Lymph nodes are obtained during the surgery and embedded in paraffin blocks for pathologic evaluation and storage. The single most important prognostic factor for most solid tumors is the presence of histologically detectable regional lymph node metastases. However, a significant proportion of node-negative patients will develop distant metastasis. Systemic dissemination may take place by routes other than lymphatic spread; the presence of bone marrow occult metastases in node-negative patients demonstrates this (8). Nevertheless, a proportion of node-negative patients without the evidence of bone marrow metastases will experience recurrence. It has become clear that another possible site for occult tumor spread in histologically node-negative patients is the regional lymph nodes.

Gusterson and Ott (9) have calculated that a pathologist has only a 1% chance of identifying a metastatic focus of cancer of a diameter of three cells in cross-section occupying a lymph node by routine histopathologic examination. It has also been clearly shown that re-examination of lymph node sections initially considered negative for tumor after routine histopathologic screening frequently show metastatic deposits (10). The studies on detection of occult tumor cells in lymph nodes can be classified into two major categories: (a) detection of metastasis after more intensive histologicl examination of the lymph node, including analysis of multiple serial sections, and (b) studies that use immunohistochemistry or molecular techniques to take advantage of the differential expression of antigens and markers between normal lymph node constituents and epithelial carcinoma cells to detect lymph node occult metastatic cells.

Cell Enrichment Methods

For detection of occult tumor cells from bone marrow or peripheral blood, enrichment methods are used in order to enhance the sensitivity of detection. Density gradient separation and immunomagnetic separation are the two most commonly employed techniques for occult tumor cell enrichment. A more recent microtechnology uses a cell size-based sieving method.

Cell Density-based Enrichment

The most established tumor cell enrichment from bone marrow and peripheral blood samples is cell density gradient centrifugation on the Ficoll-Hypaque solution (11). The basis of this cell separation assay is the differential migration of the cells during centrifugation according to their buoyant density, which results in the separation of different cell types into distinct layers. This method has been employed in most key clinical trials evaluating bone marrow aspirates for presence of single tumor cells (12,13). A variation of density gradient centrifugation is the OncoQuick (Greiner Bio-One GmbH, Frickenhausen, Germany) (14) assay, which has a porous barrier that separates the lower compartment with separation medium from the sample, prior to centrifugation. Following buoyant density gradient centrifugation, the buffy coat that contains the enriched tumor cells along with the mononuclear lymphocytes can be easily aspirated, leaving red blood cells and granulocytes partitioned below the porous barrier plug.

Antibody-based Enrichment

The enrichment by antibody-based methods relies on the expression of specific antigens on the cell surface of epithelial tumor cells or mononuclear hematopoietic cells. The magnetic separation involves either positive selection via direct epithelial tumor cell capture or negative selection by hematopoietic cell depletion. The antibodies employed in the positive selection methods target the epithelial tumor cell surface markers, such as epithelial cell adhesion molecule (15), while those used in negative selection assays are directed against the surface markers expressed abundantly in hematopoietic cells of different lineages, CD45 (16) for lymphocytes, and glycophorin for erythrocytes. Antibodies are coupled to magnetic particles by either direct functionalization or through DNA linkers.

There are multiple methods used to enrich target tumor cells. Most common is the column format, in which the target (or nontarget) cells are attached to magnetized particles that are then further separated by technologies such as the magnetic automated cell sorter system (Miltenyi Biotec, Bergisch Gladbach, Germany) or immunomagnetic particle-based separation techniques like Dynabeads (Dynal, Oslo, Norway) or RosetteSep (Stem Cell Technologies, Vancouver, Canada). When interacting with samples for the positive selection assays, the antibody-coated ferromagnetic beads enable magnetic capture of tumor cells (17). Recently there have been reports of studies that have used panels of monoclonal antibodies to improve (18) recovery rates in model systems, and consequently have detected more patients with disseminated tumor cells. This may also help make the magnetic separation more efficient by alleviating the dependence on a single marker such as epithelial cell adhesion molecule or a few markers that are known to be variably expressed among some primary tumor cells (19,20). Immunomagnetic enrichment strategies are nevertheless limited by the fact that carcinoma cells with absent or low target antigen expression may be missed by these methods. Furthermore, subpopulations of hematopoietic cells also express epithelial markers and co-purify with tumor cells in the sample (21,22).

Novel Emerging Technologies for Tumor Cell Enrichment

None of the methods described is considered very efficient. With recent advances in the manufacture of microdevices, many of the emerging technologies are using the promise of labor-saving, cost-effective, and time-efficient processing by developing miniaturized lab-on-a-chip diagnostic systems. Several microdevices are currently in development for cell enrichment and isolation integrated with downstream genetic as well as protein expression analyses. Dielectrophoresis is a method capable of isolating cancer cells in blood by exploiting the difference in dielectric property, which varies across different cell types (23,24). Circulating epithelial tumor cells are generally larger than hematopoietic cells in the peripheral blood (25–27), a property that is increasingly used for the separation of tumor cells from the background cells. A possible drawback of these techniques is that there is the possibility that some cells, which are smaller than pore diameter, may get lost. We have built a prototype using microfabricated membrane for enrichment of circulating tumor cells in blood based on size (U.S. patent pending), which will soon be clinically tested.

Analytical Methods

The origin from tumor of the enriched cells must be confirmed. This can be achieved by either morphologic or molecular assessment. The morphologic assessment typically requires an experienced pathologist while the molecular assays may transfer the decision to a molecular biologist.

Morphologic Analysis Using Immunohistochemistry and Immunocytochemistry

Following pioneering studies at the Ludwig Institute for Cancer Research (LICR) and Royal Marsden Hospital in London, England (5), a number of groups have used immunohistochemical procedures to identify disseminated tumor cells in the bone marrow and lymph nodes of patients with cancer. While many of the initial studies focused on breast cancer (5,28–31), tumors from other organs, such as colon (32–34), prostate (35–39) and lung (40–44) have also been investigated.

Antibodies

Immunohistochemical methods are based on the ability of monoclonal antibodies to distinguish between cells of different histogenesis (i.e., epithelial cancer cells vs. the hematopoietic and stromal cells of the bone marrow, peripheral blood, and lymph nodes). The most widely used monoclonal antibodies to detect occult tumor cells are antibodies to "epithelial-specific" antigens. These antibodies do not react with normal hematopoietic or stromal cells present in the bone marrow, peripheral blood, or lymph nodes. None of the antibodies used in any study is specific for cancer; all react with normal and malignant epithelial cells. They are useful because they can identify an extrinsic population of epithelial cells in compartments where there are normally no such elements. The antibodies used fall into two general classes: (i) those reactive with cell surface antigens, and (ii) those reactive with cytostructural antigens.

Among antibodies to cell surface molecules, those to epithelial membrane antigen have been widely used; these have been reported to react with plasma cells (45), which could result in false-positive staining. Antibodies reactive against cytoplasmic structural antigens are mostly directed against low-molecular-weight cytokeratin intermediate filament proteins, which detect extrinsic cells of epithelial origin in the bone marrow (2,3,30).

Because of antigenic heterogeneity in all tissues (including malignant neoplasms), none of the antigens being detected is expressed in all of the cells in any given lesion. In order to minimize this problem and to ensure identification of the maximum number of extrinsic epithelial cells, we have used a cocktail of two anti-cytokeratin antibodies, AE1 and CAM5.2, which in combination recognize the predominant intermediate filament proteins in simple epithelial cells (46). The specificities of the antibodies used in all of the studies have been well characterized; they are all specific for epithelial cells (41). Minimal cross-reactivity has been observed with normal or neoplastic hematopoietic cells. This feature is critical because the assay is based on the differential antigenic expression of epithelial versus bone marrow mononuclear cells.

Visualization of antigen-positive cells has been performed using light microscopy either manually or by automated methods or indirect immunofluorescence methods. Light microscopic visualization uses the immunoperoxidase and immunoalkaline phosphatase systems to develop color in the positive cells. These methods give good results (3,5,46) (Figures 4.1 and 4.2). Not only do they provide a permanent record, but they also allow cytologic evaluation of the cells.

Sensitivity

In patients with early-stage cancers, the concentration of extrinsic epithelial cells is presumably quite low; these cells cannot be detected by routine imaging procedures, biochemical determinations, or even cytologic examination of the bone marrow. The

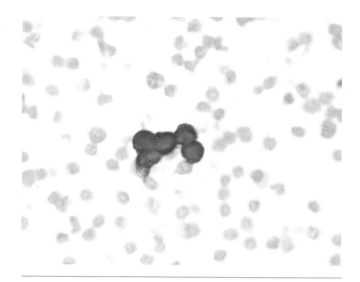

Figure 4.1 Immunohistochemical staining with monoclonal antibodies to cytokeratin (AE1 and CAM 5.2), showing three cancer cells in the bone marrow of a patient with early-stage breast cancer (magnification ×40). (See Color insert.)

reported sensitivity of the immunohistochemical method ranges from the detection of one epithelial cell in 10^3 to that of one to five epithelial cells in a 10^6 hematopoietic cells (28,29,46). The limits of detection of our methods has been studied using a model system in which the breast cancer cell lines MCF-7 and MDA-MB-468 were diluted in bone marrow cells of normal donors (29,31,46). These studies demonstrate that by using the methods described here (immunofluorescence, immunoalkaline phosphatase, or immunoperoxidase), as few as two to five extrinsic epithelial cells can be detected in a background of one million bone marrow mononuclear cells (28,29,46).

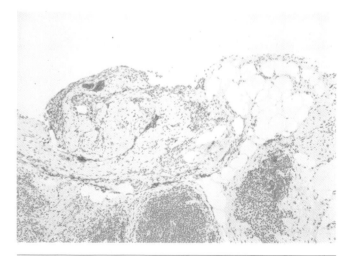

Figure 4.2 Immunohistochemical staining with monoclonal antibodies to cytokeratin (AE1 and CAM 5.2), showing a cluster of cancer cells in the lymph nodes of a patient with early-stage non–small cell lung cancer (magnification ×10).

Protein Markers—Analysis Using Quantum Dots

This is a relatively nascent and promising field, so far only a select few laboratories are examining this rather expensive approach. Quantum dots are nanometer-sized semiconductor particles with useful optical properties, such as fluorescence tunable by size and composition of the nanoparticles, where narrow and symmetric emission is coupled with broad excitation profiles that allow for single excitation light source. In comparison with the traditional organic dyes, quantum dots have remarkable photostability and bright intensity (47). With emission spectra as narrow as 12 nm (full width at half maximum), quantum dots minimize spectral overlap between different colors, making them an ideal label for multiplexing (48). With the ability to simultaneously study multiple protein markers by linking quantum dots of different color with specific antibodies, each disseminated tumor cell can be further characterized molecularly,

as shown in figure 4.3 of an example of a breast cancer cell line MCF-7.

Automated Detection of Disseminated Tumor Cells

Although immunohistochemical methods are extremely sensitive, manual microscopic screening of rare positive (i.e., antigen expressing) tumor cells is labor-intensive, time-consuming, and requires much expertise. Automated slide screening may facilitate the routine use of immunohistochemical methods to detect occult metastases. Based on our previous research in the detection of occult tumor cells in the bone marrow (2,31,44,46), we have tested the sensitivity, accuracy, and reproducibility of the Automated Cellular Imaging System (ACIS; Clarient Inc., Aliso Viejo, CA) (49) to detect these cells in the bone marrow. The automated system is controlled via an event-detection software program. In addition, the software allows the

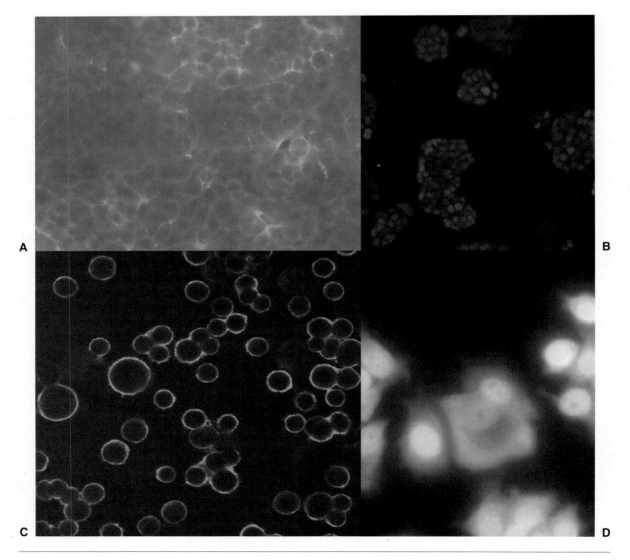

Figure 4.3 QD staining on MCF-7 ceil lines. **A.** EPCAM (Qp 565), **B.** Ki-67 (QD 655), **C.** HER2/neu (Qp 355), and **D.** three-color staining using quantum dots: orange = cytokeratin, red = epithelial cell adhesion molecule (EpCAM), turquoise = DAPI. (See color plates.)

microscope to be used in a manual mode. The microscope scans the entire specimen on the slide in an x and y plane, and identifies all positive events. A positive event is determined by previously programmed criteria based on specific instructions concerning size and color threshold. All positive events initially selected are re-examined at a higher power in order to save suspicious images for review. Questionable cells can be localized on the slides by the system, and the investigator can review the cell. During review, the investigator identifies the true positive, suspicious, and negative cells. The images of the negative cells can be deleted so that only the true positive and suspicious images are retained in memory. The results are automatically quantitated and can be stored permanently on optical disks, external hard drives, or hard copies can be printed. We have compared this method to our standard, clinically validated manual methods for detecting rare tumor cells in bone marrow and blood (49). Evaluation of the sensitivity, accuracy, and reproducibility of automated system was based on a comparison between results obtained by manual and automated screening methods. The results of our studies have shown that the sensitivity of the automated system is virtually identical to manual methods.

Flow Cytometric Analysis

Further separation of different cell types, which is based on different expression of cell surface antigens, is made possible by flow cytometry. Briefly, after incubation of cells with different antigens, cell suspension is subjected to flow cytometry. Although it may have a limited role in disseminated tumor cell enrichment, flow cytometry has mostly been used for analysis of cells, following enrichment by other methods (50).

Molecular Analysis Using Qualitative Reverse Transcriptase-Polymerase Chain Reaction

The molecular method usually employed for detection of disseminated tumor cells in bone marrow, lymph nodes, and peripheral blood is reverse transcriptase-polymerase chain reaction (RT-PCR), which differentiates gene expression between epithelial and lymphoid cells to identify epithelial cancer cells. RT-PCR entails the isolation and reverse-transcription of epithelial-specific messenger RNA to complementary-DNA (cDNA), and thereafter, involves PCR-based amplification of the cDNA template between specific primers. This results in a several thousand-fold amplification of the signal, and makes the method theoretically extremely sensitive. The drawbacks of the method include the chance of low-level epithelial gene expression from lymphoid cells that could result in high background, and the inability to employ morphologic criteria to confirm the presence of metastatic cells. Some of the studies have compared the immunocytochemistry-based detection with RT-PCR for sensitivity and concluded that RT-PCR may provide enhancement in detection, provided the target markers are sufficiently specific. Unfortunately, most of the molecular targets used in these RT-PCR assays have been shown to lack the requisite specificity because of illegitimate expression in nontarget hematopoietic cells (51), in addition to the variability in expression of the target genes even among the disseminated tumor cells.

We have evaluated the specificity of carcinoembryonic antigen, cytokeratin 19 (CK19), cytokeratin 20 (CK20), gastroin-testinal tumor-associated antigen 733.2 (GA 733.2), and mucin-1 (MUC-1) in the blood of healthy donors and lymph nodes from patients without cancer by RT-PCR. CK 20 was the only mRNA marker not detected in lymph nodes or blood from patients without cancer. This indicates clear limitation of the application of PCR techniques for the detection of disseminated tumor cells (52).

Since the first study by Smith and colleagues (53) in 1991, many authors have reported molecular diagnoses of disseminated tumor cells in the lymph nodes (54–56), bone marrow (57), and peripheral blood (58) in patients with various cancers.

Analysis Using Real-time Quantitative Reverse Transcriptase PCR

Real-time quantitative RT-PCR (q-RT-PCR) has the capability to greatly improve the detection of disseminated tumor cells because it combines high sensitivity with high throughput capability and provides quantitative information on gene expression (59,60). For the detection of disseminated tumor cells, the amplification of tumor-associated and/or tissue-specific or epithelium-restricted mRNA expression has usually been evaluated. Recently, the combination of different mRNA markers has been suggested to improve sensitivity in detecting occult tumor cells (61–64).

Although q-RT-PCR provides potentially higher sensitivity (down to one tumor cell in 10^7 normal cells) (65), enhanced detection is associated with a higher false-positive rate. The potential for quantitation of the low-level background transcription allows the definition of cutoff values for marker expression in background tissue, thus improving the specificity. Despite the claims of many publications, the sometimes unacceptably high false-positive rates of q-RT-PCR remain a problem.

Therefore, the density gradient and/or immunomagnetic tumor cell enrichment strategies are essential preparatory steps in disseminated tumor cells detection and purification, which can improve both sensitivity and specificity by eliminating mononuclear cells (66,67). Nevertheless, currently used enrichment techniques are all associated with loss of target cells to varying degrees and sensitivity of q-RT-PCR may be restrained by this fact as well.

Detection of Occult Tumor Cells in the Bone Marrow of Patients with Breast Cancer

The majority of patients with newly diagnosed breast cancer have operable disease, and these patients are considered potentially curable. However, 35% to 40% of these patients with no evidence of metastasis at the time of diagnosis develop recurrent disease after primary therapy. The most reliable prognostic parameters (lymph node status and tumor size) cannot predict which particular individuals will progress. As a result, several groups have recommended adjuvant treatment for patients with lymph node-negative disease. Although this is controversial (as the majority of node-negative patients will be clinically cured without adjuvant therapy), it is in this group of patients who have disseminated tumor cells that adjuvant therapy should be most successful. It would be of great value, therefore, to be able to further discriminate and identify those patients with early-stage disease who are most likely to recur. Detection of disseminated

Table 4.1

Antibodies Used to Detect Breast Cancer-Disseminated Tumor Cells

Type of Antigen	Specific Antigen	References
Cell surface antigen	EMA	Redding et al. (5)
		Mansi et al. (168)
	MBr 1	Porro et al. (81)
	17-1A	Schlimok et al. (3)
	T16, C26	Cote et al. (2)
Cytostructural antigens	Cytokeratin intermediate filament (e.g., AE1, CAM 5-2, A45-B/B3)	Cote et al. (2)
		Ellis et al. (30)
		Naume et al. (17)

EMA, epithelial membrane antigen.

tumor cells in these patients could be extremely beneficial in determining prognosis and in making treatment decisions.

Bone marrow is the single most common site of breast cancer metastasis, and up to 80% of patients with recurrent tumors will develop bony metastases at some point during evolution of their disease (68); it is also the most frequent initial site of clinically detectable breast cancer metastasis (69). Tumor cells are estimated to be present in the bone marrow of 10% to 45% of patients with primary operable breast cancer (2,5,31,70,71), and 10% to 70% of patients with metastatic breast cancer. As with most cancers, the most widely used method to detect disseminated tumor cells is immunohistochemistry.

Molecular methods to detect disseminated tumor cells are theoretically more sensitive and provide the possibility of automation. Datta et al. (72) used conventional PCR for keratin 19 transcript to identify cancer cells in the bone marrow and peripheral blood of breast cancer patients. Slade et al. (57) have recently shown the utility of real-time PCR analysis of keratin 19 in bone marrow and blood of early breast cancer patients at follow-up, after receiving adjuvant therapy. Another group has demonstrated the utility of real-time RT-PCR for keratin 19 and mammaglobin for detection of disseminated tumor cells to bone marrow of early breast cancer patients, with higher sensitivity as immunohistochemistry, and with great concordance in detection (73).

Nevertheless, because immunohistochemistry is the most widely used (and currently the most reliable) method for the detection of disseminated tumor cells in the bone marrow in breast cancer patients, we have summarized the results from several groups performing immunohistochemical assays using monoclonal antibodies (Table 4.1). In spite of the differences in techniques, antibodies, and patient populations among all the studies, it is striking that disseminated tumor cells in the bone marrow were detected in all of the studies.

Clinical Significance

Disseminated tumor cells to bone marrow have been correlated with known predictors of prognosis in several studies (70). The presence of disseminated tumor cells in the bone marrow has been correlated with pathologic tumor, node, and metastasis (TNM) stage in breast cancer. In our study, 23% of patients with stage I cancer, 38% of patients with stage II cancer, and 50% of patients with stage III cancer had extrinsic cells in the bone marrow (2). In the original study from the Ludwig Institute (5), the presence of bone marrow-disseminated tumor cells was correlated with the tumor stage ($p = 0.05$), and vascular invasion ($p < 0.01$), both of which are known predictors of poor prognosis.

Several studies have shown that the presence of disseminated tumor cells in the bone marrow identifies a population of patients at high risk for recurrence. The results of important trials are listed in Table 4.2. All the studies in Table 4.2 (31,71,74–80) demonstrate uniformly that patients with disseminated tumor cells in bone marrow have significantly higher recurrence rate as compared with patients in whom no disseminated tumor cells are detected. Finally, several studies have shown the

Table 4.2

Detection of Bone Marrow-Disseminated Tumor Cells (DTCBM) in Patients with Early-Stage Breast Cancer

Studies Performed by	No. of Patients	Clinical Follow-up (years)	% Patients Recurring (no.)		p Value
			DTCBM-Negative	DTCBM-Positive	
Dearnaley et al. (79), 1991	39	9.5	31 (8/26)	85 (11/13)	<0.05
Mansi et al. (74), 1999	350	12.5	25 (64/261)	48 (43/89)	<0.05
Cote et al. (31), 1991	49	2*	16 (5/31)	54 (7/13)	<0.04
Diel et al. (77), 1992	211	2	3 (4/130)	27 (22/81)	0.0001
Diel et al. (78), 1996	727	3	8 (34/412)	35 (109/315)	<0.001
Braun et al. (12), 2000	552	3.2	8 (28/353)	39 (79/199)	<0.001
Gebauer et al. (76), 2001	393	6	20 (46/227)	35 (59/166)	<0.001
Gerber et al. (75), 2001	554	4.5	9 (26/304)	24 (43/180)	0.0001
Wiedswang et al. (71), 2003	817	4	13.3 (94/709)	30.6 (33/108)	<0.001

independence of tumor cell dissemination to lymph nodes and bone marrow (2,8,77–82).

Recently published pooled analysis by Braun et al. (70) that involved 4,703 patients with early-stage breast cancer with 10-year follow-up demonstrates again that presence of disseminated tumor cells in the bone marrow at the time of diagnosis is associated with poor prognosis, poor overall survival, and breast-cancer-specific survival as well as poor disease-free survival and distant disease-free survival. This large study provides definitive evidence that the detection of disseminated tumor cells in the bone marrow by immunohistochemical methods is prognostically important. The presence of bone marrow-disseminated tumor cells predicts a higher risk for recurrence in bone as well as in other distant sites.

Of particular importance in all of these findings is the fact that the presence of disseminated tumor cells in the bone marrow identifies patients with node-negative disease who are at a higher risk for recurrence (31); this subset of patients can therefore be the target of more aggressive adjuvant therapy. Based on this evidence, the groups of patients could be stratified in three groups: (i) those with very low recurrence rates (lymph node-negative, bone marrow-negative), (ii) those with moderate rates of recurrence (lymph node-negative, bone marrow-positive, and lymph node-positive, bone marrow-negative), and (iii) those with high recurrence rates (lymph node-positive, bone marrow-positive) (Figure 4.4) (31,70,77,78,82). In addition, some studies have recently shown that disseminated tumor cells persist in bone marrow after adjuvant chemotherapy (57) and repeated bone marrow aspiration can be used to predict outcome in breast cancer patients (83).

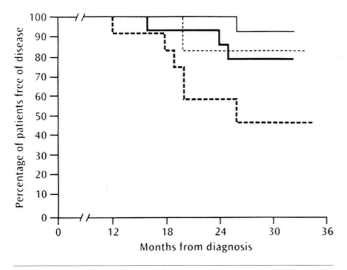

Figure 4.4 Disease free interval of patients with breast cancer according to bone marrow and axillary lymph node status. Patients who were lymph node-positive, bone marrow-positive (- - - - -, thick line) had a significantly shorter time to recurrence than patients who were lymph node-negative (—, thin line), $p <0.04$. Patients who were lymph node-negative, bone marrow-positive (- - - - -, thin line), and lymph node-positive, bone marrow-negative (—, thick line) had intermediate time to recurrence.

Another interesting finding from our studies (31) is that the number of carcinoma cells detected in the bone marrow (the bone marrow tumor burden) was significantly associated with disease recurrence. Patients with occult tumor cells who did not have recurrence had on an average fewer extrinsic cells in their marrow than those who had a recurrence (15 vs. 43 cells, respectively). The estimated 2-year recurrence rate of the 13 patients with 10 or more cells was significantly higher (46%) than that of the 36 patients with less than 10 cells (6%, $p <0.006$).

Detection of Occult Metastases in the Lymph Nodes of Patients with Breast Cancer

A subset of node-negative patients without evidence of bone marrow occult metastases will also experience recurrence. The axillary lymph nodes are, therefore, another possible site for occult tumor spread in node-negative breast cancer patients. Axillary lymph node metastases can be detected by serial sectioning, immunohistochemistry, or RT-PCR methods. Studies undertaken to detect occult lymph node metastases by routine histologic methods have generally been performed by cutting serial sections from all paraffin blocks containing lymph nodes, followed by routine staining and microscopic review. Between 7% and 33% of previously node-negative cases convert to node-positive after review (84). Several investigators have used immunohistochemistry to detect occult lymph node metastases in patients with breast cancer. Most studies have used antibodies specific for low-molecular-weight intermediate filament proteins to distinguish the epithelial tumor deposits from normal node elements. In our own studies, we have used a cocktail of two antikeratin antibodies, AE1 and Cam5.2. Although antibodies to cytokeratins have been reported to react with dendritic reticulum cells (with the possibility of producing false-positive results), this has not been a significant problem in our own experience. As with the bone marrow, the morphologic evaluation of the "positive" cells is critical; cells that do not possess the morphologic characteristics of malignant epithelial cells are not considered tumor cells in our studies. In most studies using one or two sections for immunohistochemical assessment per block, the conversion rate to node-positive is 10% to 12% (85).

As in the case of immunohistochemistry, for detection of occult lymph node metastases by RT-PCR, epithelial-specific gene expression is used to distinguish between epithelial (cancer) cells and lymphoid cells. A number of potential markers have become available with advances in molecular oncology. Keratin 19, keratins 8 and 18, mucin 1 (MUC-1), and β-human chorionic gonadotropin are few examples that have been used to breast cancer cells metastatic to the lymph nodes (86–89). Recent use of multimarker assay and real-time PCR has been promising; nevertheless, the results still have to be validated in prospective large clinical trials (88,90).

Clinical Significance of Occult Lymph Node Metastases in Patients with Breast Cancer

Although virtually all studies have demonstrated that lymph node metastases can be overlooked, there is a surprising disagreement about the prognostic importance of these occult tumor deposits. Many of the initial studies have found that the presence of occult lymph node metastases does not influence the recurrence rates in a statistically significant way (91–96). In order to begin to understand this, a few basic observations need to be made. Many earlier studies have involved fewer than 100 patients; in fact, some have involved even fewer than 50 patients. Cote and Groshen have demonstrated that, even if the finding of occult lymph node metastases is prognostically important, there is no possibility that studies of the clinical impact of occult lymph node metastases involving few patients will provide statistically significant data (unpublished observation, 1994), a fact that first was clearly pointed out by Fisher et al. (97): "It has been mathematically estimated that differences in survival of 10 percent, if indeed they occur between the two groups [true lymph node negative versus occult lymph node positive], would require a study of approximately 1400 cases." Therefore, studies involving a few patients are not suitable to address the issue of prognostic significance of occult lymph node metastases.

Investigators from the LICR and International Breast Cancer study group have performed a definitive study of the importance of occult lymph node metastases in patients with node-negative breast cancer (98). They examined serial sections of 921 node-negative breast cancer patients by routine histologic methods. Nine percent of these patients were found to have occult lymph node metastases; these patients had a poorer disease-free ($p = 0.003$) and overall survival ($p = 0.002$) after 5-year median follow-up, compared with patients whose nodes remained negative after serial sectioning. Six-year median follow-up data give even more conclusive evidence of the prognostic significance of occult lymph node metastases (84). Another large-scale study was performed by de Mascarel et al. (99) with a median follow-up of 7 years. These investigators studied the lymph nodes from 1,121 patients with primary operable breast cancer, by serial macroscopic sectioning; they found single occult lymph node metastases in 120 patients. A significant difference in recurrence ($p = 0.005$) and survival ($p = 0.04$) was found between node-negative patients and those with single occult metastases. However, in multivariate analysis using the Cox model, occult metastases were not a predicting factor. This apparent difference may be related to menopausal status. Reassessment of the results showed these occult metastases were associated with significantly poor disease-free and overall survival in postmenopausal patients but not in premenopausal patients (100). Immunohistochemically detected occult lymph node metastases remained an independent and highly significant predictor of recurrence, even after control for tumor grade, tumor size, estrogen-receptor status, vascular invasion, and treatment ($p = 0.007$) in this patient group.

Although there is ample evidence showing that occult lymph node metastases can be detected in a substantial proportion of node-negative patients and that the presence of such deposits is probably prognostically significant, the best method for detecting these deposits is not yet clear. Re-examination of multiple serial sections is laborious, time-consuming, and expensive. Immunohistochemical assays, on the other hand, are more sensitive and certainly less laborious. Definitive comparative analyses are now ongoing; results from these studies suggest that immunohistochemical methods may be superior to histologic re-examination of lymph node serial sections.

In order to provide a definitive answer and to evaluate the role and clinical significance of disseminated tumor cells in the bone marrow and lymph nodes of patients with early-stage breast cancer, the American College of Surgeons Oncology Group (ACOSOG) conducted a multicenter cooperative group trial. Patients were enrolled by the ACOSOG and our laboratory provided the scientific nucleus to support the clinical trials. In this capacity, the laboratory has processed, stained, and stored bone marrows and lymph nodes for both studies and provided pathologic interpretations. Aims included identification and quantification of disseminated tumor cells and correlation of the presence of these tumor cells with intermediate markers of tumor progression, and ultimately with recurrence and survival. Sentinel lymph nodes and bone marrow specimens from >3,600 patients with early-stage breast cancer have been collected and analyzed. This study has been closed for enrollment and results remain blinded.

Detection of Disseminated Tumor Cells in Peripheral Blood of Breast Cancer Patients

Efforts to detect circulating tumor cells in the peripheral blood have paralleled those for analysis of bone marrow. In an early study, Redding et al. (5) found the yield of tumor cells from peripheral blood to be extremely low. Many investigators have attempted to isolate these cells using the Ficoll-Hypaque density gradient method. However, this method is time-consuming, labor-intensive, and has a recovery rate of only about 68% (101). Therefore, alternative enrichment techniques have been attempted (15,17), and only recently, a positive clinical trial has been reported using an automated immunomagnetic tumor cell enrichment, demonstrating the significant prognostic value of presence of circulating tumor cells in peripheral blood of metastatic breast cancer patients (102). In this study, patients with five or more circulating tumor cells did worse than patients with fewer than five circulating tumor cells ($p = 0.0014$). Circulating tumor cells present in blood both before and after initiation of therapy were strong independent prognostic factors. The strength of this study, therefore, is the demonstration of a cutoff level for prognostic significance, influencing the outcome of patients, and the utility of detection of circulating tumor cells to monitor therapeutic efficacy (102,103). Although the method for circulating tumor cell enrichment from peripheral blood of cancer patients employed in this trial cannot yet be regarded as a definitive assay standard technology, the study demonstrates that with more effective circulating tumor cell enrichment, peripheral blood represents a suitable source of patient material to be analyzed for assessment of early metastatic dissemination. A more reliable and effective enrichment technique could therefore enable us to analyze blood of early-stage cancer patients and find the significance comparable with analysis using bone marrow, a more invasively obtained clinical resource.

Particularly in peripheral blood, PCR assays have been used to detect circulating tumor cells. Mostly, these studies have used keratin 19 and/or breast-specific markers for detection of circulating tumor cells. Smith et al. (104) have shown that circulating carcinoma cells are frequently found in patients with metastatic breast cancer by quantitative PCR for keratin 19, parallel to immunocytochemistry. In the majority of patients, cancer cell numbers as evaluated by quantitative PCR or immunocytochemistry reflected the outcome of systemic treatment, the results of quantitative PCR were more commonly in agreement with response to treatment than immunocytochemical methods (104). Stathopoulou et al. (105) have also demonstrated the utility of keratin 19 as a marker for detection of circulating tumor cells, using a highly sensitive and specific method, showing that it can be used for high-throughput continuous monitoring and quantification of circulating epithelial cells in the peripheral blood of breast cancer patients.

Another marker used for detection of circulating tumor cells in peripheral blood of breast cancer patients is mammaglobin, used as a single marker (106,107), or in a combination of markers (62,108,109). Results from trials using quantitative PCR techniques are encouraging. However, if more markers are used, costs still represent a barrier of implementation into clinical routine.

DISSEMINATED TUMOR CELLS: BIOLOGIC PROPERTIES

Recently, there have been efforts made to characterize the biology of detected disseminated tumor cells, and to demonstrate that these cells harbor malignant potential. Genetic characterization of single cytokeratin-positive tumor cells that were detected in bone marrow of patients with early breast cancer has been attempted (109,110). A recently published article on the genomic changes of disseminated tumor cells by Schardt (109,111) demonstrates that genetic changes found in disseminated tumor cells match early changes in breast cancer primary tumors and indicate that dissemination may happen even before the tumor has become malignant. These findings may have substantial impact on the future of breast cancer disease, although this is yet to be proven.

Recently, global gene expression profiling of circulating tumor cells in peripheral blood from breast, colon, and prostate cancer patients with metastatic disease has been published (112). Some other tumor-associated antigens like uPAR (113) or ERBB2 (HER2/neu) have also been used to characterize these cells (114).

Muller et al. (115) have shown that circulating tumor cells have low proliferative activity by analyzing them for expression of Ki-67. This finding indicates the reason for insensitivity of the circulating tumor cells to chemotherapeutics that target proliferating cells and most probably correlates with the theory of cancer stem cells (116) (see later discussion). Studies based on the immunohistochemical analysis of the cells have already given insight into the phenotypic characterization of the tumor cell. However, these analyses may be improved by employing quantum dots, which will allow for simultaneous evaluation of three or more markers in the same setting. Profiling of the circulating tumor cells at the mRNA level is restricted because of the previously described problem of rarity of these cells on the background of high number of hematopoietic cells.

There has been accumulating evidence that breast cancers arise from breast cancer stem cells, a small subpopulation of tumor cells that are able to divide indefinitely and generate different clones of tumor cells (116). These findings have also had an impact on the research of disseminated tumor cells, and efforts are underway to characterize these cells for stem cell properties. We have examined bone marrows from patients with early

breast cancer previously confirmed to have CK-positive cells for the prevalence of putative stem cell phenotype (CD44$^+$CD24$^-$) within the CK-positive cells. CD44 is a cell adhesion molecule known to be expressed in most cell types and has been associated with stem cells in normal breast tissue (117). It has been suggested also as a homing factor to bone marrow (118). Although the role of CD24 has not yet been well understood, recent literature suggests that expression of CD24 reduces stromal cell-derived factor-1-mediated migration and signaling via CXCR4 in breast cancer cell lines with enhanced CD24 expression, suppressing their metastatic potential. On the contrary, the metastatic potential of CD24 cells is increased as evidenced by siRNA inhibition (119). Surprisingly, we have identified such a phenotype (CD44$^+$CD24$^-$) in all patients among their disseminated tumor cells. This finding may have an impact on future research of occult tumor cells as well as therapeutic impact (120).

All these findings support the "seed and soil" theory proposed by Paget (121). However, whereas the seed element of the theory has been extensively explored, the soil element still remains largely an enigma. Microenvironment appears to play as important role in the biology of disseminated tumor cells, and the insight into it represents a significant challenge for the scientific community.

Detection of Disseminated Tumor Cells in the Bone Marrow of Patients with Lung Cancer

Although lung cancer is the second most common form of cancer, it is estimated to be the leading cause of cancer deaths in both men and women in the United States for 2008 (122). Once a tumor has developed, surgery (either alone or in combination with adjuvant therapy) represents the only potentially curative modality of treatment (123,124). Of the four major histologic types of lung cancer (squamous, adenocarcinoma, large cell, small cell), only small cell carcinoma is generally considered refractory to surgical therapy. However, small cell carcinoma accounts for approximately 20% of lung tumors overall (125); thus, 80% of lung cancers would be potentially curable by surgery if detected early enough.

The use of the TNM staging system and the staging map of the mediastinal lymph nodes is a major indicator of the curative potential and prognosis of lung cancer (126,127). For non–small cell lung cancer, accurate staging of disease has greater prognostic significance than cell type. Patients with T1N0M0 (stage I) lung cancer treated with surgical resection have an anticipated 5-year survival rate of 60% to 85%. For larger carcinomas such as T2N0M0 (stage I), patients have a 50% to 60% 5-year survival rate. However, survival rates decrease dramatically with increasing stage of disease, particularly related to the presence of metastases in regional lymph nodes. In the case of stage III lung cancer, when completely resected, survival rate varies between 3% and 13% (123).

The ability to detect the earliest spread of lung cancer would identify several important groups of patients, including those with low-stage (stage I) disease who have evidence of disseminated tumor cells and who may, therefore, benefit from adjuvant systemic treatment. In addition, among patients with locally advanced (stage III) disease, patients without disseminated tumor cells may be identified who may benefit more from aggressive local (surgical) control of their tumor.

Significance of Bone Marrow Disseminated Tumor Cells in Patients with Lung Cancer

The earliest study by Frew et al. (43) did not show any advantage of using immunohistochemistry to detect disseminated tumor cells in the bone marrow of patients with non–small cell lung cancer over routine histopathologic examination. Pantel et al. (40) observed that bone marrow-disseminated tumor cells could be detected in up to 21.9% (18 of 82 cases) of operable non–small cell lung cancer. The detection of bone marrow-disseminated tumor cells was significantly associated with size and histologic grade of the primary carcinoma. However, the association with metastatic involvement of regional lymph nodes as determined by routine histologic staining was weaker. This supports the view that hematogenous spread of lung cancer cells represents an event distinct from regional spread of tumor (to lymph nodes). They observed that the presence of bone marrow-disseminated tumor cells in patients with non–small cell lung cancer was significantly associated with the development of metastatic disease.

We have shown that bone marrow-disseminated tumor cells can be detected in a substantial proportion of patients with lung cancer who show no clinical evidence of systemic metastasis, including patients with the earliest stage of disease (stage I) (44). The rate of detection of bone marrow-disseminated tumor cells was associated with stage of disease; 29% of patients with stage I or II and 46% of patients with stage III disease had detectable bone marrow-disseminated tumor cells. The presence of bone marrow occult tumor cells was significantly associated with higher recurrence rates and a shorter time to recurrence for patients with primary localized (stage I-III) non–small cell lung cancer (35.1 vs. 7.3 months, $p = 0.0009$). Similar results were seen in comparisons of bone marrow status to overall survival. Although the presence of bone marrow occult metastases was related to stage of disease, it was independent of stage in predicting recurrence. These results for stage I lung cancer have

been confirmed in a more recent trial in which both lymph nodes and bone marrow have been analyzed (128).

Parallel to ACOSOG Z0010 (see earlier discussion), the ACOSOG Z0040 clinical trial was performed; the aims included identification and quantification of the disseminated tumor cells in the bone marrow and lymph nodes of patients with early-stage non–small cell lung carcinoma and the determination of whether the presence of disseminated tumor cells is associated with clinical outcome. In addition, novel imaging and molecular methods for the detection and characterization of the biology of disseminated tumor cells in early-stage lung cancer were developed. Nearly 900 bone marrow and lymph node specimens from patients with primary lung cancer have been collected and are being analyzed.

Other studies demonstrating the importance of detection of occult tumor cells in non–small cell lung cancer are listed in Table 4.3. Ohgami et al. (129) also performed immunostaining of p53 protein in the corresponding primary tumors and showed that overexpression of p53 was associated with positivity of the tumor cells in the bone marrow. According to the published studies, the presence of disseminated tumor cells in bone marrow appears to be a clinically important and independent predictor of recurrence and survival in patients with non–small cell lung carcinoma.

Small cell lung cancer has a high propensity for metastasis, both to regional lymph nodes and to distant sites, and primary surgical therapy (even in combination with chemotherapy and radiation therapy) is not considered a viable therapeutic option. In order to identify patients who may most benefit from adjuvant therapy, studies to detect disseminated tumor cells have been undertaken. Leonard et al. (42) showed that disseminated tumor cells in bone marrow could be detected in 8 of 12 (67%) cases of small cell lung cancer. Moreover, recurrences were observed in seven of eight (88%) of patients with detectable bone marrow disseminated tumor cells, and three of four (75%) of patients with no detectable disseminated tumor cells (Table 4.3). In a later study by Pasini et al. (130), 108 bone marrow samples were taken from 60 patients with small cell lung cancer and stained with Ab MUC1 using the immunohistochemical method. They

---

Table 4.3

Detection of Bone Marrow-Disseminated Tumor Cells (DTCBM) in Lung Cancer

Studies Performed by	No. of Patients	Antibody	% Patients Recurring (no.)		p Value
			DTCBM-Negative	DTCBM-Positive	
Pantel et al. (40), 1993	82	CK 18	37 (15/41)	67 (10/15)	DTCBM-positive associated with skeletal metastases = 0.0004; associated with shorter recurrence-free survival
Pantel et al. (41), 1996	139	CK 18	35 (19/54)	75 (9/12)	
Cote et al. (44), 1995	43	CK	23 (6/26)	76 (13/17)	
Ohgami et al. (129), 1997	39	CK 18	62 (24/39)	38 (15/39)	
Leonard et al. (42), 1990	12	EMA, CK	75 (3/4)	88 (7/8)	

EMA, epithelial membrane antigen; CK, cytokeratin.

were able to detect positive cells in 23 patients (38%). In 16 of these patients there were more than 10 positive cells or clumps of cells in aspirates (14 patients) or a positive bone marrow biopsy (2 patients). This group of patients had a poorer median survival (5.5 vs. 11 months, $p = 0.01$) than those with negative bone marrow samples or less than 10 positive cells in the aspirates.

Detection of Disseminated Tumor Cells in Lymph Nodes in Patients with Lung Cancer

Surprisingly few studies have been done on the significance of lymph node occult metastases. Chen et al. (131) used the polyclonal antikeratin antibody to demonstrate that keratin-positive cells could be detected in the regional lymph nodes of 38 of 60 (63%) cases with node-negative non–small cell lung cancer. The median survival of patients with occult metastases was shorter than that of patients whose nodes contained no tumor, although this finding did not reach the level of statistical significance. Passlick et al. (132) used the monoclonal antibody Ber-Ep4 (also called *EpCAM*) against two glycoproteins of 34 and 49 kd, present on the surface and cytoplasm of epithelial cells (133), to study the regional lymph nodes of 72 patients with node-negative non–small cell lung cancer. They found that 11 of 72 (15.3%) of patients demonstrated positively staining cells in the lymph nodes. The detection of occult metastatic cells was positively correlated with a shorter disease-free survival, while no correlation was obtained with grade, size of tumor, or the presence of occult bone marrow metastases. These results were confirmed in an ongoing study analyzing a total of 565 lymph nodes harvested from 125 patients with completely resected non–small cell lung cancer staged as pathologic (p) T1-4 N0-2 M0 by conventional histopathology (134). Another smaller study has recently confirmed these findings (135). Few studies have demonstrated the utility of RT-PCR methods to prove the clinical significance of tumor cells disseminated to regional lymph nodes in lung cancer patients (136–138).

Detection of Disseminated Tumor Cells in Bone Marrow of Patients with Prostate Cancer

Carcinoma of the prostate is the most common malignancy and the third leading cause of cancer-related death in men (122). Five-year relative survival varies with stage at diagnosis from 80% or more when malignancy is confined to the prostate to about 25% where metastases are present (139). The most frequent site of distant metastasis is the axial skeleton. Of those patients who develop metastasis, median survival time is 2.5 to 3 years. Patients with apparently localized prostate cancer who relapse following radical prostatectomy are presumed to have undetected occult metastatic dissemination at initial presentation. The ability to identify this group of patients could modify therapy aimed at local control of disease, and might form the basis for administration of adjuvant therapy early in the disease process.

Conventional microscopic examination of bone marrow aspirates in patients with operable (stage A-C) prostate cancer is of limited utility (140,141). Using an immunohistochemical method that identifies epithelial cells, Mansi et al. (142) demonstrated that 13% of patients with operable prostate cancer had occult tumor cells in the bone marrow, while 73% of cases with

confirmed metastatic disease had detectable bone marrow occult tumor cells. Oberneder et al. (36) were able to detect CK18-positive cells in the bone marrow samples of 33% of patients with stage N0M0 prostate cancer; the incidence of occult tumor cells showed a significant correlation with established risk factors, such as local tumor extent, distant metastases, and tumor differentiation. In our own study (39), we used a panel of monoclonal antibodies that recognize epithelial cell-specific membrane and cytoskeletal antigens in an immunofluorescence assay. We found that 22% cases with localized disease and 36% of cases with metastatic prostate cancer, including 100% of patients with bony metastases, had antigen-positive cells in the bone marrow. The serum prostate-specific antigen (PSA) level, a parameter used widely to detect residual/recurrent disease, appeared to correlate with the presence of occult metastases. In addition, the number of antigen-positive cells detected appears to correlate with the stage of disease.

Efforts are underway to use molecular methods to detect occult metastatic cells in patients with prostate cancer, where it is particularly advantageous to use RT-PCR because antigens such as PSA are considered to be specific to prostate tissue; any positive result is expected to be from circulating prostate cancer cells. Several studies have demonstrated the utility of RT-PCR for PSA to detect cells disseminated to bone marrow (37,143–145). Smith et al. (146) demonstrated PSA mRNA in epithelial and leukemia cell lines, as well as blood. The low level of expression of PSA mRNA in blood cells may interfere with PCR methods to detect prostate cancer occult metastases.

In general, from 13% to 38% patients with apparently localized prostate cancer have been shown to have detectable occult metastatic cells in the bone marrow using a variety of technologies. The best criterion regarding the malignant nature of the occult tumor cells is whether they were present in patients who ultimately developed recurrent disease. Whether this is the case with prostate cancer remains to be determined through more extensive studies and clinical follow-up.

Detection of Disseminated Tumor Cells in Lymph Nodes of Patients with Prostate Cancer

As previously indicated, a subset of patients with prostate cancer who undergo radical prostatectomy will suffer recurrence, even in the absence of clinically or pathologically detectable regional or systemic metastases.

The highest recurrence and progression rates in patients with regionally confined disease occur among those with pathologic stage C (pT3N0) tumors, that is, tumors with no histologic evidence of lymph node metastases (147). Recurrence in these cases is presumably by occult spread of tumor. The detection of regional or systemic spread of tumor at its earliest stages might therefore identify patients at the greatest risk for recurrence and progression of disease.

Pathologic analyses using routine histochemical methods can detect lymph node metastases in 10% to 15% of patients undergoing surgery for clinical stages A to C (T1 to T3). The extent of pelvic lymph node involvement has been shown to correlate with disease progression and death, with increasing rates of each with single, multiple, and gross nodal involvement (148–151).

Thus, the detection of regional lymph node metastases is crucial to predict the outcome in patients with prostate cancer.

Initial studies (148,150) performed to detect pelvic lymph node occult metastases in prostate cancer patients involved small and heterogeneous population of patients with prostate cancer (clinical and pathologic stages A through D). These studies concluded that occult lymph node metastases are found in a small percentage of patients (approximately 3%) with prostate cancer and suggested that the immunohistochemical detection of occult lymph node metastases is neither cost-effective nor practical. To define more completely the incidence of lymph node occult metastases in prostate cancer, we performed a larger study involving a pathologically homogenous group of patients with operable prostate cancer at high risk for recurrence (stage pT3N0); that is, tumors with extracapsular spread of tumor but no histologic evidence of lymph node metastases. Occult tumor cells were found in 24 of 180 patients (13.3%). The presence of occult tumor cells was significantly associated with increased recurrence and decreased survival compared with patients without occult tumor cells ($p < 0.001$ and $p = 0.019$, respectively). The presence of occult lymph node metastases was an independent predictor of recurrence and death in a multivariable analysis (152).

Detection of Occult Tumor Cells in the Bone Marrow in Patients with Colorectal Cancer

Colorectal carcinoma is one of the most common malignancies in the Western world, and still shows an increasing incidence. Despite advances in early detection, the 5-year survival rate of patients with resectable tumors is about 70% (122). Identification of the subset of patients in whom the primary tumor has metastasized would have considerable significance.

Several investigators have examined the clinical significance of detecting disseminated tumor cells in the bone marrow of patients with colorectal cancer, even though colorectal cancer rarely involves the skeleton as the metastatic site. Schlimok et al. (33) found cytokeratin-positive cells in 27% (42 of 156) of cases with Dukes stage A to D colorectal cancer. Using double-labeling techniques, they also found that 20% to 50% of the disseminated tumor cells expressed proliferation-associated antigens. Lindeman et al. (34) found that patients with bone marrow-disseminated tumor cells had shorter recurrence-free intervals than those without ($p = 0.0084$), and that detection of disseminated tumor cells was an independent indicator of disease relapse ($p = 0.0035$). Recurrence rates of patients with disseminated tumor cells to bone marrow were higher than of those without disseminated tumor cells. Subsequent to these studies, other investigators have found disseminated tumor cells in the bone marrow of patients with colorectal cancer by any of the available means (153–157).

The discrepancy between clinically rare bony metastasis and the frequently detected disseminated tumor cells in bone marrow in colon cancer has been the subject of much speculation. According to the original concept of Paget (121), Schlimok et al. (33) suggested that although the tumor cells are capable of proliferating and developing into metastatic deposits, the microenvironment (in this case, the bone marrow) also determines whether the tumor cells will proliferate. Although overt metastases may not develop in the skeleton, the disseminative capability of metastatic cells from an individual tumor is demonstrated by their presence in the bone marrow.

Detection of Occult Tumor Cells in Lymph Nodes of Patients with Colorectal Cancer

For prognosis of colorectal cancer, TNM and Dukes staging are considered the most important in clinical practice (158,159). A central point in staging is the involvement of the regional lymph nodes with metastatic tumor cells. Approximately 25% of patients with Dukes stage B carcinoma (i.e., no histologic evidence of lymph node metastases) die within 5 years and it is obvious that in these patients microscopic dissemination of their tumor had occurred at the time of initial diagnosis. Detection of these microscopic tumor deposits that are undetectable by routine histopathology may be of great relevance in diagnosing tumors.

Immunohistochemical detection of occult metastatic cells in patients with localized disease (Dukes stage B) has been demonstrated by several investigators. Most of the studies showed the presence of occult metastases in the regional lymph nodes in a substantial proportion of patients with localized colorectal cancer, but not all studies show prognostic significance of finding these occult metastases (160–162). Greenson et al. (163), however, showed that the presence of cytokeratin-positive cells within the lymph nodes correlated with a significantly poorer prognosis. Mescoli et al. (159) evaluated the prevalence of occult tumor cells in regional lymph nodes from 309 colorectal cancer patients and demonstrated that more than 50% of pN0 patients have occult tumor cells in mesenteric lymph nodes. Occult tumor cells status correlated significantly with both cancer stage and vascular cancer invasion; however, their clinicopathologic impact still remains to be prospectively evaluated.

Detection of Occult Metastases in Other Cancers

The presence of occult bone marrow metastases or circulating tumor cells has been studied for a variety of solid tumors. These are listed in Table 4.4.

Neuroblastoma is the most common extracranial solid tumor in childhood (164). Although the prognosis of this malignancy has improved with advances in medical management, the overall 5-year survival rate is currently only 55%. Evaluation of bone marrow by standard cytologic analysis is a routine and important component of clinical staging. Morphologic distinction between tumor cells and primitive lymphoblasts can be difficult; therefore, immunohistochemical methods have been employed to detect circulating malignant cells. Important trials are listed in Table 4.4.

The prognosis of patients with melanoma is influenced by the presence of malignant involvement of regional lymph nodes; the survival rate is significantly decreased when the lymph nodes are involved. Prophylactic regional lymph node dissection is recommended for patients with intermediate-thickness melanomas (0.76 to 4 mm). The presence of lymph node metastases is an important criterion in determining the appropriate adjuvant therapy. Because of the prognostic and therapeutic implications, it is important to identify occult lymph node metastases in patients

Table 4.4

Detection of Disseminated Tumor Cells (DTC) to Bone Marrow (BM) in Various Cancers

Tumor	Method	Target Gene/Antigen	% of Patients with DTC in BM (no.)	References
Neuroblastoma	IHC	Neuroblastoma-specific antigen	66 (131/197)	Moss et al. (169)
	RT-PCR	Tyrosine hydroxylase	NA	Naito et al. (170)
	RT-PCR	PGP 9.5	44 (8/18)	Mattano et al. (171)
Uveal melanoma	RT-PCR	Tyrosinase	50 (3/6)	Tobal et al. (172)
Ovarian cancer	IHC	Cytokeratin	24 (12/50)	Cain et al. (173)
Pancreatic cancer	IHC	CEA, Mucin	58 (15/26)	Juhl et al. (154)
Gastric cancer	IHC	CEA, Mucin	25 (9/36)	Juhl et al. (154)
Cervical cancer	RT-PCR	HPV E6/E7	91 (10/11)	Czegledy et al. (174)

IHC, immunohistochemistry; RT-PCR, reverse transcriptase-polymerase chain reaction; CEA, carcinoembryonic antigen.

with melanoma. Several studies have addressed the question of the presence of occult tumor cells in regional lymph nodes of melanoma patients, showing that the incidence of occult metastases was correlated with known predictors of prognosis and associated with a poorer survival (165,166). A multiple-marker q-RT assay has been proven to upstage histopathology-negative sentinel lymph nodes, and determine a group with enhanced risk for recurrence and death of disease (167).

SUMMARY AND FUTURE PROSPECTS

The concept of occult metastases has existed for more than 4 decades. Over the years, investigators have attempted to improve techniques for detecting occult metastatic cells, and to attribute clinical significance to the detection of such occult metastases. The majority of the work has been done in breast cancer, but an increasing body of literature exists on occult metastases detection in other cancers.

Occult metastases in the bone marrow have been shown to be of prognostic significance in a variety of malignancies, for example, breast, lung, and colorectal cancer and neuroblastoma. On the other hand, there has been a surprising disagreement about the prognostic importance of occult lymph node metastases, especially in breast cancer, although, increasingly, more studies are showing a clinical significance of detecting such occult metastases. Similarly, in colorectal cancer, the prognostic significance of occult lymph node metastases has not been shown conclusively. In lung cancer, prostate cancer, and in melanoma, detection of occult lymph node metastases has been shown to be of prognostic importance.

The presence of occult metastases (in the lymph nodes and/or bone marrow) may define not only patients who are at higher risk for recurrence and death at worse prognosis, but may also identify biologically distinct mechanisms of tumor spread (e.g., lymphatic vs. vascular dissemination). Use of techniques to detect and characterize occult tumor cells may also allow us to identify biologically important population of cells, that is, those cells constituting the earliest metastatic population of tumor cells. Thus, techniques that identify occult metastases may

be valuable in furthering our understanding of the events regulating tumor dissemination.

The detection of tumor cells circulating in peripheral blood has been of increasing importance. The barriers coming from inefficient detection techniques have slowed down the progress of the field of circulating tumor cells in particular. However, these problems seem to be addressed with recent technical advances. As already pointed out in the discussion of cell enrichment, we have attempted to address the technical problems of detection of circulating tumor cells by development of a microdevice for capture of tumor cells on a background of hematopoietic cells. We very much hope that it is one way that the detection of circulating tumor cells in breast cancer patients and patients with other cancers promises will gain on importance in the future.

Improvement in the value of disseminated tumor cell detection assays will come from methods that not just capture and count, but actually characterize the phenotype and genotype of these cells. The characterization of subclones, such as stem cells, will be of definitive importance.

A new concept that is emerging in the staging of cancers is the TNnMm classification, where the traditional T (tumor), N (node), and M (metastasis) may be complemented by n and m (nodal and systemic occult metastases). With larger studies on prognostic significance of occult metastases, either in bone marrow or lymph nodes, this staging may be applied clinically, and the estimates of outcome for populations of patients may be narrowed down to those for subpopulations of patients (i.e., those with or without occult metastases). Similarly, in the future, treatment decisions may be based on the detection of occult metastases.

REFERENCES

1. Cote RJ. Occult metastases: real harm or false alarm? *J Thor and Cardivasc Surg.* 2003;126:332–333.
2. Cote RJ, Rosen PP, Hakes TB, et al. Monoclonal antibodies detect occult breast carcinoma metastases in bone marrow of patients with early-stage disease. *Am J Surg Pathol.* 1988;12:333–40.
3. Schlimok G, Funke I, Holzman B, et al. Micrometastatic cancer cells in bone marrow: In vitro detection with anticytokeratin and

in vivo anti-17-1A monoclonal antibody. *Proc Natl Acad Sci U S A.* 1987;84:8672.

4. Dearnaley DP, Sloan JP, Imrie S, et al. Detection of isolated mammary carcinoma cells in marrow of patients with primary breast cancer. *J R Soc Med.* 1983;76:359.

5. Redding WH, Monaghan P, Imrie SF. Detection of micrometastases in patients with primary breast cancer. *Lancet.* 1983:1271–1274.

6. Pantel K, Brakenhoff RH. Dissecting the metastatic cascade. *Nat Rev Cancer.* 2004;4(6):448–456.

7. Pierga JY, Bonneton C, Vincent-Salomon A, et al. Clinical significance of immunocytochemical detection of tumor cells using digital microscopy in peripheral blood and bone marrow of breast cancer patients. *Clin Cancer Res.* 2004;10(4):1392–1400.

8. Trocciola SM, Hoda S, Osborne MP, et al. Do bone marrow micrometastases correlate with sentinel lymph node metastases in breast cancer patients? *J Am Coll Surg.* 2005;200(5):720–725; discussion 5–6.

9. Gusterson BA, Ott R. Occult axillary lymph node micrometastases in breast cancer. *Lancet.* 1990;336:434–435.

10. Neville AM. Breast cancer micrometastases in lymph nodes and bone marrow are prognostically important. *Ann Oncol.* 1989;2:13–14.

11. Pantel K, Schlimok G, Angstwurm M, et al. Methodological analysis of immunocytochemical screening for disseminated epithelial tumor cells in bone marrow. *J Hematother.* 1994;3:165–173.

12. Braun S, Pantel K, Muller P, et al. Cytokeratin-positive cells in the bone marrow and survival of patients with stage I, II, or III breast cancer. *New Engl J Med.* 2000;342(8):525–533.

13. Braun S, Naume B. Circulating and disseminated tumor cells. *J Clin Oncol.* 2005;23(8):1623–1626.

14. Rosenberg R, Gertler R, Friederichs J, et al. Comparison of two density gradient centrifugation systems for the enrichment of disseminated tumor cells in blood. *Cytometry.* 2002;49(4):150–158.

15. Witzig TE, Bossy B, Kimlinger T, et al. Detection of circulating cytokeratin-positive cells in the blood of breast cancer patients using immunomagnetic enrichment and digital microscopy. *Clin Cancer Res.* 2002;8(5):1085–1091.

16. Naume B, Borgen E, Nesland JM, et al. Increased sensitivity for detection of micrometastases in bone-marrow/peripheral-blood stem-cell products from breast-cancer patients by negative immunomagnetic separation. *Int J Cancer.* 1998;78:556–560.

17. Naume B, Borgen E, Beiske K, et al. Immunomagnetic techniques for the enrichment and detection of isolated breast carcinoma cells in bone marrow and peripheral blood. *J Hematother.* 1997;6:103–114.

18. Woelfle U, Breit E, Zafrakas K, et al. Bi-specific immunomagnetic enrichment of micrometastatic tumour cell clusters from bone marrow of cancer patients. *J Immunol Methods.* 2005;300(1–2):136–145.

19. Went PT, Lugli A, Meier S, et al. Frequent EpCam protein expression in human carcinomas. *Hum Pathol.* 2004;35(1):122–128.

20. Gottschalk J, Korves M, Skotzek-Konrad B, Goebel S, Cervos-Navarro J. Dysembryoplastic neuroepithelial micro-tumor in a 75-year-old patient with long-standing epilepsy. *Clin Neuropathol.* 1993;12(3):175–178.

21. Raynor M, Stephenson SA, Walsh DC, et al. Optimisation of the RT-PCR detection of immunomagnetically enriched carcinoma cells. *BMC Cancer.* 2002;2:14.

22. de Cremoux P, Extra JM, Denis MG, et al. Detection of MUC1-expressing mammary carcinoma cells in the peripheral blood of breast cancer patients by real-time polymerase chain reaction. *Clin Cancer Res.* 2000;6(8):3117–3122.

23. Huang Y, Yang J, Wang XB, et al. The removal of human breast cancer cells from hematopoietic CD34+ stem cells by dielectrophoretic field-flow-fractionation. *J Hematother Stem Cell Res.* 1999;8(5):481–490.

24. Cheng J, Sheldon EL, Wu L, et al. Isolation of cultured cervical carcinoma cells mixed with peripheral blood cells on a bioelectronic chip. *Anal Chem.* 1998;70:2321–2326.

25. Vona G, Sabile A, Louha M, et al. Isolation by size of epithelial tumor cells: a new method for the immunomorphological and molecular characterization of circulating tumor cells. *Am J Pathol.* 2000;156(1):57–63.

26. Mohamed H, McCurdy LD, Szarowski DH, et al. Development of a rare cell fractionation device: application for cancer detection. *IEEE Trans Nanobioscience.* 2004;3(4):251–256.

27. Kahn HJ, Presta A, Yang LY, et al. Enumeration of circulating tumor cells in the blood of breast cancer patients after filtration enrichment: correlation with disease stage. *Breast Cancer Res Treat.* 2004;86(3):237–247.

28. Osborne MP, Wong GY, Asina S, et al. Sensitivity of immunocytochemical detection of breast cancer cells in human bone marrow. *Cancer Res.* 1991;51:2706.

29. Osborne MP, Asina S, Wong GY. Immunofluorescent monoclonal antibody detection of breast cancer in bone marrow: sensitivity in a model system. *Cancer Res.* 1989;49:2510.

30. Ellis G, Fergusson M, Yamanaka E. Monoclonal antibodies for detection of occult carcinoma cells in bone marrow of breast cancer patients. *Cancer.* 1989;63:2509–2514.

31. Cote RJ, Rosen PP, Lesser ML, Old LJ, Osborne MP. Prediction of early relapse in patients with operable breast cancer by detection of occult bone marrow micrometastases. *J Clin Oncol.* 1991;9(10):1749–1756.

32. Silly H, Samonigg H, Stoger H, et al. Micrometastatic tumor cells in bone marrow in colorectal carcinoma. *Lancet.* 1992;340:1288.

33. Schlimok G, Funke I, Bock B, et al. Epithelial tumor cells in bone marrow of patients with colorectal cancer: immunocytochemical detection, phenotypic characterization, and prognostic significance. *J Clin Oncol.* 1990;8:831–837.

34. Lindeman F, Schlimok G, Dirschedl P, et al. Prognostic significance of micrometastatic tumor cells in bone marrow of colorectal cancer patients. *Lancet.* 1992;340:685–689.

35. Wood DPJ, Banks ER, Humphreys S, et al. Sensitivity of immunohistochemistry and polymerase chain reaction in detecting prostate cancer cells in the bone marrow. *J Histochem Cytochem.* 1994;42:505–511.

36. Oberneder R, Riesenberg R, Kriegmair M, et al. Immunocytochemical detection and phenotypic characterization of micrometastatic tumour cells in bone marrow of patients with prostate cancer. *Urol Res.* 1994;22:3–8.

37. Moreno JG, Croce CM, Fischer R, et al. Detection of hematogenous micrometastases in patients with prostate cancer. *Cancer Res.* 1992;52:6110–6112.

38. Mansi JL, Mesker WE, McDonnell T, et al. Automated screening for micrometastases in bone marrow smears. *J Immunol Methods.* 1988;112:105.

39. Bretton PR, Melamed MR, Fair WR, Cote RJ. Detection of occult micrometastases in the bone marrow of patients with prostate carcinoma. *Prostate.* 1994:108–114.

40. Pantel K, Izbicki JR, Angstwurm M, et al. Immunocytological detection of bone marrow micrometastasis in operable non-small cell lung cancer. *Cancer Res.* 1993;53:1027–1031.

41. Pantel K, Isbicki J, Passlick B, et al. Frequency and prognostic significance of isolated tumour cells in bone marrow of patients with non-small cell lung cancer without overt metastases. *Lancet.* 1996;347:649–653.

42. Leonard RCF, Duncan LW, Hay FG. Immunocytological detection of residual marrow disease at clinical remission predicts metastatic relapse in small cell lung cancer. *Cancer Res.* 1990;50:6545–6548.

43. Frew AJ, Ralkaier N, Ghosh AK, et al. Immunohistochemistry in the detection of bone marrow micrometastases in patients with primary lung cancer. *Br J Cancer.* 1986;53:555–556.

44. Cote RJ, Beattie EJ, Chaiwun B, et al. Detection of occult bone marrow metastases in patients with operable lung carcinoma. *Ann Surg.* 1995;222:415–425.

45. Boo K, Cheng SA. A morphological and immunohistochemical study of plasma cell proliferative lesions. *Malasian J Pathol.* 1992;14:45–48.

46. Chaiwun B, Saad AD, Chen S-C, et al. Immunohistochemical detection of occult carcinoma in bone marrow and blood. *Diag Oncol.* 1992;2:267.

47. Gao X, Nie S. Molecular profiling of single cells and tissue specimens with quantum dots. *Trends Biotechnol.* 2003;21(9):371–373.

48. Arya H, Kaul Z, Wadhwa R, et al. Quantum dots in bioimaging: Revolution by the small. *Biochem Biophys Res Commun.* 2005;22;329(4):1173–1177.

49. Bauer KD, de la Torre-Bueno J, Diel IJ, et al. Reliable and sensitive analysis of occult bone marrow metastases using automated cellular imaging. *Clin Cancer Res.* 2000;6:3552–3559.

50. Racila E, Euhus D, Weiss AJ, et al. Detection and characterization of carcinoma cells in the blood. *Proc Natl Acad Sci USA.* 1998;95:4589–4594.

51. Pelkey TJ, Frierson HF, Jr., Bruns DE. Molecular and immunological detection of circulating tumor cells and micrometastases from solid tumors. *Clin Chem.* 1996;42(9):1369–1381.

52. Bostick PJ, Chatterjee S, Chi DD, et al. Limitations of specific reverse-transcriptase polymerase chain reaction markers in the detection of metastases in the lymph nodes and blood of breast cancer patients. *J Clin Oncol.* 1998;16(8):2632–2640.

53. Smith B, Selby P, Southgate J, et al. Detection of melanoma cells in peripheral blood by means of reverse transcriptase and polymerase chain reaction. *Lancet.* 1991;338(8777):1227–1229.

54. Wallace MB, Block M, Hoffman BJ, et al. Detection of telomerase expression in mediastinal lymph nodes of patients with lung cancer. *Am J Respir Crit Care Med.* 2003;167(12):1670–1675.

55. Sakaguchi M, Virmani A, Dudak MW, et al. Clinical relevance of reverse transcriptase-polymerase chain reaction for the detection of axillary lymph node metastases in breast cancer. *Ann Surg Oncol.* 2003;10(2):117–125.

56. Blaheta HJ, Ellwanger U, Schittek B, et al. Examination of regional lymph nodes by sentinel node biopsy and molecular analysis provides new staging facilities in primary cutaneous melanoma. *J Invest Dermatol.* 2000;114:637–642.

57. Slade MJ, Singh A, Smith BM, et al. Persistence of bone marrow micrometastases in patients receiving adjuvant therapy for breast cancer: results at 4 years. *Int J Cancer.* 2005;114(1):94–100.

58. Wharton RQ, Jonas SK, Glover C, et al. Increased detection of circulating tumor cells in the blood of colorectal carcinoma patients using two reverse transcription-PCR assays and multiple blood samples. *Clin Cancer Res.* 1999;5(12):4158–4163.

59. Bustin SA, Benes V, Nolan T, Pfaffl MW. Quantitative real-time RT-PCR–a perspective. *J Mol Endocrinol.* 2005;34(3):597–601.

60. Bernard PS, Wittwer CT. Real-time PCR technology for cancer diagnostics. *Clin Chem.* 2002;48(8):1178–1185.

61. Zehentner BK, Persing DH, Deme A, et al. Mammaglobin as a novel breast cancer biomarker: multigene reverse transcription-PCR assay and sandwich ELISA. *Clin Chem.* 2004;50(11):2069–2076.

62. Schuster R, Max N, Mann B, et al. Quantitative real-time RT-PCR for detection of disseminated tumor cells in peripheral blood of patients with colorectal cancer using different mRNA markers. *Int J Cancer.* 2004;108(2):219–227.

63. Ring AE, Zabaglo L, Ormerod MG, et al. Detection of circulating epithelial cells in the blood of patients with breast cancer: comparison of three techniques. *Br J Cancer.* 2005;92:906–912.

64. Koyanagi K, Kuo C, Nakagawa T, et al. Multimarker quantitative real-time PCR detection of circulating melanoma cells in peripheral blood: relation to disease stage in melanoma patients. *Clin Chem.* 2005;51(6):981–988.

65. Houghton RL, Dillon DC, Molesh DA, et al. Transcriptional complementarity in breast cancer: application to detection of circulating tumor cells. *Mol Diagn.* 2001;6(2):79–91.

66. Choesmel V, Pierga JY, Nos C, et al. Enrichment methods to detect bone marrow micrometastases in breast carcinoma patients: clinical relevance. *Breast Cancer Res.* 2004;6(5):R556–R570.

67. Choesmel V, Anract P, Hoifodt H, et al. A relevant immuno-magnetic assay to detect and characterize epithelial cell adhesion molecule-positive cells in bone marrow from patients with breast carcinoma: immunomagnetic purification of micrometastases. *Cancer.* 2004;101(4):693–703.

68. Theriult RL, Hortobagy GN. Bone metastasis in breast cancer. *Anticancer Drugs.* 1992;3:455–462.

69. Body JJ. Metastatic bone disease: clinical and therapeutic aspects. *Bone.* 1992;13(Suppl:):857–862.

70. Braun S, Vogl FD, Naume B, et al. A pooled analysis of bone marrow micrometastasis in breast cancer. *New Engl J Med.* 2005;353:793–802.

71. Wiedswang G, Borgen E, Karesen R, et al. Detection of isolated tumor cells in bone marrow is an independent prognostic factor in breast cancer. *J Clin Oncol.* 2003;21(18):3469–3478.

72. Datta YH, Adams PT, Drobski WR, et al. Sensitive detection of occult breast cancer by reverse-transcriptase polymerase chain reaction. *J Clin Oncol.* 1994;12:475–482.

73. Benoy IH, Elst H, Van der Auwera I, et al. Real-time RT-PCR correlates with immunocytochemistry for the detection of disseminated epithelial cells in bone marrow aspirates of patients with breast cancer. *Br J Cancer.* 2004;91(10):1813–1820.

74. Mansi JL, Gogas H, Bliss JM, et al. Outcome of primary-breast-cancer patients with micrometastases: a long-term follow-up. *Lancet.* 1999;354(9174):197–202.

75. Gerber B, Krause A, Muller H, et al. Simultaneous immunohistochemical detection of tumor cells in lymph nodes and bone marrow aspirates in breast cancer and its correlation with other prognostic factors. *J Clin Oncol.* 2001;19(4):960–971.

76. Gebauer G, Fehm T, Merkle E, et al. Epithelial cells in bone marrow of breast cancer patients at time of primary surgery: clinical outcome during long-term follow-up. *J Clin Oncol.* 2001;19(16):3669–3674.

77. Diel IJ, Kaufman M, Goener R, et al. Detection of tumor cells in bone marrow of patients with primary breast cancer: a prognostic factor for distant metastases. *J Clin Oncol.* 1992;10:1534–1539.

78. Diel IJ, Kaufman M, Costa SD, et al. Micrometastatic breast cancer cells in bone marrow at primary surgery: prognostic value in comparison with nodal status. *J Natl Cancer Instit.* 1996;88(22):1652–1658.

79. Dearnaley DP, Ormerod MG, Sloane JP. Micrometastases in breast cancer: long-term follow-up of the first patient cohort. *Eur J Cancer.* 1991;27:236.

80. Braun S, Pantel K, Muller P, et al. Cytokeratin-postive cells in the bone marrow and survival of patients with stage I, II, or III breast cancer. *New Engl J Med.* 2000;342(8):525–533.

81. Porro G, Menard S, Tagliabue E, et al. Monoclonal antibody detection of carcinoma cells in bone marrow biopsy specimens from breast cancer patients. *Cancer.* 1988;61:2407.

82. Mansi JL, Easton U, Berger JC, et al. Bone marrow micrometastases in primary breast cancer: prognostic significance after six years' follow-up. *Eur J Cancer*. 1991;27:1552.

83. Drageset V, Nesland JM, Erikstein B, et al. Monitoring of disseminated tumor cells in bone marrow in high-risk breast cancer patients treated with high-dose chemotherapy. *Int J Cancer*. 2005.

84. Neville AM, Price KN, Gelber RD, et al. Axillary lymph node micrometastases and breast cancer. *Lancet*. 1991;337(8749):110.

85. Sakorafas GH, Geraghty J, Pavlakis G. The clinical significance of axillary lymph node micrometastases in breast cancer. *Eur J Surg Oncol*. 2004;30(8):807–816.

86. Schoenfeld A, Luqmani Y, Smith D, et al. Detection of breast cancer micrometastases in axillary nodes using polymerase chain reaction. *Cancer Res*. 1994;54:2986–2990.

87. Hoon DS, Sarantou T, Doi F, et al. Detection of metastatic breast cancer by beta-hCG polymerase chain reaction. *Int J Cancer*. 1996;69(5):369–374.

88. Mitas M, Mikhitarian K, Walters C, et al. Quantitative real-time RT-PCR detection of breast cancer micrometastasis using a multigene marker panel. *Int J Cancer*. 2001;93:162–171.

89. Noguchi S, Aihara T, Motomura K, et al. Detection of breast cancer micrometastases in axillary lymph nodes by means of reverse transcriptase-polymerase chain reaction. Comparison between MUC1 mRNA and keratin 19 mRNA amplification. *Am J Surg Pathol*. 1996;148:649–656.

90. Gillanders WE, Mikhitarian K, Hebert R, et al. Molecular detection of micrometastatic breast cancer in histopathology-negative axillary lymph nodes correlates with traditional predictors of prognosis: an interim analysis of a prospective multi-institutional cohort study. *Ann Surg*. 2004;239(6):828–837; discussion 37–40.

91. Bussolati G, Gugliotta P, Morra Z, et al. The immunohistochemical detection of lymph node micrometastases from infiltrating lobular carcinoma of the breast. *Br J Cancer*. 1986;54:631–636.

92. Byrne J, Waldron R, McAvinchy D, et al. The use of monoclonal antibodies for the histological detection of mammary axillary micrometastases. *Eur J Surg Oncol*. 1987;13:409.

93. Cote RJ, Taylor CR. Immunomicroscopy: a diagnostic tool for the surgical pathologist. In: Taylor CR, Cote RJ, eds. *Tumors of the Breast*. Philadelphia: WB Saunders. 1994;200–236.

94. Elson CE, Kufe D, Johnston WW. Immunohistochemical detection and significance of axillary lymph node micrometastases in breast cancer– a study of 97 cases. *Anal Quant Cytol Histol*. 1993:171–178.

95. Pickren JW. Significance of occult metastases. A study of breast cancer. *Cancer*. 1961;14:1266–1271.

96. Wilkinson EJ, Hause LL, Hoffman RG, et al. Occult axillary lymph node metastases in invasive breast carcinoma: characteristics of the primary tumor and the significance of metastases. *Path Ann*. 1982;17:67–91.

97. Fisher ER, Saminoss S, Lee CH, et al. Detection and significance of occult axillary node metastases in patients with invasive breast cancer. *Cancer*. 1978;42:2025–2031.

98. International (LUDWIG) Breast Cancer Study Group. Prognostic importance of occult lymph node micrometastases from breast cancers. *Lancet*. 1990;335:1565–1568.

99. de Mascarel I, Bonichon F, Coindre JM, et al. Prognostic significance of breast cancer axillary lymph node micrometastases assessed by two special techniques: reevaluation with longer follow-up. *Br J Cancer*. 1992;66:523–527.

100. Cote RJ, Peterson HF, Chaiwun B, et al. Role of immunohistochemical detection of lymph-node metastases in management of breast cancer. *Lancet*. 1999;354(9182):896–900.

101. Lara O, Tong X, Zborowski M, et al. Enrichment of rare cancer cells through depletion of normal cells using density and flow-through, immunomagnetic cell separation. *Exp Hematol*. 2004;32:891–904.

102. Cristofanilli M, Budd GT, Ellis MJ, et al. Circulating tumor cells, disease progression, and survival in metastatic breast cancer. *New Engl J Med*. 2004 Aug 19;351(8):781–791.

103. Cristofanilli M, Hayes DF, Budd GT, et al. Circulating tumor cells: a novel prognostic factor for newly diagnosed metastatic breast cancer. *J Clin Oncol*. 2005;23(7):1420–1430.

104. Smith BM, Slade MJ, English J, et al. Response of circulating tumor cells to systemic therapy in patients with metastatic breast cancer: comparison of quantitative polymerase chain reaction and immunocytochemical techniques. *J Clin Oncol*. 2000;18(7):1432–1439.

105. Stathopoulou A, Mavroudis D, Perraki M, et al. Molecular detection of cancer cells in the peripheral blood of patients with breast cancer: comparison of CK-19, CEA,and maspin as detection markers. *Anticancer Res*. 2003;23(2C):1883–1890.

106. Zach O, Kasparu H, Wagner H, et al. Mammaglobin as a marker for the detection of tumor cells in the peripheral blood of breast cancer patients. *Ann Ny Acad Sci*. 2000;923:343–345.

107. Zach O, Lutz D. Mammaglobin remains a useful marker for the detection of breast cancer cells in peripheral blood. *J Clin Oncol*. 2005;23(13):3160.

108. Reinholz MM, Nibbe A, Jonart LM, et al. Evaluation of a panel of tumor markers for molecular detection of circulating cancer cells in women with suspected breast cancer. *Clin Cancer Res*. 2005;11:3722–3732.

109. Klein CA, Seidl S, Petat-Dutter K, et al. Combined transcriptome and genome analysis of single micrometastatic cells. *Nat Biotechnol*. 2002;20(4):387–392.

110. Schmidt-Kittler O, Ragg T, Daskalakis A, et al. From latent disseminated cells to overt metastasis: genetic analysis of systemic breast cancer progression. *Proc Natl Acad Sci U S A*. 2003;100(13):7737–7742.

111. Schardt JA, Meyer M, Hartmann CH, et al. Genomic analysis of single cytokeratin-positive cells from bone marrow reveals early mutational events in breast cancer. *Cancer Cell*. 2005;8(3):227–239.

112. Smirnov DA, Zweitzig DR, Foulk BW, et al. Global gene expression profiling of circulating tumor cells. *Cancer Res*. 2005 15;65(12):4993–4997.

113. Heiss MM, Allgayer H, Gruetzner KU, et al. Individual development and uPA-receptor expression of disseminated tumour cells in bone marrow: a reference to early systemic disease in solid cancer. *Nat Med*. 1995;1(10):1035–1039.

114. Braun S, Schlimok G, Heumos I, et al. erbB2 overexpression on occult metastatic cells in bone marrow predicts poor clinical outcome of stage I-III breast cancer patients. *Cancer Res*. 2001;61:1890–1895.

115. Muller V, Stahmann N, Riethdorf S, et al. Circulating tumor cells in breast cancer: correlation to bone marrow micrometastases, heterogeneous response to systemic therapy and low proliferative activity. *Clin Cancer Res*. 2005;11:3678–3685.

116. Al-Hajj M, Wicha MS, Benito-Hernandez A, et al. Prospective identification of tumorigenic breast cancer cells. *Proc Natl Acad Sci U S A*. 2003;100(7):3983–3988.

117. Hebbard L, Steffen A, Zawadzki V, et al. CD44 expression and regulation during mammary gland development and function. *J Cell Sci*. 2000;113 (Pt 14):2619–2630.

118. Draffin JE, McFarlane S, Hill A, Johnston PG, Waugh DJ. CD44 potentiates the adherence of metastatic prostate and breast cancer cells to bone marrow endothelial cells. *Cancer Res*. 2004;64(16):5702–5711.

119. Schabath H, Runz S, Joumaa S, et al. CD24 affects CXCR4 function in pre-B lymphocytes and breast carcinoma cells. *J Cell Sci.* 2006;119(Pt 2):314–325.

120. Balic M, Lin H, Young L, et al. Most early disseminated cancer cells detected in bone marrow of breast cancer patients have a putative breast cancer stem cell phenotype. *Clin Cancer Res.* 2006;12(19):5615–5621.

121. Paget S. The distribution of secondary growths in cancer cells of the breast. *Lancet.* 1989;1:571–573.

122. Jemal A, Siegel R, Ward E, et al. Cancer statistics, 2008. *CA Cancer J Clin.* 2008;58(2):71–96.

123. Bernstein ED, Herbert SM, Hanna NH. Chemotherapy and radiotherapy in the treatment of resectable non-small-cell lung cancer. *Ann Surg Oncol.* 2006;13:291–301.

124. Minna JD, Pass H, Gladstein EJ, et al. Cancer of the lung. In: DeVita VT, Hellman S, Rosenberg SA, eds. *Cancer, Principles and Practice of Oncology.* Philadelphia: JB Lippincott; 1989:591–705.

125. Rosenow EC, Carr DT. Bronchogenic carcinoma. *Ca Cancer J Clin.* 1979;29:233–246.

126. Beahrs EC, Henson DE, Hutter RVP, et al. American Joint Committee in Cancer Manual for Staging Cancer. 3rd ed. Philadelphia: J.B. Lippincott; 1988.

127. Mountain CF. The international system for staging lung cancer. *Semin Surg Oncol.* 2000;18(2):106–115.

128. Osaki T, Oyama T, Gu C-D, et al. Prognostic impact of micrometastatic tumor cells in the lymph nodes and bone marrow of patients with completely resected stage I non-small-cell lung cancer. *J Clin Oncol.* 2002;20(13):2930–2936.

129. Ohgami A, Tetsuya M, Kenji S, et al. Micrometastatic tumor cells in the bone marrow of patients with non-small cell lung cancer. *Ann Thorac Surg.* 1997;64:363–367.

130. Pasini F, Pelosi G, Verlato G, et al. Positive immunostaining with MuC1 of bone marrow aspirate predicts poor outcome in patients with small-cell lung cancer. *Annal Oncol.* 1998;9:181–185.

131. Chen ZL, Perez S, Holmes EC, et al. Frequency and distribution of occult micrometastases in lymph node of patients with non-small cell lung cancer. *J Natl Cancer Inst.* 1993;85:493–498.

132. Passlick B, Izbicki JR, Kubuschak B, et al. Immunohistochemical assessment of individual tumor cells in lymph nodes of patients with non-small cell lung cancer. *J Clin Oncol.* 1994;12:1827–1832.

133. Latza U, Niedobitek G, Schwarting R, et al. New monoclonal antibody which distinguishes epithelia from mesothelia. *J Clin Path.* 1990;43:213–219.

134. Hosch SB, Scheunemann P, Izbicki JR. Minimal residual disease in non-small-cell lung cancer. *Semin Surg Oncol.* 2001 Jun;20(4):278–281.

135. Tezel C, Ersev AA, Kiral H, et al. The impact of immunohistochemical detection of positive lymph nodes in early stage lung cancer. *Thorac Cardiovasc Surg.* 2006;54(2):124–128.

136. Ge MJ, Wu QC, Wang M, et al. Detection of disseminated lung cancer cells in regional lymph nodes by assay of CK19 reverse transcriptase polymerase chain reaction and its clinical significance. *J Cancer Res Clin Oncol.* 2005;131(10):662–668.

137. Wang XT, Sienel W, Eggeling S, et al. Detection of disseminated tumor cells in mediastinoscopic lymph node biopsies and lymphadenectomy specimens of patients with NSCLC by quantitative RT-PCR. *Eur J Cardiothorac Surg.* 2005;28(1):26–32.

138. Xi L, Coello MC, Litle VR, et al. A combination of molecular markers accurately detects lymph node metastasis in non-small cell lung cancer patients. *Clin Cancer Res.* 2006;12(8):2484–2491.

139. Bracarda S, de Cobelli O, Greco C, et al. Cancer of the prostate. *Crit Rev Oncol Hematol.* 2005;56(3):379–396.

140. Clifton JA, Phillip RJ, Ludovic E, et al. Bone marrow and carcinoma of the prostate. *Am J Med Sci.* 1952;224:121–130.

141. Nelson CMK, Boatman DL, Flocks RH. Bone marrow examination in carcinoma of the prostate. *J Urol.* 1973;109:667–670.

142. Mansi JL, Berger U, Wilson P, et al. Detection of tumor cells in bone marrow of patients with prostatic carcinoma by immunocytochemical techniques. *J Urol.* 1988;139:545–548.

143. Wood DPJ, Banks ER, Humphreys S, et al. Identification of bone marrow micrometastases in patients with prostate cancer. *Cancer.* 1994;74:2533–2540.

144. Katz AE, Olsson CA, Raffo AJ, et al. Molecular staging of prostate cancer with the use of an enhanced reverse-transcriptase polymerase chain reaction assay. *Urology.* 1994;43:765–775.

145. Israeli RS, Miller WH, Su SL, et al. Sensitive nested reverse transcriptase polymerase chain reaction detection of circulating prostatic tumor cells: comparison of prostate specific membrane antigen and prostate specific antigen based assays. *Cancer Res.* 1994;54(24):6306–6310.

146. Smith MR, Biggar S, Hussain M. Prostate-specific antigen messenger RNA is expressed in non-prostate cells: implications for detection of micrometastases. *Cancer Res.* 1999 1995;55(12):2640–2644.

147. Freeman jA, Lieskovsky G, Cook DW, et al. Radical retropubic prostatectomy and post-operative radiation for pathologic stage C (PCN0) prostate cancer from 1976-1989: intermediate findings. *J Urol.* 1993;149:1029.

148. Gomella LG, White JL, McCue PA, et al. Screening for occult nodal metastasis in localized carcinoma of the prostate. *J Urol.* 1993;149:776–778.

149. Gross HJ, Verwer B, Houck D, et al. Model study detecting breast cancer cells in peripheral blood mononuclear cells at frequencies as low as 10-7. *Proc Natl Acad Sci USA.* 1995;92:537–541.

150. Moul JW, Lewis DJ, Ross AA, et al. Immunohistologic detection of prostate cancer pelvic lymph node micrometastases: correlation to pre-operative serum prostate-specific antigen. *Urology.* 1994;43:68.

151. Prout GRJ, Heaney JA, Griffith PP, et al. Nodal involvement as a prognostic indicator in patients with prostatic carcinoma. *J Urol.* 1980;124:226.

152. Pagliarulo V, Hawes D, Brands FH, et al. Detection of Occult Lymph Node Metastases in Locally Advanced Node-Negative Prostate Cancer. *J Clin Oncol.* 2006;24(18):2735–2742.

153. Gerhard M, Juhl H, Kalthoff H, et al. Specific detection of carcinoembryonic antigen-expressing tumor cells in bone marrow aspirates by polymerase chain reaction. *J Clin Oncol.* 1994;12:725–729.

154. Juhl H, Stritzel M, Wroblewski A, et al. Immunocytochemical detection of micrometastatic cells: comparative evalution of findings in the peritoneal cavity and the bone marrow of gastric, colorectal and pancreatic cancer patients. *Int J Cancer.* 1994;57:330–335.

155. O'Sullivan GC, Collins JK, Kelly J, et al. Micrometastases: marker of metastatic potential or evidence of residual disease? *Gut.* 1997;40(4):512–515.

156. Soeth E, Vogel I, Roder C, et al. Comparative analysis of bone marrow and venous blood isolates from gastrointestinal cancer patients for the detection of disseminated tumor cells using reverse transcription PCR. *Cancer Res.* 1997;57:3106–3110.

157. Weitz J, Koch M, Kienle P, et al. Detection of hematogenic tumor cell dissemination in patients undergoing resection of liver metastases of colorectal cancer. *Ann Surg.* 2000;232(1):66–72.

158. Greene FL. Staging of colon and rectal cancer: from endoscopy to molecular markers. *Surg Endosc.* 2006;20 Suppl 2:S475–S478.

159. Mescoli C, Rugge M, Pucciarelli S, et al. High prevalence of isolated tumor cells in regional lymph nodes from PN0 colorectal cancer. *J Clin Pathol.* 2006;59(8):870–874.

160. Cutait R, Alves VAF, Lopez LC, et al. Restaging of colorectal cancer based on the identification of lymph node micrometastases through immunoperoxidase staining of CEA and cytokeratins. *Dis Colon Rectum.* 1991;34:917–922.

161. Jeffers MD, O'Dowd GM, Mulcahy H, et al. The prognostic significance of immunohistochemically detected lymph node micrometastases in colorectal cancer. *J Pathol.* 1994;172:183–187.

162. Florentine B, Ettekal B, Leichman CG, et al. Prognostic importance of occult lymph node metastases detected by cytokeratin immunohistochemical techniques in stage II colon cancer. *Proceedings of ASCO 1996, Abstract No. 507.* 1996.

163. Greenson JK, Isenhart CE, Rice R, et al. Identification of occult micrometastases in pericolic lymph nodes of Duke's B colorectal cancer patients using monoclonal antibodies against cytokeratins and CC49. *Cancer.* 1994;73:563–569.

164. Stiller CA, Parkin DM. International variations in the incidence of neuroblastoma. *Int J Cancer.* 1992;52(4):538–543.

165. Cochran AJ, Wen DR, Morton DL. Occult tumor cells in the lymph nodes of patients with pathological stage I malignant melanoma. *Ann J Surg Pathol.* 1988;12:6118–6120.

166. Heller R, King B, Backey P, et al. Identification of submicroscopic lymph node metastases in patients with malignant melanoma. *Semin Surg Oncol.* 1993;9:285–289.

167. Takeuchi H, Morton DL, Kuo C, et al. Prognostic significance of molecular upstaging of paraffin-embedded sentinel lymph nodes in melanoma patients. *J Clin Oncol.* 2004;22(13):2671–2680.

168. Mansi JL, Berger U, Easton D, et al. Micrometastases in bone marrow in patients with primary breast cancer: evaluation as an early predictor of bone metastases. *Br Med J.* 1987;295:1093–1096.

169. Moss TJ, Reynolds CP, Sather SN, et al. Prognostic value of immunohistochemical detection of bone marrow metastases in neuroblastoma. *New Engl J Med.* 1991;324:219–226.

170. Naito H, Kuzumaki N, Uchino J, al. e. Detection of tyrosine hydroxylase mRNA and minimal neuroblastoma cells by reverse transcriptase polymerase chain reaction. *Eur J Cancer.* 1991;27:762–765.

171. Mattano LAJ, Moss TJ, Emerson SG. Sensitive detection of rare circulating neuroblastoma cells by reverse transcriptase polymerase chain reaction. *Cancer Res.* 1992;52:4701–4705.

172. Tobal K, Sherman LS, Foss AJE, et al. Detection of melanocytes from uveal melanoma in peripheral blood using polymerase chain reaction. *Invest Ophthalmol Vis Sci.* 1993;34:2622–2625.

173. Cain JM, Ellis GA, Collins C, et al. Bone marrow involvement in epithelial ovarian cancer by immunohistochemical assessment. *Gynaecologic Oncol.* 1990;38:442–445.

174. Czegledy J, Iosif C, Hansson BG, et al. Can a test for E6/E7 transcripts of human papillomavirus type 16 serve as a diagnostic tool for the detection of micrometastases in cervical cancer? *Int J Cancer.* 1995;64:211–215.

COMMENTARY
Anneke Q. van Hoesel and David S. B. Hoon

Tumor behavior and disease outcome vary among patients with the same stage of early malignant disease. This observation has led to efforts to characterize and stage malignant disease more meticulously, with the aim to identify early-stage patients who are at high risk of developing recurrent disease and therefore might benefit from postoperative adjuvant therapy. The lack of means to further define the risk of recurrence for individual patients with early disease can lead to undertreatment of high-risk patients or overtreatment of low-risk patients.

Ultrastaging techniques that identify micrometastasis or minimal residual disease show promise for improving the staging of melanoma, breast cancer, and other solid cancers. Examination of regional nodes can reveal regional micrometastasis. Tumor cells can be found in peripheral blood and bone marrow in a portion of some early-stage breast cancer patients with or without evidence of lymph node macro- or micrometastasis. This suggests that systemic metastasis does not necessarily occur subsequent to the development of lymphatic spread in breast cancer (1). Rather, progression and dissemination can be viewed as a function of unique tumor characteristics and tumor-host dynamics. Therefore, multiple studies have focused on the prognostic implications of minimal disease in both the regional lymph node compartment and in peripheral blood and bone marrow.

In the chapter by Drs. Balic, Hawes, Neville, and Cote, the authors give a comprehensive review on methods used for the detection of occult metastasis, and describe the relevance of ultrastaging in several types of solid cancer by discussing recent relevant papers. This commentary aims to provide additional insight into recently developed ultrastaging techniques, in particular molecular techniques. Furthermore, we address new dilemmas in clinical decision making that have arisen from the development of ultrastaging techniques, using breast cancer and melanoma as examples.

OCCULT METASTASIS: DEFINITION

Occult metastasis is a broad term that encompasses isolated tumor cells (ITCs) and micrometastases defined by different approaches. Thus, it can refer to a focus of tumor not identified during routine histopathologic examination, such as macrometastasis not revealed by hematoxylin and eosin (H&E) staining of a bisected axillary lymph node from a patient with breast cancer. Occult metastasis also may refer to a tumor focus that is clinically occult, such as a metastasis in nonenlarged lymph nodes of a patient with prostate cancer. Finally, occult metastasis may refer to circulating tumor cells (CTCs) in the blood, tumor cells in the bone marrow, or micrometastatic deposits in lymph nodes. These distinctions are important for accurate interpretation of the literature on occult metastasis and disease outcome. Some studies that discuss occult LN metastases are not necessarily limited to tumor cells, but may include "occult" micrometastases (2,3).

SAMPLING AND SECTIONING OF LYMPH NODES

Currently, there is no consensus on screening and sampling of regional lymph nodes. The implementation of available American Joint Committee on Cancer nomenclature (4) and techniques used to assess for minimal nodal involvement vary widely between health centers. It is not surprising that both the detection method (conventional H&E versus immunohistochemistry [IHC]) and the technique employed for lymph node sampling affect the rate of a positive finding. Sampling variations involve not only the number of lymph nodes submitted for pathologic evaluation, but also the volume per node (the entire node vs. half of a bisected node), the number of blocks per node, the number of sections per submitted block, and the thickness of the interval between each evaluated section level within the node. In a study of 49 patients with primary resected melanoma with a Breslow thickness ≥1.5 mm and negative sentinel lymph nodes (SLNs) on routine pathologic assessment (single slide H&E assessment of one face of a bivalved lymph node), metastases were detected in 71% of the patients using levels of 250-μm intervals and IHC with antibodies against S100 and HMB-45 (5).

For melanoma, routine IHC staining is recommended, and the yield can be further improved by serial sections. Several breast cancer studies demonstrate that IHC staining of serial sections increases detection of micrometastasis by 9% to 52% (6–8). In the American Society of Clinical Oncology Guideline Recommendations for SLN biopsy in early-stage breast cancer, it is stated that the use of IHC with antibodies against cytokeratin (CK) can result in upstaging of approximately 10% of patients with apparent negative nodes (9). However, the clinical importance of negative-to-positive conversion for metastases detected only by IHC is unknown, and there is insufficient evidence to implement anti-CK IHC as a routine screening technique for SLNs. H&E verification for all micrometastases found by IHC is recommended by the College of American Pathologists (10).

Implementation of the SLN biopsy has reduced the number of lymph nodes that need to undergo histopathologic evaluation. This allows for extensive sectioning and CK IHC, which otherwise would have been too costly and labor-intensive. To further reduce cost and man-hours, several groups have studied the performance of automated cell imaging systems in comparison with pathologist performance. The recent National Surgical Adjuvant Breast and Bowel Project (NSABP) Protocol B-32 quality assurance study found no difference in accuracy and detection rate for lymph node metastases >0.1mm (11).

LYMPH NODE MICROMETASTASIS IN BREAST CANCER: CONTROVERSIES

It is widely agreed that the presence of nodal micrometastasis in breast cancer is prognostically unfavorable. This is substantiated by the latest American Joint Committee on Cancer guidelines, in which nodal micrometastases, defined as a metastatic deposits >0.2 mm but not >2.0 mm, are classified as pN1mi. Multiple studies have indeed shown a statistically significant correlation between micrometastasis and shorter disease-free survival and increased relative risk of death (6,12,13). However, the correlation between micrometastasis and worse outcome is not always evident after multivariate analysis. Several studies have suggested that the current cutoff point of 2.0 mm for the definition of micrometastasis is suboptimal, while a cutoff closer to 1.0 mm may carry more clinical relevance (13). Data col-

lected by Fisher and colleagues (14) suggest that patients with micrometastases larger than 1.3 mm have a significantly poorer prognosis than patients with smaller micrometastases.

SENTINEL LYMPH NODE AND MICROMETASTASIS IN BREAST CANCER

The establishment of SLN biopsy as standard of care for the assessment of nodal disease in patients without palpable lymph nodes allows routine use of serial sectioning and IHC, which in turn has increased detection of metastases, particularly micrometastases. As a result, an increasing number of patients are diagnosed with positive SLNs. Thus, a new dilemma is introduced: should the finding of ITCs, defined as a cluster of IHC-positive cells ≤0.2 mm (pN0(i+)), or micrometastasis in the SLN prompt axillary lymph node dissection (ALND)? Studies show that 6% to 35% of patients with SLN micrometastasis have additional positive lymph nodes in the ALND specimen, depending on screening and sampling techniques (15,16). Metastasis has been reported in non-SLNs of approximately 10% of patients with an ITC-positive SLN (9,17). Involvement of non-SLNs occurs more often in patients with T2 and T3 tumors than in patients with T1 tumors (16). Langer et al. (18) studied a prospective cohort of patients who underwent SLN biopsy for early-stage breast cancer. The SLN was step-sectioned and evaluated by H&E and IHC. Only patients with SLN macrometastasis underwent ALND of levels I and II; patients with negative SLN or SLN micrometastasis received no further surgical treatment. After a median follow-up of 42 months, no axillary recurrences had occurred in the latter group, and all patients with micrometastases were disease-free. The authors suggest that ALND need not be performed in patients with early breast cancer and micrometastasis in the SLN. However, further trials are needed to provide more clarity.

In a multicenter study, Houvenaeghel and colleagues (19) examined potential predictive factors for non-SLN involvement in 700 patients who underwent ALND for SLN micrometastasis. On multivariate analysis, three factors seemed predictive: T category, mode of detection (H&E or IHC), and presence or absence of lymphovascular infiltration. The size of SLN micrometastasis (smaller or larger than 0.2 mm in diameter) was not a predictive factor. Authors conclude that ALND could be omitted in patients with T1a and T1b tumors. The American Society of Clinical Oncology recommends routine ALND for all patients with SLN micrometastasis but not ITC, regardless of screening method used for detection. Three ongoing clinical trials may provide an answer to the controversy. The NSABP B-32 phase III randomized trial compares ALND with SLN biopsy in clinically node-negative patients. The primary aim of this study is to determine whether regional and distant disease control is equivalent for SLN biopsy and ALND; the secondary aim is to evaluate survival of patients with occult SLN metastasis (20). The American College of Surgeons Oncology Group Z0010 trial is a prognostic study of SLN and bone marrow micrometastasis in women with clinical T1 or T2 N0 M0 breast cancer, and is now closed for enrollment (21). The International Breast

Cancer Study Group-23-01 trial is a phase III randomized study of surgical resection with or without completion ALND in women with SLN micrometastases (22). Patients may receive adjuvant therapy.

SENTINEL LYMPH NODE ISOLATED TUMOR CELLS AND BREAST CANCER

A difficulty in diagnosing ITC is the problem of identifying false-positive findings. Carter and colleagues (23) have described that benign breast epithelial cells can be found in the sinus of axillary lymph nodes. Epithelial cells can travel to the peripheral sinus via a mechanism called *benign transport*. Work performed by Diaz and colleagues (24) suggests that breast massage prior to SLN biopsy increases the chance of finding epithelial cells and cell clusters smaller than 0.2 mm without histologic evidence of malignant activity in the SLN. In addition, procedures such as core biopsy, fine-needle aspiration, and wire localization can cause displacement of epithelial cells into lymphatic spaces (25). Bleiweiss et al. (26) observed that papillary lesions or intraductal papilloma are particularly prone to fragmentation and can contribute to false-positive findings. Thus, both benign and malignant epithelial cells can be transported to the lymph node, and, unfortunately, comparison of the cytologic features of the primary lesion and the observed epithelial cells may not be sufficient to distinguish between true ITC metastasis and benign epithelial cells. In addition, the prognostic value of confirmed ITC in lymph nodes remains unknown.

REVERSE TRANSCRIPTION POLYMERASE CHAIN REACTION FOR DETECTION OF LYMPH NODE METASTASIS IN BREAST CANCER

Reverse transcription-polymerase chain reaction (RT-PCR) has been developed into a sensitive and sophisticated method to detect lymph node metastases. In the past, the use of CK or epithelial markers has led to ambiguous results because of background expression in noncancerous cells. Introduction of better molecular markers and quantitative RT-PCR (qRT) has minimized this problem and significantly changed the field of molecular diagnostics. Validation of cycle threshold (Ct) cutoff values has made it possible to use markers that are overexpressed in cancer tissue as compared with normal tissue. In all cases, the choice of the Ct cutoff value should be determined by the study's objective, as the Ct value selected will affect the false-negative and false-positive rates. The use of multiple markers rather than single markers compensates for heterogeneity of marker expression in tumor cells.

The GeneSearch BLN assay (Veridex, Warren, NJ) is a Food and Drug Administration-approved method for the detection of SLN metastasis >0.2 mm in breast cancer using RT-PCR. Markers used for this assay are CK19 and mammaglobin, both expressed in breast tissue but not in nodal tissue. Porphobilinogen deaminase is expressed in nodal tissue and is used as inter-nal control. The assay was validated comparing the results with histopathologic evaluation on IHC staining, and Ct cutoffs were chosen to achieve a minimum specificity of 95% compared with the histologic result. The performance with the chosen cutoffs was tested in a 274-subject data set; the sensitivity was 91.1% and the specificity 95.9% (27).

Our group hypothesized that presence of CTCs may be predictive for lymph node status in patients with early-stage breast cancer (28). To test this hypothesis, we developed a qRT assay using 3 mRNA markers with an established role in breast cancer: STC-1 and GalNacT, which are both overexpressed in breast cancer as compared with normal breast epithelia, and the tumor-specific marker MAGE-A3, which is expressed by several tumor types, including breast cancer. To test this assay, peripheral blood was obtained from 90 female early-stage breast cancer patients immediately before surgical tumor resection with SLN biopsy or ALND. Blood was also obtained from 39 healthy female volunteers. The detection of two or more biomarkers was an independent predictor for the presence of lymph node metastasis on multivariate analysis. The only other independent predictor of axillary lymph node metastasis was lymphovascular invasion. The calculated receiver operating characteristic curve for these two predictors combined showed an area under the curve of 0.84. Furthermore, the detection of biomarkers was correlated with the number of metastases and the number of involved nodes. The number of detected biomarkers was correlated with the presence of non-SLN nodes in addition to SLN nodes ($p = 0.0004$). No CTC biomarker was detected in the blood of the 39 healthy volunteers.

Improvements in data analysis and selection of tumor- and tissue-specific markers have made quantitative RT-PCR a valuable and sensitive asset to the arsenal of tools available for the diagnosis of occult lymph node metastasis in breast cancer, to be used in addition to routine techniques. New, rapid, high-throughput PCR instruments are being developed that enable assessment of markers in just one hour.

CIRCULATING TUMOR CELLS IN BREAST CANCER

To form distant metastases, tumor cells have to enter the circulation in order to travel to the site of metastasis. Therefore, the presence of CTCs would theoretically be a meaningful predictor of distance metastasis, although not all patients with CTCs will develop metastatic disease.

The CellSearch Circulating Tumor Cell Kit (Veridex) is a commercially available kit intended for the enumeration of CTCs of epithelial origin in whole blood. This method uses an enrichment step with magnetic beads specific for the epithelial cell adhesion molecule (EpCAM), and cells are labeled with a fluorescent nucleic acid dye. Cells are then counted with the CellSpotter Analyzer. Epithelial cells are distinguished from leukocytes with the use of fluorescence-labeled monoclonal antibodies directed against CK8, CK18, and CK19-phycoerythrin, and CD45-allophycocyan, respectively. A validation study shows that a CTC count of five or more per 7.5 mL of blood is predictive of shorter progression-free and overall survival (OS) in patients with metastatic breast cancer (29). Healthy female donors ($n = 145$) and female donors with benign breast lesions or nonmalignant conditions ($n = 200$) had a mean CTC count of 0.1 ± 0.9 per 7.5 mL of whole blood; none of these control donors' CTC count exceeded 2 CTC. A recent study investigating the intra- and inter-assay precision and inter-instrument accordance concludes that the CellSearch system is suitable for routine clinical laboratory assessment of CTC counts in patients with metastatic breast cancer (30). Hayes et al. (31) report that CTC counts at each follow-up time during therapy of metastatic breast cancer are useful to monitor the response to therapy, and may be used to guide clinical decisions concerning continuation of the therapeutic regimen. The clinical significance of CTC enumeration using the CellSearch system remains to be elucidated for early-stage breast cancer and other epithelial malignancies.

MOLECULAR STAGING OF MELANOMA

Metastasis to regional lymph nodes is one of the most important prognostic factors in early-stage melanoma. Research has been performed to determine the value of molecular staging in melanoma, for both lymph nodes and CTCs in blood. Our group demonstrated that molecular detection of metastases in early-stage melanoma patients with histologic negative SLNs is an independent prognostic factor of disease outcome in both frozen and paraffin-embedded lymph node tissue (32,33). To assess for presence of melanoma cells in paraffin-embedded lymph nodes of 215 patients, we used four qRT markers (MART-1, MAGE-A3, GalNacT, and PAX3) that have a role in independent biological pathways and are either tumor-specific (i.e., not present in benign tissue, nor in benign nevi and melanocytes) or overexpressed in melanoma. Detection of one or more markers was related to disease recurrence and poor OS. The median follow-up in this study was 60.4 months. Studies that failed to show predictive value for molecular upstaging are often not quantitative or use one single marker (34). Multiple markers may improve the reliability of molecular diagnostics as it compensates for heterogeneity in marker expression among malignant cells. Mocellin et al. (35) undertook a systemic review and meta-analysis of 22 studies assessing SLN molecular ultrastaging. The meta-analysis included 4,019 patients with stage I/II cutaneous melanoma who underwent SLN biopsy. A positive PCR result was associated with worse overall and disease-free survival ($p = 0.002$ and $p < 0.0001$, respectively). The authors concluded that PCR detection of SLN metastasis seems a powerful tool. However, they point out that their meta-analysis includes heterogeneous studies in terms of study design, and more studies are warranted.

CIRCULATING TUMOR CELLS IN MELANOMA

The clinical importance of CTCs in solid cancers is most well studied in melanoma. PCR techniques were first applied in melanoma to detect CTCs using a marker for tyrosinase mRNA,

a gene specific for melanocytes that retains its expression after malignant transformation. Although many studies have investigated whether PCR detection of CTCs could assist in predicting distant metastasis, there is currently no consensus. Mocellin et al. (36) performed a systemic review and meta-analysis of 53 CTC studies, enrolling 5,433 patients with stage I to IV cutaneous melanoma. CTC status correlated with TNM stage ($p < 0.0001$), progression-free survival ($p < 0.0001$, hazard ratio 2.45, 95% CI 1.78–3.38) and OS ($p < 0.0001$, hazard ratio 2.42, 95% CI 1.7–3.45). These results were similar for univariate and multivariate analysis, and applying the "leave-one-out" procedure revealed that no single study was responsible for heterogeneity. Differences in results between studies seem to depend largely on technical variables (type and number of markers, timing of blood withdrawal, method of isolation of blood cell fractions, use of cell enrichment, use of cutoff values for PCR analysis). The authors remark that the CTC positivity rates for stage I and II exceeded expectations, and were in discrepancy with the survival rates for these groups (32% to 41.7%; 10% to 33% 5-year mortality rates). These data suggest that there is a high false-positivity rate for PCR-based detection methods. However, this problem can be effectively eradicated by the use of qRT with cutoff values. Furthermore, some studies experience lower sensitivity than others. The use of multiple markers may be helpful to address this shortcoming. The authors concluded that it is too early for clinical implementation of molecular assessment of CTCs for cutaneous melanoma patients. However, the results of the meta-analysis should be regarded as encouraging, and multicenter prospective studies are warranted.

Our group monitored circulating melanoma cells during neoadjuvant biochemotherapy in patients with stage III melanoma (37). Blood samples were collected from 63 patients enrolled in a multicenter phase II trial of biochemotherapy, and presence of CTC was assessed for four consecutive time points during treatment, the first time point being the preoperative baseline measurement. CTCs were assessed by qRT-PCR for expression of melanoma-specific markers MART-1, GalNAc-T, PAX3, and MAGE-A3. After median follow-up of 30.4 months, 70% of patients were clinically disease-free. In relapse-free patients, the number of detected markers significantly decreased during treatment ($p < 0.0001$), whereas marker detection after treatment was associated with relapse and worse OS ($p < 0.0001$). The number of markers detected after treatment was a significant independent factor for OS in multivariate analysis ($p = 0.003$). Monitoring CTCs may be useful as a predictor for therapy response and OS in other systemic melanoma treatments.

CONCLUSION

Ultrastaging for minimal residual disease in regional lymph nodes, blood, and bone marrow shows promise for improved prediction of disease outcome in patients with solid cancers. Recently developed techniques, such as qRT-PCR, have greatly contributed to the surge in studies assessing clinical importance of minimal residual disease in several types of cancer. Additionally, the assessment of molecular biomarkers provides insight into molecular and cellular mechanisms that are crucial for tumor behavior and disease outcome. Before ultrastaging is used to guide decisions in patient treatment, further research is warranted to elucidate dilemmas that are illustrated in this commentary.

Although ultrastaging techniques are often criticized for their costliness, improved staging with good prognostic biomarkers may ultimately lead to cost reduction because of optimized and individualized cancer treatment. In turn, optimized treatment may enhance quality of life for cancer patients.

REFERENCES

1. Langer I, Guller U, Koechli OR, et al. Association of the presence of bone marrow micrometastases with the sentinel lymph node status in 410 early stage breast cancer patients: results of the Swiss Multicenter Study. *Ann Surg Oncol.* 2007;14:1896–1903.
2. Cote RJ, Peterson HF, Chaiwun B, et al. Role of immunohistochemical detection of lymph-node metastases in management of breast cancer. International Breast Cancer Study Group. *Lancet.* 1999;354: 896–900.
3. Nasser IA, Lee AK, Bosari S, et al. Occult lymph node metastases in "Node-negative" breast carcinoma. *Hum Pathol.* 1993;24:950–957.
4. Greene FL, Page DL, Fleming ID, et al. *AJCC Cancer Staging Manual*, 6th ed. New York: Springer-Verlag. 2002;421.
5. Spanknebel K, Coit DG, Bieligk SC, et al. Characterization of micrometastatic disease in melanoma sentinel lymph nodes by enhanced pathology. *Am J Surg Pathol.* 2005;29:305–317.
6. de Mascarel I, Bonichon F, Coindre JM, et al. Prognostic significance of breast cancer axillary lymph node micrometastases assessed by two special techniques: reevaluation with longer follow-up. *Br J Cancer.* 1992;66:523–527.
7. Chagpar A, Middleton LP, Sahin AA, et al. Clinical outcome of patients with lymph node-negative breast carcinoma who have sentinel lymph node micrometastases detected by immunohistochemistry. *Cancer.* 2005;103:1581–1586.
8. Rydén L, Chebil G, Sjöström L, et al. Determination of sentinel Lymph node (SLN) status in primary breast cancer by prospective use of immunohistochemistry increases the rate of micrometastases and isolated tumour cells: analysis of 174 patients after SLN biopsy. *Eur J Surg Oncol.* 2007;33:33–38.
9. Lyman GH, Giuliano AE, Somerfield MR, et al. American Society of Clinical Oncology guideline recommendations for sentinel lymph node biopsy in early-stage breast cancer. *J Clin Oncol.* 2005;23:7703–7720.
10. Fitzgibbons PL, Page DL, Weaver D, et al. Prognostic factors in breast cancer. College of American Pathologists Consensus Statement 1999. *Arch Pathol Lab Med.* 2000;124:966–978.
11. Weaver DL, Krag DN, Manna EA, et al. Detection of occult sentinel lymph node micrometastases by immunohistochemistry in breast cancer. An NSABP protocol B-32 quality assurance study. *Cancer.* 2006;107:661–667.
12. Kuijt GP, Voogd AC, van de Poll-Franse LV, et al. The prognostic significance of axillary lymph-node micrometastases in breast cancer patients. *Eur J Surg Oncol.* 2005;31:500–505.
13. Colleoni M, Rotmensz N, Peruzzotti G, et al. Size of breast cancer metastases in axillary lymph nodes: clinical relevance of minimal lymph node involvement. *J Clin Oncol.* 2005;23:1379–1389.
14. Fisher ER, Palekar A, Rockette H, et al. Pathologic findings from the National Surgical Adjuvant Breast Project (Protocol No. 4). V. Significance of axillary nodal micro- and macrometastases. *Cancer.* 1978;42:2032–2038.
15. Fournier K, Schiller A, Perry RR, et al. Micrometastasis in the sentinel lymph node of breast cancer does not mandate completion axillary dissection. *Ann Surg.* 2004;239:859–865.
16. den Bakker MA, van Weeszenberg A, de Kanter AY, et al. Non-sentinel lymph node involvement in patients with breast cancer and sentinel node micrometastasis; too early to abandon axillary clearance. *J Clin Pathol.* 2002;55:932–935.
17. Turner RR, Chu KU, Qi K, et al. Pathologic features associated with nonsentinel lymph node metastases in patients with metastatic breast carcinoma in a sentinel lymph node. *Cancer.* 2000;89:574–581.
18. Langer I, Marti WR, Guller U, et al. Axillary recurrence rate in breast cancer patients with negative sentinel lymph node (SLN) or SLN micrometastases: prospective analysis of 150 patients after SLN biopsy. *Ann Surg.* 2005;241:152–158.
19. Houvenaeghel G, Nos C, Mignotte H, et al. Micrometastases in sentinel lymph node in a multicentric study: predictive factors of nonsentinel lymph node involvement–Groupe des Chirurgiens de la Federation des Centres de Lutte Contre le Cancer. *J Clin Oncol.* 2006;24:1814–1822.
20. A randomized, phase iii clinical trial to compare sentinel node resection to conventional axillary dissection in clinically node-negative breast cancer patients. http://www.nsabp.pitt.edu/B-32.asp. Accessed 09/01/2007.
21. A prognostic study of sentinel node and bone marrow micrometastases in women with clinical T1 or T2 N0 M0. htpps://www.acosog.org/studies/closed.jsp. Accessed 09/01/2007.
22. Phase III randomized study of surgical resection with or without axillary lymph node dissection in women with clinically node-negative breast cancer with sentinel node micrometastases. http://www.cancer.gov/clinicaltrials/IBCSG-23-01. Accessed 09/01/2007.
23. Carter BA, Jensen RA, Simpson JF, et al. Benign transport of breast epithelium into axillary lymph nodes after biopsy. *Am J Clin Pathol.* 2000;113:259–265.
24. Diaz NM, Cox CE, Ebert M, et al. Benign mechanical transport of breast epithelial cells to sentinel lymph nodes. *Am J Surg Pathol.* 2004;28:1641–1645.
25. Moore KH, Thaler HT, Tan LK, et al. Immunohistochemically detected tumor cells in the sentinel lymph nodes of patients with breast carcinoma: biologic metastasis or procedural artifact? *Cancer.* 2004;100:929–934.
26. Bleiweiss IJ, Nagi CS, Jaffer S. Axillary sentinel lymph nodes can be falsely positive due to iatrogenic displacement and transport of benign epithelial cells in patients with breast carcinoma. *J Clin Oncol.* 2006;24:2013–2018.
27. GeneSearch BLN assay, information for physicians. http://www.veridex.com/pdf/VX10048-BLN_Information_for_Physicians.pdf. Accessed 09/01/2007.
28. Nakagawa T, Martinez SR, Goto Y, et al. Detection of circulating tumor cells in early-stage breast cancer metastasis to axillary lymph nodes. *Clin Cancer Res.* 2007;13:4105–4110.
29. Cristofanilli M, Budd GT, Ellis MJ, et al. Circulating tumor cells, disease progression, and survival in metastatic breast cancer. *N Engl J Med.* 2004;351:781–791.
30. Riethdorf S, Fritsche H, Muller V, et al. Detection of circulating tumor cells in peripheral blood of patients with metastatic breast cancer: a validation study of the CellSearch system. *Clin Cancer Res.* 2007;13:920–928.
31. Hayes DF, Cristofanilli M, Budd GT, et al. Circulating tumor cells at each follow-up time point during therapy of metastatic breast cancer patients predict progression-free and overall survival. *Clin Cancer Res.* 2006;12(14 Pt 1):4218–4224.
32. Takeuchi H, Morton DL, Kuo C, et al. Prognostic significance of molecular upstaging of paraffin-embedded sentinel

lymph nodes in melanoma patients. *J Clin Oncol.* 2004;22:2671–2680.

33. Kuo CT, Hoon DS, Takeuchi H, et al. Prediction of disease outcome in melanoma patients by molecular analysis of paraffin-embedded sentinel lymph nodes. *J Clin Oncol.* 2003;21:3566–3572.

34. Kammula US, Ghossein R, Bhattacharya S, et al. Serial follow-up and the prognostic significance of reverse transcriptase-polymerase chain reaction–staged sentinel lymph nodes from melanoma patients. *J Clin Oncol.* 2004;22:3989–3996.

35. Mocellin S, Hoon DS, Pilati P, et al. Sentinel lymph node molecular ultrastaging in patients with melanoma: a systematic review and meta-analysis of prognosis. *J Clin Oncol.* 2007;25:1588–1595.

36. Mocellin S, Hoon D, Ambrosi A, et al. The prognostic value of circulating tumor cells in patients with melanoma: a systematic review and meta-analysis. *Clin Cancer Res.* 2006;12:4605–4613.

37. Koyanagi K, O'Day SJ, Gonzalez R, et al. Serial monitoring of circulating melanoma cells during neoadjuvant biochemotherapy for stage III melanoma: outcome prediction in a multicenter trial. *J Clin Oncol.* 2005;23:8057–8064.

5

Hematopoietic Stem Cell Transplants for Solid Tumors

David I. Kuperman and John F. DiPersio

For more than 30 years, hematopoietic stem cell transplants (SCTs) have been used to treat malignancies. SCT is potentially curative for acute myelogenous leukemia, acute lymphocytic leukemia, non-Hodgkin lymphoma, and Hodgkin disease. With the success of this therapy in hematologic malignancies, there has been significant interest in their use for solid tumors. SCT has been reported in the treatment of breast cancer, germ cell tumors, ovarian cancers, renal cell cancer, and other solid malignancies with varying degrees of success.

SCT can be divided into two types: autologous and allogenic. In autologous SCTs, a patient's own stem cells are collected and returned to the patient following high-dose chemotherapy. The rational for autologous SCTs is that most solid tumors are at least moderately responsive to cytotoxic chemotherapy. Some solid tumors such as germ cell tumors, early-stage lung cancers, and nonmetastatic cancers of the head and neck may even be cured with combination chemotherapy or chemotherapy combined with radiation. In vivo and in vitro experiments have shown that as the dose of a chemotherapeutic is increased, more cancer cells are killed (1,2). Several early randomized studies of breast, testicular, and ovarian cancer have also demonstrated the relationship between increasing dosage of chemotherapy and efficacy for cancer cell death (3–5).

Unfortunately, there is a limit to how much the dose of chemotherapy medication may be increased because of the toxicity of the treatment. There is a class of chemotherapeutics (i.e., alkylating agents) whose primary dose-limiting toxicity is marrow suppression. The alkylating agents include such medications as cyclophosphamide, melphalan, and thiotepa (6). Autologous SCTs allow patients to receive much higher doses of these chemotherapies by giving an autologous stem cell "rescue" to prevent prolonged pancytopenia. It is also possible to give multiple cycles of high-dose chemotherapy followed by SCT. This approach is called *tandem transplant* and has been used for some solid tumors.

Allogenic transplants consist of giving HLA-compatible or partially compatible donor stem cells to the patient following chemotherapy. The source of the stem cells is most commonly a sibling, a matched unrelated donor, or unrelated cord blood. Allogenic transplants are different from autologous transplants in that they fundamentally alter the patient's immune system and this may lead to immune-mediated destruction of the cancer via the infused T cells. This is called the *graft-versus-tumor effect*. This effect is most clearly demonstrated in chronic myelogenous leukemia and acute myelogenous leukemia although it has been demonstrated in other hematologic and solid tumors. In multiple randomized trials, allogenic SCT has been shown to provide patients with hematologic malignancies the greatest disease-free survival (DFS). Its ability to eradicate the malignant clone is greater than after autologous SCTs but is associated with higher rates of treatment-related toxicities and mortality (7,8). This can only be accounted for by a beneficial graft-versus-tumor effect and a detrimental graft-versus-host effect .

Some tumors such as renal cell carcinoma have shown to be responsive to immune-modulation therapy such as interferon or interleukin-2 (9,10). Given allogenic SCTs may also lead to a beneficial immune effect; there has been significant interest in allogenic transplants for renal cell cancer.

Chemotherapy and often radiation are given to the patient prior to an SCT. This is called *conditioning*. Intensive conditioning can result in the destruction of a patient's hematopoietic ability (myeloablative conditioning) and reduced intensity or nonmyeloablative conditioning regimens primarily target the recipient's immune system, thereby limiting systemic toxicity and treatment-related mortality. Reduced intensity conditioning transplants have allowed for stem cell transplantation in older and medically infirmed patients, those who could not tolerate the toxicity of a fully myeloablative conditioning regimen.

Stem cells used for transplant can be derived from either bone marrow or from stem cells "mobilized" into the peripheral blood. Stem cells can be mobilized into the peripheral circulation by growth factors (e.g., granulocyte-stimulating factor). The stem cells can be cryogenically preserved for storage prior to transplant.

The morbidity and mortality from the transplant depends on the type of transplant performed. Infections, mucositis, thrombocytopenia, anemia, and severe neutropenia are common after autologous SCT. Autologous transplants carried significant morbidity, but advances in supportive care have reduced treatment-related mortality to <5% in most centers.

An allogenic SCT has many of the same acute toxicities as an autologous transplant but with the added toxicities associated with graft-versus-host disease (GVHD) and the medicines used to treat or prevent it. GVHD can be semantically divided into acute and chronic GVHD. Acute GVHD begins before day 100 following allogenic SCT (11). The organ systems most commonly affected by acute GVHD include the skin, liver, and gastrointestinal track. Chronic GVHD begins after day 100 and involves the skin, eyes, mucous membrane, and lungs. Acute GVHD can be reduced in incidence and severity by the prophylactic use of immune-suppressive agents such as methotrexate, cyclosporine, tacrolimus, rapamycin, and prednisone.

Allogenic SCTs have a significantly higher mortality. One third of patients will die from transplant-related toxicities (infection or GVHD) in spite of the implementation of the best GVHD and infectious prophylaxis and the best HLA-matched donor (7,8).

BREAST CANCER

SCT for breast cancer has been the subject of many studies since the late 1980s. Breast cancer is the most common cancer in women and the third most frequent cause of cancer death (12). Although breast tumors are usually sensitive to chemotherapy, it is not possible to cure metastatic breast cancer with conventional-dose chemotherapy. Many patients with locally advanced breast cancer will demonstrate tumor recurrence despite aggressive surgery, radiation, hormone therapy, and chemotherapy. Given breast cancer's sensitivity to chemotherapy, it has been considered an ideal target for high-dose chemotherapy coupled with autologous stem cell rescue.

The general strategy in patients with breast cancer has been to administer several cycles of conventional-dose chemotherapy to determine the chemotherapy responsiveness prior to proceeding to autologous SCT. If the patient did not achieve at least a partial tumor response, there was little benefit from transplant.

Metastatic Breast Cancer

The initial phase I and II studies were very encouraging that high-dose chemotherapy with autologous SCT was superior to standard-dose chemotherapy for metastatic breast cancer. In a retrospective study evaluating the available phase I and II trials published in the late 1980s, an 80% response rate was reported (13). This exciting preliminary data led to the frequent use of autologous SCTs for the treatment of metastatic breast cancer. More than 41,000 women underwent the procedure, with most being treated off an institution review board-approved clinical trial (14).

Randomized trials of high-dose chemotherapy for metastatic breast cancer have not been as encouraging (Table 5.1). The first randomized trial was published by Bezwoda et al. (15) in 1995. In this report, 90 patients were randomized to either six to eight cycles of conventional-dose cyclophosphamide, mitoxantrone, and etoposide or two cycles of the same drugs at much higher doses together with autologous stem cell rescue given after each cycle of high-dose therapy. The results of this trial were positive. At 3 years following treatment, 18% of patients in the high-dose arm were alive compared with only 4% of patients who were given the conventional dose. Unfortunately, the results of this trial could never be repeated, and on further investigation fraud was suspected. This trial was retracted by the editors of the *Journal of Clinical Oncology* in 2001.

The next randomized trial using high-dose chemotherapy with stem cell rescue was published by Staudtmeir et al. (16) in 1999. In this trial, 553 patients with metastatic breast caner were treated with six cycles of fluorouracil (5-FU), doxorubicin, and cyclophosphamide (FAC) or cyclophosphamide, methotrexate, and 5-FU (CMF), depending on dose of anthracycline received

in prior adjuvant therapy. Those who responded to chemotherapy were then randomized to high-dose chemotherapy with carboplatin, cyclophosphamide, and thiotepa followed by SCT or up to 2 years of standard-dose CMF. Of the original 553 patients, 296 responded to the initial chemotherapy. Forty-seven percent of patients had partial responses and 11% had complete responses. Unfortunately, there was a significant dropout rate and thus only 184 entered the randomized portion of the trial. The mortality in the high-dose chemotherapy/autologous transplant arm was approximately 1%. The overall survival and the progression-free survival were not significantly different at 3 years.

The PEGASE 3 trial randomized 180 patients with metastatic breast cancer who had objective response to four cycles of conventional-dose chemotherapy to either high-dose chemotherapy with autologous stem cell rescue or observation (17). At 1 year following randomization, the progression-free survival was 46% in the high dose and 19% in the observation arm, respectively ($p = 0.0001$). The 3-year overall survival, however, was not significantly different.

In the PEGASE 4 trial, patients who had a partial or complete response to initial chemotherapy were randomized to receive either high-dose chemotherapy with cyclophosphamide, melphalan, and mitoxantrone followed by autologous stem cell rescue versus two to four cycles of conventional therapy (18). The high-dose chemotherapy arm had a statically significantly longer time to progression (12 months vs. 6 months). There was also a significantly improved overall survival with 36.8% of patients alive at 5 years in the high-dose chemotherapy group as opposed to 13.8% of those who received conventional-dose chemotherapy.

Crump et al. (19) treated women with four cycles of conventional chemotherapy followed by either more conventional chemotherapy or high-dose chemotherapy with autologous stem cell rescue. Two hundred nine women were randomized into the treatment arms. Once again, event-free survival was greater in the high-dose arm but the overall survival was not different between the two arms.

Several groups have also attempted multiple cycles of high-dose chemotherapy (tandem transplantation) with the hope of improving survival of patients with metastatic breast cancer (Table 5.1). Crown et al. (20) treated 110 patients with 4 cycles of standard-dose chemotherapy for 4 cycles and then randomized them to either continued standard-dose chemotherapy or 2 cycles of high-dose chemotherapy with autologous stem cell rescue. The event-free survival was significantly greater in the high-dose arm but the overall survival was the same between the two groups. Schmid et al. (21) randomized 93 women to either 2 cycles of upfront high-dose chemotherapy or conventional chemotherapy. In this trial, there was no difference in either progression-free or overall survival.

A meta-analysis of the available randomized trials was published by Farquhar et al. (14). Six trials were analyzed consisting of 438 women who had received high-dose SCT with autologous stem cell rescue and 412 were randomized to conventional treatment. There was no statistically significant difference in overall survival. At 5 years there was a significant difference in progression-free survival favoring the high-dose group. There was a prolongation in progression-free survival at 5 years but it

Table 5.1

High-Dose Therapy with Autologous Stem Cell Transplant For Metastatic Breast Cancer

Reference	No. of Patients Randomized	Design	Statistically Significant Increase in the Time to Progression- or Event-Free Survival in Favor of High-Dose Therapy	Statistically Significant Increase in the Overall Survival in Favor of High-Dose Therapy Survival in Favor of High-Dose Therapy
Staudtmeir et al. (16)	184	High-dose chemotherapy following CR or PR to standard chemotherapy versus further standard chemotherapy	No	No
Biron et al. (17) (PEGASE 03 trial)	180	High-dose chemotherapy following CR or PR to observation	Yes	No
Lotz et al. (18) (PEGASE 04 trial)	61	High-dose chemotherapy following CR or PR to standard chemotherapy versus further standard chemotherapy	Yes	Yes
Crump et al. (19)	209	High-dose chemotherapy following CR or PR to standard chemotherapy versus further standard chemotherapy	Yes	No
Crown et al. (20)	110	2 cycles of high-dose chemotherapy following CR or PR to standard chemotherapy versus further standard chemotherapy	Yes	No
Schmid et al. (21)	93	2 cycles of high-dose . versus further standard chemotherapy	No	No

CR, complete response; PR, partial response.

was barely statically significant. Per the investigator, one more relapse would have made the results not significantly different.

Overall, high-dose chemotherapy with autologous SCT for metastatic breast cancer has not proved to be a viable therapeutic alternative. There is no prolongation of overall survival but there seems to be some modest increase in progression-free survival when compared with standard-dose chemotherapy. This comes at the cost of increased toxicity in the peritransplant period. At this time, high-dose chemotherapy with autologous stem cell rescue should only be performed in the context of a clinical trial.

Adjuvant Therapy for Breast Cancer

Nonmetastatic breast cancer is a disease treated with multimodality therapy. Surgical removal of the breast mass and af-fected lymph nodes is the cornerstone of breast cancer therapy. Adjuvant treatment may consist of radiation, chemotherapy, and endocrine therapy to reduce the rate of relapse. Despite this aggressive multimodality approach, many women will relapse and will die from their breast cancer. The women at highest risk are those with either positive margins or multiple positive lymph nodes. The risk of relapse for a 65-year-old woman with an estrogen and progesterone receptor-positive and HER2/neu gene non-amplified 1-cm tumor and node-negative disease treated with conventional chemotherapy and endocrine treatment is 6.2%, 16.1% for one to three positive nodes, 27.7% for four to nine positive nodes, and 61.1% for more than nine positive nodes (22). Because of this significant relapse rate, it has been thought that the addition of high-dose chemotherapy with autologous SCT may offer a better prognosis.

There are a number of reasons to consider that the addition of high-dose therapy with autologous stem cell rescue would be beneficial for breast cancer patients receiving adjuvant therapy. The first is that these patients have a minimal disease burden. Several studies have suggested that those with the least disease burden receive the greatest benefit from high-dose chemotherapy (2). Second, these patients had received minimal prior chemotherapy. This means that the tumor would have less opportunity to develop chemotherapy resistance and the patient would be in better overall condition to tolerate the therapy.

Early phase II trials were encouraging. Peters et al. (23) treated 102 patients with stage II/III breast cancer and at least ten positive lymph nodes. The patients received four cycles of standard-dose adjuvant chemotherapy followed by high-dose cyclophosphamide, cisplatin, and BCNU (STAMP V) and then SCT. The 5-year event-free survival was 72%. Historical controls had a 5-year event-free survival of 25%. The therapy-related mortality, however, was significant (12%). This might have been partly due to the lack of hematopoietic growth factors when this study was performed (1989–1991) as well as BCNU-induced pulmonary toxicity.

High-dose therapy has also been performed in inflammatory breast cancer. Adkins et al. (24) retrospectively analyzed 47 patients with stage IIIB inflammatory breast cancer treated with high-dose chemotherapy and autologous stem cell rescue as part of multimodality therapy. At 4 years, the DFS and overall survival were 51.3% and 51.7%, respectively, which compared favorably with to those treated with conventional chemotherapy. Ayash et al. (25) also examined women with stage III inflammatory breast cancer. In their trial, 50 patients had high-dose chemotherapy added to their multimodality therapy. The high-dose chemotherapy was given either before mastectomy (40 patients) or following the surgery (10). The estimated DFS at 30 months was 64%. The DFS was best for those patients who achieved a pathologic complete response at the time of mastectomy. None of those seven patients had relapsed at 30 months. Somlo et al. (26) treated 120 patients with stage IIIB with either single or tandem transplants. A statistically significant benefit in relapse-free survival was seen in the patients who received tandem transplants as opposed to single cycles of high-dose chemotherapy ($p = 0.049$).

Several phase III trials have been performed to test the benefit of high-dose chemotherapy in the adjuvant setting. Tallman et al. (27) randomly assigned 540 woman with resected stage II/III breast cancer who had at least 10 positive axillary lymph nodes to either six cycles of standard-dose adjuvant chemotherapy with cyclophosphamide, doxorubicin, and 5-FU (CAF) or six cycles of CAF followed by high-dose cyclophosphamide and thiotepa followed by autologous SCT. Patients also received radiation and tamoxifen, if indicated, following completion of their chemotherapy (standard dose or high dose). The transplant-related mortality was <2%. In the 417 patients who strictly met treatment criteria, there was a prolongation in DFS at 5 years (55% vs. 45%, $p = 0.045$). Thus, prolongation in DFS did not translate into a benefit in overall survival.

Rodenhuis et al. (28) randomized 885 women with stage II/III breast cancer with at least four positive lymph nodes positive to standard adjuvant therapy or high-dose chemotherapy. The standard-dose arm received 5-FU, epirubicin, and cyclophosphamide (FEC) for five cycles. Five cycles of FEC followed by high-dose cyclophosphamide, thiotepa, and carboplatin and autologous stem cell rescue was given to the study group. Patients received radiation and tamoxifen, if indicated, following completion of their chemotherapy (standard dose or high dose). The transplant-related mortality was <1%. At 5 years, the event-free survival was not significantly different. When only the patients with more than 10 positive lymph nodes were examined, the event-free survival was higher in the high-dose arm (61% vs. 51%, $p = 0.05$). Overall survival was not different between the two groups.

High-dose chemotherapy with autologous SCT seems to increase event-free survival for patients at very high risk for relapse. However, it does not increase overall survival. The applicability of these data at the present time is unclear. There have been significant advances in adjuvant therapy since the time when these trials were performed. Taxanes and aromatase inhibitors added to adjuvant chemotherapy have shown significant benefit (29,30). Trastuzumab has been very beneficial for *HER2/neu*-amplified tumors (31). Further trials are necessary to determine the applicability of high-dose chemotherapy.

GERM CELL CANCER

More than 80% of patients presenting with metastatic germ cell cancer can be cured with first-line chemotherapy (32). It is also one of the few recurrent solid tumors that can be cured with salvage chemotherapy. Vinblastine, ifosfamide, and cisplatin (VIP) is one of the most common salvage regimens and has been reported to have a complete response rate of 50% with a 32% long-term survival rate. Given the chemosensitivity of this cancer, it has been thought that the opportunity for cure could be improved with more intense chemotherapy.

The initial studies of high-dose chemotherapy with autologous stem cell rescue demonstrated that it has activity in those patients who had been heavily pretreated. Nichols et al. (33) reported a phase I/II trial of high-dose carboplatin and etoposide followed by autologous stem cell rescue in 33 patients with heavily pretreated testicular cancer. Forty-four percent of patients had a response to therapy, with 24% achieving a complete response. Four of the patients maintained a complete response for more than 1 year.

Bhatia et al. (34) published the University of Indiana's experience with salvage high-dose chemotherapy and autologous stem cell rescue for testicular cancer. Between 1992 and 1998, 65 patients with either relapsed or primary refractory testicular cancer were given two cycles of high-dose carboplatin and etoposide followed each time by autologous stem cell rescue. Some of the patients received one to three cycles of standard-dose salvage chemotherapy prior to high-dose therapy and many also received maintenance oral etoposide following the therapy. Complete responses were achieved in 43% of patients and an additional 20% were rendered disease-free by salvage surgery. At a median follow-up of 39 months 57% of patients had no evidence of disease. The median survival had not been reached when the results were published in 2000. There were no treatment-related deaths.

Beyer et al. (35) performed a matched pair analysis of high-dose chemotherapy with autologous SCT compared with conventional dose chemotherapy. The analysis suggested an overall survival benefit of 9% to 11% over standard chemotherapy.

Several phase III trials comparing high-dose salvage with standard dose are currently ongoing. One phase III trial has been completed. Rosti et al. (36) randomized 280 patients with relapsed or primary refractory testicular or extragonadal germ cell tumors to either four courses of standard-dose VIP or VIEP (vincristine, ifosfamide, etoposide, and cisplatin) or three cycles of these regimens plus one cycle of high-dose carboplatin, etoposide, and cyclophosphamide with autologous stem cell rescue. The high-dose arm was more toxic than the conventional-dose arm. There were nine treatment-related deaths in those patients receiving high-dose chemotherapy as compared with two in the standard-dose arm. The complete response rate was 41% in the standard-dose arm and 44% in the high-dose arm. The 3-year survival rate was 53% in both arms.

The role of autologous transplant as salvage in germ cell cancer remains unclear. Currently, the National Comprehensive Cancer Network recommends high-dose chemotherapy with autologous stem rescue as salvage for patients with poor risk disease (37). We await the results of the other phase III trials comparing tandem transplants with standard salvage.

A phase III trial was recently presented using high-dose chemotherapy as first-line therapy for patients with intermediate- or poor-risk germ cell tumors. Bajorin et al. (38) randomized 219 previously untreated patients with International Germ Cell Cancer Collaborative group intermediate- or poor-risk germ cell tumors to four cycles of standard-dose bleomycin, etoposide, and cisplatin (BEP) or two cycles of BEP and two cycles of high-dose carboplatin, etoposide, and cyclophosphamide with autologous stem cell rescue. There was no significant difference in complete response or survival between the two arms. High-dose chemotherapy, therefore, is not recommended as initial treatment of patients with germ cell cancer.

NEUROBLASTOMA

Neuroblastoma is one of the most common solid tumors in children (39). It is a chemosensitive tumor. High-dose chemotherapy has been shown to improve outcomes.

A number of phase II trials have been performed using high-dose chemotherapy to treat metastatic neuroblastoma. Most have shown a long-term survival of 28% to 33% (39–41). This is superior to historical control of 10% to 15% (39).

The largest prospective trial of high-dose chemotherapy versus standard chemotherapy was performed by Matthay et al. (42). In this trial, 539 patients with high-risk neuroblastoma were treated with standard-dose cisplatin, doxorubicin, etoposide, and cyclophosphamide for five cycles plus surgery and radiotherapy for those with gross disease. The patients who did not progress on this therapy were randomly assigned to another three courses of the previously mentioned chemotherapy or to high-dose therapy. The high-dose therapy consisted of carboplatin, etoposide, melphalan, and total-body irradiation with autologous stem cell rescue. The 3-year event-free survival was significantly higher with the high-dose arm (34% vs. 22%, $p = 0.034$). The treatment-related mortality was equal in both arms.

High-dose chemotherapy has become part of the standard therapy for patients with high-risk neuroblastoma.

OVARIAN CANCER

Ovarian cancer is a chemotherapy-sensitive tumor. There is also evidence that dose intensification leads to better outcomes (5). High-dose chemotherapy followed by autologous SCT had been suggested to be a potentially useful therapy for ovarian cancer.

The initial phase II trials showed impressive complete response rates for high-dose chemotherapy with autologous stem cell rescue. Stiff et al. (43) retrospectively reviewed 100 ovarian cancer patients with relapsed or refractory disease who were treated with high-dose chemotherapy. The overall response rate was 85%, with a complete response rate of 43%. For patients with platinum-sensitive disease, the complete response rate was even higher (73%). The duration of the complete response was short, with only 14% of patients free of disease at 1 year.

The phase III trials of high-dose chemotherapy for ovarian cancer have not shown benefit. Ledermann et al. (44) assigned 149 women with optimally debulked stage III or IV ovarian cancer to either standard-dose chemotherapy with platinum and paclitaxel or high-dose chemotherapy with autologous stem cell rescue. Patients in the high-dose arm received two cycles of standard-dose cyclophosphamide and paclitaxel, during which stem cells were collected. This was followed by three cycles of high-dose chemotherapy, each with stem cell rescue. The morbidity of the high-dose arm was low (1.3%). At a median follow-up of 36 months, there was no significant difference in overall survival or disease-free survival.

Cure et al. (45) compared high-dose chemotherapy with standard-dose chemotherapy as consolidation for patients with minimal disease following initial chemotherapy. In this study, there was no difference in overall or disease-free survival.

Given the lack of benefit in clinical trials, high-dose chemotherapy with autologous SCT is no longer considered to be an appropriate therapy for patients with ovarian cancer.

SMALL CELL LUNG CANCER

Small cell lung cancer accounts for approximately 25% of lung cancers (12). It is a chemosensitive tumor with a first-line chemotherapy response rate of approximately 50% and a complete response rate of 10% to 15% in metastatic disease (46). Unfortunately, relapse is almost universal for patients with extensive disease. The prognosis for limited-stage small cell cancer is also poor, with a 5-year survival of approximately 12% with conventional chemotherapy and radiation therapy (47). The chemosensitivity and poor prognosis has led to significant interest in high-dose chemotherapy.

Two approaches to high-dose chemotherapy tested in phase III trials were late intensification and early intensification. In a late intensification approach, patients who respond to standard-dose chemotherapy receive a consolidation cycle of high-dose chemotherapy to keep them in remission. In an early intensification approach, patients receive high-dose chemotherapy as a part of initial therapy.

Humblet et al. (48) tested a late consolidation approach in the early 1980s. In this trial, 101 patients with either limited- or extensive-stage small cell lung cancer received five cycles of standard-dose methotrexate, vincristine, cyclophosphamide, doxorubicin, cisplatin, and etoposide as well as prophylactic radiation to the brain. Forty-five patients who had at least a partial response were randomized to a cycle of high-dose or standard-dose cyclophosphamide, BCNU, and etoposide. The high-dose chemotherapy was able to induce more complete responses (39% following standard chemotherapy to 79% following high-dose therapy). The relapse-free survival was longer in the high-dose arm when compared with the standard-dose arm (28 weeks vs. 10 weeks, $p = 0.002$). The median overall survival, however, was not statistically significant between the two groups. It was thought the high transplant-related mortality (17%) was one of reasons why the improvement in relapse-free survival did not translate into an improvement in overall survival.

Leyvraz et al. (49) used an early intensification approach. In this trial, 145 with limited- or extensive-stage small cell cancer were randomized to six cycles of standard-dose ifosfamide, carboplatin, and etoposide or two cycles of epirubicin/paclitaxel followed by three cycles of high-dose ifosfamide, carboplatin, and etoposide with stem cell support. There was no significant difference in response rate, progression-free survival, or overall survival between the two arms.

Thus far, the randomized trials have not been favorable for either early or late intensification for small cell lung cancer. Therefore, it is not a recommended therapy.

AUTOLOGOUS TRANSPLANTS FOR OTHER SOLID TUMORS

High-dose chemotherapy has been used to treat a variety of other tumors including Ewing sarcoma, Wilms tumor, and medulloblastomas (50–54). The reports in these tumors are mostly case series or small phase II trials with no randomized phase III trials completed at this time. The results of high-dose chemotherapy in Ewing sarcoma have been mixed. Laurence et al. (50) retrospectively analyzed 46 patients with poor-risk Ewing sarcoma, 22 of whom had metastatic disease treated with high-dose chemotherapy as part of multimodality therapy. The 5-year overall survival was 34% for those with metastatic disease and 71% for those with locally advanced disease. With standard chemotherapy, the 5-year survival for metastatic disease and locally advance disease was <25% and <60%, respectively. The results of Myers et al. (51) were not as promising. In this prospective trial, 23 patients with metastatic Ewing carcinoma were given five cycles of standard-induction chemotherapy (cyclophosphamide, doxorubicin, and vincristine, alternating with ifosfamide and etoposide) and then local therapy. They had consolidation with high-dose chemotherapy and total-body irradiation with autologous stem cell rescue. The 2-year event-free survival was only 24%. Currently, a phase III trial comparing standard chemotherapy with high-dose chemotherapy is accruing (EURO-EWING-INTERGROUP-EE99).

High-dose chemotherapy has been used for children with Wilms tumor. Campbell et al. (52) treated 13 children with relapsed Wilms tumors with either one or two cycles of high-dose

Table 5.2

Current Recommendations for High-Dose Chemotherapy with Autologous Stem Cell Rescue in Solid Tumors

Tumor	Recommendations
Breast cancer	Not recommended outside of clinical trial
Neuroblastoma	Recommended as salvage therapy
Germ cell	Recommended as salvage therapy
Ovarian cancer	Not recommended
Small cell lung cancer	Not recommended

chemotherapy with autologous stem cell rescue. The overall survival at 4 years was 73%. Pein et al. (53) transplanted 29 patients with relapsed Wilms tumor and two with high-risk anaplastic Wilms tumor in first CR. The overall survival was 60% at 3 years. The patients who were transplanted earlier in their disease course (i.e., in second complete response or partial response) had a significantly better DFS.

In order to improve survival, patients with medulloblastomas have been treated with high-dose chemotherapy. Gajjar et al. (54) treated 134 patients with newly diagnosed medulloblastoma. These patients received resection, risk-adapted radiation (higher doses for the "high risk group," i.e., those with residual tumors >1.5 cm or metastasis with in the neural axis), and four cycles of high-dose chemotherapy with stem cell rescue. This trial had an improved survival versus historical controls, with a 5-year overall survival of 85% in the average-risk group and 70% for the high-risk group. This continues to be an active area of research.

Current recommendations for autologous stem cell rescue in solid tumors are outlined in Table 5.2.

ALLOGENIC STEM CELL TRANSPLANTS FOR SOLID TUMORS

Given that the majority of metastatic cancers are incurable with chemotherapy, there has been interest in allogenic SCTs. The hope has been that there would be a graft-versus-tumor effect in solid tumors like that seen in leukemias. Also, the less toxic nonmyeloablative conditioning regimens have made allogenic transplants more feasible for solid tumors. Allogenic SCTs have been attempted for several tumor types including colon cancer (55), breast cancer (55–57), cholangiocarcinoma (55), osteosarcoma (58), and renal cell cancer (55,59–61). The studies thus far consist of case reports or small case series. The most extensively studied is renal cell carcinoma.

Renal cell cancer has been a tempting target for allogenic stem cell transplantation. It has been shown to be sensitive to immune-oriented therapies. T lymphocytes have been isolated from some renal cell cancers that are cytotoxic to the tumor. Spontaneous remissions are known to occur. The immune modulators interleukin-2 and interferon-alpha have led to responses in approximately 20% of patients with renal cell carcinoma (10).

The first case series of renal cell cancer patients treated with allogenic SCTs was published by Childs et al. (59). In this case series, 19 consecutive patients with refractory metastatic renal cell carcinoma were given allogenic SCTs from HLA-compatible siblings. The conditioning consisted of a nonmyeloablative regimen of cyclophosphamide, fludarabine, and antithymocyte globulin. Cyclosporine was used for GVHD prophylaxis. For patients who did not achieve full donor T-cell chimerism (100% of T cells being of donor origin) or who had progressive disease, three donor lymphocyte infusions were administered following transplant.

The results were impressive. Ten of the 19 patients had at least a partial response to the transplant. Three patients had complete responses. Two patients died from treatment-related mortality. One patient died from sepsis and the other from severe GVHD.

The results of this trial strongly suggest the presence of a graft-versus-tumor effect in renal cell carcinoma. First, renal cell cancer is not responsive to the chemotherapy used for the conditioning regimen. Second, the best predictor of response was the presence of GVHD indicating an immunologically active graft. Third, response occurred only after complete donor chimerism was obtained and with removal of immune suppression.

Rini et al. (60), Bregni et al. (57), Hentschke et al. (55), and Massenkeil et al. (61) also treated renal cell cancer with nonmyeloablative-conditioned allogenic stem transplants. These small cases series of 7 to 15 patients showed that some patients do have responses to transplants. Further studies of allogenic stem cell transplantation in renal cell carcinoma are in progress.

CONCLUSION

The results of hematopoietic SCTs for solid tumors have been disappointing. The initial phase II trials were very encouraging. Unfortunately, with the exception of neuroblastoma, SCTs have not been shown to prolong survival in randomized clinical trials. These results illustrate the necessity for randomized trials comparing new therapies with the standard of care.

REFERENCES

1. Frei E III, Teicher BA, Holden SA, et al. Preclinical studies and clinical correlation of the effect of alkylating dose. *Cancer Res.* 1988;48:6417–6423.
2. Frei E III, Antman K, Teicher BA, et al. Bone marrow autotransplantation for solid tumors—prospects. *J Clin Oncol.* 1989;7:515–526.
3. Wood W, Budman D, Korzun A, et al. Dose and dose intensity of adjuvant chemotherapy for stage II node positive breast cancer. *N Engl J Med.* 1994;330:1253–1259.
4. Sampson MK, Rivkin SE, Jones SE, et al. Dose-response and dose-survival advantage for high versus low doses of cisplatin combined with vinblastine and bleomycin in disseminated testicular cancer: a Southwest Oncology Group study. *Cancer.* 1984;53:1029–1035.
5. Kaye SB, Lewis CR, Paul J, et al. Randomized study of two doses of cisplatin with cyclophosphamide in epithelial ovarian cancer. *Lancet.* 1992;340:329–333.
6. Chabner BA, Amrein PC, Drucker BJ, et al. Antineoplastic agents. In: Goodman and Gilman's *The Pharmacological Basis of Therapeutics.* 11th ed. McGraw-Hill. 2006;1315–1405.
7. Cassileth PA, Harrington DP, Applebaum FR, et al. Chemotherapy compared with autologous or allogeneic bone marrow transplantation in the management of acute myeloid leukemia in first remission. *N Engl J Med.* 1998;339:1649–1656.
8. Zittoun RA, Mandelli F, Willemze R, et al. Autologous or allogeneic bone marrow transplantation compared with intensive chemotherapy in acute myelogenous leukemia. *N Engl J Med.* 1995;332:217–223.
9. Fyfe G, Fisher RI, Rosenberg SA, et al. Results of treatment of 255 patients with metastatic renal cell carcinoma who received high-dose recombinant interleukin-2 therapy. *J Clin Oncol.* 1995;13:688–696.
10. Negrier S, Escudier B, Lasset C, et al. Recombinant human interleukin-2, recombinant human interferon alfa-2a, or both in metastatic renal-cell carcinoma. Groupe Francais d'Immunoherapie. *N Engl J Med.* 1998;338:1272–1278.
11. Couriel D. Acute graft-versus-host disease: pathophysiology, clinical manifestations, and management. *Cancer.* 2004;101:1936–1946.
12. Jemal A, Siegel R, Ward E, et al. Cancer statistics, 2006. *CA Cancer J Clin.* 2006;56:106–130.
13. Antman K, Gale P. Advanced breast cancer: high-dose chemotherapy and bone marrow autotransplants. *Ann Intern Med.* 1988;108:570–574.
14. Farquhar C, Marjoribanks J, Basser R, et al. High dose chemotherapy and autologous bone marrow or stem cell transplantation versus conventional chemotherapy for women with metastatic breast cancer. *Cochrane Database Syst Rev.* 2005;3:CD003142.
15. Bezwoda WR, Seymore L, Dansey R. High-dose chemotherapy with hematopoietic rescue as a primary treatment for metastatic breast cancer: a randomized trial. *J Clin Oncol.* 1995;13:2483–2489.
16. Staudtmier EA, O'Neill A, Goldstein LJ, et al. Conventional-dose chemotherapy compared with high-dose chemotherapy with autologous hematopoietic stem-cell transplantation for metastatic breast cancer. *N Engl J Med.* 2000;342:1069–1076.
17. Biron P, Durand M, Roche H, et al. High dose thiotepa (TTP) cyclophosphamide (CPM) and stem cell transplantation after 4 FEC 100 compared with 4 FEC alone allowed a better disease free survival but the same overall survival in first line chemotherapy for metastatic breast cancer. Results of the PEGASE 03 French Protocole [abstract]. *Proc Am Soc Clin Oncol.* 2002;21:167.
18. Lotz JP, Cure H, Janvier M, et al. High-dose chemotherapy with haematopoietic stem cell transplantation for metastatic breast cancer patients: final results of the French multicentric randomized CMA/PEGASE 04 Protocol. *Eur J Cancer.* 2005;41:71–80.
19. Crump M, Gluck S, Stewart D, et al. A randomized trial of high-dose chemotherapy (HDCT) with autologous peripheral blood stem cell support (AHPCT) compared to standard chemotherapy in women with metastatic breast cancer: a National Cancer Institute of Canada (NCIC) Clinical Trials Group study [abstract]. *Proc Am Soc Clin Oncol.* 2001;20:21.
20. Crown J, Pey L, Lind M, et al. Superiority of tandem high-dose chemotherapy (HDC) versus optimized conventionally-dosed chemotherapy (CDC) in patients with metastatic breast cancer (MBC): the International Randomized Breast Cancer Dose Intensity Study (IBDIS 1) [abstract]. *Proc Am Soc Clin Oncol.* 2003;22:23.
21. Schmid P, Schippinger W, Nitsch T, et alia. Up-front tandem high-dose chemotherapy compared with doxorubicin and paclitaxel in metastatic breast cancer: results of a randomized trial. *J Clin Oncol.* 2005;23:432–440.
22. Adjuventonline. www.adjuventonline.com.
23. Peters WP, Ross M, Vredenburgh JJ, et al. High dose chemotherapy and autologous bone marrow support as consolidation after

standard-dose adjuvant therapy for high-risk breast cancer [abstract]. *Proc Am Soc Clin Oncol.* 1995;14:90.

24. Adkins D, Brown R, Trinkhaus, et al. Outcomes of high-dose chemotherapy and autologous stem-cell transplantation in stage IIIB inflammatory breast cancer. *J Clin Oncol.* 1999;17:2006–2014.

25. Ayash LJ, Elias A, Ibrahim J, et al. High-dose multimodality therapy with autologous stem-cell support for stage IIIB breast carcinoma. *J Clin Oncol.* 1998;16:1000–1007.

26. Somlo G, Frankel P, Chow W, et al. Prognostic indicators and survival in patients with stage IIIB inflammatory breast carcinoma after dose intense chemotherapy. *J Clin Oncol.* 2004;22:1839–1848.

27. Tallman MS, Gray R, Robert NJ, et al. Conventional adjuvant chemotherapy with or without high-dose chemotherapy with autologous stem-cell transplantation in high-risk breast cancer. *N Engl J Med.* 2003;349:17–26.

28. Rodenhuis S, Bontebal M, Beex LVAM, et al. High-dose chemotherapy with hematopoietic stem-cell rescue for high-risk breast cancer. *N Engl J Med.* 2003;349:7–16.

29. Henderson IC, Berry DA, Demetri GD, et al. Improved outcomes from adding sequential Paclitaxel but not from escalating Doxorubicin dose in an adjuvant chemotherapy regimen for patients with node-positive primary breast cancer. *J Clin Oncol.* 2003;21:976–983.

30. Thurlimann B, Keshaviah A, Coates AS, et al. A comparison of letrozole and tamoxifen in postmenopausal women with early breast cancer. *N Engl J Med.* 2005;353:2747–2757.

31. Romond EH, Perez EA, Bryant J, et al. Trastuzumab plus adjuvant chemotherapy for operable HER2-positive breast cancer. *N Engl J Med.* 2005;353:1673–1684.

32. Loehrer PJ Sr, Gonin R, Nichols CR, et al. Vinblastine plus ifosfamide plus cisplatin as initial salvage therapy in recurrent germ cell tumor. *J Clin Oncol.* 1998;16:2500–2504.

33. Nichols CR, Anderson J, Lazarus HM, et al. High-dose carboplatin and etoposide with autologous bone marrow transplantation in refractory germ cell cancer: an Eastern Cooperative Oncology Group protocol. *J Clin Oncol.* 1992;10:558–563.

34. Bhatia S, Abonour R, Porcu P, et al. High-dose chemotherapy as initial salvage chemotherapy in patients with relapsed testicular cancer. *J Clin Oncol.* 2000;18:3346–3351.

35. Beyer J, Stenning S, Gerl A, et al. High-dose versus conventional-dose chemotherapy as first-salvage treatment in patients with non-seminomatous germ-cell tumors: a matched-pair analysis. *Ann Oncol.* 2002;13:599–605.

36. Rosti G, Pico JL, Wandt H, et al. High-dose chemotherapy (HDC) in the salvage treatment of patients failing first-line platinum chemotherapy for advanced germ cell tumors (GCT); first results of a prospective randomized trial of the European Group for Blood and Marrow Transplantation (EBMT): IT-94 study. *Proc Am Soc Clin Oncol.* 2002; 21: Abstract 716.

37. National Comprehensive Cancer Network (www.nccn.org)

38. Bajorin DF, Nichols CR, Margolin KA, et al. Phase III trial of conventional-dose chemotherapy alone or with high-dose chemotherapy for metastatic germ cell tumors (GCT) patients (PTS): a cooperative group trial by Memorial Sloan-Kettering Cancer Center, ECOG, SWOG, and CALGB. J Clin Oncol. 2006;24:4510.

39. Hale GA. Autologous stem cell transplantation for pediatric solid tumors. *Expert Rev Anticancer Ther.* 2005;5:835–846.

40. Verdeguer A, Munoz A, Canete A, et al. Long-term results of high-dose chemotherapy and autologous stem cell rescue for high risk neuroblastoma patients: a report of the Spanish working party for BMT in children. *Pediatr Hematol Oncol.* 2004;321:495–504.

41. Harmann O, Valteau-Couanet D, Vassal G, et al. Prognostic factors in metastatic neuroblastoma over 1 year of age treated with high-dose chemotherapy and stem cell transplantation: a multivariate analysis in 218 patients treated in a single institution. *Bone Marrow Transplant.* 1999;23:789–795.

42. Matthay KK, Villablanca JG, Seeger RC, et al. Treatment of high-risk neuroblastoma with intensive chemotherapy, radiotherapy, autologous bone marrow transplantation, and 13-cis-retinoic acid. Children's Cancer Group. *N Engl J Med.* 1999;341:1165–1173.

43. Stiff PJ, Bayer R, Kerger C, et al. High dose chemotherapy with autologous transplantation for persistent/relapsed ovarian carcinoma. A multivariant analysis of survival of 100 consecutively treated patients. *J Clin Oncol.* 1997;15:1309–1317.

44. Ledermann, JA, Frickhofen, N, Wandt, H, et al. A phase III randomized trial of sequential high dose chemotherapy (HDC) with peripheral blood stem cell support or standard dose Chemotherapy (SDC) for first-line treatment of ovarian cancer. *J Clin Oncol.* 2005;23:456s.

45. Cure H, Battista, C, Guastalla, JP, et al. Phase III randomized trial of high-dose chemotherapy and peripheral blood stem cell support as consolidation in patients with advanced ovarian cancer: 5-year follow-up of GINECO/FNCLCC/SFGM-TC study [abstract]. *Proc Am Soc Clin Oncol.* 2004;23:449.

46. Skarlos DV, Samantas E, Kosmidis P, et al. Randomized comparison of etoposide-cisplatin vs. etoposide-carboplatin and irradiation in small-cell lung cancer. A Hellenic Co-operative Oncology Group study. *Ann Oncol.* 1994;5:601–607.

47. Janne PA, Freidlin B, Saxman S, et al. Twenty-five years of clinical research for patients with limited-stage small cell lung carcinoma in North America. *Cancer.* 2002;95:1528–1538.

48. Humblet Y, Symann M, Bosly A, et al. Late intensification chemotherapy with autologous bone marrow transplantation in selected small-cell carcinoma of the lung: a randomized study. *J Clin Oncol.* 1987;5:1864–1873.

49. Leyvraz S, Pampallona S, Martinelli G, et al. Randomized phase III study of high-dose sequential chemotherapy (CT) supported by peripheral blood progenitor cells (PBPC) for the treatment of small cell lung cancer (SCLC): Results of the EBMT Random-ICE trial. *J Clin Oncol.* 2006;24: Abstract 7064.

50. Laurence V, Pierga JY, Barthier S, et al. Long-term follow up of high-dose chemotherapy with autologous stem cell rescue in adults with Ewing tumor. *Am J Clin Oncol* 2005; 28: 301–309.

51. Myers PA, Krailo MD, Ladanyi M, et al. High-dose melphlan, etoposide, total-body irradiation, and autologous stem-cell reconstitution as consolidation therapy for high-risk Ewing sarcoma does not improve prognosis. *J Clin Oncol.* 2001;19:2812–2820.

52. Campbell AD, Cohn SL, Reynolds M, et al. Treatment of relapsed Wilm tumor with high-dose therapy and autologous hematopoietic stem cell rescue: the experience at Children's Memorial Hospital. *J Clin Oncol.* 2004;22:2885–2890.

53. Pein F, Michon J, Valteau-Couanet D, et al. High-dose melphalan, etoposide, and carboplatin followed by autologous stem-cell rescue in pediatric high-risk recurrent Wilm tumors: a French Society of Pediatric Oncology study. *J Clin Oncol.* 1998;16:3295–3301.

54. Gajjar A, Chintaqumpala M, Ashley D, et al. Risk-adapted craniospinal radiotherapy followed by high-dose chemotherapy and stem-cell rescue in children with newly diagnosed medulloblastoma (St Jude Medulloblastoma-96): long-term results from a prospective, multicentre trial. *Lancet Oncol.* 2006;7:813–820.

55. Hentschke P, Barkholt L, Uzunel M, et al. Low-intensity conditioning and hematopoietic stem cell transplantation in patients with renal and colon carcinoma. *Bone Marrow Transplant.* 2003;31:253–261.

56. Bregni M, Fleischhauer K, Bernardi M, et al. Bone marrow mammoglobin expression as a marker of graft-versus-tumor effect after reduced intensity allografting for advanced breast cancer. *Bone Marrow Transplant.* 2006;37:311–315.

57. Bregni M, Dodero A, Peccatori J, et al. Nonmyeloablative conditioning followed by hematopoietic cell allografting and donor lymphocyte infusions for patients with metastatic renal and breast cancer. *Blood.* 2002;99:4234–4236.

58. Kounami S, Nakayama K, Yoshiyama M, et al. Non-myeloablative allogenic peripheral blood stem cell transplantation in a patient with refractory osteosarcoma. *Pediatr Transplant.* 2005;9:342–345.

59. Childs R, Chernoff A, Contentin N, et al. Regression of metastatic renal-cell carcinoma after nonmyeloablative allogeneic peripheral-blood stem-cell transplantation. *N Engl J Med.* 2000;343:750–758.

60. Rini B, Zimmerman T, Stadler W, et al. Allogenic stem-cell transplantation of renal cell cancer after nonmyeloablative chemotherapy: feasibility, engraftment, and clinical results. *J Clin Oncol.* 2002; 20:2017–2024.

61. Massenkeil G, Roigas J, Nagy M, et al. Nonmyeloablative stem cell transplantation in metastatic renal cell carcinoma: delayed graft-versus-tumor effect is associated with chimerism conversion but transplantation has high toxicity. *Bone Marrow Transplant.* 2004;34:309–316.

COMMENTARY
Michael Lill and Stephen W. Lim

The two methods of stem cell transplantation, *autologous transplantation* and *allogenic transplantation,* are associated with two different rationales in the treatment of solid tumor malignancies.

AUTOLOGOUS TRANSPLANTATION

Autologous transplantation is employed as a component of a therapeutic strategy to provide dose intensification of chemotherapy. The drugs prescribed are agents that are primarily myelotoxic, and the autologous stem cells are used as a method of rescue from the side effects of the high doses of chemotherapy. This approach depends on the theory that resistance of tumor cells to chemotherapy may be overcome by increasing the dose of chemotherapy. Autologous transplantation is used only in connection with chemotherapy that has myelosuppression as the main dose limiting toxicity. Much of the rationale for autologous transplantation was developed for the treatment of hematologic malignancies, leukemias, and lymphomas, in which alkylating agents play a key role in therapy. Alkylating agents all have predominantly myelotoxicity and can be dose-escalated quite dramatically. However, alkylating drugs may not necessarily be the best chemotherapeutic agents for solid tumor malignancies. For example, colorectal cancer is a malignancy in which alkylating agents play no role in therapy, either in the adjuvant or metastatic setting. Dose-limiting toxicities of drugs active against colorectal cancer are mainly nonhematologic and there is, therefore, no rationale for the use of dose intensification together with hematopoietic stem cell rescue.

Theoretical concerns about autologous transplantation mainly revolve around tumor cell contamination of the transplant product, early mortality, and delayed side effects of treatment (myelodysplastic syndrome and secondary malignancies).

ALLOGENIC TRANSPLANTATION

Allogenic transplantation may or may not incorporate dose intensification. Its value relies to a large extent on the concept of graft versus malignancy, an immunologically mediated attack on tumor cells. Allogenic transplantation, even when nonmyeloablative conditioning is used, is bedeviled by a relatively high rate of early transplant-related mortality due to infection and acute graft-versus-host disease, substantial risks of long-term morbidity from chronic graft-versus-host disease, the need for prolonged immunosuppression, and the difficulty in identifying donors.

SELECTION OF PATIENTS FOR TRANSPLANTATION

The clinical state of the patient at the time of transplant needs to be considered. One can conceptualize the role of transplant in a neoadjuvant setting, an adjuvant setting, or as a treatment for relapsed or metastatic disease. Clearly, the risk-benefit ratio for an expensive and moderately high-risk procedure will be altered depending on the status of the patient. In general, one would not wish to offer transplant to patients with tumors associated with a favorable prognosis with conventional therapy, even in the setting of the relatively low mortality rate associated with autologous peripheral blood stem cell transplantation. Similarly, if it could be shown to be helpful, one would be prepared to offer either autologous or even allogenic transplantation to a patient with a relapsed metastatic solid tumor.

ASSESSING THE EFFICACY OF TRANSPLANTATION

Among the difficulties in designing trials to determine the worth of transplantation in the management of solid tumors is the observation that most patients with nonmetastatic disease are cured primarily by surgery, and patients at high risk of relapse, the most suitable candidates for entry into a clinical trial, are not easily identified prospectively.

Studies of transplantation for solid tumors generally consist of several types: the single institution phase I/II study, the registry study, and the randomized phase III study. Each of these approaches has substantial limitations. Single-institution studies can suffer from local experience that cannot be generalized to a national population, selection biases that are difficult to adjust for, and a tendency to report only positive results. Registry studies rely on reporting of outcome data from multiple transplant teams around the world. These studies are enormously helpful in describing outcomes of transplants for different diseases, but not so useful in comparing different treatment strategies for a specific disease, for example, high-dose chemotherapy versus standard approaches. There are a number of fundamental problems with registry studies that can only be partially compensated for using statistical adjustments. Staging of disease can be different between different reporting institutions. Chemotherapeutic conditioning regimens are often different for the same disease. All patients transplanted at each institution are reported, so there is avoidance of selective reporting, but not all potentially eligible patients are reported. This leads to the possibility of selection bias in the patient population. This bias can potentially operate in both directions; that is, only the best performance-status patients are transplanted or only the highest risk patients are transplanted. Additionally, there are staging biases that occur when one is trying to transplant a patient. Transplant patients get more extensive imaging studies performed, which typically result in upstaging, which has the paradoxical effect of improving prognosis in patients in both lower and more advanced stages.

Phase III transplant studies often suffer from small numbers and, hence, are not powered to detect clinically significant differences. Randomization is important and helps with unidentified biases, and intent-to-treat analysis is also accepted as an important tool for generalization of trial results to a population of patients. However, when one includes a group of patients who may not benefit from the procedure (see later discussion), and one also includes patients randomized to receive a transplant but who do not receive a transplant, and patients randomized to not receive a transplant but who do receive a transplant, then the classic problem of transplant trials, which is one of small numbers, becomes even more significant.

TRANSPLANTATION IN THE MANAGEMENT OF BREAST CANCER

The role of transplantation for solid tumors is most clearly exemplified by the dramatic alterations in the frequency of high-dose chemotherapy and autologous transplantation for the treatment of breast cancer. In a very short time, this procedure became the treatment of choice for high-risk breast cancer and for chemotherapy-sensitive metastatic breast cancer. During the 1990s, breast cancer became the commonest indication for transplantation in North America and worldwide. Within another very short time, the entire field moved on, and breast cancer now constitutes a very unusual indication for transplantation. What happened?

The issue of stem cell transplantation for breast cancer is not quite as straightforward as has been outlined by the authors, and remains controversial. Several studies continue to support the use of high-dose chemotherapy and some more recent studies provide a rationale for the use of allogenic transplantation.

The authors provide the historical background and rationale for the use of high-dose chemotherapy and autologous stem cell transplantation for breast cancer. There is clearly a dose-response effect of chemotherapy on breast cancer, and there are certainly very high-risk subgroups of patients who can be prospectively identified and potentially treated with high-dose chemotherapy. The authors also outline various pitfalls associated with this approach and they discuss the apparently negative outcome of some of the trials. They do not, however, address the reason for the lack of overall survival advantage, nor do they analyze in detail some of the more positive studies, particularly in the context of study size and duration of follow-up. A brief review of some of the studies that have determined standards of care in breast cancer is warranted in order to place the transplant studies in context.

Studies of adjuvant chemotherapy and hormonal therapy generally require the enrollment of 1,000 to 3,000 patients in order to demonstrate a statistically significant difference in outcome. The outcome difference is typically reported as *relative risk reduction*. This method of analysis has the effect of increasing the apparent efficacy of the intervention, while de-emphasizing the number of patients of who have to be treated without benefit in order to achieve a benefit in a small but statistically significant group of patients. Finally, the studies of hormonal therapy did not show an overall survival benefit until a median follow-up of 8 years, and this survival benefit was preceded by a divergence in the relapse-free survival.

There have been a number of randomized studies of high-dose chemotherapy for breast cancer, most of which have been too small to be able to show a difference in survival, if one existed. The studies of Bezwoda et al. (1,2) were fraudulent, but it is not logical to dismiss a treatment because two of the positive studies have been shown to be fraudulent, although certainly it requires one to re-examine the data (1–6).

Perhaps the most compelling trial of autologous transplantation in breast cancer is The Netherlands study, reported by Rodenhuis et al. (7,8), particularly as it matures with follow-up. This is the largest randomized study and it is a very representative study, as it enrolled a substantial fraction of all the available women who met the entrance criteria in The Netherlands. This study demonstrates several interesting phenomena that complicate the interpretation of transplant studies. When it was initially reported with a small number of patients, there was a strong survival advantage to transplant versus standard therapy. As more patients were enrolled, the survival advantage disappeared, underlining the problems of small studies. Planned analyses with a median follow-up of 57 months failed to show any overall survival or relapse-free survival benefit for patients with four to ten involved lymph nodes. However, the data did reveal an improvement in relapse-free survival for those with more than ten involved nodes (61% vs. 51%, $p = 0.05$). This improvement appeared to be confined to the *HER2/neu*-negative group of patients (7). Longer-term follow-up at 84 months confirmed that this improvement was not seen in the *HER2/neu*-positive subset of patients. Conversely, the group with *HER2/neu*-negative disease had a clear relapse-free advantage (71.5% vs. 59.1% at 5 years, $p = 0.002$) and, more importantly, an overall survival advantage (78.2% vs. 71% at 5 years, $p = 0.02$) (8). It is known that *HER2/neu*-positive breast cancer is relatively resistant to alkylating agents, and alkylating agents are the mainstay of high-dose chemotherapy regimens. If these initial observations are confirmed, it will make interpretation of prior breast cancer transplant trials even more difficult, as none of the studies had routinely measured or excluded patients with *HER2/neu* breast cancer. Failure to consider the *HER2/neu* status further diminished the possibility of these trials to show a statistically significant difference in outcome in the overall population enrolled in the study, and to have diminished the power of the study to detect a difference in the *HER2/neu*-negative patient population.

In support of The Netherlands study, a German multicenter phase III trial reported by Nitz et al. (9), which employed a different transplant strategy involving tandem courses of high-dose chemotherapy with autologous blood stem cell support very early in the course of adjuvant treatment for a very high-risk group of patients, has demonstrated both a disease-free and an overall survival benefit for the high-dose chemotherapy approach. In this study, 403 patients with high-risk breast cancer (more than nine involved lymph nodes) were randomized to either two courses of dose-dense epirubicin/cyclophosphamide followed by rapidly cycled tandem courses of high-dose chemotherapy versus a moderately intensive standard chemotherapy approach of six cycles of dose-dense epirubicin/cyclophosphamide and three cycles of accelerated cyclophosphamide, methotrexate, and fluorouracil. The mean number of lymph nodes involved was 17.6 and median follow-up was 48.6 months. Event-free survival at 4 years was 60% for the high-dose chemotherapy arm and 44% for standard chemotherapy arm ($p = 0.00069$), and overall survival was 75% versus 70% ($p = 0.02$) (9).

These results from the study by Nitz et al. (9) are very similar to the results reported by Rodenhuis et al. in the group of patients with more than ten lymph nodes involved, and are supportive of the concept that it may be possible to identify a subgroup of sufficiently high-risk breast cancer patients who would benefit from a high-dose chemotherapy strategy. Additionally, the German trial suggests that it is possible that some of the negative reports on outcome from high-dose chemotherapy for breast cancer were not employing the optimal high-dose strategy.

There are a number of other legitimate criticisms about the studies of high-dose therapy and breast cancer. The most usual criticism is that the standard chemotherapy arm is not the current standard of care. The transplant studies have not included taxanes in the chemotherapy only arm and did not incorporate Herceptin (trastuzumab) or aromatase inhibitors. This is a fair criticism, but it does make it very difficult to design a clinical study. The standard of care evolves continuously. A transplant study takes time to design and then accrue sufficient patients for meaningful analysis, and then patients need to be followed long enough for relapse-free survival to translate into an overall survival benefit. By the time an overall survival benefit is demonstrated, any study is going to be confronted with the accusation that it has not been proven against the most current standard of care.

An additional problem for the interpretation of breast cancer transplant trials has been the unexpected good outcome of patients treated with chemotherapy alone. The transplant patients have done as well as they were expected to do, based on previous phase II studies. The nontransplant patients have done much better than expected, which then leads to additional potential problems with the power of the studies to identify clinically significant differences.

One of the larger negative studies of transplantation for breast cancer has a somewhat different problem in interpretation: high early mortality in the transplant arm (10). The regimen used (thiotepa and cyclophosphamide) was particularly toxic, with a relatively high early mortality in the transplant group, which made it unlikely that any moderate benefit could be observed in the transplant group. The transplant-related mortality (TRM) in this study was 9 patients of 254 analyzed and 214 actually transplanted. This rate of TRM is unacceptably high for an autologous transplant and unacceptably high for use as an adjuvant approach to the treatment of cancer. Of note, the TRM decreased substantially after the use of mobilized peripheral blood stem cells (10).

An additional criticism often leveled against transplant strategies has been a financial one. Transplant is a very intensive treatment approach with significant morbidity and cost, and it requires treatment at tertiary care centers with experience in the management of the complications of the procedure. However, the cost of an autologous transplant has remained fairly stable, or even decreased, over many years, whereas the cost of all the other drugs involved in the treatment of cancer generally has continued to increase. It is not clear that transplant is necessarily more expensive than prolonged treatment with any of the new small-molecule tyrosine kinase inhibitors or any of the monoclonal antibody strategies, particularly as they start being applied in the adjuvant setting to larger numbers of patients for longer periods of time and even start being used in a maintenance strategy.

It is unlikely that high-dose chemotherapy with transplant will be employed for any large group of breast cancer patients in the future. It is possible that subgroups may be identified who will benefit from transplant, but these subgroups will then need to be prospectively evaluated in a randomized trial against a standard of care, modern adjuvant chemotherapy program. Assessment of outcome will probably require acceptance of disease-free survival as the primary end point, as the ability of salvage therapies to prolong life continues to expand. Such studies will also need to incorporate quality-of-life assessments to determine if an abbreviated course of treatment culminating in a transplant is perhaps better tolerated than a more prolonged course of conventional chemotherapy. Additionally, a pharmacoeconomic component should also be incorporated. It is unlikely that such studies will be done, as the psychological momentum in the field, both among patients and among breast cancer specialists, has moved strongly away from any role for high-dose chemotherapy in the treatment of breast cancer.

REFERENCES

1. Bezwoda WR, Seymour L, Dansey RD. High-dose chemotherapy with hematopoietic rescue as primary treatment for metastatic breast cancer: a randomized trial. *J Clin Oncol.* 1995;13:2483–2489.
2. Bezwoda WR. High-dose chemotherapy with hematopoietic rescue in breast cancer: from theory to practice. *Cancer Chemother Pharmacol.* 1997;40(Suppl):S79–87.
3. Armand JP. The Bezwoda affair [in French]. *Bull Cancer.* 2000;87: 363–364.
4. Horton R. After Bezwoda. *Lancet.* 2000;355:942–943.
5. Sledge GW Jr. Why big lies matter: lessons from the Bezwoda affair. *Medscape Womens Health.* 2000;5:4.
6. Weiss RB, Rifkin RM, Stewart FM, et al. High-dose chemotherapy for high-risk primary breast cancer: an on-site review of the Bezwoda study. *Lancet.* 2000;355:999–1003.
7. Rodenhuis S, Bontenbal M, Beex LV, et al. High-dose chemotherapy with hematopoietic stem-cell rescue for high-risk breast cancer. *New Engl J Med.* 2003;349:7–16.

8. Rodenhuis S, Bontenbal M, van Hoesel QG, et al. Efficacy of high-dose alkylating chemotherapy in HER2/neu-negative breast cancer. *Ann Oncol.* 2006;17:588–596.

9. Nitz UA, Mohrmann S, Fischer J, et al. Comparison of rapidly cycled tandem high-dose chemotherapy plus peripheral-blood stem-cell support versus dose-dense conventional chemotherapy for adjuvant treatment of high-risk breast cancer: results of a multicentre phase III trial. *Lancet.* 2005;366:1935–1944.

10. Tallman MS, Gray R, Robert NJ, et al. Conventional adjuvant chemotherapy with or without high-dose chemotherapy and autologous stem-cell transplantation in high-risk breast cancer. *New Engl J Med.* 2003;349:17–26.

6

Intraperitoneal Drug Therapy for Intra-Abdominal Spread of Cancer

Elliot Newman, Mustafa Hussain, and Franco M. Muggia

Tumors arising in the ovaries and in the gastrointestinal (GI) tract—particularly mucinous tumors of appendiceal origin—have a high incidence of intraperitoneal (IP) spread as the most prominent manifestation of disease. Following resection of the primary site, many of the GI tumors may, in fact, initially show little tendency to invade adjacent organs or spread beyond the abdomen. In particular, low-grade adenocarcinomas that produce vast amounts of mucin, have a clinical picture consisting solely of serosal spread, giving rise to the entity known as *pseudomyxoma peritonei*.

Gynecologic oncologists have emphasized the pattern of spread shared by most epithelial ovarian cancers, and have incorporated cytology from washings, "blind" biopsies from selected peritoneal sites, and omentectomy as part of routine initial surgical staging. After more than a decade of phase I and phase II studies, finally phase III studies have established the role of IP cisplatin in upfront treatment of advanced epithelial ovarian carcinoma (1–3). On the other hand, surgical oncologists have seldom addressed peritoneal spread of cancer in their therapeutic trials. Routine oophorectomy at the time of colectomy for bowel cancers beyond T1 stage occurring in women is still controversial; preliminary data suggest a possible recurrence-free survival advantage (4). The role of IP-directed therapy in other GI malignancies (gastric, appendiceal) has occasionally been tested over the past few years (5–7). This chapter provides information on the type of IP-directed therapies that should be considered for such circumstances and emphasizes how clinical trials beyond pilot studies are required to establish a role for IP therapy. Such data should be applicable not only to gynecologic cancers, but also to primary peritoneal malignancies, to GI malignancies including pancreatic and biliary tract cancers, and to the occasional metastatic malignancy, such as some breast and endometrial cancers that at times share a predominant peritoneal spread. Although the focus to date has been IP drug therapy, the IP route is also being explored as a mode for the delivery of different genetic material (i.e., gene therapy) (8,9), immune modulators (10), radioimmunoconjugates, other targeted therapies, and physical modalities such as hyperthermia.

Drugs administered intraperitoneally have been studied primarily to determine their "pharmacologic advantage" at peritoneal surfaces versus what could be achieved in tumor capillaries by their systemic administration at maximally tolerated doses. This pharmacologic advantage is usually expressed as a ratio of drug exposure (AUC: area-under-the curve of concentration × time) in the peritoneal fluid (IP) over the plasma (PL) drug exposure. Occasionally, the ratio of peak levels in peritoneal fluid and in plasma has also been compared, because such levels may be predictive of certain toxicities. The pharmacologic advantage for a given drug at the recommended IP doses is expressed by:

$$IP\ pharmacologic\ advantage = AUC_{IP}/AUC_{PL}$$

Maximal exposure of all peritoneal surfaces is ensured by delivering the drug in large volumes, usually 2 L, but best standardized as 1 L/m^2, so as to avoid painful overfilling individuals that are small.

Despite many pharmacologic studies, however, IP drug delivery has not been widely adopted into surgical practice. This chapter begins with a historical perspective and a discussion of issues regarding the IP delivery of specific drugs, followed by a review of the status of IP therapy in ovarian, colon, other GI, and gastric cancers.

HISTORICAL PERSPECTIVE

IP chemotherapy has had a firm pharmacologic basis rooted in studies initially carried out at the National Cancer Institute and subsequently at the University of California at San Diego, The Netherlands Cancer Institute, Memorial Sloan-Kettering Cancer Center, New York University, University of Southern California (USC), among other institutions. These studies were initially performed in a small number of patients and primarily of a pharmacologic nature; moreover, response assessment in peritoneal disease was often difficult. Therefore, demonstration of benefit from IP chemotherapy obtained with various drugs and combinations has remained largely uncertain for most circumstances in which this treatment might be applicable.

Studies in the late 1970s by Dedrick, Myers, Collins, DeVita, and other colleagues at the National Cancer Institute (United States) first worked out the pharmacologic principles of IP chemotherapy (11,12). The studies from the outset were directed to the management of minimal residual ovarian cancer. Its original modeling used timed "dwells" of large (2-L) volumes of fluid containing the selected drug. Subsequent principles were extended by Howell and his coworkers (13,14) in gynecologic oncology at the University of California, San Diego, who introduced implantable IP devices, concepts of systemic neutralization, combination chemotherapy, and the first claim for a role of IP cisplatin in the treatment of ovarian cancer. Cisplatin's lack of schedule dependency eliminated the need for the cumbersome dwell (often not feasible because of outflow obstruction) and it became used alone or in combination with other cytotoxic drugs given in one volume (usually 2 L) of dialysate every 3 weeks. The study of King et al. (15) also first suggested therapeutic benefit from IP cytosine arabinoside, a drug not otherwise active by the systemic route. Speyer and colleagues (16,17) first studied 5-fluorouracil (5-FU) and described the nonlinear pharmacokinetics of systemic exposure (e.g., plasma AUCs) resulting from IP administration. With Sugarbaker et al. (18), they demonstrated an effect of 5-FU in decreasing peritoneal recurrences of colon cancer (although with no survival advantage) and in controlling the regrowth of pseudomyxoma peritonei after aggressive debulking. In 1985, at a meeting of the Gastrointestinal Tumor Study Group (19), Myers hypothesized that IP floxuridine (FUDR) would have very favorable pharmacologic characteristics for IP administration. This hypothesis generated the studies conducted at New York University and at the University of Southern California (20–22) and subsequently taken up by the Southwest Oncology Group, in a randomized phase II study testing IP consolidation with FUDR or mitoxantrone following positive second-look laparotomies for ovarian cancer (23).

Phase III studies of IP cisplatin by cooperative groups were designed after 1986, but did not yield definitive analyses until a decade later. A consistent advantage for an arm containing IP over intravenous (IV) cisplatin for the progression-free survival of epithelial ovarian cancer was documented by Alberts et al. (1), and in two subsequent studies by the Gynecologic Oncology Group (2,3). For other drugs or regimens, the rationale for the use of IP-administered drugs in minimal residual disease has not evolved much beyond phase I and pharmacologic studies. The clinical information for these other regimens is mostly confined to issues of tolerance and short-term outcome as determined by a subsequent reassessment laparotomy.

ISSUES IN INTRAPERITONEAL DRUG DELIVERY

Drug-Related Variables

In addition to important pharmacologic properties that determine the pharmacologic advantage of IP over systemic drug administration, there are other important and poorly understood variables in the selection of a drug for IP therapy. Slow clearance from the peritoneal cavity leading to prolonged IP exposure has been advocated as an attractive feature favoring IP paclitaxel (24–26). On the other hand, diffusivity (penetrance) into tumors and into juxtaperitoneal lymphatics is likely to be drug-(27) and tumor-dependent: the type of spread of malignant disease may affect the therapeutic results to be achieved. Such issues have been studied in some animal models, and cisplatin has been identified as having better penetrance than carboplatin into tumor nodules (28) and doxorubicin as having minimal penetrance (29). Cannulation of the thoracic duct in rabbits has indicated that high concentrations are achieved following IP administration of carboplatin and 5-FU, but not etoposide (30). Other drugs that have been or are under study are oxaliplatin, gemcitabine, irinotecan, the antifolates methotrexate and pemetrexed, and topotecan, alone or in combination with cisplatin.

Scheduling

Scheduling has been almost universally single dose and intermittent because it was most practical for cisplatin, but it may not be optimal for antimetabolites, podophyllotoxins (etoposide or teniposide), or topoisomerase I inhibitors. Paclitaxel was initially introduced in the usual once every 3 weeks schedule (24), but subsequently given at lower doses on a weekly schedule to improve peritoneal tolerance (25). Obvious chemical peritonitis may affect the ability to administer a drug repeatedly and this has been seen with doxorubicin (29), mitoxantrone (23), as well as paclitaxel (24). However, subclinical changes in peritoneal permeability may occur as a result of treatment and affect drug pharmacokinetics and the pharmacologic advantages in subsequent cycles. Such changes have been documented with the otherwise well-tolerated fluoropyrimidines (21,31).

Catheter Complications

Catheter complications such as obstruction, bleeding, or perforation into a viscus may follow chemical peritonitis: they occurred at a much greater rate with mitoxantrone than with FUDR in a randomized study (23). In the presence of left colon resection, complications were higher in the recent GOG trial (3,32). Also with any invasive procedure, they are more likely to occur following multiple surgeries and/or a weakened state.

Tumor Sensitivity

Tumor sensitivity has been the overriding rationale in IP drug selection. For example, IP cisplatin is the major drug used for ovarian cancer despite a pharmacologic advantage between 10- and 20-fold, which is not as remarkable as for many other drugs. However, the pharmacologic advantage does lend support to the use of some drugs that play little or no role by the systemic route. Cytarabine has yielded well-documented remissions in platinum-resistant ovarian cancer, presumably because of its three-log pharmacologic advantage despite playing no role by the systemic route (15).

Intraperitoneal (local) Dose-Limiting Factors

IP dose-limiting factors vary with drugs and may differ from toxicities resulting from their systemic administration. Catheter complications, as noted earlier, are in part drug-related (23) and dose-limiting certain drugs are associated with local toxicity (24). Again, cisplatin is not representative of many other drugs: the same dosing by the IP or IV route yields virtually identical toxicities (the exception perhaps being lesser ototoxicity for IP cisplatin) (1). At the other end of the spectrum, for fluoropyrimidines, systemic toxicity from IP drug administration becomes evident only when the capacity of the liver to thoroughly metabolize the drugs is exceeded, a feature subject to marked interindividual variation in maximum tolerated dose. Therefore, consistent systemic effects from IP fluoropyrimidines may require the concomitant administration of systemic fluoropyrimidine therapy. A similar situation is applicable to drugs causing clinical chemical peritonitis precluding IP doses associated with adequate systemic levels.

Disease-Related Variables

As already noted, the intrinsic susceptibility of ovarian cancer to platinum compounds renders IP cisplatin the preferred drug for treatment selection in this disease. Interest in IP paclitaxel has been generated for the same reason (in addition to its prolonged half-life in the peritoneal cavity). For colon or appendiceal cancer metastases, in addition to platinums, the fluoropyrimidines and topoisomerase I inhibitors are the drugs of major interest. In gastric cancer, fluoropyrimidines and platinums, and more recently taxanes, are believed to play a role. The type of disease in the peritoneum is also likely to be a key factor in both drug-regimen selection and treatment outcome: diffusely microscopic disease or many nodules with tumor volumes not exceeding 5 mm are the best targets for IP drug therapy. Such features may assume even greater importance when biological agents are included. The Gynecologic Oncology Group identified a category of patients with poor outcome following IP alpha interferon therapy: these were patients who were deemed platinum-resistant (i.e., evidence of unresponsiveness to this initial therapy or regrowth of disease within 6 months) and/or diffuse rather than patchy peritoneal seeding (33). Disease exceeding 1 cm in cross-sectional area would not be expected to preferentially yield to IP therapy vis-à-vis systemic drug administration. Moreover, in such patients, the interval between treatments may be crucial, because the circumstances for optimal therapy become progressively more unfavorable if the tumor is allowed to grow between treatment cycles.

Technique/Catheter-Related Factors

Catheters for IP drug administration evolved from experience with peritoneal dialysis, but their use for cancer treatment soon faced other issues related to prior surgeries, recent surgical exploration and resections, dynamic changes in the peritoneum as a result of drug effects, and propensity to complications related to chemical peritonitis (23).

Outflow Obstruction

Outflow obstruction is a common problem that probably results from peritoneal tissue growing into and partially blocking the catheter opening. Controversy exists whether this may be more common when catheters with multiple openings are used.

Blockage and Maldistribution

More serious are total blockage and/or maldistribution of the infused fluid into a small loculated pocket rather than throughout the peritoneal cavity. Unfortunately, factors predisposing to such occurrences or methods to avoid them have been inadequately studied. Multiple surgeries and resections certainly increase the incidence of complications. Erosions of the catheter opening into the site of bowel anastomoses or into a partially blocked ureter have been recorded by the authors. As noted earlier, some drugs, such as mitoxantrone in one randomized trial (23), may be associated with a greater frequency of problems.

Leakage

With repetitive daily dosing, perhaps related to back pressure, leakage of fluid at the needle site or subcutaneously around the port has occurred. Unless the drug is a vesicant, this complication, although troublesome, is seldom serious. However, it often reflects either needle malposition, distal obstruction with backflow around the catheter back to its connecting point at the port, or loculation—but not defective ports.

Placement of the Catheter Tip

Placement of the catheter in some areas, such as infradiaphragmatic surfaces, is done only rarely, but in our experience may have a greater propensity for malfunction. We have noted a tendency toward bleeding on lavaging a catheter that had been placed on the pancreatic head upon gastrectomy and lymph node dissection for gastric cancer. Also, the placement of multiple catheters may be counterproductive because factors leading one catheter to malfunction frequently lead to obstruction in the other.

Catheter Maintenance

Catheter maintenance, especially during early postoperative periods, may be important. Initially, frequent irrigations were advised and routinely carried out. Whereas this may not be necessary, early use of the catheter is recommended. Outflow obstruction was less frequent with the Tenckhoff catheter than with implantable ones, and this may just be a function of the frequent flushing that is routinely carried out with the Tenckhoff catheter. Following uneventful use for several cycles of IP therapy, flushing the catheter every 6 weeks has been sufficient to maintain its function if it is deemed desirable not to remove it immediately after the completion of contemplated therapy.

Type of Catheter

The type of catheter, that is, one with multiple openings rather than only a distal opening, and/or valvelike openings, may also have an impact on complication rates, but data are not available. A Groshong-type collapsible tip may be advantageous in preventing growth into the catheter. On the other hand, multiple openings have been noted to become occluded by peritoneal connective tissue growing into the catheter, which, upon its removal, resembles a centipede. IP therapy may also be delivered via percutaneously introduced catheters. Repeat administration, however, is labor-intensive for the operator and often difficult for the patient.

Timing of Intraperitoneal Delivery

The use of IP drugs immediately following resection for colon cancer (18) or pseudomyxoma peritonei (34) has been advocated by Sugarbaker and has been used following gastrectomy by Japanese and Korean surgeons (35–38). The hypothesis underlying such treatment is that optimal exposure occurs at a time before adhesions have a chance to occur and lead to sanctuaries where the IP drugs cannot adequately reach. Conversely, a one-time exposure to chemotherapy, even at the "optimal" time, may seldom prove effective. Nevertheless, when a radical debulking is carried out, only the perioperative administration of IP drugs may be feasible.

Prevention of Adhesions: Icodextrin

At present no studies have been published providing outcome in patients with cancer using icodextrin, a high-molecular-weight carrier solution, capable of slowing down the egress of fluid from the peritoneal cavity. Pharmacologic studies are ongoing and should spur subsequent development.

Distribution Studies

Distribution studies using IP contrast (in addition to standard IV and oral contrast) with computerized tomography have been routinely employed in some institutions for the purpose of obtaining baseline pretreatment staging/disease-assessment information and of confirming adequate distribution for IP drug delivery (39). Such a step is a wise investment during the initial testing of IP regimens and in guiding treatment for special circumstances, such as for patients not recently reassessed surgically that may have unsuspected metastatic sites. Other techniques for assessing distribution have included the introduction of radionuclides and magnetic resonance imaging with saline administration (39–41).

Complications

Perforations, bleeding, and infection are fortunately an uncommon occurrence in experienced hands (32). Trained nurses, backed by physicians within reach when problems are encoun-

tered, are the key aspect in minimizing the occurrence of complications, and their severity. An unusual complication of massive upper GI bleeding triggered by the first dose of IP drug administration was encountered in one of our gastric cancer trials: this occurred 29 days after partial gastrectomy with subsequent angiograms showing an aneurysmal dilatation of the left gastric artery and erosion into the duodenum.

SPECIFIC MODALITIES OF INTRAPERITONEAL THERAPY

Table 6.1 (42–57) lists chemotherapeutic drugs that have had some evaluation for their potential when given via the IP route. Most of these remain in the experimental realm, and only those drugs that have current therapeutic relevance are described in detail.

Fluoropyrimidines

We have outlined why the deoxyribose of 5-FU, FUDR, is the preferred fluoropyrimidine for IP administration (20,21). Although the two drugs share many pharmacologic properties

Table 6.1

The Pharmacologic Advantage[a] and Tolerance of Intraperitoneal (IP) Drugs

Agent (Reference)	AUC IP/Plasma	Local Toxicity	Systemic Dose-Limiting Toxicities/Other
Cisplatin (14)	12	+/−	Emesis, renal
Carboplatin (42,43)	6–10	−	Bone marrow
Melphalan (44,45)	65	−	Bone marrow
Thiotepa (46)	4	−	Bone marrow
Mitomycin C (47)	32	+ + +	Peritonitis, bone marrow
Doxorubicin (29)	400	+ +	Peritonitis
Mitoxantrone (48,49)	1,400	+ +	Peritonitis, catheter occlusions
Methotrexate (50)	92	+	Bone marrow
Fluorouracil (16)	376	+ +	Peritonitis, bone marrow
Floxuridine (20)	>1,000	−	Stomatitis
Cytarabine (15)	300–1,000	+ +	Bone marrow
Etoposide (51–53)	65	−	Alopecia, bone marrow
Paclitaxel (24,25)	—	+ +	Neuropathy
Docetaxel (54)	—	+/−	Bone marrow
Gemcitabine (55)	—	−	Bone marrow[b]
9-aminocamptothecin (56)	7.6–16.5	−	Bone marrow
Topotecan (57)	—	−	Bone marrow
Oxaliplatin[c]	NR	+ + +	Abdominal pain
Pemetrexed[d]	NR	NR	NR

AUC, area under the curve; NR, not reported; +/−, occasional toxicity; +, ++, + + +, grade of toxicity.
[a] See definition in introductory section of chapter. Numbers refer to this ratio and therefore do not have the customary units for concentration or AUC.
[b] In combination with cisplatin.
[c] Personal communication, L. Saltz (2005).
[d] Ongoing trial; personal communication, E. Poplin and J. Bertino 2007–8.

and FUDR actually yields substantial IP and plasma levels of 5-FU, they differ in their potency for surface cytotoxicity, their solubility in slightly acidic pH, and the extent of their hepatic (first-pass) metabolism. In all these characteristics, FUDR is more advantageous for IP administration, and a tolerable dose schedule has been devised and tested in both multi-institutional and other single-institution studies. However, 5-FU has been the subject of more clinical studies (see "Clinical Settings for Intraperitoneal Therapy"), probably because of cost and drug availability issues. The systemic toxicities from both drugs are identical, and relate to plasma levels resulting in mucosal and marrow toxicities. Sclerosing peritonitis, however, has been reported for 5-FU (58). Efforts to enhance their therapeutic effects have included modulating their action with IP leucovorin (folinic acid) (21,22) or by concurrent IV hydroxyurea (59), supplementing systemic exposure by concurrent IV 5-FU, or by combining them with IP cisplatin (60). The millimolar concentrations in the peritoneal cavity for either fluoropyrimidine should be cytotoxic to most tumor cells and unlikely to be enhanced further through folate modulation.

Platinum Compounds

Cisplatin is the drug that has received the widest trial via the IP route. IP cisplatin has been advocated in ovarian cancer in patients in complete clinical remission following the initial induction (currently after systemic carboplatin and paclitaxel) (61). At the University of Southern California, it has also been used postoperatively (together with FUDR) following a neoadjuvant systemic regimen of 5-FU plus cisplatin and curative gastrectomy for gastric cancer (62). The toxicities of IP cisplatin are dose-related and analogous dose per dose with systemic administration. Peak plasma levels of the drug are lower after IP administration, and a slightly improved tolerance for IP cisplatin over IV cisplatin has been noted in a randomized study (1). In patients with pre-existing neuropathy, partial substitution of cisplatin by carboplatin may allow the maintenance of dose intensity of a platinum regimen at a cost of slightly greater myelosuppression from carboplatin (60). Local signs and symptoms are generally mild with either platinum; however, subcutaneous extravasation from a malfunctioning delivery system has resulted in sloughing of the abdominal wall. Sodium thiosulfate IV has been given to protect against the nephrotoxicity of IP cisplatin in doses of up to 200 mg/m^2, but this maneuver renders the treatment more complex and its usefulness remains to be established (13,63). Cisplatin has often been given in combination with other drugs such as cytarabine (64), bleomycin (65), or etoposide (51), or as part of chemoimmunotherapy with interferon (33), but the contribution of the other drugs has been uncertain and the popularity of many of these regimens has waned. Trials of IP cisplatin with local hyperthermia have been difficult, in part because of erratic renal toxicity. Carboplatin IP has been combined with hyperthermia in order to avoid such potential aggravation of nephrotoxicity (66). IP carboplatin has also been combined with IP etoposide (67) or IP FUDR (60).

Other Chemotherapeutic Drugs

The taxane paclitaxel is currently attracting interest for possible IP use in gynecologic cancer (3,24–26). Mitomycin C IP is sub-

jectively not well tolerated, but has been extensively used during operations for gastric cancer in Japan, alone or with hyperthermia (36,47). Cytarabine is an antimetabolite with little activity against solid tumors, but concentrations achievable in the peritoneal cavity have shown activity in clinical studies, including patients with ovarian cancer (15,64). Both topotecan and gemcitabine are currently being investigated in phase I trials for their possible role in IP therapy. A number of drugs such as bleomycin and mitoxantrone have been given for the palliation of ascites, but this does not necessarily recommend their use as an adjuvant to surgery and for the containment and/or eradication of peritoneal metastases.

Other Modalities

Cytokines and Biologicals

Cytokines such as interferon-alpha (33) and interferon-gamma (68) have been given intraperitoneally in several clinical studies, and positive results in ovarian cancer have stimulated subsequent trials alone and in combination with cisplatin. Direct cytotoxicity or indirect antiangiogenic actions have been postulated to explain these therapeutic effects. Interleukin-2 was initially given with lymphokine-activated killer cells and subsequently by itself in several trials (10). Peritoneal fibrosis was a major problem, but interest has rekindled in view of some long-term survival since the largest trial with this agent. Monoclonal antibodies tagged with radionuclides have had extensive trial in ovarian cancer (69), but their role remains uncertain, even though delivery of radioactivity and the physics of the radionuclide used (yttrium, rhenium) have considerable theoretical advantages over colloidal solutions of ^{32}P.

Hyperthermia

Hyperthermia may be provided by radiofrequency to the abdomen containing fluid plus drugs (66), or may be achieved, usually intraoperatively, by administering warm dialysate (70). It has been extensively used in Japan and Korea.

Gene Therapy

Gene therapy by the IP route has been tested in animal models (8,9), and clinical trials are ongoing as planned using the herpes simplex thymidine kinase gene transduction, and relying on the "bystander effect" also killing nontransduced cells following the administration of ganciclovir. Another approach already in phase II and III trials combined with chemotherapy in ovarian cancer is the use of p53 transduction following the rationale that chemoresistance is mediated in part by p53 mutations. Phase III trials of such an approach were terminated early by the sponsor (Schering-Plough) and the results have not been published.

CLINICAL SETTINGS FOR INTRAPERITONEAL THERAPY

Ovarian Cancer

Several phase III trials demonstrated an advantage of the IP route: (a) INT 0051 demonstrated that optimally debulked (defined in this study, initiated in 1985, as ≤2 cm greatest diameter of residual lesions) stage III ovarian cancer patients treated with IP cisplatin (100 mg/m2) at 3-week intervals, had a better outcome than those treated with IV cisplatin at the same dose and schedule (both groups also received IV cyclophosphamide) (1). The median survival on the IP arm was 49 months, as compared to 41 months on the IV arm. (b) GOG No. 114, which used IP cisplatin and IV paclitaxel following IV carboplatin induction in its "dose-intense" arm to be compared with the "standard" arm of IV cisplatin and paclitaxel (2). (c) GOG 172 is the most recent study that was published demonstrating an advantage in median survival from 49 months following IV cisplatin + paclitaxel versus 67 months following IP cisplatin and also IP paclitaxel added to IV paclitaxel. (d) The European Organization for Research and Treatment of Cancer favoring IP cisplatin consolidation versus observation in patients with negative reassessment after first-line chemotherapy, but differences were not significant possibly due to closure before meeting its accrual goals. (e) A study by the Gruppo Oncologico Nord-Ovest (GONO) comparing IV cyclophosphamide, epirubicin, and cisplatin versus the same with the cisplatin IP. This study was interrupted early because of poor compliance with the IP regimen (and reliance on repeated percutaneous placement); it showed an advantage of progression-free survival for the IP arm, even if the median number of IP courses was two.

Of interest is Southwest Oncology Group study no. 8835, which used a randomized phase II selection design comparing it to IP mitoxantrone, for patients with <1 cm residual disease at second-look laparotomy. In this study, catheter complications or abdominal pain leading to treatment discontinuation occurred in 12 of 39 patients taking mitoxantrone, versus 3 of 28 patients taking FUDR. The high incidence of complications associated with IP mitoxantrone had not been attributable to the drug in preceding studies. The randomized phase II design not only selected FUDR for further study based on a superior time-to-failure (median of 24 months vs. 11 months for mitoxantrone), but also improved the interpretation of toxicologic findings (23).

Over the past few years new drugs emerging for the treatment of recurrent epithelial ovarian cancer are being explored for their potential role in IP consolidation, often in combination with a platinum. These include paclitaxel (24–26) and docetaxel, topoisomerase I inhibitors such as topotecan, irinotecan and 9-aminocamptothecin, and gemcitabine, among others.

Colorectal Carcinoma

The treatment of colorectal cancer over the last decade has changed through introduction of new treatments as well as refinements in diagnosis and surgery. In addition, pharmacologic principles are helping us to optimize the use of the available anticancer drugs. Many questions need to be addressed through clinical trials, and how to deal with peritoneal carcinomatosis deserving special attention since IP therapy, particularly with fluoropyrimidines and cisplatin, opens potential rational approaches for dealing with small or microscopic peritoneal metastases. The initial observations in the randomized study of Sugarbaker and colleagues (18) support an effect of these drugs on peritoneal disease.

Peritoneal carcinomatosis of colorectal origin is present in approximately 10% of patients at the time of diagnosis of the primary, and isolated recurrences to the peritoneum are found in 8% to 25% of patients (71–73). The minority of patients with peritoneal carcinomatosis are 5-year survivors, and reported median survivals are in the 6-month range. Systemic therapies, until recently, have not had an impact on these survival rates, and patients were given little chance of long-term survival (74–77). This attitude, however, has changed in recent times as more aggressive locoregional treatment strategies to treat cancer have been introduced. Isolated metastatic recurrences to liver, lung, and other sites are now routinely resected with 20% to 25% cure rates (78). Cytoreductive surgery for isolated peritoneal metastases followed by IP chemotherapy was pursued in the 1980s by Sugarbaker et al. (79) and further adopted by a number of medical centers worldwide. More than 20 studies have been reported looking at the value of this approach to improving outcome in peritoneal carcinomatosis, with the majority being nonrandomized and retrospective in nature (73). Some studies were confined to colorectal cancer, while others included appendiceal tumors. IP chemotherapy was mostly delivered intraoperatively but in some instances also postoperatively. Mitomycin C, 5-FU, and cisplatin were usually part of the drug regimens, and often with hyperthermia. Such a variety of treatment approaches makes a uniform conclusion difficult, but overall median survivals has ranged from 12 to 32 months and 5-year survival from 17% to 30%, suggesting an improvement over historical reports (73).

A randomized trial from The Netherlands lends further support to this locoregional approach. Verwaal et al. (80) reported a nearly twofold increase in median survival (22.3 months vs. 12.6 months) in those patients treated with aggressive cytoreduction and heated IP mitomycin C chemotherapy compared with those treated with systemic therapy and palliative surgery only. To date it is the only successfully completed randomized trial supporting the value of aggressive surgery followed by IP chemotherapy. One other attempt at a randomized trial from France was unsuccessful and closed prematurely because of poor accrual (81). Predictors of outcome following the diagnosis of peritoneal carcinomatosis commonly include the extent of disease and completeness of resection; the less disease at presentation, and the more successful the cytoreduction, the better the survival. These therapies however, are not without complications. Morbidity rates of up to 50% and mortality rates of 19% have been reported (82–84). At present, the data on using IP chemotherapy after aggressive cytoreductive surgery in peritoneal carcinomatosis of colorectal origin is provocative, but needs to be substantiated by at least one other randomized clinical trial.

Pseudomyxoma Peritonei

Pseudomyxoma peritonei is a relatively rare disease with an incidence of approximately 1/1,000,000 per year. The diagnosis is classically made incidentally at laparotomy with the discovery of copious mucinous ascites with peritoneal implants (85). This process arises most often from a mucinous neoplasm of the appendix; however, it has also been associated with mucinous tumors of the ovary, colon, pancreas, and stomach (86). The natural history of the disease has been somewhat controversial in the literature largely because of nomenclature and inconsistency in histologic categorization. Patients presenting with mucinous ascites have been given the diagnosis of pseudomyxoma but the histology of their disease may vary from a low-grade mucinous neoplasm to high-grade adenocarcinoma. This is significant because patients with low-grade disease have a 5-year survival of 84% versus 6.7% of those with high-grade disease (87). Beyond this striking heterogeneity, randomized prospective data defining optimal treatment strategies tailored to histology and prognostic factors are lacking. Several retrospective analyses and pilot trials have been reported, but no comparative data favoring one approach over another exist.

Borrowing from the gynecologic experience with ovarian malignancy with similar clinical course, serial debulking surgical therapy with or without chemotherapy has been the mainstay of treatment. Serial debulking aims at reducing the tumor burden to the extent that it can reduce symptoms, improving GI function and potentially leading to an improved survival. The use of systemic therapy has been associated with very transient responses seldom exceeding 3 or 4 months. Moreover, prolongation of the disease-free interval after cytoreductive surgery has never clearly been shown because of the lack of randomized data (88).

Both retrospective and nonrandomized prospective reports on the use of IP therapy as an adjunct to surgery exist, but the data have limited usefulness. For example, Guner et al. (89) reported a series of 28 patients who underwent surgical debulking followed by IP chemotherapy. Only 40% were able to undergo macroscopically complete resections. Fifteen patients received cisplatin, six received mitomycin C, and seven received 5-FU. Survival was linked to low tumor volume and complete resection (p <0.05) and complications rate were linked to length and extent of surgery. No conclusion could be reached about the use of IP chemotherapy, and no mention was made of histologic features that predict a better outcome (89). In a larger retrospective analysis from Memorial Sloan-Kettering, 98 patients treated between 1980 and 2002 were reviewed. A median survival of 9.8 years was reported for all patients and better outcome was linked with low-grade histology (p <0.001) and complete gross cytoreduction during at least one of the operations (p <0.001). Although 59% received systemic and 31% received IP chemotherapy, neither conferred a survival advantage (90).

Sugarbaker (91) has published most extensively on this subject and endorses aggressive early surgical treatment of pseudomyxoma peritonei in specialty centers (see Chapter 14). He advocates complete stripping of all peritoneal surfaces along with any organ resection that bears a tumor, omentectomy, gastrectomy, splenectomy, colectomy, hysterectomy and liver resection. Intraoperative peritoneal chemotherapy, usually with 35 mg/m$_2$ of mitomycin C, follows in a solution heated to 42°C. The elevated temperature presumably allows for better drug penetration into mucin, and is also tumoricidal by itself. Another ascribed benefit is counteracting hypothermia that may occur during a 10-hour surgical procedure (86). An IP catheter is left in place during the first 5 postoperative days for the administration of IP 5-FU. The underlying principle in this regimen is to expose any residual tumor cells to the chemotherapeutic agent prior to deposition of fibrin that may interfere with the optimal exposure to the IP drug. Systemic chemotherapy is reserved for patients with evidence of high-grade disease that has a potential to spread outside the peritoneum. In the experience of

Sugarbaker and Chang (92) with 385 patients followed for 37.6 months, improved survival was linked with complete cytoreduction, low-grade histology (p <0.0001), and not having had prior extensive surgery (p <0.001) (92). The complication rate was reported at 20% to 50% and was closely associated with the number of prior surgeries. Patients with prior debulking procedures are more likely to have anastomotic leaks and fistulas. There is also a mortality of 2% to 10% associated with the described procedure. Although neutropenia and catheter complications are reported, IP chemotherapy is not seen as a significant source of morbidity. With this treatment strategy, Sugarbaker reports an overall 5-year survival of 75% and a projected 10-year survival of 70%. When examining the low-grade adenomucinosis histologic subtype, with complete cytoreduction 5-year survival is >85% (91,92).

Similar findings are reported by the team at The Netherlands Cancer Institute in a retrospective series of 103 patients using aggressive cytoreduction and heated intraoperative mitomycin C. The 5-year survival was 72% in patients with low-grade histology but the overall complication rate was as high as 54%. It was hypothesized that IP chemotherapy interferes with healing at serosal injuries and indirectly contributes to abscesses, anastomotic leaks, or fistulas (93). A small study of 11 patients with 26-month follow-up also suggests a survival advantage from IP therapy (94). Interpretation of these experiences is clouded by the report of Miner et al. (90) that the subset of patients with low-grade disease treated with serial debulking have a survival similar to that of Sugarbaker (91,92). Many obstacles exist in obtaining randomized data in this rare disease entity, but the role of IP chemotherapy in relation to disease biology (whether low- or high-grade disease) and the value of serial debulking are important questions begging for answers.

Gastric Cancer

After local lymph node metastasis, peritoneal seeding is the most common site for tumor deposits in gastric cancer (95). Despite initial R0 resection, peritoneal metastasis develops in 60% of cases with T3 and T4 tumors, and 10% to 20% of patients with gastric cancer have peritoneal deposits at presentation (96). Therefore, treatment strategies specifically designed to target peritoneal disease could potentially lengthen survival.

Protocols using chemotherapy alone as adjuvant or neoadjuvant have shown limited clinical benefit (97). On the other hand, combination therapy with chemoradiation has recently shown promising results (98). IP chemotherapy as a strategy in this setting has some attractive theoretical features, exposing higher doses for longer duration to peritoneal surfaces. In addition, agents can be absorbed directly into the portal circulation attaining higher drug levels in the liver, a common site of metastasis. The liver also detoxifies drugs, thus limiting morbidity (99). This has prompted trials with IP therapy used perioperatively as described by Sugarbaker (79) or in repeated cycles postoperative as currently being tested by New York University, USC (99), and Memorial Sloan Kettering (58).

Initial studies with IP cisplatin failed to demonstrate any survival benefit (100) while in Japan mitomycin C appeared to have yielded better results. Hagiwara et al. (101) reported a 3-year survival advantage with IP chemotherapy in combination with surgery over surgery alone (p <0.01). An attempt to repeat these findings by a multicentered Austrian group closed early secondary to unacceptable surgical complication rate (102).

The timing of the IP treatment has been debated by Sugarbaker (79), who has hypothesized that fibrin deposition beginning in the postoperative period prevents optimal exposure of malignant cells in the peritoneum to drugs. Early postoperative IP chemotherapy (EPIC) is a treatment modality that aims to access free malignant cells in the peritoneum prior to fibrin deposition, namely with treatment beginning on postoperative day 1. The protocol of Yu et al. (103), with mitomycin C 10 mg/m^2 on postoperative day 1 followed by 5-FU at 700 mg/m^2 for the next 4 days each, was studied in 248 randomized patients during gastric resection. Five-year survival was 54.2 % in treatment group versus 40.1% in the surgery-only group ($p = 0.03$). EPIC was an independent and statistically significant predictor of survival. Incidence of peritoneal recurrence was 15% in the EPIC group and 29% in control ($p = 0.043$). Complications such as infection and bleeding were higher in the EPIC group, but this was not statistically significant. Patients with serosal invasion (T3 or greater) had the most dramatic benefit from the EPIC, with 5-year survival being 51% versus 25.6% ($p = 0.0007$) (103).

Another means of perioperative IP intervention is continuous hyperthermic peritoneal perfusion. In this method, an expander is attached to the abdomen after surgical resection with high-flow catheters infusing heated mitomycin C designed to optimize IP drug exposure to peritoneal tumors. Yonemura et al. (104) reported a significant improvement in survival in T3 or greater lesions with no increase in morbidity or mortality using this technique. Yonemura et al. (105), borrowing from Sugarbaker (79), has further targeted peritoneal disease with a very aggressive combination of preoperative IP chemotherapy, gastrectomy, lymph node dissection, left upper quadrant evisceration, peritonectomy, and postoperative IP chemotherapy. Complete removal of tumor is an important component of this therapy, and is the most significant predictor of survival. Therefore, in the setting of known locally advanced disease, Yonemura et al. (96) have advocated preoperative IP chemotherapy as a means to improve the possibility of cytoreduction. The regimen consists of 40 mg of docetaxel and 150 mg of carboplatin weekly in 500 mL of saline given in to the peritoneum. In patients with ascites, the drugs are administered directly into peritoneal fluid. Patients also receive neoadjuvant systemic therapy with methotrexate and 5-FU. In 12 of 17 patients, the effluent had no detectable tumor RNA. Fifty-eight percent of these 12 patients achieved complete cytoreduction with surgery, whereas none of the remaining 5 could go on to R0 resections. This suggested that response to IP chemotherapy led to more complete resections, and thereby an improved survival (96).

At our institution, we have investigated IP FUDR and cisplatin in combination with systemic therapy for locally advanced disease in two pilot studies: (a) following neoadjuvant chemotherapy (99) and (b) as an additive to adjuvant chemoradiation, which is currently the standard regimen for gastric cancer in the United States (D. Cohen, unpublished). The selection of IP FUDR for further study as a consolidation treatment in gastric cancer was partly based on vast experience at the University of Southern California in phase I and pharmacologic studies,

and subsequently in a pilot program of neoadjuvant therapy, gastrectomy, and IP consolidation (106). Tolerance to repeated daily for three courses of FUDR by itself or with leucovorin was initially established and IP FUDR with cisplatin without leucovorin was then used for postoperative consolidation in resected gastric cancer. The USC trial yielded a very favorable median survival exceeding 4 years, compared with <1 year for historical controls of resected gastric cancer patients over a 2-year period at the Los Angeles County-USC Medical Center (106).

In 1998 we initiated a phase II trial looking at the role of neoadjuvant CPT-11 and cisplatin for locally advanced gastric adenocarcinoma followed by resection and IP chemotherapy. As this trial was started prior to the reporting of the Intergroup trial results (98), adjuvant chemoradiation was not included. The rationale behind a neoadjuvant trial includes better ability to deliver therapy, to downstage disease, and to identify those patients whole aggressive disease progresses during the neoadjuvant treatment. This latter group of patients would not likely benefit from surgical resection and are only operated on in the setting of symptoms. In our neoadjuvant phase II study, we had 32 patients who demonstrated T3, T4, TN1, or TN2 disease on preoperative staging. They received two cycles of irinotecan 75 mg/m^2 with cisplatin 25 mg/m^2/week for 4 weeks followed by a 2-week break. Twenty-nine patients went on to surgical resection, with R0 resection possible in 25 patients. Half of the patients had evidence of tumor downstaging. Adjuvant postoperative IP chemotherapy consisted of FUDR 3 g × 3 days plus IP cisplatin 60 mg/m^2 on day 3. There were three catheter-related complications with minimal grade 3 or 4 morbidity associated with IP therapy. Toxicity was noted in patients with induction neoadjuvant chemotherapy, with 10 hospitalizations. Grade 4 toxicity was rare and there were no treatment-related deaths. Median overall survival in the cohort of 32 patients was 36.5 months from the start of treatment, with a median follow-up of 28 months. Among the 25 patients with R0 resection, median overall survival was 48 months, after median follow-up of 35 months. These preliminary results are encouraging and are certainly comparable with those of the Intergroup study, which used chemoradiation in the adjuvant setting (99). Our findings are supported by another recent phase II trial of 38 patients completed at Memorial Sloan-Kettering (107).

Although not yet widely adopted, IP chemotherapy may emerge as an important component to the multimodality treatment of gastric cancer. There is good evidence that IP chemotherapy may benefit patients with locally advanced disease both in the neoadjuvant and adjuvant setting with less toxicity than conventional therapy. In most of the studies, however, complete cytoreduction remains the most important predictor of favorable outcome.

CONCLUSION

It is hoped that the recent confirmation of the value of IP therapy in the treatment of ovarian cancer will lead to further trials and technical developments. Specifically in ovarian cancer, studies are looking into the pharmacologic properties of carboplatin, paclitaxel, and topotecan when given by the IP route. These drugs may play a role not only in first-line therapy, but also in consolidation. The experience with FUDR, and previously with cytosine arabinoside, suggests that pharmacologic advantages and repeated administration may lead to remarkable therapeutic effects with drugs that are not usually employed in the disease in question. The near absence of chemical peritonitis may be another prerequisite. In addition, not only the pharmacologic advantage provided by concentrations at the peritoneal surfaces but also a sustained, high concentration in juxtaperitoneal lymphatics may be responsible for lasting antitumor effects. Strategies should test IP consolidation with cisplatin coupled with topotecan in the presence of persistent disease at the time of initial reassessment. With 50% recurrences at 5 years, patients presenting with stage III disease who obtain pathologic complete responses should be targets for IP consolidation.

Similarly, in cancer of gastric origin, the neoadjuvant approach followed by surgery and IP consolidation should be tested in randomized clinical trials versus no IP consolidation. Such studies are important as they potentially are applicable to a wider group of patients presenting with clinically locally advanced disease, as opposed to adjuvant treatments that are applicable only to those with curative resections. In colorectal cancer, awareness of peritoneal disease and the potential for IP drug administration to achieve its eradication must be enhanced in order to stimulate adjuvant trials including IP therapy in patients at high risk for recurrence.

The evolution of IP drug administration (Table 6.1) into a useful treatment modality has been long and arduous. The pharmacologic basis underlying such treatment is still evolving to address issues of drug penetrance and possible immunologic mechanisms; as a result, the optimal circumstances for therapeutic effects in ovarian cancer and in other cancers with prominent peritoneal spread remain far from clear. Nevertheless, recent randomized phase II and III trials provide new, important reference points: cisplatin is better tolerated and has greater efficacy by the IP than the IV route in small-volume residual disease; FUDR is well tolerated on a daily × three schedule and has shown promising antitumor activity by itself and in combination with cisplatin for gastric and ovarian cancers. Biological approaches need to extend beyond phase I to supplement chemotherapeutic approaches. It is important for surgical oncologists to be aware of the results achievable with IP therapy, and to consider IP port placement in appropriate curative and palliative surgical settings.

REFERENCES

1. Alberts DS, Liu PY, Hannigan EV, et al. Intraperitoneal cisplatin plus intravenous cyclophosphamide versus intravenous cisplatin plus intravenous cyclophosphamide for stage III ovarian cancer. *N Engl J Med.* 1996;335:1950–1955.
2. Markman M, Bundy BN, Alberts DS, et al. Phase III trial of standard dose intravenous paclitaxel and intraperitoneal cisplatin in small-volume stage III ovarian carcinoma: an intergroup study of the Gynecologic Oncology Group, southwestern Oncology Group, and Eastern Cooperative Oncology Group. *J Clin Oncol.* 2001;19:1001–1007.
3. Armstrong DK, Bundy B, Wenzel L, et al; Gynecologic Oncology Group. Intraperitoneal cisplatin and paclitaxel in ovarian cancer. *N Engl J Med.* 2006;5;354:34–43.
4. Young-Fadok TM, Wolff BG, Nivatvongs S, et al. Prophylactic oophorectomy in colorectal carcinoma: preliminary results of a randomized, prospective trial. *Dis Colon Rectum.* 1998;41:277–285.
5. Sugarbaker PH. Patient selection and treatment of peritoneal carcinomatosis from colorectal and appendiceal cancer. *World J Surg.* 1995;19:235–240.
6. Rosen HR, Jatzko G, Repse S, et al. Adjuvant intraperitoneal chemotherapy with carbon-adsorbed mitomycin in patients with gastric cancer: results of a randomized multicenter trial of the Austrian Working Group for Surgical Oncology. *J Clin Oncol.* 1998;16:2733–2738.
7. Crookes P, Leichman CG, Leichman L, et al. Systemic chemotherapy for gastric carcinoma followed by postoperative intraperitoneal therapy: a final report. *Cancer.* 1997;79:1767–1775.
8. Cao G, Kuriyama S, Gao J, et al. Effective and safe gene therapy for colorectal carcinoma using the cytosine deaminase gene directed by the carcinoembryonic antigen promoter. *Gene Ther.* 1999;6:83–90.
9. Misawa T, Chiang MH, Pandit L, et al. Development of systemic immunologic responses against hepatic metastases during gene therapy for peritoneal carcinomatosis with retroviral HS-tk and ganciclovir. *J Gastrointest Surg.* 1997;1:527–533.
10. Edwards RP, Gooding W, Lembensky BC, et al. Comparison of toxicity and survival following intraperitoneal recombinant interleukin-2 for persistent ovarian cancer after platinum: twenty-four-hour versus 7-day infusion. *J Clin Oncol.* 1997;5:3399–3407.
11. Dedrick RL, Myers CE, Bungay PM, DeVita VT Jr. Pharmacokinetic rationale for peritoneal drug administration in the treatment of ovarian cancer. *Cancer Treat Rep.* 1978;62:1–11.
12. Myers CE, Collins JM. Pharmacology of intraperitoneal chemotherapy. *Cancer Invest.* 1983;1:395–407.
13. Howell SB, Zimm S, Markman M, et al. Long-term survival of advanced refractory ovarian carcinoma patients with small-volume disease treated with intraperitoneal chemotherapy. *J Clin Oncol.* 1987;5:1607–1612.
14. Howell SB, Pfeiffle CL, Wung WE, et al. Intraperitoneal cisplatin with systemic thiosulfate protection. *Ann Intern Med.* 1982;97:845–851.
15. King ME, Pfeiffle CE, Howell SB. Intraperitoneal cytosine arabinoside therapy in ovarian carcinoma. *J Clin Oncol.* 1984;2:662–669.
16. Speyer JL, Sugarbaker PH, Collins JM, et al. Portal levels and hepatic clearance of 5-fluorouracil after intraperitoneal administration in humans. *Cancer Res.* 1981;41:1916–1922.
17. Speyer JL, Collins JM, Dedrick RL, et al. Phase I and pharmacological studies of 5-fluorouracil administered intraperitoneally. *Cancer Res.* 1980;40:567–572.
18. Sugarbaker PH, Gianola FJ, Speyer JL, et al. Prospective, randomized trial of intravenous versus intraperitoneal 5-fluorouracil in patients with advanced primary colon or rectal cancer. *Surgery.* 1985;98:414–422.
19. Gastrointestinal Tumor Study Group. Workshop on Intraperitoneal Chemotherapy, Orlando, Florida. *Semin Oncol.* 1985;12(Suppl 4):1–115.
20. Muggia FM, Chan KK, Russell C, et al. Phase I and pharmacologic evaluation of intraperitoneal 5-fluoro-2'-deoxyuridine. *Cancer Chemother Pharmacol.* 1991;28:241–250.
21. Muggia FM, Tulpule A, Retzios A, et al. Intraperitoneal 5-fluoro-2'-deoxyuridine with escalating doses of leucovorin: pharmacology and clinical tolerance. *Invest New Drugs.* 1994;12:197–206.
22. Israel VK, Jiang C, Muggia FM, et al. Intraperitoneal 5-fluoro-2'deoxyuridine (FUDR) and (S)-leucovorin for disease predominantly confined to the peritoneal cavity: a pharmacokinetic and toxicity study. *Cancer Chemother Pharmacol.* 1995;37:32–38.

23. Muggia FM, Liu PY, Alberts DS, et al. Intraperitoneal mitoxantrone or floxuridine: effects on time-to-failure and survival in patients with minimal residual ovarian cancer after second-look laparotomy—a randomized Phase II study by the Southwest Oncology Group. *Gynecol Oncol.* 1996;61:395–402.

24. Markman M, Rowinsky E, Hakes T, et al. Phase I trial of intraperitoneal taxol: a Gynecologic Oncology Group study. *J Clin Oncol.* 1992;10:1485–1491.

25. Francis P, Rowinsky E, Schneider J, et al. Phase I feasibility and pharmacologic study of weekly intraperitoneal paclitaxel: a Gynecologic Oncology Group pilot study. *J Clin Oncol.* 1995;13:2961–2967.

26. Markman M, Brady MF, Spirtos NM, et al. Phase II trial of intraperitoneal paclitaxel in carcinoma of the ovary, tube, and peritoneum: a Gynecologic Oncology Group study. *J Clin Oncol.* 1998;16:2620–2624.

27. Dedrick RL, Flessner MF. Pharmacokinetic problems in peritoneal drug administration: tissue penentration and surface exposure. *J Natl Cancer Inst.* 1997;89:480–487.

28. Los G, Mutsaers PH, Lenglet WJ, et al. Platinum distribution in intraperitoneal tumors after intraperitoneal cisplatin treatment. *Cancer Chemother Pharmacol.* 1990;25:389–394.

29. Ozols RF, Locker GY, Doroshow JH, et al. Pharmacokinetics of adriamycin and tissue penetration in murine ovarian cancer. *Cancer Res.* 1979;39:3209–3214.

30. Lindner P, Heath DD, Shalinsky DR, et al. Regional lymphatic drug exposure following intraperitoneal administration of 5-fluorouracil, carboplatin, and etoposide. *Surg Oncol.* 1993;2:105–112.

31. Sugarbaker PH, Klecker RW, Gianola FJ, et al. Prolonged treatment schedules with intraperitoneal 5-fluorouracil diminish the local-regional nature of drug distribution. *Am J Clin Oncol.* 1986;9:1–7.

32. Markman M, Walker JL. Intraperitoneal chemotherapy of ovarian cancer: a review, with a focus on practical aspects of treatment. *J Clin Oncol.* 2006;24(6):988–994.

33. Markman M, Berek JS, Blessing JA, et al. Characteristics of patients with small-volume residual ovarian cancer unresponsive to cisplatin-based IP chemotherapy: lessons learned from a Gyneclogic Oncology Group phase II trial of IP cisplatin and recombinant alpha-interferon. *Gynecol Oncol.* 1992;45:3–8.

34. Sugarbaker PH. Pseudomyxoma peritonei. *Cancer Treat Rev.* 1986;81:105–119.

35. Jinnai D, Higashi H. Extended radical operation with preoperative chemotherapy for gastric cancer. In: Hirayama T, ed. *Cancer in Asia.* Baltimore: University Park Press. 1976;111–119.

36. Hagiwara A, Takahashi T, Kojima O, et al. Prophylaxis with carbon-absorbed mitomycin against peritoneal recurrence of gastric cancer. *Lancet.* 1992;339:629–631.

37. Tsujitani S, Okuyama T, Watanabe A, et al. Intraperitoneal cisplatin during surgery for gastric cancer and peritoneal seeding. *Anticancer Res.* 1993;13:1831–4.

38. Yu W, Whang I, Suh I, et al. Prospective randomized trial of early postoperative intraperitoneal chemotherapy as an adjuvant to respectable gastric cancer. *Ann Surg.* 1998;228:347–354.

39. Muggia FM, LePoidevin E, Jeffers S, et al. Intraperitoneal therapy for ovarian cancer: analysis of fluid distribution by computerized tomography. *Ann Oncol.* 1992;149–154.

40. Wahl RL, Gyves J, Gross BH, et al. SPECT of the peritoneal cavity: method for delineating intraperitoneal fluid distribution. *Am J Roentgenol.* 1989;152:1205–1210.

41. Magre GR, Terk M, Colletti P, et al. Saline MR peritoneography. *Am J Roentgenol.* 1989;152:1205–1210.

42. Speyer JL, Beller U, Colombo N, et al. Intraperitoneal carboplatin: favorable results in women with minimal residual ovarian cancer after cisplatin therapy. *J Clin Oncol* 1990;8:1335–1340.

43. DeGregorio MW, Lum BL, Holleran WM, et al. Preliminary observations of intraperitoneal carboplatin pharmacokinetics during a phase I study of the Northern California Oncology Group. *Cancer Chemother Pharmacol* 1988;18:235–240.

44. Piccart MJ, Abrams J, Dodion PF, et al. Intraperitoneal chemotherapy with cisplatin and melphalan. *J Natl Cancer Inst.* 1988;80(14):1118–1124.

45. Howell SB, Pfeifle CE, Olshen RA. Intraperitoneal chemotherapy with melphalan. *Ann Intern Med.* 1984;101(1):14–18.

46. Feun LG, Blessing JA, Major FJ, et al. A Phase II study of intraperitoneal cisplatin and thiotepa in residual ovarian carcinoma: a Gynecologic Oncology Group study. *Gynecol Oncol.* 1998;7(3):410–415.

47. Rosen HR, Jatzko G, Repse S, et al. Adjuvant intraperitoneal chemotherapy with carbon-adsorbed mitomycin in patients with gastric cancer: results of a randomized multicenter trial of the Austrian Working Group for surgical Oncology. *J Clin Oncol.* 1998;16:2733–2738.

48. Alberts DS, Surwit EA, Peng YM, et al. Phase I clinical and pharmacokinetic study of mitoxantrone given to patients by intraperitoneal administration. *Cancer Res.* 1988;48:5874–5877.

49. Blochl-Daum B, Eichler HG, Rainer H, et al. Escalating dose regimen of intraperitoneal mitoxantrone: phase I study –clinical and pharmacokinetics evaluation. *Eur J Cancer Clin Oncol.* 1988;241:1133–1138.

50. Jones RB, Collins JM, Myers CE, et al. High volume intraperitoneal chemotherapy with methotrexate in patients with cancer. *Cancer Res.* 1981;41:55–59.

51. Howell SB, Kirmani S, Lucas WE, et al. A Phase II trial of intraperitoneal cisplatin and etoposide for primary treatment of ovarian epithelial cancer. *J Clin Oncol.* 1990;8:137–145.

52. Muggia FM, Russell C. New chemotherapies for ovarian cancer: systemic and intraperitoneal podophyllotoxins. *Cancer.* 1991;(Suppl);67:225–230.

53. O'Dwyer PJ, LaCreta FP, Daugherty JP, et al. Phase I pharmacokinetic study of intraperitoneal etoposide. *Cancer Res.* 1991;51(8):2041–2046.

54. Morgan RJ Jr, Doroshow JH, Synold T, et al. Phase I trial of intraperitoneal docetaxel in the treatment of advanced malignancies primarily confined to the peritoneal cavity: dose-limiting toxicity and pharmacokinetics. *Clin Cancer Res.* 2003;9(16 Pt 1):5896–5901.

55. Sabbatini P, Aghajanian C, Leitao M, et al. Intraperitoneal cisplatin with intraperitoneal gemcitabine in patients with epithelial ovarian cancer: results of a Phase I/II trial. *Clin Cancer Res.* 2004;10(9):2962–2967.

56. Muggia FM, Liebes L, Hazarika M, et al. Phase I and pharmacologic study of i.p. 9-aminocamptothecin given as six fractions over 14 days. *Anticancer Drugs.* 2002;13(8):819–825.

57. Plaxe SC, Christen RD, O'Quigley J, et al. Phase I and pharmacokinetic study of intraperitoneal topotecan. *Invest New Drugs.* 1998;16:147–152.

58. Kelsen D, Karpeh M, Schwartz G, et al. Neoadjuvant therapy of high-risk gastric cancer: a Phase II trial of preoperative FAMTX and postoperative intraperitoneal fluorouracil-cisplatin plus intravenous fluorouracil. *J Clin Oncol.* 1996;14:1818–1828.

59. Garcia AA, Muggia FM, Spears CP, et al. Phase I and pharmacologic study of i.v. hydroxyurea infusion given with i.p. 5-fluoro-2'-deoxyuridine and leucovorin. *Anticancer Drugs.* 2001;12:505–511.

60. Muggia FM, Jeffers S, Muderspach L, et al. Phase I/II study of intraperitoneal floxuridine and platinums (cisplatin and/or carboplatin). *Gynecol Oncol.* 1997;66:290–294.

61. Markman M. Intraperitoneal cisplatin chemotherapy in the management of ovarian carcinoma. *Semin Oncol.* 1989;16:79–82.

62. Leichman L, Silberman H, Leichman CG, et al. Preoperative systemic chemotherapy followed by adjuvant postoperative intraperitoneal therapy gastric cancer: a University of Southern California pilot program. *J Clin Oncol.* 1992;10:1933–1942.

63. Howell SB, Pfeiffle CE, Wung WE, Olshen RA. Intraperitoneal cis-diamminedichloroplatinum with systemic thiosulfate protection. *Cancer Res.* 1983;43:1426–1431.

64. Markman M, Hakes T, Reichman B, et al. Intraperitoneal cisplatin and cytarabine in the treatment of refractory or recurrent ovarian carcinoma. *J Clin Oncol.* 1991;9:204–210.

65. Piver SM, Recio FO, Baker TJ, Driscoll D. Evaluation of survival after second-line intraperitoneal cisplatin-based chemotherapy for advanced ovarian carcinoma. *Cancer.* 1994;73:1693–1698.

66. Formenti SC, Shrivastava PN, Sapozink M, et al. Abdomino-pelvic hyperthermia and intraperitoneal carboplatin in epithelial ovarian cancer: feasibility, tolerance and pharmacology. *Int J Radiat Oncol Biol Phys.* 1996;35:993–1001.

67. Muggia FM, Groshen S, Russell C, et al P. Intraperitoneal carboplatin and etoposide for persistent epithelial ovarian cancer after platinum-based regimens. *Gynecol Oncol.* 1993;50(2):232–238.

68. Allavena P, Peccatori F, Maggioni D, et al. Intraperitoneal recombinant gamma-interferon in patients with recurrent ascitic ovarian carcinoma; modulation of cytotoxicity and cytokine production in tumor-associated effectors and of major histocompatibility antigen expression on tumor cells. *Cancer Res.* 1990;50:7318–7323.

69. Epenetos AA, Hooker G, Krausz T, et al. Antibody-guided irradiation of malignant ascites in ovarian cancer: a new therapeutic method possessing specificity against cancer cells. *Obstet Gynecol.* 1986;68:715–745.

70. Fujimoto S, Takahashi M, Kobayashi K, et al. Cytohistologic assessment of antitumor effects of intraperitoneal hyperthermic perfusion with mitomycin C for patients with gastric cancer with peritoneal metastasis. *Cancer.* 1992;70:2754–2760.

71. Brodsky JT, Cohen AM. Peritoneal seeding following potentially curative resection of colonic carcinoma: Implications for adjuvant treatment. *Dis Colon Rectum.* 1991;34: 723–727.

72. De Bree E, Witkamo AJ, Zoetmulder FA. Intraperitoneal chemotherapy for colorectal cancer. Review Article. *J Surg Oncol.* 2002;79:49–61.

73. Koppe MJ, Boerman OC, Oyen WJ, et al. Peritoneal carcinomatosis of colorectal origin: incidence and current treatment strategies. *Ann Surg.* 2006;243:212–222.

74. Chu DZ, Lang NP, Thompson C, et al. Peritoneal carcinomatosis in nongynecologic malignancy. A prospective study of prognostic factors. *Cancer.* 1989 Jan 15;63(2):364–367.

75. Sadeghi B, Arvieux C, Glehen O, et al. Peritoneal carcinomatosis from non-gynecologic malignancies: results of the EVOCAPE 1 multicentric prospective study. *Cancer.* 2000;88(2):358–363.

76. Jayne DG, Fook S, Loi C, et al. Peritoneal carcinomatosis from colorectal cancer. *Br J Surg.* 2002;89(12):1545–1550.

77. Gertsch P. A historical perspective on colorectal liver metastases and peritoneal carcinomatosis: similar results, different treatments. *Surg Oncol Clin N Am.* 2003;12(3):531–541.

78. Wei AC, Greig PD, Grant D, et al. Survival after hepatic resection for colorectal metastases: a 10-year experience. *Ann Surg Oncol.* 2006;13(5):668–676.

79. Sugarbaker PH, Cuniffe W, Belliveau JF, et al Rationale for perioperative intraperitoneal chemotherapy as a surgical adjuvant for gastrointestinal malignancy. *Reg Cancer Treat.* 1988;1:66–79.

80. Verwaal VJ, van Ruth S, de Bree E, et al. Randomized trial of cytoreduction and hyperthermic intraperitoneal chemotherapy versus systemic chemotherapy and palliative surgery in patients with peritoneal carcinomatosis of colorectal cancer. *J Clin Oncol.* 2003;21(20):3737–3743.

81. Elias, DM, Pocard M. Treatment and prevention of peritoneal carcinomatosis from colon cancer. *Surg Oncol Clin N Am.* 2003;12:543–559.

82. Esquivel J, Vidal-Jove J, Steves MA, Sugarbaker PH. Morbidity and mortality of cytoreductive surgery and intraperitoneal chemotherapy. *Surgery.* 1993;113(6):631–636.

83. Jacquet P, Stephens AD, Averbach AM, et al. Analysis of morbidity and mortality in 60 patients with peritoneal carcinomatosis treated by cytoreductive surgery and heated intraoperative intraperitoneal chemotherapy. *Cancer.* 1996;77(12):2622–2629.

84. Verwaal VJ, van Tinteren H, Ruth SV, et al. Toxicity of cytoreductive surgery and hyperthermic intra-peritoneal chemotherapy. *J Surg Oncol.* 2004 Feb;85(2):61–67.

85. Fann JI, Vierra M, Fisher D, et al. Pseudomyxoma Peritonei. *Surg Gynecol Obstet.* 1993;177:441–447.

86. Moran BJ, Cecil TD. The etiology, clinical presentation, and management of pseudomyxoma peritonei. *Surg Oncol Clin N Am.* 2003;12:585–603.

87. Ronnett BM, Zahn CM, Kurman RJ, et al. Disseminated peritoneal adenomucinosis and peritoneal mucinous carcinomatosis. A clinicopathologic analysis of 109 cases with emphasis on distinguishing pathologic features, site of origin, prognosis, and relationship to "pseudomyxoma peritonei." *Am J Surg Pathol.* 1995:19(12):1390–408.

88. Gough DB, Donohue JH, Schutt AJ, et al. Pseudomyxoma Peritonei. Long-term patient survival with an aggressive regional approach. *Ann Surg.* 1994;219(2):112–19.

89. Guner Z, Schmidt U, Dahlke MH, et al. Cytoreductive surgery and intraperitoneal chemotherapy for pseudomyxoma peritonei. *Int J Colorectal Dis.* 2005;20:155–160.

90. Miner TJ, Shia J, Jacques DP, et al. Long-term survival following treatment of pseudomyxoma peritonei: An analysis of surgical therapy. *Ann Surg.* 2005;241(2):300–308.

91. Sugarbaker, PH. New standard of care for appendiceal epithelial neoplasms and pseudomyxoma peritonei syndrome? *Lancet Oncology.* 2006;7:69–76.

92. Sugarbaker PH, Chang D. Results of treatment of 385 patients with peritoneal surface spread of appendiceal malignancy. *Ann Surg Oncol.* 1999;6(8):727–731.

93. Smeenk RM, Verwaal VJ, Zoetmulder FA. Toxicity and mortality of cytoreduction and intraoperative hyperthermic intraperitoneal chemotherapy in pseudomyxoma peritonei–a report of 103 procedures. *Eur J Surg Oncol.* 2006;32(2):186–190.

94. Butterworth SA, Panton ON, Klassen DJ, et al. Morbidity and mortality associated with intraperitoneal chemotherapy for pseudomyxoma peritonei. *Am J Surg.* 2002;183(5):529–532.

95. Douglass, HO Jr. Adjuvant therapy of gastric cancer: Have we made any progress? *Ann Oncol.* 1994;1:244–251.

96. Yonemura Y, Bandou E, Kinoshita K, et al. Effective therapy for peritoneal dissemination in gastric cancer. *Surg Oncol Clin N Am.* 2003;12(3):635–648.

97. Gonzalez, RJ, Mansfield PF. Adjuvant and Neoadjuvant therapy for gastric cancer. *Surg Clin N Am.* 2005;85:1033–1051.

98. Macdonald JS, Smalley SR, Benedetti J, et al. Chemoradiotherapy after surgery compared with surgery alone for adenocarcinoma of the stomach or gastroesophageal junction. *N Engl J Med.* 2001;345(10):725–730.

99. Newman E, Potmesil M, Ryan T, et al. Neoadjuvant chemotherapy, surgery, and adjuvant intraperitoneal chemotherapy in patients with locally advanced gastric or gastroesophageal junction carcinoma: a phase II study. *Semin Oncol.* 2005;32(6 Suppl 9):S97–S100.

100. Sautner T, Hofbauer F, Depisch D, et al. Adjuvant intraperitoneal cisplatin chemotherapy does not improve long-term survival after surgery for advanced gastric cancer. *J Clin Oncol.* 1994;12(5):970–974.

101. Hagiwara A, Takahashi T, Kojima O, et al. Prophylaxis with carbon-adsorbed mitomycin against peritoneal recurrence of gastric cancer. *Lancet.* 1992;339:629–631.

102. Rosen HR, Jatzko G, Repse S, et al. Adjuvant intraperitoneal chemotherapy with carbon-adsorbed mitomycin in patients with gastric cancer: Results of a randomized multicenter trail of the Austrian Working Group for Surgical Oncology. *J Clin Oncol.* 1998;16:2733–2738.

103. Yu W, Whang I, Chung HY, et al. Indications for early postoperative intraperitoneal chemotherapy of advanced gastric cancer: results of a prospective randomized trial. *World J Surg.* 2001;25:985–990.

104. Yonemura Y, de Aretxabala X, Fujimura T, et al. Intraoperative chemohyperthermic peritoneal perfusion as an adjuvant to gastric cancer: final results of a randomized controlled trial. *Hepatogastroenterology.* 2001;48(42):1776–1782.

105. Yonemura Y, Kamamura T, Nojima N, et al. Postoperative results of left upper abdominal evisceration for advanced gastric cancer. *Hepatogastroenterology.* 2000:47:571–574.

106. Crookes P, Leichman CG, Leichman L, et al. Systemic chemotherapy for gastric carcinoma followed by postoperative intraperitoneal therapy: a final report. *Cancer.* 1997;79(9):1767–1775.

107. Brenner B, Shah M, Karpeh M, et al. A phase II trial of neoadjuvant cisplatin-fluorouracil followed by postoperative intraperitoneal floxuridine-leucovorin in patients with locally advanced gastric cancer. *Ann Oncol.* 2006 Sep;17(9):1404–1411.

COMMENTARY
John J. Kavanagh, Jr.

Intraperitoneal antineoplastics have been used for approximately 25 years. The principles of such use have been elucidated by Dedrick et al. (1) in a classic article describing the pharmacokinetic theoretical rationale. These principles led to mathematical calculations of favorable differential exposure of neoplastic cells in the peritoneum compared with concentrations obtained in the systemic circulation. However, it is implicit in this construct that the optimal compound would have a linear dose-response curve, evidence of synergy if used in combination, immediate cytotoxic activity without intermediary metabolism, and exit from the peritoneal cavity that is slow, but on occurring results in rapid clearance, thereby minimizing systemic toxicity. There is the obvious pragmatic counterpart that the compound should not have characteristics that result in poor patient compliance, and it should be able to be given in a repeated fashion, with minimal pain and inflammatory peritonitis. Unfortunately, no such "ideal" compound presently exists.

The term *intraperitoneal* therapy actually may be inappropriate. The consensus is that the peritoneal cavity is a dynamic environment where compounds diffuse directly across the peritoneal surface, are preferentially absorbed into the lymphatic system, and also enter the portal venous circulation (2,3). These issues make the actual contribution of the intraperitoneal (IP) modality a conundrum. This is particularly true in the adjunctive therapies of gastric cancer, in which lymphatic metastases are considered of paramount importance. Unfortunately, there is very limited information on the newer compounds as to their disposition by the three major routes. Therefore, it becomes very difficult to attribute a positive outcome to a concentration-related phenomena or a simple modification of the area-under-the-curve in the systemic sense. As we use nonclassic chemotherapy agents, pharmacy-modified drugs, or biologics, understanding the pharmacodynamics will become essential in developing rational clinical strategies.

A second aspect of IP chemotherapy as discussed by Dr. Newman and his colleagues is the mechanics. Over the years, a multitude of infusates, volumes, and catheter devices have been used with this modality. Previous trials were handicapped by catheter-related problems and an inability to evaluate the suitability of the peritoneal cavity for therapy. However, technical advances in catheter technology, increased surgical experience in the placement of such devices, and the utilization of computerized tomography or radionuclide scanning for evaluation of the peritoneal cavity have allowed the proper treatment and selection of patients. Many early trials must be considered compromised because of the lack of the evolution of these factors (4–6). Although not mentioned in Chapter 6, the careful education of the patient and all medical personnel is crucial to the success of the trials. In addition, established standardized protocols of catheter care, administration of compounds, and reporting of complications are a sine qua non of minimizing complications.

As the years have progressed, certain tumor types commonly associated with residual disease after surgery seem to warrant further study. The depth of penetration of the classic chemotherapy agents in the tumor tissue is 3 mm or less. As pointed out in the chapter, there is little evidence to substantiate the treatment of so-called bulky disease with an IP modality. From the information available, one would have to assume that an advantage gained in the latter situation is from an incidental phenomenon other than direct tumor-drug interaction (i.e., systemic absorption).

Several tumor types continue to be attractive for IP therapy. Patients with epithelial ovarian cancer who have minimal or no residual disease after primary surgery and/or chemotherapy seem an ideal group. This can be intellectually justified as a result of the cooperative trial conducted by the Southwest Oncology Group and the Gynecologic Oncology Group (GOG 104 trial) in which approximately 600 patients were randomized to receive either intravenous or IP cisplatin, with both arms receiving intravenous cyclophosphamide. There was an improvement of 8 months' survival for the intraperitoneally treated patients (7).

In a subsequent trial (GOG 114) (8), 462 patients were randomized to receive either intravenous cisplatin plus paclitaxel for six cycles or two cycles of high-dose carboplatin (AUC 9) every 28 days for two courses followed by six cycles of IP cisplatin plus intravenous paclitaxel. Patients in the IP arm had a borderline statistically significant improvement in overall survival and experienced greater significant toxicity. These results led to the conclusion that the IP experimental arm was not appropriate for routine clinical use. Also, the higher doses of carboplatin may have contributed to the positive findings in the IP arm.

Following this, the GOG embarked on another randomized study (GOG 172) (9) that incorporated a taxane in both arms of the study. Patients with stage III ovarian or primary peritoneal cancer with no residual mass >1 cm were randomized to receive intravenous paclitaxel and cisplatin versus intravenous paclitaxel on day 1 followed by IP cisplatin on day 2 and IP paclitaxel on day 8. Among the 415 eligible patients, there was a significant prolongation of overall survival, representing the IP treatment arm (16 months' survival advantage: 66 vs. 50 months' survival; $p = 0.03$). However, this analysis is not based on a true intention-to-treat analysis, the difference with respect to progression-free survival was even smaller, and comparisons for progression-free survival were marginal ($p = 0.05$). One of the main problems of IP therapy is significant toxicity, which limits administration. In this study only 42% of patients received six cycles of the designated IP therapy, 8% of patients failed to receive any IP therapy, and 38% of patients received only one or two cycles. It is difficult to conclude that two cycles of IP therapy in a third of patients really contributed to the results. Nevertheless, the results of this study justify discussing the potential clinical benefit and offering combined intravenous and IP chemotherapy to appropriate patients. Future studies should focus on more functional, less toxic, regimens and newer agents, particularly targeted therapies. In addition, newer analyzed surrogates of success should be pursued.

A tumor that warrants a creative IP approach is pseudomyxoma peritonei. There is no established systemic therapy. In the initial stages of this disease, surgical cytoreduction is often optimal. Patients usually die of disease that is confined strictly to the peritoneum and require multiple surgeries to remove the mucinous deposits. Yet, there is very little information in the literature, and there has been no focused effort to conduct pilot trials with this disease when a new IP modality is reported. Nonrandomized trials appear to offer benefit by combining radical peritoneal resection plus IP chemotherapy plus or minus hyperthermia. However, the actual improvement is clouded by favorable patient selection, limited numbers of centers skilled in the therapy, nonrandomized trial design, and high complication rates. One may conclude it is a reasonable choice for an occasional patient. A therapeutic advance in this disease could result in a significant clinical benefit to patients who have the misfortune to have indolent progressive recurrences after their primary diagnosis.

The utilization of IP therapy in gastric cancer is somewhat perplexing. The chapter nicely summarizes the conflicting therapy data about the subject. It should be noted that most studies use some other form of adjunctive therapy in addition to the intra-abdominal treatment. However, if the trend toward lower IP recurrence is seen in such patients, then there is the possibility of a palliative advance. One must consider that, pending the

discovery of a more active agent in the disease, the utilization of an IP approach will be limited (10).

Another tumor that has not been well studied and yet may be a logical area of endeavor is mesothelioma. Although an uncommon disease, surgical resection is a possibility in the primary setting. In addition, if there were a means of inducing a significant cytotoxic tumor reduction, a secondary or delayed surgical approach could be helpful. The tumor often remains confined to the intra-abdominal cavity with a slowly advancing course. Pilot trials in this area could be of great potential benefit to this subset of patients.

A crucial issue that is indirectly approached in the chapter is the issue of trial design. Critics of intra-abdominal chemotherapy correctly point out that most trials have either been single-arm or randomized with insufficient power to detect meaningful differences. Often, systemic therapy is also administered. However, in fairness, this criticism of the historical experience does not prove negativity; there are simply inadequate definitive trial data. The somewhat unexpected results of the IP platinum trial in ovarian cancer by the cooperative groups demonstrated the importance of careful prospective planning of these clinical studies (7).

The final critical issue in considering an IP approach is that of agent selection. Clearly because of scientific limitations the work has largely involved classic chemotherapy agents. However, it is difficult to imagine that this is the future of developmental therapies. Indeed, compounds that have pharmacologic modifications, such as liposomal doxorubicin or polyglutamated paclitaxel, may increase activity, and/or modify toxicity. These modified agents and others that are selectively taken up and retained by cancer cells (*selective uptake retention compounds*) are obvious choices for IP experimentation. Monoclonal antibodies are another area of obvious interest. The reference provided within the chapter is that of an earlier radioisotope of murine origin (11). Clearly, we have advanced in terms of the technology of humanized antibodies and multiple active components on the antibody. The difficulty will be in determining the appropriate volumes of disease to be treated and the trial designs necessary to prove efficacy. The general consensus in ovarian cancer is that such therapy would be best suited to those patients with minimal or no detectable residual tumor. Also to be considered are the biological therapies, which include IP cytokines and cellular therapies. As published by Freedman and associates (12), the IP cavity represents a rich environment of cytokines and cellular expression. Indeed it may be that an autologous tumor vaccine coupled with a cytokine would be the optimal intra-abdominal approach, solving both the local therapeutic issue along with inducing a systemic response (12).

Another rapidly advancing area of experimental antineoplastic therapy concerns compounds that target molecular end points. These would include such drugs as tyrosine kinase inhibitors. A difficult issue in the evaluation of such drugs is how to determine their surrogate end point efficacy, that is, the positive molecular change that parallels the clinical response. Perhaps such an approach would have an advantage in IP therapy in view of the available technology for repeated access for the analysis of the constituents of the abdominal microenvironment. Indeed, the so-called molecular compounds may provide an ideal opportunity for a better understanding in cellular and molecular kinetics of the intra-abdominal environment of neoplasms.

In summary, Dr. Newman and his colleagues have provided a very reasonable and well-balanced overview of intraperitoneally administered therapies. One must recognize that despite the sound theoretical foundation there has been no compound found that equals the ideal model. Many investigators have contributed to the evolution of what is now a functional, although relatively cumbersome, form of therapy. The results of various trials now justify a continuation of the modality in an investigational setting. A consensus has been reached that gross abdominal cancer does not benefit from this approach. Tumor types that appear to be most promising are epithelial ovarian cancer, gastric cancer, pseudomyxoma peritonei, and possibly intra-abdominal mesotheliomas. The outcome of randomized cooperative group trials in ovarian cancer (GOG172) makes the application of an IP modality an evidence-based alternative in selected patients. Research in this area should now be a high priority.

REFERENCES

1. Dedrick RL, Myers CE, Bungay PM, et al. Pharmacokinetic rationale for peritoneal drug administration in the treatment of ovarian cancer. *Cancer Treat Rep.* 1978;62:1–11.
2. Wolf BE, Sugarbaker PH. Intraperitoneal chemotherapy and immunotherapy. *Recent Results Cancer Res.* 1988;110:254–273.
3. Sugarbaker PH, Cunliffe WJ, Belliveau J, et al. Rationale for integrating early postoperative intraperitoneal chemotherapy into the surgical treatment of gastrointestinal cancer. *Semin Oncol.* 1989;16(Suppl 6):83–97.
4. Piccart MJ, Speyer JL, Markman M, et al. Intraperitoneal chemotherapy: technical experience at five institutions. *Semin Oncol.* 1985;12(Suppl 4):90–96.
5. Muggia FM, LePoidevin E, Jeffers S, et al. Intraperitoneal therapy for ovarian cancer: analysis of fluid distribution by computerized tomography. *Ann Oncol.* 1992;3:149–154.
6. Wahl RL, Gyves J, Gross BH, et al. SPECT of the peritoneal cavity: method for delineating intraperitoneal fluid distribution. *AJR Am J Roentgenol.* 1989;152:1205–1210.
7. Alberts DS, Liu PY, Hannigan EV, et al. Intraperitoneal cisplatin plus intravenous cycylophosphamide versus intravenous cisplatin plus intravenous cyclophosphamide for stage III ovarian cancer. *N Engl J Med.* 1996;335:1950–1955.
8. Markman M, Bundy BN, Alberts DS, et al. Phase III trial of standard dose intravenous paclitaxel and intraperitoneal cisplatin in small-volume stage III ovarian carcinoma: an intergroup study of the Gynecologic Oncology Group, southwestern Oncology Group, and Eastern Cooperative Oncology Group. *J Clin Oncol.* 2001;19:1001–1007.
9. Armstrong DK, Bundy B, Wenzel L, et al; Gynecologic Oncology Group. Intraperitoneal cisplatin and paclitaxel in ovarian cancer. *N Engl J Med.* 2006;5;354:34–43.
10. Kelsen D, Karpeh M, Schwartz G, et al. Neoadjuvant therapy of high-risk gastric cancer: a phase II trial of preoperative FAMTX and postoperative intraperitoneal fluorouracil-cisplatin plus intravenous fluorouracil. *J Clin Oncol.* 1996;14:1818–1828.
11. Epenetos AA, Hooker G, Krausz T, et al. Antibody-guided irradiation of malignant ascites in ovarian cancer: a new therapeutic method possessing specificity against cancer cells. *Obstet Gynecol.* 1986;68:71S–74S.
12. Freedman RS, Kudelka AJ, Kavanagh JJ, et al. Clinical and biological effects of intraperitoneal injections of recombinant interferon-Υ recombinant interleukin 2 with or without tumor-infiltrating lymphocytes in patients with ovarian or peritoneal carcinoma. *Clin Cancer Res.* 2000;6:2268–2278.

7

Antibodies and Their Conjugates for the Targeted Therapy of Cancer

Robert M. Sharkey and David M. Goldenberg

Over the past 10 or more years, there has been a radical change in the way many cancers are detected and treated. Although surgery, chemotherapy and radiation therapy remain the primary modes of therapy, advances in molecular biology and immunology have begun to show how new targeted drugs and biological agents can complement existing treatments, and in some instances, offer new options. There are a number of different kinds of biological-based therapies (cellular and noncellular, such as peptides and antibodies), but this chapter will focus primarily on the development and use of antibodies and their conjugates for cancer treatment. Since we have >30 years experience in preclinical and clinical development of antibody-based targeting strategies for cancer detection and therapy, we hope to provide our experience and insights into the complexities of this technology, and the prospects for its potential contributions to improved therapies of the future.

ANTIBODIES: A NATURAL DEFENDER

Proteins, collectively known as *immunoglobulins*, are found in the serum of vertebrate animals, and while differing in their composition, they all have a common function of identifying and removing foreign substances before they are pathogenic. These proteins have evolved extensively; in humans, there are five different classes and multiple subclasses of immunoglobulins that are commonly referred to as *antibodies*. Because immunoglobulin G (IgG) has been the most frequently used antibody in cancer therapeutics, our discussion will focus on this protein.

IgG is a relatively large serum protein of about 150,000 daltons, with a highly evolved structure-function relationship. IgGs share the same basic structure, being composed of pairs of heavy and light polypeptide chains that are assembled to form in a Y-shaped structure (Figure 7.1). Each heavy chain pairs with a light chain to form one "arm" of an IgG. Each heavy and light polypeptide chain can be divided into separate domains, with the heavy chain composed of one variable and three constant domains (VH and CH1, CH2, CH3), and the light chain containing one variable and one constant domain (VL and CL). The composition of the constant regions is highly conserved. As the name implies, the variable region of the heavy and light chains is highly adaptable, changing to conform to the programmed specificity dictated by the antigen that stimulated the immune response. Most often there are three complementarity-determining regions (CDRs) in each of the heavy and light chains that actually are responsible for binding to the antigen. The CDRs give an antibody its unique structure, and the other portion of the variable domain forms the framework that sculpts the conformation of the CDRs for optimal binding. The CDRs are molded to bind with just a small segment of the antigen known as the *epitope*. The specificity is defined more by the three-dimensional structure of the epitope than by its chemical composition. Depending on the size and complexity of the antigen, multiple unique epitope structures are presented on the surface of the antigen molecule to which a unique antibody can be formed. Most of the time, the epitope is presented only once in a given antigen, but occasionally there are repeating epitope structures within an antigen molecule. Interestingly, immunoglobulins have evolved to have multiple arms, providing them with the capacity to bind to more than one epitope, thereby cross-linking two antigen molecules. In a typical immune response, multiple antibodies can cause extensive cross-linking, forming larger-sized lattices of an antigen, or form clusters from single cells that are more easily identified by immune cells.

Antibodies are formed within plasma cells that are derived from B cells and have a diverse capacity to bind to a variety of compounds. In nature, an antibody response is characterized by a *polyclonal* response, meaning that it involves the formation of many antibodies, each reacting with a unique epitope structure, and each being derived from unique B cells. The clonality of the B cells reactive to a unique substance gives rise to the ability to isolate individual antibody-forming cells (or clones) from the spleen of an immunized mouse. Using a process known as *hybridization*, where the immunized murine B cells are fused with an immortalized murine myeloma cell line, a *hybridoma* cell line is formed that is capable of producing a *monoclonal antibody (MAb)*. A MAb is defined by its ability to bind highly specifically to a well-defined, specific epitope. The MAb hybridoma technique, for which Köhler and Milstein (1) received a Nobel prize, has had a profound impact on the development of immunology and molecular biology, revolutionizing the field of immunotherapy. Over the years, antibodies have been the focus of extensive molecular engineering in order to improve their clinical use. For example, murine MAbs of clinical interest are engineered to remove a significant portion of the murine component by substituting human IgG components (2–6). The first of these molecular constructs were chimeric antibodies, where the VL and VH regions of the murine antibody were spliced onto the human IgG, making a molecule that is ~67% human and 33% murine IgG. Taking this process to the next step,

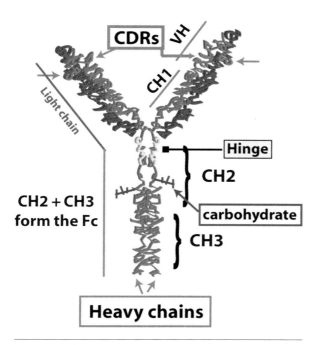

Figure 7.1 Schematic model of an immunoglobulin (Ig) G molecule. An IgG is composed of four polypeptide chains, two heavy (H) and two light (L) chains. Disulfide bridges within a hinge region hold the two heavy chains together, and each heavy chain is associated with a light chain. The heavy and light chains are divided into domains, the CH3, CH2, CH1, and VH for the heavy chain and CL and VL for the light chains. Each chain has domains that are highly conserved among IgG molecules (constant regions, C), and one region that is variable (V). Within the variable region of each chain exists several highly variable regions known as the complementarity-determining regions (CDRs), which form a three-dimensional structure that binds to the epitope of an antigen. The VH and VL regions of the molecule are referred to as the Fv region. The CH2 and CH3 portion of the IgG is referred to as the Fc portion. An IgG is also glycosylated, most often in the CH2 domain.

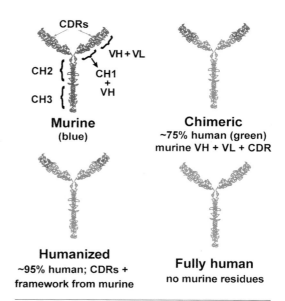

Figure 7.2 Humanizing an antibody by molecular engineering. Splicing the variable light and heavy chains of a murine immunoglobulin (Ig) G to a human IgG (CH3, CH2, CH1, VH) forms a chimeric IgG that is ~75% human IgG with the remaining portion being donated from the mouse IgG. For a humanized IgG, only the complementarity-determining regions (CDRs) from the murine IgG are taken, along with a few residues that help form the CDRs sequences in the right molecular shape to bind to the antigen (i.e., the framework regions). These sequences are spliced on VL and VH of a human IgG, making the resulting product about 95% human, with ~5% of the residues coming from the murine. A fully human IgG has the CDRs and framework from a human IgG. These molecules can be obtained from transgenic mice that are bred specifically to produce human rather than mouse IgG.

antibodies were further "demoused" by grafting only the CDR regions from the murine MAb, along with some of the surrounding framework regions to maintain CDR conformation, onto a human IgG, essentially making a molecule with ~5% of its sequence from the parental murine MAb (Figure 7.2). More recent advances have made available, either by genetic or phage-display methods, fully human MAbs that have now entered clinical practice or trials (5,7). Such engineered MAbs greatly reduce the immunogenicity of antibodies, allowing multiple injections to be given, while the human Fc enhances the interaction with other immune system elements, such as complement and effector cells.

Although the specificity of antibody-binding is determined by its variable regions and CDRs, the heavy chain constant regions also possess important properties. The CH2 and CH3 domains comprise the Fc portion of the IgG molecule. This portion can bind to Fc receptor-bearing cells (most notably other immune cells), and is responsible for binding components of the complement cascade. Thus, while one end of an antibody

binds to an antigen, for example, on the surface of a foreign cell, the other end, the Fc portion, can interact with other components of the immune system to attack and destroy this cell. These two attack mechanisms are referred to as *antibody-dependent cellular cytotoxicity* (ADCC) and *complement-mediated* or *complement-dependent cytotoxicity* (CMC or CDC) (Figure 7.3). ADCC involves the recognition of the antibody by immune cells that engage the antibody-marked cells and either through their direct action, or through the recruitment of other cell types, leads to the death of the tagged cell. CDC is a process in which a cascade of different complement proteins become activated, usually when several IgGs are in close proximity to each other, with one direct outcome being cell lysis, or indirectly being responsible for attracting other immune cells to this location for effector cell function.

ADCC and CDC were once thought to be the only mechanisms by which antibodies could kill cells or invading organisms. However, the antibody's ability to bind to at least two epitopes provides yet another mechanism. Cells need to interact with

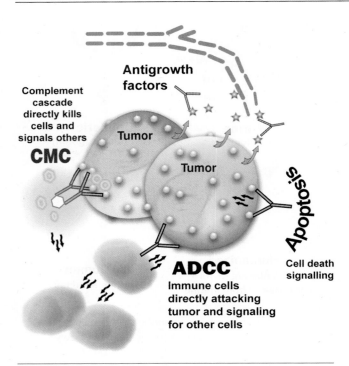

Figure 7.3 Schematic representation of the various mechanisms by which unconjugated (naked) antibodies can kill cells. The more traditional mechanisms are antibody-dependent cellular cytotoxicity (ADCC) and complement-mediated or complement-dependent cytotoxicity (CMC or CDC) where cellular or noncellular components of the immune system identify antibodies bound to the surface of a tumor cell. Certain antigens on the surface of cells when bound by an antibody send signals inside the cell that activate apoptosis that can lead to cell death. Other antibodies can bind factors that can have an impact on the growth of tumors. In this example, vascular endothelial growth factor (VEGF) is produced by tumors to stimulate the growth of vascular endothelial cells to provide a blood supply to the tumor. Antibodies can inhibit this process by either binding to the soluble VEGF or to its receptor.

their environment, and as such they display a wide array of receptors on their surface that can transmit messages to the inside of the cell. Some of these signals can cause a cell to undergo a process known as programmed cell death, or *apoptosis*. Perhaps one of the best-known examples of an antibody inducing apoptosis is the anti-CD20 antibody, rituximab (Rituxan:Genentech and Biogen IDEC) that is approved for the treatment of non-Hodgkin lymphoma (NHL) and rheumatoid arthritis (8). Rituximab binds to CD20, a B-cell surface protein. When rituximab binds to two CD20 molecules, this triggers the CD20 molecules to move within the membrane in what are known as *lipid rafts*, and this then transmits a signal inside the cell that initiates a cascade of events that lead to apoptosis (9). In vitro studies most often show that only a small proportion of the cells actually die as a consequence of this signaling event, but this level can be increased considerably when rituximab is cross-linked by other anti-antibodies (10,11). It is unlikely that rituximab becomes cross-linked by naturally occurring anti-antibodies in patients, but cross-linking can occur when the Fc portion of cell-bound

antibody is bound by immune cells through their Fc gamma receptors (FcγR). Thus, the binding of other immune cells to rituximab can initiate a more potent killing signal. Because cells frequently have alternative pathways for critical functions, interrupting a single signaling pathway alone might not be sufficient to ensure cell death, but because cells undergoing apoptosis are more susceptible to chemotherapy and radiation therapy, it is not surprising that antibodies that are proapoptotic are often best used to augment the antitumor effects of other standard forms of cytotoxic therapy (9,12–16). Trastuzumab (anti-*HER2/neu*; Herceptin:Genentech) and cetuximab (anti-epidermal growth factor receptor, EGFR; Erbitux:Bristol-Myers Squibb) and panitumumab (Vectibix, a fully human anti-EGFR antibody:Amgen) also have the ability to inhibit cell proliferation by apoptosis (17–20).

As our knowledge of cell biology continues to grow, there is an increasing awareness of the importance of various receptors and their cell functions. Interfering with the ability of a ligand to bind to a receptor by either binding the ligand or the receptor in a competitive manner can potentially interrupt critical cell processes that can either kill the cell or inhibit its ability to influence other cells. Bevacizumab (Avastin:Genentech) is a good example of this. Bevacizumab binds to vascular endothelial growth factor (VEGF) (21). VEGF is produced by a number of tumors to promote vascular formation. By binding to VEGF, bevacizumab prevents it from interacting with endothelial cells to form new blood vessels required for expanded tumor growth (Figure 7.3) (21,22). Other antibodies are being developed against other angiogenic cellular receptors (e.g., VEGFR-1 and VEGFR-2) that at least in preclinical testing show promising antitumor activity (23–26).

Antibodies can also be used to modulate immune responses. Antibodies to the cytotoxic T-cell lymphocyte-associated antigen-4 (CTLA-4) stimulate T-cell immune responses by blocking the inhibitory effects of CTLA-4, thus enhancing tumor rejection (27). However, release of this innate inhibitory mechanism can also increase the risk of autoimmunity (28). An evaluation of the changing phenotypes of the lymphocyte population in patients receiving anti-CTLA-4 therapy revealed that the antitumor activity was likely due to an activation of CD4+ and CD8+ effector cells, rather than a depletion or inhibition of the T-regulatory cells to which the anti-CTLA-4 binds (29). Two human anti-CTLA-4 antibodies are currently in clinical trials (MDX-010, or ipilimumab, and CP-675,206:Bristol-Myers Squibb and Medarex), with evidence that they may have activity in melanoma (30–32). There are already a number of antibodies used or being studied as therapeutic agents in cancer, as well as immunosuppressive agents in autoimmune diseases (e.g., alemtuzumab, daclizumab, infliximab, rituximab, and epratuzumab) (33–45). Antibodies also can block molecules associated with cell adhesion, thereby inhibiting tumor metastasis (46–49). With all these diverse mechanisms of action, there are a number of opportunities for further expanding the repertoire of antibody-based therapeutics.

THERAPY WITH UNCONJUGATED ANTIBODIES

Serotherapy is a concept that can be traced back to the 1890s, when it was first realized that resistance to infectious disease could be transferred from one animal to another through their serum (50). In 1895, Hericourt and Richet (51) immunized dogs with a human sarcoma and then transferred the serum to patients. These studies prefaced the "magic bullet" concept of Paul Ehrlich, in 1908, that "toxins" could be targeted to cancer and other diseases (52). Although interest in serotherapy continued, an evaluation of the potential therapeutic effects of unconjugated antibodies in cancer began in earnest in the early 1980s, after murine MAbs became available (1). Initial trials were performed in colorectal cancer, melanoma, and hematologic malignancies (53–60). With insufficient efficacy and the immunogenicity of the foreign murine MAbs, most of these studies were terminated, and interest in serotherapy waned. Fortunately, some investigators persevered.

An excellent lesson on the tribulations of the development of an antibody product between an academic group and industry is that of alemtuzumab (Campath, Berlex, and Genzyme) (61). Alemtuzumab (anti-CD52 humanized MAb) is one of the earliest and protracted developments of an antibody ultimately commercialized. It took >20 years from the development of the first rat immunoglobulin against CD52, changing the immunoglobulin type, and then finally developing a humanized, recombinant form, and involved several commercial firms during this time. Chemotherapy-refractive chronic lymphocytic leukemia (CLL) was the indication finally approved in 2001. Alemtuzumab, like other antibodies proven effective in hematologic malignancies, is also being applied to other conditions for which immunosuppressive therapy is beneficial (62,63).

As with any therapeutic product, efficacy and specificity depend on finding the right target. Antibodies have the extraordinary ability to be produced against diverse molecules, even reacting with multiple epitopes on a single molecule. This provides investigators with an important tool for identifying cell products so they can begin the process of sorting out those that might have therapeutic promise. In some instances, antibodies are the lead compounds in identifying suitable targets. For example, the biological consequences of binding EGRF were first studied with an antibody (64), but as the underlying mechanism and structures of compounds involved in these signaling pathways evolved, peptides, such as gefitinib (Iressa:Astra Zeneca) and erlotinib (Tarceva:Genentech), were developed and shown to also inhibit this pathway (65). While acting on the same signaling pathway, these agents bind to different sites, suggesting that combinations of peptide tyrosine kinase inhibitors with cetuximab or other EGFR antibodies could augment antitumor responses (66,67). Other binding proteins based on nonimmunoglobulin (antibody mimetic) structures are also providing new tools for designing biologically active molecules (68–70), and the modeling of the structure of an antibody-binding site can provide a basis on which synthetic selective high-affinity ligands can be prepared (71). These types of compounds could have certain advantages over antibodies, but antibodies will likely continue to dominate the clinical arena in the near future.

While today's high-throughput genomics and proteomics are busy searching libraries of gene products for candidate targets, much of this work is still empirical, yet occasionally successful. For unconjugated antibody therapy, rituximab is the most prominent example of an unprecedented success of antibody therapy, and is credited for the current widespread interest in antibody-based therapeutics. Unlike the earlier murine MAbs,

rituximab is a chimeric antibody, which not only reduced its immunogenicity, but improved its effector function associated by having a human Fc structure. For example, only the chimeric rituximab, not its parental murine anti-CD20 IgG (2B8), was shown to have ADCC activity in vitro against follicular lymphoma isolated from patients (72). Rituximab was initially approved as a monotherapy for relapsed or refractory low-grade, follicular B-cell NHL, having an overall response rate of 48% (~10% were complete responses) with a median duration of 11.8 months (73). Because CD20 is expressed only on premature and mature B cells and not on early progenitor cells of the bone marrow, rituximab induces a depletion of only CD-positive normal B cells as well as malignant B cells. The major side effects of rituximab occur during or shortly after its infusion, and are thought to be associated with the activation of complement pathways. Other less common side effects include symptoms associated with tumor lysis syndrome, severe mucocutaneous reactions, renal toxicity, cardiac arrhythmias, hypersensitivity reactions, and reactivation of hepatitis B (primarily when used in combination with chemotherapy) (73).

Unique among cancer treatments, 40% of the responsive patients retreated with rituximab could again respond with a similar duration (74). Extending the duration of rituximab therapy improves the response rate, particularly the number of complete responses and its duration. However, whether given as a maintenance regimen or retreating at the first sign of progression, the time to chemotherapy was the same (75). With both approaches having equal benefit, retreatment is generally favored because of the higher expense of maintenance regimens. Despite the success of rituximab as a monotherapy, there are still a number of patients who do not respond to the initial treatment, and over time, many of those who do respond will relapse. In an attempt to improve outcome, rituximab has been combined with chemotherapy regimens, including CHOP, CVP, and MCP, as frontline treatments with very promising results in not only follicular B-cell lymphomas, but also diffuse large cell B-cell lymphomas (76–82). Based on data from three randomized, controlled, multicenter studies in France and elsewhere, where rituximab was combined with CHOP or other anthracycline-based chemotherapy-induction regimens for patients with diffuse large cell B-cell lymphoma, the Food and Drug Administration (FDA), in February 2006, approved this treatment as frontline therapy. In each study, the overall survival benefit was improved in the rituximab-containing arms across all subgroups, including age (i.e., ≥60 and <60 years of age), gender, and disease prognostic variables. Even in CLL, where initial testing of rituximab was disappointing, dose intensification and combinations with chemotherapy have provided significant improvements in response (83,84). Rituximab has also been approved recently in combination with chemotherapy (CVP) as an initial therapy of patients with follicular, or indolent, lymphoma. Early clinical studies combining rituximab with a humanized anti-CD22, epratuzumab suggested the potential for additional benefit, particularly in patients with diffuse large cell B-cell lymphomas (85–88). Phase I/II studies have also assessed the possible role of an anti-CD80 IgG (galiximab:Biogen Idec), a hybrid human/primate MAb, as a monotherapy in NHL (89,90), leading to phase III trials that are underway.

Considerable attention has been given to understanding the mechanisms of action of rituximab. As mentioned earlier, rituximab has CDC, ADCC, and apoptotic (signaling) activities, with the former two mechanisms believed to have the greatest impact, but there are conflicting views regarding which of these two pathways contributes the most to response (9,10,91–98). Studies in transgenic and other mouse models have supported the importance of the Fc receptor-mediated mechanism of action for rituximab (99,100). These efforts have contributed in part to a better understanding of the role of various Fc receptors found on a variety of immune effector cells (e.g., B cells, neutrophils, natural killer cells, and monocytes), on the clearance of B cells (as in the case of rituximab), as well as the plasma half-life of antibodies (101–103). Not only do the various Fc receptors influence binding, but the absence of certain carbohydrates on the Fc portion of the IgG can affect both ADCC and CDC (103,104). Cartron et al. (105) found that the expression of the homozygous Fc gamma RIIIa receptor (CD16) 158V genotype correlated with a higher response rate to rituximab, but it did not have an impact on the progression-free survival. Others found a similar correlation, and also noted a higher response rate correlated independently with the homozygous expression of the Fc

gamma RIIa histidine/histidine genotype, particularly when assessing the response status ≥ 6 months from treatment (72). By unraveling the molecular basis for antibody cytotoxicity, not only can more effective antibodies be designed, but a more rational approach for combinations to enhance activity can be pursued. For example, granulocyte colony-stimulating factor up-regulates CD64 (FcγRI), which can enhance the binding of neutrophils and monocytes to B cells coated with rituximab (106). Interleukin (IL)-12 has a similar stimulatory effect in mouse models (107), and more recently has been applied clinically, but with only modest results when given concomitantly with rituximab (108).

Immunotherapy is not restricted to hematologic malignancies, but includes diverse target antigens and receptors having different biological functions (Table 7.1). Trastuzumab is an anti-HER2/neu antibody that has had a major impact on the therapy of breast cancer, and is used alone and in combination with drugs (19,109–111). *HER2/neu* is overexpressed on a proportion of breast and other cancers, and trastuzumab binds with an extracellular epitope of this target molecule. About 15% of

Table 7.1

Antibodies Approved for Use in Cancer Detection and Treatment in the United States

Generic Name	Trade Name	Agent/Target	Cancer Indication	Approval
Unconjugated				
Rituximab	Rituxan	Chimeric anti-CD20 IgG$_1$	B-cell lymphoma	1997
Trastuzumab	Herceptin	Humanized anti-HER2 IgG$_1$	Breast	1998
Alemtuzumab	Campath-1H	Humanized anti-CD52	CLL	2001
Cetuximab	Erbitux	Chimeric anti-EGFR	Colorectal Head/neck	2004 2006
Bevacizumab	Avastin	Chimeric anti-VEGF	Colorectal NSCLC	2004 2006
Panitumumab	Vectibix	Human anti-EGFR	Colorectal	2006
Radioconjugates				
Satumomab pendetide[a,b]	OncoScint	^{111}In-murine anti-TAG-72 IgG	Colorectal, ovarian	1992
Nofetumomab merpentan[a,b]	Verluma	^{99m}Tc-murine anti-EGP-1 Fab'	SCLC	1996
Arcitumomab[a,b]	CEA-Scan	^{99m}Tc-murine anti-CEA Fab'	Colorectal	1996
Capromab pendetide[a]	ProstaScint	^{111}In-murine anti-PSMA	Prostate	1996
Ibritumomab tiuxetan	Zevalin	^{90}Y-murine anti-CD20 IgG + rituximab	Follicular B-cell lymphoma	2002
Tositumomab	Bexxar	^{131}I-murine anti-CD20 IgG + unlabeled tositumomab	Follicular B-cell lymphoma	2003
Drug conjugates				
Gemtuzumab ozogamicin	Mylotarg	Humanized anti-CD33 IgG$_4$ calicheamicin conjugate	AML	2000

IgG, immunoglobulin G; CLL, chronic lymphocytic leukemia; EGFR, epidermal growth factor receptor; VEGF, vascular endothelial growth factor; NSCLC, non–small cell lung cancer; CEA, carcinoembryonic antigen; EGP, epithelial glycoprotein; SCLC, small cell lung cancer; PSMA, prostate-specific membrane antigen; AML, acute myelogenous leukemia.
[a] Cancer imaging agents.
[b] No longer commercially available.

women whose tumors overexpress HER2/neu respond to trastuzumab, but its efficacy is clearly best when used in combination with chemotherapy, where a 25% increase in the median survival to 29 months has been reported (109). Further, the addition of this antibody to adjuvant chemotherapy for breast cancer has improved survival markedly (111). Because only a portion of breast cancer patients overexpress *HER2/neu* and respond to trastuzumab, selection of suitable patients is important. New data are emerging that suggest that trastuzumab treatment after adjuvant chemotherapy can have a significant benefit compared with observation, particularly in the rate of distant recurrence (110).

As a member of a family of receptor tyrosine kinases, the binding of HER2 by trastuzumab can interrupt intracellular signaling and affect tumor cell growth, but it has also been shown to have antiangiogenic properties (112). Although these properties may be important underlying mechanisms of action, other evidence suggests that the activity of trastuzumab is principally governed by ADCC (113). However, trastuzumab combined with chemotherapy improves response rates, despite the immunosuppressive activity of the chemotherapy, and trastuzumab's activity is enhanced when combined with other, nonantibody, erb inhibitors, such as gefitinib and erlotinib, all of which suggest that its ability to interfere with signaling is important (114). Because HER2 is a member of a family of growth factors known as the neuregulins/heregulin, which is expressed in multiple neuronal and nonneuronal tissues in embryos and adult animals (115,116), including the heart, it is not surprising that cardiomyopathy has been associated with trastuzumab, particularly when combined with paclitaxel and anthracyclines (117,118).

EGFR is also overexpressed in many solid cancers, and when bound by its ligand, cell growth is stimulated. However, when engaged by an EGFR-specific antibody, receptor phosphorylation is decreased and cell growth is inhibited. The chimeric antibody against EGFR, cetuximab, also has an effect on neovascularization (119–121). Cetuximab was initially approved for use in combination with irinotecan for patients who are refractive to irinotecan-based therapies, or as a single agent for patients who are intolerant to irinotecan-based regimens. This initial approval was based on overall objective responses, but there was no evidence of increased survival. More recently, it was approved for the treatment of squamous cell head and neck cancers in combination with radiation, or as a single agent in patients for whom platinum-based therapy failed. In this indication, the combination of radiation with cetuximab resulted in a significantly improved median duration of locoregional control (24.4 vs. 14.9 months), and a median duration of survival from 29.3 to 49.0 months (18,122). Beside the usual risks associated with antibody infusions, the major toxicity of cetuximab is an acne-form rash and other skin reactions in most patients, with ~10% of these being severe. There is evidence suggesting that the intensity of the skin rash is associated with its antitumor response and even survival benefit (123). As indicated in Table 7.2, other EGFR antibodies are also in development. Panitumumab (20) was approved recently for patients who failed fluoropyrimidine-, oxaliplatin-, and irinotecan-containing chemotherapy regimens, based on a randomized trial comparing panitumumab with best supportive care, where panitumumab improved progression-free survival from 60 to 96 days. Eight percent of the patients treated with panitumumab had a partial response lasting 17 weeks, but there was no significant improvement in overall survival.

Rather than binding to the cellular receptor, bevacizumab binds to VEGF, preventing it from binding to its receptor found on the vascular endothelium. Although preclinical studies indicated that anti-VEGF antibodies were active alone, as well

Table 7.2

Partial Listing of Anticancer Antibodies in Advanced Clinical Testing

Generic Name	Agent/Target	Cancer
Apolizumab	Human anti-HLA-DR	CLL, NHL
Chimeric 14.18	Chimeric antiganglioside (GD2) IgG	Neuroblastoma, melanoma
Cotara	Radiolabeled chimeric anti-TNT	Lung, glioma
Epratuzumab	Humanized anti-CD22	NHL
Galiximab	Humanized anti-CD80	NHL
HuMax-CD4	Fully human anti-CD4	CTCL
Lumiliximab	Humanized anti-CD23 (FcεRII)	CLL
MDX-010	Anti-CTLA-4	Melanoma
Matuzumab	Humanized anti-EGFR	CRC, NSCLC, pancreatic
Oregovomab	Murine anti-CA-125	Ovarian
Pertuzumab	Humanized anti-HER-2	Breast, prostate, ovarian
Rencarex	Chimeric anti-G250 IgG	Kidney
Vitaxin	Humanized anti-αvβ3 integrin	Melanoma, prostate

CLL, chronic lymphocytic leukemia; NHL, non-Hodgkin lymphoma; IgG, immunoglobulin G; CTCL, cutaneous T-cell lymphoma; EGFR, epidermal growth factor receptor; CRC, colorectal cancer; NSCLC, non–small cell lung cancer.

as in combination with radiation (124,125), clinically, bevacizumab has only been approved for use in combination with chemotherapy (e.g., irinotecan + 5-fluorouracil + leucovorin) (21,126). In this setting, the combination was found to increase objective responses, median time to progression, and survival in patients with metastatic colorectal cancer, as compared with chemotherapy alone. It is currently being studied clinically in other colorectal cancer settings (127,128), and was approved recently for use in non–small cell lung cancer (nonsquamous type) in combination with paclitaxel and carboplatin, providing a statistically significant ~2-month survival advantage, and also improvements in the time to progression and response rate (129). Additional studies are being pursued in renal cell, pancreatic, and breast cancers (130), as well as a number of other malignancies. As might be expected, bevacizumab may cause gastrointestinal perforations and delayed wound healing, as well as hemorrhagic events (primarily seen in small cell lung cancer

trials, in which bevacizumab is not approved). Arterial thromboembolic events (e.g., cerebral infarction, transient ischemic attacks, myocardial infarction, angina) and proteinuria also have been reported (131).

IMMUNOCONJUGATES

Antibodies can also function as carriers of cytotoxic substances, such as radioisotopes, drugs, and toxins (Figure 7.4). Most often in preclinical testing, antibody conjugates are found to be far more potent than the unlabeled antibody, but as one might expect, they also are more toxic to normal organ systems. In NHL, anti-CD20 radioconjugates have superior antitumor activity as compared with their unconjugated antibody counterparts, but there is increased, but manageable, hematologic toxicity (132,133). These preclinical and clinical findings are strong

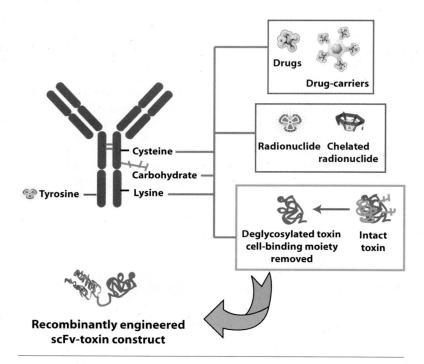

Figure 7.4 Antibody conjugates. Radioconjugates and drug conjugates are formed chemically, usually by linking the drug or radionuclide to lysine or by a sulfhydryl linkage chemistry. The radionuclide or drug can be attached directly or to an intermediate, such as a chelate that is used to capture radiometals, or dextrans that can be preloaded with multiple drug molecules before being coupled to an antibody. If these amino acid residues are found close enough to the complementarity-determining regions, antigen binding can be impaired. However, coupling a drug or radionuclide to the carbohydrate of the antibody generally ensures the coupling does not interfere with antigen binding, because the carbohydrate is typically far enough away from the antigen-binding portion of the molecule. Toxins had previously been chemically coupled to antibodies, most often after modifying the natural toxin to remove residues that are responsible for the toxin's natural ability to bind cells. Today, however, immunotoxins are prepared by recombinant engineering that fuses the active portion of the toxin molecule to an antibody or one of its engineered fragments, such as an scFv.

incentives to continue to pursue immunoconjugates for cancer therapy.

Radionuclides

Radiolabeled antibodies were the first group of immunoconjugates to be examined in the 1950s (134,135). The early investigators truly laid the foundations to this field, developing techniques to illustrate antibody targeting with only crudely purified immunoglobulins. It was not until the late 1970s when antibody targeting with an ^{131}I-labeled antibody to a human cancer antigen, carcinoembryonic antigen, provided the first clinical evidence that radioactivity could be selectively delivered to human tumors for cancer detection (136), and later for therapy in an experimental model (137). Early therapy trials integrated a relatively low dose of a radiolabeled antibody into a standard chemotherapy and radiation regimen (138), but this did not allow an analysis of the potential value of the radiolabeled antibody alone. The emphasis in clinical studies through most of the early 1980s was in cancer detection, but investigators slowly began to evaluate therapy with radiolabeled antibodies alone (139–141). The first clinical milestone in *radioimmunotherapy* (RAIT) came with the report by DeNardo et al. (142) that radiolabeled antibody therapy alone could elicit responses in patients with B-cell lymphomas, which stimulated the development of other antibodies to B-cell lymphomas, ultimately leading to the approval of two radiolabeled anti-CD20 antibodies for the treatment of NHL.

Whereas external-beam radiation delivers a localized beam of high-dose-rate radiation for short bursts that are divided over several weeks, RAIT is typically given as an intravenous injection, attempting to deliver low-dose radiation to tumor deposits throughout the body. It can take 1 to 2 days before a radiolabeled IgG reaches its maximum uptake in a tumor. Peak uptake is typically <0.01% of the total injected dose per gram of tumor, but the radioactivity deposited in the tumor can be detected several weeks later (143). The low uptake and slow kinetics of radiolabeled IgG targeting not only means that the radiation-absorbed dose delivered by RAIT occurs at a much lower dose rate than external-beam irradiation, but that it is continually present for a period of time defined by the physical half-life of the radionuclide and the biological half-life of the antibody residing in the tumor. This continuous, low-dose-rate radiation exposure can be as effective as intermittent, high-dose-rate radiation (144,145).

Because radionuclide-labeled IgG remains in the blood for an extended period of time, the highly radiosensitive red marrow is continuously exposed to the radiation, resulting in dose-limiting myelosuppression. At least for the more radiosensitive hematologic malignancies, the radiation-absorbed dose delivered at the maximum tolerated dose of a radiolabeled IgG can elicit significant antitumor responses. However, for solid tumors that are more radioresistant, the maximum tolerated dose is insufficient to result in clinically significant antitumor activity when administered as single doses. In an attempt to reduce the time spent in the blood, investigators turned to smaller forms of the antibodies, such as a F(ab')2 or Fab', and more recently, molecularly engineered antibody subfragments (Figure 7.5). These fragments have more favorable pharmacokinetic

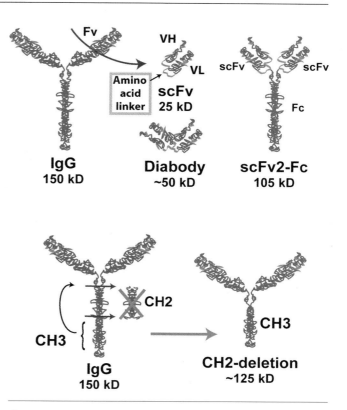

Figure 7.5 Representative forms of recombinant antibody proteins. Single chains (scFv) are formed by isolating the VH and VL polypeptide chains that make up the Fv region of an immunoglobulin (Ig) G. An scFv has only one binding site for an antigen. These chains are linked together with a short (~15 to 18) amino acid linker. If the amino acid linker is shortened, the scFvs will self-associate a form a diabody that has two binding sites. A number of different molecular constructs are made using scFvs tethered together in some manner. One such molecule shown is composed of two scFvs that are tethered to an intact Fc portion of an IgG. A CH2-deletion molecule fuses the CH3 region with the CH1 region.

properties, which improve tumor-blood ratios (146). As a consequence of their more rapid blood clearance, the fraction of the injected activity delivered to the tumor is lower with an antibody fragment than an IgG, but because hematologic toxicity is reduced, higher activities can be administered. There have been reports of improved therapeutic responses using smaller-sized antibodies, but these frequently are cleared from the blood by renal filtration, and as a result, many radionuclides (e.g., radiometals) become trapped in substantially higher concentrations in the kidneys than in the tumor (147–149). Thus, while the renally filtered radiolabeled fragments reduce the risk of hematologic toxicity, because the radiation dose required to kill tumors is higher than the limit tolerated to the kidney, radiometal-labeled antibody fragments are unable to provide the therapeutic window required for solid tumors. Whereas radiometal-labeled antibody fragments are retained in the kidneys, radioiodine is not, and therefore a favorable therapeutic window can be achieved with radioiodinated antibody fragments (150).

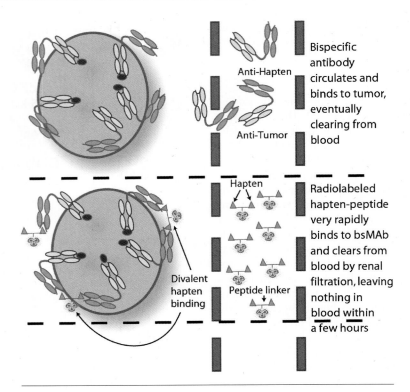

Figure 7.6 Bispecific antibody pretargeting of radionuclides. A bispecific antibody (bsMAb) is an antibody composed of two different binding specificities, one directed to a tumor antigen, the other to a hapten. The unconjugated bsMAb is injected in the bloodstream, and in time (a few days) it has bound to the tumor and cleared from the blood. The next step is the injection of the radiolabeled hapten-peptide. This molecule is very small and able to enter the extravascular space within minutes of injection. When it encounters the anti–hapten-binding portion of the bsMAb bound to a tumor cell, it too will be bound, while the unbound peptide is quickly eliminated from the body by urinary excretion. Pretargeting methods permit exceptionally high tumor-blood ratios within a few hours of the radiolabeled hapten-peptide injection, and tumor uptake can be as high as a directly radiolabeled IgG.

Multistep *pretargeting* methods, such as those using bispecific antibodies, represent a promising new method for imaging and therapy (Figure 7.6) (151). A bispecific antibody has at least one arm that binds to the tumor antigen, while a second binds to a hapten. The hapten is typically incorporated in a small peptide that can be radiolabeled. The unlabeled bispecific antibody is first given time to circulate and bind to the tumor cells, and once it has cleared from the blood and nontargeted tissues, the radiolabeled peptide is given. The small-sized radiolabeled peptide enters the extravascular space very quickly, where it can bind to the other arm of the bispecific antibody found on the tumor cells. Within minutes, the rest of the peptide clears from the blood, typically being removed from the body by urinary excretion within a few hours, leaving behind only the peptide that localizes to the bispecific antibody bound to the tumor. This method has been shown in preclinical testing to improve tumor-blood ratios by as much as 40-fold, with tumor uptake increased by as much as tenfold compared with a directly radiolabeled antibody fragment (152,153). This same method can increase the total radiation dose to tumors by 1.5-fold and can also increase the dose rate threefold, resulting in improved antitumor responses (154). Importantly, too, the radiolabeled peptide does not have as high an accretion in the kidney as with a directly radiolabeled antibody fragments, and therefore the tumor-kidney ratios provide a favorable therapeutic window.

Advances in molecular engineering have greatly enhanced the ability to provide uniform and highly novel pretargeting agents (155,156). Several pretargeting approaches have been studied, each showing improved tumor/blood ratios, as well as improving therapy when compared with directly radiolabeled antibodies (157). Dosimetry data from a pilot clinical study with ^{90}Y-biotin pretargeted by a new recombinant streptavidin-anti-TAG-72 antibody are promising, and in other indications, such as medullary thyroid cancer and glioma, encouraging therapeutic results using pretargeting methods have been reported (158–160).

Table 7.3 lists some of the more commonly used radionuclides conjugated to antibodies for cancer treatment.

Table 7.3				
Physical Properties of Several Radionuclides Used for Radioimmunotherapy				
Radionuclide	Emission	Half-life*	Range[a]	Approximate No. of Cell Diameters[b]
^{90}Yttrium	β	64.1 h	4.0–11.3 mm	400 to 1,100
^{188}Rhenium	β	17.0 h	1.9–10.4 mm	200 to 1,000
^{131}Iodine	β	8.0 d	0.08–2.3 mm	10 to 230
^{67}Copper	β	61.9 d	0.05–2.1 mm	5 to 210
^{177}Lutetium	β	6.7 d	0.04–1.8 mm	4 to 180
^{211}Astatine	α	7.2 h	60 μm	6
^{213}Bismuth	α	46 min	84 μm	8
^{125}Iodine	Auger	60.5 d	<100 nm	(1)
^{111}Indium	Auger	3.0 d	<100 nm	(1)

[a] As reported by Kassis et al. (161).
[b] Assuming a tumor cell is ~10 mcm in diameter.

Radionuclide selection is most often dictated by tumor size. Medium-energy beta-emitters, such as ^{131}I (~0.5 MeV) and ^{177}Lu (~0.8 MeV), can traverse ~1.0 mm, while high-energy beta-emitters, such as ^{90}Y or ^{188}Re (~2.1 MeV), can penetrate up to 11 mm, making it possible for beta-emitters to kill across several hundred cells, a property known as a *bystander*, or *cross-fire*, effect (161). This property is an important advantage for radioconjugates as compared with other immunoconjugates, as they can be therapeutically active even with problematic heterogeneous antigen expression, tumor architecture, or other factors. Although higher-energy beta-emitters have the potential of killing cells across a longer path length, the absorbed fraction is higher for the lower-energy beta-emitters (i.e., probability of hitting the nuclear DNA), making them more efficient killers. Alpha-emitters, such as ^{213}Bi and ^{211}At, traverse only a few cell diameters, but an alpha particle is also more potent than a low-energy beta particle, requiring fewer "hits" to damage cellular processes (161). Low-energy electrons, such as Auger emitters produced by ^{125}I, ^{67}Ga, or ^{111}In, have to be in close contact, preferably inside a cell or in the nucleus, to exert a cytotoxic effect. As one might expect, beta-emitters are best applied in situations in which tumors are ≥0.5 cm in diameter; otherwise, a substantial portion of the energy from the radioactive decay will be absorbed in the surrounding normal tissue. The alpha and low-energy electron emitters are best applied when the disease burden is smaller, more localized, or where there may be single or small clusters of cells (e.g., leukemia, malignant ascites) (162,163).

Two anti-CD20 IgG-radioconjugates are currently FDA-approved for the treatment of indolent and transformed forms of NHL, ^{90}Y-ibritumomab tiuxetan (Zevalin:Cell Therapeutics) and ^{131}I-tositumomab (Bexxar:Glaxo Smith Kline) (164). Both improve the objective response rate when compared with the unlabeled anti-CD20 antibody used in conjunction with the treatment (132,133). Although objective response rates were significantly improved, the pivotal trial comparing ^{90}Y-ibritumomab tiuxetan to rituximab did not show a statistical improvement in the duration of the response. However, continued follow-up has shown the complete responses, which were more prevalent

with ^{90}Y-ibritumomab tiuxetan, have also been more durable (165,166). Durable responses have also been reported with ^{131}I-tositumomab, and importantly, there is evidence that when used as a frontline therapy, it is better tolerated and may improve responses compared with standard chemotherapy (167–169). Clinical studies are also beginning to evaluate the use of ^{90}Y-ibritumomab tiuxetan as a frontline treatment, and other studies are showing that these treatments do not preclude patients from receiving additional cytotoxic therapies (170–172). Although more randomized clinical trials to assess efficacy and long-term follow-up to assess the risk for late toxicities (e.g., myelodysplasia) are needed (173), it is impressive that a single treatment with a radiolabeled antibody that has fewer side effects than chemotherapy given over several months can provide such a significant benefit. New efforts are underway to explore the use of these agents in other clinical indications, and new radioconjugates are being examined in lymphoma and leukemia (174–185).

The application of RAIT to solid tumors has been more challenging. These tumors are more radioresistant, which is the most likely reason why RAIT has not been as successful, because the targeting of a variety of solid tumors is as good, if not better, than that seen in lymphoma. Despite efforts to increase the administered radiation dose by using bone marrow or peripheral stem cell support, and even combining high-dose radioimmunotherapy with chemotherapy, clinically significant antitumor responses in solid tumors remain elusive (143). A phase III trial in lung cancer has indicated some success in advanced solid tumors (186), but for the most part, as first emphasized in animal model testing, RAIT is more likely to succeed when the disease burden is minimal or used in an adjuvant treatment (187–189). Early clinical studies appear to corroborate these preclinical findings, at least in colorectal cancer, where RAIT postsalvage resection of colorectal liver metastases indicated a doubling of the survival time compared with historical or contemporaneous controls (190). Additionally, clinical studies are applying radiolabeled antibodies for intracompartmental treatments, such as intracranial and intraperitoneal therapies, where it may be possible to increase the accessibility and amount of antibody targeted to tumors in these regional areas (191–195).

Preclinical studies have shown that nontherapeutic doses of chemotherapy can enhance the effects of RAIT, while other studies have shown relatively small doses of radiolabeled antibodies can enhance the therapeutic activity of a standard chemotherapy regimen (196–200). The reduced hematologic toxicity associated with pretargeting approaches should allow radioconjugates to be combined more readily with cytotoxic drugs (201,202). In addition, combinations with unconjugated antibodies, such as cetuximab, that can enhance the tumor's radiosensitivity, may be another option against EGFR-positive tumors (203–207). Thus, while challenges remain for antibody-targeted radionuclides in solid tumors, recent preclinical and initial clinical studies are encouraging.

Drug Immunoconjugates

The first evidence that an antibody-drug conjugate had activity against cancer was reported by Mathé et al. (208), who linked methotrexate to the globulin fraction of a hamster antiserum directed against the mouse leukemia L1210 cell line to protect mice from subsequent inoculation with L1210 cells. The first and only drug conjugate to be approved was gemtuzumab ozogamicin (Mylotarg:Wyeth), a humanized anti-CD33 IgG linked to calicheamicin, for the treatment of relapsed acute myelocytic leukemia in adults ≥60 years of age (209). The prospects of it as a frontline treatment, in combination with chemotherapy, and expanding its indications to include pediatric cancer patients, are under evaluation (210–215). Besides the standard precautions for side effects associated with its infusion, other primary side effects include complications associated with severe hematologic toxicity, mucositis, as well as hepatotoxicity (hyperbilirubinemia, elevated alanine aminotransferase, aspartate aminotransferase, and bilirubin).

Drug conjugates must be made chemically, with the conjugate retaining the binding activity of the antibody, as well as the biological activity of the drug (Figure 7.4). Drugs may be coupled directly to an antibody or to inert carriers, such as dextrans or amino acid polymers, which have been used increase the drug-substitution level of the conjugate (216). A careful balance between optimizing the level of drug substitution to maximum potency, while preserving the antigen-binding ability, as well as the antibody's pharmacokinetic and distribution properties, needs to be maintained. The conjugation method must allow the drug to separate from the antibody in an active form, but it cannot prematurely dissociate before reaching the tumor. Because the conjugate needs to be internalized to offer its highest potency, target selection is very important. Interestingly, gemtuzumab ozogamicin has been shown to be active even in CD33-negative cell lines, but this is because these cells are highly endocytic, allowing the conjugate to be internalized without the conjugate having to bind to the cell (217). When a drug conjugate is internalized, the drug must be liberated from the antibody in order to regain its activity. Separation of the drug from the antibody generally occurs in the lysosomes. Ineffective trafficking and drug separation inside the cell can have a profound impact on the potency of the conjugate. Drugs are often coupled to antibody with linkages that can only be cleaved in the acidic milieu of the lysosomes (216). Preclinical studies typically have found that conjugation

of a drug to an antibody alters the drug's pharmacodynamics, essentially "detoxifying" it. This has allowed drugs that otherwise would be far too toxic for human use alone (i.e., *ultratoxic drugs*) to be tested as antibody-drug conjugates. Current clinical trials with drug conjugates almost exclusively use drugs that are far more potent than most chemotherapeutic agents, and other highly potent agents also are under development (218–223).

Leukemias are a particularly attractive target for immunoconjugate therapy as the individual cells are readily available in the bloodstream and marrow. Because drugs must get inside the cell to be active, a target that is actively internalized could be more important than the target's relative abundance. For example, immunoconjugates against CD74, which is found in low density on B cells, T cells, monocytes, lymphomas, myelomas, and certain carcinomas, have been reported to be a highly efficient carrier for drugs, toxins, and radionuclides because it is readily recycled (224–226). There were hopes that antibody-drug conjugates might overcome drug resistance by bypassing the P-glycoprotein mechanism for extruding drugs (227). Unfortunately, this has not been realized, but studies have suggested that it might be possible under certain circumstances (228,229).

Pretargeting approaches have also been applied to drugs. Most often referred to as ADEPT (antibody-directed enzyme prodrug therapy), this strategy first targets an antibody-enzyme conjugate to the tumor (230). Once the conjugate is sufficiently cleared from the blood, a prodrug, which is not biologically active, is given. The prodrug is converted to an active form by the enzyme and then released as an active drug. Enzymatic conversion of the prodrug continues, resulting in locally increased levels of the active drug. The ADEPT method has been tested extensively in preclinical models, as well as in phase I clinical studies. These initial studies found the conjugate's immunogenicity and slow clearance of the antibody-enzyme conjugate from the blood to be obstacles, but preclinical studies suggest that these problems may be overcome in the near future (231–233). There are still a number of challenges to be met, but new agents are being developed that will likely lead to expanded clinical evaluation of drug immunoconjugates.

Toxin Immunoconjugates

Except for denileukin diftitox, which is a modified diphtheria toxin coupled to IL-2 for the treatment of cutaneous T-cell lymphoma, no other immunotoxins have been approved for clinical use, but there have been a number of clinical trials with a variety of toxins conjugated to antibodies (234–242).

Toxins are truly ultratoxic agents, requiring relatively few copies to kill the cell as compared with most drugs, but they face the same delivery issues as a drug conjugate. Most toxins used to prepare antibody-toxin conjugates are ribosomal inactivating proteins that interfere with the reading of messenger RNA, thereby disrupting protein synthesis (243). Most are natural proteins derived from plants, bacteria, or fungi, and therefore are foreign to patients who readily develop an immune response to these proteins (244). The possible exception is RNase, which can be derived from human sources (245). Because toxins have their own means for binding to cells, the cell-binding portion must be separated from the active portion of the toxin to improve targeting specificity (Figure 7.4) (246). As proteins, toxins are amenable to recombinant production as antibody (or other biological targeting substance, such as IL-2 or other cytokines) toxin fusion proteins (242,247).

Clinical studies in patients with B-cell lymphoma using a chemically conjugated deglycosylated ricin A chain and either an anti-CD19 or an anti-CD22 murine IgG found doses to be limited by a vascular leak syndrome (consisting of edema, tachycardia, dyspnea, weakness, and myalgia) (248,249). Insights into the molecular structure of the active ricin A chain have revealed a motif that is responsible for binding to endothelial cells, which could be an important determinant in the development of dose-limiting vascular leak syndrome (250).

A recombinant anti-CD22 × Pseudomonas exotoxin has been highly effective in patients with hairy cell leukemia, while not being as effective in NHL or CLL (236,251). In hairy cell leukemia, clinical benefit (86% complete response rate with a median duration of 36 months) was observed after a single cycle of conjugate treatment at a dose level of 40 mcg/kg every other day × 3, with the most common toxicities being hypoalbuminemia, transaminase elevations, fatigue, and edema, but a reversible hemolytic uremic syndrome requiring plasmapheresis was observed in several patients. This conjugate's activity in hairy cell leukemia with manageable toxicity is an exciting new development for immunotoxin conjugates.

Similar to the experience with other immunoconjugates, solid tumors remain a formidable challenge for therapy with immunotoxins. An immunotoxin prepared as a recombinant Pseudomonas exotoxin × anti-Lewis-Y antibody (BR96) was tested in 46 patients with Lewis-Y–positive tumors, with no objective responses (252). Gastrointestinal toxicity was dose-limiting, but this was likely because of the cross-reactivity of BR96 with normal gastrointestinal epithelium (253). This is another lesson in how challenging it can be to select the right target for a targeted therapy.

ECONOMIC CONSIDERATIONS

Perhaps one of the more perplexing future issues for most biologically based therapeutics is not the question of whether these targeting strategies will improve treatment, but how our health systems will cope with the high cost of these treatments. Unconjugated MAbs in particular are often found to be more effective when used in combination with other therapeutic agents, including other antibodies. Not all patients are responsive, presumably because of differences in the receptors being targeted, and therefore molecular testing will become part of the paradigm of biological therapy in order to choose drugs on an individual patient basis. Because these can be prescribed over several months, the costs can challenge the heath care system and third-party payers (254–256). Because antibody-based treatments generally have fewer and milder side effects compared with conventional chemotherapy, patients are more able to maintain their lifestyle while receiving these treatments, and thus this might offset some of the pharmacoeconomic concerns of these treatments.

CONCLUSIONS

Antibodies and immunoconjugates are gaining a significant and expanding role in the therapy of cancer. Because patients generally tolerate antibody treatments with minimal side effects,

as compared with many other cancer treatment modalities, immunotherapy with antibodies represents an exciting opportunity for combining with standard modalities, such as chemotherapy, as well as combinations between diverse biological agents, including antibody combinations in NHL therapy (86) and the combination of an anti-EGFR and anti-VEGF antibody with chemotherapy in metastatic colorectal cancer (20,257,258). As we learn more about how cancer and other diseased cells function, undoubtedly unconjugated antibodies will be used to disrupt these functions by targeting important sites or regulators of cell proliferation and metabolism. The use of antibodies to target radionuclides, drugs, and toxins is expanding to become the next generation of MAb-based products for cancer therapy. At least in the case of targeted radionuclides, clinical studies have shown that the immunoconjugates are more effective than immunotherapy with the antibody alone, which highlights the enhanced efficacy achieved when a cytotoxic agent is targeted by an antibody that is also active.

Over the past 25 years, great strides have been made for developing new, selective, therapeutic strategies, based on the evolution of various antibody forms and an identification of new cellular targets. As new target molecules and receptors on tumor cells are identified in the future, the experiences gained with the use of current immunoconjugates will enable a more rapid translation to clinical evaluation and use when next-generation antibodies and immunoconjugates are developed.

REFERENCES

1. Köhler G, Milstein C. Continuous cultures of fused cells secreting antibody of predefined specificity. *Nature*. 1975;256:495–497.
2. Morrison SL, Johnson MJ, Herzenberg LA, et al. Chimeric human antibody molecules: mouse antigen-binding domains with human constant region domains. *Proc Natl Acad Sci U S A*. 1984;81:6851–6855.
3. Jones PT, Dear PH, Foote J, et al. Replacing the complementarity-determining regions in a human antibody with those from a mouse. *Nature*. 1986;321:522–525.
4. Kim SJ, Park Y, Hong HJ. Antibody engineering for the development of therapeutic antibodies. *Mol Cells*. 2005;20:17–29.
5. Weiner LM. Fully human therapeutic monoclonal antibodies. *J Immunother*. 2006;29:1–9.
6. Qu Z, Griffiths GL, Wegener WA, et al. Development of humanized antibodies as cancer therapeutics. *Methods*. 2005;36:84–95.
7. Moroney S, Plückthun A. *Modern Antibody Technology: The Impact on Drug Development*, Vol V, Weinheim, Germany: Wiley-VCH Verlag GmbH & Co KGaA, 2005;1147–1186.
8. Looney RJ. B cell-targeted therapy for rheumatoid arthritis: an update on the evidence. *Drugs*. 2006;66:625–639.
9. Jazirehi AR, Bonavida B. Cellular and molecular signal transduction pathways modulated by rituximab (Rituxan, anti-CD20 mAb) in non-Hodgkin's lymphoma: implications in chemosensitization and therapeutic intervention. *Oncogene*. 2005;24:2121–2143.
10. Shan D, Ledbetter JA, Press OW. Apoptosis of malignant human B cells by ligation of CD20 with monoclonal antibodies. *Blood*. 1998;91:1644–1652.
11. Zhang N, Khawli LA, Hu P, et al. Generation of rituximab polymer may cause hyper-cross-linking-induced apoptosis in non-Hodgkin's lymphomas. *Clin Cancer Res*. 2005;11:5971–5980.
12. Czuczman MS. Immunochemotherapy in indolent non-Hodgkin's lymphoma. *Semin Oncol*. 2002;29:11–17.

13. Marty M, Cognetti F, Maraninchi D, et al. Randomized phase II trial of the efficacy and safety of trastuzumab combined with docetaxel in patients with human epidermal growth factor receptor 2-positive metastatic breast cancer administered as first-line treatment: the M77001 study group. *J Clin Oncol.* 2005;23:4265–4274.

14. Raben D, Helfrich B, Chan DC, et al. The effects of cetuximab alone and in combination with radiation and/or chemotherapy in lung cancer. *Clin Cancer Res.* 2005;11:795–805.

15. Chan A, Martin M, Untch M, et al. Vinorelbine plus trastuzumab combination as first-line therapy for HER 2-positive metastatic breast cancer patients: an international phase II trial. *Br J Cancer.* 2006;95:788–793.

16. Robert N, Leyland-Jones B, Asmar L, et al. Randomized phase III study of trastuzumab, paclitaxel, and carboplatin compared with trastuzumab and paclitaxel in women with HER-2-overexpressing metastatic breast cancer. *J Clin Oncol.* 2006;24:2786–2792.

17. Ghobrial IM, Witzig TE, Adjei AA. Targeting apoptosis pathways in cancer therapy. *CA Cancer J Clin.* 2005;55:178–194.

18. Bianco R, Daniele G, Ciardiello F, et al. Monoclonal antibodies targeting the epidermal growth factor receptor. *Curr Drug Targets.* 2005;6:275–287.

19. Meric-Bernstam F, Hung MC. Advances in targeting human epidermal growth factor receptor-2 signaling for cancer therapy. *Clin Cancer Res.* 2006;12:6326–6330.

20. Saif MW, Cohenuram M. Role of panitumumab in the management of metastatic colorectal cancer. *Clin Colorectal Cancer.* 2006;6:118–124.

21. Ferrara N, Hillan KJ, Novotny W. Bevacizumab (Avastin), a humanized anti-VEGF monoclonal antibody for cancer therapy. *Biochem Biophys Res Commun.* 2005;333:328–335.

22. Herbst RS. Therapeutic options to target angiogenesis in human malignancies. *Expert Opin Emerg Drugs.* 2006;11:635–650.

23. Hansen-Algenstaedt N, Stoll BR, Padera TP, et al. Tumor oxygenation in hormone-dependent tumors during vascular endothelial growth factor receptor-2 blockade, hormone ablation, and chemotherapy. *Cancer Res.* 2000;60:4556–4560.

24. Ribatti D, Vacca A. Novel therapeutic approaches targeting vascular endothelial growth factor and its receptors in haematological malignancies. *Curr Cancer Drug Targets.* 2005;5:573-578.

25. Wu Y, Zhong Z, Huber J, et al. Anti-vascular endothelial growth factor receptor-1 antagonist antibody as a therapeutic agent for cancer. *Clin Cancer Res.* 2006;12:6573–6584.

26. Roberts N, Kloos B, Cassella M, et al. Inhibition of VEGFR-3 activation with the antagonistic antibody more potently suppresses lymph node and distant metastases than inactivation of VEGFR-2. *Cancer Res.* 2006;66:2650–2657.

27. Leach DR, Krummel MF, Allison JP. Enhancement of antitumor immunity by CTLA-4 blockade. *Science.* 1996;271:1734–1736.

28. Kapadia D, Fong L. CTLA-4 blockade: autoimmunity as treatment. *J Clin Oncol.* 2005;23:8926–8928.

29. Maker AV, Attia P, Rosenberg SA. Analysis of the cellular mechanism of antitumor responses and autoimmunity in patients treated with CTLA-4 blockade. *J Immunol.* 2005;175:7746–7754.

30. Maker AV, Phan GQ, Attia P, et al. Tumor regression and autoimmunity in patients treated with cytotoxic T lymphocyte-associated antigen 4 blockade and interleukin 2: a phase I/II study. *Ann Surg Oncol.* 2005;12:1005–1016.

31. Attia P, Phan GQ, Maker AV, et al. Autoimmunity correlates with tumor regression in patients with metastatic melanoma treated with anti-cytotoxic T-lymphocyte antigen-4. *J Clin Oncol.* 2005;23:6043–6053.

32. Maker AV, Yang JC, Sherry RM, et al. Intrapatient dose escalation of anti-CTLA-4 antibody in patients with metastatic melanoma. *J Immunother.* 2006;29:455–463.

33. Rutgeerts P, Van Assche G, Vermeire S. Review article: Infliximab therapy for inflammatory bowel disease—seven years on. *Aliment Pharmacol Ther.* 2006;23:451–463.

34. Bordigoni P, Dimicoli S, Clement L, et al. Daclizumab, an efficient treatment for steroid-refractory acute graft-versus-host disease. *Br J Haematol.* 2006;135:382–385.

35. Cree B. Emerging monoclonal antibody therapies for multiple sclerosis. *Neurologist.* 2006;12:171–178.

36. Van Assche G, Sandborn WJ, Feagan BG, et al. Daclizumab, a humanised monoclonal antibody to the interleukin 2 receptor (CD25), for the treatment of moderately to severely active ulcerative colitis: a randomised, double blind, placebo controlled, dose ranging trial. *Gut.* 2006;55:1568–1574.

37. Cuppoletti A, Perez-Villa F, Vallejos I, et al. Experience with single-dose daclizumab in the prevention of acute rejection in heart transplantation. *Transplant Proc.* 2005;37:4036–4038.

38. Kleyn CE, Griffiths CE. Infliximab for the treatment of psoriasis. *Expert Opin Biol Ther.* 2006;6:797–805.

39. Steinfeld SD, Youinou P. Epratuzumab (humanised anti-CD22 antibody) in autoimmune diseases. *Expert Opin Biol Ther.* 2006;6:943–949.

40. Steinfeld SD, Tant L, Burmester GR, et al. Epratuzumab (humanised anti-CD22 antibody) in primary Sjögren's syndrome: an open-label phase I/II study. *Arthritis Res Ther.* 2006;8:R129.

41. Dorner T, Kaufmann J, Wegener WA, et al. Initial clinical trial of epratuzumab (humanized anti-CD22 antibody) for immunotherapy of systemic lupus erythematosus. *Arthritis Res Ther.* 2006; 8:R74.

42. Smith KG, Jones RB, Burns SM, et al. Long-term comparison of rituximab treatment for refractory systemic lupus erythematosus and vasculitis: Remission, relapse, and re-treatment. *Arthritis Rheum.* 2006;54:2970–2982.

43. Emery P, Fleischmann R, Filipowicz-Sosnowska A, et al. The efficacy and safety of rituximab in patients with active rheumatoid arthritis despite methotrexate treatment: results of a phase IIB randomized, double-blind, placebo-controlled, dose-ranging trial. *Arthritis Rheum.* 2006;54:1390–1400.

44. Cox AL, Thompson SA, Jones JL, et al. Lymphocyte homeostasis following therapeutic lymphocyte depletion in multiple sclerosis. *Eur J Immunol.* 2005;35:3332–3342.

45. Coles AJ, Cox A, Le Page E, et al. The window of therapeutic opportunity in multiple sclerosis: evidence from monoclonal antibody therapy. *J Neurol.* 2006;253:98–108.

46. Ilantzis C, DeMarte L, Screaton RA, et al. Deregulated expression of the human tumor marker CEA and CEA family member CEACAM6 disrupts tissue architecture and blocks colonocyte differentiation. *Neoplasia.* 2002;4:151–163.

47. Felding-Habermann B, Lerner RA, Lillo A, et al. Combinatorial antibody libraries from cancer patients yield ligand-mimetic Arg-Gly-Asp-containing immunoglobulins that inhibit breast cancer metastasis. *Proc Natl Acad Sci U S A.* 2004;101:17210–17215.

48. Blumenthal RD, Osorio L, Hayes MK, et al. Carcinoembryonic antigen antibody inhibits lung metastasis and augments chemotherapy in a human colonic carcinoma xenograft. *Cancer Immunol Immunother.* 2005;54:315–27.

49. Khalili P, Arakelian A, Chen G, et al. Effect of Herceptin on the development and progression of skeletal metastases in a xenograft model of human breast cancer. *Oncogene.* 2005;24:6657–6666.

50. von Behring E, Kitasato S. [The mechanism of diphtheria immunity and tetanus immunity in animals. 1890]. *Mol Immunol.* 1991;28:1317, 9–20.

51. Hericourt J, Richet CR. 'Physologie pathologique'—de la serotherapie dans le traitement du cancer. *Comptes Rendus Hebd Seanc Acad Sci (Paris)* 1895;120:567–569.

52. Himmelweit F *The Collected Papers of Paul Ehrlich*, Vol. 3, p. 56. London: Pergamon. 1960.

53. Nadler LM, Stashenko P, Hardy R, et al. Serotherapy of a patient with a monoclonal antibody directed against a human lymphoma-associated antigen. *Cancer Res.* 1980;40:3147–3154.

54. Miller RA, Maloney DG, Warnke R, et al. Treatment of B-cell lymphoma with monoclonal anti-idiotype antibody. *N Engl J Med.* 1982;306:517–522.

55. Sears HF, Atkinson B, Mattis J, et al. Phase-I clinical trial of monoclonal antibody in treatment of gastrointestinal tumours. *Lancet.* 1982;1:762–765.

56. Foon KA, Schroff RW, Bunn PA, et al. Effects of monoclonal antibody therapy in patients with chronic lymphocytic leukemia. *Blood.* 1984;64:1085–1093.

57. Meeker TC, Lowder J, Maloney DG, et al. A clinical trial of anti-idiotype therapy for B cell malignancy. *Blood.* 1985;65:1349–1363.

58. Sears HF, Herlyn D, Steplewski Z, et al. Phase II clinical trial of a murine monoclonal antibody cytotoxic for gastrointestinal adenocarcinoma. *Cancer Res.* 1985;45:5910–5913.

59. Houghton AN, Mintzer D, Cordon-Cardo C, et al. Mouse monoclonal IgG3 antibody detecting GD3 ganglioside: a phase I trial in patients with malignant melanoma. *Proc Natl Acad Sci U S A.* 1985;82:1242–1246.

60. Goodman GE, Beaumier P, Hellstrom I, et al. Pilot trial of murine monoclonal antibodies in patients with advanced melanoma. *J Clin Oncol.* 1985;3:340–352.

61. Waldmann H, Hale G. CAMPATH: from concept to clinic. *Philos Trans R Soc Lond B Biol Sci.* 2005;360:1707–1711.

62. Magliocca JF, Knechtle SJ. The evolving role of alemtuzumab (Campath-1H) for immunosuppressive therapy in organ transplantation. *Transpl Int.* 2006;19:705–714.

63. Morris PJ, Russell NK. Alemtuzumab (Campath-1H): a systematic review in organ transplantation. *Transplantation.* 2006;81:1361–1367.

64. Gill GN, Kawamoto T, Cochet C, et al. Monoclonal anti-epidermal growth factor receptor antibodies which are inhibitors of epidermal growth factor binding and antagonists of epidermal growth factor binding and antagonists of epidermal growth factor-stimulated tyrosine protein kinase activity. *J Biol Chem.* 1984;259:7755–7760.

65. Albanell J, Gascon P. Small molecules with EGFR-TK inhibitor activity. *Curr Drug Targets.* 2005;6:259–274.

66. Matar P, Rojo F, Cassia R, et al. Combined epidermal growth factor receptor targeting with the tyrosine kinase inhibitor gefitinib (ZD1839) and the monoclonal antibody cetuximab (IMC-C225): superiority over single-agent receptor targeting. *Clin Cancer Res.* 2004;10:6487–6501.

67. Jimeno A, Rubio-Viqueira B, Amador ML, et al. Epidermal growth factor receptor dynamics influences response to epidermal growth factor receptor targeted agents. *Cancer Res.* 2005;65:3003–3010.

68. Riemer AB, Klinger M, Wagner S, et al. Generation of Peptide mimics of the epitope recognized by trastuzumab on the oncogenic protein Her-2/neu. *J Immunol.* 2004;173:394–401.

69. Holliger P, Hudson PJ. Engineered antibody fragments and the rise of single domains. *Nat Biotechnol.* 2005;23:1126–1136.

70. Binz HK, Amstutz P, Pluckthun A. Engineering novel binding proteins from nonimmunoglobulin domains. *Nat Biotechnol.* 2005;23:1257–1268.

71. Hok S, Natarajan A, Perkins J, et al. Chemistry and radiochemistry of selective high affinity ligands (SHALs) designed to targeted non-Hodgkin's lymphoma and leukemia. *Cancer Biother Radiopharm.* 2006;21:392.

72. Weng WK, Levy R. Two immunoglobulin G fragment C receptor polymorphisms independently predict response to rituximab in patients with follicular lymphoma. *J Clin Oncol.* 2003;21:3940–3947.

73. Grillo-Lopez AJ, White CA, Varns C, et al. Overview of the clinical development of rituximab: first monoclonal antibody approved for the treatment of lymphoma. *Semin Oncol.* 1999;26:66–73.

74. Davis TA, Grillo-Lopez AJ, White CA, et al. Rituximab anti-CD20 monoclonal antibody therapy in non-Hodgkin's lymphoma: safety and efficacy of re-treatment. *J Clin Oncol.* 2000;18:3135–3143.

75. Hainsworth JD, Litchy S, Shaffer DW, et al. Maximizing therapeutic benefit of rituximab: maintenance therapy versus re-treatment at progression in patients with indolent non-Hodgkin's lymphoma–a randomized phase II trial of the Minnie Pearl Cancer Research Network. *J Clin Oncol.* 2005;23:1088–1095.

76. Coiffier B, Lepage E, Briere J, et al. CHOP chemotherapy plus rituximab compared with CHOP alone in elderly patients with diffuse large-B-cell lymphoma. *N Engl J Med.* 2002;346:235–242.

77. Coiffier B. Standard treatment of advanced-stage diffuse large B-cell lymphoma. *Semin Hematol.* 2006;43:213–220.

78. Forstpointner R, Unterhalt M, Dreyling M, et al. Maintenance therapy with rituximab leads to a significant prolongation of response duration after salvage therapy with a combination of rituximab, fludarabine, cyclophosphamide and mitoxantrone (R-FCM) in patients with relapsed and refractory follicular and mantle cell lymphomas—results of a prospective randomized study of the German low grade lymphoma study group (GLSG). *Blood.* 2006;108:4003–4008.

79. Held G, Poschel V, Pfreundschuh M. Rituximab for the treatment of diffuse large B-cell lymphomas. *Expert Rev Anticancer Ther.* 2006;6:1175–1186.

80. Nickenig C, Dreyling M, Hoster E, et al. Combined cyclophosphamide, vincristine, doxorubicin, and prednisone (CHOP) improves response rates but not survival and has lower hematologic toxicity compared with combined mitoxantrone, chlorambucil, and prednisone (MCP) in follicular and mantle cell lymphomas: results of a prospective randomized trial of the German Low-Grade Lymphoma Study Group. *Cancer.* 2006;107:1014–1022.

81. Tomita N, Kodama F, Oshima R, et al. Phase II study of CHOP-GR therapy for advanced-stage follicular lymphoma. *Leuk Lymphoma.* 2006;47:1041–1047.

82. Tam CS, Wolf M, Prince HM, et al. Fludarabine, cyclophosphamide, and rituximab for the treatment of patients with chronic lymphocytic leukemia or indolent non-Hodgkin lymphoma. *Cancer.* 2006;106:2412–2420.

83. Byrd JC, Murphy T, Howard RS, et al. Rituximab using a thrice weekly dosing schedule in B-cell chronic lymphocytic leukemia and small lymphocytic lymphoma demonstrates clinical activity and acceptable toxicity. *J Clin Oncol.* 2001;19:2153–2164.

84. O'Brien SM, Kantarjian H, Thomas DA, et al. Rituximab dose-escalation trial in chronic lymphocytic leukemia. *J Clin Oncol.* 2001;19:2165–2170.

85. Leonard JP, Coleman M, Ketas JC, et al. Epratuzumab, a humanized anti-CD22 antibody, in aggressive non-Hodgkin's lymphoma: phase I/II clinical trial results. *Clin Cancer Res.* 2004;10:5327–5334.

86. Leonard JP, Coleman M, Ketas J, et al. Combination antibody therapy with epratuzumab and rituximab in relapsed or refractory non-Hodgkin's lymphoma. *J Clin Oncol.* 2005;23:5044–5051.

87. Strauss SJ, Morschhauser F, Rech J, et al. Multicenter phase II trial of immunotherapy with the humanized anti-CD22 antibody, epratuzumab, in combination with rituximab, in refractory or recurrent non-Hodgkin's lymphoma. *J Clin Oncol.* 2006;24:3880–3886.

88. Goldenberg DM. Epratuzumab in the therapy of oncological and immunological diseases. *Expert Rev Anticancer Ther.* 2006;6:1341–1353.

89. Younes A, Hariharan K, Allen RS, Leigh BR. Initial trials of anti-CD80 monoclonal antibody (Galiximab) therapy for patients with relapsed or refractory follicular lymphoma. *Clin Lymphoma.* 2003;3:257–259.

90. Czuczman MS, Thall A, Witzig TE, et al. Phase I/II study of galiximab, an anti-CD80 antibody, for relapsed or refractory follicular lymphoma. *J Clin Oncol.* 2005;23:4390–4398.

91. Reff ME, Carner K, Chambers KS, et al. Depletion of B cells in vivo by a chimeric mouse human monoclonal antibody to CD20. *Blood.* 1994;83:435–445.

92. Golay J, Zaffaroni L, Vaccari T, et al. Biologic response of B lymphoma cells to antiCD20 monoclonal antibody rituximab in vitro: CD55 and CD59 regulate complement-mediated cell lysis. *Blood.* 2000;95:3900–3908.

93. Treon SP, Mitsiades C, Mitsiades N, et al. Tumor cell expression of CD59 is associated with resistance to CD20 serotherapy in patients with B-cell malignancies. *J Immunother.* 2001;24:263–271.

94. Golay J, Lazzari M, Facchinetti V, et al. CD20 levels determine the in vitro susceptibility to rituximab and complement of B-cell chronic lymphocytic leukemia: further regulation by CD55 and CD59. *Blood.* 2001;98:3383–3389.

95. Weng WK, Levy R. Expression of complement inhibitors CD46, CD55, and CD59 on tumor cells does not predict clinical outcome after rituximab treatment in follicular non-Hodgkin lymphoma. *Blood.* 2001;98:1352–1357.

96. Treon SP, Pilarski LM, Belch AR, et al. CD20-directed serotherapy in patients with multiple myeloma: biologic considerations and therapeutic applications. *J Immunother.* 2002;25:72–81.

97. Manches O, Lui G, Chaperot L, et al. In vitro mechanisms of action of rituximab on primary non-Hodgkin lymphomas. *Blood.* 2003;101:949–954.

98. Pescovitz MD. Rituximab, an anti-CD20 monoclonal antibody: history and mechanism of action. *Am J Transplant.* 2006;6:859–866.

99. Hernandez-Ilizaliturri FJ, Jupudy V, Ostberg J, et al. Neutrophils contribute to the biological antitumor activity of rituximab in a non-Hodgkin's lymphoma severe combined immunodeficiency mouse model. *Clin Cancer Res.* 2003;9:5866–5873.

100. Uchida J, Hamaguchi Y, Oliver JA, et al. The innate mononuclear phagocyte network depletes B lymphocytes through Fc receptor-dependent mechanisms during anti-CD20 antibody immunotherapy. *J Exp Med.* 2004;199:1659–1669.

101. Presta LG. Selection, design, and engineering of therapeutic antibodies. *J Allergy Clin Immunol.* 2005;116:731–736.

102. Petkova SB, Akilesh S, Sproule TJ, et al. Enhanced half-life of genetically engineered human IgG1 antibodies in a humanized FcRn mouse model: potential application in humorally mediated autoimmune disease. *Int Immunol.* 2006.

103. Presta LG. Engineering of therapeutic antibodies to minimize immunogenicity and optimize function. *Adv Drug Deliv Rev.* 2006;58:640–656.

104. Hodoniczky J, Zheng YZ, James DC. Control of recombinant monoclonal antibody effector functions by Fc N-glycan remodeling in vitro. *Biotechnol Prog.* 2005;21:1644–1652.

105. Cartron G, Dacheux L, Salles G, et al. Therapeutic activity of humanized anti-CD20 monoclonal antibody and polymorphism in IgG Fc receptor FcgammaRIIIa gene. *Blood.* 2002;99:754–758.

106. Kakinoki Y, Kubota H, Yamamoto Y. CD64 surface expression on neutrophils and monocytes is significantly up-regulated after stimulation with granulocyte colony-stimulating factor during CHOP chemotherapy for patients with non-Hodgkin's lymphoma. *Int J Hematol.* 2004;79:55–62.

107. Ansell SM. Adding cytokines to monoclonal antibody therapy: does the concurrent administration of interleukin-12 add to the efficacy of rituximab in B-cell non-hodgkin lymphoma? *Leuk Lymphoma.* 2003;44:1309–1315.

108. Ansell SM, Geyer SM, Maurer MJ, et al. Randomized phase II study of interleukin-12 in combination with rituximab in previously treated non-Hodgkin's lymphoma patients. *Clin Cancer Res.* 2006;12:6056–6063.

109. Slamon DJ, Leyland-Jones B, Shak S, et al. Use of chemotherapy plus a monoclonal antibody against HER2 for metastatic breast cancer that overexpresses HER2. *N Engl J Med.* 2001;344:783–792.

110. Piccart-Gebhart MJ, Procter M, Leyland-Jones B, et al. Trastuzumab after adjuvant chemotherapy in HER2-positive breast cancer. *N Engl J Med.* 2005;353:1659–1672.

111. Romond EH, Perez EA, Bryant J, et al. Trastuzumab plus adjuvant chemotherapy for operable HER2-positive breast cancer. *N Engl J Med.* 2005;353:1673–1684.

112. Izumi Y, Xu L, di Tomaso E, et al. Tumour biology: herceptin acts as an anti-angiogenic cocktail. *Nature.* 2002;416:279–280.

113. Gennari R, Menard S, Fagnoni F, et al. Pilot study of the mechanism of action of preoperative trastuzumab in patients with primary operable breast tumors overexpressing HER2. *Clin Cancer Res.* 2004;10:5650–5655.

114. Warburton C, Dragowska WH, Gelmon K, et al. Treatment of HER-2/neu overexpressing breast cancer xenograft models with trastuzumab (Herceptin) and gefitinib (ZD1839): drug combination effects on tumor growth, HER-2/neu and epidermal growth factor receptor expression, and viable hypoxic cell fraction. *Clin Cancer Res.* 2004;10:2512–2524.

115. Garratt AN, Ozcelik C, Birchmeier C. ErbB2 pathways in heart and neural diseases. *Trends Cardiovasc Med.* 2003;13:80–86.

116. Negro A, Brar BK, Lee KF. Essential roles of Her2/erbB2 in cardiac development and function. *Recent Prog Horm Res.* 2004;59:1–12.

117. Ewer MS, Vooletich MT, Durand JB, et al. Reversibility of trastuzumab-related cardiotoxicity: new insights based on clinical course and response to medical treatment. *J Clin Oncol.* 2005;23:7820–7826.

118. Tan-Chiu E, Yothers G, Romond E, et al. Assessment of cardiac dysfunction in a randomized trial comparing doxorubicin and cyclophosphamide followed by paclitaxel, with or without trastuzumab as adjuvant therapy in node-positive, human epidermal growth factor receptor 2-overexpressing breast cancer: NSABP B-31. *J Clin Oncol.* 2005;23:7811–7819.

119. Perrotte P, Matsumoto T, Inoue K, et al. Anti-epidermal growth factor receptor antibody C225 inhibits angiogenesis in human transitional cell carcinoma growing orthotopically in nude mice. *Clin Cancer Res.* 1999;5:257–265.

120. Karashima T, Sweeney P, Slaton JW, et al. Inhibition of angiogenesis by the antiepidermal growth factor receptor antibody ImClone C225 in androgen-independent prostate cancer growing orthotopically in nude mice. *Clin Cancer Res.* 2002;8:1253–1264.

121. Vincenzi B, Santini D, Russo A, et al. Angiogenesis modifications related with cetuximab plus irinotecan as anticancer treatment in advanced colorectal cancer patients. *Ann Oncol.* 2006;17:835–841.

122. Bonner JA, Harari PM, Giralt J, et al. Radiotherapy plus cetuximab for squamous-cell carcinoma of the head and neck. *N Engl J Med.* 2006;354:567–578.

123. Perez-Soler R, Saltz L. Cutaneous adverse effects with HER1/EGFR-targeted agents: is there a silver lining? *J Clin Oncol.* 2005;23:5235–5246.

124. Kanai T, Konno H, Tanaka T, et al. Anti-tumor and anti-metastatic effects of human-vascular-endothelial-growth-factor-neutralizing antibody on human colon and gastric carcinoma xenotransplanted orthotopically into nude mice. *Int J Cancer.* 1998;77:933–936.

125. Gorski DH, Beckett MA, Jaskowiak NT, et al. Blockage of the vascular endothelial growth factor stress response increases the antitumor effects of ionizing radiation. *Cancer Res.* 1999;59:3374–3378.

126. Hurwitz H, Fehrenbacher L, Novotny W, et al. Bevacizumab plus irinotecan, fluorouracil, and leucovorin for metastatic colorectal cancer. *N Engl J Med.* 2004;350:2335–2342.

127. Diaz-Rubio E, Schmoll HJ. The future development of bevacizumab in colorectal cancer. *Oncology.* 2005;69(Suppl 3):34–45.

128. Hurwitz HI, Fehrenbacher L, Hainsworth JD, et al. Bevacizumab in combination with fluorouracil and leucovorin: an active regimen for first-line metastatic colorectal cancer. *J Clin Oncol.* 2005;23:3502–3508.

129. Morgensztern D, Govindan R. Clinical trials of antiangiogenic therapy in non-small cell lung cancer: focus on bevacizumab and ZD6474. *Expert Rev Anticancer Ther.* 2006;6:545–551.

130. de Gramont A, Van Cutsem E. Investigating the potential of bevacizumab in other indications: metastatic renal cell, non-small cell lung, pancreatic and breast cancer. *Oncology.* 2005;69(Suppl 3):46–56.

131. Gordon MS, Cunningham D. Managing patients treated with bevacizumab combination therapy. *Oncology.* 2005;69(Suppl 3): 25–33.

132. Witzig TE, Gordon LI, Cabanillas F, et al. Randomized controlled trial of yttrium-90-labeled ibritumomab tiuxetan radioimmunotherapy versus rituximab immunotherapy for patients with relapsed or refractory low-grade, follicular, or transformed B-cell non-Hodgkin's lymphoma. *J Clin Oncol.* 2002;20:2453–2463.

133. Davis TA, Kaminski MS, Leonard JP, et al. The radioisotope contributes significantly to the activity of radioimmunotherapy. *Clin Cancer Res.* 2004;10:7792–7798.

134. Bale WF, Spar IL. Studies directed toward the use of antibodies as carriers of radioactivity for therapy. *Adv Biol Med Phys.* 1957;5:285–356.

135. Silverstein AM. Labeled antigens and antibodies: the evolution of magic markers and magic bullets. *Nat Immunol.* 2004;5:1211–1217.

136. Goldenberg DM, DeLand F, Kim E, et al. Use of radiolabeled antibodies to carcinoembryonic antigen for the detection and localization of diverse cancers by external photoscanning. *N Engl J Med.* 1978;298:1384–1386.

137. Goldenberg DM, Gaffar SA, Bennett SJ, et al. Experimental radioimmunotherapy of a xenografted human colonic tumor (GW-39) producing carcinoembryonic antigen. *Cancer Res.* 1981;41:4354–4360.

138. Order SE, Klein JL, Ettinger D, et al. Phase I-II study of radiolabeled antibody integrated in the treatment of primary hepatic malignancies. *Int J Radiat Oncol Biol Phys.* 1980;6:703–710.

139. Carrasquillo JA, Krohn KA, Beaumier P, et al. Diagnosis of and therapy for solid tumors with radiolabeled antibodies and immune fragments. *Cancer Treat Rep.* 1984;68:317–328.

140. Montz R, Klapdor R, Rothe B, Heller M. Immunoscintigraphy and radioimmunotherapy in patients with pancreatic carcinoma. *Nuklearmedizin.* 1986;25:239–244.

141. Goldenberg DM. Targeting of cancer with radiolabeled antibodies. Prospects for imaging and therapy. *Arch Pathol Lab Med.* 1988;112:580–587.

142. DeNardo SJ, DeNardo GL, O'Grady LF, et al. Treatment of a patient with B cell lymphoma by I-131 LYM-1 monoclonal antibodies. *Int J Biol Markers.* 1987;2:49–53.

143. Sharkey RM, Goldenberg DM. Perspectives on cancer therapy with radiolabeled monoclonal antibodies. *J Nucl Med.* 2005;46 Suppl 1: 115S–127S.

144. Buchsbaum DJ, Roberson PL. Experimental radioimmunotherapy: biological effectiveness and comparison with external beam radiation. *Recent Results Cancer Res.* 1996;141:9–18.

145. Hernandez MC, Knox SJ. Radiobiology of radioimmunotherapy: targeting CD20 B-cell antigen in non-Hodgkin's lymphoma. *Int J Radiat Oncol Biol Phys.* 2004;59:1274–1287.

146. Kenanova V, Wu AM. Tailoring antibodies for radionuclide delivery. *Expert Opin Drug Deliv.* 2006;3:53–70.

147. Behr TM, Behe M, Stabin MG, et al. High-linear energy transfer (LET) alpha versus low-LET beta emitters in radioimmunotherapy of solid tumors: therapeutic efficacy and dose-limiting toxicity of ^{213}Bi- versus ^{90}Y-labeled CO17-1A Fab' fragments in a human colonic cancer model. *Cancer Res.* 1999;59:2635–2643.

148. Buchegger F, Mach JP, Folli S, et al. Higher efficiency of ^{131}I-labeled anticarcinoembryonic antigen-monoclonal antibody F(ab')2 as compared to intact antibodies in radioimmunotherapy of established human colon carcinoma grafted in nude mice. *Recent Results Cancer Res.* 1996;141:19–35.

149. Behr TM, Blumenthal RD, Memtsoudis S, et al. Cure of metastatic human colonic cancer in mice with radiolabeled monoclonal antibody fragments. *Clin Cancer Res.* 2000;6:4900–4907.

150. Sharkey RM, Motta-Hennessy C, Pawlyk D, et al. Biodistribution and radiation dose estimates for yttrium-and iodine-labeled monoclonal antibody IgG and fragments in nude mice bearing human colonic tumor xenografts. *Cancer Res.* 1990;50:2330–2336.

151. Sharkey RM, Karacay H, Cardillo TM, et al. Improving the delivery of radionuclides for imaging and therapy of cancer using pretargeting methods. *Clin Cancer Res.* 2005;11:7109s–7121s.

152. Sharkey RM, Cardillo TM, Rossi EA, et al. Signal amplification in molecular imaging by pretargeting a multivalent, bispecific antibody. *Nat Med.* 2005;11:1250–1255.

153. McBride WJ, Zanzonico P, Sharkey RM, et al. Bispecific antibody pretargeting PET (immunoPET) with an ^{124}I-labeled hapten-peptide. *J Nucl Med.* 2006;47:1678–1688.

154. Karacay H, Brard PY, Sharkey RM, et al. Therapeutic advantage of pretargeted radioimmunotherapy using a recombinant bispecific antibody in a human colon cancer xenograft. *Clin Cancer Res.* 2005;11:7879–7885.

155. Rossi EA, Goldenberg DM, Cardillo TM, et al. Stably tethered multifunctional structures of defined composition made by the dock and lock method for use in cancer targeting. *Proc Natl Acad Sci U S A.* 2006;103:6841–6846.

156. Pagel JM, Lin Y, Hedin N, et al. Comparison of a tetravalent single-chain antibodystreptavidin fusion protein and an antibody-streptavidin chemical conjugate for pretargeted anti-CD20 radioimmunotherapy of B-cell lymphomas. *Blood.* 2006;108:328–336.

157. Sharkey RM, Goldenberg DM. Advances in radioimmunotherapy in the age of molecular engineering and pretargeting. *Cancer Invest.* 2006;24:82–97.

158. Shen S, Forero A, LoBuglio AF, et al. Patient-specific dosimetry of pretargeted radioimmunotherapy using CC49 fusion protein in patients with gastrointestinal malignancies. *J Nucl Med.* 2005;46:642–651.

159. Goldenberg DM, Sharkey RM, Paganelli G, et al. Antibody pretargeting advances cancer radioimmunodetection and radioimmunotherapy. *J Clin Oncol.* 2006;24:823–834.

160. Chatal JF, Campion L, Kraeber-Bodere F, et al. Survival improvement in patients with medullary thyroid carcinoma who undergo pretargeted anti-carcinoembryonic-antigen radioimmunotherapy: a collaborative study with the French Endocrine Tumor Group. *J Clin Oncol.* 2006;24:1705–1711.

161. Kassis AI, Adelstein SJ. Radiobiologic principles in radionuclide therapy. *J Nucl Med.* 2005;46 Suppl 1:4S–12S.

162. Michel RB, Brechbiel MW, Mattes MJ. A comparison of 4 radionuclides conjugated to antibodies for single-cell kill. *J Nucl Med.* 2003;44:632–640.

163. Kotzerke J, Bunjes D, Scheinberg DA. Radioimmunoconjugates in acute leukemia treatment: the future is radiant. *Bone Marrow Transplant.* 2005;36:1021–1026.

164. Sharkey RM, Burton J, Goldenberg DM. Radioimmunotherapy of non-Hodgkin's lymphoma: a critical appraisal. *Expert Rev Clin Immunol.* 2005;1:47–62.

165. Gordon LI, Molina A, Witzig T, et al. Durable responses after ibritumomab tiuxetan radioimmunotherapy for CD20+ B-cell lymphoma: long-term follow-up of a phase 1/2 study. *Blood.* 2004; 103:4429–4431.

166. Gordon LI, Witzig T, Molina A, et al. Yttrium 90-labeled ibritumomab tiuxetan radioimmunotherapy produces high response rates and durable remissions in patients with previously treated B-cell lymphoma. *Clin Lymphoma.* 2004;5:98–101.

167. Fisher RI, Kaminski MS, Wahl RL, et al. Tositumomab and iodine-131 tositumomab produces durable complete remissions in a subset of heavily pretreated patients with low-grade and transformed non-Hodgkin's lymphomas. *J Clin Oncol.* 2005;23:7565–7573.

168. Kaminski MS, Tuck M, Estes J, et al. ^{131}I-tositumomab therapy as initial treatment for follicular lymphoma. *N Engl J Med.* 2005; 352:441–449.

169. Buchegger F, Antonescu C, Delaloye AB, et al. Long-term complete responses after ^{131}I tositumomab therapy for relapsed or refractory indolent non-Hodgkin's lymphoma. *Br J Cancer.* 2006;94:1770–1776.

170. Ansell SM, Ristow KM, Habermann TM, et al. Subsequent chemotherapy regimens are well tolerated after radioimmunotherapy with yttrium-90 ibritumomab tiuxetan for non-Hodgkin's lymphoma. *J Clin Oncol.* 2002;20:3885–3890.

171. Sweetenham JW, Dicke K, Arcaroli J, et al. Efficacy and safety of yttrium-90 (^{90}Y) ibritumomab tiuxetan (Zevalin®) therapy with rituximab maintenance in patients with untreated low-grade follicular lymphoma. *ASH Annual Meeting Abstracts.* 2004;104: Abstract 2633.

172. Kaminski MS, Radford JA, Gregory SA, et al. Re-treatment with I-131 tositumomab in patients with non-Hodgkin's lymphoma who had previously responded to I-131 tositumomab. *J Clin Oncol.* 2005;23:7985–7993.

173. Connors JM. Radioimmunotherapy—hot new treatment for lymphoma. *N Engl J Med.* 2005;352:496–498.

174. Sharkey RM, Brenner A, Burton J, et al. Radioimmunotherapy of non-Hodgkin's lymphoma with ^{90}Y-DOTA humanized anti-CD22 IgG (^{90}Y-Epratuzumab): do tumor targeting and dosimetry predict therapeutic response? *J Nucl Med.* 2003;44:2000–2018.

175. Fisher RI. Overview of Southwest Oncology Group Clinical Trials in non-Hodgkin Lymphoma. S0016. A phase III trial of CHOP vs CHOP + rituximab vs CHOP + iodine131-labeled monoclonal anti-B1 antibody (tositumomab) for treatment of newly diagnosed follicular NHL. *Clin Adv Hematol Oncol.* 2005;3:544–546.

176. Leonard JP, Coleman M, Kostakoglu L, et al. Abbreviated chemotherapy with fludarabine followed by tositumomab and iodine I 131 tositumomab for untreated follicular lymphoma. *J Clin Oncol.* 2005;23:5696–5704.

177. Bennett JM, Kaminski MS, Leonard JP, et al. Assessment of treatment-related myelodysplastic syndromes and acute myeloid leukemia in patients with non-Hodgkin lymphoma treated with tositumomab and iodine I131 tositumomab. *Blood.* 2005;105: 4576–4582.

178. Inwards DJ, Cilley JC, Winter JN. Radioimmunotherapeutic strategies in autologous hematopoietic stem-cell transplantation for malignant lymphoma. *Best Pract Res Clin Haematol.* 2006;19: 669–684.

179. Jacobs SA, Vidnovic N, Joyce J, et al. Full-dose ^{90}Y ibritumomab tiuxetan therapy is safe in patients with prior myeloablative chemotherapy. *Clin Cancer Res.* 2005;11:7146s–7150s.

180. Nademanee A, Forman S, Molina A, et al. A phase 1/2 trial of high-dose yttrium-90-ibritumomab tiuxetan in combination with high-dose etoposide and cyclophosphamide followed by autologous stem cell transplantation in patients with poor-risk or relapsed non-Hodgkin lymphoma. *Blood.* 2005;106:2896–2902.

181. Dosik AD, Coleman M, Kostakoglu L, et al. Subsequent therapy can be administered after tositumomab and iodine I-131 tositumomab for non-Hodgkin lymphoma. *Cancer.* 2006;106:616–622.

182. Meredith RF. Ongoing investigations and new uses of radioimmunotherapy in the treatment of non-Hodgkin's lymphoma. *Int J Radiat Oncol Biol Phys.* 2006;66:S23–S29.

183. Weigert O, Illidge T, Hiddemann W, et al. Recommendations for the use of yttrium-90 ibritumomab tiuxetan in malignant lymphoma. *Cancer.* 2006;107:686–695.

184. Justice TE, Martenson JA, Wiseman GA, et al. Safety and efficacy of external beam radiation therapy for non-Hodgkin lymphoma in patients with prior ^{90}Y ibritumomab tiuxetan radioimmunotherapy. *Cancer.* 2006;107:433–438.

185. Fietz T, Uharek L, Gentilini C, et al. Allogeneic hematopoietic cell transplantation following conditioning with 90Y-ibritumomab-tiuxetan. *Leuk Lymphoma.* 2006;47:59–63.

186. Chen S, Yu L, Jiang C, et al. Pivotal study of iodine-131-labeled chimeric tumor necrosis treatment radioimmunotherapy in patients with advanced lung cancer. *J Clin Oncol.* 2005;23:1538–1547.

187. Sharkey RM, Pykett MJ, Siegel JA, et al. Radioimmunotherapy of the GW-39 human colonic tumor xenograft with ^{131}I-labeled murine monoclonal antibody to carcinoembryonic antigen. *Cancer Res.* 1987;47:5672–5677.

188. Sharkey RM, Weadock KS, Natale A, et al. Successful radioimmunotherapy for lung metastasis of human colonic cancer in nude mice. *J Natl Cancer Inst.* 1991;83:627–632.

189. Blumenthal RD, Sharkey RM, Haywood L, et al. Targeted therapy of athymic mice bearing GW-39 human colonic cancer micrometastases with ^{131}I-labeled monoclonal antibodies. *Cancer Res.* 1992;52:6036–6044.

190. Liersch T, Meller J, Kulle B, et al. Phase II trial of carcinoembryonic antigen radioimmunotherapy with ^{131}I-labetuzumab after salvage resection of colorectal metastases in the liver: five-year safety and efficacy results. *J Clin Oncol.* 2005;23:6763–6770.

191. Alvarez RD, Partridge EE, Khazaeli MB, et al. Intraperitoneal radioimmunotherapy of ovarian cancer with ^{177}Lu-CC49: a phase I/II study. *Gynecol Oncol.* 1997;65:94–101.

192. Mahe MA, Fumoleau P, Fabbro M, et al. A phase II study of intraperitoneal radioimmunotherapy with iodine-131-labeled monoclonal antibody OC-125 in patients with residual ovarian carcinoma. *Clin Cancer Res.* 1999;5:3249s–3253s.

193. Alvarez RD, Huh WK, Khazaeli MB, et al. A Phase I study of combined modality ^{90}Yttrium-CC49 intraperitoneal radioimmunotherapy for ovarian cancer. *Clin Cancer Res.* 2002;8:2806–2811.

194. Reardon DA, Quinn JA, Akabani G, et al. Novel human IgG2b/murine chimeric antitenascin monoclonal antibody construct radiolabeled with ^{131}I and administered into the surgically created resection cavity of patients with malignant glioma: phase I trial results. *J Nucl Med.* 2006;47:912–918.

195. Reardon DA, Akabani G, Coleman RE, et al. Salvage radioimmunotherapy with murine iodine-131-labeled antitenascin monoclonal antibody 81C6 for patients with recurrent primary and metastatic malignant brain tumors: phase II study results. *J Clin Oncol.* 2006;24:115–122.

196. DeNardo SJ, Richman CM, Kukis DL, et al. Synergistic therapy of breast cancer with Y-90-chimeric L6 and paclitaxel in the xenografted mouse model: development of a clinical protocol. *Anticancer Res.* 1998;18:4011–4018.

197. Gold DV, Schutsky K, Modrak D, et al. Low-dose radioimmunotherapy (^{90}YPAM4) combined with gemcitabine for the treatment of experimental pancreatic cancer. *Clin Cancer Res.* 2003;9:3929S–3937S.

198. Wong JY, Shibata S, Williams LE, et al. A Phase I trial of ^{90}Y-anticarcinoembryonic antigen chimeric T84.66 radioimmunotherapy with 5-fluorouracil in patients with metastatic colorectal cancer. *Clin Cancer Res.* 2003;9:5842–5852.

199. Richman CM, DeNardo SJ, O'Donnell RT, et al. High-dose radioimmunotherapy combined with fixed, low-dose paclitaxel in metastatic prostate and breast cancer by using a MUC-1 monoclonal antibody, m170, linked to indium-111/yttrium-90 via a cathepsin cleavable linker with cyclosporine to prevent human anti-mouse antibody. *Clin Cancer Res.* 2005;11:5920–5927.

200. Crow DM, Williams L, Colcher D, et al. Combined radioimmunotherapy and chemotherapy of breast tumors with Y-90-labeled anti-Her2 and anti-CEA antibodies with taxol. *Bioconjug Chem.* 2005;16:1117–1125.

201. Kraeber-Bodere F, Sai-Maurel C, Campion L, et al. Enhanced antitumor activity of combined pretargeted radioimmunotherapy and paclitaxel in medullary thyroid cancer xenograft. *Mol Cancer Ther.* 2002;1:267–274.

202. Graves SS, Dearstyne E, Lin Y, et al. Combination therapy with Pretarget CC49 radioimmunotherapy and gemcitabine prolongs tumor doubling time in a murine xenograft model of colon cancer more effectively than either monotherapy. *Clin Cancer Res.* 2003;9:3712–3721.

203. van Gog FB, Brakenhoff RH, Stigter-van Walsum M, et al. Perspectives of combined radioimmunotherapy and anti-EGFR antibody therapy for the treatment of residual head and neck cancer. *Int J Cancer.* 1998;77:13–18.

204. Wygoda Z, Tarnawski R, Brady L, et al. Simultaneous radiotherapy and radioimmunotherapy of malignant gliomas with anti-EGFR antibody labelled with iodine 125. Preliminary results. *Nucl Med Rev Cent East Eur.* 2002;5:29–33.

205. Baumann M, Krause M. Targeting the epidermal growth factor receptor in radiotherapy: radiobiological mechanisms, preclinical and clinical results. *Radiother Oncol.* 2004;72:257–266.

206. Wygoda Z, Kula D, Bierzynska-Macyszyn G, et al. Use of monoclonal anti-EGFR antibody in the radioimmunotherapy of malignant gliomas in the context of EGFR expression in grade III and IV tumors. *Hybridoma (Larchmt).* 2006;25:125–132.

207. Carlsson J, Ren ZP, Wester K, et al. Planning for intracavitary anti-EGFR radionuclide therapy of gliomas. Literature review and data on EGFR expression. *J Neurooncol.* 2006;77:33–45.

208. Mathé G, Loc TB, Bernard J. Effet sur la leucémie 1210 de la souris d'une combinaison par diazotation d'A-méthoptérine et de γ-globulines de hamsters porteurs de cette leucémie par hétérogreffe. *C R Acad Sci (Paris).* 1958;246:1626–1628.

209. Bross PF, Beitz J, Chen G, et al. Approval summary: gemtuzumab ozogamicin in relapsed acute myeloid leukemia. *Clin Cancer Res.* 2001;7:1490–1496.

210. Amadori S, Suciu S, Willemze R, et al. Sequential administration of gemtuzumab ozogamicin and conventional chemotherapy as first line therapy in elderly patients with acute myeloid leukemia: a phase II study (AML-15) of the EORTC and GIMEMA leukemia groups. *Haematologica.* 2004;89:950–956.

211. Amadori S, Suciu S, Stasi R, et al. Gemtuzumab ozogamicin (Mylotarg) as single-agent treatment for frail patients 61 years of age and older with acute myeloid leukemia: final results of AML-15B, a phase 2 study of the European Organisation for Research and Treatment of Cancer and Gruppo Italiano Malattie Ematologiche dell'Adulto Leukemia Groups. *Leukemia.* 2005;19:1768–1773.

212. Larson RA, Sievers EL, Stadtmauer EA, et al. Final report of the efficacy and safety of gemtuzumab ozogamicin (Mylotarg) in patients with CD33-positive acute myeloid leukemia in first recurrence. *Cancer.* 2005;104:1442–1452.

213. Roman E, Cooney E, Harrison L, et al. Preliminary results of the safety of immunotherapy with gemtuzumab ozogamicin following reduced intensity allogeneic stem cell transplant in children with CD33+ acute myeloid leukemia. *Clin Cancer Res.* 2005;11:7164s–7170s.

214. Nabhan C, Rundhaugen LM, Riley MB, et al. Phase II pilot trial of gemtuzumab ozogamicin (GO) as first line therapy in acute myeloid leukemia patients age 65 or older. *Leuk Res.* 2005;29:53–57.

215. Brethon B, Auvrignon A, Galambrun C, et al. Efficacy and tolerability of gemtuzumab ozogamicin (anti-CD33 monoclonal antibody, CMA-676, Mylotarg) in children with relapsed/refractory myeloid leukemia. *BMC Cancer.* 2006;6:172.

216. Wu AM, Senter PD. Arming antibodies: prospects and challenges for immunoconjugates. *Nat Biotechnol.* 2005;23:1137–1146.

217. Jedema I, Barge RM, van der Velden VH, et al. Internalization and cell cycle-dependent killing of leukemic cells by Gemtuzumab Ozogamicin: rationale for efficacy in CD33-negative malignancies with endocytic capacity. *Leukemia.* 2004;18:316–325.

218. Lambert JM. Drug-conjugated monoclonal antibodies for the treatment of cancer. *Curr Opin Pharmacol.* 2005;5:543–549.

219. Fang L, Battisti RF, Cheng H, et al. Enzyme specific activation of benzoquinone ansamycin prodrugs using HuCC49DeltaCH2-beta-galactosidase conjugates. *J Med Chem.* 2006;49:6290–6297.

220. Smith LM, Nesterova A, Alley SC, et al. Potent cytotoxicity of an auristatin-containing antibody-drug conjugate targeting melanoma cells expressing melanotransferrin/p97. *Mol Cancer Ther.* 2006;5:1474–1482.

221. Law CL, Gordon KA, Toki BE, et al. Lymphocyte activation antigen CD70 expressed by renal cell carcinoma is a potential therapeutic target for anti-CD70 antibody-drug conjugates. *Cancer Res.* 2006;66:2328–2337.

222. Sutherland MS, Sanderson RJ, Gordon KA, et al. Lysosomal trafficking and cysteine protease metabolism confer target-specific cytotoxicity by peptide-linked anti-CD30-auristatin conjugates. *J Biol Chem.* 2006;281:10540–10547.

223. Ma D, Hopf CE, Malewicz AD, et al. Potent antitumor activity of an auristatinconjugated, fully human monoclonal antibody to prostate-specific membrane antigen. *Clin Cancer Res.* 2006;12:2591–2596.

224. Govindan SV, Goldenberg DM, Elsamra SE, et al. Radionuclides linked to a CD74 antibody as therapeutic agents for B-cell lymphoma: comparison of Auger electron emitters with beta-particle emitters. *J Nucl Med.* 2000;41:2089–2097.

225. Griffiths GL, Mattes MJ, Stein R, et al. Cure of SCID mice bearing human B-lymphoma xenografts by an anti-CD74 antibody-anthracycline drug conjugate. *Clin Cancer Res.* 2003;9:6567–6571.

226. Chang CH, Sapra P, Vanama SS, et al. Effective therapy of human lymphoma xenografts with a novel recombinant ribonuclease/ anti-CD74 humanized IgG4 antibody immunotoxin. *Blood.* 2005;106:4308–4314.

227. Leslie EM, Deeley RG, Cole SP. Multidrug resistance proteins: role of P-glycoprotein, MRP1, MRP2, and BCRP (ABCG2) in tissue defense. *Toxicol Appl Pharmacol.* 2005;204:216–237.

228. Naito K, Takeshita A, Shigeno K, et al. Calicheamicin-conjugated humanized anti-CD33 monoclonal antibody (gemtuzumab zogamicin, CMA-676) shows cytocidal effect on CD33-positive leukemia cell lines, but is inactive on P-glycoprotein-expressing sublines. *Leukemia.* 2000;14:1436–1443.

229. Hamann PR, Hinman LM, Beyer CF, et al. An anti-MUC1 antibody-calicheamicin conjugate for treatment of solid tumors. Choice of linker and overcoming drug resistance. *Bioconjug Chem.* 2005;16:346–353.

230. Bagshawe KD. Antibody-directed enzyme prodrug therapy (ADEPT) for cancer. *Expert Rev Anticancer Ther.* 2006;6:1421–1431.

231. Francis RJ, Sharma SK, Springer C, et al. A phase I trial of antibody directed enzyme prodrug therapy (ADEPT) in patients with advanced colorectal carcinoma or other CEA producing tumours. *Br J Cancer.* 2002;87:600–607.

232. Mayer A, Sharma SK, Tolner B, et al. Modifying an immunogenic epitope on a therapeutic protein: a step towards an improved system for antibody-directed enzyme prodrug therapy (ADEPT). *Br J Cancer.* 2004;90:2402–2410.

233. Mayer A, Francis RJ, Sharma SK, et al. A Phase I study of single administration of antibody-directed enzyme prodrug therapy with the recombinant anti-carcinoembryonic antigen antibody-enzyme fusion protein MFECP1 and a bis-iodo phenol mustard prodrug. *Clin Cancer Res.* 2006;12:6509–6516.

234. Saleh MN, Sugarman S, Murray J, et al. Phase I trial of the anti-Lewis Y drug immunoconjugate BR96-doxorubicin in patients with lewis Y-expressing epithelial tumors. *J Clin Oncol.* 2000;18:2282–2292.

235. Messmann RA, Vitetta ES, Headlee D, et al. A phase I study of combination therapy with immunotoxins IgG-HD37-deglycosylated ricin A chain (dgA) and IgG-RFB4-dgA (Combotox) in patients with refractory CD19+, CD22+ B cell lymphoma. *Clin Cancer Res.* 2000;6:1302–1313.

236. Kreitman RJ, Wilson WH, White JD, et al. Phase I trial of recombinant immunotoxin anti-Tac(Fv)-PE38 (LMB-2) in patients with hematologic malignancies. *J Clin Oncol.* 2000;18:1622–1636.

237. Schnell R, Vitetta E, Schindler J, et al. Treatment of refractory Hodgkin's lymphoma patients with an anti-CD25 ricin A-chain immunotoxin. *Leukemia.* 2000;14:129–135.

238. Weber FW, Floeth F, Asher A, et al. Local convection enhanced delivery of IL4-Pseudomonas exotoxin (NBI-3001) for treatment of patients with recurrent malignant glioma. *Acta Neurochir Suppl.* 2003;88:93–103.

239. Schnell R, Borchmann P, Staak JO, et al. Clinical evaluation of ricin A-chain immunotoxins in patients with Hodgkin's lymphoma. *Ann Oncol.* 2003;14:729–736.

240. Azemar M, Djahansouzi S, Jager E, et al. Regression of cutaneous tumor lesions in patients intratumorally injected with a recombinant single-chain antibody-toxin targeted to ErbB2/HER2. *Breast Cancer Res Treat.* 2003;82:155–164.

241. Kreitman RJ, Squires DR, Stetler-Stevenson M, et al. Phase I trial of recombinant immunotoxin RFB4(dsFv)-PE38 (BL22) in patients with B-cell malignancies. *J Clin Oncol.* 2005;23:6719–6729.

242. Kreitman RJ, Pastan I. Immunotoxins in the treatment of hematologic malignancies. *Curr Drug Targets.* 2006;7:1301–1311.

243. Frankel AE, Kreitman RJ, Sausville EA. Targeted toxins. *Clin Cancer Res.* 2000;6:326–334.

244. Newton DL, Hansen HJ, Mikulski SM, et al. Potent and specific antitumor effects of an anti-CD22-targeted cytotoxic ribonucle-ase: potential for the treatment of non-Hodgkin lymphoma. *Blood.* 2001;97:528–535.

245. Gadina M, Newton DL, Rybak SM, et al. Humanized immunotoxins. *Ther Immunol.* 1994;1:59–64.

246. Vitetta ES, Fulton RJ, May RD, et al. Redesigning nature's poisons to create anti-tumor reagents. *Science* 1987;238:1098–1104.

247. Shimamura T, Husain SR, Puri RK. The IL-4 and IL-13 pseudomonas exotoxins: new hope for brain tumor therapy. *Neurosurg Focus.* 2006;20:E11.

248. Amlot PL, Stone MJ, Cunningham D, et al. A phase I study of an anti-CD22-deglycosylated ricin A chain immunotoxin in the treatment of B-cell lymphomas resistant to conventional therapy. *Blood.* 1993;82:2624–2633.

249. Sausville EA, Headlee D, Stetler-Stevenson M, et al. Continuous infusion of the anti-CD22 immunotoxin IgG-RFB4-SMPT-dgA in patients with B-cell lymphoma: a phase I study. *Blood.* 1995;85:3457–3465.

250. Smallshaw JE, Ghetie V, Rizo J, et al. Genetic engineering of an immunotoxin to eliminate pulmonary vascular leak in mice. *Nat Biotechnol.* 2003;21:387–391.

251. Kreitman RJ, Wilson WH, Bergeron K, et al. Efficacy of the anti-CD22 recombinant immunotoxin BL22 in chemotherapy-resistant hairy-cell leukemia. *N Engl J Med.* 2001;345:241–247.

252. Posey JA, Khazaeli MB, Bookman MA, et al. A phase I trial of the single-chain immunotoxin SGN-10 (BR96 sFv-PE40) in patients with advanced solid tumors. *Clin Cancer Res.* 2002;8:3092–3099.

253. Hellstrom I, Garrigues HJ, Garrigues U, et al. Highly tumor-reactive, internalizing, mouse monoclonal antibodies to Le(y)-related cell surface antigens. *Cancer Res.* 1990;50:2183–2190.

254. Pettengell R, Linch D. Position paper on the therapeutic use of rituximab in CD20-positive diffuse large B-cell non-Hodgkin's lymphoma. *Br J Haematol.* 2003;121:44–48.

255. Wittes RE Cancer weapons, out of reach. *The Washington Post.* June 28, 2004:A23.

256. Uyl-de Groot CA, Giaccone G. Health economics: can we afford an unrestricted use of new biological agents in gastrointestinal oncology? *Curr Opin Oncol.* 2005;17:392–396.

257. Saif MW. Targeted agents for adjuvant therapy of colon cancer. *Clin Colorectal Cancer.* 2006;6:46–51.

258. Rajpal S, Venook AP. Targeted therapy in colorectal cancer. *Clin Adv Hematol Oncol.* 2006;4:124–132.

COMMENTARY
Bruce A. Chabner

Sharkey and Goldenberg, two pioneers in the development of monoclonal antibodies for cancer treatment, have elegantly reviewed the current role of this class of agents, and have proudly displayed the variety of antibodies and antibody conjugates now playing a significant role in this disease. As an observer and at times a minor participant in the development of this group of agents, it is remarkable to me how far and how fast the field has progressed in the past decade, particularly when one considers the persistent failures that characterized the first 15 years of monoclonal antibody (Mab) trials. Much of this early work was supported by grants and contracts (and by the work of intramural scientists) of the Biological Response Modifier Program of the National Cancer Institute, but the first decade of Mab trials produced little of significance: no approved drugs, few hints of clinical activity. Yet the logic of Mab therapy remained compelling, namely the exquisite ability of this class of agents to engage targets on the cell surface with absolute specificity and high affinity. Through persistence and unbending commitment, the first successes were realized in the treatment of follicular lymphoma with Rituxan in the mid-1990s, and the more recent additions of Herceptin, Avastin, Erbitux, and others followed in a steadily expanding stream of blockbuster drugs from Biotech (1). Equally impressive is the continuous refinement and broadening of the indications for each of these drugs, largely as a result of their synergy with chemotherapy and irradiation.

Although Mabs have become a staple of cancer treatment, and investment in biotechnology companies that focus on Mabs continues to expand, major questions have not been answered. The first is the ultimate value of a Mab as compared with a small molecule as a cancer drug. Perhaps without exception, no small molecule possesses the specificity of a Mab, nor matches its ability to confine its effects to the cancer cell. The toxicity profile of most Mabs, while not absolutely clean, is highly favorable, as compared with small molecules, with little promiscuous cross-reaction with alternative receptors. However, as a drug, a Mab has certain disadvantages (2). Its large size, 150,000 daltons, prevents rapid diffusion from blood vessels into the extracellular space, and through that space to the tumor cell surface. The rate of Mab diffusion, a function of size and charge, is 10 to 100 times lower than that of the average synthetic drug, which has a molecular weight of <1,000 daltons. The problem becomes even more daunting for the Mab when one considers the additional barrier presented by high intratumoral interstitial pressure, a product of the leaky vasculature of tumors. This diffusion barrier becomes increasingly more important because it limits the number of antibody molecules escaping into the interstitial space. This escape occurs at the well-vascularized periphery of a tumor. The small number of Mabs that successfully penetrate into the interstitial space must further negotiate their way through a high density of antigenic receptors to reach the poorly perfused center of the tumor. It remains to be seen whether the much more mobile small molecules, which target cell surface receptors, will eventually replace their slower Mab cousins (e.g., Herceptin and Erbitux). As Sharkey and Goldenberg discuss, antibody fragments that preserve binding specificity but penetrate tissues more effectively may be more useful in solid tumor therapy. An alternative approach would be to correct the interstitial pressure and improve diffusion rates in tumors through use of antiangiogenic drugs, which, in some clinical circumstances, appear to have an almost immediate beneficial effect on diffusion of contrast agents and a reversal of interstitial edema (3). These effects should improve the penetration and the therapeutic results of Mabs.

A second limitation of Mabs is their inability to reach intracellular targets. For inhibition of intracellular targets such as bcr-abl, or other tyrosine kinases that are critical to signal transduction in tumor cells, Mabs have no place. There is no doubt that we have not exhausted the reservoir of targets on the cell surface, but the number of unique intracellular proteins, of interest in cancer treatment, will vastly exceed those on the cell surface.

Perhaps these facts explain the relatively poorer response rates of bulky solid tumors as compared with hematologic malignancies. Thus, because of their size and their limited diffusion capacity, Mabs would seem to be at a considerable disadvantage as compared to small molecules.

An additional hurdle to the effective use of Mabs is our current incomplete understanding of how they work, and why they fail. As the authors point out, Mabs, while possessing extreme specificity for their target, have a multiplicity of antitumor effects (antibody-dependent complement-mediated cytotoxicity, antibody-dependent cellular cytotoxicity, signaling inhibition, direct apoptosis), and it is not clear which one, or several, of these is responsible for killing tumor cells. The balance likely varies from Mab to Mab and target to target. A better understanding would undoubtedly allow the improvement of current molecules, and might allow us to explain resistance to therapy. The question of mechanism of action is further complicated by the modest antitumor activity of most Mabs as single agents. We have a difficult time classifying patients as responsive or resistant. At the moment, we choose patients for therapy with a Mab based on expression of the surface target, but clearly not all patients are benefiting. Only in the case of Erbitux, and the discovery that k-ras mutant colorectal tumors do not benefit, is it possible to exclude a significant subset of nonresponsive patients (4). Even after treatment is under way, it may be difficult to determine if patients are benefiting from Mab therapy. When Mabs are components of effective regimens, are the antibodies truly killing cells or are they simply slowing tumor progression or sensitizing cells to chemotherapy? We face this question clinically in trying to decide whether to continue Herceptin or Rituxan indefinitely in the patient who displays tumor progression. There are no clear answers.

Finally, there is the problem of convenience and cost. A pill will beat an injection, all other aspects of the drug action being equal. The requirement for repeated office visits adds bother and expense. In addition, the extraordinary development and production costs of Mabs have led to inordinately high prices, out of the range of standard cytotoxic chemotherapy. Can the health care system afford to pay for the continuously expanding indications for Erbitux, Avastin, Herceptin, and other noncurative therapies for metastatic cancer (5)? Only in the adjuvant setting, and with the exception of Rituxan for non-Hodgkin lymphoma, are Mabs curing cancer.

No doubt, the field has contributed greatly to improving treatment and proving the susceptibility of cancer to cell surface attack. Further progress will depend on advances in understanding how they kill cells, how cells become resistant, and in identifying and selecting responsive patients through molecular tests prior to treatment. Thirty years after Köhler and Milstein (6), there is still a long distance to travel if these unique drugs are to realize their full promise.

REFERENCES

1. Lawrence S. Billion dollar babies—biotech drugs as blockbusters. *Nat Biotechnol.* 2007;25:380–382.
2. Scheinberg DA, Mulford DA, Jurcic JG, et al. Antibody therapies of cancer. In: Chabner BA, Longo DL, eds. *Cancer Chemotherapy & Biotherapy: Principles and Practice.* 4th ed. Philadelphia: Lippincott Williams & Wilkins; 2006:666–698.

3. Jain RK, di Tomaso E, Duda DG, et al. Angiogenesis in brain tumours. *Nat Rev Neurosci.* 2007;8:610–622.

4. Lièvre A, Bachet JB, Boige V, et al. KRAS mutations as an independent prognostic factor in patients with advanced colorectal cancer treated with cetuximab. *J Clin Oncol.* 2008;26:374–379.

5. Hillner BE, Smith TJ. Do the large benefits justify the large costs of adjuvant breast cancer trastuzumab? J Clin Oncol. 2007;25:611–613.

6. Köhler G, Milstein C. Continuous cultures of fused cells secreting antibody of predefined specificity. Nature. 1975;256: 495–497.

Computerized Tomography, Magnetic Resonance Imaging, Ultrasonography, and Positron Emission Tomography Scanning in the Evaluation and Management of Cancer Patients

Vinay A. Duddalwar and William D. Boswell

The American Cancer Society estimated that approximately 1.4 million new cancer cases were diagnosed in the United States in 2008 (1). The management of a public health problem of this magnitude requires a multidisciplinary approach to detection and management. With the remarkable advances in imaging technology in the past several decades and now the prospect of "molecular imaging" (2), the radiologist currently and in the future will continue to play a central role in all aspects of the management of patients with cancer, including diagnosing and staging the malignancy, providing treatment, monitoring the response to therapy, and providing posttreatment surveillance. In modern practice, the radiology reading room is frequently the site of multidisciplinary collaboration, with the radiologist often contributing to and even directing critical management decisions.

In this chapter, the authors assess the role of the various imaging modalities in current oncologic radiology practice. A discussion of the role of imaging in various tumors is followed by discussing the common questions posed to radiologists by surgeons managing cancer patients. This is followed by a discussion on imaging of common *Surg Oncol* emergencies and the role of interventional radiology.

WHAT INFORMATION DOES THE CANCER SURGEON NEED FROM IMAGING STUDIES?

- Can the primary tumor be demonstrated with accurate identification of any local, adjacent visceral, and serosal involvement?
- Can the relationship of the tumor with the supplying arteries and the draining veins be demonstrated?
- Can unresectable disease be accurately identified?
- Can nodal involvement be assessed and mapped so that surgical treatment may be planned?
- Can prognosis be estimated from imaging features?
- Can imaging identify patients who could be downstaged with techniques such as image-guided ablation and neoadjuvant chemotherapy?

- Can response to chemotherapy and radiotherapy be assessed?
- Can imaging identify postsurgical complications and guide and help treatment?
- Can imaging identify local recurrence?

To answer these issues satisfactorily, the radiologist needs to have adequate information including details of past treatment and surgery. Imaging techniques may have to be modified in individual cases. It is extremely helpful, and often essential, to have previous imaging studies to assure accurate interpretation of a subsequent examination.

IMAGING MODALITIES AND TECHNIQUES

Although conventional radiography and fluoroscopy still have a central role in the practice of oncologic radiology, here we focus on other modalities including ultrasound (US), computed tomography (CT), magnetic resonance imaging (MRI), and positron emission tomography (PET) scanning, newer techniques that now play a paramount role. Breast imaging is presented in Chapters 16 A, B, and C.

Ultrasonography

Ultrasonography has several significant advantages in that it uses no ionizing radiation, allows real-time visualization, is easily portable, and thus can be used intraoperatively as well as for biopsy guidance. On the downside, it is operator-dependent and has its limitations when looking at structures behind bones and gas-filled bowel loops. There has been considerable development in the field of contrast-enhanced US where contrast injected intravascularly has been used to identify and characterize lesions in the liver and other organs (Figure 8.1).

Computed Tomography

The advent of multidetector CT technology has increased the role of CT in oncologic radiology. It has the advantages of good spatial and contrast resolution, is operator-independent, and reproducible. It is the oncology imaging workhorse but is also

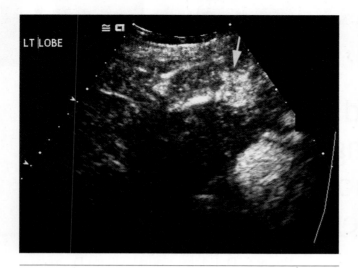

Figure 8.1 Contrast-enhanced ultrasound study: Hepatocellular carcinoma seen as a hypervascular lesion (*arrow*) in the left lobe. (Courtesy of Edward Grant, MD, University of Southern California, Los Angeles.)

used for cancer screening in virtual colonoscopy and lung screening.

The radiologist uses intravenous and enteral contrast in a variety of ways to maximize the information from the scan and to increase diagnostic confidence. Enteral contrast is used to opacify bowel to differentiate these bowel loops from fluid collections in the abdomen.

The advent of multislice technology has led to the possibility of using multiple phases with a single dose of intravenous contrast (3). A noncontrast scan is used to identify areas of calcification and hemorrhage, and as a baseline to demonstrate tumor enhancement in postcontrast scans. Scans in the arterial phase are used to generate CT angiograms and also to identify hypervascular tumors. This is followed by a scan in the venous phase, which is crucial for identifying the majority of liver lesions, and to assess the other organs. This is often followed by a delayed phase scan, which is used to demonstrate delayed washout or enhancement of lesions and to evaluate the renal excretory systems.

Another technological development is CT fluoroscopy in which continuous, real-time, low-dose CT imaging is available to improve the efficacy and speed of CT-guided interventions.

Magnetic Resonance Imaging

The advantages of MRI are that it does not use ionizing radiation, has the ability to characterize tissue, and has high soft-tissue contrast and the ability to acquire images directly in various planes. However, it is relatively complex and does not have a standard technique everywhere.

There have been numerous developments that have led to an increase in the use of MRI in oncologic radiology. Faster techniques including breath-holding sequences have made it easier to scan unstable patients. The development of specialized contrast agents such as liver-specific contrast mangafodipir trisodium (MnDPDP) has increased the accuracy of MRI. Contrast agents for the reticuloendothelial system have led to the

development of techniques such as MRI lymphography. Techniques such as MRI spectroscopy and diffusion techniques have led to increased diagnostic confidence in identifying and characterizing some neoplasms such as the prostate carcinomas.

[18]FDG Positron Emission Tomography Computed Tomography

PET with 18-fluoro-deoxy-D-glucose ([18]FDG) is discussed in detail in Chapter 9. Its advantage is the high-contrast resolution between tumors and normal tissues, making it sensitive for lesion detection, characterization, and staging. Its drawback is the lack of spatial resolution and the absence of anatomic detail. These drawbacks are significantly resolved with the fusion of the PET images with CT studies. One pitfall of PET scanning is that any inflammatory tissue or process also accumulates [18]FDG; this should be borne in mind in a postoperative study.

Postprocessing and Workstation Techniques

Most of the imaging data acquired today is volumetric, and to use all the information the data set should be viewed interactively on a workstation (3). It is difficult to reproduce three-dimensional information onto a two-dimensional axial image on film. The image data set can be viewed and interrogated using multiple window levels and widths as well as multiplanar reformations. This increases the radiologist's diagnostic confidence in the study but also increases the accuracy of the test.

Multiplanar reformations (MPRs) allow the rotation of data around any axis in real time. Specific structures can be interrogated with an optimal plane. This aids in the diagnosis of lesions on curved surfaces such as the pelvis and the limits of the abdominal cavity. Visualization is improved by using oblique, curved, and coronal reformatted images. Further postprocessing techniques include maximum-intensity projections (MIPs) and minimum-intensity projections (MinIPs) that accentuate the highest and lowest intensity structures in a given image volume, respectively. For example, MIPs are a technique used to look for lung nodules and MinIPs are used to evaluate fluid-filled ducts such as the pancreatic and biliary ducts. Other workstation techniques include volume rendering and virtual endoscopy. Most workstations now also have fusion software available for combining functional imaging such as [18]FDG PET scans with morphologic imaging such as CT scans.

Usually a combination of various techniques is needed to evaluate a data set completely. For example, a preoperative imaging study of the pancreas is often evaluated using a combination of MinIPs and MIPs for the pancreatic and biliary ducts, MIPs for evaluating the vasculature and lungs, and MPRs including curved plane reformations for evaluating local spread. However, each case is different and the radiologist might choose to add other techniques (Figure 8.2).

TUMOR STAGING AND SURVEILLANCE

Esophageal Carcinoma

There has been a significant increase in the incidence of esophageal adenocarcinoma in recent years (4–14). There are numerous predisposing factors including alcohol, smoking,

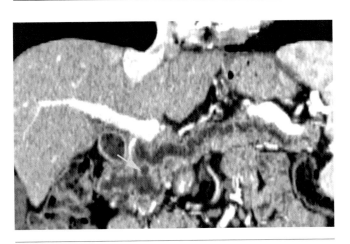

Figure 8.2 A curved plane maximum-intensity projection is an excellent method of demonstrating the pancreatic duct (*arrow*) in this case of an intraductal papillary mucinous tumor of the pancreas.

Barrett's esophagus, and achalasia. The relatively poor prognosis of esophageal carcinoma is related to both a late presentation and the lack of a true serosal cover for the esophagus. When the tumor is deeper than the mucosa, there is a significant increase in nodal disease corresponding to a poor prognosis.

Radiologic surveillance can be done by barium studies in high-risk subjects and correlated with endoscopy and endoscopic US (5). Complications such as stenosis or strictures and fistulae are well demonstrated on contrast studies.

Staging

T Stage

CT cannot determine the depth of wall invasion, and findings suggestive of early transmural spread are nonspecific (Figure 8.3). It cannot differentiate between T1 and T2 tumors. Findings

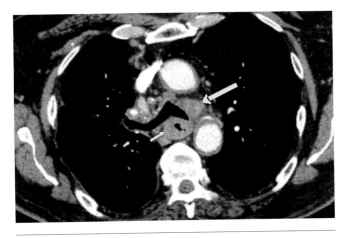

Figure 8.3 Axial contrast-enhanced computed tomography in a patient with esophageal carcinoma. The *smaller arrow* points to the eccentrically thickened esophagus at the site of the primary tumor. The *larger arrow* points to mediastinal lymphadenopathy.

suggestive of T3 diseases are obliteration or poor definition of the periesophageal fat by a tumor mass (7–10). [18]FDG PET/PET CT is poor at defining local spread (4,11,12). Involvement of adjacent organs such as the aorta and the tracheobronchial tree need to be excluded. If the mass surrounds >90 degrees of aortic circumference, aortic involvement is highly likely. Involvement of the tracheobronchial tree is suspected when a fistula is demonstrated or intraluminal tumor is demonstrated.

N Stage

CT is relatively inaccurate for determining nodal disease, with reported accuracy of 70% with a sensitivity of 40% and a specificity of 90%. The accuracy of detecting subdiaphragmatic nodal disease is higher on CT. [18]FDG PET/PET CT has the advantage of detecting metastases in normal-sized nodes (12).

M Stage

Although CT and MRI are both good at demonstrating local spread, MRI may have a advantage in demonstrating hepatic metastases (13). CT is more accurate in evaluating distant disease.

Posttreatment Surveillance

It is important to correlate any findings with the operative notes and radiotherapy to determine nonspecific changes (12,14). Often there is a small amount of pericardial or pleural fluid that may just represent postoperative or therapeutic changes. Lesions to watch out for include soft-tissue masses in the mediastinum and the abdomen, adrenal nodules, and peritoneal carcinomatosis.

Gastric Carcinoma

The advent of multiplanar and virtual endoscopic techniques has raised hopes that CT would improve the staging of stomach carcinoma (15).

Staging

T Stage

CT is better at defining invasive tumors, that is, T3 and T4 tumors with an accuracy of 85% as opposed to an accuracy of 15% for early gastric carcinoma (16). Endoscopic US is far superior in evaluating early local invasion as it can resolve individual layers of the gastric wall (17,18).

N Stage

Nodal staging using size criteria on CT is specific but not sensitive (19–23).

M Stage

CT has a significant advantage in assessing peritoneal spread and distal disease. The role of PET scans is still being assessed (24–26).

Gastrointestinal Stromal Tumors

Gastrointestinal stromal tumors are the commonest nonepithelial tumors of the gastrointestinal tract. Most of these tumors have a characteristic immunohistochemical defining feature, the c-Kit protein. These tumors are commonly found in the stomach (40% to 70%) with a progressively decreasing incidence in the small bowel, colon and rectum, esophagus, and the retroperitoneum (27,28).

Imaging features vary depending on the size and aggressiveness of the tumor. Most of the tumors are large, lobulated, and hypervascular. They may show ulceration or central necrosis and may present with bleeding. Metastatic lesions to the liver and the peritoneal cavity are common (29–34). The tumors are well demonstrated on [18]FDG-PET scans (35–38).

Posttreatment Surveillance

Surveillance is commonly carried out with CT along with [18]FDG-PET scans to resolve indeterminate issues. On contrast-enhanced CT following treatment, there is a change in the appearance of the tumor, with the tumor showing decreased vascularity or central necrosis. Posttreatment changes on [18]FDG PET scans are more rapid with a reduction in the [18]FDG uptake seen within a few days after treatment and before there is a morphologic change on CT (36,39–41) (Figure 8.4).

Colorectal Tumors

Colorectal carcinoma is the third most frequent carcinoma in the Western world. Despite recommendations from various agencies, there is a low compliance for screening. The ideal screening test should be safe, accurate, and inexpensive. Screening tests currently include fecal occult blood, barium enema, colonoscopy, and CT. There is a significant amount of interest in the role of CT/virtual colonoscopy in screening for colorectal carcinoma in view of its presumed advantages (42–44).

Staging

T Stage

The role of CT is limited because of the nonspecificity of wall thickening and pericolic stranding. It does depict local complications such as obstruction, perforation, and abscess formation (45). In the evaluation of rectal carcinomas, endoscopic US is an operator-dependent technique that provides good depiction of the depth of most tumors in the rectal wall. However, it cannot demonstrate the mesorectal fascia and has difficulties in distinguishing peritumoral fibrosis from tumor. High-spatial resolution MR using a phased array pelvic coil provides good demonstration of the tumor with accuracy between 79% and 94% in predicting T stage. MRI also demonstrates the mesorectal fascia and has a published positive predictive value of 92% of predicting the histologic status of circumferential resection margin (46,47).

N Stage

In most instances the pattern of spread is predictable. Nodal involvement is assessed with various imaging techniques as described elsewhere in this chapter (48,49) (Figure 8.5).

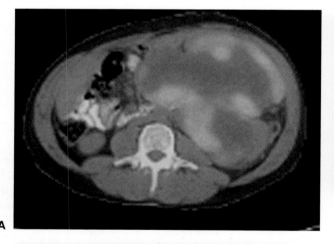

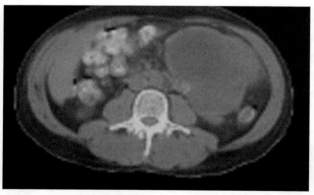

Figure 8.4 Fusion images from [18]FDG-PET-CT (18-fluoro-deoxy-D-glucose positron emission tomography-computed tomography) studies. (**A**) Large soft-tissue density mass, proven to be a gastrointestinal stromal tumor in left lower abdomen with evidence of hypermetabolism on the PET scan. (**B**) Within 2 weeks of starting imatinib therapy, the metabolic activity decreases but the size of the mass remains similar. (**C**) After 3 months there is a reduction in the size of the mass and metabolic activity.

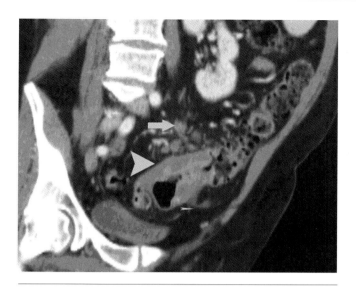

Figure 8.5 An oblique coronal image from a contrast-enhanced computed tomography scan in a patient with a sigmoid carcinoma. The *arrowhead* points to the primary tumor and the *larger arrow* points to pericolic lymphadenopathy.

M Stage

This is most commonly evaluated with CT. Common sites include the lungs, liver, and the peritoneal cavity. Radiology is crucial as preoperative chemotherapy and ablative therapy aim to increase the number of patients suitable for curative resection of metastases. On CT evaluation, hepatic metastases are usually hypovascular lesions on the parenchymal phase. Indeterminate small lesions are then further evaluated with US or MRI studies. The sensitivity of MRI studies can be further increased using hepatocyte-specific agents like mangafodipir trisodium (MnDPDP). Despite preoperative imaging, intraoperative US invariably identifies more lesions than CT and MRI and alters the surgical approach in 20% to 44% of cases (50–52).

Posttreatment Surveillance

It is imperative for the radiologist to know the details of the treatment including surgery, radiotherapy, or chemotherapy. Postoperative changes including seromas, hematomas, lymphoceles, postradiation changes, and postablation changes should be considered and correlated with the time interval from the surgery and or procedure date. It is therefore important to have a baseline scan. Any indeterminate findings should be correlated with carcinoembryonic antigen levels, and [18]FDG-PET scans and biopsies can be considered.

Local recurrence in cases of rectal carcinoma is difficult to detect clinically and the patient usually presents with pain. On CT, early recurrence is difficult to diagnose and appears as a nonspecific presacral mass. However, this needs to be differentiated from postoperative change. Other features on CT suggesting postoperative recurrence include mesorectal nodules, development of unilateral hydronephrosis, or pelvic sidewall adenopathy. On MRI, appearances are similar with difficulties in distinguishing postoperative change including fibrosis and

granulation tissue from recurrence (53).[18]FDG-PET plays a key role here because of its ability to differentiate tumor recurrence from postoperative fibrosis.

Pancreatic Carcinoma

Despite all the advances in oncology, pancreatic adenocarcinoma remains a tumor with a dismal prognosis. The challenge for radiology includes diagnosing tumors early and predicting resectability. Currently, most pancreatic adenocarcinomas are unresectable at presentation, and it is important to accurately identify those cases for which surgery will be successful. Radiologists are also involved with management of complications such as biliary obstruction and postoperative complications (54).

Staging

T Stage

Multidetector CT has revolutionized pancreatic imaging. A variety of multiplanar postprocessing techniques are used to evaluate the data set. For analyzing the vasculature, multiplanar and curved MIPs are used (55,56). Using the criterion that if ≥50% of the vessel circumference is encased by the tumor, this leads to a positive predictive value of 98% and a negative predictive value of 93% for determining arterial involvement. Similarly, venous involvement is deduced from adventitial infiltration of the venous wall leading to tethering or occlusion, with demonstration of gastrocolic varices (57,58) (Figure 8.6). Gastrointestinal tract invasion can also be assessed by the differential enhancement of normal bowel wall from tumor tissue (59,60). Endoscopic US has an increasing role to play in the imaging of pancreatic disease. While it has advantages in obtaining biopsy material, it is a technically challenging technique and cannot assess distal disease or even the supplying vessels completely (61).

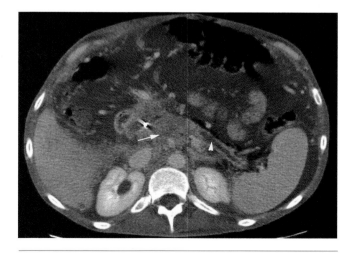

Figure 8.6 Axial contrast-enhanced computed tomography image in a case of a unresectable pancreatic carcinoma. The *arrow* denotes the primary tumor, which has invaded the celiac axis and the portal confluence, and the *arrowhead* points to the dilated pancreatic duct in the tail of the pancreas.

N Stage

The traditional criterion for lymph node involvement using a 1-cm short axis guideline for lymph nodes leads to a very low sensitivity (62). In addition there is often an element of pancreatitis in a significant number of adenocarcinomas. These could result in reactive enlargement of lymph nodes.

M Stage

This is most commonly determined with CT. Metastases to the liver are commonly seen as low density or hypovascular, with some lesions demonstrating a peripheral rim enhancement on late arterial phase imaging. The presence of ascites and peritoneal nodularity suggests peritoneal carcinomatosis (63–65).

Lung Carcinoma

CT has been used for screening for lung carcinoma in select high-risk patients. While this has resulted in early detection of lung carcinoma, there are also a high number of nodules identified that are ultimately shown to be benign. Identifying imaging features that distinguish benign from malignant nodules is the subject of new and ongoing studies (66–72).

The primary concern of surgeons treating lung carcinoma is whether the tumor is resectable. Imaging provides clinicians with information regarding type of tumor, disease extent, location, and nodal and metastatic spread. The primary modality of staging is CT, with MRI used as a problem-solving modality. In addition, PET scanning has an increasing role to play in the staging and follow-up of patients with lung carcinoma (73–80).

Staging

T Staging

It is often difficult to distinguish the tumor from distal collapsed or consolidated lung. Features that help in separating them include identifying mucus-filled bronchi and the differential enhancement of tumor from consolidation.

Extension of the tumor into the mediastinum needs multiplanar evaluation with either MRI or CT. Both appear to have similar accuracy in this respect. Indicators suggestive of resectability include: (a) <3 cm of mediastinal contact, (b) demonstration of a fat plane between the tumor and the mediastinal structures, and (c) <90 degrees of aortic contact. Imaging is better at determining resectability than nonresectability. CT studies using multidetector technology and reviewed in multiple planes on a workstation can help determine relationships with the airways and mediastinal and vascular structures. Postprocessing techniques such as virtual bronchoscopy help surgeons in planning their procedures (Figure 8.7). In the case of a peripheral tumor, diagnosing chest wall invasion can sometimes be a

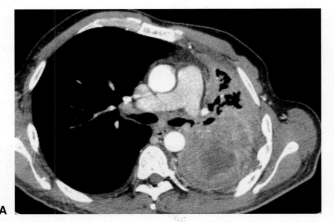

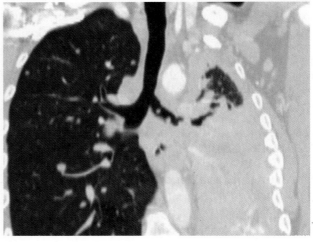

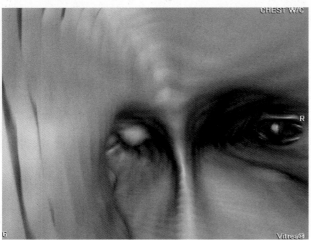

Figure 8.7 Axial contrast-enhanced computed tomography (CT) of thorax. (**A**) A heterogeneous mass is seen in the left lower lobe, extending to the left hilum with invasion of the left main bronchus. (**B**) Coronal maximum-intensity projection of the same image shows endobronchial extension of the tumor. (**C**) Virtual bronchoscopic image from the same CT study reveals endobronchial nodules (*arrow*) into the left main bronchus.

challenge because of the presence of inflammatory change or vascular engorgement (76,78,81).

N Stage

The detection of nodal disease has the same problems as elsewhere in the body, that is, difficulty in detecting metastatic disease in normal-sized nodes. Also, it is not possible to confidently diagnose reactive hyperplasia on imaging characteristics alone. There is an increasing use of [18]FDG-PET or PET-CT in these patients to determine which patients might need a mediastinoscopy. Some nodes are accessible for biopsy under CT or occasionally by endosonography (82–84).

M Stage

Common sites of metastases include the liver, adrenals, brain, and bone.

Renal Carcinoma

Recently there has been an increase in the incidence of renal carcinoma. These tumors, now accounting for about 3% of all newly diagnosed carcinomas, are often identified in asymptomatic patients who are being evaluated for other reasons (85). The radiologist contributes to treatment planning by providing critical information including tumor size and extent, relationship of the tumor with adjacent viscera and fat planes, nodal involvement, venous involvement, and adrenal and distant metastases.

Staging

T Stage

The ability of current imaging technology to depict the image data in multiple planes is especially useful in staging renal carcinoma. While accurate differentiation between Robson stage I and stage II is not needed for a radical nephrectomy, there is a need for additional information if a partial nephrectomy is contemplated. Most imaging techniques are not accurate for per-

inephric spread as they cannot differentiate accurately between perinephric spread of tumor from perinephric edema, fibrosis, or inflammatory stranding (86–88).

A single imaging test is usually sufficient to depict all the information the surgeon needs. This includes vascular supply and relationship of individual vessels to the tumor, presence of accessory vessels, and information about the collecting system, presence of nodes, and venous extension or thrombosis (89–91). Therefore, findings on imaging are among the most important factors in determining the type of surgery undertaken. It is important that the study is performed in multiple phases as different aspects of the tumor are optimally imaged in different phases. These phases include a noncontrast phase, an arterial phase that can be used to generate a CT angiogram and is also useful for identifying metastatic lesions in the liver and renal vein thrombus, a nephrographic phase that is the optimal phase for identifying tumor masses, and excretory phase to evaluate the pelvicalyceal systems, ureters, and the bladder. MRI and PET scans may provide additional or confirmatory information (Figures 8.8 and 8.9).

N Stage

As with tumors elsewhere, lymph node evaluation has the same accuracy with either CT or MRI.

M Stage

Liver metastases are typically hypervascular. Lesions may be identified on CT and MRI but lung lesions are better identified on CT.

Posttreatment Surveillance

Routine follow-up subsequent to nephrectomy should include imaging, although the timing and frequency depend on the stage of the disease and local policy.

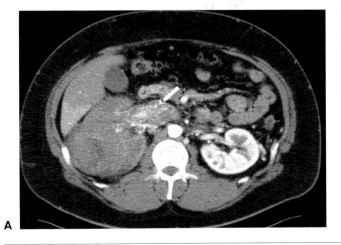
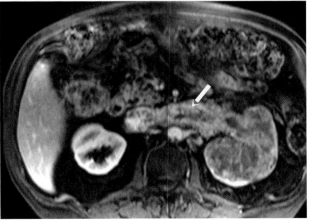

Figure 8.8 (**A**) Axial image of a contrast-enhanced computed tomography scan in a patient with a renal cell carcinoma arising from the right kidney. The *arrowhead* points to the inferior vena cava and the draining right renal vein, which are expanded by tumor thrombus. Tumor thrombus is differentiated from bland thrombus by the presence of enhancing thrombus in the arterial phase of contrast enhancement. (**B**) Axial T1-weighted magnetic resonance image following gadolinium injection in a patient with a left renal cell carcinoma with tumor thrombus extending into the left renal vein and inferior vein cava (*arrow*).

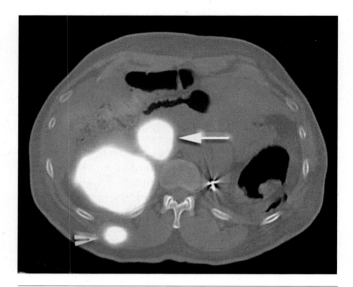

Figure 8.9 Axial fused image from an [18]FDG-PET-CT (18-fluoro-deoxy-D-glucose positron emission tomography-computed tomography) study in a patient with a renal cell carcinoma of the right kidney. The left kidney had previously been removed. A percutaneous biopsy of the right renal mass had been performed a few months before the scan was obtained. The *arrowhead* indicates a site of hypermetabolism, which was along the biopsy tract and is presumed to represent tract seeding. The *long arrow* indicates inferior vena cava invasion by tumor.

Bladder Carcinoma

Staging

T Stage

The primary tumors have traditionally been staged using cystoscopy and biopsies. However, the advent of high-resolution scans and postprocessing techniques such as virtual cystoscopy have evoked interest in using noninvasive imaging with CT or MRI (92). Bladder tumors enhance following intravenous contrast injection in the venous phase and therefore are well outlined (93,94). A smooth bladder wall suggests organ-confined disease. The use of multiplanar reconstructions including curved planes is important to demonstrate the extent of the tumor. Difficult areas include under- or overdistended bladders, tumors in diverticula, and scans following biopsies in which hemorrhage and edema can confound imaging appearances.

The role of CT and MRI is to accurately distinguish invasive bladder tumors with perivesical spread from those tumors confined to the bladder wall (95–98). Features suggesting invasive bladder carcinomas include retraction of bladder wall, infiltration into the perivesical fat, or an obvious soft-tissue mass seen outside the bladder. The demonstration of a smooth outer bladder wall at the site of the tumor suggests that the tumor is confined to the bladder. Currently it is not possible to accurately distinguish T1 and T2 tumors, that is, separate superficial from deep muscle invasion. Invasion of adjacent muscles is identified by noting masses that distort and enlarge the

muscles. MRI perhaps has a slight edge in staging early primary tumor (95).

N Stage

There is difficulty in distinguishing normal nodes from nodes with micrometastases. MRI lymphography is likely to improve nodal staging (99,100).

The role of [18]FDG-PET imaging is debated because of the low rate of hypermetabolism in nodes with metastases and the difficulty in assessing the primary tumor (101).

M Stage

Distal metastases are generally staged with CT because lung nodules, a common metastatic site, are not adequately visualized with MRI

Posttreatment Surveillance

This is generally done with CT and in selected cases with MRI (Figure 8.10).

Prostate Carcinoma

The mainstay of diagnosis for prostate carcinoma is elevated levels of prostate-specific antigen or abnormal digital rectal examination leading to histologic confirmation by transrectal US-guided biopsy.

Staging

T Stage

CT is of very limited use in evaluating the primary tumor. However, MRI can identify areas of prostatic carcinoma as areas of low signal intensity on T2-weighted images. Techniques such as endorectal coil imaging, dynamic contrast-enhanced MRI, and

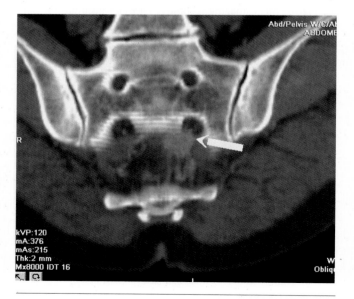

Figure 8.10 Contrast-enhanced computed tomography in a patient with previous history of transitional cell carcinoma now presenting with deep pelvic pain. Image reveals recurrent tumor causing nerve root compression (*arrow*).

MRI spectroscopy help in identifying the tumor extent and diagnosing capsular penetration (102–107).

N Stage

Lymph node staging can be performed with either CT or MRI. The first nodal group involved is usually the obturator nodes. It is unusual to find nodal disease when there is no capsule penetration. The role of MRI lymphangiography in detecting nodal disease in normal-sized nodes has been evaluated extensively (100,108).

M Stage

Distant metastases are usually evaluated with CT or bone scans.

Posttreatment Surveillance

Postoperative surveillance is usually done with CT for the assessment of distant metastases. Local recurrence is evaluated by transrectal US and MRI. Areas of concern undergo image-guided biopsy, if possible.

Testicular Tumors

Testicular tumors are primarily divided into germ cell tumors and non–germ cell tumors. Germ cell tumors are further divided into seminomas (commonest type) and the nonseminomatous germ cell tumors.

Staging

Knowledge of the patterns of spread is crucial in staging patients with testicular tumors. These tumors spread by vascular and lymphatic channels.

T Stage

Tumor staging is usually done by US alone. MRI is infrequently used (111).

N Stage

In general, right-sided tumors spread to the right-sided retroperitoneal nodes and the left-sided tumors spread to the left-sided nodes. A crossover is unusual until the nodes become bulky. Lymph node evaluation, namely the problem of identifying metastases in normal-sized nodes, is discussed elsewhere in this chapter. In general, lymph node metastases from seminomas are solid and those from nonseminomatous tumors may be heterogeneous or even cystic. Pelvic and inguinal lymphadenopathy is unusual, occurring only if there has been cryptorchidism or if there is blockage of the lymphatics by bulky nodes causing retrograde flow (112–114).

M Stage

Hematogenous spread results in spread to the lungs (115,116).

Posttreatment Surveillance

The mainstay of surveillance of these patients following resection is CT scans along with serum markers, if applicable (117–120).

Ovarian Carcinoma

The commonest ovarian tumor is of epithelial origin, with endometroid and sex cord stromal tumors forming a smaller fraction. Patients commonly present with an adnexal mass that is commonly first imaged using US. There are several features that help in distinguishing a benign from a malignant tumor. These include demonstration of irregular nodules, complex thick septations, and abnormal vascularity (121–125).

Staging

T Stage

Ultrasound scans done endovaginally are probably the best way to detect small tumors. MRI and US both can be used to characterize ovarian lesions. The extraovarian spread of tumors is better appreciated on MRI than on CT.

N Stage

Nodal assessment can be done with both MRI and CT (126–129). There is also significant interest in the use of [18]FDG-PET imaging (130).

M Stage

The primary modality of staging the tumor is CT. It can identify peritoneal implants, lymph node enlargement, and lung and liver lesions. It is important to recognize that ovarian carcinoma may spread directly into adjacent tissues, by the lymphatic or hematogenous pathways, or by the transcoelomic route. However, both CT and MRI can evaluate peritoneal disease. Contrast-enhanced studies increase the conspicuity of peritoneal nodules (131–133).

Posttreatment Surveillance

In monitoring for recurrent or residual disease, imaging is used in conjunction with laparoscopy and serum markers such as CA125. Ultrasound has a useful role in local monitoring but CT and MRI are used for monitoring the overall picture.

Retroperitoneal Tumors

The commonest modality used for identification and staging of retroperitoneal tumors is CT followed by MRI. Although differentiating retroperitoneal tumors from other abdominal tumors and processes is important, it is sometimes difficult to differentiate between subtypes of retroperitoneal tumors on imaging (134–138).

Both CT and MRI are of value in demonstrating the tumor and its extent, its relationship with adjacent viscera, vascular supply and involvement, and metastatic disease. As surgical resection of the tumor commonly includes resection of adjacent viscera, preoperative imaging should also illustrate relevant features of all regions surrounding the tumor. Because the kidney is one of the commonest organs to be resected with the primary tumor, demonstration of a normal contralateral kidney is important (Figure 8.11).

Posttreatment Surveillance

Radiographic surveillance employing CT or MRI following surgery is routinely performed because of the high incidence of recurrence. A baseline study is important to document postoperative changes (136,139).

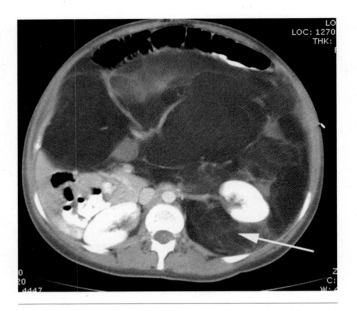

Figure 8.11 Contrast-enhanced computed tomography in a case of a retroperitoneal sarcoma. The tumor (*arrow*) has displaced the kidney anteriorly, indicating a retroperitoneal origin.

Melanoma

In the evaluation of patients with invasive melanoma, various imaging modalities are employed to assess nodal status and evidence of disseminated disease.

T Stage

The cutaneous tumor is assessed on biopsy material using the microstaging systems of Breslow and Clark. Imaging has a limited role, although CT scanning or MRI are occasionally indicated to determine local invasion of underlying vessels, nerves, muscle, or bone in thick melanomas.

N Stage

The staging of intermediate-thickness primary melanomas according to the results of sentinel node biopsy has been shown to provide important prognostic information and identifies patients with clinically occult nodal metastases whose survival can be prolonged by immediate lymphadenectomy (140). The sentinel nodes can be identified and removed by dissection in the relevant nodal basin after the peritumoral intradermal injection of a vital dye, such as isosulfan blue, or a radiocolloid, such as Tc-99m-sulfur colloid or after the injection of both markers. In many centers, a radiocolloid is injected in the nuclear medicine department 1 to 2 hours before operation and a lymphoscintogram obtained to localize the sentinel node or nodes. At operation, a gamma probe is used to identify the "hot" nodes that should be biopsied. In patients having lesions with ambiguous nodal drainage (such as the mid-back), all the potential draining regional nodal basins should be scanned after injection of the radiocolloid (141,142).

Numerous studies have demonstrated that PET scanning has a low sensitivity, 0% to 40%, for detecting sentinel node metastases, with worse results for smaller-sized lesions. It is more specific than sensitive (143).

M Stage

Symptomatic patients have imaging studies based on the clinical presentation. Routine body imaging in asymptomatic patients, including those with occult sentinel node metastases, is not indicated because disseminated disease is rarely identified (144,145). At the University of Southern California's Norris Comprehensive Cancer Center, asymptomatic patients with advanced local lesions (Breslow thickness >2 mm with ulceration or >4 mm) and those with palpable metastatic adenopathy generally undergo further preoperative staging, usually with CT-PET imaging, although there is no consensus about the indications or benefits for such systemic imaging (146).

Surveillance and Monitoring

Patients found to have additional nodal involvement on completion lymphadenectomy for a positive sentinel node may warrant systemic scanning for metastatic disease. Again, there is no consensus on the appropriate periodic surveillance of patients who remain asymptomatic after treatment of the primary locoregional disease (146).

Different modalities have different advantages in various regions of the body, and a single imaging test cannot optimally image melanoma throughout the body. Cerebral metastases are usually multiple and supratentorial. For evaluation of brain metastases, a contrast-enhanced MRI scan is more sensitive than CT. On MRI, the features are variable with only a quarter demonstrating the classic features of high signal on T1-weighted images and low signal on T2-weighted images. On CT, the features include high attenuation, perilesional edema, and enhancement on contrast injection.

Skin and soft-tissue metastases are the commonest sites for malignant melanoma, with many lesions being clinically evident. These lesions can be identified with most imaging modalities although the specificity may be low. Second echelon lymph nodes (e.g., pelvic nodes in the case of lower extremity melanomas) are evaluated adequately with all imaging modalities using characteristics described elsewhere in this chapter. Lung nodules are best identified with CT. Within the abdomen, both CT and MRI studies can be used to identify metastatic lesions (Figure 8.12). Melanoma is the commonest cause of metastases to the gastrointestinal tract including the gallbladder. Small bowel deposits can often precipitate intussusceptions and small bowel obstruction.

Lymphoma
Staging

CT is the dominant imaging modality for evaluation of lymphoma because it can demonstrate the extent of the disease, it is readily reproducible, and it can image the whole body including the lungs (Figure 8.13). CT scanning also is an excellent method of determining a site for biopsy (147–153). Compared to CT, US has its limitations in the retroperitoneum. There are no specific features of affected nodes on US. However, US is of use in evaluating focal indeterminate lesions in the liver, kidneys, or spleen. These lesions appear hypoechoic and may be lobulated (154). On MRI, appearances are nonspecific, with nodes appearing as low-to-intermediate signal intensity masses on

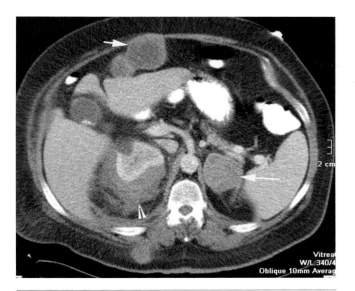

Figure 8.12 Axial image in a patient with melanoma. There are melanoma deposits in the left adrenal gland (*long arrow*), right perinephric space (*arrowhead*), peritoneal cavity (*short arrow*), and the subcutaneous tissues of the back.

T1-weighted images and are of intermediate-to-high signal intensity on T2-weighted images. Following treatment, some of the nodes may become necrotic (150,155).

All these imaging modalities, however, are limited by the difficulty in identifying disease in normal-sized nodes and

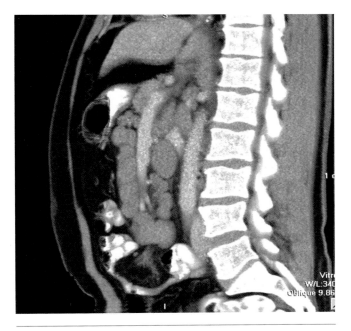

Figure 8.13 Sagittal reformatted computed tomography image in a patient of non-Hodgkin lymphoma with extensive mesenteric adenopathy. This appearance is referred to as the *burger sign,* with the nodes on either side of the superior mesenteric vessels representing the two halves of the bun.

in differentiating reactive hyperplasia from involved nodes. Theoretically, gallium 67 and PET scans using [18]FDG can identify viable tumor tissue in these two groups of nodes. However, they are both limited by the relative low spatial resolution (2 cm for gallium and 8 to 10 mm for PET scans). The use of PET-CT may change the imaging approach combining the advantages of both techniques. PET-CT has also been used to assess prognosis (156–158).

There is an increasing acceptance of image-guided percutaneous biopsy rather than open biopsy in the management of lymphoma. This can be used for diagnosis of the disease, defining the nature of a residual mass after treatment or the detection of transformation to a higher grade (159).

The evaluation of residual disease is another issue that has vexed clinicians. [18]FDG-PET scans or serial CT scans are used to differentiate fibrosis from recurrence or residual disease (158,160–162).

COMMON QUESTIONS POSED TO THE RADIOLOGIST BY THE SURGEON

Is There Peritoneal Carcinomatosis?

This is a common question put before a radiologist by oncologists, surgeons, and also other radiologists. Peritoneal carcinomatosis is not difficult to diagnose when it is obvious, but the problem arises in the early stages when it is subtle. Knowledge of the anatomy and embryology of the peritoneum, the behavior of specific tumors, recognition of the strengths and limitations of various imaging modalities, and experience play an important part in the recognition of peritoneal disease. The sensitivity of CT and MRI is similar, around 40% to 50%, although published results are for lesions larger than 2 cm (163,164). US can identify smaller lesions in the presence of ascites, although central lesions in ligaments and mesentery are easy to miss (165,166). Occasionally the site of implants is noted on barium studies. Peritoneal carcinomatosis is often difficult to identify on [18]FDG-PET as it is difficult to separate implants from bowel activity. In addition, some common mucinous tumors from the ovary and colon have low cellularity and do not exhibit significant hypermetabolism (167).

Early peritoneal implants appear as soft-tissue nodules that later coalesce to form plaques or omental cakes. All lesions are easier to identify in the presence of ascites. Some of these may enhance and may even calcify. Common sites of implants include the pelvis, the right paracolic gutter, the omentum and other ligaments, the bowel, around the liver, and the sigmoid mesocolon. Implants may be of low density and similar to ascitic fluid. Lesions could produce a scalloped appearance of the surface of liver or spleen. The omentum could appear thickened or have an infiltrated appearance (Figure 8.14). Peritoneal implants can be targeted for biopsy under either US or CT. Imaging recognition of implants is also important to assess sites for therapeutic or diagnostic paracentesis (168,169). A difficulty in assessing disease progression is the mobility of these lesions along with the omentum and bowel, so a careful review of the entire scan is necessary before commenting on particular lesions (170–172).

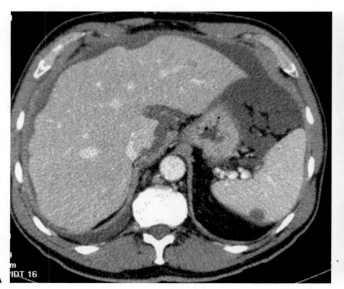
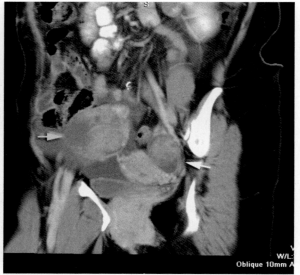

Figure 8.14 (**A**) Axial contrast-enhanced computed tomography (CT). Peritoneal carcinomatosis in a patient with colonic carcinoma. The peritoneal deposits are seen to cause a scalloped appearance on the surface of the liver and the spleen. (**B**) Oblique coronal CT image in a patient with gastric carcinoma with bilateral ovarian implants (*arrows*), the so called Krukenberg tumors.

Can We Biopsy It or Drain It?

In general, if a lesion can be seen on an imaging modality it usually can be targeted for biopsy. However, the referring physician and the radiologist should discuss the following issues: (A) the potential for tract seeding; (B) transgression of barriers such as the pleura, peritoneum, and diaphragm; and (C) transgression through organs such as the liver or bowel. The question the radiologist should ask the surgeon is, "Do you want it done?" The answer depends on the individual clinical scenario. A biopsy may be needed to stage the disease or may be needed when imaging is equivocal or conflicting. It may also be needed when residual or recurrent disease is suspected.

If a biopsy is requested, the next decision to be made is whether a fine-needle aspiration biopsy or a core biopsy is most appropriate. This depends on numerous factors including the experience of the radiologist, pathologist, or cytologist, type of tumor, and the risk of injuring nerves, vessels, or adjacent organs when using a larger-bore needle.

Guidance for the procedure can be with US, CT, MRI, fluoroscopy, or CT-fluoroscopy, the first two being the commonest. Each modality has its advantages and limitations. The advantages of US include its portability, the lack of radiation, and real-time imaging. Its drawbacks are difficulty with some deep lesions, nonvisualization because of overlying bowel, air, or bone. The drawbacks of CT include the use of ionizing radiation, and it is a relatively more time-consuming procedures. The advantages are numerous, including excellent demonstration of the tract, and high spatial and contrast resolution.

Biopsy techniques can be modified to access difficult target areas. Examples include the following. (a) Use of saline to displace vital structures. An alternative is graded compression to displace loops of bowel during US. (b) Use of curved needles. (c) Positioning the patient in a nonstandard position so

the lesion is more accessible. (d) Plugged liver biopsies in selected coagulopathic patients. An alternative is to use transjugular biopsies in which a specialized needle is passed from the internal jugular vein to the hepatic vein via the inferior vena cava. Any bleeding from the procedure would be into the patient's circulation.

The previous discussion holds true for drainages as well (Figure 8.15). An important point to consider is whether the surgeon wants an indwelling catheter placed into what could be a sterile collection. In doubtful cases, a decision could be made after aspirating the fluid and proceeding with a drain placement if the fluid appears infected.

Can We Get a Scan?

An imaging test should be performed to provide the maximum possible information for clinical decision-making and should reduce the number of inappropriate tests. There should be a strong emphasis on preventing the development of duplicate information from the use of more than one imaging technique. It is often very helpful to consult with the radiologist before ordering more tests. The radiologist may suggest modifying the technique, for example, using oral water, and additional contrast such as rectal contrast or contrast in the urinary bladder, depending on the circumstances. MRI as a modality is especially flexible and is often modified to answer the relevant question.

Imaging patients with special needs such those with renal failure, patients with hypersensitivity to contrast, and critically ill patients who are dependent on life support equipment can be performed by different methods depending on the question that needs to be answered. For example, a plain radiograph is sometimes all that is necessary to detect and evaluate a pleural effusion. A portable or limited US study is all that is necessary

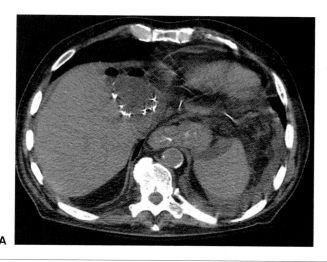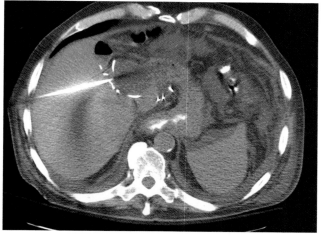

A   B

Figure 8.15 Axial computed tomography scans of the upper abdomen. (**A**) Perihepatic collection suspected to be an abscess following left hepatic resection. (**B**) The safest access to place a drain was thought to be through the right lobe of the liver.

to evaluate for biliary obstruction or obstructive uropathy or to localize fluid collections.

Why Are the Measurements Calculated on Another Recently Done Scan so Different From the Current Measurements?

This question highlights the importance of using the same techniques and radiology department, if feasible. Oncoradiology measurements are complex. The RECIST (response evaluation criteria in solid tumors) and its predecessor, the WHO criteria defined standard measurements in order to convert subjective data interpretation into quantitative data that could be tracked. While there remain unquestioned advantages in using RECIST, there are a number of areas in which there is variability in its application. These include problems in evaluating cystic metastases, ascites, difficulty in distinguishing lung lesions from adjacent areas of atelectasis, posttreatment changes in gastrointestinal stromal tumors, and difficulty in using [18]FDG-PET-CT data (173–176).

Are the Surrounding Lymph Nodes Involved?

One of the problems of current imaging techniques is that it is highly sensitive in identifying lymph nodes but not specific in determining whether the nodes are involved with metastatic foci. Traditionally, size-based criteria are used to distinguish between involved nodes and normal nodes. This strategy results in missing metastases in normal-sized nodes. On the other hand, there is an inability to distinguish reactive hyperplasia from involved nodes. This is especially important in pelvic malignancies such as prostate, rectal, and bladder carcinomas (177–179).

Features suggestive of a malignant node:

- Enlarged size
- Round rather than elongated shape
- Loss of fat in the hilum as it is replaced by malignant cells.
- Neovascularity

- Irregular contour
- Cystic or heterogeneous composition in some tumors

Imaging Modalities

Ultrasound

Although US is very good for identifying superficial nodes, it has its limitations in the pelvis and the retroperitoneum. Various criteria have been proposed, especially for thyroid carcinoma (180–182).

CT and MRI

Using size-based criteria, the sensitivity with these modalities is between 30% and 40%. Although contrast-enhanced studies occasionally maybe useful (Figure 8.16), using enhancement

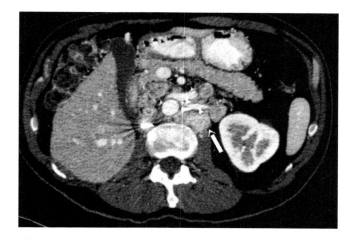

Figure 8.16 Axial contrast-enhanced computed tomography in a patient with extensive retroperitoneal lymphadenopathy. The *arrow* points to hypervascular nodes in the para-aortic group in a patient with renal cell carcinoma.

characteristics has not resulted in practical applications in everyday use.

¹⁸FDG PET

The role of PET depends on the type of cancer. Although it is extremely useful in identifying nodal metastases in lung cancer, it has limitations in urologic cancer; carcinoids, and bronchioalveolar carcinoma because of its low uptake. False-negative outcomes are possible in nodes that are smaller than 1 cm. However, the sensitivity is probably more than conventional cross-sectional imaging (183–186).

USPIO (Ultrasmall Super Paramagnetic Iron Oxide Particles) MRI Imaging

This is a technique used for intravenous MRI lymphangiography. It depends on the fact that metastases in a lymph node replace the normal phagocytic cells. On intravenous injection, USPIO tends to accumulate in lymph nodes, causing a signal loss on both T1- and T2-weighted sequences (187,188) (Figure 8.17).

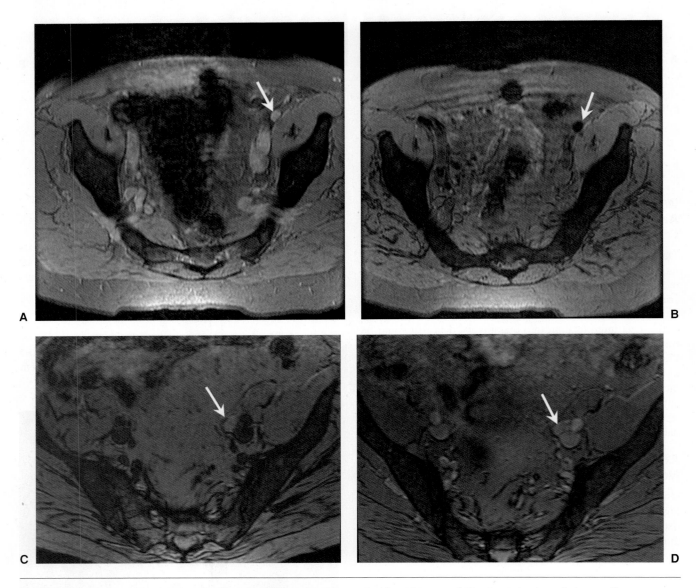

Figure 8.17 Magnetic resonance image of lymphangiography. T2-weighted axial images following injection of ultrasmall super paramagnetic iron oxide particles (USPIO). Contrast is injected intravenously and is taken up by reticuloendothelial cells in lymph nodes. Normal nodes therefore demonstrate a reduction in the intensity following USPIO. Metastatic tumor replaces the reticuloendothelial cells so there is no reduction in the intensity. (**A**) T2-weighted axial image demonstrating a prominent left external iliac node (*arrow*). (**B**) T2-weighted image. The same node demonstrates a reduction in the intensity (*arrow*) following intravenous USPIO injection and is therefore a "benign" node. (**C**) T2-weighted image. Left internal iliac node (*arrow*). (**D**) T2-weighted image following USPIO. There is no drop in the intensity of the node (*arrow*) due to replacement of the reticuloendothelial cells with metastatic cells. (Images courtesy of Mukesh Harisinghani, MD, Boston, MA.)

Lymphoscintigraphy

This nuclear medicine scan has an established role in the detection of the sentinel node or nodes in melanoma and breast carcinomas.

Histologic Confirmation

Lymph nodes can be biopsied under image guidance. Superficial nodes are well targeted by US.

Are These Small Pulmonary Nodules Likely to Represent Metastatic Disease?

Because of the widespread use of multislice CT and routine acquisition of thin sections, it is very common to demonstrate small pulmonary nodules. If calcification is demonstrated in these lesions it is likely to represent old granulomatous disease, with the exception of calcified metastases from tumors such as osteosarcoma. However, the significance of noncalcified nodules is difficult to establish. Most of these represent old granulomas or a residue of past inflammation. However, this cannot be confirmed. They are too small to biopsy and are too small to be demonstrated on an ^{18}FDG-PET study.

These nodules may be evaluated further by performing high-resolution CT of the lung, by which pattern recognition can narrow the differential diagnosis. High-resolution CT also allows the detection of lymphangitic or interstitial spread of disease.

Most oncologic radiologists approach this problem in a practical manner. In the authors' department, these nodules are documented and followed if they measure over 2 to 3 mm. If the size or number of nodules increases, then metastatic disease can be suspected. However, differential diagnoses such as inflammatory nodules and drug-induced pulmonary reactions have to be considered (189–192).

The advent of computer-aided detection programs may increase the efficiency with which these nodules are analyzed. These programs help in identifying, comparing, and characterizing multiple nodules. They aim to increase the diagnostic confidence and accuracy of the radiologist (193,194).

Is There Bowel Obstruction?

Bowel obstruction is one of the commonest surgical emergencies in oncology patients. It may be due to a number of causes including an obstructing colorectal carcinoma, a metastatic mass impinging on the bowel, a stricture complicating radiation therapy peritoneal carcinomatosis, or benign adhesions. The surgeon often asks the following questions: (a) Is there obstruction or is this a nonobstructive ileus pattern? (b) Is the obstruction complete or incomplete? (c) What is the level and the cause of obstruction?

In the postoperative period it is often difficult to differentiate between a mechanical obstruction from a paralytic ileus. CT scans, especially current multislice CT studies, are an elegant way of differentiating these conditions and also in localizing the site and cause of the obstruction. The data set is evaluated by creating multiplanar reconstructions on the CT workstation and then reviewing the data interactively (Figure 8.18). CT scans are a more efficient way of demonstrating obstruction than oral contrast studies. They offer more rapid results with the advantage of providing additional information about the other abdominal viscera (195–199).

Is the Adrenal Mass an Incidental Adenoma or Is It a Metastatic Lesion?

One result of the higher spatial resolution obtained on modern imaging is that there is an increase in the number of adrenal

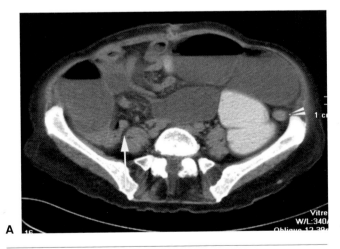
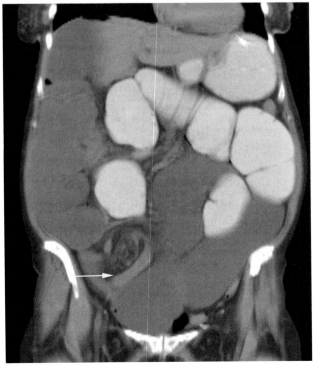

Figure 8.18 (A) Axial computed tomography (CT) image in a patient with a previously resected colonic carcinoma. The *arrow* points to the collapsed small bowel loop distal to the obstruction in this patient with small bowel obstruction due to adhesions. The *arrowhead* identifies the collapsed large bowel. **(B)** Coronal reconstruction of the same study. The level of obstruction is again seen (*arrow*). The level of bowel obstruction can be diagnosed on a CT study by using multiplanar reformations on a workstation.

nodules detected. It has been known that the adrenals are a frequent site for metastases after the lungs, liver, and the bones. In patients dying of cancer, autopsies have revealed that up to 27% of patients have adrenal metastases. The common primary tumors causing adrenal metastases include breast, bronchus, melanoma, colon, and kidney. On the other hand, it is very common to find adrenal adenomas in the normal population, with a reported incidence between 1%–8.7% (200). Conformation that an adrenal lesion is metastatic has a significant effect on the patient's treatment as it usually indicates that the patient has disseminated disease (except in an ipsilateral renal cell carcinoma). The challenge for radiologists now is to detect adrenal lesions that are small and do not necessarily enlarge the adrenal gland and also to be more specific about adrenal lesions. Applying only size criteria to adrenal glands in oncology patients results in a low positive as well as a low negative predictive value for metastases (201,202).

Accurate evaluation of an adrenal mass leads to a reduction in the number of unnecessary percutaneous biopsies and to the appropriate staging of the patient's disease. It is important to note that adrenal masses that are >3 cm are malignant in 90% to 95% of cases and, on the other hand, that bilateral adrenal enlargement does not confirm metastatic disease.

Evaluation of an Adrenal Mass

US

It is difficult to image the adrenals consistently on US and it is difficult to distinguish a metastasis from an adenoma.

CT Scan

The majority of adrenal adenomas are lipid-rich and, therefore, have a low attenuation value on unenhanced CT scans. Using a threshold of 10 Hounsfield units on a nonenhanced CT, a sensitivity of 71% and a specificity of 98% for the diagnosis of an adrenal adenoma is achieved (Figure 8.19). The exceptions to this include adrenal myelolipomas, and the very rare cases of a fat-containing pheochromocytoma or a fat-containing metastasis.

Lipid-poor adenomas can be diagnosed using a washout study on CT. This test can be applied to relatively homogenous masses with no large areas of necrosis or hemorrhage. It is based on the principle that a benign adenoma will enhance and lose its contrast (washout) faster. Based on numerous studies the following criteria are applied. (a) A washout value of >60% is associated with an 88% sensitivity and a 96% specificity for the diagnosis of an adrenal adenoma. (b) If an unenhanced scan is not available then an alternative method is to calculate the

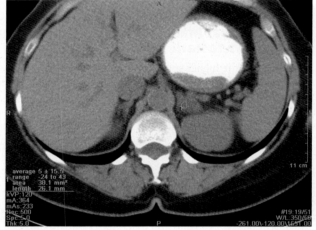

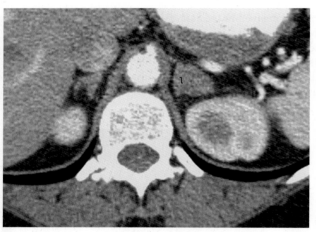

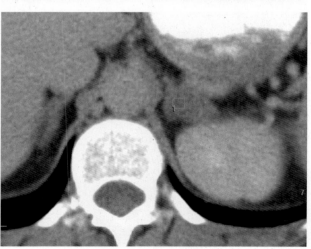

Figure 8.19 A left adrenal mass was identified in a patient with colorectal carcinoma. (**A**) The noncontrast-enhanced image reveals the nodule to have a density of 15 Hounsfield units. The nodule enhances to 84 Hounsfield units on the venous phase (**B**) and then decreases to 32 Hounsfield units on the delayed phase (**C**). These findings are indicative of a benign lesion.

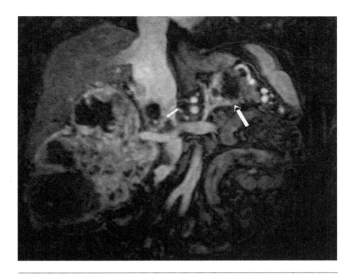

Figure 8.20 A coronal image from a T1-weighted postgadolinium study in a patient with a renal cell carcinoma. The *larger arrow* indicates the left adrenal metastasis and the *smaller arrow* identifies the tumor invading the inferior vena cava.

relative washout where a relative washout value of >40% has a sensitivity of 96% to 100% and a specificity of 100% for the diagnosis of an adrenal adenoma (202–206).

MRI

A variety of sequences are used to distinguish between benign and metastatic lesions. These include contrast-enhanced imaging, chemical shift, and fat-saturation techniques. Chemical shift imaging relies on the presence of intracellular lipid in adenomas (207–211) (Figure 8.20).

PET Scan

[18]FDG-PET imaging has a very high specificity for the diagnosis of adrenal metastases but there is a difficulty in identifying small lesions (212).

If despite all of these imaging modalities a mass remains indeterminate, it can be easily biopsied under image guidance. If the lesion proves to be metastatic, there is the option of treating isolated adrenal metastases percutaneously by various forms of ablation, including cryoablation and radiofrequency ablation (213–215).

THE ACUTE SURGICAL ABDOMEN IN ONCOLOGY PATIENTS

Imaging plays a significant part in the diagnosis and management of oncology patients who may present with an acute surgical abdomen. It is extremely important for the radiologist to be fully aware of the clinical history and previous treatment while interpreting these studies. The causes of the acute abdomen may be an incidental condition and not necessarily be related to the patient's malignant disease process (216).

An important point to consider in this situation is the fact that neutropenic patients will not mount a significant response, so the inflammatory changes that one expects to see in these patients is significantly reduced and muted.

Appendicitis

CT findings include periappendiceal inflammatory changes and an abnormal-appearing appendix (e.g., diameter >6 mm, a thickened wall, or an intraluminal appendicolith resulting in obstruction). There may be evidence of rupture or abscess formation (217–220).

Diverticulitis

There may be evidence of inflammatory changes and evidence of a pericolic collection. A colonic carcinoma may also present this way, and often it is difficult to differentiate a colorectal tumor with a pericolic collection from a diverticular abscess (221–223).

Typhlitis

The imaging features of typhlitis (neutropenic enterocolitis) include circumferential and occasionally eccentric low-attenuation colonic wall thickening and cecal distention and inflammatory stranding. Complications such as hemorrhage, pneumatosis coli, and perforation and abscess are well seen (224–226) (Figure 8.21).

Cholecystitis

The classic features noted on US include probe tenderness over the gallbladder (sonographic Murphy's sign), thickening and separation of gallbladder wall, and pericholecystic fluid (227–229) (Figure 8.22).

Wandering Spleen and Splenic Torsion

One of the causes of a wandering spleen is splenomegaly, as seen in some cases of myeloid leukemia. Following treatment, the spleen may reduce in size, leading to laxity of the splenic

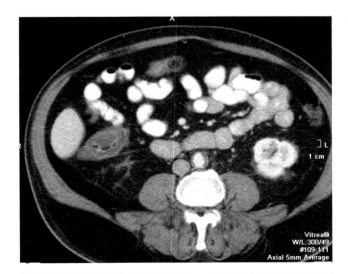

Figure 8.21 Axial image in a patient with neutropenia. There is asymmetric wall thickening of the cecum with mild pericecal inflammatory change.

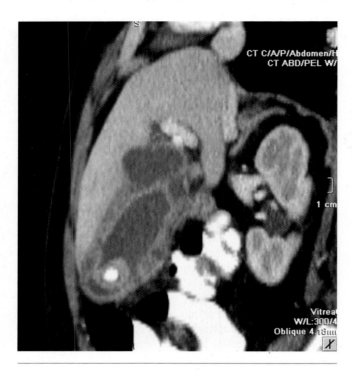

Figure 8.22 Oblique sagittal contrast-enhanced computed tomography. Abnormal thickening of the gallbladder wall in a case of calculous cholecystitis.

ligaments The spleen is now able to "wander" as well as be liable for torsion (230–232) (Figure 8.23).

Acute Abdominal Bleeding

A tumor may present with spontaneous intra-abdominal hemorrhage. Vascular hepatic tumors, such as hepatocellular carcinomas and hepatic adenomas and some vascular metastases, can present in this manner (Figure 8.24). Also, patients with renal carcinoma may occasionally have colic due to clot resulting from bleeding into the pelvicalyceal system.

Bowel Perforation

Classic signs and symptoms of perforation may be masked or be unrecognized because of the patient's condition. Perforations may be seen because of primary tumor perforation or in cases with bowel obstruction.

IMAGE-GUIDED INTERVENTION

Along with the rapid advances in imaging techniques and equipment there has been a significant increase in the scope and number of image-guided interventional techniques used in the management of oncology patients. These range from simple biopsies to treatment options such as percutaneous ablations. Some of these techniques, such as cryoablation and hepatobiliary procedures, have been dealt with elsewhere in this book.

There have been a significant number of technical advances and innovations in the development of needles, drains, and catheters. In numerous instances, discussing the case with the radiologist may result in a solution that had not been previously considered. In the postoperative state, it is important for good communication between the surgical team and radiology so that the radiologist is aware of the surgery performed. In cases in which there is an invasive procedure being considered, very often a minimally invasive way is feasible by the radiologist (233–235).

Biopsies

There have been numerous technical developments, such as new needles, better US probes, including endoscopic US probes, and CT fluoroscopy, the application of which have largely supplanted the need for open or laparoscopic biopsies. In addition, the availability of these technical advances has resulted in fewer areas heretofore deemed inaccessible for percutaneous biopsy. For example, the use of low-dose CT fluoroscopy has resulted in a significant increase in the yield of lung biopsies (236–242).

Among the newer tools available is a hand-held high-energy gamma probe that detects [18]FDG. This probe can be used intraoperatively to guide the surgeon to the site of the tissue of interest for biopsy. Thus, a lesion that is hypermetabolic on a PET scan but is not visible on a CT scan can be targeted by this technique. The patient is injected with [18]FDG. Then the lesion is targeted for biopsy under CT imaging on the basis of anatomic landmarks. The biopsy specimen is then scrutinized in the operating room for the presence of [18]FDG with the gamma probe to confirm that the correct tissue has been sampled (243).

Drainages

It has been well documented in literature that image-guided procedures including drain placement are safer than the corresponding nonguided procedures (244,245). These procedures could be either drainages of simple fluid collections such as thoracentesis or paracentesis. Many patients require indwelling drainage catheters, and these are again easier and safer to place under image guidance. In the thorax, these collections could result from the primary disease or complications of treatment resulting in empyemas or pulmonary abscesses. US- or CT-guided thoracentesis or drain placements are routinely done. Larger-bore catheters are used for sclerotherapy or complex collections. In the abdomen and the pelvis, fluid collections and abscesses may develop primarily or in the postoperative state. These are easily drained using either CT or US guidance (246–250) (Figure 8.25).

Stenting in the Gastrointestinal Tract

There are numerous palliative options for treating patients with inoperable malignancies of the gastrointestinal tract who are suffering from obstructive signs and symptoms. These include palliative surgery, radiotherapy (both external as well as intracavitary), stent placement, laser therapy, and photodynamic therapy. The choice of treatment is influenced by the fact that most of these patients have a poor prognosis with a short median survival time and the considerable morbidity and mortality rate of most surgical procedures. Oncologic therapy needs to be coordinated, and a multidisciplinary team should consider the various options and choose the most appropriate palliative measure to relieve the obstruction (251).

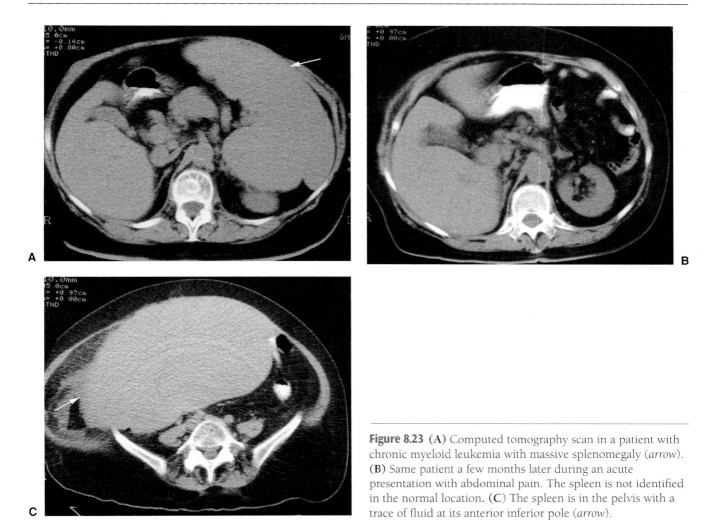

Figure 8.23 (**A**) Computed tomography scan in a patient with chronic myeloid leukemia with massive splenomegaly (*arrow*). (**B**) Same patient a few months later during an acute presentation with abdominal pain. The spleen is not identified in the normal location. (**C**) The spleen is in the pelvis with a trace of fluid at its anterior inferior pole (*arrow*).

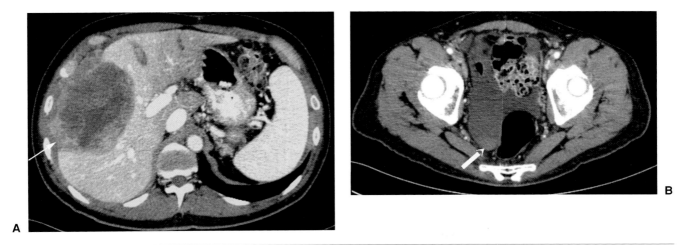

Figure 8.24 (**A**) Contrast-enhanced computed tomography of the liver. A liver mass has extended through the capsule of the liver with bleeding into the peritoneal cavity (*arrow*) as evidenced by high density (*arrow*) seen in the pelvis on image (**B**).

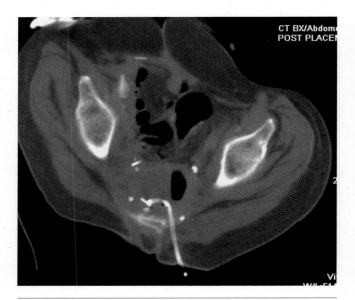

Figure 8.25 Axial contrast-enhanced computed tomography (CT) following placement of a percutaneous drain to treat a presacral collection. The drain was placed under CT guidance using a route through the greater sacrosciatic notch.

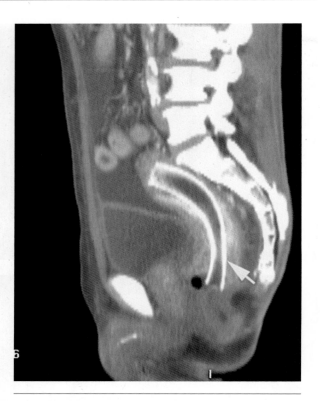

Figure 8.26 A patient with colorectal carcinoma with an obstructive lesion at the rectosigmoid (*arrow*). The obstruction was relieved by stenting.

In the upper gastrointestinal tract, stents have an important role as a palliative option in the management of esophageal carcinoma. They offer a minimally invasive method of restoring luminal patency. Newer devices with built-in antireflux devices allow stenting across the gastroesophageal junction. In cases with fistulas, such as those at anastomotic sites, covered stents that can be removed offer an alternative to extensive and difficult surgery (252–254).

Among patients with colorectal malignancy, 10% to 30% have large intestinal obstruction at presentation, with the site of obstruction commonly being in the left colon. Acute colonic obstruction is an emergency condition that can rapidly lead to perforation, metabolic and electrolyte disturbances, intestinal ischemia, and sepsis. Surgical options for colonic obstruction are either a one-stage resection and anastomosis or, more commonly, a two-stage procedure with colostomy. Emergency surgery in these patients is associated with significant morbidity and mortality (255–257). Stenting is a minimally invasive alternative choice that replaces the need for a colostomy in selected cases, with a significant number of advantages (Figure 8.26). If the patient is deemed operable, the tumor can be resected along with the stent electively after relief of the obstruction. In patients who are deemed inoperable, the stent replaces the need for a permanent colostomy. Here the minimally invasive stenting procedure is associated with improved quality of life of the terminally ill patient inasmuch as the obstruction is relieved, and the morbidity and mental stress associated with the creation and management of a stoma is obviated (257,258).

Applications in the Genitourinary Tract

One of the commonest procedures in oncologic image-guided intervention is the percutaneous nephrostomy. It is commonly used to relieve urinary tract obstruction prior to stenting or is used for urinary diversion.

Therapeutic arterial embolization is an option in the management of renal and pelvic malignancies. This technique can be used to control pain and also to reduce the size and vascularity of the tumor, thereby facilitating resection and reducing intraoperative blood loss. Radiologic techniques can also be used to dilate postoperative strictures, such as those following prostatectomy.

Ablation Techniques

Various image-guided ablative techniques have been developed to treat an array of tumors, including treatment with drugs, such as percutaneous ethanol injection; thermal energy, including radiofrequency, microwave, laser, and high-intensity focused US; ionizing radiation, such as brachytherapy; photodynamic and laser therapy; and cryoablation (Figure 8.27). These techniques have been used to manage primary as well as secondary tumors. The choice of the technique depends on the individual patient and tumor as well as operator experience. These treatment modalities are often combined with surgery or other systemic therapy (259).

Other Applications in the Thorax

Additional applications of image-guided intervention in the thorax include placement of central venous access ports, recanalization of veins in central venous occlusion syndromes, including thrombolysis and stenting, bronchial artery embolization in cases of intractable hemoptysis, and tracheobronchial stenting.

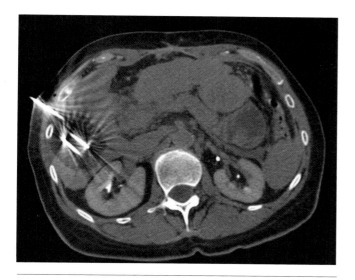

Figure 8.27 Axial computed tomography (CT) image obtained during a CT-guided cryoablation for hepatocellular carcinoma. The ice ball formed around the ablation needles is well seen. (Courtesy of Michael Katz, MD, University of Southern California, Los Angeles.)

Other Applications in the Abdomen

Various procedures to support enteral nutrition, including percutaneous gastrostomy and placement of gastrojejunostomy tubes, are routinely performed in the radiology department. Palliative procedures such as nerve plexus blocks are used to alleviate pain. Dilation of anastomotic strictures throughout the gastrointestinal tract is a well-established procedure. It can be performed on an outpatient basis and can be repeated if necessary

IMAGING FOR RADIATION ONCOLOGY

There have been dramatic advances in the delivery of radiotherapy because of the advent of conformal and intensity-modulated radiotherapy and gating technology. This has allowed the geometric shaping of the radiation beam along with modulation of its intensity. This has resulted in a reduction of the volume of otherwise normal tissue that is radiated.

The radiologist and the radiation oncologist interact in a variety of ways to provide optimum care. The radiologist assists in:

- Plotting the target volumes with the radiation oncologists
- Obtaining three-dimensional measurements of the tumor
- Providing details of adjacent viscera and tissues
- Correlating functional and morphologic imaging in selected cases
- Placing fiducial markers for radiotherapy or even placing the sources in the tumor, as in brachytherapy for the prostate and the biliary system

CONCLUSIONS

Significant developments in the management of cancer patients, including new surgical techniques, availability of a new array of potent chemotherapeutic agents, and more effective and safer radiotherapy, have been accompanied by equally dramatic advances in diagnostic and interventional radiology and imaging. Modern imaging techniques are able to provide both anatomic and functional data, which have led to an increased ability to accurately evaluate and stage malignant disease and monitor the effects of treatment in patients with cancer.

The radiologist is, therefore, an integral member of the multidisciplinary team managing the cancer patient during all stages of diagnosis and treatment.

REFERENCES

1. Jemal A, Siegel R, Ward E, et al. Cancer statistics, 2008. *CA Cancer J Clin*. 2008;58:71–96.
2. Hoffman JM, Gambhir SS. Molecular imaging: the vision and opportunity for radiology in the future. *Radiology*. 2007;244:39–47.
3. Duddalwar VA. Multislice CT angiography: a practical guide to CT angiography in vascular imaging and intervention. *Br J Radiol*. 2004;771:S27–38.
4. Alexander M, Brasic JR. The diagnosis of esophageal cancer by 2-deoxy-2-F-18 fluoro-D-glucose positron emission tomography (F-18 FDG PET). *Clinical Nuclear Medicine*. 2006;31(9):566–567.
5. Korst RJ, Altorki NK. Imaging for esophageal tumors. *Thorac.Surg.Clin*. 2004;14(1):61–69.
6. Maruyama M. Early gastrointestinal cancers. *Abdom Imaging*. 2003;28(4):456–463.
7. Lowe VJ, Booya F, Fletcher JG, et al. Comparison of positron emission tomography, computed tomography, and endoscopic ultrasound in the initial staging of patients with esophageal cancer. *Mol.Imaging Biol*. 2005;7(6):422–430.
8. Mazzeo S, Caramella D, Gennai A, et al. Multidetector CT and virtual endoscopy in the evaluation of the esophagus. *Abdom Imaging*. 2004;29(1):2–8.
9. Panebianco V, Grazhdani H, Iafrate F, et al. 3D CT protocol in the assessment of the esophageal neoplastic lesions: can it improve TNM staging? *Eur Radiol*. 2006;16:414–421.
10. Patel AN, Buenaventura PO. Current staging of esophageal carcinoma. *The Surgical Clinics of North America*. 2005;85(3):555–567.
11. Hustinx R. PET imaging in assessing gastrointestinal tumors. *Radiol Clin N Amer*. 2004;42(6):1123–39, ix.
12. Rosenbaum SJ, Stergar H, Antoch G, et al. Staging and follow-up of gastrointestinal tumors with PET/CT. *Abdom Imaging*. 2006;31(1):25–35.
13. Stein HJ, Brucher BL, Sendler A, et al. Esophageal cancer: patient evaluation and pretreatment staging. *Surg Oncol*. 2001;10:103–111.
14. Kantarci M, Polat P, Alper F, et al. Comparison of CT and MRI for the diagnosis recurrent esophageal carcinoma after operation. Diseases of the Esophagus: Official Journal of the International Society for Diseases of the Esophagus/I.S.D.E 2004;17(1):32–37.
15. Ogata I, Komohara Y, Yamashita Y, et al. CT evaluation of gastric lesions with three-dimensional display and interactive virtual endoscopy: Comparison with conventional barium study and endoscopy. *AJR Am J Roentgenol*. 1999;172(5):1263–1270.
16. Takao M, Fukuda T, Iwanaga S. Gastric cancer: Evaluation of triphasic spiral CT and radiologic-pathologic correlation. *J Comp Assist Tomography*. 1998;22:288–294.

17. Chen CH, Yang CC, Yeh YH. Preoperative staging of gastric cancer by endoscopic ultrasound: the prognostic usefulness of ascites detected by endoscopic ultrasound. *J Clin Gastroenterol.* 2002;35:321–327.

18. Lee YT, Ng EK, Hung LC, et al. Accuracy of endoscopic ultrasonography in diagnosing ascites and predicting peritoneal metastases in gastric cancer patients. *Gut.* 2005;54(11):1541–1545.

19. Adachi Y, Sakino I, Matsumata T, et al. Preoperative assessment of advanced gastric carcinoma using computed tomography. *Am J Gastroenterol.* 1997;92(5):872–875.

20. D'Elia F, Zingarelli A, Palli D, et al. Hydro-dynamic CT preoperative staging of gastric cancer: Correlation with pathological findings. A prospective study of 107 cases. *Eur Radiol.* 2000;10(12): 1877–1885.

21. Inamoto K, Kouzai K, Ueeda T, et al. CT virtual endoscopy of the stomach: Comparison study with gastric fiberscopy. *Abdom Imaging.* 2005;30(4):473–479.

22. Lee DH, Ko YT. Advanced gastric carcinoma: The role of three-dimensional and axial imaging by spiral CT. *Abdom Imaging.* 1999;24(2):111–116.

23. Yajima K, Kanda T, Ohashi M, et al. Clinical and diagnostic significance of preoperative computed tomography findings of ascites in patients with advanced gastric cancer. *Am J Surg.* 2006;192(2):185–190.

24. Zhong L, Li L, Sun JH, et al. Preoperative diagnosis of gastric cancer using 2-D magnetic resonance imaging with 3-D reconstruction techniques. *Chin J Dig Dis.* 2005;6(4):159–164.

25. Yun M, Lim JS, Noh SH, et al. Lymph node staging of gastric cancer using (18)F-FDG PET: a comparison study with CT. *J Nucl Med.* 2005;46:1582–1588.

26. Lim JS, Yun MJ, Kim MJ, et al. CT and PET in stomach cancer: Preoperative staging and monitoring of response to therapy. *Radiographics: A Review Publication of the Radiological Society of North America, Inc.* 2006;26(1):143–156.

27. Joensuu H, Fletcher C, Dimitrijevic S, et al. Management of malignant gastrointestinal stromal tumours. *Lancet Oncol.* 2002;3(11):655–664.

28. Burkill GJ, Badran M, Al-Muderis O, et al. Malignant gastrointestinal stromal tumor: Distribution, imaging features, and pattern of metastatic spread. *Radiology.* 2003;226(2):527–532.

29. Erturk SM. CT evaluation of gastrointestinal stromal tumors treated with imatinib mesylate. *AJR Am J Roentgenol.* 2005;185(5): 1366–1367.

30. Horton KM, Juluru K, Montogomery E, et al. Computed tomography imaging of gastrointestinal stromal tumors with pathology correlation. *J Comput Assist Tomography.* 2004;28(6):811–817.

31. King DM. The radiology of gastrointestinal stromal tumours (GIST). *Cancer Imaging.* 2005;5:150–156.

32. Logrono R, Bhanot P, Chaya C, et al. Imaging, morphologic, and immunohistochemical correlation in gastrointestinal stromal tumors. *Cancer.* 2006;108:257–266.

33. Amano M, Okuda T, Amano Y, et al. Magnetic resonance imaging of gastrointestinal stromal tumor in the abdomen and pelvis. *Clin Imaging.* 2006;30(2):127–131.

34. Caramella T, Schmidt S, Chevallier P, et al. MR features of gastrointestinal stromal tumors. *Clin Imaging.* 2005;29(4):251–254.

35. Rosenbaum SJ, Stergar H, Antoch G, et al. Staging and follow-up of gastrointestinal tumors with PET/CT. *Abdom Imaging.* 2006; 31(1):25–35.

36. Simo Perdigo M, Garcia Garzon JR, Soler Peter M, et al. Role of FDG PET in the staging, recurrence and treatment response to imatinib (glivec) in patients with gastrointestinal stromal tumors. *Revista Espanola De Medicina Nuclear.* 2006;25(2):80–88.

37. Choi H, Charnsangavej C, de Castro Faria S, et al. CT evaluation of the response of gastrointestinal stromal tumors after imatinib mesylate treatment: A quantitative analysis correlated with FDG PET findings. *AJR Am J Roentgenol.* 2004;183(6):1619–1628.

38. Goldstein D, Tan BS, Rossleigh M, et al. Gastrointestinal stromal tumours: Correlation of F-FDG gamma camera-based coincidence positron emission tomography with CT for the assessment of treatment response–an AGITG study. *Oncology.* 2005;69(4):326–332.

39. Shankar S, vanSonnenberg E, Desai J, et al. Gastrointestinal stromal tumor: new nodule-within-a-mass pattern of recurrence after partial response to imatinib mesylate. *Radiology.* 2005;235:892–898.

40. Stroszczynski C, Jost D, Reichardt P, et al. Follow-up of gastrointestinal stromal tumours (GIST) during treatment with imatinib mesylate by abdominal MRI. *Eur Radiol.* 2005;15(12):2448–2456.

41. Vanel D, Albiter M, Shapeero L, et al. Role of computed tomography in the follow-up of hepatic and peritoneal metastases of GIST under imatinib mesylate treatment: A prospective study of 54 patients. *Eur J Radiol.* 2005;54(1):118–123.

42. Chung DJ, Huh KC, Choi WJ, et al. CT colonography using 16-MDCT in the evaluation of colorectal cancer. *AJR Am J Roentgenol.* 2005;184(1):98–103.

43. Geenen RW, Hussain SM, Cademartiri F, et al. CT and MR colonography: Scanning techniques, postprocessing, and emphasis on polyp detection. *Radiographics: A Review Publication of the Radiological Society of North America, Inc.* 2004;24(1):e18.

44. Iannaccone R, Laghi A, Catalano C, et al. Detection of colorectal lesions: Lower-dose multi-detector row helical CT colonography compared with conventional colonoscopy. *Radiology.* 2003;229(3):775–781.

45. Zerhouni EA, Rutter C, Hamilton SR, et al. CT and MR imaging in the staging of colorectal carcinoma: report of the radiology diagnostic oncology group II. *Radiology.* 1996;200:443–451.

46. Burton S, Brown G, Daniels I, et al. MRI identified prognostic features of tumors in distal sigmoid, rectosigmoid, and upper rectum: Treatment with radiotherapy and chemotherapy. *Inter J Radiat Oncol Biol Phys.* 2006;65(2):445–451.

47. Burton S, Brown G, Daniels IR, et al. Royal Marsden Hospital, Colorectal Cancer Network. MRI directed multidisciplinary team preoperative treatment strategy: The way to eliminate positive circumferential margins? *Br J Cancer.* 2006;94(3):351–357.

48. Bipat S, Glas AS, Slors FJ, et al. Rectal cancer: Local staging and assessment of lymph node involvement with endoluminal US, CT, and MR imaging–a meta-analysis. *Radiology.* 2004;232(3):773–783.

49. Kobayashi M, Morishita S, Okabayashi T, et al. Preoperative assessment of vascular anatomy of inferior mesenteric artery by volume-rendered 3D-CT for laparoscopic lymph node dissection with left colic artery preservation in lower sigmoid and rectal cancer. *World J Gastroentrol: WJG.* 2006;12(4):553–555.

50. Cervone A, Sardi A, Conaway GL, et al. Intraoperative ultrasound (IOUS) is essential in the management of metastatic colorectal lesions. *Am Surg.* 2000;66:611–615.

51. Bipat S, van Leeuwen MS, Comans EF, et al. Colorectal liver metastases: CT, MR imaging, and PET for diagnosis–meta-analysis. *Radiology.* 2005;237:123–131.

52. Sahani DV, Kalva SP, Fischman AJ, et al. Detection of liver metastases from adenocarcinoma of the colon and pancreas: comparison of mangafodipir tri-sodium enhanced liver MRI and whole-body FDG PET. *AJR. Am J Roentgenol.* 2005;185:239–46.

53. Lahaye MJ, Engelen SM, Nelemans PJ, et al. Imaging for predicting the risk factors–the circumferential resection margin and nodal

disease–of local recurrence in rectal cancer: A meta-analysis. *Semin Ultrasound CT MR.* 2005;26(4):259–268.

54. Jeffrey RB. Pancreatic malignancy. In:Husband JE, Reznek RH, eds. *Imaging in Oncology.* 2nd ed. London: Taylor and Francis; 2004: 325–342.

55. Vargas R, Nino-Murcia M, Trueblood W, et al. MDCT in pancreatic adenocarcinoma: Prediction of vascular invasion and resectability using a multiphasic technique with curved planar reformations. *AJR. Am J Roentgenol.* 2004;182(2):419–425.

56. Valls C, Andia E, Sanchez A, et al. Dual-phase helical CT of pancreatic adenocarcinoma: Assessment of resectability before surgery. *AJR. Am J Roentgenol.* 2002;178(4):821–826.

57. Lu DS, Reber HA, Krasny RM, et al. Local staging of pancreatic cancer: Criteria for unresectability of major vessels as revealed by pancreatic-phase, thin-section helical CT. *AJR. Am J Roentgenol.* 1997;168(6):1439–1443.

58. Arslan A, Buanes T, Geitung JT. Pancreatic carcinoma: MR, MR angiography and dynamic helical CT in the evaluation of vascular invasion. *Eur J Radiol.* 2001;38:151–159.

59. Mehmet Erturk S, Ichikawa T, Sou H, et al. Pancreatic adenocarcinoma: MDCT versus MRI in the detection and assessment of locoregional extension. *J Comput Assist Tomography.* 2006;30(4):583–590.

60. Nishiharu T, Yamashita Y, Abe Y, et al. Local extension of pancreatic carcinoma: Assessment with thin-section helical CT versus with breath-hold fast MR imaging–ROC analysis. *Radiology.* 1999;212(2):445–452.

61. Mitsuhashi T, Ghafari S, Chang CY, et al. Endoscopic ultrasound-guided fine needle aspiration of the pancreas: Cytomorphological evaluation with emphasis on adequacy assessment, diagnostic criteria and contamination from the gastrointestinal tract. *Cytopathology: Official Journal of the British Society for Clinical Cytology.* 2006;17(1):34–41.

62. Roche CJ, Hughes ML, Garvey CJ, et al. CT and pathologic assessment of prospective nodal staging in patients with ductal adenocarcinoma of the head of the pancreas. *AJR. Am J Roentgenol.* 2003;180(2):475–480.

63. Ishiguchi T, Ota T, Naganawa S, et al. CT and MR imaging of pancreatic cancer. *Hepatogastroenterology.* 2001;48:923–927.

64. Heinrich S, Goerres GW, Schafer M, et al. Positron emission tomography/computed tomography influences on the management of resectable pancreatic cancer and its cost-effectiveness. *Ann Surg.* 2005;242(2):235–243.

65. Fletcher JG, Wiersema MJ, Farrell MA, et al. Pancreatic malignancy: Value of arterial, pancreatic, and hepatic phase imaging with multi-detector row CT. *Radiology.* 2003;229(1):81–90.

66. Aberle DR, Gamsu G, Henschke CI, et al. A consensus statement of the society of thoracic radiology: Screening for lung cancer with helical computed tomography. *J Thorac Imag.* 2001;16(1): 65–68.

67. Diederich S, Wormanns D. Impact of low-dose CT on lung cancer screening. *Lung Cancer (Amsterdam, Netherlands).* 2004;45 Suppl 2:S13–9.

68. Hartman TE, Swensen SJ. CT screening for lung cancer. *Semin Roentgenol.* 2005;40(2):193–196.

69. Jacobson FL. Multidetector-row CT of lung cancer screening. *Semin Roentgenol.* 2003;38(2):168–175.

70. Yankelevitz D, Henschke CI. State-of-the-art screening for lung cancer: (part 2): CT scanning. *Thorac Surg Clin.* 2004;14(1):53–59.

71. Lindell RM, Hartman TE, Swensen SJ, et al. Lung cancer screening experience: a retrospective review of PET in 22 non-small cell lung carcinomas detected on screening chest CT in a high-risk population. *AJR Am J Roentgenol.* 2005;185:126–131.

72. Swensen SJ, Jett JR, Hartman TE, et al. CT screening for lung cancer: Five-year prospective experience. *Radiology.* 2005;235(1): 259–265.

73. Quint LE, Francis IR. Radiologic staging of lung cancer. *J Thorac Imag.* 1999;14(4):235–246.

74. Passlick B. Initial surgical staging of lung cancer. *Lung Cancer (Amsterdam, Netherlands).* 2003;42 Suppl 1:S21–5.

75. Schrevens L, Lorent N, Dooms C, et al. The role of PET scan in diagnosis, staging, and management of non-small cell lung cancer. *The Oncologist.* 2004;9(6):633–643.

76. Bonomo L, Ciccotosto C, Guidotti A, et al. Lung cancer staging: The role of computed tomography and magnetic resonance imaging. *Eur J Radiol.* 1996;23(1):35–45.

77. Broderick LS, Tarver RD, Conces DJ, Jr, et al. Imaging of lung cancer: Old and new. *Semin Oncol.* 1997;24(4):411–418.

78. Chern MS, Wu MH, Chang CY. CT and MRI for staging of locally advanced non-small cell lung cancer. *Lung Cancer (Amsterdam, Netherlands).* 2003;42 Suppl 2:S5–8.

79. Detterbeck FC, Falen S, Rivera MP, et al. Seeking a home for a PET, part 2: Defining the appropriate place for positron emission tomography imaging in the staging of patients with suspected lung cancer. *Chest.* 2004;125(6):2300–2308.

80. Grover FL. The role of CT and MRI in staging of the mediastinum.*Chest.* 1994;106(6 Suppl):391S–396S.

81. Haberkorn U, Schoenberg SO. Imaging of lung cancer with CT, MRT and PET. *Lung Cancer (Amsterdam, Netherlands).* 2001;34 Suppl 3:S13–23.

82. Kramer H, Groen HJ. Current concepts in the mediastinal lymph node staging of nonsmall cell lung cancer. *Ann Surg.* 2003;238(2): 180–188.

83. Gould MK, Kuschner WG, Rydzak CE, et al. Test performance of positron emission tomography and computed tomography for mediastinal staging in patients with non-small-cell lung cancer: A meta-analysis. *Ann Intern Med.* 2003;139(11):879–892.

84. Franzius C. FDG PET: Advantages for staging the mediastinum? *Lung Cancer (Amsterdam, Netherlands).* 2004;45 Suppl 2:S69–74.

85. Heidenreich A, Ravery V. European Society of Oncological Urology. Preoperative imaging in renal cell cancer. *World J Urol.* 2004;22(5):307–315.

86. Walter C, Kruessell M, Gindele A, et al. Imaging of renal lesions: Evaluation of fast MRI and helical CT. *Br J Radiol.* 2003;76(910): 696–703.

87. Hallscheidt PJ, Bock M, Riedasch G, et al. Diagnostic accuracy of staging renal cell carcinomas using multidetector-row computed tomography and magnetic resonance imaging: a prospective study with histopathologic correlation. *J Comput Assist Tomogr.* 2004;28:333–339.

88. Reznek RH. Imaging in the staging of renal cell carcinoma. *Eur Radiol.* 1996;6(2):120–128.

89. Gupta NP, Ansari MS, Khaitan A, et al. Impact of imaging and thrombus level in management of renal cell carcinoma extending to veins. *Urologia Internationalis.* 2004;72(2):129–134.

90. Hallscheidt PJ, Fink C, Haferkamp A, et al. Preoperative staging of renal cell carcinoma with inferior vena cava thrombus using multidetector CT and MRI: Prospective study with histopathological correlation. *J Comput Assist Tomography.* 2005;29(1):64–68.

91. Tuite DJ, Geoghegan T, McCauley G, et al. Three-dimensional gadolinium-enhanced magnetic resonance breath-hold FLASH imaging in the diagnosis and staging of renal cell carcinoma. *Clin Radiol.* 2006;61(1):23–30.

92. Beer A, Saar B, Zantl N, et al. MR cystography for bladder tumor detection. *Eur Radiol.* 2004;14(12):2311–2319.

93. Kim JK, Park SY, Ahn HJ, et al. Bladder cancer: Analysis of multidetector row helical CT enhancement pattern and accuracy in

tumor detection and perivesical staging. *Radiology*. 2004;231(3): 725–731.

94. Tekes A, Kamel I, Imam K, et al. Dynamic MRI of bladder cancer: Evaluation of staging accuracy. *AJR Am J Roentgenol*. 2005;184: 121–127.

95. Husband JE, Koh DM. Bladder cancer. In: Husband JE, Reznek RH, eds. *Imaging in Oncology*. 2nd ed. London, UK: Taylor and Francis; 2004:343–374.

96. Mallampati GK, Siegelman ES. MR imaging of the bladder. *Mag Reson Imaging Clin N Am*. 2004;12(3):545–55, vii.

97. Ng CS. Radiologic diagnosis and staging of renal and bladder cancer. *Semin Roentgenol*. 2006;41(2):121–138.

98. Wong-You-Cheong JJ, Woodward PJ, Manning MA, et al. From the archives of the AFIP: Neoplasms of the urinary bladder: Radiologic-pathologic correlation. *Radiographics: A Review Publication of the Radiological Society of North America, Inc*. 2006;26(2): 553–580.

99. Montie JE. Urinary bladder cancer: Preoperative nodal staging with ferumoxtran-10-enhanced MR imaging. *J Urol*. 2005;174(3): 870–871.

100. Deserno W, Harisinghani MG, Barentsz JO. MR lymphography. In: Husband JE Reznek RH, eds. *Imaging in Oncology*. 2nd ed. London, UK: Taylor and Francis; 2004:1375–1390.

101. Drieskens O, Oyen R, Van Poppel H, et al. FDG-PET for preoperative staging of bladder cancer. *Eur J Nucl Med Mol Imaging*. 2005;32:1412–1417.

102. D'Amico AV, Whittington R, Malkowicz SB, et al. Critical analysis of the ability of the endorectal coil magnetic resonance imaging scan to predict pathologic stage, margin status, and postoperative prostate-specific antigen failure in patients with clinically organ-confined prostate cancer. *J Clin Oncol Off J Am Soc Clin Oncol*. 1996;14(6):1770–1777.

103. Futterer JJ, Engelbrecht MR, Huisman HJ, et al. Staging prostate cancer with dynamic contrast-enhanced endorectal MR imaging prior to radical prostatectomy: Experienced versus less experienced readers. *Radiology*. 2005;237(2):541–549.

104. Futterer JJ, Heijmink SW, Scheenen TW, et al. Prostate cancer: Local staging at 3-T endorectal MR imaging–early experience. *Radiology*. 2006;238(1):184–191.

105. Gerst SR, Touijer AK, Guillonneau B, et al. The importance of MRI evaluation in the preoperative work-up of prostate cancer. *Nat Clin Pract Urol* 2005;2(11):565–71; quiz 572.

106. Husband JE, Sohaib SA. Prostate cancer. In: Husband JE, Reznek RH, eds. *Imaging in Oncology*. 2nd ed. London, UK: Taylor and Francis; 2004:375–400.

107. Hricak H. MR imaging and MR spectroscopic imaging in the pretreatment evaluation of prostate cancer. *Br J Radiol*. 2005;78 Spec No 2:S103–11.

108. Wang L, Hricak H, Kattan MW, et al. Combined endorectal and phased-array MRI in the prediction of pelvic lymph node metastasis in prostate cancer. *AJR Am J Roentgenol*. 2006;186: 743–748.

109. Sala E, Eberhardt SC, Akin O, et al. Endorectal MR imaging before salvage prostatectomy: Tumor localization and staging. *Radiology*. 2006;238(1):176–183.

110. Nudell DM, Wefer AE, Hricak H, et al. Imaging for recurrent prostate cancer. *Radiol Clin N Amer*. 2000;38(1):213–229.

111. Woodward PJ, Sohaey R, O'Donoghue MJ, et al. From the archives of the AFIP: Tumors and tumorlike lesions of the testis: Radiologic-pathologic correlation. *Radiographics: A Review Publication of the Radiological Society of North America, Inc*. 2002;22(1): 189–216.

112. Daugaard G, Karas V, Sommer P. Inguinal metastases from testicular cancer. *BJU International*. 2006;97(4):724–726.

113. Dixon AK, Ellis M, Sikora K. Computed tomography of testicular tumours: Distribution of abdominal lymphadenopathy. *Clin Radiol*. 1986;37(6):519–523.

114. Mason MD, Featherstone T, Olliff J, et al. Inguinal and iliac lymph node involvement in germ cell tumours of the testis: Implications for radiological investigation and for therapy. *Clinical Oncology (Royal College of Radiologists (Great Britain))*. 1991;3(3):147–150.

115. White PM, Adamson DJ, Howard GC, et al. Imaging of the thorax in the management of germ cell testicular tumours. *Clin Radiol*.1999;54:207–211.

116. Williams MP, Husband JE. Computed tomography scanning and post-lymphangiogram radiography in the follow-up of patients with metastatic testicular cancer. *Clin Radiol*. 1989;40(1): 47–50.

117. Wright AR, White PM. Testicular cancer–who needs surveillance pelvic CT? *Clin Radiol*. 1999;54(1):78.

118. Spermon JR, De Geus-Oei LF, Kiemeney LA, et al. The role of (18)fluoro-2-deoxyglucose positron emission tomography in initial staging and re-staging after chemotherapy for testicular germ cell tumours. *BJU International*. 2002;89(6):549–556.

119. Harvey ML, Geldart TR, Duell R, et al. Routine computerised tomographic scans of the thorax in surveillance of stage I testicular non-seminomatous germ-cell cancer–a necessary risk? *Ann Oncol Off J Euro Soc Med Oncol / ESMO*. 2002;13(2):237–242.

120. Alexandre J, Fizazi K, Mahe C, et al. Stage I non-seminomatous germ-cell tumours of the testis: Identification of a subgroup of patients with a very low risk of relapse. *Eur J Cancer(Oxford, England: 1990)*. 2001;37(5):576–582.

121. Forstner R, Hricak H, White S. CT and MRI of ovarian cancer. *Abdom Imaging*. 1995;20:2–8.

122. Spencer JA. A multidisciplinary approach to ovarian cancer at diagnosis. *Br J Radiol*. 2005;78:S94–102.

123. Brown DL, Zou KH, Tempany CM, et al. Primary versus secondary ovarian malignancy: Imaging findings of adnexal masses in the radiology diagnostic oncology group study. *Radiology*. 2001;219(1):213–218.

124. Togashi K. Ovarian cancer: The clinical role of US, CT, and MRI. *Eur Radiol*. 2003;13 Suppl 4:L87–104.

125. Umemoto M, Shiota M, Shimono T, et al. Preoperative diagnosis of ovarian tumors, focusing on the solid area based on diagnostic imaging. *J Obstet Gynaecol Res*. 2006;32(2):195–201.

126. Tempany CM, Zou KH, Silverman SG, et al. Staging of advanced ovarian cancer: Comparison of imaging modalities–report from the radiological diagnostic oncology group. *Radiology*. 2000; 215(3):761–767.

127. Mata JM, Inaraja L, Rams A, et al. CT findings in metastatic ovarian tumors from gastrointestinal tract neoplasms (krukenberg tumors). *Gastro Radiol*. 1988;13(3):242–246.

128. Choi HJ, Lee JH, Kang S, et al. Contrast-enhanced CT for differentiation of ovarian metastasis from gastrointestinal tract cancer: Stomach cancer versus colon cancer. *AJR. Am J Roentgenol*. 2006;187(3):741–745.

129. Choi HJ, Lee JH, Seo SS, et al. Computed tomography findings of ovarian metastases from colon cancer: comparison with primary malignant ovarian tumors. *J Comput Assist Tomogr*. 2005;29: 69–73.

130. Gontier E, Wartski M, Guinebretiere JM, et al. 18F-FDG PET/CT in a patient with lymph node metastasis from ovarian adenocarcinoma. *AJR. Am J Roentgenol*. 2006;187(3):W285–289.

131. Buy JN, Moss AA, Ghossain MA, et al. Peritoneal implants from ovarian tumors: CT findings. *Radiology*. 1988;169(3):691–694.

132. Coakley FV. Staging ovarian cancer: Role of imaging. *Radiol Clin N Amer*. 2002;40(3):609–636.

133. Coakley FV, Choi PH, Gougoutas CA, et al. Peritoneal metastases: Detection with spiral CT in patients with ovarian cancer. *Radiology.* 2002;223(2):495–499.

134. Neville A, Herts BR. CT characteristics of primary retroperitoneal neoplasms. *Crit Rev Comput Tomograph.* 2004;45(4):247–270.

135. Nakashima J, Ueno M, Nakamura K, et al. Differential diagnosis of primary benign and malignant retroperitoneal tumors. *Int J Urol Off J Japan Urol Assoc.* 1997;4(5):441–446.

136. Nishino M, Hayakawa K, Minami M, et al. Primary retroperitoneal neoplasms: CT and MR imaging findings with anatomic and pathologic diagnostic clues. *Radiographics.* 2003;23:45–57.

137. Papanicolaou N, Yoder IC, Lee MJ. Primary retroperitoneal neoplasms: How close can we come in making the correct diagnosis. *Urol Radiol.* 1992;14(3):221–228.

138. Choi BI, Chi JG, Kim SH, et al. MR imaging of retroperitoneal teratoma: Correlation with CT and pathology. *J Comput Assist Tomography.* 1989;13(6):1083–1086.

139. Lane RH, Stephens DH, Reiman HM. Primary retroperitoneal neoplasms: CT findings in 90 cases with clinical and pathologic correlation. *AJR. Am J Roentgenol.* 1989;152(1):83–89.

140. Morton DL, Thompson JF, Cochran AJ, et al. Sentinel-node biopsy or nodal observation in melanoma. *N Engl J Med.* 2006;355:1307–1317.

141. Cecchi R, De Gaudio C, Buralli L, et al. Lymphatic mapping and sentinel lymph node biopsy in the management of primary cutaneous melanoma: Report of a single-centre experience. *Tumori.* 2006;92(2):113–117.

142. Scarsbrook AF, Ganeshan A, Bradley KM. Pearls and pitfalls of radionuclide imaging of the lymphatic system. Part 1: Sentinel node lymphoscintigraphy in malignant melanoma. *Brit J Radiol.* 2007;80:132–139.

143. Belhocine T, Pierard G, De Labrassinne M, et al. Staging of regional nodes in AJCC stage I and II melanoma: 18FDG PET imaging versus sentinel node detection. *Oncologist.* 2002;7:271–278.

144. Aloia TA, Gershenwald JE, Andtbacka RH, et al. Utility of computed tomography and magnetic resonance imaging staging before completion lymphadenectomy in patients with sentinel lymph node-positive melanoma. *J Clin Oncol.* 2006;24(18):2858–2865.

145. Miranda EP, Gertner M, Wall J, et al. Routine imaging of asymptomatic melanoma patients with metastasis to sentinel lymph nodes rarely identifies systemic disease. *Arch Surg*(Chicago, Ill.: 1960) 2004;139(8):831–836; discussion 836–837.

146. Grasee EA, Wagner JD. Update on diagnostic imaging for melanoma. *Facial Plast. Surg. Clin. North. Am.* 2003;11(1):49–60.

147. Blackledge G, Best JJ, Crowther D, et al. Computed tomography (CT) in the staging of patients with hodgkin's disease: A report on 136 patients. *Clin Radiol.* 1980;31(2):143–147.

148. Earl HM, Sutcliffe SB, Fry IK, et al. Computerised tomographic (CT) abdominal scanning in hodgkin's disease. *Clin Radiol.* 1980;31(2):149–153.

149. Ellert J, Kreel L. The role of computed tomography in the initial staging and subsequent management of the lymphomas. *J Comput Assist Tomography.* 1980;4(3):368–391.

150. Gossmann A, Eich HT, Engert A, et al. CT and MR imaging in Hodgkin's disease–present and future. *Eur J Haematol Suppl.* 2005;66:83–89.

151. Guadagnolo BA, Punglia RS, Kuntz KM, et al. Cost-effectiveness analysis of computerized tomography in the routine follow-up of patients after primary treatment for hodgkin's disease. *J Clin Oncol Off J Am Soc Clin Oncol.* 2006;24(25):4116–4122.

152. Vinnicombe SJ, Reznek RH. Computerised tomography in the staging of hodgkin's disease and non-hodgkin's lymphoma. *Eur J Nucl Med Mol Imag.* 2003;30 Suppl 1:S42–55.

153. Sohaib SA, Turner B, Hanson JA, et al. CT assessment of tumour response to treatment: Comparison of linear, cross-sectional and volumetric measures of tumour size. *Br J Radiol.* 2000;73(875):1178–1184.

154. Munker R, Stengel A, Stabler A, et al. Diagnostic accuracy of ultrasound and computed tomography in the staging of hodgkin's disease. verification by laparotomy in 100 cases. *Cancer.* 1995;76(8):1460–1466.

155. Skillings JR, Bramwell V, Nicholson RL, et al. A prospective study of magnetic resonance imaging in lymphoma staging. *Cancer.* 1991;67(7):1838–1843.

156. Castellucci P, Zinzani P, Pourdehnad M, et al. 18F-FDG PET in malignant lymphoma: Significance of positive findings. *Eur J Nucl Med Mol Imag.* 2005;32(7):749–756.

157. Blum RH, Seymour JF, Wirth A, et al. Frequent impact of [18F]fluorodeoxyglucose positron emission tomography on the staging and management of patients with indolent non-Hodgkin's lymphoma. *Clin Lymphoma.* 2003;4:43–49.

158. Guay C, Lepine M, Verreault J, et al. Prognostic value of PET using 18F-FDG in hodgkin's disease for posttreatment evaluation. *J Nucl Med Off Pub Soc Nucl Med.* 2003;44(8):1225–1231.

159. Pappa VI, Hussain HK, Reznek RH, et al. Role of image-guided core-needle biopsy in the management of patients with lymphoma. *J Clin Oncol Off J Am Soc Clin Oncol.* 1996;14(9):2427–2430.

160. Naumann R, Vaic A, Beuthien-Baumann B, et al. Prognostic value of positron emission tomography in the evaluation of post-treatment residual mass in patients with hodgkin's disease and non-hodgkin's lymphoma. *Br J Haematol.* 2001;115(4):793–800.

161. Rigacci L, Castagnoli A, Dini C, et al. 18FDG-positron emission tomography in post treatment evaluation of residual mass in hodgkin's lymphoma: Long-term results. *Oncol Report.* 2005;14(5):1209–1214.

162. Dittmann H, Sokler M, Kollmannsberger C, et al. Comparison of 18FDG-PET with CT scans in the evaluation of patients with residual and recurrent Hodgkin's lymphoma. *Oncol Rep.* 2001;8:1393–1399.

163. Coakley FV, Choi PH, Gougoutas CA, et al. Peritoneal metastases: Detection with spiral CT in patients with ovarian cancer. *Radiology.* 2002;223(2):495–499.

164. Kurtz AB, Tsimikas JV, Tempany CM, et al. Diagnosis and staging of ovarian cancer: Comparative values of doppler and conventional US, CT, and MR imaging correlated with surgery and histopathologic analysis—report of the radiology diagnostic oncology group. *Radiology.* 1999;212(1):19–27.

165. Goerg C, Schwerk WB. Peritoneal carcinomatosis with ascites. *AJR. Am J Roentgenol.* 1991;156(6):1185–1187.

166. Goerg C, Schwerk WB. Malignant ascites: Sonographic signs of peritoneal carcinomatosis. *Eur J Cancer* (Oxford, England: 1990). 1991;27(6):720–723.

167. Drieskens O, Stroobants S, Gysen M, et al. Positron emission tomography with FDG in the detection of peritoneal and retroperitoneal metastases of ovarian cancer. *Gynecol Obstet Invest.* 2003;55(3):130–134.

168. Pombo F, Rodriguez E, Martin R, et al. CT-guided core-needle biopsy in omental pathology. *Acta Radiol.* 1997;38:978–981.

169. Spencer JA, Anderson K, Weston M, et al. Image guided biopsy in the management of cancer of the ovary. *Cancer Imag.* 2006;6:144–147.

170. Pannu HK, Horton KM, Fishman EK. Thin section dual-phase multidetector-row computed tomography detection of peritoneal metastases in gynecologic cancers. *J Comput Assist Tomography.* 2003;27(3):333–340.

171. Yajima K, Kanda T, Ohashi M, et al. Clinical and diagnostic significance of preoperative computed tomography findings of ascites in patients with advanced gastric cancer. *Am J Surg.* 2006;192(2):185–190.

172. Idelevich E, Kashtan H, Mavor E, et al. Small bowel obstruction caused by secondary tumors. *Surg Oncol.* 2006;15(1):29–32.

173. Jaffe CC. Measures of response: RECIST, WHO, and new alternatives. *J Clin Oncol Off J Am Soc Clin Oncol.* 2006;24(20):3245–3251.

174. Husband JE, Schwartz LH, Spencer J, et al. International Cancer Imaging Society. Evaluation of the response to treatment of solid tumours—a consensus statement of the international cancer imaging society. *Br J Cancer.* 2004;90(12):2256–2260.

175. Tuma RS. Sometimes size doesn't matter: reevaluating RECIST and tumor response rate endpoints. *J Natl Cancer Inst.* 2006;98:1272–1274.

176. Sohaib SA, Turner B, Hanson JA, et al. CT assessment of tumour response to treatment: Comparison of linear, cross-sectional and volumetric measures of tumour size. *Br J Radiol.* 2000;73(875):1178–1184.

177. Wunderbaldinger P. Problems and prospects of modern lymph node imaging. *Eur J Radiol.* 2006;58(3):325–337.

178. Scheidler J, Hricak H, Yu KK, et al. Radiological evaluation of lymph node metastases in patients with cervical cancer. A meta-analysis. *JAMA.* 1997;278(13):1096–1101.

179. Luciani A, Itti E, Rahmouni A, et al. Lymph node imaging: Basic principles. *Eur J Radiol.* 2006;58(3):338–344.

180. Krestan C, Herneth AM, Formanek M, et al. Modern imaging lymph node staging of the head and neck region. *Eur J Radiol.* 2006;58(3):360–366.

181. Ahuja AT, Ying M. Sonographic evaluation of cervical lymph nodes. *AJR. Am J Roentgenol.* 2005;184(5):1691–1699.

182. Ahuja AT, Ying M. Evaluation of cervical lymph node vascularity: a comparison of colour doppler, power doppler and 3-D power Doppler sonography. *Ultrasound Med Biol.* 2004;30:1557–1564.

183. Crippa F, Gerali A, Alessi A, et al. FDG-PET for axillary lymph node staging in primary breast cancer. *Eur J Nucl Med Mol Imag.* 2004;31 Suppl 1:S97–102.

184. Jeong HS, Baek CH, Son YI, et al. Integrated 18F-FDG PET/CT for the initial evaluation of cervical node level of patients with papillary thyroid carcinoma: Comparison with ultrasound and contrast-enhanced CT. *Clin Endocrinol.* 2006;65(3):402–407.

185. Yasufuku K, Nakajima T, Motoori K, et al. Comparison of endobronchial ultrasound, positron emission tomography, and CT for lymph node staging of lung cancer. *Chest.* 2006;130(3):710–718.

186. Williams AD, Cousins C, Soutter WP, et al. Detection of pelvic lymph node metastases in gynecologic malignancy: A comparison of CT, MR imaging, and positron emission tomography. *AJR. Am J Roentgenol.* 2001;177(2):343–348.

187. Rasheed S, Guenther T, Talbot I, et al. USPIO—enhanced rectal cancer specimen MRI: How well does it correlate with node identification at histopathology? *Colorect Dis* 2006;8(8):721.

188. Saokar A, Braschi M, Harisinghani MG. Lymphotrophic nanoparticle enhanced MR imaging (LNMRI) for lymph node imaging. *Abdom Imaging.* 2006;31(6):660–667.

189. Libby DM, Smith JP, Altorki NK, et al. Managing the small pulmonary nodule discovered by CT. *Chest.* 2004;125(4):1522–1529.

190. Munden RF, Hess KR. "Ditzels" on chest CT: Survey of members of the society of thoracic radiology. *AJR. Am J Roentgenol.* 2001;176(6):1363–1369.

191. Prosch H, Strasser G, Oschatz E, et al. Management of patients with small pulmonary nodules: A survey of radiologists, pulmonologists, and thoracic surgeons. *AJR. Am J Roentgenol.* 2006;187(1):143–148.

192. Gietema HA, Wang Y, Xu D, et al. Pulmonary nodules detected at lung cancer screening: Interobserver variability of semiautomated volume measurements. *Radiology.* 2006;241(1):251–257.

193. Li F, Li Q, Engelmann R, et al. Improving radiologists' recommendations with computer-aided diagnosis for management of small nodules detected by CT. *Acad Radiol.* 2006;13(8):943–950.

194. Awai K, Murao K, Ozawa A, et al. Pulmonary nodules at chest CT: Effect of computer-aided diagnosis on radiologists' detection performance. *Radiology.* 2004;230(2):347–352.

195. Aufort S, Charra L, Lesnik A, et al. Multidetector CT of bowel obstruction: value of post-processing. *Eur Radiol.* 2005;15:2323–2329.

196. Idelevich E, Kashtan H, Mavor E, et al. Small bowel obstruction caused by secondary tumors. *Surg Oncol.* 2006;15(1):29–32.

197. Kwek JW, Iyer RB. Recurrent ovarian cancer: Spectrum of imaging findings. *AJR. Am J Roentgenol.* 2006;187(1):99–104.

198. Petrovic B, Nikolaidis P, Hammond NA, et al. Identification of adhesions on CT in small-bowel obstruction. *Emerg Radiol.* 2006;12(3):88–93; discussion 94–95.

199. Sinha R, Verma R. Multidetector row computed tomography in bowel obstruction. part 2. large bowel obstruction. *Clin Radiol.* 2005;60(10):1068–1075.

200. Barzon L, Sonino N, Fallo F, et al. Prevalence and natural history of adrenal incidentalomas. *Eur J Endocrinol.* 2003;149(4):273–285.

201. McNicholas MM, Lee MJ, Mayo-Smith WW, et al. An imaging algorithm for the differential diagnosis of adrenal adenomas and metastases. *AJR. Am J Roentgenol.* 1995;165(6):1453–1459.

202. Nwariaku FE, Champine J, Kim LT, et al. Radiologic characterization of adrenal masses: The role of computed tomography—derived attenuation values. *Surgery.* 2001;130(6):1068–1071.

203. Blake MA, Kalra MK, Sweeney AT, et al. Distinguishing benign from malignant adrenal masses: multi-detector row CT protocol with 10-minute delay. *Radiology.* 2006;238:578–585.

204. Caoili EM, Korobkin M, Francis IR, et al. Delayed enhanced CT of lipid-poor adrenal adenomas. *AJR. Am J Roentgenol.* 2000;175(5):1411–1415.

205. Caoili EM, Korobkin M, Francis IR, et al. Adrenal masses: Characterization with combined unenhanced and delayed enhanced CT. *Radiology.* 2002;222(3):629–633.

206. Korobkin M, Brodeur FJ, Yutzy GG, et al. Differentiation of adrenal adenomas from nonadenomas using CT attenuation values. *AJR. Am J Roentgenol.* 1996;166(3):531–536.

207. Bilbey JH, McLoughlin RF, Kurkjian PS, et al. MR imaging of adrenal masses: Value of chemical-shift imaging for distinguishing adenomas from other tumors. *AJR. Am J Roentgenol.* 1995;164(3):637–642.

208. Honigschnabl S, Gallo S, Niederle B, et al. How accurate is MR imaging in characterisation of adrenal masses: Update of a long-term study. *Eur J Radiol.* 2002;41(2):113–122.

209. Korobkin M, Giordano TJ, Brodeur FJ, et al. Adrenal adenomas: Relationship between histologic lipid and CT and MR findings. *Radiology.* 1996;200(3):743–747.

210. Mayo-Smith WW, Lee MJ, McNicholas MM, et al. Characterization of adrenal masses (<5 cm) by use of chemical shift MR imaging: observer performance versus quantitative measures. *AJR Am J Roentgenol.* 1995;165:91–95.

211. Savci G, Yazici Z, Sahin N, et al. Value of chemical shift subtraction MRI in characterization of adrenal masses. *AJR. Am J Roentgenol.* 2006;186(1):130–135.

212. Metser U, Miller E, Lerman H, et al. 18F-FDG PET/CT in the evaluation of adrenal masses. *J Nucl Med.* 2006;47(1):32–37.

213. Harisinghani MG, Maher MM, Hahn PF, et al. Predictive value of benign percutaneous adrenal biopsies in oncology patients. *Clin Radiol.* 2002;57(10):898–901.

214. Lumachi F, Borsato S, Brandes AA, et al. Fine-needle aspiration cytology of adrenal masses in noncancer patients: Clinicoradiologic and histologic correlations in functioning and nonfunctioning tumors. *Cancer.* 2001;93(5):323–329.

215. Saboorian MH, Katz RL, Charnsangavej C. Fine needle aspiration cytology of primary and metastatic lesions of the adrenal gland. A series of 188 biopsies with radiologic correlation. *Acta Cytologica.* 1995;39(5):843–851.

216. Pandey M, Mathew A, Geetha N, et al. Acute abdomen in patients receiving chemotherapy. *Indian J Cancer.* 2001;38(2–4):68–6971.

217. Doria AS, Moineddin R, Kellenberger CJ, et al. US or CT for diagnosis of appendicitis in children and adults? A meta-analysis. *Radiology.* 2006;241(1):83–94.

218. Hoeffel C, Crema MD, Belkacem A, et al. Multi-detector row CT: Spectrum of diseases involving the ileocecal area. *Radiographics.* 2006;26(5):1373–1390.

219. Keyzer C, Zalcman M, De Maertelaer V, et al. Comparison of US and unenhanced multi-detector row CT in patients suspected of having acute appendicitis. *Radiology.* 2005;236(2):527–534.

220. Pinto Leite N, Pereira JM, Cunha R, et al. CT evaluation of appendicitis and its complications: Imaging techniques and key diagnostic findings. *AJR. Am J Roentgenol.* 2005;185(2):406–417.

221. Siewert B, Tye G, Kruskal J, et al. Impact of CT-guided drainage in the treatment of diverticular abscesses: Size matters. *AJR. Am J Roentgenol.* 2006;186(3):680–686.

222. Kaiser AM, Jiang JK, Lake JP, et al. The management of complicated diverticulitis and the role of computed tomography. *Am J Gastroenterol.* 2005;100(4):910–917.

223. Zaidi E, Daly B. CT and clinical features of acute diverticulitis in an urban U.S. population: rising frequency in young, obese adults. *AJR Am J Roentgenol.* 2006;187:689–694.

224. Taylor AJ, Dodds WJ, Gonyo JE, et al. Typhlitis in adults. *Gastro Radiol.* 1985;10(4):363–369.

225. Lea JW, Jr, Masys DR, Shackford SR, et al. Typhlitis: A treatable complication of acute leukemia therapy. *Caner Clin Trial.* 1980;3(4):355–362.

226. Hoeffel C, Crema MD, Belkacem A, et al. Multi-detector row CT: Spectrum of diseases involving the ileocecal area. *Radiographics.* 2006;26(5):1373–1390.

227. Alobaidi M, Gupta R, Jafri SZ, et al. Current trends in imaging evaluation of acute cholecystitis. *Emerg Radiol.* 2004;10(5):256–258.

228. De Vargas Macciucca M, Lanciotti S, De Cicco ML, et al. Ultrasonographic and spiral CT evaluation of simple and complicated acute cholecystitis: Diagnostic protocol assessment based on personal experience and review of the literature. *La Radiologia Medica.* 2006;111(2):167–180.

229. Fidler J, Paulson EK, Layfield L. CT evaluation of acute cholecystitis: Findings and usefulness in diagnosis. *AJR. Am J Roentgenol.* 1996;166(5):1085–1088.

230. Yilmaz C, Esen OS, Colak A, et al. Torsion of a wandering spleen associated with portal vein thrombosis. *J Ultrasound Med.* 2005;24(3):379–382.

231. Tucker ON, Smith J, Fenlon HM, et al. Recurrent torsion of a wandering spleen. *Am J Surg.* 2004;188:96–97.

232. Bakir B, Poyanli A, Yekeler E, et al. Acute torsion of a wandering spleen: Imaging findings. *Abdom Imaging.* 2004;29(6):707–709.

233. Gupta S. Role of image-guided percutaneous needle biopsy in cancer staging. *Semin Roentgenol.* 2006;41(2):78–90.

234. Haaga JR. Interventional CT: 30 years' experience. *Eur Radiol.* 2005;15 Suppl 4:D116–20.

235. Winters SR, Paulson EK. Ultrasound guided biopsy: what's new? *Ultrasound Q.* 2005;21:19–25.

236. Benamore RE, Scott K, Richards CJ, et al. Image-guided pleural biopsy: Diagnostic yield and complications. *Clin Radiol.* 2006;61(8):700–705.

237. Bialecki ES, Ezenekwe AM, Brunt EM, et al. Comparison of liver biopsy and noninvasive methods for diagnosis of hepatocellular carcinoma. *Clin Gastroenterol. Hepatol.* 2006;4(3):361–368.

238. Diederich S, Padge B, Vossas U, et al. Application of a single needle type for all image-guided biopsies: Results of 100 consecutive core biopsies in various organs using a novel tri-axial, end-cut needle. *Cancer Imaging.* 2006;6:43–50.

239. Fichtinger G, Deguet A, Fischer G, et al. Image overlay for CT-guided needle insertions. *Comp Aid Surg.* 2005;10(4):241–255.

240. Hemalatha AL, Divya P, Mamatha R. Image-directed percutaneous FNAC of ovarian neoplasms. *Indian J Pathol Microbiol.* 2005;48:305–309.

241. Romics I. Ultrasound guided biopsy, a gold standard diagnostical test of the prostate cancer. *Acta Chirurgica Iugoslavica.* 2005;52(4):23–26.

242. Shah RB, Bakshi N, Hafez KS, et al. Image-guided biopsy in the evaluation of renal mass lesions in contemporary urological practice: Indications, adequacy, clinical impact, and limitations of the pathological diagnosis. *Human Pathol.* 2005;36(12):1309–1315.

243. Gulec SA, Daghighian F, Essner R. PET-probe: Evaluation of technical performance and clinical utility of a handheld high-energy gamma probe in oncologic surgery. *Ann Surg Oncol.* 2006 Jul 24 (published online):DOI:10.1245.

244. Brusciano L, Maffettone V, Napolitano V, et al. Management of colorectal emergencies: Percutaneous abscess drainage. *Annali Italiani Di Chirurgia.* 2004;75(5):593–597.

245. Maher MM, Gervais DA, Kalra MK, et al. The inaccessible or undrainable abscess: How to drain it. *Radiographics.* 2004;24(3):717–735.

246. Harisinghani MG, Gervais DA, Hahn PF, et al. CT-guided transgluteal drainage of deep pelvic abscesses: Indications, technique, procedure-related complications, and clinical outcome. *Radiographics.* 2002;22(6):1353–1367.

247. Moulton JS. Image-guided management of complicated pleural fluid collections. *Radiol Clin N Am.* 2000;38:345–374.

248. Moulton JS. Image-guided drainage techniques. *Semin Respiratory Infect.* 1999;14(1):59–72.

249. Khurrum Baig M, Hua Zhao R, Batista O, et al. Percutaneous postoperative intra-abdominal abscess drainage after elective colorectal surgery. *Technique Coloproctol.* 2002;6(3):159–164.

250. Men S, Akhan O, Koroglu M. Percutaneous drainage of abdominal abcess. *Eur J Radiol.* 2002;43(3):204–218.

251. Adler DG, Merwat SN. Endoscopic approaches for palliation of luminal gastrointestinal obstruction. *Gastroenterol Clin N Am.* 2006;35(1):65–82, viii.

252. Siersema PD. Therapeutic esophageal interventions for dysphagia and bleeding. *Curr Opin Gastroenterol.* 2006;22(4):442–447.

253. Wenger U, Johnsson E, Arnelo U, et al. An antireflux stent versus conventional stents for palliation of distal esophageal or cardia cancer: A randomized clinical study. *Surg Endoscop.* 2006.

254. Peters JH, Craanen ME, van der Peet DL, et al. Self-expanding metal stents for the treatment of intrathoracic esophageal anastomotic leaks following esophagectomy. *Am J Gastroenterol.* 2006;101:1393–1395.

255. Athreya S, Moss J, Urquhart G, et al. Colorectal stenting for colonic obstruction: The indications, complications, effectiveness and outcome-5-year review. *Eur J Radiol.* 2006;60(1):91–94.

256. Baik SH, Kim NK, Cho HW, et al. Clinical outcomes of metallic stent insertion for obstructive colorectal cancer. *Hepato-Gastroenterology*. 2006;53(68):183–187.

257. Parker MC. Colorectal stenting. *Br J Surg.* 2006;93(8):907–908.

258. Silva RA, Mesquita N, Brandao C, et al. Safety and efficacy of large-diameter esophageal metal stents. *Endoscopy.* 2006;38(7):756.

259. Kettenbach J, Jolesz FA. Editorial comment on percutaneous tumor ablation. *Eur J Radiol.* 2006;59:131–132.

COMMENTARY
Lawrence H. Schwartz

The role of imaging in oncology can be broadly divided into four categories: lesion detection, lesion characterization, staging, and assessment of therapeutic response. All of these are critical for the surgical oncologist. However, with the recent vast proliferation of imaging studies and the identification of incidental lesions on these studies, it is increasingly critical to appropriately characterize abnormalities seen at imaging. For instance, many incidental lesions are detected on screening examinations or in the workup and evaluation of a primary neoplasm. There are a myriad of modalities and imaging techniques within these modalities that may be used for characterization purposes. However, the role of imaging for characterization varies greatly depending on the specific lesion to be characterized, in terms of its initial appearance and location within the body. The radiologic workup and evaluation of a solitary pulmonary nodule may differ from multiple pulmonary nodules, which clearly differ from an adnexal mass. The remaining portions of this commentary will explore and contrast lesion characterization in different clinical and radiologic settings.

PULMONARY NODULES

Accurate characterization of a pulmonary nodule, frequently found on routine imaging for surveillance or workup of a primary neoplasm, presents a major diagnostic dilemma for radiologists and surgeons. The frequency of detection and need for a characterization of pulmonary nodules has increased dramatically as the volume of diagnostic imaging studies has increased over the decades. For instance, in the United States, more than 150,000 pulmonary nodules are identified each year on conventional chest radiography, and even in screening studies, up to 69% of patients screened with low-dose computed tomography (CT) scan demonstrate indeterminate pulmonary nodules (1,2). For the surgical oncologist, accurately characterizing a pulmonary nodule can greatly change a preoperative patient's stage of disease, and therefore the surgical procedure that may be performed. The time-honored tradition of follow-up to assess interval growth of a pulmonary nodule is of less value to the surgical oncologist because an immediate decision regarding staging and the optimal operative approach needs to be taken.

The two most commonly used techniques for characterizing pulmonary nodules are multislice CT and [18]FDG (18-fluoro-deoxy-D-glucose)/positron emission tomography (PET). Noninvasive characterization of pulmonary nodules on multislice CT evaluates certain characteristics of the nodule including margins, density, and internal characterizations. Malignant neoplasms tend to have spiculated or lobulated borders, while calcification distributed in a homogenous laminated central or "popcorn" pattern is usually associated with benign disease, such as in granulomatous disease or hamartomas (3). Imaging with [18]FDG/PET has provided another perhaps more sensitive and specific method for lung nodular characterization. In the past, the major role of PET scanning for thoracic disease was for staging lung cancer, or assessing response to therapy including the identification of tumor recurrence. However, with newer multislice hybrid (combined) PET/CT scanners, nodules detected on CT may be easily correlated with the metabolic information provided by the FDG/PET portion of the scan. PET scan has been found to be 80% to 95% sensitive and specific for characterizing nodules as malignant (4–7). Contemporary FDG/PET scanners have a false-negative rate because of the small pulmonary nodules. It is highly likely that with improved spatial resolution this will be less of a problem. False-positive diagnoses on FDG/PET may be related to more active infectious processes, which tend to have a high *standard uptake value* similar to malignancies. Frequently, these can be differentiated on the basis of morphologic characteristics on the multislice CT as well as actual quantitative FDG/PET values (8).

Finally, contrast-enhanced nodule CT characterization has been suggested as another means of characterizing pulmonary nodules. In general, FDG/PET is preferred because of its higher specificity and only slightly reduced sensitivity than contrast-enhanced CT scan for evaluating pulmonary nodules (9).

ADRENAL MASSES

Adrenal masses are also quite common in the oncologic patient population, including those patients with lung cancer as well as with other primary neoplasms. Adrenal pathology may be characterized based on the hormonal function of the adrenal glands as well as appearance on imaging studies. Hyperfunctioning adrenal status may indicate Conn or Cushing syndrome. Hypofunctional status may be of idiopathic cause from Addison disease or certain destructive bilateral adrenal pathologies. The basic approach to characterizing adrenal masses found at imaging actually begins with appropriate clinical history surrounding the pathology detected. For instance, a small adrenal lesion found in a patient who has hypertension should be evaluated with imaging in a different manner than a large, irregular adrenal mass found incidentally. The most common clinical setting for contemporary evaluation of an adrenal mass is the mass discovered in patients with normal adrenal function, usually incidentally. In the past, these lesions required invasive procedures such as biopsy or venous sampling. However, contemporary imaging with CT, magnetic resonance imaging (MRI), and nuclear studies obviate the need for these invasive techniques.

CT scan is the preferred imaging modality to evaluate the adrenal glands. CT scanning is fast, readily available, and offers the highest spatial resolution of any of the standard imaging modalities available. With contemporary CT scanning, CT slices may be obtained with 3- or 4-mm slice thicknesses, which reduces partial volume averaging and actually improves the accuracy of density measurements for many small adrenal lesions. Contrast-enhanced CT scan with delayed imaging may also help to characterize adrenal masses, especially those adenomas that do not have a high fat content. It is the high levels of intracellular lipid within adrenal adenomas that allow characterization of adenomas through the use of density (Hounsfield unit) reading on CT scan or MRI fat-suppression techniques.

MRI adds additional value to characterizing adrenal lesions, and the spatial resolution of MRI is generally adequate for characterizing even smaller adrenal lesions <1 cm. MRI uses chemical shift imaging where adenomas show a decreased signal on opposed phase imaging relative to in-phase imaging due to their fat content (10).

Ultrasound poorly characterizes adrenal masses and therefore plays relatively little role in the characterization of solid adrenal lesions. There are several nuclear radiotracers that may add quite specific information that is useful in characterizing adrenal lesions. For instance, metaiodobenzylguanidine (MIBG) has high specificity for pheochromocytomas. Recently, FDG/PET scanning combined with CT has been useful for characterizing adrenal masses based on the Hounsfield unit data on the CT portion of the examination and the standard uptake value on the PET portion of the examination (11). However, no comparison between MRI and FDG has been performed. Therefore, there are multiple outstanding modalities that may be used to noninvasively characterize adrenal masses, and perhaps the remaining challenge is to identify the optimal, cost-effective algorithm for the workup of such masses.

SMALL LIVER LESIONS

Small liver lesions are frequently found both in patients with primary tumors as well as those patients without neoplasm (12,13). Characterization of these lesions is most commonly performed with MRI. Within the radiology literature, there is abundant information concerning the performance of individual MRI pulse sequences for characterizing liver lesions. Overall, MRI is quite effective. In patients with no history of malignancy or without chronic liver disease, the probability of malignancy in small hepatic lesions, <1 cm, is relatively low. In this setting, patients may benefit simply from follow-up. However, in patients with a known diagnosis of malignancy or chronic liver disease, workup with contrast-enhanced MRI is valuable. MRI is especially useful for excluding the possibility of malignancy, and in selected cases for characterizing benign lesions such as cysts, hemangiomas, focal nodular hyperplasia, and hepatic adenomas. Standard morphologic criteria used on any imaging modality may help delineate and characterize primary hepatic neoplasms such as hepatocellular carcinoma and intrahepatic cholangiocarcinoma from metastatic disease. However, even with MRI, the ability for MRI to distinguish the site of origin of hepatic metastases is quite limited.

SMALL PANCREATIC LESIONS

Pancreatic imaging is most commonly used for staging patients with known pancreatic cancer preoperatively or in the assessment of pancreatitis. Again, with the increased utility of diagnostic imaging, more small pancreatic lesions are being incidentally detected. These small pancreatic lesions, usually cystic, require further evaluation and characterization. Both multidetector CT scanning and MRI are useful in this regard. The most difficult of pancreatic lesions to characterize are the cystic neoplasms of the pancreas. Benign microcystic serous adenomas are characterized as being composed of multiple small cysts that may or may not have a central calcification. These are benign and, in general, surgical intervention is not warranted. However, the cyst walls in serous cystadenomas may enhance, and when the cysts are tiny and innumerable, the overall lesion appears to "enhance" because of the cyst wall. This may give a false impression of the nature of the lesion and further evaluation with MRI is warranted. Macrocystic or mucinous pancreatic tumors generally consist of a single or multiple cystic lesions that tend to be larger in size than microcystic lesions. Mucinous lesions are premalignant and undergo malignant degeneration with the development of soft-tissue masses.

Recently, much has been written on the subject of intraductal papillary mucinous tumors as a distinct type of cystic pancreatic neoplasm. At endoscopy, mucin is generally seen at the pancreatic duct opening. At imaging, intraductal papillary mucinous tumors may exhibit diffuse enlargement of the pancreatic duct or focal cystic masses in continuity with the pancreatic duct. Probably the most difficult pancreatic cystic lesion to characterize is the intraductal papillary mucinous neoplasm (IPMN). This tumor was first described by Ohashi et al. (14) in 1982 and was further defined by the World Health Organization in 1996 as an intraductal papillary mucin-producing neoplasm arising in the main pancreatic duct or one of its major branches. Because IPMN represents a wide spectrum of diseases ranging from benign neoplasms to tumors with large components of invasive carcinoma, the radiologic appearance is quite variable. IPMN, characterized by cystic dilatation of the main or branches of the pancreatic duct, has been reported to represent 17% to 25% of resections of pancreatic neoplasms at major medical institutions.

With increasing recognition of this disorder, IPMNs have been characterized into four main groups on the basis of the degree of atypica: IPMN adenoma, IPMN borderline, IPMN with carcinoma in situ, and IPMN with invasive carcinoma. The surgical treatment of choice for IPMN is also somewhat controversial. This relates to imaging characterization especially of recurrences. Increasingly, patients are undergoing resection for IPMN, and it is critical to not only recognize its primary appearance but the appearance of tumor recurrence. Recurrences of IMPN have an even more variable appearance than do primary lesions. They may appear as unilocular cystic lesions or as simply solid masses. There is also very little correlation between margin status and location of recurrence.

Unfortunately, there is significant overlap in the imaging appearance of these various cystic pancreatic neoplasms. Some features such as the calcification within the cyst, enhancement of the cyst wall, and location within the pancreas help to differentiate or characterize mucinous and serous lesions. The problem of pancreatic lesion characterization is further confounded by non-neoplastic conditions such as pancreatic pseudocysts, which are also in the differential of cystic lesions. In some cases, therefore, clinical history of pancreatitis or the presence of pancreatic calcifications suggestive of chronic pancreatitis may help in distinguishing and characterizing lesions (15).

RENAL MASSES

As with other lesions, the widespread use of ultrasound, CT/MRI, and abdominal imaging has led to a dramatic increase in the detection of renal masses (16). To further characterize these masses, CT or MRI may be performed. Both CT and MRI are excellent for characterizing masses that contain fat. However, neither technique can fully distinguish or characterize benign from malignant lesions, especially those that do not contain fat. Most studies generally show equal performance of CT and MRI for characterization. However, complicated renal cysts, one of the more interesting renal lesions, may be better characterized with CT because of its improved spatial resolution. Also, enhanced spatial resolution of CT allows for better preoperative planning if indeed a lesion is characterized as being surgical in nature and requiring further therapeutic intervention.

The classic renal cystic mass classification was created by Bosniak and evolved over time, principally on the basis of criteria based on CT (17). The Bosniak classification is an effective tool for renal mass classification and divides cystic lesions into four categories. Category I refers to benign simple cysts with thin hairline walls that do not contain calcifications or solid components. Bosniak type II cystic lesions may contain a few hairline septa but are generally not measurable, and a few tiny calcifications may be present in the wall or septa. Also included in Bosniak II cystic lesions are uniformly high attenuating lesions that are <3 cm in size but which are sharply marginated and do not enhance. Type IIF, the F indicating follow-up is needed, are cysts that contain multiple thin septa that have minimal thickening and may contain calcifications that are slightly thick or nodular. These nonenhancing lesions are also thought to be benign but need to be followed to prove their size stability. Type III lesions are cystic masses with thick, irregular or smooth walls in which there is clear contrast enhancement demonstrated on CT. These masses require surgical intervention in most cases as neoplasms cannot be excluded. Type IV lesions are clearly malignant cystic masses that meet all the criteria of type III lesions but also contain distinct enhancing soft-tissue components.

In the past, the utility of ultrasound was generally thought of for its simple diagnosis of cystic lesion. However, ultrasound increasingly can be used to characterize renal masses as well. This is especially the case with the development of second-generation contrast agents that contain micro bubbles of gas. With this new contrast, ultrasound as a modality has become even more sensitive and specific to renal lesion characterization (17).

REFERENCES

1. Ost D, Fein AM, Feinsilver SH. Clinical practice: the solitary pulmonary nodule. *N Engl J Med.* 2003;348:2535–2542.
2. Swensen SJ, Jettt JR, Hartman TR, et al. Lung cancer screening with CT: Mayo Clinic experience. *Radiology.* 2003;226:756–761.
3. Ko JP. Lung nodule detection and characterization with multi-slice CT. *J Thorac Imaging.* 2005;20:196–209.
4. Patz EF, Lowe VJ, Hoffman JM, et al. Focal pulmonary abnormalities: Evaluation with F-18 fluorodeoxyglucose PET scanning. *Radiology.* 1993;188:487–490.
5. Gupta NC, Maloof J, Gunel E. Probability of malignancy in solitary pulmonary nodules using fluorine-18-FDG and PET. *J Nucl Med.* 1996;37:943–948.
6. Herder GJ, Golding RP, Hoekstra OS, et al. The performance of (18)F-fluorodeoxyglucose positron emission tomography in small solitary pulmonary nodules. *Eur J Nucl Med Mol Imaging.* 2004;31:1231–1236.
7. Dewan NA, Gupta NC, Redepenning LS, et al. Diagnostic efficacy of PET-FDG imaging in solitary pulmonary nodules. Potential role in evaluation and management. *Chest.* 1993;104:997–1002.
8. Kim SK, Allen-Auerbach M, Goldin J, et al. Accuracy of PET/CT in characterization of solitary pulmonary lesions. *J Nucl Med.* 2007;48:214–220.
9. Christensen JA, Nathan MA, Mullan BP, et al. Characterization of the solitary pulmonary nodule: 18F-FDG PET versus nodule-enhancement CT. *AJR Am J Roentgenol.* 2006;187:1361–1367.
10. Lockhart ME, Smith JK, Kenney PJ. Imaging of adrenal masses. *Eur J Radiol.* 2002;41:95–112.
11. Blake MA, Slattery JMA, Kalra MK, et al. Adrenal lesions: characterization with fused PET/CT image in patients with proved or suspected malignancy—initial experience. *Radiology.* 2006;238:970–977.
12. Jones EC, Chezmar JL, Nelson RC, et al. The frequency and significance of small (less than or equal to 15 mm) hepatic lesions detected by CT. *AJR Am J Roentgenol.* 1992;158:535–539.
13. Schwartz LH, Gandras EJ, Colangelo SM, et al. Prevalence and importance of small hepatic lesions found at CT in patients with cancer. *Radiology.* 1999;210:71–74.
14. Ohashi K, Murakami Y, Murayama M, et al. Four cases of mucous secreting pancreatic cancer. *Prog Dig Endosc.* 1982;20:348–351.
15. Scheiman JM. Management of cystic lesions of the pancreas. *J Gastrointest Surg.* 2008;12:405–407.
16. Masood J., Lane T., Koye B, et al. Renal cell carcinoma: incidental detection during routine ultrasonography in men presenting with lower urinary tract symptoms. *Br J Urol Int.* 2001;88:671–674.
17. Ascenti G, Maziotti S, Zimbaro G, et al. Complex cystic renal masses: characterization with contrast-enhanced US. *Radiology.* 2007;243:158–165.

9

Role of Positron Emission Tomography and Positron Emission Tomography-Computerized Tomography in Oncology

Hossein Jadvar

We are currently witnessing an evolution from the current nonspecific imaging methods toward patient-specific imaging evaluation based on morphologic, physiologic, molecular, and genetic markers of cancer. This evolution is stimulated through the use of multimodality imaging systems and "smart" specific imaging agents for achieving the key tasks of accurate diagnosis, staging, treatment planning, treatment response prediction and evaluation, restaging, surveillance, and prognosis in individual patients. It has become clear that the morphologic diagnostic imaging information (e.g., computed tomography [CT] or magnetic resonance imaging [MRI]) can be complemented significantly with the functional imaging information in a synergistic way, leading to increased diagnostic confidence. The impetus for this notion has been facilitated by the rapid emergence of positron emission tomography (PET) and more recently integrated positron emission tomography-computed tomography (PET-CT) in the clinical arena. PET-CT provides important complementary, and not competitive, diagnostic information by allowing precise localization of metabolic abnormalities and accurate metabolic characterization of normal and abnormal structures. PET-CT fusion imaging will also be essential with the development of more specific radiotracers in view of the little nonspecific background landmarks. Moreover, attenuation correction allows for quantitative imaging assessment, which may increasingly become clinically important.

Current evidence indicates that PET with the commonly used radiolabeled glucose analog [F-18]-2-fluoro-2-deoxy-D-glucose (^{18}FDG) is 8% to 43% more accurate than conventional workup and morphologic imaging for the diagnosis, staging, restaging, and evaluation of treatment response in many cancers. PET also affects the clinical management by upstaging or downstaging the disease in 20% to 40% of patients in a cost-effective manner (1–5). There has also emerged sufficient evidence in support of the diagnostic utility and advantage of hybrid PET-CT imaging systems over individual CT and PET studies (6–19). This chapter reviews the clinical utility of ^{18}FDG-PET and PET-CT in the imaging evaluation and management of a number of major cancers with an emphasis on those cancer types that may benefit from surgical treatment.

PET-CT FUNDAMENTALS

Radioisotopes with enough energy may undergo positron decay. A positron is positively charged and is the antiparticle that corresponds to the negatively charged electron. The positron decays with a half-time that is defined as the amount of time it takes for the activity to decrease to one half of the original activity. As the positron follows a jagged path through tissue, it loses energy and eventually the antimatter positron and the electron annihilate each other, giving rise to two gamma rays, each with energy of 511 keV, traveling in nearly opposite directions.

Two detectors placed on opposite sides of the patient can record the two gamma rays at nearly the same time, a condition known as *in coincidence*. A PET scanner detects these coincident events to form a "functional" image. PET can be combined with a CT scanner that provides the "structural" image into a hybrid machine that superimposes the functional and structural images into a fused image. The CT scan can also be used to provide information needed for attenuation correction, which is important for image quantitation. Current PET-CT scanners have a common bed, which travels from the PET gantry to the CT gantry. Further details on the physics of positron decay, PET-CT instrumentation, image reconstruction, and potential artifacts are discussed elsewhere (20–27).

TUMOR GLUCOSE METABOLISM

Warburg et al. (28) noticed that malignant cells tend to prefer glucose over free fatty acids in order to supply their increased energy needs. If the malignant cells are hypoxic, they will use anaerobic metabolism, which necessitates more glucose than aerobic metabolism. Many cancers are associated with a high glucose metabolic rate. It has been found that the glucose analog 2-deoxy-D-glucose can be labeled with the positron emitter F-18 (half-life of 110 minutes) to form ^{18}FDG for measuring glucose metabolism. ^{18}FDG accumulates in cells in proportion to glucose metabolism. PET with ^{18}FDG as the radiotracer then reflects the relative distribution of glucose metabolic activity.

Glucose transporters in the cell membrane facilitate the transport of glucose and ^{18}FDG across the cell membrane. Glucose and ^{18}FDG are phosphorylated by hexokinase. The enzymes that further metabolize glucose-6-phosphate cannot use ^{18}FDG-6-phosphate as a substrate and ^{18}FDG-6-phosphate is trapped in the cell. The conversion of glucose-6-phospate or ^{18}FDG-6-phosphate back to glucose or ^{18}FDG, respectively, is performed by phosphatase. Except for normal liver tissue and some hepatocellular carcinomas, most tissues including cancer have little phosphatase activity. The facilitative glucose transporters (GLUT) are the mainstay vehicle for glucose uptake into cells. GLUT1 is the most important for cancer imaging with ^{18}FDG PET because it is often overexpressed in tumor cells. There is also often an overexpression and activity of hexokinase in malignant cells. Although most malignancies result in high ^{18}FDG accumulation, ^{18}FDG uptake is not specific for cancer as it is well known that other physiologic (e.g., thymus and physis in children, brown adipose tissue, working muscle), benign (e.g., adenoma), and disease conditions (e.g., infection and inflammation) may also result in high ^{18}FDG accumulation. ^{18}FDG is excreted in the urine, which can pose a problem for imaging the urinary system or structures adjacent to the urinary system.

General patient instruction for oncologic imaging is fasting for 4 to 6 hours prior to scanning. This is because hyperglycemia may result in a potential false-negative study as glucose and ^{18}FDG compete for cellular uptake. For the diabetic patient, it may be helpful to schedule an early afternoon imaging session with instruction to follow a normal schedule in the morning but skipping lunch. Figure 9.1 shows a normal ^{18}FDG PET-CT scan.

Attenuation correction allows image quantification. A relatively simple semiquantitative parameter that is often used is the standardized uptake value (SUV), which is defined as:

$$SUV = \text{decay-corrected radioactivity in ROI (cps/pixel)}$$
$$\times \text{ calibration factor (mCi/g/cps/pixel)/}$$
$$\text{injected dose (mCi)/patient weight (g)}$$

where ROI refers to region of interest on the PET image, often the tumor, and the decay-corrected dose is the injected dose that is decay-corrected from the time of injection to the time of scan (29). If the PET scanner has been calibrated, then SUV can be determined at the time of image interpretation by entering the patient weight, the administered dose, and the time the dose was measured at the beginning of the imaging acquisition. Often mean SUV, maximum SUV, or both, over a region of interest are reported. The SUV would be one if the activity was uniformly distributed over the whole body. There are modifications that can be made to this SUV formula by normalizing for lean body mass or body surface area rather than the total body weight, which may be preferable and more accurate in some patients (e.g., pediatric and obese patients). The SUV is useful when comparing specific regions of interest longitudinally (e.g., during treatment) using the same camera system in the same patient and at the same time after dose administration.

BRAIN TUMORS

Gliomas (astrocytoma, oligodendrogliomas, ependymomas) in adults comprise >90% of the primary brain tumors. Higher grade of tumor reflects increasing degree of malignancy. Structural imaging modalities such as CT and MRI are commonly performed to delineate the location, size, and vascularity of the tumor, which is often heterogeneous with intermixed areas of low- and high-grade neoplastic cells, hemorrhage, and necrosis. Primary treatment involves surgical resection followed by observation, adjuvant external-beam radiotherapy, radiosurgery, brachytherapy, or chemotherapy. Anatomic imaging is limited in differentiating residual or recurrent tumor from posttherapy structural alterations. Functional imaging such as PET has proved to be useful in this clinical context (30,31). Although many radiotracers have been employed with PET in the imaging evaluation of brain tumors, as with other tumors, we concentrate on ^{18}FDG, which has been the most commonly used radiotracer.

Corticosteroids, which may be employed in patients with brain tumors for symptomatic relief of cerebral edema, can result in diminished brain glucose utilization independent of concurrent anticonvulsant medication, blood glucose level, and cerebral atrophy (32). Sedatives may also reduce cerebral glucose metabolism (33).

^{18}FDG is administered intravenously while the patient rests in a quiet room with dim lights and minimal environmental stimulation during the uptake phase of 30 to 40 minutes before start of the imaging acquisition. Cerebral cortical and subcortical gray matter and the cerebellar cortex demonstrate physiologic high glucose metabolism. The metabolic activity of a lesion is compared relative to the physiologic low activity of the white matter with the centrum semiovale of the contralateral cerebral hemisphere used as reference. High-grade tumors demonstrate

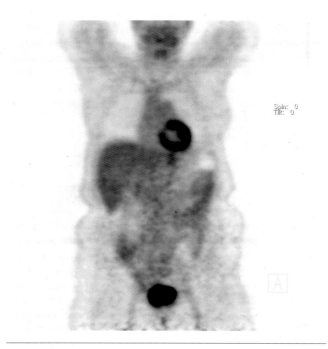

Figure 9.1 Normal ^{18}FDG positron emission tomography scan. The coronal image shows the normal biodistribution of ^{18}FDG with relatively intense cardiac and bladder urine activities.

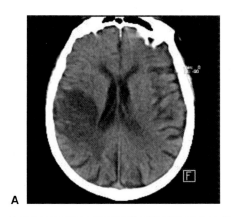 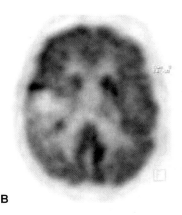 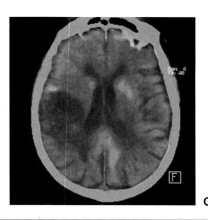

A   B   C

Figure 9.2 Recurrent brain tumor. (**A**) Computed tomography (CT; *left panel*), (**B**) positron emission tomograpy (PET; *middle panel*), and (**C**) fused PET and CT images (*right panel*) demonstrate hypermetabolic recurrent tumor at the anterolateral and the posteromedial margins of the hypoattenuated surgical basin in the right parietal lobe.

hypermetabolism and low-grade tumors show less than, equal to, or slightly higher than white matter metabolic activity.

Cerebellar diaschisis may also be seen with asymmetric cerebellar hemispheric hypometabolism contralateral to the remote primary supratentorial cerebral tumor. The mechanism of this observation is an interruption of the corticopontocerebellar pathway from the cerebral hemispheres through the ipsilateral pons to the opposite cerebellar cortex. There is no clinical correlate to the cerebellar diaschisis and it may be reversible in patients with stroke, but often remains persistent in patients with brain tumors (34).

[18]FDG-PET has been shown to be useful in grading tumors, directing biopsy site and resection, assessing for malignant transformation of low-grade tumors, evaluating treatment response, and assessing for cerebral metastases (Figure 9.2) (35–44). A study from the Massachusetts General Hospital in Boston tabulated the referral indications for 75 patients with glioma (45). The range of indications included pretherapeutic baseline studies for treatment monitoring (1%), mapping of hypermetabolic regions before surgery or biopsy (2%), mapping of hypermetabolic regions before radiotherapy (2%), postsurgical evaluation for residual tumor (2%), assessment of the malignancy of the mass as a substitute for biopsy (11%), and distinguishing between radiation necrosis and recurrent tumor (87%).

It is not entirely clear when after therapy to perform a [18]FDG-PET scan to assess for response, but reduction in lesion glucose metabolism as proxy for favorable response may be seen in as early as 1 week after chemotherapy. Similar to histopathologic analysis, the [18]FDG-PET imaging detection of residual or recurrent tumor after high doses of local radiation with gamma knife may occasionally be difficult because of the intense inflammatory response, which is induced as a result of the pathologic injury of radiation necrosis.

HEAD AND NECK CANCER

Head and neck cancers are associated with excess alcohol ingestion and tobacco use. The most common histology is squa-

mous cell carcinoma, with cervical lymph nodes representing the major site of metastases. In a minority of patients with cervical lymph node metastases, the site of the head and neck primary tumor remains unknown despite comprehensive diagnostic evaluation.

Diagnostic imaging evaluation includes chest roentgenography, CT, and/or MRI of the head and neck, followed by panendoscopy and biopsies. Approximately 80% of cancers are located in the base of the tongue or the tonsillar fossa. Management options depend on the extent of disease and may include surgery and radiation therapy for early disease and chemotherapy for advanced disease. Functional imaging with [18]FDG-PET has been shown to be useful in the detection of the primary tumor site in patients with metastatic cervical lymphadenopathy, initial staging, discrimination of posttherapy structural changes from residual and recurrent disease, assessment of tumor response to therapy, detection of synchronous lung lesions, and in prognostication (46–52).

In preparing patients for the PET study, oral diazepam (5 to 10 mg orally) may be given 30 minutes to 1 hour prior to intravenous [18]FDG injection to reduce physiologic skeletal muscle uptake that may mimic or obscure nodal disease. Patients are instructed not to chew, talk, and move the head or dry swallow excessively during the [18]FDG uptake phase. Drinking a glass of water prior to imaging will diminish the retained salivary activity in the mouth and upper esophagus. Comfortable, warm ambient room temperature will reduce tracer uptake in brown fat. Dental metallic implants can cause artifacts in attenuation-corrected images obtained with a hybrid PET-CT imaging system (53). Examination of the non–attenuation-corrected PET images helps in the recognition of this artifact. Awareness of the physiologic biodistribution of [18]FDG in the head and neck is also important (54). Palatine tonsils and adenoids may display relatively high symmetric hypermetabolism, especially in children and young adults. [18]FDG localizations in the normal laryngeal tissue and the salivary glands are symmetric and typically low. False-positive findings may result from inflammation or infection. False-negative findings may be the result of small or superficial (submucosal) tumors.

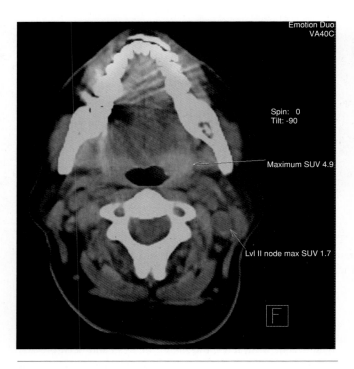

Figure 9.3 Head and neck cancer. The fused positron emission-computed tomography image shows a hypermetabolic left tonsil squamous cell carcinoma (maximum standardized uptake value [SUV] = 4.9) and an enlarged hypermetabolic regional left level II cervical metastatic node (maximum SUV = 1.7).

Squamous cell carcinoma is highly [18]FDG-avid (Figure 9.3). [18]FDG-PET complements structural imaging in accurately detecting the presence and extent of primary tumor and regional nodal metastases, especially in borderline or normal-sized nodes (50). Unsuspected distant metastases may also be detected, which may alter clinical management (55,56). In a study of 48 patients with advanced head and neck cancer, PET was able to assess lymph node involvement, distant metastases, and second primaries in a single imaging study and resulted in changes in clinical management in 8% of patients (57). PET has also been shown to be useful in localizing the site of occult primary tumor in patients with metastatic cervical adenopathy. In another study, the impact of [18]FDG-PET in the management of occult primary head and neck tumors was investigated in 16 patients with metastatic cervical lymphadenopathy. PET demonstrated sensitivity, specificity, and positive and negative predictive values of 62%, 66%, 62%, and 62%, respectively, in localizing the primary tumor site, which impacted the treatment plans in 53% of these patients (58).

The treatment-related structural alterations and edema reduce the accuracy of anatomic imaging modalities. [18]FDG-PET has been shown to be more sensitive and specific than both CT and MRI in this clinical setting (49,59). Because of intense radiation-induced inflammatory reaction, PET scanning after a delay of at least 12 weeks from the completion of radiation therapy seems to be necessary in order to reduce false-positive results (60). A decline in [18]FDG accumulation has been shown to

be correlated with favorable treatment response, improved local control, and longer survival (48). Lesions that demonstrate persistent high [18]FDG uptake indicate resistant disease that may require modification in therapeutic approach (47).

The clinical experience with PET-CT in the imaging evaluation of patients with head and neck cancer is currently limited. However, PET-CT appears to be superior to PET, and probably also to PET and CT viewed side by side (61,62). In particular, PET-CT may be widely used for treatment planning for radiation therapy (63). PET-CT has the potential for reducing tissue misses, to minimize the dose of ionizing radiation applied to nontarget areas, and to incorporate both anatomic and metabolic features of cancer into the three-dimensional conformal radiation therapy planning, which may then affect treatment outcome favorably. A recent prospective [18]FDG-PET-CT study of 24 patients with head and neck tumors showed that the PET-CT impacts the degree of confidence in anatomic localization of lesions by 51% and improves interobserver agreement (64).

THYROID CANCER

The usual presentation of thyroid cancer is a palpable nodule or a cervical lymph node discovered on physical examination. Dominant nodules in multinodular goiter, nodules that are increasing in size, and thyroid nodules in men convey greater risk for cancer. The prognosis of thyroid cancer is affected by many factors including gender, age, histology, and extent of disease. Thyroid carcinomas arise from follicular epithelium (papillary, follicular, anaplastic) or from parafollicular cells (medullary). Rare thyroid cancers include lymphoma and squamous cell carcinoma. Initial diagnosis is usually made by needle aspiration or biopsy.

The normal thyroid gland typically demonstrates no or low [18]FDG accumulation. Focal hypermetabolism may indicate benign autonomous nodules or otherwise unknown malignancy. Overexpression of GLUT1 on the cell membrane of thyroid neoplasms has been shown to be closely related to more aggressive biological behavior (65). In patients with thyroid cancer, the standard therapy is thyroidectomy followed by radioiodine (I-131) ablation. Patients are followed for evidence of recurrent or metastatic disease based on serial physical examination and monitoring of serum thyroglobulin (Tg) level. It has been noted that occasionally the diagnostic radioiodine scan may be negative in view of high clinical suspicion for disease (e.g., high Tg level or abnormal physical findings). In these situations, other nuclear studies have been employed using Tc-99m tetrofosmin, Tc-99m sestamibi, In-111 octreotide, thallium-201, and [18]FDG. While well-differentiated thyroid cancer may show low [18]FDG uptake and good iodine avidity but poorly differentiated malignancy and tumors such as anaplastic carcinoma and Hurthle cell carcinoma tend to demonstrate high [18]FDG accumulation and no iodine accumulation ("flip-flop" phenomenon) (66).

Many studies have now documented the diagnostic utility of [18]FDG-PET in localizing the non–iodine-avid metastases in up to 70% of patients and it is most promising at Tg levels of >10 mcg/L (67–76). The localization of disease may be amenable to local surgical or radiotherapeutic intervention without resort to systemic therapy (77). Although earlier studies showed that the capacity of [18]FDG-PET in localizing disease may not depend on

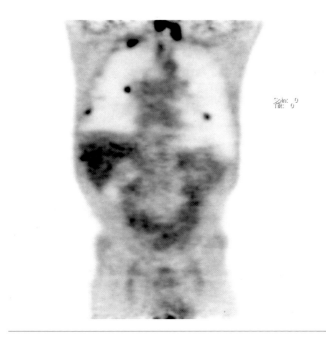

Figure 9.4 Metastatic medullary thyroid cancer. The coronal positron emission tomography image shows intensely hypermetabolic primary thyroid tumor and pulmonary metastatic disease in a patient with elevated serum calcitonin level.

the presence of high serum thyroid-stimulating hormone (TSH) level, recent reports indicate that endogenous TSH stimulation or exogenous recombinant TSH (rhTSH) stimulation improve the detectability of occult thyroid metastases with [18]FDG-PET in comparison with scans performed on TSH suppression (78–80). [18]FDG-PET has also been shown to have prognostic utility. Patients with positive PET studies, high rates of [18]FDG accumulation in the lesions, and overall high volume of [18]FDG-avid disease (>125 mL) have reduced survival in comparison to those patients without these findings (81). In patients with medullary thyroid cancer, [18]FDG-PET has been shown to be the most sensitive and specific single modality for localizing metastases in the clinical setting of increased serum calcitonin level (Figure 9.4) (82). Recent studies have also demonstrated the utility of the combined PET-CT imaging systems for the diagnosis and anatomic localization of recurrent and metastatic thyroid cancer (83).

In summary, it is expected that [18]FDG-PET will continue to have a growing role in the imaging assessment of patients with thyroid cancer, specifically in thyroidectomized patients with rising serum Tg level and negative radioiodine scan.

ESOPHAGEAL CANCER

Esophageal cancer accounts for about 4% of all digestive tract cancers. The distal esophagus is most often involved and the overall prognosis is generally poor. The diagnostic procedures include esophagoscopy with biopsy. Squamous cell carcinoma accounts for two thirds of esophageal carcinomas. Adenocarcinoma is the second most common histology and usually

arises from Barrett esophagus. Other less common malignancies include sarcoma, primary melanoma, and oat cell carcinoma (apudoma). CT and endoscopic ultrasound are the mainstays in the clinical staging of esophageal carcinoma. However, imaging evaluation with CT is not a reliable index of resectability. Surgical resection and radiation therapy remain the standard treatment for patients with esophageal carcinoma. Aggressive surgical intervention provides for a chance of cure, and radiation therapy offers palliation for obstructive symptoms. Chemotherapy may also be considered for metastatic disease.

Primary esophageal carcinoma is highly [18]FDG-avid, which is correlated with increased GLUT1 expression in the tumor (84,85). However, small cancers may be missed, especially in the gastroesophageal junction where there may be mild physiologic [18]FDG accumulation. The diagnostic performance of [18]FDG-PET may not be significantly different from that for CT in the initial staging of esophageal cancer (86). The ability of [18]FDG-PET in detecting locoregional lymph node metastases depends on many factors, including the tumor volume in the lymph node, the node size, and the background metabolic activity. PET has relatively low sensitivity (about 30% to 50%) but relatively high specificity (about 90%) in detecting local invasion and locoregional lymph node metastases (87). Combination of PET and endoscopic ultrasound with fine-needle aspiration biopsy is suggested as the most cost-effective staging procedure for patients with esophageal cancer (88).

[18]FDG-PET is most useful in assessing for recurrent and distant metastatic disease (89). Combination of conventional methods and PET is most helpful in characterizing anastomotic recurrences. PET is more sensitive than, and as specific as, CT for the detection of systemic metastatic disease and may detect distant metastases in up to 10% to 20% of patients who were not identified with CT (90). Pooled sensitivity and specificity for detection of locoregional metastases have been reported to be 51% (95% confidence interval [CI]: 34%–69%) and 84% (95% CI: 76%–91%), respectively. For distant metastases, pooled sensitivity and specificity are 67% (95% CI: 58%–76%) and 97% (95% CI: 90%–100%), respectively (91). PET may provide additional diagnostic information over CT, which may lead to management changes in nearly 14% to 30% of patients (92). In one study, [18]FDG-PET was the only modality that predicted intended curative resection that could have avoided unnecessary surgeries in up to 38% of patients with esophageal cancer who were initially considered eligible for curative resection based on conventional methods (93).

False-positive results may occur in patients with benign strictures after dilation and with esophagitis (94). The diagnostic utility of [18]FDG-PET in monitoring histopathologic tumor response to therapy, such as neoadjuvant radiotherapy and chemotherapy, has also been reported (Figure 9.5) (95). Responders show a decline in lesion [18]FDG accumulation and nonresponders show minimal decline or no significant change in [18]FDG uptake. The PET evidence of response is associated with a longer disease-free period and better overall survival in comparison with nonresponders, who have worse prognosis (96). The recently developed hybrid PET-CT imaging system has also been shown to be helpful in improving diagnostic accuracy and confidence by providing both structural and metabolic diagnostic information in this clinical setting (97).

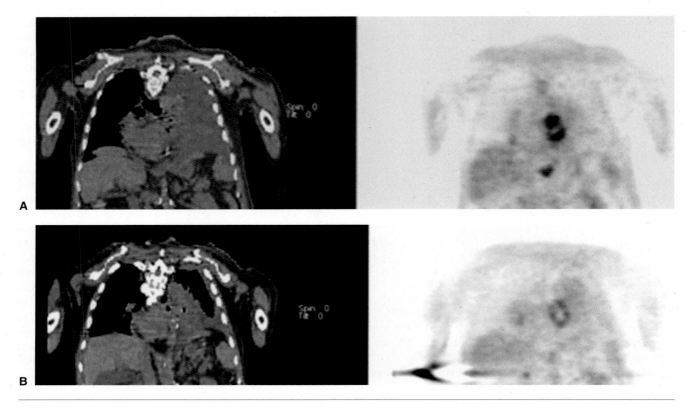

Figure 9.5 Esophageal cancer. (**A**) Pretreatment coronal computed tomography (CT; *left*) and coronal positron emission tomography (PET; *right*) show distal primary esophageal adenocarcinoma with regional hiatal metastatic lymphadenopathy. (**B**) Posttreatment coronal CT (*left*) and coronal PET (*right*) show decline in the metabolic activities of the primary tumor and the metastatic lymph nodes compatible with a favorable treatment response.

In summary, [18]FDG-PET improves staging and restaging of patients with esophageal cancer and allows for an objective assessment of tumor response to treatment while offering important prognostic information.

LUNG CANCER

Lung cancer is the foremost cause of cancer death in both sexes in the United States, with most cases attributable to smoking. Common histologies include squamous cell cancer, adenocarcinoma, bronchioloalveolar cancer (a subtype of adenocarcinoma), large cell cancer, and small cell cancer. Squamous cell cancer is located more centrally and tends to cavitate. Adenocarcinoma is located more peripherally. Lung cancer is also categorized into non–small cell cancer and small cell in view of the significant difference between their therapies and prognosis.

Normal lung displays low metabolism. Most lung cancers are generally very hypermetabolic (with SUV >2.5), except some tumor types such as bronchioloalveolar carcinoma and carcinoid that can be less [18]FDG-avid and falsely negative (98,99). An early clinical use of [18]FDG-PET was in characterizing solitary pulmonary nodule (SPN). A pulmonary nodule is smaller than 3 cm and surrounded by aerated lung. A lesion larger than 3 cm is referred to as *pulmonary mass*. Despite this definition and how the lesion may be initially discovered (e.g., incidental, screening, symptom-related workup), [18]FDG-PET is used to determine noninvasively if the lesion is likely malignant or benign. The ability of PET to detect and characterize pulmonary lesions generally depends on the tumor type, grade, size, noise, and the metabolic activities of the background and adjacent structures. With dedicated PET or hybrid PET-CT systems, lesions as small as 5 to 7 mm may be detected and characterized with optimal conditions (e.g., low noise and background activities, no motion). [18]FDG-PET has high sensitivity (about 97%) and a lower specificity (about 78%) in detecting malignant SPN (100). The lower positive predictive value is due to potential false-positive results that may occur primarily with inflammation and infection. Granulomatous disease is a common cause of false-positive results. In the current clinical practice a hypometabolic SPN with a sufficient size (relative to the spatial resolution of the imaging system) is considered benign and is followed with serial anatomic imaging (e.g., chest radiography or CT) to evaluate for interval changes. A hypermetabolic SPN is presumed malignant and will need tissue sampling despite potential for false-positive results, although metabolically active nonmalignant conditions may then be treated accordingly (Figure 9.6).

The use of [18]FDG-PET in staging lung cancer is now a common practice. The metabolic information improves the CT-based size criteria for nodal staging. This is because [18]FDG-PET can detect tumor deposits in nodes smaller than the typical CT criteria for a positive mediastinal node (short axis size >1 cm), or exclude tumor in large nodes (e.g., scarred or edematous after treatment). However, this size-based criterion is known to

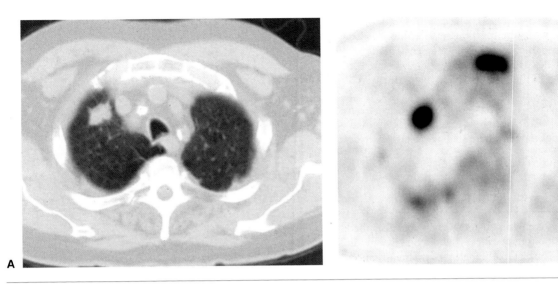

Figure 9.6 Lung cancer. Axial computed tomography (**A**) and positron emission tomography (**B**) images show an intensely hypermetabolic primary lung cancer in the right lung apex with osseous metastases involving the manubrium and ribs.

be very inaccurate. [18]FDG-PET can both identify positive nodes that are smaller in size, and identify negative nodes that are large in size (101). The important task of [18]FDG-PET and PET-CT is to separate resectable from nonresectable cancer based on accurate staging of disease (102,103). Detection of contralateral mediastinal or distant disease generally precludes surgical management (104). [18]FDG-PET may also increase the biopsy yield by directing the biopsy to the most metabolically active portion of the lesion. In a systematic review and meta-analysis of studies comparing [18]FDG-PET and CT evaluation of mediastinal lymph nodes in lung cancer, pooled sensitivity and specificity were 85% and 90% for PET and 61% and 79% for CT, respectively. [18]FDG-PET was more sensitive but less specific in enlarged lymph nodes (sensitivity of 100%, specificity of 78%) that in normal-sized nodes (sensitivity of 82%, specificity of 93%) (105). Recently it has also been shown that integrated PET-CT can provide significant diagnostic information beyond that available by conventional visual correlation of separate PET and CT scans in a substantial number of patients (106). [18]FDG-PET has also been found to improve the preoperative imaging evaluation of patients with proven or suspected lung metastases from other malignancies, altering the surgical management in about 21% of these patients (107).

[18]FDG-PET, and particularly PET-CT, may have an important role in radiation treatment planning in lung cancer by improving port and dose determinations (108,109). The goal is to improve local control by maximizing radiation to the metabolically active portions of the tumor while sparing normal adjacent tissues. [18]FDG-PET has been considerably useful in differentiating posttreatment structural changes from residual or recurrent tumor and in detecting potential second new primaries. Detection of new second primaries allows early treatment similar to the initial primary while salvage therapies can be employed for localized recurrent lung cancer (110). Hicks et al. (111) reported a sensitivity of 98% and a specificity of 82% in detecting recurrent disease in patients with suspected relapse after definitive therapy.

[18]FDG-PET scan also had an impact on clinical management in 63% of patients. Other studies have corroborated the change in clinical management in a significant number of patients with lung cancer, primarily through avoiding unnecessary diagnostic procedures and surgeries and by initiating previously unplanned therapies (112–114). In general, a short-term change in management may have an important effect on long-term outcome while allocating health care resources and dollars more effectively.

A major utility of [18]FDG-PET is in providing an objective imaging-based tool for monitoring therapy response in cancer. A decline in tumor metabolism is associated with favorable treatment response. Surgery may be considered in some patients with stage IIIB disease when [18]FDG-PET documents good treatment response to neoadjuvant chemotherapy and radiotherapy. Early decline in lesion metabolism during chemotherapy may also suggest overall good response after the completion of the treatment cycles (115). Despite this, however, the optimal time for PET scanning after completion of treatment remains undefined. In general, the longest wait is after radiation therapy because radiation is associated with a relatively marked inflammatory reaction and healing, which are hypermetabolic and cannot be readily distinguished from residual or recurrent tumor. Nevertheless, PET typically may be performed >3 months after radiotherapy when the inflammatory reaction largely subsides.

[18]FDG-PET may also provide important prognostic information (116). A retrospective study of 155 patients with lung cancer showed that the 118 patients with an SUV <10 had a median survival 24.6 months and the 37 patients with an SUV >10 had a median survival of 11.4 months (117). Multivariate analysis showed that SUV provided independent prognostic information when compared with clinical stage and lesion size. Similar findings have been reported by other investigators. In one study, patients with lesion SUV ≤5 had significantly longer disease-free survival, than those with lesion SUV >5 (88% vs. 17%, respectively) (118). Another investigation showed that patients with tumor SUV ≥7 had 6.3 times the 5-year mortality

of those with tumor SUV <7 (119). The prognostic information provided by SUV may stem from the relationship between [18]FDG avidity and tumor biological behavior (such as grade and proliferation) (120). [18]FDG-PET has also been shown to be cost-effective when inserted in the diagnostic imaging evaluation of patient with non–small cell lung cancer (121).

In summary, [18]FDG-PET has a major role in the diagnostic imaging evaluation of patients with lung cancer through providing important information on accurate staging, restaging, treatment evaluation, and prognosis.

BREAST CANCER

Breast cancer is the most common cancer in women in the United States. The lifetime risk of breast cancer is about one in eight in the American women. The histopathologic types of breast cancer include ductal adenocarcinoma, lobular carcinoma, lymphoma, sarcoma, and Paget disease of the nipple. Mammography and ultrasound are currently the principal imaging modalities for screening. Mammography has low specificity, and although it is relatively sensitive for detecting suspicious lesions in fatty breasts, it has lower sensitivity in detecting lesions in dense and augmented breasts. Breast MRI has also been employed for characterization of breast lesions and for determination of tumor relationship to the axillary and supraclavicular neurovascular structures. Scintimammography with Tc-99m sestamibi may be helpful in the evaluation of radiographically dense breasts. Bone scintigraphy is useful for the detection of osseous metastatic disease. There has also been a fast-growing utilization of preoperative mapping of the sentinel lymph node(s) with scintigraphy in order to stage the axilla to avoid complete axillary nodal dissection with its associated potential morbidity (e.g., chronic pain, numbness, lymphedema).

[18]FDG-PET and to a lesser extent PET-CT have been evaluated for diagnosis, staging, restaging, and monitoring therapy response in patients with breast cancer (Figure 9.7) (122–132). Although the current data suggest that [18]FDG-PET may have limited diagnostic utility in the detection of small primary tumors, in staging the axilla, and in detecting blastic osseous metastatic lesions, PET has superiority over conventional imaging in detecting distant metastases and recurrent disease, and in monitoring therapy response.

Although few studies have demonstrated overexpression of GLUT1 in untreated primary breast cancer, others have reported no clear relationship between tumor [18]FDG uptake and GLUT1 or Hexokinase-II overexpression (133,134). [18]FDG localization is significantly higher in ductal carcinoma than in lobular (median SUV 5.6 for infiltrating ductal carcinomas vs. 3.8 for lobular carcinomas) (135,136). Breast density and hormonal status affect the [18]FDG uptake in the breast tissue. Dense breasts demonstrate higher [18]FDG uptake than nondense breasts. However, the highest SUV observed in dense breasts is relatively low at about 1.4 (137).

Lactating breast shows high [18]FDG localization that appears to be related to suckling. The high [18]FDG uptake in the breast, however, may impede tumor detection in this subset of patients. Similarly, acute or chronic infectious mastitis and postsurgical hemorrhagic mastitis may lead to breast hypermetabolism.

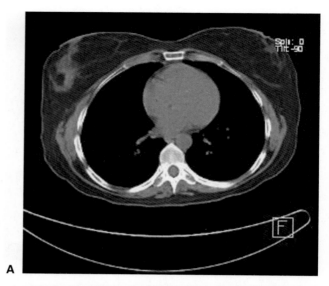

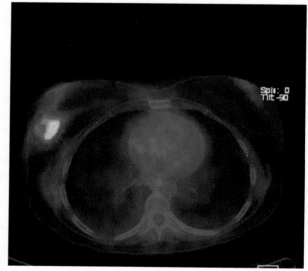

Figure 9.7 Breast cancer. (**A**) Axial computed tomography (CT; *top*) and (**B**) fused position emission tomography-CT (*bottom*) images show a hypermetabolic infiltrating ductal carcinoma in the right breast.

Mammography and ultrasound remain the main diagnostic imaging tools for the diagnosis of primary breast cancer. However, the metabolic information provided by [18]FDG-PET may be useful in the noninvasive characterization of the indeterminate lesions. The development of the new combined PET and radiographic imaging systems (a positron emission mammography device mounted on a stereotactic x-ray mammography system) and the positron-sensitive probe may help in discriminating between benign and malignant breast masses, in guiding biopsy, and in reducing costly surgical procedures (138,139). PET is also useful in the evaluation of patients with augmented breasts in whom the other traditional diagnostic imaging techniques may be inconclusive (140). For the diagnosis of breast cancer, lesion detectability appears to increase with the more delayed scan time of 3 hours than the usual scan time of 1 to 1.5 hours (93% vs. 83%, respectively) after the intravenous administration of [18]FDG. It is also of note that false-positive PET may occur in specific conditions such as fibroadenoma, but this is similar to the case with Tc-99m sestamibi imaging. However, in general it appears that SUV of benign lesion is lower than that of the malignant lesion, although there is significant overlap. [18]FDG-PET has also been found to be useful in the imaging evaluation of selected patients with high-risk operable breast cancer by offering higher specificity (fewer false-positive results) than conventional imaging studies (141).

[18]FDG-PET has limited sensitivity in staging the axilla in patients with early breast cancer with a false-negative rate that may approach over 20% (142,143). A recent prospective multicenter study of axillary nodal staging with [18]FDG-PET demonstrated mean sensitivity, specificity, and positive and negative predictive values of 61%, 80%, 62%, and 79%, respectively (144). [18]FDG-PET appears to be a specific method for staging the axilla such that sentinel lymph node biopsy or axillary lymph node dissection may be avoided in patients with positive axilla on the PET study (145,146). The overall sensitivity and specificity for the detection of the axillary metastases on [18]FDG-PET does not appear to be related to the SUV of the primary carcinoma (147). The differences among studies in the reported diagnostic performance of PET in relation to axillary nodal staging are likely because of several factors including differences in the tumor type, the prevalence of disease in the study population, the imaging method, and the image interpretation criteria. However, detection of micrometastases and small tumor-infiltrated lymph nodes is limited by the spatial resolution of the current PET imaging systems (148).

[18]FDG-PET has also been reported to be a useful tool in the evaluation of patients with suspected metastatic plexopathy, particularly if the other imaging studies are unremarkable (149,150). PET can also differentiate between radiation-induced plexopathy and metastatic plexopathy. [18]FDG-PET has been found helpful in the evaluation of patients with inflammatory breast cancer. Mammography usually demonstrates parenchymal distortion, diffuse increased density, and skin thickening. On [18]FDG-PET, the diffuse pattern of breast [18]FDG uptake reflects the dermal lymphatic spread of the malignancy. In another uncommon malignancy, cystic infiltrating ductal carcinoma, PET shows intense focal [18]FDG localization in the solid component and a ringlike increased uptake corresponding to the wall of the cystic component of the tumor.

[18]FDG-PET has been demonstrated to be accurate in the diagnosis of recurrent and metastatic disease not recognized by conventional imaging methods (151–154). In a study comparing [18]FDG-PET and MRI for detecting recurrent disease, the sensitivity and specificity were 79% and 100% for MRI and 94% and 72% for PET. Additional unknown metastases were detected by whole-body PET in a few patients, which influenced the clinical management (155). A comparative study of [18]FDG-PET and conventional imaging in patients with clinical suspicion of local recurrence or distant metastatic disease demonstrated sensitivity, specificity, and positive and negative predictive values of 97%, 82%, 87%, and 96% for [18]FDG-PET in comparison with 84%, 60%, 73%, and 75% for conventional imaging. [18]FDG-PET upstaged the disease in 10% and downstaged the disease in 13%

of patients and led to a change in therapeutic management in 21% of patients (156). PET is also more sensitive than serum tumor markers (CA15-3 and carcinoembryonic antigen [CEA]) in detecting relapsed breast cancer (157–159). In a recent study of 46 women with elevated serum tumor markers 1 to 21 years after their initial diagnosis and treatment of breast cancer, PET-CT had a higher sensitivity (81% vs. 59%) and specificity (76% vs. 47%) than CT in detecting tumor recurrence. PET-CT also affected the clinical management 51% of these patients (160). [18]FDG-PET has been compared with bone scan in the detection of osseous metastases. PET and bone scan appear to offer similar sensitivity in this regard, but PET provides a specificity advantage over bone scan (161). Bone metastases of the osteolytic or mixed type are usually better visualized on PET than the sclerotic bony lesions. In general, [18]FDG-PET may impact the clinical stage and management of about 30% of patients with suspected recurrent and metastatic breast cancer (162).

[18]FDG-PET has been shown to be useful in the assessment of therapy response in patients with breast cancer by demonstrating decline in the tumor glucose metabolism with successful chemotherapy in correlation with decline in serum tumor markers. In one study, the median SUV of the lesions of patients who responded to chemotherapy decreased from 7.7 at baseline to 5.7 after the first chemotherapy course to 1.2 at the end of the chemotherapy regimen (163). In patients with stable disease as the best response, no significant decrease in tumor glucose SUV was noted in comparison to the baseline level (163). A complete response may be predicted after the first course of chemotherapy with a sensitivity of 90% to 100% and a specificity of 74% to 85% by SUV decrease below half that on the baseline pretreatment scan (164,165). Moreover, [18]FDG-PET has been demonstrated to be useful in evaluating response to the new therapies such as stereotactic interstitial laser therapy, which is emerging as a promising alternative to surgery for treating early-stage breast cancer (166).

PET can also stratify the clinical outcome more accurately than conventional imaging such that a negative PET predicts longer disease-free survival in comparison to a positive PET. [18]FDG-PET can provide quantitative metabolic information that may be used to predict overall and relapse-free survival in patients with breast cancer. Patients with lesions that demonstrate high [18]FDG uptake have significantly poorer prognoses than those with lesions that have low [18]FDG uptake (167,168).

COLORECTAL CANCER

Colorectal cancer is the third most common malignancy in the United States. The predisposing conditions include familial polyposis and ulcerative colitis. Digital rectal examination, fecal occult blood test, and endoscopy are used for screening. Barium enema and/or the recently developed CT colonography may also be employed for the imaging evaluation of patients with suspected colorectal cancer. The most common histology is adenocarcinoma with the tumor spread from the primary site to adjacent lymph nodes and further up to the mesenteric lymph node chain. Low rectal and anal cancers tend to spread laterally to perineal and inguinal nodes. Primary tumor is usually removed as local symptoms are relieved, which can enhance the quality of life.

Palliative radiation therapy is used in unresectable tumors with excessive bleeding. Chemotherapy has been employed for palliation and as radiation sensitizer. In postoperative patients, an elevated serum CEA level suggests recurrent and/or metastatic disease. The most common sites of metastases include the liver, lung, and brain. Resection of isolated metastases is associated with improved survival.

The utility of [18]FDG-PET in colorectal carcinoma has been studied relatively extensively (Figure 9.8) (169–175). For preoperative diagnosis, both CT and [18]FDG-PET may miss the involvement of the local lymph nodes. However, [18]FDG-PET is superior to CT for detecting liver metastases (pooled sensitivity and specificity of 88% and 96% for PET, and 83% and 84% for CT, respectively), affecting clinical management in 32% of patients (176). The detection of the primary tumor by PET depends on the size of the tumor and the background activity. Colon may occasionally demonstrate high [18]FDG localization. However, focal intense hypermetabolism is highly suspicious for neoplasms that may include carcinoma, although focal inflammation and infection can have similar appearance (177). False-negative findings may also result in subcentimeter and mucinous tumors.

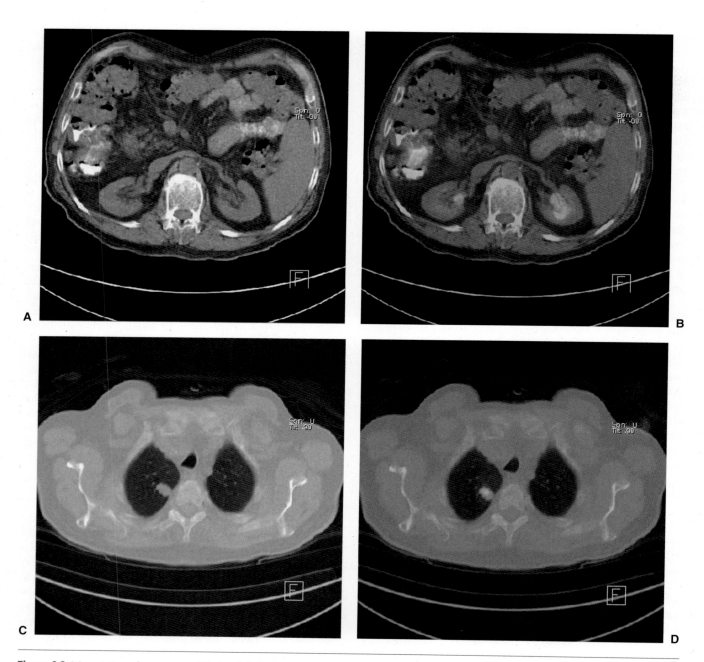

Figure 9.8 Metastatic colon cancer. (**A**) Axial abdomen computed tomography (CT; *top left*) (**B**) and fused position emission tomography (PET)-CT (*top right*) show the primary cecal tumor. (**C**) The axial chest CT (*bottom left*) (**D**) and fused PET-CT (*bottom right*) images show the metastatic deposit in the right lung apex.

[18]FDG-PET is mainly useful in the restaging of colorectal cancer for detection of recurrence and metastatic disease (178,179). Cancer tends to recur in up to one third of patients within 2 years after the primary curative therapy. In patients with elevated or increasing serum CEA level, imaging is used to localize the site of recurrence and/or metastasis. CT may miss both hepatic and extrahepatic metastases in a significant number of patients and cannot differentiate postsurgical anatomic alterations from tumor recurrence. Combined functional and structural imaging provides valuable complementary information on localization and characterization of lesions. In one study of 22 patients with abnormal CEA levels and normal conventional imaging, [18]FDG-PET displayed a positive predictive value of 89% and a negative predictive value of 100% for tumor detection (180). A recent meta-analysis synthesizing the findings of 11 peer-reviewed articles in 281 patients reported an overall sensitivity of 97% (95% CI: 95%–99%) and a specificity of 76% (95% CI: 64%–88%) for [18]FDG-PET in detecting recurrent colorectal cancer throughout the whole body. An overall [18]FDG-PET–directed change in management of 29% (95% CI: 25%–34%) was also reported (181). In another study, a survey of referring physicians indicated that [18]FDG-PET had a major impact on the management of their patients with a change in clinical stage in 42% and a change in clinical management in >60% of patients with colorectal cancer (182).

[18]FDG-PET is also cost-effective when inserted in the diagnostic imaging evaluation of patients with colorectal cancer. In one study of patients undergoing preoperative restaging, [18]FDG-PET resulted in substantial potential savings primarily as a result of detecting nonresectable disease and thereby avoiding unnecessary surgery (183,184). In a blinded prospective comparative study of [18]FDG-PET and CEA scan (99mTc-labeled arcitumomab) with surgical exploration as "gold standard," [18]FDG-PET scans predicted unresectable disease in 90% of patients and CEA scans failed to predict unresectable disease in any patient. In patients found to have resectable disease or disease that could be treated with regional therapy, [18]FDG-PET scan prediction rate was 81% and that of CEA scan was only 13% (185).

[18]FDG-PET has been shown to be useful in monitoring tumor response to treatment. Lesions that show decline in [18]FDG uptake after therapy demonstrate favorable response, while presence of residual [18]FDG uptake can lead to additional treatment (186–189). Radiation therapy is often associated with intense inflammatory reaction, which hinders detection of residual cancer with [18]FDG-PET performed early after completion of therapy. Although the exact time course of the [18]FDG uptake in relation to the postradiation inflammatory reaction remains undefined, presence of hypermetabolism several months (e.g., >6 months) after the completion of the radiotherapy raises the suspicion for residual cancer.

In summary, [18]FDG-PET is complementary to CT for preoperative staging at the time of initial diagnosis and is particularly indicated for restaging in patients with suspected recurrent and metastatic disease based on elevated or rising serum CEA level. PET is also useful for differentiating posttreatment changes from residual/recurrent cancer and in monitoring tumor response to therapy. [18]FDG-PET can have significant impact on the clinical management of recurrent colorectal cancer in a cost-effective manner.

MELANOMA

Melanoma develops from the malignant transformation of the melanocyte that produces the pigment melanin. Melanoma is a potentially curable disease if discovered at an early stage. Diagnosis is established by biopsy, either excisional or by a core-punch technique. Important histopathologic factors include the lesion thickness (Breslow's microstaging) and level of invasion (Clark's microstaging). Melanoma can metastasize to almost any organ site, with the regional lymph nodes, lung, liver, bone, and brain as the more common sites. Surgical treatments include wide lesion excision for early-stage disease, excision of the regional nodes as directed by mapping the sentinel lymph node, and resection of accessible isolated distant metastases. Radiotherapy is considered for bone, brain, skin, and soft-tissue metastases. There is a lack of effective chemotherapy but immunotherapy with a variety of biological agents has been employed for metastatic disease.

The optimal management of melanoma depends on the accurate staging of disease, and in that sense [18]FDG-PET is evolving as a standard diagnostic imaging tool in patients with melanoma (190–194). Whole-body [18]FDG-PET is cost-effective in the imaging evaluation of patients at high risk for metastatic disease (Breslow thickness >1.5 cm) (195). [18]FDG-PET impacts the clinical management by detecting unknown metastases prior to planned surgery (which may be cancelled or altered), by prompting other treatment protocols (e.g., radiotherapy, immunotherapy), and can also be useful in objective imaging evaluation of treatment response (196–198). From the referring physician's perspective, [18]FDG-PET has a major impact on the management of patients with melanoma by either downstaging or upstaging the disease, leading to changes in treatment strategy in up to 53% of patients (199). However, false-positive results may occur with other benign and malignant lesions, and with infection and inflammation (200). False-negative results may occur with small-volume disease (including micrometastases) because of spatial resolution limitations (201–203). Sensitivities of 22% and 100% have been reported for PET and sentinel node biopsy, respectively, for detecting lymph node metastasis in melanoma ≥1 mm Breslow thickness. In one study, the sensitivity threshold for detection of nodal metastases was 90% for tumor volume ≥78 mm^3 and only 14% for tumor volumes <78 mm^3 (204). In another similar study, PET detected 100% of metastases ≥10 mm, 83% of metastases 6 to 10 mm, and only 23% of metastases ≤5 mm. [18]FDG-PET can reliably detect lymph node tumor deposits greater than approximately 80 mm^3 volume, which is most likely to occur in patients with stage III and IV disease, and therefore PET cannot substitute for sentinel lymph node mapping and tissue sampling (205).

[18]FDG-PET offers a diagnostic advantage over CT for the detection of recurrent and metastatic disease (Figure 9.9) (206). In a retrospective study of 104 patients with primary or recurrent melanoma who had a median follow-up of 24 months, the sensitivity and specificity were 84% (95% CI: 78%–89%) and 97% (95% CI: 95%–99%), respectively, for PET, and 58% (95% CI: 49%–66%) and 70% (95% CI: 51%–84%), respectively, for CT. The sensitivity of CT increased to 69% (95% CI: 59%–77%), still lower than that for PET, when sites not routinely evaluated by CT were excluded from comparative analysis (207).

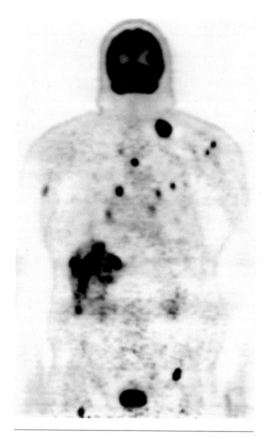

Figure 9.9 Metastatic melanoma. Coronal position emission tomography image shows numerous hypermetabolic metastatic deposits including panlobar involvement of the liver.

In another study that reviewed the published literature between 1980 and 2000, an overall sensitivity of 74% to 100% and specificity of 67% to 100% were reported. PET was considered particularly valuable when surgical intervention was being considered and for clarification of the abnormal radiologic findings at follow-up (208). In a meta-analysis of the diagnostic accuracy of ^{18}FDG-PET in cutaneous melanoma that included 11 studies, the pooled sensitivity and specificity of PET were reported to be 79% (95% CI: 66%–99%) and 86% (95% CI: 78%–95%). Subgroup analysis revealed that PET was more accurate for systemic staging than for regional staging (209). In another similar meta-analysis of 13 ^{18}FDG-PET studies, an overall sensitivity of 92% (95% CI: 88%–96%), and an overall specificity of 90% (95% CI: 83%–96%) were reported for detection of recurrent melanoma. The overall PET-directed change in management was 22% (210).

In summary, ^{18}FDG-PET provides an accurate imaging tool for surveying the whole body in patients with melanoma and is superior to CT for the detection of metastatic disease. Although PET cannot detect micrometastases, this is a common current limitation with any clinical imaging modality. In patients at high risk for metastases (Breslow thickness >1.5 mm), PET may be performed first to assess for possible distant metastatic disease. In patients with negative findings on PET studies, sentinel lymph node mapping and tissue sampling may be performed to evaluate

for micrometastatic nodal disease. In patients with PET demonstration of metastatic disease, management decisions may be made in a cost-effective manner without additional diagnostic workup.

SUMMARY

PET and PET-CT have now emerged not only as important research tools but also as significant diagnostic imaging systems in clinical medicine. There is little doubt that in the near future PET and PET-CT will become even more essential clinical imaging tools in oncology. PET and PET-CT will aid in the evolution from the current nonspecific imaging methods toward patient-specific imaging evaluation based on morphologic, physiologic, molecular, and genetic markers of disease. Ultimately, the use of multimodality imaging systems such as PET-CT and the expected forthcoming PET-MRI as well as development of "smart" specific imaging agents will achieve the key tasks of accurate diagnosis, staging, restaging, treatment planning, treatment response prediction and evaluation, surveillance, and prognosis in individual patients with cancer.

REFERENCES

1. Phelps ME. PET: the merging of biology and imaging into molecular imaging. *J Nucl Med.* 2000;41:661–681.
2. Oriuchi N, Higuchi T, Ishikita T, et al. Present role and future prospects of positron emission tomography in clinical oncology. *Cancer Sci.* 2006;97:1291–1297.
3. Czernin J, Allen-Auerbach M, Schelbert HR. Improvements in cancer staging with PET/CT: literature-based evidence as of September 2006. *J Nucl Med.* 2007;48(Suppl 1):78S–88S.
4. Delbeke D, Coleman RE, Cuiberteau MJ, et al. Procedure guideline for tumor imaging with 18F-FDG PET/CT. *J Nucl Med.* 2006; 47:885–895.
5. Gambhir SS, Czernin J, Schwimmer J, et al. A tabulated summary of the FDG PET literature. *J Nucl Med.* 2001;42(5 Suppl): 1S–93S.
6. Gambhir SS. Molecular imaging of cancer with positron emission tomography. *Nat Rev Cancer.* 2002;2:683–693.
7. Weber WA, Figlin R. Monitoring cancer treatment with PET/CT: does it make a difference? *J Nucl Med.* 2007;48(Suppl 1): 36S–44S.
8. Jarritt PH, Carson KJ, Hounsell AR, et al. The role of PET-CT scanning in radiotherapy planning. *Br J Radiol.* 2006;79 Spec No 1:S27–S35.
9. Endo K, Oriuchi N, Higuchi T, et al. PET and PET/CT using 18F-FDG in the diagnosis and management of cancer patients. *Int J Clin Oncol.* 2006;11:286–296.
10. Shankar LK, Hoffman JM, Bacharach S, et al. Consensus recommendation for the use of 18F-FDG PET as an indicator of therapeutic response in patients in National Cancer Institute Trials. *J Nucl Med.* 2006;47:1059–1066.
11. Blodgett TM, McCook BM, Federle MP. Positron emission tomography/computed tomography: protocol issues and options. *Semin Nucl Med.* 2006;36:157–168.
12. Messa C, Di Muzio N, Picchio M, et al. PET/CT and radiotherapy. *Q J Nucl Med Mol Imaging.* 2006;50:4–14.
13. von Schulthess GK, Steinert HC, Hany TF. Integrated PET/CT: current applications and future directions. *Radiology.* 2006;238:405–422.

14. Ell PJ. The contribution of PET/CT to improved patient management. *Br J Radiol.* 2006;79:32–36.

15. Beyer T, Townsend DW, Blodgett TM. Dual-modality PET/CT tomography for clinical oncology. *Q J Nucl Med.* 2002;46:24–34.

16. Cohade C, Wahl RL. Applications of positron emission tomography/computed tomography image fusion in clinical positron emission tomography: clinical use, interpretation methods, diagnostic improvements. *Semin Nucl Med.* 2003;33:228–237.

17. Delbeke D, Martin WH. Metabolic imaging with FDG: a primer. *Cancer J.* 2004;10:201–213.

18. Siegel BA, Dehdashti F. Oncologic PET/CT: current status and controversies. *Eur Radiol.* 2005;15 Suppl 4:D127–D132.

19. Wong TZ, Paulson EK, Nelson RC, et al. Practical approach to diagnostic CT combined with PET. *Am J Roentgenol AJR.* 2007;188: 622–629.

20. Jadvar H, Parker JA. *Clinical PET and PET-CT.* London: Springer-Verlag. 2005.

21. Blodgett TM, Meltzer CC, Townsend DW. PET/CT: form and function. *Radiology.* 2007;242:360–385.

22. Blodgett TM, Casagranda B, Townsend DW, et al. Issues, controversies, and clinical utility of combined PET-CT scanning: what is the interpreting physician facing? *AJR Am J Rontgenol.* 2005;184(Suppl):S138–S145.

23. Mawlawi O, Pan T, Macapinlac HA. PET/CT imaging techniques, considerations, and artifacts. *J Thorac Imaging.* 2006;21:99–110.

24. Antoch G, Freudenberg LS, Egelhof T, et al. Focal tracer uptake: a potential in contrast-enhanced dual-modality PET/CT scans. *J Nucl Med.* 2002;43:1339–1342.

25. Seemann MD. PET/CT: fundamental principles. *Eur J Med Res.* 2004;9:241–246.

26. Townsend DW. From 3-D positron emission tomography to 3-D positron emission tomography/computed tomography: What did we learn? *Mol Imaging Biol.* 2004;6(5):275–290.

27. Yau YY, Chan WS, Tam YM, et al. Application of intravenous contrast in PET-CT: does it really introduce significant attenuation correction error? *J Nucl Med.* 2005;46:283–291.

28. Warburg O, Wind F, Neglers E. On the metabolism of tumors in the body. In: Warburg O, ed. *Metabolism of tumors.* London: Constabel, 1930:254–270.

29. Wang Y, Chiu E, Rosenberg J, et al. Standardized uptake value atlas: characterization of physiological 2-deoxy-2-[F-18]fluoro-D-glucose uptake in normal tissues. *Mol Imaging Biol.* 2007;9:83–90.

30. Coleman RE, Hoffman JM, Hanson MW, et al. Clinical application of PET for the evaluation of brain tumors. *J Nucl Med.* 1991;32:616–622.

31. Wong TZ, van der Westhuizen GJ, Coleman RE. Positron emission tomography imaging of brain tumors. *Neuroimaging Clin N Am.* 2002;12:615–626.

32. Fulham MJ, Brunetti A, Aloj L, et al. Decreased cerebral glucose metabolism in patients with brain tumors: an effect of corticosteroids. *J Neurosurg.* 1995;83:657–664.

33. Blacklock JB, Oldfield EH, Di Chiro G, et al. Effect of barbiturate coma on glucose utilization in normal brain versus glioma. Positron emission tomography studies. *J Neurosurg.* 1987;67: 71–75.

34. Patronas NJ, Di Chiro G, Smith BH, et al. Depressed cerebellar glucose metabolism in supratentorial tumors. *Brain Res.* 1984;291:93–101.

35. De Witte O, Lefranc F, Levivier M, et al. FDG-PET as a prognostic factor in high-grade astrocytoma. *J Neurooncol.* 2000;49: 157–163.

36. De Witte O, Levivier M, Violon P, et al. Prognostic value positron emission tomography with [18F]fluoro-2-deoxy-D-glucose in the low-grade glioma. *Neurosurgery.* 1996;39:470–476.

37. Francavilla TL, Miletich RS, Di Chiro G, et al. Positron emission tomography in the detection of malignant degeneration of low-grade gliomas. *Neurosurgery.* 1989;24:1–5.

38. Griffeth LK, Rich KM, Dehdashti F, et al. Brain metastases from non-central nervous system tumors: evaluation with PET. *Radiology.* 1993;186:37–44.

39. Holzer T, Herholz K, Jeske J, et al. FDG PET as a prognostic indicator in radiochemotherapy of glioblastoma. *J Comput Assisted Tomogr.* 1993;17:681–687.

40. Levivier M, Goldman S, Pirotte B, et al. Diagnostic yield of stereotactic brain biopsy guided by positron emission tomography with [18F]fluorodeoxyglucose. *J Neurosurg.* 1995;82:445–452.

41. Langleben DD, Segall GM. PET in differentiation of recurrent brain tumor from radiation injury. *J Nucl Med.* 2000;41:1861–1867.

42. Mirzaei S, Knoll P, Kohn H. Diagnosis of recurrent astrocytoma with fluorodeoxyglucose F18 PET scanning. *N Engl J Med.* 2001;344:2030–2031.

43. Padma MV, Said S, Jacobs M, et al. Prediction of pathology and survival by FDG PET in gliomas. *J Neurooncol.* 2003;64:227–237.

44. Tralins KS, Douglas JG, Stelzer KJ, et al. Volumetric analysis of 18F-FDG PET in glioblastoma multiforme: prognostic information and possible role in definition of target volumes in radiation dose escalation. *J Nucl Med.* 2002;43:1667–1673.

45. Deshmukh A, Scott JA, Palmer EL, et al. Impact of fluorodeoxyglucose positron emission tomography on the clinical management of patients with glioma. *Clin Nucl Med.* 1996;21:720–725.

46. Chisin R, Macapinlac HA. The indications of FDG-PET in neck oncology. *Radiol Clin North Am.* 2000;38:999–1012.

47. Lowe VJ, Dunphy FR, Varvares M, et al. Evaluation of chemotherapy response in patients with advanced head and neck cancer using [F-18]fluorodeoxyglucose positron emission tomography. *Head Neck.* 1997;19:666–674.

48. Brun E, Kjellen E, Tennvall J, et al. FDG PET studies during treatment: prediction of therapy outcome in head and neck squamous cell carcinoma. *Head Neck.* 2002;24:127–135.

49. Lapela M, Grenman R, Kurki T, et al. Head and neck cancer: detection of recurrence with PET and 2-[F-18]fluoro-2-deoxy-D-glucose. *Radiology.* 1995;197:205–211.

50. Hannah A, Scott AM, Tochon-Danguy H, et al. Evaluation of 18 F-fluorodeoxyglucose positron emission tomography and computed tomography with histopathologic correlation in the initial staging of head and neck cancer. *Ann Surg.* 2002;236:208–217.

51. Greven KM, Williams DW 3rd, McGuirt WF Sr, et al. Serial positron emission tomography scans following radiation therapy of patients with head and neck cancer. *Head Neck.* 2001;23:942–946.

52. Wax MK, Myers LL, Gabalski EC, et al. Positron emission tomography in the evaluation of synchronous lung lesions in patients with untreated head and neck cancer. *Arch Otolaryngol Head Neck Surg.* 2002;128:703–707.

53. Goerres GW, Hany TF, Kamel E, et al. Head and neck imaging with PET and PET/CT: artifacts from dental metallic implants. *Eur J Nucl Med Mol Imaging.* 2002;29(3):367–370.

54. Goerres GW, Von Schulthess GK, Hany TF. Positron emission tomography and PET-CT of the head and neck: FDG uptake in normal anatomy, in benign lesions, and in changes resulting from treatment. *AJR Am J Roentgenol.* 2002;179:1337–1343.

55. Johansen J, Eigtved A, Buchwald C, et al. Implication of 18F-fluoro-2-deoxy-D-glucose positron emission tomography on management of carcinoma of unknown primary in the head and neck: a Danish cohort study. *Laryngoscope.* 2002;112:2009–2014.

56. Regelink G, Brouwer J, de Bree R, et al. Detection of unknown primary tumors and distant metastases in patients with cervical

metastases: value of FDG-PET versus conventional modalities. *Eur J Nucl Med Mol Imaging*. 2002;29:1024–1030.

57. Schmid DT, Stoeckli SJ, Bandhauer F, et al. Impact of positron emission tomography on the initial staging and therapy in locoregional advanced squamous cell carcinoma of the head and neck. *Laryngoscope*. 2003;113:888–891.

58. Wong WL, Saunders M. The impact of FDG PET on the management of occult primary head and neck tumors. *Clin Oncol (R Coll Radiol)*. 2003;15:461–466.

59. Ware RE, Matthews JP, Hicks RJ, et al. Usefulness of fluorine-18 fluorodeoxyglucose positron emission tomography in patients with a residual structural abnormality after definitive treatment for squamous cell carcinoma of the head and neck. *Head Neck*. 2004;26:1008–1017.

60. Porceddu SV, Jarmolowski E, Hicks RJ, et al. Utility of positron emission tomography for the detection of disease in residual neck nodes after chemoradiotherapy in head and neck cancer. *Head Neck*. 2005;27:175–181.

61. Fukui MB, Blodgett TM, Meltzer CC. PET/CT imaging in recurrent head and neck cancer. *Semin Ultrasound CT MR*. 2003;24(3):157–163.

62. Goerres GW, von Schulthess GK, Steinert HC. Why most PET of lung and head and neck will be PET-CT? *J Nucl Med*. 2004;45(Suppl 1): 665–715.

63. Ciernik IF, Dizendorf E, Baumert BG, et al. Radiation treatment planning with an integrated positron emission and computer tomography (PET/CT): a feasibility study. *Int J Radiat Oncol Biol Phys*. 2003;57:853–863.

64. Syed R, Bomanji JB, Nagabhushan N, et al. Impact of combined (18)F-FDG PET/CT in head and neck tumors. *Br J Cancer*. 2005;92:1046–1050.

65. Schonberger J, Ruschoff J, Grimm D, et al. Glucose transporter 1 gene expression is related to thyroid neoplasms with an unfavorable prognosis: an immunohistochemical study. *Thyroid*. 2002;12:747–754.

66. Khan N, Oriuchi N, Higuchi T, et al. PET in the follow-up of differentiated thyroid cancer. *Br J Radiol*. 2003;76:690–695.

67. Conti PS, Durski JM, Bacqai F, et al. Imaging of locally recurrent and metastatic thyroid cancer with positron emission tomography. *Thyroid*. 1999;9:797–804.

68. Frilling A, Tecklenborg K, Gorges R, et al. Preoperative diagnostic value of [(18)F] fluorodeoxyglucose positron emission tomography in patients with radioiodine-negative recurrent well-differentiated thyroid carcinoma. *Ann Surg*. 2001;234:804–811.

69. Grunwald F, Kalicke T, Feine U, et al. Fluorine-18 fluorodeoxyglucose positron emission tomography in thyroid cancer: results of a multicenter study. *Eur J Nucl Med*. 1999;26:1547–1552.

70. Helal BO, Merlet P, Toubert ME, et al. Clinical impact of (18)F-FDG PET in thyroid carcinoma patients with elevated thyroglobulin levels and negative (131)I scanning results after therapy. *J Nucl Med*. 2001;42:1464–1469.

71. Jadvar H, McDougall IR, Segall GM. Evaluation of suspected recurrent papillary thyroid carcinoma with [18F]fluorodeoxyglucose positron emission tomography. *Nucl Med Commun*. 1998;19:547–554.

72. McDougall IR, Davidson J, Segall GM. Positron emission tomography of the thyroid, with an emphasis on thyroid cancer. *Nucl Med Commun*. 2001;22:485–492.

73. Muros MA, Llamas-Elvira JM, Ramirez-Navarro A, et al. Utility of fluorine-18-fluorodeoxyglucose positron emission tomography in differentiated thyroid carcinoma with negative radioiodine scans and elevated serum thyroglobulin levels. *Am J Surg*. 2000;179:457–461.

74. Wang W, Macapinlac H, Larson SM, et al. [18F]-2-fluor-2-deoxy-D-glucose positron emission tomography localizes residual thyroid cancer in patients with negative diagnostic (131I) whole body scans and elevated serum thyroglobulin levels. *J Clin Endocrinol Metab*. 1999;84:2291–2302.

75. Larson SM, Robbins R. Positron emission tomography in thyroid cancer management. *Semin Roentgenol*. 2002;37:169–174.

76. Lind P, Kresnik E, Kumnig G, et al. 18F-FDG-PET in the follow-up of thyroid cancer. *Acta Med Austriaca*. 2003;30:17–21.

77. Kraeber-Bodere F, Cariou B, Curtet C, et al. Feasibility and benefit of fluorine 18-fluoro-2-deoxyglucose-guided surgery in the management of radioiodine-negative differentiated thyroid carcinoma metastases. *Surgery*. 2005;138:1176–1182.

78. Moog F, Linke R, Manthey N, et al. Influence of thyroid-stimulating hormone levels on uptake of FDG in recurrent and metastatic differentiated thyroid carcinoma. *J Nucl Med*. 2000;41:1989–1995.

79. van Tol KM, Jager PL, Piers DA, et al. Better yield of (18)fluorodeoxyglucose-positron emission tomography in patients with metastatic differentiated thyroid carcinoma during thyrotropin stimulation. *Thyroid*. 2002;12:381–387.

80. Petrich T, Borner AR, Otto D, et al. Influence of rhTSH on [(18)F]fluorodeoxyglucose uptake by differentiated thyroid carcinoma. *Eur J Nucl Med Mol Imaging*. 2002;29:641–647.

81. Wang W, Larson SM, Fazzari M, et al. Prognsotic value of [18F]fluorodeoxyglucose positron emission tomographic scanning in patients with thyroid cancer. *J Clin Endocrinol Metab*. 2000;85:1107–1113.

82. Diehl M, Risse JH, Brandt-Mainz K, et al. Fluorine-18 fluorodeoxyglucose positron emission tomography in medullary thyroid cancer: results of a multicenter study. *Eur J Nucl Med*. 2001;28:1671–1676.

83. Zimmer LA, McCook B, Meltzer C, et al. Combined positron emission tomography/computed tomography imaging of recurrent thyroid cancer. *Otolaryngol Head Neck Surg*. 2003;128:178–184.

84. Kato H, Takita J, Miyazaki M, et al. Correlation of 18-F-fluorodeoxyglucose (FDG) accumulation with glucose transporter (Glut-1) expression in esophageal in esophageal squamous cell carcinoma. *Anticancer Res*. 2003;23:3263–3272.

85. Tohma T, Okazumi S, Makino H, et al. Relationship between glucose transporter, hexokinase and FDG-PET in esophageal cancer. *Hepatogastroenterol*. 2005;52:486–490.

86. Wren SM, Stijns P, Srinivas S. Positron emission tomography in the initial staging esophageal cancer. *Arch Surg*. 2002;137:1001–1006.

87. Yoon YC, Lee KS, Shim YM, et al. Metastasis to regional lymph nodes in patients with esophageal squamous cell carcinoma: CT versus FDG-PET for presurgical detection prospective study. *Radiology*. 2003;227:764–770.

88. Wallace MB, Nietert PJ, Earle C, et al. An analysis of multiple staging management strategies for carcinoma of the esophagus: computed tomography, endoscopic ultrasound, positron emission tomography, and thoracoscopy/laparoscopy. *Ann Thorac Surg*. 2002;74:1026–1032.

89. Liberale G, van Lathem JL, Gay F, et al. The role of PET scan in the preoperative management of esophageal cancer. *Eur J Surg Oncol*. 2004;30:942–947.

90. Kneist W, Schreckenberger M, Bartenstein P, et al. Prospective evaluation of positron emission tomography in the preoperative staging of esophageal carcinoma. *Arch Surg*. 2004;139:1043–1049.

91. van Westreenen HL, Westerterp M, Bossuyt PM, et al. Systematic review of the staging performance of 18F-fluorodeoxyglucose positron emission tomography in esophageal cancer. *J Clin Oncol*. 2004;22:3805–3812.

92. Flamen P, Lerut A, van Cutsem E, et al. The utility of positron emission tomography for the diagnosis and staging of recurrent esophageal cancer. *J Thorac Cardiovasc Surg.* 2000;120:1085–1092.

93. van Westreenen HL, Heeren PA, van Dullemen HM, et al. Positron emission tomography with F-18-fluorodeoxyglucose in a combined staging strategy of esophageal cancer prevents unnecessary surgical explorations. *J Gastrointest Surg.* 2005;9:44–61.

94. van Westreenen HL, Heeren PA, Jager PL, et al. Pitfalls of positive findings in staging esophageal cancer with F-18-fluorodeoxyglucose positron emission tomography. *Ann Surg Oncol.* 2003;10:1100–1105.

95. Brucher BL, Weber W, Bauer M, et al. Neoadjuvant therapy of esophageal squamous cell carcinoma: Response evaluation by positron emission tomography. *Ann Surg.* 2001;233:300–309.

96. Choi JY, Jang HJ, Shim YM, et al. 18F-FDG-PET in patients with esophageal squamous cell carcinoma undergoing curative surgery: Prognostic implications. *J Nucl Med.* 2004;45:1843–1850.

97. Jadvar H, Henderson RW, Conti PS. 2-Deoxy-2-[F-18]Fluoro-D-glucose positron emission tomography/computed tomography imaging evaluation of esophageal cancer. *Mol Imaging Biol.* 2006;8(3):193–200.

98. Jadvar H, Segall GM. False-negative fluorine-18-FDG PET in metastatic carcinoid. *J Nucl Med.* 1997;38(9):1382–1383.

99. Yap CS, Schiepers C, Fishbein MC, et al. FDG-PET imaging in lung cancer: how sensitive is it for bronchioloalveolar carcinoma? *Eur J Nucl Med Mol Imaging.* 2002;29(9):1166–1173.

100. Gould MK, Maclean CC, Kuschner WG, et al. Accuracy of positron emission tomography for diagnosis of pulmonary nodules and mass lesions: a meta-analysis. *JAMA.* 2001;285(7):914–924.

101. de Langen AJ, Raijmakers P, Riphagen I, et al. The size of mediastinal lymph nodes nad its relation with metastatic involvement: a meta-analysis. *Eur J Cardiothorac Surg.* 2006;29:26–29.

102. Bruzzi JF, Munden RF. PET/CT imaging of lung cancer. *J Thorac Imaging.* 2006;21:123–136.

103. Pieterman RM, van Putten JW, Meuzelaar EL, et al. Preoperative staging of non-small cell lung cancer with positron emission tomography. *New Engl J Med.* 2000;343:254–261.

104. Salminen E, Mac Manus M. Impact of FDG-labeled positron emission tomography imaging on the management of non-small-cell lung cancer. *Ann Med.* 2001;33:404–409.

105. Gould MK, Kuschner WG, Rydzak CE, et al. Test performance of positron emission tomography and computed tomography for mediastinal staging in patients with non-small cell lung cancer: a meta-analysis. *Ann Intern Med* 139:879–892.

106. Lardinias D, Weder W, Hany TF, et al. Staging of non-small cell lung cancer with integrated positron emission tomography and computed tomography. *New Engl J Med.* 2003;348:2500–2507.

107. Pastorino U, Veronesi G, landoni C, et al. Fluorodeoxyglucose positron emission tomography improves preoperative staging of resectable lung metastasis. *J Thorac Cardiovasc Surg.* 2003;126:1906–1910.

108. MacManus MP, Hicks RJ, Ball DL, et al. F-18 fluorodeoxyglucose positron emission tomography staging in radical radiotherapy candidates with nonsmall cell lung carcinoma: powerful correlation with survival and high impact on treatment. *Cancer.* 2001;92:886–895.

109. Nestle U, Hellwig D, Fleckenstein J, et al. Comparison of early pulmonary changes in 18FDG-PET and CT after combined radiochemotherapy for advanced non-small-cell lung cancer: a study in 15 patients. *Front Radiat Ther Oncol.* 2002;37:26–33.

110. Hellwiq D, Groschel A, Graeter TP, et al. Diagnostic performance and prognostic impact of FDG PET in suspected recurrence of surgically treated non-small cell lung cancer. *Eur J Nucl Med Mol Imaging.* 2006;33:13–21.

111. Hicks RJ, Kalff V, MacManus MP, et al. The utility of (18)F-FDG PET for suspected recurrent non-small cell lung cancer after potentially curative therapy: impact on management and prognostic stratification. *J Nucl Med.* 2001;42(11):1605–1613.

112. Keidar Z, Haim N, Guralnik L, et al. PET/CT using 18F-FDG in suspected lung cancer recurrence: diagnostic value and impact on patient management. *J Nucl Med.* 2004;45:1640–1646.

113. Kalff V, Hicks RJ, MacManus MP, et al. Clinical impact of (18)F fluorodeoxyglucose positron emission tomography in patients with non-small-cell lung cancer: a prospective study. *J Clin Oncol.* 2001;19(1):111–118.

114. Seltzer MA, Yap CS, Silverman DH, et al. The impact of PET on the management of lung cancer: the referring physician's perspective. *J Nucl Med.* 2002;43(6):752–756.

115. Weber WA, Petersen V, Schmidt B, et al. Positron emission tomography in non-small-cell lung cancer: prediction of response to chemotherapy by quantitative assessment of glucose use. *J Clin Oncol.* 2003;21(14):2651–2657.

116. Pandit N, Gonen M, Krug L, et al. Prognostic value of [18F]FDG-PET imaging in small cell lung cancer. *Eur J Nucl Med Mol Imaging.* 2003;30(1):78–84.

117. Ahuja V, Coleman RE, Herndon J, et al. The prognostic significance of fluorodeoxyglucose positron emission tomography imaging for patients with non-small cell lung carcinoma. *Cancer.* 1998;83:918–924.

118. Higashi K, Ueda Y, Arisaka Y, et al. 18F-FDG uptake as a biologic prognostic factor for recurrence in patients with surgically resected non-small cell lung cancer. *J Nucl Med.* 2002;43(1):39–45.

119. Jeong HJ, Min JJ, Park JM, et al. Determination of the prognostic value of [(18)F]fluorodeoxyglucose uptake by using positron emission tomography in patients with non-small cell lung cancer. *Nucl Med Commun.* 2002;23(9):865–870.

120. Duhaylongsod FG, Lowe VJ, Patz EF, Jr., et al. Lung tumor growth correlates with glucose metabolism measured by fluoride-18 fluorodeoxyglucose positron emission tomography. *Ann Thorac Surg.* 1995;60(5):1348–1352.

121. Gambhir SS, Hoh CK, Phelps ME, et al. Decision tree sensitivity analysis for cost-effectiveness of FDG-PET in the staging and management of non-small-cell lung carcinoma. *J Nucl Med.* 1996;37(9):1428–1436.

122. Quon A, Gambhir SS. FDG PET and beyond: molecular breast cancer imaging. *J Clin Oncol.* 2005;23:1664–1673.

123. Zangheri B, Messa C, Picchio M, et al. PET/CT and breast cancer. *Eur J Nucl Med Mol Imaging.* 2004;31 Suppl 1:S135–S142.

124. Wu D, Gambhir SS. Positron emission tomography in diagnosis and management of invasive breast cancer: current status and future perspectives. *Clin Breast Cancer.* 2003;4 Suppl 1:S55–S63.

125. Bassa P, Kim EE, Inoue T, et al. Evaluation of preoperative chemotherapy using PET with fluorine-18-deoxyglucose in breast cancer.*J Nucl Med.* 1996;37:931–938.

126. Bombardieri E, Crippa F. PET imaging in breast cancer. *Q J Nucl Med.* 2001;45:245–256.

127. Crowe JP Jr, Adler LP, Shenk RR, et al. Positron emission tomography and breast masses: comparison with clinical, mammographic and pathological findings. *Ann Surg Oncol.* 1994;1:132–140.

128. Flanagan FL, Dehdashti F, Siegel BA. PET in breast cancer. *Semin Nucl Med.* 1998;28:290–302.

129. Hoh CK, Schipers C. 18-FDG imaging in breast cancer. *Semin Nucl Med.* 1999;29:49–56.

130. Rose C, Dose J, Avril N. Positron emission tomography for the diagnosis of breast cancer. *Nucl Med Commun.* 2002;23:613–618.

131. Tse NY, Hoh CK, Hawkins RA, et al. The application of positron emission tomographic imaging with fluorodeoxyglucose to the evaluation of breast disease. *Ann Surg.* 1992;216: 27–34.

132. Wahl RL. Current status of PET in breast cancer imaging, staging, and therapy. *Semin Roentgenol.* 2001;36:250–260.

133. Avril N, Menzel M, Dose J, et al. Glucose metabolism of breast cancer assessed by 18F-FDG PET: histologic and immunohistochemical tissue analysis. *J Nucl Med.* 2001;42:9–16.

134. Brown RS, Goodman TM, Zasadny KR, et al. Expression of hexokinase II and Glut-1 in untreated human breast cancer. *Nucl Med Biol.* 2002;29:443–453.

135. Avril N, Rose CA, Schelling M, et al. Breast imaging with positron emission tomography and fluorine-18 fluorodeoxyglucose: use and limitations. *J Clin Oncol.* 2000;18:3495–3502.

136. Buck A, Schirrmeister H, Kuhn T, et al. FDG uptake in breast cancer: correlation with biological and clinical prognostic parameters. *Eur J Nucl Med Mol Imaging.* 2002;29:1317–1323.

137. Vranjesevic D, Schiepers C, Silverman DH, et al. Relationship between 18F-FDG uptake and breast density in women with normal breast tissue. *J Nucl Med.* 2003;44:1238–1242.

138. Adler LP, Weinberg IN, Bradbury MS, et al. Method for combined FDG-PET and radiographic imaging of primary breast cancers. *Breast J.* 2003;9:163–166.

139. Raylman RR, Majewski S, Weisenberger AG, et al. Positron emission mammography-guided breast biopsy. *J Nucl Med.* 2001; 42:960–966.

140. Wahl RL, Helvie MA, Chang AE, et al. Detection of breast cancer in women after augmentation mammoplasty using fluorine-18-fluorodeoxyglucose PET. *J Nucl Med.* 1994;35:872–875.

141. Port ER, Yeung H, Gonen M, et al. 18F-2-fluoro-2-deoxy-D-glucose positron emission tomography scanning affects surgical management in selected patients with high risk, operable breast carcinoma. *Ann Surg Oncol.* 2006;13:677–684.

142. Avril N, Dose J, Janicke F, et al. Assessment of axillary lymph node involvement in breast cancer patients with positron emission tomography using radiolabeled 2-(fluorine-18)-fluoro-2-deoxy-D-glucose. *J Natl Cancer Inst.* 1996;88:1204–1209.

143. Scirrmeister H, Kuhn T, Guhlmann A, et al. Fluorine-18 2-deoxy-2-fluoro-D-glucose PET in the preoperative staging of breast cancer: comparison with the standard staging procedures. *Eur J Nucl Med.* 2001;28:351–358.

144. Wahl RL, Siegel BA, Coleman RE, et al. Prospective multi-center study of axillary nodal staging by positron emission tomography in breast cancer: a report of the staging breast cancer with PET study group. *J Clin Oncol.* 2004;22:277–285.

145. Greco M, Crippa M, Agresti R, et al. Axillary lymph node staging in breast cancer by 2-fluoro-2-deoxy-D-glucose positron emission tomography: clinical evaluation and alternative management. *J Natl Cancer Inst.* 2001;93:630–635.

146. Barranger E, Grahek D, Antoine M, et al. Evaluation of fluorodeoxyglucose positron emission tomography in the detection of axillary lymph node metastases in patients with early-stage breast cancer. *Ann Surg Oncol.* 2003;10:622–627.

147. Crippa F, Agresti R, Seregni E, et al. Prospective evaluation of fluorine-18-FDG PET in presurgical staging of the axilla in breast cancer. *J Nucl Med.* 1998;39:4–8.

148. van der Hoeven JJ, Hoekstra OS, Comans EF, et al. Determinants of diagnostic performance of [F-18]fluorodeoxyglucose positron emission tomography for axillary staging in breast cancer. *Ann Surg.* 2002;236:619–624.

149. Ahmad A, Barrington S, Maisey M, et al. use of positron emission tomography in evaluation of brachial plexopathy in breast cancer patients. *Br J Cancer.* 1999;478–482.

150. Eubank WB, Mankoff DA, Vesselle HJ, et al. Detection of locoregional and distant recurrences in breast cancer patients by using FDG PET. *Radiographics.* 2002;22:5–17.

151. Bender H, Kirst J, Palmedo H, et al. Value of 18fluorodeoxyglucose positron emission tomography in the staging of recurrent breast carcinoma. *Anticancer Res.* 1997;17:1687–1692.

152. Dose J, Bleckmann C, Bachmann S, et al. Comparison of fluorodeoxyglucose positron emission tomography and "conventional diagnostic procedures" for the detection of distant metastases in breast cancer patients. *Nucl Med Commun.* 2002;23:857–864.

153. Jadvar H, Epstein A, Conti PS. Evaluation of suspected recurrent and metastatic breast carcinoma with ^{18}F-FDG PET. *J Nucl Med.* 2003;44(5 Suppl):170P.

154. Moon DH, Maddahi J, Silverman DH, et al. Accuracy of whole-body fluorine-18-FDG PET for the detection of recurrent or metastatic breast carcinoma. *J Nucl Med.* 1998;39:431–435.

155. Goerres GW, Miche SC, Fehr MK, et al. Follow-up of women with breast cancer: comparison between MRI and FDG PET. *Eur Radiol.* 2003;13:1633–1644.

156. Gallowitsch HJ, Kresnik E, gasser J, et al. F-18 fluorodeoxyglucose positron emission tomography in the diagnosis of tumor recurrence and metastases in the follow-up of patients with breast carcinoma: a comparison to conventional imaging. *Invest Radiol.* 2003;38:250–256.

157. Kamel EM, Wyss MT, Fehr MK, et al. [18F]-Fluorodeoxyglucose positron emission tomography in patients with suspected recurrence of breast cancer. *J Cancer Res Clin Oncol.* 2003;129: 147–153.

158. Siggelkow W, Zimmy M, Faridi A, et al. The value of positron emission tomography in the follow-up for breast cancer. *Anticancer Res.* 2003;23:1859–1867.

159. Suarez M, Perez-Castejon MJ, Jimenez A, et al. Early diagnosis of recurrent breast cancer with FDG-PET in patients with progressive elevation of serum tumor markers. *Q J Nucl Med.* 2002;46:113–121.

160. Radan L, Ben Haim S, bar-Shalom R, et al. The role of FDG PET-CT in suspected recurrence of breast cancer. *Cancer.* 2006;107:2545–2551.

161. Yang SN, Liang JA, Lin FJ, et al. Comparing whole body [18F]-2-deoxyglucose positron emission tomography and technetium-99m methylene diphosphonate bone scan to detect bone metastases in patients with breast cancer. *J Cancer Res Oncol.* 2002;128:325–328.

162. Yap CS, Seltzer MA, Schiepers C, et al. Impact of whole-body 18F-FDG PET on staging and managing patients with breast cancer: the referring physician's perspective. *J Nucl Med.* 2001;42:1334–1337.

163. Gennari A, Donati S, Salvadori B, et al. Role of 2-[18F]-fluorodeoxyglucose (FDG) positron emission tomography (PET) in the early assessment of response to chemotherapy in metastatic breast cancer patients. *Clin Breast Cancer.* 2000;1:156–161.

164. Schelling M, Avril N, Nahrig J, et al. Positron emission tomography using [(18)F]fluorodeoxyglucose for monitoring primary chemotherapy in breast cancer. *J Clin Oncol.* 2000;18:1689–1695.

165. Smith IC, Welch AE, Hutcheon AW, et al. Positron emission tomography using [(18)F]-fluorodeoxy-D-glucose to predict the pathologic response of breast cancer to primary chemotherapy. *J Clin Oncol.* 2000;18:1676–1688.

166. Nair N, Ali A, Dowlatshahi K, et al. Positron emission tomography with fluorine-18 fluorodeoxyglucose to evaluate response of early breast carcinoma treated with stereotactic interstitial laser therapy. *Clin Nucl Med.* 2000;25:505–507.

167. Oshida M, Uno K, Suzuki M, et al. Predicting the prognoses of breast carcinoma patients with positron emission tomography

using 2-deoxy-2-fluoro[18F]-D-glucose. *Cancer*. 1998;82:2227–2234.

168. Vranjesevic D, Filmont JE, Meta J, et al. Whole-body (18)F-FDG PET and conventional imaging for predicting outcome in previously treated breast cancer patients. *J Nucl Med*. 2002;43:325–329.

169. de Geus-Oei LF, Ruers TJ, Punt CJ, et al. FDG-PET in colorectal cancer. *Cancer Imaging*. 2006;6:S71–S81.

170. Delbeke D, Martin WH. PET and PET-CT for evaluation of colorectal carcinoma. *Semin Nucl Med*. 2004;34:209–223.

171. Abdel-Nabi H, Doerr RJ, Lamonica DM, et al. Staging of primary colorectal carcinoma with fluorine-18 fluorodeoxyglucose whole-body PET: correlation with histopathologic and CT findings. *Radiology*. 1998;206:755–760.

172. Falk PM, Gupta NC, Thorson AG, et al. Positron emission tomography for preoperative staging of colorectal carcinoma. *Dis Colon Rectum*. 1994;37:153–156.

173. Schiepers C, Penninckx F, De Vadder N, et al. Contribution of PET in the diagnosis of recurrent colorectal cancer: comparison with conventional imaging. *Eur J Surg Oncol*. 1995;21:517–522.

174. Staib L, Schirrmeister H, Reske SN, et al. Is (18F)F-fluorodeoxyglucose positron emission tomography in recurrent colorectal cancer a contribution to surgical decision making? *Am J Surg*. 2000;180:1–5.

175. Vitola JV, Delbeke D, Sandler MP, et al. Positron emission tomography to stage metastatic colorectal carcinoma to the liver. *Am J Surg*. 1996;171:21–26.

176. Wiering B, Krabbe PF, Jager GJ, et al. The impact of fluor-18-deoxyglucose-positron emission tomography in the management of colorectal liver metastases. *Cancer*. 2005;104:2658–2670.

177. Tatlidil R, Jadvar H, Bading JR, et al. Incidental colonic [F-18] fluorodeoxyglucose uptake: correlation with colonoscopy and histopathology. *Radiology*. 2002;224:783–787.

178. Beets G, Penninckx F, Schiepers C, et al. Clinical value of whole-body positron emission tomography with [18F] fluorodeoxyglucose in recurrent colorectal cancer. *Br J Surg*. 1994;81:1666–1670.

179. Imdahl A, Reinhardt MJ, Nitzsche EU, et al. Impact of 18F-FDG positron emission tomography for decision making in colorectal cancer recurrences. *Arch Surg*. 2000;385:129–134.

180. Flanagan FL, Dehdashti F, Ogunbiyi OA, et al. Utility of FDG PET for investigating unexplained plasma CEA elevation in patients with colorectal cancer. *Ann Surg*. 1998;227:319–323.

181. Huebner RH, Park KC, Shepherd JE, et al. A meta-analysis of the literature for whole-body FDG PET detection of recurrent colorectal cancer. *J Nucl Med*. 2000;41:1177–1189.

182. Meta J, Seltzer M, Schiepers C, et al. Impact of 18F-FDG PET on managing patients with colorectal cancer: the referring physician's perspective. *J Nucl Med*. 2001;42:586–590.

183. Valk PE, Abella-Columna E, Haseman MK, et al. Whole-body PET imaging with F-18-fluorodeoxyglucose in management of recurrent colorectal cancer. *Arch Surg*. 1999;134:503–511.

184. Gambhir SS, Valk P, Shepherd J, et al. Cost effective analysis modeling of the role of FDG PET in the management of patients with recurrent colorectal cancer. *J Nucl Med*. 1997;38:90P.

185. Libutti SK, Alexander HR Jr, Choyke P, et al. A prospective study of 2-[18F] fluoro-2-deoxy-D-glucose/positron emission tomography scan, 99mTc-labeled arcitumomab (CEA-scan), and blind second-look laparotomy for detecting colon cancer recurrence in patients with increasing carcinoembryonic antigen levels. *Ann Surg Oncol*. 2001;8:779–786.

186. Donckier V, Van Laethem JL, Goldman S, et al. [F-18]fluorodeoxyglucose positron emission tomography as a tool for early recognition of incomplete tumor destruction after radiofrequency ablation for liver metastases. *J Surg Oncol*. 2003;84:215–223.

187. Findlay M, Young H, Cunningham D, et al. Noninvasive monitoring of tumor metabolism using fluorodeoxyglucose and positron emission tomography in colorectal cancer liver metastases: correlation with tumor response to fluorouracil. *J Clin Oncol*. 1996;14:700–708.

188. Guillem J, Calle J, Akhurst T, et al. Preoperative assessment of primary rectal cancer response to preoperative radiation and chemotherapy using 18-fluorodeoxyglucose positron emission tomography. *Dis Colon Rectum*. 2000;43:18–24.

189. Vitola JV, Delbeke D, Meranze SG, et al. Positron emission tomography with F-18-fluorodeoxyglucose to evaluate the results of hepatic chemoembolization. *Cancer*. 1996;78:2216–2222.

190. Holder WD Jr, White RL Jr, Zuger JH, et al. Effectiveness of positron emission tomography for the detection of melanoma metastases. *Ann Surg*. 1998;227:764–769.

191. Macfarlane DJ, Sondak V, Johnson T, Wahl RL. Prospective evaluation of 2-[18F]-2-deoxy-D-glucose positron emission tomography in staging of regional lymph nodes in patients with cutaneous malignant melanoma. *J Clin Oncol*. 1998;16:1770–1776.

192. Rinne D, Baum RP, Hor G, et al. Primary staging and follow-up of high risk melanoma patients with whole-body 18F-fluorodeoxyglucose positron emission tomography: results of a prospective study of 100 patients. *Cancer*. 1998;82:1664–1671.

193. Stas M, Stroobants S, Dupont P, et al. 18-FDG PET scan in the staging of recurrent melanoma: additional value and therapeutic impact. *Melanoma Res*. 2002;12:479–490.

194. Tyler DS, Onaitis M, Kherani A, et al. Positron emission tomography scanning in malignant melanoma. *Cancer*. 2000;89:1019–1025.

195. Boni R, Huch-Boni RA, Steinert H, et al. Early detection of melanoma metastasis using fluorodeoxyglucose F 18 positron emission tomography. *Arch Dermatol*. 1996;132:875–876.

196. Bastiaannet E, Oyen WJ, Meijer S, et al. Impact of [18F]-fluorodeoxyglucose positron emission tomography on surgical management of melanoma patients. *Br J Surg*. 2006;93:243–249.

197. Gulec SA, Faries MB, Lee CC, et al. The role of fluorine-18 deoxyglucose positron emission tomography in the management of patients with metastatic melanoma: impact on surgical decision making. *Clin Nucl Med*. 2003;28:961–965.

198. Jadvar H, Johnson DL, Segall GM. The effect of fluorine-18 fluorodeoxyglucose positron emission tomography on the management of cutaneous malignant melanoma. *Clin Nucl Med*. 2000;25:48–51.

199. Wong C, Silverman DH, Seltzer M, et al. The impact of 2-deoxy-2[18F]fluoro-D-glucose whole body positron emission tomography for managing patients with melanoma: the referring physician's perspective. *Mol Imaging Biol*. 2002;4:185–190.

200. Boni R, Boni RA, Steinert H, et al. Staging of metastatic melanoma by whole-body positron emission tomography using 2-fluorine-18-fluoro-2-deoxy-D-glucose. *Br J Derm*. 1995;132:556–562.

201. Acland KM, Healy C, Calonje E, et al. Comparison of positron emission tomography scanning and sentinel node biopsy in the detection of micrometastases of primary cutaneous malignant melanoma. *J Clin Oncol*. 2001;19:2674–2678.

202. Belhocine T, Pierard G, De Labrassinne M, et al. Staging of regional nodes in AJCC stage I and II melanoma: 18FDG PET imaging versus sentinel node detection. *Oncologist*. 2002;7:271–278.

203. Havenga K, Cobben DC, Oyen WJ, et al. Fluorodeoxyglucose-positron emission tomography and sentinel lymph node biopsy in staging primary cutaneous melanoma. *Eur J Surg Oncol*. 2003;29:662–664.

204. Wagner JD, Schauwecker DS, Davidson D, et al. FDG-PET sensitivity for melanoma lymph node metastases is dependent on tumor volume. *J Surg Oncol*. 2001;77:237–242.

205. Crippa F, Leutner M, Belli F, et al. What kind of lymph node metastases can FDG PET detect? A clinical study in melanoma. *J Nucl Med.* 2000;41:1491–1494.
206. Mijnhout GS, Comans EF, Raijmakers P, et al. Reproducibility and clinical value of 18F-fluorodeoxyglucose positron emission tomography in recurrent melanoma. *Nucl Med Commun.* 2002;23:475–481.
207. Swetter SM, Carroll LA, Johnson DL, et al. Positron emission tomography is superior to computed tomography for metastatic detection in melanoma patients. *Ann Surg Oncol.* 2002;9:646–653.
208. Prichard RS, Hill AD, Skehan SJ, et al. Positron emission tomography for staging and management of malignant melanoma. *Br J Surg.* 2002;89:389–396.
209. Mijnhout GS, Hoekstra OS, van Tulder MW, et al. Systematic review of the diagnostic accuracy of (18)F-fluorodeoxyglucose positron emission tomography in melanoma patients. *Cancer.* 2001;91:1530–1542.
210. Schwimmer J, Essner R, Patel A, et al. A review of the literature for whole-body FDG PET in the management of patients with melanoma. *Q J Nucl Med.* 2000;44:153–167.

COMMENTARY
Alan D. Waxman

The chapter by Dr. Hossein Jadvar is an outstanding contribution to the field of molecular imaging in cancer. The chapter discusses the clinical management of several cancer types as well as discussing the fundamentals of positron emission tomography-computed tomography (PET-CT) in a way that can be understood by all those who read this chapter, whether or not they are molecular imagers.

BRAIN TUMORS

The section on brain tumors discusses the value of [F-18]-2-fluoro-2-deoxy-D-glucose (FDG)-PET in the assessment of primary brain tumors. As stated, the chapter concentrates mainly on the use of FDG, which has been the most commonly used radiopharmaceutical. Other radiopharmaceuticals such as carbon-11 methionine have been shown to be of interest in that the extent of tumor infiltration of the brain is more accurately determined with methionine than with FDG (1). The carbon-11 compounds are not practical in that a cyclotron must be in the vicinity because of the short half-life (12 minutes).

The diminished brain glucose utilization of tumors due to medications such as steroids, anticonvulsants, and certain sedatives may hamper accurate scanning. In addition, Dr. Jadvar points out that cortical atrophy and blood glucose levels are critical factors that have an impact in achieving optimal FDG-PET scans of the brain. As in other areas of FDG-PET imaging, patient preparation prior to FDG injection is critical in obtaining a quality study.

Occasionally, patients demonstrate neurologic signs and symptoms that mimic a neurodegenerative process. Careful observation of the cortical distribution, especially in older patients, may demonstrate a scan pattern consistent with a neurodegen-

erative process such as Alzheimer disease, Lewy body disease, or frontal temporal dementia. It is therefore important to include the brain in the scan in patients with cognitive or other central nervous system symptoms. A screening brain scan may be done initially as part of the whole-body scan; however, if detailed information is desired, a different protocol should be used to carefully evaluate the brain.

HEAD AND NECK CANCER

Dr. Jadvar discusses the need to adequately prepare the patient for evaluation of the head and neck region. Especially important is the need to keep the patient isolated and away from friends or relatives during the uptake phase of the FDG study. Patients have a tendency to engage in conversations, which may alter the scan pattern because of muscular activity, especially muscles that support the movement of the vocal cords.

At the Cedars-Sinai Medical Center, we have found that a dual interpretation of head and neck studies by a specially trained radiologist (usually a neuroradiologist) is extremely rewarding when precise knowledge of anatomy is critical in the final interpretation in the combined FDG-PET. We have also noted that a hybrid PET-CT appears to be superior to a stand-alone PET image fused with a separately acquired CT image because of the more precise registration of images.

In addition to the avoidance of a cold environment to reduce the brown fat activity in or around the neck region, avoidance of nicotine as well as ephedrine-containing compounds is important. Animal studies have demonstrated a significant additive effect of nicotine and ephedrine in activating brown fat (2). The use of beta blockers may reduce FDG uptake in brown fat tissue (3).

THYROID CANCER

Dr. Jadvar's section on thyroid cancer is extremely well written and thorough. It has been well described that the FDG-PET scan is extremely valuable in patients who have a negative findings on a radioiodine scan in the presence of a high or rising serum thyroglobulin level. In our experience, the combined use of ultrasound along with the PET-CT gives optimum results with regard to defining a specific focus of thyroid cancer in the neck.

Ultrasound-guided biopsies are critical in determining whether a small lymph node contains thyroid cancer. If the cellular content is insufficient for pathologic diagnosis it is often possible to make a smear of the fluid and tissue, which can subsequently be stained for thyroglobulin. In this way we have identified with certainty areas of suspicious FDG activity that may or may not correlate with small lymph nodes on CT scan. An ultrasound of the suspicious area often yields desired results.

Thyroid cancer may be incidentally discovered on whole-body PET-CT studies performed for other disease processes. Focal increase of FDG in the thyroid is often associated with primary or metastatic thyroid tumors (4,5).

ESOPHAGEAL CANCER

In our institution, patients with esophageal cancer routinely undergo FDG-PET scanning for staging and restaging disease and to follow response to therapy. Because of the nonspecific nature of FDG-PET, inflammatory changes of the esophagus may be confused with tumor involvement. The combined use of PET with CT using hybrid technology has helped to alleviate some of the problems of false-positive results previously noted. However, inflammatory esophagitis and physiologic activity often seen in the gastroesophageal junction may still be confusing.

FDG-PET has a high sensitivity in detecting metastatic sites in subjects with esophageal cancer and is excellent in following response to chemotherapy. Efficacy of a given chemotherapeutic protocol may be assessed by obtaining a baseline PET study prior to initiating chemotherapy and repeating the study after two or three cycles. In this way, FDG-PET may facilitate choice of the optimal chemotherapeutic regimen

LUNG CANCER

One of the earliest approved applications for FDG-PET was in the evaluation of the pulmonary nodule. The main purpose was to determine whether a nodule seen on CT was benign or malignant. Arbitrary cutoffs have been suggested, with several reports stating that a standardized uptake value (SUV) >2.5 was malignant, and <2.5 was benign. Today we know that this simplistic approach is inappropriate. In general, the higher the SUV, the greater the likelihood for malignancy. There are many malignancies that exhibit low SUV values. These include extremely well-differentiated adenocarcinomas, bronchoalveolar carcinomas, carcinoid tumors, and tumors that have been "stunned" because of prior chemotherapy or radiation. Conversely, many benign lesions, mainly inflammatory or infected, will demonstrate high SUV values.

It is now evident that the best approach to evaluate pulmonary nodules is to use a hybrid system with a combined FDG-CT capability. Nodules as small as 4 mm have been detected using FDG-PET because they may be sufficiently different from surrounding background activity of the lung when the nodule on CT is viewed in a fused or precisely aligned manner with the PET study.

Staging of lung cancer has proved to be extremely useful. Staging is more accurate when a combined FDG-CT modality is used in order to determine whether activity in the hilar or mediastinal region has a CT correlate suggesting enlargement of a lymph node or an adjacent mass. It has been demonstrated that the likelihood of metastatic involvement of hilar or mediastinal lymph nodes is enhanced significantly when the PET scan is compared with the size of the hilar or mediastinal nodes. PET is the dominant factor in determining whether malignancy is present, with size as a secondary factor. The highest probability for malignancy is in patients with enlarged (>10 mm) lymph nodes with positive findings on FDG-PET scan. Multiple scattered nodules involving the hilar and mediastinal structures are most often related to a granulomatous process including sarcoid, tuberculosis, or old fungal disease.

Dr. Jadvar discusses the prognostic value of FDG-PET in evaluating pulmonary masses or nodules. The precise SUV to determine prognosis is difficult to define. Multiple levels, varying from SUVs of 5 to 10, have been suggested to define poor prognosis. As in determining the malignant status of a nodule, the higher the SUV, the more likely the patient will have a poor clinical outcome.

BREAST CANCER

The use of FDG-PET in the detection of breast cancer has been well documented. Dr. Jadvar correctly points out that PET imaging with FDG is superior to conventional imaging in detecting distant metastasis and recurrent disease and in monitoring therapeutic response.

Contrary to previous reports, it has been recently demonstrated that FDG-PET may play an important role in evaluating the axilla in patients with breast cancer (6–9). In a recent series from our institution (6), we found that an FDG-avid lymph node with an SUV of >2.0 had malignant spread to that lymph node with a specificity of a 100%. However, sensitivity in this series for detecting axillary metastases was quite low (76%) because of multiple lymph nodes with microscopic metastases not detectable using PET technology. These results suggest that lymph node positive studies with an SUV >2.0 may allow the surgeon to omit sentinel node biopsy and proceed directly to axillary dissection. This approach also would eliminate the need for axillary lymphoscintigraphy and blue dye injection.

Prone imaging of the breast may be superior to the conventional supine imaging techniques in that the breast is elongated in this position and questionable areas of abnormality in the extreme posterior portion of the breast are separated from the chest wall. Imaging in this position significantly enhances detection of focal abnormalities in this portion of the breast.

Primary imaging of the breast tumor with FDG-PET does not appear to offer any advantages over the use of magnetic resonance imaging (MRI) techniques, especially when gadolinium is used in a dynamic mode to evaluate wash-in and wash-out curves of the tumor in order to differentiate a benign from a malignant lesion.

Many patients are staged with FDG-PET after a biopsy of the breast lesion confirms the presence of cancer. However, evaluation of the biopsy site is unreliable because it has been demonstrated that the biopsy procedure itself will result in increased activity in the region because of healing and inflammation. This phenomenon may last months, and if sutures are placed within the breast, the area may be falsely positive for years.

COLORECTAL CANCER

Dr. Jadvar correctly points out that FDG-PET, especially with PET-CT, is extremely useful in the evaluation of patients with colorectal cancer.

We have encountered two areas of difficulty in the use of PET or PET-CT in evaluating patients with colorectal cancer. Liver metastases may be isointense within the liver, resulting in a PET scan that may be read as revealing no evidence for hepatic metastases. It is imperative, therefore, that the PET scan be interpreted in the light of the findings observed on other imaging studies, such as MRI, CT, or ultrasound. If a lesion in the liver is >20 mm, there should be an accompanying reduction of activity in the liver, if the lesion is benign, without increased metabolic activity. However, tumors may be active but not more active than surrounding normal hepatic uptake. If equal activity is seen in lesions >20 mm, the study should be considered as positive and not normal.

Findings in the rectal region are often difficult to interpret as many patients free of tumor will have increased activity in this area from inflammation from a variety of causes. The problem is partially but not completely solved by the use of PET-CT. When there is no rectal wall thickening there may be some FDG-PET accumulation from inflammation. However, when the rectal wall is thickened, even without the presence of a mass, tumor must be considered, especially if the original tumor was in this region. Patients who have undergone radiation therapy of the colon and/or rectal area often have significant areas of increased PET activity from an ongoing inflammatory response.

MELANOMA

Melanoma has been demonstrated to have one of the highest tumor-to-background ratios using FDG-PET when compared with all other tumors. It is an excellent indicator for metastatic or distant disease. Because melanoma can spread to any part of the body, including the distal extremities, it has been suggested that the patient undergo a true whole-body scan from the top of the head to the toes. Recent studies have disputed this approach, stating that in a large series of melanoma patients studied the additional benefit for evaluating the legs was <1% (10). Despite the controversy, at our institution we are continuing to perform true whole-body scans.

SARCOMA

The use of FDG-PET in evaluating patients with sarcoma is growing an importance. A baseline study in patients with osteosarcoma or chondrosarcoma may be important in determining whether the patient has distant metastases at the time of initial discovery. Staging and restaging after chemotherapy and prior to surgery is important, and the routine use of postoperative FDG-PET has proven useful in determining tumor recurrence or late-appearing metastatic disease (11,12).

Overall, the use of FDG-PET in sarcoma has been demonstrated to be useful to surgeons, along with MRI and/or CT, in defining the best surgical plan and overall therapy using chemotherapy or radiation therapy in conjunction with a surgical approach (13).

PANCREATIC CANCER

FDG-PET has been demonstrated to be useful in detection and staging in patients with adenocarcinoma of the pancreas. Initial staging may be important in determining which patients may be candidates for extensive pancreatic surgery such as a Whipple procedure. Patients with limited disease at the time of discovery are unusual, but surgical expiration with intent to cure should be considered in the presence of an FDG-PET scan in which no tumor extension is demonstrated beyond the initial pancreatic lesion.

New chemotherapeutic agents are now available with a significant antitumor activity in patients with pancreatic cancer.

Surgery with intent to cure followed by chemotherapy may result in a higher incidence of cure and enhanced disease-free survivals (14).

NEUROENDOCRINE TUMORS

The use of FDG-PET accompanied by octreotide scans are often useful in selecting patients who may be successfully treated using a surgical approach. Patients with carcinoid or pancreatic neuroendocrine tumors with a highly positive FDG-PET scan tend to have a poorer prognosis than those patients with lower FDG activity. Often patients with low FDG activity have extremely high somatostatin receptor content with highly positive octreotide scans. The combination of octreotide scans and PET scans may be important in determining a rational strategy for treating these patients (15,16).

Patients who have metastatic neuroendocrine tumors to the liver are not precluded from having aggressive surgery with debulking of the liver in order to prolong a high quality of life for the individual patient.

SUMMARY

In summary, Dr. Jadvar has written a chapter discussing FDG-PET scanning in patients with cancer that is directed to the surgical subspecialties. It is extremely thorough and well written. He has demonstrated that FDG-PET is extremely useful in the evaluation of patients with cancer who are surgical candidates or who have had surgery and are being followed to determine surgical outcomes. The use of the hybrid systems performing PET and PET-CT have dramatically improved the diagnostic accuracy for both PET and CT. New radiopharmaceuticals for PET with the intention of looking at cell proliferation, amino acid metabolism, or cell receptor status are currently being evaluated and are expected to add to the diversity of molecular imaging in the near future.

REFERENCES

1. Kracht LW, Miletic H, Busch S, et al. Delineation of brain tumor extent with [^{11}C] $^{L-}$ methionine positron emission tomography. *Clin Cancer Res.* 2004;:7163–7170.
2. Baba S, Tatsumi M, Ishimori T, et al. Effect of nicotine and ephedrine on the accumulation of 18F-FDG in brown adipose tissue. *J Nucl Med.* 2007;48:981–986.
3. Tatsumi M, Engles JM, Ishimori T, et al. Intense (18) F-FDG uptake in brown fat can be reduced pharmacologically. *J Nucl Med.* 2004;45:1189–1193.
4. Yi JG, Marom EM, Munden RF, et al. Focal uptake of fluorodeoxyglucose by the thyroid in patients undergoing initial disease staging with combined PET/CT for non-small cell lung cancer. *Radiology.* 2005;236:271–275.
5. Van den Bruel A, Maes A, De Potter T, et al. Clinical relevance of thyroid fluorodeoxyglucose whole body positron emission tomography incidentaloma. *J Clin Endocrinol Metab.* 2002;87:1517–1520.
6. Chung A, Hagiike M, Fujimoto K, et al. Preoperative FDG-PET scan detects axillary metastases in patients with breast cancer. *Arch Surg.* 2006;141:783–789.

7. Crippa F, Gerali A, Alessi A, et al. FDG-PET for axillary lymph node staging in primary breast cancer. *Eur J Nucl Med Mol Imaging.* 2004;31(Suppl 1):S97–102.

8. Barranger E, Grahek D, Antoine M, et al. Evaluation of fluorodeoxyglucose positron emission tomography in the detection of axillary node metastases in patients with early-stage breast cancer. *Ann Surg Oncol.* 2003;10:622–627.

9. Veronesi U, De Cicco C, Galimberti VE, et al. A comparatve study on the value of FDG-PET and sentinel node biopsy to identify occult axillary metastases. *Ann Oncol.* 2007;18:473–478.

10. Loffler M, Weckesser M, Franzius CH, et al. Malignant melanoma and ^{18}F-FDG-PET: should the whole body scan include the legs? *Nuklearmedizin.* 2003;42:167–172.

11. Folpe AL, Lyles RH, Sprouse JT, et al. (F-18) Fluorodeoxyglucose positron emission tomography as a predictor of pathologic grade and other prognostic variables in bone and soft tissue sarcoma. *Clin Cancer Res.* 2000;6:1279–1287.

12. Brenner W, Bohuslavizki KH, Eary JF. PET imaging of osteosarcoma. *J Nucl Med.* 2003;44:930–942.

13. Ioannidis JPA, Lau J. ^{18}F-FDG PET for the diagnosis and grading of soft-tissue sarcoma: a meta-analysis. *J Nucl Med.* 2003;44:717–724.

14. Maldonado A, Gonzalez F, Tamames S, et al. The Role of 18F-FDG PET/CT in the evaluation of pancreatic lesions. *J Nucl Med.* 2007;48(Suppl 2): Abstract 26P.

15. Krenning EP, Kwekkeboom DJ, Bakker WH, et al. Somatostatin receptor scintigraphy with [^{111}In-DTPA-D-Phe[1]] and [^{123}I-Tyr[3]] octreotide: the Rotterdam experience with more than 1000 patients. *Eur J Nucl Med.* 1993;20:716–731.

16. de Herder WW, Hofland LJ, van der Lely AJ, et al. Somatostatin receptors in gastroentero-pancreatic neuroendocrine tumours. *Endocrine-Related Cancer.* 2003;10:451–458.

10

Organ Transplantation and Malignancy

Steven D. Colquhoun and Andrew S. Klein

The first successful organ transplant was performed over 50 years ago and since then the evolution in both the art and science of transplantation has been remarkable. Improvements in surgical techniques, knowledge of immunology and immunosuppression, understanding of disease processes, prophylaxis against infection, and a general sophistication of pre- and post-transplant patient management have all contributed dramatically to the advances in transplantation. In 1984, Congress passed the *National Organ Transplant Act* and under its authority, the *United Network for Organ Sharing* (UNOS), the *Organ Procurement and Transplant Network* (OPTN), administered by UNOS, and the transplant community have worked continuously to improve awareness of organ donation, increase the availability of organs for transplantation, and optimize organ allocation. In the present era, kidney, pancreas, liver, heart, lung, small bowel, and almost every conceivable combination of multiorgan transplants have been performed with success. Technical considerations no longer represent major obstacles to patients in need. For those fortunate enough to receive organs, outcomes have become excellent, with 1-year patient survival approaching or exceeding 90% for most organs (Table 10.1). In the United States, as in most of the world, transplantation has become the standard of care for selected patients with end-stage organ failure. In the last 20 years almost 400,000 individuals in this country have received organ transplants and more than half are alive today. Currently in the United States there are over 100,000 individuals waiting for transplants of various organs (Table 10.2) With this volume of activity, there is now an overwhelming likelihood that "nontransplant" physicians will encounter either patients who have already received an organ transplant, or those who may be future candidates. Currently, all physicians must have some familiarity with the central issues, indications, and limitations of organ transplantation. For the surgical oncologist, there are additional issues and concerns, as well as some fascinating and instructive aspects in the simultaneous consideration of immunosuppression and malignancy. Indeed, surgical oncology and transplantation overlap in a number of areas, obligating physicians in each discipline to maintain an understanding of the problems common to both. The two areas of greatest interest include the treatment of malignancy with organ transplantation and the consequences of immunosuppression on the development of malignancy.

TRANSPLANTATION FOR THE TREATMENT OF MALIGNANCY

In general, the utilization of organ transplantation for the treatment of malignancy is extremely limited. With rare exceptions, kidney, pancreas, small bowel, heart, and lung transplants are *not* performed as a treatment for malignancy. The presence of any microscopic residual tends to flourish under the influence of immunosuppression. "Pouring gasoline on a fire" is the most commonly used analogy. Even if the risks to an individual might be less with transplantation when compared with alternatives, such practices are precluded by the extreme shortage of organs and the need for optimal outcomes. The most important exception is that of liver transplantation for a primary hepatic malignancy under circumstances in which all disease will be removed with the explanted organ. Of the two most common primary hepatic malignancies, liver transplants are performed with frequency only for the treatment of hepatocellular carcinoma.

Hepatocellular Carcinoma

The common denominator for most patients presenting with hepatocellular carcinoma (HCC) is a significant underlying parenchymal liver disease. Cirrhosis per se is a premalignant condition, with an incidence of HCC of between 1% and 4% per year (1). In fact, no more than 15% of HCC occurs in *non*cirrhotic individuals (2). Although some causes of liver disease have a stronger association than others, a patient with cirrhosis from any cause remains at risk. Patients in particular jeopardy are those with hemochromatosis, tyrosinemia, and α_1-antitrypsin deficiency, but even the much more common diagnoses of hepatitis B and C have a several hundred-fold increased relative risk (3,4).

Hepatitis C is by far the most frequent indication for liver transplantation in the United States, accounting for approximately 40% of activity at most centers. Although not all patients with hepatitis C progress in the same manner, the average interval from acquisition of the virus to cirrhosis and then tumor is often protracted and in the range of 18 to 20 years. Hepatitis B is an hepatotrophic DNA virus that contributes nearly 15% of U.S. transplant activity. Hepatitis B is one of the exceptions in which tumor development can be related to the direct interactions of the virus on the host hepatocytes, and some patients may present with tumor even in the absence of frank cirrhosis (5). The malignant degeneration of a pre-existing hepatic adenoma represents another, albeit rare, exception to the rule associating HCC with cirrhosis (6).

For most liver transplant programs in the United States, the diagnosis of HCC is based on the findings of high-quality imaging studies in the proper context. Magnetic resonance imaging or spiral contrast-enhanced computed tomography (CT) is the best modality. A hypervascular lesion found in the setting of cirrhosis, with or without an elevated alpha-fetoprotein, will usually suffice. Lipiodol uptake on either CT imaging or angiography

Table 10.1

Transplant Patient Survival Rates (%)[a]

Organ	Survival		
	1 Year	3 Years	5 Years
Heart	87.8	80.2	74.4
Kidney			
Deceased donor	94.8	88.4	80.6
Living donor	98.0	94.7	90.3
Liver	86.9	78.9	73.6
Pancreas	96.7	91.9	88.1
Lung	84.0	68.0	52.6
Intestine	81.0	67.4	43.6

Source: Organ Procurement and Transplantation Network (www.optn.org)
Data as of May 1, 2007.

may also be used. Biopsies of suspected HCC lesions are usually avoided because of the risks of bleeding, issues of percutaneous access, sampling errors, and finally, anecdotal reports of needle tract seeding and recurrences after transplantation (7). Although a number of studies have documented the accuracy of HCC diagnosis in the absence of a biopsy, a biopsy is still justified in equivocal circumstances (8).

The intuitive appeal of transplantation in the treatment of HCC is that it removes both the disease and its underlying cause. In general, fewer than 15% of patients presenting with HCC are found to be candidates for surgical resection because of the limitations imposed by their background liver disease (9). Even when feasible, surgical resection leaves diseased liver in situ, which tends to give rise to new tumors with remarkable frequency, often >20% per year (10). It is best to consider HCC to be essentially a multifocal disease, with the afflicted liver representing "fertile soil" for new tumor growth. Liver transplantation removes all presently detectable, subclinical, and "future" tumors.

In the earliest days of liver transplantation, a number of patients with advanced HCC were transplanted. Such patients

Table 10.2

U.S. Transplant Waiting List[a]

Organ	No.
Kidney	78,482
Liver	15,728
Pancreas	1,552
Kidney/pancreas	2,242
Heart	2,775
Lung	2,006
Heart/lung	83
Intestine	216
All candidates	100,841

[a]As of February 24, 2009. All candidates will be less that the sum due to candidates waiting for multiple organs.
Source: Organ Procurement and Transplantation Network (www.optn.org)

Table 10.3

Hepatocellular Carcinoma: Eligibility Criteria for Liver Transplantation

Milan Criteria (12)	UCSF Criteria (13)
1 tumor ≤ 5 cm	1 tumor ≤ 6.5 cm
or	or
Up to 3 tumors, none >3 cm	Multiple tumors, none >4.5 cm and total tumor diameter ≤8 cm

UCSF, University of California at San Francisco.

often had extensive tumor, but relatively well-compensated cirrhosis, making them a better surgical risk for the then new, difficult, and high-risk procedure. The outcomes for tumor patients in that pre-1990 era were generally dismal. A summary of the early outcomes found 2-year actuarial survival of 22.5% for those with TMN stage III/IV disease, with the longest survivor at only 31 months (11). However, as liver transplantation evolved and was performed in greater numbers, it was appreciated that many patients with incidental tumors, or known lower stage tumors, fared very well. In contrast, those with stage I/II disease had a 4-year survival of 75%. Ultimately, a set of limits on size and number of lesions was developed and adopted as a guiding standard (12). The *Milan Criteria*, as they came to be known, were adopted by UNOS for directing organ allocation in the United States. The details of the Milan Criteria and the UNOS staging system are shown in Tables 10.3. and 10.4 (12,13)

The current UNOS/OPTN organ allocation algorithm for livers is based on the *Model for End-Stage Liver Disease* (MELD) (14). This is an objective scheme that prioritizes patients according to the severity of their liver disease. A continuous score between 6 and 40 is generated using a formula that includes only three blood tests: total bilirubin, serum creatinine, and the prothrombin time expressed as the international normalized

Table 10.4

UNOS-Modified TNM Staging System (14)

T1	1 nodule ≤ 1.9 cm
T2	One nodule 2.0–5.0 cm; two or three nodules, all < 3.0 cm
T3	One nodule > 5.0 cm; two or three nodules, at least one > 3.0 cm
T4a	Four or more nodules, any size
T4b	T2, T3, or T4a with gross intrahepatic portal or hepatic vein involvement
Stage	
I	T1
II	T2
III	T3
IVA1	T4a
IVA2	T4b
IVB	Any N1, any M1

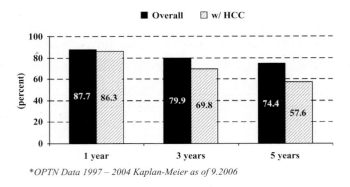

Figure 10.1 United States liver transplant survival: overall and for hepatocellular carcinoma (HCC) at 1, 3, and 5 years. Survival estimates by Kaplan-Meier method as of September, 2006 based on 1997–2004 data from the Organ Procurement and Transplantation Network (14).

ratio (INR). In patients with HCC, tumor progression will often surpass that of the cirrhosis. Additional MELD points are given for those patients with stage II HCC with automatic increases awarded at defined time intervals until the patient receives a transplant, or until the tumor progresses beyond acceptable criteria. Patients with stage I disease are thought to be too early to prioritize, and those with stage III or IV disease do not fare well enough to justify utilization of scarce organs. With the institution of the MELD allocation system in February 2002, the percentage of patients transplanted in the United States with HCC increased from about 3% to almost 20% by 2004. Recent U.S. liver transplant survival statistics include those patients transplanted between 1997 and 2004. Overall 1-, 3-, and 5-year survivals are 87.7%, 79.9%, and 74.4%, respectively, while those for HCC patients are 86.3%, 69.8%, and 57.6% (Figure 10.1) (14). Many studies have shown disease-free survival for HCC patients treated with resection to be in the range of only 27% to 40% at 5 years (15, 16). Given the fact that most HCC transplant recipients are by definition beyond surgical resection, such results seem even more respectable. It is the general expectation of the transplant community that outcomes for all patients, including those with HCC, will continue to improve. However, as with any surgical intervention, patient selection is critical.

Despite the good results afforded by adherence to the *Milan Criteria*, there have been recommendations to expand eligibility to patients with more extensive disease. Recently, a new set of expanded eligibility criteria, the *University of California San Francisco Criteria* (Table 10.3) has been advocated and appears to be associated with equally favorable results (13).

Cholangiocarcinoma

Cholangiocarcinoma (CCA) is a frustrating disease in both diagnosis and treatment. Although it occurs in a peripheral, intrahepatic form, a more common presentation is that of central, perihilar, and extrahepatic ductal involvement. In the United States there is an increasing incidence, now estimated at 3000 to 4000 per year, with high rates among patients with primary sclerosing cholangitis (PSC). A primary disease of the biliary tree, PSC can lead to cirrhosis and end-stage liver failure, and such patients are commonly treated and evaluated at transplant centers. A prominent confounding diagnostic dilemma is that benign PSC-related

strictures can mimic CCA, and distinguishing benign, dysplastic and malignant lesions can be challenging or impossible (17).

As with HCC, most early efforts to transplant patients with CCA met with extremely poor results (18,19). When arising in the hilar and extrahepatic ducts, local perineural, submucosal, and lymphatic extension can be difficult to detect, but will recur with rapid aggression under the influence of immunosuppression. For these reasons, known CCA continues to be considered a contraindication to liver transplantation at most centers (20). However, as with HCC, several studies have documented that patients transplanted with incidental CCA found in the explanted organs often had excellent long-term survival (21). Even more recently, 5-year survival rates approaching 80% have been reported among a highly select group of patients treated with neoadjuvant chemoradiation followed by transplantation (22,23). Rea et al. (24) reported that such preoperative therapy followed by liver transplantation was more effective than resection for node-negative hilar cholangiocarcinoma.

Currently, UNOS/OPTN is giving consideration to the allowance of additional MELD points to select patients with CCA in a manner similar to those given to patients with HCC (14). Patients given points in this way would be required to be participants in a clinical trial. It seems certain that the details of proper patient selection and treatment will soon extend liver transplantation to the more routine treatment of CCA.

Epithelioid Hemangioendothelioma

Epithelioid hemangioendothelioma is a rare, low-grade vascular neoplasm of endothelial origin with an unpredictable malignant potential that can occur in the liver and other visceral organs (25). Hepatic epithelioid hemangioendothelioma (HEHE) has an incidence of <0.1 per 100,000 and has no proven associations or etiologic factors (26). It does appear more commonly in women (3:2) and it has been related to past oral contraceptive use, trauma, and vinyl chloride exposure (27). The diagnosis of HEHE can be problematic, and confusion with other tumors can often lead to a misdiagnosis (28). Imaging can mimic HCC and other lesions, and immunohistology is usually required to distinguish HEHE from, for example, metastatic adenocarcinoma. Clinical presentation can be quite variable as can the size, number, and location of tumors. The course of HEHE is highly unpredictable, but almost always progressive. Long-term survival has been reported, even in the presence of metastatic disease.

Because of its rarity and unpredictable nature, the optimal treatment of HEHE remains unclear. Systemic chemotherapy is generally ineffective, and surgical resection is often precluded by the location or multiplicity of lesions. This has led to the utilization of total hepatectomy with orthotopic liver transplantation (OLT) for many patients. However, when considering transplantation for the treatment of a low-grade malignancy, the need for immunosuppression presents a dilemma: introducing the potential for converting an otherwise slowly advancing tumor to one that is rapidly progressive. Combinations of locoregional interventions have also yet to be fully explored. For example, a recent case report has described the use of preoperative adjuvant therapy with hepatic arterial chemoembolization (HACE) followed by liver transplantation (29). Explant pathology indicated HACE led to significant necrosis and an overall 50% reduction in tumor burden. As expected with such an uncommon disease, the reports thus far have been almost exclusively small, single-center retrospective reviews, but a role for liver transplantation in the treatment of this disease has clearly evolved.

A comprehensive review of the literature dating to the first description of HEHE has been published (26). So far it appears that liver transplantation has been the most often-employed treatment option (44.8%), with "no treatment" (24.8%) placing a distant second. To date, surgical resection has been used in <10% of all reported cases of HEHE. The 1- and 5-year patient survival with liver transplantation has been 96% and 54.5%, respectively, while no treatment has resulted in survivals of 73.3% and 30%, respectively. For those few treated with surgical resection, 1- and 5-year survivals have been 100% and 75%. As with HCC and CCA, liver transplantation may remain the best option for well-selected patients.

Carcinoid and Other Neuroendocrine Tumors

From the time they were first described, carcinoid and related neuroendocrine tumors (NET) have been appreciated to be more indolent than other malignancies. Although metastatic, liver transplantation has been used with some success to treat such tumors. However, when discussing the treatment of NET there can be many confounding issues, such as nomenclature and accuracy of diagnosis, nonfunctional versus functional tumors and, if present, the severity of the patient's symptoms. The optimal use of imaging—including CT, magnetic resonance imaging, positron emission tomography, endoscopic ultrasound, and octreotide scanning—can be challenging, while identification and elimination of the primary lesion can often be problematic. In addition, a number of both systemic and locoregional alternative treatment options now exist. These include combinations of somatostatins, interferon, resection, ablative technologies, and chemoembolization. Finally, as with HEHE, the use of transplantation as an alternative must be weighed against the probability of an otherwise slowly advancing disease transforming into one that is more aggressive with immunosuppression.

Relative to HCC and CCA, the early transplant experience with NETs was encouraging with some long-term survivors (30,31). A review of the world's literature up to 1994 revealed only 30 patients transplanted for NETs with a 1-year survival of 52%, and a death rate of 17% in the first year related to tumor recurrence. Caution and great attention to individual patient selection was emphasized (32). A subsequent larger study of 103 patients found overall survival at 2 and 5 years to be 60% and 47%, respectively, but with a disease-free survival of only 24%. Not surprisingly, a poorer prognosis was associated with those patients requiring foregut resection or a Whipple procedure at the time of transplantation (33). A number of studies have since observed better survival among those transplanted with carcinoid disease over other NETs (34,35). A report of 19 highly selected patients transplanted under protocol at the Mayo Clinic included an estimated 2-year survival of 87% with disease recurrence in the same period of 23% (36). A low proliferate index (Ki67 <10%) and a diagnosis of carcinoid were found to be important positive prognostic factors. Other more recent studies have reported less impressive survivals (37).

With continued experience, the ever-increasing shortage of organs, and the evolution of other treatment options, liver transplantation for metastatic carcinoid disease remains uncommon. To date, only about 160 cases have been reported worldwide

(37). Liver transplantation may continue to play a small role in the treatment of hepatic metastases of NET, but alternatives should first be considered. Presently, aggressive nontransplant management of hepatic NET using combinations of resection, ablation, and HACE, can achieve 5-year survivals of 72% (38). At this time, transplantation could be appropriate for a young, otherwise healthy patient with carcinoid disease in whom the primary has been controlled, there is no extrahepatic spread, other alternatives have failed or are unavailable, and who suffers from significant symptomatic hormone-related syndromes, mass effect, or other sequelae such as portal hypertension. Ideally, a Ki67 proliferative index should be low (<10%). Under certain favorable circumstances, excellent palliation and even cure has been achieved with OLT in such patients. However, utilization of the scarce resource of deceased donor organs must be considered. Each organ transplanted into one individual is an organ denied to another. The use and impact of living donor liver transplantation on such patients will be interesting to follow and raises many additional ethical questions.

Other Hepatic Malignancies
Sarcoma

An early report from the Cincinnati Transplant Tumor Registry of patients transplanted for either hemangiosarcoma or epithelioid endotheliosarcoma found the longest survivor to be 27 months (39). The most recent U.S. data from the Israel Penn International Transplant Tumor Registry (IPITTR) identified a total of 19 patients treated with transplantation for sarcoma (40). Six patients had primary and 13 had metastatic disease. Recurrence was essentially universal, with a median survival of 6 months and a 5-year survival of 5%. Unless performed in the context of a new experimental protocol, primary or metastatic hepatic sarcoma remains an unacceptable indication for transplantation (41,42).

Biliary Cystadenocarcinoma

Biliary cystadenocarcinoma is another rare condition, associated with Caroli disease, for which there are anecdotal reports of successful treatment with liver transplantation. Insufficient information exists regarding long-term follow-up, and transplantation appears to be an inappropriate treatment option (42).

Premalignant and Unresectable Benign Disease

A number of histologically benign conditions have been treated with liver transplantation, including those that are premalignant, or effectively malignant, in their impact on the patient. These include the three most common benign hepatic tumors: adenoma, focal nodular hyperplasia, and giant cavernous hemangioma. Because adenomas have the potential for spontaneous life-threatening hemorrhage and malignant degeneration, there is an obvious appeal to considering transplantation when lesions are otherwise unresectable. A number of transplant centers have reported this uncommon indication for OLT and, as expected, patients generally do well (43,44). Other anecdotal reports continue to appear, documenting unusual circumstances in which liver transplantation has been used to treat patients with both focal nodular hyperplasia and hemangioma (45,46). Over the last 2 decades other, even more uncommon, benign conditions have also been treated with transplantation, including mesenchymal hamartoma, hemangioma with Kasabach-Merritt syndrome, inflammatory pseudotumor, and massive hepatic lymphangiomatosis (43). Currently, the likelihood of acquiring an organ for a non–life-threatening indication is negligible. Nevertheless, the national UNOS/OPTN database does track the diagnosis of "benign neoplasm" among liver transplant recipients (14). Between 1997 and 2004, 1-year survival was 86% (N = 56), 3-year survival 82% (N = 720), and 5-year survival was 70.8% (N = 49).

For the sake of completeness, the most common histologically benign condition appropriately treated with liver transplantation is that of symptomatic, massive hepatomegaly due to adult polycystic liver disease. There is a frequent association with polycystic kidney disease, often leading to dual-organ transplantation. In appropriately selected patients, liver transplantation can provide excellent outcomes with a dramatic resolution to a dramatic problem (47).

MALIGNANCY AS A RESULT OF TRANSPLANTATION

Modern immunology and solid organ transplantation have co-evolved, each vitally important to the development of the other. Beginning with the earliest efforts to prevent organ rejection, an appreciation for the profound interaction between the immune system and malignancy also developed. The true magnitude of this relationship was dramatically illustrated when an early organ recipient succumbed to a donor's malignancy, establishing that immunosuppression can facilitate transplantation of more than just an organ (48). Over time, immunosuppression was found to be a risk for both incidence and aggression of certain de novo tumors, as well as affecting outcomes of common sporadic cancers (Figure 10.2 and Tables 10.5 and 10.6).

De Novo Malignancy After Transplantation

By the late 1960s it was appreciated that transplant recipients appeared to be at an increased risk for developing certain lymphomas (49,50). Within a few years, observations expanded to include other neoplasms of the viscera, skin, and cervix (51). It has now long been recognized that the predominant tumors found in transplant recipients include lymphomas, carcinoma

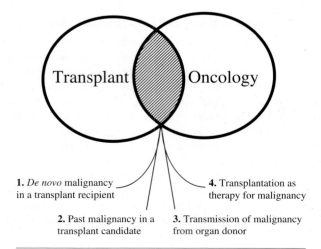

1. *De novo* malignancy in a transplant recipient

2. Past malignancy in a transplant candidate

3. Transmission of malignancy from organ donor

4. Transplantation as therapy for malignancy

Figure 10.2 Interplay between transplantation, immunology, and oncology.

Table 10.5

De Novo Malignancy after Transplantation: Relative Incidence of Some Specific Tumors

	General Population	Transplant Recipients
Lymphoma	5%	24%
Lip cancer	0.2%	6%
Kaposi's sarcoma	Negligible	6%
Anogenital	0.4%	3.5%
Hepatobiliary	1.5%	2.4%
Other Sarcomas	0.5%	1.8%

of the skin and lips, carcinoma of the vulva and perineum, and Kaposi sarcoma (KS), among others (52) (Table 10.5).

As immunosuppressive therapies have become increasingly sophisticated, some patterns of malignancy have also changed. As with other aspects of transplantation, data regarding post-transplant malignancy vary somewhat by era (50). Differences in the incidence of malignancy between different periods may reflect a multitude of changes, including not only the availability and action of specific drugs, evolution of therapeutic combinations and strategies, but also improved outcomes with longer survivals, inclusion of older recipients, and better screening. Currently, the overall incidence of de novo malignancy among transplant recipients is in the range of 2% per year (53).

Skin Cancer

Nonmelanoma

The most recent report from the IPITTR reconfirms that skin cancer is the most common malignancy among transplant recipients, with the median interval from transplant to diagnosis of just over 4 years (54). In contrast to the general population, those with squamous cell cancer (SCC) outnumber those with basal cell cancer by almost 2:1, with a 9% incidence of either local or nodal spread. In this study, cancer-related death for those with SCC was 8%, clearly illustrating a more aggressive behavior under the influence of immunosuppression. Many other published reports support similar findings. Recent results from the national renal transplant database in Ireland found up to a 200-fold increased risk for skin cancer among recipients when compared

Table 10.6

Immunosuppression Related Malignancy

Proposed Mechanisms

1) Direct carcinogenic effects of immunosuppressants
2) Facilitation of oncogenic viral mechanisms
3) Sensitization to environmental carcinogens
4) Diminished immune surveillance
5) Chronic antigenic stimulation: hyperplasia to neoplasia
6) Impaired immunoregulation /unrestrained lymphoid proliferation
7) Decreased interferons / altered cytokine milieu

with an age-matched nontransplant population (55). The risk for an invasive SCC in that study was 82-fold higher than nontransplant controls. Because of patterns of sun exposure, >50% of such tumors can involve the head and neck, further complicating therapeutic options (56).

Melanoma

The American Cancer Society estimates that the lifetime risk of developing invasive melanoma in the United States is on the order of 2% (57). The incidence of melanoma in transplant patients is consistently higher than that seen in the general population, with several retrospective reviews suggesting up to a fivefold increase in the incidence of malignant melanoma occurring among transplant recipients (58).

Merkel Cell

Merkel cell carcinoma is a rare, aggressive cutaneous malignancy of the elderly with both epithelial and neuroendocrine elements. The head and neck, followed by the upper extremities, are the most common sites. This tumor is dramatically more common in transplant recipients, who account for 8% of all reported cases (59). Many present with disseminated disease, and overall 5-year survival has been reported to be as low as 46%.

Posttransplant Lymphoproliferative Disorders

Both inherited and acquired forms of immunodeficiency are associated with an increased incidence of lymphoma. It is not surprising, then, that pharmacologic immunosuppression has the same association, and a posttransplant lymphoproliferative disorder (PTLD) is well described in this setting. PTLD is a non-Hodgkin B-cell lymphoma with an Epstein-Barr virus association similar to that of Burkett's lymphoma, and probably the same pathophysiology as AIDS-associated B-cell lymphoma (60,61). However, PTLD differs from non-Hodgkin lymphoma in the general population in several ways. PTLD has higher incidence of extranodal distribution (≥24% vs. nearly 70%) and CNS involvement (1% vs. ≤28%), where it may be confined (62). Finally, the transplanted organ is involved in about 20% of cases (63). PTLD occurs rather unpredictably, although the incidence is highest within the first year after transplant. It is generally associated with more potent immunosuppressive regimens and higher cumulative doses. PTLD is therefore more likely to afflict patients who have undergone intensive therapy for episodes of rejection, or who have received aggressive antibody induction therapy.

With progress and the development of more potent immunosuppressive agents, the incidence of PTLD initially increased from the earliest observations. With increased awareness of the disease and its causes, the incidence now appears to have at least stabilized (50,64). With varying immunosuppressant strategies, there are differences in the incidence of PTLD among recipients of different organs: kidney recipients about 1%; liver recipients, 2.7%; heart, 3.3%; and heart/lung, 3.8%. The incidence among small bowel transplant recipients is highest at about 20% (61). Currently, the overall incidence of PTLD remains at between 2% and 5% of all organ transplant recipients (64,65). Although PTLD in transplant patients can frequently be fatal, outcomes are highly dependant on specific circumstances. Greater awareness, newer agents, and better immunosuppressive strategies will likely lead to a lower incidence of this disease. More effective means of diagnosis, pre-emptive interventions, and better treatment strategies have combined to reduce the impact of this disease and improve survival.

Kaposi Sarcoma

Although KS was largely an obscure medical oddity prior to the onset of the AIDS epidemic, it was already appreciated to occur with increased frequency in transplant recipients (66). By 1979 an epidemiologic study found up to a 500-fold increase in KS among renal transplant recipients (67). In 1997 the Cincinnati Transplant Tumor Registry reported an overall 5.7% incidence of KS in transplant recipients, with a rising incidence from 3% to 10% with the use of cyclosporine (68). The majority of KS lesions in transplant recipients involve only the skin, with rare conjunctival or mucosal involvement, and less common visceral disease. On average, KS appears around 21 months after transplantation. As with the classic form, KS is more common in recipients with a Mediterranean or Middle Eastern background (68). The etiology of KS has long been suspected to be at least partly due to viral infection. More recently the herpes virus HSV-8 has become strongly implicated. Complete clinical remission of KS has recently been reported by changing from the calcineurin inhibitor cyclosporine to the mTOR (mammalian target of rapamycin) inhibitor sirolimus (69).

Other Sarcomas

There is some evidence to suggest an increased incidence of sarcomas other than KS in transplant recipients (70). Fibrous histiocytoma, fibrosarcomas, rhabdomyosarcoma, and hemangiosarcoma have been seen with greater-than-expected frequencies. Similar observations have been made in patients with human immunodeficiency virus-related AIDS.

Sporadic Tumors

Aside from skin cancer and lymphoma, the incidence of sporadic malignancies common among the general population was long thought to be no higher among transplant recipients (71,72). More recently, such tumors have been found to occur in kidney transplant recipients with roughly twice the expected frequency (58). In any event, when such tumors do occur, they tend to behave much more aggressively, and are associated with much lower overall survival rates (73).

According to the IPITTR, transplant recipients with Duke C colorectal disease were found to be younger and had a 5-year survival of only 20% compared with 65% for similar patients found in the National Cancer Institute Surveillance, Epidemiology, and End Results (SEER) database. In another small study of 395 transplant recipients, 1% were found to have developed de novo gastrointestinal tumors over a 12-year period, with a 75% mortality despite optimal therapy (74). The incidence and stage at diagnosis of breast cancer among posttransplant recipients does not appear to be significantly different than that of the general population. However, for those presenting with stage III or IV disease, survival does appear relatively lower, suggesting a more aggressive course (50,75).

Immunosuppression and Malignancy

Although undeniable evidence implicates immunosuppressive drugs in the development of tumors following transplantation, the exact mechanisms by which they facilitate malignancies remain unclear. Possibilities include diminished immuno-surveillance, facilitation of viral oncogenesis, increased sensitivity to environmental carcinogens, chronic antigenic stimulation with hyperplasia, or a host of effects at the cellular level (71) (Table 10.6). It seems likely that none are mutually exclusive, but rather the overall effect is multifactorial.

For many years, the incidence of malignancy increased along with the potency of available drugs. Several studies have documented an increased incidence of malignancy among patients treated with cyclosporine- versus azathioprine-based immunosuppression regimens (50). A strong, dose-dependant association exists between the use of the monoclonal antibody OKT3 and the incidence PTLD (76). However, no significant differences have been identified between the two calcineurin inhibitors, cyclosporine and tacrolimus (77). Drugs implicated as possible direct carcinogens include those now rarely used, such as azathioprine (AZA) and cyclophosphamide, but also include cyclosporine (71). Mycophenolate mofetil may actually have a reduced association with malignancy over AZA, which it has now largely replaced (78). Because drugs are most often used in combination, no single agent can be exonerated.

Perhaps the most significant change on the topic of immunosuppression and malignancy has been the relatively recent introduction of the drug rapamycin, and other mTOR agents (79). Early experimental data suggested a possible antitumor effect in animals, and this has been supported by some clinical observations (50,80,81). The most compelling data thus far are from the Organ Procurement and Transplantation Network (OPTN) database (82). This multivariate analysis of 33,249 U.S. patients in the database revealed a significantly lower de novo malignancy rate for mTOR-based (0.60%) versus calcineurin-based (1.81%) therapy. Although not always used as a primary agent, many transplant programs may use such an agent when a de novo or recurrent tumor arises in a transplant recipient.

Pre-existing Malignancy in Transplant Candidates

The candidate with a history of malignancy presents one of the most difficult aspects of transplantation. The risks of a recurrent neoplasm in the immunosuppressed environment must be weighed against the alternatives without a transplant. Although it seems unlikely that immunosuppression per se will alter the risk of recurrence, there seems little doubt that it will alter the consequences. The type, grade, stage, and disease-free interval all must be considered. The direct, life-saving nature of heart, lung, or liver transplants must be distinguished from those that are not. The likelihood of recurrence must also be considered in light of the ongoing organ shortage; an organ used in one individual is an organ denied to another. In 1997, Israel Penn (83) categorized various pre-existing malignancies in transplant candidates into categories of low, intermediate, and high risk, based on the likelihood of recurrence after transplantation) (Table 10.7) Since that time there has been very little additional information to guide waiting-time decisions. The most recent comprehensive review is summarized in table 10.8 (72). Given that optimal therapy has been rendered, small (<5 cm) RCCs, as well as in situ tumors in general, should require no specific waiting time. In optimal circumstances, carcinoma of the prostate should elicit a 2-year wait prior to transplant. In gen-

Table 10.7

Tumor Recurrence Following Transplant

Low (0% to 10%)	Intermediate (11% to 22%)	High (≥23%)
Incidental renal cell (1%)	Lymphoma (11%)	Breast (23%)
Uterine (4%)	Wilms (13%)	Bladder (29%)
Testicular tumors (5%)	Prostate (18%)	Renal cell (27%)
Uterine cervix (6%)	Colon (21%)	Sarcoma (29%)
Papillary thyroid (7%)	Melanoma (21%)	Skin cancer (53%) Myeloma (67%)

From Penn I. Evaluation of transplant candidates with pre-existing malignancies. *Ann Transplant.* 1997;2:14–17.

eral, invasive carcinoma of the breast and lymphoma in most all cases will be at high risk for recurrence, regardless of the wait (72,84). Until the availability of better data, decisions regarding pretransplant waiting times in patients with a prior history of malignancy must be tailored to individual circumstances.

Recipient Death from Malignancy

One final approach to comprehending the impact of malignancy on transplant recipients is to look at long-term outcomes and causes of death. Among long-term survivors after heart transplantation, malignancy is now the leading cause of death (85). According to the University of Pittsburgh experience, malignancy was the second-leading cause of death among liver transplant recipients, following cardiovascular complications (86). Indeed, a recent editorial headlined "will all liver transplantation patients eventually die from cancer?" (87). Similar statistics can be found for other organs as well. Clearly, posttransplant malignancy is a complex issue of major impact.

Donor Transmission

A number of early reports documented the disastrous potential to transmit malignancy with a transplanted organ (48,88). Failure to elicit a prior history of a malignancy or an unrecognized lesion in a deceased donor has led to the transmission of a broad variety of tumors (89). Treatment options always include immunosuppression dose reduction but, if feasible as with kidney or pancreas transplants, these drugs can be completely discontinued with removal of the organs. Even diffuse metastases have been reported to resolve in the absence of ongoing immunosuppression (88). Organs from deceased donors with primary CNS malignancies have been knowingly used, given the low incidence of extracranial spread. A recent OPTN/UNOS report of 650 organs from donors with a history of such tumors failed to show any recipients with a transmitted malignancy (90). Given the increasing shortage of organs, further assessment of the risks may allow expansion of the donor pool into this previously avoided area.

SUMMARY

No other field of medicine has undergone more dramatic changes in the last 50 years than that of organ transplantation.

Table 10.8

Prior Malignancy: Recommended Wait Times for Transplant Candidates

Malignancy	Recommended Wait (years)
Incidental renal cell	None
Basal cell	None
Bladder (in situ)	None
Cervical (in situ)	None
Lymphoma	2
Prostate	2
Thyroid	2
Testicular	2
Renal cell	2
Bladder	2
Colorectal	0–5 (depending on stage)
Breast	2–5 (depending on stage)
Melanoma	2–5 (depending on stage)

Adapted from Girndt M, Kohler H. Waiting time for patients with history of malignant disease before listing for organ transplantation. *Transplantation.* 2005;80(1 Suppl):S167–S170.

Malignancy among transplant candidates, recipients, and donors continues to be an area of major significance. Continued experience and research in the areas common to both surgical oncology and transplantation will, without doubt, provide the foundations for future successes in the treatment of malignancy.

REFERENCES

1. Schafer DF, Sorrell MF. Hepatocellular carcinoma. *Lancet.* 1999;353:1253–1257.
2. Kew MC, Popper H. Relationship between hepatocellular carcinoma and cirrhosis. *Semin Liver Dis.* 1984;4:136–146.
3. Levrero M. Viral hepatitis and liver cancer: the case of hepatitis C. *Oncogene.* 2006;25:3834–3847.
4. Raimondo G, Balsano C, Craxi A, et al. Occult hepatitis B virus infection. *Dig Liver Dis.* 2000;32:822–826.
5. Kremsdorf D, Soussan P, Paterlini-Brechot P, et al. Hepatitis B virus-related hepatocellular carcinoma: paradigms for viral-related human carcinogenesis. *Oncogene.* 2006;25:3823–3833.
6. Burri E, Steuerwald M, Cathomas G, et al. Hepatocellular carcinoma in a liver-cell adenoma within a non-cirrhotic liver. *Eur J Gastroenterol Hepatol.* 2006;18:437–441.
7. Saborido BP, Diaz JC, de Los Galanes SJ, et al. Does preoperative fine needle aspiration-biopsy produce tumor recurrence in patients following liver transplantation for hepatocellular carcinoma? *Transplant Proc.* 2005;37:3874–3877.
8. Torzilli G, Minagawa M, Takayama T, et al. Accurate preoperative evaluation of liver mass lesions without fine-needle biopsy. *Hepatology.* 1999;30:889–893.
9. Bismuth H, Majno PE, Adam R. Liver transplantation for hepatocellular carcinoma. *Semin Liver Dis.* 1999;19:311–322.
10. Nagasue N, Uchida M, Makino Y, et al. Incidence and factors associated with intrahepatic recurrence following resection of hepatocellular carcinoma. *Gastroenterology.* 1993;105:488–494.
11. Olthoff KM, Millis JM, Rosove MH, et al. Is liver transplantation justified for the treatment of hepatic malignancies? *Arch Surg.* 1990;125:1261–1268.
12. Mazzaferro V, Regalia E, Doci R, et al. Liver transplantation for the treatment of small hepatocellular carcinomas in patients with cirrhosis. *N Engl J Med.* 1996;334:693–699.
13. Yao FY, Ferrell L, Bass NM, et al. Liver transplantation for hepatocellular carcinoma: comparison of the proposed UCSF criteria with the Milan criteria and the Pittsburgh modified TNM criteria. *Liver Transpl.* 2002;8:765–774.
14. Organ Procurement and Transplant Network: http://www.optn.org
15. Fan ST, Ng IO, Poon RT, et al. Hepatectomy for hepatocellular carcinoma: the surgeon's role in long-term survival. *Arch Surg.* 1999;134:1124–1130.
16. Blumgart LH, Fong Y. Hepatobiliary cancer. *Semin Surg Oncol.* 2000;19:83.
17. LaRusso NF, Shneider BL, Black D, et al. Primary sclerosing cholangitis: summary of a workshop. *Hepatology.* 2006;44:746–764.
18. Herbener T, Zajko AB, Koneru B, et al. Recurrent cholangiocarcinoma in the biliary tree after liver transplantation. *Radiology.* 1988;169:641–642.
19. Goldstein RM, Stone M, Tillery GW, et al. Is liver transplantation indicated for cholangiocarcinoma? *Am J Surg.* 1993;166:768–772.
20. Meyer CG, Penn I, James L. Liver transplantation for cholangiocarcinoma: results in 207 patients. *Transplantation.* 2000;69:1633–1637.
21. Shimoda M, Farmer DG, Colquhoun SD, et al. Liver transplantation for cholangiocellular carcinoma: analysis of a single-center experience and review of the literature. *Liver Transpl.* 2001;7:1023–1033.
22. Sudan D, DeRoover A, Chinnakotla S, et al. Radiochemotherapy and transplantation allow long-term survival for nonresectable hilar cholangiocarcinoma. *Am J Transplant.* 2002;2:774–779.
23. Heimbach JK, Gores GJ, Haddock MG, et al. Liver transplantation for unresectable perihilar cholangiocarcinoma. *Semin Liver Dis.* 2004;24:201–207.
24. Rea DJ, Heimbach JK, Rosen CB, et al. Liver transplantation with neoadjuvant chemoradiation is more effective than resection for hilar cholangiocarcinoma. *Ann Surg.* 2005;242:451–458; discussion 458–61.
25. Makhlouf HR, Ishak KG, Goodman ZD. Epithelioid hemangioendothelioma of the liver: a clinicopathologic study of 137 cases. *Cancer.* 1999;85:562–582.
26. Mehrabi A, Kashfi A, Fonouni H, et al. Primary malignant hepatic epithelioid hemangioendothelioma: a comprehensive review of the literature with emphasis on the surgical therapy. *Cancer* 2006; 107:2108-21.
27. Gelin M, Van de Stadt J, Rickaert F, et al. Epithelioid hemangioendothelioma of the liver following contact with vinyl chloride. Recurrence after orthotopic liver transplantation. *J Hepatol.* 1989;8:99–106.
28. Demetris AJ, Minervini M, Raikow RB, et al. Hepatic epithelioid hemangioendothelioma: biological questions based on pattern of recurrence in an allograft and tumor immunophenotype. *Am J Surg Pathol.* 1997;21:263–270.
29. St Peter SD, Moss AA, Huettl EA, et al. Chemoembolization followed by orthotopic liver transplant for epithelioid hemangioendothelioma. *Clin Transplant.* 2003;17:549–553.
30. Arnold JC, O'Grady JG, Bird GL, et al. Liver transplantation for primary and secondary hepatic apudomas. *Br J Surg.* 1989;76:248–249.
31. Makowka L, Tzakis AG, Mazzaferro V, et al. Transplantation of the liver for metastatic endocrine tumors of the intestine and pancreas. *Surg Gynecol Obstet.* 1989;168:107–111.
32. Bechstein WO, Neuhaus P. Liver transplantation for hepatic metastases of neuroendocrine tumors. *Ann N Y Acad Sci.* 1994;733:507–514.

33. Lehnert T. Liver transplantation for metastatic neuroendocrine carcinoma: an analysis of 103 patients. *Transplantation.* 1998;66:1307–1312.

34. Routley D, Ramage JK, McPeake J, et al. Orthotopic liver transplantation in the treatment of metastatic neuroendocrine tumors of the liver. *Liver Transpl Surg.* 1995;1:118–121.

35. Le Treut YP, Grégoire E, Belghiti J, et al. Results of liver transplantation in the treatment of metastatic neuroendocrine tumors. A 31-case French multicentric report. *Ann Surg.* 1997;225:355–364.

36. van Vilsteren FG, Baskin-Bey ES, Nagorney DM, et al. Liver transplantation for gastroenteropancreatic neuroendocrine cancers: defining selection criteria to improve survival. *Liver Transpl.* 2006;12:448–456.

37. Frilling A, Malago M, Weber F, et al. Liver transplantation for patients with metastatic endocrine tumors: single-center experience with 15 patients. *Liver Transpl.* 2006;12:1089–1096.

38. Touzios JG, Kiely JM, Pitt SC, et al. Neuroendocrine hepatic metastases: does aggressive management improve survival? *Ann Surg.* 2005;241:776–785.

39. Penn I. Hepatic transplantation for primary and metastatic cancers of the liver. *Surgery.* 1991;110:726–735.

40. Husted TL, Neff G, Thomas MJ, et al. Liver transplantation for primary or metastatic sarcoma to the liver. *Am J Transplant.* 2006;6:392–397.

41. Testa G, Klintmalm GB. Liver transplantation for primary and metastatic liver cancers. *Ann Transplant.* 1997;2:19–21.

42. O'Grady JG. Treatment options for other hepatic malignancies. *Liver Transpl.* 2000;6(6 Suppl 2):S23–S29.

43. Tepetes K, Selby R, Webb M, et al. Orthotopic liver transplantation for benign hepatic neoplasms. *Arch Surg.* 1995;130:153–156.

44. Mueller J. Keeffe EB, Esquivel CO. Liver transplantation for treatment of giant hepatocellular adenomas. *Liver Transpl Surg.* 1995;1:99–102.

45. Fujita S, Mekeel KL, Fujikawa T, et al. Liver-occupying focal nodular hyperplasia and adenomatosis associated with intrahepatic portal vein agenesis requiring orthotopic liver transplantation. *Transplantation.* 2006;81:490–492.

46. Ferraz AA, Sette MJ, Maia M, et al. Liver transplant for the treatment of giant hepatic hemangioma. *Liver Transpl.* 2004;10:1436–1437.

47. Ueno T, Barri YM, Netto GJ, et al. Liver and kidney transplantation for polycystic liver and kidney-renal function and outcome. *Transplantation.* 2006;82:501–507.

48. McIntosh D, McPhaul J, Peterson E, et al. Homotransplantation of a cadaver neoplasm and a renal homograft. JAMA 1965; 192: 1171-3.

49. Penn I, Hammond W, Brettschneider L, et al. Malignant lymphomas in transplantation patients. *Transplant Proc.* 1969;1:106–112.

50. Kauffman HM, Cherikh WS, McBride MA, et al. Post-transplant de novo malignancies in renal transplant recipients: the past and present. *Transpl Int.* 2006;19:607–620.

51. Penn I, Halgrimson CG, Starzl TE. De novo malignant tumors in organ transplant recipients. *Transplant Proc.* 1971;3:773–778.

52. Penn I, Cancers in renal transplant recipients. *Adv Ren Replace Ther.* 2000;7:147–156.

53. Kauffman HM. Malignancies in organ transplant recipients. *J Surg Oncol.* 2006;94:431–433.

54. Buell JF, Hanaway MJ, Thomas M, et al. Skin cancer following transplantation: the Israel Penn International Transplant Tumor Registry experience. *Transplant Proc.* 2005;37:962–963.

55. Moloney FJ, Comber H, O'Lorcain P, et al. A population-based study of skin cancer incidence and prevalence in renal transplant recipients. *Br J Dermatol.* 2006;154:498–504.

56. Gourin CG, Terris DJ. Head and neck cancer in transplant recipients. *Curr Opin Otolaryngol Head Neck Surg.* 2004;12:122–126.

57. Jemal A, Siegel R, Ward E, et al. Cancer statistics, 2008. *CA Cancer J Clin* 2008; 58: 71–96.

58. Kasiske BL, Snyder J, Gilbedrtson D, Wang C. Cancer after kidney transplantation in the United States. *Am J Transplant.* 2004;4:905–913.

59. Buell JF, Trofe J, Hanaway MJ, et al. Immunosuppression and Merkel cell cancer. *Transplant Proc.* 2002;34:1780–1781.

60. Babcock GJ, Decker LL, Freeman RB, et al. Epstein-Barr virus-infected resting memory B cells, not proliferating lymphoblasts, accumulate in the peripheral blood of immunosuppressed patients. *J Exp Med.* 1999;190:567–576.

61. Gottschalk S, Rooney CM, Heslop HE. Post-transplant lymphoproliferative disorders. *Annu Rev Med.* 2005;56:29–44.

62. Buell JF, Gross TG, Hanaway MJ, et al. Posttransplant lymphoproliferative disorder: significance of central nervous system involvement. *Transplant Proc.* 2005;37:954–955.

63. Penn I. Cancers complicating organ transplantation. *N Engl J Med.* 1990;323:1767–1769.

64. Aucejo F, Rofaiel G, Miller C. Who is at risk for post-transplant lymphoproliferative disorders (PTLD) after liver transplantation? *J Hepatol.* 2006;44:19–23.

65. Nalosnik MA, Rao AS, Furukawa H, et al. Autologous lymphokine-activated killer cell therapy of lymphoproliferative disorders arising in organ transplant recipients. *Transplant Proc.* 1997;29:1905–1906.

66. Siegel JH, Janis R, Alper JC, et al. Disseminated visceral Kaposi's sarcoma. Appearance after human renal homograft operation. *JAMA.* 1969;207:1493–1496.

67. Harwood AR, Osoba D, Hofstader SL, et al. Kaposi's sarcoma in recipients of renal transplants. *Am J Med.* 1979;67:759–765.

68. Penn I. Kaposi's sarcoma in transplant recipients. *Transplantation.* 1997;64:669–673.

69. Stallone G, Schena A, Infante B, et al. Sirolimus for Kaposi's sarcoma in renal-transplant recipients. *N Engl J Med.* 2005;352:1317–1323.

70. Penn I. Sarcomas in organ allograft recipients. *Transplantation.* 1995;60:1485–1491.

71. Penn I. Posttransplant malignancies. *Transplant Proc.* 1999;31:1260–1262.

72. Girndt M, Kohler H. Waiting time for patients with history of malignant disease before listing for organ transplantation. *Transplantation.* 2005;80(1 Suppl):S167–S170.

73. Buell JF, Papaconstantinou HT, Skalow B, et al. De novo colorectal cancer: five-year survival is markedly lower in transplant recipients compared with the general population. *Transplant Proc.* 2005;37:960–961.

74. Adani GL, Baccarani U, Lorenzin D, et al. De novo gastrointestinal tumours after renal transplantation: role of CMV and EBV viruses. *Clin Transpl.* 2006;20:457–460.

75. Buell JF, Hanaway MJ, Trofe J, et al. De novo breast cancer in renal transplant recipients. *Transplant Proc.* 2002;34:1778–1779.

76. Swinnen LJ, Costanzo-Nordin MR, Fisher SG, et al. Increased incidence of lymphoproliferative disorder after immunosuppression with the monoclonal antibody OKT3 in cardiac-transplant recipients. *N Engl J Med.* 1990;323:1723–1728.

77. Madalosso C, de Souza NF Jr, Listrup DM, et al. Cytomegalovirus and its association with hepatic artery thrombosis after liver transplantation. *Transplantation.* 1998;66:294–297.

78. David KM, Morris JA, Steffen BJ, et al. Mycophenolate mofetil vs. azathioprine is associated with decreased acute rejection, late acute rejection, and risk for cardiovascular death in renal transplant recipients with pre-transplant diabetes. *Clin Transpl.* 2005;19:279–285.

79. Law BK. Rapamycin: an anti-cancer immunosuppressant? *Crit Rev Oncol Hematol.* 2005;56:47–60.

80. Buell JF, Gross TG, Woodle ES. Malignancy after transplantation. *Transplantation.* 2005;80(2 Suppl):S254–S264.

81. Kahan BD, Yakupoglu YK, Schoenberg L, et al. Low incidence of malignancy among sirolimus/cyclosporine-treated renal transplant recipients. *Transplantation.* 2005;80:749–758.

82. Kauffman HM, Cherikh WS, Cheng Y, et al. Maintenance immunosuppression with target-of-rapamycin inhibitors is associated with a reduced incidence of de novo malignancies. *Transplantation.* 2005;80:883–889.

83. Penn I. Evaluation of transplant candidates with pre-existing malignancies. *Ann Transplant.* 1997;2:14–17.

84. Kasiske BL, Cangro CB, Hariharan S, et al. The evaluation of renal transplantation candidates: clinical practice guidelines. *Am J Transplant.* 2001;1(Suppl 2):3–95.

85. Hauptman PJ, Mehra MR. It is time to stop ignoring malignancy in heart transplantation: a call to arms. *J Heart Lung Transplant.* 2005;24:1111–1113.

86. Fung JJ, Jain A, Kwak EJ, et al. De novo malignancies after liver transplantation: a major cause of late death. *Liver Transpl.* 2001;7(11 Suppl 1):S109–S118.

87. Sanchez W, Talwalkar JA, Gores GJ. "Will all liver transplantation patients eventually die from cancer?" *J Hepatol.* 2006;44:13–18.

88. Colquhoun SD, Robert ME, Shaked A, et al. Transmission of CNS malignancy by organ transplantation. *Transplantation.* 1994;57:970–974.

89. Kauffman HM, McBride MA, Delmonico FL. First report of the United Network for Organ Sharing Transplant Tumor Registry: donors with a history of cancer. *Transplantation.* 2000;70:1747–1751.

90. Kauffman HM, McBride MA, Cherikh WS, et al. Transplant tumor registry: donors with central nervous system tumors1. *Transplantation.* 2002;73:579–582.

COMMENTARY
John P. Duffy and Ronald W. Busuttil

The first successful orthotopic liver transplantation (OLT) in humans was performed for primary hepatic malignancy on July 23, 1967, by Thomas E. Starzl, who replaced the liver in a 19-month-old girl who had hepatocellular carcinoma (HCC) (1). The patient survived 13 months after the operation before succumbing to disease recurrence and dissemination (1). Since this first experience, many advances have been made in transplant techniques and medical management of these patients, producing improved short- and long-term graft and patient outcomes (2). Despite these improvements, overall outcomes remain significantly lower for patients transplanted for HCC compared with those with end-stage liver disease but free of hepatic malignancy (2).

LIVER TRANSPLANTATION FOR HEPATOCELLULAR CARCINOMA

The management of the patient with end-stage liver disease and HCC remains the central and most important issue concerning OLT for malignancy today. The incidence of HCC in the United States has nearly doubled over the last 2 decades, and an estimated 8,500 to 11,000 new cases of HCC occur annually in the United States (3,4). This increase has been attributed to infections with hepatitis C virus from the 1970s and 1980s, and hepatitis C virus-associated HCC is expected to further double within the next 20 years (5,6). Although *overall* outcomes are indeed somewhat lower, major improvements in OLT for *selected*

patients with HCC have been clearly accomplished. Today, patients with limited tumors can expect posttransplant survival rates similar to patients with benign disease such as Laennec's cirrhosis or chronic hepatitis C infection.

Achievement of such outcomes relies heavily on several key components of peritransplant care: (a) accurate radiographic delineation of disease extent, (b) early listing for patients with disease extent within the Milan criteria, (c) effective locoregional therapy prior to transplantation, and (d) en bloc resection of all intrahepatic disease. With optimal management of these components, better outcomes have been achieved in patients with measured expansion of existing criteria. Ultimately, outcomes appear to be influenced by the microscopic biology of the individual tumors; as a result, successful OLT for HCC arises from thorough evaluation of patients and tumors, a process that truly enmeshes the bench and the bedside.

Preoperative Delineation of the Extent of HCC

Appropriate selection of OLT recipients is paramount to successful treatment of HCC with hepatic allografts, still today a precious and scarce resource. Pretransplant assessment of the liver typically involves imaging with computerized tomography and magnetic resonance imaging (7). Most series, however, demonstrate that radiographic data underestimate tumor extent in approximately 20% of cases. Preoperative imaging is necessary to document tumor size and number, as well as to rule out any absolute contraindications to liver transplantation including extrahepatic disease spread, tumor-related portal vein thrombosis, and encasement of the hepatoduodenal ligament. Patients with disease extent resting within the Milan criteria have been shown to have superior posttransplant outcomes compared with patients with HCC beyond these criteria, and are therefore recommended as transplant candidates (8,9). It is important to note that the Milan outcomes are based on disease extent determined through preoperative imaging, whereas, until recently, data for expanded University of California, San Francisco (UCSF) criteria have been based on explant pathologic assessment (10,11).

Listing for Liver Transplantation

Patients with HCC within Milan criteria are listed for transplantation. The Model for End-Stage Liver Disease (MELD) scoring system introduced in 2002 now offers priority for patients with HCC within conventional Milan criteria (12). Early United Network for Organ Sharing (UNOS) data indicate that implementation of MELD scores prioritizing OLT for HCC has resulted in more OLTs for HCC, decreased mortality while awaiting OLT, as well as decreased time on the waiting list (13). In 2003, priority scoring for HCC was reduced from 24 to 20 for stage I tumors (one tumor ≤1.9 cm) and from 29 to 24 for stage II tumors (single tumor 2 to 5 cm or three or less tumors, none larger than 3 cm) (14). This shift in MELD priority scoring has not had an impact on survival on the waiting list and has not lengthened time awaiting OLT on a national basis, but it has produced regional differences in these two factors (14). In the University of California, Los Angeles (UCLA) experience, patients transplanted in the MELD era have had improved posttransplant survival rates compared with patients transplanted pre-MELD (15).

Locoregional Therapy for HCC

Despite MELD priority scoring, disease progression and dissemination on the waiting list remain real possibilities for patients with HCC. Locoregional therapies, including radiofrequency ablation (RFA) and transarterial chemoembolization, have been shown to be effective "bridging" techniques, limiting HCC progression prior to OLT (16,17). The UCLA experience with RFA for HCC prior to OLT has proven to be effective treatment before OLT, as it limited the dropout rate from OLT candidacy to only 5.8% and contributed to post-OLT survival rates of 85% and 76% at 1 and 3 years after transplant (17). However, in multivariate analysis of 467 patients transplanted at UCLA for HCC, preoperative locoregional therapy did not independently impact posttransplant survival (15). Other investigators have also demonstrated no significant effect of locoregional therapy on posttransplant survival, particularly in the MELD era (18). This is thought to be secondary to shorter waiting times prior to OLT and increased rates of transplantation for HCC. Nevertheless, the majority of the evidence indicates that RFA and transarterial chemoembolization can effectively treat patients with HCC and enable them to remain as appropriate OLT candidates. More prospective data are necessary in this important area, especially as locoregional technology continues to evolve.

Expansion of HCC Criteria for Liver Transplantation

Over the past quarter century, OLT has been established as a durable therapy for end-stage liver disease (2,19). OLT appears ideally suited for HCC as it provides complete oncologic resection and correction of the underlying liver dysfunction. As stated by Colquhoun and Klein, early experience with OLT for HCC resulted in poor posttransplant survival and high recurrence rates that were attributed to suboptimal patient selection (20–23). In 1991, Ringe et al. (20) found 3- and 5-year survival of 15% after 61 transplants, 80% of which demonstrated tumor size >5 cm. Furthermore, Iwatsuki et al. (21) and Moreno et al. (22) found 3- and 5-year survival rates <50% after transplantation of advanced stage tumors, with >50% in each study having multifocal disease. Recurrence rates were high in both of these studies, at 43% and 54%, respectively (21,22). In 1996, Mazzaferro and colleagues (8) reported improved results with OLT in patients with a single tumor ≤5 cm or no more than three tumors, each no larger than 3 cm. For patients meeting the Milan criteria, overall and recurrence-free survivals were 85% and 92%, respectively, and overall recurrence rate was 8% at 4-year follow-up (8). As the Milan criteria consistently have been associated with improved survival (8,9,24), they are currently used by UNOS and Medicare to guide patient selection for cadaveric OLT for HCC. Restrictive criteria in the United States, where around 20,000 patients await OLT and donor organs number only 5,000 per year consistently, can result in prolonged waiting time for OLT, and a case dropout rate of up to 20% to 50% (25). For many transplant surgeons, there remains concern that the current guidelines are too restrictive and eliminate potential favorable recipients from the best current treatment for HCC.

More recent studies have proposed expanded criteria to offer OLT to a broader group of patients with HCC (10,26,27).

Using explant pathologic data, Yao and coworkers (10) at UCSF reported 5-year posttransplant survival of 75% in patients with tumors as large as 6.5 cm and cumulative tumor burden ≤8 cm. These results have been challenged because of a small sample size and use of explant pathology, rather than preoperative imaging, as the determinant for tumor stage. The Barcelona Clinic Liver Cancer Group has developed systems based on tumor stage, liver function, physical status, and cancer-related symptoms to select OLT candidates with emphasis on dropout rate and intention-to-treat analyses (25,28,29). The Barcelona group expanded criteria include one tumor <7 cm, three tumors <5 cm, five tumors <3 cm, or down-staging to conventional Milan criteria with pretransplant adjuvant therapies (25,28,29). Using this approach, the Barcelona group has achieved 5-year posttransplant survival in excess of 50%, significantly greater than the 20% survival seen with palliative therapy alone (25). Despite such promising results, the role of OLT for tumors beyond the conventional Milan criteria remains controversial.

We recently analyzed the 22-year experience at UCLA with OLT for HCC in 467 patients (15). We evaluated tumor extent through both preoperative imaging and explant pathologic data, and examined their impact on posttransplant survival. By imaging and explant criteria, patients meeting Milan criteria had similar post-OLT survival rates compared with patients meeting UCSF criteria, and both groups had significantly improved survival versus patients with HCCs beyond the UCSF criteria. On multivariate analysis, increased tumor number, lymphovascular invasion, and poor differentiation were found to independently predict poorer survival after OLT for HCC (15). These determinants have been associated with poor outcome in prior series and serve to underscore the crucial principle that tumor biology determines outcome after OLT for HCC. The multinational database analysis from Onaca et al. (11) also showed good results for some expanded tumors, with 5-year survival above 60% for patients with two to four tumors from 3 to 5 cm. Some tumors, even large or extensive ones, exhibit less aggressive biology than do others.

Tumor Biology

The current challenge for liver transplant surgeons, therefore, is to identify a reliable method for assessing tumor biology prior to OLT. Although tumor size and number remain the cornerstones of current clinical practice, they comprise merely crude surrogates for tumors' microscopic biology. This realization may suggest routine pre-OLT tumor biopsy for potential candidates, but risks of tumor dissemination and associated hemorrhage remain real concerns. Promising noninvasive methods for identifying tumor characteristics include molecular imaging, using magnetic resonance with angiogenic factor labeling to identify tumor neoangiogenesis (29). Shirabe and coworkers (30) have measured des-gamma-carboxy-prothrombin in serum of patients with HCC and found elevated levels to have 75% sensitivity and 85% specificity for microvascular invasion. Some advocate for routine biopsy in order to perform HCC genotyping to identify additional prognostic factors and aid in pretransplant staging (31). This remains a fertile area for future investigation; for the near future, preoperative imaging will continue to be used as the main method for evaluating tumor extent and, ultimately, in determining candidacy for OLT.

LIVER TRANSPLANTATION FOR OTHER MALIGNANCIES AND METASTASES

Currently, the only indication for OLT for metastatic tumor involves indolent, well-differentiated neuroendocrine gastrointestinal metastases (32). Liver transplantation for metastatic colorectal cancer metastases has been discouraged since reports in 1994 demonstrated high recurrence rates (33). Some progress has been made in OLT for cholangiocarcinoma, however. Investigators at the Mayo Clinic have demonstrated improved results after OLT for cholangiocarcinomas pretreated with chemotherapy and radiation (34). As results for hepatic resection for colorectal metastases have improved alongside chemotherapeutic advancements, perhaps similar expansion of OLT for highly select patients with colorectal metastases remains possible. Such expansion of OLT for colorectal metastases will require enrollment of select patients into treatment protocol, precise management of immunosuppression, and close follow-up. Currently, we do not perform OLT for patients with metastatic colorectal disease; however, we support re-evaluation and further investigation of OLT in this group of patients.

REFERENCES

1. Starzl TE, Groth CG, Brettschneider L, et al. Orthotopic homotransplantation of the human liver. *Ann Surg.* 1968;168:392–415.
2. Busuttil RW, Farmer DG, Yersiz H, et al. Analysis of long-term outcomes of 3200 liver transplantations over two decades: a single-center experience. *Ann Surg.* 2005;241:905–916.
3. El Serag HB, Mason AC. Rising incidence of hepatocellular carcinoma in the United States. *N Engl J Med.* 1999;340:745–750.
4. El Serag HB. Hepatocellular carcinoma: recent trends in the United States. *Gastroenterology.* 2004;127:S27–34.
5. Davis GL, Albright JE, Cook SF, et al. Projecting future complications of chronic hepatitis C in the United States. *Liver Transpl.* 2003; 9:331–338.
6. Barazani Y, Hiatt JR, Tong MJ, et al. Chronic viral hepatitis and hepatocellular carcinoma. *World J Surg.* 2007;31:1243–1248.
7. Shetty K, Timmins K, Brensinger C, et al. Liver transplantation for hepatocellular carcinoma: validation of present selection criteria in predicting outcome. *Liver Transpl.* 2004;10:911–918.
8. Mazzaferro V, Regalia E, Doci R, et al. Liver transplantation for the treatment of small hepatocellular carcinomas in patients with cirrhosis. *N Engl J Med.* 1996;334:693–699.
9. Regalia E, Coppa J, Pulvirenti A, et al. Liver transplantation for small hepatocellular carcinoma in cirrhosis: analysis of our experience. *Transplant Proc.* 2001;33:1442–1444.
10. Yao FY, Ferrell L, Bass NM, et al. Liver transplantation for hepatocellular carcinoma: expansion of the tumor size limits does not adversely impact survival. *Hepatology.* 2001;33:1394–1403.
11. Onaca N, Davis GL Goldstein RM, et al. Expanded criteria for liver transplantation in patients with hepatocellular carcinoma: a report from the International Registry of Hepatic Tumors in Liver Transplantation. *Liver Transpl.* 2007;13:391–399.
12. Kamath PS, Wiesner RH, Malinchoc M, et al. A model to predict survival in patients with end stage liver disease. *Hepatology.* 2001; 33:464–470.
13. Sharma P, Balan V, Hernandez JL, et al. Liver transplantation for hepatocellular carcinoma: the MELD impact. *Liver Transpl.* 2004;10:36–41.
14. Sharma P, Harper AM, Hernandez JL, et al. Reduced priority MELD score for hepatocellular carcinoma does not adversely impact candidate survival awaiting transplantation. *Am J Transplant.* 2006;6:1957–1962.
15. Duffy JP, Vardanian A, Benjamin E, et al. Liver transplantation criteria for hepatocellular carcinoma should be expanded: a 22-year experience with 467 patients at UCLA. *Ann Surg.* 2007;246:502–509.
16. Yao FY, Kinkhabwala M, LaBerge JM, et al. The impact of preoperative loco-regional therapy on outcome after liver transplantation for hepatocellular carcinoma. *Am J Transplant.* 2005;5:795–804.
17. Lu DSK, Yu NC, Raman SS, et al. Percutaneous radio frequency ablation of hepatocellular carcinoma as a bridge to liver transplantation. *Hepatology.* 2005;41:1130–1137.
18. Porrett PM, Peterman H, Rosen M, et al. Lack of benefit of pretransplant locoregional hepatic therapy for hepatocellular cancer in the current MELD era. *Liver Transpl.* 2006;12:665–673.
19. Roberts MS, Angus DC, Bryce CL, et al. Survival after liver transplantation in the United States: a disease-specific analysis of the UNOS database. *Liver Transpl.* 2004;10:886–897.
20. Ringe B, Pichlmayr R, Wittekind C, et al. Surgical treatment of hepatocellular carcinoma: experience with liver resection and transplantation in 198 patients. *World J Surg.* 1991;15:270–285.
21. Iwatsuki S, Starzl TE, Sheahan DG, et al. Hepatic resection versus transplantation for hepatocellular carcinoma. *Ann Surg.* 1991; 214:221–228.
22. Moreno P, Juarrieta E, Figueras J, et al. Orthotopic liver transplantation: treatment of choice in cirrhotic patients with hepatocellular carcinoma? *Transplant Proc.* 1995;27:2296–2298.
23. Van Thiel DH, Carr B, Iwatsuki S, et al. The 11-year Pittsburgh experience with liver transplantation for hepatocellular carcinoma: 1981–1991. *J Surg Oncol Suppl.* 1993;3:78–82.
24. Merli M, Nicolini G, Gentili F, et al. Predictive factors of outcome after liver transplantation in patients with cirrhosis and hepatocellular carcinoma. *Transplant Proc.* 2005;37:2535–2540.
25. Llovet JM, Burroughs A, Bruix J. Hepatocellular carcinoma. *Lancet.* 2003;362:1907–1917.
26. Roayaie S, Frischer JS, Emre SH, et al. Long-term results with multimodal adjuvant therapy and liver transplantation for the treatment of hepatocellular carcinomas larger than 5 centimeters. *Ann Surg.* 2002;235:533–539.
27. Fernandez JA, Robles R, Marin C, et al. Can we expand the indications for liver transplantation among hepatocellular carcinoma patients with increased tumor size? *Transplant Proc.* 2003;35:1818–1820.
28. Llovet JM, Bruix J, Fuster J, et al. Liver transplantation for small hepatocellular carcinoma: the tumor-node-metastasis classification does not have prognostic power. *Hepatology.* 1998;27:1572–1577.
29. Llovet JM, Fuster J, Bruix J, Barcelona-Clinic Liver Cancer Group. The Barcelona approach: diagnosis, staging, and treatment of hepatocellular carcinoma. *Liver Transpl.* 2004;10:S115–120.
30. Anderson SA, Rader RK, Westlin WF, et al. Magnetic resonance contrast enhancement of neovasculature with alpha-v-beta-3 targeted nanoparticles. *Mag Res Med.* 2000;44:433–439.
31. Shirabe K, Itoh S, Yoshizumi T, et al. The predictors of microvascular invasion in candidates for liver transplantation with hepatocellular carcinoma-with special reference to the serum levels of des-gamma-carboxy prothrombin. *J Surg Oncol.* 2007;95:235–240.
32. Marsh JW, Finkelstein SD, Demetris AJ, et al. Genotyping of hepatocellular carcinoma in liver transplant recipients adds predictive power for determining recurrence-free survival. *Liver Transpl.* 2003;9:664–671.
33. Fernandez JA, Robles R, Marin C, et al. Role of liver transplantation in the management of metastatic neuroendocrine tumors. *Transplant Proc.* 2003;35:1832–1833.
34. Muhlbacher F, Huk I, Steininger R, et al. Is orthotopic liver transplantation a feasible treatment for secondary cancer of the liver? *Transplant Proc.* 1991;23:1567–68.
35. Heimbach JK, Gores GJ, Haddock MG, et al. Predictors of disease recurrence following neoadjuvant chemoradiotherapy and liver transplantation for unresectable perihilar cholangiocarcinoma. *Transplantation.* 2006;82:1703–1707.

11

Minimally Invasive Surgery for Cancer

Sarah J. Lee, Yuichiro Ito, and Edward H. Phillips

Laparoscopy is a technology that has evolved from a limited diagnostic tool in the early 1900s (Figure 11.1), to techniques that encompass complex therapeutic modalities (1). Although improvements in insufflation and light transmission have been important, the development of the miniature charged-coupled device camera, which allows high-quality images to be displayed on monitors, was the major advancement that allowed a group of surgeons to work together on complex procedures. The rapid adoption of laparoscopic procedures led to questions and controversy regarding the application of laparoscopic techniques to the management of malignancy. For example, does laparoscopy worsen tumor outcomes by fragmenting cancer cells, promoting implantation, and spread? Does the loss of tactile sense limit the quality of oncologic surgery? Are the laparoscopic benefits of decreased pain, hospital stay, and earlier return to activity achieved at the expense of a worsened oncologic outcome? Or is there decreased stress response and improved maintenance of immune competence during laparoscopy as compared with laparotomy, and does this effect the oncologic outcome?

This chapter will focus on evidence-based results and guidelines to help surgeons understand the physiologic changes that occur during laparoscopy and the role that laparoscopic techniques play in the management of patients with malignancy.

PHYSIOLOGY OF PNEUMOPERITONEUM

Pulmonary

Carbon dioxide is the usual gas of choice for pneumoperitoneum because of its safety profile and low cost. It does not support combustion and absorbs readily, making it less likely than oxygen to have deleterious effects if gas embolism occurs. It is also readily absorbed by the peritoneum, and diffuses well into lungs, allowing levels to be monitored by the anesthesiologist (2). Compensation for hypercarbia can then be made through changes in minute ventilation. If unable to correct for hypercarbia, acidosis may ensue and the effects of both acidosis and hypercarbia can cause cardiac disturbances (3). Patients with underlying lung diseases that alter gas exchange need to be closely monitored for such complications during laparoscopy.

Compliance of the lungs is decreased, and peak inspiratory pressure is increased by pneumoperitoneum, which is usually set at approximately 15 mm Hg. Additionally, laparoscopy often requires positioning changes that may include the Trendelenberg position. Most people tolerate this threefold increase from the resting abdominal pressure without respiratory compro-

mise, but certain patient populations will have compliance problems. Obese patients, for example, comprise about 30% of the American population, and they already start at a higher resting abdominal pressure of 9 to 10 mm Hg. The changes in peak inspiratory pressure and compliance can be dramatic during pneumoperitoneum in these patients. However, ventilator changes can usually compensate because alveolar gas exchange itself is not altered by pneumoperitoneum (4).

Recognized, but rare, complications of pneumoperitoneum include gas embolism, pneumothorax, subcutaneous emphysema, and pneumomediastinum. Gas embolism should be suspected if there is sudden bradycardia, cyanosis, a decrease in the end-tidal carbon dioxide ($ETCO_2$), and cardiovascular collapse occurring during or soon after insufflation. Treatment includes left lateral decubitus positioning, release of pneumoperitoneum, and supportive management of cardiorespiratory abnormalities. Signs of pneumothorax intraoperatively include subcutaneous emphysema, increased $ETCO_2$, decreased compliance, and hypoxemia. Treatment includes release of pneumoperitoneum and hyperventilation, with tube thoracostomy or conservative management, depending on patient status. Subcutaneous emphysema and pneumomediastinum are usually a result of pneumothorax or improper insufflation into the subcutaneous tissue. Signs include palpable crepitus, usually noted first in the periorbital area, and an increase in $ETCO_2$ (5). If no compressive airway compromise is evident, the patient can be managed expectantly with resolution of the crepitus over days.

Cardiac

As pneumoperitoneum is established, an acute vasovagal response can occur, with hypotension and bradycardia. Once pneumoperitoneum is obtained, heart rate and mean arterial pressure actually increase, but studies using Swan-Ganz catheterization and transesophageal echocardiography have shown a decrease in cardiac output (3). Pneumoperitoneum decreases preload secondary to decreased venous return and increases afterload due to increased systemic vascular resistance. These effects on cardiac output may be transient in patients with healthy cardiovascular status because the body compensates for the physiologic changes induced during laparoscopy (6). Patients with underlying cardiovascular disease do not always have this ability. Specifically, patients with malignancy are frequently dehydrated from poor oral intake, side effects of treatments, and bowel preparation. Volume depletion augments the deleterious effects of pneumoperitoneum on the cardiovascular system.

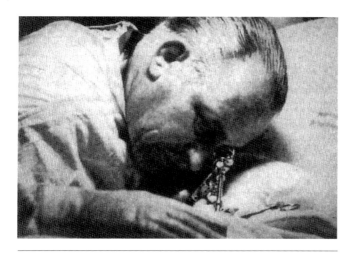

Figure 11.1 Heinz Kalk during laparoscopy in 1951. Courtesy of Dr. George Berci.

Visceral Blood Flow

Decreased cardiac output systemically causes decreased perfusion to the visceral organs. Additionally, perfusion pressure to the abdominal organs depends on the difference between the mean arterial pressure and the pressure in the surrounding cavity. In the case of pneumoperitoneum, the abdominal compartment pressure increases by 2 to 3 times the normal resting levels. The effects are diminished mesenteric blood flow and reduced portal vein flow. Moreover, the pressure itself has been postulated to cause a reflexive release of the splanchnic vasoconstrictor arginine vasopressin (AVP), measured in animal models at 5 times normal levels (2). Decreased visceral blood flow has very little clinical significance in the majority of people; however, subpopulations of patients with underlying liver, small bowel, or renal disease may have more pronounced clinical consequences (7).

Thromboembolic

Oncology patients are hypercoagulable and at increased risk of venous thrombosis. Pneumoperitoneum further increases this risk by causing a decrease in venous return. Studies have shown significant decreases in femoral vein blood flow velocity with pneumoperitoneum, especially combined with reverse Trendelenberg positioning (4). Sequential compression devices were shown to decrease this flow difference, even returning most healthy patients to baseline levels. Obese patients, as an exception, did not return to baseline flow even with sequential compression device use. Despite these risks, patients having minimally invasive procedures are usually mobile postoperatively earlier than patients who undergo laparotomy. Therefore, it has never been definitively demonstrated that patients having laparoscopic surgery rather than laparotomy are at higher risk of thromboembolic events.

Central Nervous System

Intracranial pressure has been shown in animal models to increase by 7 mm Hg during pneumoperitoneum (3). Animal studies have shown this increase remains present after controlling for hypercarbia and acidosis, and therefore is primarily re-

lated to pneumoperitoneum itself (8). Trendelenberg, a common position used during laparoscopy, further increases the intracranial pressure. Pneumoperitoneum and positioning effects may be prohibitive issues in patients with central nervous system pathology.

Immune System

Laparoscopic surgery has been shown to cause a less intense inflammatory reaction than traditional surgery. A prospective, randomized trial studied the levels of interleukin (IL)-6, IL-8, and tumor necrosis factor in the peritoneal fluid and serum of patients who underwent either laparoscopic or open colon resection for cancer. Both groups demonstrated much higher levels of these inflammatory cytokines in the peritoneum than in the serum, but serum levels were significantly lower in the laparoscopic group as early as 2 hours after surgery (9). The difference between the groups diminished during the course of the postoperative period.

One factor involved in the blunted inflammatory response seems to be the nature of the gas used for pneumoperitoneum. Macrophages, one of the most abundant and earliest responding inflammatory cells in the peritoneal cavity, have been studied under conditions of pressure and carbon dioxide exposure to simulate laparoscopy. Exposure of these cells to various gases have shown that cells in a carbon dioxide environment produce significantly less tumor necrosis factor and IL-1 than those incubated in helium or air. The cells were also more acidic, which was shown to independently decrease the release of these inflammatory mediators, as well as superoxide production. Therefore, both the exposure of these cells to carbon dioxide and the resultant acidification influenced the diminished inflammatory response (10,11). Production of these substances returned to baseline within 12 to 24 hours.

Other studies have sought to compare the immune response difference between conventional and laparoscopic surgery. In the same prospective, randomized study of colon cancer previously mentioned, C-reactive protein, leukocyte counts, leukocyte subpopulations, and expression of HLA-DR on monocytes were measured before and after surgery. Significant findings included slightly earlier normalization of white blood cell count and total lymphocyte levels in the laparoscopic group, slightly earlier restoration of HLA-DR measurements, and earlier normalization of natural killer cell counts (9). Another study evaluated rat cell-mediated immunity by monitoring skin reactions to an antigen before and after laparoscopic-assisted or conventional resection of the cecum. The laparoscopic-assisted colon removal group had better preservation of the cell-mediated immune response to skin testing even to postoperative day 4 (12).

The importance of understanding the relationship between laparoscopy and the immune system is to find potential links between how these differences might affect the behavior of tumors. Immunosuppression is a recognized risk factor for cancer development, and blunting this consequence of surgery may improve the oncologic outcome. A murine model study in 1995 showed that rats with tumor cell implantation had increased growth of tumor after laparotomy compared with laparoscopy (13). Further studies are needed to fully elucidate the complex relationships between surgical techniques and cancer outcomes.

LAPAROSCOPIC TECHNIQUES IN CANCER DIAGNOSIS AND TREATMENT

Basic Instrumentation

Although not necessary for success, specially designed operating room suites, with high-technology cameras, ceiling-mounted monitors, and recording devices make performing and documenting advanced laparoscopic procedures comfortable and convenient. Even if access to these amenities is limited, the basic requirements to perform laparoscopy include insufflation, light source, charged coupled device camera, laparoscope, monitors, and laparoscopic working ports. Additionally, biopsy needles, forceps, suction, irrigation, and cautery are necessary.

For more advanced procedures, angled telescopes increase visualization around structures, such as the dome of the liver, Morrison's pouch, and the pelvis. Properly securing the patient to the operating table allows manipulation of position and better visualization. Examining the small and large intestines must be done gently with atraumatic graspers to avoid enterotomies. Needle drivers or assisted suturing devices, laparoscopic staplers, and clips aid in the division of structures and hemostasis. A device that combines suction, cautery, and irrigation has proven useful in biopsy and dissection, as well as achieving hemostasis, by partially hiding the hook cautery in the tubing then suctioning the bleeding tissue as cautery is applied (14). Laparoscopic ultrasound is a very useful tool, allowing visualization of masses, nodes, and relationships of these to anatomic structures.

Diagnostic Laparoscopy and Biopsy

Although computed tomography (CT) scans and other diagnostic imaging studies continue to improve, laparoscopy still provides information that previously could be obtained only by laparotomy. Imaging can underestimate the tumor burden; as a result, the finding of carcinomatosis (Figure 11.2) when a large incision is used subjects the patient to a significant amount of pain, hospital stay, and healing time before other treatment options can be considered. Indications for diagnostic laparoscopy include finding and diagnosing lesions that may be missed by imaging, identifying positive nodes, assessing liver involvement, and determining resectability. Diagnostic laparoscopy has proven especially useful in management of gastric, pancreatic, ovarian, and esophageal cancer (15–19). A thorough inspection includes evaluating the liver, then retracting the left lobe to fully visualize the anterior stomach, opening the gastrohepatic ligament to see the celiac axis and lesser curvature of the stomach, dividing the greater omentum to evaluate the posterior stomach wall and anterior pancreas, looking over the spleen, running the small and large bowel taking note of the mesentery, studying the pelvic organs, and visualizing the peritoneum and diaphragmatic surfaces. Ultrasound is also indicated for full laparoscopic evaluation, adding information regarding the liver, pancreas, vessels, and nodal basins.

Tissue diagnosis is an important component of oncologic staging and treatment planning. Options include image-guided biopsy, endoscopic-guided biopsy, or surgical biopsy. The benefits of laparoscopic biopsy include excellent visualization, avoidance of injury to viscera, ability to obtain adequate tissue, and achievement of hemostasis. In addition, it can be performed on an outpatient basis .The main disadvantage is the need for general anesthesia.

Pancreas

Surgical treatment for pancreatic adenocarcinoma should begin with diagnostic laparoscopy. Prognosis is often dismal, and stratifying patients who will benefit from surgical excision is an important determination. The Whipple procedure generally requires a laparotomy, but it is frequently aborted because of the finding of unsuspected metastatic disease or locally advanced disease. Performing diagnostic laparoscopy significantly decreases the number of laparotomies performed for unresectable disease by 33% to 65%. The addition of laparoscopic ultrasound also increases the sensitivity of predicting respectability (Table 11.1) (15,16,20)

Laparoscopic pancreaticoduodenectomy has been described, but it is exceedingly difficult to gain appropriate exposure and safely handle major vessels that are deep in the retroperitoneum (21). Even in the hands of experts, operative times average 8 to 10 hours and there has been no benefit shown in terms of hospital stay. There is also a significant conversion rate (40%) (22).

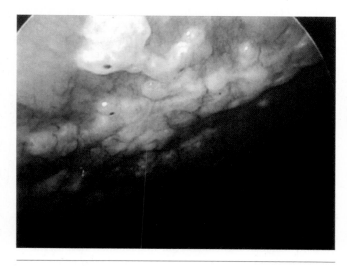

Figure 11.2 Carcinomatosis. Tumor implants on peritoneum as viewed through laparoscope.

Table 11.1

Predicting Resectability in Pancreatic Cancer (%)

Result	CT Scan[20] (N = 213)	Laparoscopy[15] (N = 115)	Laparoscopy and Intraoperative Ultrasound[16] (N = 90)
Resectable (%)	67	91	98
Treatment alteration	N/A	38	14

CT, computed tomography.

Even if the pancreatic tumor is found to be unresectable, laparoscopic biliary and/or enteric bypass is an appropriate palliative procedure. Results of laparoscopic bypass in 14 patients compared with 14 case controls who underwent open bypass demonstrated improved morbidity (7% vs. 43%), mortality (0% vs. 29%), and length of hospital stay (9 vs. 21 days) (23). In addition, endoscopic palliative procedures, namely stent placement in gastrointestinal obstruction and biliary obstruction, have shown good results with little morbidity and mortality in patients who often have life expectancy in the range of months. However, the risk of needing endoscopic stent replacement, of stent migration, gastrointestinal obstruction, or stent erosion becomes more likely with time. Patients with a life expectancy longer than 6 months, or unsuccessful endoscopic intervention, may require operative bypass for palliation (24). Minimally invasive techniques have diminished the significant morbidity and mortality of open operative bypass and make it a feasible option. Also, thoracoscopic splanchnicectomy can address the debilitating pain often experienced by patients with pancreatic cancer. Even unilateral thoracic splanchnicectomy significantly improves pain in 80% to 90% of patients, with resultant improved quality of life (25).

Distal and subtotal pancreatectomy with negative margins can be performed laparoscopically for body and tail tumors or cystic neoplasms. Enucleation of appropriate neuroendocrine tumors is another laparoscopic option. Hepatic metastases of neuroendocrine tumors can be palliated with laparoscopic resection or guided radiofrequency ablation under the same anesthetic. Complications of laparoscopic pancreatic resection are much the same as open laparotomy, including pancreatic fistula; thus, drainage principles should be the same. Other reported complications include bleeding, intra-abdominal infection, and wound infection. It is difficult to draw definitive conclusions from the literature regarding laparoscopic results for treatment of pancreatic malignancy as most large series combine their results for both benign and malignant tumors and include all areas of the pancreas. Long-term data on tumor recurrence and comparisons of survival with traditional open procedures are not yet available (21,26–28).

Stomach

Expertise with foregut laparoscopic techniques as well as endoscopic skills, such as endoscopic ultrasound, has led to advances in the management of gastric cancer. Laparoscopic wedge resection and intragastric mucosal resection are options for early gastric cancer. If the tumor invades only the mucosa, the risk of lymph node involvement is just 1% to 3%, but this increases to 11% to 20% for those tumors that reach the submucosa (29). Wedge resection uses endoscopy for localization (Figure 11.3) and laparoscopy for elevating the tumor to the anterior abdominal wall and stapling a wedge of stomach. The intragastric mucosal resection technique (Figure 11.4) again uses endoscopy for localization, but also to insufflate the stomach and allow passage of trocars, first through the abdominal wall, then directly through the anterior stomach wall. Once trocars are intragastric, the mucosal and submucosal layers are removed around and under the tumor (30).

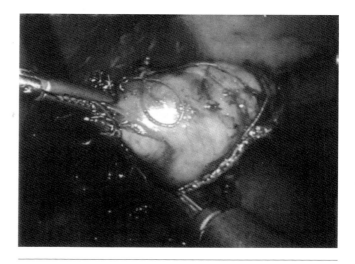

Figure 11.3 Wedge gastric resection. Laparoscopic removal of a lesion in stomach using staplers.

Gastric cancers with increased risk of lymph node involvement demand more extensive resection. These include raised (>25 mm) or ulcerated (>15 mm) tumors, previous positive margins after less invasive resections, submucosal invasion, or evidence of perigastric lymph node metastasis. Even some tumors that invade only the mucosa may require more extensive resection if they are in a position or of a size that make the previously described techniques difficult. Distal tumors can be handled laparoscopically with distal or subtotal gastrectomy and gastroenterostomy. Dividing the right gastroepiploic artery at the pancreatic surface and dividing the left and right gastric arteries allows significant lymph node dissection, including the pyloric, left cardiac and superior gastric nodes, hepatic artery nodes, and along the lesser curvature (30). Even division of the left gastric artery and removal of related nodes is feasible laparoscopically as long as the proximal remnant is left in continuity with the short gastric vessels.

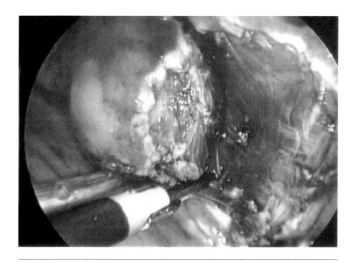

Figure 11.4 Intragastric mucosal resection. View of lesion removal process using trocars placed into the stomach lumen.

Laparoscopic total gastrectomy is appropriate for more proximal lesions. Celiac and splenic nodes can be removed as more extensive vessel ligation is carried out. The esophagus is mobilized, vagus nerves divided, and reconstruction carried out with the aid of a circular stapler to a Roux-en-Y limb of jejunum (30).

Studies comparing open and laparoscopic management of gastric cancer show they are equivalent. A randomized, prospective series comparing 29 open subtotal gastrectomies with 30 laparoscopic gastrectomies demonstrated similar morbidity, mortality, and disease-free survival, while hospital stay and resumption of oral intake were improved in the laparoscopic group (31). The number of lymph nodes retrieved and margin status were similar in both groups. Another prospective study included 11 patients undergoing open total gastrectomy compared with 8 patients who had undergone laparoscopic total gastrectomy. Again, lymph node harvest and margins were not compromised with the laparoscopic technique. Complications were diminished, especially noting two splenectomies performed during open total gastrectomy for splenic injury and bleeding (32).

Gastrointestinal stromal tumors (GIST) are highly vascular, friable tumors. The same principles as those that guide open GIST resection should be followed for laparoscopic resection. Specifically, care must be taken not to handle the tumor and to prevent breaking or bleeding. Margins of 1 to 2 cm should be obtained, and en bloc resection of other involved tissue and structures may be necessary. This tumor spreads hematogenously, so extensive lymph node dissection is not required (33).

Spleen

Staging laparotomy for Hodgkin lymphoma used to be performed more frequently; however, with improved imaging and improved treatment, the need for surgical staging has decreased from 85% of patients to 5% (34). Laparoscopic technique is now preferred in the rare cases in which surgical staging for Hodgkin lymphoma is indicated as it is less painful, and is associated with less respiratory complication and shorter hospital stay compared with laparotomy.

Other lymphomas rarely require splenectomy unless the diagnosis is unclear or if palliation is required for symptoms related to hypersplenism (35). The myeloproliferative diseases occasionally require splenectomy for symptom control, to decrease transfusion requirements, and to improve quality of life. Primary malignancies of the spleen such as angiosarcoma, plasmacytoma, and malignant fibrous histiocytoma are treatable by laparoscopic splenectomy if there is no evidence of invasion. Splenectomy is also infrequently performed for metastatic disease, usually ovarian cancer (Figure 11.5) (36). Splenic biopsy is also possible via laparoscopy. Contraindications to laparoscopic splenectomy include ascites, portal hypertension, and coagulopathy. Spleen size is a relative contraindication, but the size at which laparoscopic technique becomes too difficult varies with surgeon experience and comfort. Even large spleens can be extracted in a bag after morcellation. Embolization preoperatively is occasionally used to decrease the size and blood supply to the spleen (37).

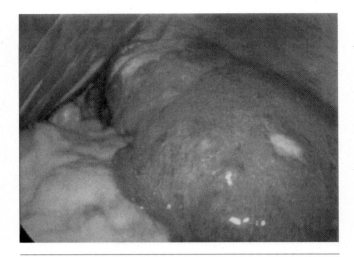

Figure 11.5 Splenic metastasis. Lesions are visible on the splenic surface.

Colon and Rectum

Recent prospective, randomized studies proving equivalent oncologic outcomes of laparoscopic and open colon cancer resection have finally allowed widespread acceptance of these techniques in the treatment of colon cancer. Retrospective studies demonstrated equivalent oncologic results, while confirming the generally accepted laparoscopic benefits of earlier discharge and diet resumption. In a retrospective study from Cedars-Sinai Medical Center in Los Angeles (38), the results of laparoscopic colectomy in 80 patients were compared with results observed among 90 patients who underwent open colectomy for treatment of colorectal cancer. The authors reported that operative time was equivalent in the laparoscopic and open groups (laparoscopic, 161 minutes; open, 163 minutes; $p = 0.94$). Blood loss was less for the laparoscopic group (laparoscopic, 104 mL; open, 184 mL; $p = 0.001$), and resumption of oral intake was earlier (laparoscopic, 3.9 days; open, 4.9 days; $p = 0.001$), but length of hospitalization was similar. Mean lymph node yield in the laparoscopic group was 12 compared with 16 in the open group ($p = 0.16$). Rates of morbidity, recurrence, and survival were similar in both groups, and no port-site recurrences occurred among patients managed laparoscopically.

The *Clinical Outcomes of Surgical Therapy* (COST) study group conducted a multi-institutional randomized trial designed to test the hypothesis that disease-free and overall survival are equivalent among patients undergoing laparoscopic-assisted or open colectomy for colon cancer (39). Eight hundred seventy-two patients with curable colon cancer were randomly assigned to undergo laparoscopic-assisted or open colectomy. Patients were followed a median of 7 years (range, 5 to 10 years). Disease-free 5-year survival (open, 68.4%; laparoscopic, 69.2%; $p = 0.94$) and overall 5-year survival (open, 74.6%; laparoscopic, 76.4%; $p = 0.93$) were similar for the two groups. Overall recurrence rates also were similar for the two groups (open, 21.8%; laparoscopic, 19.4%; $p = 0.25$). The recurrences observed were distributed similarly between the two treatment groups, and the sites of first recurrence were distributed similarly between the treatment arms (open: wound, 0.5%; liver, 5.8%; lung, 4.6%; other, 8.4%; laparoscopic: wound, 0.9%; liver, 5.5%; lung, 4.6%; other, 6.1%). The COST study group concluded that laparoscopic colectomy for curable colon cancer is not inferior to open surgery.

Lacy and colleagues (40) at the University of Barcelona conducted a randomized trial designed to compare the long-term outcome of laparoscopy-assisted colectomy (LAC) and open colectomy (OC) in the management of nonmetastatic colon cancer. Data derived from the management of 219 patients entered into the trial were analyzed according the intention-to-treat principle. The median follow-up was 95 months. The mean number of lymph nodes resected (11.1 with LAC vs. 10.7 with OC, $p = 0.70$) and the presence of metastatic lymphadenopathy ($p = 0.70$) were similar in both arms of the study.

When patients were stratified according to tumor stage, the probabilities of overall survival ($p = 0.048$), cancer-related survival ($p = 0.02$), and freedom from recurrence ($p = 0.048$) were significantly higher in the LAC group compared with OC for stage III tumors. The superiority of LAC over OC regarding these variables was exclusively due to significant differences in patients with stage III tumors; the probability curves in patients with stage I and II tumors were identical in each of these parameters for both therapeutic approaches. The authors were unable to clarify the mechanisms by which LAC could achieve a better survival rate compared with the OC group, why this advantage in survival was limited to patients with stage III colon cancer, and why these results have not been reproduced in other trials. The authors speculate that the observed advantage may be due to preserved cellular immunity, attenuated stress and inflammatory response, minimal tumor handling, and lower complication rate in patients treated by laparoscopically.

There exist many techniques for minimally invasive colorectal cancer removal, including laparoscopic colectomy, LAC, laparoscopic abdominoperineal resection, and transanal endoscopic microsurgery (41). All are reported, but it should be noted that results of equivalency trials for laparoscopic and open procedures do involve experienced surgeons, and inexperienced surgeons should learn the laparoscopic technique by treating patients with benign disease before applying this technique to cancer patients.

Small Intestine

Small intestinal cancer accounts for only 2% of malignancies, with the two most common cancers being adenocarcinoma and carcinoid. Therefore, it is not surprising that only sporadic literature exists on the laparoscopic treatment of these tumors. No large comparative studies are available comparing laparoscopic and open small bowel resection for malignancy. However, extrapolating laparoscopic experience from other organs, laparoscopy should be equal as long as the same basic principles are followed. Laparoscopy can also be used for diagnosis of lesions suspected by symptoms, imaging modalities, or capsule imaging.

Adenocarcinoma of the duodenum has a better prognosis than pancreatic adenocarcinoma, and the Whipple procedure should be performed as appropriate. As described previously,

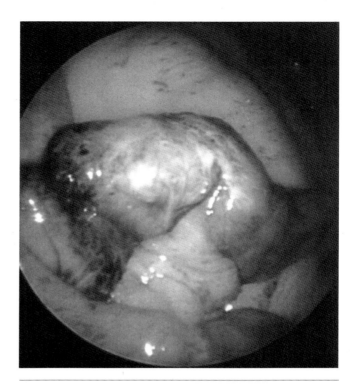

Figure 11.6 Small bowel gastrointestinal stromal tumor, as seen via laparoscope.

the laparoscopic Whipple operation is a lengthy, exceedingly difficult procedure that even laparoscopic experts think may not be worth pursuing (21,22). The more distal an adenocarcinoma presents in the small bowel, the worse the prognosis. If the patient has positive nodes, 5-year survival is only in the 10% to 15% range. Therefore, the guiding principles of curative resection are en bloc small bowel and mesenteric resection with 6-inch margins. Resection is still recommended for palliation to prevent obstruction and bleeding; however, extensive resection should not be pursued at the expense of major organs or the superior mesenteric vessels as this will not improve survival and will diminish quality of life. Lymphoma of the small bowel is treated similarly. GIST tumors of the small bowel do not require mesenteric dissection for lymph nodes as this is not the usual mode of spread (Figure 11.6) (42). Patients with carcinoid tumors of the small bowel require a complete examination of the entire small bowel to look for other primary carcinoids, which occur in 30% of these patients (42). Duodenal carcinoids are less aggressive than their more distal counterparts, which have an increased risk of metastatic disease; therefore, a thorough exploration of the abdominal cavity should be undertaken. If metastatic disease is found that is amenable to resection, palliative benefit can be obtained.

Liver

The role of laparoscopy in the management of liver tumors includes biopsy, palliative measures including radiofrequency ablation, and tumor resection (Figure 11.7). Controlling bleeding from the liver parenchyma is more difficult laparoscopically and has been the limiting factor in major advancements. However,

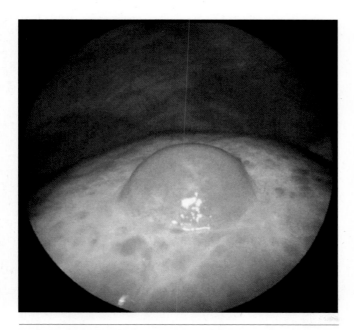

Figure 11.7 Hepatic tumor. A mass protruding from liver may be amenable to diagnostic or therapeutic interventions laparoscopically.

as technology has improved, laparoscopic techniques have become a viable option for the treatment of primary hepatocellular carcinoma and for metastatic disease to the liver. As in laparotomy, the patient must have adequate liver reserve to tolerate a resection and have acceptable coagulation studies. Laparoscopy best accesses the laterally located and surface neoplasms; therefore, knowing the exact location of the tumor preoperatively is more important when using laparoscopy as opposed to conventional liver surgery. Hand-assisted laparoscopic hepatic resection may help reach more posterior lesions, and also provides a rapid method of hemostasis (direct pressure) if needed. The hand-assistance port can then be the site of specimen retrieval (43). Controlling blood loss, which is technically challenging even during open resection, is an important consideration. Hemostatic laparoscopic tools—such as clip appliers, articulating staplers, coagulation and dissection combined instruments, and hemostatic glues and films—can be used to diminish blood loss. Finally, the pneumoperitoneum during dissection and transection of relatively large veins increases the risk of carbon dioxide embolism. For this reason, some surgeons recommend abdominal wall-lifting measures instead of pneumoperitoneum to provide working space during parenchyma division (43).

Liver transplantation is often the only available option for treatment of advanced hepatocellular carcinoma, and early work is being performed by specialists in applying laparoscopic techniques to transplantation. If laparoscopic, living donor, partial hepatectomy were to become a low-risk procedure, the severe liver shortage for potential transplant recipients may be ameliorated.

Biliary System

The use of laparoscopy for the treatment of gallbladder cancer is usually an incidental event. Typically, a laparoscopic cholecystectomy is done for what is thought to be benign disease, but cancer is found in the specimen. If the tumor is confined to the mucosa, then no further treatment is warranted. However, if the tumor is greater than stage IA (invasion of lamina propria or muscle layer) on analysis or margins are positive, then a radical operation should be performed. There is currently no evidence to support a laparoscopic attempt at this procedure. To the contrary, reports have shown a very high rate of tumor dissemination in gallbladder cancer that was inadvertently violated during laparoscopic cholecystectomy. Of ten patients referred to a major cancer institute for gallbladder cancer that was diagnosed after laparoscopic cholecystectomy, seven patients had disease that precluded curative resection at a mean of only 30 days following the original procedure (44).

Gallbladder cancer should be considered in patients whose preoperative studies reveal a gallbladder polyp, a calcified gallbladder, a mass in the gallbladder >1 cm diameter, or loss of the normal gallbladder/liver interface. In these cases, the surgeon must avoid any violation of the tumor and have a low threshold for opening and performing the appropriate cancer operation. Five-year survival for T1A lesions treated with laparoscopic cholecystectomy is 100%; these are the only lesions for which no further treatment is needed (45,46). Biliary cancers other than T1A lesions are aggressive, and diagnostic laparoscopy can be a useful tool to assess for resectability and avoid laparotomy in inappropriate patients.

Adrenal Gland

Laparoscopic adrenalectomy is an acceptable option for the treatment of an adrenal mass as long as no preoperative evidence of invasion exists. Although any tumor larger than 6 cm is at increased risk of being malignant and needs to be treated as such with complete excision, tumors up to 10 to 12 cm have been resected laparoscopically. The main consideration is that incomplete excision dramatically decreases the survival of patients with adrenocortical carcinoma. Therefore, if proper excision without tumor fracture cannot be done laparoscopically, the patient should be opened. Isolated metastatic disease to the adrenal gland when the primary has been controlled is another consideration for laparoscopic adrenalectomy. Analyzing combined series of laparoscopic adrenalectomy for malignancy showed that in 63 patients, there were no positive margins, 13% had local recurrence, 3% had port-site metastasis, and 22% had distant metastasis. Although not prospective, this compares favorably to data reported for open adrenalectomy (47).

Esophagus

Laparoscopy has been used to stage esophageal cancer and to assess for surgical feasibility. Sensitivity of staging laparoscopy compared with CT scan was 71% versus 14% for detecting peritoneal metastasis, 78% versus 55% for lymph nodes, and 86% versus 71% for liver metastasis (48).

Laparoscopic fundoplication for the treatment of low-grade Barrett disease related to gastroesophageal reflux may be considered a cancer-preventive procedure. Patients with Barrett esophagus (BE) are at increased risk of developing adenocarcinoma. Reflux of gastric acid mixed with bile salts and pancreatic enzymes is the cause of Barrett changes to the esophagus. Although medical treatment may diminish the symptoms and acid content of the reflux, it does not prevent reflux events. In theory, therefore, surgical prevention of reflux would decrease these changes. In a study of 49 patients with biopsy-proven BE who underwent laparoscopic fundoplication and were then followed with esophagogastroduodenoscopy (EGD) after surgery, 18% had regression of the BE and 6% had decreased BE. Of note, six of these patients had low-grade dysplasia on preoperative EGD. In this group, four had no dysplasia postoperatively, one was unchanged, and one patient actually progressed to carcinoma in situ (49). The fact that the majority improved, but some remained unchanged or even worsened, is similar to results seen in many series. For this reason, the general consensus is that response is unpredictable, and patients are still at risk for development of adenocarcinoma, requiring EGD surveillance. Further studies are needed to elucidate this relationship.

When treatment of esophageal cancer via transhiatal esophagectomy was accepted, this represented a less invasive technique than the standard Ivor-Lewis resection. Laparoscopy and thoracoscopy have allowed even less invasive treatment options for esophageal cancer. a single institution reported their results in a series of 222 minimally invasive esophagectomies and although their technique changed from laparoscopic transhiatal to combined laparoscopic and thoracoscopic mobilization for improved nodal dissection, the results showed decreased mortality, shorter hospital stay, and equivalent oncologic factors as most reported open series (50). This is a very advanced minimally invasive operation. Robotic-assisted minimally invasive esophagectomy is now being attempted and reported with encouraging results. The robot has multiarticulated arms, three-dimensional optics, and motion scaling that some surgeons have found very helpful in this precise procedure, even allowing what may prove to be oncologically equivalent results without needing a thoracic portion of the operation (51,52).

Pediatric Malignancy

Minimally invasive techniques have been used in many areas of pediatric surgery, and its utility extends to the diagnosis and treatment of malignancy. Most pediatric solid tumors are treated with a multimodality approach, so tissue diagnosis in the least morbid manner is desirable. Many of these children also undergo many procedures throughout their treatment; thus, minimizing pain, hospital stay, immune system stress, and adhesions is of great benefit.

A single-institution retrospective study evaluated its experience on pediatric oncologic patients. There were no mortality, and the complication rate was 5%, including two liver hematomas and one bowel perforation during adhesiolysis. The conversion rate to open was 29%, noted mostly in the thoracoscopic group when the masses, which are often quite small in the pediatric population, were unable to be located. The authors note that they have diminished their conversion rate with preoperative needle localization (53).

Reported experiences to date indicate that minimally invasive techniques are safe and effective in children with cancer. Because of tumor biology, however, a consensus committee of pediatric surgical oncology leaders has stated that metastatic osteogenic sarcoma to the lung is not appropriate for thoracoscopy as there are often more lesions found by palpation than are seen on preoperative scans. Resectable Wilms tumor is another exception to laparoscopy as tumor spillage or seeding during biopsy or laparoscopy led to up-staging and the need for more aggressive adjuvant therapy (53).

Lung

Although this chapter has focused on laparoscopy, video-assisted thoracic surgery (VATS) has been a breakthrough in the management of patients with lung cancer. VATS has decreased postoperative pain and morbidity associated with thoracotomy, while still allowing anatomic dissection and division of vessels and bronchi, and adequate retrieval of lymph nodes. In combining several retrospective series of VATS lobectomy and pneumonectomy, results were found to be equal or better than standard thoracotomy in terms of lymph node retrieval and survival. Wound recurrence was 0.3%, mortality 0.5%, complications 10% to 21%, conversion 10%, and length of stay 4.6 days (54).

Kidney

The two advances that have led to increased use of minimally invasive techniques in the management of renal tumors are improvement in laparoscopic technology and the increased use of imaging, which has identified numerous asymptomatic, incidental lesions. Since the 1990s, the mean renal tumor size has decreased by 32% (55). The gold standard for the treatment of renal cancer is radical nephrectomy, and this is being done laparoscopically via a transperitoneal approach with or without hand assist, or by the retroperitoneal approach. As smaller tumors were found, laparoscopic partial nephrectomy has been developed to preserve as much renal function as possible. Problems with this method include risk of positive margins, hemorrhage, and damage to the collecting system. In a large series comparing 200 patients who underwent laparoscopic or open partial nephrectomy, the laparoscopic group had 3% positive margins, while none were found in the open group. The laparoscopic group also had more intraoperative complications, mainly related to hemorrhage, but it had better recovery data (56).

Tissue ablation techniques such as cryoablation, radiofrequency ablation, and high-intensity focused ultrasound have also been used, usually for small tumors in patients who are elderly or too infirm to undergo a more extensive operation. There are serious questions regarding the adequacy of these treatments for cancer, and outcome data are not yet available. Follow-up of these patients is also ill-defined because of the lack of data (55).

Prostate

Laparoscopic radical prostatectomy is an established technique for treating prostate cancer. Advantages include the magnification of nerves and visualization of the urethrovesical anastomosis. It can be done intraperitoneally (most common) or extraperitoneally, usually in cases in which there was previous abdominal or pelvic surgery. The operation is not comfortable for the surgeon and is technically demanding. Robotic assistance has been used to aid the urologist by providing better angles to sew the anastomosis in a more ergonomic fashion. Oncologic principles are the same for any of the methods of performing radical prostatectomy, and results to date show fairly equivalent results. There is a steep learning curve cited throughout the literature; thus, the literature must be interpreted knowing that experienced surgeons are the ones whose results are being cited (57,58). Localized prostate cancer can also be treated with even less invasive methods such as transurethral ultrasound-guided cryotherapy or high-intensity focused ultrasound. Each method has its own potential complications, but both are designed to decrease the incontinence and impotence rates seen with standard radical prostatectomy (57).

Bladder

Laparoscopic radical cystectomy and urinary diversion is a field in its infancy. Technically demanding and time-consuming, experience is growing slowly in large centers. Early results are encouraging and work continues to make improvements in the technique and outcomes (59,60).

Peritoneum

Primary peritoneal cancer histologically resembles and responds to treatment like ovarian epithelial tumors, but the presentation is peritoneal with minimal or no involvement of the ovaries. It can even occur in women who have previously had bilateral oophorectomy for benign disease. Because of the similarities, treatment is also similar, involving debulking surgery, total abdominal hysterectomy, bilateral oophorectomy, and chemotherapy (61). Intraperitoneal administration of chemotherapy has also shown improved outcomes (62). Even with this aggressive treatment plan, median survival is 16 to 24 months. The role of laparoscopy is accepted for staging and biopsy to rule out metastatic disease, most commonly from the ovary, pancreas, or stomach. If it is truly a primary peritoneal cancer, then prognosis is related to the adequacy of cytoreduction, usually performed by laparotomy.

Gynecology

Laparoscopy has become useful to the gynecologic oncologists in the staging and treatment of early cervical and endometrial cancers. Laparoscopic lymphadenectomy of the pelvic and retroperitoneal nodal basins has made laparoscopic-vaginal radical hysterectomy or purely laparoscopic radical hysterectomy possibilities. In young women with early cervical cancers, laparoscopic pelvic lymphadenectomy with radical vaginal trachelectomy is a modification of radical hysterectomy that preserves fertility potential. Studies have shown fairly equal recurrence rates, and 30 births in these patients have been reported (63). Although no evidence exists to conclusively prove that laparoscopic techniques provide equivalent oncologic outcomes, the Gynecologic Oncology Group is working on providing data evaluating laparoscopic radical hysterectomy.

Staging of ovarian malignancy is also an accepted role for laparoscopy, which aids in selecting patients for immediate cytoreduction versus those who will receive neoadjuvant chemotherapy. CT imaging and CA 125 serum levels have positive predictive values for resectable patients of only approximately 68% (64). Laparoscopy saves patients from laparotomy in 36% to 50% of cases (63). However, laparoscopy is not generally recommended for the actual treatment of ovarian cancer because inadequate cytoreduction and puncture or breakage of ovarian cancer is associated with worse outcomes.

PORT-SITE RECURRENCE

Some may argue that the loss of direct tactile feedback in laparoscopy does not allow sufficient exploration of the abdominal cavity for metastasis, small synchronous lesions, or other pathology. However, this is a limitation that partly has been overcome with improved laparoscopic skill, better instrumentation, visualization, and imaging techniques. Early reports of port-site metastasis occurring in 21% of cases were probably due to inexperience, flaws in technique, and poor instrumentation. However, these reports and other anecdotal concerns regarding tumor seeding and port-site metastasis provoked many trials studying the effects of abdominal pressure and carbon dioxide insufflation on tumor cells. The underlying concern was whether combining pneumoperitoneum with tissue damage promoted an environment that allowed dissemination of malignant cells and a tissue matrix for their adherence. One study was of rats with tumor cells injected into the abdominal cavity and then subjected to 16 mm Hg carbon dioxide pressure, 4 mm Hg, or no insufflation. Eleven days after the experiment, the rats were examined for tumor at autopsy. The higher pressure group had significantly higher tumor load than the other two groups (65). However, another study was of tumor cells injected intra-abdominally into rats, which were then divided into four groups: gasless laparoscopy, pneumoperitoneum at 8 mm Hg pressure, laparotomy, and control. When these rats were examined at autopsy, there was no significant difference between any of the surgical groups, but all surgical groups had increased abdominal wall tumor burden compared with the control group (66).

In studies involving patients, it appears that port-site recurrences are not statistically different between laparoscopic and open groups, both showing ~1% occurrence. One large review of 1,650 diagnostic laparoscopic procedures for upper gastrointestinal tumors revealed only 0.79% of the procedures led to a port-site recurrence after surgery. Of all patients who had an open procedure after laparoscopy, 0.86% (9 of 1,040) developed an open incision recurrence. It should be noted, however, that 62% of the patients with wound recurrence in the diagnostic laparoscopy group were found to have metastatic disease at the time of surgery. This supports the fact that wound recurrences, whether occurring after laparoscopy or laparotomy, may be more related to tumor biology and extent of disease than to the method of surgical management (67). Another large study of wound recurrence after laparoscopic colon resection in 480 patients found the rate to 1.1%.

SUMMARY

In summary, as instrumentation improves and surgeons gain additional experience with advanced laparoscopic techniques, the indications for the laparoscopic treatment of malignancy will continue to expand and provide our patients the benefits of the laparoscopic approach, without compromising, and possibly improving, the oncologic outcome.

REFERENCES

1. Berci G. History of pneumoperitoneum. In: Rosenthal RJ, Friedman RL, Phillips EH, eds. *The pathophysiology of pneumoperitoneum.* Berlin: Springer; 1998:1–6.

2. Lacy A, Sala Blanch X, Visa J. Alternative gases in laparoscopic surgery. In: Rosenthal RJ, Friedman RL, Phillips EH, eds. *The Pathophysiology of Pneumoperitoneum.* Berlin: Springer; 1998:7–17.

3. Ouellette JR, Ko AS, Lefor AT. The physiologic effects of laparoscopy: applications in oncology. *Cancer J.* 2005;11:2–9.

4. Nguyen NT, Wolfe BM. The physiologic effects of pneumoperitoneum in the morbidly obese. *Ann Surg.* 2005;241:219–226.

5. Lowham AS, Filipi CJ, Tomonaga T. Pneumoperitoneum related complications: diagnosis and treatment. In: Rosenthal RJ, Friedman RL, Phillips EH, eds. *The Pathophysiology of Pneumoperitoneum.* Berlin: Springer; 1998:131–146.

6. Zuckerman RS, Heneghan S. The duration of hemodynamic depression during laparoscopic cholecystectomy. *Surg Endosc.* 2002;16:1233–1236.

7. Eleftheriadis E, Kotzampassi K. Influence of pneumoperitoneum on the mesenteric circulation. In: Rosenthal RJ, Friedman RL, Phillips EH, eds. *The Pathophysiology of Pneumoperitoneum.* Berlin: Springer; 1998:49–61.

8. Rosenthal RI, Hiatt JA, Phillips EH, et al. Pneumoperitoneum related changes in intracranial pressure: observations in a large animal model. *Surg Endosc.* 1997;11:376–380.

9. Wu FP, Sietses C, von Blomberg BM, et al. Systemic and peritoneal inflammatory response after laparoscopic or conventional colon resection in cancer patients: a prospective, randomized trial. *Dis Colon Rectum.* 2003;46:147–155.

10. West MA, Hackam DJ, Baker J, et al. Mechanism of decreased In vitro murine macrophage cytokine release after exposure to carbon dioxide. *Ann Surg.* 1997;226:179–190.

11. Kapernik G, Avinoach E, Grossman Y, et al. The effect of high partial pressure of carbon dioxide environment on metabolism of human peritoneal cells. *Am J Obstet Gynecol.* 1998;179:1503–1510.

12. Allendoy JD, Bessler M, Whelan RL, et al. Better preservation of immune function after laparoscopic-assisted vs. open bowel resection in a murine model. *Dis Colon Rectum.* 1996;39:567–572.

13. Allendorf JD, Bessler M, Kayton ML, et al. Increased tumor establishment and growth after laparotomy vs laparoscopy in a murine model. *Arch Surg.* 1995;130:649–653.

14. Paz-Partlow M. Basic instrumentation and troubleshooting. In: Phillips EH, Rosental RJ, eds. *Operative Strategies in Laparoscopic Surgery.* Berlin: Springer: 1995:3–9.

15. Conlon KC, Dougherty E, Klimstra DS, et al. The value of minimal access surgery in the staging of patients with potentially resectable peripancreatic malignancy. *Ann Surg.* 1996;223:134–140.

16. Minnard EA, Conlon KC, Hoos A, et al. Laparoscopic ultrasound enhances standard laparoscopy in the staging of pancreatic cancer. *Ann Surg.* 1998;228:182–187.

17. Burke EC, Karpeh MS, Conlon KC, et al. Laparoscopy in the management of gastric adenocarcinoma. *Ann Surg.* 1997;225:262–267.

18. Espat NJ, Brennan MF, Conlon KC. Patients with laparoscopically staged unresectable pancreatic adenocarcinoma do not require subsequent surgical biliary or gastric bypass. *J Am Coll Surg.* 1999;188:649–655.

19. Krasna MJ. Advances in staging of esophageal carcinoma. *Chest.* 1998;113:107S–111S.

20. Freeny PC, Traverso LW, Ryan JA. Diagnosis and staging of pancreatic adenocarcinoma with dynamic computed tomography. *Am J Surg.* 1993;165:600–606.

21. Tseng D, Sheppard BC, Hunter JG. New approaches to the minimally invasive treatment of pancreatic cancer. *Cancer J.* 2005;11:43–51.

22. Gagner M, Pomp A. Laparoscopic pancreatic resection: is it worthwhile? *J Gastrointest Surg.* 1997;1:20–26.

23. Rothin MA, Schob O, Weber M. Laparoscopic gastro- and hepaticojejunostomy for palliation of pancreatic cancer: a case controlled study. *Surg Endosc.* 1999;13:1065–1069.

24. Maire F, Hammel P, Ponsot P, et al. Long-term outcome of biliary and duodenal stents in palliative treatment of patients with unresectable adenocarcinoma of the head of pancreas. *Am J Gastroenterol.* 2006;101:735–742.

25. Leksowski, K. Thoracoscopic splanchnicectomy for control of intractable pain due to advanced pancreatic cancer. *Surg Endosc.* 2001;15:129–131.

26. Azimuddin K, Chamberlain RS. The surgical management of pancreatic neuroendocrine tumors. *Surg Clin North Am.* 2001;81:511–525.

27. Edwin B, Mala T, Mathisen O, et al. Laparoscopic resection of the pancreas: a feasibility study of the short-term outcome. *Surg Endosc.* 2004;18:407–411.

28. Dulucq JL, Wintringer P, Stabilini C, et al. Are major laparoscopic pancreatic resections worthwhile? A prospective study of 32 patients in a single institution. *Surg Endosc.* 2005;19:1028–1034.

29. Kunisaki C, Shimada H, Takahashi M, et al. Prognostic factors in early gastric cancer. *Hepatogastroenterology.* 2001;48:294–298.

30. Otsuka K, Murakami M, Aoki T, et al. Minimally invasive treatment of stomach cancer. *Cancer J.* 2005;11:18–25.

31. Huscher CG, Mingoli A, Sgarzini G, et al. Laparoscopic versus open subtotal gastrectomy for distal gastric cancer: five-year results of a randomized prospective trial. *Ann Surg.* 2005;241:232–237.

32. Dulucq JL, Wintringer P, Stabilini C, et al. Laparoscopic and open gastric resections for malignant lesions: a prospective comparative study. *Surg Endosc.* 2005;19:933–938.

33. DeMatteo RP, Brennan MF. Gastrointestinal stromal tumors. In: Cameron JL, ed. *Current Surgical Therapy,* 8th ed. Philadelphia: Elsevier Mosby; 2004:100–103.

34. Urba WJ, Longo DL. Hodgkin's disease. *N Engl J Med.* 1992;326:678–687.

35. Phillips EH, Korman JE, Friedman R. Laparoscopic splenectomy. In: Hiatt JR, Phillips EH, Morgenstern L, eds. *Surgical Diseases of the Spleen.* Berlin: Springer; 1997:211–232.

36. Lee SS, Morgenstern L, Phillips EH, et al. Splenectomy for splenic metastases: a changing clinical spectrum. *Ann Surg.* 2000;66:837–840.

37. Burch M, Misra M, Phillips EH. Splenic malignancy: a minimally invasive approach. *Cancer J.* 2005;11:36–42.

38. Khalili TM, Fleshner PR, Hiatt JR, et al. Colorectal cancer: comparison of laparoscopic with open approaches. *Dis Colon Rectum.* 1998;41:832–837.

39. Fleshman J, Sargent DJ, Green E, et al. Laparoscopic colectomy for cancer is not inferior to open surgery based on 5-year data from the Cost Study Group trial. *Ann Surg.* 2007;246:655–662.

40. Lacy, AM, Delgado S, Castells, A, et al. The long-term results of a randomized clinical trial of laparoscopy-assisted versus open surgery for colon cancer. *Ann Surg.* 2008;248:1–7.

41. Phillips EH, Franklin M, Carroll BJ, et al. Laparoscopic colectomy. *Ann Surg.* 1992;216:703–707.

42. Scheri RP, Drebin JA. Small bowel tumors. In: Cameron JL, ed. *Current Surgical Therapy.* 8th ed. Philadelphia: Elsevier Mosby; 2004:120–124.

43. Fujita F, Fujita R, Kanematsu T. New approaches to the minimally invasive treatment of liver cancer. *Cancer J.* 2005;11:52–56.

44. Fong Y, Brennan MF, Turnbull A, et al. Gallbladder cancer discovered during laparoscopic surgery. Potential for iatrogenic tumor dissemination. *Arch Surg.* 1993;128:1054–1056.

45. Kim EK, Lee SK, Kim WW. Does laparoscopic surgery have a role in the treatment of gallbladder cancer? *J Hepatobiliary Pancreat Surg.* 2002;9:559–563.

46. Russel SE, Zinner MJ. Tumors of the gallbladder. In: Cameron JL, ed. *Current Surgical Therapy.* 8th ed. Philadelphia: Elsevier Mosby; 2004:439–444.

47. Sturgeon C, Kebebew E. Laparoscopic adrenalectomy for malignancy. *Surg Clin North Am.* 2004;84:755–774.

48. Bonavina L, Incarbone R, Lattuada E, et al. Preoperative laparoscopy in management of patients with carcinoma of the esophagus and of the esophagogastric junction. *J Surg Oncol.* 1997;65:171–174.

49. Abbas AE, Deschamps C, Cassivi SD, et al. Barrett's esophagus: the role of laparoscopic fundoplication. *Ann Thorac Surg.* 2004;77:393–396.

50. Luketich JD, Alvelo-Rivera M, Buenaventura PO, et al. Minimally invasive esophagectomy: outcomes in 222 patients. *Ann Surg.* 2003;238:486–495.

51. Horgan S, Berger RA, Elli EF, et al. Robotic-assisted minimally invasive transhiatal esophagectomy. *Am Surg.* 2003;69:624–626.

52. Espat NJ, Jacobsen G, Horgan S, et al. Minimally invasive treatment of esophageal cancer: laparoscopic staging to robotic esophagectomy. *Cancer J.* 2005;11:10–17.

53. Spurbeck WW, Davidoff AM, Lobe TE, et al. Minimally invasive surgery in pediatric cancer patients. *Ann Surg Oncol.* 2004;11:340–343.

54. McKenna RJ Jr. New approaches to the minimally invasive treatment of lung cancer. *Cancer J.* 2005;11:73–76.

55. Trabulsi EJ, Kalra P, Gomella LG. New approaches to the minimally invasive treatment of kidney tumors. *Cancer J.* 2005;11:57–63.

56. Gill IS, Matin SF, Desai MM, et al. Comparative analysis of laparoscopic versus open partial nephrectomy for renal tumors in 200 patients. *J Urol.* 2003;170:64–68.

57. Akduman B, Barqawi AB, Crawford ED. Minimally invasive surgery in prostate cancer: current and future perspectives. *Cancer J.* 2005;11:355–361.

58. Smith JA Jr, Herrell SD. Robotic-assisted laparoscopic prostatectomy: do minimally invasive approaches offer significant advantages? *J Clin Oncol.* 2005;23:8170–8175.

59. Puppo P, Naselli A. Laparoscopic radical cystectomy. *Curr Urol Rep.* 2005;6:106–108.

60. Moinzadeh A, Gill IS. Laparoscopic radical cystectomy with urinary diversion. *Curr Opin Urol.* 2004;14:83–87.

61. Menczer J, Chetrit A, Barda G, et al. Primary peritoneal carcinoma: uterine involvement and hysterectomy. *Gynecol Oncol.* 2006;100:565–569.

62. Sarnaik AA, Sussman JJ, Ahmad SA, et al. Technology of intraperitoneal chemotherapy administration: a survey of techniques with a review of morbidity and mortality. *Surg Oncol Clin North Am.* 2003;12:849–863.

63. Abu-Rustum NR. Laparoscopy 2003: oncologic perspective. *Clin Obstet Gynecol.* 2003;46:61–69.

64. Rouzier R, Pomel C. Update on the role of laparoscopy in the treatment of gynaecological malignancy. *Curr Opin Obstet Gynecol.* 2005;17:77–82.

65. Whittich P, Steyerberg EW, Simons SH, et al. Intraperitoneal tumor growth is influenced by pressure of carbon dioxide pneumoperitoneum. *Surg Endosc.* 2000;14:817–819.

66. Lecuru F, Agostini A, Camatte S, et al. Impact of pneumoperitoneum on tumor growth. *Surg Endosc.* 2002;16:1170–1174.

67. Shoup M, Brennan MF, Karpeh MS, et al. Port site metastasis after diagnostic laparoscopy for upper gastrointestinal tract malignancies: an uncommon entity. *Ann Surg Oncol.* 2002;9:632–636.

68. Vukasin P, Ortega AE, Greene FL, et al. Wound recurrence following laparoscopic colon cancer resection. Results of the American Society of Colon and Rectal Surgeons Laparoscopic Registry. *Dis Colon Rectum.* 1996;39:S20–S23.

COMMENTARY 1
David A. Kooby

Authors Lee, Ito, and Phillips have prepared an excellent review of the issues surrounding minimally invasive surgery (MIS) and cancer. They walk the reader through the history, physiology, potential advantages, and potential concerns of laparoscopic management of malignant disease. The report is unbiased and comprehensive. Individual operations are discussed for all the major organ sites, and relevant supporting data are provided, when available. Like any well-prepared piece of writing on a controversial topic, the chapter raises more questions than it answers.

First and foremost, surgeons treating cancer must be well versed in cancer management. They must adhere to basic principles of assessment, resection, and reconstruction, without sacrificing surgical margins, nodal assessment, and patient survival for the sake of perceived benefit or marketing. The motto "just because you *can*, does not mean you *should*" rings true for anyone performing these procedures. This having been said, innovation and progress require some degree of risk.

Few will argue the accepted benefits of laparoscopic cholecystectomy, minimally invasive bariatric surgery, and laparoscopic or endoscopic antireflux procedures; however, this was not always the case. One of the earliest experiences with laparoscopic cholecystectomy was scorned by surgical pundits. The reward for innovation, in this case, was the end of a pioneering surgical career following a bile duct injury well into the surgeon's experience (1). Today, even those who initially snubbed this approach to gallbladder removal now have come to understand its merits.

This commentary addresses some of the points made in the preceding text chapter, and delves into issues tangential to it. Rather than rehash specific procedures, various technical and theoretical issues are explored, with the goal of providing a balanced complement to the work of the authors. As a disclosure, the author of this commentary is a surgical oncologist with experience in both open and minimally invasive approaches to neoplasms of the gastrointestinal tract, hematologic, and endocrine organs, and who has witnessed both the wonders and hazards of treating cancer with minimally invasive techniques.

IMMUNE FUNCTION

Surgical procedures induce stress (2). The more involved the procedure the more stress to the patient, and the more intense the stress response, both locally and systemically. Stress may be associated with impaired host response to neoplastic disease (3,4). Human and animal data abound regarding the assuaging influences of MIS on immune response, a concept that the authors illustrated quite well.

The purported benefit in systemic immunity associated with MIS may be offset by inhibitory effects on locoregional immune function. Direct drying effects of prolonged CO_2 exposure, as well as inhibitory effects on intraperitoneal macrophage tumor necrosis factor-α production, may induce locoregional immune-suppression (5). In response to such concerns, alternatives to CO_2 gas insufflation are used by some centers. Two such alternatives include gasless laparoscopy with abdominal wall lifters, and insufflation with alternative gases, such as helium (6,7). Currently, most centers are still using CO_2 insufflation, as it is inexpensive and readily available.

The key question is how animal models and human laboratory data translate to clinical outcome for the patients. We must turn to existing adequately powered, prospective, randomized, controlled trials to attempt to answer this question. There are few that satisfy these criteria. Evidence of infection (wound or other) is the most obvious, clinically relevant, surrogate marker of immunity following surgery. In both the *Clinical Outcomes of Surgical Therapy (COST)* trial for laparoscopically assisted versus open colectomy for cancer and the open mesh versus laparoscopic mesh repair of inguinal hernia trials reported in the *New England Journal of Medicine*, there were no differences in early or late infective complications between comparison groups (8,9). However, in the hernia trial there were significantly more complications overall in the laparoscopic arm. This does not prove that immunity is not protected with MIS approaches, but may indicate that the translated clinical benefit is subtle if at all.

LAPAROSCOPIC RESECTION FOR CANCER

All cancer resections consist of at least two stages, an assessment phase wherein the surgeon inspects to determine resectability and a destructive phase wherein the tumor or tumor-bearing organ is removed. In cases involving hollow organs, a third stage (reconstructive phase) is added. For example, a pancreaticoduodenectomy for cancer will start with an inspection of abdominal cavity for peritoneal or hepatic metastases or extensive local invasion of unresectable structures, such as the hepatic or superior mesenteric arteries. If these findings are not overtly present, then a destructive phase ensues, with division of the bile duct, intestinal tract, pancreatic neck, and retroperitoneal margin to permit extirpation of disease. Finally, a reconstructive phase involves anastomoses between the intestine and the pancreas, bile duct and stomach or duodenum. Techniques for performing these operations with MIS techniques are well described (10). Technical and theoretical considerations of each phase are discussed.

Diagnostic Laparoscopy (Assessment Phase)

Some institutions advocate diagnostic laparoscopy (DL) for assessment in certain abdominal cancers, primarily to avoid laparotomy in unresectable patients (11–15). Although this approach seems logical, there are certain caveats: the operating room staff may be confused as to whether to open instruments for the main procedure, adding time and expense; bile duct hamartomas and mesothelial proliferation on peritoneal surfaces are often exaggerated by magnification and can mimic malignancy, and yield may be less than that prior to recent advances in imaging technology allowing more accurate preoperative assessment. At what cutoff point does the change in management suggest a benefit to DL? Do we hedge our bet and perform this portion of the procedure in patients in whom we are less enthusiastic about proceeding with operation (elderly with comorbid factors)? Is a 10% yield enough to say it is worthwhile? Selective use of DL is probably warranted. Certain tumors with a high propensity for peritoneal spread should still have this done at the outset (e.g., gastric and gallbladder cancers).

Another approach is to perform DL on multiple patients on a single operative day with no intention off proceeding with resection that same day. Subsequently, patients amenable to resection are brought back for resection at a separate setting. This seems plausible; however, many patients travel long distances and the extra travel time, longer wait, and additional anesthetic exposure limit enthusiasm for this approach.

In addition to looking for metastases, DL can provide assessment of liver quality, presence of ascites, and varices not noted on preoperative imaging, obviating unnecessary incisions in poor candidates. This, in turn, allows such patients to leave the hospital sooner and proceed with the next level of care.

Resection (Destructive Phase)

Regarding the destructive phase in which the tumor is removed, there are numerous potential pitfalls. The obvious one is obtaining inadequate tumor-free margins. Absence of tactile feedback, compromised visibility, limited degrees of freedom or articulation, equipment limitations, and less experience with proper technique are all cited as potential problems with this portion of the operation (16–18). Limited randomized data exist to comment on these issues. The best data are again in colon cancer. The COST trial demonstrated no difference in margin and node dissection (mean number of nodes was 12 in both groups), but this trial did not evaluate rectal cancer. In the United Kingdom Medical Research Council's randomized trial, *Conventional versus Laparoscopic-Assisted Surgery in Colorectal Cancer (UK MRC CLAS-ICC)*, conventional and laparoscopic-assisted surgery were compared in patients with cancer of the colon and rectum. Overall, there were no differences in long-term outcomes (3-year overall survival, disease-free survival, local recurrence, or quality of life). However, higher positivity of the circumferential resection margin was reported after laparoscopic anterior resection, but this finding did not translate into an increased incidence of local recurrence. The authors concluded that (a) successful laparoscopic-assisted surgery for colon cancer is as effective as open surgery in terms of oncologic outcomes and preservation of quality of life, and (b) long-term outcomes for patients with rectal cancer were similar in those undergoing abdominoperineal resection and anterior resection (19). In a cautionary word, the National Comprehensive Cancer Network (NCCN) recommended that laparoscopic surgery for rectal cancer generally be performed in the context of a randomized trial.

Only limited data on margin status for pancreatic, hepatic, and gastric resections exist, as no large multicenter randomized trials have been performed comparing open and laparoscopic technique for tumors involving these organs.

Hand-assisted laparoscopic surgery is a newer, hybrid technique in which a hand port is introduced into the abdomen through a small incision, thereby allowing the surgeon to palpate the tumor and better assess the margins of resection. In contrast to minimally invasive bariatric and antireflux surgery, in oncologic surgery an incision is almost always necessary to extract the tumor specimen. The hand-port incision serves as an excellent specimen extraction site.

A word on lymphadenectomy: there is no randomized proof to demonstrate a clear-cut survival advantage for extended lymphadenectomy in most cancers. Having stated this point, it is becoming increasingly clear that a powerful association exists between the ratios of positive nodes evaluated to the total number evaluated, with a lower ratio being associated with better prognosis stage for stage (20–24). Perhaps there is better tumor clearance, but it does make sense that patients with lower ratios are more accurately staged. It is impossible to stage a patient with colon cancer as IIIB if only three nodes were evaluated in the specimen (25), and if the nodal harvest is inferior laparoscopically, then we must be cautious about using this approach.

In the COST trial, the mean lymph node count for both groups was 12 (which is the minimum number necessary for adequate staging according to the American Joint Committee on Cancer and the NCCN). Obviously, the onus falls on both the surgeon and the pathologist to ensure adequate evaluation, but assuming the pathologists were performing the same routine evaluation, the key variable in this study was the surgical approach. Can this be translated to gastric cancer? The answer is no. In a colon cancer dissection, the nodes are resected en bloc with the named vessels, while in gastric cancer the celiac axis and splenic artery are preserved, making laparoscopic harvest more challenging. We simply need more data to reach a more general conclusion on this point.

Anastomosis (Reconstructive Phase)

Finally, there is the reconstructive phase for any hollow organ tumor resection. Again, for MIS for colon cancer, the anastomosis is most often performed in an extracorporeal fashion, hence the term *laparoscopically assisted*, although it can be done entirely laparoscopically. Patients experience complications, such as anastomotic leaks, at our hands. This is a surgical fact of life. However, it is easier to accept complications following an operation performed according to "standard of care" or "best common practice." This is a complex issue that all surgeons performing these procedures must face and accept. Perhaps the overall complication rate is less or will improve with experience, but it is clear that the number of bile duct injuries rose with the laparoscopic cholecystectomy boom (26), and that laparoscopic inguinal hernia repair was associated with an increase in "life-threatening" complications over the standard open mesh repair in the Veterans Affairs cooperative trial (9).

EDUCATIONAL AND FINANCIAL CONSIDERATIONS

There is no doubt that surgical training is dramatically altered by MIS. In these days of the ever-shrinking reimbursement for services rendered, surgeons are forced to see more patients and operate 4 to 5 days a week to cover expenses. Many academic centers limit operating room availability in the mid- to late afternoon based on personnel restrictions, and pressure mounts to get cases done. Taking residents through complex MIS cancer operations can be time-consuming and challenging. Furthermore, many programs now have MIS fellowships, and cases that were once routine, open mid-level procedures are being performed by fellows. Many articles evaluate the time and expense associated with MIS (27,28).

CONCLUSIONS

As surgeons, we must remember that laparoscopy is a method and not an operation. Few properly powered randomized trials exist to prove the purported benefits, thus proper disclosure to patients and referring doctors must be provided. Referring physicians can be the worst offenders, as they may send marginal candidates to surgeons who are comfortable with MIS under the guise that it is less dangerous to remove a pancreatic tumor if it can be done laparoscopically. All patients and treating surgeons must adopt the attitude that if visualization, tension, or other technical limitations prohibit proper performance, the case must be converted to open, or not even attempted laparoscopically, in the best interests of the individual patient.

With regard to the future, a few pioneering surgeons are removing gallbladders, appendixes, and other organs via transgastric, transvaginal, and transrectal approaches with the aid of complex endoscopes equipped with extra working channels. This approach termed *NOTES* for *Natural Orifice Transluminal Endoscopic Surgery* (29,30) leaves the patient without any abdominal incisions whatsoever. Although not yet a standard approach by any means, NOTES may seem about as ridiculous to many members of the surgical community as laparoscopic cholecystectomy, cardiopulmonary bypass, cell phones, or traveling to the moon once seemed. As far as the role for NOTES in cancer therapy, only time will tell.

REFERENCES

1. Litynski GS. Erich Mühe and the rejection of laparoscopic cholecystectomy (1985): a surgeon ahead of his time. *JSLS.* 1998;2:341–346.
2. Fink PF. The role of cytokines as mediators of the inflammatory response. In: Townsend CM, Beauchamp RD, Evers BM, eds. *Sabiston Textbook of Surgery.* Philadelphia: WB Saunders;2001:28–44.
3. Carter JJ, Whelan RL. The immunologic consequences of laparoscopy in oncology. *Surg Oncol Clin North Am.* 2001;10:655–677.
4. Hartley JE, Mehigan BJ, Monson JR. Alterations in the immune system and tumor growth in laparoscopy. *Surg Endosc.* 2001;15:305–313.
5. Lee SW, Feingold DL, Carter JJ, et al. Peritoneal macrophage and blood monocyte functions after open and laparoscopic-assisted cecectomy in rats. *Surg Endosc.* 2003;17:1996–2002.

6. Neuhaus SJ, Watson DI, Ellis T, et al. Metabolic and immunologic consequences of laparoscopy with helium or carbon dioxide insufflation: a randomized clinical study. *ANZ J Surg.* 2001;71:447–452.

7. Kim WW, Jeon HM, Park SC, et al. Comparison of immune preservation between CO2 pneumoperitoneum and gasless abdominal lift laparoscopy. *JSLS.* 2002;6:11–15.

8. Clinical Outcomes of Surgical Therapy Study Group. A comparison of laparoscopically assisted and open colectomy for colon cancer. *N Engl J Med.* 2004;350:2050–2059.

9. Neumayer L, Giobbie-Harder A, Jonasson O, et al. Open mesh versus laparoscopic mesh repair of inguinal hernia. *N Engl J Med.* 2004;350:1819–1827.

10. Kooby DA, Fong Y. Laparoscopic and liver surgery. In: *Mastery of Laparoscopic and Endoscopic Surgery.* 2nd ed. Philadelphia: Lippincott Williams & Wilkins; 2004.

11. D'Angelica M, Fong Y, Weber S, et al. The role of staging laparoscopy in hepatobiliary malignancy: prospective analysis of 401 cases. *Ann Surg Oncol.* 2003;10:183–189.

12. Conlon KC, Dougherty E, Klimstra DS, et al. The value of minimal access surgery in the staging of patients with potentially resectable peripancreatic malignancy. *Ann Surg.* 1996;223:134–140.

13. Weitz J, D'Angelica M, Jarnagin W, et al. Selective use of diagnostic laparoscopy prior to planned hepatectomy for patients with hepatocellular carcinoma. *Surgery.* 2004;135:273–281.

14. Bartlett DL, Fong Y, Fortner JG, et al. Long-term results after resection for gallbladder cancer. Implications for staging and management. *Ann Surg.* 1996;224:639–646.

15. Burke EC, Karpeh MS, Conlon KC, et al. Laparoscopy in the management of gastric adenocarcinoma. *Ann Surg.* 1997;225:262–267.

16. Miyazawa M, Oishi T, Isobe Y, et al. Laparoscopic-assisted hepatectomy (LAH) for the treatment of hepatocellular carcinoma. *Surg Laparosc Endosc Percutan Tech.* 2000;10:404–408.

17. Koea J, Gane E, McCall J. Laparoscopic hepatectomy for hepatocellular carcinoma: a caution. *ANZ J Surg.* 2005;75:86–88.

18. Kooby DA. Laparoscopic surgery for cancer: historical, theoretical, and technical considerations. *Oncology (Huntington).* 2006;20:917–928.

19. Jayne DG, Guillou PJ, Thorpe H, et al; UK MRC CLASICC Trial Group. Randomized trial of laparoscopic-assisted resection of colorectal carcinoma: 3-year results of the UK MRC CLASICC Trial Group. *J Clin Oncol.* 2007;25):3061–3068.

20. Ding YB, Chen GY, Xia JG, et al. Correlation of tumor-positive ratio and number of perigastric lymph nodes with prognosis of patients with surgically-removed gastric carcinoma. *World J Gastroenterol.* 2004;10:182–185.

21. Moorman PG, Hamza A, Marks JR, et al. Prognostic significance of the number of lymph nodes examined in patients with lymph node-negative breast carcinoma. *Cancer.* 2001;91:2258–2262.

22. Berger AC, Watson JC, Ross EA, et al. The metastatic/examined lymph node ratio is an important prognostic factor after pancreaticoduodenectomy for pancreatic adenocarcinoma. *Am Surg.* 2004;70:235–240.

23. Prandi M, Lionetto R, Bini A, et al. Prognostic evaluation of stage B colon cancer patients is improved by an adequate lymphadenectomy: results of a secondary analysis of a large scale adjuvant trial. *Ann Surg.* 2002;235:458–463.

24. Voordeckers M, Vinh-Hung V, Van de Steene J, et al. The lymph node ratio as prognostic factor in node-positive breast cancer. *Radiother Oncol.* 2004;70:225–230.

25. Johnson PM, Porter GA, Ricciardi R, Baxter NN. Increasing negative lymph node count is independently associated with improved long-term survival in stage IIIB and IIIC colon cancer. *J Clin Oncol.* 2006;24(22):3570–3575.

26. Way LW, Stewart L, Gantert W, et al. Causes and prevention of laparoscopic bile duct injuries: analysis of 252 cases from a human factors and cognitive psychology perspective. *Ann Surg.* 2003;237:460–469.

27. Senagore AJ, Brannigan A, Kiran RP, et al. Diagnosis-related group assignment in laparoscopic and open colectomy: financial implications for payer and provider. *Dis Colon Rectum.* 2005;48:1016–1020.

28. Braga M, Vignali A, Zuliani W, et al. Laparoscopic versus open colorectal surgery: cost-benefit analysis in a single-center randomized trial. *Ann Surg.* 2005;242:890–895.

29. Rattner D, Hawes RH. Notes: Gathering momentum. *Surg Endosc.* 2006;20:711–712.

30. McGee MF, Rosen MJ, Marks J, et al. A primer on natural orifice transluminal endoscopic surgery: building a new paradigm. *Surg Innov.* 2006;13:86–93.

COMMENTARY 2
George Berci, Masanobu Hagiike, and Leo A. Gordon

"Endoscopy" (looking inside), was mentioned at the time of Hippocrates. At that time, the rectum and the vagina were the first organs to be inspected as both orifices have external access. A very simple speculum was used with reflecting light (sunlight) to inspect these areas. Is it not ironic that the one of the oldest uses of endoscopy was vaginal as we face the newest use of endoscopy: natural orifice transluminal endoscopic surgery (NOTES)?

The endoscopic challenge has been threefold: obtain reliable access, obtain reliable lighting, and maintain the access during manipulation. In 1806, Philippe Bozzini (1) developed the first light conductor. This was a candle encased in housing with an eyepiece on one side. He designed multiple tubes of various diameters to introduce into certain orifices. He used reflected light to provide vision. Bozzini's colleagues became envious and jealous because many patients requested his help by word of mouth. Perhaps Bozzini was clairvoyant, anticipating the patient-driven early days of laparoscopic cholecystectomy.

In 1867 Desormeaux (2) subsequently developed an endoscope. This tube was illuminated by a mixture of alcohol and turpentine. The beam of the light was reflected by a mirror. He examined the vagina, bladder, and urethra with this instrument; however, the heat production of this lighting system was significant. Approximately 10 years later, a break-through in endoscopy was created by a general practitioner, Maximillian Nitze (3). In 1879, he developed the first telescope. Tiny lenses were placed in a tube in certain intervals by spacers. This system was used for the next several decades in many disciplines as the "telescope for endoscopy."

Because many inventors of this period were primarily interested in diseases of the urinary bladder, a rudimentary cystoscope emerged. The illumination in the first prototype of a cystoscope was a platinum wire in glass housing. The wire was heated to create light. Simultaneously, though, the device needed to be cooled by means of circulating water. A few years later, Edison discovered the filament globe. A miniature lamp was immediately developed in Vienna and was incorporated into the cystoscope.

Mikulicz (4), in 1881, employed a similar system and, with his optical designer Leiter, developed a longer version of the instrument. This had an angulated tip to be used as a gastroscope. He described three major physiological movements of the stomach: peristalsis, respiration, and transmission of aortic pulsation. At the turn of the century, Nitze improved the system by developing the first photo cystoscope; he also published an atlas of the pathology of the urinary bladder.

The Nitze-type telescope provided the impetus to look into the abdominal and thoracic cavities. The system consisted of small lenses placed into a tube with a 90-degree (right-angled) direction with a narrow viewing angle and a tiny electric globe at the tip, which had to be carefully handled because of the heat. If the image were dim and the rheostat turned up, the globe easily burned out.

EARLY HISTORY OF LAPAROSCOPY

Kelling (5), in 1923, was the first to recommend a procedure called *Koelioskopie*, or coelioscopy. He was originally interested in gastric and duodenal ulcer bleeding and thought that by performing a pneumoperitoneum, compression of the stomach could be achieved and the bleeding thus arrested. In the interim, there were a few experiments done by Ott (6), a gynecologist in St. Petersburg, who used a speculum for illumination.

In our opinion, the most important work was performed 13 years after Kelling's report by a Swedish internist named Jacobeaus (7). Regarding instrumentation, he tried to change the optic to a straightforward one instead of the lateral view. He used trocars for penetrating the abdominal wall. He was very clever because the first patients were selected with ascitic fluid where the penetration into the abdominal cavity was safer and easier. He published 17 cases in 1910. He also extended his activities into the thoracic cavity where tuberculous exudates were common. The introduction of air was allegedly therapeutic. He was also able to lyse pleural adhesions.

In 1911 an assistant surgeon at Johns Hopkins, Bernheim, allegedly without knowing of the work by Kelling and Jacobeaus, inserted a proctoscope through the abdominal wall and used an electric headlamp for illumination. He employed pneumoperitoneum. In those earlier times, room air was used with or without an air filter (8).

Korbsch described in greater detail the laparoscopic technique with heavy premedication and sedation using the Nitze cystoscope modified by Jacobaeus. Unfortunately, in 1922, he did not find too many followers. Fervers (9), in 1933, employed the cystoscope after creating a pneumoperitoneum. He described it as a very simple process without any complications. Patients received morphine before and sometimes with an intravenous drip during the procedure. He used an operating room table on which he could change the position of the patient. Local anesthesia was generously employed. A detailed technique described how penetration of the various layers of the abdominal wall was sensed by the penetrating needle resistance, and finally aspira-

tion of air bubbles indicated that the abdominal cavity was entered. Sometimes yellowish fluid was obtained, indicating that the intestine was violated. He continued with the procedure, changing the needle position, and observed the patient. No severe symptoms were noted after the procedure. He was among the early investigators who mentioned oxygen or CO_2 gas for insufflation; thus, some of the originators already considered CO_2 despite the fact that coagulation was not employed at that time. Fervers had already described small endoscopic procedures for transection of adhesions. In one case he used oxygen and a heat element, a so-called cold coagulation probe. A "small explosion" occurred in the abdominal cavity. The patient was observed and survived. There were primitive coagulation probes employed at that time and the conclusion was that room air should be used instead of oxygen.

The real promoter and pioneer in laparoscopy was the hepatologist named Kalk (10), who in 1951 published a monograph of 2,000 laparoscopies performed with local anesthesia without mortality. Three complications occurred, only one of which required exploration. He used filtered air and trocars and created a "street map" for the safe introduction of the pneumoperitoneum needles as well as the trocar penetrations. He made significant changes in the existing optical system, which was originally a lateral 90-degree view and was very cumbersome for viewing and created a number of blind spots in the abdominal cavity.

Kalk collaborated with manufacturers to make a 130-degree for-oblique view telescope. This produced better overall observation of the abdominal cavity (Figure 11C.1). Patients were sedated and local anesthesia applied. He was the originator of the second trocar approach through which a needle, a manipulator, biopsy forceps, scissors, and other instruments including coagulation could be employed.

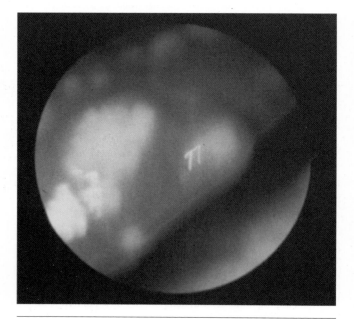

Figure 11C.1. Liver metastases. Primary was in the colon. Photograph was taken in 1959 with a modified Kalk (Nitze) telescope. Note the small size of the organ and the image quality.

The next milestone in the safe approach to pneumoperitoneum was the spring-loaded pneumoperitoneum needle developed by Veress (11) in 1938. He initially used it for air insufflation in the thoracic cavity in cases of lower lobe tuberculous cases and to evacuate pleural fluids. The needle had a blunt side-hole stylet that would retract into the needle during the introduction because of a spring on the other end. If resistance were lost during the advancement through the abdominal wall, the spring pushed the blunt end forward into the abdominal cavity.

John Ruddock (12), a cardiologist, modified the optics of Kalk's for-oblique view telescope. He also designed accessory instruments. In 1937 he published 500 cases with a mortality of 0.2 % and a diagnostic accuracy of 92%. His comments were prescient: "The internist must share the responsibility on fruitless laparotomies performed for diagnostic purposes and should use all the ancillary procedures at this disposal before you recommend diagnostic laparotomy in order to make an intra abdominal diagnosis . . ."

In 1957 Ruddock (13) published over 5,000 peritoneoscopic examinations in the *Surgical Clinics of North America*. He premedicated and observed the patients before each procedure. Biopsies were performed to compare the visual appearance with the pathologic diagnosis. Complications were uncommon. In ten cases, he punctured the bowel with the needle or with a trocar. There was one mortality from hemorrhage from a liver biopsy in a patient with extensive metastatic liver disease. Despite the impressive experience, the acceptance of the procedure was minimal.

THE REFORMATION OF ENDOSCOPY

Berci (14) started using laparoscopy for staging abdominal malignancies, evaluation of liver disease, and problematic abdominal dilemmas in 1962. Many refinements were made, but the major issues were limited vision and problems with the technique, instrumentation, and documentation. There were three major developments that contributed to the wider acceptance of endoscopic procedures: optics, illumination, and television.

Optics

A new era of laparoscopy was created by the introduction of a new rod lens invention by Hopkins (15). A smaller scope with a brighter image, a wider viewing angle, less peripheral distortions, and better color responses resulted in improved orientation and perception (Figure 11C.2). This optical improvement opened a new era for endoscopy and its extension to other disciplines.

Illumination

Illumination was always a problem because more light in general meant more heat. Using larger globes with higher intensity and placing the globe externally, the endoscope was separated from the light source and made it possible to use a flexible fiber light cord as a light conductor (16).

Television

With the introduction of television, it became obvious that observing an image through an eyepiece with a monocular view

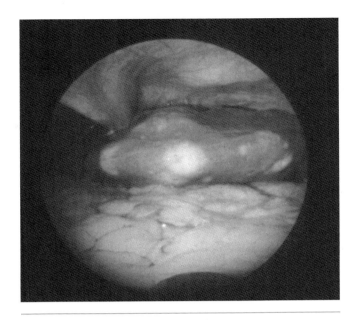

Figure 11C.2. Left lobe of the liver with metastases from a sigmoid colon carcinoma. Photograph was taken with the Hopkins laparoscope. Note the size and improvements of the image quality (such as resolution, size of object, and color display).

was inferior to an enlarged magnified view of the anatomy observed from a convenient distance with both eyes on a larger screen. Even in earlier times, laparoscopy needed four hands if biopsies or small operations were performed. Coordinated movements of the assistant are a necessity. Berci and Davids (17) developed a miniature black and white endoscopic camera and performed the first teleconference from the hospital to a meeting in 1962. Needless to say, the monochrome interpretation was not accepted.

Soulas (18), a French bronchoscopist, published the first televised bronchoscopy in 1957 using a 140-poundstudio Orthicon camera. Advances followed, leading to a televised choledochoscopy during biliary surgery in 1980 (19,20). This was followed by gynecologic laparoscopic procedures in 1984. When laparoscopy was introduced on the West Coast in 1970, only the gynecologists were interested in learning more about the technique. It took approximately 10 to 12 years before general surgeons became interested in the technique and created a "revolution" of laparoscopic surgery. This revolution was hastened by the introduction and refinement of laparoscopic cholecystectomy.

There is no doubt that without a more efficient optical system, improved illumination, and television display, there would be no minimally invasive surgery. Today, a large part of general abdominal, thoracic, gynecologic, and other surgical disciplines are performed under laparoscopic settings. The advantages for the patient are obvious. Minimally invasive surgery depends on the education and training of surgeons, competency of the operator, and further progress in technology. These advances have made it possible to intrude into some areas of oncology without exploring the patient.

CLINICAL LAPAROSCOPY FOR THE SURGICAL ONCOLOGIST

Instrumentation

Every standard laparoscopic cholecystectomy set can be used for diagnostic laparoscopy in the oncologic setting. The operator has to check only whether the following instruments are present:

1. Biopsy cup-forceps
2. Hook-punch biopsy forceps
3. Flat-punch forceps
4. Aspiration cannula to remove fluid
5. An insulated suction coagulation device for hemostasis

Documentation

A videotape recorder and a printer for color photos are standard in the majority of operating theaters where laparoscopic cholecystectomy is performed. In previous years, many surgeons routinely videotaped all procedures performed through the laparoscope. Because this procedure (which was unique in 1990) is now a matter of routine, standard videotaping is not usually performed. Video documentation, however, may be helpful to the pathologist. Such documentation may guide radiation treatment. The teaching aspects of such documentation are clear.

Anesthesia

The type of anesthesia depends on the patient's general condition, underlying diseases, and the surgeon's experience. Diagnostic laparoscopy may be performed under local anesthesia with sedation if an anesthesiologist is present. High-pressure pneumoperitoneum may be avoided. One of the appealing aspects of diagnostic laparoscopy under local anesthesia is that it can be performed safely in the high-risk patient.

Indications

Operative laparoscopy in the oncologic setting provides the surgical oncologist a direct method of identifying intra-abdominal disease. It can bypass many time-consuming and low-yield investigative studies.

Liver Disease

Both lobes of the liver can be well visualized using laparoscopy. Asymmetry of appearance between lobes may give an indication of intraparenchymal disease. Dilated veins in the omentum or parietal peritoneum may signify portal hypertension. The laparoscopic surgeon can perform a liver biopsy in a safer manner than can be done in the standard blind percutaneous fashion. Bleeding or oozing may be controlled by compression or by coagulation. The biopsy site can be more accurately selected.

Suspected Liver Tumors

Cirrhotic patients have a higher incidence of hepatocellular carcinomas. Sometimes these tumors originate from a normal-appearing liver. The value of laparoscopy in these patients hinges on the fact that smaller lesions may be missed by computed tomography. Multicentricity may be detected laparoscopically.

Suspected Metastases

If the clinical picture indicates dissemination of a primary lesion, laparoscopy can help to define this problem. Laparoscopically targeted biopsies yield larger tissue samples for the pathologist.

Palpable Mass

Intra-abdominal masses that are palpable on physical examination may be specifically defined laparoscopically. They may be extrahepatic. Retroperitoneal tumors protruding into the abdominal cavity may be better defined. Given the risk of venous bleeding with percutaneous biopsy, laparoscopy affords a safer method of biopsy in the patient with venous compression secondary to malignant disease.

Ascites of Unknown Origin

Radiologic examinations are impaired when large fluid volumes are present in the abdomen. Laparoscopy affords many benefits for the patient who has ascites of unknown origin. When performing laparoscopy in this setting, it is helpful to place the pneumoperitoneum needle parallel to the abdominal wall after insertion. This maneuver avoids creating bubbles in the ascitic fluid. These bubbles may interfere with visibility.

In the patient with dilated periumbilical veins, alternative sites of needle and trocar placement should be considered. During laparoscopy in the patient with ascites, usually a few milliliters of ascitic fluid are withdrawn to indicate that the needle is in the proper place. Trocars are placed after installation of the pneumoperitoneum.

Unfortunately, ascites does not provide a "protective cushion." A small pneumoperitoneum is still required. The Veress pneumoperitoneum needle should be kept parallel with the abdominal wall after penetration of the abdominal wall to avoid creation of a bubble in the ascitic fluid. Because the intestines are gas-filled, they float on top of the ascitic fluid, presenting the risk of enteric perforation. Once the telescope has been successfully introduced above the fluid level of ascites, another small incision may he made for additional trocar placement. The patient is placed in a reverse Trendelenburg position, and the ascitic fluid is removed by suction. It is possible to evacuate several liters of fluid at this time. Anesthetic management is key to ensuring the hemodynamic stability of the patient. Once the ascitic fluid has been removed, the liver and other viscera may be visualized. The cirrhotic liver may be seen. The undersurface of the liver may be examined by using additional instruments. Metastatic lesions may be discovered in the parietal peritoneum, falciform ligament, or even on the serosa of the intestine or stomach. It is suggested that trocar sites in patients with ascites be closed with fascial sutures and subcutaneous sutures to the skin. Laparoscopy in the patient with ascites of unknown origin will usually reveal the diagnosis.

Staging

One of the major issues in laparoscopy in oncology is the value of this procedure in staging the patient. Carcinoma of the pancreas is a good example. In approximately one third of cases of pancreatic cancer there is peritoneal involvement at the time of diagnosis. At this stage, computed tomographic scanning or ultrasound is not sensitive enough to detect small nodules on the parietal peritoneum or the diaphragm. It is helpful to perform laparoscopy prior to any major oncologic procedure. If the patient is brought to surgery for resection, laparoscopy should be performed prior to laparotomy. This approach to pancreatic cancer can save the patient a full laparotomy with its attendant prolonged hospitalization.

Non-Hodgkin lymphoma, with its widespread appearance, can easily be seen and biopsied. In Hodgkin lymphoma, multiple liver biopsies can be performed on both lobes. This affords a larger sample for the pathologist. Larger lymph nodes presenting in the mesentery may also be biopsied. The assessment of splenic involvement in Hodgkin lymphoma is controversial.

Patient Selection
Cardiorespiratory Disease

Significant cardiac disease or recent myocardial infarction may prevent the performance of laparoscopy. Compensated disease is usually not an absolute contraindication if the patient has been properly evaluated and is meticulously monitored. Severe chronic obstructive pulmonary disease should also be evaluated prior to the procedure.

Previous Abdominal Surgery

In the patient with previous abdominal surgery, it is essential that the puncture site be carefully selected and tested prior to the installation of the pneumoperitoneum. A precise history of the patient's previous surgery is important in assessing the extent of intra-abdominal adhesions.

Contraindications to Laparoscopy
Mechanical or Paralytic ileus

There is widening experience with laparoscopy in the patient with bowel obstruction or ileus. The greatest danger is perforation of dilated intestinal loops. Laparoscopy in this situation depends on the expertise of the surgeon and the severity of the ileus or obstruction.

Blood Dyscrasias and Coagulopathies

Hematologic abnormalities should be assessed and corrected prior to laparoscopy. There are large variations in the extent and severity of such coagulopathies, and each case should be individually evaluated. Special attention should be paid to aspirin intake and other platelet inhibitors.

Obesity

The obese patient presents several technical problems to the oncologic laparoscopist. It may he difficult to obtain pneumoperitoneum using the closed technique. The technique may be changed to open laparoscopy, using a Hasson trocar. It is essential that longer instruments be available in the truly morbidly obese patient.

Technical Suggestions for the Surgical Oncologist

The technique of operative laparoscopy has been described elsewhere; however, several points regarding the oncologic patient are worth mentioning. In sick or cachectic patients, the grade of CO_2 installation should be slow (1 to 1.5 L/min). Such patients may develop hemodynamic changes if there is sudden interference with venous return or a vasovagal reflex due to sudden tension on the diaphragm. In cases of hypertension or other problems occurring during pneumoperitoneum, the surgeon should stop the pneumoperitoneum and deflate the abdomen. The same evacuation of pneumoperitoneum should occur if the trocar has been placed and a problem is identified by the anesthesiologist. Usually the problem disappears, and the pneumoperitoneum may be attempted again at a slower rate. The usual pressure for such laparoscopies is in the 15 to l7 mm Hg range.

Operative laparoscopy is done in the supine position. If ascites is present or a better view of the liver is required, the reverse Trendelenburg position may facilitate observation. After the laparoscopy is completed, the abdominal cavity should be examined for bleeding as well as for evidence of organ injury. Trocar sites are usually infiltrated with local anesthesia to decrease postoperative pain and should be meticulously closed with a few subcutaneous stitches to avoid leakage. In the nonoperated abdomen, the pneumoperitoneum is usually instilled subumbilically. Needle aspiration is performed. The saline drop test is also performed to assure free flow at the tip of the needle. If a palpable mass is present in the midline, the needle may be placed in any number of lateral positions.

Current operative laparoscopy offers significant advantages for the patient suspected of harboring a malignancy. Laparoscopy is an effective tool in the surgical oncologist's armamentarium. The ongoing refinement of laparoscopic instruments coupled with advances in imaging and computer technology place operative laparoscopy at the center of surgical oncology.

REFERENCES

1. Bozzini PH. Lichtleiter, eine Erfindung zur Anschauung innerer Teile und Krankheiten. *J Prak Heilk.* 24:107.
2. Desormeaux AJ. Endoscope and its application to the diagnosis and treatment of affections of the genitourinary passages. *Chicago Med J.* 1867.
3. Nitze M. Beobachtungs und Untersuchungsmethode fur Harnrohre Harnblase und Rectum. *Wien Med Wochenschr.* 1879;24:651.
4. Mikulicz J. Uber Gastroskopie und Osophagoskopie. *Wien Med Presse.* 1881;45:1405.
5. Kelling G. Zur Colioskpie und Gastroskopie. *Arch Klin Chir.* 1923;126:226–228.
6. Ott D. Illumination of the abdomen (ventroscopia) [in Russian]. *J Akush i Zhensk Boliez.* 1901;15:1045–1049.
7. Jacobaeus HC. Ueber die Moglichkeit die Zystoskopie bei Untersuchung seroser Hohlungen anzuwenden. *Munch Med Wochenschr.* 1910;57:2090–2092.
8. Davis CJ. A history of endoscopic surgery. *Surg Laparosc Endosc.* 1992;2:16–23.
9. Fervers C. Die Laparoskopie mit dem Cystoskop. *Med Klin.* 1933;29:1042–1045.
10. Kalk H, Bruhl W. *Leitfaden der Laparoscopie.* Stuttgart: Thieme; 1951.
11. Veress J. Neus Instrument zur Ausfuhrung von Brust-oder Bauchpunktionen und Pheumonthoraxbehandlung. *Deutsche med Wochenschr.* 1938;64:1480–1481.
12. Ruddock JC. Peritoneoscopy. *Surg Gynecol Obstet.* 1937;65:623–639.

13. Ruddock JC: Peritoneoscopy: a critical clinical review. *Surg Clin North Am.* 1957;37:1249–1260.
14. Berci, G. Peritoneoscopy. *Br. Med J.* 1962;1:562–564.
15. Hopkins HH. Optical principles of the endoscope. In: Berci G, ed. *Endoscopy.* New York: Appleton-Century Crofts; 1976:3–27.
16. Olson V. Light Sources. In: Berci G, ed. *Endoscopy.* New York: Appleton-Century-Crofts; 1976.
17. Berci G, Davids J. Endoscopy and televison. *Br Med J.* 1962;1: 1610–1613.
18. Soulas A. Televised bronchoscopy. *Presse Med.* 1956;64:97.
19. Berci G, Shulman AG, Morgenstern L, et al. Television choledochoscopy. *Surg Gynecol Obstet.* 1985;160:176–177.
20. Berci G, Cuschieri A. *Practical Laparoscopy.* London: Bailliere Tindall; 1986.

12

Radiation Therapy:
An Overview of Recent Advances and Future Innovations

Bernard S. Lewinsky and Robert P. Zimmermann

One hundred ten years ago, in Chicago, Illinois, Emile Grubbe treated the first patient with breast cancer using the energy that later became known as roentgen rays or x-rays (1). In the ensuing century, much has changed in the application and use of this form of energy, and the radiobiologic principles of this modality have been fully developed and tested in the laboratory. In fact, the basis of all modern radiation effects on tumors and normal tissues has been studied both in vitro and in animal models prior to clinical application, exemplifying what we now term *translational evidence-based medicine*.

In 1898, Madame Curie discovered radium 226 and developed methods for using the energy from radium for the treatment of malignancies. Higher energy x-ray tubes were developed subsequently, leading to the orthovoltage era. In the early 1950s and 1960s, technological advances led to the use of higher energy sources like cobalt 60 and the development of the higher-energy machines, linear accelerators, that introduced the megavoltage era.

Whereas higher energy machines were thought to be one of the "answers" to the cure of cancer, it was soon realized that normal tissue tolerance was the limiting factor regardless of the energy of the beam. Consequently, the technical innovations in radiation oncology in the last decade have been aimed at improving the therapeutic index. These efforts have led to the development of new, sophisticated computer software, hardware, and equipment that allow for the deposition of this energy into defined targets while avoiding as much normal tissue damage as possible. Through better targeting of the tumor as a result of advanced radiologic and nuclear medicine innovations and by limiting normal tissue damage, higher doses of radiation can be safely delivered. Ultimately, these higher tumor doses should lead to a higher rate of tumor control. Thus, the aim in radiation oncology is to control the tumors by targeting them for destruction with minimal adjacent tissue damage.

The current techniques and potential innovations in the pipeline in the field of radiotherapy are reviewed in this chapter, emphasizing the benefits and limitations of this modality of antitumor therapy.

ADVANCES IN EXTERNAL-BEAM RADIOTHERAPY

Much as the development of megavoltage linear accelerators led to dramatic improvements in treatment 40 years ago, current improvements in computerized planning and sophisticated treatment delivery are changing the face of radiotherapy today. The transition from superficial radiation treatments to deeply penetrating megavoltage beams came at a very high price because of the lack of understanding of the energy deposition in tissues associated with the higher beams compared with the superficial treatments. Pioneer radiation oncologists used the skin as a guide to radiation effect, prescribing doses that would lead to erythema, thus the "erythema dose" prescription. When cobalt 60 was introduced, it took some time to understand why the erythema dose was more difficult to achieve. Yet, the patients were treated to "erythema doses." Acute and long-term skin and organ reactions and complications ensued, marring the reputation of cobalt 60 machines forever. Once it was understood that the dose was deposited deeper in the tissues because of the energy of cobalt 60 (approximately 1.2 MeV), and the doses were correctly prescribed at depth, the complication rates diminished.

In the past, dosimetry and planning were done by hand; many man-hours were needed to produce a plan. Treatment plans were designed to inform the radiation oncologist what was to be done but not necessarily how it should best be accomplished. A set of depth-dose curves was available for each machine, and the radiation physicist would create the radiation distribution map known as the treatment plan. Computerization of the process allowed the instantaneous creation of more elaborate plans. The introduction of computer technology in radiology with the development of the computed tomographic (CT) imaging allowed more exact identification of the organs and malignant structures that needed to be irradiated. Adding the more advanced power of modern computers led to the three-dimensional (3D) representation of tumors and the ability to "see" tumors and their surrounding organs in three dimensions. Multiple radiation beams could be set up to focus on the tumor and conform to the size and shape of the target. This type of treatment is known as *3D-conformal radiotherapy*. The modern era of treatment planning thus began just a few years ago.

Building on the foundation of 3D conformal radiotherapy, current advancements allow even more precise treatment with better sparing of normal tissues. This section provides a guide through the array of acronyms used to describe the latest radiation modalities. Treatments are now routinely planned on the basis of CT images, which are often combined with magnetic resonance images (MRIs) or even positron emission tomography (PET). The use of PET/CT scans brings the planning and delivery of the radiation dose to a tumor into a totally new dimension. Not only can the beam be concentrated on the metabolically active tumor, but normal tissue (such as atelectatic lung) can also be deliberately avoided, thus sparing vital function.

Intensity-modulated radiation therapy (IMRT) is a technique wherein the radiation beam can be shaped to deliver homogeneous doses of radiation to the target while at the same time minimizing the dose, and therefore the damage, to adjacent normal tissues. With these more precise treatments, verification by image guidance has become more important. *Image-guided radiation therapy* (IGRT) can be done with ultrasound images, stereoscopic x-rays, or CT.

The next phase in the evolution of these technologies is *adaptive radiotherapy* (ART) or *dynamic adaptive radiotherapy* (DART). With ART, radiation doses are recalculated daily before treatment based on real-time patient and tumor anatomy. This allows continual sparing of tissues that may have otherwise moved into the high-dose region because of tumor shrinkage or organ motion between fractions.

Another frontier is the development of stereotactic targeting of both brain targets and extracranial sites for radiosurgery. Single-fraction *stereotactic radiosurgery* is commonly used now in the brain for both benign and malignant brain tumors. This technology is now being adapted to allow treatment of lung and liver tumors using either a single fraction or in three to five high-dose fractions. The latter has been termed *hypofractionated stereotactic radiotherapy*.

ADVANCES IN RADIOTHERAPY PLANNING

Originally, radiation therapy ports were set up clinically, based on the radiation oncologist's knowledge of surface anatomy and how this related to internal anatomy. High-energy x-ray images called *port films* could be taken to verify adequate coverage of the target and document the area treated. Subsequently, treatment simulators were developed to allow fluoroscopic imaging of the planned portal using the same laser coordinates and collimator settings as the linear accelerators. Initially, hand blocks were used to shield areas within the rectangular field that did not need to be treated. Later, custom lead-alloy blocks were developed to allow more precise shielding of normal structures. For treatment of abdominal and pelvic tumors, contrast material was used to help delineate the targets and guide the placement of these blocks. Currently, radiotherapy treatment planning is based on CT. CT-based planning is used for 3D conformal therapy, IMRT, and even ART. CT-based planning is so pervasive in current practice that many radiotherapy departments have eliminated conventional simulators in favor of dedicated CT simulation for all patients.

Three-dimensional conformal therapy begins with the radiation oncologist delineating the target volumes on CT images. Adjacent normal tissues can also be contoured so that the dose to these organs can be accurately determined. Next, a series of fixed beams are set up to treat the target. Computer-designed custom blocking is then constructed to conform to the shape of the target volume as seen from each individual field. This type of blocking is done around the "beam's eye view" of the tumor. The beams are oriented in such a way as to minimize the exposure to normal tissues. Adjacent organs can be blocked, but only to the extent that less margin around the tumor is added on the side that abuts the structure to be shielded.

IMRT is a major technologic advance over 3D conformal radiotherapy. One major difference is that the radiation beam is divided into hundreds of sections called *beamlets*, each of which can be individually controlled or modulated. The key component of IMRT is *inverse planning*. Instead of blocking based on the shape of the tumor, the beam intensity is adjusted or modulated within the various beamlets that make up each port in order to produce the desired dose coverage and, more importantly, normal tissue sparing. The radiation oncologist contours the targets and normal structures in much more detail than with 3D conformal therapy. He or she then defines the acceptable target coverage and desired normal tissue dose limits. Variables that can be adjusted include the minimum dose, maximum dose, and various dose-volume histogram limits. For example, the radiation oncologist may prescribe a minimum prostate dose of 79 Gy with a maximum dose of 81 Gy and a maximum rectal dose of 65 Gy. The software then works backward through a process called inverse planning to determine the appropriate treatment intensity needed through each part of the field to achieve the desired result. Priorities and penalty values can be adjusted to help guide the computer to meet the goals set up by the physician. Not surprisingly, compromises sometimes need to be made. In order to achieve strict sparing of some tissues, inhomogeneities ("hot spots") within the tumor may be needed. The radiation oncologist weighs the relative importance of each of these factors in selecting a final IMRT plan.

As new imaging technologies become more prevalent, these are being incorporated into radiation therapy planning systems. For example, MR scans give much better images of certain regions than CT scans. This is true in the brain, head and neck, and even the prostate. Most systems now allow oncologists to fuse CT and MR images to allow for more accurate treatment planning. This method preserves the geometric accuracy of CT scans and allows precise visualization of soft tissues as seen on MR.

Another new imaging technology that has been incorporated into treatment planning is PET. Increasingly, PET scans are being obtained as part of combined PET/CT imaging, in which information about metabolic activity is overlaid on CT scan images. Combined PET/CT imaging is extremely helpful in defining target volumes for radiation therapy. For example, PET scan-negative lymph node targets can be treated with lower doses of radiation, or may not need to be treated at all. The activity on a PET scan, quantitated as *standard uptake value*, may also give information about the dose needed to control a particular tumor. It is predicted that in the future, planning systems will be able to routinely incorporate PET/CT data and other metabolic information into the planning process so that radiotherapy doses can be tailored to individual levels of PET activity to achieve a given probability of controlling the cancer. In addition, PET scan activity could be monitored during treatment to determine the response and allow changes to be made.

IMAGE GUIDANCE

Historically, radiation fields were set up clinically and port films were used to document the treatment area and allow the treating physician to make any needed shifts or changes in the field to be treated. Beginning in the late 1980s, *electronic portal imaging devices* (EPID) were introduced into clinical practice. These systems use digital images to document treatment fields, and images can be acquired on a daily basis during the actual treatment in order to ensure that the field remains in precisely the same area as was initially planned. However, portal imaging does not allow tumor visualization nor can it account for organ motion.

As advancements in radiation treatment planning have allowed for more precise dosing of tumors, it has become more important to understand and adjust for organ motion between and even during treatments. Prior to image guidance, one strategy to account for organ motion was to add a margin of up to 2 cm around the actual targets. This avoids a motion-related "geographic miss," but results in surrounding normal tissues receiving the full dose of radiation. When the intended tumor dose exceeds the tolerance dose of adjacent organs, adding a large margin around the target will result in unacceptable normal tissue toxicity. Image guidance addresses this problem.

Real-time imaging at the time of treatment is used to visualize the target organ and thus minimize the margin needed to be applied to account for organ motion. Several different imaging modalities can be used to guide precision radiotherapy including ultrasound, stereoscopic kilovoltage x-rays, and both kilovoltage and megavoltage CT. In certain cases, implanted fiducial markers (usually gold seeds or coils) are used. With respiratory gating, chest wall and lung motion are monitored during treatment to prevent underdosing of tumors. ART is a new technology that tracks not only organ position but also organ shape. Various forms of image guidance are enabling radiation oncologists to escalate tumor doses beyond the tolerance of adjacent normal tissues with precision and confidence.

Ultrasound Guidance

Daily ultrasound imaging of the prostate to guide radiation therapy has been used since 1998 and is probably the first widely used form of image guidance. The first commercially available system was the *B-mode Acquisition and Targeting System* (BAT), developed by the NOMOS Corporation (Best Nomos, Sewickley, PA). With this system, which "sees" the target in the same angle that the beam is delivered, the radiation therapist uses a handheld ultrasound probe to obtain axial and sagittal images of the target in the treatment room prior to therapy. The software then overlays the ultrasound images onto the CT scan used for treatment planning and the images are moved until they are aligned. Thereafter, the software calculates the shift needed to align the patient in the correct position. The system is accurate to within millimeters (2–6).

Ultrasound systems were initially used to localize the prostate, but their use is now being expanded to other sites including breast, pancreas, and liver cancers (7,8). Since the release of the BAT (from Best Nomos) system, several other ultrasound-based systems have been approved by the U.S. Food and Drug Administration and are used for ultrasound-based IGRT. These include the SonArray system from Varian (Best Nomos, Palo Alto,

CA), the ExacTrac Ultrasound from BrainLAB (BrainLAB, Inc., Westchester, IL), and the I-Beam system from CMS (Elekta AB, Stockholm, Sweden).

Stereoscopic X-Ray

EPIDs based on amorphous silicon technology were originally designed to provide filmless port images to document the radiation fields. These detectors have now been adapted to allow stereoscopic localization of the radiation target. Orthogonal kilovoltage x-rays can be used to verify and adjust patient setup on the treatment table prior to each fraction being delivered. For soft-tissue targets such as the prostate, an implanted fiducial marker or seed is used to visualize the location of the target. Compared with ultrasound-based IGRT, implanted seed marker prostate localization shows less variability and may result in less significant daily shifts (9). This may allow tighter expansion margins when this form of IGRT is used, resulting in less damage to the surrounding tissues.

Cone Beam Computed Tomography

Perhaps the gold standard for image guidance prior to radiotherapy is to perform a daily CT scan with the patient in the treatment position. The first systems to attempt this used a CT scanner "on rails," which could move into position around the actual treatment couch in the linear accelerator (LINAC) vault (10,11). Because it was not very practical, CT on rails system has not been widely implemented. Recently, a method of performing cone beam CT reconstructions has been developed using the EPID detectors that are already in place at many centers. This technology is part of what some vendors have called "on-board imaging" or OBI. With cone beam CT scanning, the gantry of the treatment unit rotates 360 degrees and acquires a limited kilovoltage CT image through the treatment area. The patient's position can then be matched to the treatment planning CT scan and an adjustment can be made to achieve optimal target coverage (12–14).

Megavoltage Computed Tomography

The term *megavoltage* applies to x-ray photon energies that exceed one million electron volts or 1 MeV. X-ray energies in this range are used for radiation therapy. Megavoltage CT refers to a CT image that has been reconstructed from data acquired during a scan using the LINAC itself as the source of x-rays. A separate kilovoltage (diagnostic energy) x-ray source is not used. The advantage to using megavoltage CT is that it does not require a separate kilovoltage x-ray source to be integrated into the gantry. The potential disadvantage is that megavoltage images, like port films, lack the contrast of regular x-rays, which makes these images more difficult to read. This is because of the physical properties of the megavoltage x-rays. Current advances in computerized image processing have made megavoltage scans suitable for IGRT.

Currently, the TomoTherapy Hi-Art system (TomoTherapy, Inc. Madison, WI) uses megavoltage CT to acquire pretreatment CT images using the same 6-MeV beam used for treatment. The resulting TomoImage is registered to the planning CT scan and patient shift is generated. In addition to linear shifts, the system allows for changes in the table roll as well. After the physician

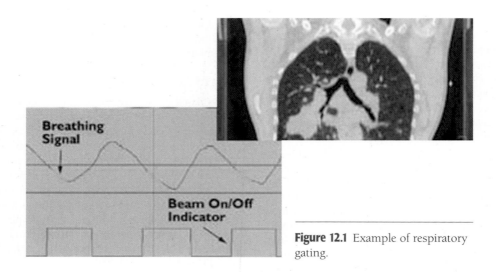

Figure 12.1 Example of respiratory gating.

approves the shift, the machine itself then automatically shifts the patient into the correct position prior to treatment (15–17).

Megavoltage CT capability has also been developed for other LINACs equipped with EPID detectors (18). The quality of the scans is expected to improve with time in this rapidly developing technology.

Respiratory Gating

Organ motion during respiration presents a problem for thoracic and abdominal malignancies treated with precision radiation therapy. As the diaphragm moves during inspiration and expiration, lung and abdominal tumors move as well. In the lung, this motion is most problematic in the middle and lower lobes. One solution to this problem has been to add a large craniocaudal margin to the planning volume to account for the respiratory excursion. The extra margin leads to the treatment of more normal tissues and increases the risk of complications. This is particularly important in the thorax, given that the lung is very sensitive to even low doses of radiation and the volume of lung tissue receiving 20 Gy should be kept at 20% or less.

One solution to this problem is to have the patient use a breath-hold technique. However, respiratory gating is a new technology that offers another solution to this problem (19–21). During this process, organ motion during the respiratory cycle is tracked and studied. Special software is used to allow treatment only during the portion of the respiratory cycle when there is less motion. Respiration is monitored during treatment using either x-ray images or a camera that detects abdominal wall motion. This technique typically requires a significant amount of patient training and cooperation (22). This process is illustrated in Figure 12.1. Several studies have shown significant dosimetric benefits compared with conventional nongated treatment (23,24). In one study, respiratory gating resulted in a reduction in the proportion of the tumor receiving less than the prescribed dose from 33% down to 9% (25). The studies also showed significant sparing of normal lung tissue (23,24). However, there have been no randomized clinical trials comparing the outcome of conventional radiotherapy with respiratory-gated treatment for lung cancer.

Adaptive Radiotherapy

One of the latest advancements in image guidance is adaptive radiotherapy (ART). Not only is organ motion tracked, but the actual organ shape is also recorded. Using CT images, the contours of the target and normal structures are captured and automatically deformed or adjusted prior to treatment. The treatment is then adapted to account for the actual shapes of the target and critical structures on that given day (26,27).

ART is most suited to treatment of targets whose size and shape are likely to change from day to day or from week to week. One example of this is prostate cancer. The position and shape of prostate varies from day to day depending on the contents of the bladder and especially the rectum. If the rectum is full of air and pushing the prostate anteriorly, more of the rectum may have received higher doses of radiation than anticipated. Similar changes can occur with daily variations in bladder content (28,29).

Currently, image guidance can be used to detect such changes and make manual adjustments to ensure adequate target coverage or minimize the dose to normal tissues (Figure 12.2). In the future, this process will be automatic. The prostate and rectal contours will be deformable and will be registered prior to daily treatment. The system will then replan the treatment so that it is optimized for that patient on that day according to the inverse plan parameters. This concept also applies to tumors that shrink during treatment as they respond to radiotherapy. We might expect significant shrinkage with lymphomas, small cell carcinomas, and possibly head and neck malignancies. ART limits damage to normal tissues adjacent to shrinking lung or head and neck tumors in a way that was never before possible.

SPECIALIZED RADIOTHERAPY DELIVERY SYSTEMS

There are several radiation therapy delivery systems that are used for specialized indications. Many of these are used to deliver highly focused radiation therapy to lesions involving the brain, lungs, or liver. Examples of this include the Gamma Knife (Elekta AB, Stockholm, Sweden), CyberKnife (Accuracy, Inc.,

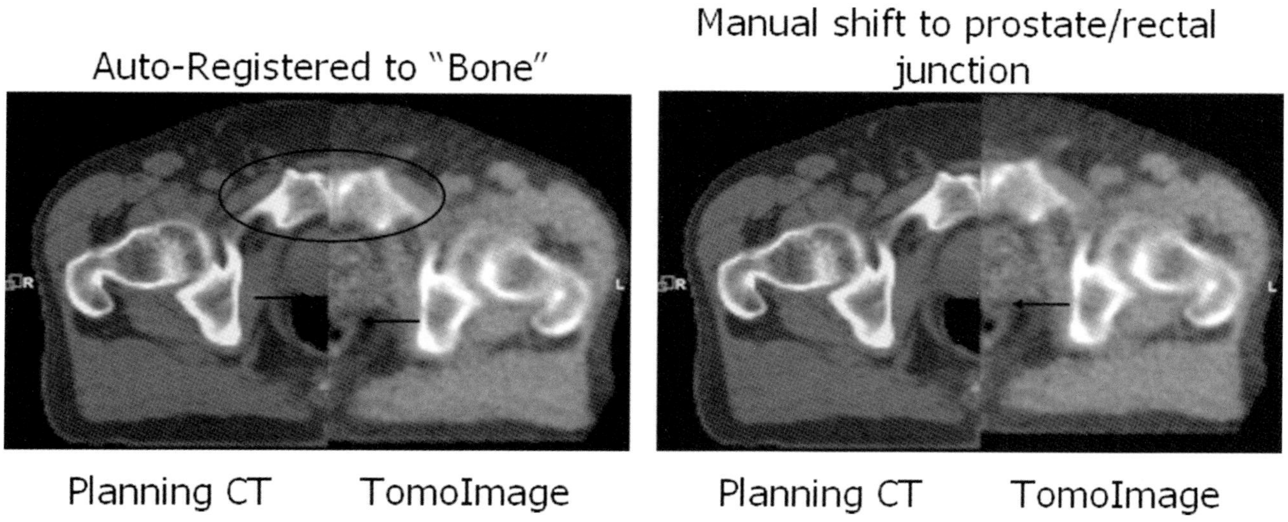

Figure 12.2 Adaptive radiotherapy: manual shift to align field to prostate/rectal interface.

Sunnyvale, CA), and a variety of LINAC-based radiosurgery systems. Helical Tomotherapy is a system in which radiotherapy is delivered while the patient moves through the treatment tube, which looks much like a diagnostic CT scanner. Patients can also be scanned prior to therapy, allowing for IGRT and eventually ART. There are also several proton treatment facilities around the world that offer this very specialized form of particle therapy. The unique physical properties of protons allow for very precise dose distributions. This type of therapy is well suited to treatment of tumors adjacent to critical structures. Protons are also well suited to treatment of pediatric malignancies because of the low dose to surrounding tissues.

Intraoperative Radiation Therapy

An obvious extension of radiation therapy technology includes the possibility of local electron beam therapy at the time of surgery. Intraoperative radiation therapy has been used in many trials but because of the enormous expense of building a radiation vault in or adjacent to a surgical operating suite, this modality is available only in a few institutions. The biologic principle is to deliver a single large dose of electron beam therapy to the tumor bed. The hope is that no further radiation will be needed to achieve the goal of eliminating local recurrences. New equipment is being developed that can deliver local superficial radiation that does not require the extensive shielding that a conventional LINAC requires. The consequence of having smaller machines, if they are found to be effective, is the limitless application in the clinical use of these units. Greater cooperation between surgeon and radiation oncologist will be necessary to take advantage of this modality.

Gamma Knife

The first system for stereotactic radiosurgery was invented by neurosurgeon Lars Leksell, MD, and was installed at the Karolinska Institute in Stockholm, Sweden, in 1968. He called this system the *Gamma Knife*. This form of noninvasive brain surgery has now been widely accepted as a less morbid alternative to open surgery in the treatment of brain metastases (30), as well as

numerous benign brain lesions including arteriovenous malformations (31), vestibular schwannomas (32), meningiomas (33), and pituitary adenomas (34). This 1-day treatment is usually delivered on an outpatient basis.

The Gamma Knife system uses 201 cobalt 60 sources that are all focused on a single isocenter. Lesions up to 3.5 cm can be treated using different-sized cylindrical collimators that are used to focus the gamma rays. A stereotactic localization ring is secured to the cranium during pretreatment CT scanning and treatment. This allows accurate 3D localization of the target. The accuracy of the system is <1 mm, which allows obliteration of the target while sparing adjacent normal brain tissue. There are currently more than 100 Gamma Knife centers in the United States and more than double that number of installations worldwide. To date, over 350,000 patients have been treated with this system.

Linear Accelerator-Based Radiosurgery

The limited availability of Gamma Knife units in some areas led to the development of LINAC-based systems to deliver single fraction radiosurgery to the brain (35). LINACs were initially fitted with cylindrical collimators to produce a "pencil beam" of radiation, which was then aimed at an intracranial target. The accelerator then delivered a series of treatment arcs at different table angles and resulting in a spherical dose distribution that is very similar to what is seen with GammaKnife treatment. Currently, most LINAC-based radiosurgery systems use mini-multileaf collimators to focus the radiation beam. These movable leafs can shape the target more accurately and allow the treatment of irregular targets using a single isocenter. Although there are vocal proponents of both LINAC-based systems and the Gamma Knife, both are capable of providing submillimeter accuracy with similar dose distributions and steep falloff (36).

CyberKnife

Robotics and image guidance have been incorporated into the CyberKnife system. A small LINAC in the head of the unit is controlled by a series of robotic arms with six degrees freedom.

This produces an extremely precise isodose volume that can be used to treat both intracranial and extracranial lesions. The system is able to track, detect, and correct for tumor and patient movement throughout the treatment (37).

TomoTherapy Hi Art

Tomotherapy Inc. has developed an integrated system for planning and delivery of precise image-guided, intensity-modulated radiation therapy (IGRT/IMRT). The system uses a megavoltage LINAC mounted in the gantry of a ring similar to a CT scanner. Using the treatment unit itself, a megavoltage CT scan is then obtained and compared with the pretreatment diagnostic CT used for planning. Craniocaudal, lateral, and vertical adjustments are then made to achieve the desired positioning. Because dose can be delivered from any angle along the gantry, the system gives better dose distributions than systems using five or seven fixed gantry angles to deliver "step and shoot" IMRT. The system is ideally suited to deliver ART (38) and is also capable of both intracranial and extracranial stereotactic radiosurgery.

Proton Therapy

Protons are nuclear particles with unique physical properties that allow excellent sparing of normal tissues adjacent to tumors. They differ from x-rays or photons in that there is much less exit dose after the beam has passed through the target. Protons are slightly more effective in "killing" (biological effectiveness) than photons but the drawbacks listed here limit their use. Protons are well suited for treating small lesions such as brain tumors and prostate cancers (39–41). They are also being used to treat pediatric malignancies, given the importance in limiting collateral radiation damage in children (42). Further improvement of the dose distributions is possible with intensity-modulated proton therapy that uses inverse planning. The main limitations to proton therapy are the limited number of treatment facilities, the high cost of the equipment and therefore the therapy, and the inability to treat large tumor volumes. To overcome the latter, proton therapy is frequently combined with conventional radiation therapy when regional lymphatics need to be treated.

BRACHYTHERAPY

The placement of radioactive materials into either organ tissues or cavities became known as *brachycurietherapy*, whereas the use of larger quantities of radioactive materials to treat patients at a distance was known as *telecurietherapy*. The latter evolved into *external-beam therapy* with the development of artificially produced radiation machines; the former is now known as *brachytherapy*.

In the early years of brachytherapy, sources were maintained in storage vaults or "Radium Safe," and custodians were employed to prepare the appropriate sources or applicators for each patient. As the incidental exposure to personnel and other patients became a concern because of the higher than expected leukemia rates in these custodians, equipment was developed to remotely deliver the sources to the patient's tumor treatment areas. With computer control, we now have a variety of delivery systems that allow for the intricate and precise treatment of various organs.

By virtue of the source strength, two modalities have become the most commonly used radioactive treatment methods: *low-dose-rate radiation* (LDR) and *high-dose-rate radiation* (HDR).

Low-Dose-Rate Radiation

The most commonly used isotopes for this type of treatment are radium 226, cesium 137, iridium 192, iodine 131, iodine 125, phosphorous 32, palladium 103a, and gold 198. The energies of the various isotopes vary considerably, and the radiation characteristics are specific for each isotope, thus providing the armamentarium for the radiation oncologist. One of the earliest reported uses of LDR was by a British surgeon, Sir Geoffrey Keynes, who published the successful use of radium needles for the treatment of breast cancer in 1937 (43). "Low dose rate" implies that the radiation deposition is slow, with treatment times ranging in days, weeks, or months.

The radioactive material can be prepared in various forms. In the early years, the radioactive material, mainly radium 226 or cesium 137, were encased in a needle that was then implanted into the tumor area. Calculations were then performed on the needles as they were distributed in the tissues. The treatment time to deliver the planned dose was calculated, and the implant was then removed at the appropriate time. Because the total dose in all volume implants is usually calculated at the perimeter of the tumor volume, the dose in the center of the volume is much higher. This physical factor is the main reason that the implanted tumor has a high likelihood of being destroyed. Defining the radiosensitivity and the actual extent of the tumor remains challenging.

The use of radioactive needles with its inherent high exposure to physicians and health care givers led to the development of afterloading techniques for both LDR and HDR treatments. Plastic catheters are introduced into tumor areas, the volume is defined, appropriate calculations are made, and then radioactive sources are ordered. These are then afterloaded into the catheters and the dose of radiation is given by leaving the source in place for the appropriate length of time. Cancers in various anatomic areas such as the head and neck, breast, prostate, extremities, and even intra-abdominal sites can be treated in this fashion.

Radioactive liquid gold 198 was used in the early years of brachytherapy for the local treatment of prostate cancer (44). The difficulties of containment, contamination, and dosimetry of this material made it less than ideal for wide clinical application. Small (0.75 × 3 mm) titanium seeds were developed that contain small quantities of either iodine 125 or palladium 103 isotopes. The strength of the material and the volume of the implanted organ determine the number of seeds required. Ultrasound guidance has allowed the placement of the seeds spatially in the prostate to deliver a high dose of radiation over a period of time ranging from 4 to 12 months, depending on the half-life of the isotope.

The half-life of an isotope is unique for each specific isotope. It is the time it takes for the radioactive material to decay to one-half its original strength. Thus, in approximately four half-lives, the majority of the dose is delivered to the implanted volume. Seed implants have been used in various sites, but because of dosimetry and safety reasons, prostate cancer is the most ideal malignancy treated in this manner. For a short period of time, pancreatic cancer was treated with seed implants. However, there was no impact on survival or local control; thus, this modality for pancreatic cancer has largely been abandoned.

High-Dose-Rate Radiation

Afterloading technology provided equipment that is capable of remotely delivering a very intense and hot source of iridium 192 to the implanted catheters in the tumor or target tissues. Because the source is strong, the dose delivery time is greatly reduced. This approach is known as *high-dose-rate brachytherapy*. More importantly, the exposure to hospital personnel and staff is markedly reduced. A 10 (or more) Curie source of iridium 192 is welded onto a chain that is guided into the implanted catheters by a remotely controlled and computerized system.

Brachytherapy for Breast Cancer

After segmental mastectomy, rows of Teflon catheters are placed into the tumor bed in single or multiple planes to provide intense doses of radiation to the volume designated as the area of highest risk of recurrence. This technique initially was devised to add a "boost" to the tumor-bearing area in a short period of time in conjunction with external-beam radiation. The potential long-term side effects include fibrosis and skin changes that may diminish the cosmetic advantage of breast-conservation therapy. The increased use of radiomimetic chemotherapy either neoadjuvantly or postoperatively may further increase the development of soft tissue changes.

Recently, brachytherapy employing this technique of catheter insertion has been used to treat the tumor cavity and surrounding tissue as the primary mode of adjuvant radiation therapy. Two fractions per day are given for 5 days as the only treatment to the tumor bed. In order to simplify the technique of brachytherapy, the MammoSite (Cytyc Corporation, Marlborough, MA) inflatable balloon technique was introduced. Here a balloon is inserted and inflated in the tumor cavity either under direct vision in the operating room immediately following segmental resection, or percutaneously employing ultrasound guidance within several days after operation. The catheter to which the balloon is connected is attached to a HDR transfer tube and after dose calculations are completed, 10 fractions of radiation are given in a fashion similar to that previously described. Again, adjuvant chemotherapy may influence the final cosmetic outcome.

Brachytherapy for Prostate Cancer

The advent of the prostate ultrasound technology led to the development of both LDR techniques with seeds or catheters and HDR techniques with varying dose schedules. These techniques were developed to deliver very precise and accurate doses to the prostate either as a boost or as primary treatment. Because of the location of the prostate (between bladder and rectum) and because of the high doses required to sterilize the prostate, the primary treatment of prostate cancer with HDR as monotherapy has seen limited use and is still considered to be experimental.

The most common technique is to combine external beam to 45 or 50.4 Gy to the surrounding tissues (and may include pelvic nodes, if indicated) followed by an implant HDR boost to the prostate. In our facility, we deliver three 6-Gy fractions over

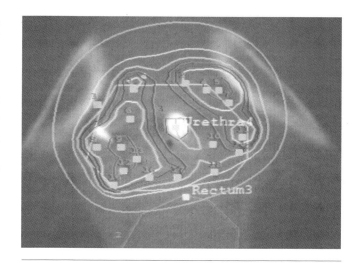

Figure 12.3 Isodose distribution of prostate as rendered on computed tomography planning film. (See color plates.)

a 36-hour period. The advantage of this technique is that the seminal vesicles can be implanted if there is disease extending into that area (Figures 12.3 to 12.6).

Although the future of this brachytherapy technique depends on comparisons with IMRT technology, this approach is very attractive in the treatment of prostate cancer because of the intensity of the radiation dose and the higher doses actually delivered to the tumor itself. With the advent of tumor mapping in the prostate with MRI-spectroscopy, the location of the tumor can be identified and additional "miniboost" doses can be added to that area simultaneously in the same treatment process (45).

Brachytherapy for Other Tumors

Wherever catheters and applicators can technically be placed, HDR brachytherapy can be delivered. To avoid missing an opportunity to provide benefit from this form of therapy, *pretreatment* consultation with a radiation oncologist is recommended

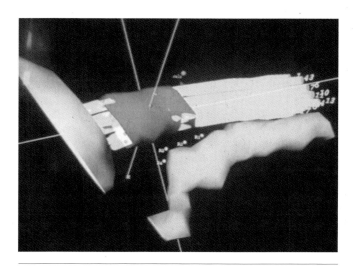

Figure 12.4 Three-dimensional reconstruction of implant from computed tomography-based dosimetry.

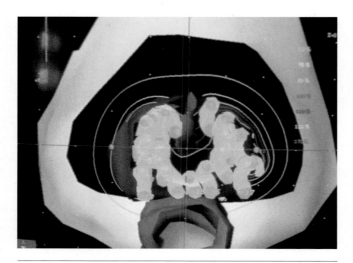

Figure 12.5 Three-dimensional reconstruction with superimposition of the dose distribution of prostate implant/high dose rate radiation.

to determine the applicability of brachytherapy in a given patient before the treatment plan is finalized. Other circumstances under which HDR techniques may be appropriate include primary treatment and retreatment of head and neck cancers, gynecologic cancers, and cancers of the esophagus, lung, and common bile duct. Brachytherapy may also be indicated in treatment of the tumor bed following resection of a soft-tissue sarcoma and in the management of large superficial skin cancers when electron or orthovoltage beams are not available.

HYPERTHERMIA

Hyperthermia has been used in conjunction with both radiation and chemotherapy when it appears to enhance the efficacy of both modalities (46). Hyperthermia causes the collapse of

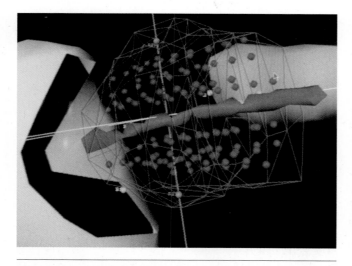

Figure 12.6 Spatial orientation of the source stops in the individual catheters during high-dose-rate delivery of the prescribed dose to the prostate.

tumor neovascularity and in turn increases the effectiveness of ionizing radiation. The tumor is heated by either microwaves or ultrasound to 42°C for a minimum of 45 to 50 minutes every 72 hours. Hyperthermia has not been approved for primary treatment of cancer except for superficial recurrences of malignant melanoma. Melanoma is highly sensitive to heat, and the combination of heat and radiation can be very effective (47). Unfortunately, most recurrences are systemic and deep, rather than superficial. For all other tumors, hyperthermia is used as a salvage modality when previous radiation already has been given. The use of low doses of radiation with hyperthermia (e.g., 300 cGy 2/week for 10 fractions plus heat) is equivalent to approximately 4,000 cGy of conventional therapy.

Unfortunately, clinically applicable technology to deliver heat to deep organs or sites is not currently available. In addition, the inability to measure temperature accurately in the tumor has impeded progress in this field. Several systems are under development to deliver heat to deeply seated sites and measure temperature, but these systems currently remain highly experimental and technical, so that hyperthermia in this setting is generally restricted to use in research institutions under strict guidelines.

Tumors that are currently best suited for hyperthermia need to be superficial, relatively small in size, and readily measured. Patients with recurrences of head and neck and chest wall recurrences from previous breast cancer comprise the largest groups of patients treated with hyperthermia. Hyperthermia can be delivered through small antennae, thus making this modality an excellent complement to interstitial HDR radiotherapy in those patients who have suitable tumors.

The side effects of hyperthermia are relatively minimal. Suitable patients for this therapy must have sufficient skin sensation to allow them to perceive and report any unusual increases in temperature. Microwaves are unpredictable and can form spots of intense heat, leading to thermal burns, emphasizing the necessity for patients to be able to report any sudden changes in temperature. Thus, patients with grafts (such as TRAM flap reconstructions) are not candidates for hyperthermia because of the anesthesia and lack of sensation in the area. The incidence of thermal burns is approximately 10%. When they occur, burns are treated with local ointments and, occasionally, resection of the damaged area.

TREATMENT WITH RADIOPHARMACEUTICALS

An array of radiopharmaceuticals has been available for many years. For the most part, these agents have been used in a palliative manner rather than for curative treatment. The most commonly used isotope is iodine 131, which has had a major impact in the management of thyroid cancer. By virtue of the natural incorporation of iodine into the cells of the thyroid, iodine 131 provides an "ideal" radiopharmaceutical that autokills the malignant cells once all normal thyroid has been ablated or resected.

Other radiopharmaceuticals that have been used include liquid radioactive gold 198 for injection into various tissues and cavities, phosphorus 32 for metastatic bone disease and intraperitoneal instillations, and strontium 90 for superficial topical treatments. The indications for use of these agents have markedly diminished with the advent of newer and less toxic agents.

Radioimmunotherapy, a new, evolving therapeutic modality, is a form of biologically targeted radiopharmaceutical treatment. Here an isotope (usually a high-energy beta-emitting isotope) is chemically bound to a target-specific monoclonal antibody or fragment. These compounds thus combine the target specificity of the humoral immune system with the cancer-killing capabilities of the high-energy isotope. The two agents that have been approved to date are yttrium 90-ibritumomab tiuxetan and iodine 131-tositumomab for the treatment of malignant B-cell lymphomas. Both target the CD-20 surface molecule on normal or malignant B-cells (48). Results to date are generally in the range of 20% to 40% complete response rates and 60% to 80% overall response rates. It should be noted, however, that these agents are currently being used in patients who have failed previous treatments and are not in de novo situations.

Future applications likely will include this technology either in combination or sequentially with chemotherapy and conventional external-beam radiation therapy. If, and when, genetically altered patterns in cells can be detected, and their genetic markers can be identified and targeted, the future use of radiation therapy in its many forms will greatly expand into the treatment of genetically altered tissues prior to frank malignant transformation.

CONCLUSIONS

Radiation oncology is a speciality that has dramatically progressed in this past century and is at the gates of another technological revolution. The current struggles, fears, and uncertainties of radiation therapy will be replaced by a confident, specific, and targeted modality that hopefully will eradicate malignant disease or even premalignant disease before the development of debilitating clinical manifestation and with minimal damage to normal tissues and structures.

REFERENCES

1. delRegato J. *Radiological Oncologists: The Unfolding of a Medical Specialty*. Reston, VA: Radiology Centenial, Inc.; 1993:241.
2. Lattanzi J, McNeely S, Pinover W, et al. A comparison of daily CT localization to a daily ultrasound-based system in prostate cancer. *Int J Radiat Oncol Biol Phys.* 1999;43:719–725.
3. Lattanzi J, McNeely S, Pinover W, et al. Ultrasound-based stereotactic guidance in prostate cancer: quantification of organ motion and set-up errors in external beam radiation therapy. *Comput Aided Surg.* 2000;5:289–295.
4. Morr J, DiPetrillo T, Tsai JS, et al. Implementation and utility of a daily ultrasound-based localization system with intensity-modulated radiotherapy for prostate cancer. *Int J Radiat Oncol Biol Phys.* 2002;53:1124–1129.
5. Little DJ, Dong L, Levy LB, et al. Use of portal images and BAT ultrasonography to measure setup error and organ motion for prostate IMRT: implications for treatment margins. *Int J Radiat Oncol Biol Phys.* 2003;56:1218–1224.
6. Langen KM, Pouliot J, Anezinos C, et al. Evaluation of ultrasound-based prostate localization for image-guided radiotherapy. *Int J Radiat Oncol Biol Phys.* 2003;57:635–644.
7. Fuss M, Salter BJ, Cavanaugh SX, et al. Daily ultrasound-based image-guided targeting for radiotherapy of upper abdominal malignancies. *Int J Radiat Oncol Biol Phys.* 2004;59:1245–1256.
8. Kuban DA, Dong L Cheung R, et al. Ultrasound-based localization. *Semin Radiat Oncol.* 2005;15:180–191.
9. Scarbrough TJ, Golden NM, Ting JY, et al. Comparison of ultrasound and implanted seed marker prostate localization methods: implications for image guided radiotherapy. *Int J Radiat Oncol Biol Phys.* 2006;65:378–387.
10. Cheng CW, Wong J, Grimm L, et al. Commissioning and clinical implementation of a sliding gantry CT scanner installed in an existing treatment room and early clinical experience for precise tumor localization. *Am J Clin Oncol.* 2003;26(3):e28–e36.
11. Ma CM, Paskalcv K. In-room CT technique for image-guided radiation therapy. *Med Dosim.* 2006;31(1):30–39.
12. Letourneau D, Wong JW, Oldham M, et al. Cone-beam-CT guided radiation therapy: technical implementation. *Radiother Oncol.* 2005 Jun;75(3):279–286.
13. Yin FF, Guan H, Lu W. A technique for on-board CT reconstruction using both kilovoltage and megavoltage beam projections for 3D treatment verification. *Med Phys.* 2005;32:2819–1826.
14. McBain CA, Henry AM, Sykes J, et al. X-ray volumetric imaging in image-guided radiotherapy: the new standard in on-treatment imaging. *Int J Radiat Oncol Biol Phys.* 2006;64:625–634.
15. Mackie TR, Kapatoes J, Ruchala K, et al. Image guidance for precise conformal radiotherapy. *Int J Radiat Oncol Biol Phys.* 2003;56:89–105.
16. Forrest LJ, Mackie TR, Ruchala K, T et al. The utility of megavoltage computed tomography images from a helical tomotherapy system for setup verification purposes. *Int J Radiat Oncol Biol Phys.* 2004;60:1639–1644.
17. Meeks SL, Harmon JF Jr, Langen KM, et al. Performance characterization of megavoltage computed tomography imaging on a helical tomotherapy unit. *Med Phys.* 2005;32:2673–2681.
18. Morin O, Gillis A, Chen J, et al. Megavoltage cone-beam CT: system description and clinical applications. *Med Dosim.* 2006;31:51–61.
19. Berson AM, Emery R, Rodriguez L, et al. Clinical experience using respiratory gated radiation therapy: comparison of free-breathing and breath-hold techniques. *Int J Radiat Oncol Biol Phys.* 2004;60:419–426.
20. Mageras GS, Yorke E. Deep inspiration breath hold and respiratory gating strategies for reducing organ motion in radiation treatment. *Semin Radiat Oncol.* 2004;14:65–75.
21. Rosenzweig KE, Yorke E, Amols H, et al. Tumor motion control in the treatment of non small cell lung cancer. *Cancer Invest.* 2005;23:129–133.
22. Kini VR, Vedam SS, Keall PJ, et al. Patient training in respiratory-gated radiotherapy. *Med Dosim.* 2003;28:7–11.
23. Butler LE, Forster KM, Stevens CW, et al. Dosimetric benefits of respiratory gating: a preliminary study. *J Appl Clin Med Phys.* 2004;5:16–24.
24. Underberg RW, van Sornsen de Koste JR, Lagerwaard FJ, et al. A dosimetric analysis of respiration-gated radiotherapy in patients with stage III lung cancer. *Radiat Oncol.* 2006;1:8.
25. Dietrich L, Tucking T, Nill S, et al. Compensation for respiratory motion by gated radiotherapy: an experimental study. *Phys Med Biol.* 2005;50:2405–2414.
26. Wu C, Jeraij R, Olivera GH, et al. Re-optimization in adaptive radiotherapy. *Phys Med Biol.* 2002;47:3181–3195.

27. Yan D, Lockman D, Martinez A, et al. Computed tomography guided management of interfractional patient variation. *Semin Radiat Oncol.* 2005;15:168–179.

28. Song W, Schaly B, Bauman G, et al. Image-guided adaptive radiation therapy (IGART): radiobiological and dose escalation considerations for localized carcinoma of the prostate. *Med Phys.* 2005;32:2193–2203.

29. Wu Q, Liang J, Yan D. Application of dose compensation in image-guided radiotherapy of prostate cancer. *Phys Med Biol.* 2006;51:1405–1419.

30. Mehta MP, Tsao MN, Whelan TJ, et al. The American Society for Therapeutic Radiology and Oncology (ASTRO) evidence-based review of the role of radiosurgery for brain metastases. *Int J Radiat Oncol Biol Phys.* 2005;63:37–46.

31. Maruyama K, Kondziolka D, Niranjan A, et al. Stereotactic radiosurgery for brainstem arteriovenous malformations: factors affecting outcome. *J Neurosurg.* 2004;100:407–413.

32. Lunsford LD, Niranjan A, Flickinger JC, et al. Radiosurgery of vestibular schwannomas: summary of experience in 829 cases. *J Neurosurg.* 2005;102(Suppl):195–199.

33. Kondziolka D, Niranjan A, Lunsford LD, et al. Stereotactic radiosurgery for meningiomas. *Neurosurg Clin North Am.* 1999;10:317–325.

34. Sheehan JP, Jagannathan J, Pouratian N, et al. Stereotactic radiosurgery for pituitary adenomas: a review of the literature and our experience. *Front Horm Res.* 2006;34:185–205.

35. Ulm AJ, Friedman WA, Bova FJ, et al. Linear accelerator radiosurgery in the treatment of brain metastases. *Neurosurgery.* 2004;55:1076–1085.

36. Solberg TD, Goetsch, SJ, Selch MT, et al. Functional stereotactic radiosurgery involving a dedicated linear accelerator and gamma unit: a comparison study. *J Neurosurg.* 2004;101(Suppl 3):373–380.

37. Welch WC, Gerszten PC. Accuray CyberKnife image-guided radiosurgical system. *Expert Rev Med Devices.* 2005;2:141–147.

38. Welsh JS, Patel RR, Ritter MA, et al. Helical tomotherapy: an innovative technology and approach to radiation therapy. *Technol Cancer Res Treat.* 2002;1:311–316.

39. Levin WP, Kooy H, Loeffler JS, et al. Proton beam therapy. *Br J Cancer.* 2005;93:849–854.

40. Cox JD. Proton beam radiation therapy in the treatment of cancer. *Clin Adv Hematol Oncol.* 2004;2:355–356.

41. Suit H, Goldberg S, Niemierko A, et al. Proton beams to replace photon beams in radical dose treatments. *Acta Oncol.* 2003;42:800–808.

42. Wilson VC, McDononough J, Tochner Z. Proton beam irradiation in pediatric oncology: an overview. *J Pediatr Hematol Oncol.* 2005;27:444–448.

43. Keynes G. Conservative treatment of cancer of the breast. *Br Med J.* 1937;2:643–647.

44. Elkins HD, Flocks RH, Culp DA. Evaluation of the use of colloidal radioactive gold in the treatment of prostatic carcinoma. *Radiology.* 1958;70:386–389.

45. Pickett B, Kurhanewicz J, Puliot J, et al. Three-dimensional conformal external beam radiotherapy compared with permanent prostate seed implantation in low-risk prostate cancer based on endorectal magnetic resonance spectroscopy imaging and specific antigen level. *Int J Radiat Oncol Biol Phys.* 2006;65:65–72.

46. Falk MH, Issels RD. Hyperthermia in oncology. *Int J Hyperthermia.* 2001;17:1–18.

47. Overgaard J, Gonzales D, Huslhof MCCM, et al. Randomized trial of hyperthermia as adjuvant to radiotherapy for recurrent or metastatic malignant melanoma. *Lancet.* 1995;345:540–543.

48. Pohlman B, Sweetenham J, Macklis RM. Review of clinical radioimmunotherapy. *Expert Rev Anticancer Ther.* 2006;6:445–461.

COMMENTARY
Oscar E. Streeter, Jr., and Janelle L. Park

Relatively recent improvements in imaging technology have given rise to great advances in the field of *radiation therapy*, with the ability to improve the delivery of tumoricidal doses while sparing the adjacent critical normal tissues. In radiation oncology, this is ultimately the limiting factor—delivering as much dose as possible to the tumor while simultaneously sparing the adjacent normal tissues to the greatest extent possible (1). With rapidly advancing technology, the delivery of ionizing radiation can only continue to dramatically improve with time.

ADVANCES IN EXTERNAL-BEAM RADIOTHERAPY

At present, a majority of radiation therapy plans are created using computed tomography (CT) images. The images, taken in the axial plane, are transmitted to radiation therapy treatment-planning computers. The target and adjacent critical normal structures are outlined on each slice. The two-dimensional slices are then summated and used to re-create the patient and outlined structures into three-dimensional volumes.

Three-dimensional conformal radiation therapy (3D-CRT) implies that CT images were used in creating a treatment plan that closely conforms to the target, while blocking as much of the adjacent normal tissues as possible. A subset of 3D-CRT is intensity-modulated radiation therapy (IMRT). IMRT, also CT-image based, often employs the use of a multileaf collimator, with motor-driven thin blocking leaves located in the treatment head of the linear accelerator. The location of the leaves is not static with a given field, and the leaves' positions are changed during administration of dose for one particular beam. This allows the creation of beamlets, in which, although the gantry position is unchanged, the leaf position is changed during the course of treatment for a given field. Thus, greater conformity to the target is possible using IMRT, which primarily provides decreased incidence and severity of side effects. This in turn may allow the administration of greater total dose to the tumor itself (2).

One caution to keep in mind: although IMRT is more technologically advanced than 3D-CRT, this does not necessarily automatically equate that it is superior. Although most commonly IMRT provides the superior plan, it is not always a universal truth, and sometimes with careful planning and evaluation, 3D-CRT may actually derive the "better" treatment plan. The radiation oncologist should carefully consider the various pros and cons of different treatment plans, and select the plan with the "best" dosimetry. An additional question, that has yet to be answered in radiation oncology trials, is whether the physics improvement of new technology result in an improved clinical outcome (3). One area of question is whether IMRT actually results in improved clinical outcomes over 3D-CRT is in the radiation treatment of prostate cancer, an organ centrally located, ideal for both the less expensive and less treatment planning and treatment intensive therapy of IMRT (4).

ADVANCES IN RADIOTHERAPY PLANNING

CT-based radiation therapy treatment planning has provided the ability to "see" the tumor and normal adjacent surrounding tissues in real three-dimensional space. With CT-based radiation therapy planning, nomenclature was developed in order to describe the target volume. The International Commission on Radiation Units and Measures (ICRU) Reports 50 and 62 provide the foundations by which radiation oncologists define the target volumes (5,6).

ICRU Report 50 established the definitions of gross tumor volume (GTV), clinical target volume (CTV), and planning target volume (PTV) as follows:

GTV: Gross Tumor Volume: gross extent of known malignant growth as determined by physical examination or imaging studies

CTV: Clinical Target Volume: incorporates the GTV + areas at high risk of microscopic, subclinical disease (regional nodal drainage)

PTV: Planning Target Volume: incorporates the CTV + margin for organ motion, patient motion, and daily setup errors

Subsequently, ICRU 62 refined the target volume concept by introducing the definition of an internal margin to take into account variations in size, shape, and position of the CTV. This is known as the *internal target volume* (ITV), which incorporates the CTV + margin that accounts for internal organ motion. In ICRU 62, the ITV is then expanded with a margin for daily setup errors and patient motion, and the PTV created.

Ultimately, coverage of the PTV by the prescribed dose is what is considered in evaluating any treatment plan. With 3D-CRT, the ability to generate dose-volume histograms with treatment planning arises. These essentially plot dose on the x-axis against percent volume on the y-axis, for the contoured organs. Coverage of the PTV is carefully considered, as well as careful evaluation of the amount of exposure to various normal tissue structures to different doses.

Regarding dose homogeneity, ICRU 50 recommends that dose coverage of the PTV fall within +7% and −5% of the prescribed dose. However, with current IMRT techniques, this level of homogeneity may not be attainable, and it is left to the radiation oncologist to decide whether the level of heterogeneity in a given plan is ultimately acceptable. A plan that exceeds the homogeneity constraints may still be approved, especially if the higher doses are located within areas of the PTV where a high concentration of malignant cells may be anticipated.

IMAGE GUIDANCE

Early development of image-guided radiation therapy began with electronic portal imaging devices. Digital images are taken of the patient's setup on a given day, and compared with the digitally reconstructed radiograph generated by the treatment planning system. The digital images are essentially low-quality x-ray films, and provide the opportunity to evaluate the location of the field relative to various bony landmarks; however, there is no ability to delineate or view the tumor, as the images are similar to x-ray films.

The ability to delineate daily where the target was located began with ultrasound imaging. This has been expanded now to include daily tracking of fiducial markers on x-ray imaging, as well as daily CT imaging to evaluate the location of the target and patient. With improved ability to "track" the target, this should allow tighter margins for the PTV, with decreased incidence and severity of associated side effects. In addition, this may ultimately allow increased tumor control probability with dose escalation.

RESPIRATORY GATING

With image-guided radiation therapy (IGRT), tumors with pronounced movement with respiration may be CT imaged during respiration, with "real-time" movement of the target recorded on the CT images. The radiation oncologist and physicist then create a treatment plan that allows dose delivery during selected parts of the respiratory cycle, when the target is within the open field (gated radiation therapy). This ideally decreases the chance of a "geographic miss," or having the tumor moving in and out of the field or under a block edge during treatment.

A second approach to IGRT is using the ICRU 62 definition of ITV (internal target volume). In this approach, the patient may be imaged by CT 5 days in a row, thus evaluating the variation in target location on a day-to-day basis. The CTV from each of these five scans may be summated to form a single ITV, and the ITV then expanded to provide the PTV for the treatment planning process. In this manner, daily variation in patient breathing and tumor location is accounted for, and a treatment plan is created that takes these factors into account.

SPECIALIZED RADIOTHERAPY DELIVERY SYSTEMS

Gamma Knife Stereotactic Radiosurgery

As the first system for stereotactic radiosurgery, the Gamma Knife has the longest history and established use (7). Because of the design of the system, it is limited to lesions in the brain. In addition, there are other treatment parameters that may limit its application: large tumor size, relatively low-lying lesion, and location adjacent to the optic chiasm or optic apparatus. Despite these limitations, Gamma Knife has a long-standing, well-established history in treating brain lesions. Most recently a Radiation Therapy Oncology Group study reported on the benefits of delivering a stereotactic boost after whole-brain radiation (WBRT) for patients with one to three brain metastases who had a lung primary, controlled systemic disease, and high functioning status. Patients who received a stereotactic radiosurgery boost (SBRT) were more likely to have a stable or improved Karnofsky Performance Status at 6 months' follow-up than were patients allocated to WBRT alone (43% vs, 27%, respectively; $p = 0.03$) with an improved median survival time of 6.5 versus

4.9 months ($p = 0.0393$). The interpretation showed that SBRT improved functional autonomy for all patients and survival for patients with a single unresectable brain metastasis. It is the author's conclusion that WBRT and SBRT boost should be standard treatment for patients with a single unresectable brain metastasis and considered for patients with two or three brain metastases (8).

CyberKnife Stereotactic Radiosurgery

CyberKnife allows much more freedom in delivering localized stereotactic radiation therapy. As the monoenergetic linear accelerator (6-MV photon) is mounted on a robotic arm with six degrees of freedom, the CyberKnife is not restricted to the brain, but instead is able to treat any location in the human body. In addition, there are fewer limitations in the size of lesions, and larger lesions and fields may be treated using the CyberKnife. As it is often employed in treating previously irradiated tissues, and with larger target volumes, treatment with the CyberKnife is often hypofractionated to a course of up to 5 days, as opposed to administering the prescribed dose in a single setting.

Currently, CyberKnife presents a different type of IGRT than that provided by such plans as respiratory gating. With the newest generation of CyberKnife, real-time tracking of the tumor by fiducial markers is possible during the treatment, with the machine compensating for real-time movement. Instead of turning the beam off and on as with respiratory gated IGRT, adjustments are made in real time for variations in tumor location with the head of the linear accelerator receiving feedback from infrared markers secured to a stretchable torso jacket, and it correspondingly moves up and down following the patient's respiratory inhalation and exhalation pattern. This capability to follow sine wave respiratory motion makes effective treatment of obstructive lung cancer lesions very effective with minimal toxicities (9).

Tomotherapy

Tomotherapy is perhaps one of the most interesting recent developments in radiation therapy. It is still relatively early in the clinical application of tomotherapy, and increased patient numbers and reports on long-term outcomes are eagerly awaited.

REFERENCES

1. Balter JM, Kessler ML. Imaging and alignment for image-guided radiation therapy. *J Clin Oncol.* 2007;25:931–937.
2. Galvin JM, De Neve W. Intensity modulating and other radiation therapy devices for dose painting. *J Clin Oncol.* 2007;25:924–930.
3. Lawrence TS. Think globally, act locally. *J Clin Oncol.* 2007;25: 921–923.
4. Huang D, Petrovich Z, Streeter OE. The incidence of late toxicity of six field conformal radiotherapy in the management of prostate cancer. *Radiology.* 2001;221:35–42.
5. International Commission on Radiation Units and Measurements. *ICRU Report 50: Prescribing, Recording, and Reporting Photon Beam Therapy.* Bethesda, MD: International Commission on Radiation Units and Measurements, 1993.
6. International Commission on Radiation Units and Measurements. *ICRU Report 62: Prescribing, Recording, and Reporting Photon Beam Therapy* (Supplement to ICRU Report 50). Bethesda, MD: International Commission on Radiation Units and Measurements, 1999. http://www.icru.org/n_992_4.htm.
7. Yamamoto M. Gamma Knife radiosurgery: technology, applications, and future directions. *Neurosurg Clin North Am.* 1999;10:181–202.
8. Andrews DW, Scott CB, Sperduto PW, et al. Whole brain radiation therapy with or without stereotactic radiosurgery boost for patients with one to three brain metastases: phase III results of the RTOG 9508 randomized trial. *Lancet.* 2004;363:1665–1672.
9. Kumar P, Streeter OE, Hagen J. Treatment of lung lesions is safe and effective with CyberKnife stereotactic radiotherapy: the thoracic experience at the University of Southern California. *Radiother Oncol.* 2006;81(Suppl 1):S493.

13

Surgical Consequences of Abdominal Irradiation

Leon Morgenstern

Radiation to the abdomen or pelvis administered in therapeutic doses for neoplastic disease can adversely affect the structure and function of any organ system or viscus in the path of the radiation beam (1–5). The severity of the damage incurred is determined by the radiation dose, the radiosensitivity of the tissue, the volume exposed, and a number of other factors that influence tissue vulnerability. This chapter reviews the broad spectrum of radiation injury to the intra-abdominal viscera, the factors influencing its occurrence and severity, the underlying pathologic processes, the clinical manifestations of radiation injuries, and their surgical management. Damage in tissues due to irradiation is manifested in pathologic tissue changes that are lifelong. Thus, clinical manifestations of injury, such as obstruction, ulceration, or fistulization, may occur many years after the completion of the radiotherapy. Also discussed in this chapter are preventive measures that can limit or obviate injury to vulnerable structures. Table 13.1 lists the neoplastic diseases for which abdominal or pelvic radiation therapy is often prescribed and the dosage ranges commonly employed in most treatment centers.

PREVALENCE OF RADIATION INJURY

The most widely accepted figure for radiation injury after treatment in the usual dosage range (45 Gy or 1.50 to 2.00 Gy 5 times weekly for 5 to 6 weeks) is 5%. This is often expressed as the *minimum tolerance dose* (TD 5/5), the dosage at which 5% of patents will manifest symptoms of radiation injury within 5 years after treatment (6). As dosage is increased for specific indications, such as salvage therapy in ovarian or uterine carcinoma, the prevalence of injury maybe expected to rise (7,8). The expression denoting the *maximum tolerance dose* (TD 50/5) is that dosage after which 50% of the patients treated will exhibit manifestations of injury within 5 years. Although this figure is approached in certain salvage regimens (9), no current therapeutic regimen results in such a high rate of injury.

Modern variations in radiation technique designed to lessen or minimize radiation injury include three-dimensional treatment planning, conformal radiotherapy, intensity-modulated radiotherapy, tomotherapy, hyperfractionation, and proton therapy (see Chapter 12).

ORGAN OR ORGAN SYSTEMS INVOLVED IN RADIATION INJURY AFTER ABDOMINAL IRRADIATION

The gastrointestinal tract is by far the organ system most vulnerable to abdominal irradiation. This is a function of its high rate of cell replication. It is this system that will be chiefly discussed in this chapter.

Other structures that may incur injury are the liver, pancreas, kidneys, ureter, and bladder. The surgical consequences of injuries to these structures are much less prevalent and are discussed briefly after injuries to various portions of the gastrointestinal tract.

Gastrointestinal Tract: Relative Vulnerability

The duodenum, jejunum, and ileum are the most radiosensitive segments of the gastrointestinal tract. Although the colon is moderately sensitive, significant injury to the ascending, transverse, and descending colon is relatively rare. The sigmoid colon, more likely to be included in the radiation field for pelvic malignancies, may incur significant damage. The rectum is the least radiosensitive of the gastrointestinal segments, but because it is frequently in the direct path of the radiation beam for gynecologic, prostatic, and rectal malignancies, it is often the site of significant injury.

Acute reactions are those that occur within 3 weeks to 2 months after treatment. They may include such disquieting symptoms as nausea, vomiting, and diarrhea, or more serious sequelae such as bleeding or obstruction. These are usually transitory. Late reactions denote more serious injury and are manifest from 6 months to many years after treatment.

The comparative radiation tolerances of the various components of the gastrointestinal tract are listed in Table 13.2.

Pathology of Radiation Injury to the Intestine

All elements of the intestinal wall suffer damage with ionizing radiation (10–14). The earliest injury is to the mucosa, where the cellular replication rate is the highest. The early changes are diffuse or multifocal ulceration with varying degrees of damage to the surface and crypt epithelium. These early changes seldom, if

Table 13.1

Neoplasms Treated by Abdominal Abdominopelvic Irradiation

Condition	Dose Range (Gy)
Bile duct carcinoma	30–50
Pancreatic carcinoma	45–60
Ovarian carcinoma	45–70
Uterine carcinoma	45–75 (implant)
Cervical carcinoma	45–75 (implant)
Bladder carcinoma	40–60
Rectal carcinoma	45–60
Anal carcinoma	50–75 (implant)
Prostatic carcinoma	50
Hodgkin's Disease	30–45
Seminoma	20–30
Lymphoma	3000–4500
Wilm's Tumor	45–60
Neuroblastoma	45
Rhabdomyosarcoma	45
Liposarcoma	45–70

ever, require surgical intervention. The regenerated mucosa, in all parts of the irradiated gastrointestinal tract, exhibits cells with bizarre nuclear changes, varying degrees of structural aberration. The permanently altered mucosa results in decreased absorptive capacity and increased susceptibility to mechanical injury, especially in the stomach and colon, which are subject to friction by solid contents within them. Trauma to the vulnerable mucosa may be the initiating event in the development of ulceration leading to surgical complications. In the small intestine, the villi are blunted and irregular, with altered absorptive capacity.

Radiation-induced changes in the submucosa are of greater surgical consequence than the mucosal changes. The submucosa undergoes diffuse hyalinization, and telangiectasia of lymphatic, venous, and arterial channels. Bizarre fibroblasts known as *radiation fibroblasts* are scattered in the collagenous matrix. It is the dense collagenization of the submucosa that gives the "stiffened" character to the radiation-damaged intestine.

All vascular elements, including capillaries, arteries, and veins of all sizes suffer the effects of irradiation. The principal damage is to the endothelium, which responds by intimal proliferation and progressive hyalinization, often to the point of luminal obliteration. Richter et al. (15) have postulated a decrease in endothelial anticoagulant substances, normally present in endothelium, as a factor leading to the vascular damage. Progressive endarteritic changes are responsible for the late occurrence of ischemic necrosis and segmental infarction of the bowel wall, a catastrophic complication.

The muscularis propria does not exhibit the severe changes seen in the mucosa and submucosa. There are scattered foci of collagen deposition, radiation fibroblasts, and some disruption of the normal architecture. The basic structural integrity of the muscularis, however, is not significantly altered.

Alterations of the serosal surface also have major surgical consequences. These are probably the most frequent pathologic changes encountered by the surgeon on opening the abdomen for a complication of radiotherapy. The serosa, which has a normal thickness of 1 to 2 microns, may, in its altered state measure 10 microns or more. The thickened serosa or "peel" is dense collagenous tissue, infiltrated with radiation fibroblasts. In the presence of surgically induced adhesions, the serosal reaction promotes an agglutination of adjacent loops, rendering them difficult or impossible to separate without serious risk of inadvertent enterotomy. The serosal thickening also gives the radiation-injured bowel its "parboiled" appearance, with occasional mottling due to the irregular deposition of collagen and areas of telangiectasia. The tightly coiled, agglutinated loops are most frequently encountered within or just above the pelvis. Dense fibrotic adherence to all structures within the pelvis can render the dissection extraordinarily difficult. At risk are the bladder, rectum, iliac vessels, and ureters, which may be involved in the fibrotic process or "fused" to the fibrotic peel of the affected intestinal loops. Fistulization may occur as enterocutaneous, enteroenteral, enterovesical, enterovaginal, or enterorectal fistulas.

Table 13.2

Radiation Tolerances of Parts of the Gastrointestinal Tract

Organ	Injury	Min./Max. Tolerance Dose (cGy) (TD 5/5) (TD 50/5)
Esophagus	Ulcer, stricture, perforation	6000–7500
Stomach	Ulcer, perforation	4500–5500
Small intestine	Ulcer, stricture, fistula, infarction, perforation	4500–6500
Colon	Ulcer, stricture, fistula	4500–6500
Rectum	Ulcer, stricture, fistula	5500–8000

Adapted from Rubin and Casarett.[6]

Stomach

The stomach, although not as radiosensitive as the small intestine, can be the site of sequelae that require surgical intervention. The two most frequent complications are bleeding and ulceration.

Bleeding may occur from diffuse focal erosions or small ulcerations, chiefly in the distal stomach. Beneath the atrophic mucosa, embedded in the hyalinized submucosa, lies a complex of telangiectatic vessels that are subject to exposure and erosion. Bleeding from this source is not massive but constant, requiring increasingly frequent blood replacement by transfusion. This type of intractable bleeding from diffuse injury requires surgical intervention if it does not respond to medical measures (discussed later).

Chronic gastric ulcer, manifested clinically by intractable pain and occasionally by massive bleeding episodes, also may require surgical intervention. The chronic radiation ulcer can resemble the chronic peptic ulcer, but is characterized by the typical radiation-induced changes seen on histologic examination. Bleeding, at times of massive proportions, results if a major arterial or venous vessel is exposed deep within the ulcer. The radiation-induced ulcer is most commonly seen in the distal stomach, the usual site of maximal exposure to radiation. It does not ordinarily respond to medical measures. Perforation due to radiation injury is not a frequent occurrence, although it has been reported. In contrast to the small intestine, the vascular supply of the stomach is more extensive, generally precluding infarction, necrosis, and perforation due to endovascular occlusion. The thickness of the gastric wall and decreased acid-pepsin levels are also factors in the less-than-expected incidence of free perforation from radiation-induced ulcer. Worthy of mention, however, is the perforation of the stomach that occurs following irradiation of some gastric lymphomas in which the radiosensitive neoplasm, involving the full thickness of stomach wall, is totally destroyed. The surgical consequence—free perforation of the involved stomach—is an acute abdominal catastrophe.

Gastric erosions and ulcers in the irradiated stomach are not exactly analogous to their acid-peptic counterparts in the nonirradiated stomach. A treatment for peptic ulcer earlier in the lasts century was gastric irradiation in a dosage range of 25 Gy. This effectively decreased gastric acidity by sufficient damage to the parietal cells to heal some peptic ulcers. At higher dosage levels in the irradiated stomach the acid-peptic factors are still operative, but to a lesser extent. Equally important factors favoring ulceration in the irradiated stomach are the atrophic, easily injured mucosa with its impaired reparative ability, the pre-existent hyalinization of the submucosa, and the vascular changes within the gastric wall, all accentuating the tendency to extension of the destructive process.

For bleeding or ulceration, intense medical measures should be employed before surgical treatment is undertaken. These include all current therapies such as H$_2$ blockers, omeprazole, sucralfate, and endoscopic coagulation of focal bleeding sites, where accessible. For chronic blood loss unresponsive to iron therapy, occasional transfusions are of lesser risk than major extirpative surgery, especially in elderly or debilitated patients.

When intractable pain, progressive blood loss, or episodes of massive bleeding are unmanageable with medical measures,

resection of the affected gastric segment is the surgical treatment of choice. Distal gastrectomy should include as much of the damaged stomach as possible or feasible, from the pylorus to grossly proximal normal stomach. The choice between a Billroth I or II type of reconstruction will depend on conditions at operation. Anastomoses constructed with irradiated tissues are always precarious and should be done meticulously, whether hand-sewn or stapled. Carefully done, there is no advantage of one type of anastomosis over the other. Anastomoses—whether of the Billroth I or II type—should be under no tension whatsoever. Ease of approximation without tension may influence the decision between a Billroth I and II reconstruction. Hand-sewn anastomoses should be marked at their extremities with hemoclips for ease of radiologic identification later. Postoperative nasogastric suction is advisable for 48 to 72 hours to ensure decompression of the stomach and to detect postoperative bleeding. Resumption of oral intake is not recommended before 5 days. Thereafter, progression to the usual postgastrectomy dietary regimen should be allowed as tolerated.

Small Intestine

The small intestine is the most frequent site of radiation-induced injuries that require surgical intervention within the abdomen (16,17). The indications for surgical intervention include intractable bleeding, obstruction, ulceration, fistulization, and infarction-necrosis with perforation. Any or all of these may exist alone or in combination.

Bleeding as a primary reason for operation on the irradiated small intestine is unusual, although possible, from either a focal or diffuse source. Bleeding from a unifocal site is generally due to deep ulceration into a major mesenteric vessel. An even rarer source of hemorrhage has been reported wherein a primary aortoduodenal fistula developed between the fourth portion of the duodenum and the abdominal aorta 20 years following radiotherapy and para-aortic lymph node dissection for seminoma (18).

The most common indication for surgical intervention in the irradiated small intestine is obstruction, usually occurring within 6 months to 2 years after radiotherapy, but possible even decades later. The obstructive episode may be acute, complete, and strangulating or, as more commonly encountered, multiple recurrent episodes, finally unmanageable by nonoperative therapy.

The etiologic mechanism has already been described in the discussion of the pathology of radiation injury. The hyalinized, stiffened submucosa and serosa impair motility; the presence of adhesions secondary to prior operations sets the stage for an adhesive enteropathy in which loops of bowel become entrapped in a complex of narrowed, convoluted loops, with progressive endoluminal compromise as the fibrosis advances. The initiating mechanism of individual obstructive episodes is often difficult to identify, as is also the case with nonirradiated bowel. However, once initiated, the obstructive process feeds on itself and worsens, with progressive dilatation of proximal fluid-filled loops and impaired peristaltic ability. The latter results in failure to propel the intraluminal contents distalward beyond the constricted lumina. If the obstruction is acute, complete, or strangulating, early or immediate surgical intervention is indicated. More often, the obstructive episodes are chronic, recurrent, and increasingly difficult to resolve by medical measures.

The most common site for the obstruction just described is in the pelvis because this is the site where the small bowel is subjected to most irradiation in the more commonly used regimens. It is also the site where postoperative adhesions and confinement of the small bowel within a small space predisposes to radiation injury. Similar phenomena of "agglutinated," obstructive loops may be found adherent to the anterior abdominal wall along the site of surgical incision or to the retroperitoneum, where the bowel has become adherent to deperitonealized areas. Such adhesions occur with para-aortic lymph node dissection or resection of retroperitoneal tumors.

If strangulation is not suspected on the basis of physical findings, the first therapeutic measures should be conservative. Cessation of oral intake and intubation-suction may be all that is necessary to circumvent operation when the obstruction is early or incomplete. Long intestinal tubes with a weighted bag designed to facilitate passage of the tube distalward (such as the Cantor and Miller-Abbot tubes) were effective means of intestinal decompression before the use of metallic mercury was prohibited. Barium has proved a poor substitute for mercury in the weighted bag, but it works occasionally. Nasogastric intubation is second best in this situation but may suffice to override the acute situation and avoid operation.

If operation cannot be avoided, the administration of broad-spectrum antibiotics preoperatively is recommended. Informed consent should always include possible intestinal resection and the possibility of an enteric stoma, if there is any likelihood of such a necessity in the surgeon's judgment. If the obstructive mechanism is in the pelvis or near the pelvic brim, the ureters should be catheterized.

It is best to avoid incision into heavily irradiated skin to avoid postoperative wound-healing problems. Entry into the peritoneal cavity should be exceedingly cautious to avoid inadvertent enterostomy. The laparoscopic approach to radiation-induced intestinal obstruction is not recommended.

The course of action after the offending pathology is identified depends on the individual situation. In the rare event that the obstructive mechanism is simple and involves lysis of some adhesions easily amenable to lysis, resection of bowel should be avoided. In such situations, particular attention should be paid to the possibility of small enterotomies or fistulae, which may be difficult to discern on casual inspection, but if overlooked can be catastrophic postoperatively. The long tube also served a useful purpose following lysis of adhesions, inasmuch as methylene blue could be instilled into the intestinal lumen and extravasation could be identified easily.

More commonly, the finding is one of an aggregation of tightly coiled loops, densely adherent to one another in a conglomerate mass, through which no plane can be identified. It is a mistake in this setting to proceed with lengthy, extensive, difficult lysis of adhesions, often with multiple accidental superimposed enterotomies. Even if successful, this mode of dealing with radiation-induced obstruction only sets the stage for a later intervention, which is rendered even more difficult and of greater risk to the patient. If a discrete group of involved loops can be seen and dissected from contiguous tissues as a unit, it

is preferable to resect this obstructive complex and anastomose unobstructed, relatively uninvolved bowel to its distal counterpart. If the obstructive mass is in the vicinity of the ileocecal valve, it is wiser to resect the terminal ileum and perform an ileocolic anastomosis rather than to preserve a small segment of ileum proximal to the ileocecal valve. The latter type of anastomosis does not function well. Anastomosis may be hand-sewn in the usual fashion or constructed with intestinal staplers. They may be end-to end, if the lumina are adequate, or side-to-side (functional end-to-end), depending on the operator's preference. Both reconstructions function well. The extremities of the anastomosis should be marked with hemoclips.

Bypass of the affected, obstructive loops should be performed only in the rare circumstance wherein resection poses unacceptable risks of morbidity and mortality. Leaving the bypassed, radiation-damaged intestine poses a lifelong risk for later complications.

There should be no undue hurry in discontinuing nasogastric suction in the postoperative period. Only when there is indication of effective peristalsis through the newly constructed anastomosis should oral feeding be begun, usually not before a minimum of 5 days. If delay further than 7 days is necessary for any reason before oral feeding is resumed, supplemental parenteral nutrition should be considered. In nutritionally depleted patients, parenteral nutrition should be initiated preoperatively and continued until caloric intake is adequate.

Fistulization

The radiation-damaged small intestine is prone to fistulization in a manner akin to that seen with granulomatous enteritis. Although not as common as obstruction, fistulization may occur between loops, into the colon, rectum, vagina, bladder, or through the skin. Enteroenteral fistulas in themselves need not be an indication for surgery if they are asymptomatic. Fistulas at the other sites mentioned require surgical intervention. Enterocutaneous fistulas may occur in the immediate or late postoperative period from anastomotic leaks or minute enterotomies. If the source is from a radiation-damaged loop, they rarely close spontaneously.

A principle to remember in radiation-induced enteric fistulas is that they cannot be managed by simple closure. Such closures inevitably fail; after a short, delusive, apparently successful interlude then a larger fistula usually results. The loop involved in the fistula must be resected and the bowel segments carefully approximated in the manner previously mentioned. Enterocutaneous fistulas secondary to radiation injury and associated operative procedures rarely close with nonoperative therapy, unless they are very minute. When enterocutaneous fistulas occur in the context of advanced malignancy, management by enterostomal therapy and nutritional support are kinder than an aggressive resective approach to therapy.

Ulcer

Small intestinal ulcers as a consequence of radiation are rare. They are probably due to focal vascular compromise, generally extending deep into the muscularis propria. In this setting, they may be the source of an intractable bleed, or by associated cicatrization and luminal constriction, the cause of obstruction. In either event, the indication is for segmental resection. Conservative measures are of little avail.

Infarction, Necrosis, and Perforation

This trio of complications represents the ultimate catastrophe in radiation injury to the small intestine. It is the end stage of progressive endoluminal vascular occlusion of larger feeding vessels to an intestinal segment or segments. Infarction may be in a single or multiple segments.

The natural history of infarcted intestine is well known. The sequelae are full-thickness necrosis and ultimate perforation. There is no room for expectant treatment, because the clinical picture is one of an acute abdomen with progressive sepsis. The sequence of infarction, necrosis, and perforation is usually a late complication associated with severe radiation damage. It is more frequent in the pelvis than in the upper abdomen. The only definitive treatment is by resection of the affected segment or segments.

Predisposing Factors

Among the factors that are considered conducive to radiation injury are body habitus, malnutrition, generalized vascular disease (e.g., diabetes, arteriosclerosis), concomitant chemotherapy, and rare genetic syndromes (e.g., ataxia-telangiectasia, Fanconi anemia). The most important factor by far, however, is postoperative fixation and decrease in mobility of loops by postoperative adhesions. This is most pronounced in the pelvis, in the region of the incision, and in the retroperitoneum. The pelvis is by far the most common site.

Obesity may be a contributing factor if it interferes with accurate delineation of the radiation ports and direction of the beam. Ultimately, the most potent factor influencing radiation damage is the radiation dosage. As the dose approaches levels above the 4,500 to 5,000 cGy level, increasing degrees of radiation damage can be predicted with certainty.

Although some relationship of late radiation injuries to severe symptoms encountered during the original therapy has been suspected, evidence for this is anecdotal and difficult to document. There are no convincing long-term studies to substantiate such a conclusion. On the basis of anecdotal evidence, however, it is advisable to interrupt therapy in the face of severe adverse symptoms that occur early in the treatment regimen.

Preventive Measures

Preventive measures should begin before institution of radiotherapy, principally in the operating room. Areas of peritoneal denudation should be reperitonealized as completely as possible in the pelvis and retroperitoneum. Although this does not obviate postoperative adhesions, it lessens their number and density.

Various measures have been tried to exclude the small bowel from the pelvis, all with questionable success and some with serious shortcomings. Among the simplest, if omentum is available, is the positioning of as much omentum into the pelvis as possible, with fixation to pelvic sidewalls or pelvic brim (19). However, this maneuver is helpful only if the omentum is plentiful and mobile. It is not available in some operations for pelvic malignancy, either because of prior removal or indicated removal concurrent with the operation.

The placing of packing or prosthetic devices in the pelvis to exclude the small intestine during the course of radiotherapy has not been widely accepted. Among the devices used have been plain packing, silicone prostheses (20), and foam rubber prostheses shaped to conform to and fill the pelvis. These are removed in a second stage after completion of radiotherapy. They are not recommended.

In vogue in recent years has been the construction of an absorbable mesh barrier at the pelvic brim to exclude the intestine from the pelvis (21–23). The sheet of mesh, either polyglycolic acid or polyglactin, is tacked to the edges of the pelvic inlet as tautly as possible. It has been shown to retain its tautness for sufficient time to complete the radiotherapy, after which the absorption of the material allows the small bowel to again descend into the pelvis. No convincing evidence of the effectiveness of this maneuver based on a large series of cases has been published, and the method has some disadvantages. The mesh itself is desmoplastic, inducing a dense fibrous reaction to structures with which it is in contact. This can render future operation extraordinarily difficult. Secondly, defects in the mesh barrier can and do occur, either at the sutured edges or in the substance of the mesh itself, allowing herniation of loops through dangerously small openings. Nevertheless, it is an operative maneuver still in the process of evaluation and deserves continuing consideration.

During radiotherapy, several steps have been suggested or adopted to lessen the likelihood of injury. It is now routine in a number of treatment centers to perform a small bowel series with a mixture of barium and gastrografin during the planning simulation of therapy. With predetermined knowledge of areas of small bowel fixation, it is possible to alter position, ports, and radiation fields, or to interpose blocks or other barriers to avoid, if possible, direct irradiation of fixed immobile loops.

Hyperfractionation of radiation treatments (e.g., divided doses twice daily rather than a single dose daily) has had limited acceptance in a few centers only. The difficult logistics of multiple daily treatments for a questionable benefit ratio has not yet justified a more generalized use of fractionation.

The history of radioprotective agents has not been encouraging. Among the classes of drugs used have been the thiophosphates, prostaglandin antagonists, antiproteases, and antioxidants. None of these has proven dependable. The latest drug that does show some promise is amifostine (24,25), a cytoprotective agent now used as an adjunct in cancer chemotherapy and radiation therapy. It is administered only by the intravenous route. Favorable results have been reported.

The use of elemental diets, total parenteral nutrition, cholestyramine, and other nutrition modifiers have not been shown to be unequivocally useful.

Colon and Rectum

The ascending, transverse, and descending colon are seldom the site of radiation damage except in instances of extreme radiosensitivity or unusually high dosage. The sigmoid and rectosigmoid colon, however, may suffer the same sequelae and surgical consequences as indicated for the small intestine, but with much less frequency. Conditions in which the rectosigmoid or sigmoid may be damaged during radiotherapy are in management of gynecologic malignancies and carcinoma of the rectum, anal canal, and prostate.

The rectum is the most frequently injured segment of the lower gastrointestinal tract, despite its lesser sensitivity to radiation damage as compared with the small intestine (26). The vulnerability of the rectum is a consequence of its fixation, its high exposure to the radiation beam, and the frequent use of booster dosages in the treatment of pelvic malignancies (27).

The most frequently encountered consequence of radiation injury to the rectum is bleeding. Radiation proctitis is best diagnosed by proctoscopy and is recognized by the granular, hyperemic, and friable rectal mucosa. Such proctitis occurring soon after the initiation of therapy is usually well managed by topical therapy or endoscopic treatment of focal bleeding points with laser or electrocoagulative therapy. Late, persistent, or chronic proctitis is more difficult to manage. Pain, tenesmus, and steady blood loss may require surgical intervention in addition to all medical measures.

There are many topical agents useful in radiation proctitis that may be effective in controlling mild or moderate cases. These include sucralfate (28), hydrocortisone enemas, sodium pentosanpolysulfate (PPS), and even formalin (29). Severe proctitis may not be relieved and may require fecal diversion, although colostomy alone may still not fully alleviate symptoms or control blood loss. Focal ulceration with bleeding has been managed successfully with laser or electrocoagulation. Medical measures as previously mentioned should also be employed concurrently. Hyperbaric oxygen therapy has been advocated recently in the treatment of radiation injury, with some reports of beneficial results (30,31).

In order of severity, the next major complication in the rectum is the chronic rectal ulcer. These are characteristically on the anterior rectal wall, shallow in depth, circumscribed by a zone of induration, and exhibiting a necrotic grayish-yellow base. The ulcer may bleed or give rise to severe pain. Conversely, they may be entirely asymptomatic. Most ulcers respond to topical therapy in time, but others may require fecal diversion.

Radiation-induced strictures may be found in the rectum or rectosigmoid as a consequence of ulceration with healing or more diffuse circumferential injury. Neoplastic involvement should always be suspected and sought endoscopically during study of the stricture. Strictures of early onset usually have an acute inflammatory component that will respond to nonsurgical measures. Higher grade strictures of later onset require fecal diversion or an extirpative procedure.

Rectovaginal fistula is the most common fistula that complicates radiation injury to the rectum. More severe grades of fistulization involve the bladder, buttocks, and even the retroperitoneum. Radiation-induced fistulas do not respond to nonoperative measures. The least extensive surgical procedure is a diverting colostomy, which may result in the healing of the less severe cases. The more severe cases require complex reconstructive tissue transfer procedures for permanent cure in addition to fecal diversion, if permanent closure of the fistula is to be obtained.

Proctectomy and Colostomy

The radiation-damaged rectum, whether involved with intractable bleeding, ulceration, stricture, or fistula may require proc-

tectomy as the definitive procedure. Low rectal anastomoses in the presence of radiation injury are always precarious, and in the majority of instances should be protected with a proximal colostomy.

If the colostomy is performed in the sigmoid colon, which is generally the most easily accessible and best functional site for such a stoma, there is likelihood that the sigmoid may also have been in the path of the radiation beam. Special attention must therefore be given to the creation of the stoma to avoid serious complications.

If at all possible, the stoma should not be placed in an area of skin that has been irradiated. The colonic mucosa should not be sutured flush with the abdominal wall but at least 2 or 3 cm should be allowed to protrude as a rosette. Stomata within irradiated bowel have a great tendency to retract and segmental or circumferential necrosis may occur if there has been vascular compromise or there is tension on the exteriorized bowel.

The rules of postoperative colostomy care then pertain as usual. The stoma should be observed daily for circulatory sufficiency and viability. Excessive digital examination and dilatation should be avoided.

Damage to Other Intra-Abdominal or Retroperitoneal Structures

Collateral damage secondary to radiation to organs or structures outside the gastrointestinal tract during abdominal radiation are rarely of surgical consequence.

The liver, pancreas, kidneys, and bone marrow may be affected to a greater or lesser degree, depending on the radiation dosage absorbed by them. For a detailed discussion of the effects on these organs, the reader is referred to other sources (1,2,4,5).

MAXIMS IN THE MANAGEMENT OF RADIATION ENTEROPATHY

1. Operation should always be a measure of last resort.
2. Optimal nutritional status should be achieved preoperatively.
3. Incision into heavily irradiated areas of skin should be avoided. Dilated bowel should be decompressed preoperatively, by long tube if possible.
4. Antibiotic bowel preparation should be done preoperatively and broad-spectrum parenteral antibiotics should be given postoperatively.
5. Resection of severely damaged bowel is more definitive than bypass, but judgment at the time of operation should determine this decision.
6. Excessive adhesiolysis should be avoided. It rarely is definitive treatment for obstructive enteropathy; it may aggravate it and risks fistula formation.
7. Hand-sewn, stapled, end-to-end, or side-to-side anastomoses are equally effective, but each requires meticulous fashioning. Anastomoses in radiation-damaged bowel are precarious.

8. Anastomosis should be identifiable either by staple lines in stapled anastomoses or by hemoclips in hand-sewn anastomoses.

9. Oral feeding should be delayed until effective peristalsis returns and the anastomosis is functional. A minimum 5-day delay is recommended.

10. Low rectal anastomoses in irradiated bowel should be protected against leaks with a proximal colostomy for maximum safety.

11. Intestinal stomas made with irradiated bowel or in irradiated skin are prone to complications. An ample segment should be exteriorized.

12. Radiation-induced fistulas rarely respond to nonoperative therapy or simple closure. Resection or tissue transfer is usually necessary. Bypass exclusion is an option, although it is less desirable.

REFERENCES

1. Trott K-R, Herrmann T. Radiation effects on abdominal organs. In: Scherer E, Streffer C, Trott K-R, eds. *Medical Radiology.* New York: Springer-Verlag; 1991:313–346.
2. Fajardo LF. Sequelae. Morphology of radiation effects on normal tissues. In: Perez CA, Brady LW, eds. *Principles and Practice of Radiation Oncology,* 2nd ed. Philadelphia: JB Lippincott; 1992:50–63, 114–123.
3. Cox JD, Ang KKE, eds. *Radiation Oncology: Rationale, Technique, Results.* St. Louis: Mosby; 2003.
4. Mettler FA Jr, Upton AC, ed. *Medical Effects of Ionizing Radiation.* 2nd ed. Philadelphia: WB Saunders; 1995:1–23, 214–295,375–383.
5. Coia LR, Myerson RJ, Tepper JE. Late effects of radiation therapy on the gastrointestinal tract. *Int J Radiat Oncol Biol Phys.* 1995;31:1213–1236.
6. Rubin P, Casarett G. A direction for clinical radiation pathology: the tolerance dose. In: Vaeth JM, ed. *Frontiers of Radiation Therapy and Oncology.* Vol 6. Baltimore: University Park Press; 1972:1–16.
7. Hacker NF, Berek JS, Burnison CM, et al. Whole abdominal radiation as salvage therapy for epithelial ovarian cancer. *Obstet Gynecol.* 1985;65:60–66.
8. Reddy S, Lee M-S, Yordan E, et al. Salvage whole abdomen radiation therapy: its role in ovarian cancer. *Int J Radiat Oncol Biol Phys.* 1993;27:879–884.
9. Fine BA, Hempling RE, Piver MS, et al. Severe radiation morbidity in carcinoma of the cervix: impact of pretherapy surgical staging and previous surgery. *Int J Radiat Oncol Biol Phys.* 1995;31:717–723.
10. Warren S, Friedman NB. Pathology and pathologic diagnosis of radiation lesions in the gastrointestinal tract. Am J Pathol. 1942;18:499–513.
11. White DC. Intestines. In: White DC, ed. *An Atlas of Radiation Histopathology.* Technical Information Center, Office of Public Affairs, US Energy Research and Development Administration, Washington, DC; 1975:141–160.
12. Berthrong M, Fajardo LF. Radiation injury in surgical pathology. Part II. Alimentary tract. Am J Surg Pathol. 1981;5:153–178.
13. Fajardo LF. General morphology of radiation injury. In: *Pathology of Radiation Injury.* New York: Masson; 1982:6–14.
14. Berthrong M. Pathologic changes secondary to radiation. *World J Surg.* 1986;10:155–170.
15. Richter KK, Fink LM, Hughes BM, et al. Differential effect of radiation on endothelial cell function in rectal cancer and normal rectum. *Am J Surg.* 1998;176:642–647.
16. Morgenstern L, Thompson R, Friedman NB. The modern enigma of radiation enteropathy: sequelae and solutions. *Am J Surg.* 1977;134:166–172.
17. Morgenstern L, Hart M, Lugo D, et al. Changing aspects of radiation enteropathy. *Arch Surg.* 1985;120:1225–1228.
18. Kalman DR, Barnard GF, Massimi GJ, et al. Primary aortoduodenal fistula after radiotherapy. *Am J Gastroenterol.* 1995;90:1148–1150.
19. O'Leary DP. Use of the greater omentum in colorectal surgery. *Dis Col Rectum.* 1999;42:533–539.
20. Sezur A, Martella L, Abbou C, et al. Small intestine protection from radiation by means of a removable adapted prosthesis. *Am J Surg.* 1999;178:22–25.
21. Devereaux DF, Chandler JJ, Eisenstat T, et al. Efficacy of an absorbable mesh in keeping the small bowel out of the human pelvis following surgery. *Surg Gynecol Obstet.* 1984;159:162–163.
22. Dasmahapatra KS, Anangur PS. The use of biodegradable mesh to prevent radiation associated small-bowel injury. *Arch Surg.* 1991;126:366–369.
23. Bazan A, Hontanilla B. The use of the rectus abdominis muscle and a vicryl mesh to protect the small intestine and the rectus in radiation treatments to the lower pelvis. *Plastic Recon Surg.* 1999;103:746–747.
24. Sasse AD, Clark LG, Sasse EC, et al. Amifostine reduces side effects and improves complete response rate during radiotherapy: results of a meta-analysis. *Int J Radiat Oncol Biol Phys.* 2006;64:784–791.
25. Kouvaris JR, Kouloulias VE, Vlahos LJ. Amifostine : the first selective-target and broad-sectrum radioprotector. *Oncologist.* 2007;12:738–747.
26. Otchy DP, Nelson H. Radiation injuries of the colon and rectum. *Surg Clin North Am.* 1993;73:1017–1035.
27. Ogino I, Kitamura T, Okamoto N, et al. Late rectal complication following high dose rate intracavitary brachytherapy in cancer of the cervix. *Int J Radiat Oncol Biol Phys.* 1995;31:725–734.
28. Kochhar R, Sriram PVJ, Sharma SC, et al. Natural history of late radiation proctosigmoiditis treated with topical sucralfate suspension. *Dig Dis Sci.* 1999;44:973–978.
29. Rubinstein E, Ibsen T, Rasmussen RB. Formalin treatment of radiation-induced hemorrhagic proctitis. *Am J Gastroenterol.* 1986;81:44–45.
30. Girnius S, Cersonsky N, Gesell L, et al. Treatment of refractory radiation-induced hemorrhagic proctitis with hyperbaric oxygen therapy. *Am J Clin Oncol.* 2006;29:588–592.
31. Nakabayashi M, Beard C, Kelly SM, et al. Treatment of radiation-induced rectal ulcer with hyperbaric oxygen therapy in a man with prostate cancer. *Urol Oncol.* 2006;24:503–508.

COMMENTARY
Christopher M. Rose and Leslie Botnick

Professor Morgenstern has written an authoritative chapter describing the distressing consequences of radiation injury to the abdomen and the approaches to palliate these problems. He points out that although predisposing factors such as obesity and diabetes may increase the risk of late radiation injury, high radiation dose is the single factor most likely to produce this injury. It is clear that both radiation dose and technique do matter. Developments allowing for a more precise and differential delivery of radiation as well as an increased understanding of the molecular mechanisms of radiation injury have created new strategies to prevent or minimize morbidity in an era in which combined modality surgery, radiation, and chemotherapy are resulting in both increased local control and longer survival. The latter salutary effects allow time for the manifestations of chronic radiation injury to appear.

In 2001, Denham et al. (1) proposed a new formulation to categorize radiation injury to normal tissues, not merely as a semantic issue but as a means to develop interventions to avert injury or minimize its development. Rather than categorizing all injury as "early," arising from damage to target epithelial stem cells, and "late," resulting from either slowly turning over stem cells or vascular injury, the newer categorization holds that ionizing radiation results in three interacting effects: *cytocidal effects,* *indirect effects,* and *functional effects.* All three categories can lead to acute and chronic injury. Cytocidal effects relate to direct DNA damage and then depletion of the stem cell compartments of both epithelial and supporting stromal cells. Depending on the size of the stem cell compartment and the rate of renewal, these effects could occur early (as in the mucosa of the intestine) or late (as in piecemeal necrosis of hepatocytes). Indirect effects are reactive phenomena that occur as a result of injury to supporting tissues. The classic example is parenchymal cell depletion due to hypoxia caused by vascular injury. However, indirect effects also include such phenomena as the "bystander" effect and tissue reactions to cell lethality resulting in the elaboration of vasoactive, procoagulant, and inflammatory mediators, including cytokines, growth factors, and chemokines. These phenomena are referred to as the *consequential mechanisms* of delayed injury. Current research has focused on an understanding of these inflammatory cascades and the creation of small molecule inhibitors and modifiers in an attempt to prevent such "consequential" radiation damage that leads to the final common pathway of increased collagen deposition, sometimes called *adverse tissue remodeling.*

The third category, functional effects, includes manifestations not easily characterized as cytocidal or indirect. They result from nonlethal effects on different intra- and extracellular molecules and changes in gene expression in irradiated cells leading, for example, to direct inactivation of anticoagulant molecules (resulting in thrombin deposition), activation of latent growth factors, and activation of proteases. Documented examples of these functional effects include activation of protein kinase C and the inflammatory cytokines AP-1 and NK $\kappa\beta$; inactivation of thrombomodulin and α_1-antitrypsin; activation of transforming growth factor-β; increased phospholipase A2 activity; and decreased endothelial nitric oxide synthetase (NOS), prostacyclin-2, and transgluaminase. These activities can be inhibited or ameliorated in the laboratory, leading to decreased manifestations of chronic injury.

In this formulation, chronic radiation injury occurs through a complex interaction that involves all three types of effects and is organ-, radiation dose-, and radiation volume-specific. The progressive parenchymal atrophy, vascular sclerosis, and fibrosis noted by Morgenstern as the hallmark of chronic abdominal radiation injury develops as a combination of cytocidal effects

on parenchymal and endothelial cells, functional effects that promote increased coagulation, inflammation, and extracellular thrombin and collagen deposition (adverse tissue remodeling), and indirect effects due to devascularization.

In this commentary we focus primarily on physical strategies to decrease the radiation dose to normal tissues or to decrease the effects of such exposure. An understanding of the complex interplay between cytocidal, indirect, and functional effects should lead to a host of pharmacologic interventions that hopefully will reduce the incidence of chronic abdominal radiation injury (2). The pathobiology of small intestine toxicity can be diagrammed as follows:

Reactive oxidative species (ROS)-induced cytocidal injury
→ enterocyte depletion → mucosal barrier breakdown
→ secretory diarrhea → bacterial translocation
→ adverse tissue remodeling

Each step along the pathway to excessive scar formation can be inhibited. Radioprotector agents such as amifostine, vitamin E, and other sulfhydryl compounds decrease ROS injury. Epithelial growth factors and gastrointestinal (GI) peptides can counteract enterocyte depletion. Modulators of intraluminal factors, such as resin bile salt binders and soluble fiber, can ameliorate damage caused by mucosal barrier breakdown. Immunomodulators and cytokine modulators are being developed to downregulate the exuberant migration of small round cells into the injured mucosa. Antidiarrheal agents are used today to decrease the secretory diarrhea that follows mucositis. Antibiotics and probiotics are also being tested to regularize the normal flora of the gut. Finally, agents such as pentoxiphyllin are known to inhibit the activity of transforming growth factor-β and actually decrease the density of fibrotic tissue in irradiated sites. The task of the clinical oncology team will be to develop prevention and avoidance strategies, as well as to test new radioprotector agents.

Modern concepts of dose-response relationships for predicting chronic normal tissue injury include an appreciation of how the probability of injury varies with volume and daily dose as well as total dose. Different organs manifest different volume effects depending on whether their functional subunits (FSUs) are arranged in series or in parallel. If FSUs are arranged in series (e.g., small intestine), low dose to a large volume may be innocuous but high dose to a small volume may be hazardous. Therefore, there is a small volume effect. Previous concepts of dose tolerance such as D5/D50 as described in Chapter 13 pertain to these types of organs. However when the FSUs are arranged in parallel (e.g., liver and kidney) low doses to a large volume that subtends many FSUs can be hazardous and a high dose to a small volume may be innocuous. Thus, there is a large volume effect. Three-dimensional (3D) conformal therapy and intensity-modulated radiotherapy (IMRT) allow for the full dose to be delivered to the tumor while limiting the dose to normal tissues. By keeping the daily dose lower than 100 cGy sublethal damage repair protects the normal tissues in a manner not predicted by total dose calculations.

Much descriptive and retrospective research in radiotherapy in the past 10 years has elucidated these dose-volume relationships in order to create guidelines for dose deposition to normal tissues adjacent to tumors that require very high doses. The formulation that radiation oncologists use to express these relationships is the *cumulative dose-volume histogram* (DVH). The organ-specific DVH graph delineates what proportion of the target organ can receive what amount of radiation. DVH analysis is a standard exercise in the evaluation of both 3D conformal and intensity-modulated treatment planning.

Two illustrative examples are studies using 3D conformal radiation for the treatment of primary liver and biliary tract tumors (3) and IMRT of gynecologic cancers (4). Dawson and associates (3) from the University of Michigan were able to demonstrate the "parallel" nature of liver FSUs and a large-volume effect. In their series of 203 patients receiving liver radiotherapy, only 19 developed radiation-induced liver disease. Patients with small and medium-sized hepatomas and biliary carcinomas tolerated doses of radiation of 60 to 66 Gy at 150 cGy twice daily, far higher than tolerance doses estimated by previous D5/D50 calculations. For all 203 patients studied, after a threshold mean liver dose of 30 Gy (below which no patient developed radiation-induced liver disease), the probability of injury increased by approximately 4%/Gy increase in the mean dose.

Similarly, although the volume effect was much smaller, Mundt and associates (4) at the University of Chicago in treating patients with gynecologic malignancies with IMRT were able to give more than the 45 to 50 Gy predicted by standard dose tolerance tables to small intestine. Their patients experienced 30% less grade II acute GI toxicity and no significant chronic GI toxicity compared with patients undergoing standard 3D conformal whole-pelvic irradiation. Dose-volume constraints were employed in their inverse treatment planning process for IMRT that prevented maximum doses of >49 Gy to small amounts of intestine, and no more than 40% of the small intestine could receive >32 Gy.

The most efficient strategies for prevention of chronic radiation injury include either the minimization or the avoidance of irradiation of sensitive normal tissue. Mak and associates (5) from the MD Anderson Cancer Center have described the use of an open tabletop device combined with bladder compression that moves the small bowel out of the treatment field when patients are treated in the prone position. This method that has been adopted by many radiation oncology departments reduces the rate of small bowel obstruction in patients treated with radical surgery and postoperative radiotherapy for gynecologic and cancers of the rectum and rectosigmoid. This technique is facile, reproducible, and does not require patient compliance.

The revolution in tumor imaging has also been important in ameliorating radiation injury. Computed tomography (CT)/positron emission tomography studies coupled with direct imaging of anal and colorectal tumors by endorectal ultrasound have allowed for better estimation of depth of tumor penetration and peritumoral nodal enlargement. Patients who previously were treated postoperatively now can be treated preoperatively. The volume of tissue irradiated can be reduced, loops of small bowel that might be fixed by perioperative scarring can be mobilized out of the field by the methods previously described, and sophisticated IMRT or 3D planning can steer the radiation dose away from the bystander normal bowel to the region of the tumor or to the more radioresistant bladder. In the upper abdomen, neoadjuvant chemoradiation strategies for muscle-penetrating gastric and T3 category pancreatic cancer have allowed for smaller and targeted treatment volumes that include the primary tumor, a peritumoral margin to capture direct tumor extension, and the immediately adjacent lymph node groups at risk for metastatic dissemination. This approach is to be compared with the alternative postoperative approach that requires surgical identification of patients who might benefit from chemoradiation, but also requires radiation to be delivered to the tumor bed, the appropriate nodal groups, and the anastamosis. Although the volume to be treated is similar in the pelvis, postoperative irradiation to upper abdominal (stomach and pancreas) sites results in a much larger volume of small intestine subtended in the radiation beam. As long as the preoperative radiation dose to the anastamotic region is kept <50 Gy, there is no evidence that anastamotic leaks or postoperative peritonitis rates are higher than when the treatment is given postoperatively.

Previous radiation approaches using large anterior and posterior portals, 200-cGy fractions, lack of CT-based planning, and primarily postoperative treatment resulted in the distressing complications described in this chapter. The use of bile salt binders, radioprotectors, CT-based planning, differential dose planning via 3D conformal and IMRT approaches, prone positioning with an open tabletop, and identification of normal tissues to be avoided by the radiation beam can decrease side effects and allow for dose escalation and chemotherapy to decrease the volume of resections and increase cure rates. Cooperative preoperative treatment planning by the surgeon, medical oncologist, and radiation oncologist at tumor boards and multidisciplinary conferences provides the best opportunity to reduce complications and increase cure.

REFERENCES

1. Denham JW, Hauer-Jensen M, Peters LJ. Is it time for a new formalism to categorize normal tissue radiation injury? *Int J Radiat Oncol Biol Phys.* 2001;50:1105–1106.

2. Vujaskovic Z. Radiation-induced normal tissue damage. Paper presented at: the American Society for Therapeutic Radiology and Oncology Spring Refresher Course; March 2007; Chicago, IL.

3. Dawson LA, Normolle D, Balter JM, et al. Analysis of radiation-induced liver disease using the Lyman NTCP model. *Int J Radiat Oncol Biol Phys.* 2002;53:810–821.

4. Mundt AJ, Lujan AE, Rotmensch J, et al. Intensity-modulated whole pelvic radiotherapy in women with gynecologic malignancies. *Int J Radiat Oncol Biol Phys.* 2002;52:1330–1337.

5. Mak AC, Rich TA, Schultheiss TE, et al. Late complications of postoperative radiation therapy for cancer of the rectum and rectosigmoid. *Int J Radiat Oncol Biol.* 1994;28:597–560.

14

Peritoneal Carcinomatosis, Sarcomatosis, and Mesothelioma: Surgical Responsibilities

Paul H. Sugarbaker

As surgical oncology expanded in the midst of a technological revolution in patient care, this discipline accepted responsibilities not only for the resection of primary tumor but also the surgical management of metastatic disease. For gastrointestinal cancer, early success with this new concept was with complete resection of locally recurrent colon and rectal cancer (1,2). Then the resection of isolated liver metastases from the same disease was shown to be of benefit to a selected group of patients (3). Aggressive management strategies to bring about long-term survival to patients with peritoneal surface malignancy have been pioneered at the Washington Cancer Institute (4). Treatment of abdominal and pelvic malignancies that disseminate to peritoneal surfaces has grown out of extensive experience with appendiceal cancer. Appendiceal cancer became the paradigm for successful treatment of peritoneal carcinomatosis (5). This review presents the background, the technique for cytoreduction, the standardized regional chemotherapy currently in use, and the results of treatment of peritoneal surface malignancy. The selection factors leading to long-term benefit with acceptable morbidity and mortality will be a central focus. The peritoneal surface malignancies to be discussed include appendix cancer and pseudomyxoma peritonei, colon cancer with carcinomatosis, gastric cancer with carcinomatosis, abdominopelvic sarcoma with sarcomatosis, and primary peritoneal surface malignancy including peritoneal mesothelioma, papillary serous cancer, and primary peritoneal adenocarcinoma. A discussion regarding palliative treatments for debilitating ascites is included.

PRINCIPLES OF MANAGEMENT

The successful treatment of peritoneal surface malignancy requires a combined approach that uses cytoreductive surgery and perioperative intraperitoneal chemotherapy. In addition, proper patient selection is mandatory. Complete resection of all visible malignancy is essential for treatment of peritoneal surface malignancy to result in long-term survival. Up to six peritonectomy procedures may be required (6). The visceral and parietal peritonectomy procedures that one must use to adequately resect all visible evidence of disease are illustrated in the next section. Their utilization depends on the distribution and extent of invasion of the malignancy disseminated within the peritoneal space.

Normal peritoneum is not excised, only that which is implanted by cancer.

Peritonectomy Procedures

If a surgeon elects to manage patients with peritoneal surface malignancy, a requirement is for the surgeon to be knowledgeable regarding the dissemination of cancer on peritoneal surfaces. It is imperative that the surgeon develop the technical skills and be proficient in dissection using electrosurgery.

Rationale for Peritonectomy Procedures

Peritonectomy procedures are necessary if one is to successfully treat peritoneal surface malignancies with curative intent. Peritonectomy procedures are used in the areas of visible cancer progression in an attempt to leave the patient with only microscopic residual disease. Isolated tumor nodules are removed using electroevaporation; involvement of the visceral peritoneum frequently requires resection of a portion of the stomach, small intestine, or colorectum. Layering of cancer on a peritoneal surface or a portion of the bowel requires peritonectomy or bowel resection for complete removal.

Locations of Peritoneal Surface Malignancy

Peritoneal surface malignancy tends to involve the visceral peritoneum in greatest volume at three definite sites (7). These are sites where the bowel is anchored to the retroperitoneum and peristalsis causes less motion of the visceral peritoneal surface. The rectosigmoid colon, as it emerges from the pelvis, is a nonmobile portion of the bowel. Also, it is located in a dependent site and therefore is frequently layered by carcinomatosis. Usually a complete pelvic peritonectomy requires stripping of the abdominal sidewalls, the peritoneum overlying the bladder, the cul-de-sac, and the rectosigmoid colon. The ileocecal valve is another area where there is limited mobility. Resection of the terminal ileum and a small portion of the right colon are often necessary. A final site often requiring resection is the antrum of the stomach, which is fixed to the retroperitoneum at the pylorus. Tumor coming into the foramen of Winslow accumulates in the subpyloric space and may cause intestinal obstruction as a result of gastric outlet obstruction. Large volumes of tumor in the lesser omentum combined with disease in the subpyloric space may cause a confluence of disease that requires a total gastrectomy for complete cytoreduction.

Electroevaporative Surgery

In order to adequately perform cytoreductive surgery, the surgeon must use electrosurgery. Peritonectomies and visceral resections using the traditional scissor and knife dissection will unnecessarily disseminate a large number of tumor cells within the abdomen. High-voltage electrosurgery leaves a margin of heat necrosis that is devoid of viable malignant cells. Not only does electroevaporation of tumor and normal tissue at the margins of resection minimize the likelihood of persistent disease, but also it minimizes blood loss. In the absence of electrosurgery, profuse bleeding from stripped peritoneal surfaces may occur; this may be especially prominent during the intraperitoneal wash with chemotherapy.

The Peritoneum as a First Line of Defense in Carcinomatosis

Cancer surgery in the absence of perioperative intraperitoneal chemotherapy may actually harm patients in the long run rather than help them. If peritoneal surface malignancy is present, cancer resection without intraperitoneal chemotherapy will cause tumor cells to become implanted within a deeper layer of the abdomen and pelvis. As cancer progresses this may contribute to obstruction of vital structures such as the ureter or common bile duct. Also, deep involvement of the pelvic sidewall and tissues along vascular structures will occur. If surgeons attempt to treat peritoneal surface malignancy, they must become thoroughly familiar with the techniques of intraperitoneal chemotherapy. Complete cytoreduction combined with aggressive perioperative intraperitoneal chemotherapy and proper patient selection are the three essential requirements of treatment for peritoneal surface malignancy.

Position and Incision

The patient is placed in the supine position with the gluteal fold advanced to the end of the operating table to allow full access to the perineum during the surgical procedure (Figure 14.1). In the lithotomy position the weight of the legs must be directed to the soles of the feet. Myonecrosis within the gastrocnemius muscle may occur unless the legs are protected properly.

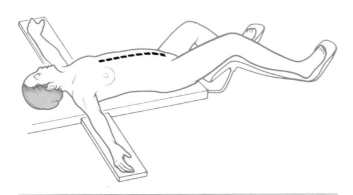

Figure 14.1 Modified lithotomy position and maximal midline incision for cytoreductive surgery. (Modified from ref. 6.)

Abdominal skin preparation is from midchest to midthigh. The external genitalia are prepared in male patients and a vaginal preparation is used in female patients. A Foley catheter is placed and a silastic 18-gauge nasogastric sump tube is placed within the stomach.

Abdominal Exposure, Greater Omentectomy, and Splenectomy

The abdomen is opened through a midline incision from xiphoid to pubis. Generous abdominal exposure is achieved through the use of a Thompson Self-Retaining Retractor (Thompson Surgical Instruments, Inc., Traverse City, MI; Figure 14.2). The standard tool used to dissect tumor on peritoneal surfaces from the normal tissues is a 3-mm ball-tipped electrosurgical handpiece (Valleylab, Boulder, CO). The ball-tipped instrument is placed at the interface of tumor and normal tissues. The focal point for further dissection is placed on strong traction. The electrosurgical generator is used on pure cut at high voltage. Electroevaporative surgery is used cautiously for tumor removal on tubular structures, especially the ureters, small bowel, and colon.

Using ball-tipped electrosurgery on pure cut creates a large volume of plume because of the electroevaporation (carbonization) of tissue. To maintain visualization of the operative field and to preserve a smoke-free atmosphere, a smoke filtration unit is used. The vacuum tip is maintained 2 to 3 inches from the field of dissection whenever electrosurgery is performed.

To free the midabdomen of a large volume of tumor, the greater omentectomy-splenectomy is performed. The greater omentum is elevated and then separated from the transverse colon using electrosurgery. This dissection continues beneath the peritoneum that covers the transverse mesocolon in order to expose the lower border of the pancreas. The branches of the gastroepiploic arcade to the greater curvature of the stomach are clamped, ligated, and divided. Also, the short gastric vessels are transected. With traction on the spleen, the peritoneum superior to the pancreas is stripped from the gland using electrosurgery. This freely exposes the splenic artery and vein at the tail of the pancreas. These vessels are ligated in continuity and proximally suture ligated.

Left Subphrenic Peritonectomy

To begin the peritonectomy procedure in the left upper quadrant, the epigastric fat and peritoneum at the edge of the abdominal incision is stripped off the posterior rectus sheath (Figure 14.3). Strong traction is exerted on the tumor specimen throughout the left upper quadrant in order to separate tumor from the diaphragmatic muscle, the left adrenal gland, and the superior half of perirenal fat. The splenic flexure of the colon is severed from the left abdominal gutter and moved medially by dividing the peritoneum along the line of Toldt. Dissection beneath the hemidiaphragm muscle must be performed with ball-tipped electrosurgery, not by blunt dissection. Numerous blood vessels between the diaphragm muscle and its peritoneal surface must be electrocoagulated before their transection or unnecessary bleeding will occur as the divided blood vessels retract into the muscle of the diaphragm. The plane of dissection is defined using ball-tipped electrosurgery on pure cut, but all blood vessels are electrocoagulated before their division.

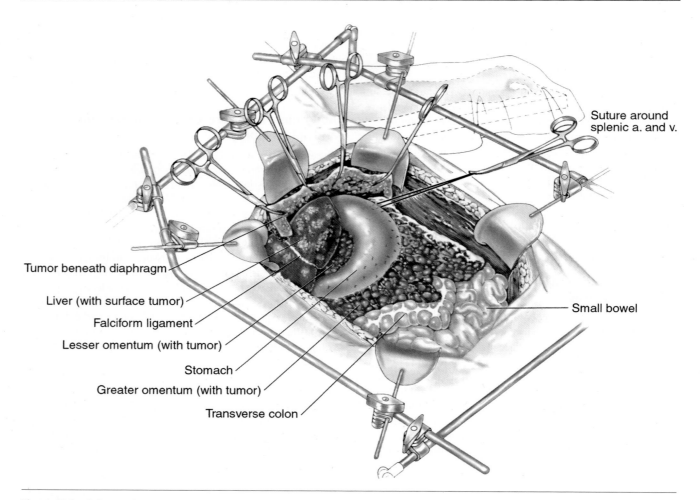

Figure 14.2 Abdominal exposure using a self-retaining retractor, complete greater omentectomy, and splenectomy. (Modified from ref. 6.)

Labels on figure:
Suture around splenic a. and v.
Tumor beneath diaphragm
Liver (with surface tumor)
Falciform ligament
Lesser omentum (with tumor)
Stomach
Greater omentum (with tumor)
Transverse colon
Small bowel

Left Subphrenic Peritonectomy Completed

When the left upper quadrant peritonectomy is completed, the stomach may be reflected medially (Figure 14.4). Numerous branches of the gastroepiploic arteries that have been ligated are evident. The left adrenal gland, pancreas, and left perinephric fat are visualized completely, as is the anterior surface of the transverse mesocolon. The surgeon must avoid the right and left gastric artery and vein to preserve the vascular supply to the stomach.

Right Subphrenic Peritonectomy

Peritoneum is stripped from the right posterior rectus sheath to begin the peritonectomy in the right upper quadrant of the abdomen (Figure 14.5). Strong traction on the specimen is used to elevate the hemidiaphragm into the operative field. Again, ball-tipped electrosurgery on pure cut is used to dissect at the interface of tumor and normal tissue. Coagulation current is used to divide the blood vessels as they are encountered and before they bleed.

Stripping of Tumor from Glisson's Capsule

The stripping of tumor from the right hemidiaphragm continues until the bare area of the liver is encountered (Figure 14.6). At

that point, tumor on the superior surface of the liver is electroevaporated until the liver surface is cleared. With ball-tipped electroevaporative dissection, a thick layer of tumor may be lifted off the liver surface by moving beneath Glisson's capsule with electrosurgical dissection. Isolated patches of tumor on the liver surface are electroevaporated with the distal 2 cm of the ball tip bent and stripped of insulation ("hockey-stick" configuration). Ball-tipped electrosurgery is also used to extirpate tumor from attachments of the falciform ligament and round ligament.

Tumor from beneath the right hemidiaphragm, from the right subhepatic space, and from the surface of the liver forms an envelope as it is removed en bloc. The dissection is greatly facilitated if the tumor specimen is maintained intact. The dissection continues laterally on the right to encounter the perirenal fat covering the right kidney. Also, the right adrenal gland is visualized and carefully avoided as tumor is stripped from the right subhepatic space. Care is taken not to traumatize the vena cava or to disrupt the caudate lobe veins that pass between the vena cava and segment I of the liver.

Completed Right Subphrenic Peritonectomy

One can visualize the completed right subphrenic peritonectomy with strong upward traction on the right costal margin by the

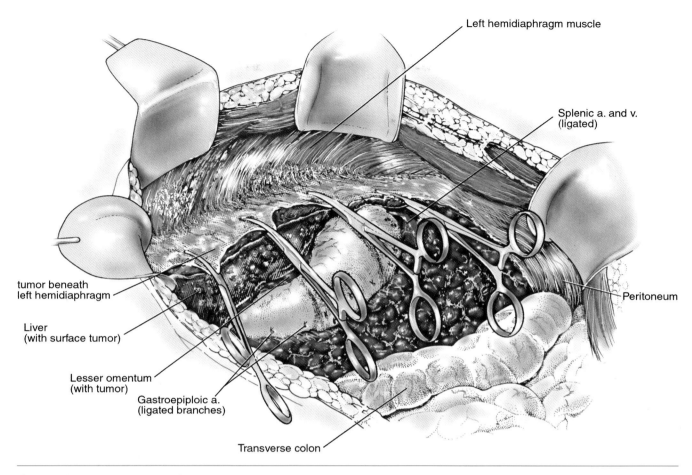

Figure 14.3 Peritoneal stripping from the left diaphragm. (Modified from ref. 6.)

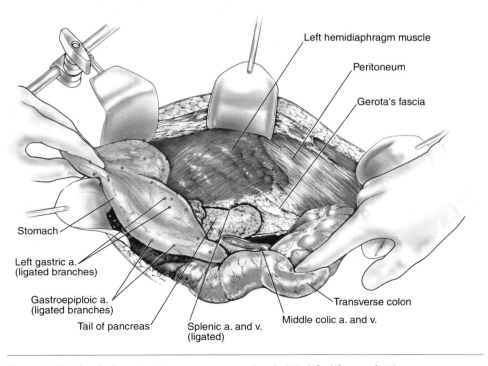

Figure 14.4 Left subphrenic peritonectomy completed. (Modified from ref. 6.)

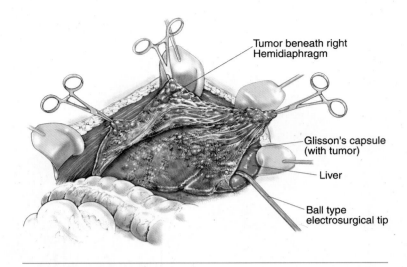

Tumor beneath right Hemidiaphragm

Glisson's capsule (with tumor)

Liver

Ball type electrosurgical tip

Figure 14.5 Peritoneal stripping of the undersurface of the right hemidiaphragm. (Modified from ref. 6.)

self-retaining retractor and medial displacement of the right liver (Figure 14.7). The anterior branches of the phrenic artery and vein on the hemidiaphragm are seen and have been preserved. The right hepatic vein and the vena cava below have been exposed. The right subhepatic space including the right adrenal gland and perirenal fat covering the right kidney constitutes the base of the dissection.

If the malignancy is invasive, tumor is densely adherent to the tendinous central portion of the left or right hemidiaphragm. If this occurs, the normal tissue infiltrated by tumor must be resected. This usually requires an elliptical excision of a portion of the hemidiaphragm on either the right or the left side. The defect in the diaphragm is closed with interrupted sutures after the intraoperative chemotherapy of both chest and abdomen is completed.

Lesser Omentectomy and Cholecystectomy with Stripping of the Hepatoduodenal Ligament

The gallbladder is removed in a routine fashion from its fundus toward the cystic artery and cystic duct. These structures are ligated and divided. The hepatoduodenal ligament is characteristically heavily layered with tumor. Using strong traction, the cancerous tissue that coats the porta hepatis is bluntly stripped from the base of the gallbladder bed toward the duodenum (Figure 14.8). The right gastric artery going to the lesser omental arcade is preserved. To continue resection of the lesser omentum, the surgeon separates the gastrohepatic ligament from the fissure that divides liver segments II, III, and IV from segment I. Ball-tipped electrosurgery is used to electroevaporate tumor from the surface of the caudate process. Care is taken not to traumatize the

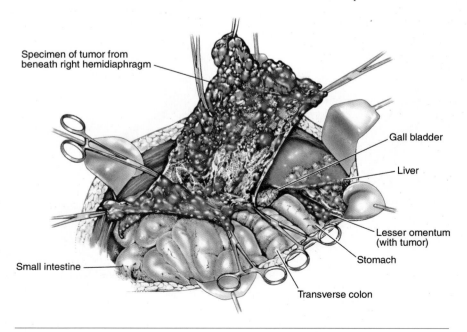

Specimen of tumor from beneath right hemidiaphragm

Gall bladder

Liver

Lesser omentum (with tumor)

Stomach

Small intestine

Transverse colon

Figure 14.6 Stripping of tumor from Glisson's capsule. (Modified from ref. 6.)

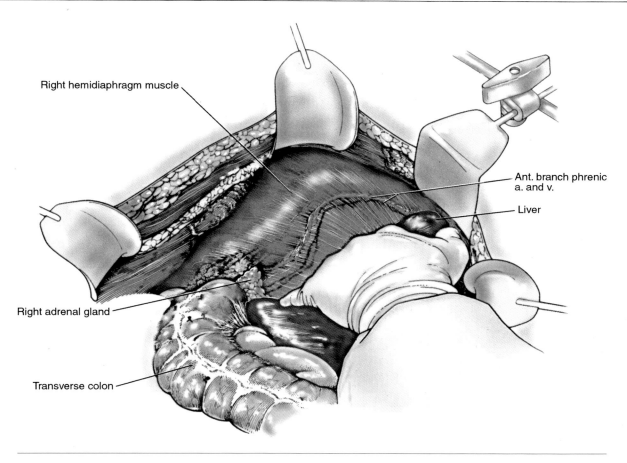

Figure 14.7 Completed right subphrenic peritonectomy. (Modified from ref. 6.)

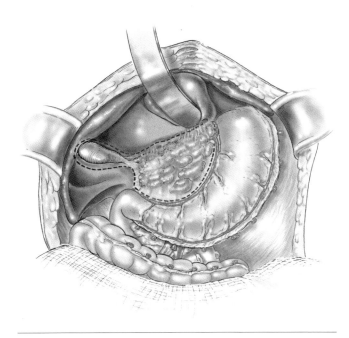

Figure 14.8 Lesser omentectomy and cholecystectomy with stripping of the porta hepatis. (Modified from ref. 6.)

anterior surface of the caudate process, for this can result in excessive and needless blood loss. The segmental blood supply to the caudate lobe is located on the anterior surface of this segment of the liver, and hemorrhage may occur with only superficial trauma. Also, care must be taken to avoid the left hepatic artery that may arise from the left gastric artery and cross through the hepatogastric fissure.

Stripping of the Omental Bursa

As one clears the left side of liver segment I of tumor, the vena cava is visualized beneath. To begin to strip the omental bursa, strong traction is maintained on the tumor and ball-tipped electrosurgery is used to divide the fibrous tissue between liver segment I and the vena cava (Figure 14.9). The phrenoesophageal ligament is incised in order for the peritoneum to be elevated away from the crus of the right hemidiaphragm. The common hepatic artery and the left gastric artery are skeletonized and lymph nodes in this are region avoided. The branches of the left gastric artery and vein are identified and avoided. Tumor and lesser omental fat are separated from the lesser omental arcade by compressing tissue between the thumb and index finger. The major branches of the left gastric artery to the lesser curvature of the stomach are preserved to provide blood supply to the stomach.

The surgeon dissects in a clockwise direction along the lesser curvature of the stomach, attempting to preserve the arcade between the right and left gastric arteries. Care is taken to preserve as much omental fat as possible, attempting to remove

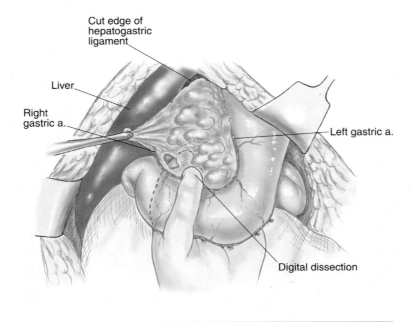

Figure 14.9 Stripping of the omental bursa. (Modified from ref. 6.)

tumor tissue only. One attempts to spare the anterior vagus nerve going toward the antrum of the stomach.

Complete Pelvic Peritonectomy

The tumor-bearing peritoneum is stripped from the posterior surface of the lower abdominal incision, exposing the rectus muscle. The muscular surface of the bladder is revealed as ball-tipped electrosurgery strips peritoneum and preperitoneal fat from this structure. The urachus must be divided and is then elevated on a clamp as the leading point for this dissection (Figure 14.10). In the female, the round ligaments are divided as they enter the internal inguinal ring.

The peritoneal incision around the pelvis is connected to the peritoneal incisions of the right and left paracolic sulci. The right and left ureters are identified and preserved. In women, the right and left ovarian veins are ligated at the level of the lower pole of the kidney and divided. A linear stapler is used to divide the sigmoid colon just above the limits of the pelvic tumor. The vascular supply of the distal portion of the bowel is traced back to its origin on the aorta. The inferior mesenteric artery is suture ligated and divided. This allows one to pack all the viscera, including the proximal sigmoid colon, in the upper abdomen.

Resection of Rectosigmoid Colon and cul-de-sac of Douglas

Electrosurgery is used to dissect at the limits of the mesorectum. The surgeon works in a centripetal fashion. Extraperitoneal ligation of the uterine arteries is performed just above the ureter and close to the base of the bladder (Figure 14.11). The bladder is dissected away from the cervix and the vagina is entered. The vaginal cuff anterior and posterior to the cervix is transected using electrosurgery, and the rectovaginal septum is entered. The perirectal fat is divided beneath the peritoneal reflection so that all tumor that occupies the cul-de-sac is removed intact with the specimen. The rectal musculature is skeletonized using electro-

surgery so that a stapler can be used to close off the rectal stump. The rectum is sharply divided above the stapler.

Vaginal Closure and Low Colorectal Anastomosis

One of the few suture repairs performed prior to the intraoperative chemotherapy is the closure of the vaginal cuff. If

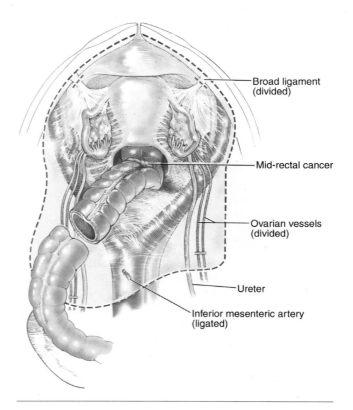

Figure 14.10 Complete pelvic peritonectomy. (Modified from ref. 6.)

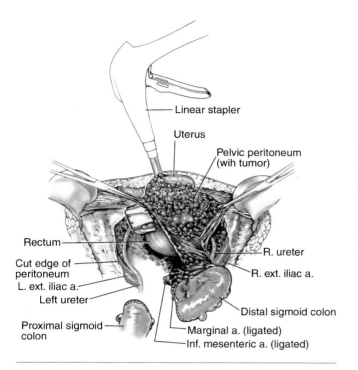

Figure 14.11 Resection of rectosigmoid colon and cul-de-sac of Douglas. L. ext., left external; R. ext., right external; Inf., inferior. (Modified from ref. 6.)

one fails to close the vaginal cuff, chemotherapy solution will leak from the vagina. The circular stapled colorectal anastomosis occurs after the intraoperative chemotherapy has been completed. A circular stapling device is passed into the rectum, and the trochar penetrates the staple line (Figure 14.12). A purse-string applier is used to secure the staple anvil in the proximal sigmoid colon. The body of the circular stapler and anvil are mated and the stapler is activated to complete the low colorectal anastomosis.

Descending Colon Mobilization for a Tension-Free Low Colorectal Anastomosis

An absolute requirement for a complication-free low colorectal anastomosis is the absence of tension on the staple line. Adequate mobilization of the entire left colon is needed, and several steps may be required to accomplish this. The inferior mesenteric artery is ligated on the aorta, and then its individual branches are resected as they arise from this vascular trunk. The Y-configuration of the sigmoidal vessels is converted to a V-configuration to keep the intermediate arcade intact. The inferior mesenteric vein is divided as it courses around the duodenum. The mesentery of the transverse colon and splenic flexure are completely elevated from the perirenal fat surrounding the left kidney. Taking care to avoid the left ureter, the surgeon divides the left colon mesentery from all its retroperitoneal attachments. These maneuvers allow the junction of the sigmoid and descending colon to reach to the low rectum or anus for a tension-free anastomosis. Redundant descending colon should fall into the hollow of the sacrum.

To assess the stapled colorectal anastomosis, the proximal and distal tissue rings are examined for completeness. Air is insufflated into the rectum with a water-filled pelvis to check for an airtight circle of staples. Two hands should easily pass beneath the sigmoid colon to ensure there is no tension on the stapled anastomosis. A rectal examination is done to check for staple-line bleeding at the anastomosis.

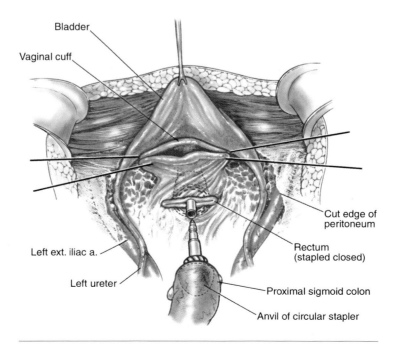

Figure 14.12 Vaginal closure and low colorectal anastomosis. ext., external. (Modified from ref. 6.)

Tubes and Drains Required for Intraoperative and Early Postoperative Intraperitoneal Chemotherapy

Four closed-suction drains are placed in the dependent portions of the abdomen. This includes one in the right subhepatic space, one in the left subdiaphragmatic space, and two in the pelvis. A Tenckhoff catheter is placed through the abdominal wall and positioned within the abdomen at the site that is thought to be the area of greatest risk for recurrence. All transabdominal drains and tubes are secured to the skin in a watertight fashion with a purse-string suture. Temperature probes are placed at the inflow site (Tenckhoff catheter) and at a remote site. The temperature probes are removed after the intraoperative chemotherapy has been completed but all closed-suction drains are retained. Right angle thoracostomy tubes (Deknatel, Floral Park, NY) are inserted on both the right and left side to prevent abdominal fluid from accumulating in the chest as a result of the subphrenic peritonectomy.

Rationale for Perioperative Intraperitoneal Chemotherapy

Cancers that occur within the abdomen or pelvis will disseminate by three different routes. These are hematogenous metastases, lymphatic metastases, and spread through the peritoneal space to surfaces within the abdomen and pelvis. In a substantial number of patients with abdominal or pelvic malignancy, surgical treatment failure is isolated to the resection site or to peritoneal surfaces. This suggests that effective treatment of peritoneal surface malignancy may have an impact on the survival of these cancer patients. Also it would eliminate a leading cause of suffering in patients with these malignancies. Prior to the use of cytoreductive surgery and intraperitoneal chemotherapy these conditions were uniformly fatal, eventually resulting in intestinal obstruction. Occasionally, patients with low-grade malignancies such as pseudomyxoma peritonei and cystic mesothelioma have survived for several years, but all reports of end results show a fatal outcome.

Current technology for the administration of intraperitoneal chemotherapy demands that it be used as an integral part of the surgical procedure. Several crucial technological modifications of chemotherapy administration are required. First, an intraperitoneal rather than an intravenous route for chemotherapy is used. The intraperitoneal route, when properly used, will allow uniform distribution of a high concentration of anticancer therapy at the site of the malignancy. This is achieved by the surgeon intraoperatively manipulating the intestinal contents to uniformly distribute the chemotherapy. In the early postoperative period, the patient's position is repeatedly changed to assist gravity in maintaining an optimal chemotherapy distribution.

Secondly, the chemotherapy administration is timed so that all of the malignancy, except for microscopic residual disease, will have been removed prior to the chemotherapy treatments. This means that the limited penetration of chemotherapy into tissues, which is approximately 1 mm, will be adequate to eradicate all tumor cells. Also, the chemotherapy will be used prior to the construction of any anastomosis. This means that suture line recurrences should also be eliminated. Finally, because all adhesions were resected during cytoreduction, there will be no surfaces in the abdomen or pelvis excluded by scar tissue from contact with chemotherapy solutions.

The combined treatments of cytoreductive surgery and intraperitoneal chemotherapy must be used as early in the natural history of the cancer as is possible. No longer can the clinician wait for the patient with peritoneal carcinomatosis to become symptomatic to begin treatments. The treatment of patients with an invasive malignancy that has a wide distribution of a large mass of cancer will not produce long-term benefits. Peritoneal surface malignancy can be cured, but an optimal result requires that these aggressive treatments be initiated in a timely fashion.

Peritoneal Plasma Barrier

Intraperitoneal chemotherapy gives high response rates within the abdomen because the "peritoneal plasma barrier" provides dose-intensive therapy. Many chemotherapy agents are large-molecular-weight substances so that they are confined to the abdominal cavity for long periods (8). This means that the exposure of peritoneal surfaces to pharmacologically active molecules can be greatly increased by giving the drugs via the intraperitoneal route rather than the intravenous route.

For the chemotherapy agents used to treat peritoneal carcinomatosis or peritoneal sarcomatosis, the area under the curve ratios of intraperitoneal to intravenous exposure are favorable. Table 14.1 presents the area under the curve (intraperitoneal/intravenous) for the drugs in routine clinical use in patients with peritoneal seeding. In our studies, these include 5-fluorouracil, mitomycin C, doxorubicin, cisplatin, paclitaxel, and gemcitabine.

One should not assume that the intraperitoneal administration of chemotherapy eliminates their systemic toxicities. Although the drugs are sequestered within the peritoneal space, they eventually are cleared into the systemic circulation. For this reason, the safe doses of most drugs instilled into the peritoneal cavity are identical to the intravenous dose. The exceptions are drugs with hepatic metabolism such as 5-fluorouracil and gemcitabine. An increased dose of approximately 50% is usually

---

Table 14.1

Area Under the Curve (Concentration of Drug Times the Duration of Exposure) Ratios of Peritoneal Surface Exposure to Systemic Exposure for Drugs Used to Treat Intra-Abdominal Cancer

Drug	Molecular Weight	Area Under the Curve Ratio
5-Fluorouracil	130	250
Mitomycin C	334	75
Doxorubicin	544	500
Cisplatin	300	20
Paclitaxel	808	1,000
Gemcitabine	263	50

possible with 5-fluorouracil. The dose for a 5-day course of intravenous 5-fluorouracil is approximately 500 mg/m^2; for intraperitoneal 5-fluorouracil, the dose is 750 mg/m^2 per day. This increase (approximately 50%) in the dose of 5-fluorouracil is of great advantage in treating peritoneal carcinomatosis.

Tumor Cell Entrapment

Tumor cell entrapment may explain the rapid progression of peritoneal surface malignancy in patients who undergo treatment using surgery alone. This theory relates the high incidence and rapid progression of peritoneal surface implantation to fibrin entrapment of intra-abdominal tumor emboli on traumatized peritoneal surfaces and progression of these entrapped tumor cells through growth factors involved in the wound-healing process. Tumor cell entrapment may cause a high incidence of surgical treatment failure in patients treated for primary gastrointestinal cancer. Also, the reimplantation of malignant cells into peritonectomized surfaces in a reoperative setting must be expected unless intraperitoneal chemotherapy is used.

In order to eradicate implantation of tumor cells on abdominal and pelvic surfaces, the abdominal cavity is flooded with chemotherapy in a large volume of fluid during the operation as heated intraoperative intraperitoneal chemotherapy and in the postoperative period as early postoperative intraperitoneal chemotherapy.

Prior Limited Benefits with Intraperitoneal Chemotherapy

The use of intraperitoneal chemotherapy in the past has met with limited success and acceptance by oncologists. There have been three major impediments to greater benefits. Intracavitary instillation allows very *limited penetration* of drug into tumor nodules. Only the outermost layer (approximately 1 mm) of a cancer nodule is penetrated by the chemotherapy. This means that only minute tumor nodules can be definitely treated. In most trials, oncologists have attempted to treat established disease, and this improper selection of patients has resulted in disappointment with intraperitoneal drug use. Microscopic residual disease is the ideal target for intraperitoneal chemotherapy protocols.

A second cause for disappointment with intraperitoneal chemotherapy is a *nonuniform drug distribution*. A majority of patients treated by drug instillation into the abdomen or pelvis have had prior surgery, which invariably causes scarring between peritoneal surfaces. The adhesions create multiple barriers to the free access of fluid. Although the instillation of a large volume of fluid will partially overcome the problems created by adhesions, large surface areas frequently will have no access to chemotherapy. Limited access from adhesions is impossible to predict and may increase with repeated instillations of chemotherapy.

Not only do adhesions interfere with chemotherapy distribution, they also sequester cancer cells away from chemotherapy. Surgery causes fibrin deposits on surfaces that have been traumatized by the cancer resection. Free intraperitoneal cancer cells become trapped within the fibrin. The fibrin is infiltrated by platelets, neutrophils, and monocytes as part of the wound-healing process. As collagen is laid down, the tumor cells are entrapped within scar tissue. The scar tissue is dense and is not penetrated by intraperitoneal chemotherapy.

Nonuniform drug distribution may be caused by gravity. Intraperitoneal fluid does not uniformly distribute itself to anterior peritoneal surfaces. Gravity pulls the fluid to dependent areas especially the pelvis, paracolic gutters, and the right retrohepatic space. Unless the patient actively pursues frequent changes in position, the surfaces between bowel loops and the anterior abdominal wall will remain relatively untreated.

A final obstacle to success with the administration of intraperitoneal chemotherapy encountered in the past is the *difficulty and dangers* of *long-term peritoneal access*. There has been no technical solution to the requirement for reliable access to the peritoneal space. Repeated installations of large volumes of chemotherapy solution cause great inconvenience and can result in a large number of serious complications. Whether the oncologist chooses repeated paracentesis or an indwelling catheter, complications such as pain on instillation, bowel perforation, instillation into soft tissues, or inability to infuse or drain occur repeatedly. At this time, prolonged peritoneal access is a technical challenge without a known solution.

The limitations of penetration, distribution, and repeated access have led to the development of surgically directed chemotherapy. All visible abdominal or pelvic cancer should be completely extirpated by surgery. Then in the operating room, a high dose of heated chemotherapy is delivered with manual distribution to eradicate tiny tumor nodules and microscopic cancer cells. This means that all abdominal and pelvic components of the cancer, including persistent peritoneal surface malignancy, are eliminated. Systemic components of the disease now become the responsibility of the medical oncologist.

Patient Selection for Treatment

The greatest impediment to lasting benefits from intraperitoneal chemotherapy should be attributed to improper patient selection. A great number of patients with advanced intra-abdominal disease have been treated with minimal benefit. Excluding patients with pseudomyxoma peritonei, extensive cytoreductive surgery and aggressive intraperitoneal chemotherapy is not likely to produce a lasting benefit. Rapid recurrence of peritoneal surface cancer combined with progression of lymph nodal or systemic disease, are likely to interrupt long-term survival in these patients. Patients who benefit must have minimal peritoneal surface disease isolated to peritoneal surfaces so that complete cytoreduction can occur. Uniform access to chemotherapy is required so that complete eradication of disease can occur. In the natural history of this disease early initiation of treatment has a great bearing on the benefits achieved. Asymptomatic patients with small-volume peritoneal surface malignancy must be selected for the combined treatment.

Clinical Assessments of Peritoneal Surface Malignancy

In the past, peritoneal carcinomatosis was considered to be a fatal disease process. The only assessment used was either carcinomatosis *present* with a presumed fatal outcome *or* carcinomatosis *absent* with curative treatment options available. Currently, there are four important clinical assessments of peritoneal surface malignancy that need to be used to select patients who will benefit from treatment protocols. These assessments are (a) the histopathology to assess the invasive character of the malignancy, (b) the preoperative computed tomography (CT) scan of abdomen and pelvis, (c) the Peritoneal Cancer Index, and (d) the completeness of cytoreduction score.

Histopathology to Assess Invasive Character

The biological aggressiveness of a peritoneal surface malignancy will have profound influence on its treatment options. Noninvasive tumors such as pseudomyxoma peritonei showing adenomucinosis or mesothelioma with nuclear diameter <31 millimicrons may have extensive spread on peritoneal surfaces and yet be completely resectable by peritonectomy procedures. Also, these noninvasive malignancies are extremely unlikely to metastasize by lymphatics to lymph nodes and by the blood to liver and other systemic sites. Therefore, protocols for cytoreductive surgery and intraperitoneal chemotherapy may have a curative intent in patients with a large mass of widely disseminated pseudomyxoma peritonei and well-differentiated peritoneal mesothelioma (9,10). Also, some low-grade sarcomas despite extensive disease progression may be aggressively treated with cure as a goal using cytoreductive surgery and intraperitoneal chemotherapy. Pathology review and an assessment of the invasive or nonaggressive nature of a malignancy are essential to treatment planning.

Preoperative Computed Tomography Scan

The preoperative CT scan of chest, abdomen, and pelvis may be of great value in planning treatments for peritoneal surface malignancy. Systemic metastases can be clinically excluded and pleural surface spread ruled out. Unfortunately, the CT scan should be regarded as an inaccurate test by which to quantitate intestinal type of peritoneal carcinomatosis from adenocarcinoma (11). The malignant tissue progresses on the peritoneal surfaces and its shape conforms to the normal contours of the abdominopelvic structures. This is quite different from the metastatic process in the liver or lung that progresses as three-dimensional tumor nodules and can be accurately assessed by CT.

However, the CT scan has been of great help in locating and quantitating mucinous adenocarcinoma within the peritoneal cavity (12). These tumors produce large volumes of mucoid material that is readily distinguished by shape and by density from normal structures. Using two distinctive radiologic criteria, those patients with a high likelihood for complete cytoreduction can be selected from those with nonresectable malignancy. This keeps patients who are unlikely to benefit from undergoing cytoreductive surgical procedures from which little or no benefit occurs. The two radiologic criteria found to be most useful are segmental obstruction of small bowel and presence of tumor nodules >5 cm in diameter on small bowel surfaces or directly adjacent to small bowel mesentery of jejunum and upper ileum.

These criteria reflect radiologically the biology of the mucinous adenocarcinoma. Obstructed segments of bowel signal an invasive character of malignancy on small bowel surfaces that would be unlikely to be completely cytoreduced. Mucinous cancer on small bowel or small bowel mesentery indicates that the mucinous cancer is no longer redistributed. This means that

small bowel surfaces or small bowel mesentery will have residual disease after cytoreduction because these surfaces are impossible to peritonectomize.

The CT scan is also of great help in the identification of nodules of recurrent sarcoma and sarcomatosis. The recurrences on peritoneal surfaces are nodular and are the result of fibrin entrapment of traumatically disseminated sarcoma cells. In a CT scan with maximal filling of bowel with oral contrast, even small 1-cm nodular sarcoma recurrences are imaged.

Peritoneal Cancer Index

The third assessment of peritoneal surface malignancy is the Peritoneal Cancer Index. This is a clinical integration of both peritoneal implant size and distribution of nodules on the peritoneal surface (Figure 14.13). It should be used in the decision-making process as the abdomen is completely explored. To arrive at a score, the size of intraperitoneal nodules must be assessed. The lesion size (LS) score should be used. An LS-0 score means that no malignant deposits are visualized. An LS-1 score signifies tumor nodules <0.5 cm are present. The number of nodules is not scored, only the size of the largest nodule. An LS-2 score signifies tumor nodules between 0.5 and 5.0 cm are present. LS-3 signifies tumor nodules >5.0 cm in any dimension are present. If there is a confluence of tumor, the lesion size is scored as 3.

In order to assess the distribution of peritoneal surface disease, the abdominopelvic regions are used. For each of these 13 regions, an LS score is determined. The summation of the LS score in each of the 13 abdominopelvic regions is the Peritoneal Cancer Index for that patient. A maximal score is 39 (13 × 3).

The Peritoneal Cancer Index has been validated to date in three separate situations. First, Steller (13) and colleagues used it successfully to quantitate intraperitoneal tumor in a murine peritoneal carcinomatosis model. Gomez and coworkers (14) showed that the Peritoneal Cancer Index could be used to predict long-term survival in patients with peritoneal carcinomatosis from colon cancer undergoing a second cytoreduction. Berthet and coworkers (15) showed that the Peritoneal Cancer Index predicted benefits for treatment of peritoneal sarcomatosis from recurrent visceral or parietal sarcoma. In both of these clinical studies, patients with a favorable prognosis had a score of <13.

There are some exceptions to the rules established for the use of the Peritoneal Cancer Index. First, noninvasive malignancy on peritoneal surfaces may be completely cytoreduced even though the Index is up to 39. Diseases such as pseudomyxoma peritonei, low-nuclear-grade peritoneal mesothelioma, and grade 1 sarcoma are in this category. With these minimally invasive tumors, the status of the abdomen and pelvis after cytoreduction may have no relationship to its status at the time of abdominal exploration. In other words, even though the surgeons may find an abdomen with a Peritoneal Cancer Index of 39, it can be converted to an index of 0 by cytoreduction. In these diseases, the prognosis will only be related to the condition of the abdomen after the cytoreduction (completeness of cytoreduction score).

A second caveat for the Peritoneal Cancer Index regards cancer at crucial anatomic sites. For example, invasive cancer not cleanly resected on the common bile duct will result in a poor prognosis despite a low Peritoneal Cancer Index. Invasion

Peritoneal Cancer Index

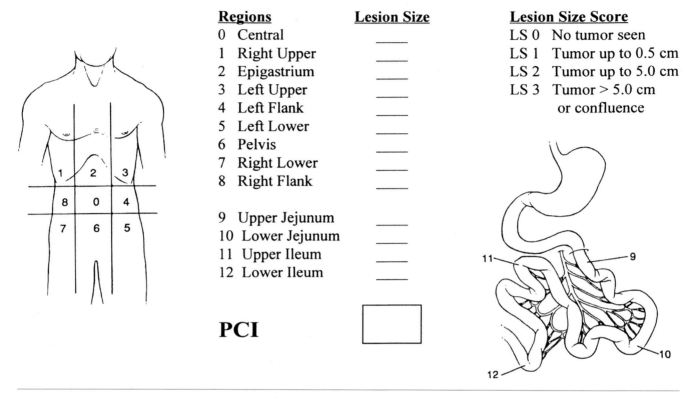

Figure 14.13 Peritoneal Cancer Index (PCI) is a composite score of lesion size 0 to 3 in abdominopelvic regions 0 to 12.

of the base of the bladder or unresectable disease on a pelvic side wall may, by itself, result in residual invasive cancer after cytoreduction and result in a poor prognosis. Also, unresectable cancer at numerous sites on the small bowel may by itself confer a poor prognosis. In other words, invasive cancer at crucial anatomic sites may function as systemic disease in assessing prognosis with invasive cancer. Because long-term survival can occur only in patients with a complete cytoreduction, residual disease at anatomically crucial sites may override a favorable score with the Peritoneal Cancer Index.

Completeness of Cytoreduction Score

The most definitive assessment to be used to assess prognosis with peritoneal surface malignancy is the completeness of cytoreduction (CC) score. This information is of less value to the surgeon in planning treatments than the Peritoneal Cancer Index. The CC score is not available until after the cytoreduction is complete, whereas the Peritoneal Cancer Index is available at the time of abdominal exploration. If during exploration it becomes obvious that cytoreduction will not be complete, the surgeon may decide that a palliative debulking, which will provide symptomatic relief, is appropriate and discontinue plans for an aggressive cytoreduction with intraperitoneal chemotherapy. In both noninvasive and invasive peritoneal surface malignancy, the CC score is the major prognostic indicator. It has been shown to

function with accuracy in pseudomyxoma peritonei, peritoneal carcinomatosis from colon cancer, sarcomatosis, and peritoneal mesothelioma (15–18).

For gastrointestinal cancer the CC score has been defined as follows: A CC-0 score indicates that no peritoneal seeding was exposed during the complete exploration. A CC-1 score indicates that tumor nodules persisting after cytoreduction are <2.5 mm. This is a nodule size thought to be penetrable by intracavity chemotherapy and would therefore be designated a complete cytoreduction. A CC-2 score indicates tumor nodules between 2.5 mm and 2.5 cm. A CC-3 score indicates tumor nodules >2.5 cm or a confluence of unresectable tumor nodules at any site within the abdomen or pelvis. CC-2 and CC-3 cytoreduction scores are considered incomplete.

Current Method for Delivery of Intraperitoneal Chemotherapy

Heated Intraoperative Intraperitoneal Chemotherapy Administration

In the operating room, heated intraoperative intraperitoneal chemotherapy is used. Thermal targeting is part of the optimizing process and is used to bring dose intensity to the abdominal and pelvic surfaces. Hyperthermia with intraperitoneal chemotherapy has several advantages. First, heat by itself has more toxicity for cancerous tissue than for normal tissue. This predominant effect on cancer increases as the vascularity of the malignancy decreases. Second, hyperthermia increases the penetration of chemotherapy into tissues. As tissues soften in response to heat, the elevated interstitial pressure of a tumor mass may decrease and allow improved drug penetration. Third, and probably most important, heat increases the cytotoxicity of selected chemotherapy agents. This synergism occurs only at the interface of heat and body tissue at the peritoneal surface. The rationale for using heated chemotherapy as a surgically directed modality in the operating room is presented in Table 14.2.

After the cancer resection is complete and prior to performing any anastomoses, the Tenckhoff catheter and closed suction drains are placed through the abdominal wall and made watertight with a purse-string suture at the skin. Temperature probes are secured to the skin edge. Using a long running no. 2 monofilament suture, the skin edges are secured to the self-retaining retractor. A plastic sheet is incorporated into these sutures to create a covering for the abdominal cavity. A slit in the plastic cover is made to allow the surgeon's double-gloved hand access to the abdomen and pelvis. During the 90 minutes of perfusion, all the anatomic structures within the peritoneal cavity are uniformly exposed to heat and to chemotherapy. The surgeon continuously manipulates all viscera to eliminate adherence of peritoneal surfaces. Roller pumps force the chemotherapy solution into the abdomen through the Tenckhoff catheter and pull it out through the drains. A heat exchanger keeps the fluid being infused at 42°C to 46°C to maintain the intraperitoneal fluid at 41°C to 42°C. The smoke evacuator is used to pull air from beneath the plastic cover through activated charcoal, preventing contamination of air in the operating room by chemotherapy aerosols.

After the intraoperative perfusion is complete, the abdomen is suctioned dry of fluid. The abdomen is then reopened, retrac-

---

Table 14.2

Rationale for the Use of Heated Intraoperative Intraperitoneal Chemotherapy

Heat increases drug penetration into tissue.

Heat increases the cytotoxicity of selected chemotherapy agents.

Heat has an antitumor effect by itself.

Intraoperative chemotherapy allows manual distribution of drug and heat uniformly to all surfaces of the abdomen and pelvis.

Renal toxicities of chemotherapy given in the operating room can be avoided by careful monitoring of urine output during chemotherapy perfusion.

The time that elapses during the heated perfusion allows a normalization of many physiologic parameters (e.g., temperature, blood clotting, hemodynamic).

Access to the peritoneal cavity over 90 minutes allows time for manicure of tumor nodules from small bowel surfaces and a mechanical disruption of cancer from within blood clots and fibrin accumulations.

Table 14.3

Standardized Orders for Heated Intraoperative Intraperitoneal Chemotherapy

For pseudomyxoma peritonei, adenocarcinoma from appendiceal and colonic cancer

1. Add mitomycin _____ mg to 2 L of 1.5% peritoneal dialysis solution.
2. Add doxorubicin _____ mg to the same 2 L of 1.5% peritoneal dialysis solution.
3. Dose of mitomycin C and for doxorubicin is 15 mg/m^2 for each chemotherapy agent.
4. Add _____ mg 5-fluorouracil (400 mg/m^2) and leucovorin _____ mg (20 mg/m^2) to separate bags of 250 mL normal saline. Begin rapid IV infusion of both drugs simultaneous with IP chemotherapy.

For sarcoma, ovarian cancer, and mesothelioma

1. Add cisplatin _____ mg to 2 L of 1.5% peritoneal dialysis solution. The dose of cisplatin is 50 mg/m^2.
2. Add doxorubicin _____ mg to the same 2 L of 1.5% peritoneal dialysis solution. The dose of doxorubicin is 15 mg/m^2.

IV, intravenous; IP, intraperitoneal.

---

tors repositioned, and reconstructive surgery is performed. It should be re-emphasized that no suture lines are constructed until after the chemotherapy perfusion is complete. One exception to this rule is closure of the vaginal cuff to prevent intraperitoneal chemotherapy leakage. The standardized orders for heated intraoperative intraperitoneal chemotherapy are given in Table 14.3.

Mitomycin C and doxorubicin are used intraoperatively to treat appendiceal, colonic, and gastric cancer. Occasionally, patients with pancreatic cancer or small bowel adenocarcinoma may be appropriate for this drug. It is appropriate for patients with ovarian cancer who have cisplatin neuropathy.

A combination of doxorubicin and cisplatin is used to treat sarcomatosis, peritoneal mesothelioma, and ovarian cancer. Also, papillary serous cancer and primary peritoneal adenocarcinoma are treated with the doxorubicin and cisplatin regimen.

Early Postoperative Intraperitoneal 5-Fluorouracil

The standardized orders for early postoperative intraperitoneal 5-fluorouracil are presented in Table 14.4. After the patient stabilizes postoperatively, and after the drainage from the immediate postoperative abdominal lavage is no longer blood stained, the 5-fluorouracil instillation occurs. The patients treated are those with carcinomatosis from adenocarcinoma. In some patients who have extensive small bowel trauma from lysis of adhesions, the early postoperative instillation of 5-fluorouracil is withheld for fear of fistula formation.

Adjuvant Treatment with Intravenous Mitomycin C and Intraperitoneal 5-Fluorouracil

Patients should be carefully selected to receive additional cycles of intraperitoneal chemotherapy. Intestinal adhesions are

Table 14.4

Early Postoperative Intraperitoneal Chemotherapy with 5-Fluorouracil

Postoperative Days 1–4

1. Add to ___ mL 1.5% dextrose peritoneal dialysis solution:
   (a) ___ mg 5-fluorouracil (650 mg/m^2; maximal dose, 1,300 mg)
   (b) 50 mEq sodium bicarbonate
2. Intraperitoneal fluid volume: 1 L for patients <2.0 m^2, 1.5 L for >2.0 m^2.
3. Drain all fluid from the abdominal cavity prior to instillation, then clamp abdominal drains.
4. Run the chemotherapy solution into the abdominal cavity through the Tenckhoff catheter as rapidly as possible. Dwell for 23 hours and drain for 1 hour prior to next instillation.
5. Use gravity to maximize intraperitoneal distribution of the 5-fluorouracil. Instill the chemotherapy with the patient in a full right lateral position. After $\frac{1}{2}$ hour, direct the patient to turn to the full left lateral position. Change position right to left every $\frac{1}{2}$ hour. If tolerated, use 10 degrees of Trendelenburg position. Continue turning for the first 6 hours after instillation of chemotherapy solution.
6. Continue to drain abdominal cavity after final dwell until Tenckhoff catheter is removed.

the most frequent contraindication to its use. Usually, adjuvant intraperitoneal chemotherapy is not recommended in patients with extensive prior peritonectomy. The treatment is directed at the small bowel surfaces and is designed to eradicate large numbers of minute peritoneal implants. Parietal peritoneal surfaces, stomach surfaces, and the large bowel can usually be completely cytoreduced. Small bowel surfaces are the most common site for residual disease that prevents the CC-0 or CC-1 cytoreduction.

Reoperative Surgery Plus Additional Intraperitoneal Chemotherapy

As the clinical data regarding treatment of peritoneal surface malignancy become available, the need for a more aggressive approach in selected patients has become clear. Peritoneal carcinomatosis from colon cancer is sometimes managed with a second-look surgery; also, patients with primary peritoneal surface malignancy, especially mesothelioma, may profit from a scheduled second-look surgery at 6 to 9 months.

At the second-look surgery, the abdomen is opened wide and all of the peritoneal surfaces are visualized with a complete takedown of all adhesions. Additional cytoreduction is performed, and additional visceral resections may be required. If a CC-1 cytoreduction can again be achieved, then the treatment with heated intraoperative intraperitoneal chemotherapy is repeated. Also, if the patient has adenocarcinoma, early postoperative intraperitoneal 5-fluorouracil is again recommended.

If it appears from the reoperation that the initial heated chemotherapy and early postoperative chemotherapy treatments were successful at most anatomic sites, then the same regimen will be employed again. If there is a "chemotherapy failure" and recurrent disease is seen in areas that have been previously peritonectomized, then a chemotherapy change would be initiated.

Indications for Heated Intraoperative Intraperitoneal Chemotherapy as an Oncologic Emergency

As a primary gastrointestinal cancer is resected, unexpected dissemination of cancer cells on peritoneal surfaces may be documented. Resections of gastrointestinal cancers may occur in which there is disruption of the cancer specimen resulting in "intraoperative tumor spill." In women, ovarian involvement of a gastrointestinal cancer indicates peritoneal contamination. A small volume of localized cancer seeding on the specimen or in the omentum that would be resected as part of the removal of the primary tumor signals generalized peritoneal contamination. Another indication would be a perforated intra-abdominal malignancy when that perforation is through the cancer itself. Positive peritoneal cytology and malignant ascites would also be considered an indication for the oncologic emergency. A majority of these patients will be recommended for a second-look surgery at 6 to 9 months after the appropriate adjuvant chemotherapy is completed.

Clinical Results of Treatment

Reliable Relief of Debilitating Ascites

Patients with a large volume of malignant ascites are frequently encountered as a cancerous process moves toward its terminal phase. This may be caused by breast cancer, gastric cancer, mucinous malignancies of the colon or appendix, and primary peritoneal surface cancers. Intraperitoneal chemotherapy is uniformly successful in eliminating the debilitating ascites (19,20). Success usually requires three or four cycles of a systemic dose of appropriate chemotherapy into the abdomen. Combinations of both systemic and intraperitoneal chemotherapy (bidirectional) are often selected. Also, Link and colleagues (21) used mitoxantrone in this clinical situation.

It is important to inform patients that intraperitoneal chemotherapy as treatment for malignant ascites is for symptomatic relief and should not be considered curative. The mass of solid tumor will remain unchanged or will progress during treatment. Only the ascites will disappear. The mechanism of action of intraperitoneal chemotherapy on large-volume malignant ascites is destruction of surface cancer. It is thought that intraperitoneal chemotherapy results in a layer of fibrosis over all malignant deposits and also on normal parietal and visceral peritoneal surfaces. This fibrotic layer of tissue prevents formation of both normal peritoneal fluid and malignant fluids.

Technique for Chemotherapy Instillation for Treatment of Malignant Ascites

The technique used for repeated instillations of intraperitoneal chemotherapy to palliate malignant ascites is crucial for success. First, paracentesis using a temporary all-purpose drain should provide access to the peritoneal space. A long-term indwelling

(Tenckhoff) catheter should not be used to provide access because of the high incidence of infection with a foreign body located within a large volume intra-abdominal fluid over a long period. Also, an intraperitoneal subcutaneous port should not be used because of difficulties it creates with drainage of intraperitoneal fluid. Repeated paracentesis is safe if CT or ultrasound is used to select the site on the abdominal wall for puncture. When the ascites is gone or greatly diminished, the paracentesis becomes more dangerous. Of course, because these treatments are palliative if the malignant ascites is greatly reduced, then these treatments are discontinued.

Schedule and Dose of Intraperitoneal Chemotherapy for Treatment of Malignant Ascites

The all-purpose drain is kept in place for 5 days. Each day, the ascites fluid is drained as completely as possible. Multiple changes in the patient's position may facilitate drainage. Then the intraperitoneal chemotherapy solution is instilled for a 23-hour dwell. For adenocarcinoma, intravenous mitomycin C and intraperitoneal 5-fluorouracil may be appropriate. In some patients a combination of cisplatin ($15 \ mg/m^2$/day) and doxorubicin ($3 \ mg/m^2$/day) are instilled. As soon as the chemotherapy solution has entered the abdomen, the patient is instructed to turn from front to back and from side to side every half hour. Alternatively, mitoxantrone can be used at $3 \ mg/m^2$/day for 5 days in a row (21). The cycle of treatments is repeated at 3-week intervals. In a few patients, persistent ascites may require a surgical procedure (debulking) in order to separate adherent bowel loops, remove bulk disease, and allow the use of a single cycle of heated intraoperative intraperitoneal chemotherapy. During the debulking the large masses of tumor are removed and any obstructing portions of bowel are resected. This generally includes the greater and lesser omentum and pedunculated tumor masses. No attempt at a complete cytoreduction is made. The responses achieved in patients who are debulked and then given intraoperative chemotherapy may be more lasting than in patients given chemotherapy only.

Treatment of Mucinous Ascites

If the intraperitoneal fluid is mucinous, it cannot be drained through a tube. Relief of mucinous ascites can only be achieved by laparotomy and manual removal of mucinous tumor. Usually a greater omentectomy is performed as part of the debulking. Liposuction apparatus may greatly facilitate evacuation of the viscous material. If the tumor mass can be reduced to a low level, then intraoperative and early postoperative intraperitoneal chemotherapy may slow the reaccumulation of mucinous tumor.

Curative Approach to Carcinomatosis
Appendiceal Cancer and Pseudomyxoma Peritonei

The paradigm for treatment of peritoneal carcinomatosis is appendiceal malignancy. Yan and colleagues (22) reviewed the experience with 863 patients from 8 institutions treated over a 15-year period. The 5-year survival was 69%. In a group of patients with adenomucinosis treated with optimal cytoreductive surgery and perioperative intraperitoneal chemotherapy, the 20-year projected survival for 307 patients was 75% (23).

Appendiceal Malignancy as a Paradigm

The concepts gained from treating peritoneal surface malignancy from an appendiceal primary tumor can be applied to the management of other gastrointestinal cancers. There are unique clinical features of the appendiceal malignancies that have facilitated the extraordinary favorable results of treatment documented with this tumor. Spread from appendiceal tumors usually occurs in the absence of lymph node and liver metastases. The primary tumor occurs within a tiny lumen. Even small tumors early in the natural history of the disease will cause appendiceal obstruction and perforation. This results in a release of tumor cells into the free peritoneal cavity. The seeding of the abdomen occurs in almost every patient before lymph node metastases or liver metastases have occurred. Second, there is a wide spectrum of invasion in which these tumors exhibit. Mucinous tumors that are minimally invasive can be totally resected using peritonectomy procedures to achieve a CC-1 cytoreduction. Third, the majority of these tumors are mucinous. The texture of the implants allows greater penetration by chemotherapy than with solid tumors. Finally, the malignancy disseminates so that all of the disease is within the regional chemotherapy field. If the intraperitoneal chemotherapy is successful in eradicating microscopic residual disease on peritoneal surfaces, the patient will be a long-term survivor. In these patients the response achieved by the intraperitoneal chemotherapy determines the outcome, assuming of course, that a CC-1 cytoreduction was possible.

The treatment strategies used included peritonectomy procedures combined with perioperative intraperitoneal chemotherapy with mitomycin C and 5-fluorouracil. Survival was significantly correlated with the invasive character of the mucinous tumor, the completeness of cytoreduction, and the prior surgical score. In contrast to most studies with gastrointestinal cancer patients, lymph node involvement was not a determinate prognostic factor in patients with peritoneal dissemination of malignancy if intraperitoneal chemotherapy was used (5).

Recently, numerous articles studying the survival of patients with carcinomatosis from colon cancer have been published. Yan and colleagues (24) critically reviewed these reports. In the 14 articles reviewed, the median survival was approximately 30 months for >1,000 patients included in the systematic review. There was a single randomized controlled study that compared cytoreductive surgery plus heated intraoperative intraperitoneal mitomycin C with a control group of patients who had surgery to relieve symptoms and systemic 5-fluorouracil (25). There was a statistically significant improvement in survival in the experimental arm. Glehen and colleagues (26) studied 506 patients from 28 different institutions. All of these patients had cytoreductive surgery with perioperative intraperitoneal chemotherapy. The median survival of the group of patients was 19 months overall and 32 months in those patients who had a complete cytoreduction. The Peritoneal Cancer Index provided valuable prognostic information in these patients by which to select for an aggressive treatment approach (Figure 14.14) (27).

Sarcomatosis

Berthet and colleagues (15) have reviewed their experience with cytoreductive surgery and intraperitoneal chemotherapy for treatment of selected patients with sarcomatosis. If the

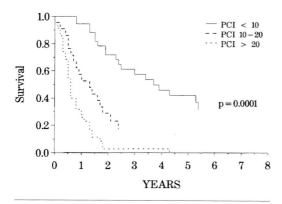

Figure 14.14 Survival of patients with peritoneal carcinomatosis from colon cancer by Peritoneal Cancer Index (PCI).

Peritoneal Cancer Index at the time of abdominal exploration was <13, there was a 75% 5-year survival. In those who had a Peritoneal Cancer Index of ≥13, the 5-year survival was only 13%. The completeness of cytoreduction was also statistically significant for an improved prognosis. Twenty-seven patients with a complete cytoreduction had a 5-year survival of 39%. Sixteen patients with a CC-2 or CC-3 resection had a survival of 14%.

Peritoneal Seeding from Gastric Cancer

Extensive studies with peritoneal seeding from gastric cancer have been conducted in Japan and Korea and a meta-analysis has been published (28). Reports from Western series are not available. Survival rates for patients in Japan with heated intraoperative intraperitoneal chemotherapy at time of gastrectomy vary from 10% to 43%. Results of treatment of a group of Western patients have not yet been reported; however, a theoretical and clinical basis for treatment has been established (29).

Primary Peritoneal Surface Malignancy

A confusing and poorly understood group of tumors that have been successfully treated with peritonectomy and perioperative intraperitoneal chemotherapy are the primary peritoneal surface malignancies. These diseases include diffuse malignant peritoneal mesothelioma. Currently, all patients are being treated with heated intraoperative cisplatin and doxorubicin and adjuvant intraperitoneal paclitaxel. Recent results show a median survival of 5 years; a marked improvement from 1 year reported just a few years ago (30).

Morbidity and Mortality of Phase II Studies

The morbidity and mortality of 356 consecutive patients who had cytoreductive surgery and heated intraoperative intraperitoneal chemotherapy for peritoneal carcinomatosis have been reported (31). In these patients, the in-hospital mortality was 2%. There were 19% of patients with grade IV complications and 11% of patients required a return to the operating room.

Alternative Approaches

Peritoneal carcinomatosis has been treated in the past with systemic chemotherapy. No long-term survivors from this treatment have been described in the literature. Palliative surgery can give temporary relief of intestinal obstruction. These efforts have always been categorized as low-value surgery because long-term survival was rarely achieved. Other therapies that include intraperitoneal immunotherapy, intraperitoneal isotopes, and intraperitoneal labeled monoclonal antibody have not shown reproducible beneficial results. In summary, alternative curative approaches to cytoreductive surgery and intraperitoneal chemotherapy for peritoneal carcinomatosis have not been reported.

Postoperative Management

The major management issue postoperatively with combined cytoreductive surgery and intraperitoneal chemotherapy is prolonged ileus. Patients may have a nasogastric tube in place with large volumes of secretions being aspirated for 2 to 4 weeks postoperatively. The length of time required for nasogastric suctioning depends on the extent of the peritonectomy procedures and the extent of prior abdominal adhesions requiring lysis.

A life-threatening postoperative complication is the fistula. These are almost always sidewall perforations of the small bowel, but colon and stomach perforations have occurred. Patients need to be made aware of the possibility of a fistula before cytoreductive surgery and intraperitoneal chemotherapy are contemplated. As previously mentioned, the anastomotic leak rate is low.

Pancreatitis occurs in approximately 30% of patients who have an extensive upper abdominal cytoreduction. Prolonged nutritional support, antibiotics, and CT to drain peripancreatic fluid collections may be necessary. The process is self-limited but may cause fever and persistent nausea for several weeks postoperatively.

Following these treatments, the patient is usually maintained on parenteral feeding for 2 to 4 weeks. Approximately 20% of patients, especially those who have had extensive prior surgery or who have a short bowel, will need parenteral feeding for several months after they leave the hospital.

ETHICAL CONSIDERATION IN CLINICAL STUDIES WITH PERITONEAL SURFACE MALIGNANCY

The sequence of events that should accompany a new program in peritoneal surface malignancy has not yet been defined. The requirements for formal institutional review board approval will vary from one institution to another. Guidelines for an evolution of treatment strategies that allow for reliable clinical research may occur as follows:

Without exception, adjuvant intraperitoneal chemotherapy studies in patients with primary gastrointestinal cancer must be randomized and require review by a research board. An exception to the need for randomization is resected pancreatic cancer. Also, when a group first attempts to initiate treatment plans with intraperitoneal chemotherapy, the learning curve associated with a new technology is best approached by a start-up protocol approved by an institutional review board. This forces the group to standardize the methods and familiarize themselves with the experience of others. Selection criteria to treat patients with a reasonable likelihood of benefit must be determined. An omnibus protocol is suggested that allows aggressive cytoreduction and perioperative intraperitoneal chemotherapy in patients without systemic dissemination and with small-volume peritoneal seeding from peritoneal carcinomatosis, peritoneal sarcomatosis, and mesothelioma. This omnibus protocol should be used for a limited time to treat 10 to 20 patients.

Formal protocols should not be required for the treatment of debilitating ascites because of the marked quality-of-life benefits demonstrated (32). Also, long-term survival of patients with peritoneal surface malignancy that has a small volume and limited distribution has been established. After completing the start-up protocols, treatment of this group of patients by an oncologic team that has demonstrated experience should proceed without the need for further institutional review board approval. The peritoneal surface spread of most gastrointestinal cancers that have a low Peritoneal Cancer Index and that after surgery have a CC score of 0 or 1 should be routinely treated according to standardized intraperitoneal chemotherapy protocols. Treatment of peritoneal carcinomatosis, sarcomatosis, and mesothelioma definitively at the time of initial diagnosis will always be preferred over treatment of recurrence.

REFERENCES

1. Gunderson LL, Sosin H. Areas of failure found at reoperation (second or symptomatic look) following "curative surgery" for adenocarcinoma of the rectum: clinicopathologic correlation and implications for adjuvant therapy. *Cancer.* 1974;34:1278–292.
2. Sugarbaker PH. Surgical management of locally recurrent and metastatic colorectal cancer. In: Karakousis CP, Copeland EM, Bland QUI, eds. *Atlas of Surgical Oncology.* Philadelphia: Saunders; 1995:671–692.
3. Sugarbaker PH, Hughes KA. Surgery for colorectal metastasis to liver. In: Wanebo H, ed. *Colorectal Cancer.* St. Louis: Mosby-Year Book; 1993:405–413.
4. Sugarbaker PH. *Peritoneal Carcinomatosis: Principles of Management.* Boston: Kluwer, 1996.
5. Sugarbaker PH. Results of treatment of 385 patients with peritoneal surface spread of appendiceal malignancy. *Ann Surg Oncol* 1999;6:727–731.
6. Sugarbaker PH. Peritonectomy procedures. *Surg Oncol Clin North Am* 2003;12:703–727.
7. Carmignani P, Sugarbaker TA, Bromley CM, et al. Intraperitoneal cancer dissemination: mechanisms of the patterns of spread. *Cancer Metastasis Rev.* 2003;22:465–472.
8. Sugarbaker PH, Graves T, DeBruijn EA, et al. Rationale for early postoperative intraperitoneal chemotherapy (EPIC) in patients with advanced gastrointestinal cancer. *Cancer Res.* 1990;50:5790–5794.
9. Ronnett BM, Zahn CM, Kurman RJ, et al. Disseminated peritoneal adenomucinosis and peritoneal mucinous carcinomatosis: a clinicopathologic analysis of 109 cases with emphasis on distinguishing pathologic features, site of origin, prognosis, and relationship to "pseudomyxoma peritonei." *Am J Surg Pathol.* 1995;19:1390–1408.
10. Cerruto CA, Brun EA, Sugarbaker PH. Prognostic significance of histo-morphologic parameters in diffuse malignant peritoneal mesothelioma. *Arch Pathol Lab Med.* 2006;130:1654–1661.
11. Jacquet P, Jelinek JS, Steves MA, et al. Evaluation of computer tomography in patients with peritoneal carcinomatosis. *Cancer.* 1993;72:1631–1636.
12. Jacquet P, Jelinek JS, Chang D, et al. Abdominal computed tomographic scan in the selection of patients with mucinous peritoneal carcinomatosis for cytoreductive surgery. *J Am Coll Surg.* 1995; 181:530–538.
13. Steller EP. Comparison of four scoring methods for an intraperitoneal immunotherapy model. *Enhancement and Abrogation: Modifications of Host Immune Influence IL-2 and LAK Cell Immunotherapy* [dissertation]. Rotterdam, the Netherlands: Erasmus University Rotterdam; 1988.
14. Gomez Portilla A, Sugarbaker PH, Chang D. Second-look surgery after cytoreductive and intraperitoneal chemotherapy for peritoneal carcinomatosis from colorectal cancer: Analysis of prognostic features. *World J Surg.* 1999;23:23–29.
15. Berthet B, Sugarbaker TA, Chang D, et al. Quantitative methodologies for selection of patients with recurrent abdominopelvic sarcoma for treatment. *Eur J Cancer.* 1999;35:413–419.
16. Sugarbaker PH, Ronnett BM, Archer A, et al. Management of pseudomyxoma peritonei of appendiceal origin. *Adv Surg.* 1997;30:233–280.
17. Sebbag G, Yan H, Shmookler BM, et al. Results of treatment of 33 patients with peritoneal mesothelioma. *Br J Surg.* 2000;87:1587–1593.
18. Sugarbaker PH. Successful management of microscopic residual disease in large bowel cancer. *Cancer Chemother Pharmaco* 1999;43(Suppl):S15–S25.
19. Gilly FN, Sayag, AC, Carry PY, et al. Intraperitoneal chemohyperthermia (CHIP): A new therapy in the treatment of the peritoneal seedings. *Int Surg.* 1991;76:164–167.
20. Fujimoto S, Shrestha RD, Kokubun M, et al. Intraperitoneal hyperthermic perfusion combined with surgery effective for gastric cancer patients with peritoneal seeding. *Ann Surg.* 1988;208:36–41.
21. Link K, Roitman M, Holtappels M, et al. Intraperitoneal chemotherapy with mitoxantrone in malignant ascites. *Surg Oncol Clin North Am.* 2003;12:865–872.
22. Yan TD, Black D, Savady R, et al. A systematic review on the efficacy of cytoreductive surgery and perioperative intraperitoneal chemotherapy for pseudomyxoma peritonei. *Ann Surg Oncol.* 2007;14:484–492.
23. Sugarbaker PH: Are there curative options to peritoneal carcinomatosis [editorial]? *Ann Surg.* 2005;242:748–750.
24. Yan TD, Savady R, Black D, et al. A systematic review of cytoreductive surgery combined with perioperative intraperitoneal chemotherapy for colorectal peritoneal carcinomatosis. *J Clin Oncol.* 2006;24:4011–4019.
25. Verwaal VJ, van Ruth S, de Bree E, et al. Randomized trial of cytoreduction and hyperthermic intraperitoneal chemotherapy versus systemic chemotherapy and palliative surgery in patients with peritoneal carcinomatosis of colorectal origin. *J Clin Oncol.* 2003;21:3737–3743.
26. Glehen O, Mithieux F, Osinsky D, et al. Surgery combined with peritonectomy procedures and intraperitoneal chemohyperthermia in abdominal cancers with peritoneal carcinomatosis: a phase II study. *J Clin Oncol.* 2003;21:799–806.
27. Pestieau SR, Sugarbaker PH. Treatment of primary colon cancer with peritoneal carcinomatosis: a comparison of concomitant versus delayed management. *Dis Colon Rectum.* 2000;43:1341–1348.
28. Xu DZ, Zhan YQ, Sun XW, et al. Meta-analysis of intraperitoneal chemotherapy for gastric cancer. *World J Gastroenterol.* 2004;10:2727–2730.
29. Sugarbaker PH, Yu W, Yonemura Y. Gastrectomy, peritonectomy and perioperative intraperitoneal chemotherapy: the evolution of treatment strategies for advanced gastric cancer. *Semin Surg Oncol.* 2003;21:233–248.
30. Sugarbaker PH, Welch L, Mohamed F, et al. A review of peritoneal mesothelioma at the Washington Cancer Institute. *Surg Oncol Clin North Am.* 2003;12:605–621.

31. Sugarbaker PH, Alderman R, Edwards G, et al. Prospective morbidity and mortality assessment of cytoreductive surgery plus perioperative intraperitoneal chemotherapy to treat peritoneal dissemination of appendiceal mucinous malignancy. *Ann Surg Oncol.* 2006;13:635–644.

32. McQuellon RP, Loggie BW, Fleming RA, et al. Quality of life after intraperitoneal hyperthermic chemotherapy (IPHC) for peritoneal carcinomatosis. *Eur J Surg Oncol.* 2001;27:65–73.

COMMENTARY
Shishir K. Maithel and Yuman Fong

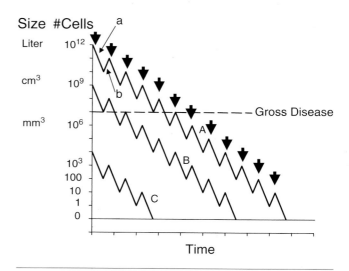

Figure 14C.1. Log-kill hypothesis. Line a illustrates the size of the log kill with each dose (*thick arrow*) of chemotherapy. Line b shows the regrowth of tumor prior to the next dose. Lines A, B, and C refer to progressively smaller initial tumor volume. The percentage of cells killed each time is greatest for the smaller tumor volume (C), resulting in the best chance for a cure.

EVOLUTION OF SURGICAL CYTOREDUCTION FOR CANCER

The goal of most cancer operations is complete eradication of disease in an attempt for cure. In the past, only highly selected patients were offered surgical cytoreduction or "debulking," which can be defined as planned incomplete resection of tumor. There are many theoretical and practical justifications for this procedure. Cytoreduction can improve quality of life in patients with bulky, symptomatic tumors. Reducing tumor burden may decrease the tumor's immunosuppressive effects and improve response to systemic therapies (1,2). Tumor volume reduction may prevent further metastases. Until recently, despite these reasons, most cytoreductive procedures have been reserved for patients with very slow-growing tumors or patients with symptomatic tumors.

A number of factors have combined to stimulate interest in and extend the indications for cytoreductive surgery. First and foremost is the increasing safety of even the most extensive operative procedures (3). Ablative procedures have also become safe and effective alternatives to extended resections (4). In addition, renewed interest results from the increasingly effective chemotherapy and biologic treatments for cancer, which are converting many initially unresectable patients to the realm of surgical therapy. Currently, surgical cytoreduction is based on the concept that safe debulking of gross disease by resection or ablation can be combined with chemotherapy and/or radiation to result in improved outcome.

In his text, Dr. Sugarbaker has discussed the role of peritoneal cytoreduction and regional therapy. The goal of this commentary is to highlight other evolving paradigms for cytoreductive surgery.

CYTOREDUCTIVE SURGERY WITH RESIDUAL MICROSCOPIC DISEASE, FOLLOWED BY ADJUVANT THERAPY

A general principle of chemotherapy is that the potential for cure is inversely proportional to tumor burden. This is because chemotherapeutic agents appear to kill a constant fraction of cells after each dose, rather than a specific number of cells (1) (Figure 14C.1). According to this log-kill hypothesis, reducing the initial tumor volume improves the likelihood that repeated cycles of chemotherapy will reduce the number of viable tumor cells toward the end point of zero.

Thus, the most common scenario in the application of cytoreductive surgery is resection of all visible tumor in patients with lesions associated with a high risk of residual microscopic disease. Surgery is followed by adjuvant chemotherapy and/or radiation therapy. This is typified by patients with lymphatic metastases from cancers such as esophageal cancer, colorectal cancer, or breast cancer. Because chemotherapy or radiation therapy generally will not completely eradicate gross disease, the hope is that surgical resections along with regional lymphadenectomy will reduce the bulk of tumor to a level potentially treatable by chemotherapy, thereby producing either a long disease-free period or potential cure. This is illustrated in Figure 14C.2A. Surgery (depicted by x in Figure 14C.2) eliminates all gross disease. In these cases, clinical-pathologic parameters such as node positivity, primary tumor size, or persistently abnormal tumor markers indicate a high risk for recurrence. Patients are therefore placed on a limited course of adjuvant chemotherapy. These treatments, when effective, can eliminate microscopic residual and result in cure.

CYTOREDUCTION WITH RESIDUAL SMALL VOLUME GROSS DISEASE, FOLLOWED BY HIGHLY EFFECTIVE ADJUVANT CHEMOTHERAPY

In some cancers, the chemotherapeutic agents are so effective that even gross residual disease can be treated for survival benefit.

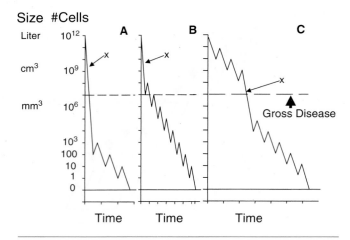

Figure 14C.2. Various roles of surgical resection or cytoreduction in the multimodality care of the cancer patient. **Panel A** is the classic schema of a patient undergoing surgical resection (x) followed by multiple courses of potentially curative adjuvant chemotherapy. **Panel B** represents cytoreductive surgery (x) to a level of minimal gross disease, followed by effective chemotherapy that reduces tumor to levels below clinical detectability. **Panel C** illustrates the use of initial induction chemotherapy, followed by subsequent cytoreduction (x), and finishing with consolidation chemotherapy.

The prototypic disease for this scenario is ovarian cancer. In this cancer, surgery is required to reduce the bulk of disease to a level at which the chemotherapy can be expected to be the most effective. This is a disease in which it is proven that cytoreduction to tumor bulk of 1 to 2 cm^3 can be combined with effective adjuvant chemotherapy to produce survival benefit (5). This paradigm is depicted in Figure 14C.2B. Reducing the total tumor volume to be treated also substantially diminishes the chances of cancer cells developing drug resistance, an event that increases directly with the number of cancer cells and the time it takes to complete treatment (1).

SURGICAL CYTOREDUCTION AFTER EFFECTIVE SYSTEMIC CHEMOTHERAPY OR BIOLOGIC THERAPY

There have been such improvements in systemic therapies in the last 2 decades that many patients with advanced-stage non-resectable disease are now treated with sufficient reduction of disease to be subsequently considered for surgical resection. The prototypic disease in this category is germ cell tumor. Chemotherapy is so effective that patients with extensive retroperitoneal nodal disease, liver disease, lung disease, and even brain metastases can be restored to a status amenable to potentially curative surgical cytoreduction (6). The justification for aggressive multiorgan resections after systemic therapy is clear. Over 80% of patients treated with chemotherapy, followed by orchiectomy, retroperitoneal node dissection, and even liver, lung, and brain metastasectomy can be cured. The concept is that chemotherapy can produce such effective tumor debulking

that final cytoreduction by surgery is both possible and useful. It should be noted that chemotherapy can also produce dedifferentiation of tumor to a chemoresistant phenotype (teratoma) that requires resection.

Recent improved chemotherapy regimens have also produced similar downstaging of patients with metastatic colorectal cancer to the liver who then benefit from subsequent effective cytoreduction. In the largest series reported to date, 20% of patients with initially unresectable colorectal cancer to the liver were found to have sufficient reduction of cancer bulk to allow for subsequent hepatic resection. After resection, 30% of patients were found to be long-term survivors (7).

Improvements in biologic therapies have also contributed to favorable results employing this strategy. The discovery that gastrointestinal stromal tumors may be characterized by c-Kit mutation and sensitive to treatment by imatinib mesylate (Gleevec) brought an effective therapy to many patients with previously untreatable disease. Most patients with advanced disease are still not being cured by biologic therapies alone. Many are, however, and return to the surgeon after Gleevec therapy with potentially resectable tumor and are being treated with surgery (8). Whether such cytoreductive surgery after induction biologic therapy ultimately will be curative or palliative awaits longer follow-up and reporting.

The myriad of effective chemotherapies, biologic therapies, and hormonal therapies for breast cancer has moved some advanced-stage patients into the realm of effective surgical cytoreduction. Some patients with bone, liver, nodal, and lung metastases who have responded to aggressive systemic therapy can be considered for cytoreductive surgery for the residual disease, followed by consolidative postoperative systemic therapy. Generally, a long period of observation on systemic therapy is conducted before engaging in such radical cytoreductive surgery. The ultimate results of such combined therapies await future reporting.

The schema for this general strategy is illustrated in Figure 14C.2C. In disease in which systemic treatment is so effective as to produce immediate and dramatic reduction of tumors in patients with advanced disease, surgical resection aims to complete the gross eradication of disease. In cases of hepatic colorectal metastases or gastrointestinal stromal tumors, it may allow a subsequent finite course of systemic therapy to be more effective treatment of microscopic residual disease. Cytoreduction may also allow a holiday from potentially toxic and expensive systemic therapy. In the case of breast cancer, response to systemic therapy over a sustained period allows the hope that resection of gross residual disease can be curative and can be followed by less toxic hormonal therapy.

CYTOREDUCTION FOR SLOW-GROWING TUMOR

There are a number of tumors in which cytoreductive surgery is beneficial because of the slow growth of the tumor. Typical tumors in this category are well-differentiated liposarcomas, hepatocellular carcinomas, and neuroendocrine tumors. The concept is that if a tumor is sufficiently slow growing, the morbidity of the cytoreductive procedure will be justified by

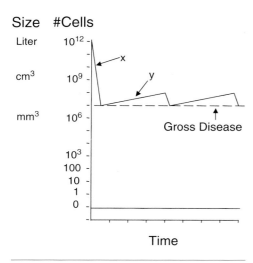

Figure 14C.3. Cytoreduction for slow-growing tumors. Cytoreduction is depicted by line x. A long period may pass before regrowth of the tumor (y) to significant levels. At that time, further cytoreduction may be performed by resection or ablation.

a long period of symptom-free survival. This is illustrated in Figure 14C.3.

In the case of retroperitoneal liposarcomas, not only are the primary tumors slow growing, but they are also very resistant to systemic therapies. This tumor also rarely produces hematogenous or lymphatic metastases so that mortality is due to local progression. Cytoreduction may not only alleviate symptoms and reduce the volume of tumor that may undergo high-grade dedifferentiation, but it also may increase survival (9). Hepatocellular carcinoma is another chemoresistant tumor that can be effectively treated by cytoreduction in the form of surgery, embolization, or thermoablation (10,11).

For neuroendocrine tumors, cytoreduction is beneficial even after the tumor has metastasized (12). Liver metastases can be treated with either resection or ablation of liver tumors with clinical benefit. In particular, patients with hormonal symptoms have a high likelihood of symptomatic relief (13). For bulky disease, surgical resection can result in a durable response.

CONCLUSIONS

Indications for surgical cytoreduction are expanding. At one time, incomplete resections were offered only to patients with significant symptoms as a palliative therapy. With increasingly safe procedures, patients with classically slow-growing tumors, or tumors that in specific cases prove to be slow growing through long-term follow-up, are now offered cytoreductive surgery. The goals of such safe debulking procedures are to bring about prolonged symptom-free survival, as well as allow holidays from potentially toxic systemic therapy.

Recent improvements in systemic and regional chemotherapy have further expanded indications. Combined systemic and surgical therapies are increasingly used as effective therapies

for tumors previously thought to be unresectable. In many of the newer indications for surgical cytoreduction, patients are generally first treated with chemotherapy and/or biologic therapies. After a tumoricidal effect is seen, patients are offered optimum cytoreductive resection of residual tumor, usually followed by additional chemotherapy. This allows a waiting period on chemotherapy for observation of the biologic behavior of the tumor.

Even with the recent major improvements in systemic therapies, it is clear that for solid tumors chemotherapies and biologic treatments are unlikely to be curative for a patient with bulky disease. A decade ago, there were predictions that improving systemic therapies would make surgery obsolete. On the contrary, our increasingly effective systemic therapies have not eliminated the need for surgical procedures, but rather increased the role of surgery in the treatment of many malignancies. Surgeons are no longer asked to perform only palliative operations in patients with stage IV disease but are consulted under suitable circumstances to perform potentially curative cytoreductive surgery, often as a component of a multidisciplinary treatment program.

REFERENCES

1. Muss HB. Chemotherapy of gynecologic cancer. In: Deppe G, ed. *Principles of Cancer Chemotherapy.* Philadelphia: Wiley-Liss; 1990:1– 40.
2. Pollock RE, Roth JA. Cancer-induced immunosuppression: implications for therapy? *Semin Surg Oncol.* 1989;5:414–419.
3. Jarnagin WR, Gonen M, Fong Y, et al. Improvement in perioperative outcome after hepatic resection: analysis of 1,803 consecutive cases over the past decade. *Ann Surg.* 2002;236:397–406.
4. Decadt B, Siriwardena AK. Radiofrequency ablation of liver tumours: systematic review. *Lancet Oncol.* 2004;5:550–560.
5. Curtin JP, Shapiro F. Adjuvant therapy in gynecologic malignances. Ovarian, cervical, and endometrial cancer. *Surg Oncol Clin North Am.* 1997;6:813–830.
6. Carver BS, Shayegan B, Serio A, et al. Long-term clinical outcome after postchemotherapy retroperitoneal lymph node dissection in men with residual teratoma. *J Clin Oncol.* 2007;25:1033–1037.
7. Adam R, Delvart V, Pascal G, et al. Rescue surgery for unresectable colorectal liver metastases downstaged by chemotherapy: a model to predict long-term survival. *Ann Surg.* 2004;240:644–657.
8. Verweij J, van OA, Blay JY, et al. Imatinib mesylate (STI-571 Glivec, Gleevec) is an active agent for gastrointestinal stromal tumours, but does not yield responses in other soft-tissue sarcomas that are unselected for a molecular target. Results from an EORTC Soft Tissue and Bone Sarcoma Group phase II study. *Eur J Cancer.* 2003;39:2006– 2011.
9. Shibata D, Lewis JJ, Leung DH, et al. Is there a role for incomplete resection in the management of retroperitoneal liposarcomas? *J Am Coll Surg.* 2001;193:373–379.
10. Livraghi T. Radiofrequency ablation, PEIT, and TACE for hepatocellular carcinoma. *J Hepatobiliary Pancreat Surg.* 2003;10:67–76.
11. Covey AM, Maluccio MA, Schubert J, et al. Particle embolization of recurrent hepatocellular carcinoma after hepatectomy. *Cancer.* 2006;106:2181–2189.
12. Janson ET, Oberg K. Malignant neuroendocrine tumors. *Cancer Chemother Biol Response Modif.* 2002;20:463–470.
13. Que FG, Sarmiento JM, Nagorney DM. Hepatic surgery for metastatic gastrointestinal neuroendocrine tumors. *Adv Exp Med Biol.* 2006;574:43–56.

15

Cancer and Pregnancy

Kristine E. Calhoun, Gary N. Mann, and Benjamin O. Anderson

Although the co-existence of cancer and pregnancy is thought to be a rare event, population data suggest that it complicates up to 1 in 1,000 pregnancies worldwide (1,2), with malignancy being the second most common cause of death among women in their reproductive years (3,4). As more women delay the onset of childbearing in much of the westernized world, mostly because of the pursuit of educational and professional endeavors, it is believed that the incidence of pregnancy-associated cancer will increase concordantly. Given the relative rarity of pregnancy-associated cancer, it is not surprising that the majority of available literature involves case reports or small retrospective series data. The lack of prospective, randomized control trial data with large numbers of patients means there is often a lack of consensus as to the standard of care with which these individuals should be treated (5).

When a woman is diagnosed with cancer during pregnancy, a multitude of ethical, psychological, and medical issues must all be dealt with concurrently. Not surprisingly, conflicting issues between maternal and fetal health can arise. In these situations, women must deal with a life-giving and a life-threatening condition simultaneously, having to make treatment decisions that may benefit one "patient" while harming the other (5). The personal and practical challenges of treating the patient with pregnancy-associated malignancy should not be underestimated, as the well-being of both the mother and developing fetus must be addressed under one unified therapeutic plan. As the number of women affected by pregnancy-associated malignancy increases, the number of physicians who will need to deal with these complex cases will increase as well.

Although nearly all types of cancer can complicate pregnancy, breast, cervical and thyroid carcinoma, melanoma, lymphoma, and leukemia are the malignancies most commonly diagnosed in the gravid female (6–8). A detailed review of all pregnancy-associated malignancies is beyond the scope of this review. Instead, this chapter provides an in-depth analysis of pregnancy-associated breast cancer, followed by a more limited summary of pregnancy-associated melanoma. The management strategies of these two diseases illustrate the approaches that can be employed with other less common pregnancy-associated malignancies.

BREAST CANCER AND PREGNANCY

Breast cancer occurs in up to 1 in 3,000 pregnancies (9,10) and is second only to cervical cancer among the malignancies diagnosed during gestation. Approximately 3% of all women diagnosed with breast cancer will fit the criteria of pregnancy-associated disease (3,11). Traditionally, pregnancy-associated breast cancer has been defined as any malignancy diagnosed either during gestation itself, within 1 year of delivery, or at any time during lactation (12–14). Pregnant women diagnosed with breast cancer typically range in age from 32 to 38 years (10,13). As more women delay first pregnancy into this age range, it is believed that the incidence of breast cancer during pregnancy will increase accordingly.

Clinical Presentation

Most women diagnosed with pregnancy-associated breast cancer present with a painless mass or breast thickening that fails to resolve (15,16). The pregnant female who presents with a picture consistent with inflammatory cancer is the exception, not the rule (17). Given the changes in breast density and size that accompany pregnancy, the presence of a mass may erroneously be thought to represent normal physiologic changes. Therefore, small masses may be difficult to detect within a rapidly enlarging breast. A thorough baseline breast history and clinical breast examination should be conducted at the first obstetric visit to minimize the impact that these physiologic changes may have on future examinations (18). Furthermore, any asymmetric, focal dominant masses identified during pregnancy should be evaluated and followed during pregnancy. Such findings should not be assumed to be "normal" changes in the absence of objective evaluation and surveillance.

Diagnostic delay is common among patients found to have pregnancy-associated breast cancer. Delays ranging from 2 to 15 months have been documented, with an average of 5 to 7 months being routine (3,17). Unfortunately, delayed diagnosis is associated with an increased likelihood of axillary metastases. Previous investigations have reported an increase in axillary disease of 5.1% when a diagnostic delay of 6 months exists (9,19). The risk of disease progression during pregnancy increases the importance of investigating any new breast mass identified during pregnancy.

Diagnostic Imaging
Mammography

When a pregnant woman presents with a palpable mass, diagnostic workup should be undertaken with imaging that is appropriate based on the clinical findings. Despite belief to the contrary, mammography with appropriate abdominal shielding can be performed safely during any stage of gestation. Standard bilateral mammography exposes the mother to 200 to 400 mGy of radiation, which translates into <0.5 mGy of radiation exposure to the embryo/fetus (20,21). This exposure is well below

10 mGy, the threshold that has been demonstrated to increase the risk of fetal malformation by 1% (22). Although mammography can be performed safely in the pregnant patient, it may be of limited benefit secondary to the physiologic changes of pregnancy that increase breast density. As the pregnancy progresses, breast glandularity and water content both increase, which subsequently decreases the sensitivity of mammographic examination (6,23). Despite these potential shortcomings, mammography should be included as part of the imaging workup for any newly detected breast mass during pregnancy, as it provides an initial "road map" for the clinician and radiologist in evaluating the breast.

Breast Ultrasound

Ultrasound is more accurate than mammography in evaluating localized palpable breast masses in the dense gravid breast, and does so without exposing the developing fetus to ionizing radiation. Ultrasound is especially useful for differentiating cystic from solid lesions and can be performed rapidly (10,24). In addition, ultrasound may be useful in assessing the axilla of the pregnant individual with a new diagnosis of cancer. If abnormal nodes are observed sonographically, needle biopsy may be pursued, thus eliminating the need for an invasive procedure such as sentinel node biopsy.

Breast Magnetic Resonance Imaging

In general, contrast-enhanced breast magnetic resonance imaging (MRI) is contraindicated during pregnancy (9). Although MRI does not expose the fetus to ionizing radiation, the contrast agent gadolinium, which is required for breast MRI imaging, is a category C drug that crosses the placental membrane and has been shown to cause fetal malformations in animal models (25–27). The high-energy magnetic fields of MRI may place the fetus at risk from tissue heating and cavitation (tissue damage caused by high temperatures that form secondary to the collapse of microvacuum pockets) (17,25). These facts, coupled with a lack of studies investigating MRI during pregnancy, have led the majority of radiologists to argue against the use of MRI as an imaging modality in the pregnant patient (28), especially during the first trimester.

Tissue Diagnosis

Even when diagnostic imaging fails to show a discrete abnormality at the site of a dominant palpable mass in the breast or axilla during pregnancy, percutaneous tissue sampling should be strongly considered in order to complete the "triple test" for clinical breast evaluation (29). Although either fine-needle aspiration (FNA) or core needle biopsy can be pursued, FNA may be difficult to perform and more challenging to interpret during pregnancy (10,30). The pathologist who will be interpreting the FNA specimen should be informed that the patient is pregnant, because the hyperproliferative changes of pregnancy can be misinterpreted (9). Consultation with a dedicated breast pathologist familiar with the physiologic changes of the gravid breast may improve diagnostic accuracy when interpreting these tissue samples.

Because FNA samples obtained during pregnancy can be particularly challenging to interpret, core needle biopsy has been advocated as a preferable alternative for obtaining tissue diagnosis. Although core biopsy may allow more accurate diagnosis by providing histologic rather than cytologic samples, the amount of tissue removed with this larger-bore needle biopsy can increase the risk of both hematoma or, in the lactating patient, milk fistula formation (12,31). Prior to performing core biopsy in a lactating individual, the patient should be encouraged to fully empty the breast and be informed that if a milk fistula develops, she may need to discontinue breast-feeding prematurely (9). Finally, women undergoing core biopsy during pregnancy should have pressure dressings applied to decrease the risk of significant bleeding in the breast.

Prior to accepting the results of a needle sampling as "benign," the surgeon must confirm that the histologic and/or cytologic findings are concordant with the clinical presentation of the palpable mass. Open surgical biopsy should be considered in the event of discordant findings between the imaging and needle biopsy results. Excisional biopsy, or incisional biopsy in the presence of an extremely large mass, can be safely performed under local anesthetic and has an accuracy that matches that when performed in the nonpregnant female (18,32). As with core biopsy, cessation of lactation and emptying the breast of milk prior to biopsy is recommended, and particular attention to hemostasis is suggested to decrease the risk of hematoma formation in the hypervascular gravid breast.

Staging Workup

Metastatic workup studies should be used sparingly in pregnant patients and be limited to those individuals in whom metastases are suspected on the basis of clinical symptoms and/or advanced stage at presentation (6). The use of ionizing radiation must be balanced against the potential that beneficial information will be gained from the examination. The risk of fetal malformation and loss increases when the fetus is exposed to levels of radiation above 5 to 10 rad (0.05 to 0.1 Gy), especially during the first and second trimesters (9,33). In general, radiation exposure during the pre- or postimplantation stage (0 to 8 days) may lead to spontaneous abortion, while irradiation during organogenesis can cause fetal malformations, intrauterine growth delay, microcephaly, and/or mental retardation (11). Mental retardation is largely dose- and trimester-dependent, with the risk increased at doses of 0.06 to 0.31 Gy at 8 to 15 weeks and at 0.28 Gy at 16 to 25 weeks (34).

Fortunately, some imaging studies can safely be performed during pregnancy. To evaluate for lung involvement, standard chest radiography can be obtained with appropriate abdominal shielding without exposing the fetus to unnecessary risk (9). Routine laboratory investigations can be safely pursued, although it should be remembered that elevations of alkaline phosphatase are normal during pregnancy, while elevations of other liver enzymes are not (9). Bone scans and abdominal computed tomography imaging should only be undertaken in the symptomatic patient, as computed tomography scanning may expose the fetus to as much as 0.09 Gy of radiation (35). If there is a clinical suspicion for intra-abdominal disease, ultrasound is the preferred initial study. Although a modified "low-dose" bone scan for use in pregnant females has been described, using 10 mCi of technichium-99 in place of the usual 20-mCi dose, the general consensus is that bone scan should not be undertaken in the gravid female (18). If there is a high suspicion of bony involvement, noncontrast MRI may be considered.

Pathology

Despite initial reports suggesting that the biology of cancer diagnosed during pregnancy differed from that of tumors identified in a nongestational state, this hypothesis has not been clinically confirmed. Pregnancy-associated breast cancers are histologically similar to tumors from age-matched controls, with upward of 75% of patients in both groups being diagnosed with invasive ductal carcinoma (36–39). The percentage of poorly differentiated cancers has been reported to be as high as 80% in some series (11,39), but this rate is thought to be similar to age-matched controls.

Pregnancy-associated breast cancer is commonly estrogen receptor (ER) and progesterone receptor (PR) negative. Most studies report that fewer than 25% of all breast carcinomas diagnosed during pregnancy are ER- or PR-positive (40–42). Although many premenopausal women diagnosed with breast cancer have hormone receptor-negative cancers, the percentage of ER-negative tumors appears to be even higher among pregnant patients compared with age-matched controls (39,43). Theoretically, ER and PR receptors may be down-regulated secondary to the high circulating levels of steroid hormones during pregnancy (44,45). Nonhormonal growth factors such as insulinlike growth factor-1 could also be involved in the pathogenesis of breast cancer (46). It also appears that *HER2/neu* overexpression may be more common among pregnancy-associated females (47). One study described a *HER2/neu* overexpression rate of 58% (48), well above the commonly reported rate of 15% to 20% identified in typical breast cancer.

Family History and Genetics

Women with a positive family history of breast cancer and/or a genetic predisposing mutation may account for a higher percentage of pregnancy-associated breast cancers. Women with *BRCA1* and/or *BRCA2* genetic mutations have been found to be overrepresented among women with breast cancer diagnosed during pregnancy (49,50). Elevated levels of circulating estrogens or other circulating growth factors during gestation may accelerate the growth of breast cancers initially formed through the malignant transformation induced by genetic predisposition. Family history in the absence of a known genetic alteration may, in and of itself, increase an individual's risk of pregnancy-associated malignancy, although the exact relationship between genetics and breast cancer diagnosed during pregnancy has yet to be determined.

Therapy

Algorithms for the management of pregnancy-related breast cancer are presented in Table 15.1 and Figure 15.1.

Surgical Treatment

Despite a fear that general anesthesia could cause unacceptable maternal and fetal complications, administration of anesthesia even during the first trimester has not been shown to increase the rate of congenital abnormalities (18,51). Although an association with low birth weight, secondary to prematurity and

Table 15.1

Algorithm for Treatment of the Pregnant Breast Cancer Patient

First Trimester
Inoperable, large primary, or nodal disease
  Yes:
    Start systemic therapy after end of first trimester
    Surgery
    Delivery
    Radiotherapy
    Endocrine therapy

  No:
    Surgery
    Chemotherapy (if indicated)
    Delivery
    Radiotherapy
    Endocrine Therapy

Second and/or Third Trimester
Inoperable, large primary, or nodal involvement
  Yes:
    Chemotherapy
    Delivery
    Surgery (may be before delivery)
    Adjuvant therapy as indicated
    Radiotherapy
    Endocrine Therapy

  No:
    Surgery
    Delivery (after 35 weeks)
    Adjuvant therapy as indicated
    Radiotherapy
    Endocrine therapy

Adapted from Loibl S, von Minckwitz G, Gwyn K, et al. Breast cancer during pregnancy: international recommendations from an expert meeting. *Cancer.* 2006;106:237–246.

intrauterine growth retardation, has been reported by some following anesthetic administration (51), other studies have refuted this finding and suggest that birth outcomes are equivalent among women who have and have not undergone anesthesia (52). Performing surgery after the 12th week of gestation is preferable, if possible, because of the lower risk of spontaneous abortion (53). Given that a clear link with anesthesia and preterm labor has been identified, maternal/fetal monitoring is recommended for any woman with a potentially viable fetus. Maternal issues such as delayed gastric emptying, increases in heart rate, cardiac output, platelets, and total blood volume must all be considered when subjecting the pregnant female to general anesthesia (54).

Breast-Conserving Therapy

Previously, women diagnosed with pregnancy-associated breast cancer were treated universally with modified radical mastectomy. Mastectomy eliminates the need for whole-breast

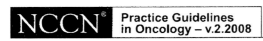 | **Practice Guidelines in Oncology – v.2.2008** | **Breast Cancer During Pregnancy**

CLINICAL PRESENTATION   PRIMARY TREATMENT[a]   ADJUVANT TREATMENT[a]

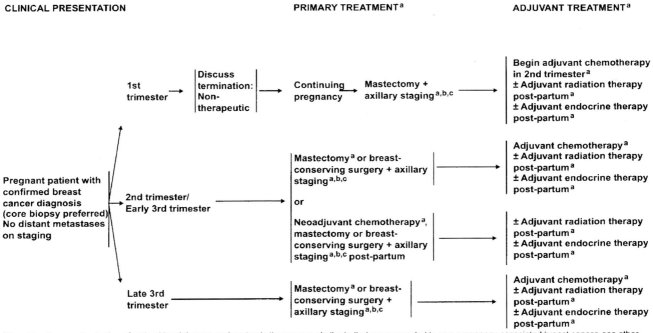

[a]Considerations and selection of optimal local therapy and systemic therapy are similar to that recommended in non-pregnancy associated breast cancer, see other
  sections of this guideline. Chemotherapy should not be administered during the first trimester of pregnancy and radiation therapy should not be administered during any
  trimester of pregnancy. Most experience with chemotherapy during pregnancy for breast cancer is from regimens that utilize various combinations of doxorubicin,
  cyclophosphamide and fluorouracil. Consideration for post-partum chemotherapy are the same as for non-pregnancy associated breast cancer.
[b]See Surgical Axillary Lymph Node Staging (BINV-C).
[c]Due to limited data the use of isosulfan blue in pregnancy, and to the possibility of teratogenic effects of methylene blue dye, these colloids should not be used in
  pregnant patients.

| Note: All recommendations are category 2A unless otherwise indicated. |
| Clinical Trials: NCCN believes that the best management of any cancer patient is in a clinical trial. Participation in clinical trials is especially encouraged. |

Figure 15.1 Recommendations by the National Comprehensive Cancer Network for the management of breast cancer during pregnancy. (From *NCCN Practice Guidelines, Breast Cancer*, Vol. 2, 2008.)

radiation, which is contraindicated during all stages of pregnancy. More recently, the requirement that every pregnant female diagnosed with breast cancer undergo mastectomy has been questioned, especially when the woman is diagnosed during the second or third trimester. Breast-conservation therapy is a reasonable option for women diagnosed late in the third trimester in that adjuvant radiotherapy can be provided following delivery and still be started within the acceptable time frame after surgery. Women in the second trimester who require chemotherapy can undergo segmental mastectomy followed by chemotherapy and then again receive timely radiotherapy following delivery (55,56).

The issue of whether breast conservation is reasonable for women diagnosed during the first trimester remains unclear, given the potential for unacceptable delays between surgery, delivery, and definitive radiation. As such, the majority of patients diagnosed during the first trimester undergo mastectomy (13). Individualizing treatment plans, however, is of the utmost importance, as even those women diagnosed during the first trimester may be considered for conserving therapy in some circumstances (20). Although large numbers are lacking, small series of pregnant patients treated with breast-conserving therapy have demonstrated similar outcomes in terms of disease-free and overall survival when compared with women treated with mastectomy (55,57). The surgical criteria for breast-conservation therapy in the pregnant female should be identical to those in the nonpregnant individual.

Axillary Staging

The necessity for routine axillary lymph node dissection rather than initial sentinel node analysis for nodal staging in pregnancy-associated breast cancers has recently been challenged. Although sentinel node dissection has become standard of care for axillary staging in the nongravid patient, its use during pregnancy has been more controversial. No large series has investigated the use of sentinel node during pregnancy, and as such, the majority of reports in the literature are small series or case reports. Isosulfan blue dye is a category C agent that has not been studied in pregnancy and is contraindicated as a mapping agent in the gravid patient (20,58). As such, vital blue dyes should not be used when attempting sentinel node procedures in the pregnant female.

In contrast, the use of radioisotope appears to expose the developing fetus to minimal radiation and is thought to be safe. Based on limited data, the maximum dose of radiation that the developing fetus will potentially be exposed to is 4.3 mGy, a figure well below the threshold of 50 mGy thought to be detrimental (58–61). Any decision to pursue sentinel node biopsy should be undertaken only after appropriate counseling, but the procedure does appear to be safe based on limited available data. At our institution, we offer sentinel node dissection using a reduced dose of technichium-99, but only in the second and third trimesters. If the presence of nodal metastases can be established by another modality, such as with axillary ultrasound and percutaneous needle sampling, sentinel node biopsy can be avoided. Women with documented axillary involvement should undergo a standard axillary lymphadenectomy at the time of definitive breast surgery.

Systemic Chemotherapy

Chemotherapy during the first trimester is contraindicated because of an unacceptably high risk of detrimental fetal effects. One classic study demonstrated the risk of congenital malformation from chemotherapy exposure during the first trimester to be as high as 16% (62). Systemic therapy administered during, or after, the second trimester is associated with a congenital malformation rate of 3%, a figure identical to the frequency seen among the general pregnant population not receiving chemotherapy (20,63). All chemotherapeutic agents can potentially cross the placenta, so fetal anemia is a possibility (9). Intrauterine monitoring for evidence of fetal distress is advised. As newborns have a limited capacity to metabolize and eliminate these drugs, it is advisable to avoid chemotherapy after the 35th week of gestation to avoid transient neutropenia and other complications in the newborn (35,64). Women treated with chemotherapy postpartum should be counseled against breast-feeding, as all commonly used agents are expressed in breast milk.

Most agents currently used to treat women with breast cancer appear to be safe after the first trimester. In a landmark study, investigators at the MD Anderson Cancer Center used a regimen of fluorouracil, cyclophosphamide, and doxorubicin (FAC) every 3 to 4 weeks after the first trimester. No birth defects were identified, the median age of delivery was 38 weeks, and the only significant complications were preterm delivery, low birth weight, and transient neutropenia (9,35). As such, anthracycline-based regimens are believed to be safe and are among the most commonly used chemotherapy drugs during pregnancy.

Limited data suggest that the taxanes and targeted biological therapies such as Herceptin have limited toxicity during pregnancy (9,15,20). Nonetheless, most investigators argue against their routine use during pregnancy until more definitive data regarding safety profiles are available (65). Because HER2/neu expression is high in embryonic tissues and it has been reported that Herceptin can cross the placenta in animal models, use of the drug is generally avoided until after delivery (11,15). Methotrexate should not be used during pregnancy because of its ability to induce spontaneous abortion, as well as aminopterin syndrome (cranial dysostosis), especially when administered during the first trimester (15,66).

Fortunately, infants exposed to chemotherapy in utero appear to experience few side effects. Occasional complications can occur, and include preterm delivery, low birth weight, intrauterine growth retardation, transient tachypnea of the newborn, and transient leukopenia (9). Avoidance of chemotherapy after the 35th week of pregnancy can help to minimize newborn complications. Delayed side effects manifesting in older children exposed to chemotherapy in utero appear to be limited. One study of 84 children (age range, 6 to 29 years) born after in utero exposure reported no derangements in physical, psychological, and/or neurologic development (67). Additional follow-up with larger numbers are needed, but preliminary results indicate that children with fetal exposure to chemotherapy develop normally.

Hormonal Therapy

Tamoxifen is the only endocrine agent approved for use in the premenopausal female with breast cancer. Unfortunately, tamoxifen exposure has been associated with fetal anomalies in both animal and human models, suggesting that tamoxifen is contraindicated during pregnancy (9). Fetal anomalies including ambiguous genitalia, craniofacial defects, and Goldenhar syndrome, which is characterized by oculoauriculovertebral dysplasia, have been reported (68–70). Most physicians delay tamoxifen therapy until after delivery has occurred. When given postpartum, breast-feeding is contraindicated as the drug is expressed in breast milk.

Adjuvant Radiation Therapy

Whole-breast radiation is contraindicated during all stages of pregnancy and should only be initiated after delivery. Prior to demonstrating that neoadjuvant chemotherapy is safe during the second and third trimesters of pregnancy, inability to administer radiation therapy was the primary reason all women with pregnancy-associated breast cancer underwent mastectomy instead of breast-conserving surgery.

Standard whole-breast radiotherapy involves the use of 5,000 to 6,000 rad (50 to 60 Gy) of radiation (20). The amount of fetal exposure depends on the trimester and position of the gravid uterus, and is due to internal scatter of radiation from the mother, a phenomenon that can not be overcome with abdominal shielding (18). It is believed that the degree of exposure is between 2 and 7.6 rad (0.02 and 0.076 Gy) during the first trimester, 2.2 and 24.6 rad (0.022 and 0.246 Gy) during the second trimester, and may be as high as 200 rad (2 Gy) during the third trimester (12,22). The risk of malformation and loss increases when the fetus is exposed to levels of radiation above 5 to 10 rad (0.05 to 0.1 Gy), especially during early pregnancy (9,33). Mental retardation is dose- and trimester-dependent and the risk increases with doses of 0.06 to 0.31 Gy at 8 to 15 weeks and 0.28 Gy at 16 to 25 weeks (34). Expected exposures during both the second and third trimesters are above these figures, and as such irradiation during pregnancy can not be safely recommended.

Therapeutic Abortion

Historically, when a pregnant woman was diagnosed with breast cancer, termination of the pregnancy was routinely recommended. It was erroneously believed that termination would improve survival. Multiple studies have refuted this hypothesis, demonstrating no difference in outcome between women electing to undergo termination and those who kept their pregnancy (17,18). Today, abortion is reserved for those individuals with exceptionally dire circumstances who are not expected to survive to delivery, or for those women with an absolute requirement for chemotherapy during the first trimester. Discussion of selective termination should be provided on a case-by-case basis, but in general, abortion is not required.

Maternal Prognosis

Pregnancy-associated breast cancers were previously thought to have universally poor outcomes. In the 1940s, a classic study by Haagensen and Stout (71) indicated that the 5-year survival for these women was dismal and no better than 8.6%. Older studies suggested that women with pregnancy-associated breast cancer should receive only palliative treatment. More recent data have challenged these findings, and indicate that women with breast cancer diagnosed during pregnancy have similar stage-for-stage survival as their nonpregnant counterparts (9,10,14,18,72) (Table 15.2). Additional studies have also found that women with pregnancy-associated breast cancer are more likely to present with advanced disease and are less likely to be diagnosed as stage I (64,73).

Fetal/Newborn Issues

When a woman is diagnosed with breast cancer during pregnancy, her treatment team must deal with not one, but two patients, simultaneously. Of paramount importance is the inclusion of an obstetrician/gynecologist with experience in high-risk pregnancies on the multidisciplinary treatment team. Standard prenatal care is advised, with an ultrasound recommended prior to the initiation of therapy to ensure accurate gestational age and confirm that the fetus appears normal and viable (20). The fetus should be reassessed after every cycle of chemotherapy, and any evidence of intrauterine growth retardation or anemia should be investigated with an ultrasound of the cord vessels. Any later trimester maternal surgical procedures should be accompanied by fetal monitoring, especially in the case of a viable or potentially viable fetus. Chemotherapy should be held after the 35th

Table 15.2

Maternal Survival (%) for Women with Pregnancy-Associated Breast Cancer versus Controls

	5 Years	10 Years
Pregnancy-associated		
Node-negative	82	77
Node-positive	47	25
Control		
Node-negative	82	75
Node-positive	59	41

Adapted from Petrek JA, Dukoff R, Rogatko A. Prognosis of pregnancy associated breast cancer. *Cancer.* 1991;67:869–872.

week of gestation, or within 3 weeks of planned delivery, to avoid newborn anemia and/or neutropenia.

Delivery can be vaginal or via caesarian section, and is reasonable at any time once fetal maturation has been established. These women should be delivered at a hospital with appropriate neonatal support (20). The placenta should be sent for complete pathologic examination, as metastatic involvement has been sporadically reported (64,74,75). Fortunately, metastatic spread of breast cancer to the fetus itself has never been documented (76). These infants may be at an increased risk of intrauterine growth retardation, low birth rate, and preterm delivery (3,17). If the mother is to receive additional chemotherapy or adjuvant hormonal therapy following delivery, breast-feeding is contraindicated, although after a washout period of 2 to 4 weeks following the last dose of drug, it is permissible.

Pregnancy After Breast Cancer

Traditionally, pregnancy has been discouraged following a diagnosis of breast cancer because of fears that high levels of gestational hormones would negatively impact both recurrence risk and overall survival. The links between female sex steroid hormones, reproductive factors, and mammary carcinogenesis are well known. The risk of developing breast cancer is lowered by a number of factors that decrease an individual's exposure to unopposed estrogens. Late menarche, early natural menopause, multiparity, and young age at first pregnancy all appear to be protective against breast cancer development (77). Knowledge of this link between female hormones and mammary carcinogenesis contributed to the belief that pregnancy should be discouraged, or at least delayed, for a minimum of 2 years following successful treatment, if pursued. Fears related to the stimulation of dormant micrometastases by gestational hormones were largely responsible for these recommendations (78,79). The hypothesis that pregnancy contributes to recurrence and systemic dissemination of breast cancer, however, has been challenged by a number of studies published during the last 20 years. In fact, no series has demonstrated a link between pregnancy and decreased survival.

As more women defer childbearing, increasing numbers of physicians can expect to be approached by premenopausal females inquiring as to the advisability of pregnancy following breast cancer treatment. In addition to questions related to overall survival, the impact of adjuvant treatments such as radiation therapy and systemic chemotherapy on mother and infant, as well as questions of timing of the pregnancy, all become important when discussing subsequent pregnancy in a breast cancer survivor.

The Impact of Therapy on Fertility

Surgery is thought to have a minimal impact on an individual's subsequent reproductive capabilities, although women treated with segmental mastectomy may lose the ability to breast-feed from the affected side. Similarly, radiation can result in diminished lactation from the ipsilateral breast, thereby resulting in an inability to sustain breast-feeding (80). Neither surgery nor radiation, however, has been shown to negatively impact an individual's subsequent ability to become pregnant or produce a viable infant.

Although local treatment has no apparent deleterious effects on fertility, the same is not true for adjuvant chemotherapy. One of the most dreaded consequences that can occur when chemotherapy is administered to a premenopausal female who desires preservation of fertility is premature ovarian failure. Chemotherapeutic agents are believed to impair follicular growth and maturation, produce postmenopausal levels of follicle-stimulating hormone, luteinizing hormone, and estradiol, and ultimately result in irregular menses and amenorrhea (81,82). Although all chemotherapy agents currently used to treat breast cancer can produce these effects, medications such as cyclophosphamide and doxorubicin appear to be the most likely culprits because of their propensity to act on undeveloped oocytes or be toxic to the germinal epithelium, respectively (83).

Premature ovarian failure appears dependent on the individual's age at the time of treatment and the total cumulative dose of medication received. Although permanent amenorrhea is unlikely among women younger than 35 years of age, the incidence increases above the age of 40 and is generally irreversible among older women (82). Roughly 10% of women younger than 35 years will be rendered permanently amenorrheic after completion of systemic chemotherapy (84). This risk rises as the total dose of chemotherapy increases, with higher doses required to produce infertility in younger females (82). Regardless of age, all premenopausal females treated with systemic chemotherapy should be counseled that therapy may produce permanent amenorrhea. Goserelin can be used to suppress ovarian function during chemotherapy to protect subsequent ovarian viability in nonpregnant premenopausal patients, but this method could not employed during pregnancy without interfering with normal gestational development (85).

Although chemotherapy can induce early menopause, these systemic agents do not appear to have a negative impact on infants born to breast cancer survivors who do retain their fertility. Higher rates of congenital abnormalities have not been identified when infants born to women with a history of breast cancer are compared with normal controls (86). These findings are not surprising, given the fact that chemotherapy can be safely given to gravid patients in the second or third trimester of pregnancy. Although the number of infants born to breast cancer survivors is limited, these offspring do not appear to be at an increased risk for malformations or other health problems.

The Impact of Pregnancy on Survival

Provided that fertility is preserved, it is reasonable to anticipate that some premenopausal breast cancer survivors may wish to discuss the advisability of pursing a future pregnancy. One of the most important issues to discuss with each individual is the impact that this subsequent pregnancy may have on overall survival. A number of population-based and case control studies published since the 1950s have dealt directly with this subject and form the basis for recommendations regarding pregnancy after a breast cancer diagnosis (81). Despite fears of activation of dormant micrometastases by systemic gestational hormones, no study has shown pregnancy after a diagnosis of breast cancer to be detrimental to survival. Instead of impacting negatively on survival, a number of publications have actually suggested that

a subsequent live birth may actually confer a survival advantage to these women.

One such study to suggest equal, if not superior, survival rates for women with a history of breast cancer who went on to deliver a child versus those who did not was published by Sankila and colleagues (87) in 1994. These investigators identified 91 survivors between 1967 and 1989 who delivered an infant at least 10 months after a breast cancer diagnosis. The cases were matched to 471 controls without evidence of a subsequent pregnancy. Overall, women who became pregnant had superior survival compared with the control group (92% vs. 60% 10-year survival rates for cases vs. controls, respectively), although six cancer-related deaths did still occur among those who successfully delivered a child. The authors hypothesized that a "healthy mother effect" helped explain these findings, suggesting the existence of an inherent selection bias whereby only those females who feel well and have no evidence of ongoing cancer issues elect to pursue pregnancy. Since publication of the healthy mother effect theory, additional studies have supported the hypothesis that pregnancy following breast cancer treatment does not negatively impact on long-term survival (88–90). All three of these investigations confirmed that women who become pregnant after a diagnosis of breast cancer do not have evidence of poorer survival than controls.

Interestingly, several studies have actually supported the initial findings set forth by Sankila et al., suggesting that pregnancy following a diagnosis of breast cancer may in fact confer a survival advantage. A population-based study from Denmark found that 173 female breast cancer survivors who delivered a full-term infant had a nonsignificantly reduced risk of dying (relative risk, 0.55) compared with matched controls (91), while two additional investigations also support this phenomenon. The first revealed that at 5 and 10 years, the survival of the cases was superior to the controls, with 5-year rates of 85% and 10-year rates of 74% for the cases (92). The most recent study reported that women who gave birth at least 10 months after diagnosis had a significantly reduced risk of death compared with controls (93).

Although the available data suggest that pregnancy after a diagnosis of breast cancer is not detrimental to overall survival, and may in fact be protective, these studies are not without limitations. The publications are all retrospective in nature, have small sample sizes, and are likely to have some degree of recall bias, thereby leading to potential underreporting and failure to capture all women who actually do become pregnant after a diagnosis of breast cancer (81,82,90). By underestimating the true denominator population of those who become pregnant, it is possible that selection bias may be introduced. Despite this bias, there are no prospective, randomized trials designed to address this question and it is doubtful that they ever will be designed. Although likely biased, the available retrospective studies can at least be used to reassure women interested in pursuing pregnancy after treatment of breast cancer that, at a minimum, childbirth will not lead to adverse cancer outcomes.

Hypotheses to Explain Survival

Attempts to explain the finding that pregnancy does not have a detrimental effect on survival following breast cancer treatment have largely been explained by the hypotheses of (a) the healthy mother effect and (b) the fetal antigen theory. The healthy mother effect is believed to occur among breast cancer survivors whereby only those women who feel well will pursue a subsequent pregnancy (87). Patient self-selection occurs, with only those individuals who are doing well in terms of disease outcomes electing to pursue pregnancy. Therefore, it is difficult to determine whether the survival benefit that some breast cancer patients seem to enjoy following pregnancy is related to some unknown biological effect of the pregnancy itself or instead to this possible selection bias.

An actual biological phenomenon has been proposed to explain these findings. Termed the *fetal antigen hypothesis,* this theory states that protective immunization may occur during pregnancy. Based on the principle that fetal and breast cancer cells share common antigens, it is believed that the pregnant female develops isoimmunization against breast carcinoma cells (77,94). Fetal antigens are believed to stimulate the women's immune system to generate cellular and humoral responses against her cancer and thus keep micrometastatic tumor cells controlled. If true, this theory may help explain why the feared outcome of stimulation of dormant disease does not occur during exposure to high levels of gestational hormones.

Issues Specific to Pregnancy Following Breast Cancer

If a premenopausal woman decides to pursue childbirth after breast cancer treatment, questions as to the optimal timing of this subsequent pregnancy may arise. Traditionally, it was believed that women who delivered within 1 year of their cancer diagnosis had worse outcomes than women with no further episodes of fertility or those who waited for extended periods of time (95). This was thought to relate to the diagnostic delays that often occur during pregnancy and lactation.

The majority of investigators therefore subscribe to the belief that fertility should only be pursued once the patient had passed her 2-year cancer diagnosis anniversary. By deferring pregnancy during the first 2 years, when statistically the majority of recurrences and/or systemic relapses will develop, women with less aggressive tumors and better prognoses will proclaim themselves (77). A classic study by Clark and Reid (96) found that waiting up to 2 years to become pregnant improved survival rates from 54% to 78% compared with individuals who became pregnant within 6 months of therapy completion. Regardless of the exact length of time that passes between diagnosis and pregnancy, it seems prudent to allow some time to elapse in order to gauge each individual's response to therapy.

An additional issue that should be addressed with each patient who pursues pregnancy is the apparent increased risk of spontaneous abortion. Miscarriage rates as high as 29% have recently been reported in the literature (89,90). It has been hypothesized that advanced maternal age and/or alterations of hormone profiles related to adjuvant therapy may be responsible for these findings, thus making these women less able to support a pregnancy to term. Although the majority of women in one study who experienced a miscarriage ultimately went on to deliver a viable term infant (89), the possibility that these women may have more difficulty sustaining a pregnancy does exist.

A final issue that may arise with the breast cancer survivor who wishes to become pregnant is the issue of the safety of assisted fertility. Given that premature ovarian failure can result from adjuvant chemotherapy, women with breast cancer may inquire as to the feasibility of in vitro fertilization (IVF) followed by cryopreservation of embryos. Although the data are limited, IVF does not appear to confer an increased risk of breast cancer over an individual's lifetime (97). Furthermore, preliminary studies suggest that ovarian stimulation and subsequent IVF prior to the administration of systemic chemotherapy do not have a negative impact on overall breast cancer survival (98). Although more sophisticated procedures such as oocyte freezing and ovarian tissue banking are still considered experimental, the use of assisted fertility technologies will likely become more prevalent as the number of premenopausal women with breast cancer who have delayed their fertility continues to increase.

MELANOMA AND PREGNANCY

Pregnancy-associated melanoma shares many similarities with pregnancy-associated breast cancer. It appears that the presentation of melanoma is similar among pregnant and nonpregnant females, even in terms of primary site location (6). Any change in the size, pigmentation, or symmetry of a nevus during pregnancy mandates investigation, as the majority of lesions will develop in pre-existing areas. One issue that may contribute to diagnostic delay, which is a common finding with melanoma, is pregnancy-associated hyperpigmentation (99). Most women experience at least some element of this condition, which may make subtle changes in a nevus difficult to interpret. Patients should be instructed in the importance of monitoring their moles and report any changes, no matter how minor, to a provider.

Any suspicious skin lesion warrants investigation with tissue sampling. As with the nonpregnant population, biopsy is recommended and can be performed safely during any trimester, either with or without anesthesia. Historically, it was believed that women with pregnancy-associated melanoma tended to present with thicker lesions than nonpregnant individuals (100–102), while more recent studies have reported no difference in tumor thickness between gravid and nongravid patients (103, 104). This is a significant finding, as tumor thickness is the most important determinant of overall survival among melanoma patients.

Surgery remains the most common treatment modality for pregnant women diagnosed with melanoma. As with any melanoma patient, margin status is of paramount importance. Extrapolating from the breast cancer literature, sentinel node staging can be offered to the gravid female using radioisotope only, as isosulfan blue remains a category C drug and is contraindicated during pregnancy. One alternative endorsed by some authors is to perform wide local excision during pregnancy and delay sentinel node mapping until after delivery to avoid the issues of fetal exposure to radioisotope (1). There is insufficient evidence at the current time regarding the use of biologic therapy during pregnancy (103), so agents such as interferon are not recommended.

Therapeutic abortion is no longer believed to be necessary when a pregnant woman is diagnosed with melanoma, as it has never been shown that termination of pregnancy results in regression of the primary lesion (105–107). Melanoma diagnosed during pregnancy appears to have a similar prognosis to those cases diagnosed during the nongravid state, when the primary is matched for age, stage, and anatomic site (6), although again, much like with breast cancer, delay in diagnosis often translates into a more advanced stage at presentation. Systemic staging should be limited to those women who are symptomatic and at highest risk for having metastatic disease.

Infants born to women with melanoma during pregnancy are at risk for disease transmission, as metastases to the placenta have been reported most frequently with this disease state (6). It is mandatory that the placenta be examined for evidence of implants, and if discovered, the newborn should be monitored for signs of disease development. Unfortunately, there have been at least four cases of fetal death from melanoma among the handful of infants found to develop the disease secondary to in utero exposure (74).

Women were traditionally counseled to avoid pregnancy for up to 3 years following a diagnosis of melanoma because of a fear that increased levels of hormones would lead to stimulation of dormant micrometastatic disease (103). This hypothesis has been challenged, and although a delay in future fertility events may allow for a better determination of overall disease outcome, 3 years may be excessive for women with early-stage, favorable primaries. Finally, given fears of microscopic disease stimulation, females with a previous history of melanoma historically have been counseled to avoid oral contraceptives (108). This belief, too, has been found to be incorrect and monitored oral contraceptive use is now thought to be acceptable.

CONCLUSIONS

Breast Cancer

Breast cancer complicates up to 1 in 3,000 pregnancies. Most women present with a painless mass often erroneously believed to represent normal pregnancy-associated changes, so diagnostic delays are common. Any dominant mass should undergo diagnostic workup to include imaging and histology. Mammography can safely be done with abdominal shielding, although ultrasound is more sensitive and has the added benefit of no ionizing radiation exposure. Breast MRI is contraindicated. Staging workup should be limited to individuals with a high likelihood of metastatic disease.

Palpable masses should undergo biopsy. FNA is acceptable, although a core biopsy can provide more complete information. Open diagnostic surgical biopsy may be necessary. The majority of pregnancy-associated breast cancers are of a ductal variety, poorly differentiated, and receptor-negative, with a higher percentage of HER2/neu-positive lesions.

Therapy should be individualized. Surgery traditionally involved use of the modified radical mastectomy. Breast conservation can be considered for those women who would be candidates for lumpectomy if not pregnant, especially if other therapies will allow radiation to be delayed until after delivery. Sentinel node biopsy can be performed after the first trimester

with radioisotope only. Chemotherapy is safe after the first trimester, while tamoxifen is contraindicated. Whole-breast radiation should be delayed until after delivery because of issues regarding fetal malformations and loss. Therapeutic abortion is no longer recommended, as it has never been shown to improve outcome.

These women have outcomes similar to nonpregnant, age-matched controls, while infants born to women with breast cancer are at an increased risk for intrauterine growth retardation and preterm delivery. Long-term results, however, suggest that these children develop normally.

As more women delay childbearing, the number of individuals treated for breast cancer who are expected to desire fertility following treatment will increase. Adjuvant systemic chemotherapy may induce premature ovarian failure. Fortunately, women who do give birth appear to have infants with no increased risk of congenital malformations. Women with a history of breast cancer who become pregnant are at an increased risk for spontaneous abortion. More concerning may be the fear that a subsequent pregnancy may have a negative impact on survival. Historically, women diagnosed with breast cancer were advised against future episodes of fertility by an unfounded fear that unopposed gestational hormones could stimulate growth of dormant metastatic cells, subsequent recurrence, and death. Available data argue against this belief, and many have suggested that subsequent pregnancy is protective, perhaps because of an immune mechanism.

Melanoma

Pregnancy-associated melanoma shares many similarities with pregnancy-associated breast cancer and complicates nearly 3 of every 1,000 pregnancies. Any change in a pre-existing nevus during pregnancy mandates investigation. As with breast cancer, diagnostic delay is common. A suspicious skin lesion warrants investigation with tissue sampling. Recent studies have refuted the belief that pregnancy-associated melanoma tends to present with thicker lesions. Surgery involves wide local excision, and sentinel node staging can safely be offered using radioisotope only. Biologic therapy is not recommended during pregnancy. Therapeutic abortion does not result in regression of the primary lesion. Pregnancy-associated melanoma appears to have a similar prognosis to that diagnosed in nonpregnant females, when matched for age, stage, and anatomic site. Women were traditionally counseled to avoid pregnancy for up to 3 years following a diagnosis of melanoma, although this recommendation has been challenged.

Infants exposed to melanoma in utero are at risk for melanoma transmission, as placental implants have been reported. The placenta should be examined for evidence of involvement and the newborn monitored for signs of disease development. There have been at least four cases of fetal death from melanoma among infants who developed the disease following fetal exposure.

SUMMARY

The co-existence of cancer and pregnancy is a rare event. Although nearly all types of cancer have been reported, breast carcinoma and melanoma, as well as cervical cancer, lymphoma, leukemia, and thyroid carcinoma are the malignancies most commonly associated with the gravid female. As more women delay childbearing, the incidence of pregnancy-associated cancer will increase. There is often a lack of consensus as to the standard of care with which these individuals should be treated. Women diagnosed with cancer during pregnancy experience a multitude of ethical, psychological, and medical issues, dealing with a life-giving and a life-threatening condition simultaneously. The difficulty of treating the patient with pregnancy-associated malignancy should not be underscored, as the well-being of both mother and fetus must be addressed simultaneously.

REFERENCES

1. Jacobs IA, Chang CK, Salti GI. Coexistence of pregnancy and cancer. *Am Surg.* 2004;70:1025–1029.
2. Antonelli NM, Doters DJ, Katz VL, et al. Cancer in pregnancy: a review of the literature. *Obstet Gynecol Surv.* 1996;51:125–134.
3. Weisz B, Schiff E, Lishner M. Cancer in Pregnancy: Maternal and Fetal Implications. *Human Reprod Update.* 2001;7(4):384–393.
4. Murphey GP (ed.). Ca-Cancer Statistics. 1999. CA 49:20–21.
5. Oduncu FS, Phil MA, Kimmig R, et al. Cancer in pregnancy: maternal-fetal conflict. *J Cancer Res Clin Oncol.* 2003;129:133–146.
6. Lishner M. Cancer in Pregnancy. *Ann Oncol.* 2003;14 Suppl 3; iii31–iii36.
7. Sait KH, Ashour A, Rajabi M. Pregnancy outcome in non-gynecological cancer. *Arch Gynecol Obstet.* 2005;271:346–349.
8. Cunningham FG, Gant NF, Leveno KJ, et al. Neoplastic diseases. In: Williams Obstetrics. 21st ed. New York: McGraw-Hill; 2001: 1439–1459.
9. Woo JC, Yu T, Hurd TC. Breast cancer in pregnancy. A literature review. *Arch Surg.* 2003;138:91–98.
10. Keleher AJ, Teriault RL, Gwyn, KM. Multidisciplinary management of breast cancer concurrent with pregnancy. *J Am Coll Surg.* 2001;194:54–64.
11. Ring AE, Smith IE, Ellis PA. Breast cancer and pregnancy. *Ann Oncol.* 2005;16:1855–1860.
12. Gemignani ML, Petrek JA. Pregnancy-associated breast cancer: diagnosis and treatment. *Breast J.* 2000;6:68–73.
13. Rosenkranz KM, Lucci A. Surgical treatment of pregnancy associated breast cancer. *Breast Disease.* 2006;23:87–93.
14. Petrek JA, Dukoff R, Rogatko A. Prognosis of pregnancy associated breast cancer. *Cancer.* 1991;67:869–872.
15. Kelly HL, Collichio FA, Dees EC. Concomitant pregnancy and breast cancer: options for systemic therapy. *Breast Disease.* 2006; 23:95–101.
16. Sorosky JI, Scott-Conner CE. Breast disease complicating pregnancy. *Obstet Gynecol Clin North Am.* 1998;25:353–363.
17. Pavlidis N, Pentheroudakis G. The pregnant mother with breast cancer: diagnostic and therapeutic management. *Cancer Treat Rev.* 2005;31:439–447.
18. Psyrri, Burtness. Breast cancer and pregnancy. *Cancer J.* 2005; 11(2):83–95.
19. Nettleton J, Long J, Kuban D, et al. Breast cancer during pregnancy: quantifying the risk of treatment delay. *Obstet Gynecol.* 1996;87:414–418.
20. Loibl S, von Minckwitz G, Gwyn K, et al. Breast cancer during pregnancy: international recommendations from an expert meeting. *Cancer.* 2006;106(2):237–246.
21. Liberman L, Giess CS, Dershaw DD, et al. Imaging of pregnancy-associated breast cancer.*Radiology.* 1994;191:245–248.
22. Mazonakis M, Varveris H, Damilakis J, et al. Radiation dose to conceptus resulting from tangential breast irradiation. *Int J Radiat Oncol Biol Phys.* 2003;55:386–391.
23. Barnavon Y, Wallack MK. Management of the pregnant patient with carcinoma of the breast. *Surg Gynecol Obstet.* 1990;171:347–352.
24. Carol EH, Conner S, Schorr S. The diagnosis and management of breast problems during pregnancy and lactation. *Am J Surg.* 1995;170:401–404.
25. Nicklas A, Baker M. Imaging strategies in pregnant cancer patients. *Semin Oncol.* 2000;27:623–632.
26. Garel C, Brisse H, Sebag G, et al. Magnetic resonance imaging of the fetus. *Pediatr Radiol.* 1998;28:201–211.
27. Pelsang R. Diagnostic imaging modalities during pregnancy. *Obstet Gynecol Clin North Am.* 1998;25:287–300.
28. Kanal E. Pregnancy and the safety of magnetic resonance imaging. *Magn Reson Imaging Clin North Am.* 1994;2:309–317.
29. Vetto JT, Pommier RF, Shih RL, et al. Breast fine-needle aspirates with scant cellularity are clinically useful. *Am J Surg.* 2005; 189:621–625.
30. Novotny DB, Maygarden SJ, Shermer RW, et al. Fine needle aspiration of benign and malignant breast masses associated with pregnancy. *Acta Cytol.* 1991;35:676–686.
31. Schackmuth EM, Harlow CL, Norton LW. Milk fistula: a complication after core biopsy. *Am J Roentgenol.* 1993;61:961–962.
32. Byrd BF, Bayer DS, Robertson JC, et al. Treatment of breast tumors associated with pregnancy and lactation. *Ann Surg.* 1962; 155:940–947.
33. Mayr N, Wen BC, Saw C. Radiation therapy during pregnancy. *Obstet Gynecol Clin North Am.* 1998;25:301–321.
34. Otake M, Schull WJ, Lee J. Threshold for radiation-related severe mental retardation in prenatally exposed A-bomb survivors: A Reanalysis. *Int J Radiat Biol.* 1996;70:755–763.
35. Osei EK, Faulkner K. Fetal doses from radiological examinations. *Br J Radiol.* 1999;72:773–780.
36. Berry DL, Theriault RL, Holmes FA, et al. Management of breast cancer during pregnancy using a standardized protocol. *J Clin Oncol.* 1999;17:855–861.
37. Ring AE, Smith IE, Jones A, et al. Chemotherapy for breast cancer during pregnancy: an 18 year experience from five London teaching hospitals. *J Clin Oncol.* 2005;23:1492–1497.
38. Giacalone PL, Laffargue F, Benos P. Chemotherapy for breast carcinoma during pregnancy: a French national survey. *Cancer.* 1999;86:2266–2272.
39. Bonnier P, Romain S, Dilhuydy JM, et al. Influence of pregnancy on the outcome of breast cancer: a case control study. *Int J Cancer.* 1997;72:720–727.
40. Shousha S. Breast carcinoma presenting during or shortly after pregnancy and lactation. *Arch Pathol Lab Med.* 2000;124:1053–1060.
41. Merkel DE. Pregnancy and breast cancer. *Semin Surg Oncol.* 1996;12:370–375.
42. Wallack MC, Wolf JA Jr, Bedwinek J, et al. Gestational carcinoma of the female breast. *Curr Probl Cancer.* 1983;7:1–58.
43. Aziz S, Perez S, Khan S, et al. Case control study of novel prognostic markers and disease outcome in pregnancy/lactation-associated breast carcinoma. *Pathol Res Pract.* 2003;199: 15–21.
44. Horowitz KB, McGuire WL. Nuclear mechanisms of estrogen action. *J Bio Chem.* 1978;253:8185–8191.
45. Hoover HC Jr. Breast cancer during pregnancy and lactation. *Surg Clin North Am.* 1990;70:1151–1162.

46. Thordarson G, Slusher N, Leong H, et al. Insulin-like growth factor (IGF-1) obliterates the pregnancy-associated protection against mammary carcinogenesis in rats: evidence that IGF-1 enhances cancer progression through estrogen receptor-alpha activation via the mitogen-activated protein kinase pathway. *Breast Cancer Res.* 2004;6:R423–R436.

47. Reed W, Hannisadl E, Skovlund E, et al. Pregnancy and breast cancer: a population-based study. *Virchows Arch.* 2003;443:44–50.

48. Elledge RM, Ciocca DR, Langone G, et al. Estrogen receptor, progesterone receptor, and her2/neu protein in breast cancers from pregnant patients. *Cancer.* 1993;71:2499–2506.

49. Shen T, Vortmeyer AO, Zhuang Z, et al. High Frequency of allelic loss of BRCA 2 gene in pregnancy-associated breast carcinoma. *J Natl Cancer Institute.* 1999;91:1686–1687.

50. Johannsson O, Loman N, Borg A, et al. Pregnancy-associated breast cancer in BRCA1 and BRCA2 germline mutation carriers. *Lancet.* 1998;352:1359–1360.

51. Mazze RI, Kallen B. Reproductive outcome after anesthesia and operation during pregnancy: a registry of 5405 cases. *Am J Obstet Gynecol.* 1989;161:1178–1185.

52. Duncan PG, Pope WD, Cohen MM, et al. Fetal risk of anesthesia and surgery during pregnancy. *Anesthesiology.* 1986;64:790.

53. Tummers P, De Sutter P, Dhont M. Risk of spontaneous abortion in singleton and twin pregnancies after IVF/ICSI. *Hum Reprod.* 2003;18:1720–1723.

54. Gianopouous JG. Establishing the criteria for anesthesia and other precautions for surgery during pregnancy. *Surg Clin North Am.* 1995;75:33.

55. Kuerer HM, Gwyn K, Ames FC, et al. Conservative surgery and chemotherapy for breast carcinoma during pregnancy. *Surgery.* 2002;131:108–110.

56. Kaufman M, von Minckwitz G, Smith R, et al. International expert panel on the use of primary (preoperative) systemic treatment of operable breast cancer: review and recommendations. *J Clin Oncol.* 2003;21:2600–2608.

57. Kuerer HM, Cunningham JD, Bleiweiss IJ, et al. Conservative surgery for breast carcinoma associated with pregnancy. *Breast J.* 1998;4:171–176.

58. Keleher A, Wendt R, Delpassand E, et al. The safety of lymphatic mapping in pregnant breast cancer patients using Tc-99 sulfur colloid. *Breast J.* 2004;10(6):492–495.

59. Mondi MM, Cuenca RE, Ollila DW, et al. Sentinel lymph node biopsy during pregnancy: initial clinical experience. *Ann Surg Oncol.* 2007;14:218–221.

60. Gentilini O, Cremonesi M, Trifiro G, et al. Safety of sentinel node biopsy in pregnant patients with breast cancer. *Ann Oncol.* 2004;15:1348–1351.

61. Morita ET, Chang J, Leong SPL. Principles and controversies in lymphoscintigraphy with emphasis on breast cancer. *Surg Clin North Am.* 2000;80:1721–1739.

62. Doll D, Ringenberg Q, Yarbro J. Antineoplastic agents and pregnancy. *Semin Oncol.* 1989;16:337–346.

63. Kalter H, Warkany J. Congenital malformations. *N Engl J Med.* 1983;308:424–431.

64. Zemlickis D, Lishner M, Degendorfer P, et al. Maternal and fetal outcome after breast cancer in pregnancy. *Am J Obstet Gynecol.* 1992;166:781–787.

65. Hahn KME, Johnson PH, Gordon N, et al. Treatment of pregnant breast cancer patients and outcomes of children exposed to chemotherapy in utero. *Cancer.* 2006;107:1219–1226.

66. Cardonick E, Iacobucci A. Use of chemotherapy during human pregnancy. *Lancet Oncol.* 2004;5:283–291.

67. Aviles A, Neri N. Hematological malignancies and pregnancy: a final report of 84 children who received chemotherapy in utero. *Clin Lymphoma.* 2001;2:173–177.

68. Saunders CM. Breast Cancer in Pregnancy. In: Shaugn O'Brien P, MacLean A eds., *Hormones and Cancer.* London: Royal College of Obstetricians and Gynecologists Press. 1999;312–321.

69. Tewari K, Bonebrake RG, Asrat T, et al. Ambiguous genitalia in infant exposed to tamoxifen in utero. *Lancet.* 1997;350:183.

70. Cullins SL, Pridjian G, Sutherland CM. Goldenhar's syndrome associated with tamoxifen given to the mother during gestation. *JAMA.* 1994;271:1905–1906.

71. Haagensen CD, Stout AP. Carcinoma of the breast: criteria of operability. *Ann Surg.* 1943;118:859–870.

72. Gemignani ML, Petrek JA. Breast cancer during pregnancy: diagnostic and therapeutic dilemmas. *Adv Surg.* 2000;34:273–286.

73. Anderson BO, Petrek JA, Byrd DR, et al. Pregnancy influences breast cancer stage at diagnosis in women 30 years of age and younger. *Ann Surg Oncol.* 1996;3:204–211.

74. Dildy GA, Moise KJ, Carpenter RJ, et al. Maternal malignancy metastatic to the products of conception: a review. *Obstet Gynecol Surv.* 1989;44:535–540.

75. Potter JF, Schoeneman M. Metastasis of maternal cancer to the placenta and fetus. *Cancer.* 1970;25:380–388.

76. Brahim BE, Mrad K, Driss M, et al. Placental metastasis of breast cancer. *Gynecol Obstet Fertil.* 2001;29:545–548.

77. Averette HE, Mirhashemi R, Moffat FL. Pregnancy after breast carcinoma. The ultimate medical challenge. *Cancer.* 1999;85:2301–2304.

78. Petrek JA. Pregnancy safety after breast cancer. *Cancer Suppl.* 1994;74:528–531.

79. Gemignani ML, Petrek JA. Pregnancy after breast cancer. *Cancer Control.* 1999;6:272–276.

80. Dow KH, Harris JR, Roy C. Pregnancy after breast conserving surgery and radiation therapy for breast cancer. *J Natl Cancer Inst Monogr.* 1994;16:131–137.

81. Upponi SS, Ahmad F, Whitaker IS, et al. Pregnancy after breast cancer. *Eur J Cancer* 2003;39:736–741.

82. Surbone A, Petrek JA. Childbearing issues in breast carcinoma survivors. *Cancer.* 1997;79:1271–1278.

83. Collichio FA, Agnello R, Staltzer J. Pregnancy after breast cancer: from psychosocial issues through conception. *Oncology.* 1998;12:759–769.

84. Sutton R, Buzdar AU, Hortobagyi GN. Pregnancy and offspring after adjuvant chemotherapy in breast cancer patients. *Cancer.* 1977;39:1403–1407.

85. Del Mastro L, Catzeddu T, Boni L, et al. Prevention of chemotherapy-induced menopause by temporary ovarian suppression with goserelin in young, early breast cancer patients. *Ann Oncol.* 2006;17:74–78.

86. Mulvihill JJ, McKeen EA, Rosner F, et al. Pregnancy outcome in cancer patients. *Cancer.* 1987;60:1143–1150.

87. Sankila R, Heinavaara S, Hakulinen T. Survival of breast cancer patients after subsequent term pregnancy: "healthy mother effect." *Am J Obstet Gynecol.* 1994;170:818–823.

88. Malamos NA, Stathopoulos GP, Keramopoulos A, et al. Pregnancy and offspring after the appearance of breast cancer. *Oncology.* 1996;53:471–475.

89. Velentgas P, Daling JR, Malone KE, et al. Pregnancy after breast carcinoma. outcomes and influence on mortality. *Cancer.* 1999;85:2424–2432.

90. Blakely LJ, Buzdarm AU, Lozada JA, et al. Effects of pregnancy after treatment for breast carcinoma on survival and risk of recurrence. *Cancer.* 2004;100(3):465–469.

91. Kroman N, Jensen M-B, Melbye M, et al. Should women be advised against pregnancy after breast-cancer treatment? *Lancet.* 1997;350:319–322.

92. Gelber S, Coates AS, Goldhirsch A, et al. Effect of pregnancy on overall survival after the diagnosis of early-stage breast cancer. *J Clin Oncol.* 2001;19:1671–1675.

93. Mueller BA, Simon MS, Deapen D, et al. Childbearing and survival after breast carcinoma in young women. *Cancer.* 2003;98:1131–1140.

94. Surbone A, Petrek JA. Pregnancy after breast cancer. The relationship of pregnancy to breast cancer development and progression. *Crit Rev Oncol Hematol.* 1998;27:169–178.

95. Kroman N, Mouridsen HT. Prognostic influence of pregnancy before, around, and after diagnosis of breast cancer. *Breast.* 2003;12:516–521.

96. Clark FM, Reid JM. Carcinoma of the breast in pregnancy and lactation. *International J Radiat Oncol Biol Phys.* 1978;4:693–698.

97. Venn A, Watson L, Bruinsma F, et al. Risk of cancer after use of fertility drugs with in-vitro fertilization. *Lancet.* 1999;354:1586–1590.

98. Oktay K, Buyuk E, Libertella N, et al. Fertility preservation in breast cancer patients: a prospective controlled comparison of ovarian stimulation with tamoxifen and letrozole for embryo cryopreservation. *J Clin Oncol.* 2005;23:4347–4253.

99. Errickson CV, Matus NR. Skin disorders of pregnancy. *Am Fam Physician.* 1994;49:605–610.

100. MacKie RM, Bufalino R, Morabito A, et al. Lack of effect of pregnancy on outcome of melanoma: the World Health Organisation programme. *Lancet.* 1991;337:653–655.

101. Roberts DL, Antsey AV, Barlow RJ, et al. UK guidelines for the management of cutaneous melanoma. *Br J Dermatol.* 2002;146:7–17.

102. Travers RL, Sober AJ, Berwick M, et al. Increased thickness of pregnancy-associated melanoma. *Br J Dermatol.* 1995;132:876–883.

103. Lens MB, Rosdahl I, Ahlbom A, et al. Effect of pregnancy on survival in women with cutaneous malignant melanoma. *J Clin Oncol.* 2004;22:4369–4375.

104. O'Meara AT, Cress R, Xing G, et al. Malignant melanoma in pregnancy: a population-based evaluation. *Cancer.* 2005;103:1217–1226.

105. Kirkwood JM, Strawderm MH, Ernstoff MS, et al. Interferon adjuvant therapy of high-risk resected cutaneous melanoma: ECOG trial EST 1684. *J Clin Oncol.* 1996;14:7–17.

106. Derek JW, Strassner HT. Melanoma in pregnancy. *Clin Obstet Gynecol.* 1990;33:782–791.

107. Colburn DS, Nathason L, Belilos E. Pregnancy and malignant melanoma. *Semin Oncol.* 1989;16:377–387.

108. Daryanani D, Plukker JT, De Hullu JA, et al. Pregnancy and Early-Stage Melanoma. *Cancer.* 2003;97:2248–2253.

COMMENTARY
Philomena McAndrew

Although cancer during pregnancy or reproductive years is an uncommon occurrence, it is likely to be seen with more frequency with concomitant increasing age of childbearing. Besides the initial devastating emotional impact of the diagnosis, there are multiple issues that the patient and health care team must consider for the long-term well-being of the woman and current or future pregnancies.

I will discuss the issues that play a major role in decision making regarding choice of cancer therapy for women of reproductive age, the effect of systemic therapy on fertility and premature ovarian failure, and current options for fertility preservation.

SYSTEMIC THERAPY IN YOUNG WOMEN WITH CANCER

More than 13,000 women under age 45 are diagnosed with leukemia and lymphoma per year in the United States (1). Fifteen percent of breast cancers occur in women younger than 45 years, with nearly 1,400 under 40 years of age (2,3). During the last decade, mortality from breast cancer has declined, with the largest benefit thought to be related to adjuvant systemic therapy, especially among younger women (4). There are many issues to consider in the recommendation of type of adjuvant systemic in young women with breast cancer, including hormone receptor status and metastatic risk of the tumor based on staging and other biologic features (grade, *HER2/neu* status). Ongoing clinical trials have been designed to compare the benefits of ovarian suppression or ovarian ablation with current regimens employing chemotherapy or tamoxifen. These trials include the SOFT trial (Suppression of Ovarian Function Trial); the TEXT trial (Tamoxifen and Exemestane Trial); and the Perche Trial (Premenopausal Endocrine Responsive Chemotherapy Trial).

The risk of amenorrhea following chemotherapy varies based on the age of the patient and the type and dose of chemotherapy (5). Several reports have suggested premature ovarian failure rates of 30% to 100% in women younger than 40 years of age receiving chemotherapy for hematologic malignancies (6–12). In a Web-based survey, 29% of women stated that fertility concerns influenced their treatment decisions (11).

Having more specific information as to the benefits of systemic chemotherapy and/or adjuvant hormonal therapy via predictive models (Adjuvant! Online *www.adjuvantonline.com*) or genomic profiling of tumors (Oncotype Dx, Genomic Health, Redwood City, CA and MammaPrint, Agendia, Huntington Beach, CA) can aid women with concerns of childbearing or other long-term effects of premature ovarian failure to better understand the additional benefits conferred by the specific treatment modality (13–15). Many women believe that they had not been adequately informed of the risk of infertility prior to beginning systemic treatment. In one study polling 657 premenopausal women with breast cancer, 27% of patients had no discussion with their physician regarding impact of therapy on fertility, only 51% believed that their fertility issues were adequately addressed, and only 17% of patients had met with a fertility specialist (11). It has also been noted that receiving menopause-related information at the time of diagnosis of cancer and during and following therapy may be at least as important as receiving fertility-related information (16). These data suggest that there is a need for better communication addressing these concerns in premenopausal women with newly diagnosed cancer. An excellent monograph published in the *Journal of the National Cancer Institute* has an in-depth discussion regarding various aspects of the topic of fertility and cancer, including legal and ethical issues, third-party reproduction, and issues facing women with *BRCA* mutations (17).

Although chemotherapy-induced ovarian ablation is beneficial for patients with hormone receptor-positive breast cancers, it may be unexpected and an unfortunate consequence for women wishing future pregnancies, especially for those with hormonally unresponsive tumors who, therefore, will receive no benefit from induced estrogen deficiency.

THE IMPACT OF CHEMOTHERAPEUTIC AGENTS AND SYSTEMIC ENDOCRINE THERAPY ON OVARIAN FUNCTION

The gonadal failure associated with cancer therapy is related to both the specific modality of therapy (surgery, radiation, cytotoxic chemotherapy, endocrine therapy) and the age of the individual at the time of treatment. Specific data are available regarding both short-term amenorrhea and risk of permanent premature ovarian failure in women treated for cancer. The physiologic effects of premature ovarian failure have also included osteopenia, atherosclerosis, vasomotor and genitourinary symptoms, as well as psychological distress (18–21).

THE NATURAL PROCESS OF OOCYTE DEPLETION

The ovaries contain a fixed number of primordial follicles at birth, which constitute the ovarian reserve. The female infant has approximately 6 million oocytes at 20 weeks' gestation, which are reduced to 1 to 2 million at birth. There are 25,000 oocytes present by age 37, and 1,000 remain at menopause (average age, 51 years) (22,23). In normal women at about age 37 an accelerated atresia of oocytes begins, and not only the number but the quality of the oocytes fall below a critical level, which leads to higher rate of aneuploidy and greater risk of spontaneous abortion (24,25). Premature ovarian failure (under age 40) occurs in 1% of the general population and may be influenced by familial predisposition as well as environmental and toxic exposures.

CHEMOTHERAPY-INDUCED OVARIAN DAMAGE AND OVARIAN FAILURE

Chemotherapy causes depletion of the primordial follicle pool in a drug- and dose-dependent manner (26). Alkylating agents are significantly gonadotoxic as they are not cell cycle-specific and can damage resting primordial cycles. Anthracyclines and taxanes contribute to the risk of premature ovarian failure. Tamoxifen does not cause the loss of primordial follicles in reproductive-age women but treatment with this drug may result in a 5-year delay in attempting pregnancy. A major weakness of many studies that have reported on the impact of chemotherapy on fertility have used resumption of menses as a surrogate for fertility, but it is recognized that this is not an indication that fertility has been preserved.

One year after starting cytotoxic therapy, amenorrhea can be seen in up to 5% of women under age 30, nearly 40% of 40-year-old women, and 80% of 45-year-old women who were previously experiencing regular menses prior to chemotherapy (12,27).

The definitions of drug-induced amenorrhea and menopause are not consistent throughout the literature, with some studies using the lack of menses at 3 to 12 months from the cessation of chemotherapy, and others have used infertility or estradiol and follicle-stimulating hormone (FSH) levels as indicators of premature ovarian failure or menopause (12,13).

ADJUVANT ENDOCRINE THERAPY AND OVARIAN FUNCTION

Amenorrhea is not synonymous with lack of ovarian function, especially during tamoxifen therapy. Tamoxifen-induced amenorrhea may obscure the presence of hyperactive ovaries by a positive feedback mechanism. In a study evaluating the effects of tamoxifen following chemotherapy in premenopausal patients with breast cancer (28), 114 patients underwent serial measurements of serum FSH and estradiol and transvaginal ultrasonography. After high-dose chemotherapy (51 patients), all women developed amenorrhea and a postmenopausal hormone status as defined by a serum estradiol level of <10 pmol/L and FSH >30, irrespective of presence or absence of menses. In 63 patients receiving standard-dose chemotherapy, 21 developed amenorrhea. In 27 patients with premenopausal hormone levels, 19 developed ovarian cysts, despite amenorrhea in 12 patients (29). Higher estradiol levels were noted in patients with ovarian cysts. A diminution of hot flashes in some women despite ongoing amenorrhea suggests estrogenic effect is overriding the tamoxifen.

These findings have significant implications in that these patients thought to be postmenopausal are not candidates for aromatase inhibitor (AI) therapy even though they remain persistently amenorrheic. By administering such women an AI they will not only be receiving ineffective therapy but may be at risk of unplanned pregnancy. Smith et al. (30) identified 45 women ≥40 years old with chemotherapy-induced amenorrhea and biochemically proven menopause who were treated with an AI either first line (n = 16), after 1 to 3 years of tamoxifen (n = 20), or after 5 years of tamoxifen (n = 9). Twelve of the 45 patients (27%) had recovery of ovarian function with two not regaining menstruation (one with pregnancy without prior menses; the other with estradiol levels >1,500 pmol/L with diminished vasomotor symptoms). The median age was 44 years, with a range of 40 to 50 years, and median duration of amenorrhea prior to recovery of ovarian function was 12 months (range, 4 to 59 months). This is in contrast to 0% to 11% of women >40 years with chemotherapy-induced amenorrhea regaining spontaneous menses, suggesting AIs may increase the incidence of ovarian recovery.

Recent guidelines have been suggested for the use of AI after chemotherapy-induced menopause (30):

1. Women younger than 40 years should not receive an AI alone. If estrogen depletion is the desired endocrine strategy, this should be by ovarian function suppression (oophorectomy or chemical suppression with a gonadotropin-releasing hormone [GNRH] agonist) concomitant with an AI.

2. In women >40 years, measurement of the baseline estradiol and gonadotropin levels and accurate monitoring of serial levels should be performed.

   a. If baseline levels are in the premenopausal range (normal gonadotropin and estradiol >20 pmol/L) the patient should be treated with tamoxifen alone, ovarian suppression/ablation plus tamoxifen, or ovarian suppression/ablation plus an AI.

   b. If baseline levels suggest menopause (elevated gonadotropin and estradiol <10 pmol/L) an AI may be considered but serial monitoring should be continued for 6 months. Estradiol levels should remain below 10 pmol/L to ensure effective therapy. Rising estradiol levels require ovarian suppression/ablation or switching to tamoxifen therapy.

3. For women >40 years for whom monitoring is not available or acceptable, tamoxifen is the preferred endocrine therapy. In this setting, AIs should be used with caution and with concurrent ovarian suppression or ablation.

FERTILITY PRESERVATION IN WOMEN UNDERGOING CANCER THERAPY

There are two approaches currently used to improve the possibility of fertility preservation in women undergoing chemotherapy: (a) Coadministration of a GNRH analogue with chemotherapy and (b) assisted reproduction. At this writing, there have been no completed prospective, randomized clinical trials that have validated either clinical efficacy or safety of either method in women who have undergone chemotherapy.

The American Society of Clinical Oncology has recently published a consensus panel report on guidelines for recommendations on fertility preservation in cancer patients in an effort to encourage discussion of these issues with patients facing treatment (31). Ongoing trials in Italy (32,33), the United States (34), and Germany are evaluating fertility preservation in breast cancer as well as lupus (35). Patients should be encouraged to participate in such trials and registries to allow for further delineation of the benefits of these methods.

GNRH Agonist Treatment

Because dividing cells are known to be more sensitive to the cytotoxic effects of alkylating agents than cells at rest, it has been suggested that the inhibition of the pituitary-gonadal axis would reduce oogenesis, making the germinal epithelium less susceptible to the effects of chemotherapy (36). Pretreatment with GNRH agonists (leuprolide, buserelin, goserelin) has been shown to inhibit chemotherapy-induced depletion of ovarian follicles in rats, but the human ovary has lower concentrations of GNRH receptors and may not have the same response (36,37). The concept of creating a prepubertal state to preserve ovarian function was suggested from long-term studies of girls who were treated with chemotherapy for Hodgkin lymphoma and were found to have a 13% incidence of premature ovarian failure, in contrast to 25% to 50% of similarly treated adults (36–38).

The possibility of administering an adjuvant treatment that may reduce ovarian damage is appealing. Although thee are a number of studies that have shown improvement in resumption or preservation of menstrual function (34,38–44), there has been

a lack of randomized controlled trials, follow-up has been short term, and published studies have not addressed whether fertility had been preserved (26,45,46). There has been some concern raised as to the safety of GNRH analogues in cancer patients (46,47), but there are no compelling clinical data to support a harmful effect on either cancer or pregnancy outcome.

Assisted Reproductive Technology

Recent advances in assisted reproductive technology allow for banking of oocytes, embryos, and ovarian tissue prior to exposure to systemic cytotoxic therapy. The appropriate options for an individual woman depend on the patient's age, type of treatment, diagnosis, the time available before beginning cancer therapy, and the possibility that the cancer may have metastasized to her ovaries (26).

Embryo Cryopreservation

Embryo cryopreservation is the most established technique that has been used for fertility preservation in women (26). Initially, 10 to 14 days of ovarian stimulation is given from the beginning of the menstrual cycle; next, eggs are harvested, then in vitro fertilization is performed with partner or donor sperm, and subsequently the embryo is frozen for later implantation. This technique yields a higher number of embryos per cycle in contrast to natural cycle retrieval (1.6 vs. 0.6), and, therefore, a higher possibility of an eventual pregnancy. Although this is an outpatient procedure, there are significant costs as well as a delay in the initiation of systemic therapy.

There are no data to either suggest safety or risk of ovarian stimulation in women with hormone-responsive tumors. Recently, newer techniques of ovarian stimulation using FSH and tamoxifen or an AI are being used that appear to give even higher yields (46,48). Live birth rates after embryo cryopreservation depend on the patient's age and the number of embryos cryopreserved, and may be lower than fresh embryos. There has been no increased recurrence of breast cancer noted in women who have undergone stimulation with FSH and tamoxifen and letrozole. The initial pregnancy rates using this technique are encouraging.

Oocyte Cryopreservation

Harvesting and freezing of unfertilized eggs is still investigational, with small case series and reports (47,49,50), but this procedure may be an option especially for patients with ethical or religious objections to embryo freezing, or for patients with no available partner and who do not wish to use banked donor sperm (26). Oocytes appear to be more prone to damage during cryopreservation than embryos and may lead to overall lower rates of pregnancy. Further research is being done to improve the efficiency of this technique and should be conducted only under institutional review board-approved protocols in experienced centers. As of 2008, over 900 oocyte cryopreservation babies have been born with no apparent increase in congenital anomalies (50).

Ovarian Tissue Cryopreservation and Transplantation

Ovarian tissue cryopreservation is currently investigational. This procedure does not require the delay in cancer treatment necessary in techniques that use ovarian stimulation and may be performed at any time during the menstrual cycle. Reimplantation of the thawed tissue can occur after the completion of cancer therapy. Ovarian cryopreservation is the only fertility-sparing option in children. There are a few reports of pregnancies and live births but the ischemia experienced by the ovarian tissue after transplantation because of the time necessary for revascularization leads to partial fibrosis and loss of a significant percentage of primordial follicles. The possibility of residual tumor cells in revascularizing transplanted ovarian tissue remains a concern in patients who are at risk of ovarian metastases (26).

Donor Eggs and Surrogacy

In vitro fertilization with donor eggs is an alternative for fertility in patients with premature ovarian failure, with success rates of >60% per embryo transfer. This method allows for the use of partner sperm for fertilization. Gestational surrogacy has become more available and can be the most appropriate option for patients who have undergone hysterectomy or who are at high risk of cancer recurrence and require prolonged endocrine therapy (26,44).

SUMMARY

Many young patients who are diagnosed with cancer are at risk for premature ovarian failure and subnormal fertility, even with resumption of menstruation. Patients often miss an opportunity for preservation of their fertility because of the anxiety surrounding their diagnosis and sense of urgency to begin treatment. Women who are diagnosed with cancer during childbearing years can experience profound and persistent physical and psychological sequelae as a result of therapy, especially when reproductive concerns have not been addressed prior to treatment. Although professional organizations such as the American Society for Reproductive Medicine, and patient advocacy groups like Fertile Hope, Susan G. Komen for the Cure, and the Lance Armstrong Foundation provide information, resources, and support, it is the responsibility of the health care providers to discuss these issues and inform their patients of the risk of infertility, premature ovarian failure, and menopause associated with treatment. These young individuals require this input to make educated decisions regarding their cancer therapy and reproductive future.

REFERENCES

1. Ries LAG, Eisner MP, Kosary CL, (eds). *SEER Cancer Statistics Review, 1975–2000.* Bethesda, MD: National Cancer Institute; 2003. http://seer.cancer.gov/csr/1975_2000/. Accessed October 15, 2008.
2. Hankey BF, Miller B, Curtis R, et al. Trends in breast cancer in younger women in contrast to older women. *J Natl Cancer Inst Monogr.* 1994;16:7–14.
3. American Cancer Society. *Breast Cancer Facts and Figures 2003–2004.* Atlanta: American Cancer Society; 2003.
4. Chu KC, Tarone RE, Kessler LG, et al. Recent trends in US Breast cancer incidence, survival, and mortality rates. *J Natl Cancer Inst.* 1996;88:1571–1579.
5. Blumfeld Z. Gender difference: fertility preservation in young women but not in men exposed to gonadotoxic chemotherapy. *Minvera Endocrinol.* 2007;32:23–34.
6. Pereyra Pacheco B, Mendez Ribas JM, Milone G, et al. Use of GnRH analogs for functional protection of the ovary and preservation of fertility during cancer treatment in adolescents: a preliminary report. *Gynecol Oncol.* 2001;81:391–397.
7. Castelo-Branco C, Nomdedeu B, Camus A, et al. Use of gonadotropin-releasing hormone agonists in patients with Hodgkin's disease for preservation of ovarian function and reduction of gonadotoxicity related to chemotherapy. *Fertil Steril.* 2007;87:702–705.
8. Del Mastro L, Catzeddu T, Boni L, et al. Prevention of chemotherapy-induced menopause by temporary ovarian suppression with goserelin in young, early breast cancer patients. *Ann Oncol.* 2006;17:74–78.
9. Recchia F, Saggio G, Amiconi G, et al. Gonadotropin-releasing hormone analogues added to adjuvant chemotherapy protect ovarian function and improve clinical outcomes in young women with early breast carcinoma. *Cancer.* 2006;106:514–523.
10. Fox KR, Scaialla J, Moore H. Preventing chemotherapy-related amenorrhea using leuprolide during adjuvant chemotherapy for early-stage breast cancer [abstr 50]. *Proc Am Soc Clin Oncol.* 2003;22:13.
11. Partridge AH, Gelber S, Peppercorn J, et al. Web-based survey of fertility issues in young women with breast cancer. *J Clin Oncol.* 2004;22:4174–4183.
12. Walshe JMJ, Denduluri N, Swain SM. Amenorrhea in premenopausal women after adjuvant chemotherapy for breast cancer. *Clin Oncol.* 2006;24:5769–5779.
13. Ravdin PM, Siminoff AL, Davis GJ, et al. Computer program to assist in making decisions about adjuvant therapy for women with early breast cancer. *J Clin Oncol.* 2001;19:980–991.
14. Paik S, Shak S, Tang G, et al. A multigene assay to predict recurrence of tamoxifen-treated, node-negative breast cancer. *N Engl J Med.* 2004;351:2817–2826.
15. Van de Vijver MJ, He Yd, van 't Veer LJ, et al. A gene-expression signature as a predictor of survival in breast cancer. *N Engl J Med.* 2002;347:1999–2009.
16. Thewes B, Meiser B, Taylor A, et al. Fertility and menopause-related information needs of younger women with a diagnosis of early breast cancer. *J Clin Oncol.* 2005;235155–5165.
17. Schover LR (ed.). Parenthood after cancer: today's options and tomorrow's hope. *J Natl Cancer Inst Monogr.* 2005;34:1–113.
18. Vehmanen L, Elomaa I, Blomqvist C, et al. Tamoxifen treatment after adjuvant chemotherapy has opposite effects on bone mineral density in premenopausal patients depending on menstrual status. *J Clin Oncol.* 2006;24:675–680.
19. Saarto T, Blomqvist C, Ehnholm C, et al. Effect of chemotherapy-induced castration on serum lipids and apoproteins in premenopausal women with node-positive breast cancer. *J Clin Endocrinol Metab.* 1996;81:2253–2257.
20. Sverrisdottir A, Fornander T, Jacobsson H, et al. Bone mineral density among premenopausal women with early breast cancer in a randomized trial of adjuvant endocrine therapy. *J Clin Oncol.* 2004;22:3694–3699.
21. Vehmanen L, Saarto T, Blomqvist C, et al. Tamoxifen treatment reverses the adverse effects of chemotherapy-induced ovarian failure on serum lipids. *Br J Cancer.* 2004;91:476–481.
22. Faddy MJ, Gosden RG, Gougeon A, et al. Accelerated disappearance of ovarian follicles in mid-life: implications for forecasting menopause. *Hum Reprod.* 1992;7:1342–1346.
23. Gougeon A, Ecochard R, Thalabard JC. Age-related changes of the population of human ovarian follicles: increase in the disappearance rate of non-growing and early-growing follicles in aging women. *Biol Reprod.* 1994;50:653–663.
24. Lobo RA. Potential options for preservation of fertility in women. *N Engl J Med.* 2005;353:64–73.

25. Benadiva CA, Kligman I, Munne S. Aneuploidy 16 in human embryos increases significantly with maternal age. *Fertil Steril.* 1996;66:248–255.

26. Sonmezer M, Oktay K. Fertility preservation in young women undergoing breast cancer therapy. *Oncologist.* 2006;11:422–434.

27. Goodwin PJ. Options for preservation of fertility in women. *N Engl J Med.* 2005;353:1418–1420.

28. Mourits MJ, de Vries EG, Willemse PH, et al. Ovarian cysts in women receiving tamoxifen for breast cancer. *Br J Cancer.* 1999;79:1761–1764.

29. Mourits MJ, de Vries EG, ten Hoor KA, et al. Beware of amenorrhea during tamoxifen: it may be a wolf in sheep's clothing. *J Clin Oncol.* 2007;25:3787–3788.

30. Smith IE, Dowsett M, Yap YS, et al. Adjuvant aromatase inhibitors for early breast cancer after chemotherapy-induced amenorrhea: caution and suggested guidelines. *J Clin Oncol.* 2006;24:2444–2447.

31. Lee SJ, Schover LR, Partridge AH, et al. American Society of Clinical Oncology recommendations on fertility preservation in cancer patients. *J Clin Oncol.* 2006;24:2917–2932.

32. Del Mastro L, Venturini M. Fertility preservation strategies for breast cancer patients. *J Clin Oncol.* 2006;24:4220–4221.

33. Gruppo Italiano Mammella. Triptorelin in preventing early menopause in premenopausal women who are receiving chemotherapy for stage i, stage ii, or stage iii breast cancer that has been removed by surgery [identifier NCT 00311636]. Bethesda, MD: National Cancer Institute. http://clinicaltrials.gov. Accessed October 7, 2007.

34. SWOG/Intergroup. Goserelin in preventing ovarian failure in women receiving chemotherapy for breast cancer [identifier NCT 00068601]. Bethesda, MD: National Cancer Institute. http://clinicaltrials.gov. Accessed October 7, 2007.

35. Manger K, Wildt L, Kalden JR, et al. Prevention of gonadal toxicity and preservation of gonadal function and fertility in young women with systemic lupus erythematosus treated by cyclophosphamide: the PREGO-Study. *Autoimmun Rev.* 2006;5:269–272.

36. Blumenfeld Z, Avivi I, Ritter M, et al. Preservation of fertility and ovarian function and minimizing chemotherapy-induced gonadotoxicity in young women. *J Soc Gynecol Investig.* 1999;6:229–239.

37. Blumenfeld Z, Eckman A. Preservation of fertility and ovarian function and minimization of chemotherapy-induced gonadotoxicity in young women by GnRH-a. *J Natl Cancer Inst Monogr.* 2005;34:40–43.

38. Blumenfeld Z. Ovarian rescue/protection from chemotherapeutic agents. *J Soc Gynecol Investig.* 2001;8(1 Suppl Proceedings):S60–64.

39. Recchia F, Sica G, De Filippis S, et al. Goserelin as ovarian protection in the adjuvant treatment of premenopausal breast cancer: a phase II pilot study. *Anticancer Drugs.* 2002;13:417–424.

40. Urruticoechea A, Arnedos M, Walsh G, et al. Ovarian protection with goserelin during adjuvant chemotherapy for pre-menopausal women with early breast cancer (EBC). *Breast Cancer Res Treat.* 2004;(Suppl 1):S229.

41. Moore HCF, Theriault RL. Commentary: ovarian function does not equal fertility does not equal babies. *Oncologist.* 2007;12:1067–1069.

42. Oktay K, Sönmezer M, Öktem O, et al. Absence of conclusive evidence for the safety and efficacy of gonadotropin-releasing hormone analogue treatment in protecting against chemotherapy-induced gonadal injury. *Oncologist.* 2007;12:1055–1066.

43. Wildiers H, Neven P, Amant F, et al. Fertility preservation in (breast) cancer patients: is it safe? *J Clin Oncol.* 2006;24:5335–5336.

44. Roberts JE, Oktay K. Fertility preservation: a comprehensive approach to the young woman with cancer. *J Natl Cancer Inst Monogr.* 2005;34:57–59.

45. Oktay K, Buyuk E, Davis O, et al. Fertility preservation in breast cancer patients: IVF and embryo cryopreservation after ovarian stimulation with tamoxifen. *Hum Reprod.* 2003;18:90–95.

46. Oktay K. Further evidence on the safety and success of ovarian stimulation with letrozole and tamoxifen in breast cancer patients undergoing in vitro fertilization to cryopreserve their embryos for fertility preservation. *J Clin Oncol.* 2005;23:3858–3859.

47. Oktay K, Cil AP, Bang H. Efficiency of oocyte cryopreservation: a meta-analysis. *Fertil Steril.* 2006;86:70–80.

48. Oktay K, Buyuk E, Libertella, N, et al. Fertility preservation in breast cancer patients: a prospective controlled comparison of ovarian stimulation with tamoxifen and letrozole for embryo cryopreservation. *J Clin Oncol.* 2005;23:4259–4261.

49. Chang HJ, Suh CS. Fertility preservation for women with malignancies: current developments of cryopreservation. *J Gynecol Oncol.* 2008;19:99–107.

50. Noyes N, Porcu E, Borini A. Over 900 oocyte cryopreservation babies born with no apparent increase in congenital anomalies. *Reprod Biomed Online.* 2009;18:769–776.

16

Breast Imaging

Chapter 16A
Mammography

Early Detection of Breast Cancer Challenges Current Standards of Care

László Tabár, Peter B. Dean, H. H. Tony Chen, Stephen W. Duffy, Amy Ming-Fang Yen, and Sherry Yueh-Hsia Chiu

We live in an era when both the incidence of breast cancer and mortality from the disease show changes that the previous generation of physicians has not experienced. Although we lack a definitive explanation for the steady increase in incidence in all age subgroups, also among younger women (there was a 58% increase in incidence in two counties in Sweden during the past 20 years in the age group 20 to 39), ours is the first generation of physicians able to provide a significantly better outcome for breast cancer patients (1). During the past few decades a significant improvement in recognizing the histologic tumor features at the time of diagnosis has been brought about by early detection, creating a revolutionary new situation for those involved in the diagnosis and treatment of breast cancer patients.

The establishment of the Swedish Cancer and Death Registry in 1958 has made possible an accurate analysis of breast cancer incidence and mortality over several decades. Figure16A.1 shows the steady increase in breast cancer *incidence* during the past 40 years in Dalarna County, prior to screening and during the screening epoch. The similarity of the breast cancer incidence among women who attended screening at regular intervals during the 20-year screening epoch and among the contemporaneous women who declined mammographic screening indicates that "over diagnosis" appears to play little if any role in the steady increase of breast cancer incidence.

...ear screening epoch, all women in the age ...s received invitations to mammographic ...tervals. The majority of them (about 85%) ...n and attended screening. This group is ...eening. All breast cancers detected in the ...at screening or during the interscreening ...in Figure 16A.1. Women who declined screening belong to the "unexposed" group. Both groups were treated according to the same nationwide therapeutic guidelines. The outcome of cases diagnosed in the group exposed to screening (i.e., screen-detected and interval cancers combined) can be compared with the outcome of cases diagnosed in the unexposed group, and both of them can be compared with breast cancer death in the era prior to screening. Comparison of patient outcome between the contemporaneous groups enables us to assess the individual impact of early detection on breast cancer mortality among 40- to 69-year-old women in the population. Adjustment for selection bias improves the reliability of these data. The combined effect of all the other changes on breast cancer mortality, such as increased patient awareness, the use of modern therapeutic methods, adjuvant endocrine and cytotoxic chemotherapy included, and so forth, can be estimated among the contemporaneous 40- to 69-year-old women who declined the screening that was offered to them at regular intervals (1,2).

Figure 16A.1 also shows that the breast cancer *mortality* trend *has changed* after the introduction of screening. In the group exposed to screening, a 45% to 50% significant decrease in disease-specific mortality was observed as compared with the breast cancer death rate prior to screening. By lowering the diagnostic threshold through screening, the malignant process is arrested at a certain time point in the preclinical detectable phase. This results in a decrease in the advanced cancer rate and a significant decrease in premature death from the disease. On the other hand, as Figure 16A.1 clearly demonstrates, no significant improvement in the outcome of breast cancer patients could be demonstrated in the unexposed group, compared with women prior to screening, despite extensive use of modern therapeutic regimens. Based on earlier publications, (3–6) a similar conclusion has been reached: "The portions of the female population that did not participate in mammographic screening had essentially unchanged or only very minor improvements in mortality compared with previous years, despite widespread use of adjuvant systemic chemotherapy and hormonal therapy, particularly in young patients, patients over 70, or in patients with advanced disease" (7).

This conclusion is supported by statistics in the following population subgroups: women aged 20 to 39 years who were never screened but who were treated according to the prevailing standard of care showed no significant decrease in breast cancer mortality (relative risk [RR], 0.73; 95% confidence interval [CI]: 0.50-1.06); in age group of 40 to 49 years the unscreened women had a 19% nonsignificant decrease in mortality from breast cancer during the screening epoch (RR, 0.81; 95% CI: 0.60-1.09), while those who attended screening had a 48% highly significant decrease in breast cancer death (RR, 0.52; 95% CI: 0.40-0.67).

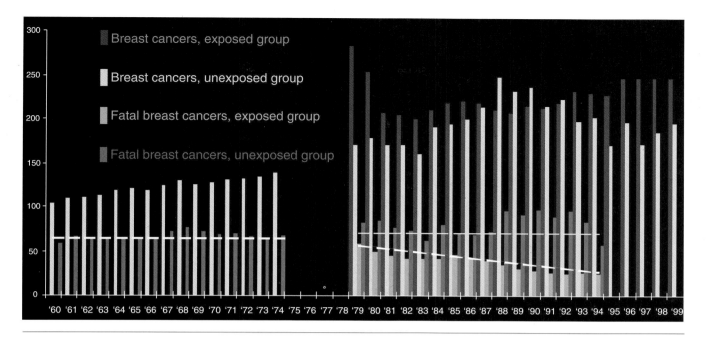

Figure 16A.1. Incidence of *all* breast cancers and *ultimately fatal* breast cancers before screening (1960–1974) *and* among women exposed *and* not exposed to screening during the screening epoch (1979–1999) (5-year moving average). Dalarna County, Sweden. Age group, 40 to 69 years at diagnosis; follow-up until December 31, 2003. (See color plates.)

There was a significant 44% reduction in breast cancer mortality among those women in the age group 40 to 69 years who attended screening at regular intervals and 16% in those not exposed to screening (1).

The long-term survival of all breast cancer patients aged 40 to 69 years at diagnosis in the entire population of two Swedish counties is demonstrated in Figure 16A.2. During the 20-year period prior to screening, fewer than half of the breast cancer patients survived the disease. The introduction of mammographic screening has led to a significant improvement in the outcome of breast cancer patients who attended screening regularly. The contemporaneous women who declined screening, but who received modern therapeutic regimens, had relatively little improvement in survival compared with the outcome of breast cancer patients diagnosed before screening was introduced. After the introduction of service screening in Dalarna County, Sweden, the 17-year follow-up showed 82% disease-specific survival in the group exposed to screening as opposed to 50% disease-specific survival in the group that declined to participate (Figure 16A.3).

In conclusion, women who never have been screened had either no improvement (8) or only a slightly better outcome (1,9) from breast cancer than women in the prescreening period. This indicates the impact attributable to all changes that occurred during 2 decades, the use of modern treatment regimens included. The corresponding outcome in women who attended organized service screening in Sweden was of a much greater magnitude, indicating that most of the 45% to 50% mortality reduction in these women can be attributed to early detection and treatment in an early stage (9). Based on the nationwide screening in the Netherlands, Vervoort et al. (10) concluded that there is a reduction in breast cancer mortality related to adjuvant therapy (7%), while the reduction related to screening "may be three to

four times as large" according to their estimation. Paci et al. (11) evaluated two population-based Italian screening programs and concluded that: "Early diagnosis, not differential treatment, explains better survival in service screening." The following observation adds further confirmation to these findings: "In Europe, countries that do not have population screening still have breast cancer fatality rates of 50%, whereas countries with population screening have markedly reduced breast cancer mortality" (7). An excellent example is comparison of the breast cancer mortality in Denmark and Sweden. Both countries follow the same therapeutic guidelines to treat breast cancer. Sweden has one of the *lowest* breast cancer mortality rates in Europe, whereas Denmark has one of the *highest* breast cancer mortality rates in Europe. There has been organized nationwide screening in Sweden since 1986, but there is still no nationwide mammography screening in Denmark. There can be no doubt that the implementation of organized nationwide screening could dramatically decrease breast cancer death in Denmark.

REVISING THE STANDARD OF CARE THROUGH A CRITICAL EVALUATION OF THE SCIENTIFIC EVIDENCE

The results of hospital-based clinical therapy trials evaluating the impact of adjuvant therapeutic regimens on disease-specific survival cannot be directly applied as a mortality benefit in a population. This is because the absolute benefit is restricted to only a fraction of all breast cancer patients in the population and has relatively little influence on the total number of breast cancer deaths in that given population. On the other hand, regular

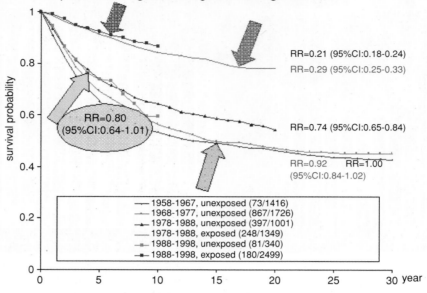

Figure 16A.2. Cumulative survival of women 40 to 69 years old at diagnosis in Kopparberg (W) and Östergötland (E) counties, Sweden. The 20-year disease-specific survival (diagnosis between 1958–1967 and 1968–1977) can be compared with the outcome of breast cancer patients who attended screening ("exposed" group diagnosed between 1977–1988 and 1989–1998) and with the outcome of those who did not attend screening ("unexposed") during the screening era. Women in the unexposed group had a survival curve very similar to those who were diagnosed prior to screening. RR, relative risk; CI, confidence interval.

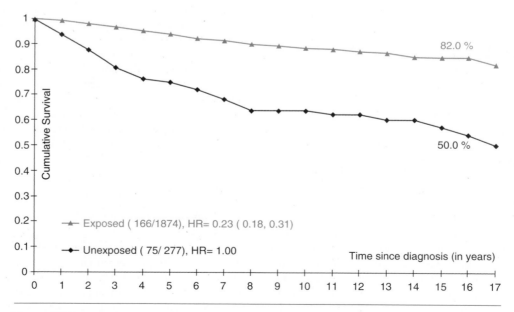

Figure 16A.3. Cumulative survival by exposure status in women aged 40 to 69 years invited to screening after 1986 in Dalarna County, Sweden, and followed until December 31, 2003. HR, hazard ratio.

mammographic screening has an impact on all those who attend, who comprise most of the eligible women in a given population (e.g., 70% to 90% in the organized nationwide screening in Sweden (9) and 85% of women over 40 years of age in the state of Rhode Island (7). The outcome measure of population-based organized screening is mortality from breast cancer in that entire population, which is quite different from survival in a minority of all cases of breast cancer as measured in hospital-based clinical therapy trials.

Molecular biology is offering us new insights into the potential impact of adjuvant chemotherapy on breast cancer. Pawitan et al. (12) concluded in their recent publication: "Using the expression profiles of 64 genes we developed a prognostication of breast cancer patients after surgery. We identified that *almost three-quarters of early breast cancer patients might not benefit from adjuvant therapy* because of superior outcome or because of failing to respond to current adjuvant therapy." The success of the randomized controlled mammography screening trials in demonstrating a significant decrease in mortality from breast cancer has given us convincing evidence that breast cancer is not systemic from its inception (13). This evidence contradicts the theory of Fisher (14) and undermines the justification for systemic therapy in most screen-detected cancers, as they are still localized to the breast and can be cured by local treatment alone. The widespread use of mammographic screening leads to the detection of an ever-increasing number of 1- to 14-mm invasive cancers, which has prompted Cady and Chung (7) to conclude: "The possibility of simplified therapy with decreased rates of mastectomy, less need for radiotherapy, and less need for chemotherapy are reasonable choices for patients with smaller cancers. Thus, the decreasing size and nodal involvement of screen-detected cancers have the potential to allow still more simplified therapy, especially in older women who have estrogen receptor–positive cancer. The reduction in the need for radiation and systemic adjuvant chemotherapy, which are both expensive and toxic, is made possible by detecting highly curable T1a and T1b breast cancers."

Mammographic screening causes a significant shift in tumor size distribution from predominantly large to predominantly small. Figure 16A.4.1 demonstrates the tumor size distribution during three consecutive time periods among women unexposed to screening. Although the average tumor size remains large, because the tumors are self-detected, there is a tendency toward smaller tumor diameter in the service screening era, most probably because of increased awareness. Figure 16A.4.2 shows the tumor size distribution among women exposed to screening in the screening era. A highly significant shift can be observed toward the nonpalpable size ranges compared with the pre-screening epoch. In Figure 16A.4.3 the tumor size range of the combined exposed and unexposed groups is demonstrated. The shift toward smaller size, although less pronounced, is still highly significant relative to the prescreening era. Figures 16A.4.2 and 16A.4.3 illustrate the effect of *participation in* versus *invitation to* mammography screening on tumor size.

Mammographic screening has a significant impact on axillary node status as shown in Figures 16A.5.1 through 16A.5.3. There is no demonstrable difference in node status among the unexposed groups during the three consecutive eras (Figure 16A.5.1). Figure 16A.5.2 shows the highly significant improvement in axillary node status among women exposed to screening. The improvement in axillary node status is less marked when the exposed and unexposed groups are combined, but this improvement is still highly significant (Figure 16A.5.3).

The death rate from breast cancer cannot be reduced without first decreasing the rate of advanced cancers. The incidence of advanced cancers thus serves as the most predictive measure of success or failure of a screening program. High-quality mammographic screening has a significant impact on tumor stage distribution, as shown in Figures 16A.6.1 through 16A.6.3. There is a slight improvement in the stage distribution among women in the unexposed group during the screening epoch (Figure 16A.6.1). Figure 16A.6.2 shows the highly significant improvement in tumor stage distribution among women exposed

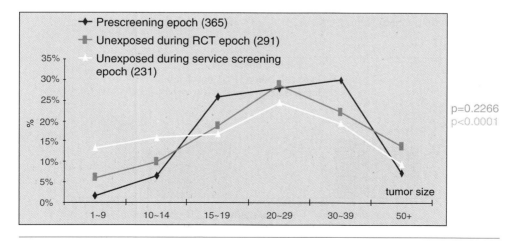

Figure 16A.4.1. Tumor size distribution among women unexposed to screening during the randomized controlled trial (RCT) and service screening epochs compared with the prescreening epoch.

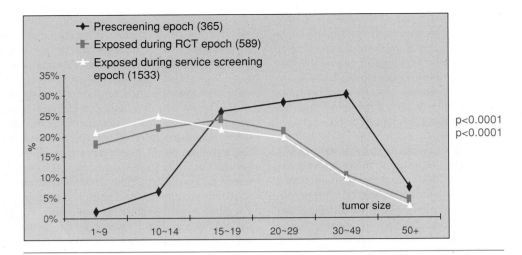

Figure 16A.4.2. Tumor size distribution among women exposed to screening during the randomized controlled trial (RCT) and service screening epochs compared with the prescreening epoch.

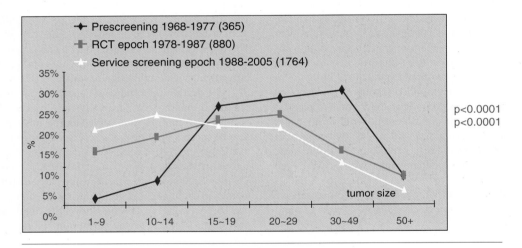

Figure 16A.4.3. Tumor size distribution among women exposed and unexposed groups combined during the randomized controlled trial (RCT) and service screening epochs compared with the prescreening epoch.

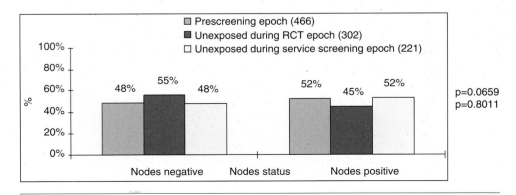

Figure 16A.5.1. Axillary node status among women unexposed to screening during the randomized controlled trial (RCT) and service screening epochs compared with the prescreening epoch.

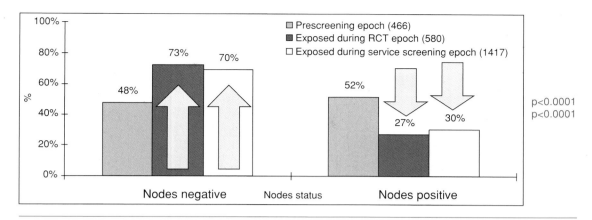

Figure 16A.5.2. Axillary node status among women exposed to screening during the randomized controlled trial (RCT) and service screening epochs compared with the prescreening epoch.

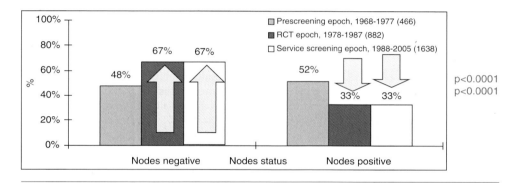

Figure 16A.5.3. Axillary node status among women exposed and unexposed combined during the randomized controlled trial (RCT) and service screening epochs compared with the prescreening epoch.

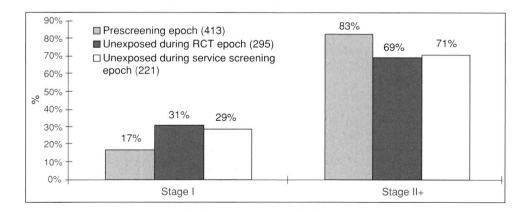

Figure 16A.6.1. Tumor stage among women unexposed to screening during the randomized controlled trial (RCT) and service screening epochs compared with the prescreening epoch.

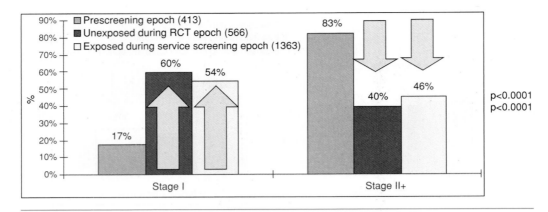

Figure 16A.6.2. Tumor stage among women exposed to screening during the randomized controlled trial (RCT) and service screening epochs compared with the prescreening epoch.

to screening. The improvement is less marked, but still significant when the exposed and unexposed groups are combined (Figure 16A.6.3).

THE NEW ERA IN THE DIAGNOSIS AND MANAGEMENT OF BREAST CANCER

The regular use of high-quality mammography performed at sufficiently frequent intervals has brought about a shift in the balance of breast cancer cases from mainly palpable, advanced cancers to mainly small, impalpable cases that are still localized to the breast. High-quality mammography screening detects tumors that are often 5 mm to 15 mm in size, of which only 20% are grade 3 and approximately 5% to 15% are node-positive. This predominance of early-stage disease has brought about a new era in the diagnosis and treatment of breast cancer. We are experiencing a paradigm shift in controlling the disease as our main task is to prevent the development of advanced cancer by arresting the disease process through early detection and treatment in the early phase. Earlier diagnosis creates a new situation in which both the diagnostic and the therapeutic team mem-

bers encounter previously uncommon situations. Our goal is to improve the benefit/risk ratio by avoiding under- and overtreatment as well as under- and overdiagnosis. Guidelines for the treatment of breast cancer detected at screening, when most cases are still localized to the breast, should not be based on trial results obtained from palpable, clinically diagnosed cancers. Using the established methods for treating palpable cancers on mammographically detected, nonpalpable lesions carries a considerable risk of overtreatment because the histologic prognostic parameters do not reliably predict the outcome of 1- to 14-mm invasive breast cancers (15). This potential risk is demonstrated by the following study: 988 consecutive invasive breast cancers of size 1 to 14 mm were diagnosed and treated between 1977 and 2003 in women aged 40 to 69 years in Dalarna County, Sweden, and followed for up to 26 years. Of these, 440 were in the size category of 1 to 9 mm, and had a 90% long-term breast cancer-specific survival. The remaining 548 cancers were in the size range 10 to 14 mm. The 26-year disease-specific survival was 88%. Despite the excellent prognosis for the majority of patients with small breast carcinomas, a small number of women still died from T1a and T1b tumors within a few years after diagnosis.

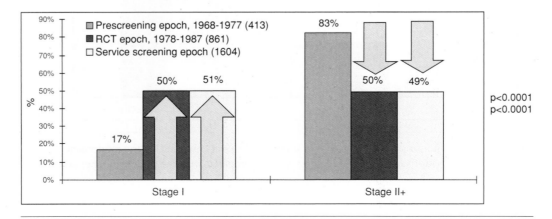

Figure 16A.6.3. Tumor stage among women exposed and unexposed combined during the randomized controlled trial (RCT) and service screening epochs compared with the prescreening epoch.

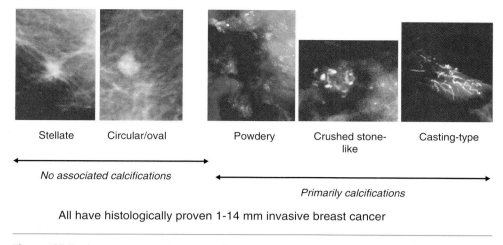

Stellate   Circular/oval   Powdery   Crushed stone-   Casting-type
                                            like

No associated calcifications

Primarily calcifications

All have histologically proven 1-14 mm invasive breast cancer

Figure 16A.7. The mammographic tumor features of 1- to 14-mm invasive breast cancers.

When searching for features common to the few fatal cases, we found that neither axillary node status nor histologic malignancy grade could reliably discriminate the fatal cases from the cases with excellent prognosis within the T1a and T1b category. Given that the mammographic image is a reflection of the underlying histology, we have searched for mammographic tumor features that might have prognostic value. The radiologic images of 1- to 14-mm invasive breast carcinomas can be classified into five separate categories (Figure 16A.7). The frequency of mammographic tumor features in tumor size 1 to 9 mm, 10 to 14 mm, and 1 to 14 mm are shown in Figures 16A.8.1, Figure 16A.8.2, and Figure 16A.8.3, respectively.

The unreliability of the axillary node status in predicting the long-term outcome of women with 1- to 9-mm and 10- to 14-mm invasive breast cancers is demonstrated in Figures 16A.9.1 through 16A.9.4. Also, the mammographic tumor features are shown in relation to the long-term patient outcome. The surprising finding shown in these figures is the consistently poor outcome of women with 1- to 14-mm invasive cancer, regardless

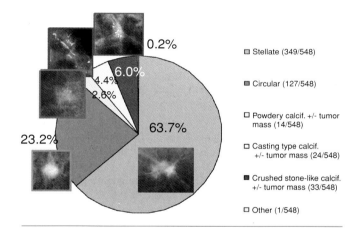

0.2%
6.0%
4.4%
2.6%
23.2%
63.7%

□ Stellate (349/548)

■ Circular (127/548)

□ Powdery calcif. +/- tumor mass (14/548)

□ Casting type calcif. +/- tumor mass (24/548)

■ Crushed stone-like calcif. +/- tumor mass (33/548)

□ Other (1/548)

Figure 16A.8.2. Frequency (%) of mammographic tumor features in women aged 40 to 69 years with 10- to 14-mm breast cancer. calcif., calcification. (See color plates.)

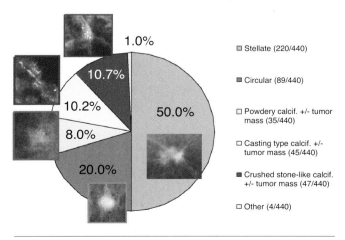

1.0%
10.7%
10.2%
8.0%
20.0%
50.0%

■ Stellate (220/440)

■ Circular (89/440)

□ Powdery calcif. +/- tumor mass (35/440)

□ Casting type calcif. +/- tumor mass (45/440)

■ Crushed stone-like calcif. +/- tumor mass (47/440)

□ Other (4/440)

Figure 16A.8.1. Frequency (%) of mammographic tumor features in women aged 40 to 69 years with 1- to 9-mm breast cancer. calcif., calcification. (See color plates.)

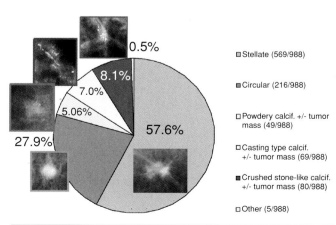

0.5%
8.1%
7.0%
5.06%
27.9%
57.6%

■ Stellate (569/988)

■ Circular (216/988)

□ Powdery calcif. +/- tumor mass (49/988)

□ Casting type calcif. +/- tumor mass (69/988)

■ Crushed stone-like calcif. +/- tumor mass (80/988)

□ Other (5/988)

Figure 16A.8.3. Frequency (%) of mammographic tumor features in women aged 40 to 69 years with 1- to 14-mm breast cancer. calcif., calcification. (See color plates.)

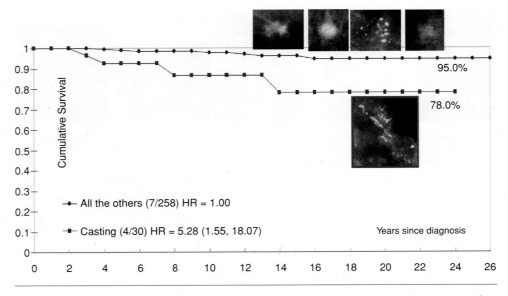

Figure 16A.9.1. Cumulative survival of women with 1- to 9-mm node-negative breast cancer by mammographic tumor features. HR, hazard ratio.

of node status, in which the mammographic image shows casting type calcifications. Most women with 1- to 14-mm invasive breast cancers will have excellent long-term survival, even those with node-positive 1- to 9-mm invasive tumors, provided that there are no associated casting type calcifications. These findings demonstrate the unreliability of node status as a prognostic factor in very small tumors.

The unreliability of the histologic malignancy grade in predicting the long-term outcome of women with 1- to 9-mm and 10- to 14-mm invasive breast cancers is demonstrated in Figures 16A.10.1 through 16A10.6. One would expect that women with grade 3 tumors would have poor long-term outcome, but there

was a 100% disease-specific survival in the 1- to 9-mm tumor size range. Even at the size range of 10 to 14 mm, half of the grade 3 tumors had a 100% 24-year survival rate.

The surprisingly different long-term survival curves of women with 1- to 9-mm grade 3 and grade 2 invasive breast cancers causes us to *critically evaluate* our present knowledge about the value of histologic malignancy grade as a prognostic factor. Although axillary node status and malignancy grade are well-established and reliable prognostic factors in tumors >20 mm, they seem to lose this predictive value with decreasing tumor size. The explanation for the failure of histologic malignancy grade to predict the long-term outcome in 1- to 14-mm invasive

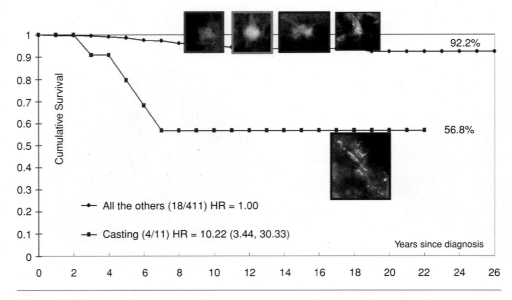

Figure 16A.9.2. Cumulative survival of women with 10- to 14-mm node-negative breast cancer by mammographic tumor features. HR, hazard ratio.

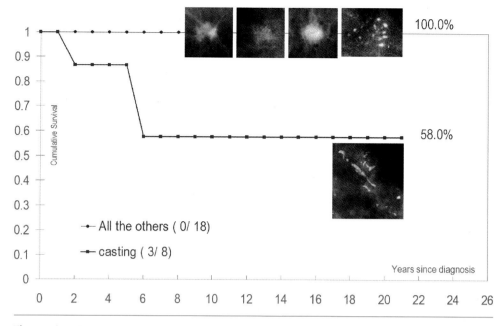

Figure 16A.9.3. Cumulative survival of women with 1- to 9-mm node-positive breast cancer by mammographic tumor features.

cancers is based on the following observation: women with 1- to 9-mm grade 2 *stellate tumors* without calcifications had 100% 26-year survival. The poor outcome of T1a and T1b cancers is restricted to those cases that are associated with casting-type calcifications representing extensive grade 3 ductal carcinoma in situ (DCIS) (Figure 16A.11). Surprisingly, the associated invasive tumors are most often grade 2 and not grade 3, as might be expected (Figures 16A.12.1 and 16A.12.2).

Our interpretation of these findings is as follows: (a) Women with 1- to 9-mm grade 2 invasive carcinomas without associated casting-type calcifications have excellent long-term survival. (b) When 1- to 14-mm invasive cancers are associated with casting-type calcifications, it is the large tumor burden contained within the area with casting-type calcifications that must be responsible for the poor outcome. (c) The malignant process producing the casting-type calcifications is generally classified as

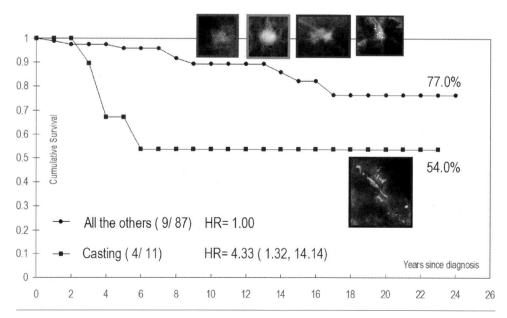

Figure 16A.9.4. Cumulative survival of women with 10- to 14-mm node-positive breast cancer by mammographic tumor features. HR, hazard ratio.

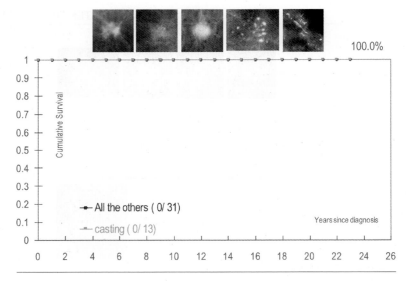

100.0%

Figure 16A.10.1. Cumulative survival of women with 1- to 9-mm grade 3 invasive breast cancer by mammographic tumor features.

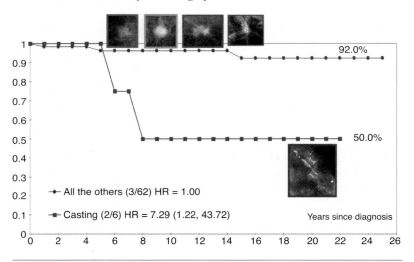

All the others (0/ 31)

casting (0/ 13)

Years since diagnosis

92.0%

50.0%

All the others (3/62) HR = 1.00

Casting (2/6) HR = 7.29 (1.22, 43.72)

Years since diagnosis

Figure 16A.10.2. Cumulative survival of women with 10- to 14-mm grade 3 invasive breast cancer by mammographic tumor features. HR, hazard ratio.

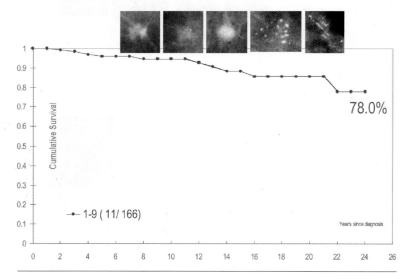

78.0%

1-9 (11/ 166)

Years since diagnosis

Figure 16A.10.3. Cumulative survival of all women with 1- to 9-mm grade 2 invasive breast cancer by mammographic tumor features.

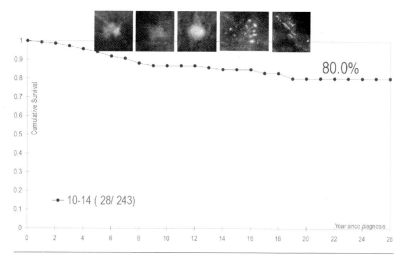

Figure 16A.10.4. Cumulative survival of all women with 10- to 14-mm grade 2 invasive breast cancer by mammographic tumor features.

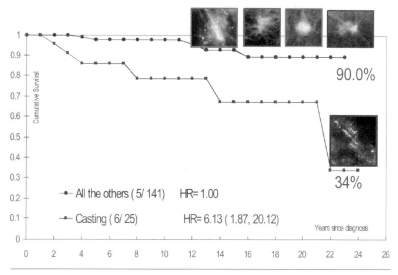

Figure 16A.10.5. Cumulative survival of women with 1- to 9-mm grade 2 invasive breast cancer by mammographic tumor features. HR, hazard ratio.

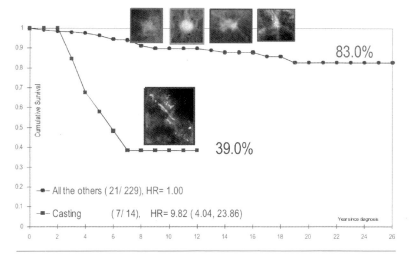

Figure 16A.10.6. Cumulative survival of women with 10- to 14-mm grade 2 invasive breast cancer by mammographic tumor features. HR, hazard ratio.

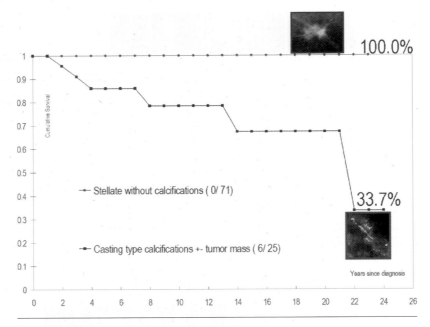

Figure 16A.11. Cumulative survival of women with 1- to 9-mm grade 2 stellate invasive breast cancer. Women with solitary 1- to 9-mm stellate lesion without associated calcifications had a 100% 26-year survival. Women with identical size and grade invasive tumors that are associated with casting-type calcifications had a 34% 26-year survival.

grade 3 DCIS at histologic examination. (d) We propose that the casting-type calcifications represent both an in situ carcinoma (when the cancer cells are confined within the pre-existing duct system), but also represent a "duct-forming, high-grade invasive carcinoma," in which the cancer cells are localized within the newly formed ducts, mimicking the adjacent in situ process. The presence of extensive periductal desmoplastic reaction and periductal lymphocytic infiltration on conventional hematoxylin and eosin histologic staining distinguishes the newly formed ducts from the pre-existing ducts. Also, overexpression

of tenascin immunohistochemical staining highlights the newly formed ducts. We suggest that the term *duct neogenesis* be used to describe this process. (e) Consequently, the presence of high-grade invasive duct-forming carcinoma distributed over a several centimeter-sized region in the breast can explain the high rate of fatality in these cases. (f) The associated tiny grade 2 invasive carcinoma is not responsible for the high rate of fatality, as similar invasive tumors of similar size, histologic grade, and node status have excellent long-term survival in the absence of casting-type calcifications.

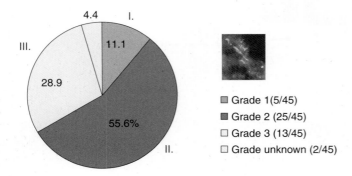

Figure 16A.12.1. Distribution of histologic grade in 1- to 9-mm invasive tumors associated with casting-type calcifications. Roman numerals in circle graph indicate histologic grade. Arabic numbers are percentages. (See color plates.)

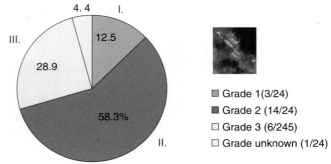

Figure 16A.12.2. Distribution of histologic grade in 10- to 14-mm invasive tumors associated with casting-type calcifications. Roman numerals in circle graph indicate histologic grade. Arabic numbers are percentages. (See color plates.)

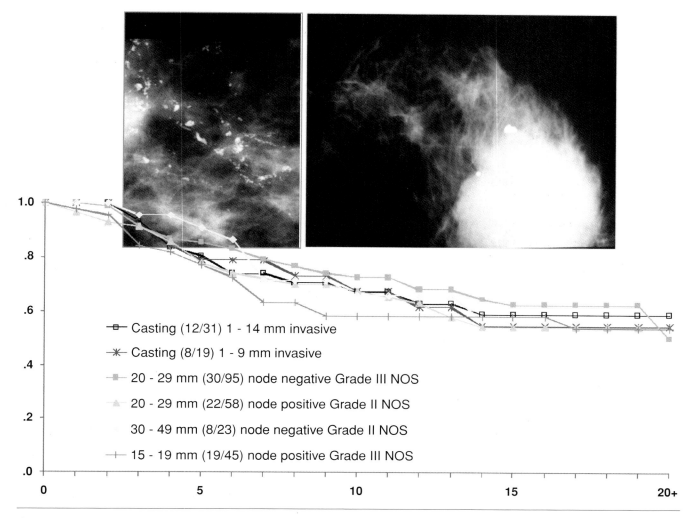

Figure 16A.12.3. Comparison of long-term survival curves of advanced breast cancers with the long-term survival patients with of 1- to 9-mm and 1- to 14-mm invasive breast cancers associated with casting-type calcifications. Age group, 40 to 74 years; Dalarna County, Sweden; follow-up to December 31, 1998. NOS, not otherwise specified.

MANAGEMENT OF 1- TO 14-MM INVASIVE BREAST CANCERS WILL BE MORE APPROPRIATE WHEN MAMMOGRAPHIC TUMOR FEATURES ARE TAKEN INTO ACCOUNT TO DISTINGUISH BREAST CANCERS WITH SIGNIFICANTLY DIFFERENT PROGNOSIS

Current breast cancer patient management guidelines are based on survival curves taking into account the known first- and second-generation histologic prognostic factors. This approach was developed from experience with palpable breast cancers. Unfortunately, as has been delineated here, these histologic prognostic factors cannot reliably distinguish the cases with excellent prognosis from those few with a surprisingly poor prognosis relative to their histologic features.

An analysis of the five mammographic tumor features has shown these features to be a highly reliable prognostic tool for predicting the long-term outcome of 1- to 14-mm invasive breast cancers (15). Half of the 1- to 9-mm fatal breast cancer cases shared a single, easily recognizable mammographic feature: casting-type calcifications. Even though this subset composed only 10.0% of the T1a and T1b size ranges, it accounted for 50% of the breast cancer deaths in this size range. The 26-year survival of 1- to 9-mm and 10- to 14-mm cases associated with casting-type calcifications was 49% and 54%, respectively. These results suggest that T1a and T1b tumors as well as 10- to 14-mm tumors that are associated with casting-type calcifications should belong to a more advanced-stage category, reflecting their clinical behavior. This can be seen from Figure 16A.12.3, in which women with advanced tumors have long-term survival curves that are nearly identical to those of the 1- to 14-mm invasive tumors associated with casting-type calcifications. This comparison supports our conclusion that the casting-type calcifications represent a large invasive malignant process comparable in behavior with other advanced, fatal cancers. As the preceding survival curves demonstrate, it is not the 1- to 14-mm grade 2 invasive carcinoma that is responsible for the poor prognosis. Thus, the clinical practice giving preference to the tiny grade 2 invasive carcinoma instead of the associated high-volume grade 3 malignant process, which is responsible for the poor outcome, is misleading.

A CALL FOR REVISING THE CURRENT TNM BREAST CANCER STAGING SYSTEM

Breast cancers are detected in ever-increasing numbers at ever-smaller sizes because of the widespread application of screening mammography. Most 1- to 14-mm invasive breast cancers have excellent long-term prognosis without adjuvant therapy, but there exists a small subset of 1- to 14-mm breast cancers with unexpectedly poor prognosis for this size category, despite adjuvant therapy. Separating 1- to 14-mm invasive breast cancers into these two categories with a high degree of accuracy would have two advantages: the group with excellent outcome after surgery alone could be spared much adjuvant therapy, and the group with poor prognosis could be selected for more appropriate treatment. The current TNM classification fails to distinguish these two groups from each other.

We propose to improve on the current clinical practice of classifying and predicting the long-term outcome of small, 1- to 14-mm invasive breast cancers using morphologic criteria based *only* on histopathologic examination. We suggest a modification of the current TNM cancer staging system to incorporate the use of five specific mammographic tumor features to classify 1- to 14-mm invasive breast cancers into distinct, easily classifiable subgroups with either very good or very poor prognosis (15). The method uses currently available high-quality mammography, either digital or screen/film, and follows a clearly defined protocol. Published results on 1- to 9-mm invasive tumors have demonstrated the capability of classification by mammographic tumor features to successfully discriminate the T1a and T1b invasive carcinomas into five subgroups, four of which have a 26-year disease-specific survival ranging from 90% to 100%, regardless of histologic malignancy grade or axillary node status. The remaining subgroup, an easily recognizable entity, is characterized by the presence of casting-type calcifications on the mammogram. The casting-type calcifications are produced by grade 3 DCIS, and when associated with a T1a or T1b invasive carcinoma, the 26-year disease-specific survival was 49%; the corresponding survival in the size range 10 to 14 mm was 54%. This subgroup of 1- to 14-mm invasive cancers, comprising 7% of all invasive breast tumors, acts as if it were a much larger and more malignant tumor. We propose that this subgroup should be separately classified in the TNM cancer staging system.

Integration of the mammographic tumor features into the TNM cancer staging system will enable practicing physicians to more accurately distinguish between the 1- to 14-mm invasive breast cancers with extremely good long-term prognosis versus those cases with unexpectedly poor prognosis, and thus provide more specifically targeted therapy, also avoiding overtreatment.

Our proposal addresses a critical barrier to improvements in the current treatment guidelines for screen-detected 1- to 14-mm invasive cancers. The problem is that the associated small focus (foci) of invasive, generally grade 2 carcinoma is currently the determining component for the TNM classification of this breast cancer subtype. This is misleading and fails to account for the frequent, extensive lymph vessel invasion and poor outcome, especially because similar size and grade stellate tumors without associated casting-type calcifications have a 99% 24-year disease-specific survival. Our proposed method provides a more precise estimate of outcome to individual women with small, 1- to 14-mm invasive breast cancers.

To date, there are three confirmatory studies showing that the presence of casting-type microcalcifications on a mammogram is a reliable predictor for poor prognosis in women with small invasive breast carcinomas (16–18). The imaging, histologic, and prognostic aspects of this deceptive breast cancer subtype have been recently reviewed in further detail by Tabar and associates (19).

SUMMARY

Most women with 1- to 14-mm invasive breast cancer have excellent long-term disease-specific survival. However, there is a small, well-defined group of breast cancers with fatal outcome that have been customarily relegated to the T1a-T1b category, despite their poor long-term survival, which is similar to the outcome of cancers that are 30 to 50 mm in diameter. Obviously, the long-term outcome curves of this fatal subgroup of T1a-T1b cancers indicate that we are dealing with a much larger tumor burden than the size range of 1 to 14 mm would indicate.

This should alert us to the possibility that the current breast cancer classification system is not adequately serving its purpose. This group of fatal cancers is characterized by the combination of a 1- to 14-mm typically grade 2 invasive cancer and a large, high-grade in situ component with casting-type calcifications on the mammogram, which, however, may act as a large, poorly differentiated invasive carcinoma, explaining the high fatality rate among these cases. The primary characteristic feature of this breast cancer subtype is its mammographic appearance.

REFERENCES

1. Tabar L, Yen MF, Vitak B, et al. Mammography service screening and mortality in breast cancer patients: 20-year follow-up before and after introduction of screening. *Lancet.* 2003;361:1405–1410.
2. Duffy, SW, Tabar, L, Chen H-H, et al. The impact of organized mammography service screening on breast carcinoma mortality in seven swedish counties: a collaborative evaluation. *Cancer.* 2002;95:458–469.
3. Pisani P, Forman D. Declining mortality from breast cancer in Yorkshire, 1983–1998: extent and causes. *Br J Cancer.* 2004;90:652–656.
4. Otto SJ, Fracheboud J, Looman CW, et al. National Evaluation Team for Breast Cancer Screening. Initiation of population-based mammography screening in Dutch municipalities and effect on breast-cancer mortality: a systematic review. *Lancet.* 2003;361:1411–1417.
5. Randolph WM, Goodwin JS, Mahnken JD, et al. Regular mammography use is associated with elimination of age-related disparities

in size and stage of breast cancer at diagnosis. *Ann Intern Med.* 2002;137:783–790.

6. Tabar L, Vitak B, Chen HH, et al. Beyond randomized controlled trials: organized mammographic screening substantially reduces breast carcinoma mortality. *Cancer.* 2001;91:1724 –1731.

7. Cady B, Chung M. Mammographic screening: no longer controversial [editorial]. *Am J Clin Oncol.* 2005:28:1–4.

8. Parvinen I, Helenius H, Pylkkänen L, et al. Service screening mammography reduces breast cancer mortality among elderly women in Turku. *J Med Screen.* 2006;13:34–40.

9. Duffy SW, Tabar L, Chen H-H, et al. Reduction in breast cancer mortality from organized service screening with mammography: 1. Further confirmation with extended data. The Swedish Organized Service Screening Evaluation Group. *Cancer Epidemiol Biomarkers Prev* 2006;15(1):45–51.

10. Vervoort MM, Draisma G, Fracheboud J, et al. Trends in the usage of adjuvant systemic therapy for breast cancer in the Netherlands and its effect on mortality. *Br J Cancer.* 200419;91:242–247.

11. Paci E, Ponti A, Zappa M, et al. Early diagnosis, not differential treatment, explains better survival in service screening. *Eur J Cancer.* 2005;41:2728–2734.

12. Pawitan Y, Bjöhle J, Amler L, et al. Gene expression profiling spares early breast cancer patients from adjuvant therapy: derived and validated in two population-based cohorts. *Breast Cancer Res.* 2005:7:R953–R964.

13. Tabar L, Fagerberg G, Day NE, et al. Breast cancer treatment and natural history: new insights from results of screening. *Lancet.* 1992; 339:412–414.

14. Fisher B. Laboratory and clinical research in breast cancer—a personal adventure: the David A. Karnofsky memorial lecture. *Cancer Res.* 1980;40:3863–3874.

15. Tabar L, Chen HH, Yen MF, et al. Mammographic tumor features can predict long-term outcomes reliably in women with 1-14-mm invasive breast carcinoma. *Cancer.* 2004;101:1745–1759.

16. Thurfjell E, Thurfjell MG, Lindgren A. Mammographic finding as predictor of survival in 1-9 mm invasive breast cancers. worse prognosis for cases presenting as calcifications alone. *Breast Cancer Res Trea.* 2001;67:177–180.

17. Zunzunegui RG, Chung MA, Oruwari J, et al. Casting-type calcifications with invasion and high-grade ductal carcinoma in situ: a more aggressive disease? *Arch Surg.* 2003;138:537–540.

18. Peacock C, Given-Wilson RM, Duffy SW. Mammographic casting-type calcification associated with small screen-detected invasive breast cancers: is this a reliable prognostic indicator? *Clin Radiol.* 2004;59:165–170.

19. Tabar L, Tot T, Dean PB. *Breast Cancer: Early Detection with Mammography. Casting Type Calcifications: Sign of a Subtype with Deceptive Features.* Stuttgart: Georg Thieme Verlag, 2007.

COMMENTARY
Blake Cady

This chapter highlights a well-recognized aspect of breast cancer in the contemporary environment. Dr. Tabár points out the increasingly favorable results from women who are actually screened by mammography in the two-county area of Sweden, where a randomized clinical trial was carried out in previous years. From this extensively studied population, as well as the literature review from other areas, Dr. Tabár has shown that there are dramatic changes in breast cancer presentation and management as a result of population-wide mammographic screening. The impact of screening on mortality has been minimized by reports that fail to recognize that the hypothesis of randomized control trials of mammographic screening is that if women are *offered* mammographic screening, mortality will be reduced. These were no trials of mortality reduction of women who actually *received* mammographic screening. The population trials demonstrated that approximately 15% to 20% of women in the experimental group (received invitation to mammographic screening) did not obtain mammograms, and roughly the same proportion of the control group (not invited) did receive mammograms. A reasonable conclusion is that the 31% reduction in mortality demonstrated probably understated the effect of actually obtaining mammographic screening by about 50%. That assumption is confirmed by Dr. Tabár's survival and mortality data of women who actually received mammographic screening in the Swedish two-county area compared with the previous decades when mammographic screening was not available.

From 1958 to 1977, before any screening was available, roughly half of breast cancer patients had died of disease by 20 years. During the 20 years of the screening era, 50% of the women in the randomized trial were actually screened but 85% actually received mammograms during the service screening era (all women offered mammographic screening). The survival curves, demonstrated in Figures 16A.2 and 16A.3 of Dr. Tabár's chapter, indicate that there is over an 80% survival rate at 15 years in patient's actually screened by mammography, compared with 50% in patients not screened. Thus, a dramatic 60% reduction in breast cancer mortality occurs in patients actually receiving mammographic screening compared with those not screened.

It should be emphasized that, in the Swedish two-county area, mammographic screening occurs at a 24- to 30-month median interval, and interval cancers became palpable in 39% of patients. The size and node positivity rate of patients screened at 1- or 2-year intervals, in contrast to 30-month intervals, indicate that with yearly screening intervals, 84% of cancers are discovered by mammography and the median diameter of nonpalpable cancers is only 10 mm and node metastases occur in only 13%. Only 16% of cancers are interval palpable cancers (1). When screening occurs every 2 years, the median cancer diameter is 13 mm, and only 17% of patients have positive nodes. With 2-year screening, 26% of patients have interval palpable cancers (1). The survival curves presented by Dr. Tabár of patients actually screened includes the 39% who appear with palpable interval cancers between scheduled screens. Thus, one can imagine the even more dramatic improvements in breast cancer mortality reduction that can be achieved by yearly screening, with far fewer interval cancers (2).

Unfortunately, yearly screening is the exception rather than the rule in the United States, and the median interval between "yearly" screens is about 16 months (3). Most distressing is that only a small proportion of patients actually complete yearly screening over a 10-year period (3). A quarter of patients who have an initial screening mammogram may never return for further mammograms and only a minority adhere to yearly screening recommendations. Thus, patients miss the opportunity of much smaller size, very low positive node rate, lowered incidence of grade 3 tumors, and lowered risk of poorer prognosis interval palpable cancers.

From a public health point of view, it can be seen vividly in Dr. Tabár's data that the primary control of breast cancer mortality today should be extensive mammographic screening. Dr. Tabár also shows that patients who do not undergo screening but who get contemporary systemic chemotherapy management have little change in mortality risk compared with the premammographic screening era. The women who do not get screened consisted those under the age of 40 who are not offered screening, as well as patients of screening age who chose not to be screened. These patients have a long-term mortality from breast cancer that does not differ significantly from women prior to the development of mammographic screening. Dr. Tabár makes the case that for control of breast cancer in developed countries today it is more important, in terms of reduction of breast cancer mortality, to offer extensive screening than it is to offer adjuvant chemotherapy or hormonal therapy. It is more important to interrupt the progressive disease course by screening detection of nonpalpable small cancers than it is to use contemporary systemic adjuvant therapy in poor prognosis patients with larger palpable cancers. This conclusion has been borne out in analysis of the effect of screening and systemic therapy in Holland where Dutch authors concluded that 80% of the 35% reduction (28%) in mortality of breast cancer in Holland has been the result of mammographic screening compared with 20% of the reduction (7%) results from the utilization of modern systemic chemotherapy and hormonal therapy (4).

This chapter by Dr. Tabár emphasizes that from a public health point of view, it is more important to invest in mammographic screening, particularly yearly screening, than it is in continued drug development for control of poor prognosis cancers. Systemic chemotherapy and hormonal therapy have accomplished a great deal for individual patients with poor prognosis, but from the public health point of view—that is, when considering mortality from breast cancer in the entire population—more resources should be devoted to extensive mammographic screening, particularly among socioeconomically disadvantaged women. To "pick up the pieces" after the appearance of palpable cancers in women who are not regularly participating in mammographic screening by use of adjuvant systemic therapy is more expensive and less effective.

In an analysis of patients who died of breast cancer in the state of Rhode Island, 75% had either never been screened or were not following a regular screening program (2). These unscreened women made up only 15% to 20% of the population yet incurred the great majority (75%) of the mortality, despite the use of modern therapeutic regimens. Only 25% of breast cancer deaths occurred in the 80% of patients regularly screened even if only at 2-year intervals. The screened women mortality outcome also included, of course, the palpable interval cancers that arose after a previous negative mammogram and have a larger size, higher node positivity rate, more rapid growth, and a poor prognosis even though the patients do obtain regular mammographic screening.

The conclusion from Dr. Tabár is that the great majority of women detected by mammographic screening have a disease prognosis so good (because of the small size and few node metas-

tases) they do not require adjuvant systemic therapy. One major task of contemporary breast cancer management is to avoid overtreatment of the majority of patients with excellent prognosis while not undertreating patients with palpable cancers and more aggressive growth patterns.

Surgeons must appreciate the much earlier disease presentation and the need for rethinking routine adjuvant treatments, as groups of high-risk patients can be carefully defined either through mammographic calcification characteristics (5), or by size, node metastases, high grade, or other traditional poor prognostic features such as lymphovascular involvement. Dr. Tabár's chapter emphasizes the critical role that surgeons play in control of contemporary breast cancer and their need to help their patients make the most rational use of multidisciplinary integrated therapy incorporating appropriate systemic therapy as well as appropriate radiotherapy. The great majority of mammographically discovered, small, estrogen receptor-positive breast cancer patients are older (median age, ±65 years). Radiation therapy may have little to offer in terms of local control as demonstrated by two recently published randomized control trials of older women with smaller cancers (6,7). Adequate surgical margins do need to be obtained, however, to decrease the need for radiation after breast-conserving surgery.

The larger lesson for surgical oncologists is that opportunities for appropriate screening should not be overlooked. For instance, data from Japan in screening for gastric cancer is essentially identical in overall accomplishments as that seen with breast cancer (8). Opportunities for screening common cancers include melanoma (most contemporary melanoma is extremely early in presentation) and colorectal carcinoma, for which reports indicate that 75% or more of deaths could be averted by screening with either occult fecal blood testing or colonoscopy with removal of precancerous polyps (9). Detection of head and neck cancers, a priority of dentists, has also led to far earlier disease and less radical therapy. Prostate cancer screening is still somewhat controversial as proof of decreased mortality on the basis of screening has not yet been completely resolved. Many cancers do not lend themselves to screening because of their obscure nature, aggressive behavior, anatomic location, or aggressive growth behavior without a prolonged phase of preliminary growth. Lung, pancreatic, and ovarian cancers do not lend themselves to screening. This highlights the major advances that can be made by screening for cancers with a biological progressive growth phase that can be interrupted in an accessible target organ.

A message not included in Dr. Tabár's chapter is that the frequent precancerous ductal carcinoma in situ that is screen-detected and excised, will lead to a reduction in the incidence of later invasive breast cancer over a long period of time, as precursor ductal carcinoma in situ lesions are obliterated successively over many years of screening (10,11). This situation has already been demonstrated in cervix cancer for which regular elimination of preinvasive lesions has systematically occurred for decades, resulting in far fewer invasive cancers and many fewer deaths. In colorectal cancers the consistent elimination of precancerous polyps has demonstrably lowered the incidence of cancer itself as well as the mortality rate.

Thus, population screening by mammography has not only dramatically improved the survival of breast cancer patients and mortality from the disease in the population, but holds the promise of actually reducing the incidence of invasive breast cancer significantly over longer periods of time (12). Dramatically illustrated in this chapter are the many opportunities for more conservative surgery and the appreciation of the risk of overtreatment of many breast cancer patients today.

REFERENCES

1. Hunt KA, Rosen EL, Sickles E. Outcome analysis for women undergoing annual versus biennial screening mammography: a review of 24,211 examinations. *AJR Am J Roentgenol.* 1999;173:285–289.
2. Spencer DB, Potter JE, Chung MA, et al. Mammographic screening and disease presentation of breast cancer patients who die of disease. *Breast J.* 2004;10:298–303.
3. Blanchard K, Colbert JA, Puri D, et al. Mammographic screening: patterns of use and estimated impact on breast carcinoma survival. *Cancer.* 2004;101:495–507.
4. Vervoort MM, Draisma G, Fracheboud J, et al. Trends in the usage of adjuvant systemic therapy for breast cancer in the Netherlands and its effect on mortality. *Br J Cancer.* 2004;91:242–247.
5. Zunzunegui RG, Chung MA, Oruwari J, et al. Casting-type calcifications with invasion and high-grade ductal carcinoma in situ. *Arch Surg.* 2003;138:537–540.
6. Fyles AW, McCready DR, Manchul LA, et al. Tamoxifen with or without breast irradiation in women 50 years of age or older with early breast cancer. *N Engl J Med.* 2004;351:963–970.
7. Hughes KS, Schnaper LA, Berry D, et al. Lumpectomy plus tamoxifen with or without irradiation in women 70 years of age or older with early breast cancer. *N Engl J Med.* 2004;351:971–977.
8. Kunisaki C, Ishino J, Nakajima S, et al. Outcomes of mass screening for gastric carcinoma. *Ann Surg Oncol.* 2006;13:221–228.
9. Battat AC, Rouse RV, Dempsey L, et al. Institutional commitment for rectal cancer screening results in earlier-stage cancers on diagnosis. *Ann Surg Oncol.* 2004;11:970–976.
10. Cady B, Chung MA. The prevention of invasive breast carcinoma. *Cancer.* 2004;101:2147–2151.
11. McCann J, Treasure P, Duffy S. Modelling the impact of detecting and treating ductal carcinoma in situ in a breast screening programme. *J Med Screen.* 2004;11:117–125.
12. Coburn NG, Chung MA, Fulton J, et al. Decreased breast cancer tumor size, stage, and mortality in Rhode Island: an example of a well-screened population. *Cancer Control.* 2004;11:222–230.

Chapter 16B
Ultrasonography:

Performance and Clinical Applications

Pulin A. Sheth, Linda Hovanessian Larsen, Yuri Parisky, and Dennis R. Holmes

Ultrasound plays a central role in the evaluation and management of benign and malignant breast conditions. Until recently, breast ultrasound largely remained a tool of radiologists; however, surgeons are increasingly recognizing the diverse applications of ultrasound in the management of breast abnormalities and the value of incorporating this technology into their armamentarium. The acquisition of skills in ultrasonography has been facilitated by educational programs sponsored by the American College of Surgeons, the American College of Radiology, and the American Society of Breast Surgeons. In this chapter we present the basic principles of breast ultrasonography and its evolving application in surgical practice.

The American College of Radiology (ACR) Practice Guideline for the Performance of the Breast Ultrasound Examination (1) lists appropriate indications for breast sonography to include, but not be limited to, the following:

1. Evaluation and characterization of palpable masses and other breast related signs and/or symptoms.
2. Evaluation of suspected or apparent abnormalities detected on other imaging studies, such as mammography or magnetic resonance imaging.
3. Initial imaging evaluation of palpable masses in women under 30 years of age and in lactating and pregnant women.
4. Evaluation of problems associated with breast implants.
5. Evaluation of breasts with microcalcifications and/or architectural distortion suspicious for malignancy or highly suggestive of malignancy in a setting of dense fibroglandular tissue, for detection of an underlying mass that may be obscured on the mammogram.
6. Guidance of breast biopsy and other interventional procedures.
7. Treatment planning for radiation therapy.

The role of "screening" ultrasonography has heretofore been unestablished. However, as a result of studies suggesting an improved yield of cancer detection when screening mammography is supplemented by ultrasonography in high-risk women with dense breasts (2,3), a clinical trial, the American College of Radiology Imaging Network (ACRIN) 6666 trial (4), was undertaken to assess the worth of screening ultrasonography in conjunction with mammography. This prospective, randomized, multicenter trial was designed to compare the diagnostic yield of screening breast mammography plus ultrasound with mammography alone in women at increased risk of breast cancer. A total of 2,809 women at least 25 years of age who were deemed at increased risk of breast cancer were enrolled in the trial (4). Risk factors considered were personal history of breast cancer; lifetime risk ≥25% by Gail or Claus model; 5-year Gail model risk of ≥2.5% or ≥1.7% and extremely dense breasts; atypical ductal or lobular hyperplasia; lobular carcinoma in situ; atypical papilloma; mutation in *BRCA1* or *BRCA2* gene; and history of chest, mediastinal, or axillary irradiation.

In this study, supplemental ultrasound was associated with a 55% increase in diagnosing breast cancer compared with mammography alone. The diagnostic yield for mammography was 7.6 per 1,000 women screened and increased to 11.8 per 1,000 for combined mammography plus ultrasound. Thus, the supplemental yield was 4.2 per 1,000 women screened (95% confidence interval, 1.1-7.2 per 1,000; $p = 0.003$ that supplemental yield is 0). Unfortunately, analysis of the data also confirmed that the positive predictive value of screening ultrasound was low. Of 233 women for whom biopsy was recommended based on a suspicious ultrasound finding, only 20 (8.6%) were diagnosed with breast cancer. Thus, 91.4% of all suspicious ultrasound findings identified were due to benign changes (4,5). Consequently, the value of the improved diagnostic yield observed must be weighed against the cost and patient anxiety associated with a high false-positive rate leading to many biopsies, in retrospect, unnecessary.

TECHNICAL FACTORS

The technical requirements for the appropriate performance of breast ultrasound equal or exceed those for ultrasonography of other parts of the body (6). The American College of Radiology and American College of Surgeons have established minimum technical requirements for sonographic hardware. Use of a 7-MHz (or greater) center frequency transducer, high-resolution near field capability, and linear array multifocal electronic refocusing are just a few of the necessary elements for the appropriate performance of breast ultrasound and are currently found on most state-of-the-art ultrasound units. The emergence of small, portable, and affordable ultrasound units has made ownership a practical venture for the practicing surgeon.

Patient Positioning

Patients should be scanned in the supine or supine-oblique position, with the breast of interest closest to the examiner and raised slightly relative to the contralateral breast. The ipsilateral arm should be elevated and placed behind the patient's head. This maneuver flattens the breast and optimally exposes the upper outer quadrant and axilla to sonographic scrutiny. Conversely, reverse oblique positioning may better expose the medial aspect of the breast, especially in women with large or pendulous breasts. On occasion, the target palpable lesion may only be appreciated on physical examination when the patient is in the upright position. In this instance, ultrasound may be performed with the patient upright. Positioning for interventional procedures is dictated by the location of the lesion and the procedure to be performed. Medial lesions are often best approached from the contralateral side.

Scanning Technique

It is advisable for the examiner to have an assistant present during the examination who can assume responsibility for annotating and recording the ultrasonographic images. In patients with known physical findings, the physical examination is repeated by the ultrasonographer and directly correlated with the area to be imaged. Scanning the area of concern must be performed in at least two orthogonal planes, most commonly longitudinal and transverse. However, radial and antiradial scanning provides optimal evaluation of ductal anatomy and conforms to the natural anatomic distribution of lobular tissue. Imaging behind the nipple-areolar complex can be difficult and may be facilitated by the examiner using his or her free hand to gently compress and elevate the region while simultaneously scanning with the transducer positioned perpendicular to the chest wall. Lesions that are superficial, such as epidermal inclusion cysts, are best imaged with the use of commercially available standoff pads, which bring the focal zone closer to the skin.

Lesion Documentation

Once an abnormality is detected ultrasonographically, it should be determined whether it correlates with the physical finding, or is an incidental finding. All lesions must be documented and measured with electronic calipers in two orthogonal planes. The location of the lesion should be noted, including laterality, distance from a fixed landmark (nipple, visible scar), and clock position. Simple orientation, such as upper outer quadrant, is discouraged as it may hamper reproducibility and follow-up.

Although there is no accepted standard for documentation of multiple similar lesions in a specific region of interest, good practice requires establishing that all the lesions observed are in fact similar ultrasonographically, and dimensions of the largest lesions should be documented. This scenario is common in women with cysts and fibroadenomas, but may also occur with multiple foci of malignancy.

Documentation of negative findings is particularly important from a medicolegal standpoint. A negative targeted ultrasonographic examination with appropriately documented images (coupled with a mammogram with negative findings when indicated) validates the impression of a negative examination.

ANATOMY

The breast can be divided histologically into fat, fibrous, and glandular tissues. Fat and fibrous tissues comprise the stromal component. The proportion of fat varies from patient to patient but generally increases with age. Fibrous tissue includes the Cooper's ligaments, interlobular dense fibrous tissue, and less dense intralobular fibrous tissue. Composition differences between the interlobular and intralobular fibrous tissue account for variations in sonographic appearance.

The female breast contains approximately five to ten lobes (7), each of which empties into a primary major duct that dilates to form a lactiferous sinus before terminating in the nipple. Peripherally, each major duct branches into successively smaller divisions, ultimately terminating in a lobule—the milk-bearing component of the breast. The terminal ductolobular unit (TDLU) is the site of the majority of physiologic and pathologic processes within the breast. The contents of the axilla include vascular structures, lymph nodes, and nerves, all embedded in adipose tissue. Normal breast tissue overlies and interdigitates with the inferior portion of the axillary compartment, forming the axillary tail of Spence. Occasionally, ectopic (accessory) breast tissue may also overlie the axilla.

SONOGRAPHIC ANATOMY

The differential sonographic appearance of normal and abnormal breast tissue is a function of transmission, reflection, and refraction of sound by acoustically dissimilar tissues. Echogenic tissue reflects sound waves back to the transducer, an effect that is represented electronically as a bright signal on the ultrasound monitor; the greater the reflection, the brighter the image. Anechoic tissue reflects no sound waves back to the transducer. The resulting effect is a dark image. The most echogenic structures in the breasts are calcium deposits, dense fibrous tissue, and fibrous capsular tissue of certain structures. The most anechoic structures are fluid-filled simple cysts, ducts, and blood vessels. Between the two extremes is a spectrum of normal structures and pathologic lesions of varying echogenicities.

The breast may be divided sonographically into three distinct compartments or zones progressing from superficial to deep: the subcutaneous zone, the mammary zone, and the retromammary zone. The subcutaneous zone is bordered by the skin anteriorly and the superficial layer of the superficial fascia posteriorly. This zone contains fat, the suspensory (Cooper's) ligaments, vasculature and occasional ectopic ducts, and glandular tissue. The mammary zone contains virtually all of the ductal structures, lobules, and TDLUs, in addition to fat and fibrous tissues. Almost all breast pathology occurs in this zone, which is bordered anteriorly by the superficial layer of the superficial fascia and posteriorly by the deep layer of the superficial fascia. The retromammary zone, containing almost exclusively fat and fibrous tissue, lies between the deep layer of the superficial fascia and the fascia of the pectoralis major muscle. This zone is more evident on mammography, as it can be separated from the chest wall with correct mammographic positioning. In the supine patient, the retromammary zone is dependant, and often compressed against the chest wall by the weight of the breast. It is argued that lesions that appear to originate in this zone actually are an extension of disease from the mammary zone. Malignancy that extends to the chest wall passes through the retromammary zone by direct extension.

LESION CHARACTERIZATION

Lesions encountered during performance of breast ultrasound require diligent characterization. The features that should be observed and recorded include lesion location, size, shape, orientation, margin definition, internal echogenicity, and posterior attenuation characteristics. A sonographic lexicon has been developed to describe findings seen on ultrasound imaging and should be used regardless of whether the scan was performed by a radiologist or surgeon (8). All significant findings should be correlated with the physical examination to ascertain whether a palpable lesion truly corresponds to the ultrasonographic abnormality. The common, important sonographic features of breast disease are described later. A more comprehensive description of the sonographic appearances of benign and malignant breast lesions is available in excellent reference texts and imaging atlases (6,9,10).

The sonographic appearance of axillary lymph nodes is similar to that of lymph nodes elsewhere in the body: reniform shape, gently lobulated hypoechoic cortex, and an echogenic central fatty hilum (Figure 16B.1). Diseased nodes may demonstrate one or more of the following: round shape, marked hypoechogenicity, loss or compression of the fatty hilum, thickened irregular cortex, extranodal spread, and marked increase in size (Figure 16B.2). Suspect axillary, supraclavicular, or internal mammary lymph nodes can be readily biopsied under ultrasound guidance. Benign intramammary lymph nodes may be found in the mammary zone of the breast, most commonly in the upper outer quadrant. These are incidental normal structures generally <1 cm in size. With careful sonographic scrutiny, an echogenic hilum can almost always be detected.

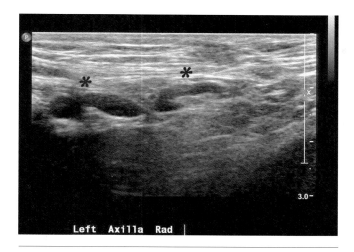

Figure 16B.1. Normal axillary lymph nodes. Two adjacent axillary nodes (*) demonstrating typical sonographic appearance.

The most commonly encountered benign lesions of the breast include cysts and fibroadenomas. These lesions often occur in the younger population and frequently present as a smooth palpable mass or an incidental mass detected during screening mammography. Fibroadenomas are generally painless (unless large) while cysts can on occasion be tender or painful. Cysts are formed from marked dilatation of a TDLU. *Simple cysts* have strict criteria for sonographic classification, and if adhered to, can be categorized as such with virtually 100% certainty. Classification as a simple cyst depends on excellent technique and appropriate adjustment of sonographic focus and gain. The contents of a simple cyst are anechoic. These lesions have thin, well-circumscribed margins and enhanced through-transmission that

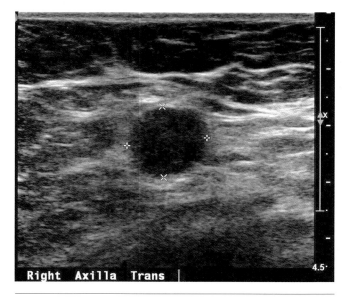

Figure 16B.2. Abnormal axillary lymph node. Note the rounded shape and loss of the echogenic (bright) fatty hilum. Nodal metastasis was confirmed on needle biopsy.

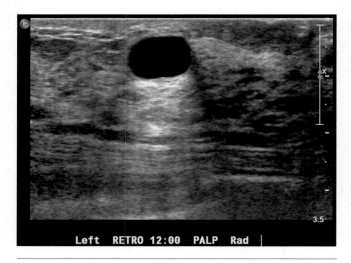

Figure 16B.3. Simple cyst. This palpable mass satisfies all the sonographic criteria for classification as a simple cyst.

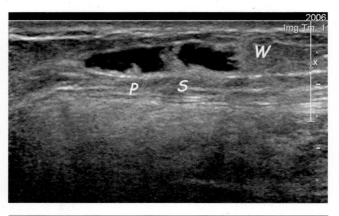

Figure 16B.4. Complex cystic mass. Thickened irregular wall (*w*), thick septations (*s*), and papillary excrescences (*p*) are seen in this lesion, a histologically confirmed malignant high-grade lymphoma.

produces a bright signal immediately posterior to the cyst (Figure 16B.3). The posterior wall has a thin bright reflector representing the interface of fluid and breast tissue. Each of these criteria must be present to classify the cyst as "simple." Thin dark lines extending posteriorly from the lateral edges of the cyst (edge refraction) is a normal artifact related to the shape of the lesion and should not be mistaken for central posterior shadowing. Occasionally, one may encounter a small grapelike cluster of cysts, commonly referred to as *clustered microcysts*, which are invariably benign (11).

Internal echoes can occur in otherwise simple cysts as a result of cellular debris, blood products, protein, or cholesterol. These lesions can be characterized as *complicated cysts* (due to the presence of the internal echoes) so long as all of the remaining strict criteria of a simple cyst are met. Such complicated cysts are being observed with increasing frequency as ultrasound resolution improves with advances in technology. The likelihood of a complicated cyst being malignant, especially in the background of multiple *simple cysts,* is exceedingly rare, as demonstrated in a study by Berg et al. (11). On the contrary, *a complex cyst* has both cystic and solid components, and characteristics such as a thick perceptible wall, thick (>0.5 mm) septations, distinct mural nodule, or papillary excrescences (Figure 16B.4). These lesions warrant biopsy because up to 30% are malignant (11) Although intracystic papillary lesions account for a very small percentage of all breast cancers (<1 %), recognition of such lesions is important.

Solid lesions pose a problem for both surgeons and radiologists. Some have suggested that all solid breast lesions be biopsied, given the overlap of certain sonographic features between benign and malignant (Figure 16B.5). Others argue that we should be more selective in determining which lesions are biopsied, citing the preponderance of benign lesions relative to malignant and the potential harm and costs of unnecessary biopsies. Current thinking has substantially evolved since Donegan (12) advocated "removal of every solid mass." In 1995, Stavros et al. (13) published a large series in which all solid breast masses were prospectively characterized as benign, malignant, or inde-

terminate using strict sonographic criteria. This study affirmed that there are certain sonographic characteristics suggesting benignity that have >98% negative predictive value, thus obviating the need for immediate biopsy (Table 16B.1).

Fibroadenomas commonly appear as smooth, round-to-oval, isoechoic, or slightly hypoechoic masses. As they increase in size they may contain up to one to three gentle macrolobulations (Figure 16B.6). Posterior enhancement characteristics are variable. There is often visualized a thin echogenic pseudo-capsule, a surface cleft or thin linear echogenic septa coursing through it (Figure 16B.7). The long axis is always parallel to the chest wall. Most importantly, there should be no specific malignant characteristics (Table 16B.2). Such lesions may be safely followed in the short interval (generally 6 months) for demonstration of stability. The caveat is that there is strict adherence to the criteria for benignity; if there is even one exception in the ultrasonographic appearance, tissue sampling is warranted. The rare cystosarcoma phyllodes tumor may be sonographically indistinguishable from a fibroadenoma. In general, they tend to be larger (>3 cm) and demonstrate more rapid growth. Truly echogenic (fat-containing) lesions are invariably benign. These include hamartomas, lipomas, intramammary lymph nodes, oil cysts, and galactoceles. Benign hemangiomas of the breast have also been described as having a uniform echogenic appearance. Other benign masses of the breast have variable and nonspecific appearances and include pseudoangiomatous stromal hyperplasia, desmoid tumors, and benign fibrous lesions of the breast. Fat necrosis and radial sclerosing lesions are best evaluated with mammography.

In contrast to those features suggestive of benignity, Stavros et al. (13) have also identified characteristics that are strongly suggestive of malignancy (Table 16B.2). Recognizing these characteristic features facilitates appropriate differential management of various solid masses. The imaging appearances reflect the underlying pathophysiology of the lesion and the biology of the host response. Densely packed tumor cells dampen the transmitted sound waves, which produces the appearance of lesion hypoechogenicity and posterior acoustic shadowing. Unregulated

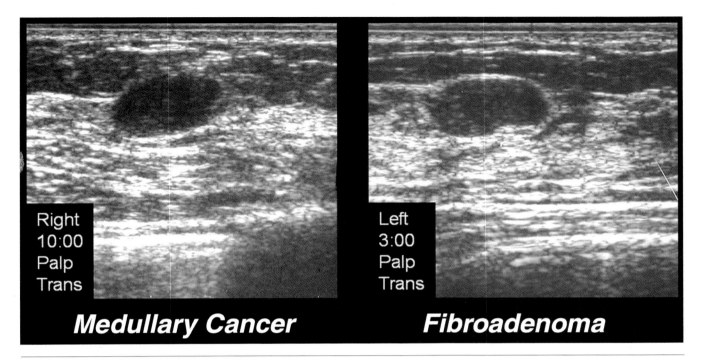

Medullary Cancer   **Fibroadenoma**

Figure 16B.5. Similar-appearing solid masses. This patient presented with bilateral the palpable masses visualized here. Both masses underwent ultrasound-guided biopsy. Biopsy of the breast mass on the left revealed a medullary carcinoma and the breast mass on the right was consistent histologically with a benign fibroadenoma. (Courtesy of Lawrence Bassett.)

tumor growth into the surrounding tissues results in an irregular shape with angular, microlobulated, or spiculated margins (Figure 16B.8). The multiple tiny interfaces between the invading tumor spicules and host tissues create multiple reflective echoes forming a thick echogenic halo around the mass. Desmoplastic reaction in the surrounding tissues may cause parenchymal distortion, fascial tenting, and/or skin changes such as thickening, tethering, or retraction. As these tumors arise from the TDLU one may see duct extension or a branching pattern. Invasive lobular cancer tends to infiltrate the breast widely in a single-file manner with minimal desmoplastic reaction. As a result, a discrete mass is often absent on ultrasound. Occasionally, nonspecific shadowing may be present in the area. Coupled with a palpable or mammographic asymmetry, this may be the only clue to the diagnosis. Although less common, invasive cancers can present as a circumscribed mass or masses. These

include medullary, mucinous, and papillary carcinomas; lymphomas; and metastatic deposits. Mucinous tumors are particularly problematic as they may be mistaken on cursory examination for benign cysts, given their predominant fluid (mucinous) content.

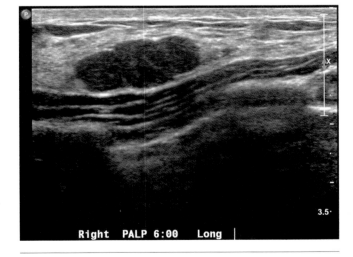

Right PALP 6:00 Long

Figure 16B.6. Lobulated fibroadenoma. This biopsy-proven fibroadenoma demonstrates smooth, gentle lobulations characteristic of this lesion. Note also that there is an abrupt transition with the parenchyma, commonly referred to as a *pseudocapsule*, and the long axis is parallel to the chest wall (the plan of least resistance).

Table 16B.1
Ultrasound Characteristics Suggestive of Benignity[a]
Hyperechoic
Three or fewer lobulations
Ellipsoid shape
Thin echogenic capsule

[a] Adapted from Stavros AT, ed. *Breast Ultrasound.* 1st ed. Philadelphia: Lippincott Williams & Wilkins; 2003.

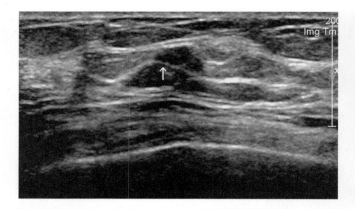

Figure 16B.7. Thin septation within a fibroadenoma. Thin linear septations (*arrow*) may be seen coursing through benign fibroadenomas. Although this would not be seen within malignant cancers, one may mistake this for a fat lobule.

Patients with lesions that are regarded as highly suspicious for malignancy should undergo additional ultrasonographic interrogation to include the surrounding ipsilateral breast and axilla. This is particularly important in women with dense breasts. Evaluation of adjacent tissues is recommended to assess for possible multifocal or multicentric disease, which may significantly impact surgical treatment (Figure 16B.9). If additional suspicious breast lesions or more extensive malignant breast disease is detected by ultrasonography, the extent of disease can be mapped out appropriately with ultrasound-guided localization or biopsies. If an abnormal axillary lymph node is detected, confirmation of malignant involvement by ultrasound-guided fine-needle aspiration (FNA) or core needle biopsy will allow the surgeon to proceed directly to axillary dissection rather than sentinel node biopsy. However, if sonography shows normal-appearing lymph nodes, or ultrasound-guided FNA or core needle biopsy is negative, the surgeon should not be deterred from a sentinel lymph node procedure that would have otherwise been performed (14).

Table 16B.2
Ultrasound Characteristics Suggestive of Malignancy[a]
Spiculated Capsule
Taller-than-wide
Angular margins
Posterior shadowing
Branch pattern
Markedly hypoechoic
Microcalcifications
Duct extension
Microlobulations

[a] Adapted from Stavros AT, ed. *Breast Ultrasound.* 1st ed. Philadelphia: Lippincott Williams & Wilkins; 2003.

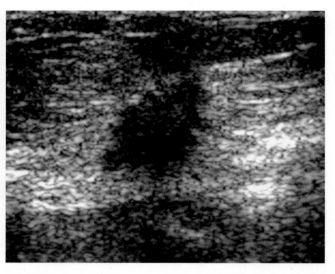

Figure 16B.8. Malignant tumor. Typical appearance for an invasive breast cancer. Notice the irregular shape and spiculated margin with the surrounding tissue. The mass is also growing perpendicular and not parallel to the chest wall.

BREAST INTERVENTION USING ULTRASOUND GUIDANCE

The Radiologist's Perspective

The cost, comfort, availability, and accuracy of breast ultrasound have brought this modality to the front lines in the management of breast disease. The widening applicability of ultrasound, from simple cyst aspirations, to percutaneous core biopsies, to guided placement of localizing wires, catheters, and treatment delivery

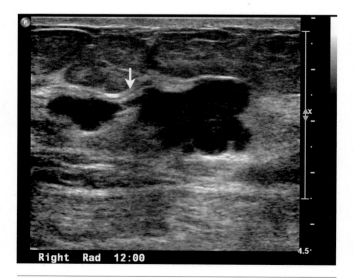

Figure 16B.9. Multifocal invasive breast cancer. The two adjacent masses appear to be connected by a small bridge of tumor (*arrow*); however, only the larger mass was palpable and mammographically apparent.

devices, has led Kaufman (15) to assert that "ultrasound may be the gateway to the future of breast care."

The following briefly describes some of the more common applications of ultrasound-guided intervention employed at the Harold E. and Henrietta C. Lee Breast Center at the USC/Norris Comprehensive Cancer Center.

Cyst Aspiration

Simple or incidental complicated cysts typically do not require intervention unless the patient wishes symptomatic relief or reassurance. A palpable complicated cyst, seroma, or possible abscess may initially undergo ultrasound-guided aspiration. When the fluid obtained is characteristic of a benign cyst (i.e., nonbloody), it can be discarded without further analysis. The cyst should be completely aspirated under direct ultrasound visualization. If there is evidence of an intracystic mass, further intervention is needed. Some perform a pneumocystogram (instillation of air) into the cyst following aspiration for mammographic correlation and potentially to decrease the incidence of cyst recurrence.

Fine-Needle Aspiration Cytology

In the appropriate hands, FNA biopsy is a safe and effective means of obtaining a rapid cytologic diagnosis in select clinical situations. Greater accuracy is achieved with both expert technique and interpretation by an experienced cytopathologist. This technique is most often used in the evaluation of suspect axillary or supraclavicular lymph nodes in patients with known primary breast cancer (Figure 16B.10). A diagnosis of axillary nodal metastasis makes sentinel lymph node biopsy unnecessary

and leads directly to the performance of a formal axillary dissection. In addition, an FNA diagnosis of metastasis may guide the medical and radiation oncologist to appropriate neoadjuvant or adjuvant therapy.

Ultrasound-guided FNA can also be used to evaluate a patient with isolated axillary adenopathy, to establish a diagnosis of benign disease (such as infection or reactive lymphadenopathy), lymphoma, or metastasis from an unknown primary.

With adequate sampling of a breast lesion, an FNA biopsy can establish the diagnosis of malignancy and provide information on hormone receptor status and *HER2/neu* expression. However, when compared with core needle biopsy, FNA is less reliable in establishing a specific benign diagnosis and can not accurately differentiate in situ malignancy from invasive disease.

Percutaneous Core Needle Biopsy

Percutaneous core needle biopsy is the procedure of choice for establishing the diagnosis of image-detected breast abnormalities. This method of tissue sampling is less invasive, less traumatic, less disfiguring, and less costly than open surgical biopsy. Furthermore, when applying sound principles, the overall accuracy and false-negative rates are comparable. A major goal of modern breast medicine is to minimize the number of patients with benign lesions who undergo open surgical breast biopsies for diagnosis (14). When a diagnosis of cancer has been made preoperatively, incisions can be planned, definitive surgery can be performed, and clear margins are more likely to be obtained. Core biopsies are performed under ultrasound guidance for most ultrasound-visible lesions. Surgical biopsy is indicated in cases of insufficient sampling of the lesion, discordant findings on imaging-histologic correlation, and when certain high-risk lesions are detected in the core biopsy material, such as atypical ductal or lobular hyperplasia, lobular carcinoma in situ, radial scar, and papillary lesions.

Instrumentation used to obtain minimally invasive core needle biopsies can be broadly divided into three categories: 14-gauge spring-loaded needles, 12- to 7-gauge vacuum-assisted or rotational devices, and a large core tissue-acquisition apparatus. The 14-gauge needle acquires approximately 20 mg of tissue per core while the 11-gauge vacuum-assisted breast biopsy (VABB) device obtains approximately 100 mg/core. The volume of the needle varies inversely with the gauge so that as the needle gauge decreases, the volume of tissue excised increases. A large-core tissue acquisitions apparatus, such as the *Intact Breast Lesion Excisio System* (Intact, Natick, MA), can obtain a single tissue specimen ranging in size from 0.8 g up to 3.0 g, using mammographic or ultrasound guidance. The rate of major complications does not significantly rise with the use of larger acquisition devices, but there is a slight increase in risk of bleeding, which is usually minor. Sufficient tissue is obtained with 14-gauge core needles in patients with large masses in which sampling errors are less of an issue. VABB is preferred over 14-gauge needles for most image-detected abnormalities warranting histologic confirmation (Figure 16B.11). Atypical ductal hyperplasia and ductal carcinoma in situ have been shown to have decreased upstaging at surgical excision with VABB versus 14-gauge core biopsy (16). Larger tissue acquisition methods may have a role in cases of atypical ductal hyperplasia, lobular carcinoma in situ, small papillary and intracystic lesions (lesions that may be totally

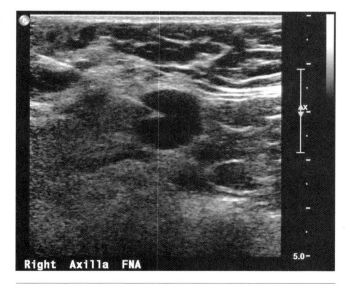

Figure 16B.10. Fine-needle aspiration (FNA) biopsy of abnormal axillary lymph node. This patient has a known ipsilateral invasive cancer and a normal clinical examination of the axilla. Ultrasound revealed an abnormal axillary lymph node (see Figure 16B.2). FNA biopsy confirmed metastatic disease, saving the patient an unnecessary sentinel lymph node procedure. Note the tip of the biopsy needle in the center of the lesion.

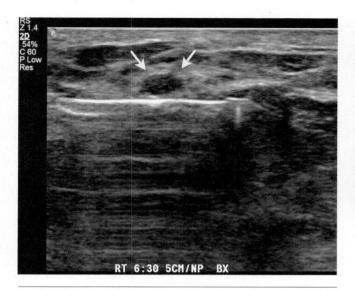

Figure 16B.11. Vacuum-assisted breast biopsy (VABB). Ultrasound guidance can be used to sample a palpable or nonpalpable image-detected lesion (*arrows*) with great accuracy, low cost, and low morbidity. VABB is preferred over spring-loaded devices for small lesions.

captured), and other high-risk proliferative lesions as it better maintains the three-dimensional architecture and provides the pathologist with a larger intact piece of tissue for evaluation.

A biopsy clip compatible with the biopsy method chosen should be deployed at the conclusion of these procedures. The biopsy clip serves several important functions. It confirms that the lesion of interest has, in fact, been sampled; it marks the site of a lesion that may have been entirely removed at the time of biopsy; it targets an abnormality seen on only one imaging modality; or it can be used to target a known cancer prior to neoadjuvant chemotherapy. Clips are generally made of stainless steel or titanium, may contain gel foam, bovine, or porcine collagen for hemostasis, and come in various shapes. Deploying different shape clips is helpful in distinguishing lesions when more than one abnormality in the same breast is being biopsied.

Wire Localization

Ultrasound-visible lesions are often best localized using ultrasound guidance, the exception being the presence of associated suspicious microcalcifications visible only on mammography. The procedure under ultrasound guidance is often faster than under mammographic guidance, and is easier for patients to more fully cooperate as it is a more comfortable approach. Furthermore, with ultrasound the patient, the breast, and the lesion more closely simulate the positions they will assume on the operating room table. This results in more flexibility in orientation of the wires to accommodate the individual surgical approach. Finally, there is the added advantage of real-time visualization of needle placement and wire deployment in relation to the target lesion, skin, chest wall, and implant, if present (Figure 16B.12). Postprocedural mammograms are always obtained to facilitate orientation of the wires in relation to the lesion for the operating surgeon. Specimen ultrasound may be easily performed for

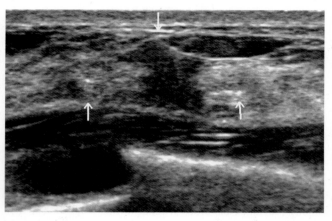

Figure 16B.12. Ultrasound-guided wire localization. This biopsy-proven invasive cancer (*upper arrow*) was better visualized and localized on ultrasound. Two wires are placed on either side of the mass under real-time visualization to bracket the tumor. The wires are seen in cross-section as two tiny white dots (*lower arrows*).

lesions visible only by ultrasound to confirm lesion capture and margin assessment.

Complications from Image-Guided Procedures

Serious complications requiring immediate treatment or intervention are exceedingly rare. Minor complications occur occasionally and include vasovagal reactions, infection, hematoma, clip malfunction or displacement, and inadequate sampling. Additional reported complications include implant rupture, uncontrolled bleeding, skin necrosis, pneumothorax, pseudoaneurysm, milk fistula, and Mandor's disease. Patients receiving anticoagulation therapy are at some increase risk of developing a hematoma or ecchymosis following needle biopsy. Ideally, the coagulation status should be returned to normal, and substances that impair coagulation such as aspirin, nonsteroidal anti-inflammatory agents, fish oil supplements, and some Chinese herbal medicines, should be stopped approximately a week before the biopsy. When this is unsafe to do, biopsy may proceed with the patient's understanding of the possibility of some, usually minor, bleeding.

Postbiopsy Care and Instructions

Following core biopsies, direct continuous compression is applied over the biopsy site (not the skin entry site) until hemostasis is obtained. At our institution, we place a circumferential elastic dressing for continuous added pressure for 24 to 48 hours. Patients are advised to refrain from strenuous activity, bathing or soaking the biopsy site, or resuming anticoagulants, aspirin, and related medications (if safe) for several days.

Clinical-Radiologic-Pathologic Correlation

Establishing clinical-radiologic-pathologic concordance ("the triple test") is mandatory to minimize false-negative FNA and core biopsy results. Thus, highly suspicious lesions on physical examination or imaging that yield a core biopsy finding of non-specific benign changes or normal breast tissue require further tissue sampling or excision.

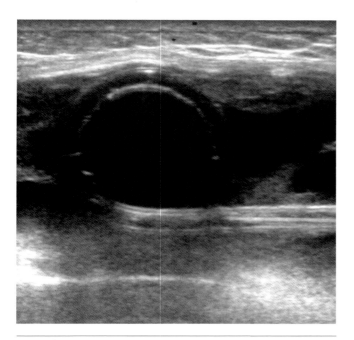

Figure 16B.13. Seroma drainage. A pigtail drainage catheter was safely placed under ultrasound guidance into an enlarging postoperative seroma.

Additional Ultrasound-Guided Procedures

Ultrasound guidance can be used for aspiration and catheter placement in the management of seromas and abscesses (Figure 16B.13). Ultrasound guidance has also been employed for the postoperative placement of a Mammosite brachytherapy balloon catheter (Hologic, Inc., Marlborough, MA) or similar apparatus within the segmental mastectomy (lumpectomy) cavity for delivery of accelerated partial breast irradiation (Figure 16B.14). Ultrasound is currently being used in image-guided percutaneous cryoablation of histologically proven benign breast lesions, most commonly small palpable and nonpalpable fibroadenomas (17,18).

OFFICE-BASED AND PERIOPERATIVE USES OF BREAST ULTRASOUND

The Surgeon's Perspective

Evaluation of the Palpable Breast Mass

The patient with a palpable mass is a common clinical presentation in surgical office practice. Ultrasound is the imaging modality of choice for patients younger than 30 years of age or if the patient has had a negative mammogram in the prior 6 months. In general, young patients should not have mammography as the initial examination. Complicated cysts and symptomatic simple cysts may be aspirated in the office with ultrasound guidance. Solid lesions may be confirmed histologically. A dilemma arises when the ultrasonographic examination is negative in the setting of a physical finding. Here, the surgeon must decide if a needle biopsy is warranted, if expectant management or serial examination should be employed, or if the patient should be sent for evaluation by a radiologist. As a rule, surgeons should maintain

a low threshold for seeking radiologic consultation under these circumstances.

Management of the Inflamed Breast

Ultrasound plays an essential role in the management of the inflamed breast, permitting distinction between mastitis (edema and no mass), inflammatory breast cancer (edema and a solid mass), and a breast abscess (minimal or localized edema and a fluid-containing mass). For the patients with a solid mass, ultrasound-guided core biopsy may be used to establish a diagnosis of malignancy. For the patient with a suspected breast abscess, ultrasound-guided aspiration may be employed diagnostically to confirm the clinical impression and provide fluid for microbiological studies. Complete aspiration of breast abscesses under ultrasound guidance is now used therapeutically as the preferred method for initial management of small (<3 cm) breast abscesses (19,20). For larger or recurrent breast abscesses, placement of a large-gauge drainage catheter under ultrasound guidance (in conjunction with antibiotic therapy) allows ongoing drainage, thus obviating the need for open surgical drainage in many instances.

Management of Postoperative Seromas

Although palpation-guided aspiration has been standard practice in the management of seromas following mastectomy, lumpectomy, or axillary dissection, surgeons with ultrasound experience recognize the advantages of ultrasound-guided seroma aspiration to ensure safe and complete evacuation. Ultrasound may also be used to guide optimal placement of a seroma drainage catheter if needed for recurrent collections. In addition, ultrasound of the surgical site enables distinction between seroma, hematoma, and edema, which aids the surgeon in wound management.

Placement of Brachytherapy Catheters

For patients undergoing brachytherapy using a balloon catheter system, ultrasound is very useful in localizing the postlumpectomy cavity, in evaluating the bridge of tissue between the skin surface and the surgical cavity, in guiding placement of the brachytherapy balloon catheter, and in assessing balloon catheter symmetry (21).

Percutaneous Excision of Fibroadenomas

Fibroadenomas with classic features may be monitored with serial ultrasound examinations to confirm stability. Alternatively, ultrasound may be used to perform ultrasound-guided core needle biopsy to confirm the clinical impression. For the patient desiring fibroadenoma removal, a larger-gauge vacuum-assisted core biopsy device may be used to achieve piecemeal, minimally invasive, percutaneous excision of the lesion (22). Although this procedure may not eliminate every fragment of the fibroadenoma, wholesale debulking of the fibroadenoma will confirm the diagnosis and accomplish removal of a symptomatic or anxiety-provoking palpable mass. Additionally, surgeons and radiologists are now exploring the use of vacuum-assisted core biopsy as an alternative to open surgical excisional biopsy of other benign breast masses (e.g., papillomas and atypical

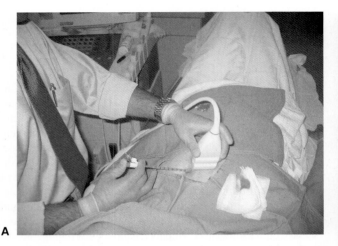

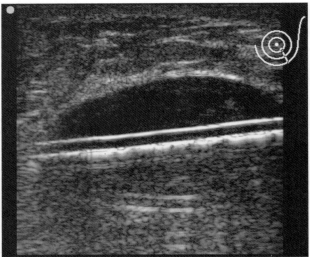

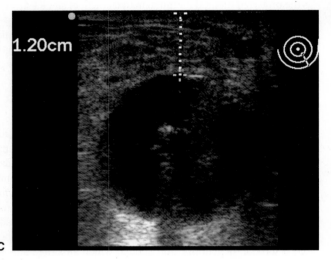

Figure 16B.14. Mammosite brachytherapy balloon catheter placement. Ultrasound is ideally suited for identification and evaluation of the lumpectomy cavity for Mammosite-accelerated partial breast irradiation therapy. Ultrasound can be used for percutaneous placement (**A**) and evaluation of the balloon catheter with longitudinal (**B**) and transverse (**C**) images.

lesions). Initial results are promising in selected cases, but there is presently insufficient data to support replacement of open surgical biopsy with vacuum-assisted core biopsy for the management of these conditions.

Cryoablation of Fibroadenomas

Percutaneous cryoablation is a minimally invasive technique that achieves tissue necrosis by alternately freezing and thawing tissues (23). The cryoablation procedure uses ultrasound to guide positioning of the cryoprobe and to allow real-time assessment of the cryoablation process. Ultrasound may also be used following treatment to monitor resorption of the cryoablated fibroadenoma (24). The American Society of Breast Surgeons has endorsed cryoablation as a safe and effective management option for fibroadenomas measuring ≤3 cm in diameter (25).

Staging and Treatment Planning

In patients with breast cancer, preoperative staging and treatment planning may be expedited by the use of axillary ultrasound. Manual examination of the axilla is notoriously unreliable in assessing the presence and nature of adenopathy. However, ultrasound is a highly accurate technique for evaluating

lymph nodes, both in patients with or without clinically apparent adenopathy. Ultrasound-guided, preoperative biopsy of abnormal-appearing axillary nodes may obviate the need for sentinel node analysis prior to full axillary lymphadenectomy, as previously discussed.

Intraoperative Uses of Breast Ultrasound

For palpable, ultrasound-visible masses treated with open surgical excision, intraoperative ultrasound (IOUS) is a helpful adjunct, especially when open excision is performed under local anesthesia. Indeed, most surgeons have experienced a few moments of anxiety when an obviously palpable breast mass became significantly more difficult to palpate after injection of the local anesthetic. Ultrasound used intraoperatively will ensure easy identification of an ultrasound-visible mass and facilitate efficient localization and excision (26).

Intraoperative localization of nonpalpable, ultrasound-visible masses can significantly improve the accuracy and efficiency of wide local excision whether or not localizing wires are used (27). IOUS enables a more direct approach to the breast mass as the lesion is localized within the breast in the surgical position. This aids placement of the incision and minimizes excessive dissection that sometimes results from suboptimal placement of localizing wires. In addition, intraoperative localization using ultrasound allows for convenient surgical scheduling without dependence on radiologists for placement of localizing wires, which can be inserted, if necessary, by the surgeon in the operating room rather than in the radiology suite. Intraoperative localization also eliminates the need for mammography following wire placement performed in the radiology suite (28).

IOUS permits in vivo assessment and planning of surgical margins to confirm adequate distance from the edge of the tumor prior to incising breast parenchyma. Following resection, ultrasound of the surgical specimen verifies excision of the breast cancer as well as reconfirms the width of the surgical margins (29). If a wider margin in needed, resection of additional tissue can be performed prior to wound closure. Additionally, in the setting of dense breasts, tumor desmoplasia, or postbiopsy induration when discrete tumor margins may not be readily palpated, IOUS permits accurate determination of lesion location and dimensions, potentially minimizing resection of excessive tissue in an effort to obtain clear margins. For patients requiring tumor re-excision for positive margins of resection, ultrasound evaluation of the postlumpectomy seroma facilitates re-excision without disruption of the lumpectomy cavity and spillage of seroma contents, especially because the location of the skin incision does not always correspond exactly with the location of the lumpectomy cavity.

CONCLUSION

The ability to perform and interpret ultrasound is an increasingly important skill for surgeons involved in the management of breast disease. In addition to its central role in the diagnostic evaluation of benign and malignant breast conditions, ultrasonography forms the foundation of a growing number of interventional procedures involved in the preoperative, intraoperative, and postoperative care of patients. The availability of small, affordable, portable ultrasound units has made ultrasound ownership a practical venture for many surgeons and has allowed ultrasound to move beyond the radiology department to find usage in physician offices, outpatient facilities, and in the operating room.

REFERENCES

1. ACR Practice Guideline for the Performance of a Breast Ultrasound Examination. Revised October 1, 2007. http://www.acr.org. Accessed May 13, 2009.
2. Kolb TM, Lichy J, Newhouse JH. Comparison of the performance of screening mammography, physical examination, and breast US and evaluation of factors that influence them: an analysis of 27,825 patient evaluations. *Radiology.* 2002;225:165–175.
3. Berg WA. Supplemental screening sonography in dense breasts. *Radiol Clin North Am.* 2004;42:845–851.
4. Berg WA, Blume JD, Cormack JB, et al. Combined screening with ultrasound and mammography vs. mammography alone in women at elevated risk of breast cancer. *JAMA.* 2008;299:2151–2163.
5. Kuhl CK. The "coming of age" of nonmammographic screening for breast cancer. *JAMA.* 2008;299:2203–2205.
6. Stavros AT, ed. *Breast Ultrasound.* 1st ed. Philadelphia: Lippincott Williams & Wilkins; 2003.
7. Love SM, Barsky SH. Anatomy of the nipple and breast ducts revisited. *Cancer.* 2004;101:1947–1957.
8. American College of Radiology (ACR). ACR BI-RADS—Ultrasound. *ACR Breast Imaging Reporting and Data System, Breast Imaging Atlas.* Reston, VA: American College of Radiology; 2003.
9. Bassett L, ed. *Diagnosis of Diseases of the Breast.* 2nd ed. Philadelphia: Saunders; 2004.
10. Hashimoto DB. *Breast Imaging: A Correlative Atlas.* New York: Thieme; 2003.
11. Berg WA, Campassi CI, Ioffe OB. Cystic lesions of the breast: sonographic-pathologic correlation. *Radiology.* 2003;227:183–191.
12. Donegan WL. Evaluation of a palpable breast mass. *N Engl J Med.* 1992;327:937–942.
13. Stavros AT, Thickman D, Rapp CL, et al. Solid breast nodules: use of sonography to distinguish between benign and malignant lesions. *Radiology.* 1995;196:123–134.
14. Silverstein MJ, Lagios MD, Recht A, et al. Image-detected breast cancer: state of the art diagnosis and treatment. *J Am Coll Surg.* 2005;201:586–597.
15. Kaufman CS. Breast ultrasound: current use, future vision. *General Surgery News.* 2004:15–19.
16. Jackman RJ. Stereotactic vacuum-assisted breast biopsy in 2874 patients: a multicenter study. *Cancer.* 2004;101:430–431.
17. Kaufman CS, Littrup PJ, Freman-Gibb LA, et al. Office-based cryoablation of breast fibroadenomas: 12-month followup. *J Am Coll Surg.* 2004;198:914–923.
18. Littrup PJ, Freeman-Gibb L, Andea A, et al. Cryotherapy for breast fibroadenomas. *Radiology.* 2005;234:63–72.
19. Berna-Serna JD, Madrigal M, Berna-Serna JD. Percutaneous management of breast abscesses. An experience of 39 cases. *Ultrasound Med Biol.* 2004;30:1–6.
20. Christensen AF, Al-Suliman N, Nielsen KR, et al. Ultrasound-guided drainage of breast abscesses: results in 151 patients. *Br J Radiol.* 2005;78:186–188.
21. Zannis VJ, Walker LC, Barclay-White B, et al. Postoperative ultrasound-guided percutaneous placement of a new breast brachytherapy balloon catheter. *Am J Surg.* 2003;186:383–385.
22. Sperber F, Blank A, Metser U, et al. Diagnosis and treatment of breast fibroadenomas by ultrasound-guided vacuum-assisted biopsy. *Arch Surg.* 2003;138:796–800.
23. Kaufman CS, Bachman B, Littrup PJ, et al. Office-based ultrasound-guided cryoablation of breast fibroadenomas. *Am J Surg.* 2002;184:394–400.
24. Kaufman CS, Bachman B, Littrup PJ, et al. Cryoablation treatment of benign breast lesions with 12-month follow-up. *Am J Surg.* 2004;188:340–348.
25. American Society of Breast Surgeons. Position Statement on Ablative and Percutaneous Treatment of Breast Cancer. 2002. www.breastsurgeons.org. Accessed May 13, 2009.
26. Buman SJ, Clark DA. Breast intraoperative ultrasound: prospective study in 112 patients with impalpable lesions. *ANZ J Surg.* 2005;75:124–127.
27. Kolpattil S, Crotch-Harvey M. Improved accuracy of wire-guided breast surgery with supplementary ultrasound. *Eur J Radiol.* 2006;60:414–417.
28. Kaufman CS. Intraoperative ultrasonography guidance is accurate and efficient according to results in 100 breast cancer patients. *Am J Surg.* 2003;186:378–382.

29. Mesurolle B, El-Khoury M, Hori D, et al. Sonography of postexcision specimens of nonpalpable breast lesions: value, limitations, and description of a method. *AJR Am J Roentgenol.* 2006;186:1014–1024.

COMMENTARY
Mark A. Gittleman

Drs. Sheth, Larsen, Parisky, and Holmes have written an excellent chapter on the performance and clinical applications of breast ultrasound, a procedure of critical importance to the surgeon caring for patients undergoing evaluation of the breast.

PRACTICE GUIDELINES

In addition to the American College of Radiology and the American Institute of Ultrasound in Medicine, the American Society of Breast Surgeons (ASBS) has developed practice guidelines for the performance of breast ultrasound, available on its Web site, www.breastsurgeons.org. The ASBS lists the following indications for breast ultrasound:

- Identification and characterization of palpable abnormalities noted on clinical breast examination
- Identification and characterization of localized breast symptoms, such as breast pain, fullness, and nipple discharge
- Identification and characterization of nonpalpable abnormalities detected on other breast-imaging modalities
- Guidance for invasive procedures
- Evaluation and assessment of the breast after surgical or medical therapy
- Preoperative evaluation of the breast and axilla in patients with a confirmed malignant lesion

The authors have reviewed the findings of the American College of Radiology Imaging Network (ACRIN) 6666 trial indicating the increased diagnostic yield associated with the addition of whole-breast ultrasonography to routine screening mammography in women at increased risk for breast cancer (1). In current practice, breast ultrasound most commonly is employed as a focused examination directed toward an area of the breast of clinical interest. Such "diagnostic" ultrasound examinations are indicated for patients with a specific complaint of pain or mass in a specific area of the breast, those with palpable findings, such as increased tissue density or a mass in a particular area of the breast, or those who have mammographic findings suggesting asymmetry, densities, or masses.

TRAINING AND CERTIFICATION IN BREAST ULTRASOUND

Many practicing surgeons have not had formal training in ultrasound (or specifically breast ultrasound) during residency training. Although the Residency Review Committee for General Surgery has mandated that training in ultrasound should be an integral part of surgical residency programs, there has been inconsistent compliance with this requirement. Additionally, in the more than 30 currently existing breast surgical fellowship programs, training and experience in the practical application of breast ultrasound likewise has been less than adequate. Most fellowship-trained breast surgeons have had only an observational experience with breast ultrasound. Many surgeons, both those in practice and those recently trained, have found it necessary to obtain additional training in breast ultrasound. In addition to the educational programs as mentioned by the authors sponsored by the American College of Surgeons and the American College of Radiology, the ASBS offers educational programs in basic and advanced breast ultrasound for the practicing surgeon.

In 2000, the ASBS developed a *Breast Ultrasound Certification Program* for surgeons. The following minimum prerequisites for surgeons who may choose to undertake breast ultrasound certification are:

- Current certification by the American Board of Surgery or American Osteopathic Board of Surgery
- Documentation of an appropriate level of training and a minimum of 1 year of experience in the performance and interpretation of breast ultrasound
- Documented performance of no fewer than 100 breast ultrasound examinations per year with review of a minimum of 100 mammography examinations annually that include the authenticated reports. These must include a minimum of 80 diagnostic and 20 interventional examinations.
- Documented completion of 15 AMA Category 1 containing medical education credits in breast ultrasound toward the AMA Physician's Recognition Award. At least 7 credits in breast ultrasound in the 12 months prior to application must be included.

The purpose of the ASBS Breast Ultrasound Certification Program is to demonstrate competency in the performance and interpretation of breast ultrasound examinations by surgeons. Certification in breast ultrasound is becoming increasingly more important for surgeons in order to demonstrate to third-party payers, to referring physicians, and to patients not only the value of having the breast ultrasound examination performed as part of the clinical breast evaluation by the practicing surgeon, but that it is being performed in a competent manner.

ARE SURGEONS CURRENTLY PERFORMING BREAST ULTRASOUND?

At the 2007 annual ASBS meeting, a poll was taken asking the question whether breast ultrasound examinations were performed in the individual surgeons' practices; 364 or 78% responded yes and 104 or 22% responded no. Interestingly, 144 surgeons in the audience said they planned to apply for certification.

PERFORMANCE OF BREAST ULTRASOUND BY THE SURGEON

It is critically important for the surgeon breast ultrasonographer to perform the examination in real time as opposed to relying on the review of images acquired by a technologist. Optimal correlation of the physical findings and mammographic findings is accomplished in this manner. Additionally, providing immediate feedback to the patient allays the anxiety of waiting for a report of the results at a later date in the case of a normal or benign finding and expedites management in the case of an abnormal finding.

The recognition and identification of normal ultrasound anatomy is easily learned by the surgeon as a result of experience with clinical breast evaluation and knowledge of the three-dimensional anatomy acquired from experience in the operating room in the performance of various breast surgical procedures. Therefore, it is relatively easy for the surgeon to apply the known surgical anatomy of the breast to the two-dimensional image created on the ultrasound monitor. Likewise, using the standard sonographic lexicon, as described by the authors, surgeons can form an immediate impression of an ultrasound-detected lesion, when combining this information with the physical and mammographic findings.

INTERVENTION

Generally, an abnormal finding is an indication for some type of intervention, except in the case of an asymptomatic patient whose focal abnormality within the breast represents a simple cyst, or in the case of a solid mass of long standing and known to be stable over a series of prior imaging studies. Complicated cysts can be aspirated to determine their benign nature, assuming the cyst completely disappears following aspiration and that nonbloody fluid is obtained. Should no fluid be obtained on attempted aspiration, the lesion represents a solid mass and therefore biopsy is recommended. Complex masses and other solid masses should undergo ultrasound-guided needle biopsy for diagnosis.

INDICATIONS FOR INTERVENTIONAL PROCEDURES

The ASBS currently lists the following indications for office-based interventional procedures:

- Cyst aspiration
- Fine-needle aspiration cytology
- Core needle biopsy with various devices
- Placement of marking clips or guide wires
- Placement of brachytherapy devices
- Targeted breast tissue ablation
- Other similar procedures

Prior to the acquisition of ultrasound skills by surgeons, palpable masses were subjected to core needle biopsy or fine-needle aspiration without ultrasound guidance. This is to be discouraged as the actual position of the interventional device within the abnormality can be more certainly documented with ultrasound guidance. This will lead to less concern about possible discordance between the expected results based on imaging and the cytology or histology of the specimen. Therefore, ultrasound guidance is recommended for the placement of interventional devices for both palpable and nonpalpable breast abnormalities.

As mentioned by the authors, when a lesion in the breast is of concern for malignancy, the ipsilateral axilla should likewise be scanned to determine whether there is any ultrasonic evidence of involvement of the axillary lymph nodes. If abnormal axillary lymph nodes are noted, fine-needle aspiration or core biopsy of the lymph nodes can be performed at the same time as the interventional biopsy of the breast mass. This will obviously aid in treatment planning concerning the necessity for sentinel node biopsy and the need for axillary dissection without prior sentinel node biopsy.

When performing intervention for a solid breast mass, fine-needle aspiration or core biopsy can determine whether or not a malignancy is present. However, core biopsy is preferred as it is extremely difficult, if not impossible, to determine the difference between an in situ and an invasive lesion with fine-needle aspiration. Additionally, there is often not enough material to determine ER/PR (estrogen/progestin receptor) status and *HER2/neu* expression on fine-needle aspiration specimens compared with core needle biopsy specimens.

The authors correctly emphasize that percutaneous core needle biopsy is the procedure of choice for establishing a diagnosis of image-detected and palpable breast abnormalities. Open surgical biopsy, however, is indicated for a patient who desires complete removal of an abnormality highly likely to be benign, such as in a young woman with a palpable, benign-appearing lesion consistent with a fibroadenoma, who wishes complete excision rather than core sampling.

The authors describe various biopsy devices available for interventional procedures under ultrasound guidance and state the various reasons for preference of vacuum-assisted breast biopsy instruments over 14-gauge needles for most abnormalities. Likewise, the recommendation for placing the marking clip or image-detected abnormality at the biopsy site is appropriately emphasized. Even for large lesions subjected to biopsy, which could otherwise be easily detected after biopsy without a marking clip present, the marking clip is extremely helpful should the patient undergo neoadjuvant chemotherapy, and a complete clinical response is noted making the location of the previously detected abnormality now more difficult to identify.

When comparing stereotactic image-guided biopsy with ultrasound-guided biopsy, a stereotactic biopsy is the modality of choice for suspicious or indeterminate microcalcifications without an associated mass noted on mammogram. Additionally, stereotactic biopsy is indicated for the nonpalpable, image-detected mass, which has no ultrasonographic correlate. However, should a solid breast mass be noted both on mammogram and ultrasound, ultrasound-guided biopsy is preferred for the reasons noted by the authors.

In the operating room, ultrasound is indicated for planning the surgical excision of an area of concern with or without the placement of a hook wire needle localization device; assessment of the adequacy of surgical excision of both palpable and nonpalpable lesions following their removal; and to facilitate other procedures, for example, ultrasound guidance for ablative procedures.

DOCUMENTATION REQUIREMENT

All ultrasound examinations, including both diagnostic and ultrasound guidance procedures, require recorded images to be stored in the hard copy or electronic format. In addition, a written interpretation of all ultrasound studies should be kept in the patient's record, either as a separate stand-alone document or incorporated into the clinical progress notes.

INTEGRATION OF BREAST ULTRASOUND INTO THE SURGICAL PRACTICE: HOW TO GET STARTED

Certain practical and logistical concerns must be addressed by the surgeon ultrasonographer when incorporating breast ultrasound into office practice. Other than the training aspects previously covered, the surgeon must select the appropriate ultrasound equipment for its intended use. If the surgeon will be performing only breast ultrasound, a relatively basic system with a single transducer is sufficient. The appropriate transducer for breast evaluation is commonly referred to as a *small parts transducer* consisting of an electronically focused linear array of elements with a frequency of 7.5 MHz or greater. Most present-day transducers for breast ultrasound provide a range of frequencies from 7.5 to 12 or 13 MHz. Colon Doppler is not necessary for breast imaging; however, should the surgeon also wish to use the ultrasound equipment for vascular imaging, color Doppler is necessary. The price range for the equipment adequate for breast ultrasound in the surgeon's office ranges from $25,000 to $50,000.

The surgeon ultrasonographer must also decide where the examinations are to be performed. If the ultrasound procedures are to be performed in a fixed location in a single examination room in the surgeon's office, then a cart-based system is a good consideration. However, should there be a need for portability bringing the ultrasound machine into various examinations rooms in the office and/or for transporting the ultrasound machine to various hospital operating rooms or ambulatory surgical centers, then consideration should be given to a portable system, many of which are currently available.

The examination room in the surgeon's office might need to be modified to accommodate the ultrasound equipment and various ancillary equipment. In addition to the examination table, the room should have an x-ray view box, a work light, a Mayo-type stand to place equipment for interventional procedures, an ultrasound gel warmer, and storage cabinets for supplies (such as all the various equipment needed for interventional procedures, including core needle biopsy devices and sterile supplies). A waste basket and a disposal container for sharps are also necessary. Documentation devices such as a thermal printer and a plan for storage of the documented procedures need to be provided. Informed consent forms and a written description of the operative procedures should be developed and available for use.

When beginning the process of performing breast ultrasound examinations, it is best to perform the procedure on patients who have recently had a breast ultrasound evaluation and whose images are available. The surgeon ultrasonographer can compare the results obtained during the procedure with those already obtained at the outside imaging facility. Following a reasonable number of evaluations done in this manner, typically 10 to 15, the surgeon should then perform breast diagnostic ultrasound in patients who have not yet had this evaluation. The patient may or may not be sent for an outside ultrasound following that procedure to compare evaluations. In this manner, confidence in the performance of the procedure will be attained and the surgeon ultrasonographer will feel increasingly more comfortable performing the evaluations for his or her patients.

Prior to performing any interventional breast ultrasound procedures, practicing with a phantom model should be performed to gain the necessary skills in developing the hand/eye coordination necessary for these procedures.

Initially, interventional procedures should be performed for palpable cysts with ultrasound guidance. When these have been performed successfully, ultrasound biopsy of larger lesions should be the next step. After acquiring these skills, then smaller nonpalpable lesions (<1 cm) can be biopsied. The surgeon will need to determine which interventional devices to use and choose among the vast array of breast biopsy devices that are currently available. Whenever a biopsy is performed, the placement of a marker at the biopsy site should be done.

Periodic reviews of the cases performed, the results obtained, and resolution of any discrepancy due to nonconformance must be done.

The skills necessary to perform breast ultrasound procedures are not difficult to acquire and should be attainable by most practicing clinical surgeons.

SUMMARY

Ultrasound has become an essential component of breast evaluation in the office practice of surgery. Incorporating breast ultrasound into clinical practice leads to a more complete evaluation of the patient's breast complaints, a more secure diagnostic impression, and allows for breast interventional procedures when indicated. All surgeons involved in the care of breast patients can and should incorporate breast ultrasound into their practices.

REFERENCE

1. Berg WA, Blume JD, Cormack JB, et al. Combined screening with ultrasound and mammography vs mammography alone in women at elevated risk of breast cancer. *JAMA.* 2008;299:2151–2163.

SUGGESTED READINGS

Harness JK, Wisher DB. *Ultrasound in Surgical Practice: Basic Principles and Clinical Applications.* New York: John Wiley & Sons; 2001.

Staren ED. *Ultrasound for the Surgeon.* Philadelphia: Lippincott-Raven; 1997.

Whitworth P, Mabry CD. *Ultrasound in Surgical Practice.* Vol. 1. Bothell, WA: SonoSite; 2004.

Chapter 16C
The Role of Magnetic Resonance Imaging in the Assessment and Diagnosis of Breast Cancer

Constance D. Lehman, Wendy DeMartini, and Nola Hylton

In this chapter we share our evidence-based recommendations for the appropriate use of magnetic resonance imaging (MRI) of the breast in surgical oncology practice. We review the history of breast MRI, compare mammography and MRI in the detection and evaluation of breast cancer, and describe the appropriate patient populations who may benefit from breast MRI. We conclude with a review of the key components of a high-quality breast MRI program.

Over the past 2 decades, results from a substantial number of clinical trials have been published on the performance of breast MRI in select patient populations. These studies provide useful information to guide informed decision making and clarify the potential benefits and the potential harms of incorporating breast MRI into a surgical oncology practice. By reviewing these studies, it is our hope to clarify how MRI can best be used in the treatment of women with a current breast cancer and in those at high risk for breast cancer.

HISTORY OF BREAST MRI

Since the 1980s, MRI has been widely accepted as the preferred imaging tool for multiple clinical indications in orthopaedic surgery and neurosurgery. However, its application to breast imaging has been slower to develop. Although some of the very first images of the body produced with MRI were of the breast (1), it took many years for investigators to clarify that contrast agents such as gadolinium were required to distinguish benign from malignant tissue in the breast. Over 2 decades of subsequent investigation further clarified techniques for obtaining consistent, accurate, and high-quality diagnostic breast MR images.

Since 2000, there has been general agreement that both high temporal and high spatial resolution are important to obtain information about both the pharmacokinetics and the morphology of breast lesions, and the technology to provide both high spatial and high temporal resolution is now widely commercially available.

Unlike mammography, MRI does not use ionizing radiation to create images of the breast. Although mammography relies on differences in x-ray attenuation values of malignant and benign breast tissue to detect cancers, MRI capitalizes instead on differences in microvessel density and permeability of malignant versus benign breast tissue. Another distinction in these two imaging techniques is that mammography results in two-dimensional images while MRI provides data in three dimensions. Although

mammography performance in the United States is regulated through the Mammography Quality Standards Act (2), there is currently no comparable oversight of performance of breast MRI.

Advantages of mammography include its relatively short examination time, low cost, and wide availability. Although the diagnostic accuracy of mammography varies based on technique used (film screen vs. digital), skill of the interpreting radiologist, and density of the breast tissue, overall, mammography is the sole imaging tool that has been proven to reduce breast cancer mortality when used for screening (3–5). Mammography has also been shown to improve surgical outcomes when used as a diagnostic tool in patients prior to breast cancer surgery (6). Disadvantages are its weaker performance in women with dense breast tissue, premenopausal women, and women receiving hormone replacement.

Breast MRI has several advantages, including its very high sensitivity and ability to detect cancers that are occult to mammography and ultrasound. Disadvantages include its relatively higher cost, longer scan time (approximately 30 minutes for most protocols), and lower availability. Two additional significant current challenges of breast MRI are lack of detailed standards to guide the performance of high-quality breast MRI and a paucity of clinical trials designed to measure the impact of breast MRI on long-term outcomes.

CLINICAL APPLICATIONS FOR BREAST MRI

Based on results from a large body of clinical research, the two patient populations most likely to benefit from breast MRI are (a) women with a recent diagnosis of breast cancer (who undergo diagnostic MRI in conjunction with clinical evaluation, diagnostic mammography, and ultrasound when indicated), and (b) women at high risk for breast cancer (who undergo screening MRI in conjunction with clinical evaluation and screening mammography).

Presurgical Evaluation

For the patient recently diagnosed with breast cancer, the most pressing decision is often how best to surgically manage the index breast cancer. The choice between breast conservation and mastectomy relies heavily on the extent of disease within the breast. It is logical that determining the true extent of disease within the breast prior to surgical planning is important to the surgeon and patient. What is the true size of the cancer? Does it involve one or more quadrants? Is it purely in situ carcinoma or is there also invasive disease? Numerous clinical trials demonstrate that MRI more accurately defines the true extent and type of disease in the breast than mammography alone or the combination of mammography and ultrasound.

Extent of Disease in the Ipsilateral Breast

Harms et al. (7) were the first authors to publish results on the sensitivity of MRI when used in the preoperative evaluation of patients with breast cancer. They studied 30 women undergoing mastectomy for lesions suspicious for malignancy based on

Table 16C.1

Frequency of Magnetic Resonance Imaging (MRI)-Detected Unsuspected Malignancy in the Ipsilateral Breast in Patients with a Recent Diagnosis of Breast Cancer

First Author, Year (Ref.)	No. of Malignant Cases	No. (%) with Additional Unsuspected Ipsilateral MRI Malignancy	No. (%) Multifocal	No. (%) Multicentric
Harms, 1993 (7)	29 breasts	10 (34)	3 (10)	7 (24)
Orel, 1995 (12)	64 women	13 (20)	NA	NA
Mumtaz, 1997 (11)	92 breasts	11 (12)	1 (1)	10 (11)
Fischer, 1999 (9)	336 women	54 (16)	30 (9)	24 (7)
Bedrosian, 2003 (8)	267 women	49 (18)	NA	NA
Liberman, 2003 (10)	70 women	19 (27)	14 (20)	5 (7)
Schelfout, 2004 (13)	170 women	33 (19)	12 (7)	17 (10)
Schnall (IBMC), 2005 (14)	423 women	41 (10)	NA	NA
Total	1,451	230 (16)	60 (9[a])	63 (9[a])

NA, not available; IBMC, International Breast Magnetic Resonance Consortium.

[a] Percent of 697 cases from the studies reporting multifocality and multicentricity.

clinical findings or conventional imaging. Preoperative breast MRI was performed in all patients and the images were compared with the serially sectioned mastectomy specimens. MRI detected additional unsuspected malignancy in 34% of women with breast cancer. Since that publication, numerous single- and multicenter trials have been performed investigating the utility of MRI for determining the extent of disease in the ipsilateral breast (Table 16C.1) (7–14).

The rationale for determining whether breast MRI could identify otherwise unsuspected malignancy was based on the recognized limitations of existing clinical and imaging tools in assessing the full extent of malignancy prior to surgery. Publications since the 1950s regarding the pathologic evaluation of mastectomy specimens have reported additional unsuspected sites of cancer in the ipsilateral breast in 20% to 60% of patients (15–22). Additionally, recurrence rates after breast conservation continue to be reported as high as 35% in women who do not receive radiation and 13% in women who do receive radiation (23,24). These reports prompted investigators to explore the accuracy of MRI for evaluation of extent of disease in women with a recent breast cancer diagnosis, with the goals of improving the likelihood of clear margins at the first lumpectomy and reducing recurrences. Given that women who have received radiation treatment after breast conservation must undergo mastectomy if a recurrence is diagnosed, investigators hoped that by removing the disease burden more completely initially through a more extensive surgery to encompass the disease but still preserve the breast, subsequent mastectomies might be reduced. The goals were to decrease the costs and morbidity associated with breast cancer treatment by reducing the number of operations required to achieve clear margins, reducing recurrence rates, and potentially improving survival.

The published studies when combined have evaluated MRI in approximately 1,500 cases of newly diagnosed breast can-

cer. All have found that MRI identifies otherwise unsuspected additional malignancy in the ipsilateral breast (Table 16C.1; Figure 16C.1). The reported frequency of additional MRI-detected disease ranges from 10% to 34%, with an average of 16%. In the subset of studies that assessed in detail the full extent of the additional malignancy, multifocal disease was found in 9% of the women studied, and multicentric disease was found in an additional 9%.

In addition to the research demonstrating improved local staging of disease, several studies have assessed the impact of this improved MRI staging on surgical planning and management. All are relatively small studies, and comparison of the results is challenging because the study designs vary. Overall, the studies have evaluated approximately 1,200 women considered breast-conservation candidates prior to MRI. Additional MRI-detected malignancy in the ipsilateral breast resulted in changes in the surgical management in 6% to 26% of patients, with an average of 16% (Table 16C.2) (8,9,12,13,25–27). For example, in their study of 64 patients who underwent MRI prior to excisional biopsy of suspicious breast lesions, Orel et al. (12) found that MRI appropriately changed the surgical management in 7 patients (11%). The MRI-prompted changes were a wider excision at lumpectomy in two patients and a change from breast conservation to mastectomy in five patients. Schelfout et al. (13) studied 170 women with suspicious breast lesions who had preoperative breast MRI, and categorized changes in management due to MRI as necessary or unnecessary. They found that necessary alterations in surgical management were made in 42 patients (25%), with 24 requiring wider excision lumpectomy and 18 changed from breast conservation to mastectomy.

It is important to clarify that the published studies to date address the diagnostic accuracy of MRI for extent of disease and the impact of MRI on surgical planning. Investigations of long-term outcomes such as reduction in positive margins in

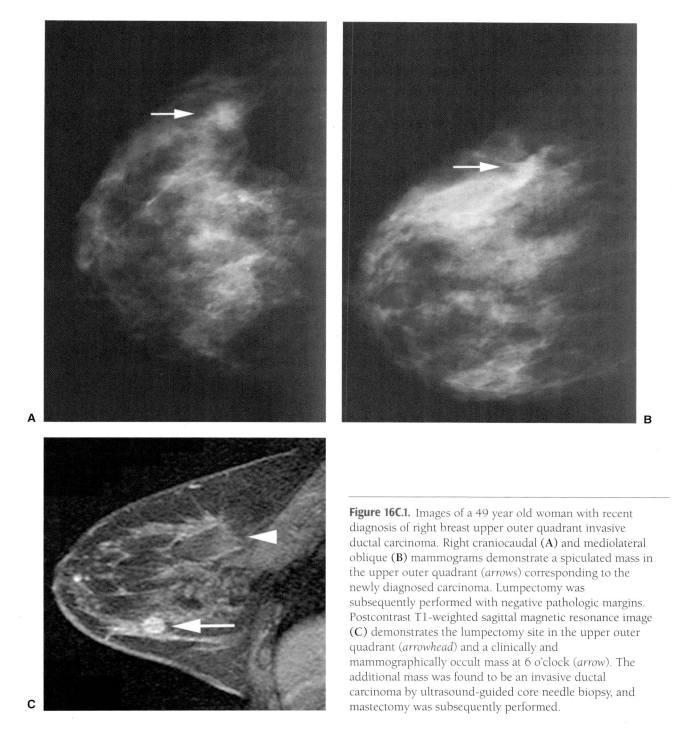

Figure 16C.1. Images of a 49 year old woman with recent diagnosis of right breast upper outer quadrant invasive ductal carcinoma. Right craniocaudal (**A**) and mediolateral oblique (**B**) mammograms demonstrate a spiculated mass in the upper outer quadrant (*arrows*) corresponding to the newly diagnosed carcinoma. Lumpectomy was subsequently performed with negative pathologic margins. Postcontrast T1-weighted sagittal magnetic resonance image (**C**) demonstrates the lumpectomy site in the upper outer quadrant (*arrowhead*) and a clinically and mammographically occult mass at 6 o'clock (*arrow*). The additional mass was found to be an invasive ductal carcinoma by ultrasound-guided core needle biopsy, and mastectomy was subsequently performed.

breast-conservation patients or reduction in recurrence rates have not yet been reported. Although Fischer et al. (28) reported lower recurrence rates in women who received preoperative MRI compared with those who did not, the treatment and control groups were not matched and the women who received MRI had tumors that were less advanced than the tumors in women who did not receive preoperative MRI. As such, it is not clear whether the differences in recurrence rates between the patient groups in the study were truly due to the preoperative MRI.

Although most acknowledge that MRI better defines the true extent of malignancy compared with mammography and ultrasound, questions remain as to whether this improvement is found in all women or only those with certain tumor histologies, such as invasive lobular carcinoma. Berg et al. (27) wondered if ultrasound used in conjunction with mammography might perform as well as MRI in extent of disease evaluation in certain subgroups. In their study of 111 women with a recent breast cancer diagnosis, the accuracy of MRI, ultrasound, and

Table 16C.2

Frequency of Impact on Surgical Management of Magnetic Resonance Imaging (MRI)-Detected Malignancy in the Ipsilateral Breast in Patients with a Recent Diagnosis of Breast Cancer

First Author, Year (Ref.)	No. of Malignant Cases	No. (%) with Additional Ipsilateral MRI Malignancy Impacting Surgical Management[a]
Orel, 1995 (12)	64	7 (11)
Fischer, 1999 (9)	336	51 (15)
Tan, 1999 (25)	83	5 (6)
Tillman, 2002 (26)	207	18 (9)
Bedrosian, 2003 (8)	267	49 (18)
Shelfout, 2004 (13)	170	42 (25)
Berg, 2004 (27)	111	29 (26)
Total	1,238	201 (16)

[a] MRI malignancy resulting in change from planned breast conservation to mastectomy or from planned breast conservation to conservation with wider excision.

mammography were compared for different index cancer histologies. They found that clinical breast examination, MRI, and mammography were the best combination of imaging tools in defining extent of disease across all histologies, and that MRI was particularly helpful in defining extent of lobular carcinoma. Of particular interest, although historically MRI had been described as a poor method to evaluate ductal carcinoma in situ (DCIS), the study by Berg et al. found MRI to be the most accurate method of determining the true extent of DCIS when compared with mammography and/or ultrasound.

Others have wondered if MRI might be useful in women with more dense breast tissue but not so in women with fatty breast tissue. This hypothesis is logical as mammography is most challenged in women with dense breast tissue. In the study by Berg et al., MRI did not provide added benefit over mammography in women with fatty breast tissue. However, this result has not been replicated in other studies. In a study by Tan et al. (25) neither index tumor histology nor breast density were significant predictors of improved performance with breast MRI.

Postsurgical Evaluation

Current standards recommend achieving clear margins when in situ and invasive carcinoma are surgically excised. In >10% of patients, the first attempt at surgical excision is unsuccessful (12,29). Although MRI is best used prior to the initial breast surgery, it may be useful when positive margins are identified at surgery. In these cases MRI can be used to better define the extent of residual disease before returning to the operating room.

It can be challenging to distinguish between residual disease and postoperative change adjacent to the surgical site on breast MRI. It is important to recognize that the purpose of postsurgical evaluation MRI is not to evaluate the area of the surgical margins, as re-excision is required based on the positive pathologic margins regardless of the results of breast MRI. The purpose of the postsurgical MRI is to identify unsuspected disease distant

from the surgical margins and to assess the extent to which the residual disease may extend from the margin. Thus, the MRI should be performed without delay after surgery as (a) the enhancement of the surgical margin can persist for many months after surgery and (b) the purpose is not to evaluate the margins themselves but areas distant from the surgical cavity.

Disease in the Contralateral Breast

Some physicians have questioned whether additional MRI-detected disease in the ipsilateral breast is clinically relevant, hypothesizing that such residual disease will be treated by radiation therapy. However, several clinical trials have demonstrated MRI detects otherwise occult disease in the contralateral breast, which would not be influenced by radiation treatment to the breast with known cancer. Overall, the published trials suggest that about 4% of women with a current unilateral breast cancer diagnosis have contralateral cancer that can be diagnosed if breast MRI is incorporated in the diagnostic workup prior to surgical planning (Table 16C.3; Figure 16C.2) (9,27,30–37).

Lehman et al. (37) recently published the results of the American College of Radiology Imaging Network (ACRIN) trial 6667. In this trial, representing the largest series of patients studied to date, 969 women with newly diagnosed unilateral breast cancer were enrolled. MRI detected clinically and mammographically occult breast cancer in the contralateral breast in 30 (3.1%) of the women studied. The cancers detected by MRI in this trial were early-stage lesions. Forty percent were DCIS. The invasive tumors had a mean diameter of 10.9 mm and were all node-negative; 94% of the lesions were staged T1 and 6% at T2.

As with the studies regarding extent of disease in the ipsilateral breast, the investigations of MRI of the contralateral breast did not find significant differences in the detection rates in specific subgroups of patients. Specifically, the improved accuracy of breast MRI in diagnosing contralateral disease was not limited to women with dense breast tissue or with certain cancer histologies (e.g., lobular carcinoma).

Table 16C.3

Cancer Yield of Magnetic Resonance Imaging (MRI) in Studies Screening the Contralateral Breast of Women with Recent Diagnosis of Breast Cancer

First Author, Year (Ref.)	Mean Age in Years (Range)	Recommendations for Biopsy in Contralateral Breast/Total No. Screened	No. of Cancers Detected in Contralateral Breast/ Total No. Screened	Cancer Yield from MRI Alone (%)
Rieber, 1997 (30)	—	NA	3/34	3 (9%)
Fischer, 1999 (9)	54 (21–89)	NA	19/463	15 (3%)
Slanetz, 2002 (31)	49 (34–78)	10/17 (29%)	4/17	4 (24%)
Liberman, 2003 (32)	48 (28–79)	72/223 (32%)	12/223	12 (5%)
Lee, 2003 (33)	50 (22–78)	15/182 (8%)	7/182	7 (4%)
Viehweg, 2004 (34)	—	NA	11/119	4 (3%)
Berg, 2004 (27)	49 (26–81)	NA	10/111	3 (3%)
Pediconi, 2005 (35)	52 (35–78)	14/50 (28%)	11/50	11 (22%)
Lehman (IBMC), 2005 (36)	52 (31–79)	12/103 (12%)	4/103	4 (4%)
Lehman (ACRIN), 2007 (37)	53	135/969 (13.9%)	33/969	30 (3%)
Total			114/2,271	93 (4%)

NA, not available; IBMC, International Breast Magnetic Resonance Consortium; ACRIN, American College of Radiology Imaging Network.

Axillary Adenopathy with Unknown Primary Site

Rarely, women present with adenocarcinoma metastases in the axillary lymph nodes without a clinically or mammographically identified primary source of cancer, a clinical presentation that accounts for <1% of reported breast cancers (38) and is clinically challenging. If the primary cannot be found, adenocarci-noma in the axillary lymph nodes is presumed to be from an ipsilateral breast primary and mastectomy has been typically recommended. If the primary can be found, mastectomy may be avoided and breast conservation performed. In several published trials, MRI accurately identified the primary cancer in the majority of patients presenting with axillary adenopathy, unknown primary. Overall, approximately 59% of women with this

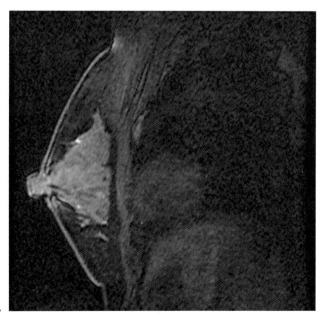

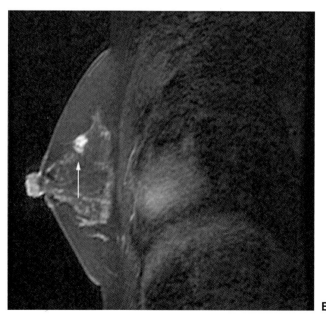

A   B

Figure 16C.2. Images of a 52-year-old woman with recent diagnosis of right breast cancer. Left mammogram (not shown) was negative. Pre (**A**) and post (**B**) contrast-enhanced sagittal magnetic resonance images of the left breast reveal an 8-mm enhancing mass at 12 o'clock in the left breast (*arrow*). Core needle biopsy confirmed infiltrating ductal carcinoma. Final pathology from lumpectomy demonstrated an 8-mm infiltrating ductal carcinoma, sentinel lymph node-negative.

Table 16C.4

Breast Magnetic Resonance (MR) Imaging for Detection of Occult Breast Cancer in Patients with Axillary Adenopathy, Unknown Primary

First Author, Year (Ref.)	No.	MR Detection Rate No. (%)
Stomper, 1999 (38)	8	2/8 (25)
Henry-Tillman, 1999 (39)	8	8/8 (100)
Orel, 1999 (40)	22	19/22 (86)
Obdeijn, 2000 (41)	20	8/20 (40)
Olson, 2000 (42)	40	28/40 (70)
Buchanan, 2005 (43)	64	31/64 (48)
Total	162	96/162 (59)

clinical scenario will have the primary identified in the breast by MRI (Table 16C.4; Figure 16C.3), allowing them to pursue more appropriate and focused therapy for the breast malignancy (38–43).

Evaluating Response to Neoadjuvant Chemotherapy

The randomized trial National Surgical Adjuvant Breast Project (NSABP) B18 compared preoperative and postoperative chemotherapy for women with operable breast cancer and found no statistically significant difference in overall survival or disease-free survival between the two groups (44,45). However, more patients in the preoperative group were able to receive lumpectomies, particularly patients with large tumors. A further advantage of preoperative or neoadjuvant chemotherapy was the opportunity to observe the primary tumor response, not possible in the postoperative group. In the preoperative group, the primary tumor response to chemotherapy was found to correlate with survival outcomes. The results from NSABP B18 and other studies comparing pre- and postoperative surgery have led to greater use of preoperative chemotherapy for women with operable breast cancer, especially those desiring a lumpectomy but with tumors too large at presentation for breast-conservative surgery.

MRI is effective for staging the primary tumor extent both before and after chemotherapy. Preoperative MRI often reveals more extensive disease than indicated by physical examination or mammography, suggesting that neoadjuvant chemotherapy may be appropriate. MRI can also be used to monitor the tumor response during treatment and to restage disease extent following treatment and before surgery.

MRI for Assessing Residual Disease

MRI can be used to measure residual disease after chemotherapy, although a higher rate of false-negative findings occurs with treated versus untreated tumors. This is caused by decreased contrast uptake as a result of the antiangiogenic effect of treatment, or due to partial volume averaging that can occur when the residual disease is distributed diffusely. Several studies have compared MRI with mammography, ultrasound, and/or clinical examination for estimation of residual disease extent following chemotherapy, with most reporting better correlation of MRI with histopathologic residual disease size than the other imaging modalities or clinical examination (46–54).

Other studies using breast MRI to assess response to treatment have reported both under- and overestimation of residual disease size, with a tendency for MRI to underestimate residual disease extent in tumors with significant response. The study by Partridge et al. (47) suggested that the accuracy of breast MRI for evaluating residual disease is improved if interpreted relative to the disease extent at baseline and using relaxed enhancement criteria for detecting residual tumor.

MRI for Monitoring Tumor Response

If MRI is performed before and after neoadjuvant chemotherapy, objective tumor response can be assessed by applying guidelines developed by the *Response Evaluation Criteria in Solid Tumors (RECIST) Group* (55). Figure 16C.4 shows examples of prechemotherapy and postchemotherapy images for three patients showing different degrees of response on MRI. Several studies compared MRI measurements of tumor response with that measured clinically. MRI-determined rates of complete response, partial response, or no response correlated well with response measurements by standard clinical assessment (46,51,53,54).

Other studies have explored the usefulness of MRI performed early in treatment for predicting the eventual overall clinical or histopathologic tumor response (56–63). These studies evaluated size and morphologic measurements by MRI as well as functional parameters related to the pharmacokinetics of contrast agent uptake. Cheung et al. (59) found that an early tumor size reduction, measured after the first course of treatment, correlated with response. Pickles et al. (57) found that early changes in tumor volume and pharmacokinetic parameters were significantly different between responding and nonresponding patients. Martincich and colleagues (56) found that reductions in both tumor volume and contrast uptake after two cycles of treatment were associated with a major histopathologic response. Several studies found correlations between the initial morphologic patterns of breast tumors on MRI and their likelihood of response to treatment (62–64). Esserman et al. (63) classified tumor morphology according to the degree of tumor containment and found that well-circumscribed tumors demonstrated the highest percentage of complete responses and underwent breast conservation at a higher rate. Murata and colleagues (62) used a similar classification and also found an association between those tumors of a solitary nodular type at presentation and the likelihood of achieving a pathologic complete response with treatment.

These studies and others suggest a role for MRI in characterizing the response of breast tumors to neoadjuvant chemotherapy. Imaging techniques that quantitatively assess response, both morphologically and functionally, are being integrated into oncologic clinical trials to test their ability to measure the effects of treatment and to explore the value of imaging measurements for predicting treatment benefit. The data provided by clinical trials will hopefully help to determine the most effective imaging approaches for monitoring patients during treatment.

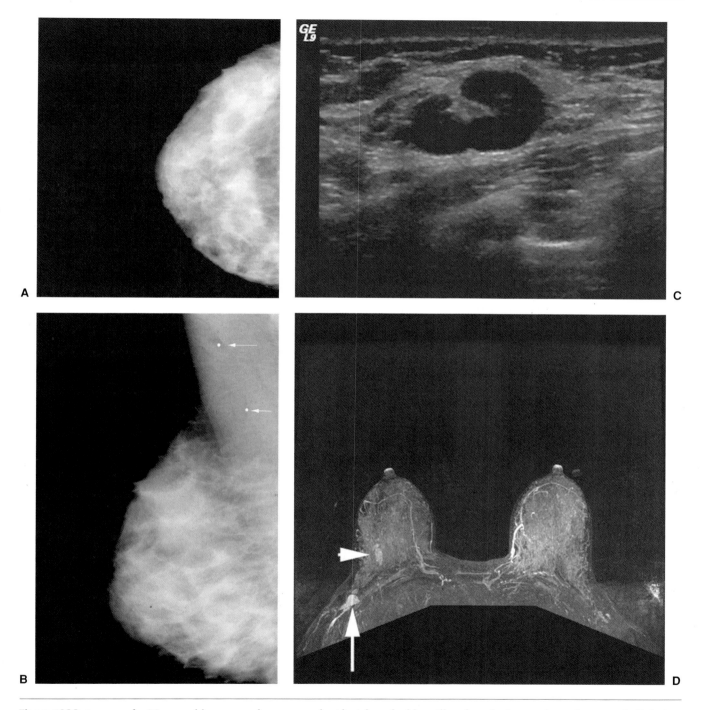

Figure 16C.3. Images of a 39-year-old woman who presented with right palpable axillary lymphadenopathy and a normal clinical breast examination. Right craniocaudal (**A**) and mediolateral oblique (**B**) mammograms demonstrate no abnormality. BB markers overlie the site of the palpable abnormality in the axilla (*arrows*), but the lymph nodes are not included on the images because of their posterior location. Ultrasound of the right axilla (**C**) demonstrates an abnormal axillary lymph node. Ultrasound-guided core biopsy demonstrated poorly differentiated adenocarcinoma. Axial maximum intensity projection (**D**) from postcontrast T1-weighted fat-suppressed magnetic resonance images demonstrate an 18-mm mass in the right breast upper outer quadrant (*arrowhead*) and the known right axillary adenopathy (*arrow*). The mass was found to be the primary invasive ductal carcinoma by ultrasound-guided core needle biopsy, and lumpectomy was subsequently performed.

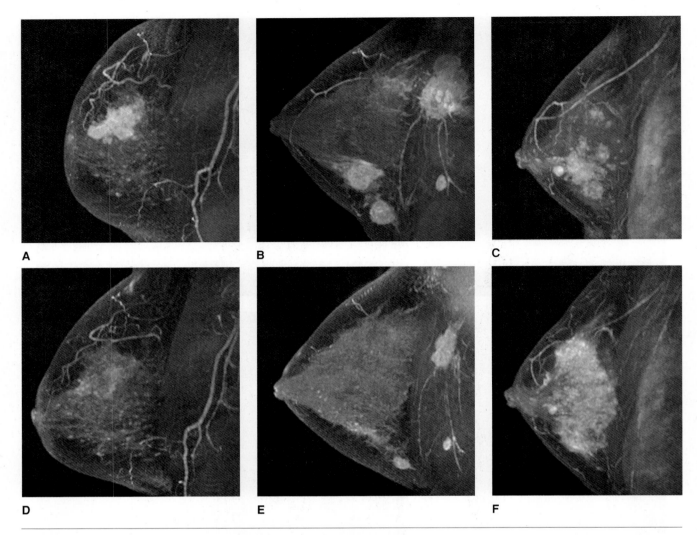

Figure 16C.4. Prechemotherapy (**top row, A through C**) and postchemotherapy (**bottom row, D through F**) maximum intensity projection images are shown for three patients demonstrating varying degrees of tumor response. The images shown in the left column (A and D) are for a patient with an excellent tumor response, center column (B and E) are for a patient showing a partial response in the breast and axilla, and right column (C and F) are for a patient whose tumor progressed on treatment.

Posttherapy Follow-up of Patients With a Personal History of Breast Cancer

Once a patient has successfully completed therapy, is there a continued role for breast MRI? There are no studies reporting results from continued screening of women with a personal history of breast cancer. Understandably, women who have been treated for breast cancer but never had an MRI as part of their workup may wonder if MRI might demonstrate residual occult disease in the ipsilateral or contralateral breast. This is reasonable given the benefits of MRI previously described. However, whether continued annual MR evaluation of these patients is beneficial or not is unknown.

There is a good deal of literature on the benefits of MRI in screening women at high risk for breast cancer. Most of the studies published include women with a known genetic mutation and those who have >25% lifetime risk based primarily on family history (65–73). In these studies, MRI consistently demonstrates higher sensitivity in detecting breast cancers compared with mammography or to mammography and ultrasound (Table 16C.5; Figure 16C.5). Overall, approximately 30 otherwise occult cancers will be diagnosed in every 1,000 high-risk women screened. The reported risks of false-positive findings when screening these women with MRI varied across studies but were within acceptable limits with approximately 5% of women undergoing benign biopsy and 30% of biopsies performed yielding cancer.

In 2003, the American Cancer Society (ACS) published its update of breast cancer screening recommendations, suggesting that high-risk women and their clinicians consider MRI or ultrasound as complements to screening mammography. Because of data published since that time, the most recent report by the ACS on screening for breast cancer in high-risk women recommends that screening MRI be performed in addition to mammography. These "high-risk" women include women with

Comparative Sensitivity of Screening Mammography (Mam), Ultrasound (US), and Magnetic Resonance Imaging (MRI) in Women at Increased Risk for Breast Cancer

First Author (Ref.), Site	Study Design[a]	Follow-up (months)	Mean Age in Years (Range)	No. of Cancers Detected/Total No. Screened	Sensitivity (%) Mam	Sensitivity (%) MRI	Sensitivity (%) US	Cancer Yield from MRI Alone (%) [Confidence Interval][a]	Biopsies Recommended as a Result of MRI	PPV of Biopsies Performed Based on MRI (%)
Kuhl (65), Germany	P	Varied 24–84	42 (27–59)	8.1% (43/529)	33% (14/43)	91% (39/43)	40% (17/43)	19/529 (3.6%) [2.2%, 5.6%]	78/529 (14.7%)	50
Warner (66), Canada	P	36	47 (26–65)	9.3% (22/236)	36% (8/22)	77% (17/22)	33% (7/21)	7/236 (3.0%)[b] [1.7%, 7.1%]	37/236 (15.7%)	46
Podo (Italian Multi-Center Project) (67), Italy	P	24	46 (25–77)	7.6% (8/105)	13% (1/8)	100% (8/8)	13% (1/8)	7/105 (6.7%) [2.7%, 13.3%]	9/105 (8.6%)	89
Tilanus-Linthorst (68), Netherlands	P	12	42 (22–68)	2.8% (3/109)	0%	100% (3/3)	—	3/109 (2.8%) [0.6%, 7.8%]	5/109 (4.6%)	60
Morris (69), USA	R	None	50[c] (23–82)	3.8% (14/367)	0[d]	100%	—	14/367 (3.8%) [2.1%, 6.3%]	59/367 (15.8%)	24
Kriege (MRI Screening Study Group) (70), Netherlands[e]	P	33	40 (19–72)	2.4% (45/1909)	40% (18/45)	71% (32/45)	—	22/1909 (1.2%) [1.1%, 2.4%]	56/1909 (2.9%)	57
Lehman (IBMC) (71), International	P	None	45 (26–86)	1.1% (4/367)	25% (1/4)	100% (4/4)	—	3/367 (0.8%) [0.2%, 2.4%]	23/367 (6.3%)	17
Leach (MARIBS) (73), UK	P	Varied 0–72	40 (31–55)	5.1% (33/649)	40% (14/35)[f]	77% (27/35)	—	19/649 (2.9%) [1.7%–4.5%]	—	25
Lehman (IBMC) (72), USA	P	None	46 (25–72)	3.5% (6/171)	33% (1/6)	100% (2/6)	17% (6/6)	4/171 (2.3%) [0.6%, 6%]	14/171 (8.2%)	42

PPV, positive predictive value; P, prospective; R, retrospective; IBMC, International Breast Magnetic Resonance Consortium; MARIBS, Magnetic Resonance Imaging in Breast Screening.

[a]Exact binomial confidence intervals.

[b]One patient who had an MRI only cancer in this study did not receive ultrasound.

[c]Reported median.

[d]To be included in this study, subjects had to have a negative mammogram.

[e]The results are shown for 45 of the 50 cancers diagnosed. Five cases were omitted that did not have all imaging performed.

[f]Two cancers in the study were identified as "interval" and were not detected by either screening examination.

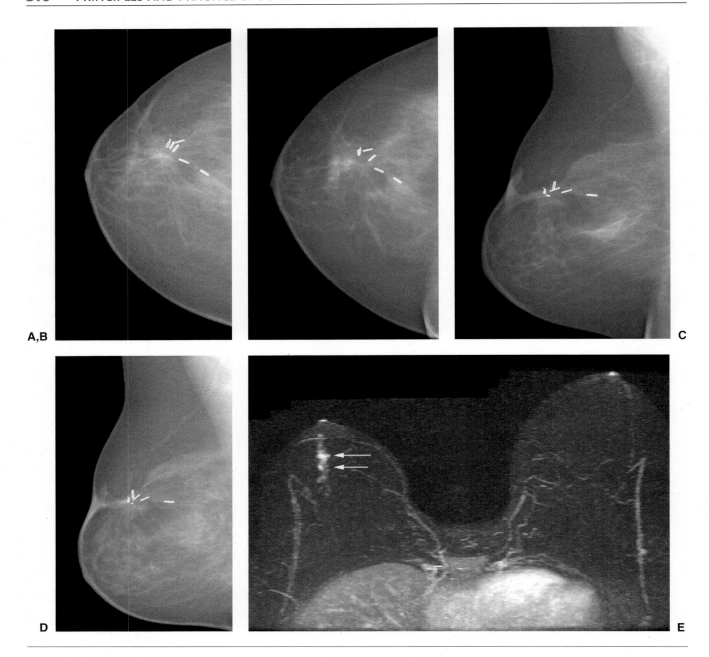

Figure 16C.5. Images of a 36-year-old woman with personal history of right breast cancer 3 years ago, status postlumpectomy with widely negative margins. Routine mammography demonstrated no change in the appearance of the surgical site on prior (**A**) and current (**B**) craniocaudal view mammograms or on prior (**C**) and current (**D**) medial lateral oblique view mammograms. However, axial maximum intensity projection from postcontrast T1-weighted fat-suppressed magnetic resonace (MR) images (**E**) shows clumped enhancement in linear distribution (*arrows*). MRI-guided needle biopsy confirmed high-grade ductal carcinoma in situ and subsequent mastectomy found focus of invasive ductal carcinoma.

a known genetic mutation, women who have not been tested but who have a first-degree relative with a known mutation, women with a 20 to 25% or greater lifetime risk of breast cancer as determined by currently available risk assessment tools, and women who received chest irradiation between the ages of 10 and 30 (74). The ACS does not consider the currently available data sufficient to make clear recommendations for screening MRI in women with a personal history of breast cancer, women with dense breast tissue, or women with prior benign biopsy (in-

cluding atypical ductal hyperplasia, lobular carcinoma in situ, and atypical lobular hyperplasia). The ACS recommends against screening MRI in average-risk women.

POTENTIAL HARM ASSOCIATED WITH BREAST MRI

Although many acknowledge that additional disease can be seen when MRI is used preoperatively and that screening MRI can detect more cancers at an earlier stage in women at high risk, there are important concerns regarding the use of breast MRI. One such apprehension is that MRI will lead to unnecessary mastectomies. There are two scenarios where this might occur. The first is when a false-positive MRI finding causes a patient to opt for a mastectomy rather than breast-conserving therapy. For example, when a patient hears there is a finding on the MRI and changes her mind from breast conservation to mastectomy, only to find after the mastectomy that the suspicious area on the MRI was benign. It is hoped that these scenarios can be avoided with (a) appropriate counseling before and after the breast MRI and (b) clear understanding of the need for histologic confirmation of suspicious lesions on MRI prior to surgical planning decisions.

The second scenario that can lead to a potentially unnecessary mastectomy is the patient who is initially a breast-conservation candidate, but the MRI reveals additional malignancy that leads to a change in surgical plans to mastectomy. Although the MRI findings are confirmed malignancy in this case, some have opined that it is possible that this additional disease is not clinically important. Perhaps the patient's disease would be treated appropriately with radiation therapy, avoiding a mastectomy. Or perhaps the disease would never progress to become clinically significant.

Until trials are performed that evaluate impact on morbidity or mortality, how can we counsel our patients? One option is to recommend against MRI in the absence of randomized clinical trials with mortality as an end point. We believe this is not practical as many of our decisions in medicine must be made without this level of information. And the clinical trial results to date are clear in demonstrating that MRI will detect significant invasive disease occult on mammography and ultrasound. The hypothesis that the additional disease is not "clinically significant" is questionable as our current understanding of breast cancer leads us to obtain clear surgical margins in order to reduce the risk of recurrence and improve long-term outcomes. Given our current understanding of breast cancer, it appears prudent to use the technology we currently have to most accurately diagnose the true extent of disease prior to surgical planning.

How can we use this technology appropriately? First, we must have a clear understanding of both the potential benefits and harms of breast MRI. The benefits include earlier detection in high-risk women, more accurate assessment of the true extent of disease in women with a current breast cancer diagnosis, and more accurate assessment of response to therapy. These benefits have the potential to reduce morbidity and mortality associated with breast cancer. The harms include false-positive examinations that lead to unnecessary biopsies, delays in treatment, added financial costs, and possibly unnecessary mastectomies.

COMPONENTS OF A HIGH-QUALITY BREAST MRI PROGRAM

Over the past decade, there has been significant progress in developing consensus over what constitutes a high-quality breast MR examination. The American College of Radiology is developing a voluntary accreditation program that will allow sites that comply with established standards to demonstrate the quality of their program through ACR accreditation. Guidelines for performing high-quality MRI include the following:

- 1.5 T or greater magnet strength
- Dedicated bilateral breast coil
- One T1-weighted precontrast series and one "bright fluid" precontrast series
- At least two postcontrast T1-weighted series
- High spatial resolution defined as <3.0 mm slice thickness and <1.0 mm by <1.0 mm in-plane pixel size
- High temporal resolution as defined by <4 minutes for each postcontrast series
- Acceptable method of eliminating the high signal from fat, either through subtraction methods or software methods of suppressing the fat signal

All MRI examinations should be evaluated in conjunction with other breast images, including mammography and ultrasound images.

OUR CURRENT RECOMMENDATIONS

In our practices, we use breast MRI predominantly in (a) patients with a recent history of breast cancer to evaluate the true extent of disease in the known cancer breast and to identify possible contralateral disease and (b) patients who are at high risk for breast cancer as a complement to screening mammography. We also recommend breast MRI in all patients with axillary adenopathy from an unknown primary site, and we use MRI selectively in patients undergoing neoadjuvant chemotherapy.

We stress the importance of a complete mammographic and sonographic evaluation of all patients with a recent breast cancer diagnosis prior to breast MRI and stress the importance of using MRI as a complement, not a replacement, to thorough evaluation with traditional imaging. MRI is not used to determine whether or not a suspicious mammographic or sonographic lesion should be biopsied. For all lesions, and particularly for calcifications, the management must be determined by the appearance on mammography and a decision to biopsy should not be "overruled" by a negative MRI.

Although in some practices the MRI is performed in patients with suspicious lesions prior to needle biopsy, we recommend confirmation of malignancy by core needle biopsy before the MRI is obtained. Once a patient is diagnosed with a malignancy (DCIS or invasive carcinoma) then MRI is recommended for evaluation of disease extent. If additional lesions distant from the known cancer are identified on diagnostic mammography or ultrasound, we typically perform the MRI prior to additional biopsies. In that way, we can have a thorough imaging workup in the known cancer patient before planning the logical steps in further tissue sampling. We place significant importance on tissue confirmation of suspicious MRI lesions, emphasizing that although MRI is a very sensitive imaging tool, all suspicious lesions are not malignant and tissue confirmation is essential prior to changing surgical management. This is important to reduce "unnecessary mastectomies" in which patients or their clinicians prematurely opt for mastectomy only to find that the additional suspicious enhancement was only benign proliferative or fibroadenomatous change within the breast.

FUTURE OF BREAST MRI

Research to clarify optimal acquisition protocols for breast MRI is needed. Recent work in breast MRI in 3-Tesla magnets is very exciting and holds promise for even higher spatial and temporal resolution and further improvements in image quality. In the future, novel contrast agents may provide more sensitive and more specific discrimination of benign from malignant lesions. In vivo functional measurements of tumor biology using contrast-enhanced MRI, diffusion-weighted MRI, or MR spectroscopy may yield markers that can be used to predict response to treatment more accurately and earlier in treatment.

Based on the past 3 decades of research, it is clear that MRI plays an important role in the management of women at high risk for breast cancer and in those with a current breast cancer diagnosis. There is significant work to be done to optimize the application and performance of breast MRI. Further research on long-term outcomes is needed and partnerships between imaging and treatment trials are encouraged in order that the application of this exciting and powerful imaging tool is used most appropriately.

REFERENCES

1. Mansfield P, Morris PG, Ordidge R, et al. Carcinoma of the breast imaged by nuclear magnetic resonance (NMR). *Br J Radiol* 1979;52:242–243.
2. Houn F, Elliott ML, McCrohan JL. The Mammography Quality Standards Act of 1992. History and philosophy. *Radiol Clin North Am.* 1995;33:1059–1065.
3. *Saving Women's Lives: Integration and Innovation: A Framework for Progress in Early Detection and Diagnosis of Breast Cancer.* Washington, DC: National Acadamies Press; 2005.
4. Fletcher SW, Elmore JG. Clinical practice. Mammographic screening for breast cancer. *N Engl J Med.* 2003;348:1672–1680.
5. Humphrey LL, Helfand M, Chan BK, et al. Breast cancer screening: a summary of the evidence for the U.S. Preventive Services Task Force. *Ann Intern Med.* 2002;137:347–360.
6. Morrow M, Schmidt R, Hassett C. Patient selection for breast conservation therapy with magnification mammography. *Surgery.* 1995;118:621–626.
7. Harms SE, Flamig DP, Hesley KL, et al. MR imaging of the breast with rotating delivery of excitation off resonance: clinical experience with pathologic correlation. *Radiology.* 1993;187:493–501.
8. Bedrosian I, Mick R, Orel SG, et al. Changes in the surgical management of patients with breast carcinoma based on preoperative magnetic resonance imaging. *Cancer.* 2003;98:468–473.
9. Fischer U, Kopka L, Grabbe E. Breast carcinoma: effect of preoperative contrast-enhanced MR imaging on the therapeutic approach. *Radiology.* 1999;213:881–888.
10. Liberman L, Morris EA, Dershaw DD, et al. MR imaging of the ipsilateral breast in women with percutaneously proven breast cancer. *AJR Am J Roentgenol.* 2003;180:901–910.
11. Mumtaz H, Hall-Craggs MA, Davidson T, et al. Staging of symptomatic primary breast cancer with MR imaging. *AJR Am J Roentgenol.* 1997;169:417–424.
12. Orel SG, Schnall MD, Powell CM, et al. Staging of suspected breast cancer: effect of MR imaging and MR-guided biopsy. *Radiology.* 1995;196:115–122.
13. Schelfout K, Van Goethem M, Kersschot E, et al. Contrast-enhanced MR imaging of breast lesions and effect on treatment. *Eur J Surg Oncol.* 2004;30:501–507.
14. Schnall MD, Blume J, Bluemke DA, et al. MRI detection of distinct incidental cancer in women with primary breast cancer studied in IBMC 6883. *J Surg Oncol.* 2005;92:32–38.
15. Qualheim RE, Gall EA. Breast carcinoma with multiple sites of origin. *Cancer.* 1957;10:460–468.
16. Rosen PP, Fracchia AA, Urban JA, et al. "Residual" mammary carcinoma following simulated partial mastectomy. *Cancer.* 1975;35:739–747.
17. Lagios MD. Multicentricity of breast carcinoma demonstrated by routine correlated serial subgross and radiographic examination. *Cancer.* 1977;40:1726–1734.
18. Schwartz GF, Patchesfsky AS, Feig SA, et al. Multicentricity of nonpalpable breast cancer. *Cancer.* 1980;45:2913–2916.
19. Egan RL. Multicentric breast carcinomas: clinical-radiographic-pathologic whole organ studies and 10-year survival. *Cancer.* 1982;49:1123–1130.
20. Holland R, Veling SH, Mravunac M, et al. Histologic multifocality of Tis, T1-2 breast carcinomas. Implications for clinical trials of breast-conserving surgery. *Cancer.* 1985;56:979–990.
21. Anastassiades O, Iakovou E, Stavridou N, et al. Multicentricity in breast cancer. A study of 366 cases. *Am J Clin Pathol.* 1993;99:238–243.
22. Vaidya JS, Vyas JJ, Chinoy RF, et al. Multicentricity of breast cancer: whole-organ analysis and clinical implications. *Br J Cancer.* 1996;74:820–824.
23. Fisher ER, Dignam J, Tan-Chiu E, et al. Pathologic findings from the National Surgical Adjuvant Breast Project (NSABP) eight-year update of Protocol B-17: intraductal carcinoma. *Cancer.* 1999;86:429–438.
24. Fisher ER, Anderson S, Tan-Chiu E, et al. Fifteen-year prognostic discriminants for invasive breast carcinoma: National Surgical Adjuvant Breast and Bowel Project Protocol-06. *Cancer.* 2001;91:1679–1687.
25. Tan JE, Orel SG, Schnall MD, et al. Role of magnetic resonance imaging and magnetic resonance imaging–guided surgery in the evaluation of patients with early-stage breast cancer for breast conservation treatment. *Am J Clin Oncol.* 1999;22:414–418.
26. Tillman GF, Orel SG, Schnall MD, et al. Effect of breast magnetic resonance imaging on the clinical management of women with early-stage breast carcinoma. *J Clin Oncol.* 2002;20:3413–3423.
27. Berg WA, Gutierrez L, NessAiver MS, et al. Diagnostic accuracy of mammography, clinical examination, US, and MR imaging in preoperative assessment of breast cancer. *Radiology.* 2004;233:830–849.
28. Fischer U, Zacharine O, Baum F, et al. The influence of preoperative MRI of the breasts on recurrence rate in patients with breast cancer. *Eur Radiol.* 2004;14:1725–1731.
29. Chagpar AB, Martin RC 2nd, Hagendoorn LJ. Lumpectomy margins are affected by tumor size and histologic subtype but not by biopsy technique. *Am J Surg.* 2004;188:399–402.
30. Rieber A, Merkle E, Bohm W, et al. MRI of histologically confirmed mammary carcinoma: clinical relevance of diagnostic procedures for detection of multifocal or contralateral secondary carcinoma. *J Comput Assist Tomogr.* 1997;21:773–779.
31. Slanetz PJ, Edmister WB, Yeh ED. Occult contralateral breast carcinoma incidentally detected by breast magnetic resonance imaging. *Breast J.* 2002;8:145–148.
32. Liberman L, Morris EA, Kim CM, et al. MR imaging findings in the contralateral breast of women with recently diagnosed breast cancer. *AJR Am J Roentgenol.* 2003;180:333–341.
33. Lee SG, Orel SG, Woo IJ, et al. MR imaging screening of the contralateral breast in patients with newly diagnosed breast cancer: preliminary results. *Radiology.* 2003;226:773–778.

34. Viehweg P, Rotter K, Laniado M, et al. MR imaging of the contralateral breast in patients after breast-conserving therapy. *Eur Radiol.* 2004;14:402–408.

35. Pediconi F, Venditti F, Padula S, et al. CE-Magnetic Resonance Mammography for the evaluation of the contralateral breast in patients with diagnosed breast cancer. *Radiol Med (Torino).* 2005;110: 61–68.

36. Lehman CD, Blume JD, Thickman D, et al. Added cancer yield of MRI in screening the contralateral breast of women recently diagnosed with breast cancer: results from the International Breast Magnetic Resonance Consortium (IBMC) trial. *J Surg Oncol.* 2005;92:9–15; discussion 15–16.

37. Lehman CD, Gatsonis C, Kuhl CK, et al. MRI evaluation of the contralateral breast in women with recently diagnosed breast cancer. *N Engl J Med.* 2007;356: 1295–1303.

38. Stomper PC, Waddell BE, Edge SB, et al. Breast MRI in the Evaluation of Patients with occult primary breast carcinoma. *Breast J.* 1999;5:230–234.

39. Henry-Tillman RS, Harms SE, Westbrook KC, et al. Role of breast magnetic resonance imaging in determining breast as a source of unknown metastatic lymphadenopathy. *Am J Surg.* 1999;178:496–500.

40. Orel SG, Weinstein SP, Schnall MD, et al. Breast MR imaging in patients with axillary node metastases and unknown primary malignancy. *Radiology.* 1999;212:543–549.

41. Obdeijn IM, Brouwers-Kuyper EM, Tilanus-Linthorst MM, et al. MR imaging-guided sonography followed by fine-needle aspiration cytology in occult carcinoma of the breast. *AJR Am J Roentgenol.* 2000;174:1079–1084.

42. Olson JA, Jr., Morris EA, Van Zee KJ, et al. Magnetic resonance imaging facilitates breast conservation for occult breast cancer. *Ann Surg Oncol.* 2000;7:411–415.

43. Buchanan CL, Morris EA, Dorn PL, et al. Utility of breast magnetic resonance imaging in patients with occult primary breast cancer. *Ann Surg Oncol.* 2005;12:1045–1053.

44. Fisher B, Bryant J, Wolmark N, et al. Effect of preoperative chemotherapy on the outcome of women with operable breast cancer. *J Clin Oncol.* 1998;16:2672–2685.

45. Wolmark N, Wang J, Mamounas E, et al. Preoperative chemotherapy in patients with operable breast cancer: nine-year results from National Surgical Adjuvant Breast and Bowel Project B-18. *J Natl Cancer Inst Monogr.* 2001;30:96–102.

46. Drew PJ, Kerin MJ, Mahapatra T, et al. Evaluation of response to neoadjuvant chemoradiotherapy for locally advanced breast cancer with dynamic contrast-enhanced MRI of the breast. *Eur J Surg Oncol.* 2001;27:617–620.

47. Partridge SC, Gibbs JE, Lu Y, et al. Accuracy of MR imaging for revealing residual breast cancer in patients who have undergone neoadjuvant chemotherapy. *AJR Am J Roentgenol.* 2002;179:1193–1199.

48. Londero V, Bazzocchi M, Del Frate C, et al. Locally advanced breast cancer: comparison of mammography, sonography and MR imaging in evaluation of residual disease in women receiving neoadjuvant chemotherapy. *Eur Radiol.* 2004;14:1371–1379.

49. Yeh E, Slanetz P, Kopans DB, et al. Prospective comparison of mammography, sonography, and MRI in patients undergoing neoadjuvant chemotherapy for palpable breast cancer. *AJR Am J Roentgenol.* 2005;184:868–877.

50. Montemurro F, Martincich L, De Rosa G, et al. Dynamic contrast-enhanced MRI and sonography in patients receiving primary chemotherapy for breast cancer. *Eur Radiol.* 2005;15:1224–1233.

51. Akazawa K, Tamaki Y, Taguchi T, et al. Preoperative evaluation of residual tumor extent by three-dimensional magnetic resonance imaging in breast cancer patients treated with neoadjuvant chemotherapy. *Breast J.* 2006;12:130–137.

52. Schott AF, Roubidoux MA, Helvie MA, et al. Clinical and radiologic assessments to predict breast cancer pathologic complete response to neoadjuvant chemotherapy. *Breast Cancer Res Treat.* 2005;92:231–238.

53. Abraham DC, Jones RC, Jones SE, et al. Evaluation of neoadjuvant chemotherapeutic response of locally advanced breast cancer by magnetic resonance imaging. *Cancer.* 1996;78:91–100.

54. Balu-Maestro C, Chapellier C, Bleuse A, et al. Imaging in evaluation of response to neoadjuvant breast cancer treatment benefits of MRI. *Breast Cancer Res Treat.* 2002;72:145–152.

55. Therasse P, Arbuck SG, Eisenhauer EA, et al. New guidelines to evaluate the response to treatment in solid tumors. European Organization for Research and Treatment of Cancer, National Cancer Institute of the United States, National Cancer Institute of Canada. *J Natl Cancer Inst.* 2000;92:205–216.

56. Martincich L, Montemurro F, De Rosa G, et al. Monitoring response to primary chemotherapy in breast cancer using dynamic contrast-enhanced magnetic resonance imaging. *Breast Cancer Res Treat.* 2004;83:67–76.

57. Pickles MD, Lowry M, Manton DJ, et al. Role of dynamic contrast enhanced MRI in monitoring early response of locally advanced breast cancer to neoadjuvant chemotherapy. *Breast Cancer Res Treat.* 2005;91:1–10.

58. Padhani AR, Hayes C, Assersohn L, et al. Prediction of clinicopathologic response of breast cancer to primary chemotherapy at contrast-enhanced MR imaging: initial clinical results. *Radiology.* 2006;239:361–374.

59. Cheung YC, Chen SC, Su MY, et al. Monitoring the size and response of locally advanced breast cancers to neoadjuvant chemotherapy (weekly paclitaxel and epirubicin) with serial enhanced MRI. *Breast Cancer Res Treat.* 2003;78:51–58.

60. Manton DJ, Chaturvedi A, Hubbard A, et al. Neoadjuvant chemotherapy in breast cancer: early response prediction with quantitative MR imaging and spectroscopy. *Br J Cancer.* 2006;94: 427–435.

61. Wasser K, Klein SK, Fink C, et al. Evaluation of neoadjuvant chemotherapeutic response of breast cancer using dynamic MRI with high temporal resolution. *Eur Radiol.* 2003;13:80–87.

62. Murata Y, Ogawa Y, Yoshida S, et al. Utility of initial MRI for predicting extent of residual disease after neoadjuvant chemotherapy: analysis of 70 breast cancer patients. *Oncol Rep.* 2004;12:1257–1262.

63. Esserman L, Kaplan E, Partridge S, et al. MRI phenotype is associated with response to doxorubicin and cyclophosphamide neoadjuvant chemotherapy in stage III breast cancer. *Ann Surg Oncol.* 2001;8:549–559.

64. Martincich L, Montemurro F, Cirillo S, et al. Role of Magnetic Resonance Imaging in the prediction of tumor response in patients with locally advanced breast cancer receiving neoadjuvant chemotherapy. *Radiol Med (Torino).* 2003;106:51–58.

65. Kuhl CK, Schrading S, Leutner CC, et al. Mammography, breast ultrasound, and magnetic resonance imaging for surveillance of women at high familial risk for breast cancer. *J Clin Oncol.* 2005;23:8469–8476.

66. Warner E, Plewes DB, Hill KA, et al. Surveillance of BRCA1 and BRCA2 mutation carriers with magnetic resonance imaging, ultrasound, mammography, and clinical breast examination. *JAMA.* 2004;292:1317–1325.

67. Podo F, Sardanelli F, Canese R, et al. The Italian multi-centre project on evaluation of MRI and other imaging modalities in early detection of breast cancer in subjects at high genetic risk. *J Exp Clin Cancer Res.* 2002;21:115–124.

68. Tilanus-Linthorst MM, Obdeijn IM, Bartels KC, et al. First experiences in screening women at high risk for breast cancer with MR imaging. *Breast Cancer Res Treat.* 2000;63:53–60.

69. Morris EA, Liberman L, Ballon DJ, et al. MRI of occult breast carcinoma in a high-risk population. *AJR Am J Roentgenol.* 2003;181:619–626.

70. Kriege M, Brekelmans CT, Boetes C, et al. Efficacy of MRI and mammography for breast-cancer screening in women with a familial or genetic predisposition. *N Engl J Med.* 2004;351:427–437.

71. Lehman CD, Blume JD, Weatherall P, et al. Screening women at high risk for breast cancer with mammography and magnetic resonance imaging. *Cancer.* 2005;103:1898–1905.

72. Lehman CD, Isaacs C, Schnall MD, et al. Cancer yield of mammography, MR, and US in high risk women: prospective multi-institution breast cancer screening study. *Radiology.* 2007;244: 381–388.

73. Leach MO, Boggis CR, Dixon AK, et al. Screening with magnetic resonance imaging and mammography of a UK population at high familial risk of breast cancer: a prospective multicentre cohort study (MARIBS). *Lancet.* 2005;365:1769–1778.

74. Saslow D, Boetes C, Burke W, et al. American Cancer Society guidelines for breast screening with MRI as an adjunct to mammography. *CA Cancer J Clin.* 2007;57: 75–89.

COMMENTARY
Laurie L. Fajardo and Jeong Mi Park

Clinical decision making for applying screening tests and for managing patients with breast cancer should be based on the best current evidence, clinical expertise, and patient values. Although radiology has made important progress in the field of evidence-based medical imaging, the specialty is still behind other specialties that have been at the forefront of evidence-based medicine in the past decade. Despite our best intentions, most of what constitutes modern medical imaging practice is based on habit, anecdotes, and scientific writings that are too often fraught with biases. Best estimates suggest that only approximately 30% of what constitutes "imaging knowledge" is substantiated by reliable scientific inquiry (1). This poses problems for clinicians and radiologists when management decisions result in inefficient, cost-ineffective, inefficacious, or occasionally, even harmful care. In recent years, recognition of how the practice of medicine based on scientifically unsubstantiated concepts and methods can result in poor-quality care and poor health outcomes has led to a number of initiatives. Medical imaging has grown exponentially in the last 3 decades with the development of many promising and often noninvasive diagnostic studies and therapeutic modalities. The corresponding medical literature can be overwhelming to physicians and varies in scientific rigor and clinical applicability. Evidence-based medical practice derives from clinical research and research synthesis as the means of providing a more definitive and accurate knowledge basis for medical care. Although the roots of evidence-based medicine are in fields other than radiology, substantial efforts by our field have led to better understandings of evidence-based radiology.

The introduction and widespread use of mammography for the early detection of breast cancer undoubtedly is one of the most important recent achievements in the control of this disease. The prognosis associated with detecting and treating breast cancer while it is still localized in the breast is clearly superior to that associated with therapy provided when the disease is diagnosed at a more advanced stage. Consequently, the trend over the past decade toward diagnosis at a more favorable stage has played a major role in the reduction of the rate of death due to this disease. The age-adjusted rate of death from breast cancer in the United States was 24% lower in 2003 than it was in 1989, a decline that has been attributed principally to the role of mammography in detecting early-staged tumors and improvements in therapy (2,3).

In recent years, magnetic resonance imaging (MRI) of the breast has emerged as a new imaging tool with widely suggested applications in patients with breast cancer or at risk for developing the disease. Although there are published evidence-based recommendations for the appropriate use of breast MRI for certain applications, the evidence for its use in other suggested applications is lacking. The availability of breast MRI is increasing throughout the United States. In a recent national survey of 575 American breast-imaging practices from the membership database of the Society of Breast Imaging, 12% of practices reported they offered breast cancer screening with MRI, and 51% reported offering diagnostic evaluation of the breast with MRI (4). However, there have been concerns about the increasing use of breast MRI and the wide-ranging quality of the examinations. It is uncertain whether performance results reported in the literature can be reproduced in all centers offering MRI today. One current concern is the existence of facilities that perform breast MRI but lack the ability to perform MRI-guided breast biopsies. Recently published American Cancer Society guidelines strongly recommend against the performance of breast MRI at locations that lack the capacity to perform percutaneous, MRI-guided biopsies of lesions observed only on MRI (5).

In making recommendations on the appropriate use of breast MRI for current clinical practices, it is important that the indications be as specifically defined as possible. Broad categories such as "women with recent diagnosis of breast cancer" should be avoided and further defined by listing specific subcategories of applicability along with the scientific data and evidence on which the recommendations are based.

USE OF BREAST MRI AS A SCREENING TOOL

There is no evidence that the use of MRI alone as a screening tool is efficacious in the detection of breast cancer in women. MRI is defined only as an adjunct to mammography when used in the screening setting (i.e., for patients who are asymptomatic and undergoing routine screening evaluation). The use of MRI in this manner, as an adjunctive screening tool, constitutes a somewhat different definition of a "screening examination" than is ordinarily used in the general practice of medicine. In 2007, the American Cancer Society (ACS) published guidelines for breast screening with MRI as an adjunct to mammography, wherein the ACS Breast Cancer Advisory Group defined its specific recommendations, indicated the lifetime risk of the population to which a specific recommendation should apply, and noted the strength of the evidence supporting the various recommendations (Table 16C.1) (5). The guidelines are based on the assessment of lifetime risk of developing breast cancer as defined by the breast cancer probability (BRCAPRO) model (6,7) or other breast cancer estimation models that are largely dependent on family history, as well as on a series of studies assessing the worth of screening MRI (8–16). BRCAPRO is a statistical model for assessing the probability that an individual carries a germline deleterious mutation of the *BRCA1* and *BRCA2* genes based on an individual's family history of breast and ovarian cancer, including male breast cancer and bilateral synchronous and asynchronous diagnoses.

Thus, it is clear that careful risk assessment is required before recommending breast MRI as a screening tool adjunctive to routine mammography. When an appropriate indication exists, there is no consensus as to the timing of the screening MRI relative to the screening mammogram. Some experts advocate

---

Table 16C.1

American Cancer Society Guidelines for Breast Screening with Magnetic Resonance Imaging (MRI) as an Adjunct to Mammography

Recommend Annual MRI Screening (Based on Evidence*)
   BRCA mutation
   First-degree relative of BRCA carrier, but untested
   Lifetime risk ~20–25% or greater, as defined by
      BRCAPRO or other models that are largely dependent
      on family history

Recommend Annual MRI Screening (Based on Expert
Consensus Opinion†)
   Radiation to chest between age 10 and 30 years
   Li-Fraumeni syndrome and first-degree relatives
   Cowden and Bannayan-Riley-Ruvalcaba syndromes and
      first degree relatives

Insufficient Evidence to Recommend for or Against MRI
Screening‡
   Lifetime risk 15–20% as defined by BRCAPRO or other
      models that are largely dependent on family history
   Lobular carcinoma in situ (LCIS) or atypical lobular
      hyperplasia (ALH)
   Atypical ductal hyperplasia (ADH)
   Heterogeneously or extremely dense breast on
      mammography
   Women with a personal history of breast cancer,
      including ductal carcinoma in situ (DCIS)

Recommend Against MRI Screening (Based on Expert
Consensus Opinion)
   Women at <15% lifetime risk

---

*Evidence from nonrandomized screening trials and observational studies.
†Based on evidence of lifetime risk for breast cancer.
‡Payment should not be a barrier. Screening decisions should be made on a case-by-case basis, as there may be particular factors to support MRI. (Adapted from ref. 5.)

---

performing the MRI and mammography at the same time and others recommend staggering the MRI and the mammography screening every 6 months. For women at sufficient risk to warrant screening MRI, it is most important that MRI screening be provided in addition to, not instead of, mammography because the sensitivity and cancer yield of MRI and mammography combined is greater than for MRI alone (10–14,17–20). This finding also applies to noninvasive breast cancer. Although Kuhl et al. (21) reported that screening MRI was more sensitive than mammography in detecting pure ductal carcinoma in situ, especially lesions with high nuclear grade, other studies indicate that MRI has a poorer sensitivity for detecting microcalcifications and ductal carcinoma in situ than does mammography (8,22–25).

In 2006, Bruening et al. (25), in an analysis prepared for the Agency for Healthcare Quality and Research, evaluated various imaging techniques for women with an average risk level for breast cancer. Their findings indicated that if a woman with a suspicious lesion tests negative for breast cancer by MRI, her chance of actually having breast cancer drops from 20% to 3.8%. Thus, for every 1,000 women with an abnormal mammogram and a subsequent MRI interpreted to be negative, about 962 could have avoided an unnecessary biopsy, but 38 women would have missed cancers. It was concluded that the potential benefit of sparing patients from unnecessary biopsies did not outweigh the potential harm of missed or delayed diagnoses of breast cancer. Thus, mammography remains the most cost-effective screening modality available for the detection of early breast cancer.

Physicians recommending screening breast MRI as an adjunct to screening mammography should understand that MRI is associated with a certain false-positive rate just as screening mammography. In addition, when a "6-month follow-up" mammogram is recommended for a probably benign finding (Breast Imaging Reporting and Data Systems [BI-RADS] 3 diagnosis), the patient and the health care system incur considerably less cost than when a 6-month follow-up breast MRI is recommended for probably benign findings detected on MRI. The exact rate of BI-RADS 3 breast diagnoses on MRI has not been well characterized in the literature, but in the guidelines report of the ACS (5) it is stated that the specificity of MRI is significantly lower than that of mammography in all studies to date, resulting in more recalls and biopsies. Call-back rates for additional imaging range from 8% to 17% in the MRI screening studies, and biopsy rates range from 3% to 15%. The proportion of biopsies that are cancerous (positive predictive value) is 20% to 40% (11–15).

As provided in the data contained within Table 16C.5, the positive predictive value of biopsies performed based on abnormal MRI examinations ranges from 17% to 89% in the published literature. All of the data provided in Table 16C.5 are based on annual MRI screening, and there are few data regarding whether longer or shorter screening intervals might be more appropriate. Further, most reported data are based entirely on the first screening examination (i.e., the "prevalent screen") and there is a lack of data available for longer-term or repetitive MRI screenings (i.e., "incidence screens"). However, because MRI recommendations are for "adjunctive screening" in addition to screening mammography, it would be expected that the detection rates at both prevalent and incidence screens would be better than those for mammography alone. In a recently reported multi-center comparative study using multiple modalities to screen women at genetic-familial high risk for breast cancer, 11 breast cancers were found in 278 women in the first round and 7 breast cancers in 99 women in a second round of screening that included clinical breast examination, mammography, ultrasonography, and MRI (8). In 6 of the 18 patients (33%) cancer was detected only with breast MRI. The high sensitivity rate for MRI (94% vs. 50%, 59%, and 65% for clinical breast examination, mammography, and ultrasonography, respectively) was offset by its relatively lower positive predictive value of 63% (vs. 82%, 77%, and 65% for clinical breast examination, mammography, and ultrasonography, respectively). Of 20 false-positive findings that led to invasive diagnostic procedures, two were attributable

to the clinical breast examination, three to mammography, six to ultrasound, and nine to breast MRI. The authors did not report on their short-term interval follow-up recommendation rates in this interim report (8).

SHOULD ALL WOMEN WITH A DIAGNOSIS OF BREAST CANCER HAVE A BREAST MRI?

This question has been the center of recent discussions and debates at national surgical oncology conferences. One of the

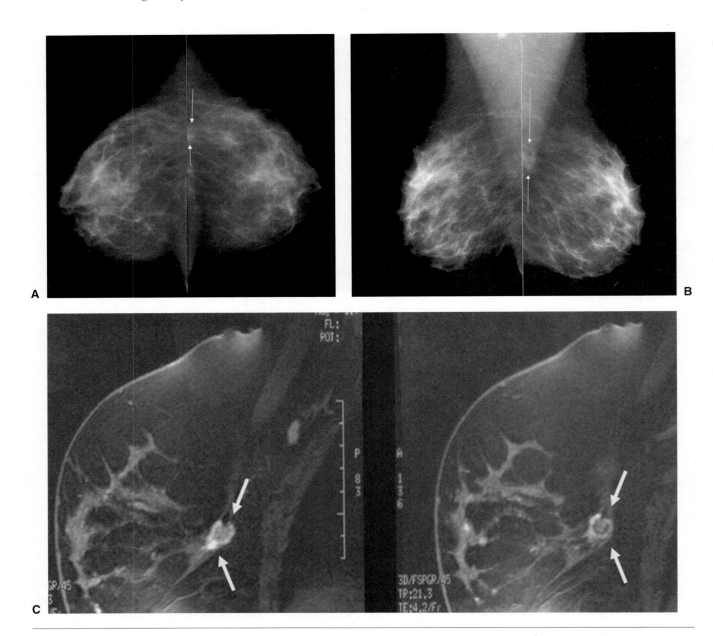

Figure 16C.1. Bilateral craniocaudal (**A**) and mediolateral oblique (**B**) mammographic images of a 52-year-old woman demonstrate vague density in the deep posterior aspect of the upper outer quadrant, left breast (*arrows*); new since mammogram of 1 year ago. Presurgical contrast-enhanced magnetic resonance image of left breast (**C**) demonstrates a suspicious, ring enhancing mass (*arrows*) proven to be infiltrating ductal carcinoma at biopsy.

difficulties in addressing the question concerns the imprecise indications in patient subpopulations often vaguely defined that might be considered for MRI. Indeed, when developing the technical applications and tools for breast MRI and its efficacious clinical applications, broadly defining patient populations into "women at high risk for breast cancer" (who undergo screening MRI as an adjunct to screening mammography) and "women with a recent diagnosis of breast cancer" (who undergo MRI for an array of indications) will likely prove suboptimal. Particularly for this latter population, MRI has been advocated for a myriad of suggested applications including: (A) to provide presurgical evaluation (Figure 16C.C1); (B) to assess extent of disease in the ipsilateral breast (Figure 16C.C2); (c) to evaluate for presence

of disease in the contralateral breast; (d) to provide postsurgical evaluation, such as evaluating for the presence of residual disease in patients with inadequately excised margins (Figure 16C.C3); (e) to investigate metastatic axillary adenopathy with unknown primary site; and (f) to evaluate tumor response to neoadjuvant chemotherapy (Figure 16C.C4) or other therapies.

Many breast surgeons believe that MRI performed for presurgical assessment of the extent of disease in the ipsilateral breast may yield information that precludes the feasibility of breast-conservation therapy or information that leads to a reduction in the occurrence of positive surgical margins when attempting primary treatment with lumpectomy. However, improved marginal status after lumpectomy has not yet been

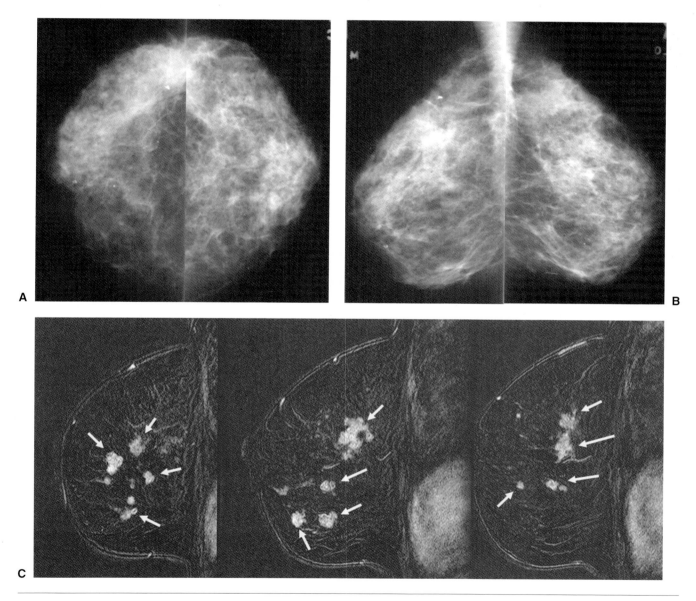

Figure 16C.2. Bilateral craniocaudal (**A**) and oblique mediolateral (**B**) mammography images show dense breast tissue with no definite abnormality in 43-year-old woman with palpable right breast mass. Contrast-enhanced magnetic resonance image of right breast (**C**) shows multiple lobulated and irregularly marginated masses (*arrows*) proven to be infiltrating lobular carcinoma on biopsy.

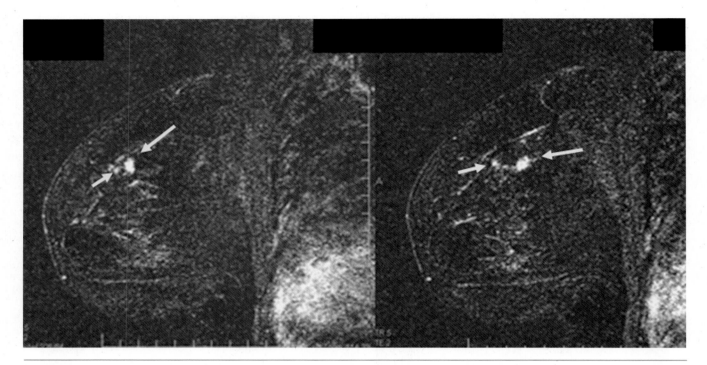

Figure 16C.3. Contrast-enhanced magnetic resonance images obtained to evaluate positive margins postoperatively show enhancing small mass and areas of enhancing nodularity (*arrows*) in surgical cavity that corresponded to area of residual ductal carcinoma on re-excision lumpectomy.

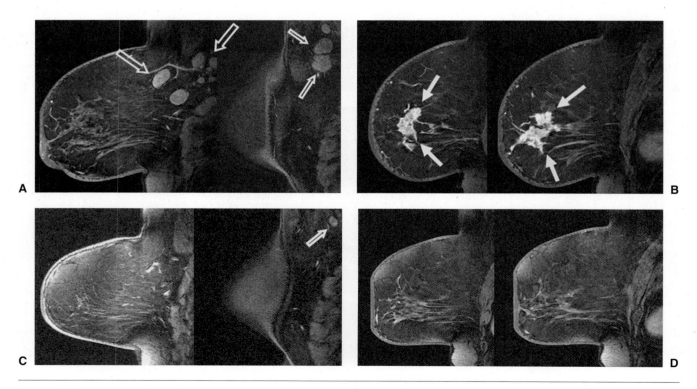

Figure 16C.4. Contrast-enhanced magnetic resonance image (MRI) **(A,B)** of 55-year-old woman with biopsy-proven ductal carcinoma prior to beginning neoadjuvant chemotherapy. Figure A shows extensive axillary adenopathy (*open arrows*) and Figure B shows enhancing, irregular mass (*arrows*). Following three cycles of chemotherapy, adenopathy is markedly reduced (*open arrow,* **C**) and mass is no longer visible on MRI **(D)**.

confirmed by data from clinical trials or other clinical studies. Similarly, some surgeons advocate preoperative MRI to detect occult contralateral disease which, if found, would allow management of both breasts at the same sitting. Lehman et al. (20) reported that MRI detected clinically and mammographically occult breast cancer in the contralateral breast in 3.1% of 969 women with recently diagnosed unilateral breast cancer.

Studies evaluating MRI for assessing response to neoadjuvant therapy have yielded mixed results. Current breast MRI technology may be ineffective in identifying complete responses to chemotherapy (and the potential of avoiding subsequent radiation therapy). Several case series reporting MRI used to evaluate tumor response to neoadjuvant chemotherapy found that the breast MRI can both overestimate and underestimate residual disease (26–28).

When breast MRI detects cancer that is not visualized on mammography or on breast sonography, the lesion must be localized and/or biopsied using MRI guidance. MRI-guided localizations and biopsies can be complex, time-consuming, and expensive because MR technology is considerably more expensive than mammography or ultrasound imaging systems.

Finally, depending on its utilization, breast MRI may not be cost-effective. Important determinants of breast MRI cost-effectiveness are (a) absolute risk for breast cancer (which may vary among specific genetic-familial aberrations), (b) mammography sensitivity (which may vary with parenchymal radiodensity), (c) MRI cost, and (d) quality of life gain from MRI (which varies with age and functional status). For instance, if all 135,000 women estimated to be newly diagnosed with breast cancer underwent breast MRI evaluations, at a cost $1,000 to $2,000 per breast MRI, an additional $135 million to $270 million in breast cancer care costs would accrue to the health care system. This would not include any additional MRI biopsies that might be recommended for abnormal scans.

Recent studies attempting to model the cost-effectiveness of breast MRI in genetically predisposed, high-risk populations have reported the incremental cost per additional cancer detected to be $27,500 to $50,900 (29). Screening strategies that incorporate annual MRI as well as annual mammography have a cost per quality-adjusted life-year (QALY) gained ranging from less than $45,000 to more than $700,000, depending on the ages selected for MRI screening and the specific *BRCA* mutation. Relative to screening with mammography alone, the cost per QALY gained by adding MRI from ages 35 to 54 years is $55,420 for *BRCA1* mutation carriers, $130,695 for *BRCA2* mutation carriers, and $98,454 for *BRCA2* mutation carriers who have mammographically dense breasts (30). Clearly, more work identifying the potential benefits of breast MRI needs to be done so that costs-per-life year saved and costs per QALY saved can be calculated.

SUMMARY

Recommendations regarding guidelines for incorporating breast MRI as a screening and/or evaluation tool for women at risk for or with a diagnosis of breast cancer are based on current evidence from recent clinical trials. However, there is currently a lack of solid outcome data to substantiate all suggested applications for breast MRI presented and discussed in published overviews and review articles. There are still no detailed data analyses on types of cancers, stage of disease, recurrence or survival rates, and lead-time bias. In summary, prior to adopting routine performance of breast MRI to evaluate all women with breast cancer, more substantial evidence of clinical benefit is needed, such as reduced recurrence rates (ipsilateral and contralateral) and improved overall- and disease-free survival. Imaging researchers must link future studies evaluating breast-imaging technologies like breast MRI to therapy trials with acceptable outcomes such as the impact of breast MRI on treatment decisions and survival.

REFERENCES

1. Fajardo LF, Berg WA, Smith RA. Breast imaging. In: Medina LS, Blackmore CC, eds. *Evidence-Based Imaging: Optimizing Imaging in Patient Care.* New York: Springer Science and Business Media; 2006:28–56, 2006.
2. Ries L, Harkins D, Krapcho M, et al, eds. *SEER Cancer Statistics Review, 1975-2003.* Bethesda, MD: National Cancer Institute; 2006.
3. Tabar L, Vitak B, Chen HH, et al. Beyond randomized controlled trials: organized mammographic screening substantially reduced breast cancer mortality. *Cancer.* 2001;91:1724–1731.
4. Farria DM, Schmidt ME, Monsees BS, et al. Professional and economic factors affecting access to mammography: a crisis today or tomorrow? Results from a national survey. *Cancer.* 2005;104:491–498.
5. Saslow D, Boetes CB, Burke W, et al. American Cancer Society guidelines for breast screening with MRI as an adjunct to mammography. *CA Cancer J Clin.* 2007;57:75–89.
6. Parmigiani G, Berry DA, Aguilar O. Determining carrier probabilities for breast cancer-susceptibility genes BRCA1 and BRCA2. *Am J Hum Genet.* 1998;62:145–158.
7. Berry DA, Parmigiani G, Sanchez J, et al. Probability of carrying a mutation of breast-ovarian cancer gene BRCA1 based on family history. *J Natl Cancer Inst.* 1997;89:227–238.
8. Sardanelli F, Podo F, Giuliano D, et al. Multicenter comparative multimodality surveillance of women at genetic-familial high risk for breast cancer (HIBCRIT Study): interim results. *Radiology.* 2007; 242:698–715.
9. Sardanelli F, Podo F. Breast MR imaging in women at high-risk for breast cancer. Is something changing in early breast cancer detection? *Eur Radiol.* 2007;17:873–887.
10. Port ER, Park A, Borgen PI, et al. Results of MRI screening for breast cancer in high-risk patients with LCIS and atypical hyperplasia. *Ann Surg Oncol.* 2007;14:1051–1057.
11. Lehman CD, Blume JD, Weatherall P, et al. Screening women at high risk for breast cancer with mammography and magnetic resonance imaging. *Cancer.* 2005;103:1898–1905.
12. Leach MO, Boggis CR, Dixon AK, et al. Screening with magnetic resonance imaging and mammography of a UK population with high familial risk of breast cancer: a prospective multicentre cohort study (MARIBS). *Lancet.* 2005;365:1769–1778.
13. Kuhl CS, Schrading S, Leutner CC, et al. Mammography, breast ultrasound and magnetic resonance imaging for surveillance of women at high familial risk for breast cancer. *J Clin Oncol.* 2005; 23:8469–8476.
14. Kriege M, Brekelmans CT, Boetes C, et al. Efficacy of MRI and mammography for breast cancer screening in women with a familial or genetic predisposition. *N Engl J Med.* 2004;351:427–437.

15. Warner E, Plewes DB, Hill KA, et al. Surveillance of BRCA1 and BRCA2 mutation carriers with magnetic resonance imaging, ultrasound, mammography and clinical breast examination. *JAMA.* 2004;292:1317–1325.

16. Kuhl CK, Schmultzler RK, Leutner CC, et al. Breast MR imaging screening in 192 women proved or suspected to be carriers of a breast cancer susceptibility gene: preliminary results. *Radiology.* 2000;215:267–279.

17. Lehman CD, Isaacs C, Schnall MD, et al. Cancer yield of mammography, MRI, and ultrasound in high risk women: prospective multi-institution breast cancer screening study. *Radiology.* 2007;244:381–388.

18. Morris EA, Liberman L, Ballon DJ, et al. MRI of occult breast carcinoma in a high-risk population. *AJR Am J Roentgenol.* 2003;181:619–626.

19. Podo F, Sardanelli F, Canese R, et al. The Italian multi-centre project on evaluation of MRI and other imaging modalities in early detection of breast cancer in subjects at high genetic risk. *J Exp Clin Cancer Res.* 2002;21:115–124.

20. Lehman CD, Gatsonis C, Kuhl CK, et al. MRI evaluation of the contralateral breast in women with recently diagnosed breast cancer. *N Engl J Med.* 2007;356:1295–1303.

21. Kuhl CK, Schrading S, Bieling NB, et al. MRI for diagnosis of pure ductal carcinoma in situ: a prospective observational study. *Lancet.* 2007;370:485–92.

22. Bazzocchi M, Zuiani C, Panizza P, et al. Contract-enhanced breast MRI in patients with suspicious microcalcifications on mammography: results of a multicenter trial. *AJR Am J Roentgenol.* 2006;186:1723–1732.

23. Tchiknavorian X, Perruchio S, Agin P, et al. Retrospective analysis of 561 breast magnetic resonance imaging (MRI): the largest study to date. *J Clin Oncol.* 2004;22(14S):712.

24. Boetes C, Strijik SP, Holland R. False-negative MR imaging of malignant breast tumors. *Eur Radiol.* 1997;7:1231–1234.

25. Bruening W, Launders J, Pinkney N, et al. *Effectiveness of Noninvasive Diagnostic Tests for Breast Abnormalities.* Comparative Effectiveness Review No. 2. Rockville, MD: Agency for Healthcare Research and Quality (AHRQ); 2006. AHRQ Publication No. 06-EHC005-EF.

26. Kwong MS, Chung GG, Horvath LJ, et al. Postchemotherapy MRI overestimates residual disease compared with histopathology in responders to neoadjuvant therapy for locally advanced breast cancer. *Cancer J.* 2006;12:212–221.

27. Nakamura S, Ishiyama M, Tsunoda-Shimizu H. Magnetic resonance mammography has limited ability to estimate pathological complete remission after primary chemotherapy or radiofrequency ablation therapy. *Breast Cancer.* 2007;14:123–130.

28. Chen JH, Mehta RS, Carpenter PM, et al. Magnetic resonance imaging in predicting pathological response of triple negative breast cancer following neoadjuvant chemotherapy. *J Clin Oncol.* 2007;25:5667–5669.

29. National Institute for Clinical Excellence (NICE), National Collaborating Centre for Primary Care. Familial breast cancer—the classification and care of women at risk of familial breast cancer in primary, secondary, and tertiary care. Partial update. Draft for consultation. May 2006. Available at: http://www.nice.org.uk/download.aspx?o= 317667. Accessed December 17, 2007.

30. Plevritis SK, Kurian AW, Sigal BM, et al. Cost-effectiveness of screening BRCA 1/2 carriers with breast magnetic resonance imaging. *JAMA.* 2006;295: 2374–2384.

17

Non-invasive and Premalignant Neoplasms of the Breast

Chapter 17A
Breast Cancer: Ductal Carcinoma in Situ:

Treatment Controversies and Oncoplastic Surgery

Melvin J. Silverstein

Ductal carcinoma in situ (DCIS) of the breast is a heterogeneous group of lesions with diverse malignant potential and a range of controversial treatment options. It is the most rapidly growing subgroup in the breast cancer family of disease, with more than 62,000 new cases diagnosed in the United States during 2006 (21% of all new cases of breast cancer) (1). Most new cases (>90%) are nonpalpable and discovered mammographically.

It is now well appreciated that DCIS is a stage in the neoplastic continuum in which most of the molecular changes that characterize invasive breast cancer are already present (2). All that remains on the way to invasion are quantitative changes in the expression of genes that have already been altered. Genes that may play a role in invasion control a number of functions, including angiogenesis, adhesion, cell motility, the composition of extracellular matrix, and more. To date, genes that are uniquely associated with invasion have not been identified. DCIS is clearly the precursor lesion for most invasive breast cancers but not all DCIS lesions have the time or the genetic ability to progress to become invasive breast cancer (3–5).

Therapy for DCIS ranges from simple excision to various forms of wider excision (e.g., segmental resection, quadrant resection, oncoplastic resection), all of which may or may not be followed by radiation therapy. When breast preservation is not feasible, total mastectomy, with or without immediate reconstruction, is generally performed.

Because DCIS is a heterogeneous group of lesions rather than a single entity (6,7) and because patients have a wide range of personal needs that must be considered during treatment selection, it is clear that no single approach will be appropriate for all forms of the disease or for all patients. At the current time, treatment decisions are based on a variety of measurable parameters (e.g., tumor extent, margin width, nuclear grade, comedo-type architecture, age), physician experience and bias, and on randomized trial data, which suggest that *all* conservatively treated patients should be managed with postexcisional radiation therapy.

THE CHANGING NATURE OF DUCTAL CARCINOMA IN SITU

There have been dramatic changes in the past 20 years that have affected DCIS. Before mammography was common, DCIS was rare, representing <1% of all breast cancer (8). Today, DCIS is common, representing 22% of all newly diagnosed cases and as much as 30% to 50% of cases of breast cancer diagnosed by mammography (1,9–13).

Previously, most patients with DCIS presented with clinical symptoms, such as breast mass, bloody nipple discharge, or Paget disease (14,15). Today, most lesions are nonpalpable and generally detected by mammography alone.

Until approximately 20 years ago, the treatment for most patients with DCIS was mastectomy. Today, almost 75% of newly diagnosed patients with DCIS are treated with breast preservation (16). In the past, when mastectomy was common, reconstruction was uncommon; if it was performed, it was generally done as a delayed procedure. Today, reconstruction for patients with DCIS treated by mastectomy is common; when it is performed, it is generally done immediately, at the time of mastectomy. In the past, when a mastectomy was performed, large amounts of skin were discarded. Today, it is considered perfectly safe to perform a skin-sparing mastectomy for DCIS. In the past, there was little confusion. All breast cancers were considered essentially the same and mastectomy was the only treatment. Today, all breast cancers are different and there is a range of acceptable treatments for every lesion. For those patients who choose breast conservation, there continues to be a debate as to whether radiation therapy is necessary in every case. These changes were brought about by a number of factors. Most important were increased mammographic utilization and the acceptance of breast-conservation therapy for invasive breast cancer.

The widespread use of mammography changed the way DCIS was detected. In addition, it changed the nature of the disease detected by allowing us to enter the neoplastic continuum at an earlier time. It is interesting to note the impact that mammography had on The Breast Center in Van Nuys, California, in terms of the number of DCIS cases diagnosed and the way they were diagnosed (17).

From 1979 to 1981, the Van Nuys Group treated a total of only 15 patients with DCIS, 5 per year. Only two lesions (13%) were nonpalpable and detected by mammography. In other words, 13 patients (87%) presented with clinically apparent disease. Two state-of-the-art mammography units and a full-time experienced radiologist were added in 1982 and the number of new DCIS cases increased to more than 30 per year, most of them nonpalpable. When a third machine was added in 1987, the number of new cases increased to 40 new cases per year. In 1994, the Van Nuys Group added a fourth mammography machine and a prone stereotactic biopsy unit. Analysis of the entire series of 1,236 patients through December 2005 shows that 1,081 lesions (87%) were nonpalpable (subclinical). If we look at only those diagnosed during the past 5 years at University of Southern California (USC)/Norris Cancer Center, 95% were nonpalpable.

The second factor that changed how we think about DCIS was the acceptance of breast-conservation therapy (lumpectomy, axillary node dissection, and radiation therapy) for patients with invasive breast cancer. Until 1980, the treatment for most patients with any form of breast cancer was generally mastectomy. Since that time, numerous prospective randomized trials have shown an equivalent rate of survival for selected patients with invasive breast cancer treated with breast-conservation therapy (18–22). Based on these results, it made little sense to continue treating less aggressive DCIS with mastectomy while treating more aggressive invasive breast cancer with breast preservation.

Current data suggest that many patients with DCIS can be successfully treated with breast preservation, with or without radiation therapy. This chapter will show how easily available data can be used to help in the complex treatment selection process.

PATHOLOGY

Classification

Although there is no universally accepted histopathologic classification, most pathologists divide DCIS into five architectural subtypes (papillary, micropapillary, cribriform, solid, and comedo), often comparing the first four (noncomedo) with comedo (6,13,23). Comedo DCIS is frequently associated with high nuclear grade (6,13,23,24) aneuploidy, a higher proliferation rate (25), *HER2/neu* gene amplification or protein overexpression (26–30), and clinically more aggressive behavior (31–34). Noncomedo lesions tend to be just the opposite.

The division by architecture alone, comedo versus noncomedo, is an oversimplification and does not work if the purpose of the division is to sort the patients into those with a high risk of local recurrence versus those with a low risk. It is not uncommon for high nuclear grade noncomedo lesions to express markers similar to those of high-grade comedo lesions and to have a risk of local recurrence similar to comedo lesions. Adding to the confusion is the fact that mixtures of various architectural subtypes within a single biopsy specimen are common. In my personal series, >70% of all lesions had significant amounts of two or more architectural subtypes, making division into a predominant architectural subtype problematic.

Regarding comedo DCIS, there is no uniform agreement among pathologists of exactly how much comedo DCIS needs to be present to consider the lesion a comedo DCIS. Although it is clear that lesions exhibiting a predominant high-grade comedo DCIS pattern are generally more aggressive and more likely to recur if treated conservatively than low-grade noncomedo lesions. Architectural subtyping does not reflect current biologic thinking. Rather, it is the concept of nuclear grading that has assumed importance. Nuclear grade is a better biologic predictor than architecture; therefore, it has emerged as a key histopathologic factor for identifying aggressive behavior (31,34–38). In 1995, the Van Nuys Group introduced a new pathologic DCIS classification (39) based on the presence or absence of high nuclear grade and comedo-type necrosis (the Van Nuys classification).

The Van Nuys Group chose high nuclear grade as the most important factor in their classification because there was general agreement that patients with high nuclear grade lesions were more likely to experience recurrence at a higher rate and in a shorter time period after breast conservation than patients with low nuclear grade lesions (31,34,37,40–42). Comedo-type necrosis was chosen because its presence also suggests a poorer prognosis (43,44) and it is easy to recognize (45).

The pathologist, using standardized criteria as noted later, first determines whether the lesion is high nuclear grade (nuclear grade 3) or non–high nuclear grade (nuclear grades 1 or 2). Then the presence or absence of necrosis is assessed in the non–high-grade lesions. This results in three groups (Figure 17A.1).

Nuclear grade is scored by previously described methods (39). Essentially, low-grade nuclei (grade 1) are defined as nuclei one to one and one-half red blood cells in diameter with diffuse chromatin and unapparent nucleoli. Intermediate nuclei (grade 2) are defined as nuclei one to two red blood cells in diameter with coarse chromatin and infrequent nucleoli. High-grade nuclei (grade 3) are defined as nuclei with a diameter greater than two red blood cells, with vesicular chromatin, and one or more nucleoli.

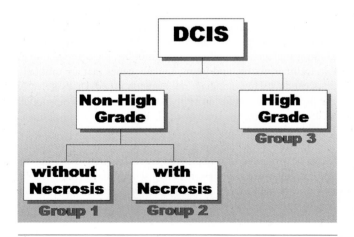

Figure 17A.1. Van Nuys ductal carcinoma in situ (DCIS) classification. DCIS patients are separated in high nuclear grade and non–high nuclear grade. Non–high nuclear grade cases are then separated by the presence or absence of necrosis. Lesions in group 3 (high nuclear grade) may or may not show necrosis.

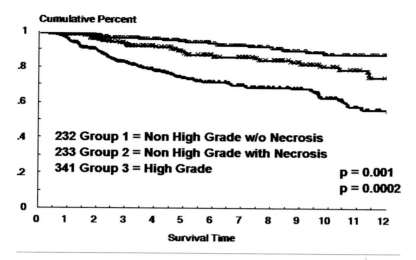

Figure 17A.2. Probability of local recurrence-free survival for 806 breast conservation patients using Van Nuys ductal carcinoma in situ pathologic classification (both p <0.01).

In the Van Nuys classification, no requirement is made for a minimum or specific amount of high nuclear grade DCIS, nor is there any requirement for a minimum amount of comedo-type necrosis. Occasional desquamated or individually necrotic cells are ignored and are not scored as comedo-type necrosis.

The most difficult part of most classifications is nuclear grading, particularly the intermediate-grade lesions. The subtleties of the intermediate-grade lesion are not important to the Van Nuys classification; only nuclear grade 3 needs be recognized. The cells must be large and pleomorphic, lack architectural differentiation and polarity, have prominent nucleoli and coarse clumped chromatin, and generally show mitoses (39,43).

The Van Nuys classification is useful because it divides DCIS into three different biologic groups with different risks of local recurrence after breast-conservation therapy (Figure 17A.2). This pathologic classification, when combined with tumor size, age, and margin status, is an integral part of the USC/Van Nuys Prognostic Index (USC/VNPI), a system that will be discussed in detail.

Progression to Invasive Breast Cancer

Which DCIS lesions will become invasive and when will that happen? These are the most important questions in the DCIS field today. Currently, there is intense molecular genetic study and knowledge regarding the progression of normal breast epithelium through hyperplastic and atypical hyperplastic changes to DCIS and then to invasive breast cancer. Most of the genetic and epigenetic changes present in invasive breast cancer are already present in DCIS. To date, no genes uniquely associated with invasive cancer have been identified (2,16). As DCIS progresses to invasive breast cancer, quantitative changes in the expression of genes related to angiogenesis, adhesion, cell motility, and the composition of the extracellular matrix may occur (2,16). Using gene array technology, researchers are attempting to identify high-risk patterns who will require quicker and more aggressive treatment.

Because most patients with DCIS have been treated with mastectomy, knowledge of the natural history of this disease is relatively scant. In a study of 110 consecutive, medicolegal autopsies of young and middle-aged women between the ages of 20 and 54 years, 14% were found to have DCIS (46), suggesting that the subclinical prevalence of DCIS is significantly higher than the clinical expression of the disease.

The studies of Page et al. (47), Sanders et al. (48), and Rosen et al. (49) enlighten us regarding the nontreatment of DCIS. In these studies, patients with noncomedo DCIS were initially misdiagnosed as having benign lesions and therefore went untreated. Subsequently, approximately 25% to 35% of these patients developed invasive breast cancer, generally within 10 years (47,48). Had the lesions been high-grade comedo DCIS, the invasive breast cancer rate likely would have been higher than 35%. With few exceptions, in both of these studies the invasive breast carcinoma was of the ductal type and located at the site of the original DCIS. These findings and the fact that autopsy series have shown up to a 14% incidence of DCIS suggest that not all DCIS lesions progress to invasive breast cancer or become clinically significant (46,50). There is far more microscopic DCIS than clinically apparent DCIS.

Page et al. (47, 51) and Sanders et al. (48) recently updated their series. Of 28 women with low-grade DCIS misdiagnosed with benign lesions and treated with biopsy between 1950 and 1968, 11 patients have had recurrence locally with invasive breast cancer (39%). Eight patients developed recurrence within the first 12 years. The remaining three were diagnosed over 23 to 42 years. Five patients developed metastatic breast cancer (18%) and died from the disease within 7 years of developing invasive breast cancer. These recurrence and mortality rates, at first glance, seem alarming. However, they are only slightly worse than what can be expected with long-term follow-up of patients with lobular carcinoma in situ, a disease that most clinicians are willing to treat with careful clinical follow-up. In addition, these patients were treated with biopsy only. No attempt was made to excise these lesions with a clear surgical margin. The natural history of low-grade DCIS can extend over 40 years and is markedly different from that of high-grade DCIS.

Microinvasion

The incidence of microinvasion is difficult to quantitate because until recently there was no formal and universally accepted definition of exactly what constitutes microinvasion. The 1997 edition of *The Manual for Cancer Staging* (5th edition) carried the first official definition of what is now classified as pT1mic and reads as follows: "Microinvasion is the extension of cancer cells beyond the basement membrane into adjacent tissues with no focus more than 0.1 cm in greatest dimension. When there are multiple foci of microinvasion the size of only the largest focus is used to classify the microinvasion (do not use the sum of all individual foci). The presence of multiple foci of microinvasion should be noted, as it is with multiple larger invasive carcinomas."

The reported incidence of occult invasion (invasive disease at mastectomy in patients with a biopsy diagnosis of DCIS) varies greatly, ranging from as little as 2% to as much as 21% (52). This problem was addressed in the investigations of Lagios et al. (31). They performed a meticulous serial subgross dissection correlated with specimen radiography. Occult invasion was found in 13 of 111 mastectomy specimens from patients who had initially undergone excisional biopsy of DCIS. All occult invasive cancers were associated with DCIS >45 mm in diameter; the incidence of occult invasion approached 50% for DCIS >55 mm. In the study of Gump et al. (53), foci of occult invasion were found in 11% of patients with palpable DCIS but in no patients with clinically occult DCIS. These results suggest a correlation between the size of the DCIS lesion and the incidence of occult invasion. Clearly, as the size of the DCIS lesion increases, microinvasion and occult invasion become more likely.

If even the smallest amount of invasion is found, the lesion should not be classified as DCIS. It is a T1mic (if the largest invasive component is ≤1 mm) with an extensive intraductal component. If the invasive component is 1.1 to 5 mm, it is a T1a lesion with an extensive intraductal component. If there is only a single focus of invasion, these patients do quite well. When there are many tiny foci of invasion, these patients have a poorer prognosis than expected. Unfortunately, the TNM staging system does not have a T category that fully reflects their malignant potential as they are classified by their largest single focus of invasion (10).

Multicentricity and Multifocality of Ductal Carcinoma in Situ

Multicentricity is generally defined as DCIS in a quadrant other than the quadrant in which the original DCIS (index quadrant) was diagnosed. There must be normal breast tissue separating the two foci. However, definitions of multicentricity vary among investigators. Hence, the reported incidence of multicentricity also varies. Rates from zero to 78% (7,49,54,55), averaging about 30%, have been reported. Twenty years ago, the 30% average rate of multicentricity was used by surgeons as the rationale for mastectomy in patients with DCIS. This was incorrect.

Holland et al. (56) evaluated 82 mastectomy specimens by taking a whole-organ section every 5 mm. Each section was ra-

diographed. Paraffin blocks were made from every radiographically suspicious spot. In addition, an average of 25 blocks was taken from the quadrant containing the index cancer; random samples were taken from all other quadrants, the central subareolar area, and the nipple. The microscopic extension of each lesion was verified on the radiographs. This technique permitted a three-dimensional reconstruction of each lesion. This study demonstrated that most DCIS lesions were larger than expected (50% were >50 mm), involved more than one quadrant by continuous extension (23%), but most importantly, were unicentric (98.8%). Only one of 82 mastectomy specimens (1.2%) had "true" multicentric distribution with a separate lesion in a different quadrant. This study suggests that complete excision of a DCIS lesion is possible due to unifocality but may be extremely difficult because of larger than expected size. In an update, Holland and Faverly (57) reported whole-organ studies in 119 patients, 118 of whom had unicentric disease. This information, when combined with the fact that most local recurrences are at or near the original DCIS, suggests that the problem of multicentricity per se is not important in the DCIS treatment decision-making process.

Multifocality is defined as separate foci of DCIS within the same ductal system. The studies of Holland et al. (56), Holland and Faverly (57), and Noguchi et al. (58) suggest that a great deal of multifocality may be artifactual, resulting from looking at a three-dimensional arborizing entity in two dimensions on a glass slide. It would be analogous to saying that the branches of a tree were not connected if the branches were cut at one plane, placed separately on a slide, and viewed in cross-section (47). Multifocality may be due to small gaps of DCIS or skip areas within ducts as described by Faverly et al. (42).

DETECTION AND DIAGNOSIS

The importance of quality mammography cannot be overemphasized. Currently, most patients with DCIS (>90%) present with nonpalpable lesions. A few percent of the cases of DCIS are detected as random findings during a biopsy for a breast thickening or some other benign fibrocystic change; most lesions, however, are detected by mammography. The most common mammographic findings are microcalcifications, frequently clustered and generally without an associated soft-tissue abnormality. More than 80% of DCIS patients exhibit microcalcifications on preoperative mammography. The patterns of these microcalcifications may be focal, diffuse, or ductal, with variable size and shape. Patients with comedo DCIS tend to have "casting calcifications." These are linear, branching, and bizarre and are almost pathognomonic for comedo DCIS (59) (Figure 17A.3). Almost all comedo lesions have calcifications that can be visualized on mammography.

Thirty-seven percent of noncomedo lesions in my personal series did not have mammographic calcifications, making them more difficult to find and the patients more difficult to follow, if treated conservatively. When noncomedo lesions are calcified, they tend to have fine, granular powdery calcifications or crushed stonelike calcifications (Figure 17A.4).

A major problem confronting surgeons relates to the fact that calcifications do not always map out the entire DCIS lesion,

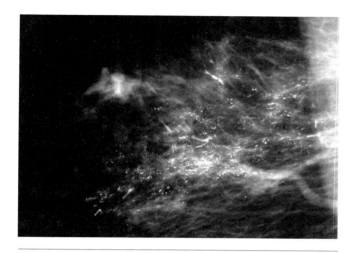

Figure 17A.3. Mediolateral mammography in a 43-year-old woman shows irregular branching calcifications. Histopathology showed high-grade comedo ductal carcinoma in situ, Van Nuys group 3.

particularly those of the noncomedo type. Even though all the calcifications are removed, in some cases noncalcified DCIS may be left behind. Conversely, in some patients, the majority of the calcifications are benign and map out a lesion bigger than the true DCIS lesion. In other words, the DCIS lesion may be smaller, larger, or the same size as the calcifications that led to its identification. Calcifications more accurately approximate the size of high-grade comedo lesions than low-grade noncomedo lesions (56).

Before mammography was common or of good quality, most DCIS was usually clinically apparent, diagnosed by palpation or inspection; it was gross disease. Gump et al. (53) divided DCIS by method of diagnosis into gross and microscopic disease. Similarly, Schwartz et al. (32) divided DCIS into two groups: clinical and subclinical. Both researchers thought patients presenting

with a palpable mass, a nipple discharge, or Paget disease of the nipple required more aggressive treatment. Schwartz et al. (32) believed that palpable DCIS should be treated as though it were an invasive lesion. They suggested that the pathologist simply has not found the area of invasion. Although it makes perfect sense to believe that the change from nonpalpable to palpable disease is a poor prognostic sign, our group has not been able to demonstrate this for DCIS. In our series, when equivalent patients (by size and nuclear grade) with palpable and nonpalpable DCIS were compared, they did not differ in the rate of local recurrence or mortality.

If a patient's mammogram shows an abnormality, most likely it will be microcalcifications, but it could be a nonpalpable mass or a subtle architectural distortion. At this point, additional radiologic workup needs to be performed. This may include compression mammography, magnification views, or ultrasonography. Magnetic resonance imaging is becoming increasingly popular to map out the size and shape of biopsy-proven DCIS lesions or invasive breast cancers.

Biopsy and Tissue Handling

If radiologic workup shows an occult lesion that requires biopsy, there are multiple approaches: fine-needle aspiration (FNA) biopsy, core biopsy (with various types and sizes of needles), and directed surgical biopsy using guide wires or radioactivity. FNA is generally of little help for nonpalpable DCIS. With FNA, it is possible to obtain cancer cells, but because there is insufficient tissue, there is no architecture. So although the cytopathologist can say that malignant cells are present, the cytopathologist generally cannot say whether the lesion is invasive. In addition, FNA of a nonpalpable lesion is difficult to perform. Because the lesion cannot be felt, the FNA must be performed under mammographic control.

Stereotactic core biopsy became widely available in the early 1990s and is now widely used. Dedicated digital tables make this a precise tool in experienced hands. Currently, large-gauge (11 gauge or larger) vacuum-assisted needles are the tools of choice for diagnosing DCIS. Ultrasound-guided biopsy also became very popular in the 1990s but is of less value for DCIS as most DCIS lesions do not present with a mass. All suspicious microcalcifications should be evaluated by ultrasound because a mass will be found in 5% to 15% of cases (9).

Open surgical biopsy should be used only if the lesion cannot be biopsied using minimally invasive techniques. This should be a rare event with current image-guided biopsy techniques (9). Needle localization segmental resection should be a critical part of the treatment, not the diagnosis.

Whenever needle localization excision is performed, whether for diagnosis or treatment, intraoperative specimen radiography and correlation with the preoperative mammogram should be performed. Margins should be inked or dyed and specimens should be serially sectioned at 3- to 4-mm intervals. The tissue sections should be arranged and processed in sequence. Pathologic reporting should include a description of all architectural subtypes, a determination of nuclear grade, an assessment of the presence or absence of necrosis, the measured size or extent of the lesion, and the margin status with measurement of the closest margin.

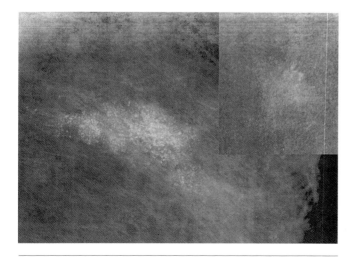

Figure 17A.4. *Left:* crushed stone-type calcifications. *Right inset:* fine granular powdery calcifications.

Tumor size should be determined by direct measurement or ocular micrometry from stained slides for smaller lesions. For larger lesions, a combination of direct measurement and estimation, based on the distribution of the lesion in a sequential series of slides, should be used. The proximity of DCIS to an inked margin should be determined by direct measurement or ocular micrometry. The closest single distance between any involved duct containing DCIS and an inked margin should be reported.

If the lesion is large and the diagnosis unproven, either stereotactic or ultrasound-guided vacuum-assisted biopsy should be the first step. If the patient is motivated for breast conservation, a multiple-wire–directed oncoplastic excision can be planned. This will give the patient her best chance at two opposing goals: clear margins and good cosmesis. The best chance at completely removing a large lesion is with a large initial excision. The best chance at good cosmesis is with a small initial excision. It is the surgeon's job to optimize these opposing goals. A large quadrant resection should not be performed unless there is histologic proof of malignancy. This type of resection may lead to breast deformity, and should the diagnosis prove to be benign, the patient will be unhappy.

Removal of nonpalpable lesions is best performed by an integrated team of surgeon, radiologist, and pathologist. The radiologist who places the wires and interprets the specimen radiograph must be experienced, as must the surgeon who removes the lesion and the pathologist who processes the tissue.

TREATMENT

For most patients with DCIS, there will be no single correct treatment. There will generally be a choice of treatments. The choices, although seemingly simple, are not simple at all. As the choices increase and become more complicated, frustration increases for both the patient and her physician (60,61).

Counseling the Patient with Biopsy-Proven Ductal Carcinoma in Situ

It is never easy to tell a patient that she has breast cancer. But is DCIS really cancer? From a biologic point of view, DCIS is unequivocally cancer. But when we think of cancer, we generally think of a disease that, if untreated, runs an inexorable course toward death. That is certainly not the case with DCIS (48). We must emphasize to the patient that she has a borderline cancerous lesion, a preinvasive lesion, which at this time is not a threat to her life. In our series of 1,236 patients with DCIS, the raw mortality rate is <1%. Numerous other DCIS series (62–65) confirm an extremely low mortality rate.

Patients often ask, why is there any mortality rate at all if DCIS is truly a noninvasive lesion? If DCIS recurs as an invasive lesion and the patient goes on to die from metastatic breast cancer, the source of the metastases is clear. But what about the patient who undergoes mastectomy and some time later develops metastatic disease, or a patient who is treated with breast preservation who never develops a local invasive recurrence but still dies of metastatic breast cancer? These latter patients probably had an invasive focus with established metastases at the time of their original treatment but the invasive focus was missed during routine histopathologic evaluation. No matter how carefully

and thoroughly a specimen in examined, it is still a sampling process and a 1- to 2-mm focus of invasion can be missed.

One of the most frequent concerns expressed by patients once a diagnosis of cancer has been made is the fear that the cancer has spread. We are able to assure patients with DCIS that no invasion was seen microscopically and the likelihood of systemic spread is minimal.

The patient needs to be educated that the term *breast cancer* encompasses a multitude of lesions of varying degrees of aggressiveness and lethal potential. The patient with DCIS needs to be reassured that she has a minimal lesion and that she is likely going to need some additional treatment, which may include surgery, radiation therapy, an antiestrogen, or some combination of these. She needs reassurance that she will not need chemotherapy, that her hair will not fall out, and that it is highly unlikely that she will die from this lesion. She will, of course, need careful clinical follow-up.

End Points for Patients with Ductal Carcinoma in Situ

When evaluating the results of treatment for patients with breast cancer, a variety of end points must be considered. Important end points include local recurrence (both invasive and DCIS), regional recurrence, distant recurrence, breast cancer-specific survival, overall survival, and quality of life. The importance of each end point varies depending on whether the patient has DCIS or invasive breast cancer.

When treating invasive cancer, the most important end points are distant recurrence and breast cancer-specific survival; in other words, living with or dying from breast cancer. For invasive breast cancer, a variety of different systemic treatments have been shown to significantly improve survival. These include a wide range of chemotherapeutic regimens and antiestrogens. Variations in local treatment do not affect survival (22,66). However, they do affect local recurrence.

DCIS is similar to invasive breast cancer in that variations in local treatment affect local recurrence, but no study to date has shown a significant difference in distant disease-free or breast cancer-specific survival, regardless of any treatment (systemic or local) and no study is likely to show a difference as there are so few breast cancer deaths in patients with pure DCIS. The most important outcome measure, breast cancer-specific survival, is essentially the same no matter what local or systemic treatment is given. Consequently, local recurrence has become the most commonly used end point when evaluating treatment for patients with DCIS.

Local recurrences are clearly important to prevent in patients treated with DCIS. They are demoralizing. They often lead to mastectomy and theoretically, if they are invasive, they upstage the patient and are a threat to life.

Following treatment for DCIS, 40% to 50% of all local recurrences are invasive. About 10% to 20% of DCIS patients who develop local invasive recurrences develop distant metastases and die from breast cancer (67,68). In the long term, this is likely to translate into a mortality rate of about 0% to 0.5% for patients treated with mastectomy, 1% to 2% for conservatively treated patients who receive radiation therapy, and 2% to 3% for patients treated with excision alone. In order to save their breasts, many patients are willing to accept this theoretic, and as of now statistically unproven, small absolute risk associated with breast conservation therapy.

Treatment Options

Mastectomy

Mastectomy is, by far, the most effective treatment available for DCIS if our goal is simply to prevent local recurrence. Most mastectomy series reveal local recurrence rates of approximately 1%, with mortality rates close to zero (69). But mastectomy is an aggressive form of treatment for patients with DCIS. It clearly provides a local recurrence benefit but only a theoretical survival benefit. It is, therefore, often difficult to justify mastectomy, particularly for otherwise healthy women with screen-detected DCIS, during an era of increasing utilization of breast conservation for invasive breast carcinoma. Mastectomy is indicated in cases of true multicentricity (multiquadrant disease) and when a unicentric DCIS lesion is too large to excise with clear margins and an acceptable cosmetic result.

Genetic positivity to one or more of the breast cancer-associated genes (*BRCA1*, *BRCA2*) is not an absolute contraindication to breast preservation but many patients who are genetically positive and who develop DCIS seriously consider bilateral mastectomy.

Breast Conservation

The most recently available Surveillance Epidemiology and End Results (SEER) data reveal that 72% of patients with DCIS are treated with breast conservation. Although breast conservation is now widely accepted as the treatment of choice for DCIS, not all patients are good candidates. Certainly, there are patients with DCIS whose local recurrence rate with breast preservation is so high (based on factors that will be discussed later in this chapter) that mastectomy is clearly a more appropriate treatment. However, the majority of women with DCIS diagnosed currently are candidates for breast conservation. Clinical trials have shown that local excision and radiation therapy in patients with negative margins can provide excellent rates of local control (62,65,70–73). However, even radiation therapy may be overly aggressive as many cases of DCIS may not recur or progress to invasive carcinoma when treated by excision alone (31,48,74–77).

Rationale for Excision Alone

There are four lines of reasoning that suggest that excision alone may be an acceptable treatment for selected patients with DCIS.

1. Anatomic: Evaluation of mastectomy specimens using the serial subgross tissue processing technique reveals that most DCIS is unicentric, meaning it involves a single breast segment and is radial in its distribution (38,42,56,57,78,79). This means that in many cases it is possible to excise the entire lesion with a segment or quadrant resection. Because DCIS, by definition, is not invasive and has not metastasized, it can be thought of in Halstedian terms. Complete excision should cure the patient without any additional therapy.

2. Biologic: Some DCIS is simply not aggressive; for example, small, well-excised, low-grade lesions bordering on atypical ductal hyperplasia. Lesions like this carry a low potential for development into an invasive lesion, about 1% per year at most (47,48,51,74,80,81). This is only slightly more than lobular carcinoma in situ, a lesion that is routinely treated with careful clinical follow-up.

3. Prospective randomized data: As will be pointed out throughout this chapter, these trials show no difference in breast cancer-specific survival, regardless of treatment after excision (62,65,73). If this is true, why not strive for the least aggressive treatment?

4. Radiotherapy may do harm: Numerous studies have shown that radiation therapy for breast cancer may increase mortality from both lung cancer and cardiovascular disease (82–86). More current radiotherapy techniques, which make use of computed tomography planning, make every attempt to spare the heart and lungs from radiation exposure, but long-term data are not available. If there is no proof that breast irradiation for patients with DCIS improves survival and there is proof that radiation therapy may cause harm, it makes perfect sense to spare patients from this potentially dangerous treatment whenever possible.

DISTANT DISEASE AND DEATH

When a patient with DCIS, previously treated by any modality, develops a local invasive recurrence, followed by distant disease and death due to breast cancer, this stepwise Halstedian progression makes sense. The patient has been upstaged by her local invasive recurrence. The invasive recurrence becomes the source of the metastatic disease and death is now a possibility.

In contrast, when a previously treated patient with DCIS develops distant disease and there has been no invasive local recurrence, a completely different sequence of events must be postulated. This sequence implies that invasive disease was present within the original lesion but was never discovered and it was already metastatic at the time of the original diagnosis. The best way to avoid missing an invasive cancer is with complete sequential tissue processing at the time the original lesion is treated. Nevertheless, even the most extensive evaluation may miss a tiny focus of invasion.

If even the tiniest invasive component is found during histopathologic evaluation, this patient can no longer be classified as having DCIS. She has invasive breast cancer and she needs to be treated as such. She will need sentinel node biopsy, and so forth, and appropriate medical oncologic consultation and aftercare.

THE PROSPECTIVE RANDOMIZED TRIALS

All of the prospective randomized trials have shown a significant reduction in local recurrence for patients treated with radiation therapy compared with excisional alone, but no trial has reported a survival benefit, regardless of treatment (62,65,70–73,87,88).

Only one trial has compared mastectomy with breast conservation for patients with DCIS and the data were only incidentally accrued. The National Surgical Adjuvant Breast Project (NSABP) performed protocol B-06, a prospective randomized trial for patients with invasive breast cancer (54,89). There were three treatment arms: total mastectomy, excision of the tumor plus radiation therapy, and excision alone. Axillary nodes were removed regardless of the treatment assignment.

During central slide review, a subgroup of 78 patients was confirmed to have pure DCIS without any evidence of invasion (54). After 83 months of follow-up, the percent of patients with local recurrences were as follows: zero for mastectomy, 7% for excision plus radiation therapy, and 43% for excision alone (90). In spite of these large differences in the rate of local recurrence for each different treatment, there was no difference among the three treatment groups in breast cancer-specific survival.

Contrary to the lack of trials comparing mastectomy with breast conservation, a number of prospective randomized trials comparing excision plus radiation therapy with excision alone for patients with DCIS are ongoing (91). Three have been published: the NSABP (protocol B-17) (70), the European Organization for Research and Treatment of Cancer (EORTC), protocol 10853 (73), and the United Kingdom, Australia, New Zealand DCIS Trial (UK Trial) (65).

The results of NSABP B-17 were updated in 1995 (88), 1998 (72), 1999 (71), and 2001 (62). In this study, more than 800 patients with DCIS excised with clear surgical margins were randomized into two groups: excision alone versus excision plus radiation therapy. The main end point of the study was local recurrence, invasive or noninvasive (DCIS). The definition of a clear margin was nontransection of the DCIS. In other words, only a fat or fibrous cell needed to be present between DCIS and the inked margin to call the margin clear. Many margins, of course, were likely much wider.

After 12 years of follow-up, there was a statistically significant, 50% decrease in local recurrence of both DCIS and invasive breast cancer in patients treated with radiation therapy. The overall local recurrence rate for patients treated by excision alone was 32% at 12 years. For patients treated with excision plus breast irradiation, it was 16%, a relative benefit of 50% (62). There was no difference in distant disease-free or overall survival in either arm. These updated data led the NSABP to confirm their 1993 position and to continue to recommend postoperative radiation therapy for all patients with DCIS who chose to save their breasts. This recommendation was clearly based primarily on the decreased local recurrence rate for those treated with radiation therapy, and secondarily on the potential survival advantage it might confer.

The early results of B-17, in favor of radiation therapy for patients with DCIS, led the NSABP to perform protocol B-24 (71). In this trial, more than 1,800 patients with DCIS were treated with excision and radiation therapy, and then randomized to receive either tamoxifen or placebo. After 7 years of follow-up, 11% of patients treated with placebo had recurred locally, whereas only 8% of those treated with tamoxifen had recurred (62). The difference, although small, was statistically significant for invasive local recurrence but not for noninvasive (DCIS) recurrence. Data presented at the 2002 San Antonio Breast Cancer Symposium suggested that the ipsilateral benefit

was seen only in estrogen receptor-positive patients (92). Again, there was no difference in distant disease-free or overall survival in either arm of the B-24 Trial.

The EORTC results were published in 2000 (73,87). This study was essentially identical to B-17 in design and margin definition. More than 1,000 patients were included. The data were updated at the San Antonio Breast Cancer Symposium in 2005 (93). After 10 years of follow-up, 15% of patients treated with excision plus radiation therapy had recurred locally compared with 26% of patients treated with excision alone, results similar to those obtained by the NSABP at the same point in their trial. As in the B-17 Trial, there was no difference in distant disease-free or overall survival in either arm of the EORTC Trial. In the initial report, there was a statistically significant increase in contralateral breast cancer in patients who were randomized to receive radiation therapy. This was not maintained when the data were updated.

The United Kingdom, Australia, New Zealand DCIS Trial (UK Trial) was published in 2003 (65). This trial, which involved more than 1,600 patients, performed a two-by-two study in which patients could be randomized into two separate trials within a trial. The patients and their doctors chose whether to be randomized in one or both studies. After excision with clear margins (same nontransection definition as the NSABP), patients were randomized to receive radiotherapy (yes or no) and/or to tamoxifen versus placebo. This yielded four subgroups: excision alone, excision plus radiation therapy, excision plus tamoxifen, and finally, excision plus radiation therapy plus tamoxifen. Those who received radiation therapy obtained a statistically significant decrease in ipsilateral breast tumor recurrence similar in magnitude to the ones shown by the NSABP and EORTC. Contrary to the findings of the NSABP, there was no significant benefit from tamoxifen. As with the NSABP and the EORTC, there was no benefit in terms of survival in any arm of the UK DCIS study.

Overall, these trials support the same conclusions. They all show that radiation therapy decreases local recurrence by a relative 50% and they all show no survival benefit, regardless of treatment. The only difference is that the NSABP B-24 Trial shows a significant decrease in local recurrence attributable to tamoxifen and the UK Trial does not.

With all the trials, as the amount of treatment increases, the rate of local recurrence decreases; but no matter how much treatment is increased, there is no improvement in survival. In fact, there could be a slight decrease in survival if there is a negative effect from radiation therapy.

LIMITATIONS OF THE PROSPECTIVE RANDOMIZED TRIALS

The randomized trials were designed to answer a single broad question: does radiation therapy decrease local recurrence? They have accomplished that goal. All have clearly shown that, overall, radiation therapy decreases local recurrence, but they cannot identify in which subgroups the benefit is so small, that the patients can be safely treated with excision alone?

Many of the parameters considered important in predicting local recurrence (e.g., tumor size, margin width, nuclear grade) were not routinely collected prospectively during the randomized DCIS trials. In addition, the trials did not specifically require the marking of margins or the measurement of margin width. The exact measurement of margin width was present in only 5% of the EORTC pathology reports (87). The NSABP did not require size measurements and many of their pathologic data were determined by retrospective slide review. In the initial NSABP report, >40% of patients had no size measurement (70). Unfortunately, if margins were not inked and tissues not completely sampled and sequentially submitted, then these predictive data can never be determined accurately by retrospective review.

The relative reduction in local recurrence seems to be the same in all three trials—about 50% for any given subgroup at any point in time. What does this relative reduction mean? If the absolute local recurrence rate is 30% at 10 years for a given subgroup of patients treated with excision alone, radiation therapy will reduce this rate by approximately 50%, leaving a group of patients with a 15% local recurrence rate at 10 years. Radiation therapy seems indicated for a subgroup with such a high local recurrence rate. But consider a more favorable subgroup, a group of patients with a 6% to 8% absolute recurrence rate at 10 years. These patients receive only a 3% to 4% absolute benefit. We must irradiate 100 women to see a 3% to 4% decrease in local recurrence. Here we must ask whether the benefits are worth the risks and costs involved and we should make every attempt possible to identify such low-risk subgroups.

Radiation therapy is expensive, time-consuming, and is accompanied by significant side effects in a small percentage of patients (e.g., cardiac, pulmonary) (91). Radiation fibrosis continues to occur but it is less common with current techniques than it was during the 1980s. Radiation fibrosis changes the texture of the breast and skin, makes mammographic follow-up more difficult, and may result in delayed diagnosis if there is a local recurrence. The use of radiation therapy for DCIS precludes its use if an invasive recurrence develops at a later date. The use of radiation therapy with its accompanying skin and vascular changes make skin-sparing mastectomy, if needed in the future, more difficult to perform.

Most importantly, if we give radiation therapy for DCIS, we must assume all of these risks and costs without any proven distant disease-free or breast cancer-specific survival benefits. The only proven benefit will be a decrease in local recurrence. It is important, therefore, to carefully examine the need for radiation therapy in all conservatively treated patients with DCIS. The NSABP has recently agreed that all patients with DCIS may not need postexcisional radiation therapy (62). The problem is how to accurately identify those patients. If we can identify subgroups of patients with DCIS in which the probability of local recurrence after excision alone is low, they may be the patients in whom the costs, risks, and side effects of radiotherapy outweigh the benefits.

In spite of the randomized data that suggest that all conservatively treated patients benefit from radiation therapy, American doctors and patients have embraced the concept of excision alone. The 1999 SEER data reveal that 72% of patients with DCIS were treated with breast conservation. Almost half of these conservatively treated patients (46%) were treated with excision alone. When all patients with DCIS are considered, 28% received mastectomy, 39% excision plus radiation therapy, and 33% were treated with excision alone. It is clear that both American doctors and American patients are not blindly following the results and the recommendations of the prospective trials.

PREDICTING LOCAL RECURRENCE IN CONSERVATIVELY TREATED PATIENTS WITH DCIS

There is now sufficient, readily available information that can aid clinicians in differentiating patients who significantly benefit from radiation therapy after excision from those who do not. These same data can point out patients who are better served by mastectomy because recurrence rates with breast conservation are unacceptably high even with the addition of radiation therapy.

Our research (39,94–97) and the research of others (31,34,37,43,44,75,76,81,88,98) has shown that various combinations of nuclear grade, the presence of comedo-type necrosis, tumor size, margin width, and age are all important factors that can be used to predict the probability of local recurrence in conservatively treated patients with DCIS.

The Original Van Nuys Prognostic Index and Its Updated Version

In 1995, the Van Nuys DCIS pathologic classification, based on nuclear grade and the presence or absence of comedonecrosis, was developed (39) (Figure 17A.1). Nuclear grade and comedo-type necrosis reflect the biology of the lesion, but neither alone nor together are they adequate as the guidelines in the treatment decision-making process. Tumor size and margin width reflect the extent of disease, the adequacy of surgical treatment, and the likelihood of residual disease, and are of paramount importance.

The challenge was to devise a system using these variables (all independently important by multivariate analysis) that would be clinically valid, therapeutically useful, and user-friendly. The original Van Nuys Prognostic Index (VNPI) (36,99) was devised in 1996 by combining tumor size, margin width, and pathologic classification (determined by nuclear grade and the presence or absence of comedo-type necrosis). All of these factors had been collected prospectively in a large series of DCIS patients who were selectively treated (nonrandomized) (100).

A score, ranging from 1 for lesions with the best prognosis to 3 for lesions with the worst prognosis, was given for each of the three prognostic predictors. The objective with all three predictors was to create three statistically different subgroups for each, using local recurrence as the marker of treatment failure. Cutoff points (e.g., what size or margin width constitutes low, intermediate, or high risk of local recurrence) were determined statistically, using the log rank test with an optimum p-value approach.

Size Score

A score of 1 was given for a small tumors ≤15 mm, 2 was given for intermediate-sized tumors 16 to 40 mm, and 3 was given for large tumors ≥41 mm in diameter. The determination of size required complete and sequential tissue processing along with mammographic/pathologic correlation Size was

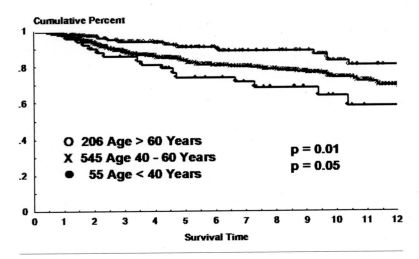

Figure 17A.5. Probability of local recurrence-free survival by age group for 806 breast conservation patients (both $p \leq 0.05$).

determined over a series of sections rather than on a single section and is the most difficult parameter to reproduce. If a 3-cm specimen is cut into 10 blocks, each block is estimated to be 3 mm thick. If a lesion measuring 5 mm in maximum diameter on a single slide appears in an out of 7 sequential blocks, it is estimated to be 21 mm (3 mm × 7) in maximum size, not 5 mm. As measured on a single slide. The maximum diameter on a single slide was the way the size was measured for most of the patients in the prospective randomized trials.

Margin Score

A score of 1 was given for widely clear tumor-free margins of ≥ 10 mm. This was often achieved by re-excision with the finding of no residual DCIS or only focal residual DCIS in the wall of the biopsy cavity. A score of 2 was given for intermediate margins of 1 to 9 mm and a score of 3 for margins <1 mm (involved or close margins).

Pathologic Classification Score

A score of 3 was given for tumors classified as group 3 (high-grade lesions), 2 for tumors classified as group 2 (non–high-grade lesions with comedo-type necrosis), and a score of 1 for tumors classified as group 1 (non–high-grade lesion without comedo-type necrosis) (39,101). The classification is diagrammed in Figure 17A.1.

The final formula for the original Van Nuys Prognostic Index (VNPI) became:

$$VNPI = pathologic\ classification\ score + margin\ score + size\ score$$

The University of Southern California/ Van Nuys Prognostic Index

By early 2001, a multivariate analysis at the University of Southern California (USC) revealed that age was also an independent prognostic factor in our database and that it should be added to the VNPI with a weight equal to that of the other factors (96,97,102).

An analysis of our local recurrence data by age revealed that the most appropriate break points for our data were between ages 39 and 40 and between ages 60 and 61 (Figure 17A.5). Based on this, a score of 3 was given to all patients 39 years old or younger, a score of 2 was given to patients aged 40 to 60, and a score of 1 was given to patients 61 or older. The new scoring system for the USC/VNPI is shown in Table 17A.1. The final formula for the USC/VNPI became:

$$USC/VNPI = pathologic\ classification\ score + margin\ score + size\ score + age\ score$$

Scores range from 4 to 12. The patients least likely to have recurrence after conservative therapy had a score of 4 (small, low-grade, well-excised lesions in older women). The patients most likely to have recurrence had a score of 12 (large, poorly excised, high-grade lesions in younger women). The probability of recurrence increased as the USC/VNPI score increased.

Updated Results Using the USC/VNPI

Through December 2005, our group treated 1,240 patients with pure DCIS. Four hundred thirty-four patients were treated with mastectomy and are not included in any analysis that uses local recurrence as the end point. Eight hundred six patients were treated with breast conservation: 496 by excision alone and 310 by excision plus radiation therapy. The average follow-up for all patients was 81 months: 79 months for mastectomy, 105 months for excision plus radiation therapy, and 65 months for excision alone.

There were 144 local failures, 42% of which were invasive. The probability of local failure was reduced, overall, by 60% if radiation therapy was given, a result almost identical with the prospective randomized trials. The local recurrence-free survival in shown by treatment in Figure 17A.6. As expected, at any point in time, mastectomy had the lowest probability of local recurrence and excision alone had the highest.

Seven patients (2.5%) treated with radiation therapy developed local recurrences and distant metastases, six of whom

Table 17A.1

The University of Southern California/Van Nuys Prognostic Index (USC/VNPI) Scoring System[a]

Score	1	2	3
Size (mm)	≤15	16–40	≥41
Margins (mm)	≥10	1–9	<1
Pathologic classification	Non–high grade without necrosis	Non–high grade with necrosis	High grade with or without necrosis
Age (years)	≥61	40–60	≤39

[a] One to three points are awarded for each of four different predictors of local breast recurrence (size, margins, pathologic classification, and age). Scores for each of the predictors are totaled to yield a USC/VNPI score ranging from a low of 4 to a high of 12.

have died from breast cancer. One patients (0.2%) treated with excision alone developed local invasive recurrence and metastatic disease and died from breast cancer. Two patients with mastectomy developed distant disease after developing local invasive recurrences. One has died from breast cancer. There is no statistical difference in breast cancer-specific survival (Figure 17A.7) or overall survival (Figure 17A.8) when patients treated with excision alone, excision plus irradiation, or mastectomy are compared.

Seventy-one additional patients have died from other causes without evidence of recurrent breast cancer. The 12-year actuarial overall survival, including deaths from all causes, is 90%. It is virtually the same for all three treatment groups and for all three USC/VNPI groups (Figure 17A.9).

The local recurrence-free survival for all 806 breast conservation patients is shown by tumor size in Figure 17A.10, by margin width in Figure 17A.11, by pathologic classification in Figure 17A.2, and by age in Figure 17A.5. The differences between every local disease-free survival curve for each of the four predictors that make up the USC/VNPI are statistically significant.

Figure 17A.12 groups patients with low (USC/VNPI = 4, 5, or 6), intermediate (USC/VNPI = 7, 8, or 9), or high (USC/VNPI = 10, 11, or 12) risks of local recurrence together. Each of these three groups is statistically different from one another.

Patients with USC/VNPI scores of 4, 5, or 6 do not show a local recurrence-free survival benefit from breast irradiation (Figure 17A.13) (p = NS). Patients with an intermediate rate of local recurrence, USC/VNPI 7, 8, or 9, are benefited by irradiation (Figure 17A.14). There is a statistically significant decrease in the probability of local recurrence, averaging 12% to 15% throughout the curves, for irradiated patients with intermediate USC/VNPI scores compared with those treated by excision alone (p = 0.02). Figure 17A.15 divides patients with a USC/VNPI of 10, 11, or 12 into those treated by excision plus irradiation and those treated by excision alone. Although the difference between the two groups is highly significant (p = 0.001), conservatively treated DCIS patients with a USC/VNPI of 10, 11, or 12 recur at an extremely high rate even with radiation therapy.

CURRENT TREATMENT TRENDS

In the current era of evidence-based medicine, it is reasonable to interpret the prospective randomized data as support for the tenet that all conservatively treated patients with DCIS should receive postexcisional radiation therapy. However, in spite of these

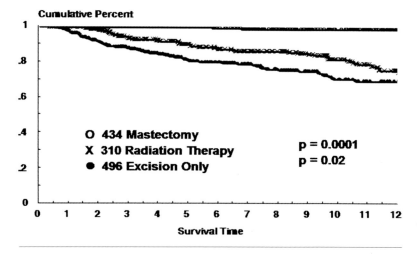

Figure 17A.6. Probability of local recurrence-free survival by treatment for 1,240 patients with ductal carcinoma in situ (p ≤0.03).

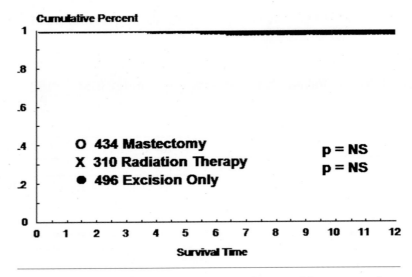

Figure 17A.7. Probability of breast cancer-specific survival by treatment for 1,240 patients with ductal carcinoma in situ ($p =$ NS [not significant]).

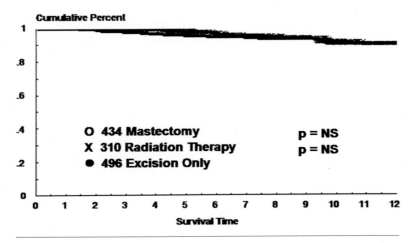

Figure 17A.8. Probability of overall survival by treatment for 1,240 patients with ductal carcinoma in situ ($p =$ NS [not significant]).

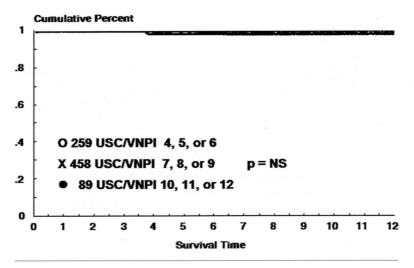

Figure 17A.9. Probability of breast cancer-specific survival for 806 breast-conservation patients grouped by Modified University of Southern California/Van Nuys Prognostic Index (USC/VNPI) score (4, 5, or 6 vs. 7, 8, or 9 vs. 10, 11, or 12) ($p =$ NS [not significant]).

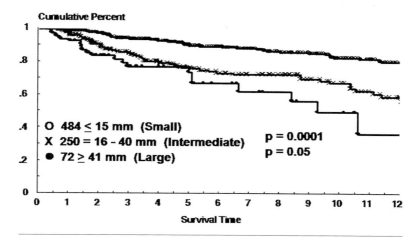

Figure 17A.10. Probability of local recurrence-free survival by tumor size for 806 breast-conservation patients (both $p \leq 0.05$).

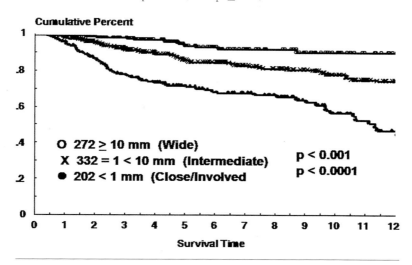

Figure 17A.11. Probability of local recurrence-free survival by margin width for 806 breast-conservation patients (both $p \leq 0.001$).

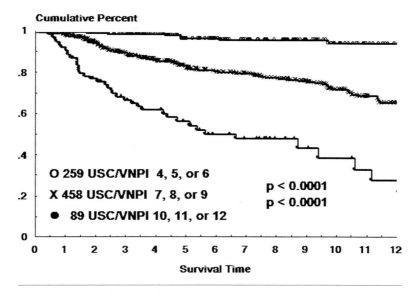

Figure 17A.12. Probability of local recurrence-free survival for 806 breast-conservation patients grouped by University of Southern California/Van Nuys Prognostic Index (USC/VNPI) score (4, 5, or 6 vs. 7, 8, or 9 vs. 10, 11, or 12) (both $p <0.00001$).

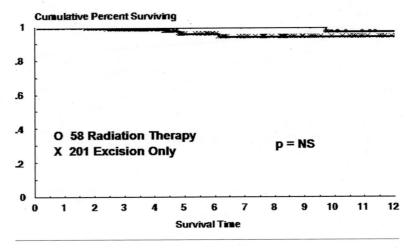

Figure 17A.13. Probability of local recurrence-free survival by treatment for 259 breast-conservation patients with University of Southern California/Van Nuys Prognostic Index scores of 4, 5, or 6 (p = NS [not significant]).

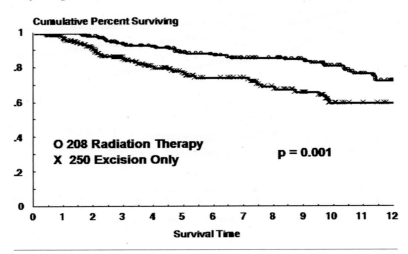

Figure 17A.14. Probability of local recurrence-free survival by treatment for 458 breast-conservation patients with University of Southern California/Van Nuys Prognostic Index scores of 7, 8, or 9 ($p \leq 0.01$).

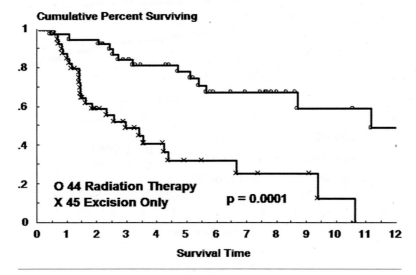

Figure 17A.15. Probability of local recurrence-free survival by treatment for 89 breast conservation patients with modified University of Southern California/Van Nuys Prognostic Index scores of 10, 11, or 12 ($p = 0.0001$).

Table 17A.2

Treatment Guidelines Based on the University of Southern California/Van Nuys Prognostic Index (USC/Van Nuys Prognostic Index)

USC/VNPI Score	Recommended Treatment
4–6	Excision only
7–9	Excision + radiation
10–12	Mastectomy

data, the number of patients with DCIS being treated with excision alone continues to increase. The 1999 SEER data revealed that approximately one third of all patients with DCIS in the United States are now being treated with excision alone (16,103).

As an aid to the complex treatment decision-making process, the USC/VNPI can be used as a staring point to suggest reasonable treatment options supported by local recurrence data. The USC/VNPI divides patients with DCIS into three groups with differing probabilities of local recurrence after breast-conserving surgery. Although there is an apparent treatment choice for each group (Table 17A.2), excision alone for patients who score 4 to 6, excision plus radiation therapy for patients who score 7 to 9, and mastectomy for those who score 10 to 12, the USC/VNPI is offered only as a guideline, a starting place for discussions with patients.

THE USE OF MARGIN WIDTH AS THE SOLE PREDICTOR OF LOCAL RECURRENCE

Determining size has always been the most difficult part of the USC/VNPI. Our method computes size over a series of sections rather than on a single slide (unless the measurement on a single slide is larger) and correlates this with the mammographic findings. For example, if a 6 × 4 mm DCIS appears in and out of 7 consecutive sections and the blocks are on average 3 mm wide, the diameter of this lesion would be recorded as a 21 mm DCIS (7 blocks × 3 mm average block width) in our database. In many other databases, it would be a 6-mm DCIS, the largest diameter on a single section.

By way of example, when the NSABP reviewed their pathologic material for the B-17 study, 75% to 90% of their cases were measured at ≤10 mm in extent (62,104). The NSABP reported tumor size as the largest diameter on a single slide. Although this is clearly the simplest and most reproducible way to measure DCIS, it is often an underestimation. Compare the NSABP sizes with our cases in which only 45% (365/806) of our conservatively treated patients had DCIS lesions measuring ≤10 mm. It is unlikely that the NSABP had twice as many smaller cases than a single group devoted to diagnosing and treating DCIS. Rather, the explanation probably lies in the way tissue was processed and the method used to estimate tumor size. In all likelihood, both groups treated tumors of similar size.

Because of the difficulty of estimating size, in 1997 we began evaluating the possibility of using margin width as the sole predictor of local recurrence, as a surrogate for the USC/VNPI (95). The rationale was based on a multivariate analysis wherein patients with margin widths <1 mm had a ninefold increase in the probability of local recurrence compared with patients who had ≥10 mm margin widths. Narrow margin width was the single most powerful predictor of local failure.

In the current data set presented here, there were 272 patients with margin widths of ≥10 mm, 13 of whom (4.8%) have developed a local recurrence (1 in the radiotherapy group and 12 within the excision-only group) (Figure 17A.16). The local recurrence benefit for radiation therapy neared significance ($p = 0.06$). In spite of this, the actuarial local recurrence rate at 12 years for those treated with excision alone was only 14%, virtually identical to that reported by the NSABP at 12 years for all patients treated with excision plus radiation therapy (62).

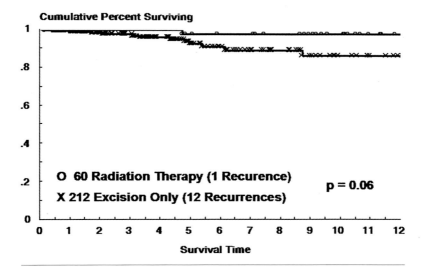

Figure 17A.16. Probability of local recurrence-free survival by treatment for 272 breast conservation patients with margins widths ≥10 mm ($p = 0.06$).

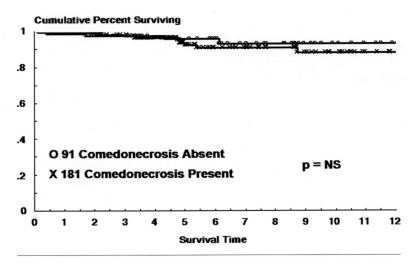

Figure 17A.17. Probability of local recurrence-free survival by the presence or absence of comedonecrosis for 272 breast-conservation patients with margins widths ≥10 mm (p = NS [not significant]).

There were 259 patients with USC/VNPI scores of 4, 5, or 6, four of whom (1.5%) have developed a local recurrence (Figure 17A.13). The USC/VNPI is a better predictor of local recurrence than margin width alone (half as many recurrences) and it should be, as it is based on five predictive factors, including margin width. Nevertheless, there are so few recurrences among patients with widely clear margins that for all practical purposes, margin width can be used by itself as a surrogate for the USC/VNPI.

Figures 17A.17 through 17A.20 evaluate local recurrence by various parameters for patients with ≥10 mm margin widths. Figure 17A.17 shows that if widely clear margins are obtained, the presence of comedonecrosis does not significantly increase the local recurrence rate. Figure 17A.18 shows that if widely clear margins are obtained, high nuclear grade (grade 3) does not significantly increase the local recurrence rate. Figure 17A.19

shows that if widely clear margins are obtained, young age does not significantly increase the local recurrence rate. Figure 17A.20 shows that if widely clear margins are obtained, large size may continue to increase the local recurrence rate, although there are too few lesions >40 mm with ≥10 mm margins (n = 14) to draw firm conclusions.

TREATMENT OF THE AXILLA FOR PATIENTS WITH DCIS

In 1986, our group suggested that axillary lymph node dissection be abandoned for DCIS (105). In 1987, the NSABP made axillary node dissection for patients with DCIS optional, at the discretion of the surgeon. Since that time, we have

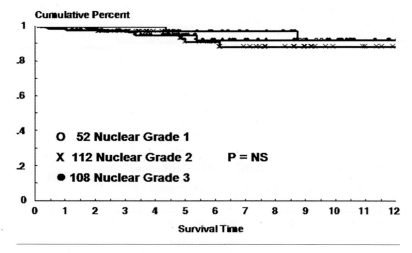

Figure 17A.18. Probability of local recurrence-free survival by nuclear grade for 272 breast-conservation patients with margins widths ≥10 mm (p = NS [not significant]).

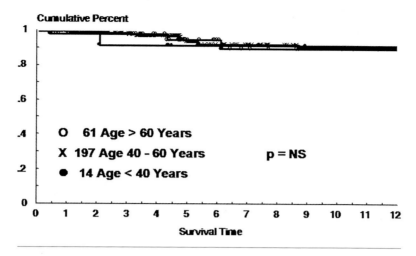

Figure 17A.19. Probability of local recurrence-free survival by age 272 breast-conservation patients with margins widths ≥10 mm ($p =$ NS [not significant]).

published a series of articles that continue to show that axillary node dissection is not indicated for patients with DCIS (94,106). To date, our group has performed a total of 571 node evaluations, 2 of which (0.5%) contained positive nodes by hematoxylin and eosin (H&E) staining. Both those patients were treated with adjuvant chemotherapy. Both were alive and well without local or distant recurrence at 8 and 10 years after their initial surgery (both had mastectomies, and invasive cancer was likely missed during the serial sectioning of their specimens).

Frykberg et al. (107), in their review of the management of DCIS, compiled the data of 9 studies with a total of 754 patients. The incidence of axillary lymph node metastasis for patients with DCIS was 1.7%. Despite these low probabilities of nodal positivity, some authors continue to advocate removal of the axillary nodes in patients with palpable or extensive DCIS

because of their belief that these patients have a higher risk of occult invasion and positive nodes.

Sentinel Node Biopsy for DCIS

Through December 2005, I have performed 171 sentinel node biopsies for patients with DCIS. All were negative by H&E; 10 (6%) were positive by immunohistochemical (IHC) assay. In every case there were only a few positive cells (range, 4 to 93). In no case were there patients upstaged to stage II nor were any treated with chemotherapy. All are alive and well without distant recurrence with follow-up ranging from 0.5 to 9.7 years (average, 2.9 years).

Not all IHC-positive cells are cancer cells. Some may merely by cytokeratin-positive debris. Their morphology must be looked at closely.

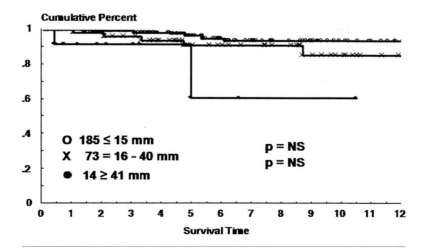

Figure 17A.20. Probability of local recurrence-free survival by tumor size for 272 breast-conservation patients with margins widths ≥10 mm ($p =$ NS [not significant]).

My policy for sentinel node biopsy in patients with DCIS is as follows. I perform it in all patients with DCIS who are undergoing a mastectomy. I perform it if the DCIS is an upper outer-quadrant lesion and the sentinel node can be easily removed through the same incision. I also remove a sentinel node if the DCIS is palpable, or larger (>4 cm on mammography).

ONCOPLASTIC RESECTION

When treating a patient with biopsy-proven DCIS, surgeons have generally made a small, cosmetically placed curvilinear incision over the area to be removed. They excised no skin, took a relatively small piece of breast tissue, accepted nontransection as the definition of clear margins, did not require complete and sequential tissue processing, and used radiation therapy routinely. But the trend is changing. During the last 20 years, my colleagues and I have developed a comprehensive multidisciplinary oncoplastic approach for DCIS (106,108,109). It requires surgical coordination with a pathologist, a radiologist, and often a plastic surgeon, and it is gaining in popularity.

Oncoplastic surgery combines sound surgical oncologic principles with plastic surgical techniques. Coordination of the two surgical disciplines may help to avoid poor cosmetic results after wide excision and may increase the number of women who can be treated with breast-conserving surgery by allowing larger breast excisions with more acceptable cosmetic results. Although this chapter is about DCIS, these techniques are applicable to patients with invasive breast cancer.

As mentioned earlier, DCIS generally involves a single breast segment and is commonly distributed in a radial fashion. Serial subgross whole-organ sectioning suggests that when margin widths exceed 10 mm the likelihood of residual disease is relatively small (57). With these facts in mind, the goal with biopsy-proven DCIS is to widely excise the entire involved ductal unit in a radial fashion in the most cosmetically acceptable way possible.

Oncoplastic resection is a therapeutic procedure, not a breast biopsy. It is performed on patients with a proven diagnosis of breast cancer. This approach was strongly supported by the 2005 Consensus Conference on Image-Detected Breast Cancer (9).

An important goal in caring for a woman with breast cancer is to go to the operating room a single time and to perform a definitive procedure that does not require reoperation. Whenever possible, the initial breast biopsy should be made using a minimally invasive percutaneous technique (9). This usually provides ample tissue for diagnosis, the rate of upgrading to invasive breast cancer is low (around 10% to 15%), and the core biopsy site is small and can be closed with a Steri-Strip.

When excising a lesion that is DCIS, the surgeon faces two opposing goals: clear margins versus an acceptable cosmetic result. From an oncologic point of view, the largest specimen possible should be removed in an attempt to achieve the widest possible margins. From a cosmetic point of view, a much smaller amount of tissue should be removed. The first attempt to remove a cancerous lesion is critical. The first excision offers the best chance to remove the entire lesion in one piece, evaluate its extent and margin status, and to achieve the best possible cosmetic result. Because more than 90% of currently diagnosed DCIS cases are grossly both nonpalpable and nonvisualizable, the surgeon essentially operates blindly. Multiple hooked wires can help define the extent of the lesion radiographically (Figure 17A.21). Using bracketing wires, the surgeon should make an

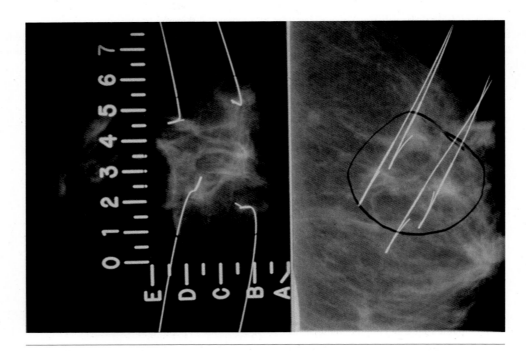

Figure 17A.21. Craniocaudal (left) and mediolateral (right) mammograms showing four wires bracketing an area of architectural distortion that turned out to be a micropapillary ductal carcinoma in situ.

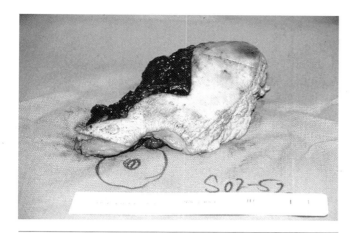

Figure 17A.22. A color-coded specimen from a hemibatwing excision. Skin, full thickness of breast, and pectoral fascia have been removed.

attempt to excise the entire lesion within a single piece of tissue. This should include overlying skin as well as pectoral fascia (Figure 17A.22).

If the specimen is removed in multiple pieces rather than a single piece, there is little likelihood of evaluating margins and size accurately. Figure 17A.23 shows an excision specimen with four additional pieces that allegedly represent the new margins. The additional pieces are too small and do not reflect the true margins of the original specimen. If one makes a judgment on margin clearance based on these small additional pieces, that judgment might very well be wrong.

Complete excision of DCIS should not be attempted using a single guide wire, as it may result in incomplete removal of

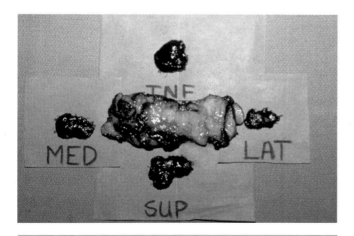

Figure 17A.23. An excision specimen with four additional pieces of tissue that allegedly represent the new margins. The additional pieces are too small and do not reflect the true margins of the original specimen. If one makes a judgment on margin clearance based on these small additional pieces, that judgment might very well be wrong. MED, medial; TNF, tumor necrosis factor; LAT, lateral; SUP, superior.

the abnormality and the need to re-excise the biopsy cavity. The bracketing wire technique, although not guaranteeing complete removal of the lesion, makes it more likely. Incomplete excisions are more probable when the mammographic abnormality does not correspond to the entire extent of the lesion. This in turn is more likely to occur in low-grade rather than high-grade lesions. The failure to perform specimen radiography in every wire-directed case may also lead to incomplete excision because the surgeon lacks immediate feedback from the radiologist as to the adequacy of the excision.

Oncoplastic Excisions

Whole-organ studies (56,57,78,79,110) have clearly demonstrated the radial nature of the disease, and this should be considered when planning the incision for resection. A curvilinear incision in the natural lines of the breast, which is very popular, often does not work for DCIS as the disease tends to extend toward the nipple. A variety of oncoplastic excisions can be designed to take advantage of the radial distribution of DCIS (Figure 17A.24).

Figure 17A.25 shows the operative procedure for a patient in whom a curvilinear lateral incision has been made in the 3 o'clock position of the left breast at another facility. The medial margin, extending toward the nipple, was positive. After mammography showed residual microcalcifications, a decision was made to re-excise the patient using a radial excision and four guide wires. The entire lateral segment down to and including the pectoralis major fascia was removed. The surrounding tissue was then undermined (Figure 17A.26). The remaining tissue was advanced with deep sutures and the breast was remodeled (Figure 17A.27).

All segmental resections should be drained for 24 to 48 hours and the wound completely closed in layers. The cosmetic result should be constantly monitored and reappraised during wound closure. This type of radial segmental resection may alter the size and shape of the breast but good cosmetic results are generally achieved (Figure 17A.28). A radial excision will not displace the nipple areola complex even though overlying skin is removed.

In contrast to the old axiom "the seroma is your friend," when performing oncoplastic breast surgery the exact opposite is true. It is best if the wound heals with as little seroma and blood as possible. Regardless of how the wound is closed, there will always be a small amount of fluid in the biopsy cavity, but this should be minimized.

Segmentectomy Using a Variety of Reduction Mammoplasty Excisions

In a fully counseled woman with a larger breast who might benefit from a reduction mammoplasty or a mastopexy, and whose DCIS is in the right position, a variety of creative reduction/mastopexy excisions can be designed that allow for complete removal of the lesion.

For lesions in the lower hemisphere of the breast, a standard reduction incision can be used (111). This allows access to lesions from 4 to 8 o'clock, going clockwise. Large amounts of breast tissue can be removed with excellent cosmetic results and generally widely clear margins.

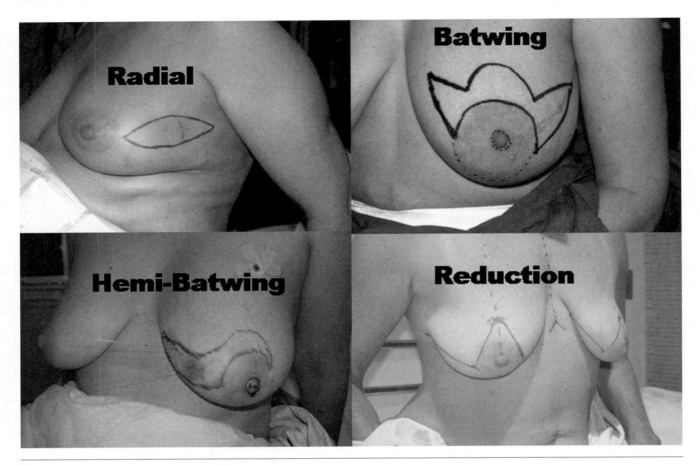

Figure 17A.24. Four different oncoplastic incisions: **Top left**, radial; **top right**, standard batwing; **bottom left**, hemibatwing; **bottom right**, standard reduction.

For lesions in the upper hemisphere (8 to 4 o'clock, going clockwise), batwing or hemibatwing excisions can be used (Figures 17.24 and 17.29 through 17.31). Both these incisions allow the lesion to be generously removed (specimens often weigh ≥200 g) while allowing recontouring the breast in a desirable fashion. When using either batwing excision, the nipple areola complex is elevated from its original position. Figures 17A.30 and 17A.31 show a patient with bilateral DCIS that was excised using bilateral hemibatwing excisions. Widely clear margins were obtained on both sides. Figure 17A.32 shows a woman whose lesion in the 12 o'clock position of the left breast was excised using a crescent mastopexy incision.

As a general rule, the contralateral breast should not be adjusted at the same time. It is best to know the final pathology and, particularly the margin status, before altering the appearance of the opposite breast. However, if the patient decides that she is willing to accept the risks of close or positive margins (that might require reoperation) and would prefer a single operation, the contralateral side can be adjusted during the same operation.

If permanent microscopic sections reveal involved margins and the residual breast is amenable to re-excision, the inflammatory response and induration should be allowed to subside before re-excision. This may take as long as 3 to 4 months. There is little chance that residual DCIS, if there is any, will progress to invasive cancer within such a short time. The cosmetic results from re-excision are routinely better after a sufficient period of wound healing and scar resolution.

Figure 17A.33 shows a patient with a large upper outer to upper central DCIS. She underwent two prior excisions through an upper central curvilinear transverse incision in natural skin lines but the inferior margin (toward the nipple) remained positive. The wound was allowed to heal for 3 additional months and re-excised, using a batwing design combined with re-excision of the old scar. This approach converted her resection to a radial segmentectomy with excellent cosmetic results (Figures 17.34 and 17.35).

Mastectomy with Immediate Reconstruction

In patients whose lesions are too large mammographically to yield clear margins and an acceptable cosmetic result, skin-sparing mastectomy with immediate reconstruction can be performed as the initial procedure. Having performed only a percutaneous minimally invasive breast biopsy, the surgeon will not be faced with a skin incision in the wrong place or a biopsy scar that needs re-excision.

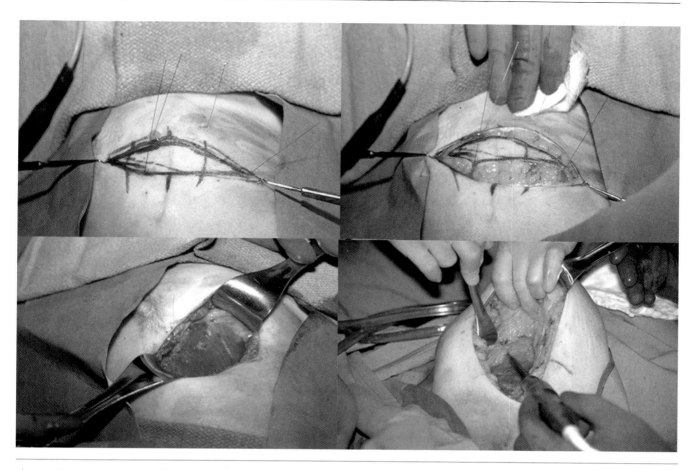

Figure 17A.25. **Top left:** A radial excision has been mapped out using four guide wires. **Top right:** The incision has been made. **Bottom left:** The entire specimen down to and including the pectoralis major fascia has been removed. **Bottom right:** The surrounding tissue is being undermined 4 to 5 cm in every direction so that it can be advanced and reshaped.

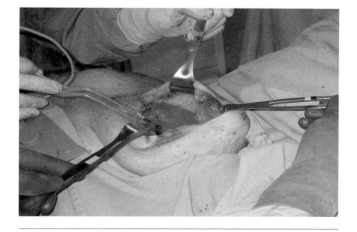

Figure 17A.26. The breast is fully undermined for a distance of 4 to 5 cm in every direction.

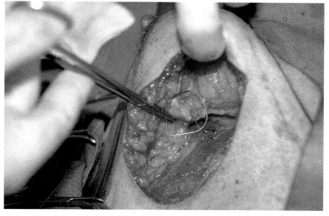

Figure 17A.27. The breast is remodeled and a layered closure is done, bringing all breast tissue together and obliterating any dead space.

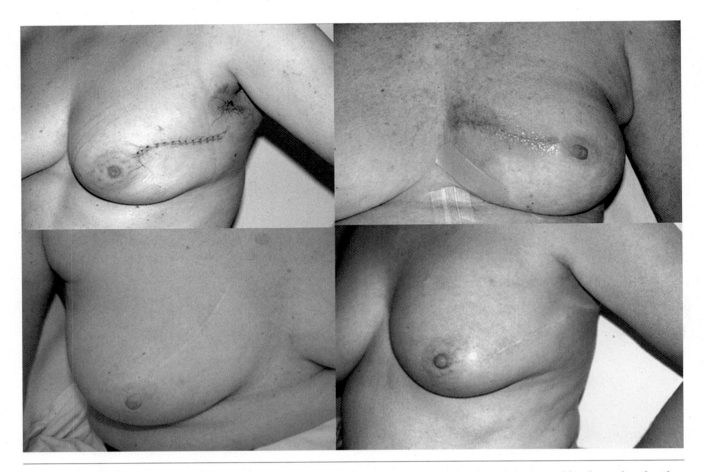

Figure 17A.28. The results of a radial excision. **Top left:** The patient is 3 days postoperatively and the wound has been closed with sutures. A sentinel node biopsy has also been performed. **Top right:** The patient is 1 day postoperatively and the wound has been closed with Dermabond (Ethicon, Inc., Cincinnati, OH). **Bottom right and left:** Both patients are more than 1 year postoperatively. The radial scars are barely visible. There has been no significant change in breast shape.

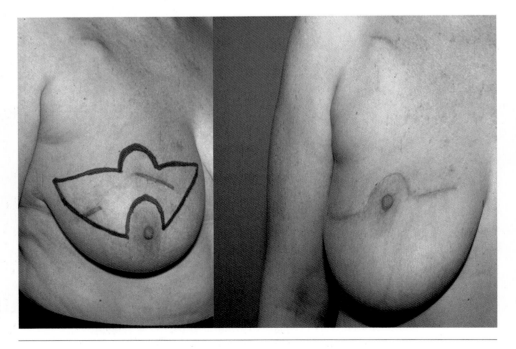

Figure 17A.29. Left: Typical batwing excision plan. The excisions can be used in any patient with a medium to large-sized breast. The wings of the excision can be designed to allow removal of lesions anywhere from the 8:00 to 4:00 position (clockwise). **Right:** Result of batwing excision 1 month postoperatively.

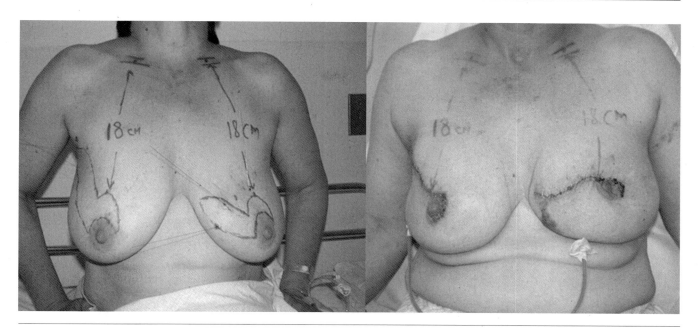

Figure 17A.30. Left: Bilateral hemibatwing excisions; preoperative bilateral segmental excision plan. The nipple is going to be raised to 18 cm below the midpoint of the clavicle on both sides. **Right:** One day postoperative result with drains in place.

Figures 17A.36 through 17A.38 show a patient with a large right-sided DCIS who underwent a right mastectomy using a standard reduction incision, immediate reconstruction of the right breast with a pedicle transverse rectus abdominis musculocutaneous (TRAM) flap, and a simultaneous contralateral left mastopexy.

Figures 17A.39 and 17A.40 show a patient who underwent a left mastectomy using a skin-sparing excision. Immediate reconstruction was performed with a free TRAM flap.

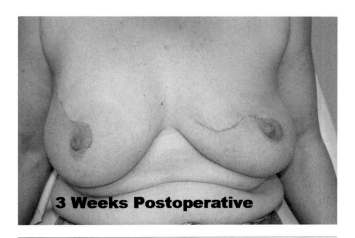

Figure 17A.31. Same patient as in Figure 30 at 3 weeks postoperative bilateral hemibatwing excisions. Both wounds will continue to improve with time.

PAGET DISEASE OF THE NIPPLE

Paget disease presents with eczematoid changes of the nipple (Figures 17.41 and 17.42). In many cases, there is an underlying lesion that may or may not be palpable. The underlying lesion may be invasive or noninvasive. After a complete mammographic workup, the nipple and, if present, the underlying lesion should be biopsied using local anesthesia. Treatment depends on many factors. If the underlying lesion is invasive, it should be excised along with the nipple areolar complex. Postexcisional radiation therapy should be given. Sentinel node biopsy or axillary dissection should be performed. The cosmetic results for central lesions are generally quite good.

If the underlying lesion is DCIS, I generally excise the nipple–areola complex with a generous wedge of breast tissue that includes the underlying lesion. If the underlying lesion is marked with microcalcifications, wires should be used to direct the resection. All edges should be color-coded or inked and the tissue should be serially sectioned and sequentially embedded. If no underlying lesion is found, I do nothing further. If an underlying DCIS is found, I use the USC/VNPI classification as a guideline for suggesting treatment. If histologic margins are involved, I either re-excise or perform a mastectomy with immediate reconstruction, depending on the size of the breast and the degree of margin involvement. I generally do not irradiate patients after complete excision with widely clear margins. Selected cases of Paget disease can be treated with nipple preservation and radiation (112). Sentinel node biopsy or complete node dissection is not indicated for Paget disease unless an underlying invasive carcinoma is found. Nipple areolar reconstruction should be delayed until permanent sections are available that

Crescent

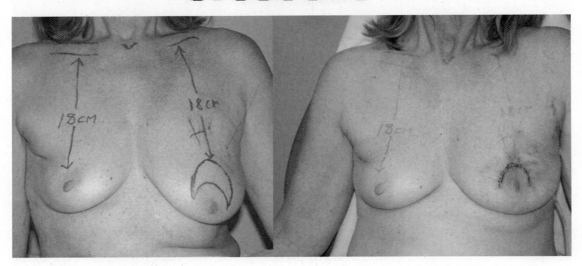

Preoperative   **1 Day Postop**

Figure 17A.32. Crescent excision.

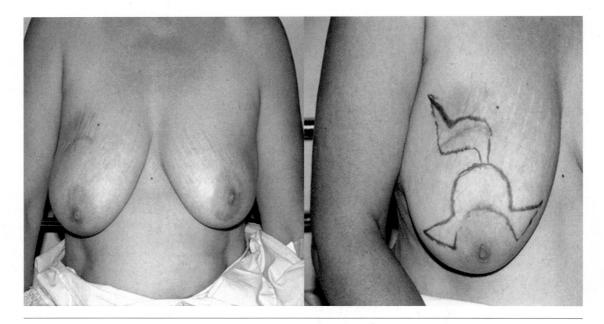

Figure 17A.33. Left: A patient who has undergone two previous excisions elsewhere through a transverse upper central incision (no skin was removed) for a large ductal carcinoma in situ. The margins were persistently positive inferiorly, toward the nipple. **Right:** Excision plan: batwing with re-excision of previous biopsy site. This will elevate the nipple areola complex and reduce the right breast in size. Fortunately, the right breast is a bit larger than the left. This excision will convert the upper transverse excision into a radial resection.

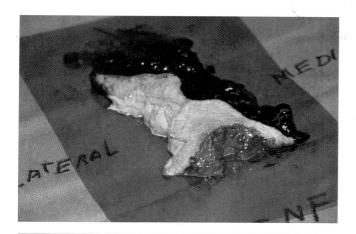

Figure 17A.34. The color-coded excision specimen for the patient in Figure 17A.33.

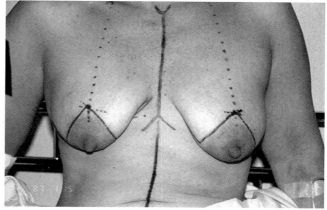

Figure 17A.36. A patient with a 70-mm right-sided ductal carcinoma in situ. Because of the large size of her lesion and the relatively small size of her breast, she was not thought to be a candidate for breast conservation. Treatment plan: A right mastectomy with sentinel node biopsy to be performed through a reduction excision, which has been mapped out. The right nipple-areola complex will be removed. A left mastopexy will be performed through a standard reduction mammoplasty incision.

show clear histologic margins and a decision has been made as to whether radiation therapy is going to be used.

SUMMARY

DCIS is now relatively common, and its frequency is increasing. Most of this is because of better and more frequent mammography by a greater proportion of the female population.

Not all microscopic DCIS will progress to clinical cancer, but if a patient has DCIS and is not treated, she is more likely to develop an ipsilateral invasive breast cancer than is a woman without DCIS.

The comedo subtype of DCIS is more aggressive and malignant in its histologic appearance and is more likely to be associated with subsequent invasive cancer than the noncomedo subtypes. Comedo DCIS is more likely to have a high S-phase, overexpress *HER2/neu*, and show increased thymidine labeling

as compared with noncomedo DCIS. Comedo DCIS treated conservatively is also more likely to recur locally than noncomedo DCIS. However, separation of DCIS into two groups by architecture is an oversimplification and does not reflect the biologic potential of the lesion as well as separation by nuclear grade and comedo-type necrosis.

Most DCIS detected today will be nonpalpable. It will be detected by mammographic calcifications. It is not uncommon for DCIS to be larger than expected by mammography, to involve more than a quadrant of the breast, and to be unicentric in its distribution.

Preoperative evaluation should include film-screen mammography with compression magnification and ultrasonography. Magnetic resonance imaging is becoming increasingly more popular. The surgeon and the radiologist should plan the excision procedure carefully. The first attempt at excision is the best chance to get a complete excision with a good cosmetic result.

Re-excisions often yield poor cosmetic results and the overall plan should be to avoid them whenever possible. In light of this, the initial breast biopsy should be an image-guided biopsy.

After the establishment of the diagnosis, the patient should be counseled. If she is motivated for breast conservation, the surgeon and radiologist should plan the procedure carefully, using multiple wires to map out the extent of the lesion.

When considering the entire population of patients with DCIS without subset analyses, the prospective randomized trials have shown that postexcisional radiation therapy can reduce the relative risk of local recurrence by about 50% for conservatively treated patients. But in some low-risk DCIS patients, the costs may outweigh the potential benefits. In spite of a relative 50% reduction in the probability of local recurrence, the absolute reduction may be only a few percent. Although local

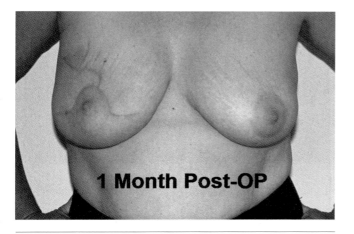

Figure 17A.35. The patient in Figure 33 at 1 month postoperatively. The symmetry is good. The shape is excellent. The scars will continue to improve and lighten.

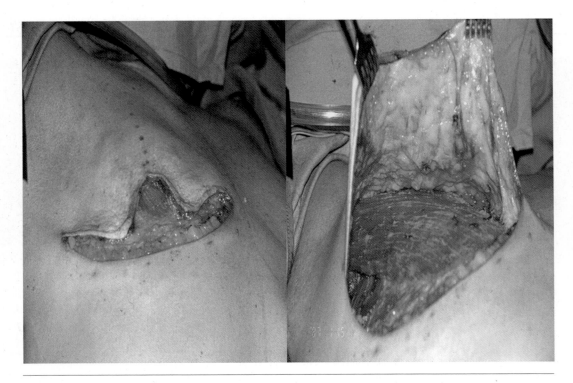

Figure 17A.37. The patient in Figure 17A.36. **Left:** The right mastectomy has been performed through a reduction mammoplasty incision. The nipple-areola complex has been removed. **Right:** Isosulfan blue, which has turned green, was used to find the sentinel lymph node and can be seen in lymphatics on the superior flap. The skin flaps are thin and viable. The pectoralis major muscle fascia has been removed with the mastectomy specimen.

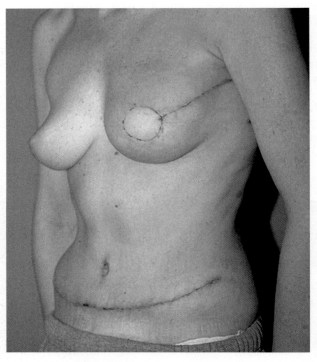

Figure 17A.39. A patient with a large ductal carcinoma in situ, which was incompletely excised at another institution using a circumareolar excision. A left mastectomy has been performed using a skin-sparing incision. The only skin removed was the nipple areola complex. The left breast has been reconstructed with a free transverse rectus abdominis musculocutaneous (TRAM) flap. The abdominal incision is visible.

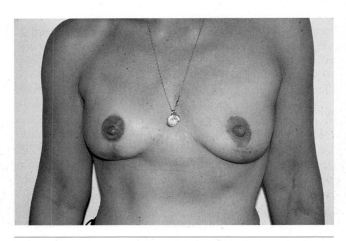

Figure 17A.38. The patient in Figure 17A.36 4 months postoperatively. The right immediate reconstruction was performed with a pedicle transverse rectus abdominis musculocutaneous (TRAM) flap. The right nipple areola has been reconstructed with a local flap and tattooing.

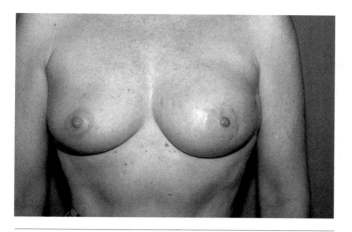

Figure 17A.40. The patient in Figure 17A.39. The left nipple areola has been reconstructed with a local flap and tattooing. Good symmetry and color match has been achieved.

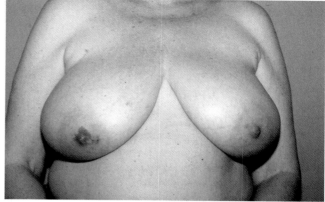

Figure 17A.42. A patient with Paget disease that has spread to the areola. The right nipple and areola complex is involved.

recurrence is extremely important, breast cancer-specific survival is the most important end point for all patients with breast cancer, including patients with DCIS, and no DCIS trial has ever shown a survival benefit for radiation therapy when compared with excision alone. Moreover, radiation therapy is not without financial and physical cost. Because of this, in recent years an increasing number of selected patients with DCIS have been treated with excision alone.

The USC/VNPI uses five independent predictors to predict the probability of local recurrence after conservative treatment for DCIS; these predictors are tumor size, margin width, nuclear grade, age, and the presence or absence of comedonecrosis. In combination, they can be used as an aid to identify subgroups of patients with extremely low probabilities of local recurrence after excision alone; for example, patients who score 4, 5, or 6 using the USC/VNPI. If size cannot be accurately determined, margin width by itself can be used as a surrogate for the USC/VNPI, although it is not quite as good.

New oncoplastic techniques that allow for more extensive excisions can be used to achieve both acceptable cosmesis and widely clear margins, alleviating the need for radiation therapy in many cases.

The decision to use excision alone as treatment for DCIS should be made only if complete and sequential tissue processing has been used and the patient has been fully informed and has participated in the treatment decision-making process.

THE FUTURE

Our knowledge of DCIS genetics and molecular biology is increasing at a remarkably rapid rate. Future studies are likely to identify markers that will allow us to differentiate DCIS with an aggressive potential from DCIS that is merely a microscopic finding. Once we can identify DCIS that will soon develop the potential to invade and metastasize from DCIS that will not, the treatment selection process will become much simpler.

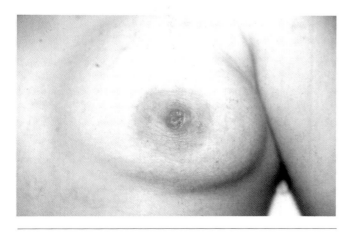

Figure 17A.41. A patient with Paget disease limited to the nipple. The left nipple is reddened and eroded.

REFERENCES

1. Jemal A, Siegel R, Ward E, et al. Cancer statistics, 2006. *CA Cancer J Clin.* 2006;56:106–130.
2. Burstein HJ, Polyak K, Wong JS, et al. Ductal carcinoma in situ of the breast. *N Engl J Med.* 2004;350:1430–1441.
3. Seth A, Kitching R, Landberg G, et al. Gene expression profiling of ductal carcinomas in situ and invasive breast tumors. *Anticancer Res.* 2003;23:2043–2051.
4. Porter D, Lahti-Domenici J, Keshaviah A, et al. Molecular markers in ductal carcinoma in situ of the breast. *Mol Cancer Res.* 2003;1:362–375.
5. Ma XS, Alunga R, Tuggle J, et al. Gene expression profiles of human breast cancer progression. *Proc Natl Acad Sci U S A.* 2003;100:5974–5979.
6. Page D, Anderson T. *Diagnostic Histopathology of the Breast.* New York: Churchill Livingstone; 1987:157–174.
7. Patchefsky A, Schwartz G, Finkelstein S, et al. Heterogeneity of intraductal carcinoma of the breast. *Cancer.* 1989;63:731–741.
8. Nemoto T, Vana J, Bedwani R, et al. Management and survival of female breast cancer: Results of a national survey by The American College of Surgeons. *Cancer.* 1980;45:2917–2924.

9. Silverstein M, Lagios M, Recht A, et al. Image-detected breast cancer: state of the art diagnosis and treatment. *J Am Coll Surg.* 2005;201:586–597.

10. Tabar L, Smith RA, Vitak B, et al. Mammographic screening: a key factor in the control of breast cancer. *Cancer J.* 2003;9(1):15–27.

11. Duffy SW, Tabar L, Smith RA. Screening for breast cancer with mammography. *Lancet.* 2001;358:2166–2168.

12. Silverstein MJ, Cohlan B, Gierson E, et al. Duct carcinoma in situ: 227 cases without microinvasion. *Eur J Cancer.* 1992;28(2/3):630–634.

13. Lagios MD. Duct carcinoma in situ: pathology and treatment. *Surg Clin North Am.* 1990;70:853–871.

14. Ashikari R, Hadju S, Robbins G. Intraductal carcinoma of the breast. *Cancer.* 1971;28:1182–1187.

15. Silverstein MJ. Ductal Carcinoma in Situ of the Breast. *Ann Rev Med.* 2000;51:17–32.

16. Baxter N, Virnig B, Durham S, et al. Trends in the treatment of ductal carcinoma in situ of the breast. *J Natl Cancer Inst.* 2004;96:443–448.

17. Silverstein MJ. The Van Nuys Breast Center—The First Free-Standing Multidisciplinary Breast Center. *Surg Oncol Clinics N Amer.* 2000;9(2):159–175.

18. Van Dongen J, Bartelink H, Fentiman I, et al. Randomized clinical trial to assess the value of breast-conserving therapy in stage I and II breast cancer, EORTC 10801 trial. *Monogr Natl Cancer Inst.* 1992;11:15–18.

19. Veronesi U, Banfi A, Salvadori B, et al. Breast conservation is the treatment of choice in small breast cancer: Long-term results of a randomized trial. *Eur J Cancer.* 1990;26:668–670.

20. Fisher B, Redmond C, Poisson R, et al. Eight-year results of a randomized clinical trial comparing total mastectomy and lumpectomy with or without radiation therapy in the treatment of breast cancer. *N Eng J Med.* 1989;320:822–828.

21. Veronesi U, Cascinelli N, Mariani L, et al. Twenty-year follow-up of a randomized study comparing breast-conserving surgery with radical mastectomy for early breast cancer. *N Engl J Med.* 2002;347:1227–1232.

22. Fisher B, Anderson S, Bryant J, et al. Twenty-year follow-up of a randomized trial comparing total mastectomy, lumpectomy, and lumpectomy plus irradiation for the treatment of invasive breast cancer. *N Engl J Med.* 2002;347:1233–1241.

23. Tavassoli F. Intraductal carcinoma, in Pathology of the breast. Tavassoli FA, Editor. Appleton and Lange: Norwalk, Connecticut. 1992;229–261.

24. Aasmundstad T, Haugen O. DNA Ploidy in intraductal breast carcinomas. *Eur J Cancer.* 1992;26:956–959.

25. Meyer J. Cell kinetics in selection and stratification of patients for adjuvant therapy of breast carcinoma. *National Cancer Institute Monograph.* 1986;1:25–28.

26. Allred D, Clark G, Molina R, et al. Overexpression of HER-2/neu and its relationship with other prognostic factors change during the progression of in situ to invasive breast cancer. *Hum Pathol.* 1992;23:974–979.

27. Barnes D, Meyer J, Gonzalez J, et al. Relationship between c-erbB-2 immunoreactivity and thymidine labelling index in breast carcinoma in situ. *Breast Cancer Res Treat.* 1991;18:11–17.

28. Bartkova J, Barnes D, Millis R, et al. Immunohistochemical demonstration of c-erbB-2 protein in mammary ductal carcinoma in situ. *Human Pathol.* 1990;21(11):1164–1167.

29. Liu E, Thor A, He M, et al. The HER2 (c-erbB-2) oncogene is frequently amplified in in situ carcinomas of the breast. *Oncogene.* 1992;7:1027–1032.

30. van de Vijver M, Peterse J, Mooi WJ, et al. Neu-protein overexpression in breast cancer: association with comedo-type ductal

31. Lagios M, Margolin F, Westdahl P, et al. Mammographically detected duct carcinoma in situ. Frequency of local recurrence following tylectomy and prognostic effect of nuclear grade on local recurrence. *Cancer.* 1989;63:619–624.

32. Schwartz G, Finkel G, Carcia J, et al. Subclinical ductal carcinoma in situ of the breast: treatment by local excision and surveillance alone. *Cancer.* 1992;70:2468–2474.

33. Silverstein MJ, Waisman J, Gierson E, et al. Radiation therapy for intraductal carcinoma: Is it an equal alternative? *Arch Surg.* 1991;126:424–428.

34. Solin L, Yeh I, Kurtz J, et al. Ductal carcinoma in situ (intraductal carcinoma) of the breast treated with breast-conserving surgery and definitive irradiation. Correlation of pathologic parameters with outcome of treatment. *Cancer.* 1993;71:2532–2542.

35. Silverstein MJ, Barth A, Waisman J, et al. Predicting local recurrence in patients with intraductal breast carcinoma (DCIS). *Proc Am Soc Clin Oncol.* 1995;14:117.

36. Silverstein MJ, Poller D, Craig P, et al. A prognostic index for ductal carcinoma in situ of the breast. *Cancer.* 1996;77:2267–2274.

37. Lagios M, Westdahl P, Margolin F, et al. Duct Carcinoma in situ: Relationship of extent of noninvasive disease to the frequency of occult invasion, multicentricity, lymph node metastases, and short-term treatment failures. *Cancer.* 1982;50:1309–1314.

38. Holland R, Peterse J, Millis R, et al. Ductal carcinoma in situ: A proposal for a new classification. *Semin Diag Pathol.* 1994;11(3):167–180.

39. Silverstein MJ, Poller D, Waisman J, et al. Prognostic classification of breast ductal carcinoma-in-situ. *Lancet.* 1995;345:1154–1157.

40. Jensen J, Handel N, Silverstein M, et al. Glandular replacement therapy (GRT) for intraductal breast carcinoma (DCIS). *Proc Am Soc Clin Oncol.* 1995;14:138.

41. Jensen J, Handel N, Silverstein M. Glandular Replacement Therapy: An argument for a combined surgical approach in the treatment of noninvasive breast cancer. *Breast Journal.* 1996;2:121–123.

42. Faverly D, Burgers L, Bult P, et al. Three dimensional imaging of mammary ductal carcinoma is situ: Clinical implications. *Semin in Diag Pathol.* 1994;11(3):193–198.

43. Poller D, Silverstein M, Galea M, et al. Ductal carcinoma in situ of the breast: a proposal for a new simplified histological classification association between cellular proliferation and c-erbB-2 protein expression. *Modern Pathology.* 1994;7:257–262.

44. Bellamy C, McDonald C, Salter D, et al. Noninvasive ductal carcinoma of the breast: the relevance of histologic categorization. *Human Pathol.* 1993;24:16–23.

45. Sloane J, Ellman R, Anderson T, et al. Consistency of histopathological reporting of breast lesions detected by breast screening: Findings of the UK national external quality assessment (EQA) scheme. *Eur J Cancer.* 1994;10:1414–1419.

46. Nielson M, Thomsen J, Primdahl S, et al. Breast cancer and atypia among young and middle-aged women; A study of 110 medicolegal autopsies. *Br J Cancer.* 1987;56:814–819.

47. Page D, Rogers L, Schuyler P, et al. The natural history of ductal carcinoma in situ of the breast. In: Silverstein MJ, Recht A, Lagios M, eds. *Ductal Carcinoma in Situ of the Breast.* Philadelphia: Lippincott Williams and Wilkins; 2002:17–21.

48. Sanders M, Schuyler P, Dupont W, et al. The natural history of low-grade ductal carcinoma in situ of the breast in women treated by biopsy only revealed over 30 years of long-term follow-up. *Cancer.* 2005;103:2481–2484.

49. Rosen P, Senie R, Schottenfeld D, et al. Noninvasive breast carcinoma: frequency of unsuspected invasion and implications for treatment. *Ann Surg.* 1979;1989:377–382.

50. Alpers C, Wellings S. The prevalence of carcinoma in situ in normal and cancer-associated breast. *Hum Pathol.* 1985;16:796–807.

51. Page D, Dupont W, Roger L, et al. Intraductal carcinoma of the breast: Follow-up after biopsy only. *Cancer.* 1982;49:751–758.

52. Schuh M, Nemoto T, Penetrante R, et al. Intraductal carcinoma: analysis of presentation, pathologic findings, and outcome of disease. *Arch Surg.* 1986;121:1303–1307.

53. Gump F, Jicha D, Ozzello L. Ductal carcinoma in situ (DCIS): A revised concept. *Surgery.* 1987;102:190–195.

54. Fisher E, Sass R, Fisher B, et al. Pathologic findings from the National surgical Adjuvant Breast Project (Protocol 6) i. Intraductal carcinoma (DCIS). *Cancer.* 1986;57:197–208.

55. Simpson T, Thirlby R, Dail D. Surgical treatment of ductal carcinoma in situ of the breast: 10 to 20 year follow-up. *Arch Surg.* 1992;127:468–472.

56. Holland R, Hendriks J, Verbeek A, et al. Extent, distribution, and mammographic/histological correlations of breast ductal carcinoma in situ. *Lancet.* 1990;335:519–522.

57. Holland R, Faverly D. *Whole Organ Studies.* In: Silverstein MJ, Recht A, Lagios M, eds. *Ductal Carcinoma in Situ of the Breast.* Philadelphia: Lippincott Williams and Wilkins; 2002.

58. Noguchi S, Aihara T, Koyama H, et al. Discrimination between multicentric and multifocal carcinomas of breast through clonal analysis. *Cancer.* 1994;74:872–877.

59. Tabar L, Dean P. Basic principles of mammographic diagnosis. *Diagn Imag Clin Med.* 1985;54:146–157.

60. Silverstein MJ. Intraductal breast carcinoma: Two decades of progress? *Am J Clin Oncol.* 1991;14(6):534–537.

61. Silverstein MJ. Noninvasive breast cancer: The dilemma of the 1990s. *Obstet Gynecol Clinics N Amer.* 1994;21(4):639–658.

62. Fisher B, Land S, Mamounas E, et al. Prevention of invasive breast cancer in women with ductal carcinoma in situ: An update of the National Surgical Adjuvant Breast and Bowel Project Experience. *Semin Oncol.* 2001;28(4):400–418.

63. Fentiman I, Fagg N, Millis R, et al. In situ ductal carcinoma of the breast: Implications of disease pattern and treatment. *Eur J Surg Oncol.* 1986;12:261–266.

64. Solin L, Kurtz J, Fourquet A, et al. Fifteen year results of breast conserving surgery and definitive breast irradiation for treatment of ductal carcinoma in situ of the breast. *J Clin Oncol.* 1996;14:754–763.

65. UK Coordinating Committee on Cancer Research (UKCCCR) Ductal Carcinoma in Situ (DCIS) Working Party, Radiotherapy and tamoxifen in women with completely excised ductal carcinoma in situ of the breast in the UK, Australia, and New Zealand: randomised controlled trial. *Lancet.* 2003;362:95–102.

66. Fisher B, Jeong J, Anderson S, et al. Twenty-five year follow-up of a randomized trial comparing radiacal mastectomy, total mastectomy, and total mastectomy followed by irradiation. *N Engl J Med.* 2002;347:567–575.

67. Silverstein MJ, Lagios M, Martino S, et al. Outcome after local recurrence in patients with ductal carcinoma in situ of the breast. *J Clin Oncol.* 1998;16:1367–1373.

68. Romero L, Klein L, Ye W, et al. Outcome after invasive recurrence in patients with ductal carcinoma in situ of the breast. *Am J Surg.* 2004;188:371–376.

69. Swain S. Ductal carcinoma in situ—incidence, presentation and guidelines to treatment. *Oncology.* 1989;3:25–42.

70. Fisher B, Costantino J, Redmond C, et al. Lumpectomy compared with lumpectomy and radiation therapy for the treatment of intraductal breast cancer. *N Engl J Med.* 1993;328:1581–1586.

71. Fisher B, Dignam J, Wolmark N, et al. Tamoxifen in treatment of intraductal breast cancer: National Surgical Adjuvant Breast and Bowel Project B-24 randomized controlled trial. *Lancet.* 1999;353:1993–2000.

72. Fisher B, Dignam J, Wolmark N, et al. Lumpectomy and radiation therapy for the treatment of intraductal breast cancer: findings from National Surgical Adjuvant Breast and Bowel Project B-17. *J Clin Oncol.* 1998;16(2):441–452.

73. Julien J, Bijker N, Fentiman I, et al. Radiotherapy in breast conserving treatment for ductal carcinoma in situ: First results of EORTC randomized phase III trial 10853. *Lancet.* 2000;355:528–533.

74. Page D, Dupont W, Rogers L, et al. Continued local recurrence of carcinoma 15-25 years after a diagnosis of low grade ductal carcinoma in situ of the breast treated only by biopsy. *Cancer.* 1995;76:1197–1200.

75. Zafrani B, Leroyer A, Fourquet A, et al. Mammographically detected ductal in situ carcinoma of the breast analyzed with a new classification. A study of 127 cases: correlation with estrogen and progesterone receptors, p53 and c-erbB-2 proteins, and proliferative activity. *Semin Diag Pathol.* 1994;11(3):208–214.

76. Schwartz G. The role of excision and surveillance alone in subclinical DCIS of the breast. *Oncology.* 1994;8:21–26.

77. Schwartz G. Treatment of Subclinical Ductal Carcinoma in Situ of the Breast by Local Excision and surveillance: An Updated Personal Experience. In: Silverstein MJ, Recht A, Lagios M, eds. *Ductal Carcinoma in Situ of the Breast.* Philadelphia: Lippincott Williams and Wilkins; 2002:308–321.

78. Holland R, Faverly D. Whole Organ Studies. Ductal Carcinoma. In: *Situ of the Breast.* Silverstein M, ed. Baltimore: Williams and Wilkins. 1997:233–240.

79. Holland R, Hendriks J. Microcalcifications associated with ductal carcinoma in situ: mammographic-pathologic correlation. *Semin Diag Pathol.* 1994;11(3):181–192.

80. Page D, Dupont W, Roger L, et al. Atypical hyperplastic lesions of the female breast. A log-term follow-up study. *Cancer.* 1985;55:2698–2708.

81. Lagios M. Controversies in diagnosis, biology, and treatment. *Breast J.* 1995;1:68–78.

82. Group, EBCTC, Favorable and unfavorable effects on long-term survival of radiotherapy for early breast cancer: an overview of the randomized trials. *Lancet.* 2006;2000:1757–1770.

83. Giordano S, Kuo Y, Freeman J, et al. Risk of cardiac death after adjuvant radiotherapy for breast cancer. *J Natl Cancer Inst.* 2005;97:419–424.

84. Darby S, McGale P, Taylor C, et al. Long-term mortality from heart disease and lung cancer after radiotherapy for early breast cancer: prospective cohort study of about 300,000 women in US SEER cancer registries. *Lancet Oncol.* 2005;6:557–565.

85. Zablotska L, Neugut A. Lung carcinoma after radiation therapy in women treated with lumpectomy or mastectomy for primary breast carcinoma. *Cancer.* 2003;97:1404–1411.

86. Darby S, McGale P, Peto R, et al. Mortality from cardiovascular disease more than 10 years after radiotherapy for breast cancer: nationwide cohort study of 90,000 Swedish women. *BMJ.* 2003;326:256–257.

87. Bijker N, Peterse J, Duchateau L, et al. Risk factors for recurrence and metastasis after breast-conserving therapy for ductal carcinoma in situ: Analysis of European Organization for Research and Treatment of Cancer Trial 10853. *J Clin Oncol.* 2001;19:2263–2271.

88. Fisher E, Constantino J, Fisher B, et al. Pathologic findings from the National Surgical Adjuvant Breast Project (NSABP) Protocol B-17. *Cancer.* 1995;75:1310–1319.

89. Fisher B, Bauer M, Margolese R, et al. Five-year results of a randomized clinical trial comparing total mastectomy and lumpectomy with or without radiation therapy in the treatment of breast cancer. *N Eng J Med.* 1985;312:665–673.

90. Fisher E, Lemming R, Andersen S, et al. Conservative management of intraductal carcinoma (DCIS) of the breast. *J Surg Oncol.* 1991;47:139–147.

91. Recht A. Randomized Trial Overview. In: Silverstein MJ, Recht A, Lagios M, eds. *Ductal Carcinoma in Situ of the Breast.* Philadelphia: Lippincott Williams and Wilkins; 2002:414–419.

92. Allred D, Bryant J, Land S, et al. Estrogen receptor expression as a predictive marker of effectiveness of tamoxifen in the treatment of DCIS: Frindings from NSABP Protocol B-24. *Breast Cancer Res Treat.* 2003;76(suppl 1):36.

93. Bijker N, Meijnen P, Peterse J, et al. Radiotherapy in breast conserving treatment for ductal carcinoma in situ: ten-year results of EORTC randomized phase III trial 10853. *Breast Cancer Research Treat.* 2005;94, Supplement 1:S7.

94. Silverstein MJ, Barth A, Poller D, et al. Ten-year results comparing mastectomy to excision and radiation therapy for ductal carcinoma in situ of the breast. *Eur J Cancer.* 1995;31A:1425–1427.

95. Silverstein MJ, Lagios M, Groshen S, et al. The influence of margin width on local control in patients with ductal carcinoma in situ (DCIS) of the breast. *N Engl J Med.* 1999;340:1455–1461.

96. Silverstein MJ, Buchanan C. Ductal carcinoma in situ: USC/Van Nuys Prognostic Index and the impact of margin status. *The Breast.* 2003;12:457–471.

97. Silverstein MJ. The University of Southern California/Van Nuys Prognostic Index for ductal carcinoma in situ of the breast. *Am J Surg.* 2003;186:337–343.

98. Ottesen G, Graversen H, Blichert-Toft M, et al. Ductal carcinoma in situ of the female breast. Short-term results of a prospective nationwide study. *Am J Surg Pathol.* 1992;16:1183–1196.

99. Silverstein MJ, Lagios M, Craig P, et al. The Van Nuys Prognostic Index for ductal carcinoma in situ. *Breast Journal.* 1996;2:38–40.

100. Silverstein MJ, Lagios M, Recht A, eds. *Ductal Carcinoma in Situ of the Breast.* 2nd ed. Philadelphia: Lippincott Williams and Wilkins; 2002.

101. Poller D, Silverstein MJ. The Van Nuys Ductal carcinoma in situ: an update. In: Silverstein MJ, Recht A, Lagios M, eds. *Ductal Carcinoma in Situ of the Breast.* Philadelphia: Lippincott Williams and Wilkins; 2002:222–233.

102. Silverstein MJ. The University of Southern California/Van Nuys Prognostic Index. In: Silverstein MJ, Recht A, Lagios M, eds. *Ductal Carcinoma in Situ of the Breast.* Philadelphia: Lippincott Williams and Wilkins; 2002:459–473.

103. Ernster VL, Barclay J, Kerlikowske K, et al. Mortality among women with ductal carcinoma in situ of the breast in population-based surveillance, epidemiology and end results program. *Arch Intern Med.* 2000;160:953–958.

104. Fisher E, Dignam J, Tan-Chie E, et al. Pathologic findings from the National Adjuvant Breast Project (NSABP) eight-year update of Protocol B-17: intraductal carcinoma. *Cancer.* 1999;86:429–438.

105. Silverstein MJ, Rosser R, Gierson E, et al. Axillary Lymph node dissection for intraductal carcinoma—is it indicated? *Cancer.* 1987;59:1819–1824.

106. Silverstein MJ. An argument against routine use of radiotherapy for ductal carcinoma in situ. *Oncology.* 2003;17(11):1511–1546.

107. Frykberg E, Masood S, Copeland E, et al. Duct carcinoma in situ of the breast. *Surg Gynecol Obstet.* 1993;177:425–440.

108. Silverstein MJ, Larsen L, Soni R, et al. Breast biopsy and oncoplastic surgery for the patient with ductal carcinoma in situ: Surgical, pathologic and radiologic issues. In: Silverstein MJ, Recht A, Lagios M, eds. *Ductal Carcinoma in Situ of the Breast.* Philadelphia: Lippincott Williams and Wilkins; 2002:185–206.

109. Anderson B, Masetti R, Silverstein M. Oncoplastic approaches to partial mastectomy: an overview of volume displacement techniques. *Lancet Oncol.* 2005;6:145–157.

110. Holland PA, Gandhi A, Knox WF, et al. The importance of complete excision in the prevention of local recurrence of ductal carcinoma in situ. *Br J Cancer.* 1998;77(1):110–114.

111. Clough K, Lewis J, Couturaud B, et al. Oncoplastic techniques allow extensive resections for breast conserving therapy of breast carcinomas. *Ann Surg.* 2003;237:26–34.

112. Stockdale A, Brierley J, Whire W, et al. Radiotherapy for Paget's disease of the nipple: a conservative alternative. *Lancet.* 1989;II:664–666.

COMMENTARY

Elisa R. Port

For the first time, in 2006, a decline in the incidence of breast cancer was reported. However, the number of cases of ductal carcinoma in situ (DCIS) continues to increase and will comprise an increasingly larger proportion of newly diagnosed cases (1). Dr. Melvin J. Silverstein provides a comprehensive chapter on the current state of the art of diagnosis and treatment of DCIS, and provides an excellent springboard for discussion of potential future directions of diagnosis and treatment. Given the increase in number of diagnosed cases of DCIS, all of which fall under the broad-based classification of "stage 0," what does the future hold with regard to improvement in diagnostic techniques and refinement in treatment? Two major technological developments that stand to affect the diagnosis and management of DCIS in the near future are magnetic resonance imaging (MRI) and tumor profiling.

As Dr. Silverstein points out, the number of diagnosed DCIS cases surged in the 1980s and early 1990s. The increased utilization of mammographic screening led to increasing detection of early-stage breast cancer, the earliest of which is DCIS. The most significant development in breast cancer diagnosis since the early 1990s has been the advent and increasing usage of breast MRI. Definitive guidelines regarding appropriate applications of MRI are evolving. Specifically, the only mention of MRI for breast cancer *screening* in the current National Comprehensive Cancer Network recommendations is its advice to consider MRI in women with known *BRCA* mutations (2). Although more data are needed to further define appropriate applications of this technology for both screening and further evaluation of patients with a known new cancer, MRI is being used liberally in most modern breast cancer practices at the discretion of the physician and the request of the patient (see Chapter 16C).

With regard to breast cancer screening in the high-risk population, MRI has been shown to detect cancer that is otherwise mammographically occult in 1% to 7% of those screened (3). Furthermore, some studies have indicated that in high-risk patients screened with MRI, cancers detected tend to be smaller and earlier stage (3,4). If approximately 25% of all mammographically detected cancer is DCIS, and MRI has been shown to potentially detect cancer at an earlier stage than mammography, a subset of patients undergoing additional screening with MRI will presumably further increase the number of cases of DCIS identified. Thus, similar to the explosion in the incidence of DCIS associated with increased use of mammography, it is highly likely that this trend of increased detection of DCIS may be further propagated by MRI.

Although the small benefit of screening MRI for selected high-risk patients is known, MRI is also associated with a substantial risk of false-positive findings, potentially leading to unnecessary biopsies, scar tissue, and anxiety (3,4). Furthermore, the detection of DCIS by MRI may further complicate our understanding of what is already a complex disease process. DCIS, as Dr. Silverstein points out, represents a panoply of diseases, ranging from diffuse lesions co-mixed with microinvasive cancer to small foci of low-grade disease that may percolate for years before becoming clinically significant. A proportion of MRI-detected DCIS may represent an entity that is very different biologically and clinically from that detected mammographically; the clinical relevance of such disease and its appropriate treatment may be different as well. For example, a small focus of DCIS detected by MRI may represent a new subtype of disease caught so early in its evolution that minimal treatment, such as wide excision alone, may prove to be sufficient. Clearly, from the standpoint of diagnosis, increasing usage of MRI for screening has the potential to have a profound effect on the diagnosis and treatment of DCIS in the near future.

Other applications of MRI, such as evaluating extent of disease in the presence of a known cancer, may also impact management for patients with DCIS. As discussed by Dr. Silverstein, Holland et al. (5) demonstrated that a significant percentage of patients (23%) with DCIS who underwent mastectomy had more extensive disease than expected, involving more than one quadrant. In addition, a certain proportion of women who undergo lumpectomy and radiation therapy have residual microscopic disease, which is effectively eradicated by radiation, as evidenced by the difference in recurrence rate between patients who undergo radiation treatment and those who do not (6). More intense imaging scrutiny of the ipsilateral breast could potentially lead to the identification of subclinical multifocality/multicentricity that otherwise might have been treated with radiation. The a priori identification of such disease could potentially alter surgical decision making regarding the appropriateness of breast-conservation therapy and lead to a higher mastectomy rate.

The second technological advance that may potentially alter the future management of DCIS is genetic profiling and analysis. The staging system for invasive breast cancer in general has undergone countless revisions. It has become more refined along the way, adapting to and accommodating new data, such as those related to the sentinel node biopsy technique and information regarding the number and extent of lymph node positivity. Conversely, the staging of DCIS, which represents a broad spectrum of pathology with different biologic potentials, remains an unrefined category designated as stage 0. Among cases of DCIS, significant interobserver variability can exist even between experienced pathologists' determinations of DCIS compared with

invasive or noncancerous lesions (7). A number of different models, such as Dr. Silverstein's Van Nuys Prognostic Index, have been proposed to refine the management of DCIS by stratifying patients into low-, medium-, and high-risk groups based on criteria such as tumor grade, size, margin width, and patient age (8). In addition, histopathology using morphologic descriptions such as papillary, cribriform, solid, and comedo has been used to describe different subtypes of DCIS. Nevertheless, treatment strategies remain essentially the same, involving more or less surgery, with or without the addition of radiation therapy.

Much work is being devoted to further characterizing subtypes of DCIS based on genetic changes and determining whether specific factors contributing to progression of DCIS to invasive cancer can be identified. The identification of such factors could lead to the development of therapeutic targets and interventions to prevent progression of disease. Over the past 5 years, high-throughput technologies have been developed that can identify and characterize genetic signature differences seen in different tumor types. Specific genetic changes, such as up-regulation or down-regulation, can now be identified and investigated for their potential roles in tumorigenesis and progression. These technologies may provide the basis for refinement of our understanding and classification of the DCIS disease process.

For example, Buerger et al. (9) used comparative genomic hybridization techniques to analyze 77 cases of cancer and demonstrated that low-grade DCIS was genetically similar to well-differentiated invasive cancer, while high-grade DCIS was more homologous with poorly differentiated breast cancer. These findings challenge our previously held hypothesis on how cancer progresses. Previously, our understanding of cancer progression involved a multistep model that proposes that, with genetic changes, benign tissue evolves into atypical hyperplasia, which then can progress to DCIS with further accumulation of genetic alterations. This multistep model proposes that if left untreated, low-grade DCIS will develop into higher-grade DCIS, and that the majority of DCIS lesions will ultimately develop into invasive cancer. By contrast, data such as these from Buerger et al. suggest that a linear progression model may not represent the only pathway of invasive cancer development. Instead, low-grade DCIS may progress directly to well-differentiated invasive cancer without passing through the stages of increasingly higher-grade stages of DCIS.

In addition to this study looking at cancer progression models, recent work has focused on genetic profiling of DCIS and the identification of specific genes of interest in cancer development and progression. Hannemann et al. (10) studied 40 specimens each of DCIS and invasive breast cancer, comparing their gene expression profiles. Genetic profiles of low-grade DCIS lesions were compared with those of high-grade DCIS cases, and cases of DCIS were compared with invasive ductal cancer. A profile of 43 genes was identified that were differentially expressed between low- and high-grade DCIS; many involved metabolic function and intercellular communication pathways. Of interest, *BCL2*, an antiapoptotic gene, was significantly up-regulated in well-differentiated DCIS compared with poorly differentiated DCIS. When comparing DCIS cases with invasive cancer cases, a profile of 35 differentially expressed genes were identified, many of which are involved in signal transduction and cellular growth.

A separate study by Schuetz et al. (11) compared genetic changes seen in DCIS and invasive cancer. This study examined fewer cases of DCIS and invasive cancer than that of Hannemann et al. (10), but to better control for the genetic variability inherent in comparing tissue from different patients, they analyzed matched pairs of microdissected DCIS and invasive cancer taken from the same patients. Their use of microdissection techniques also reduced the genetic variability resultant from contamination of pure tumors by stromal components, which is especially important given the heterogeneous nature of breast tissue. This study demonstrated up-regulation in invasive cancer of genes prominently involved in promoting invasion, such as *TWIST1* (involved in promoting epithelial-mesenchymal transition and metastasis) and *MMP11*.

The studies cited here, as well as much work in progress, provide better insight into the genetic alterations associated with DCIS. Identification of specific genes of importance in DCIS progression may lead to refinement in staging of DCIS. In addition, identifying and understanding the roles of specific genetic abnormalities may also pave the way for the development of therapeutic interventions capable of halting DCIS progression. Genetic profiling and MRI are examples of emerging modalities and technology that will undoubtedly play significant roles in how patients with DCIS are treated in the 21st century. These and other technologies represent the potential for future developments to help us better understand the pathogenesis and progression of DCIS and provide more individualized and specific treatment.

REFERENCES

1. Jemal A, Seigel R, Ward E, et al. Cancer statistics, 2007. *CA Cancer J Clin.* 2007;57:43–66.
2. The NCCN Breast Cancer Screening and Diagnosis Guidelines in Oncology (Version 1. 2007). 2006 National Comprehensive Cancer Network, Inc. http://www.nccn.org. Accessed February 26, 2007.
3. Morris EA, Liberman L, Ballon DJ, et al. MRI of occult breast carcinoma in a high-risk population. *AJR Am J Roentgenol.* 2003;181:619–626.
4. Port ER, Park A, Borgen PI, et al. Results of MRI screening for breast cancer in high-risk patients with LCIS and atypical hyperplasia. *Ann Surg Oncol.* 2007;14:1051–1057.
5. Holland R, Hendricks J, Verbeek A, et al. Extent, distribution, and mammographic/histological correlations of breast ductal carcinoma in situ. *Lancet.* 1990;335:519–522.
6. Fisher B, Anderson S, Bryant J, et al. Twenty-year follow-up of a randomized trial comparing total mastectomy, lumpectomy, and lumpectomy plus irradiation for the treatment of invasive breast cancer. *N Engl J Med.* 2002;347:1233–1241.
7. Rosai J. Borderline epithelial lesions of the breast. *Am J Surg Pathol.* 1991;15:209–221.
8. Silverstein MJ, Poller D, Waisman J, et al. Prognostic classification of breast ductal carcinoma in situ. *Lancet.* 1995;345:1154–1157.
9. Buerger H, Otterbach F, Simon R, et al. Comparative genomic hybridization of ductal carcinoma in situ of the breast-evidence of multiple genetic pathways. *J Pathol.* 1999;187:396–402.
10. Hannemann J, Velds A, Halfwerk JB, et al. Classification of ductal carcinoma in situ by gene expression profiling. *Breast Cancer Res.* 2006;8:R61.
11. Schuetz CS, Bonin M, Clare SE, et al. Progression-specific genes identified by expression profiling of matched ductal carcinomas in situ and invasive breast tumors, combining laser capture microdissection and oligonucleotide microarray analysis. *Cancer Res.* 2006;66:5278–5286.

Chapter 17B
Breast Cancer: Association with Lobular Neoplasia and Other Benign Lesions

Dennis R. Holmes

A *typical lobular hyperplasia, lobular carcinoma in situ, atypical ductal hyperplasia, intraductal papilloma,* and *radial scars* are benign lesions that may be associated with adjacent breast malignancy. Thus, special considerations in the management of these lesions are required, especially when they are detected on core needle biopsy. The issues related to lobular neoplasia are emphasized in this chapter.

LOBULAR NEOPLASIA

Atypical lobular hyperplasia (ALH) and lobular carcinoma in situ (LCIS) are proliferative lesions of the breast characterized by the accumulation of small, loosely cohesive, lobular epithelial cells resulting in marked distension of acini within the terminal-ductal lobular unit. The histopathologic distinction between ALH and LCIS is largely a matter of degree: ALH describes lobular proliferation involving up to 50% of a lobule whereas LCIS is defined as lobular proliferation involving >50% of a lobule (1). Mitoses and necrosis are usually absent in both conditions but may be present in the pleomorphic subtype of LCIS, which is morphologically similar to ductal carcinoma in situ.

LCIS was originally described by Foote and Stewart (2) as a "rare form of mammary cancer." Recognizing the "misleading and unfortunate name" of this nonmalignant process, Haagensen et al. (1) introduced the term *lobular neoplasia* to describe the spectrum of lesions ranging from minimal ALH to LCIS. Lobular neoplasia also more accurately reflects the benign clinical nature of this condition. In this discussion, lobular neoplasia (LN) will refer to ALH and LCIS, except where indicated.

LN has been widely regarded as a multicentric, multifocal, and bilateral process (1, 3–5). Multicentric and multifocal LN has been described in up to 80% of mastectomy specimens in which LN was noted, and bilateral LN has been demonstrated in as much as 35% of women from whom bilateral tissue was obtainable. However, the natural history of LN suggests an even higher frequency of bilateralism. Because of the absence of specific clinical or imaging features, LN is generally regarded as a serendipitous histologic finding in breast biopsies performed for other indications. Although most biopsies yielding a diagnosis of LN are performed to evaluate discrete imaging abnormalities (e.g., microcalcifications, architectural distortion, or masses) that are caused by discrete lesions (e.g., ductal hyperplasia of the usual type, fibrocystic changes, or adenosis), the prevailing view that LN is a purely occult phenomenon is challenged by the fact that up to 41% of LN lesions have mammographically detectable microcalcifications within affected lobules (6–9).

Because of its frequently occult nature, the true incidence of LN is unknown. The reported incidence ranges from 0.3% to 7% for ALH and 0.7% to 4.0% for LCIS based on excisional and core needle biopsy data (1, 10–13). Rising prevalence of LN has coincided with increasing use of screening mammography and minimally invasive biopsies, such as stereotactic and ultrasound-guided core needle biopsies. Most women diagnosed with LN are premenopausal, suggesting that the condition might regress after menopause (1).

Recent decades have witnessed considerable evolution in the management of LN. When originally described, LCIS was considered a malignancy of the breast for which mastectomy was required. Currently, ALH and LCIS are regarded as generalized risk factors for the development of breast malignancy in either breast, for which mastectomy is no longer considered necessary. However, there is now growing recognition of LN as a potential marker of concurrent adjacent breast malignancy, suggesting that this entity might also function as a direct precursor to breast cancer in some patients.

Is Lobular Neoplasia a Risk Factor, Precursor Lesion, or both?

The role of LN as a risk factor for breast cancer is supported by several key observations in the natural history of ALH and LCIS: (a) LN is associated with an increased risk of subsequent invasive breast cancer and ductal carcinoma in situ, (b) the elevated risk of breast malignancy substantially affects both breasts, (c) subsequent breast malignancies are commonly of the ductal type (i.e., invasive ductal carcinoma and ductal carcinoma in situ) rather than the lobular type, and (d) most patients with LN never actually develop breast cancer. Data supporting the generalized risk of breast malignancy following the diagnosis of ALH are derived from the Nashville Breast Studies and the Nurses' Health Study, which reported a 3.1- to 5.3-fold increased risk of breast cancer among study participants, and a 9.6-fold increased risk among those in whom ALH was detected premenopausally (10,14,15). LCIS has also been reported in several historical series to be associated with a 9- to 12-fold increased risk of subsequent breast malignancy (1,3,16,17). The risk appears to increase with age and corresponds to a 20% to 30% absolute risk of breast malignancy for patients followed up to 24 years.

The bilateral risk of LN-associated breast cancer is supported by the Surveillance, Epidemiology, and End Results (SEER) registry of women with a history of LCIS (18). Among 4,853 women diagnosed by or treated with partial mastectomy, the SEER registry reported virtually identical rates of ipsilateral and contralateral invasive breast cancers developing 5 to 25 years after the diagnosis of LCIS, an observation also confirmed by several other investigators (19–22). Although each of these series reported an increased incidence of invasive lobular carcinoma among women with a history of LCIS compared with the

general population, the majority of resulting carcinomas were of ductal histology rather than lobular histology. However, the majority of women with the diagnosis of LCIS remained cancer-free. Although historical data strongly support LN as a *risk factor* for breast malignancy, growing evidence also points to a compelling role for LN as a *precursor* to invasive breast cancer and ductal carcinoma in situ. In recent years, multiple series have been published reporting the coexistence of breast cancer in as many as 50% of women receiving a diagnosis of LN by core needle biopsy. These findings have led to a growing trend among surgeons, pathologists, and radiologists to recommend follow-up wide local excision of LN lesions diagnosed on core needle biopsy to rule out an associated occult malignancy (7,23,24).

Several investigators have described genetic similarities between LN and associated invasive breast carcinoma. Using comparative genomic hybridization, similar patterns of gene amplification or deletion involving chromosomes 11, 16, 17, and 22 are reported in up to 50% of LN lesions and its associated invasive carcinoma (25–30). Mutations in the E-cadherin gene, a transmembrane glycoprotein involved in cell-cell adhesion, also points to ALH and LCIS as precursors for invasive lobular carcinoma. Whereas E-cadherin is almost universally expressed in invasive ductal carcinomas and ductal carcinoma in situ, loss of E-cadherin expression occurs in >90% of LCIS and 56% of invasive lobular carcinoma (12).

Although the majority of invasive breast cancers coexisting with or diagnosed after LCIS are of ductal histology, invasive lobular carcinomas are observed much more frequently than expected in the setting of LN. For example, the SEER registry reported a higher incidence of infiltrating lobular carcinoma (23.1%) and a lower incidence of infiltrating ductal carcinoma (49.7%) in women with a history of LCIS, compared with expected rates of 6.5% for infiltrating lobular carcinoma and 71.0% for infiltrating ductal carcinoma in the general population. Similarly, other investigators reported rates of infiltrating lobular carcinoma ranging from 25% to 35% among women with a history of LCIS (1,4,21). The strong association between LCIS and infiltrating lobular carcinoma was even more convincingly expressed by Sasson et al. (31), who reported the presence of LCIS in 51% of infiltrating lobular carcinoma but only 2% of infiltrating ductal carcinoma in a series of 1,272 patients with stage I and II invasive breast cancer.

A precursor role for LCIS is also suggested by the findings in National Surgical Adjuvant Breast and Bowel Project (NSABP) Protocol B-17, a study of ductal carcinoma in situ that inadvertently included 180 patients with LCIS previously misclassified as ductal carcinoma in situ (32). Among patients initially diagnosed with LCIS, a total of 40 subsequent malignancies were reported in 12 years of follow-up, the majority occurring in the ipsilateral breast compared with the contralateral breast (n = 26 vs. n = 14). A propensity for the development of ipsilateral malignancy was also observed for LCIS in the Danish Breast Cancer Cooperative Group cohort study, and for ALH in the Nashville Breast and the Nurses' Health Studies, all of which showed a significantly higher incidence of ipsilateral malignancy following an initial diagnosis of LCIS or ALH (3,14,33). These findings are in marked contrast to SEER registry findings and suggest that LCIS may be a premalignant lesion in some patients. Of note, NSABP B-17 also reported a strikingly high incidence of infiltrating lobular carcinomas (89% ipsilateral and 75% contralateral) among subsequent breast cancers.

Considering all available data, it is reasonable to conclude that LN is both a risk factor *and* a precursor to invasive breast cancer in some patients (5). However, the degree to which LN influences risk or antecedes breast cancer may vary from one individual to another or among different histologic subtypes of LN. Although LCIS has been shown to confer a higher risk of subsequent breast malignancy compared with ALH (11), many series report similar rates of concurrent malignancy for both lesions. Some series suggest that pleomorphic LCIS may have a highest risk of coincident breast malignancy, but this relationship has not be consistently observed. Gene expression profiling or similar molecular analyses may hold the key to these unresolved issues and someday permit identification of LN lesions that are more likely to be associated with or progress to breast cancer.

Lobular Neoplasia, Atypical Ductal Hyperplasia, Intraductal Papilloma, and Radial Scar Diagnosed by Core Needle Biopsy

In 2005, the International Consensus Conference on Image Detected Breast Cancer concluded that all image-detected breast abnormalities should first be diagnosed with a core needle biopsy, using ultrasound for ultrasound-visible lesions or stereotaxis for all other nonpalpable abnormalities (34). The intent of this recommendation was to reduce the number of women undergoing unnecessary diagnostic excisional breast biopsies for benign conditions and to improve the accuracy and efficiency of management of breast malignancy. Although this objective is achieved in the majority of situations, the principle limitation of core needle biopsy is the potential of inaccurate staging due to inadequate sampling of a pathologic lesion. Thus, a core needle biopsy, which typically removes only a portion of a targeted lesion, might fail to remove a coexisting higher-grade component that might alter patient management. This problem of understaging is largely mitigated by the use of the *triple test,* a clinical management tool that assesses concordance between clinical, imaging, and pathology results. Therefore, if a core needle biopsy reveals a benign result in the setting of suspicious clinical or imaging findings, the results are considered nonconcordant and surgical excision of the lesion is required to resolve the diagnostic dilemma.

Although the triple test performs well in most scenarios, some pathologic lesions have traditionally had such high discordance between core needle biopsy and surgical excision histology that the triple test cannot be dependably used to evaluate the adequacy of core needle biopsy. The classic example of this is *atypical ductal hyperplasia* (ADH) diagnosed by core needle biopsy, which is frequently shown on surgical excision to coexist with ductal carcinoma in situ or invasive breast cancer. Based on several series (35–40) comparing core needle biopsy-diagnosed ADH and follow-up wide local excision, the accuracy of core needle biopsy has been shown to correlate with the volume of tissue removed by the biopsy device employed (Table 17B.1), such that a 14-gauge core needle biopsy revealing ADH has a 13% to 58% (35–38) rate of underdetecting an associated malignancy compared with an 11-gauge core needle biopsy, which has a 10% to 25% (37,39,40) rate of underdetection. These

Table 17B.1

Upgrade Rates for Atypical Ductal Hyperplasia, Atypical Lobular Hyperplasia, and Lobular Carcinoma in Situ Lesions (N = 96) by Stereotactic Biopsy Device[a]

Biopsy Device (<0.05)	%
14-gauge tru-cut	44
14-gauge vacuum-assisted	27
11-gauge vacuum-assisted	21
9-gauge vacuum-assisted	15

Adapted by Margenthaler JA, Duke D, Monsees BS, et al. Correlation between core biopsy and excisional biopsy in breast high-risk lesions. *Am J Surg.* 2006;192:534–537.

numbers approximate the false-negative rates for core needle biopsy-detected *intraductal papilloma* and *radial scar,* which are associated with a 14% to 18% incidence of malignancy on wide local excision (41,42). In each of these cases, the potential for a missed occult malignancy is considered sufficiently high to justify subsequent wide local excision as standard management for ADH, intraductal papilloma, and radial scar diagnosed by core needle biopsy.

LN poses a unique challenge for the triple test. Because LN is usually detected as an incidental histologic finding, imaging or clinical criteria cannot be reliably used to assess the adequacy of a clinically or imaging occult lesion. Moreover, because infiltrating lobular carcinoma, a malignancy commonly associated with LN, is also notoriously occult to clinical and imaging evaluation during its earliest stages, one cannot ensure early detection of an associated invasive lobular carcinoma. Therefore, the central question remains: should LN diagnosed on core needle biopsy routinely undergo wide local excision to rule out an associated malignancy?

Recognizing the potential for histologic understaging, surgeons, radiologists, and pathologists have begun to investigate the coexistence of breast cancer in core needle biopsy-diagnosed LN. The result has been a growing body of data demonstrating false-negative rates ranging from 7% to 31% for "pure" LN lesions initially diagnosed by 11- and 14-gauge core needle biopsies compared with wide local excision results (8,11,43,44). "Pure" LN refers to those cases of LN that are not associated with other high-risk histology (e.g., ADH and radial scar) that may be associated with breast cancer risk. Some authors suggest that lower false-negative rates can be achieved by complete percutaneous removal of imaging abnormalities or assiduous clinical, radiology, and pathology concordance (45,46). However, based on the limitations of the triple test in the setting of LN, many clinicians, but not all (45), are recommending wide local excision of LN diagnosed on core needle biopsy to avoid missing an associated adjacent occult malignancy.

This recommendation is supported by the recent report of Brem et al. (44). These authors found that 38 of 164 patients (23%) who underwent surgical excision based on a finding of LN on image-guided needle biopsy had cancer. In this series, significant sampling errors were observed regardless of the type of core biopsy device, number of specimens obtained, histologic-radiographic concordance, mammographic appearance, and apparently complete excision of the lesion as determined by imaging. These observations led the authors to call for surgical excision for all patients with the finding of LN on core or vacuum-assisted biopsy.

Presently, there are no guidelines delineating how much tissue removal constitutes adequate wide local excision following a core biopsy revealing LN. Certainly, the surgical excision should encompass the original biopsy site, any residual imaging abnormality, and some apparently normal adjacent breast tissue. The availability of large-gauge (e.g., 8-gauge) vacuum-assisted breast biopsy systems creates an opportunity to study the application of these large-volume tissue-sampling instruments as a substitute for surgical excision in some patients. However, the efficacy of this approach has yet to be established.

Lobular Neoplasia Diagnosed by Excisional Biopsy

Most of the long-term data regarding the natural history of LN is based on LN diagnosed by excisional biopsy. In this context, women who were found to have an associated occult malignancy were immediately upstaged to invasive breast cancer or ductal carcinoma in situ and managed accordingly. Consequently, most clinicians consider a surgical excisional biopsy finding of LN sufficient tissue sampling as to preclude the need for further tissue removal. Similarly, removal of LN with clear margins is also thought to be unnecessary as long as the area in question is considered adequately excised. Indeed, the only way to reliably ensure clear margins for this generally multicentric, multifocal, and bilateral condition is to perform bilateral mastectomies, an approach that would seem to be excessive given that most patients never develop a breast malignancy (5).

Consideration should also be given to the implications of LN detected incidentally at the time of breast-conserving surgery for a breast malignancy. The significance of LN in this setting was addressed by three large series, two of which showed no relationship between the presence of LN in the resection specimen and breast cancer outcome in women with stage I and II breast cancer (31,47,48). The largest of these series was a case-controlled study that showed identical local recurrence rates (13% vs. 12%) in women with and without an LCIS-associated malignancy. The third study showed a higher local recurrence rate in a cohort of women with LCIS-associated malignancy. Despite these divergent conclusions, the authors did not suggest that the finding of LCIS in association with breast malignancy should alter a woman's surgical or adjuvant therapy options or necessitate re-excision for LCIS at the surgical margins.

SUMMARY OF MANAGEMENT OF LOBULAR NEOPLASIA

Available data suggest that LN is both a risk factor and precursor to malignancy in some patients. Unfortunately, no criteria have been shown to reliably identify subsets of LN that merely indicate a future generalized risk of breast cancer in either breast, the likelihood of a concurrent ipsilateral breast malignancy, or a propensity for progression to an ipsilateral breast cancer.

To minimize the potential for an undetected malignancy, the preponderance of available data point to the merits of follow-up wide local excision to evaluate ALH and LCIS diagnosed by core needle biopsy. Such a uniform approach might seem excessively broad in an environment of personalized care based on individualized risk, but the relative infrequency of LN would minimize the number of women undergoing such "aggressive" management. For clinicians seeking a more nuanced approach for the management of core needle biopsy-detected LN, the following factors have been identified by some authors as more likely to be associated with an concurrent malignancy: the presence of pleomorphic LCIS (9,49), extensive LCIS (more than ten lobules involved in LCIS) (50), LCIS or ALH associated with a mass or residual microcalcifications (8,12), and LN associated with ADH (7,51). Unfortunately, because of small sample sizes and inconsistent inclusion and exclusion criteria, none of these factors has been shown to be independent predictors of concurrent breast malignancy.

Regardless of whether or not a surgeon or patient chooses wide local excision as initial management of core needle biopsy-proven LN, the increased risk of breast cancer warrants vigilant surveillance for concurrent or subsequent ipsilateral or bilateral breast cancer. Consequently, some clinicians recommend semi-annual clinical breast examination along with bilateral screening mammography. Currently, there are no widely accepted standard guidelines for the use of annual bilateral breast contrast-enhanced magnetic resonance imaging (MRI) in the management of patients with LN, but periodic evaluation with breast MRI is increasingly employed by many clinicians. At the University of Southern California Kenneth Norris Comprehensive Cancer Center, patients with LN are generally advised to undergo breast MRI to permit early detection of a malignancy that might initially be mammographically occult, particularly given the likelihood of higher breast density in this predominantly premenopausal population.

In addition to enhanced screening, clinicians should also discuss with each patient the potential benefits of chemoprevention based on the NSABP P-1 prevention study, which demonstrated a 54% reduction in the relative risk of an invasive breast malignancy in women with LCIS who took tamoxifen for 7 years (52). The recently reported Study of Tamoxifen and Raloxifene (STAR) P-2 Trial in postmenopausal women showed equivalent risk reduction benefits among women taking raloxifene or tamoxifen, but fewer treatment-related side effects (e.g., uterine cancer and thromboembolism) among the raloxifene-treated subjects (53).

Bilateral prophylactic mastectomy remains an option for women seeking maximal (approximately 90%) risk reduction benefits. Although many surgeons would consider bilateral prophylactic mastectomy to be overtreatment for a condition that in most cases will not progress to malignancy, this risk-reduction strategy should remain an option for appropriately counseled women. Because LN is generally considered a multifocal, multicentric, and bilateral process, there is little rational role for "preventive" breast-conserving surgery or unilateral prophylactic mastectomy. In addition, there are few or no data supporting the need for additional surgery in patients with LN diagnosed by excisional biopsy, LN at the surgical margins, or LN detected concurrently with a breast malignancy.

REFERENCES

1. Haagensen CD, Lane N, Bodian C, et al. Lobular neoplasia (so-called lobular carcinoma in situ) of the breast. *Cancer.* 1978;42:737–769.

2. Foote FW, Stewart FW. Lobular carcinoma in situ: a rare form of mammary cancer. *Am J Pathol.* 1941;17:491–495.

3. Ottesen GL, Graversen HP, Blichert-Toft M, et al. Carcinoma in situ of the female breast. 10 year followup results of a prospective nationwide study. *Breast Cancer Res Treat.* 2000;62:197–210.

4. Rosen PP, Kosloff C, Lieberman PH, et al. Lobular carcinoma in situ of the breast. Detailed analysis of 99 patients with average follow-up of 24 years. *Am J Surg Pathol.* 1978;2:225–251.

5. Anderson BO, Calhoun KE, Rosen EL. Evolving concepts in the management of lobular neoplasia. *J Natl Compr Canc Netw.* 2006; 4:511–522.

6. Crisi GM, Mandavilli S, Cronin E, et al. Invasive mammary carcinoma after immediate and short-term follow-up for lobular neoplasia on core biopsy. *Am J Surg Pathol.* 2003;27:325–333.

7. Arpino G, Allred DC, Mohsin SK, et al. Lobular neoplasia on core-needle biopsy—clinical significance. *Cancer.* 2004;101:242–250.

8. Elsheikh TM, Silverman JF. Follow-up surgical excision is indicated when breast core needle biopsies show atypical lobular hyperplasia or lobular carcinoma in situ: a correlative study of 33 patients with review of the literature. *Am J Surg Pathol.* 2005;29:534–543.

9. Georgian-Smith D, Lawton TJ. Calcifications of lobular carcinoma in situ of the breast: radiologic-pathologic correlation. *AJR Am J Roentgenol.* 2001;176:1255–1259.

10. Page DL, Schuyler PA, Dupont WD, et al. Atypical lobular hyperplasia as a unilateral predictor of breast cancer risk: a retrospective cohort study. *Lancet.* 2003;361:125–129.

11. Foster MC, Helvie MA, Gregory NE, et al. Lobular carcinoma in situ or atypical lobular hyperplasia at core-needle biopsy: is excisional biopsy necessary? *Radiology.* 2004;231:813–819.

12. Berg WA, Mrose HE, Ioffe OB, et al. Atypical lobular hyperplasia or lobular carcinoma in situ at core-needle breast biopsy. *Radiology.* 2001;218:503–509.

13. Wheeler JE, Enterline HT, Roseman JM, et al. Lobular carcinoma in situ of the breast. Long-term follow-up. *Cancer.* 1974;34: 554–563.

14. Colditz GA, Rosner B. Cumulative risk of breast cancer to age 70 years according to risk factor status: data from the Nurses' Health Study. *Am J Epidemiol.* 2000;152:950–964.

15. Marshall LM, Hunter DJ, Connolly JL, et al. Risk of breast cancer associated with atypical hyperplasia of lobular and ductal types. *Cancer Epidemiol Biomarkers Prev.* 1997;6:297–301.

16. Rosen PP. Coexistent lobular carcinoma in situ and intraductal carcinoma in a single lobular-duct unit. *Am J Surg Pathol.* 1980;4:241–246.

17. Page DL, Kidd TE Jr, Dupont WD, et al. Lobular neoplasia of the breast: higher risk for subsequent invasive cancer predicted by more extensive disease. *Hum Pathol.* 1991;22:1232–1239.

18. Chuba PJ, Hamre MR, Yap J, et al. Bilateral risk for subsequent breast cancer after lobular carcinoma-in-situ: analysis of surveillance, epidemiology, and end results data. *J Clin Oncol.* 2005;23:5534–5541.

19. Tavassoli FA, Devilee P. Tumours of the breast and female genital organs. In: Tavassoli F, ed. *World Health Organization Classification of Tumors.* Lyon, France: International Agency for Research on Cancer; 2003.

20. Andersen JA. Lobular carcinoma in situ. A long-term follow-up in 52 cases. *Acta Pathol Microbiol Scand [A].* 1974;82:519–533.

21. Andersen JA. Lobular carcinoma in situ of the breast. An approach to rational treatment. *Cancer.* 1977;39:2597–2602.

22. Millikan R. The changing face of epidemiology in the genomics era. *Epidemiology.* 2002;13:472–480.

23. Bauer VP, Ditkoff BA, Schnabel F, et al. The management of lobular neoplasia identified on percutaneous core breast biopsy. *Breast J.* 2003;9:4–9.

24. Lechner MC, Jackman RJ, Parker SH, et al. Lobular carcinoma in situ and atypical lobular hyperplasia at percutaneous core biopsy with surgical correlation: A multi-institutional study [abstract]. *Radiology.* 2000;213:106.

25. Hwang ES, DeVries S, Chew KL, et al. Patterns of chromosomal alterations in breast ductal carcinoma in situ. *Clin Cancer Res.* 2004;10:5160–5167.

26. Vos CB, ter Haar NT, Rosenberg C, et al. Genetic alterations on chromosome 16 and 17 are important features of ductal carcinoma in situ of the breast and are associated with histologic type. *Br J Cancer.* 1999;81:1410–1418.

27. Lakhani SR, Collins N, Sloane JP, et al. Loss of heterozygosity in lobular carcinoma in situ of the breast. *Clin Mol Pathol.* 1995;48:M74–M78.

28. Lishman SC, Lakhani SR. Atypical lobular hyperplasia and lobular carcinoma in situ: surgical and molecular pathology. *Histopathology.* 1999;35:195–200.

29. Lu YJ, Osin P, Lakhani SR, et al. Comparative genomic hybridization analysis of lobular carcinoma in situ and atypical lobular hyperplasia and potential roles for gains and losses of genetic material in breast neoplasia. *Cancer Res.* 1998;58:4721–4727.

30. Nayar R, Zhuang Z, Merino MJ, et al. Loss of heterozygosity on chromosome 11q13 in lobular lesions of the breast using tissue microdissection and polymerase chain reaction. *Hum Pathol.* 1997;28:277–282.

31. Sasson AR, Fowble B, Hanlon AL, et al. Lobular carcinoma in situ increases the risk of local recurrence in selected patients with stages I and II breast carcinoma treated with conservative surgery and radiation. *Cancer.* 2001;91:1862–1869.

32. Fisher ER, Land SR, Fisher B, et al. Pathologic findings from the National Surgical Adjuvant Breast and Bowel Project: twelve-year observations concerning lobular carcinoma in situ. *Cancer.* 2004;100:238–244.

33. Page DL, Dupont WD, Rogers LW, et al. Atypical hyperplastic lesions of the female breast. A long-term follow-up study. *Cancer.* 1985;55:2698–2708.

34. Silverstein MJ, Lagios MD, Recht A, et al. Image-detected breast cancer: state of the art diagnosis and treatment. *J Am Coll Surg.* 2005;201:586–597.

35. Maganini RO, Klem DA, Huston BJ, et al. Upgrade rate of core biopsy-determined atypical ductal hyperplasia by open excisional biopsy. *Am J Surg.* 2001;182:355–358.

36. Margenthaler JA, Duke D, Monsees BS, et al. Correlation between core biopsy and excisional biopsy in breast high-risk lesions. *Am J Surg.* 2006;192:534–537.

37. Jackman RJ, Marzoni FA Jr, et al. Stereotactic, automated, large-core needle biopsy of nonpalpable breast lesions: false-negative and histologic underestimation rates after long-term follow-up. *Radiology.* 1999;210:799–805.

38. Darling ML, Smith DN, Lester SC, et al. Atypical ductal hyperplasia and ductal carcinoma in situ as revealed by large-core needle breast biopsy: results of surgical excision. *AJR Am J Roentgenol.* 2000;175:1341–1346.

39. Brem RF, Behrndt VS, Sanow L, et al. Atypical ductal hyperplasia: histologic underestimation of carcinoma in tissue harvested from impalpable breast lesions using 11-gauge stereotactically guided directional vacuum-assisted biopsy. *AJR Am J Roentgenol.* 1999;172:1405–1407.

40. Winchester DJ, Bernstein JR, Jeske JM, et al. Upstaging of atypical ductal hyperplasia after vacuum-assisted 11-gauge stereotactic core needle biopsy. *Arch Surg.* 2003;138:619–622.

41. Liberman L, Tornos C, Huzian R, et al. Is surgical excision warranted after benign, concordant diagnosis of papilloma at percutaneous breast biopsy? *AJR Am J Roentgenol.* 2006;186:1328–1334.

42. López-Medina A, Cintora E, Múgica B, et al. Radial scars diagnosed at stereotactic core-needle biopsy: surgical biopsy findings. *Eur Radiol.* 2006;16:1803–1810.

43. Shin SJ, Rosen PP. Excisional biopsy should be performed if lobular carcinoma in situ is seen on needle core biopsy. *Arch Pathol Lab Med.* 2002;126:697–701.

44. Brem RF, Lechner MC, Jackman RJ, et al. Lobular neoplasia at percutaneous breast biopsy: variables associated with carcinoma at surgical excision. *AJR Am J Roentgenol.* 2008;190:637–641.

45. Nagi CS, O'Donnell JE, Tismenetsky M, et al. Lobular neoplasia on core needle biopsy does not require excision. *Cancer.* 2008;112:2152–2158.

46. Jackman RJ, Burbank F, Parker SH, et al. Atypical ductal hyperplasia diagnosed at stereotactic breast biopsy: improved reliability with 14-gauge, directional, vacuum-assisted biopsy. *Radiology.* 1997;204:485–488.

47. Abner AL, Connolly JL, Recht A, et al. The relation between the presence and extent of lobular carcinoma in situ and the risk of local recurrence for patients with infiltrating carcinoma of the breast treated with conservative surgery and radiation therapy. *Cancer.* 2000;88:1072–1077.

48. Ben-David MA, Kleer CG, Paramagul C, et al. Is lobular carcinoma in situ as a component of breast carcinoma a risk factor for local failure after breast-conserving therapy? Results of a matched pair analysis. *Cancer.* 2006;106:28–34.

49. Liberman L, Sama M, Susnik B, et al. Lobular carcinoma in situ at percutaneous breast biopsy: surgical biopsy findings. *AJR Am J Roentgenol.* 1999;173:291–299.

50. Ottesen GL, Graversen HP, Blichert-Toft M, et al. Lobular carcinoma in situ of the female breast. Short term results of a prospective nationwide study. The Danish Breast Cancer Cooperative Group. *Am J Surg Pathol.* 1993;17:14–21.

51. Renshaw AA, Derhagopian RP, Martinez P, et al. Lobular neoplasia in breast core needle biopsy specimens is associated with a low risk of ductal carcinoma in situ or invasive carcinoma on subsequent excision. *Am J Clin Pathol.* 2006;126:310–313.

52. Fisher B, Costantino JP, Wickerham DL, et al. Tamoxifen for the prevention of breast cancer: current status of the National Surgical Adjuvant Breast and Bowel Project P-1 study. *J Natl Cancer Inst.* 2005;97:1652–1662.

53. Vogel VG, Costantino JP, Wickerham DL, et al. Effects of tamoxifen vs raloxifene on the risk of developing invasive breast cancer and other disease outcomes: the NSABP Study of Tamoxifen and Raloxifene (STAR) P-2 trial. *JAMA.* 2006;295:2727–2741.

COMMENTARY
Yuri Parisky

The work of Parker, Brenner, and their colleagues (1–4) in the development of minimally invasive biopsy devices has revolutionized the diagnosis of breast lesions, especially those that are clinically occult but apparent on breast imaging. A benign finding on tissue acquired by minimally invasive biopsy devices often saves the patient an unnecessary open biopsy, and a ma-

lignant diagnosis by needle or core biopsy allows the patient the opportunity to carefully consider the range of treatment options available prior to definitive surgery.

Breast core biopsy is widely employed in the United States for sampling a broad spectrum of imaging abnormalities (5). Core biopsy results in few complications, and the procedure is associated with less disfigurement, decreased patient discomfort, and lower cost than a surgical biopsy (2,5).

Diagnoses based on the small samples of tissue acquired on core biopsies are highly accurate when the histologic findings are concordant with the clinical and imaging findings (1,2). However, surgical biopsy is required when a benign finding on core biopsy is discordant with the clinical examination or breast imaging studies and for apparently benign lesions often associated with adjacent malignancy, such as those discussed by Dr. Holmes and the subject of this commentary (1).

As mentioned by Dr. Holmes, at the 2005 International Consensus Conference on Image-Detected Breast Cancer, the expert panel concluded that a minimally invasive breast biopsy is the optimal initial tissue-acquisition method and the procedure of choice for image-detected breast abnormalities (6). Percutaneous histologic tissue-acquisition techniques include large-core biopsy (typically 12 to 14 gauge), vacuum-assisted biopsy (typically 7 to 11 gauge), and larger tissue-acquisition methods. The consensus panel considered stereotactic guidance using vacuum-assisted devices with larger diameter needles (11-gauge or less) the preferred approach for lesions presenting as microcalcifications without a mass inasmuch as this method permits contiguous and more complete tissue acquisition than achieved with smaller diameter needs. The panel further recommended ultrasonography as the preferred biopsy guidance method for lesions visible on ultrasound. For lesions ≤1 cm, percutaneous excision using a vacuum-assisted device was considered desirable because sampling errors appear to be substantially reduced and characterization of important pathologic parameters is more reliable. For lesions >1 cm, a 14-gauge core needle biopsy was considered sufficient, although even in such instances, pathologic parameters may be more reliably characterized when larger gauge needles are used. If percutaneous biopsy results in removal of the entire lesion or a substantial portion of it, the consensus panel called for the placement of a clip or other marking device at the time of biopsy.

Finally, the consensus panel strongly recommended that core biopsy specimens be interpreted by pathologists experienced in breast pathology to avoid errors in diagnosis. Interpretation by such "expert" pathologists is particularly relevant in the case of borderline lesions, such as atypical ductal or lobular hyperplasia and lobular carcinoma in situ inasmuch as Verkooijen et al. (7) found significant interobserver variability between general and expert breast pathologists in the interpretation of such lesions.

LOBULAR NEOPLASIA

This is the most controversial subject discussed by Dr. Holmes. Various studies in the literature provide opposing recommendations regarding the management of lobular neoplasia detected by core biopsy. As a practical matter, the following observations can be made:

- Lobular neoplasia (LN) is a relatively rare lesion, with no distinct mammographic or ultrasonographic findings.
- LN is discovered as an incidental finding when other lesions, most notably calcifications, are targeted for image-guided biopsy. Thus, its discovery is serendipitous.
- The diagnosis of LN depends on the skill and experience of the pathologist. Distinction from ductal lesions may require immunostaining for E-cadherin, an adhesion molecule typically expressed in ductal lesions but not in LN (8–10).
- There is no established treatment of LN, whether discovered by core biopsy or excision. Further resection or chemotherapy is of no known value in patients after surgical biopsy revealing LN, even with marginal involvement. Some data suggest use of tamoxifen for risk reduction for subsequent invasive cancer (11).
- The exact relationship between LN and coincident and subsequent invasive breast cancer is yet to be fully understood.

The issue at hand is whether to proceed with further excisional biopsy when LN is discovered on core biopsy unaccompanied by a second lesion mandating excision. There is no consensus. Various authors conclude that excision is not warranted (12–14), while others advocate routine excision (15,16). Thus, Nagi et al. (13) reported that among 45 patients with LN who underwent excisional biopsy, 42 (93%) had that lesion alone. The remaining three patients had biopsies with the following findings: atypical ductal hyperplasia (ADH) in one patient, residual lobular carcinoma in situ, and a separate minute focus of infiltrating lobular carcinoma in the second patient, and ductal carcinoma in situ (DCIS) admixed with lobular carcinoma in situ in the third patient. The authors concluded that excision of LN is unnecessary, provided that (a) careful radiographic-pathologic correlation is performed, (b) strict histologic criteria are adhered to when making the diagnosis, and (c) close radiologic and clinical follow-up is provided. In contrast, Arpino et al. (15) reported a series in which malignant disease was found in 14% (3/21) of excisional biopsy samples following the detection of LN on core biopsy. Similarly, in the series reported by Brem et al. (16), 23% of patients with LN on core biopsy had cancer on excisional biopsy. Furthermore, these authors could identify no subset of patients free of this substantial risk and, therefore, recommended excision for all of these patients.

ATYPICAL DUCTAL HYPERPLASIA

Management of ADH discovered at core biopsy has been more extensively studied than LH, perhaps because of its greater incidence and clearer association with DCIS and invasive disease on surgical excision (15,17,18). Liberman et al. (18) reported that 11 of 21 (52%) cases of ADH found on core biopsy using a 14-gauge needle were upgraded to DCIS (73%) or invasive ductal cancer (27%) on excisional biopsy. Eby and associates (17) found that even among cases of focal ADH diagnosed after 9- or 11-gauge stereotactic vacuum-assisted breast biopsies, 12.5% were upgraded after surgical biopsy. The upgrade rates were not

significantly different between the 9- and 11-gauge instruments. Nevertheless, as the volume of the tissue sampled increases with use of even larger-core biopsy needles, there is the potential for modification of the standard recommendation calling for an excision of all lesions harboring ADH on needle biopsy. For instance, if a postbiopsy mammography indicates that a small focus of calcifications harboring ADH has been completely removed with a large-bore vacuum-assisted biopsy device, either as a result of multiple samples or a single large contiguous excision sample, then the obligation to proceed with surgical excision may be obviated.

RADIAL SCARS AND COMPLEX SCLEROSING LESIONS

Radial scars are small (<10 mm) and impalpable, stellate, or spiculated lesions usually detected on mammography. Complex sclerosing lesions are larger (>10 mm) and may be palpable, but both lesions are regarded as part of a continuum. These lesions may have a radiolucent center but on imaging (including ultrasound examination) cannot be distinguished from carcinoma (19).

Appropriate management has been the subject of considerable debate. The manner in which the biopsy is performed and the pathologic results influence subsequent management. Douglas-Jones et al. (19) reported 11 false-negative needle-core biopsies among 281 cases of radial scar or complex sclerosing lesion, an incidence of 3.9%. On surgical excision, six cases revealed DCIS only, and in five cases, invasive cancer was observed. These findings led the authors to recommend routine excision of these lesions diagnosed on core biopsy. Brenner and associates (20), in a multi-institutional study, reviewed the findings after excision of 157 lesions interpreted as showing a radial scar on a core needle biopsy. Eight percent (13/157) of the radial scars subsequently excised harbored DCIS or invasive ductal cancer. However, among these cases, the incidence of malignancy was 28% (8/29) when ADH was present in the core biopsy specimen, but only 4% (5/128) when there was no associated atypia (p <0.0001). The technique and apparatus used had an impact on the false-negative rate for cancer. Malignancy was missed in 9% (5/58) of lesions biopsied with a 12- or 14-gauge spring-loaded device versus 0% (0/70) of lesions biopsied with an 11- or 14-gauge directional vacuum-assisted device (p = 0.01). False-negative results for cancer were observed in 8% (5/60) of lesions sampled with less than 12 specimens per lesion versus 0% (0/68) of lesions sampled with 12 or more specimens (p = 0.015). Lesion type, maximal lesion diameter, and type of imaging guidance (stereotactic or sonographic) were not significant factors in determining the presence of malignancy. Thus, the authors concluded that the diagnosis of radial scar based on core needle biopsy is likely to be reliable when there is no associated atypical hyperplasia at percutaneous biopsy, when the biopsy includes at least 12 specimens, and when mammographic findings are concordant with histologic findings. When the lesion diagnosed by core needle biopsy as radial scar does not meet these criteria, the authors call for excisional biopsy.

In the future it may be determined that fewer than 12 core specimens will provide an adequate tissue sample to avoid false-negative findings if needles larger that 11 gauge are employed.

PAPILLARY LESIONS

Papillary lesions are a heterogenous group of breast lesions identified histologically by the presence of a fibrovascular stalk. They include papilloma, papillomatosis, atypical papilloma, noninvasive papillary carcinoma, and invasive papillary carcinoma (21). Radiologically, these lesions can present as an architectural distortion or an abnormal density or mass. Occasionally there are associated calcifications. However, neither mammography nor ultrasonography can reliably distinguish benign from malignant lesions (22). There is a consensus that papillary lesions with atypia or those associated with foci of ADH observed on needle core biopsy require surgical excision because of a high rate of upgrading to cancer. Thus, Ashkenazi et al. (23) culled 109 cases of such lesions from various reported series and found that malignancy was observed on surgical excision in 54% (59/109).

In contrast, the appropriate management of apparently benign papillary lesions without atypia or associated ADH observed on core needle biopsy remains uncertain. Among 316 such lesions reported in various serious and regarded as benign and with mammographic concordance, only 4% (14/316) were upgraded to cancer (23). These findings suggest that excision is not necessary, and radiographic follow-up is appropriate (21,24–26). However, several recent reports indicate a much higher rate of upgrading to a final diagnosis of malignancy. Rates of upgrading reported by Ashkenazi et al. (23), Rizzo et al. (22), Skandarajah et al. (27), and Tseng et al. (28) were 20% (4/20), 10.5% (9/86), 19% (15/86), and 29% (7/24), respectively. These latter findings suggest that all papillary lesions detected on core biopsy should be excised (22,27,28).

AVOIDING SAMPLING ERRORS

The finding of malignancy on surgical excision of lesions deemed free of cancer on needle biopsy is the result of sampling errors associated with removal of small volumes of tissue. Many of the studies reporting high rates of upgrading employed small-volume core biopsy needles. These false-negative rates are likely to be reduced in future series using percutaneous biopsy apparatus, which provides larger volumes of tissue. Such sampling tools include 8- to 9-gauge vacuum-assisted core biopsy needles, the Intact Breast Lesion Excision System (Intact Medical Corporation, Natick, MA, www.intactmedical.com), or the single-specimen tissue capture device, which harvests a tissue sample of 1.5 to 2 cm, currently being evaluated by Tot and Tabar (29).

HOW I DO IT

The strategy for percutaneous biopsy of an image-detected breast lesion includes the choice of the biopsy device and the method of image guidance for the procedure. The sample obtained must be sufficient for routine histopathologic diagnosis as well as suf-

ficient for additional stains and biomarker determinations requested by the clinician or pathologist. The latter tests are particularly important when neoadjuvant therapy is planned prior to excision of a malignancy. Tumor expression of hormonal sensitivity, expression of HER2/neu, and other factors have an impact on prognosis, the choice of agents given preoperatively, and the likely response to the neoadjuvant program (30).

My selection of the image-guidance method is based on ease of access. Ultrasound guidance is quicker than stereotactic means. Real-time, ultrasonographic observation of the target lesion being traversed by the biopsy needle confirms appropriate location of the biopsy device and adequate sampling or complete removal. Although calcifications are most commonly sampled by stereotactic means, the presence of highly suspicious, pleomorphic calcifications in the setting of increasing density or possible mass or spiculation leads me to consider ultrasound scrutiny first. Hypoechoic, irregular tissue observed amid the calcifications, may represent a focus of invasion associated with DCIS, which may be specifically targeted with ultrasound-guided large-core needle biopsy. Simply targeting the calcifications by stereotactic means may not sample the focus of invasion, a circumstance that has obvious surgical management implications. Indeterminate or suspicious calcifications should be approached by stereotactic means. Masses, architectural distortion, or a persistent new asymmetric density should, after thorough mammographic workup, be evaluated by ultrasonography prior to attempt at stereotactic biopsy. Lesions, especially mammographically vague ones, may be obscured by introduced lidocaine, and frustrate stereotactic targeting. Worrisome lesions discovered by magnetic resonance imaging (MRI) necessitate focused, second-look ultrasonography directed to the area of concern identified on the MRI in order to determine if ultrasound guidance is feasible prior to proceeding with the more difficult and costly MRI-guided biopsy.

Needle selection is simple: the smaller the lesion, the larger the needle (corresponding to a smaller gauge) that is selected. An obvious ultrasonographically apparent, highly suspicious mass may be confirmed as malignant with the use of a 14-gauge core biopsy needle, provided enough tissue is obtained for additional biomarker evaluation. Calcifications should be biopsied by any of the large-core, vacuum-assisted devices available in order to ensure adequate target tissue sampling. Continued use of 14-gauge core biopsy needles for this purpose should be discouraged, given their relative insufficient sampling rates (31,32). When calcifications are targeted, specimen radiographs of all the biopsy cores should be obtained to confirm adequate sampling of the calcifications. In the case of noncalcified lesions, in which histologic architecture and abundant tissue evaluation is key to rendering a diagnosis, especially in the so-called borderline lesions, I encourage use of ultrasound-guided, large-core, vacuum-assisted biopsy devices Here I attempt to nearly completely remove small lesions.

In nearly all instances, clips should be deposited at the site of the biopsy to facilitate subsequent wire localization, if required. Nothing is more frustrating than a cancer completely responding to neoadjuvant treatment, virtually disappearing, wherein needle localization for lumpectomy becomes guesswork rather than precise bracketing with wires. Furthermore, adequately marking the site of a lesion shown to be benign memorializes the nature and location of the abnormality in subsequent imaging examinations.

REFERENCES

1. Brenner RJ, Bassett LW, Fajardo LL, et al. Stereotactic core-needle breast biopsy: a multi-institutional prospective trial. *Radiology.* 2001;218(3):866–872.
2. Parker SH, Burbank F, Jackman RJ, et al. Percutaneous large-core breast biopsy: a multi-institutional study. *Radiology.* 1994;193:359–364.
3. Parker SH, Jobe WE, Dennis MA, et al. US-guided automated large-core breast biopsy. *Radiology.* 1993;187:507–511.
4. Parker SH, Lovin JD, Jobe WE, et al. Stereotactic breast biopsy with a biopsy gun. *Radiology.* 1990;176:741–747.
5. March DE, Raslavicus A, Coughlin BF, et al. Use of breast core biopsy in the United States: results of a national survey. *AJR Am J Roentgenol.* 1997;169:697–701.
6. Silverstein MJ, Lagios MD, Recht A, et al. Image-detected breast cancer: state of the art diagnosis and treatment. *J Am Coll Surg.* 2005;201:586–597.
7. Verkooijen HM, Peterse JL, Schipper ME, et al. Interobserver variability between general and expert pathologists during the histopathological assessment of large-core needle and open biopsies of non-palpable breast lesions. *Eur J Cancer.* 2003;39:2187–2191.
8. De Leeuw WJ, Berx G, Vos CB, et al. Simultaneous loss of E-cadherin and catenins in invasive lobular breast cancer and lobular carcinoma in situ. *J Pathol.* 1997;183:404–411.
9. Jacobs TW, Pliss N, Kouria G, et al. Carcinomas in situ of the breast with indeterminate features: role of E-cadherin staining in categorization. *Am J Surg Pathol.* 2001;25:229–236.
10. Moll R, Mitze M, Frixen UH, et al. Differential loss of E-cadherin expression in infiltrating ductal and lobular breast carcinomas. *Am J Pathol.* 1993;143:1731–1742.
11. Frykberg ER. Lobular carcinoma in situ of the breast. *Breast J.* 1999;5:296–303.
12. Bauer VP, Ditkoff BA, Schnabel F, et al. The management of lobular neoplasia identified on percutaneous core breast biopsy. *Breast J.* 2003;9:4–9.
13. Nagi CS, O'Donnell JE, Tismenetsky M, et al. Lobular neoplasia on core needle biopsy does not require excision. *Cancer.* 2008;112:2152–2158.
14. Renshaw AA, Cartagena N, Derhagopian RP, et al. Lobular neoplasia in breast core needle biopsy specimens is not associated with an increased risk of ductal carcinoma in situ or invasive carcinoma. *Am J Clin Pathol.* 2002;117:797–799.
15. Arpino G, Allred DC, Mohsin SK, et al. Lobular neoplasia on core-needle biopsy: clinical significance. *Cancer.* 2004;101:242–250.
16. Brem RF, Lechner MC, Jackman RJ, et al. Lobular neoplasia at percutaneous breast biopsy: variables associated with carcinoma at surgical excision. *AJR Am J Roentgenol.* 2008;190:637–641.
17. Eby PR, Ochsner JE, Demartini WB, et al. Is surgical excision necessary for focal atypical ductal hyperplasia found at stereotactic vacuum-assisted breast biopsy? *Ann Surg Oncol.* 2008;15:3232–3238.
18. Liberman L, Cohen MA, Dershaw DD, et al. Atypical ductal hyperplasia diagnosed at stereotaxic core biopsy of breast lesions: an indication for surgical biopsy. *AJR Am J Roentgenol.* 1995;164:1111–1113.
19. Douglas-Jones AG, Denson JL, Cox AC, et al. Radial scar lesions of the breast diagnosed by needle core biopsy: analysis of cases containing occult malignancy. *J Clin Pathol.* 2007;60:295–298.
20. Brenner RJ, Jackman RJ, Parker SH, et al. Percutaneous core needle biopsy of radial scars of the breast: when is excision necessary? *AJR Am J Roentgenol.* 2002;179:1179–1184.
21. Rosen EL, Bentley RC, Baker JA, et al. Imaging-guided core needle biopsy of papillary lesions of the breast. *AJR Am J Roentgenol.* 2002;179:1185–1192.
22. Rizzo M, Lund MJ, Oprea G, et al. Surgical follow-up and clinical presentation of 142 breast papillary lesions diagnosed by ultrasound-guided core-needle biopsy. *Ann Surg Oncol.* 2008;15:1040–1047.
23. Ashkenazi I, Ferrer K, Sekosan M, et al. Papillary lesions of the breast discovered on percutaneous large core and vacuum-assisted biopsies: reliability of clinical and pathological parameters in identifying benign lesions. *Am J Surg.* 2007;194:183–188.
24. Liberman L, Bracero N, Vuolo MA, et al. Percutaneous large-core biopsy of papillary breast lesions. *AJR Am J Roentgenol.* 1999;172:331–337.
25. Sohn V, Keylock J, Arthurs Z, et al. Breast papillomas in the era of percutaneous needle biopsy. *Ann Surg Oncol.* 2007;14:2979–2984.
26. Sydnor MK, Wilson JD, Hijaz TA, et al. Underestimation of the presence of breast carcinoma in papillary lesions initially diagnosed at core-needle biopsy. *Radiology.* 2007;242:58–62.
27. Skandarajah AR, Field L, Yuen Larn Mou A, et al. Benign papilloma on core biopsy requires surgical excision. *Ann Surg Oncol.* 2008;15:2272–2277.
28. Tseng HS, Chen YL, Chen ST, et al. The management of papillary lesion of the breast by core needle biopsy. *Eur J Surg Oncol.* 2008;35:21–24.
29. Tot T, Tabar L. Papillary lesions of the breast: Histologic examination of contiguous tissue can predict the need for surgical excision. Paper presented at the 12th annual Multidisciplinary Symposium on Breast Disease; February 2007; Amelia Island, FL.
30. Colleoni M, Viale G, Zahrieh D, et al. Expression of ER, PgR, HER1, HER2, and response: a study of preoperative chemotherapy. *Ann Oncol.* 2008;19:465–472.
31. Darling ML, Smith DN, Lester SC, et al. Atypical ductal hyperplasia and ductal carcinoma in situ as revealed by large-core needle breast biopsy: results of surgical excision. *AJR Am J Roentgenol.* 2000;175:1341–1346.
32. Philpotts LE, Shaheen NA, Carter D, et al. Comparison of rebiopsy rates after stereotactic core needle biopsy of the breast with 11-gauge vacuum suction probe versus 14-gauge needle and automatic gun. *AJR Am J Roentgenol.* 1999;172:683–687.

18

Surgical Options for Stage I and II Breast Cancer

Valerie L. Staradub and Monica Morrow

Over the last 50 years, the surgical treatment of stage I and II breast cancer has evolved from the routine use of radical mastectomy to a patient-driven choice between total mastectomy with or without reconstruction and breast-conserving therapy (BCT) for the majority of patients. In this chapter, we review current selection criteria and outcomes for these procedures. In addition, we address newer approaches to local therapy including neoadjuvant therapy for operable cancer, partial breast reconstruction, and nipple-sparing mastectomy.

BREAST-CONSERVING THERAPY

Clinical Trials

In the past, a major objection to the use of BCT was the known multicentricity of breast cancer. The reported incidence of multicentricity ranges from 9% to 75% (1–3), depending on the definition employed and the techniques of pathologic examination used. The possibility of residual microscopic cancer at a distance from the primary tumor was used to argue against any surgical therapy for breast cancer other than mastectomy. The surgical component of BCT often will not remove the entire tumor in the breast, thus moderate-dose radiation must be employed to eradicate microscopic residual disease. Since 1970, there have been six major prospective randomized trials in which conservative surgery plus radiotherapy (RT) have been compared with mastectomy (Table 18.1) (4–9). These studies differed widely in patient selection criteria, the extent of the surgical procedure performed, and the techniques of irradiation used. In spite of these differences in patient selection and treatment techniques, none of these trials demonstrate a significant survival difference between patients treated by BCT (conservative surgery plus RT) versus mastectomy. In 2002, the two largest of these important trials reported 20-year follow-up data, and the lack of a significant survival difference between mastectomy and BCT was found to persist (6,9). Long-term follow-up data demonstrate only small differences in local failure rates between the two procedures, even in these early studies.

In the Milan I study, 710 women with breast tumors measuring ≤2 cm were randomized to radical mastectomy or quadrantectomy followed by RT (9). Although there was no significant difference in survival, the 20-year incidence of local recurrence after BCT was 8.8% compared with 2.3% after radical mastectomy ($p < 0.001$). In the National Surgical Adjuvant Breast and Bowel Project (NSABP) B-06 study, 1,851 women were randomized to total mastectomy, lumpectomy alone, or lumpectomy with RT (6). The 20-year local recurrence rates were 14% for

patients who underwent lumpectomy with postoperative irradiation and 10% among those who underwent mastectomy. Larger differences in local recurrence rates between BCT and mastectomy were observed in the National Cancer Institute (7) and the European Organization for Research and Treatment of Cancer (8) studies, but these studies did not require histologically negative margins after lumpectomy.

Since these early studies of BCT were conducted, local recurrence rates in the preserved breast have deceased significantly, and in more recent studies range from 2% to 6% at 10 years (10–12). Pass et al. (13) observed a decrease in 5-year actuarial local recurrence rates from 8% to 1% ($p = 0.001$) for patients treated at a single institution between 1981 and 1996. During this period, mean tumor size decreased from 2.2 cm to 1.6 cm, the number of patients with negative surgical margins increased from 74% to 97%, and the mean number of slides examined per case doubled from 10.6 to 21.1. Changes in the use of RT and adjuvant systemic therapy were also noted. The proportion of patients treated with a dose of >60 Gy to the tumor bed increased from 66% to 95%, and the use of adjuvant tamoxifen increased from 10% to 61%. Overall, the decrease in local recurrence rates appears to be multifactorial and can be attributed to improvements in the mammographic evaluation of the extent of disease, a better understanding of what constitutes an adequate surgical resection, more detailed pathologic evaluation to determine the adequacy of resection, and the widespread use of adjuvant chemotherapy and/or endocrine therapy for the majority of women with breast cancer. Ten-year rates of local failure of <7% were observed in patients in the systemic therapy arms of a recent series of NSABP trials (12), indicating that improvements in local control have translated to a wide variety of practice settings.

Contraindications to Breast-Conserving Therapy

The majority of patients with early-stage breast cancer are eligible for BCT. Absolute and relative contraindications to BCT have been defined, and regularly updated, by a joint committee of the American College of Radiology, the American College of Surgeons, the College of American Pathology, and the Society of Surgical Oncology (14). The most recent version of these guidelines is summarized in Table 18.2. Absolute contraindications are related to the inability to safely deliver RT, the inability to reduce the tumor burden to a microscopic level that is likely to be controlled by RT, or the inability to detect local recurrence. Pregnant women can never safely receive RT. However, for women diagnosed in the third trimester, RT can be

Table 18.1

Survival and Local Recurrence Results in the Modern Randomized Trials Comparing Conservative Surgery and Radiation Therapy With Mastectomy

Trial (Ref.)	Patients (n)	Follow-up (year)	Overall Survival[a] M (%)	BCT (%)	Local Recurrence M (%)	BCT (%)
Institut Gustave-Roussy (4)	179	22	50	60	10	16
Milan I (9)	701	20	41	42	2	9
NSABP B-06 (6)	1219	20	47	46	10	14
NCI (7)	237	18	58	59	6	22
EORTC (8)	874	10	66	65	12	20
Danish Breast Cancer Group (5)	904	6	82	79	4	3

M, mastectomy; BCT, breast-conserving therapy (conservative surgery plus radiation therapy); NSABP, National Surgical Adjuvant Breast and Bowel Project; NCI, National Cancer Institute; EORTC, European Organization for Research and Treatment of Cancer.
[a]None of the differences in survival were statistically significant.

delayed until after delivery. This is particularly appropriate when surgery is followed by adjuvant chemotherapy. Prior radiation therapy to the target region is another absolute contraindication to BCT. This may include prior ipsilateral breast RT, radiation therapy for ipsilateral lung cancer, and mantle irradiation for Hodgkin disease. Patients with two or more primary tumors in separate quadrants of the breast are not eligible for BCT because of a significant risk of a heavy subclinical disease burden unlikely to be controlled by RT. In patients with diffuse malignant-appearing or indeterminate calcifications, the pres-

Table 18.2

Absolute and Relative Contraindications to Breast-Conserving Therapy

Absolute contraindications
    First or second trimester of pregnancy
    Two or more primary tumors in separate quadrants of the breast
    Diffuse malignant or indeterminate-appearing microcalcifications
    History of prior radiation therapy in the breast radiation field
    Persistent positive margins after reasonable surgical attempts

Relative contraindications
    History of collagen vascular disease (i.e., lupus, scleroderma)
    Multiple tumors in one quadrant (depending on distance and breast size)
    Tumor size (relative to breast size)
    Very large or pendulous breasts (radiotherapist to evaluate feasibility of radiotherapy)

Data derived from ref. 14 Morrow M, Strom EA, Bassett LW, et al. Standard for breast conservation therapy in the management of invasive breast carcinoma. *CA Cancer J Clin.* 2002;52:277–300.

ence of malignancy cannot be reliably excluded without complete surgical resection, while clear surgical margins indicate that the residual tumor burden in the breast is likely to be controlled with RT.

The presence of a relative contraindication to breast conservation does not necessarily preclude BCT but warrants careful, and often multidisciplinary, consideration to determine eligibility. Large tumor size or small breast size alone is not a contraindication, but the size of the tumor must be weighed against the overall breast size; that is, a larger tumor can be resected from a larger breast while maintaining an acceptable cosmetic outcome, whereas even a moderate-sized tumor may not be amenable to BCT in a very small breast. Patients in this category who desire BCT should be considered for cytoreduction with preoperative chemotherapy or endocrine therapy, as discussed later in this chapter. Similarly, the presence of more than one tumor or a sizeable area of calcifications in one quadrant of the breast must be evaluated in terms of the feasibility of resection of the entire area while achieving an acceptable cosmetic result. Finally, there are some relative contraindications to radiation therapy that need to be evaluated in conjunction with the radiation oncologist. Active collagen vascular disease such as systemic lupus erythematosus or scleroderma requires special consideration, as does the presence of a mechanical device such as a pacemaker or implantable nerve-stimulating device. An especially large or pendulous breast may post a significant challenge to the radiation oncologist in terms of delivering a reproducible, homogenous dose to the treatment target.

A number of factors do not impact eligibility for BCT. Features associated with poor prognosis such as axillary metastases, high tumor grade, or the presence of lymphatic or vascular invasion, do not preclude BCT. Histology of the tumor, including infiltrating lobular carcinoma or the presence of an extensive intraductal component, is also not a contraindication as long as histologically negative margins can be obtained. Tumor location does not affect the success of BCT. Occasionally it may be necessary to resect the nipple-areolar complex (NAC) if the tumor is in a subareolar location and intimately associated with the NAC, but this approach still leaves the patient with a sensate breast mound. A strong family history of breast cancer or the presence of a known *BRCA* gene mutation is also not a contraindication to breast conservation, although these patients are at increased risk for the development a new primary tumor in either breast, and may therefore opt for a procedure to address this increased risk, such as a bilateral mastectomy.

Patient Selection for Breast-Conserving Therapy

As is apparent from the previous discussion, BCT is a procedure with well-defined contraindications that have traditionally been identified with a history, physical examination, and diagnostic mammography with or without ultrasound. Morrow et al. (15) reported that of 216 patients with ductal carcinoma in situ or stage I or II invasive cancer evaluated between 1989 and 1993 who were thought to be candidates for BCT, the procedure was successful in 210 (97%). The purpose of imaging is to identify contraindications to BCT that are not clinically apparent such as multicentricity, extensive multifocality, or diffuse calcifications. These findings are relatively infrequent in stage I and II carcinoma. Morrow et al. (16) observed multifocal or multicentric carcinoma in only 39 of 432 (9%) consecutive patients undergoing multidisciplinary evaluation. Pathology studies using standard techniques of examination of breast tissue consisting of gross inspection of the specimen and a limited number of random sections of grossly normal breast have also identified multicentric carcinoma in fewer than 15% of cases (17,18). However, the use of magnetic resonance imaging (MRI) in patients with breast cancer that appears to be localized by conventional evaluation identifies additional tumor foci in 10% to 54% of cases (19–29). Studies of MRI in localized breast cancer are summarized in Table 18.3. These findings have raised the question of whether MRI should be a routine part of the presurgical evaluation. The most common outcome when additional tumor is detected by MRI is the performance of a mastectomy that would not otherwise have been done. Bedrosian et al. (26) reported that

MRI altered surgical management in 69 of 267 patients (29%) thought to have unicentric disease by routine evaluation, with conversion from BCT to mastectomy occurring in 44 patients (16.5% of the total population, 64% of those with abnormalities detected by MRI).

The high rate of cancer detected by MRI alone is difficult to reconcile with the <7% incidence of local failure 10 years after treatment in women selected for BCT with conventional imaging discussed in the previous section (12). These disparate observations strongly suggest that the majority of the disease detected by MRI is controlled with RT. This hypothesis is supported by data from pathology studies that used serial subgross sectioning to perform detailed mapping studies of the microscopic distribution of tumor in breasts with clinically unicentric carcinoma (Table 18.4) (2,3,30–34). Multifocal or centric disease was identified in 21% to 63% of cases, and its presence was used to support the routine performance of mastectomy. In the study by Holland et al. (34), 95% of the pathologically detected tumor foci were within 4 cm of the reference tumor, a finding remarkably similar to that of Berg et al. (35), who observed that 87% of the additional tumor foci detected by MRI were within 4 cm of the reference tumor. At this time, there is no clinical evidence that the use of MRI reduces local recurrence rates after BCT or increases the number of women who have negative margins after a single operative procedure. Increased mastectomy rates and a significant number of breast biopsies and follow-up MRIs for benign abnormalities (26,35) have been observed in studies that have used this technology. Until MRI has been shown to be clinically beneficial, it should not be a routine part of the evaluation of patients for BCT.

Concerns persist about the suitability of patients with infiltrating lobular carcinoma for BCT. Lobular carcinoma is more difficult to detect mammographically than ductal carcinoma (36,37) and is more frequently multifocal/centric in its growth pattern (38). The use of MRI in women with lobular cancer is reported to identify additional tumor in as many as 60% of cases (39). Morrow et al. (40) matched 349 patients with

Table 18.3			
Detection of Multifocal/Multicentric Cancer by Magnetic Resonance Imaging			
Study (Ref.)	Year	No. of Patients	% Additional Cancer
Harms et al. (19)	1993	29	54
Boetes et al. (20)	1995	61	15
Mumtaz et al. (21)	1997	92	11
Fischer et al. (22)	1999	336	16
Drew et al. (23)	1999	178	23
Esserman et al. (28)	1999	58	10
Liberman et al. (24)	2003	70	19
Furman et al. (25)	2003	76	13
Bedrosian et al. (26)	2003	267	15
Schnall et al. (29)	2004	426	24
Deurloo et al. (27)	2005	116	18

Pathologic Studies of Multifocality/Multicentricity

Study (Ref.)	No. of Cases	Population	% Multifocal/Multicentric
Qualheim and Gall (2)	157	Not stated	54
Rosen et al. (3)	203	Invasive carcinoma	33
Egan (30)	118	Not stated	60
Schwartz et al. (31)	43	Nonpalpable cancer	44
Vaidya et al. (32)	30	Invasive carcinoma	63
Anastassiades et al. (33)	366	Invasive ≤7 cm, noninvasive	49
Holland et al. (34)	282	Clinically unicentric invasive cancer <5 cm	63

pure or mixed invasive lobular carcinoma to controls with ductal carcinoma on the basis of year of diagnoses, menopausal status, and disease stage. Patients with lobular carcinoma had larger tumors (2.6 cm vs. 2.1 cm; $p < 0.001$) and their tumors were more likely to be mammographically occult (28% vs. 10%; $p < 0.001$). BCT was successful in 84% of patients with lobular carcinoma who chose this option and 87% of those with ductal carcinoma. In a conditional logistic regression model adjusting for age and pathologic tumor size, no difference in the failure rate of BCT or the number of excisions required to obtain histologically negative margins was observed on the basis of tumor type. Local control rates after BCT do not differ between patients with lobular and ductal carcinoma (41,42), indicating that this histology should not be used as a selection factor for mastectomy.

Another area of recent interest is the suitability of the patient with a known or suspected *BRCA1/2* mutation for breast-conserving approaches. The high rates of contralateral breast cancer observed in this patient group (43) raised concern that the use of BCT in mutation carriers would result in unacceptably high rates of local recurrence. Several retrospective studies of mutation carriers treated with BCT fail to demonstrate an increase in true local recurrence compared with controls with sporadic cancer (44,45), particularly if oophorectomy has been performed (46). These women appear to have an increased risk of late recurrences occurring elsewhere in the breast, which are suggestive of new primaries (44,45), and a significant increase in contralateral cancers (43–46). Thus, known or suspected mutation carrier status is not a contraindication to BCT, but before treatment is selected the risk of subsequent cancer in the ipsilateral and the contralateral breast should be discussed in detail. In the woman known to carry a predisposition mutation, this discussion can take place at the time of diagnosis. The problem is more complex in the woman who presents with cancer and a family history, which raises the possibility of a predisposition mutation. In such a patient who desires BCT, it is important to discuss the impact that carrier status would have on the risk of second cancers and encourage the patient to undergo genetic counseling. Breast-conserving surgery is performed, and during chemotherapy, the patient undergoes genetic counseling and testing if desired. The decision about local therapy is then finalized prior to beginning RT. This approach allows the patient time for reflection and maximizes the information available to make a final decision regarding local therapy.

Extent of Surgery

A major unresolved question in breast-conserving surgery is how much normal breast tissue should be removed as part of a lumpectomy. In making this determination, the surgeon seeks to achieve a low rate of local recurrence in the breast while maintaining a good cosmetic outcome. There is no consensus on what constitutes an optimal margin of resection for a lumpectomy. In a 2002 survey of 702 radiation oncologists from North America and 431 from Europe, 46% of North American respondents and 28% of those from Europe endorsed the definition of a negative margin as no tumor cells seen on the ink. The second most common North American definition was no tumor cells at a distance <2 mm from the ink (22%), while the most common European definition was no tumor cells at a distance <5 mm from the ink (29%) (47). From a practical point of view, an appropriate negative margin is one that results in a residual tumor burden that is low enough for there to be a high likelihood of control with RT. In a review of recent NSABP trials, patients receiving adjuvant systemic therapy had local failure rates of ≤7% at 10 years in studies that required a margin consisting of tumor cells not touching the inked surface (12). It is quite clear that margins that are involved by tumor (tumor touching ink) result in a higher rate of local recurrence than those that are not involved. In a review of 5,138 patients in whom margin status was reported as positive or negative, local recurrence occurred in 15.8% of those with involved margins compared with 5.6% of those with free margins (48). However, when comparing margins of >1 mm with those >2 mm, no clear benefit was noted for the larger excision.

There are a number of factors to consider in assessing the adequacy of excision. The significance of tumor cells in proximity to a margin varies depending on which margin is approached by tumor. The anterior and posterior margins of the breast are anatomically limited. If the excision has been carried to the level of the subcutaneous fat anteriorly or to the pectoral fascia posteriorly, a close margin is of no relevance because there is no breast tissue remaining in these areas. In addition, flattening of the specimen for specimen radiography or during pathologic processing may artificially decrease anterior and posterior margins (49). In contrast, close margins in areas where additional breast tissue is present may indicate the possibility of a significant residual tumor burden. Tumor histology is also important to consider when evaluating the adequacy of resection. Schmidt-Ullrich et al. (50) have demonstrated that in patients with positive or unknown margin status, only 37% of those with infiltrating ductal carcinoma without an extensive intraductal component (EIC) had residual tumor at re-excision compared with 50% of infiltrating lobular carcinomas and 67% of infiltrating ductal tumors with an EIC. Schnitt et al. (51) also found that an EIC predicted a greater likelihood of residual tumor in re-excisions (88% EIC positive vs. 48% EIC negative; $p = 0.002$). These clinical observations are supported by the mapping studies of Holland et al. (1), in which 30% of patients with EIC-positive tumors were found to have prominent residual tumor more than 2 cm from the primary tumor, compared with only 2% of patients with EIC-negative tumors ($p <0.0001$; Figure 18.1). The extent of disease near the surgical margin is also predictive of the presence of residual tumor in the breast and the risk of local recurrence. Park et al. (52) reported a 14% risk of local recurrence in 122 patients with focally positive margins compared with 27% in those with extensively positive margins. Darvishian et al. (53) correlated the length of the margin surface involved with tumor with the presence of residual tumor in the re-excision specimen. If ≥ 1 cm of the margin was involved with tumor, 93% of patients had additional disease in the re-excision specimen. In contrast, only 17% of patients had tumor at re-excision when ≤ 5 mm of the margin surface was involved with tumor. Although these

studies included patients with margin involvement, the principles are applicable to those with close margins as well.

The final important factor to consider in evaluating the appropriate extent of resection is patient age. Younger women, defined as those under 45 or 40 years of age, have a higher risk of local recurrence than their older counterparts. After 20 years of follow-up in the Milan I trial (9), the local recurrence rate per 100 woman-years of follow-up for those age 45 years or younger was 1.05, compared with 0.34 for those age 46 to 60 years and 0.54 for those older than 60 years. A similar relationship between younger age and local recurrence was observed in the NSABP B06 trial for those younger than 35 years old (54), and in the study of Bartelink et al. (55), examining the role of a boost dose of irradiation. Retrospective studies suggest that this increased risk can be significantly reduced by obtaining widely clean margins (10,56). Neuschatz et al. (10) reported a 12-year rate of local recurrence of 19% for women under age 45 years with a negative margin of <2 mm compared with 5% for their older counterparts. In contrast, after a negative re-excision, local recurrence rates were 5% and 3%, respectively. The information discussed in this section indicates that no single negative margin width is appropriate for all patients. In the older women with a pure infiltrating ductal carcinoma and a focally close margin, re-excision is unlikely to be of benefit. In contrast, the 40-year-old patient with a tumor with an EIC and multiple margins approached by tumor is likely to benefit from re-excision.

When re-excision is undertaken, attempts to excise the entire biopsy cavity surrounded by normal breast tissue usually result in the sacrifice of unnecessary amounts of breast tissue unless the original biopsy cavity was extremely small, or enough time has elapsed that it is fibrosed and contracted. Our technique of re-excision is to excise each wall of the biopsy cavity separately, marking the new margin surface with a suture to orient the pathologist. If the initial specimen was marked with orienting sutures, re-excision is limited to the involved margins. Gibson et al. (57) compared the incidence of local recurrence in patients undergoing re-excision of the entire old biopsy cavity with those who underwent re-excision of only the positive margins and found no significant difference between groups. However, significantly less tissue was excised in the ink-directed group. The presence of residual tumor in the re-excision is not a contraindication to breast-conserving treatment. The status of the final margin should be used to determine the patient's suitability for the procedure. Kearney and Morrow (58) found that 86 of 90 patients undergoing re-excision for positive or unknown margins were satisfactory candidates for breast-conserving treatment.

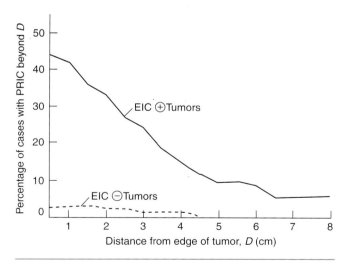

Figure 18.1 Percentage of mastectomy specimens with extensive intraductal carcinoma (EIC) at or beyond certain distances from the edge of the primary tumor. PRIC, (From Holland R, Connolly JL, Gelman R, et al. The presence of an extensive intraductal component following a limited excision correlates with prominent residual disease in the remainder of the breast. *J Clin Oncol.* 1990;8:113–118, with permission.)

EXPANDING ELIGIBILITY FOR BREAST-CONSERVING THERAPY

Based on the patient selection criteria and contraindications to BCT described elsewhere in this chapter, most women with early-stage breast cancer will be eligible for BCT. However, some will not be candidates under the conventional guidelines but may still be strongly motivated to pursue BCT. Although it is not possible to convert all patients into candidates for BCT, there are methods by which to expand patient eligibility. These generally involve either making the tumor smaller or improving the cosmetic outcome of resection of a larger area of breast tissue.

Neoadjuvant Systemic Therapy

Neoadjuvant (also called induction or primary) systemic therapy is routinely used in the treatment of locally advanced breast cancer and its use has been expanded to operable cancers. In doing so, several questions were addressed. First, is there any demonstrable survival advantage to giving systemic therapy earlier in the course of treatment, prior to surgical therapy? Second, is it possible to reduce the tumor volume to the extent that patients with large tumors relative to their breast size can undergo BCT with a cosmetically acceptable outcome? And finally, is there an increase in local recurrence rates among patients treated with neoadjuvant chemotherapy followed by BCT? Several randomized studies have addressed these questions, with one of the largest and most important being the NSABP B-18 study. In the B-18 study, 1,523 women with a palpable T1-T3 breast cancer were randomized to preoperative versus postoperative administration of four cycles of doxorubicin plus cyclophosphamide at standard doses (59–61). The clinical size of the tumor and clinical nodal status were documented prior to the initiation of treatment, and clinical complete response was defined as absence of clinical evidence of tumor in the breast or the lymph nodes at the completion of neoadjuvant chemotherapy. Clinical partial response was classified as a reduction in the size of the breast tumor by at least 50%. Clinical disease progression was considered as an increase in the size of the tumor by at least 50%, and anything else was defined as clinically stable disease. A reduction in tumor size of at least 50% occurred in 80% of patients in the neoadjuvant chemotherapy group: 36% with a clinical complete response and 44% with a clinical partial response (59). However, only 36% of the patients who had a clinical complete response to neoadjuvant chemotherapy had a complete pathologic response, an overall pathologic complete response rate of only 9%. Tumor progression occurred in 3% of patients during chemotherapy.

The B-18 study not only evaluated the clinical response to chemotherapy, but also examined whether this translated into an increase in the number of patients eligible for BCT. At randomization, approximately two thirds of the patients in both treatment groups were assessed by their treating surgeon as eligible for lumpectomy (59,60). When the initial surgical recommendation was compared with the procedure actually performed, more patients in the neoadjuvant arm actually had breast-conservation surgery. In the postoperative chemotherapy group, 66% of patients were initially proposed as candidates for BCT, and 60% ultimately received it, versus 65% proposed for and 67% receiving BCT in the neoadjuvant group ($p = 0.002$) (60). As expected, there was a higher conversion rate to BCT among patients in the neoadjuvant group who had a larger initial tumor size (for tumors ≥ 5.1 cm, 3% were initially proposed for BCT and 22% ultimately received it vs. 9% in the postoperative chemotherapy group). Overall, 27% of patients not eligible for BCT initially were able to undergo the procedure after chemotherapy. At 9 years of follow-up, there were no differences in overall survival, distant disease-free survival, or disease-free survival between the two groups (61). There was a slightly higher rate of ipsilateral breast tumor recurrence overall in the neoadjuvant chemotherapy group (10.7%) as compared with the postoperative chemotherapy group (7.6%), but this difference did not reach statistical significance ($p = 0.12$) (61). However a significant increase in local recurrence was seen in the subset of patients who became eligible for breast conservation only after neoadjuvant chemotherapy as compared with those who were candidates for lumpectomy initially (15.9% vs. 9.9%; $p = 0.04$). In a European Organization for Cancer Research and Treatment trial, 23% of patients initially requiring mastectomy were able to undergo BCT after neoadjuvant chemotherapy (62). Experience has demonstrated that patients with high tumor grade, estrogen receptor- and progesterone receptor-negative disease, and ductal rather than lobular histology are most likely to benefit from neoadjuvant therapy (63). The NSABP B27 trial (63,64) demonstrated that the addition of docetaxel to doxorubicin and cyclophosphamide preoperatively significantly increased the incidence of clinical and pathologic complete responses, while Buzdar et al. (65) found that neoadjuvant therapy with paclitaxel followed by fluorouracil, epirubicin, and cyclophosphamide with concurrent trastuzumab in patients whose tumors overexpressed *HER2* resulted in pathologic complete response in 54% of patients. These findings suggest that the optimal neoadjuvant strategy is to use the therapy that would be considered optimal in the postoperative adjuvant setting.

Patients whose tumors are estrogen receptor- and/or progesterone receptor-positive, particularly those that are low grade or occur in older women who would not otherwise receive chemotherapy, are candidates for neoadjuvant endocrine therapy. Three randomized trials have compared the effect of aromatase inhibitors with tamoxifen in postmenopausal women with estrogen receptor-positive tumors. All of the trials used ineligibility for BCT as an entry criterion. The results are shown in Table 18.5 (66–68). In all studies, the use of the aromatase inhibitor was associated with a higher rate of BCT than the use of tamoxifen.

There are advantages and disadvantages in considering neoadjuvant chemotherapy in an attempt to increase eligibility for breast conservation. When patients are treated with adjuvant chemotherapy after surgical resection of the primary tumor, there is no reliable method of measuring the responsiveness of an individual tumor to the particular treatment regimen. With neoadjuvant therapy, however, it is possible to assess clinical and pathologic response to a given treatment. Complete pathologic response to chemotherapy has been shown to be is a strong predictor of patient outcome (59,64,69). On the other hand, neoadjuvant chemotherapy requires reliance on clinical staging, which is less accurate than pathologic staging, particularly with regard to lymph node status. Lack of knowledge of the number of pathologically positive lymph nodes prior to therapy may make it difficult to determine which patients will benefit from postmastectomy RT or the use of nodal RT fields following BCT. In this circumstance, decisions about therapy should be made using a combination of the clinical stage at presentation and the pathologic stage after neoadjuvant therapy.

A major limitation to increasing the use of BCT after neoadjuvant therapy is the inability to reliably assess response using

Table 18.5

Effect of Neoadjuvant Endocrine Therapy on Eligibility for Breast-Conserving Surgery

Study (Ref.)	Trial	Duration (months)	% BCT		
			AI	Tam	p Value
Eiermann et al. (66)	Letrozole 2.5 mg vs. Tamoxifen 20 mg	4	45	35	0.022
Smith et al. (67)	Anastrozole 1 mg vs. Tamoxifen 20 mg	3	44	31	0.23
Semiglazov et al. (68)	Exemestane 25 mg vs. Tamoxifen 20 mg	3	37	20	0.05

BCT, breast-conserving therapy; AI, aromatase inhibitor; Tam, tamoxifen.

clinical and radiographic examinations. A combination of physical examination, mammography, ultrasound, and breast MRI may be employed (70), but it is not possible to definitively identify a complete pathologic response by clinical and imaging criteria alone. Thus, even in those patients with a complete clinical (and radiologic) response, lumpectomy must still be performed to evaluate for residual microscopic disease. The use of a radiologic marker placed prior to the initiation of neoadjuvant therapy will facilitate identification of the tumor site (71), and this can later be the localization target at the time of lumpectomy. Although at least 70% of patients have a partial response to neoadjuvant chemotherapy, the increases in BCT rates reported in randomized trials are relatively modest. This appears to be related both to difficulty in assessing the extent of residual tumor and the manner in which the tumor responds to therapy. Tumors can shrink in a concentric fashion, so that the area occupied by the tumor is smaller, making it relatively simple to perform a lumpectomy. Conversely, tumor cells may die in a patchy fashion, so there are fewer viable tumor cells in a fibrotic background, still occupying the same volume of tissue (72,73). This pattern of response can result in a clinical response to chemotherapy but the patient remains ineligible for BCT.

Because of the possibility of a patchy response to neoadjuvant treatment, surgery after neoadjuvant therapy should be conducted in a slightly different fashion than primary breast-conserving surgery. First, it is not necessary to resect the entire volume of tissue initially occupied by the tumor. The resection should include any residual clinical or imaging abnormality or, in the case of the patient with a clinical complete response, be centered on the marker clip. In either circumstance, a generous sample of apparently normal breast tissue should be taken to ensure that it is free of microscopic carcinoma. If pathology demonstrates no residual tumor or a unicentric residual tumor with a margin free of tumor cells for a distance of ≥2 mm, we consider the resection complete. If there is residual multifocal tumor throughout the specimen, even if the margins are negative, this should raise concerns about a significant additional tumor burden in the unresected tissue, and we perform a re-excision. If the re-excision is free of tumor, the patient is considered an appropriate candidate for RT. Positive margins, as always, are an indication for further surgery. The group at the MD Ander-

son Cancer Center retrospectively developed a recurrence score for patients undergoing surgery after neoadjuvant chemotherapy (74). Tumor morphology (no residual, unifocal, multifocal), lymphovascular space invasion, residual tumor size, and initial clinical lymph node status were used in the model. Five-year in breast recurrence rates ranged from 3% to 12% to 18% in the low-, intermediate-, and high-risk groups, respectively ($p = 0.0001$). This model has not been prospectively validated, but supports the evaluation of a combination of the amount of residual tumor, its growth pattern, and margin status when assessing the adequacy of resection. It appears that the combination of improved chemotherapy regimens and increased surgical experience with lumpectomy after neoadjuvant therapy is resulting in a decrease in local recurrence rates for patients having BCT in the neoadjuvant setting. In the NSABP B27 trial (64), local recurrence was seen in only 4.7% and 5.5% of the patients in the preoperative and postoperative taxane arms after a median follow-up of 77.9 months, compared with a 10.7% rate of local failure in the earlier B18 trial (61).

Partial Breast Reconstruction

An alternative to the use of neoadjuvant therapy to increase patient eligibility for breast conservation is to make a larger area of excision cosmetically acceptable. This can sometimes be done by partial breast reconstruction. It is important to keep in mind that partial breast reconstruction must not be allowed to interfere with the fundamental principles of breast conservation: the ability to deliver RT in a timely fashion and the ability to provide effective clinical and mammographic surveillance of the breast following treatment. Two basic strategies have been described for partial breast reconstruction following breast-conserving surgery. One is the reshaping of the existing tissue (using mammoplasty or mastopexy techniques) and the other involves use of an autologous flap. Partial reconstruction with saline or silicone implants is not feasible because of both capsule formation and the radio-opaque nature of such implants. Tissue reshaping is often accompanied by a symmetry procedure on the contralateral side to further cosmetic similarity between the two breasts (75).

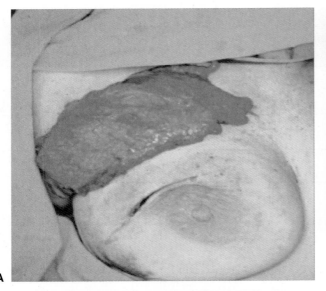

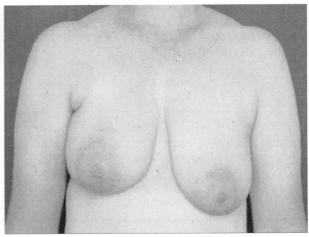

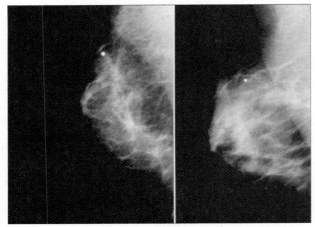

Figure 18.2 Partial breast reconstruction with latissimus dorsi flap. (**A**) Latissimus muscle pulled through axillary incision to illustrate the size of the breast defect. (**B**) Appearance of right breast 12 months after radiation. Shrinkage from radiation is not eliminated, but no defect is seen in the upper outer quadrant at the lumpectomy site. (**C**) Postoperative mammogram demonstrating radiolucency of the flap.

Of the autologous tissue flaps described for partial breast reconstruction, the latissimus dorsi flap has emerged as the most promising for several reasons, including its proximity to the site of the tumor, the flexibility in the amount of tissue that can be taken from the donor site for transfer, the relative radiolucency of the latissimus muscle, and the availability of a skin paddle if needed for reconstruction (76). Recently, Losken and colleagues (77) described the ability to endoscopically harvest the flap without incising the skin on the back, thus removing one of the most significant drawbacks to the procedure. When the latissimus dorsi flap is used for partial breast reconstruction, patients who require completion mastectomy at a later date still have several options available to them for postmastectomy reconstruction, as described elsewhere in this chapter. It is crucial to ensure negative margins in patients undergoing partial breast reconstruction prior to placement of the flap, and is usually best to do this as a two-stage procedure. The initial stage is resection of the primary tumor and sentinel node biopsy. The second stage is carried out after negative margins have been confirmed but before the postlumpectomy seroma has been resorbed and remodeled. If axillary dissection is neces-

sary, it is performed during the second-stage procedure. Partial breast reconstruction with a latissimus dorsi flap is illustrated in Figure 18.2.

Tissue reshaping and remodeling techniques do not require a second surgical site for harvest of a flap. Plastic surgery techniques such as mammoplasty can be employed to help recontour the breast following resection of a relatively large volume of tissue, usually accompanied by a contralateral symmetry procedure (78–83). In a study from Milan, 30 patients undergoing excision with breast remodeling were compared with a control group undergoing quadrantectomy, the standard procedure in Italy (79). In 2 of the 20 patients assigned to the tissue-remodeling group, partial flap reconstruction was used, and 90% of the remodeling group also had a contralateral symmetry procedure. In the quadrantectomy group, 56.7% had negative margins at the first operation, and 33.3% had close margins (≤2 mm), while 3.3% had positive margins and 6.7% had unknown margin status. In the tissue-remodeling group, 83.4% had negative margins, 13.3% had close margins (≤2 mm), and 3.3% had positive margins. Although negative margins were obtained at the first operation in a significantly higher proportion of cases in the tissue-remodeling group ($p = 0.05$), the problem of how to address positive margins once tissue remodeling has been done remains more vexing. Clough and colleagues (78) evaluated 101 consecutive patients who underwent lumpectomy with a remodeling mammoplasty over a 14-year period. All patients underwent a contralateral procedure for symmetry, either at the same operation or in a delayed fashion. The average tumor size in this group was 3.2 cm (range, 1.0 to 7.0 cm), and the mean weight of excised tissue was 222 g (range, 20 to 1,450 g). The cosmesis was considered favorable in 82%. One of the main drawbacks to this tissue-remodeling approach was evident in that 10% of patients had involved margins identified at pathology. Of those cases, half proceeded to mastectomy and half had a radiation boost to the tumor bed. Some of the patients in this study had preoperative rather than postoperative RT, and this led to higher complications rates and poorer cosmetic result than in the postoperative group. The 5-year local recurrence rate in this study was 9.4%, which compared favorably with institutional rates of local recurrence following BCT without tissue reshaping. Further work needs to be done in addressing the problem of positive margins once the original tumor bed has been reshaped to make this a widely used technique.

MASTECTOMY AND IMMEDIATE RECONSTRUCTION

The shift from radical mastectomy to modified radical mastectomy, together with advances in plastic surgical technique, has made immediate reconstruction an option for most patients who undergo mastectomy. A variety of techniques for postmastectomy reconstruction have been described (Table 18.6). Potential concerns about immediate reconstruction have included the possibility of an increased incidence of local failure, delay in the diagnosis of local failure, or delay in the administration of adjuvant therapy due to wound-healing issues. More recently, as indications for postmastectomy RT have expanded, the impact of RT on reconstruction has also become an issue.

There have been no prospective trials comparing mastectomy alone with mastectomy with immediate reconstruction,

Table 18.6

Common Types of Reconstruction after Mastectomy

Type	Advantages	Disadvantages	Contraindications
Implant	One-stage procedure Short operative time Minimal prolongation of hospitalization and recovery Low cost	Capsular contracture Implant rupture or leakage; poor cosmetic outcome in very large ptotic breasts	Irradiated skin
Tissue expander	Short operative time Low cost Hospitalization, recovery not prolonged	Multiple physician visits Rupture of implant Implant leakage	Irradiated skin
Latissimus Dorsi Flap	Reliable flap Autogenous tissue Natural contour	Donor site scar Moderate prolongation, hospitalization, and recovery Usually requires an implant	Major comorbidities
Transverse Rectus abdominis myocutaneous flap	Autogenous tissue Natural contour Abdominoplasty	Donor site scar Significant prolongation, hospitalization, and recovery Abdominal wall hernia Partial flap loss	Major comorbidities
Deep inferior epigastric perforator flap	Autogenous tissue Natural contour Abdominoplasty Muscle-sparing	Donor site scar Moderate prolongation, hospitalization, and recovery Partial flap loss Limited availability due to need for microsurgeon	Major comorbidities Active smokers
Superior gluteal artery perforator flap	Autogenous tissue Natural contour Alternative donor site	Donor site scar Moderate prolongation, hospitalization, and recovery Partial flap loss Limited availability due to need for microsurgeon	Major comorbidities

but the available retrospective data do not support concerns about the incidence or detection of local recurrence in the reconstructed patient. Petit et al. (84) compared 146 patients treated with both immediate and delayed silicone-gel implant reconstruction with a control group of patients treated with mastectomy alone. The groups were matched for age, year of diagnosis, stage, histologic tumor type, grade, and nodal status. At 10 years, 8% of the reconstructed patients had experienced local recurrence compared with 15% of the patients having mastectomy alone. In a similar study, Webster et al. (85) compared 85 patients having immediate reconstruction using a variety of techniques with 85 controls undergoing mastectomy alone who were matched for age, stage, nodal involvement, and receptor status. At 30 months, the incidence of local and distant recurrence did not differ between groups.

More recently, skin-sparing mastectomy, in which skin excision is limited to the NAC and the excisional biopsy scar (if present), has been used to preserve the skin envelope of the breast and facilitate reconstruction. Greenway and colleagues (86) retrospectively compared a single surgeon's experience with skin-sparing versus conventional mastectomy and found no difference in local, regional, or systemic recurrence at an average of 49 months among the 225 patients who had skin-sparing mastectomy with immediate reconstruction and 1,022 patients who underwent modified radical mastectomy. Kroll et al. (87) analyzed 87 patients having 100 reconstructions using a skin-sparing technique who were followed for a mean of 23 months. Two patients developed local recurrence, one of which was associated with widespread metastases. Other studies of skin-sparing mastectomy are summarized in Table 18.7 (88–93). The low rate of local failure reported in these studies is consistent with prior observations that the extent of skin removal in patients treated with mastectomy alone is not a major determinant of the risk of chest wall recurrence (94).

The effect of reconstruction on the detection of local recurrence was studied by Noone and coworkers (95) in 306 patients followed for a mean of 6.4 years. Local recurrence as the first site of treatment failure occurred in 5.2% of the group. Fourteen of the 16 recurrences were in the skin or subcutaneous fat, so detection was not effected by the presence of the reconstruction. Similar results were reported by Newman et al. (91), who noted that 22 of 23 local recurrences after skin-sparing mastectomy presented as palpable masses in the skin flap. Noone et al. (95) observed no delay in the administration of chemotherapy in patients having reconstruction, a finding also reported by Eberlein and coworkers (96).

Nipple-Sparing Mastectomy

Traditionally, skin-sparing mastectomy has included resection of the NAC. The rationale for this approach is both the risk of leaving behind malignancy with nipple preservation because of the extension of ductal tissue into the nipple and the need to leave breast tissue on the NAC to provide a blood supply. These concerns led to the current strategy of excision of the NAC followed by surgical re-creation of a nipple with tattooing for color matching. Recently, however, investigators have begun to explore the safety of nipple-sparing mastectomy (NSM) in selected cases.

There have been many studies investigating occult involvement of the NAC in patients with known breast cancer, with the reported incidence of NAC involvement ranging from 0% to 58% (97). This wide range is due to variations in tumor stage and the number of sections taken from the NAC specimen. Santini and colleagues (98) reported a study of pathologic evaluation of the NAC in 1,291 consecutive mastectomies, with a rate of NAC involvement of 12%. In 8% of cases, this was not suspected on clinical grounds. Vlajcic and colleagues (99) evaluated 108 women with unilateral breast cancer in whom 1 cm of tissue beneath the NAC was excised and sent both for frozen and permanent section. Tumor was identified in this tissue in 25 cases (23%). Of concern, false-negative frozen sections occurred in 5 of the 108 cases (4.6% of the total, 20% of the NACs with tumor involvement).

Kissin and colleagues (100) sought to identify factors that predicted a NAC negative for cancer, then used their criteria to select patients to undergo NSM. They began by evaluating the NAC in 100 mastectomy specimens. Of note, this group took only two sections from the NAC, as opposed to others who evaluated the NAC more extensively. Their prospectively developed criteria for NSM were a clinically normal nipple, a "peripheral" tumor, tumor size <5 cm, and a negative frozen section of the tissue beneath the NAC. Based on their criteria, 40 of the 60 prospectively evaluated patients were not candidates for NSM. Twenty patients ultimately had preservation of the nipple but two (10%) had full-thickness loss of the nipple postoperatively, requiring excision and skin grafting. Another two patients had

Table 18.7			
Local Recurrence after Skin-Sparing Mastectomy			
Author/s (Ref.)	No.	Stage	% LR
Medina-Franco et al. (88)	176	I-III	4.5
Carlson et al. (89)	565	0-IV	5.5
Singletary (90)	545	I-II	2.6
Newman et al. (91)	437	I-II	6.2
Gerber et al. (92)	112	0-III	5.4
Slavin et al. (93)	51	0-II	2.0

partial loss of the nipple, which healed by primary intention. Of the 18 patients with intact NACs, one patient (5.6%) had a recurrence at the site of the NAC. Gerber et al. (92) selected potential candidates for NSM who had peripherally located tumors ≤2 cm in size, no clinical evidence of nipple involvement, and clinically negative nodes. In spite of this, frozen section analysis demonstrated microscopic tumor in the subareolar tissue in 46% of 112 patients. Of the 61 patients treated by NSM, only 1 experienced a local recurrence in the NAC with a mean follow-up of 59 months. Crowe et al. (101) used selection criteria similar to those of Gerber et al. (92) and found that 16% of 37 patients with cancer had unsuspected tumor in the subareolar tissue on frozen section analysis.

These studies indicate that NSM may be a viable option in highly selected women, specifically patients with small, peripherally located, node-negative tumors with favorable histologic features. Most women in this category are candidates for BCT. Morrow et al. (16) reported that only 10% of women with T1 tumors had contraindications to BCT. In their experience, only 19% of women who were candidates for BCT opted to have a mastectomy, and only one third of these chose to undergo reconstruction. This suggests that only about 10% of women with T1 tumors would potentially choose to pursue NSM with immediate reconstruction. Based on the experience with intraoperative frozen section previously discussed (92,101), only 50% to 85% of this small group could undergo the procedure for oncologic reasons. The eligible population for NSM is further limited by the requirement that the nipple be in the appropriate position on the reconstructed breast. This is rarely the case for women with large, ptotic breasts, further limiting the application of this procedure.

There are many questions remaining to be addressed before the use of NSM can be widely adopted, such as the significance of atypical hyperplasia in the NAC and whether NSM should be used in patients whose tumor has been downstaged by neoadjuvant chemotherapy. The small number of women with cancer who are eligible for, and interested in, NSM will make it extremely difficult to obtain reliable data on the risk of local recurrence associated with this procedure. It is likely that the greatest application of NSM may be in women undergoing prophylactic mastectomy, in which the risk of future cancer development in the small amount of breast tissue retained to ensure viability of the NAC is the only oncologic concern. This is a particular worry in women at risk on the basis of *BRCA1* or *BRCA2* mutations. Ultimately, the desirability of NSM may be determined by the sensory and erectile function of the preserved nipple, an area that has not been systematically studied. Gerber et al. (92) reported "sensitivity" of the nipple areolar complex in 75% of women after NSM, while Petit et al. (102) reported complete or partial loss of sensation in the NAC in all of their patients treated with NSM and intraoperative irradiation to the preserved NAC. Partial recovery was seen in 33%, but complete recovery occurred in only 19%. This is an area worthy of further study because the function of the nipple may assist in determining what level of increased risk of local recurrence is acceptable for its preservation. In addition, the skin island placed at the site of the NAC in flap reconstruction is an important method of monitoring the viability of the flap, which is lost when the NAC is preserved.

In summary, immediate reconstruction with preservation of the skin envelope of the breast has not been shown to alter the outcome of mastectomy or to delay the administration of systemic therapy. Immediate reconstruction has the advantages of avoiding the need for a second major operative procedure and the psychological morbidity of the loss of the breast. The two major reconstructive techniques involve the use of implants or expanders or the use of myocutaneous tissue flaps to create a new breast mound. The advantages and disadvantages of the techniques are summarized in Table 18.6. Implant reconstructions are best suited for women with small-to-moderate size breasts with minimal ptosis, while flap reconstructions allow more flexibility in the size and shape of the reconstructed breast. In the past, most breast implants were filled with silicone gel. However, after uncontrolled reports suggested an increased incidence of connective tissue disease in women with silicone implants (103,104) the Food and Drug Administration declared a moratorium on their use. Since that time, several epidemiologic studies have failed to demonstrate an increased incidence of connective tissue disorders in women with implants compared with matched control populations (105,106). Silicone implants are available for use in breast cancer patients, but many patients opt for saline implants or flap reconstructions as a result of the adverse publicity surrounding silicone implants. Regardless of the reconstructive technique chosen, preservation of the skin envelope of the breast will aid the reconstructive surgeon in obtaining symmetry. From an oncologic point of view, the only skin that must be removed as part of mastectomy is the biopsy scar, with resection of the NAC remaining the standard approach. Exposure for complete removal of the breast and axillary contents can be obtained by incision rather than excision of skin (Figure 18.3).

Reconstructive choices may be influenced by the possible need for postmastectomy RT. There are a variety of strategies that have been proposed for selecting the type of reconstruction for a patient with a significant likelihood of requiring postmastectomy RT. The use of RT in patients who have been reconstructed with implants is associated with a higher risk of implant loss than in nonirradiated patients (107). However, Cordeiro et al. (108) reported that after a mean follow-up of 34 months in 68 patients

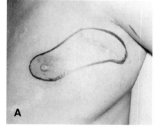 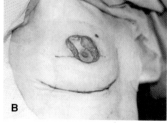

Figure 18.3 Skin-sparing mastectomy incisions incorporating nipple-areolar complex and upper outer quadrant biopsy scar **(A)** and removing very small skin paddle including nipple-areolar complex and biopsy scar **(B)**. Horizontal lines mark potential sites of skin incision for additional exposure.

reconstructed with tissue expanders or implants who received RT, 80% had good-to-excellent aesthetic results and 72% would have chosen the same form of reconstruction again. The corresponding figures for nonirradiated patients were 88% ($p =$ NS) and 85%. Implant loss occurred in 11% of patients with irradiated implants and 6% of nonirradiated patients. The finding that the majority of patients who require RT after implant reconstruction have good cosmesis and are satisfied with their reconstruction choice has led some to advocate insertion of an expander that is inflated during chemotherapy and exchanged for a permanent implant prior to RT. In patients who are satisfied with the outcome after RT, no further surgery is required. In patients with significant cosmetic deformity, a secondary flap reconstruction is performed. This approach has the advantage of allowing preservation of the breast skin and providing the patient with a breast mound during what may be a prolonged course of systemic therapy. A primary flap reconstruction is another alternative for the patient who may require postmastectomy RT. Variable outcomes have been reported for patients who receive RT after transverse rectus myocutaneous (TRAM) flap reconstruction (109–111). Complete flap loss is rare, but fat necrosis, fibrosis, and volume loss occur. As in the native breast, the full cosmetic impact may not be evident until 3 years posttreatment. A third approach is to perform sentinel node biopsy prior to mastectomy to identify patients with nodal involvement at highest risk for requiring postmastectomy RT and delay reconstruction in this subset until after the completion of oncologic therapy.

There is also evidence to suggest that the technique of RT has a significant impact on the cosmetic result in the reconstructed breast. Victor et al. (112) found that the use of bolus technique was significantly associated with poor cosmetic outcome. Anderson et al. (113) reported that the 5-year incidence of major complications after TRAM reconstruction was 0% (n = 35) and 5% after tissue expander/implant (n = 50) reconstruction followed by RT when a custom wax bolus was used for treatment. This is an area that continues to evolve, and multidisciplinary consultation between the oncologic surgeon, reconstructive surgeon, and radiation oncologist will help to ensure optimal patient outcomes.

PATIENT INVOLVEMENT IN SURGICAL DECISION MAKING

In spite of the large body of evidence discussed earlier in this chapter, supporting the use of BCT for stage I and II breast cancer, mastectomy remains a common approach to breast cancer management (114). Persistent high mastectomy rates, coupled with geographic variations in the use of BCT, have been cited as evidence of failure to involve women in the decision-making process for breast cancer surgery (115,116). A population-based study of women with ductal carcinoma in situ and stage I and II breast cancer diagnosed in 2002 and reported to the Los Angeles and Detroit Surveillance, Epidemiology, and End Results (SEER) registries was used to examine the role of patients in the selection of local therapy for breast cancer (117). In this sample of 1,844 women, 30.2% were treated by mastectomy. Most women

reported that they made the surgical decision (41.0%) or shared it with their surgeon (37.1%). Only 21.9% reported that the surgeon was the primary decision maker. Among white women, increased patient involvement was associated with higher mastectomy rates, with only 5.3% of patients whose surgeon made the treatment decision receiving mastectomy compared with 16.8% of women who shared the decision and 27.0% of women who were the primary decision makers (p <0.001). Patient concern about disease recurrence was the most influential factor in the treatment decision. Interestingly, only 50% of the patient sample were aware that survival was equal after BCT and mastectomy (118). Similar findings were observed regarding the use of immediate or early postmastectomy breast reconstruction. Only 38% of patients having a mastectomy received breast reconstruction, although 78% reported that it was discussed (119), and only 25% of patients correctly identified the lack of impact of reconstruction on local recurrence. A survey of the surgeons who treated the patient sample found that high-volume breast surgeons were more likely to favor BCT than their lower-volume counterparts (120), and experienced more conflict with patients when recommending BCT (121). These findings suggest that methods to improve patient understanding of the risks and benefits of treatment are urgently needed to allow them to partner more fully in the decision-making process.

REFERENCES

1. Holland R, Connolly JL, Gelman R, et al. The presence of an extensive intraductal component following a limited excision correlates with prominent residual disease in the remainder of the breast. *J Clin Oncol.* 1990;8:113–118.
2. Qualheim RE, Gall EA. Breast carcinoma with multiple sites of origin. *Cancer.* 1957;10(3):460–468.
3. Rosen PP, Fracchia AA, Urban JA, et al. "Residual" mammary carcinoma following simulated partial mastectomy. *Cancer.* 1975; 35(3):739–747.
4. Arriagada R, Le MG, Guinebretiere JM, et al. Late local recurrences in a randomised trial comparing conservative treatment with total mastectomy in early breast cancer patients. *Ann Oncol.* 2003; 14(11):1617–1622.
5. Blichert-Toft M, Rose C, Andersen JA, et al. Danish randomized trial comparing breast conservation therapy with mastectomy: six years of life-table analysis. Danish Breast Cancer Cooperative Group. *J Natl Cancer Inst Monogr.* 1992;(11):19–25.
6. Fisher B, Anderson S, Bryant J, et al. Twenty-year follow-up of a randomized trial comparing total mastectomy, lumpectomy, and lumpectomy plus irradiation for the treatment of invasive breast cancer. *N Engl J Med.* 2002;347(16):1233–1241.
7. Poggi MM, Danforth DN, Sciuto LC, et al. Eighteen-year results in the treatment of early breast carcinoma with mastectomy versus breast conservation therapy: the National Cancer Institute Randomized Trial. *Cancer.* 2003;98(4):697–702.
8. van Dongen JA, Voogd AC, Fentiman IS, et al. Long-term results of a randomized trial comparing breast-conserving therapy with mastectomy: European Organization for Research and Treatment of Cancer 10801 trial. *J Natl Cancer Inst.* 2000;92(14):1143–1150.
9. Veronesi U, Cascinelli N, Mariani L, et al. Twenty-year follow-up of a randomized study comparing breast-conserving surgery with radical mastectomy for early breast cancer. *N Engl J Med.* 2002; 347:1227–1232.

10. Neuschatz AC, DiPetrillo T, Safaii H, et al. Long-term follow-up of a prospective policy of margin-directed radiation dose escalation in breast-conserving therapy. *Cancer.* 2003;97(1):30–39.

11. Obedian E, Haffty BG. Negative margin status improves local control in conservatively managed breast cancer patients. *Cancer J Sci Am.* 2000;6(1):28–33.

12. Wapnir I. Survival after IBTR in NSABP Node Negative Protocols B-13, B-14, B-19, B-20 and B-23. ASCO Annual Meeting Proceedings, Vol. 23, No 16S. Orlando, FL: *J Clin Oncol.* 2005;517.

13. Pass H, Vicini FA, Kestin LL, et al. Changes in management techniques and patterns of disease recurrence over time in patients with breast carcinoma treated with breast-conserving therapy at a single institution. *Cancer.* 2004;101(4):713–720.

14. Morrow M, Strom EA, Bassett LW, et al. Standard for breast conservation therapy in the management of invasive breast carcinoma. *CA Cancer J Clin.* 2002;52(5):277–300.

15. Morrow M, Schmidt R, Hassett C. Patient selection for breast conservation therapy with magnification mammography. *Surgery.* 1995;118(4):621–626.

16. Morrow M, Bucci C, Rademaker A. Medical contraindications are not a major factor in the underutilization of breast conserving therapy. *J Am Coll Surg.* 1998;186(3):269–274.

17. Fisher ER, Gregorio R, Redmond C, et al. Pathologic findings from the National Surgical Adjuvant Breast Project (protocol no. 4). I. Observations concerning the multicentricity of mammary cancer. *Cancer.* 1975;35(1):247–254.

18. Stratton RL. Multicentricity in cancer of the breast. *J Kans Med Soc.* 1973;74:48–52.

19. Harms SE, Flamig DP, Hesley KL, et al. MR imaging of the breast with rotating delivery of excitation off resonance: clinical experience with pathologic correlation. *Radiology.* 1993;187(2):493–501.

20. Boetes C, Mus RD, Holland R, et al. Breast tumors: comparative accuracy of MR imaging relative to mammography and US for demonstrating extent. *Radiology.* 1995;197(3):743–747.

21. Mumtaz H, Hall-Craggs MA, Davidson T, et al. Staging of symptomatic primary breast cancer with MR imaging. *AJR Am J Roentgenol.* 1997;169(2):417–424.

22. Fischer U, Kopka L, Grabbe E. Breast carcinoma: effect of preoperative contrast-enhanced MR imaging on the therapeutic approach. *Radiology.* 1999;213(3):881–888.

23. Drew PJ, Turnbull LW, Chatterjee S, et al. Prospective comparison of standard triple assessment and dynamic magnetic resonance imaging of the breast for the evaluation of symptomatic breast lesions. *Ann Surg.* 1999;230(5):680–685.

24. Liberman L, Morris EA, Dershaw DD, et al. MR imaging of the ipsilateral breast in women with percutaneously proven breast cancer. *AJR Am J Roentgenol.* 2003;180(4):901–910.

25. Furman B, Gardner MS, Romilly P, et al. Effect of 0.5 Tesla magnetic resonance imaging on the surgical management of breast cancer patients. *Am J Surg.* 2003;186(4):344–347.

26. Bedrosian I, Mick R, Orel SG, et al. Changes in the surgical management of patients with breast carcinoma based on preoperative magnetic resonance imaging. *Cancer.* 2003;98(3):468–473.

27. Deurloo EE, Peterse JL, Rutgers EJ, et al. Additional breast lesions in patients eligible for breast-conserving therapy by MRI: impact on preoperative management and potential benefit of computerised analysis. *Eur J Cancer.* 2005;41:1393–1401.

28. Esserman L, Hylton N, Yassa L, et al. Utility of magnetic resonance imaging in the management of breast cancer: evidence for improved preoperative staging. *J Clin Oncol.* 1999;17(1):110–119.

29. Schnall M, Blume, J, Bluemke D, et al. MRI detection of multifocal breast carcinoma: Report from the International Breast MRI Consortium. *J Clin Oncol.* 2004;22(14s):4s (Abstract 504).

30. Egan RL. Multicentric breast carcinomas: clinical-radiographic-pathologic whole organ studies and 10-year survival. *Cancer.* 1982;49(6):1123–1130.

31. Schwartz GF, Patchesfsky AS, Feig SA, et al. Multicentricity of non-palpable breast cancer. *Cancer.* 1980;45(12):2913–2916.

32. Vaidya JS, Vyas JJ, Chinoy RF, et al. Multicentricity of breast cancer: whole-organ analysis and clinical implications. *Br J Cancer.* 1996;74(5):820–824.

33. Anastassiades O, Iakovou E, Stavridou N, et al. Multicentricity in breast cancer. A study of 366 cases. *Am J Clin Pathol.* 1993;99(3):238–243.

34. Holland R, Veling SH, Mravunac M, Hendriks JH. Histologic multifocality of Tis, T1-2 breast carcinomas. Implications for clinical trials of breast-conserving surgery. *Cancer.* 1985;56(5):979–990.

35. Berg WA, Gutierrez L, NessAiver MS, et al. Diagnostic accuracy of mammography, clinical examination, US, and MR imaging in preoperative assessment of breast cancer. *Radiology.* 2004;233(3):830–849.

36. White JR, Gustafson GS, Wimbish K, et al. Conservative surgery and radiation therapy for infiltrating lobular carcinoma of the breast. The role of preoperative mammograms in guiding treatment. *Cancer.* 1994;74:640–647.

37. Newstead GM, Baute PB, Toth HK. Invasive lobular and ductal carcinoma: mammographic findings and stage at diagnosis. *Radiology.* 1992;184(3):623–627.

38. Lesser ML, Rosen PP, Kinne DW. Multicentricity and bilaterality in invasive breast carcinoma. *Surgery.* 1982;91(2):234–240.

39. Quan ML, Sclafani L, Heerdt AS, et al. Magnetic resonance imaging detects unsuspected disease in patients with invasive lobular cancer. *Ann Surg Oncol.* 2003;10(9):1048–1053.

40. Morrow M, Keeney K, Scholtens D, et al. Selecting patients for breast-conserving therapy: the importance of lobular histology. *Cancer.* 2006;106(12):2563–2568.

41. Santiago RJ, Harris EE, Qin L, et al. Similar long-term results of breast-conservation treatment for Stage I and II invasive lobular carcinoma compared with invasive ductal carcinoma of the breast: The University of Pennsylvania experience. *Cancer.* 2005;103(12):2447–2454.

42. Singletary SE, Patel-Parekh L, Bland KI. Treatment trends in early-stage invasive lobular carcinoma: a report from the National Cancer Data Base. *Ann Surg.* 2005;242(2):281–289.

43. Verhoog LC, Brekelmans CT, Seynaeve C, et al. Survival and tumour characteristics of breast-cancer patients with germline mutations of BRCA1. *Lancet.* 1998;351(9099):316–321.

44. Haffty BG, Harrold E, Khan AJ, et al. Outcome of conservatively managed early-onset breast cancer by BRCA1/2 status. *Lancet.* 2002;359(9316):1471–1477.

45. Seynaeve C, Verhoog LC, van de Bosch LM, et al. Ipsilateral breast tumour recurrence in hereditary breast cancer following breast-conserving therapy. *Eur J Cancer.* 2004;40(8):1150–1158.

46. Pierce LJ, Levin AM, Rebbeck TR, et al. Ten-year multi-institutional results of breast-conserving surgery and radiotherapy in BRCA1/2-associated stage I/II breast cancer. *J Clin Oncol.* 2006;24:2437–2443.

47. Taghian A, Mohiuddin M, Jagsi R, et al. Current perceptions regarding surgical margin status after breast-conserving therapy: results of a survey. *Ann Surg.* 2005;241(4):629–639.

48. Singletary SE. Surgical margins in patients with early-stage breast cancer treated with breast conservation therapy. *Am J Surg.* 2002;184(5):383–393.

49. Graham RA, Homer MJ, Katz J, et al. The pancake phenomenon contributes to the inaccuracy of margin assessment in patients with breast cancer. *Am J Surg.* 2002;184(2):89–93.

50. Schmidt-Ullrich RK, Wazer DE, DiPetrillo T, et al. Breast conservation therapy for early stage breast carcinoma with outstanding 10-year locoregional control rates: a case for aggressive therapy to the tumor bearing quadrant. *Int J Radiat Oncol Biol Phys.* 1993; 27(3):545–552.

51. Schnitt SJ, Hayman J, Gelman R, et al. A prospective study of conservative surgery alone in the treatment of selected patients with stage I breast cancer. *Cancer.* 1996;77(6):1094–1100.

52. Park CC, Mitsumori M, Nixon A, et al. Outcome at 8 years after breast-conserving surgery and radiation therapy for invasive breast cancer: influence of margin status and systemic therapy on local recurrence. *J Clin Oncol.* 2000;18(8):1668–1675.

53. Darvishian F, Hajdu SI, DeRisi DC. Significance of linear extent of breast carcinoma at surgical margin. *Ann Surg Oncol.* 2003; 10(1):48–51.

54. Fisher ER, Anderson S, Redmond C, et al. Ipsilateral breast tumor recurrence and survival following lumpectomy and irradiation: pathological findings from NSABP protocol B-06. *Semin Surg Oncol.* 1992;8:161–166.

55. Bartelink H, Horiot JC, Poortmans P, et al. Recurrence rates after treatment of breast cancer with standard radiotherapy with or without additional radiation. *N Engl J Med.* 2001;345(19):1378–1387.

56. Jobsen JJ, van der Palen J, Ong F, et al. The value of a positive margin for invasive carcinoma in breast-conservative treatment in relation to local recurrence is limited to young women only. *Int J Radiat Oncol Biol Phys.* 2003;57(3):724–731.

57. Gibson GR, Lesnikoski BA, Yoo J, et al. A comparison of ink-directed and traditional whole-cavity re-excision for breast lumpectomy specimens with positive margins. *Ann Surg Oncol.* 2001;8(9):693–704.

58. Kearney TJ, Morrow M. Effect of reexcision on the success of breast-conserving surgery. *Ann Surg Oncol.* 1995;2(4):303–307.

59. Fisher B, Brown A, Mamounas E, et al. Effect of preoperative chemotherapy on local-regional disease in women with operable breast cancer: findings from National Surgical Adjuvant Breast and Bowel Project B-18. *J Clin Oncol.* 1997;15(7):2483–2493.

60. Fisher B, Bryant J, Wolmark N, et al. Effect of preoperative chemotherapy on the outcome of women with operable breast cancer. *J Clin Oncol.* 1998;16(8):2672–2685.

61. Wolmark N, Wang J, Mamounas E, et al. Preoperative chemotherapy in patients with operable breast cancer: nine-year results from National Surgical Adjuvant Breast and Bowel Project B-18. *J Natl Cancer Inst Monogr.* 2001;(30):96–102.

62. van der Hage JA, van de Velde CJ, Julien JP, et al. Preoperative chemotherapy in primary operable breast cancer: results from the European Organization for Research and Treatment of Cancer trial 10902. *J Clin Oncol.* 2001;19:4224–4237.

63. Bear HD, Anderson S, Brown A, et al. The effect on tumor response of adding sequential preoperative docetaxel to preoperative doxorubicin and cyclophosphamide: preliminary results from National Surgical Adjuvant Breast and Bowel Project Protocol B-27. *J Clin Oncol.* 2003;21(22):4165–4174.

64. Bear HD, Anderson S, Smith RE, et al. Sequential preoperative or postoperative docetaxel added to preoperative doxorubicin plus cyclophosphamide for operable breast cancer:National Surgical Adjuvant Breast and Bowel Project Protocol B-27. *J Clin Oncol.* 2006;24(13):2019–2027.

65. Buzdar AU, Ibrahim NK, Francis D, et al. Significantly higher pathologic complete remission rate after neoadjuvant therapy with trastuzumab, paclitaxel, and epirubicin chemotherapy: results of a randomized trial in human epidermal growth factor receptor 2-positive operable breast cancer. *J Clin Oncol.* 2005;23(16):3676–3685.

66. Eiermann W, Paepke S, Appfelstaedt J, et al. Preoperative treatment of postmenopausal breast cancer patients with letrozole: A randomized double-blind multicenter study. *Ann Oncol.* 2001;12(11): 1527–1532.

67. Smith IE, Dowsett M, Ebbs SR, et al. Neoadjuvant treatment of postmenopausal breast cancer with anastrozole, tamoxifen, or both in combination: the Immediate Preoperative Anastrozole, Tamoxifen, or Combined with Tamoxifen (IMPACT) multicenter double-blind randomized trial. *J Clin Oncol.* 2005;23(22):5108–5116.

68. Semiglazov V, Kletsel A, Semiglazov V, et al. Exemestane (E) vs tamoxifen (T) as neoadjuvant endocrine therapy for postmenopausal women with ER+ breast cancer (T2N1-2, T3N0-1, T4N0M0). *ASCO Meeting Abstracts.* 2005;23(16 Suppl): 530.

69. Cance WG, Carey LA, Calvo BF, et al. Long-term outcome of neoadjuvant therapy for locally advanced breast carcinoma: effective clinical downstaging allows breast preservation and predicts outstanding local control and survival. *Ann Surg.* 2002;236:295–303.

70. Yeh E, Slanetz P, Kopans DB, et al. Prospective comparison of mammography, sonography, and MRI in patients undergoing neoadjuvant chemotherapy for palpable breast cancer. *AJR Am J Roentgenol.* 2005;184(3):868–877.

71. Edeiken BS, Fornage BD, Bedi DG, et al. US-guided implantation of metallic markers for permanent localization of the tumor bed in patients with breast cancer who undergo preoperative chemotherapy. *Radiology.* 1999; 213(3):895-900.

72. Buchholz TA, Hunt KK, Whitman GJ, et al. Neoadjuvant chemotherapy for breast carcinoma: multidisciplinary considerations of benefits and risks. *Cancer.* 2003;98(6):1150–1160.

73. Veronesi U, Bonadonna G, Zurrida S, et al. Conservation surgery after primary chemotherapy in large carcinomas of the breast. *Ann Surg.* 1995;222(5):612–618.

74. Chen AM, Meric-Bernstam F, Hunt KK, et al. Breast conservation after neoadjuvant chemotherapy. *Cancer.* 2005;103(4):689–695.

75. Kronowitz SJ, Feledy JA, Hunt KK, et al. Determining the optimal approach to breast reconstruction after partial mastectomy. *Plast Reconstr Surg.* 2006;117(1):1-11; discussion 12–14.

76. Munhoz AM, Montag E, Fels KW, et al. Outcome analysis of breast-conservation surgery and immediate latissimus dorsi flap reconstruction in patients with T1 to T2 breast cancer. *Plast Reconstr Surg.* 2005;116(3):741–752.

77. Losken A, Schaefer TG, Carlson GW, et al. Immediate endoscopic latissimus dorsi flap: risk or benefit in reconstructing partial mastectomy defects. *Ann Plast Surg.* 2004;53:1–5.

78. Clough KB, Lewis JS, Couturaud B, et al. Oncoplastic techniques allow extensive resections for breast-conserving therapy of breast carcinomas. *Ann Surg.* 2003;237(1):26–34.

79. Kaur N, Petit JY, Rietjens M, et al. Comparative study of surgical margins in oncoplastic surgery and quadrantectomy in breast cancer. *Ann Surg Oncol.* 2005;12(7):539–545.

80. Clough KB, Kroll SS, Audretsch W. An approach to the repair of partial mastectomy defects. *Plast Reconstr Surg.* 1999;104(2):409–420.

81. Nos C, Fitoussi A, Bourgeois D, et al. Conservative treatment of lower pole breast cancers by bilateral mammoplasty and radiotherapy. *Eur J Surg Oncol.* 1998;24(6):508–514.

82. Baildam AD. Oncoplastic surgery of the breast. *Br J Surg.* 2002; 89(5):532–533.

83. Anderson BO, Masetti R, Silverstein MJ. Oncoplastic approaches to partial mastectomy: an overview of volume-displacement techniques. *Lancet Oncol.* 2005;6(3):145–157.

84. Petit JY, Le MG, Mouriesse H, et al. Can breast reconstruction with gel-filled silicone implants increase the risk of death and second primary cancer in patients treated by mastectomy for breast cancer? *Plast Reconstr Surg.* 1994;94(1):115–119.

85. Webster DJ, Mansel RE, Hughes LE. Immediate reconstruction of the breast after mastectomy. Is it safe? *Cancer.* 1984;53(6):1416–1419.

86. Greenway RM, Schlossberg L, Dooley WC. Fifteen-year series of skin-sparing mastectomy for stage 0 to 2 breast cancer. *Am J Surg.* 2005;190:918–922.

87. Kroll SS, Ames F, Singletary SE, Schusterman MA. The oncologic risks of skin preservation at mastectomy when combined with immediate reconstruction of the breast. *Surg Gynecol Obstet.* 1991;172(1):17–20.

88. Medina-Franco H, Vasconez LO, Fix RJ, et al. Factors associated with local recurrence after skin-sparing mastectomy and immediate breast reconstruction for invasive breast cancer. *Ann Surg.* 2002; 235(6):814–819.

89. Carlson GW, Styblo TM, Lyles RH, et al. Local recurrence after skin-sparing mastectomy: tumor biology or surgical conservatism? *Ann Surg Oncol.* 2003;10(2):108–112.

90. Singletary SE. Skin-sparing mastectomy with immediate breast reconstruction: the M. D. Anderson Cancer Center experience. *Ann Surg Oncol.* 1996;3(4):411–416.

91. Newman LA, Kuerer HM, Hunt KK, et al. Presentation, treatment, and outcome of local recurrence afterskin-sparing mastectomy and immediate breast reconstruction. *Ann Surg Oncol.* 1998; 5(7):620–626.

92. Gerber B, Krause A, Reimer T, et al. Skin-sparing mastectomy with conservation of the nipple-areola complex and autologous reconstruction is an oncologically safe procedure. *Ann Surg.* 2003; 238(1):120–127.

93. Slavin SA, Schnitt SJ, Duda RB, et al. Skin-sparing mastectomy and immediate reconstruction: oncologic risks and aesthetic results in patients with early-stage breast cancer. *Plast Reconstr Surg.* 1998;102(1):49–62.

94. Dao TL, Nemoto T. The clinical significance of skin recurrence after radical mastectomy in women with cancer of the breast. *Surg Gynecol Obstet.* 1963;117:447–453.

95. Noone RB, Frazier TG, Noone GC, et al. Recurrence of breast carcinoma following immediate reconstruction: a 13-year review. *Plast Reconstr Surg.* 1994;93:96–108.

96. Eberlein TJ, Crespo LD, Smith BL, et al. Prospective evaluation of immediate reconstruction after mastectomy. *Ann Surg.* 1993; 218(1):29–36.

97. Cense HA, Rutgers EJ, Lopes Cardozo M, Van Lanschot JJ. Nipple-sparing mastectomy in breast cancer: a viable option? *Eur J Surg Oncol.* 2001;27(6):521–526.

98. Santini D, Taffurelli M, Gelli MC, et al. Neoplastic involvement of nipple-areolar complex in invasive breast cancer. *Am J Surg.* 1989;158(5):399–403.

99. Vlajcic Z, Zic R, Stanec S, et al. Nipple-areola complex preservation: predictive factors of neoplastic nipple-areola complex invasion. *Ann Plast Surg.* 2005; 55(3):240–244.

100. Kissin MW, Kark AE. Nipple preservation during mastectomy. *Br J Surg.* 1987;74(1):58–61.

101. Crowe JP, Jr., Kim JA, Yetman R, et al. Nipple-sparing mastectomy: technique and results of 54 procedures. *Arch Surg.* 2004; 139(2):148–150.

102. Petit JY, Veronesi U, Orecchia R, et al. Nipple-sparing mastectomy in association with intra operative radiotherapy (ELIOT): a new

type of mastectomy for breast cancer treatment. *Breast Cancer Res Treat.* 2006;96(1):47–51.

103. Byron MA, Venning VA, Mowat AG. Post-mammoplasty human adjuvant disease. *Br J Rheumatol.* 1984;23(3):227–229.

104. van Nunen SA, Gatenby PA, Basten A. Post-mammoplasty connective tissue disease. *Arthritis Rheum.* 1982;25(6):694–697.

105. Gabriel SE, O'Fallon WM, Kurland LT, et al. Risk of connective-tissue diseases and other disorders after breast implantation. *N Engl J Med.* 1994;330:1697–1702.

106. Schusterman MA, Kroll SS, Reece GP, et al. Incidence of autoimmune disease in patients after breast reconstruction with silicone gel implants versus autogenous tissue: a preliminary report. *Ann Plast Surg.* 1993;31(1):1–6.

107. Barreau-Pouhaer L, Le MG, Rietjens M, et al. Risk factors for failure of immediate breast reconstruction with prosthesis after total mastectomy for breast cancer. *Cancer.* 1992;70(5):1145–1151.

108. Cordeiro PG, Pusic AL, Disa JJ, et al. Irradiation after immediate tissue expander/implant breast reconstruction: outcomes, complications, aesthetic results, and satisfaction among 156 patients. *Plast Reconstr Surg.* 2004;113(3):877–881.

109. Hunt KK, Baldwin BJ, Strom EA, et al. Feasibility of postmastectomy radiation therapy after TRAM flap breast reconstruction. *Ann Surg Oncol.* 1997;4(5):377–384.

110. Williams JK, Carlson GW, Bostwick J, 3rd, et al. The effects of radiation treatment after TRAM flap breast reconstruction. *Plast Reconstr Surg.* 1997;100(5):1153–1160.

111. Proulx GM, Loree T, Edge S, et al. Outcome with postmastectomy radiation with transverse rectus abdominis musculocutaneous flap breast reconstruction. *Am Surg.* 2002;68(5):410–413.

112. Victor SJ, Brown DM, Horwitz EM, et al. Treatment outcome with radiation therapy after breast augmentation or reconstruction in patients with primary breast carcinoma. *Cancer.* 1998;82(7): 1303–1309.

113. Anderson PR, Hanlon AL, Fowble BL, et al. Low complication rates are achievable after postmastectomy breast reconstruction and radiation therapy. *Int J Radiat Oncol Biol Phys.* 2004;59(4):1080–1087.

114. Tuttle TM, Habermann EB, Grund EH, et al. Increasing use of contralateral prophylactic mastectomy for breast cancer patients: A trend toward more aggressive surgical treatment. *J Clin Oncol.* 2007;25(33):5203–5209.

115. Wennberg JE. Unwarranted variations in healthcare delivery: implications for academic medical centres. *BMJ* 2002;325(7370): 961–964.

116. Hewitt M, Simone JV, eds. *Ensuring Quality Cancer Care.* Institute of Medicine and Commission on Life Sciences, National Research Council. Washington, DC: National Academy Press; 1999: 97.

117. Katz SJ, Lantz PM, Janz NK, et al. Patient involvement in surgery treatment decisions for breast cancer. *J Clin Oncol.* 2005;23(24): 5526–5533.

118. Katz SJ, Lantz PM, Janz NK, et al. Patterns and correlates of local therapy for women with ductal carcinoma-in-situ. *J Clin Oncol.* 2005;23(13):3001–3007.

119. Morrow M, Mujahid M, Lantz PM, et al. Correlates of breast reconstruction: results from a population-based study. *Cancer.* 2005; 104(11):2340–2346.

120. Katz SJ, Lantz PM, Janz NK, et al. Surgeon perspectives about local therapy for breast carcinoma. *Cancer.* 2005;104(9):1854–1861.

121. Opatt D, Morrow M, Hawley S, et al. Conflicts in decision-making for breast cancer surgery. *Ann Surg Oncol.* 2007;14:2463–2469.

COMMENTARY
Karen T. Lane and John A. Butler

Over 200,000 women will be diagnosed with breast cancer each year in the United States and the majority of women will have multiple options with respect to the surgical treatment of their disease. In this chapter, Drs. Staradub and Morrow provide a thorough overview of the surgical treatment of stage I and II breast cancer. There were six prospective randomized trials that led to the National Institutes of Health consensus that breast conservation provided equivalent survival to total mastectomy (1). In 2002, two of the largest trials, National Surgical Adjuvant Breast and Bowel Project (NSABP) B-06 and Milan I, reported 20-year follow-up data showing equal survival for mastectomy and breast conservation (2,3). Both studies concluded that local recurrence rates were higher for patients undergoing lumpectomy with postoperative radiation versus mastectomy. This can often be quite confusing to patients who consider recurrence of their breast cancer to be a devastating event. Therefore, it is important that the patients understand the implications of local recurrence when making a decision regarding surgery. The authors report a significant decrease in local recurrence rates for breast conservation in several recent studies when compared with earlier trials. The cause appears to be multifactorial. The widespread use of tamoxifen and, more recently, aromatase inhibitors (for postmenopausal women) has significantly reduced the recurrence rate and mortality for women with estrogen receptor-positive tumors (4,5). Tumors are identified at a smaller size because of improvements in the quality and utilization of imaging studies.

The increasing use of magnetic resonance imaging (MRI) for tumors not identified on mammogram, for infiltrating lobular carcinoma, and for patients with persistently positive margins is addressed by the authors. As they correctly indicate, the routine use of MRI is currently not warranted, as there does tend to be a number of false-positives resulting in unnecessary procedures for the patient. MRI does have a role for patients with persistently positive margins or for evaluation of the contralateral breast in a patient with a mammographically occult breast cancer. In addition, data currently being collected in patients undergoing neoadjuvant chemotherapy support MRI as a modality in determining the efficacy of chemotherapy regimens based on tumor response as assessed by sequential MRI studies.

The authors discuss the use of cytoreductive, or neoadjuvant, chemotherapy for patients with a relatively large tumor compared to breast size. The two largest studies evaluating the use of neoadjuvant chemotherapy are NSABP B-18 and the European Organization for Cancer Research and Treatment (EORTC) trial. Both trials showed that over 20% of patients were converted from mastectomy to breast-conserving therapy (6,7). Neither trial showed an overall survival benefit for neoadjuvant chemotherapy; however, patients with a pathologic complete response had improved survival. A recent study from the MD Anderson Cancer Center reviewed 109 patients who underwent segmental mastectomy after achieving a complete pathologic response with neoadjuvant chemotherapy. The local recurrence rate was 2.7% at 6 years with a 5-year recurrence-free survival of 98.1% (8). The addition of Herceptin to the neoadjuvant armamentarium has substantially improved the pathologic response rate along with other newer regimens outlined in NSABP B27 (9–11). It seems logical that as the neoadjuvant chemotherapy regimens improve, and more pathologic complete responses are obtained, a survival benefit will ultimately be identified.

The authors' thoughtful discussion regarding breast conservation after neoadjuvant chemotherapy is critical. A generous sample of breast tissue should be excised encompassing any residual clinical or imaging abnormality. A clip, placed at the time of initial tissue sampling, is helpful in guiding subsequent surgery, particularly in patients who have a complete clinical response. Again, MRI may play a role in following the tumor during neoadjuvant chemotherapy to characterize the pattern of shrinkage and to better guide the surgeon as to what tissue to remove to ensure adequate evaluation of any residual microscopic disease.

The ability to identify *BRCA1/2* mutations in a subset of patients with a strong family history of breast and ovarian cancer, cancer diagnosed at an early age, or patients with Ashkenazi-Jewish background, has resulted in further decision making for the patient. The approach the authors describe for a patient with breast cancer and a strong family history is excellent. The patient can undergo breast-conserving therapy and then receive genetic counseling and testing during chemotherapy if desired. This allows the patient sufficient time to make an informed decision regarding local therapy and proceed with either bilateral mastectomy or radiation therapy to the involved breast. Unilateral mastectomy is not a good option in this patient population because of the high risk of developing a contralateral breast cancer. If the patient opts for mastectomy, we encourage her to pursue bilateral mastectomy with immediate reconstruction. For the prophylactic mastectomy, a sentinel lymph node biopsy should be considered in these patients in case a small invasive cancer is identified in the mastectomy specimen. An alternative regimen for patients with more advanced disease (larger tumors/node positive) would be to proceed with neoadjuvant chemotherapy, during which time genetic counseling and testing could be performed. Patients could then determine the desirability of a more extensive surgical procedure before any operation is performed.

The issue of margins for breast-conserving surgery is one that continues to be debated. Current definitions of negative margins include (a) no tumor cells on ink, (b) no tumor cells within 2 mm of ink, and (c) no tumor cells within 5 mm of ink. The authors report a review of over 5,000 patients in whom positive margins had a local recurrence rate of 15.8% compared with 5.6% for negative margins (12). No difference was seen when comparing margins of 1 mm versus 2 mm. The issue is further complicated by other factors addressing the adequacy of excision. In older women, the breast tissue may be extremely fatty, and compression of the tissue for specimen radiography as well as aggressive inking of the edges may result in a falsely close or positive margin. Orientation of the specimen may not be clear to the pathologist or may be interpreted differently by the surgeon, resulting in misunderstanding with respect to the actual close or involved margin. One option is to invite the pathologist to the operating room to assess the tumor cavity and grossly examine the specimen to correctly understand the anatomic orientation. Another option would be to submit additional margins separately from areas where additional breast tissue is present. The issue of margins will continue to be discussed until there are data available to justify one approach over another. The authors make an important point about the age of the patient as a factor for extent of resection. It is known that younger women have a higher rate of local recurrence. In an elderly patient with multiple comorbidities, re-excision for a focally close margin may not be indicated. It is critical to discuss the possibility of additional surgery with the patient preoperatively so that she is not surprised and confused by the necessity of a re-excision for a close or positive margin.

The use of sentinel lymph node dissection (SLND) has widely replaced the standard axillary lymph node dissection (ALND) in patients with early-stage breast cancer. It is estimated that 65% to 75% of newly diagnosed breast cancers in the United States present with node-negative disease. Following an early study of lymphatic mapping for melanoma, Giuliano et al. (13) performed 174 lymphatic mapping procedures, injecting a dye at the primary breast cancer tumor site to follow it to the sentinel node. This sentinel node was removed followed by a standard ALND. Sentinel lymph nodes were identified in 114 of 174 cases (65.5%). In 109 of 114 cases (95.6%), axillary lymph node status was correctly represented by the sentinel lymph node status. This accuracy improved as the surgeon became more practiced in the procedure, with the last 87 procedures 100% accurate. Veronesi et al. (14) randomized 516 patients with primary breast cancer (tumor size ≤ 2 cm) to either SLND or ALND. Patients with positive sentinel lymph nodes also underwent ALND. The investigators found positive sentinel nodes in 83 of 257 patients (32.3%) in the axillary lymph node dissection group versus 92 of 259 patients (35.5%) undergoing SLND alone. Overall accuracy of the procedure was 96.9%, sensitivity was 91.2%, and specificity was 100%.

Several large U.S. studies designed to further define the role of SLND in early-stage breast cancer have just completed accrual and will provide data on survival and morbidity of SLND and ALND. NSABP B32 randomized patients to SLND plus ALND versus ALND only if the SLN was positive, which is a design similar to the Italian SLN randomized trial by Veronesi et al. (14) previously described, but with almost tenfold more patients. This trial will evaluate the accuracy of SLND compared with ALND and compare the impact on survival. The American College of Surgeons Trial ACOSOG Z00011, is a randomized trial of ALND versus no ALND in women with breast cancers <5 cm and a positive SLN. This trial will evaluate the difference ALND makes in survival and the survival benefit associated with removing the rest of the axillary basin in node-positive patients. ACOSOG Z00010 is a registry of patients undergoing SLND to assess SLN identification rates as well as short- and long-term morbidity. Surgeons participating in this observational study have demonstrated proficiency by having performed 20 SLND procedures followed by ALND, or through documented SLND training during residency or fellowship.

As with any new technology, controversies do exist with respect to the role of SLND. Pathologic evaluation using immuno-histochemistry should not dictate additional surgical treatment until there are data to show an adverse outcome if pathologists find microscopic foci of disease not visible with standard light microscopy. The role of SLND in patients who have undergone neoadjuvant chemotherapy has recently been addressed and found to be accurate in experienced hands (15). Despite the acceptance of this technique, geographic differences in the use of SLND do exist. We looked at over 34,000 women undergoing SLND in different areas of the United States. There was a significantly lower rate of SLND performed in rural communities (16). The disparity should be addressed to ensure the highest quality of care for all breast cancer patients.

Breast reconstruction is an important component of the treatment of breast cancer patients. The psychological impact of having a good cosmetic result following surgical treatment of breast cancer cannot be underestimated. The authors discuss the use of the latissimus dorsi flap for partial breast reconstruction. One consideration with this technique would be to wait until well after radiation therapy to determine the final cosmetic result and then perform the reconstruction at that point. As stressed in the chapter, obtaining negative margins is critical prior to undertaking any partial breast reconstruction. Further, the use of "oncoplastic" techniques for reshaping breast tissue after breast conservation has improved the cosmetic result for many patients. The issue of positive margins after this tissue reshaping is of real concern and will require further study.

For patients undergoing mastectomy, skin-sparing mastectomy with immediate reconstruction has become a widely used option. Certain patients may not be candidates for immediate reconstruction, including patients with inflammatory cancer, morbidly obese patients, and some patients with diabetes. For patients requiring radiation therapy, autologous flap reconstruction is usually delayed. Another recent trend has been toward the use of nipple-sparing mastectomy. The authors reviewed the limited literature, which included one study involving 1,291 mastectomy specimens with a rate of nipple-areolar complex involvement of 12% (17). We agree with the authors' conclusion that the number of patients for which this technique is a viable option is limited and the current standard of retaining the skin envelope but removing the nipple-areolar complex remains the safest option for patients with breast cancer.

The authors conclude the chapter with a discussion of the patient's involvement in decision making. This is extremely important with breast cancer, in which, unlike other types of malignancies, there are multiple viable treatment options. As stated in the chapter, the patient needs to be educated regarding the risks and benefits of the various surgical choices and have a better understanding of the issue of local recurrence versus the most important variable of survival. One important issue for the use of breast conservation is the patient's ability or willingness to receive radiation therapy to the breast when indicated. Many patients do not live in proximity to radiation centers or do not have adequate transportation for the 6-week duration of radiotherapy. This raises the issue of improving ways to deliver radiation. Currently, a partial breast irradiation trial is being conducted by the NSABP (B39). In addition, an international trial is underway to evaluate intraoperative radiotherapy for a select group of postmenopausal women with T1 tumors and negative nodal status. The rationale for these trials is based on retrospective evaluation of previous studies that revealed that recurrences elsewhere in the breast were equal between patients receiving external-beam radiation and partial breast radiotherapy (18–24). This indicates that whole-breast radiation is not preventing any additional recurrences outside the index quadrant and may be unnecessary. We will be anxiously awaiting the results of these studies in the hope that we can improve the delivery of radiation for breast cancer patients.

REFERENCES

1. National Institute of Health Consensus Development Conference. Consensus statement: treatment of early-stage breast cancer. *J Natl Cancer Inst Monogr.* 1992;11:105–116.
2. Fisher B, Anderson S, Bryant J, et al. Twenty-year follow-up of a randomized trial comparing total mastectomy, lumpectomy, and lumpectomy plus irradiation for the treatment of invasive breast cancer. *N Engl J Med.* 2002;347:1233–1241.
3. Veronesi U, Cascinelli N, Mariani L, et al. Twenty-year follow-up of a randomized study comparing breast-conserving surgery with radical mastectomy for early breast cancer. *N Engl J Med.* 2002;247:1227–1232.
4. Early Breast Cancer Trialists' Collaborative Group. Tamoxifen for early breast cancer: an overview of the randomized trials. *Lancet.* 1998;351:1451–1467.
5. Baum M, Budzar AU, Cuzick J, et al. Anastrozole alone or in combination with tamoxifen versus tamoxifen alone for adjuvant treatment of postmenopausal women with early breast cancer: first results of the ATAC randomised trial. *Lancet.* 2002;359:2131–2139.
6. Fisher B, Brown A, Mamounas E, et al. Effect of preoperative chemotherapy on local-regional disease in women with operable breast cancer: findings from National Surgical Adjuvant Breast and Bowel Project B-18. *J Clin Oncol.* 1997;15:2483–2493.
7. van der Hage JA, ven de Velde CJ, Julien JP, et al. Preoperative chemotherapy in primary operable breast cancer: results from the European Organization for Research and Treatment of Cancer trial 10902. *J Clin Oncol.* 2001;19:4224–4237.
8. Peintinger F, Symmans WF, Gonzalez-Angulo AM, et al. The safety of breast-conserving surgery in patients who achieve a complete pathologic response after neoadjuvant chemotherapy. *Cancer.* 2006;107:1248–1254.
9. Bear HD, Anderson S, Brown A, et al. The effect on tumor response of adding sequential preoperative docetaxel to preoperative doxorubicin and cyclophosphamide: preliminary results from National Surgical Adjuvant Breast and Bowel Project Protocol B-27. *J Clin Oncol.* 2003;21:4165–4174.
10. Bear HD, Anderson S, Smith RE, et al. Sequential preoperative or postoperative docetaxel added to preoperative doxorubicin plus cyclophosphamide for operable breast cancer: National Surgical Adjuvant Breast and Bowel Project Protocol B-27. *J Clin Oncol.* 2006;24:2019–2027.
11. Buzdar AU, Ibrahim NK, Francis D, et al. Significantly higher pathologic complete remission rate after neoadjuvant therapy with trastuzumab, paclitaxel, and epirubicin chemotherapy: results of a randomized trial in human epidermal growth factor receptor 2-positive operable breast cancer. *J Clin Oncol.* 2005;23:3676–3685.
12. Singletary SE. Surgical margins in patients with early-stage breast cancer treated with breast conservation therapy. *Am J Surg.* 2002;184:383–393.
13. Giuliano AE, Kirgan DM, Guenther JM, et al. Lymphatic mapping and sentinel lymphadenectomy for breast cancer. *Ann Surg.* 1994;220:391–401.
14. Veronesi U, Paganelli G, Viale G, et al. A randomized comparison of sentinel-node biopsy with routine axillary dissection in breast cancer. *N Engl J Med.* 2003;349:546–553.
15. Lang JE, Esserman LJ, Ewing CA, et al. Accuracy of sentinel lymph node biopsy following neoadjuvant chemotherapy: Effect of clinical node status at presentation. *J Am Coll Surg.* 2004;199:856–862.
16. Maggard, MA, Lane KT, O'Connell JB, et al. Beyond the Clinical Trials: How Prevalent is Sentinel Lymph Node Biopsy Performed for Breast Cancer? *Ann Surg Oncol.* 2005;12:41–47.
17. Santini D, Taffurelli M, Gelli MC, et al. Neoplastic involvement of nipple-areolar complex in invasive breast cancer. *Am J Surg.* 1989;158:399–403.
18. King TA, Bolton JS, Kuske RR, et al. Long-term results of wide-field brachytherapy as the sole method of radiation therapy after segmental mastectomy for Tis,1,2 breast cancer. *Am J Surg.* 2000;180:299–304.
19. Fisher B, Redmond C, Poisson R, et al. Eight-year results of a randomized clinical trial comparing total mastectomy and lumpectomy with or without irradiation in the treatment of breast cancer. *N Engl J Med.* 1989;320:822–828.
20. Fisher B, Anderson S, Redmond CK, et al. Reanalysis and results after 12 years of follow-up in a randomized clinical trial comparing total mastectomy with lumpectomy with or without irradiation in the treatment of breast cancer. *N Engl J Med.* 1995;333:1456–1461.
21. Crile G Jr, Esselstyn CB Jr. Factors influencing local recurrence of cancer after partial mastectomy. *Cleve Clin J Med.* 1990;57:143–146.
22. Liljegren G, Holmberg L, Adami HO, et al. Sector resection with or without postoperative radiotherapy for stage I breast cancer: five-year results of a randomized trial. Uppsala-Orebro Breast Cancer Study Group. *J Natl Cancer Inst.* 1994;86:717–722.
23. Clark RM, Whelan T, Levine M, et al. Randomized clinical trial of breast irradiation following lumpectomy and axillary dissection for node-negative breast cancer: an update. Ontario Clinical Oncology Group. *J Natl Cancer Inst.* 1996;88:1659–1664.
24. Veronesi U, Luini A, Del Vecchio M, et al. Radiotherapy after breast-preserving surgery in women with localized cancer of the breast. *N Engl J Med.* 1993;328:1587–1591.

Radiation Therapy in Breast-Conserving Therapy for Invasive Breast Cancer

Pramila Rani Anné and Walter J. Curran, Jr.

Breast-conserving therapy is a standard treatment option for eligible patients with early-stage breast cancer. Radiation therapy is added to breast-conserving surgery to treat microscopic residual disease within the breast. Several prospective, randomized trials comparing mastectomy with breast-conserving therapy have confirmed equivalent survival (1–8) (Table 19.1). Follow-up as long as 20 years has been reported (1,2). Trials comparing breast-conserving surgery alone with breast-conserving surgery plus whole-breast radiation therapy showed a substantial decrease in local recurrence with the addition of whole-breast radiation, and, as a consequence, a reduced requirement for mastectomy. These studies established the standard of breast-conserving surgery followed by whole-breast radiation (1,8–14). Based on the results of these studies, the National Cancer Institute in 1991 published the first consensus statement on early-stage disease, with a recommendation that breast-conserving therapy be a preferred option for eligible patients (15).

PATIENT SELECTION

Criteria for selecting patients for breast-conservation surgery followed by breast radiation include factors used in the original clinical trials as well as guidelines developed by the American College of Radiology and American College of Surgeons (16). The most suitable patients include those with unifocal disease with tumors ≤5 cm resected with clear margins and able to receive breast irradiation. Absolute contraindications to whole-breast irradiation include pregnancy, because of scattered radiation dose to the fetus, and prior breast radiation. The latter is relevant for patients treated with mantle radiation for Hodgkin disease as adolescents or young adults, as the risk of radiation-induced breast cancer is significant 20 to 30 years later. Diffuse malignant-appearing microcalcification within the breast is another contraindication, as it indicates a high probability of extensive disease. Relative contraindications to radiation therapy include scleroderma or similar collagen vascular diseases (but not rheumatoid arthritis), as these conditions increase radiation toxicity and fibrosis and are associated with poor cosmesis. Difficulty in complying with the provision radiation therapy, such as an inability to lie supine, is another relative contraindication.

WHOLE-BREAST IRRADIATION

Whole-breast radiation was introduced as part of breast-conserving therapy on the premise that there could be micro-scopic residual disease within the breast after segmental mastectomy ("lumpectomy"). Studies of total mastectomy specimens demonstrated that microscopic disease could extend as much as 2 to 4 cm within the breast tissue beyond the primary tumor (17). Long-term results of multiple randomized trials have now been published comparing mastectomy with breast-conserving therapy (segmental mastectomy plus whole-breast radiation) (1–8). Equivalent survival rates between the two treatment strategies have been observed (Table 19.1). The long duration of follow-up, >20 years, in the National Surgical Adjuvant Breast Project (NSABP) B-06 and Milan Cancer Institute studies (1,2), has confirmed the equivalence of the two treatments. The requirement for breast radiation has been established in randomized trials comparing breast-conserving surgery alone with breast-conserving surgery plus radiation (Table 19.2) (9–14). The survival rates were comparable, but the addition of radiotherapy was associated with a significant reduction in local recurrence. Thus, the benefit of adding radiation to breast-conserving surgery is that mastectomy and its associated cosmetic consequences can be avoided with a low local recurrence rate and no adverse impact on survival.

In 2002, Fisher et al. (1) reported the 20-year follow-up of the NSAPB B-06 randomized trial comparing total mastectomy, lumpectomy, and lumpectomy plus whole-breast radiation (50 Gy in 25 fractions) for the treatment of invasive breast cancer. Eligibility criteria included tumor size ≤4 m and microscopically negative margins of resection; that is, tumor not transected at the margin. Local recurrence was decreased from 39% to 14% by the addition of radiation after lumpectomy. However, overall survival was not statistically different.

Although the individual trials show no effect of the improved local control on survival, a recent meta-analysis based on published randomized trials suggests improved survival in patients who received breast radiation compared with breast-conserving surgery alone (18).

Because of the heterogeneity of patient and tumor characteristics in these trials, several studies have been conducted to evaluate the need for breast radiation in a subset of women with lesions associated with a low risk of recurrence. A small study from the Joint Center for Radiation Therapy of stage I patients treated with segmental mastectomy alone (without radiation or systemic therapy) was closed early because of higher than expected local failure rates (19). Larger randomized trials have also been performed (20–23). In the NSABP B-21 trial, 1,009 women with node-negative breast cancer and tumors <1 cm who

Table 19.1

Randomized Trials Comparing Mastectomy with Breast-Conserving Therapy (BCT)

Trial (Ref.)	No. of Patients	Maximum Tumor Size (cm)	Median Follow-up (years)	Overall Survival (%) (mastectomy)	Overall Survival (%) (BCT)	Local Recurrence % (BCT)	Local Recurrence % (mastectomy)
NSABP B-06 (1)	1,851	4	20	47	lumpectomy 46 lumpectomy + radiation 46	lumpectomy 39.2 lumpectomy + radiation 14.3	10.2
Milan Cancer Institute (2)	701	2	20	58.8	58.3	8.8	2.3
National Cancer Institute (3)	237	5	18.4	58	54	22	0
Institute Gustave Roussy (6)	179	2	10	79	78	4	NR
EORTC/DBCCG Pooled Results	1,772	5	9.8	67	67	9	10

NSABP, National Surgical Adjuvant Breast Project; EORTC, European Organization for the Research and Treatment of Cancer; DBCCG, Danish Breast Cancer Cooperative Group; NR, not reported.

underwent lumpectomy were randomized to receive postoperative breast radiation plus tamoxifen, breast radiation alone, or tamoxifen alone. Median follow-up was 7.3 years. Investigators were unable to identify a subgroup that did not benefit from radiation. At 8 years, the local recurrence rates were 2.85% in patients treated with radiation and tamoxifen, 9.3% in patients treated with radiation alone, and 16.5% in patients treated with

tamoxifen alone ($p < 0.01$ for all comparisons). Overall survival was equivalent for all three groups (93%, 94%, and 93%) (20). In a Canadian study, 709 women, 50 years of age and older with T1 or T2 node-negative tumors, were randomized to tamoxifen plus breast radiation versus tamoxifen alone. Median follow-up was 5.6 years. At 5 years, the local relapse rate was 0.6% on the combined group and 7.7% in the tamoxifen group

Table 19.2

Randomized Trials Comparing Breast-Conserving Surgery (BCS) with BCS and Radiation (RT)

Trial (Ref.)	No. of Patients	Maximum Tumor Size (cm)	Median Follow-up (years)	Overall Survival (%) (BCS)	Overall Survival (%) (BCS + RT)	Local Recurrence (%) (BCT)	Local Recurrence (%) (BCT + RT)
NSABP B-06 (1)	1,137	4	20	46	46	39	14
Uppsala Orebro Breast Cancer Study Group (9)	381	2	10	78	77.5	24	8.5
Milan Cancer Institute (11)	579	<2.5	9	77	82	24	6
Ontario Clinical Oncology Group (10)	837	4	7.6	76	79	35	11
Scottish Cancer Trial (12)	585	4	5.7	83	83	25	6
Swedish Breast Cancer Group (14)	1,179	5[a]	5	93	94	14	4

NSABP, National Surgical Adjuvant Breast Project.
[a]Only one patient with a tumor >3 cm.

(21). The Cancer and Leukemia Group B (CALGB) trial specifically evaluated older women. The trial randomized 636 women 70 years of age or older with T1 tumors, clinically node-negative and estrogen-receptor positive, to tamoxifen alone or tamoxifen and breast radiation. At a median follow-up of 4 years, (5 years) the local relapse rate was 4% in the tamoxifen-only group and 1% in the combined group. There was no difference in overall survival or in mastectomy rates between the groups (22). This trial suggests that select older patients may be at a sufficiently low enough risk as not to require radiation. Longer follow-up is required from these trials to determine if late local failures occur. These trials suggest that breast radiation is still the standard of care for the majority of patients with low risk breast cancer.

Technique

Whole-breast radiation is typically delivered with the patient in the supine position, either flat or at a slight angle. Optimal breast setup requires immobilization of the patient. Patients may be placed on a special device called a *breast board*, which is commercially available, or customized foam cradles may be used for each patient. The arm on the treated side is positioned over the head. The treatment setup should allow the patient to assume the same relative position each treatment day. The treatment fields are then defined. Simulation films or a computed tomography (CT) scan (CT simulation) is obtained. CT-based treatment planning is performed commonly to allow for delineation of critical structures such as the heart and lung, and also allows for optimization of dose homogeneity within the breast (24,25). Newer planning techniques involve three-dimensional (3-D) treatment planning and intensity-modulated radiation therapy.

The radiation fields are two opposed tangential fields, which encompass the breast, a portion of the chest wall, and the lower axilla. The supraclavicular fossa or regional nodal fields may be added for patients with positive axillary lymph nodes. Additional radiation limited to the region of the tumor bed is called *boost radiation*. The extent of the field is determined by the lumpectomy bed, often outlined by clips placed by the surgeon at the time of tumor excision. Boost radiation can be performed with an electron beam, brachytherapy, or minitangential photon fields.

Dose, Fractionation, and Boost Radiation

A radiation dose of 45 to 50 Gray (Gy) is delivered in 25 to 28 fractions (daily doses) Monday through Friday to the breast. Boost radiation may also be given. The dose is typically 10 to 16 Gy (higher if a there is a focally positive margin) given at 2.0 Gy per fraction. Although not included in the original breast-conserving trials, boost radiation has been used commonly to further decrease the risk of local recurrence. Two randomized trials have confirmed the benefit of a boost. A recent EORTC trial, using a 16-Gy boost, reduced the local recurrence rate from 7.3% to 4.3% at 5 years (26). Younger patients experienced the greatest benefit, as their local recurrence rates without the boost were highest. In a trial from Lyon, a 10-Gy boost was associated with a smaller but nonetheless significant reduction in local recurrence at 5 years, from 4.5% to 3.6% (27). Two smaller trials showed borderline statistical benefits from boost radiation (28,29). It should be noted that boost radiation can

have a negative impact on cosmesis (27,30) and also adds cost and time to the treatment.

Accelerated Hypofractionation

Accelerated hypofractionation is a method of whole-breast radiation in which larger daily doses are given over a shorter overall period of time. The lower total dose delivered in fewer, larger fractions is hypothesized to be at least as safe and effective as the standard treatment. Multiple randomized trials have been undertaken to test this hypothesis. In 2002, Whelan et al. (31) reported the results of a multicenter Canadian trial in which enrolled patients were randomized to 50 Gy in 25 fractions or 42.5 Gy in 16 fractions. Eligible women were node-negative and had negative resection margins. Women with a large breast size, defined as more than 25 cm of tissue thickness at the midpoint of the radiation field, were excluded. A total of 1,234 women were evaluated, and at 5-year follow-up, there was no difference in recurrence rates or cosmesis between the two groups.

In the Institute of Cancer Research trial (United Kingdom) (32,33) the investigators randomly assigned 1,410 women with invasive breast cancer (tumor stage 1–3 with a maximum of one positive node and no metastasis) who had had local tumor excision of early-stage breast cancer to receive 50 Gy radiotherapy given in 25 fractions, 39 Gy given in 13 fractions, or 42.9 Gy given in 13 fractions, all given over 5 weeks. After a median follow-up of 9.7 years, the probability of local recurrence was significantly different between the 39 Gy and 42.9 Gy arms, but not the 50 Gy arm. Thus, the risk of ipsilateral tumor relapse after 10 years was 12.1% in the 50 Gy group, 14.8% in the 39 Gy group, and 9.6% in the 42.9 Gy group. The difference between 39 Gy and 42.9 Gy groups was significant ($p = 0.027$). There was no difference in cosmesis at a minimum of 5 years of follow-up.

Despite the findings in these studies, there continues to be concern about the possible increased incidence of late fibrosis and soft-tissue complications with decreased cosmesis associated with accelerated hypofractionation (34,35). To further address the issues of local recurrence and late normal tissue effects, the United Kingdom Coordinating Committee for Cancer Research (now the National Cancer Research Institute) initiated the Standardisation of Breast Radiotherapy (START) Trials (36). Between 1998 and 2002, 2,236 women with early breast cancer (pT1-3a pN0-1 M0) at 17 centers in the United Kingdom were randomly assigned after primary surgery to receive 50 Gy in 25 fractions of 2.0 Gy versus 41.6 Gy or 39 Gy in 13 fractions of 3.2 Gy or 3.0 Gy over 5 weeks. The findings, published in 2008, indicate that after a median follow-up of 5.1 years, the rate of local-regional tumor relapse at 5 years was 3.6% after 50 Gy, 3.5% after 41.6 Gy, and 5.2% after 39 Gy. The estimated absolute differences in 5-year local-regional relapse rates compared with 50 Gy were 0.2% (95% confidence interval [CI]: −1.3% to 2.6%) after 41.6 Gy and 0.9% (95% CI: −0.8% to 3.7%) after 39 Gy. Photographic and patient self-assessments suggested lower rates of late adverse effects after 39 Gy than with 50 Gy. The investigators concluded that the data were consistent with the hypothesis that breast cancer and the dose-limiting normal tissues respond similarly to change in radiotherapy fraction size, and further that 41.6 Gy in 13 fractions was similar to the control regimen of 50 Gy in 25 fractions in terms of local-regional tumor control and late normal tissue effects.

Such shorter courses of treatment save time and cost and may be an alternative to standard fractionation in select patients. A number of countries including Canada have adopted these shorter courses of treatment.

Treatment Toxicity

Breast irradiation is well tolerated by most women. Common acute toxicity includes skin irritation, erythema, breast edema, and fatigue (37). The magnitude of these side effects depends on the size of the patient, prior chemotherapy, and extent of axillary dissection. Mild-to-moderate long-term complications are not frequent, and include breast fibrosis and lymphedema. Less common or rare late effects include radiation pneumonitis, rib fractures, brachial plexopathy, cardiac events, and second malignancies. Approximately 5% to 10% of patients may experience mild breast pain attributable to the radiation therapy. There may also be an adverse or poor cosmetic outcome in approximately 5% of patients due to breast fibrosis, scar retraction, and telangiectasia (37). Contracture of the treated breast may occur and also depends on the volume of breast tissue removed at the time of surgery. Lymphedema of the arm is now decreasing in incidence with the use of sentinel node biopsy/sampling as opposed to axillary dissection. A randomized trial of sentinel node biopsy versus standard axillary dissection reported lymphedema rates of 5% versus 13%, respectively, at 12 months after surgery (38). Lymphedema probability also increases if the regional lymph nodes receive radiation (39,40). The incidence of radiation pneumonitis is typically under 1% in patients receiving breast irradiation alone, but increases if the patient is receiving nodal irradiation or concurrent chemotherapy (41,42). Rib fractures can occur in 1% to 5% of patients, but are typically asymptomatic and found incidentally (43,44). Serious long-term effects, such as brachial plexus injury and pericarditis, are relatively rare (44–46).

Breast cancer radiotherapy regimens of the 1970s and early 1980s appreciably increased mortality from heart disease 10 to 15 years afterward, particularly in patients in whom the left breast or internal mammary nodes were treated (47–49). With the current use of 3-D CT-based treatment planning, more recent series indicate no difference in cardiac mortality at 10 years, although longer follow-up is needed (50,51). Radiation-induced second malignancies (sarcomas) are extremely rare, with the long-term risk at 0.2% at 10 years (52). The risk of lung cancer in nonsmokers is minimal with modern radiation techniques. There is a report that smokers may have a slight increase in lung cancer in the ipsilateral lung (53).

ACCELERATED PARTIAL BREAST RADIATION

Accelerated partial breast irradiation (APBI) is a newer concept in providing radiotherapy following breast-conserving surgery and is still under investigation. APBI involves the treatment of the surgical bed plus a margin of surrounding normal tissue following lumpectomy. The rationale for APBI is based on the concept, not yet rigorously proven, that in selected patients with negative margins of resection after lumpectomy, any residual microscopic disease is not disseminated throughout the remaining breast, but is usually within a 1- to 2-cm region surrounding the lumpectomy cavity (17,54–57). The rationale is further supported by the finding that when no radiation is given after lumpectomy, the overwhelming majority of local recurrences are located at or near the lumpectomy site (57). Thus, by limiting the volume of breast receiving radiation, acceleration of the dose delivery and completion of treatment in less than 5 treatment days becomes feasible.

Because standard breast radiation therapy requires daily treatment for 5 to 6.5 weeks, some patients eligible for breast-conserving surgery may nevertheless opt to have a mastectomy instead in order to avoid whole-breast radiation because of time or travel constraints; they may elect to forego radiation as part of their breast-conservation therapy; or they may be noncompliant in completing the course of whole-breast radiation (58–61). ABPI has the potential to provide more women with optimal breast-conservation therapy (surgery and radiation). However, patient selection is critical In a revised consensus statement published online in 2005 (62), the American Society of Breast Surgeons recommended the following selection criteria when considering patients for treatment with APBI as a sole form of radiation therapy outside of multi-institutional studies and institutional protocols:

- Age 45 years or older
- Invasive ductal carcinoma or ductal carcinoma in situ
- Total tumor size (invasive and ductal carcinoma in situ [DCIS]) ≤3 cm in size
- Negative microscopic surgical margins of excision
- Axillary lymph nodes/sentinel lymph node negative

Several treatment techniques are available for the delivery of APBI: multicatheter interstitial brachytherapy, intracavitary balloon catheter brachytherapy, 3-D conformal external-beam radiotherapy, and intraoperative radiotherapy.

There is currently an ongoing national phase III randomized trial (NSABP B39/RTOG 0413) (63) designed to determine whether partial breast irradiation limited to the region of the tumor bed following lumpectomy provides equivalent local tumor control in the breast compared with conventional whole-breast irradiation in the management of early-stage breast cancer. Patients randomized to receive APBI will be treated with multicatheter interstitial brachytherapy, MammoSite (Proxima Therapeutics Inc., Alpharetta, GA) balloon catheter brachytherapy, or 3-D conformal external-beam radiotherapy, at the discretion of the attending physician. Eligibility criteria include patients who have undergone lumpectomy for stage, 0, I, or II breast cancer with lesions ≤3 cm and in whom there are no more than three positive nodes.

Multicatheter Interstitial Brachytherapy

Multicatheter interstitial brachytherapy is the method of APBI for which there is the most extensive treatment experience and follow-up data (64–73). In this approach, afterloading catheters are placed through the breast tissue surrounding the lumpectomy cavity. The exact number of catheters used is determined by the size and shape of the target. Toxicities include infection, erythema, hyperpigmentation, breast pain, and edema, which diminish over time. Late effects include fat necrosis, telangiectasias, and breast fibrosis (64–69). Results from centers with conservative patient selection and acceptable quality assurance reveal excellent local control rates and satisfactory cosmesis (66).

Arthur et al. (64) recently reported the results of Radiation Therapy Oncology Group protocol 95-17, a prospective phase II cooperative group trial evaluating multicatheter brachytherapy after lumpectomy in select early-stage breast cancers. Eligibility criteria included stage I or II breast carcinoma confirmed to be <3 cm, unifocal, invasive nonlobular histology with zero to three positive axillary nodes without extracapsular extension. APBI treatment was delivered with either low-dose-rate (45 Gy in 3.5 to 5 days) or high-dose-rate (34 Gy in 10 twice-daily fractions over 5 days) brachytherapy. Median follow-up among the 66 patients in the low-dose-rate group was 6.14 years, with the 5-year estimates of in-breast, regional, and contralateral failure rates of 3%, 5%, and 2%, respectively. The 33 patients in the low-dose-rate group experienced similar results with a median follow-up of 6.22 years. The 5-year estimates of in-breast, regional, and contralateral failure rates were 6%, 0%, and 6%, respectively.

Although results appear satisfactory, this method of treatment is technically demanding, and because of the difficulty and the invasiveness of the procedure, alternative methods of dose delivery have now been developed.

Intracavitary Balloon Catheter Brachytherapy

A balloon catheter treatment device was developed to simplify the brachytherapy procedure while improving the reproducibility of the dosimetry/radiation coverage of the lumpectomy cavity. The commercially available system is the Mammosite Radiation Therapy System (Proxima Therapeutics Inc.). The catheter is located centrally within a balloon that is placed into the lumpectomy cavity and inflated. After inflation, balloon catheter placement is evaluated and final approval for treatment depends on multiple dosimetric guidelines. The device may be placed into the lumpectomy cavity at the time of surgery (open technique) or may be inserted postoperatively percutaneously under ultrasound guidance (closed technique) with comparable results (74). The postoperative, closed technique has the advantage of establishing histologic clearance of the margins of resection before introducing the catheter.

In 2007, Benitez et al. (75) reported the five results observed in 43 patients who were entered into a trial of MammoSite balloon brachytherapy. The trial was conducted to obtain clearance from the United States Food and Drug Administration and to establish the safety of the device. Criteria for entry into the study were unifocal invasive ductal carcinoma, tumor size ≤2 cm, age ≥45 years, absence of extensive intraductal component, cavity size ≥3 cm in one dimension, node-negative, and final margins negative per NSABP definition. A minimum balloon-to-skin surface distance of 5 mm was required. A dose of 34 Gy was delivered in 10 fractions over 5 days prescribed to 1 cm from the applicator surface using iridium 192 high-dose-rate brachytherapy. Among the 43 patients, the infection rate was 9.3%. Seroma formation occurred in 32.6% of patients, of which 12% were symptomatic and required aspiration. Asymptomatic fat necrosis was identified in 4 of the 43 patients, noted from time of catheter removal at 11, 14, 42, and 63 months. Good-to-excellent cosmetic outcomes were achieved in 83.3% of the 36 patients with >5 years of follow-up. Cosmetic outcomes were improved, with increased skin spacing, having statistical significance at skin spacing ≥7 mm. The only serious adverse events were two infections: mastitis and abscess. No local recurrences (either at the tumor bed or elsewhere in the breast) or regional recurrences have occurred in the 36 patients who have been followed for a median of 5.5 years.

Subsequently, the American Society of Breast Surgeons conducted the MammoSite Breast Brachytherapy Registry Trial (76,77). In 2008, 3 years of data were reported reflecting on treatment efficacy, cosmetic results, and toxicities (77). A total of 1,440 patients (1,449 cases) with early-stage breast cancer who were undergoing breast-conserving therapy were treated with the MammoSite device to deliver APBI (34 Gy in 3.4 Gy fractions). Of these, 1,255 (87%) cases had invasive breast cancer (IBC; median size = 10 mm), and 194 (13%) cases had DCIS (median size = 8 mm). Median follow-up was 30.1 months. Twenty-three (1.6%) cases developed an ipsilateral breast tumor recurrence for a 2-year actuarial rate of 1.04% (1.11% for IBC and 0.59% for DCIS). The percentages of breasts with good-to-excellent cosmetic results at 12 (n = 980), 24 (n = 752), 36 (n = 403), and 48 months (n = 67 cases) were 95%, 94%, 93%, and 93%, respectively. Symptomatic seromas occurred in 10.6% of cases, and 1.5% of cases developed fat necrosis. A subset analysis of the first 400 consecutive cases enrolled was performed (352 with IBC, 48 with DCIS). With a median follow-up of 37.5 months, the 3-year actuarial rate of ipsilateral breast tumor recurrence was 1.79%.

Three-Dimensional Conformal External-Beam Radiotherapy

This is another method of APBI that is attractive to both physicians and patients because it is noninvasive, delivers a homogeneous dose with decreased trauma to the breast compared with brachytherapy, and offers a potential reduction in normal breast tissue toxicity compared with standard whole-breast external beam radiation. There are only short-term data on studies with good quality control, but these studies reveal acceptable levels of acute toxicity (78–80).

In 2007, Vicini et al. (78) presented their ongoing clinical experience using this modality in the management of 91 patients with early-stage breast cancer treated with breast-conserving therapy. The clinical target volume consisted of the lumpectomy cavity plus a 10- to 15-mm margin. The prescribed dose was 34 or 38.5 Gy in 10 fractions given over 5 consecutive days. The median follow-up was 24 months. Twelve patients have been followed for ≥4 years, 20 for ≥3.5 years, 29 for >3.0 years, 33 for ≥2.5 years, and 46 for ≥2.0 years. No local recurrences were observed. Cosmetic results were rated as good-to-excellent in 100% of evaluable patients at ≥6 months (n = 47), 93% at 1 year (n = 43), 91% at 2 years (n = 21), and in 90% at ≥3 years (n = 10). Only two patients (3%) developed marked toxicity, which was manifest as breast pain that resolved with time.

Intraoperative Radiation Therapy

In contrast to the other approaches, intraoperative radiotherapy (IORT) offers further acceleration of dose delivery. With this approach, the entire partial breast radiation dose is delivered in one large fraction of 20 to 21 Gy at the time of surgical excision. Preliminary data from various institutions appear favorable (81–85). Veronesi et al. (83) reported their experience with IORT in the management of 590 patients. These patients, affected by unifocal breast carcinoma up to a diameter of 2.5 cm, underwent wide resection of the breast lesion followed by IORT with electrons. Most patients received 21 Gy intraoperatively, biologically equivalent to 58 to 60 Gy in standard fractionation. Patients were evaluated 1, 3, 6, and 12 months after surgery, and thereafter every 6 months, to look for early, intermediate, late complications, and other events. After a follow-up from 4 to 57 months (mean, 24 months; median, 20 months), 19 patients (3.2%) developed breast fibrosis, which was mild in 18 and severe in one, which resolved within 24 months. Three patients (0.5%) developed local recurrences, three patients developed ipsilateral carcinomas in other quadrants, and five other patients developed contralateral breast carcinoma. One patient (0.2%) died of distant metastases. The authors concluded that IORT with electrons is a safe method for treating conservatively operated breasts, avoids the long period of postoperative radiotherapy, diminishes radiation to normal tissues and organs, and reduces drastically the cost of radiotherapy. Furthermore, early results on local control and toxicity are encouraging.

The apparently salutary effects observed with IORT in these early-phase trials has led to the development of an international prospective randomized phase III trial, the Targeted Intraoperative Radiation (TARGIT) Trial, (86) to determine whether single-fraction IORT targeted to the tumor bed provides equivalent local control compared with whole-breast irradiation in patients with early-stage invasive breast cancer. Patients are randomized to receive either whole-breast irradiation or IORT. Patients randomized to conventional whole-breast irradiation receive radiotherapy postoperatively, typically beginning 1 month after breast-conserving surgery or after completing chemotherapy, if indicated. Patients randomized to IORT receive tumor bed irradiation prescribed at 20 Gy to the surgical margins using soft x-rays (50 kV) delivered with the Intrabeam Photon Radiosurgery System (Zeiss Inc., Oberkochen, Germany). The IORT may be delivered immediately after resection of the beast cancer or, alternatively, the TARGIT trial also permits IORT to be administered at a second operation after initial breast-conserving surgery or at the time of re-excision or axillary staging if not completed at the initial operation. The delivery of radiotherapy at a second operation has the advantage of allowing confirmation of the marginal status before the administration of IORT. However, repeat IORT is not permitted at a second operation to clear involved margins after having received IORT immediately after the first operation.

Inclusion criteria for the TARGIT trial include age ≥35 years and operable invasive breast cancer (T1-3, N0-1, M0) suitable for breast-conserving surgery. Exclusion criteria include multifocal, multicentric, or bilateral breast cancer (factors that might increase the risk of local recurrence); primary chemotherapy or hormonal therapy (factors that might limit visualization of the tumor dimension and increase the likelihood of re-excision); clinically positive lymph nodes (a factor that might increase the risk of local-regional recurrence); and extensive intraductal or invasive lobular cancer (factors that increase the risk of recurrence and re-excision). The accrual goal is 2,200 patients.

Investigators at the University of North Carolina are evaluating an alternative approach to delivering IORT (87,88). Here the radiation is delivered immediately *prior* to excision of the breast tumor in an effort to improve delivery to the region at risk and reduce the volume of normal tissue irradiated. In the operating room, the tumor is exposed, the IORT is delivered, and then a segmental mastectomy is performed in the usual manner.

CONCLUSIONS

Radiation therapy is an important component of breast-conserving therapy. Randomized trials have validated the role of radiation therapy for the majority of patients who receive breast conservation. The treatment is well tolerated, with very few serious long-term side effects. Future directions involve assessing newer techniques such as accelerated hypofractionation, the various forms of APBI, and intensity-modulated radiation therapy in an effort to decrease side effects and treatment time, and defining any subsets of patients who may not benefit from or require radiation therapy.

REFERENCES

1. Fisher B, Anderson S, Bryant J, et al. Twenty-year follow-up of a randomized trial comparing total mastectomy, lumpectomy, and lumpectomy plus irradiation for the treatment of invasive breast cancer. *N Engl J Med.* 2002;347:1233–1241.
2. Veronesi U, Cascinelli N, Mariani L, et al. Twenty-year follow-up of a randomized study comparing breast-conserving surgery with radical mastectomy for early breast cancer. *N Engl J Med.* 2002;347:1227–1232.
3. Poggi MM, Danforth DN, Sciuto LC, et al. Eighteen-year results in the treatment of early breast carcinoma with mastectomy versus breast conservation therapy: The National Cancer Institute Randomized Trial. *Cancer.* 2003;98:697–702.
4. Van Dongen J, Bartelink H, Fentiman I. Factors influencing local relapse and survival and results of salvage treatment after breast conserving therapy in operable breast cancer: EORTC trial 10801, breast conservation compared with mastectomy in TNM stage I and II breast cancer. *Eur J Cancer.* 1992;28A:801–805.
5. Van Dongen JA, Voogd AC, Fentiman IS, et al. Long-term results of a randomized trial comparing breast-conserving therapy with mastectomy: European Organization for Research and Treatment of Cancer 10801 trial. *J Natl Cancer Inst.* 2000;92:1143–1150.
6. Sarrazin D, Le MG, Arriagada R, et al. Ten year results of a randomized trial comparing a conservative treatment to mastectomy in early breast cancer. *Radiother Oncol.* 1989;14:177–184.
7. Blichert-Toft M, Rose CA, Anderson J. Danish randomized trial comparing breast conservation therapy with mastectomy: six years of life-table analysis, Danish Breast Cancer Cooperative Group. *J Natl Cancer Inst Monogr.* 1992;11:19–25.
8. Voogd AC, Nielsen M, Peterse JL, et al. Differences in risk factors for local and distant recurrence after breast-conserving therapy or mastectomy for stage I and II breast cancer: Pooled results of two large European randomized trials. *J Clin Oncol.* 2001;19:1688–1697.

9. Liljegren G, Holmberg L, Bergh J, et al. 10-year results after sector resection with or without postoperative radiotherapy for stage 1 breast cancer: a randomized trial. *J Clin Oncol.* 1999;17:2326–2333.

10. Clark RM, Whelan T, Levine M, et al. Randomized clinical trial of breast irradiation following lumpectomy and axillary dissection for node-negative breast cancer: an update. *J Natl Cancer Inst.* 1996;88:1659–1664.

11. Veronesi U, Marubini E, Mariani L, et al. Radiotherapy after breast-conserving surgery in small breast carcinoma: long-term results of a randomized trial. *Ann Oncol.* 2001;12:997–1003.

12. Forrest AP, Stewart HJ, Everington D, et al. Randomised controlled trial of conservation therapy for breast cancer: 6-year analysis of the Scottish trial. *Lancet.* 1996;348:708–713.

13. Holli K, Saaristo R, Isola J, et al. Lumpectomy with or without post-operative radiotherapy for breast cancer with favourable prognostic features: results of a randomized study. *Br J Cancer.* 2001;84:164–169.

14. Malström P, Holmberg L, Anderson H, et al. Breast conservation surgery, with and without radiotherapy, in women with lymph node-negative breast cancer: a randomized clinical trial in a population with access to public mammography screening. *Eur J Cancer.* 2003;39:1690–1697.

15. NIH consensus conference. Treatment of early-stage breast cancer. *JAMA.* 1991;265:391–395.

16. Morrow M, Strom EA, Bassett LW, et al. Standard for breast conservation therapy in the management of invasive breast carcinoma. *CA Cancer J Clin.* 2002;52:277–300.

17. Holland R, Veling SH, Mravunac M, et al. Histologic multifocality of Tis, T1-2 breast carcinomas. Implications for clinical trials of breast conserving surgery. *Cancer.* 1985;56:979–990.

18. Morris AD, Morris RD, Wilson JF, et al. Breast-conserving therapy vs mastectomy in early-stage breast cancer: a meta-analysis of 10-year survival. *Cancer J Sci Am.* 1997;3:6–12.

19. Schnitt SJ, Hayman J, Gelman R, et al. A prospective study of conservative surgery alone in the treatment of selected patients with stage I breast cancer. *Cancer.* 1996;77:1094–1100.

20. Fisher B, Bryant J, Dignam JJ, et al. Tamoxifen, radiation therapy, or both for prevention of ipsilateral breast tumor recurrence after lumpectomy in women with invasive breast cancers of one centimeter or less. *J Clin Oncol.* 2002;20:4141–4149.

21. Fyles A, McCready D, Manchul L, et al. Tamoxifen with or without breast irradiation in women 50 years of age or older with early breast cancer. *N Engl J Med.* 2004;351:1021–1023.

22. Hughes KS, Schnaper L, Berry D, et al. Lumpectomy plus tamoxifen with or without irradiation in women 70 years of age or older with early breast cancer. *N Engl J Med.* 2004;351:971–977.

23. Winzer KJ, Sauer R, Sauerbrei W, et al. Radiation therapy after breast-conserving surgery: First results of a randomized clinical trial in patients with low risk of recurrence. *Eur J Cancer.* 2004;40:998–1005.

24. Lichter AS, Fraass BA, Yanke B. Treatment techniques in the conservative management of breast cancer. *Semin Radiat Oncol.* 1992;2:94.

25. Das I, Cheng E, Freedman G, et al. Lung and heart dose volume analysis with CT simulator in radiation treatment of breast cancer. *Int J Radiat Oncol Biol Phys.* 1998;42:11.

26. Bartelink H, Horiot JC, Poortmans P, et al. Recurrence rates after treatment of breast cancer with standard radiotherapy with or without additional radiation. *N Engl J Med.* 2001;345:1378–1387.

27. Romestaing P, Lehingue Y, Carrie C, et al. Role of 10 Gy boost in the conservative treatment of early breast cancer: Results of a randomized clinical trial in Lyon, France. *J Clin Oncol.* 1997;15:963–968.

28. Teissier E, He'ry M, Ramaioli A, et al. Boost in conservative treatment: 6 years results of randomized trial [abstract 345]. *Breast Cancer Res Treat.* 1998;50:287.

29. Polgar C, Fodor J, Orosz Z, et al. Electron and high-dose-rate brachytherapy boost in the conservative treatment of stage I-II breast cancer. First results of the randomized Budapest boost trial. *Strahlenther Onkol.* 2002;178:615–623.

30. Vrieling C, Collette L, Fourquet A, et al. On behalf of the EORTC radiotherapy and breast cancer cooperative groups: the influence of the boost in breast-conserving therapy on cosmetic outcome in the EORTC "boost versus no boost" trial. *Int J Radiat Oncol Biol Phys.* 1999;45:677–685.

31. Whelan T, Mackenzie R, Julian J, et al. Randomized trial of breast irradiation schedules after lumpectomy with lymph node-negative breast cancer. *J Natl Cancer Inst.* 2002;94:1143–1150.

32. Yarnold J, Ashton A, Bliss J, et al. Fractionation sensitivity and dose response of late adverse effects in the breast after radiotherapy for early breast cancer: long-term results of a randomised trial. *Radiother Oncol.* 2005;75:9–17.

33. Owen JR, Ashton A, Bliss JM, et al. Effect of radiotherapy fraction size on tumour control in patients with early-stage breast cancer after local tumour excision: long-term results of a randomised trial. *Lancet Oncol.* 2006;7:467–471.

34. Harris JR. Notes on the Ontario trial in the context of breast-conserving therapy for early stage breast cancer. *J Clin Oncol.* 2000;18:43S–44S.

35. Sartor CI, Tepper JE. Is less more? Lessons in radiation schedules in breast cancer. *J Natl Cancer Inst.* 2002;94:1114–1115.

36. START Trialists' Group, Bentzen SM, Agrawal RK, et al. The UK Standardisation of Breast Radiotherapy (START) Trial A of radiotherapy hypofractionation for treatment of early breast cancer: a randomised trial. *Lancet Oncol.* 2008;9:331–341.

37. Kurtz JM, Miralbell R. Radiation therapy and breast conservation: cosmetic results and complications. *Semin Radiat Oncol.* 1992;2:125–131.

38. Mansel RE, Fallowfield L, Kissin M, et al. Randomized multicenter trial of sentinel node biopsy versus standard axillary treatment in operable breast cancer: the ALMANAC Trial. *J Natl Cancer Inst.* 2006;98:599–609.

39. Meek AG. Breast radiotherapy and lymphedema. *Cancer.* 1998;83(12 Suppl Am): 2788–2797.

40. Larson D, Weinstein M, Goldberg I, et al. Edema of the arm as a function of the extent of axillary surgery in patients with stage I-II carcinoma of the breast treated with primary radiotherapy. *Int J Radiat Oncol Biol Phys.* 1986;12:1575–1582.

41. Lingos T, Recht A, Vicini F, et al. Radiation pneumonitis in breast cancer patients treated with conservative surgery and radiation therapy. *Int J Radiat Oncol Biol Phys.* 1991;21:335.

42. Lind P, Marks L, Hardenbergh P, et al. Technical factors associated with radiation pneumonitis after local + regional radiation for breast cancer. *Int J Radiat Oncol Biol Phys.* 2002:52:137.

43. Overgaard M. Spontaneous radiation-induced rib fractures in breast cancer patients with postmastectomy radiation. A clinical radiobiological analysis of the influence of fraction size and dose-response relationships on late bone damage. *Acta Oncol.* 1988:27: 117.

44. Pierce S, Recht A, Lingos T, et al. Long-term radiation complications following conservative surgery (CS) and radiation therapy (RT) in patients with early stage breast cancer. *Int J Radiat Oncol Biol Phys.* 1992;23:915.

45. Olsen N, Pfeiffer P, Johanssen L, et al. Radiation-induced brachial plexopathy: Neurological follow-up on 161 recurrence-free breast cancer patients. *Int J Radiat Oncol Biol Phys.* 1993:26:43.

46. Powell S, Cooke J, Parsons C. Radiation-induced brachial plexus injury: follow-up of two different fractionation schedules. *Radiother Oncol.* 1990;18:213–220.

47. Paszat LF, Mackillop WJ, Groome PA, et al. Mortality from myocardial infarction after adjuvant radiotherapy for breast cancer in the surveillance, epidemiology, and end-results cancer registries. *J Clin Oncol.* 1998;16:2625–2631.

48. Rutqvist LE, Johansson H. Mortality by laterality of the primary tumour among 55,000 breast cancer patients from the Swedish Cancer Registry. *Br J Cancer.* 1990;61:866–868.

49. Darby SC, McGale P, Taylor CW, et al. Long-term mortality from heart disease and lung cancer after radiotherapy for early breast cancer: prospective cohort study of about 300,000 women in US SEER cancer registries. *Lancet Oncol.* 2005;6:557–565.

50. Giordano SH, Kuo YF, Freeman JL, et al. Risk of cardiac death after adjuvant radiotherapy for breast cancer. *J Natl Cancer Inst.* 2005;97:419–424.

51. Harris EE, Correa C, Hwang WT, et al. Late cardiac mortality and morbidity in early-stage breast cancer patients after breast-conservation treatment. *J Clin Oncol.* 2006;24:4100–4106.

52. Taghian A, de Vathaire F, Terrier P, et al. Long-term risk of sarcoma following radiation treatment for breast cancer. *Int J Radiat Oncol Biol Phys.* 1991;21:361–367.

53. Inskip PD, Stovall M, Flannery JT. Lung cancer risk and radiation dose among women treated for breast cancer. *J Natl Cancer Inst.* 1994;86:983–988.

54. Faverly D, Burgers L, Bult P, et al. Three dimensional imaging of mammary ductal carcinoma in situ: clinical implications. *Semin Diagn Pathol.* 1994;11:193–198.

55. Imamura H, Haga S, Shimizu T, et al. Relationship between the morphological and biological characteristics of intraductal components accompanying invasive ductal breast carcinoma and patient age. *Breast Cancer Res Treat.* 2000;62:177–184.

56. Ohtake T, Abe R, Kimijima I, et al. Intraductal extension of primary invasive breast carcinoma treated by breast-conservative surgery. *Cancer.* 1995;76:32–45.

57. Pawlik TM, Buchholz TA, Kuerer HM. The biologic rationale for and emerging role of accelerated partial breast irradiation for breast cancer. *J Am Coll Surg.* 2004;199:479–492.

58. Athas WF, Adams-Cameron M, Hunt WC, et al. Travel distance to radiation therapy and receipt of radiotherapy following breast-conserving surgery. *J Natl Cancer Inst.* 2000;92:269–271.

59. Du X, Freeman JL, Freeman DH, et al. Temporal and regional variation in the use of breast-conserving surgery and radiotherapy for older women with early-stage breast cancer from 1983 to 1985. *J Gerontol A Biol Sci Med Sci.* 1999;54:M474–M478.

60. Hahn CA, Marks LB, Chen DY, et al. Breast conservation rates-barriers between tertiary care and community practice. *Int J Radiat Oncol Biol Phys.* 2003;55:1196–1199.

61. Nattinger AB, Hoffmann RG, Kneusel RT, et al. Relation between appropriateness of primary therapy for early-stage breast carcinoma and increased use of breast-conserving surgery. *Lancet.* 2000;356:1148–1153.

62. American Society of Breast Surgeons. Revised consensus statement for accelerated partial breast irradiation. December 8, 2005. http://www.breastsurgeons.org.

63. A Randomized Phase III Study of Conventional Whole Breast Irradiation (WBI) Versus Partial Breast Irradiation (PBI) for Women with Stage 0, I, or II Breast Cancer (NSABP B-39/RTOG 0413). http://www.nsabp.pitt.edu.

64. Arthur DW, Winter K, Kuske RR, et al. A phase II trial of brachytherapy alone after lumpectomy for select breast cancer: tumor control and survival outcomes of RTOG 95-17. *Int J Radiat Oncol Biol Phys.* 2008;72:467–473.

65. Vicini FA, Kestin L, Chen P, et al. Limited-field radiation therapy in the management of early-stage breast cancer. *J Natl Cancer Inst.* 2003;95:1205–1210.

66. Chen PY, Vicini FA, Benitez P, et al. Long-term cosmetic results and toxicity after accelerated partial-breast irradiation: a method of radiation delivery by interstitial brachytherapy for the treatment of early-stage breast carcinoma. *Cancer.* 2006;106:991–999.

67. King TA, Bolton JS, Kuske RR, et al. Long-term results of wide-field brachytherapy as the sole method of radiation therapy after segmental mastectomy for T(is, 1,2) breast cancer. *Am J Surg.* 2000;180:299–304.

68. Arthur D, Koo D, Zwicker RD. Partial breast brachytherapy following lumpectomy: a low dose rate and high dose rate experience. *Int J Radiat Oncol Biol Phys.* 2003;56:681–689.

69. Kuske R, Winter K, Arthur D, et al. Phase II trial of brachytherapy alone following lumpectomy for select breast cancer: toxicity analysis of RTOG 95-17. *Int J Radiat Oncol Biol Phys.* 2006;65:45–51.

70. Krishnan L, Jewell WR, Tawfik OW, et al. Breast conservation therapy with tumor bed irradiation alone in a selected group of patients with stage 1 breast cancer. *Breast J.* 2001;7:91–96.

71. Cionini L, Pacini P, Marzano S. Exclusive brachytherapy after conservative surgery in cancer of the breast. *Lyon Chir.* 1993;89:128.

72. Lawenda BD, Taghian AG, Kachnic LA, et al. Dose-volume analysis of radiotherapy for T1N0 invasive breast cancer treated by local excision and partial breast irradiation by low-dose-rate interstitial implant. *Int J Radiat Oncol Biol Phys.* 2003;56:671–680.

73. Wazer DE, Berle L, Graham R, et al. Preliminary results of a phase I/II study of HDR brachytherapy alone for T1/T2 breast cancer. *Int J Radiat Oncol Biol Phys.* 2002;53:889–897.

74. Soran A, Evrensel T, Beriwal S, et al. Placement technique and the early complications of balloon breast brachytherapy: Magee-Womens Hospital Experience. *Am J Clin Oncol.* 2007;30:152–155.

75. Benitez PR, Keisch ME, Vicini F, et al. Five-year results: the initial clinical trial of MammoSite balloon brachytherapy for partial breast irradiation in early-stage breast cancer. *Am J Surg.* 2007;194:456–462.

76. Zannis V, Beitsch P, Vicini F, et al. Descriptions and outcomes of insertion techniques of a breast brachytherapy balloon catheter in 1403 patients enrolled in the American Society of Breast Surgeons MammoSite breast brachytherapy registry trial. *Am J Surg.* 2005;190:530–538.

77. Vicini F, Beitsch PD, Quiet CA, et al. Three-year analysis of treatment efficacy, cosmesis, and toxicity by the American Society of Breast Surgeons MammoSite Breast Brachytherapy Registry Trial in patients treated with accelerated partial breast irradiation (APBI). *Cancer.* 2008;112:66.

78. Vicini FA, Chen P, Wallace M, et al. Interim cosmetic results and toxicity using 3D conformal external beam radiotherapy to deliver accelerated partial breast irradiation in patients with early-stage breast cancer treated with breast-conserving therapy. *Int J Radiat Oncol Biol Phys.* 2007;69:1124–1130.

79. Formenti SC, Truong MT, Goldberg JD, et al. Prone accelerated partial breast irradiation after breast-conserving surgery: preliminary clinical results and dose-volume histogram analysis. *Int J Radiat Oncol Biol Phys.* 2004;60:493–504.

80. Vicini FA, Pass H, Wong J. A phase I/II trial to evaluate three dimensional conformal radiation therapy (3D-CRT) confined to the region of the lumpectomy cavity for stage I and II breast carcinoma. Philadelphia, PA: Radiation Therapy Oncology Group; protocol #0319, 2003.

81. Veronesi U, Gatti G, Luini A, et al. Full-dose intraoperative radiotherapy with electrons during breast-conserving surgery. *Arch Surg.* 2003;138:1253–1256.

82. Vaidya JS, Tobias JS, Baum M, et al. Intraoperative radiotherapy for breast cancer. *Lancet Oncol.* 2004;5:165–173.

83. Veronesi U, Orecchia R, Luini A, et al. Full-dose intraoperative radiotherapy with electrons during breast-conserving surgery: experience with 590 cases. Ann Surg. 2005;242:101–106.

84. Orecchia R, Luini A, Veronesi P, et al. Electron intraoperative treatment in patients with early-stage breast cancer: data up date. *Expert Rev Anticancer Ther.* 2006;6:605–611.

85. Beal K, McCormick B, Zelefsky P, et al. Single-fraction intraoperative radiotherapy for breast cancer: early cosmetic results. *Int J Radiat Oncol Biol Phys.* 2007;69:19–24.

86. Holmes DR, Baum M, Joseph D. The TARGIT trial: targeted intraoperative radiation therapy versus conventional postoperative whole-breast radiotherapy after breast-conserving surgery for the management of early-stage invasive breast cancer (a trial update). *Am J Surg.* 2007;194:507–510.

87. Stitzenberg KB, Klauber-Demore N, Chang XS, et al. In vivo intraoperative radiotherapy: a novel approach to radiotherapy for early stage breast cancer. *Ann Surg Oncol.* 2007;14:1515–1516.

88. Ollila DW, Klauber-DeMore N, Tesche LJ, et al. Feasibility of breast preserving therapy with single fraction in situ radiotherapy delivered intraoperatively. *Ann Surg Oncol.* 2007;14:660–669.

COMMENTARY
Gregory M. Chronowski and Thomas A. Buchholz

Drs. Anne and Curran provide a comprehensive and concise review of radiation therapy in breast-conserving therapy for invasive breast cancer. Their chapter provides an excellent description of the central role of radiotherapy in breast-conserving therapy for invasive carcinoma. In this commentary, we have chosen to expand on some of the themes discussed by the authors, particularly the various controversies regarding accelerated partial breast irradiation.

This is an exciting time for physicians involved in the research and care of patients with invasive breast cancer. Improvements in the surgical staging of patients with invasive breast cancer through the use of sentinel node evaluation have reduced the incidence of axillary toxicity. Improvements in systemic therapy through the use of taxanes, dose-dense scheduling, hormonal modulators, and targeted agents, such a trastuzumab, have provided important incremental benefits in outcome for breast cancer patients. Finally, advances in radiotherapy technique and fractionation scheduling have allowed for radiation to be administered with less toxicity through the use of conformal techniques that avoid the myocardium and lung, and in selected cases, with greater convenience by employing altered fractionation schedules that treat patients over a shorter period of time. Through the rational integration of all these modalities, further advances will be made in the treatment of invasive breast cancer over the next decade.

RADIOTHERAPY IMPROVES SURVIVAL IN EARLY-STAGE BREAST CANCER

The central role of radiotherapy in reducing the incidence of local recurrence has been well described by Drs. Anne and Curran (1–5). The authors correctly state that extensive analyses have never been able to document a subgroup of patients with invasive breast carcinoma who do not benefit from breast irradiation, although its benefit in older women treated with tamoxifen is small (6). For many years, the lack of a proven survival benefit associated with breast irradiation led some physicians to simply view breast irradiation as a means of reducing the subsequent need for salvage mastectomy after breast-conserving surgery. However, with the publication of the Early Breast Cancer Trialists' Collaborative Group (EBCTCG) meta-analysis on the effects of radiotherapy for early breast cancer (7) this paradigm has come into question. This large, rigorous analysis of 42,000 women treated in 11 randomized trials showed that for every four local recurrences avoided, one breast cancer death would be avoided at 15 years. From a teleologic standpoint, these data suggest that local recurrence of breast cancer is not a benign phenomenon, and that in addition to the cosmetic consequences of additional salvage surgery, local tumor recurrence can ultimately result in breast cancer mortality.

IRRADIATION OF THE HIGH AXILLA AND SUPRACLAVICULAR FOSSA

Although the benefit of radiotherapy in early breast cancer is clear, there is some controversy as to what the appropriate irradiated volume should be. Classically, radiation has been delivered to the breast alone in patients with small primary tumors and zero to three positive lymph nodes on axillary dissection. In patients with four or more positive lymph nodes, a "third field" to treat level III of the axilla and the supraclavicular fossa is commonly employed. Patients with advanced disease who undergo mastectomy routinely have the chest wall and level III of the axilla and supraclavicular fossa irradiated. In addition, in the randomized trials conducted by Ragaz et al. (8) and Overgaard et al. (9), both of which documented a survival benefit associated with postmastectomy irradiation, this region was included within the radiation treatment volume. It is important to note that these two trials included patients with one to three positive axillary nodes, although the adequacy of the axillary dissections has been criticized because of the low number of lymph nodes removed at surgery (approximately eight). Nevertheless, these trials have led some to question whether patients treated with breast-conserving surgery who have one to three positive axillary lymph nodes also might benefit from level III/supraclavicular fossa irradiation in addition to the fields used to treat the breast. This issue is being addressed in the MA20 trial (10) open in Canada, the United States, and Australia in which patients treated with breast-conserving surgery and axillary dissection with zero, one to three, and more than three positive lymph nodes are randomized to breast radiotherapy alone or breast and regional nodal irradiation, including both the level III axillary nodes and ipsilateral internal mammary lymph nodes.

ACCELERATED PARTIAL BREAST IRRADIATION

Although whole-breast radiotherapy remains the standard of care for patients with early breast cancer, whole-breast external-beam radiotherapy is associated with some disadvantages. Although the risk of complications is low and long-term cosmetic outcomes are excellent after external-beam radiotherapy, this approach to treatment can be inconvenient, as it requires patients to come for daily therapy for 5 to 6 weeks. Moreover, this inconvenience may decrease the probability for some patients to be treated with breast conservation (11). One method to shorten overall treatment time by giving larger daily doses of radiation, while at the same time achieving acceptable cosmetic outcomes and maintaining adequate local control of the primary tumor, is to decrease the volume of normal tissue within the irradiated volume. This has led to the development of accelerated partial breast irradiation (APBI) regimens. These strategies deliver radiation to the resection cavity of the breast, plus an additional margin (commonly 1 to 2 cm) of adjacent breast tissue over approximately 1 week. However, this strategy is based on the assumption that microscopic tumor does not extend far beyond the initial resection cavity. Whether this is, indeed, the case is the fundamental question regarding the suitability of APBI approaches to breast cancer. Unfortunately, the clinical and pathologic data that might provide an answer to this question are somewhat conflicting.

Drs. Anne and Curran cite the important work by Holland et al. (12) showing that microscopic disease can extend as far as 4 cm beyond the lumpectomy cavity. These data suggest that residual tumor within the breast might be missed if only 2 cm of tissue adjacent to the tumor bed were irradiated, as is done commonly with many APBI approaches. This finding suggests that a radiation approach that treats larger volumes of breast tissue, such as whole-breast irradiation, may be optimal. However, this conclusion is weakened by the fact that in the 1980s, when the report by Holland et al. (12) was published, surgical margins were not routinely analyzed after the simulated "lumpectomies" performed prior to mastectomy in their series. Had margin assessment in this series conformed to the standard of care today, it is probable that many patients in this series would not have been deemed to have an adequate lumpectomy by the presence of positive margins. These patients would, at a minimum, have required additional breast-conserving surgery, or possibly mastectomy, to achieve local tumor clearance, thus weakening the relevance of this study's findings with respect to modern APBI treatments. In addition, most of the patients in this series did not have their disease detected by mammographic screening, perhaps resulting in subtle upward stage migration compared with modern mammographically detected series. Data reported by Vaidya et al. (13) also raise theoretical concerns about the potential efficacy of APBI. These investigators analyzed mastectomy specimens and found that tumor cells were located >2 cm from the resection cavity in 47% of patients, suggesting that these cells would have been left behind if the tumor had hypothetically been resected with a 2-cm margin.

In contrast to these studies by Holland et al. (12) and Vaidya et al. (13), there are other data to suggest that tumor cells do not extend >2 cm from the lumpectomy bed. The strongest information supporting the use of APBI and the concept of irradiating only the tissue immediately surrounding the lumpectomy bed comes primarily from the numerous randomized trials of breast-conservation therapy (1–5). Among the patients randomized to undergo surgery without postoperative radiation, and who had a subsequent breast recurrence, >80% developed their recurrence within the quadrant of the breast that had harbored the initial primary tumor. It is believed that the approximately 20% of failures that occurred outside the index quadrant of the breast represented new primary tumors that would not have been prevented by whole-breast radiotherapy. Imamura et al. (14), who evaluated 253 patients with invasive breast cancer treated with either breast-conserving surgery or mastectomy, found that the mean distance of microscopic intraductal spread of tumor away from the primary tumor mass ranged from 0.25 to 1.7 cm, with greater distances of spread occurring in younger patients compared with older patients. Ohtake et al. (15), who examined 20 quadrantectomy specimens from patients with primary invasive breast cancer, likewise found that the intraductal extension of tumor away from the primary tumor mass ranged from 0.77 to 2.27 cm, with longer distances predominating in patients with comedo necrosis, microcalcifications, and marked intraductal component of primary tumor.

Ultimately, the results of RTOG 0413/NSABP B39 phase III trial (16) comparing accelerated partial-breast irradiation with whole-breast radiotherapy will provide much needed level I data that can show definitively whether local control with APBI is equivalent to that of whole-breast radiotherapy.

With the development of specialized radiotherapy delivery systems that can be placed in the operating room, intraoperative radiotherapy (IORT) has become another option for the administration of APBI, typically in a single, large fraction. A number of systems are commercially available. The Intrabeam system (Carl Zeiss Surgical GmbH, Oberkochen, Germany) uses a miniature electron beam-driven x-ray source (50 kV maximum) and is being compared in a phase III trial with whole-breast radiotherapy in the United Kingdom, Europe, the United States, and Australia. The Novac-7 system (Hitesys Inc., Latina, Italy) uses a mobile 3- to 7-MeV linear accelerator and is being evaluated in a phase III trial by the European Institute of Oncology in Milan. The results observed in a series of patients recently reported by Veronesi et al. (17) have been discussed by Drs. Anne and Curran.

The primary advantage of IORT is that all radiotherapy is administered immediately after lumpectomy, eliminating the need for subsequent outpatient therapy and maximizing patient convenience. A significant disadvantage is that all adjuvant radiotherapy is delivered before final pathologic results are available. In particular, information from the complete assessment of microscopic margins and the axillary nodal status are not routinely available prior to the administration of radiotherapy; thus, patient selection for APBI is made only on the basis of information from an intraoperative frozen section or touch preparation.

Although IORT represents the ultimate in patient convenience, the incomplete pathologic assessment prior to therapy

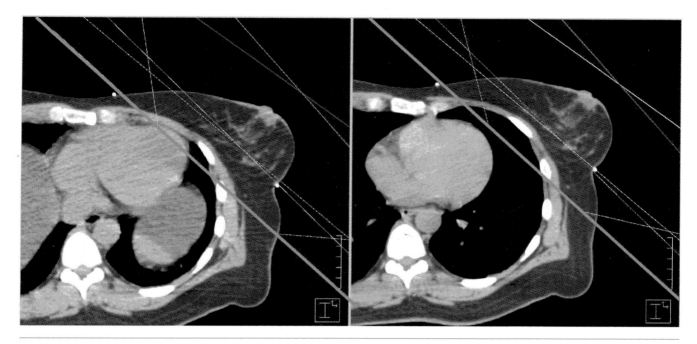

Figure 19C.1 Modern computed tomography-based treatment planning of breast cancer radiotherapy allows for sparing of the heart from the radiotherapy fields. The red line represents the posterior edge of the radiotherapy ports. The image on the left does not have the geometry of the portals optimized to spare the heart, while the image on the right has been optimized to spare the heart. (See color plates.)

has raised some concerns regarding its merits compared with other APBI approaches. The results regarding its effectiveness from large phase III trials should be available within the next few years and will better define the role of this technology in the treatment of early-stage breast cancer.

TOXICITY OF WHOLE-BREAST IRRADIATION AND ADVANCES TO MINIMIZE IT

Until the mid 1990s, most patients with breast cancer were treated using two-dimensional techniques that often exposed a portion of the myocardium to radiation in patients receiving radiotherapy for left-sided breast tumors An analysis of over 20,000 women in the United Kingdom treated with radiotherapy for breast cancer showed a 25% increase in cardiovascular mortality at 15 years in patients treated for cancer of the left breast compared with those treated for right-sided lesions (18). A study from the University of Pennsylvania (19) suggested that treatment of the left breast with radiotherapy resulted in higher rates of myocardial infarction and coronary artery disease compared with patients treated to the right breast. However, a study from Canada (20) showed no difference in cardiac morbidity or mortality between patients treated to the left or right breast compared with the general population. Two studies from our institution, MD Anderson Cancer Center (21,22) have analyzed data from the Surveillance, Epidemiology, and End Results (SEER) database, and showed an increase in mortality from ischemic heart disease in patients treated to the left breast before 1980, with a steady decrease in cardiac mortality over time, with no

difference detected in patients treated after 1980, suggesting that improvements in radiotherapy techniques have reduced, and perhaps eliminated, the risk of cardiac morbidity and mortality for patients with left-sided breast cancers.

Radiation pneumonitis is a rare complication of breast radiotherapy (23,24). However, isolated reports have suggested that its incidence is increased in patients receiving tamoxifen (25). Modern three-dimensional techniques now allow radiotherapy to be delivered to the breast while minimally irradiating the lung and avoiding the myocardium entirely (Figure 19C.1). Although long-term outcomes using these newer three-dimensional techniques are lacking, radiobiologic mathematical models suggest that these techniques have the potential to decrease the incidence of major long-term cardiac complications (26).

CONCLUSIONS

Drs. Anne and Curran have provided an excellent overview of the role of radiotherapy in invasive breast cancer treated with breast-conserving therapy We have attempted to broaden the discussion on some of the controversies regarding this complex subject, In particular, we have emphasized the important role that the optimization of local control has on outcomes in patients with early breast cancer. Accelerated partial breast irradiation has the potential to expand the use of radiotherapy in appropriate patients by maximizing patient convenience; however, caution should be exercised in adopting this relatively new modality until the results of mature phase III trials are available. Radiation oncologists continue to refine the techniques used to administer radiotherapy to the breast and draining lymphatics, both to improve local control and to reduce toxicity. It is an exciting time to be a radiation oncologist who treats patients with breast cancer, as there are many new tools under investigation in our armamentarium that hopefully will further contribute to the incremental advances in the management of breast cancer that have been made over the past decade.

REFERENCES

1. Clark RM, Whelan T, Levine M, et al. Randomized clinical trial of breast irradiation following lumpectomy and axillary dissection for node-negative breast cancer: an update. Ontario Clinical Oncology Group. *J Natl Cancer Inst.* 1996;88:1659–1664.

2. Fisher B, Anderson S, Bryant J, et al. Twenty-year follow-up of a randomized trial comparing total mastectomy, lumpectomy, and lumpectomy plus irradiation for the treatment of invasive breast cancer. *N Engl J Med.* 2002;347:1233–1241.

3. Liljegren G, Holmberg L, Bergh J, et al. 10-Year results after sector resection with or without postoperative radiotherapy for stage I breast cancer: a randomized trial. *J Clin Oncol.* 1999;17:2326–2333.

4. Uppsala-Oreboro Breast Cancer Study Group. Sector resection with or without postoperative radiotherapy for stage I breast cancer: a randomized trial. Uppsala-Orebro Breast Cancer Study Group. *J Natl Cancer Inst.* 1990;82:277–282.

5. Veronesi U, Marubini E, Mariani L, et al. Radiotherapy after breast-conserving surgery in small breast carcinoma: long-term results of a randomized trial. *Ann Oncol.* 2001;12:997–1003.

6. Winzer KJ, Sauer R, Sauerbrei W, et al. Radiation therapy after breast-conserving surgery; first results of a randomised clinical trial in patients with low risk of recurrence. *Eur J Cancer.* 2004;40:998–1005.

7. Clarke M, Collins R, Darby S, et al. Effects of radiotherapy and of differences in the extent of surgery for early breast cancer on local recurrence and 15-year survival: an overview of the randomised trials. *Lancet.* 2005;366:2087–2106.

8. Ragaz J, Jackson SM, Le N, et al. Adjuvant radiotherapy and chemotherapy in node-positive premenopausal women with breast cancer. *N Engl J Med.* 1997;337:956–962.

9. Overgaard M, Jensen MB, Overgaard J, et al. Postoperative radiotherapy in high-risk postmenopausal breast-cancer patients given adjuvant tamoxifen: Danish Breast Cancer Cooperative Group DBCG 82c randomised trial. *Lancet.* 1999;353:1641–1648.

10. Olivotto IA, Chua B, Elliott EA, et al. A clinical trial of breast radiation therapy versus breast plus regional radiation therapy in early-stage breast cancer: the MA20 trial. *Clin Breast Cancer.* 2003;4:361–363.

11. Athas WF, Adams-Cameron M, Hunt WC, et al. Travel distance to radiation therapy and receipt of radiotherapy following breast-conserving surgery. *J Natl Cancer Inst.* 2000;92:269–271.

12. Holland R, Veling SH, Mravunac M, et al. Histologic multifocality of Tis, T1-2 breast carcinomas. Implications for clinical trials of breast-conserving surgery. *Cancer.* 1985;56:979–990.

13. Vaidya JS, Vyas JJ, Chinoy RF, et al. Multicentricity of breast cancer: whole-organ analysis and clinical implications. *Br J Cancer.* 1996;74:820–824.

14. Imamura H, Haga S, Shimizu T, et al. Relationship between the morphological and biological characteristics of intraductal components accompanying invasive ductal breast carcinoma and patient age. *Breast Cancer Res Treat.* 2000;62:177–184.

15. Ohtake T, Abe R, Kimijima I, et al. Intraductal extension of primary invasive breast carcinoma treated by breast-conservative surgery. Computer graphic three-dimensional reconstruction of the mammary duct-lobular systems. *Cancer.* 1995;76:32–45.

16. A Randomized Phase III Study of Conventional Whole Breast Irradiation (WBI) Versus Partial Breast Irradiation (PBI) for Women with Stage 0, I, or II Breast Cancer (NSABP B-39/RTOG 0413). http://www.nsabp.pitt.edu. Accessed August 17, 2005.

17. Veronesi U, Orecchia R, Luini A, et al. Full-dose intraoperative radiotherapy with electrons during breast-conserving surgery: experience with 590 cases. *Ann Surg.* 2005;242:101–106.

18. Roychoudhuri R, Robinson D, Putcha V, et al. Increased cardiovascular mortality more than fifteen years after radiotherapy for breast cancer: a population-based study. *BMC Cancer.* 2007;7:9.

19. Harris EE, Correa C, Hwang WT, et al. Late cardiac mortality and morbidity in early-stage breast cancer patients after breast-conservation treatment. *J Clin Oncol.* 2006;24:4100–4106.

20. Vallis KA, Pintilie M, Chong N, et al. Assessment of coronary heart disease morbidity and mortality after radiation therapy for early breast cancer. *J Clin Oncol.* 2002;20:1036–1042.

21. Patt DA, Goodwin JS, Kuo YF, et al. Cardiac morbidity of adjuvant radiotherapy for breast cancer. *J Clin Oncol.* 2005;23:7475–7482.

22. Giordano SH, Kuo YF, Freeman JL, et al. Risk of cardiac death after adjuvant radiotherapy for breast cancer. *J Natl Cancer Inst.* 2005;97:419–424.

23. Meric F, Buchholz TA, Mirza NQ, et al. Long-term complications associated with breast-conservation surgery and radiotherapy. *Ann Surg Oncol.* 2002;9:543–549.

24. Lind PA, Marks LB, Hardenbergh PH, et al. Technical factors associated with radiation pneumonitis after local +/− regional radiation therapy for breast cancer. *Int J Radiat Oncol Biol Phys.* 2002;52:137–143.

25. Bentzen SM, Skoczylas JZ, Overgaard M, et al. Radiotherapy-related lung fibrosis enhanced by tamoxifen. *J Natl Cancer Inst.* 1996;88:918–922.

26. Louwe RJ, Wendling M, van Herk MB, et al. Three-dimensional heart dose reconstruction to estimate normal tissue complication probability after breast irradiation using portal dosimetry. *Med Phys.* 2007;34:1354–1363.

20

Adjuvant Therapy in Breast Cancer

Antony J. Charles, Vivek Roy, and Edith A. Perez

Breast cancer is the most common female cancer in the United States and is the second most common cause for cancer death after lung cancer. An estimated 182,460 new cases of invasive breast cancer are expected to occur among women and 1,990 new cases among men in the United States in 2007. An estimated 40,930 women will die from breast cancer in 2008 (1). The incidence of breast cancer increases with age, with the greatest risk being in women older than 40 years (2). The lifetime risk of developing invasive breast cancer is 1 in 8 for women in the United States (1). The 5-year survival rate for women diagnosed with invasive breast cancer in the United States is 88%, with 52% of women surviving 20 years (3).

Physicians generally offer chemotherapy if the absolute reduction in the risk of recurrence is ≥3% at 5 years (4). Individual women make very different treatment decisions given a similar scenario (5). Research has shown that women with breast cancer overestimate the value of adjuvant therapy and often will accept remarkably low degrees of net benefit (6).

THEORETICAL RATIONALE

Adjuvant therapy refers to the use of systemic therapy with curative intent, employing hormonal, chemotherapeutic, or biological agents, such as trastuzumab, following surgical resection of locoregional disease. Most breast cancers are diagnosed when they are clinically localized and are potentially curable. However, a significant proportion of tumors relapse, and distant relapses (metastases) are considered incurable. The reason for relapse is thought to be the presence of micrometastatic disease that later leads to distant treatment failures. The underlying rationale for adjuvant therapy is that because it appears that cancer cells acquire additional genetic abnormalities and resistance to therapy with advancing disease burden, chemotherapy given early in the postoperative period may be able to eradicate occult, micrometastatic disease before clinically evident metastases develop. The use of adjuvant systemic therapy is thought to be at least partly responsible for the decline in breast cancer-specific mortality (7). According to the widely held "genetic selection" model of metastasis, a small subpopulation of cells within the primary tumor acquires advantageous genetic alterations over time, which allows the cells within this subpopulation to metastasize and form new solid tumors at distant sites. However, the results of gene expression profiling of human breast carcinomas have challenged this model. DNA microarray studies show that primary breast tumors that develop metastases can be distinguished by their gene expression profiling from tumors that remain localized. These data imply that the metastatic capacity of poor prognosis tumors might be acquired by mutations at a much earlier stage of tumorigenesis than previously assumed.

ABSOLUTE VERSUS RELATIVE RISK REDUCTION

It is important to distinguish between absolute and relative risk reduction in the estimate of recurrence or death from cancer.

Figure 20.1 depicts two different treatments offered to two different populations. The first treatment, administered to population A with a 60% risk of dying, reduces the risk to 40%. The second treatment, administered to population B with a 3% risk of dying, reduces the risk to 2%. Both treatments reduce the risk by one-third. In population A, the absolute risk reduction is 20% and relative risk reduction is 33%. In population B, the relative risk reduction is also 33%, but absolute risk reduction is only 1%. If the risk of severe adverse events with chemotherapy is 10%, one would be willing to recommend chemotherapy in population A but not in population B. The same results when presented in different ways may lead to different treatment decisions. It has been shown that clinicians are less inclined to treat patients when results are presented as absolute risk reduction rather than relative risk reduction (8). Patients react similarly in that they tend to choose a treatment described in terms of relative risk reduction than absolute risk reduction (9). When risk reduction is not specified (for instance "Drug Z is 40% effective in reducing the risk of death"), "effectiveness" almost invariably refers to relative risk reduction.

RISK ASSESSMENT

Prognostic factors help to understand the natural course of disease, help to stratify the risk of recurrence, and help to assess the potential benefit of adjuvant therapy. Traditional prognostic factors in breast cancer are involvement of axillary lymph nodes, size of the primary tumor, histologic grade, estrogen and progesterone receptor expression, *HER2* status, and lymphovascular invasion. Knowledge of these prognostic factors is invaluable in estimating the efficacy of a particular treatment regimen in a given patient.

Tumor Size

Tumor size independently correlates with risk of relapse, irrespective of nodal status (10,11) (Table 20.1). The risk of relapse increases as the size of the tumor increases. Based on Surveillance Epidemiology and End Results (SEER) data from the National

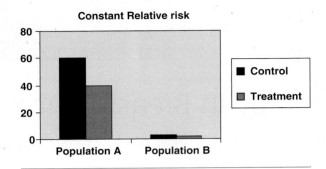

Figure 20.1 Absolute versus relative risk reduction. See text for details.

Cancer Institute, the 5-year survival rate of node-negative patients with tumors <1 cm was 100% compared with 81% in tumors >5 cm (10,11). In node-positive patients, the 5-year survival for patients with tumors <1 cm was 92.6% compared with 62.9% with tumors >5 cm.

Nodal Status

The number of positive axillary lymph nodes strongly predicts survival and relapse risk of breast cancer. The American Joint Committee on Cancer staging system for breast cancer reflects the importance of lymph nodes. The pathologic staging schema classifies pN1 disease as one to three positive lymph nodes, pN2 as four to nine positive lymph nodes, and pN3 as ten or more positive lymph nodes. Nodal status is an independent prognostic factor irrespective of tumor size (11). Even in patients with tumor size <0.5 cm, the 5-year breast cancer-specific mortality rate is 41% in patients with more than three positive lymph nodes, compared to 0.8% with no positive lymph nodes (Table 20.1) (11). There is a 4% annual relative risk of recurrence with

Table 20.1

5-Year Breast Cancer-Specific Mortality Rate (%) Based on Nodal Status and Tumor Size[a]

Tumor Size (cm)	Positive Nodes		
	0	1 to 3	>3
<0.5	0.8	4.7	41.0
0.5–0.9	1.7	6.0	45.8
1.0–1.9	4.2	13.4	32.8
2.0–2.9	7.7	16.6	36.6
3.0–3.9	13.8	21	43.1
4.0–4.9	15.4	30.2	47.4
>5.0	17.8	27.0	54.5

[a] Surveillance Epidemiology and End Results data derived from Margolese RG, Hortabagyi GN, Bucholz TA. Neoplasms of the breast. In: Kufe DW, Pollock RE, Weichselbaum RR, et al. *Cancer Medicine*, 6th ed., Hamilton, Ontario, Canada: American Cancer Society and BC Decker. 2003; 1892. This table was published in *NCCN Task Force Report 2006, Adjuvant Therapy for Breast Cancer*, Carlson RW, Brown E, Burstein HW et al., JNCCN 2006; Mar 4(Suppl I): S1–S26.

positive nodes, and the survival curves never flatten even after 20 years of follow-up.

Tumor Histology and Grade

The common breast cancers are of ductal, lobular, mixed, and medullary histologies. The "favorable" breast cancers are rare and include tubular, mucinous, cribriform, papillary, adenoid cystic, and colloid histologies. Tubular carcinomas rarely spread to axillary lymph nodes, and abundant mucin, rather than malignant cells, contribute to the size of mucinous carcinomas. Higher histologic grade is associated with a higher risk for relapse.

Lymphovascular invasion is a risk factor for local recurrence and breast cancer death, irrespective of nodal status. Even in patients with tumors <1 cm and that are node-negative, lymphovascular invasion by itself can be considered an indication for adjuvant therapy.

Hormone Receptor Status

The steroid hormone receptors, estrogen receptor (ER) and progesterone receptor (PR), are important prognostic and predictive factors. Endocrine therapies are beneficial in patients with positive hormone receptor status and less useful in patients with negative hormone receptors. Although the ER results are given as positive or negative, the ER concentration is actually a continuous variable. Endocrine responsiveness is directly proportional to the amount of receptor protein (12). Also the short-term benefit of chemotherapy may be smaller in patients with positive hormone receptors (13). Berry et al. (14) reported that absolute benefits from chemotherapy are greater in ER-negative tumors compared with ER-positive tumors: 22.8% more ER-negative patients survived to 5 years disease-free receiving chemotherapy versus 7.0% for ER-positive patients; corresponding improvements for overall survival (OS) were 16.7% versus 4.0%.

HER2 Status

Human epidermal growth factor 2 (HER2) overexpression is a newer and important predictive and prognostic factor. Overexpression of *HER2* is a poor prognostic factor.

HER2 positivity is an indication for treatment with trastuzumab, a humanized, anti-*HER2* monoclonal antibody that has produced remarkable benefits in this subgroup of patients.

GENE EXPRESSION ANALYSIS

Identifying gene expression patterns that correlate with prognosis and metastatic risk and determine the need for adjuvant therapy is an exciting new development. The two types of assays that are commercially available are the *Oncotype DX* assay (Genomic Health, Redwood City, CA) and the *MammaPrint* (Agendia, Inc., Amsterdam, the Netherlands) assay.

Oncotype DX assay is a reverse transcription polymerase chain reaction-based, 21-gene assay that can be done on formalin-fixed, paraffin-embedded breast cancer tissue (15,16). The test has been validated from tissue samples obtained from patients enrolled in the National Surgical Adjuvant Breast and Bowel Project clinical trial B-14 (NSABP B-14) as well as in a community-based study of 4,964 patients at Kaiser Permanente (17). The assay is done in node-negative, ER-positive

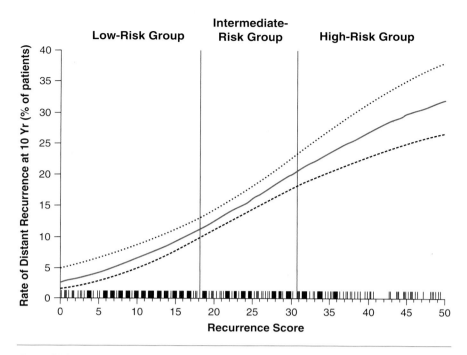

Figure 20.2 Rate of distant recurrence as a continuous function of the recurrence score. The *dashed curves* indicate the 95% confidence interval. The rug plot on the top of the x-axis shows the recurrence score for individual patients in the study. The likelihood of distant recurrence at 10 years increased continuously as the recurrence score increased (15).

breast cancer patients. It measures expression of a total of 21 genes (16 cancer and 5 reference genes) that were chosen based on their likelihood of being a predictive and prognostic factor in node-negative, ER-positive patients. Paik and associates (15) and Sparano and Paik (16) derived a *recurrence score* based on the gene expression pattern observed among 668 patients with node-negative, tamoxifen-treated breast cancer who were enrolled in NSABP B-14. The recurrence score was categorized as indicating low (<18), intermediate (19 to 30), or high (≥31) risk. Thus, the recurrence score is predictive of distant recurrence at 10 years when evaluated as a continuous variable (Figure 20.2) (15,16). Hormone therapy alone is adequate for patients with low risk, and chemotherapy is largely beneficial in patients with high risk (relative risk of 0.26). The score not only quantifies the likelihood of recurrence of breast cancer, but also predicts the magnitude of chemotherapy benefit (18).

The main limitation of the test is a lack of validation in prospective trials and the unclear role of chemotherapy in patients with intermediate scores. These issues are being addressed in the Trial Assigning IndividuaLized Options for Treatment (TailorRx), a multicenter prospective National Cancer Institute study launched in May 2006. The trial will enroll over 10,000 women at 900 sites in the United States and Canada. It is designed to determine whether adjuvant hormonal therapy alone is as effective as adjuvant hormonal therapy plus chemotherapy for women with midrange recurrence scores of 11 to 25 with early-stage ER-positive, *HER2*-negative, node-negative breast cancer (16).

The MammaPrint is a multigene DNA microarray assay developed in Netherlands that was approved by the Food and

Drug Administration in February 2007 and is based on the expression of a 70-gene signature (19). The gene signature was able to identify patients at risk for metastasis and divided them into low- and high-risk groups. The test was validated in 307 patients with a median follow-up of 13.6 years (20). In this study, patients were divided into high- and low-risk groups based on the gene signature classification and on clinical risk classifications. Patients were assigned to the gene signature low-risk group if their 5-year distant metastasis-free survival was >90%. Patients were assigned to the clinicopathologic low-risk group if their 10-year survival estimated by Adjuvant! software (http://www.adjuvantonline.com) was >88% (for ER-positive patients) or 92% (for ER-negative patients). For patients in the gene signature high-risk group, 10-year OS was 69% for patients in both the low- and high-risk clinical groups; for patients in the gene signature low-risk group, the 10-year survival rates were 88% and 89% in the low- and high-risk clinical groups, thereby demonstrating the better prognostic ability of the gene signature. The 70-gene signature outperformed the clinicopathologic risk assessment in predicting all end points: distant metastasis, disease-free survival (DFS), and OS. The need for frozen tissue to do the testing is a potential limitation of this assay.

ADJUVANT CHEMOTHERAPY

The landmark trial for adjuvant chemotherapy for breast cancer was published by Bonadonna and colleagues (21) in 1976. It showed that 12 months of chemotherapy with CMF (cyclophosphamide, methotrexate, and fluorouracil) in node-positive patients after radical mastectomy decreased relapse of breast cancer. The study results were updated in 2005, with an impressive median follow-up of 28.5 years (22). Adjuvant CMF was found to reduce the relative risk of relapse significantly (hazard ratio [HR], 0.71; $p = 0.005$) and death (HR, 0.79; $p = 0.04$). Since then, numerous trials have been conducted to find the optimum adjuvant therapy with the best therapeutic ratio.

Chemotherapy Versus no Chemotherapy

The Early Breast Cancer Trialist's Collaborative Group (EBCTCG), also called the *Oxford Review*, meets every 5 years to review data from global clinical trials (23). The final results from the year 2000 EBCTCG meta-analyses of the trials of systemic adjuvant treatments were published in 2005 and included trials that began in or before 1995 and women randomized before 1999. These analyses have provided a great deal of information on the long-term results of adjuvant therapy because it analyzed a large database of 145,000 women in 194 trials over 15 years. However, the limitation is that recent therapies like taxanes and trastuzumab are not included in the analyses. The report combines six meta-analyses: anthracycline-based versus no chemotherapy (8,000 women); CMF-based versus no chemotherapy (14,000); anthracycline-based versus CMF-based chemotherapy (14,000); about 5 years of tamoxifen versus none (15,000); about 1 to 2 years of tamoxifen versus none (33,000); and about 5 years versus 1 to 2 years of tamoxifen (18,000).

There were 22,000 women in the polychemotherapy versus no therapy trials (Figure 20.3). Polychemotherapy reduced the annual risk of relapse and death from breast cancer by 37% and 30%, respectively, in women under age 50. The absolute improvement in 15-year survival was 10% in women under age 50 and 3% in women aged 50 to 69. The most impressive finding is the divergence of the survival curves for breast cancer over time, suggesting that the benefit of adjuvant chemotherapy persists and improves well after therapy is completed. The absolute benefit for polychemotherapy versus no adjuvant chemotherapy in women <50 years old is twice as great at 15 years as at 5 years (10% vs. 4.7%).

Longer Versus Shorter Duration of Chemotherapy

In the EBCTCG analysis, there were 6,000 women in trials comparing longer versus shorter duration of chemotherapy, but only 720 were in trials that compared anthracyclines. There was little long-term gain from longer treatment (12 months compared with 6 months) with largely CMF-based regimens. Six months of CMF was superior to 3 months of CMF only in patients with ER-negative status and age <40 years in a joint analysis done in Europe (24). The usual duration of adjuvant oral CMF is 6 months and AC (Adriamycin + cyclophosphamide) is 3 months in the United States for all node-negative patients, irrespective of age or ER status.

Age, ER Status, and Nodal Status

The absolute benefit of chemotherapy appears greater in younger women, although data in older women are limited. The reasoning is that younger women tend to have ER-negative tumors, which respond better to chemotherapy. In the EBCTCG analysis, there was a 13% recurrence risk reduction in ER-negative tumors compared with 8% in ER-positive tumors in women younger than 50 years of age. Similarly, in women aged 50 to 69 years, chemotherapy reduced the recurrence risk by 10% in ER-negative tumors and 5% in ER-positive tumors. Chemotherapy can cause premature ovarian failure and amenorrhea, and this could be an added benefit in hormone-responsive tumors, beyond the antitumor effect.

The relative risk reduction was similar in both node-positive and node-negative patients in the EBCTCG analysis; however, the absolute risk reduction was higher in the node-positive group because they have a higher risk of relapse.

Anthracyclines Versus CMF

The absolute difference in survival between anthracycline-based regimens and CMF chemotherapy is about 3% at 5 years and 4% at 10 years, irrespective of age. Oral CMF is superior to intravenous CMF regimen (25). Four cycles of AC (Adriamycin and cyclophosphamide) is considered equivalent to six cycles of oral (classic) CMF, and this was first shown in the NSABP-15 study (26,27). Four cycles of AC therapy given every 3 weeks can be completed in 12 weeks compared with 6 months of oral CMF therapy, which requires more physician visits as well as longer intake of antinausea medications.

Six cycles of CEF or FEC (fluorouracil, epirubicin, and cyclophosphamide) has been shown to be superior to classic CMF regimen (28,29). However, the United States Intergroup trial 0102 with six cycles cyclophosphamide, adriamycin, and fluorouracil (CAF) did not improve DFS as a primary end point compared with six cycles CMF, although there was a slight improvement in OS with CAF (30). Given greater toxicity, CAF was not thought to be superior to CMF in this trial.

In the EBCTCG analysis, the removal of the four trials with four cycles of AC showed a significant increase in the amount of benefit (approximate 25% decrease in mortality) with anthracyclines compared with nonanthracycline therapy. Thus, there is indirect evidence in the EBCTCG analysis to show that six cycles of FAC is superior to four cycles of AC. The current NSABP 36 trial will prospectively address the question of whether six cycles of CEF is superior to that of four cycles of AC.

In summary, a 6-month course of an anthracycline-based therapy (FAC, FEC) may be superior to four cycles of AC or 6 months of oral CMF, but with the risk of increased toxicity.

TAXANES

The taxanes are among the most active agents against breast cancer. Paclitaxel is the prototype of the taxane family of antitumor drugs and was the first natural product shown to stabilize microtubules, which play a key role during mitosis. Docetaxel is a semi synthetic analog of paclitaxel and differs from it in significant ways. It is more avidly taken up by tumor cell lines than paclitaxel, and its efflux from the cells is slower (31). The potency of docetaxel, measured at the pharmacologic level by the ability to inhibit depolymerization, is twice that of paclitaxel (32).

Multiple trials have explored the role of taxanes and have shown a survival benefit with taxanes in the adjuvant setting.

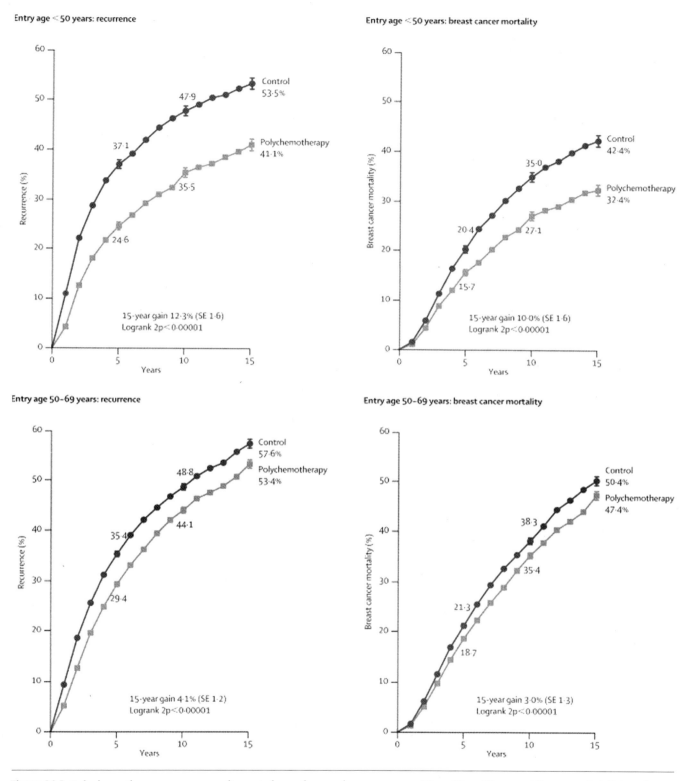

Figure 20.3 Polychemotherapy versus no adjuvant chemotherapy, by entry age, <50 or 50 to 69 years: 15-year probabilities of recurrence and of breast cancer mortality. Younger women, 35% node-positive; older women, 70% node-positive. Error bars are ± 1SE. (From Early Breast Cancer Trialist's Collaborative Group (EBCTCG). Effects of chemotherapy and hormonal therapy for early breast cancer on recurrence and 15-year survival: an overview of the randomised trials. *Lancet.* 2005;365:1687–717, with permission.)

Sequential Taxane Therapy

The CALGB 9344/Intergroup 0148 trial tested the benefit of adding paclitaxel after Adriamycin and cyclophosphamide in 3,121 patients with node-positive breast cancer. Patients were assigned randomly to receive one of three dose levels of Adriamycin (A; 60 mg/m^2, 75 mg/m^2, or 90 mg/m^2) with cyclophosphamide (C; 600 mg/m^2) with or without sequential paclitaxel (175 mg/m^2 every 3 weeks ×4) (33). At 7 years, TC was associated with improved DFS (81% TC vs. 75% AC, 20; $p = 0.031$, HR, 0.74) and superior OS (87% TC vs. 82% AC; $p = 0.032$, HR, 0.69). The paclitaxel group had significant improvement in both DFS (HR, 0.83; adjusted $p = .023$) and OS (HR, 0.82; $p = .0064$). Further subgroup analysis has shown that the benefit of paclitaxel was limited to patients with ER-negative breast cancer (14).

In the NSABP-28 study, 3,060 node-positive women were randomly assigned to receive four cycles of AC chemotherapy with or without four cycles of paclitaxel (225 mg/m^2 every 3 weeks ×4) (34). The paclitaxel group had a17% better 5-year DFS (relative risk, 0.83; $p = 0.006$) but similar OS. There was no difference between the ER-positive and -negative groups, in contrast to the results in the CALGB 9344 trial.

In the ECOG 1199 trial, 4,950 patients with node-positive or high-risk node-negative disease received AC every 3 weeks for four cycles, after which they were assigned to one of four arms: paclitaxel (80 mg/m^2) or docetaxel (35 mg/m^2) given weekly or paclitaxel (175 mg/m^2) or docetaxel (100 mg/m^2)given every 3 weeks (35). There was improved 5 year DFS and OS in the weekly paclitaxel arm compared to every 3 week paclitaxel arm.

Concurrent Taxane Therapy

In the BCIRG 001 study, 1,491 node-positive women were randomized to receive six cycles of TAC (docetaxel 75 mg/m^2, Adriamycin 50 mg/m^2, and cyclophosphamide 500 mg/m^2) versus six cycles of FAC (5-fluorouracil 500 mg/m^2 with AC in same doses as the other arm) every 3 weeks (36). With a median follow-up of 55 months, the TAC arm had 28% reduction in risk of relapse (HR, 0.72; $p = 0.001$) and 30% reduction in risk of death (HR, 0.70; $p = 0.008$) irrespective of ER status, HER2 status, menopausal status, and number of involved lymph nodes. The TAC arm had higher incidence of febrile neutropenia (24.7% vs. 2.5%) but the rates of grade 3 or 4 infection were similar (3.9 vs. 2.2); there were no deaths from infection.

The PACS-01 French study randomly assigned 1,999 node-positive women to six cycles of FEC (5-fluorouracil at 500 mg/m^2, epirubicin 100 mg/m^2, and cyclophosphamide 500 mg/m^2) versus the same regimen of FEC for three cycles followed by docetaxel at 100 mg/m^2 for three cycles (37). At a median follow-up of 60 months, the docetaxel arm had better DFS (HR, 0.83; $p = 0.041$) and OS (HR, 0.77; $p = 0.05$). This study highlighted the beneficial effects of taxanes over and above the benefits of longer duration of chemotherapy.

In the ECOG 2197 trial, 2,952 patients with node-positive or high-risk node-negative cancer were assigned to AC × 4 versus AT × 4 (docetaxel at 60 mg/m^2) (38). At 53-months median follow-up, DFS rates were similar in both groups, but three treatment-related deaths were reported in the doxorubicin/docetaxel arm. Life-threatening sepsis has also been re-

ported with the doxorubicin/docetaxel combination and is not recommended as adjuvant therapy (39). In a trial conducted by U.S. Oncology Research, Inc., 1,016 women (52% node-positive) were randomized to receive AC × 4 versus TC × 4 (docetaxel at 75 mg/m^2) every 3 weeks (40). At 5 years, TC was associated with higher DFS (86% vs. 80%; $p = 0.015$) but similar OS (90% vs. 87%; $p = 0.13$). Docetaxel/cyclophosphamide is considered as a viable adjuvant therapy alternative in patients unable to receive anthracycline, although a confirmation study would be helpful.

The previously discussed studies show that taxanes are beneficial as adjuvant therapy in node-positive breast cancer patients and high-risk (ER-negative, PR-negative) node-negative patients.

NEOADJUVANT THERAPY

Neoadjuvant (preoperative) therapy refers to the method of administering systemic chemotherapy in patients prior to surgery. It is established practice in patients with locally advanced or inflammatory breast cancer. It has potential advantages over postoperative chemotherapy. The effect on the primary tumor may decrease the extent of necessary surgery. Inoperable tumors can become operable, and patients initially thought to require mastectomy may become candidates for segmental mastectomy (lumpectomy) and, consequently, breast conservation. The ability to observe the response of tumors to a given chemotherapy regimen can allow one to discard noneffective therapies. Neoadjuvant therapy allows study of biomarkers prior to and after therapy at the time of surgery, which may serve as predictors of response to specific agents and improve the understanding of clinical response, although there is no proof that biomarkers predictive of pathologic response are the same ones that predict for DFS or OS.

NSABP B-18 was a neoadjuvant trial in which 1,523 women were assigned to four cycles of AC (AC × 4) before or after surgery (41). Preoperative therapy decreased the tumor size in 80% of women and, importantly, the breast conservation rate was higher (68% compared with 60%). At 5 years, there was no difference in relapse-free survival or OS. Rates of ipsilateral breast tumor recurrence after lumpectomy were similar in both groups.

In the NSABP B-27 trial, 2,411 women with T1-3 breast cancer (70% node-positive) were randomly assigned to one of three arms: AC × 4 followed by surgery; AC × 4 followed by surgery and then docetaxel × 4; or AC × 4 followed by docetaxel × 4 and then surgery (42). Tamoxifen was initiated concurrently with chemotherapy. At a median follow-up of 77.9 months, the addition of docetaxel did not improve DFS or OS, and a similar rate of breast-conserving therapy was noted in all arms. Pathologic complete response was doubled by the addition of preoperative docetaxel and was a significant predictor of OS regardless of treatment (HR, 0.33; $p < 0.0001$), but the docetaxel-containing arms did not have better DFS. Pathologic nodal status after chemotherapy was a significant predictor of OS ($p < 0.0001$). Concurrent use of tamoxifen may have limited the impact of adding docetaxel.

Some studies have indicated an increased incidence of in-breast recurrence after neoadjuvant therapy in patients undergoing lumpectomy instead of mastectomy at presentation. Ipsilateral breast tumor recurrence is a strong predictor for distant metastases (43). A meta-analysis of nine neoadjuvant trials involving 3,946 patients showed that neoadjuvant therapy was statistically associated with an increased risk of locoregional disease recurrences (RR = 1.22), especially in trials in which patients received radiation therapy without surgery (RR = 1.53) (44).

ADJUVANT CHEMOTHERAPY IN POSTMENOPAUSAL/OLDER WOMEN

The early EBCTCG analysis showed that there may be less benefit to adding chemotherapy to tamoxifen in older women with ER-positive cancer, although the latest analysis in 2006 invalidates this previously held notion. In node-positive women, an OS benefit for adding chemotherapy to tamoxifen was shown in two trials, NSABP 16 and Intergroup trial 0100 (45,46). Both studies used anthracycline-containing regimens. An analysis of three CALGB trials in 6,644 women with node-positive breast cancer showed more benefit for chemotherapy in ER-negative women with an OS improvement of 16.7% compared with an improvement of 4% in ER-positive women (14). In node-negative women, the benefits of chemotherapy are more conflicting. The NSABP-20 trial of 2,306 patients did not show a statistically significant survival benefit in women receiving chemotherapy over 60 years (47). In the International Breast Cancer Study Group (IBCSG) Trial IX of 1,669 patients with a median follow-up of 71 months, postmenopausal patients with lymph node-negative breast cancer benefited substantially from adjuvant chemotherapy if their cancer was ER-negative (i.e., endocrine-nonresponsive). In contrast, if their cancer was ER-positive (i.e., endocrine-responsive), they obtained no benefit from the addition of chemotherapy prior to treatment with tamoxifen (48).

The benefit of chemotherapy may be less in older women, although this concept may be biased by the reduced or less intense chemotherapy typically administered in older patients. The risk of breast cancer death as a function of stage is remarkably consistent above 40 years of age (49). However, the non–breast cancer mortality climbs rapidly after 60 years of age, thereby making breast cancer a smaller contributor to mortality in this age group. The quantitative ER levels are 2 to 3 times greater in patients aged >60 years compared with women <50 years (50). This results in improved response to hormonal therapy in older women.

DOSE-DENSE THERAPY

Dose-dense therapy refers to the method of administration of chemotherapy with a shorter interval between cycles. This is feasible with the use of hematopoietic growth factor support. In the breast cancer setting, this implies chemotherapy being administered every 2 weeks instead of every 3 weeks. The rationale is that following chemotherapy, the cytoreduced residual tumor may undergo a period of rapid exponential growth contributing to relapse (51). The more frequent administration of chemotherapy in a dose-dense schedule decreases the period available for

regrowth and is hypothesized to result in improved response rates.

The most well-studied dose-dense therapy trial was CALGB 9741, which studied 2,005 women in a 2 × 2 factorial design in node-positive breast cancer (52). The four arms were (I) sequential A × 4 (doses) → T × 4 → C × 4 with doses every 3 weeks, (II) sequential A × 4 → T × 4 → C × 4 every 2 weeks with filgrastim, (III) concurrent AC × 4 → T × 4 every 3 weeks, or (IV) concurrent AC × 4 → T × 4 every 2 weeks. At a median follow-up of 36 months, dose-dense treatment improved the primary end point, DFS (RR, 0.74; $p = 0.010$), and OS (RR, 0.69; $p = 0.013$). One hypothesis is that the improvement observed in this study was due to paclitaxel being a schedule-dependent drug. Further subset analysis has shown that the benefit was pronounced in ER-negative tumors (14).

The Italian Groupo Oncologica Nord Ovest-Mammella Intergruppo (GONO-MIG) group compared fluorouracil, epirubicin, and cyclophosphamide (FEC) every 14 days versus 21 days (53). At a median follow-up of 10.4 years, there was no statistically significant difference in the hazard of death or recurrence between the two arms. The limitation of the study was that it was underpowered for any subset analysis even though there was some evidence to suggest that the dose-dense strategy showed a 20% risk reduction in ER-negative women compared with a 2% risk reduction in ER-positive women. The epirubicin dose used was 60 mg/m^2 compared with the current standard dose of 100 mg/m^2.

METRONOMIC THERAPY

Metronomic therapy (analogous to a metronome) refers to the frequent, even daily, administration of chemotherapy at doses significantly below the maximum tolerated dose, with no prolonged drug-free intervals (54). Standard cytotoxic chemotherapy targets proliferating tumor cells and is given at the maximum tolerated dose, with the risk of significant toxicities. In contrast, metronomic therapy targets the endothelial cells of the growing vasculature of the tumor (antiangiogenic) and is better tolerated with significantly fewer toxicities (54). Despite the lower cumulative doses, the antitumor effects of metronomic dosing appear superior to conventional therapy in preclinical studies (55) and mathematical models (56). Studies are ongoing to validate this hypothesis.

TIMING OF CHEMOTHERAPY

The timing of chemotherapy after surgery is an important question. This question was addressed in a large United Kingdom trial in which the majority of patients received anthracyclines (57). A total of 1,161 patients were retrospectively analyzed and divided into two groups. The DFS and OS of the 368 patients starting chemotherapy within 21 days of surgery (group A) were compared with those of the 793 patients commencing chemotherapy ≥21 days after surgery (group B). Median follow-up time was 39 months (range, 12 to 147 months). No significant difference in 5-year DFS or 5-year OS was found between the two groups.

Another retrospective European trial looked at early initiation of adjuvant chemotherapy, ER status, and prognosis in 1,788 premenopausal, node-positive patients treated in International Breast Cancer Study Group (IBCSG) trials I, II, and VI (58). The DFS for 599 patients (84 with ER-negative tumors) who commenced adjuvant chemotherapy within 20 days (early initiation) was compared with the DFS for 1,189 patients (142 with ER-negative tumors) who started chemotherapy 21 to 86 days after surgery (conventional initiation). The median follow-up was 7.7 years. Among patients with ER-negative tumors, the 10-year DFS was 60% for the early initiation group compared with 34% for the conventional initiation group (HR, 0.49; confidence interval [CI]: 0.33-0.72; $p = 0.0003$). In contrast, early initiation of chemotherapy did not significantly improve DFS for patients with ER-positive tumors (HR, 0.93; CI: 0.79-1.10; $p = 0.40$).

Thus, it is reasonable to start adjuvant chemotherapy after allowing adequate time for surgical recovery and wound healing, but avoiding inordinate delay.

CHEMOTHERAPY AND RADIOTHERAPY SEQUENCE

The majority of patients receiving adjuvant therapy will require chemotherapy and/or radiotherapy, and their sequence is of interest. In a trial done from 1984 to 1992, 244 patients were randomized to receive chemotherapy before or after radiation (59). At a median follow-up of 135 months, no difference in OS was noted. However, patients with close microscopic resection margins (<1 mm) had a 4% local recurrence rate with initial radiation therapy compared with 32% with initial chemotherapy. Hence, the patients who would benefit the most with initial radiation are those with surgical margins of <1 mm. Chemotherapy is given first to all other patients. Concurrent chemotherapy and radiation therapy is deemed too toxic and is generally not used.

HER2/neu AND TRASTUZUMAB

HER2/neu (named from human epidermal growth factor receptor 2) is an oncogene expressed in about 20% of all breast cancers. The *ERBB2* gene family encodes for transmembrane receptor of growth factors, including the epidermal growth factors, namely *HER1, HER2, HER3,* and *HER4.* The *HER2* receptor has an intracellular and extracellular domain. The intracellular domain has tyrosine kinase activity that is responsible for signal transduction leading to cellular growth and proliferation (60). Amplification of the *HER2* oncogene on chromosome 17 causes a marked increase (up to 100 times the usual level) in the expression of *HER2* on the surface of breast tumor cells (61). *HER2*-positivity is an adverse prognostic factor associated with an aggressive course; more poorly differentiated, high-grade tumors; and relatively short disease-free intervals (62). Only about half of *HER2*-positive breast cancers express steroid hormone receptors (ER, PR), and, in addition, the receptors are in lower concentration than in *HER2*-negative tumors. This results in relative resistance to tamoxifen (61). The humanized monoclonal antibody trastuzumab (Herceptin) targets *HER2* and was initially noted to be beneficial in the setting of metastatic breast cancer (63). Subsequently, several landmark trials (described later) have proven

its efficacy in the adjuvant setting and have revolutionized the care of *HER2*-positive breast cancer. Because trastuzumab is effective only in *HER2*-positive tumors, testing for it in breast cancer has become routine.

Interactions Between Trastuzumab and Tumor Cells

HER2 serves as a coreceptor with related members of the *HER* family of tyrosine kinase–associated growth factors. Trastuzumab is a humanized monoclonal antibody that binds to *HER2* and inhibits tumor cell growth through a variety of intracellular, and possibly extracellular, mechanisms (Figure 20.4) (61).

HER2 Testing

HER2 testing can be performed on primary breast tumor tissue or metastatic specimens (64). This can be accomplished by two methods that are currently approved by the Food and Drug Administration: immunohistochemistry (IHC) and fluorescent is situ hybridization (FISH). IHC determines *HER2* expression in paraffin-embedded tissue samples using a *HER2*-specific antibody. The breast tumor specimens are stained on a semiquantitative scale from 0 (no detectable HER2 protein) to 3+ (high *HER2* expression). Tumors scored 0 to 1+ are deemed negative, and those scored 3+ are deemed positive and likely to respond to trastuzumab. Tumors with a 2+ score are deemed indeterminate and need further testing with FISH. A ratio of *HER2/ neu* to CEP 17 >2.2 by FISH is considered positive for *HER2* expression, although a ratio ≥ 2 was used in the trastuzumab trials. FISH allows quantification of gene copy number and determines *HER2* gene amplification.

The American Society of Clinical Oncologists (ASCO), in collaboration with the College of American Pathologists (CAP), released new guidelines in January 2007 to address the problematic issue of *HER2* testing, although the cut-offs recommended have not been validated in clinical trials (65). The guidelines opined that 20% of current *HER2* testing may be inaccurate. Because *HER2* testing has critical clinical implications, the panel recommends that *HER2* testing be done in a CAP-accredited laboratory or in a laboratory that meets the accreditation and proficiency testing requirements enumerated in the guidelines. The guidelines recommend the algorithms for *HER2* testing presented in Figures 20.5 and 20.6.

Adjuvant Trastuzumab Therapy

There are four major trials and a fifth, smaller Finnish trial (FinHer) (66) that have established the efficacy of trastuzumab in an adjuvant setting (Table 20.2). The four major trials, which have enrolled more than 13,000 patients, are the Herceptin Adjuvant (HERA), (67) the National Surgical Adjuvant Breast and Bowel Project (NSABP) B-31, the North Central Cancer Treatment Group (NCCTG) N9831(63), and the Breast Cancer International Research Group (BCIRG) 006 (68). All five trials enrolled patients who tested positive for gene or protein (by FISH with ratio >2 or 3+ by IHC). Patients with cardiac dysfunction were excluded, and in all trials, a minimum left ventricular ejection fraction of 50% was required. Patients' median age was 50 years, and 50% had hormone receptor-positive cancers. The

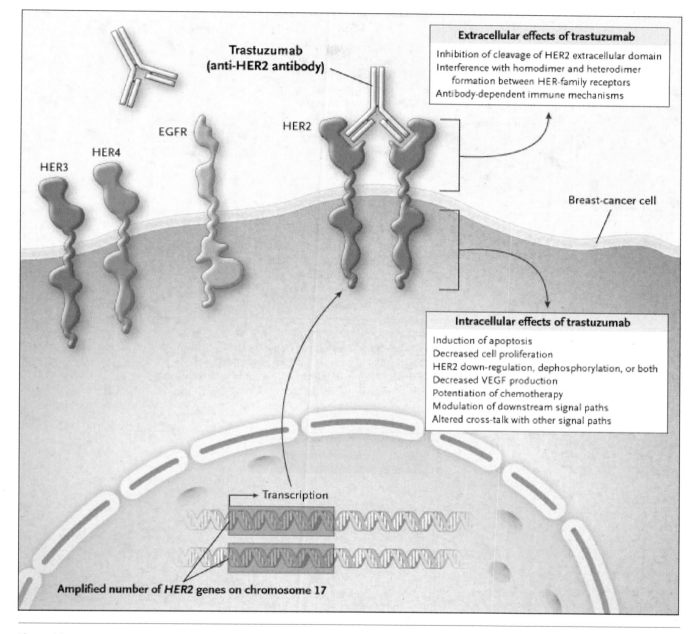

Figure 20.4 Interactions between trastuzumab and tumor cells. See text for details. (From Burstein HJ. The distinctive nature of HER2-positive breast cancers. *N Engl J Med.* 2005;353:1652–1654, with permission.)

timing of trastuzumab initiation varied between the trials. It was delayed up to 8 months in the HERA trial, up to 4 months in NSABP B31 and N9831 trials, and up to 1 month in the FinHer trial and the platinum/taxane arm of the BCIRG 006 trial. In the BCIRG 006 trial, patients received trastuzumab weekly during the two arms of the trial providing concurrent chemotherapy (AC followed by docetaxel vs. docetaxel and carboplatin) and every 3 weeks thereafter. In the third arm of the trial, patients received AC followed by docetaxel, but no trastuzumab.

Patients were dosed with trastuzumab every 3 weeks in the HERA trial and weekly in the remaining trials. The duration of trastuzumab also varied and was 9 weeks in the FinHer study,

2 years in one arm of the HERA trial, and for 1 year in the remaining trials.

A combined analysis was presented from the NCCTG N9831 and the NSABP B31 trials, with the approval of the National Cancer Institute. All of the studies consistently show about a 39% to 52% reduction in the risk of recurrence at a median follow-up of 1 to 3 years. The HERA trial update in 2007 showed a significant OS benefit (HR, 0.66; p <0.0001) after a median follow-up of 2 years (69). The combined NSABP–NCCTG analysis update presented at the 2007 conference of ASCO showed a HR of 0.49 for DFS and 0.63 for OS favoring the trastuzumab arm (70).

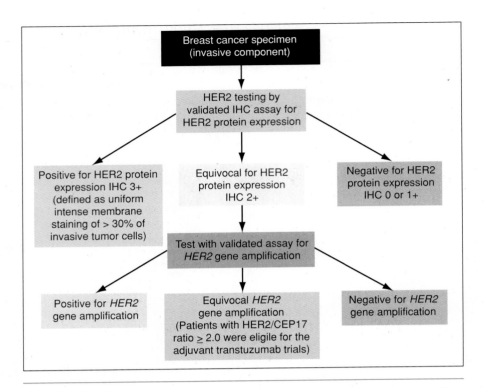

Figure 20.5 HER2 testing. Algorithm for immunohistochemistry (IHC). (From Wolff AC, Hammond MEH, Schwartz JN, et al. American Society of Clinical Oncology/College of American Pathologists guideline recommendations for human epidermal growth factor receptor 2 testing in breast cancer. *J Clin Oncol.* 2007;25:118–145, with permission.)

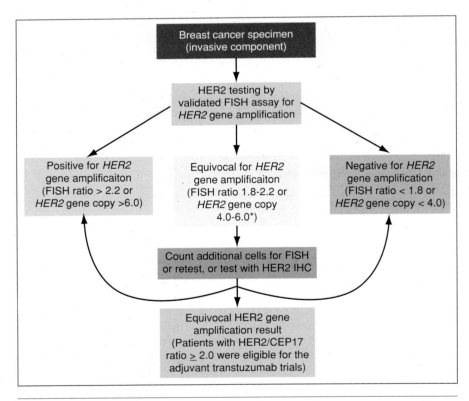

Figure 20.6 HER2 testing. Algorithm for fluorescent in situ hybridization (FISH). (From Wolff AC, Hammond MEH, Schwartz JN, et al. American Society of Clinical Oncology/College of American Pathologists guideline recommendations for human epidermal growth factor receptor 2 testing in breast cancer. *J Clin Oncol.* 2007;25:118–145, with permission.) (See color plates.)

Table 20.2

Summary of Trastuzumab (Herceptin) Trials

	HERA Control (1,693) H × 1 year (1,694)	NCCTG N9831 + NSABP 31 Control (1,679) H × 1 year (1,672)	BCIRG 006 AC-D (1,073) AC-D + H (1,074) DCp + H (1,075)	FinHer Control (115) H × 9 weeks (116)
Eligibility for high-risk node-negative	Size >1 cm	Size >1 cm	Size >2 cm	Size >2cm
Trastuzumab dosing	Every 3 weeks	Weekly	Weekly with CT, then every 3 weeks	Weekly
DFS HR	0.64	0.49	0.61/0.67	0.42[a]
DFS p value	<0.0001	<0.0001	0.000011/0.00028	0.01
OS HR	0.66	0.63	0.59/0.66	0.41
OS p value	0.0115	0.0004	0.004/0.017	0.07
Median follow-up	2 years	2.9 years	3 years	38 months

HERA, Herceptin adjuvant; H, trastuzumab (Herceptin); NCCTG, North Central Cancer Treatment Group; NSABP,
 National Surgical Adjuvant Breast and Bowel Project; BCIRG, Breast Cancer International Research Group; AC,
 Adriamycin and cyclophosphamide; D, docetaxel; Cp, carboplatin; FinHer, Finnish Herceptin; CT, chemotherapy;
 DFS, disease-free survival; HR, hazard ratio.
[a] FinHer used relapse-free survival in contrast to DFS in all other trials.

The second interim analysis of the BCIRG 006 trial was presented at the San Antonio Breast Cancer Symposium in December 2006 (71). The DFS curves for both the trastuzumab arms have met, showing an equal efficacy at a median follow-up of 3 years. This finding raises the provocative question of whether an anthracycline is needed, because the docetaxel/carboplatin/trastuzumab combination offers an alternative with possibly less cardiac toxicity and leukemogenic potential, although there was indeed slightly higher number of patients with breast cancer relapse or death in the non–anthracycline arm of this trial. The final results of the HERA trials with the longer 2-year arm are eagerly awaited.

In a retrospective analysis of the BCIRG006 data, the investigators made the intriguing observation that coamplification of the topoisomerase II-alpha gene occurs in one third of *HER2*-positive tumors (68,71). Such patients benefit with anthracycline regimens, and the ones without coamplification do not have the same benefit with anthracyclines and may be treated with nonanthracycline regimens without the risk of cardiac toxicity. These data, however, are viewed as premature and need validation before being incorporated into standard practice.

Neoadjuvant or Preoperative Trastuzumab

Several trials have explored the concept of preoperative trastuzumab, with all showing the pathologic complete response rates in the range of 18% to 25% (72,73). The highest response rates were seen in a small phase III MD Anderson Cancer Center trial (74). Patients with *HER2*-positive early-stage breast cancer were randomized to a control arm of paclitaxel × 4 every 3 weeks followed by FEC (fluorouracil, epirubicin, and cyclophosphamide) × 4 every 3 weeks. In the treatment arm, trastuzumab was added weekly to this regimen. An overall pathologic complete response rate of 26.3% in the control arm and 65.2% in

the trastuzumab arm was reported. The study was stopped prematurely after an accrual of 42 patients because of the significant difference in response rates between the trastuzumab and nontrastuzumab arms. Interestingly, epirubicin was used concurrently with trastuzumab but no severe cardiac toxicities were reported. The limitation was that tumors >5 cm were not included in the study. The high response rates can be attributed to the longer duration of chemotherapy or the concurrent use of anthracycline and trastuzumab. A proposed trial by the American College of Surgeons Oncology Group will evaluate this concept.

SIDE EFFECTS OF ADJUVANT CHEMOTHERAPY

The therapeutic ratio of chemotherapy is narrow and the benefits always need to be weighed against its short- and long-term risks. Contrary to general perception, chemotherapy-related serious adverse effects among younger women with breast cancer may be more common than reported by large clinical trials and can lead to more patient suffering and health care expenditures than previously estimated (75). In an insurance database study of 12,239 newly diagnosed breast cancer women aged 63 or younger, 4,075 received chemotherapy within the first 12 months of diagnosis. The chemotherapy-associated serious adverse events resulting in hospitalization and/or emergency department visits was 16% in this series of patients (75). The side effects need to be balanced with the clear improvements in DFS and OS demonstrated by the use of adjuvant chemotherapy.

Immediate Adverse Effects

Alopecia is nearly universal with regimens containing anthracyclines and taxanes. Nausea, vomiting, mucositis, and cytopenias related to bone marrow suppression are acute and reversible. Neutropenia can occur 10 to 14 days following chemotherapy. ASCO guidelines recommend prophylactic use of growth factors in regimens with expected incidence of neutropenia >20% (76). Two such regimens are dose-dense AC given every 2 weeks and TAC therapy. Sensory and motor neuropathies are common with taxanes and are dose-dependent and cumulative. Early recognition of the toxicities and dose reduction or delaying therapy can prevent symptomatic neuropathy. Premenopausal women gain weight with chemotherapy as a result of ovarian failure and decreased physical activity (77). Significant fatigue is also a common complaint (78). Vasomotor symptoms are also common in women receiving chemotherapy secondary to the ovarian suppression effects. The HABITS (Hormonal Replacement after Breast Cancer) trial has clearly demonstrated that estrogen-based hormone replacement therapy for vasomotor symptoms is contraindicated in women with breast cancer (79).

Long-Term Adverse Effects

Concerns have been raised about the cognitive decline in patients who receive chemotherapy, but the relationship is uncertain. Periodic surveillance has been recommended in the Canadian guidelines (80). Premature ovarian failure is more likely in women >40 years of age as well as those receiving CMF or CEF regimens (81). Chemotherapy-induced amenorrhea can be transient in young women, and these women need to be counseled on birth control as they can ovulate and become pregnant, despite the absence of menstrual cycles. There is also an increased risk of bone fractures and osteoporosis in women with breast cancer, at least in part related to premature ovarian failure; therefore, patients should be counseled about regular exercise, limiting smoking, avoiding excessive alcohol use, and the potential benefits of calcium, vitamin D, and bisphosphonates.

Secondary Leukemias

There are two different types of secondary leukemias reported with breast cancer chemotherapy and the incidence, which is related to the total cumulative dose and the agents used, is estimated to be about 1%. Radiation therapy following chemotherapy increases the risk for leukemias (82). The first type occurs with alkylating agents like cyclophosphamide in 3 to 7 years following therapy, often preceded by a myelodysplastic phase (83). The second type occurs with topoisomerase inhibitors like etoposide and anthracyclines, and develops 24 to 36 months following chemotherapy (84). This type does not have a myelodysplastic phase and is associated with the characteristic 11q23 chromosomal abnormalities. The risk for a secondary leukemia is about 1.3% with anthracyclines, compared with a 0.4% risk with CMF (50). The secondary leukemias are usually refractory to treatment and have a dismal prognosis.

Cardiac Toxicity

Cardiac toxicity is a concern with anthracyclines and now with trastuzumab. The cardiac toxicity with doxorubicin was 5% with a cumulative lifetime dose of 550 mg/m^2 in an older study done in the 1970s (85). A retrospective analysis of three trials published in 2003 showed a higher than anticipated 26% cardiac toxicity at a cumulative dose of 550 mg/m^2 and age >65 was a major risk factor (86). With these data, cardiac toxicity is now a concern at a cumulative dose of doxorubicin of >400 mg/m^2 as reported in the National Comprehensive Cancer Network (NCCN) task force report (50). Dexrazoxane, a cardioprotective agent, has been investigated and used by some physicians, although not very commonly in view of potential interferences with the antitumor activity of anthracyclines.

Historically, the risk increases in patients with history of a radiation therapy field that includes the heart. However, newer and improved radiation therapy techniques, like forward-plane intensity-modulated radiation therapy and respiratory gating, decrease the risk of cardiac toxicities.

Trastuzumab is fairly well tolerated without the usual side effects of regular chemotherapeutic agents. The principal adverse effect of trastuzumab is cardiotoxicity, which is not dose-related, in contrast to the anthracyclines (87). In various reports, the incidence of mild-to-severe symptomatic or asymptomatic cardiac dysfunction was 1.4% when trastuzumab was used as a single agent (88), 13% in patients receiving paclitaxel with trastuzumab, and 27% in patients concurrently receiving trastuzumab with an anthracycline (89). An independent review of cardiac events in seven trastuzumab trials showed age and concurrent anthracycline administration as the major risk factors (90). Hence, trastuzumab is given sequentially and not concurrently with an anthracycline. The incidence of congestive heart failure has remained at acceptable levels of 0.6% to 3.3% and most patients respond to treatment (91). Trastuzumab should be discontinued if congestive heart failure is detected and temporarily suspended for a decline in left ventricular ejection fraction of 15% or any declines that result in an ejection fraction ≤50% (64). A case series of 38 patients with trastuzumab-related cardiac dysfunction showed that 37 of these patients had recovery of left ventricular ejection fraction with cessation of trastuzumab and medical management (92). The average time for recovery of ejection fraction was 1.5 months. Twenty-five of these patients were re-treated with trastuzumab, and only three developed recurrent left ventricular dysfunction. The only other unexpected side effect in the trastuzumab adjuvant trials was interstitial pneumonitis in nine patients (two deaths) in the combined NCCTG–NSABP analysis and two fatal pneumonias in the taxotere, carboplatin, and herceptin arm of BCIRG 006 (93).

ADJUVANT HORMONAL MANIPULATION

The rationale for hormonal manipulation is to prevent estrogen-mediated cancer cell growth. This can be accomplished by blocking estrogen from binding to the receptor on target organs or by preventing estrogen production. Hormonal therapy is used only in ER-positive or PR-positive women. The intriguing report of 5% to 10% response to hormonal therapy in ER- and PR-negative women in the earlier EBCTCG analysis (94) may be related to the nonhormonal effects of tamoxifen in reducing insulinlike growth factor (95) or may be explained on the basis that the test was not sensitive enough to identify lower levels of hormonal positivity. Estrogen receptors have now been identified as two distinct subtypes: α and β. Current estrogen testing methods only detect α-receptors. Expression of ERβ has been shown as an independent marker for favorable prognosis after adjuvant tamoxifen treatment in ERα-negative breast cancer patients and involves a gene expression pattern distinct from ERα (96). This could possibly explain the tamoxifen response seen in ER-negative patients who truly could be ERβ-positive (96). The most recent EBCTCG analysis did not show a benefit in ER-negative women taking tamoxifen at 5 years (23). As a consensus, hormonal therapy is not used in ER- and PR-negative patients.

There are various approaches to reducing estrogen activity. Tamoxifen is an oral selective estrogen receptor modulator that can be used in both premenopausal and postmenopausal women and blocks estrogen binding to its receptors. However, it also has partial agonistic actions on other tissues that lead to its side effects of endometrial cancer and thromboembolism. Estrogen production can be permanently prevented by bilateral surgical oophorectomy or by irradiation to the ovaries. In addition, estrogen production can be temporarily reduced by gonadotropin-releasing hormone analogues (GnRH), such as leuprolide or goserelin. In postmenopausal women, the main site of estrogen production is in the peripheral tissues. Aromatase inhibitors (AIs) prevent conversion of androgen to estrogen by the aromatase enzyme in the peripheral tissues and are used only in postmenopausal women. If AIs are used in premenopausal women, the negative feedback of estrogen to the hypothalamus and pituitary results in increased gonadotrophin secretion, resulting in deleterious effects. The two different types of AIs are the reversibly binding steroidal inhibitors (anastrozole and letrozole) and the irreversibly binding steroidal inhibitors (exemestane and formestane).

Tamoxifen

The 2005 EBCTCG overview analysis clearly demonstrates the efficacy of 5 years of tamoxifen therapy in ER-positive women (Figure 20.7) (23). A 41% reduction in the annual breast cancer recurrence and a 34% reduction in the annual death rate was observed. The benefit of tamoxifen continued long after its discontinuation. At 15 years, the absolute reduction in recurrence risk was 12% and mortality rate was 9%. There was also a 39% risk reduction in contralateral breast cancer.

In the NSABP B-14 trial, node-negative, tamoxifen-treated patients were reassigned after 5 years to placebo or continued tamoxifen treatment (97). At the 7-year analysis, the tamoxifen arm had worse DFS (78% vs. 82%; $p = 0.03$) and OS (91% vs. 94%; $p = 0.07$). A Scottish trial with node-negative patients also showed similar worse outcomes with longer tamoxifen intake (98), and concern was raised for a twofold increase in endometrial cancer with the longer duration. However, an Eastern Cooperative Oncology Group (ECOG) trial in node-positive patients showed longer time to relapse ($p = 0.014$) with longer tamoxifen intake but no difference in OS ($p = 0.81$) (99).

Based on the EBCTCG analysis and NSABP B-14 trial, tamoxifen treatment at 20 mg daily is recommended for 5 years in ER-positive women. Patients receiving tamoxifen beyond 5 years may develop tamoxifen resistance, resulting in agonistic action

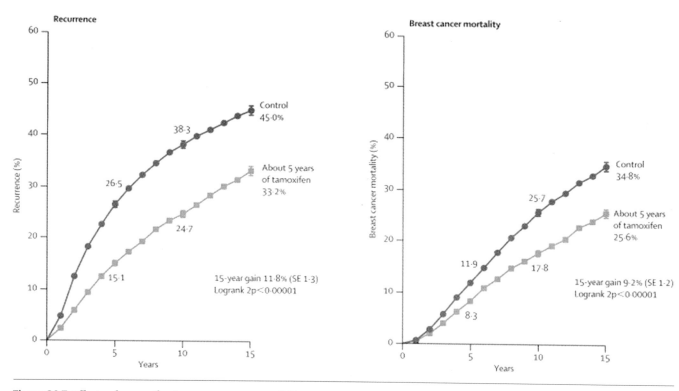

Figure 20.7 Effects of tamoxifen in estrogen receptor (ER)-positive or ER-unknown disease. Comparison of 15-year probabilities of recurrence and of breast cancer mortality among patients receiving about 5 years of tamoxifen versus no tamoxifen. Among 10,386 patients, 20% were ER-unknown and 30% were node-positive. Error bars are ±1 SE. (From Early Breast Cancer Trialists Collaborative Group (EBCTCG). Effects of chemotherapy and hormonal therapy for early breast cancer on recurrence and 15-year survival: an overview of the randomised trials. *Lancet.* 2005;365:1687–717, with permission.)

on tissues and increasing the risk of adverse events (100). The standard of care is to use tamoxifen sequentially with chemotherapy rather than use it concurrently, as supported by data from Intergroup trial (INT) 0100 (46). In this trial, at a median follow-up of 8.5 years, the DFS was 67% in the sequential arm compared with 62% in the concurrent arm. The estimated DFS advantage was 18% in the sequential arm.

Similarly, tamoxifen is typically used sequentially with radiotherapy. There are two theoretical concerns raised with concurrent use. An increased incidence of pulmonary (101) and breast fibrosis (102) has been noted with concurrent use, and tamoxifen renders cancer cells relatively radioresistant in in vitro studies. However, no significant differences in DFS or OS were noted in several retrospective studies reviewing concurrent versus sequential use of tamoxifen and radiotherapy (103,104). Hence, tamoxifen is used concurrently with radiotherapy in many clinical trials and by clinicians in practice.

Ovarian Function Suppression in Premenopausal Women

The EBCTCG analysis reviewed 15 randomized trials of premenopausal women with breast cancer who were treated with ovarian ablation by surgery, radiation, or hormonal therapy. It showed that ovarian function suppression alone reduced breast cancer recurrences and death and the effect lasted over 15 years (23). Some of the benefits of chemotherapy in premenopausal women are attributed to its effect in causing ovarian failure.

Many trials have shown no difference in outcomes between ovarian function suppression (OFS) and chemotherapy. These studies, however, were criticized for using intravenous CMF, which is considered inferior to oral CMF. The International Breast Cancer Study Group (IBCSG) trial VIII was the only trial to compare goserelin with oral CMF; the outcomes were similar in ER-positive patients, but ER-negative patients did better with oral CMF (105). Two trials have shown that the combined therapy of OFS with tamoxifen is better (106), or at least equivalent (107) to, CMF therapy. However, OFS has not been studied well against newer therapeutic agents such as anthracycline and taxanes, which are deemed superior to CMF. Currently ongoing trials of ovarian suppression may clarify many of the unanswered, intriguing questions. The Suppression of Ovarian Function Trial (SOFT) (108) addresses the issues of whether OFS adds benefit to chemotherapy in premenopausal women and whether OFS adds benefit to tamoxifen or exemestane in premenopausal women not treated with chemotherapy. The Tamoxifen and Exemestane Trial (TEXT) (109) addresses the issue of the possible superiority of AI to tamoxifen in premenopausal women treated with OFS. The Premenopausal Endocrine Responsive Chemotherapy Trial (PERCHE) (110) was aimed at determining if chemotherapy is necessary in premenopausal women receiving combined endocrine therapy but, unfortunately, low accrual forced the premature closure of this study in 2006.

Aromatase Inhibitors

AIs are currently used only in hormone-receptor positive tumors in postmenopausal women. Premenopausal women can become temporarily amenorrheic following chemotherapy, and AI can be used only if permanent menopause is established, which is usually about a year after the onset of amenorrhea. In unclear situations, tamoxifen is the preferred drug because the indiscrete use of AI in women who are not truly menopausal will deprive them of their hormonal therapy benefits.

Initial Therapy

The ATAC trial (Arimidex, Tamoxifen Alone or in Combination) compared anastrozole with tamoxifen for 5 years in 9,366 postmenopausal women with localized breast cancer (111). After a median follow-up of 68 months, anastrozole (Arimidex) significantly prolonged DFS (HR, 0.87; $p = 0.01$), time to recurrence (HR, 0.79; $p = 0.0005$), reduced distant metastases (HR, 0.86; $p = 0.04$), and contralateral breast cancers (42% reduction, $p = 0.01$), but there was no difference in OS (HR, 0.97; $p = 0.7$) between the two groups. The anastrozole arm had fewer gynecologic problems and vascular events, but arthralgia and fractures were increased. Interestingly, a retrospective analysis hypothesized that the benefit was more with anastrozole in ER-positive/PR-negative tumors than ER-positive/PR-positive tumors (HR of 0.43 vs. 0.85) (112).

The BIG 1-98 trial (113) is a randomized, phase III, double-blind trial in postmenopausal women with ER- and/or PR-positive breast cancer comparing the following four options: monotherapy with letrozole or with tamoxifen for 5 years, or sequential administration of tamoxifen for 2 years followed by letrozole for 3 years, or sequential administration of letrozole for 2 years followed by tamoxifen for 3 years. From March 1998 to March 2000, patients were randomly assigned to one of the following two arms: monotherapy with letrozole (2.5 mg daily) or tamoxifen (20 mg daily). From April 1999 to May 2003, patients were randomly assigned to all four arms. In a 2007 update with a median follow-up time of 51 months limited to patients in the monotherapy arms, 352 DFS events among 2,463 women receiving letrozole and 418 events among 2,459 women receiving tamoxifen were noted. This shows an 18% reduction in the risk of an event in favor of letrozole (HR, 0.82; CI: 0.71-0.95; $p = 0.007$), but there was no difference in OS (114).

Sequential Therapy

The Intergroup Exemestane Study (IES) (115), Italian Tamoxifen Anastrozole (ITA) Trial (DFS HR, 0.35; $p = 0.001$) (116) and the ARNO 95 trial (117) favor exemestane and anastrozole use following 2 to 3 years of tamoxifen, instead of taking tamoxifen for 5 straight years. The recent updates in 2006 from both IES (DFS HR, 0.74; $p < 0.0001$; OS HR, 0.83; $p = 0.04$) (118) and ARNO (DFS HR, 0.66; $p = 0.049$; OS HR, 0.53; $p = 0.040$) (117) show a survival benefit with sequential AI use.

Extended Therapy (beyond 5 years)

The National Cancer Institute of Canada Clinical Trials Group MA.17 trial assigned 5,187 patients after 5 years of tamoxifen therapy to an additional 5 years of treatment with letrozole or placebo (119). The study was terminated early at a median follow-up of 30 months when an interim analysis showed benefit with letrozole use (DFS of 94% with letrozole vs. 90% placebo; HR, 0.58; $p = 0.00008$). The trial was unblinded and placebo patients were offered letrozole. At unblinding, 1,655 of 2,268 placebo patients accepted letrozole. At median follow-up of 54 months, 4-year DFS was 94.3% versus 91.4% (HR, 0.64; $p = 0.00002$) favoring the letrozole arm. Letrozole was equally effective in node-positive and node-negative patients in DFS. The 4-year OS was 95.0% versus 95.1% (HR, 1.00; $p = 0.99$). There was no difference in OS, but a subgroup analysis showed an improved OS ($p = 0.038$) in node-positive patients (120). A companion study looking at the effects of letrozole on bone mineral density at 24 months showed higher risk of lumbar osteoporosis (4.1% in letrozole arm vs. 0% in placebo; $p = 0.064$) and decline in bone mineral density (hip, −3.6% vs. placebo, −0.71; $p = 0.044$ and lumbar spine −5.35% vs. placebo −0.70; $p = 0.008$) in the letrozole arm (121).

DECISION-MAKING TOOLS

Optimal decision making in consideration of an individual patient's age, comorbid conditions, and tumor characteristics requires the integration of a vast amount of data derived from multiple clinical trials. Adjuvant! (www.adjuvantonline.com) is a Web-based tool developed by Ravdin et al. (122) that addresses this need and is available free online as well as in a PDA (personal digital assistant) version. It draws on information from the SEER database of the National Cancer Institute, the Oxford Review, or the EBCTCG (Early Breast Cancer Trialists Collaborative Group), and individual clinical trial results. Adjuvant! Estimates a 10-year relapse as well as mortality rates depending on individual patient and disease characteristics. It also estimates risk reduction with chemotherapy, hormonal therapy, and combined therapy in a given scenario. The relapse estimates by Adjuvant! are higher than those derived from Oncotype Dx, as it includes local, contralateral, and distant relapses in contrast to Oncotype Dx, which predicts only distant relapse rates. The distant relapse rates correlate more closely with mortality rates. A genomic version of Adjuvant! incorporates Oncotype Dx scores into risk estimates. Adjuvant! has been validated using the British Columbia Breast Cancer Outcomes Unit (BCOU) database, derived from the management of 4,083 women diagnosed between 1989 and 1993 in British Columbia with T1-2, N0-1, M0 breast cancers (123). The predicted and observed outcomes were within 2% in most groups. The only group in which Adjuvant! overestimated survival was in women <35 years of age. Finprog (http://www.finprog.org) is another Web-based tool that tries to predict breast cancer mortality based on a database of 2,032 Finnish women (124).

NEWER THERAPEUTIC AGENTS

Lapatinib (Tykerb) is an orally active dual tyrosine kinase inhibitor of HER2 and epidermal growth factor receptor. It is active in combination with capecitabine in women with HER2-positive metastatic breast cancer that has progressed after trastuzumab therapy (125). Lapatinib has shown preliminary evidence of penetration into the central nervous system. In a case series of 39 women with HER2-positive disease and brain metastasis on trastuzumab, there was one partial responses, and seven patients were progression-free at 16 weeks (126). This agent is currently being studied in an adjuvant setting in HER2-positive breast cancers.

Bevacizumab (Avastin) is a humanized recombinant antibody that inhibits angiogenesis by binding to *vascular endothelial growth factor* (VEGF). VEGF is an angiogenic growth factor that has been implicated in various cancers, including breast, colon,

and lung cancers. A high level of VEGF tumor expression correlates with a worse prognosis in breast cancer (127). Bevacizumab with capecitabine has shown to improve response rates but not OS in heavily pretreated metastatic breast cancer (128). In a randomized, phase 3 trial, Miller et al. (129) enrolled 722 patients to compare the efficacy of paclitaxel with that of paclitaxel plus bevacizumab as initial treatment for metastatic breast cancer. Paclitaxel plus bevacizumab significantly prolonged progression-free survival as compared with paclitaxel alone (median, 11.8 vs. 5.9 months; HR for progression, 0.60; $p < 0.001$) and increased the objective response rate (36.9% vs. 21.2%; $p < 0.001$). The OS rate, however, was similar in the two groups (median, 26.7 vs. 25.2 months; HR, 0.88; $p = 0.16$).

SUMMARY RECOMMENDATIONS FOR ADJUVANT THERAPY

Guidelines of the National Comprehensive Cancer Network

The NCCN (www.nccn.org) is an alliance of 19 leading cancer centers in the United States that periodically recommends clinical practice guidelines that are applied widely in practice. NCCN recommends chemotherapy for women with breast cancer ≥1 cm in size or node-positive, irrespective of hormone status or HER2 status. The exceptions are to consider chemotherapy for tumors 0.6 to 1.0 cm if lymphovascular invasion, high nuclear grade, or high histologic grade are present. The other exception is in patients with tubular and colloid histology, when chemotherapy is recommended for tumors are ≥3 cm in size and should be considered for tumors 1 to 2.9 cm in size. Trastuzumab is added to adjuvant therapy in HER2-positive tumors that are >1 cm or node-positive. Independent of its recommendations for adjuvant chemotherapy, the NCCN recommends that patients with receptor-positive tumors receive adjuvant endocrine therapy under the following circumstances: macrometastatic nodal disease; tumors >1 cm; and tumors 0.6 to 1.0 cm if moderately or poorly differentiated or with unfavorable features or possibly with such tumors with pN1mi disease. The NCCN recommends the use of AI over tamoxifen in postmenopausal women. When both adjuvant chemotherapy and endocrine therapy are indicated, therapy should be given sequentially, with endocrine therapy following chemotherapy (130).

Recommendations of the Tenth St. Gallen International Consensus Panel

The St. Gallen (Switzerland) Expert Consensus Panel on the primary therapy of early breast cancer meets every 2 years. In the report of the tenth consensus meeting (131), convened in March 2007, the panel reaffirmed the primary importance of determining endocrine responsiveness as the first approach in selecting systemic therapy. Three categories were recognized: highly endocrine responsive, incompletely endocrine responsive, and endocrine nonresponsive tumors. The panel accepted HER2-positivity to assign trastuzumab, and noted that adjuvant trastuzumab has only been assessed together with chemotherapy. They largely endorsed previous definitions of risk categories. The features in the *low-risk category* include tumors ≤2 cm, grade 1, absence of lymphovascular invasion or HER2 gene amplification, and age ≥35 years. The *intermediate-risk category* includes node-negative disease with tumors >2 cm or other un-favorable features absent in the low-risk category. Patients with one to three positive nodes are included in this group if the tumor expresses ER and/or PR and is *HER2*-negative. Disease with one to three positive nodes without these favorable features or disease involving four or more nodes constitutes the *high-risk category*. Among *HER2*-negative patients, those highly or incompletely endocrine responsive receive endocrine therapy; chemother-apy is also given in the intermediate- and high-risk categories. *HER2*-positive patients also receive trastuzumab. All patients in the endocrine nonresponsive group receive chemotherapy with trastuzumab added if *HER2* is positive. The main difference from the NCCN guidelines is that the St. Gallen panel does not recom-mend chemotherapy for some patients with tumors 1 to 2 cm; the NCCN guidelines call for chemotherapy for tumors >1 cm.

American Society of Clinical Oncology Guidelines on Hormonal Therapy

The ASCO guidelines (132) recommend AI, either initially or fol-lowing a period of tamoxifen (if patients are already taking it for 2 to 3 years) in all postmenopausal women with ER-positive breast cancer. Tamoxifen alone for 5 years is not adequate therapy for postmenopausal women. Letrozole and anastrozole are approved for initial adjuvant therapy, and exemestane is approved for early sequential therapy after 2 to 3 years of tamoxifen. Letrozole is the only approved AI for extended adjuvant therapy after 5 years of tamoxifen (100). The NCCN recommends the use of AI over tamoxifen in postmenopausal women.

CONCLUSIONS

Adjuvant systemic therapy has clearly been shown to improve OS in breast cancer. The standard approach is to tailor the aggres-siveness of the therapy to the risk of recurrence. The expertise lies in treating only those patients who will benefit significantly from chemotherapy and avoiding its use in patients in whom only marginal benefits are likely to accrue, thereby avoiding the toxicities of therapy and huge costs to the health care system. Pa-tients need to be actively involved in decision making and need to have a clear understanding of the risks and benefits of therapy.

Adjuvant therapy has advanced from the era of CMF to anthracyclines to taxane therapy with incremental survival ben-efits. The advent of trastuzumab and newer molecular agents like lapatinib and bevacizumab has provided new opportunities. The exciting genetic advances that help to define better predictors of the efficacy of therapy and recurrence risk may soon turn a new chapter in the management of early breast cancer. The "one size fits all" approach may soon be a concept of the past. In the future, patients are likely to be treated individually on the basis of their tumor genetic profiles.

REFERENCES

1. Jemal A, Siegel R, Ward E, et al. Cancer Statistics, 2008. *CA Cancer J Clin.* 2008;58(2):71–96.
2. McPherson K, Steel CM, Dixon JM. ABC of breast diseases. Breast cancer-epidemiology, risk factors, and genetics. *BMJ.* 2000;321 (7261):624–628.
3. Ries LAG, Eisner MP, Kosary CL, et al. *SEER Cancer Statistics Review 1975–2002.* Bethesda, MD: National Cancer Institute; 2005.
4. Lippman ME, Hayes DF. Adjuvant therapy for all patients with breast cancer? *J Nat Cancer Inst.* 2001;93:80–82.
5. Simes RJ, Coates AS. Patient preferences for adjuvant chemother-apy of early breast cancer: how much benefit is needed? *Journal of the National Cancer Institute Monographs.* 2001;(30):146–152.
6. Ravdin PM, Siminoff IA, Harvey JA. Survey of breast cancer pa-tients concerning their knowledge and expectations of adjuvant therapy. *Journal of Clinical Oncology.* 1998;16(2):515–521.
7. Berry DA, Cronin KA, Plevritis SK, et al. Effect of screening and adjuvant therapy on mortality from breast cancer. [see comment]. *New England Journal of Medicine.* 2005;353(17):1784–1792.
8. Forrow L, Taylor WC, Arnold RM. Absolutely relative: how re-search results are summarized can affect treatment decisions. *Am J Med.* 1992;92:121–124.
9. Malenka DJ, Baron JA, Johansen S, et al. The framing effect of rela-tive and absolute risk. *Journal of General Internal Medicine.* 1993;8: 543–548.
10. Elkin EB, Hudis C, Begg CB, et al. The effect of changes in tumor size on breast carcinoma survival in the U.S.: 1975–1999. [see comment]. *Cancer.* 2005;104(6):1149–1157.
11. Margolese RG, Hortabagyi GN, Bucholz TA. Neoplasms of the breast. In: Kufe DW, Pollock RE, Weichselbaum RR, et al. *Cancer Medicine,* 6th ed., Hamilton, Ontario, Canada: American Cancer Society and BC Decker. 2003; 1892.
12. Bezwoda WR, Esser JD, Dansey R, et al. The value of estrogen and progesterone receptor determinations in advanced breast cancer. Estrogen receptor level but not progesterone receptor level corre-lates with response to tamoxifen. *Cancer.* 1991;68(4):867–872.
13. Goldhirsch A, Glick JH, Gelber RD, et al. Meeting Highlights: International Expert Consensus on the Primary Therapy of Early Breast Cancer 2005. *Ann Oncol.* 2005;16(10):1569–1583.
14. Berry DA, Cirrincione C, Henderson IC, et al. Estrogen-receptor status and outcomes of modern chemotherapy for patients with node-positive breast cancer. *JAMA* 2006;295:1658–1667.
15. Paik S, Shak S, Tang G, et al. A multigene assay to predict recur-rence of tamoxifen-treated, node-negative breast cancer. *N Engl J Med.* 2004;351:2817–2826.
16. Sparano JA, Paik S. Development of the 21-gene assay and its ap-plication in clinical practice and clinical trials. *J Clin Oncol.* 2008; 26:721–728.
17. Habel LA, Shak S, Jacobs MK, et al. A population-based study of tumor gene expression and risk of breast cancer death among lymph node-negative patients. *Breast Cancer Research.* 2006;8(3): R25.
18. Paik S, Tang G, Shak S, et al. Gene expression and benefit of chemotherapy in women with node-negative, estrogen receptor-positive breast cancer. [see comment]. *Journal of Clinical Oncology.* 2006;24(23):3726–3734.
19. van de Vijver MJ, He YD, van't Veer LJ, et al. A gene-expression signature as a predictor of survival in breast cancer. *New England Journal of Medicine.* 2002;347(25):1999–2009.
20. Buyse M, Loi S, van't Veer L, et al. Validation and Clinical Utility of a 70-Gene Prognostic Signature for Women With Node-Negative Breast Cancer. *J Natl Cancer Inst.* 2006;98(17):1183–1192.
21. Bonadonna G, Brusamolino E, Valagussa P, et al. Combination chemotherapy as an adjuvant treatment in operable breast cancer. *New England Journal of Medicine.* 1976;294(8):405–410.
22. Bonadonna G, Moliterni A, Zambetti M, et al. 30 years' follow up of randomised studies of adjuvant CMF in operable breast cancer: cohort study. *BMJ* 2005;330(7485):217.
23. Early Breast Cancer Trialists Collaborative Group (EBCTCG). Ef-fects of chemotherapy and hormonal therapy for early breast

cancer on recurrence and 15-year survival: an overview of the randomised trials. *Lancet.* 2005;365:1687–1717.

24. Colleoni M, Litman HJ, Castiglione-Gertsch M, et al. Duration of adjuvant chemotherapy for breast cancer: a joint analysis of two randomised trials investigating three versus six courses of CMF. *British Journal of Cancer.* 2002;86(11):1705–1714.

25. Goldhirsch A, Coates AS, Colleoni M, et al. Adjuvant chemoendocrine therapy in postmenopausal breast cancer: cyclophosphamide, methotrexate, and fluorouracil dose and schedule may make a difference. International Breast Cancer Study Group. *Journal of Clinical Oncology.* 1998;16(4):1358–1362.

26. Fisher B, Brown AM, Dimitrov NV, et al. Two months of doxorubicin-cyclophosphamide with and without interval reinduction therapy compared with 6 months of cyclophosphamide, methotrexate, and fluorouracil in positive-node breast cancer patients with tamoxifen-nonresponsive tumors: results from the National Surgical Adjuvant Breast and Bowel Project B-15. *Journal of Clinical Oncology.* 1990;8(9):1483–1496.

27. Fisher B, Anderson S, Tan-Chiu E, et al. Tamoxifen and chemotherapy for axillary node-negative, estrogen receptor-negative breast cancer: findings from National Surgical Adjuvant Breast and Bowel Project B-23. *Journal of Clinical Oncology.* 2001;19(4):931–942.

28. Coombes RC, Bliss JM, Wils J, et al. Adjuvant cyclophosphamide, methotrexate, and fluorouracil versus fluorouracil, epirubicin, and cyclophosphamide chemotherapy in premenopausal women with axillary node-positive operable breast cancer: results of a randomized trial. The International Collaborative Cancer Group. *J Clin Oncol.* 1996;14:35–45.

29. Levine MN, Pritchard KI, Bramwell VHC, et al. Randomized trial comparing cyclophosphamide, epirubicin, and fluorouracil with cyclophosphamide, methotrexate, and fluorouracil in premenopausal women with node-positive breast cancer: update of National Cancer Institute of Canada Clinical Trials Group Trial MA5. *Journal of Clinical Oncology.* 2005;23(22):5166–5170.

30. Hutchins LF, Green SJ, Ravdin PM, et al. Randomized, controlled trial of cyclophosphamide, methotrexate, and fluorouracil versus cyclophosphamide, doxorubicin, and fluorouracil with and without tamoxifen for high-risk, node-negative breast cancer: treatment results of Intergroup Protocol INT-0102. *Journal of Clinical Oncology.* 2005;23(33):8313–8321.

31. Crown J. Docetaxel: Overview of an Active Drug for Breast Cancer. *Oncologist.* 2001;6(90003):1–4.

32. Diaz JF, Andreu JM. Assembly of purified GDP-tubulin into microtubules induced by taxol and taxotere: reversibility, ligand stoichiometry, and competition. *Biochemistry.* 1993;32(11):2747–2755.

33. Henderson IC, Berry DA, Demetri GD, et al. Improved outcomes from adding sequential Paclitaxel but not from escalating Doxorubicin dose in an adjuvant chemotherapy regimen for patients with node-positive primary breast cancer. *Journal of Clinical Oncology.* 2003;21(6):976–983.

34. Mamounas EP, Bryant J, Lembersky B, et al. Paclitaxel after doxorubicin plus cyclophosphamide as adjuvant chemotherapy for node-positive breast cancer: results from NSABP B-28. *J Clin Oncol.* 2005;23:3686–3696.

35. Sparano JA, Wang M, Martino S, et al. Weekly paclitaxel in the adjuvant treatment of breast cancer. *New England Journal of Medicine.* 2008;358:1663–1671.

36. Martin M, Pienkowski T, Mackey J, et al. Adjuvant docetaxel for node-positive breast cancer. *New England Journal of Medicine.* 2005;352(22):2302–2313.

37. Roche H, Fumoleau P, Spielmann M, et al. Sequential adjuvant epirubicin-based and docetaxel chemotherapy for node-positive breast cancer patients: the FNCLCC PACS 01 Trial. *Journal of Clinical Oncology.* 2006;24(36):5664–5671.

38. Goldstein LJ, O'Neill A, Sparano J, et al. E2197: Phase III AT (doxorubicin/docetaxel) vs. AC (doxorubicin/cyclophosphamide) in the adjuvant treatment of node positive and high risk node negative breast cancer. *J Clin Oncol* (Meeting Abstracts) 2005; 23(16_suppl):512.

39. Brain EGC, Bachelot T, Serin D, et al. Life-threatening sepsis associated with adjuvant doxorubicin plus docetaxel for intermediate-risk breast cancer. *JAMA.* 2005;293:2367–2371.

40. Jones SE, Savin MA, Holmes FA, et al. Phase III trial comparing doxorubicin plus cyclophosphamide with docetaxel plus cyclophosphamide as adjuvant therapy for operable breast cancer. *Journal of Clinical Oncology.* 2006;24(34):5381–5387.

41. Fisher B, Bryant J, Wolmark N, et al. Effect of preoperative chemotherapy on the outcome of women with operable breast cancer. *Journal of Clinical Oncology.* 1998;16(8):2672–2685.

42. Bear HD, Anderson S, Smith RE, et al. Sequential preoperative or postoperative docetaxel added to preoperative doxorubicin plus cyclophosphamide for operable breast cancer: National Surgical Adjuvant Breast and Bowel Project Protocol B-27. *Journal of Clinical Oncology.* 2006;24(13):2019–2027.

43. Rouzier R, Extra JM, Carton M, et al. Primary chemotherapy for operable breast cancer: incidence and prognostic significance of ipsilateral breast tumor recurrence after breast-conserving surgery. *Journal of Clinical Oncology.* 2001;19(18):3828–3835.

44. Mauri D, Pavlidis N, Ioannidis JPA. Neoadjuvant versus adjuvant systemic treatment in breast cancer: a meta-analysis. *Journal of the National Cancer Institute.* 2005;97(3):188–194.

45. Fisher B, Redmond C, Legault-Poisson S, et al. Postoperative chemotherapy and tamoxifen compared with tamoxifen alone in the treatment of positive-node breast cancer patients aged 50 years and older with tumors responsive to tamoxifen: results from the National Surgical Adjuvant Breast and Bowel Project B-16. *Journal of Clinical Oncology.* 1990;8(6):1005–1018.

46. Albain KS, Green SJ, Ravdin PM, et al. Adjuvant chemohormonal therapy for primary breast cancer should be sequential instead of concurrent: initial results from intergroup trial 0100 (SWOG-8814) [abstract 143]. *Proc Am Soc Clin Oncol.* 2002;21.

47. Fisher B, Dignam J, Wolmark N, et al. Tamoxifen and chemotherapy for lymph node-negative, estrogen receptor-positive breast cancer. *Journal of the National Cancer Institute.* 1997;89(22):1673–1682.

48. International Breast Cancer Study Group (IBCSG). Endocrine Responsiveness and Tailoring Adjuvant Therapy for Postmenopausal Lymph Node-Negative Breast Cancer: A Randomized Trial. *J Natl Cancer Inst.* 2002;94(14):1054–1065.

49. Vinh-Hung V, Royce M. Age patterns of mortality in early breast cancer: A graphical presentation (abstract). In: San Antonio Breast Cancer Symposium; 2004 December 8–11, 2004.

50. Carlson RW, Brown E, Burstein HJ, et al. NCCN Task Force Report: Adjuvant Therapy for Breast Cancer. Journal of the National Comprehensive *Cancer Network.* 2006;4 Suppl 1:S1–S26.

51. Norton L. A Gompertzian model of human breast cancer growth. *Cancer Research.* 1988;48(24 Pt 1):7067–7071.

52. Citron ML, Berry DA, Cirrincione C, et al. Randomized trial of dose-dense versus conventionally scheduled and sequential versus concurrent combination chemotherapy as postoperative adjuvant treatment of node-positive primary breast cancer: first report of Intergroup Trial C9741/Cancer and Leukemia Group B Trial 9741. *J Clin Oncol.* 2003;21:1431–1439.

53. Venturini M, Del Mastro L, Aitini E, et al. Dose-dense adjuvant chemotherapy in early breast cancer patients: results from a randomized trial. *Journal of the National Cancer Institute.* 2005; 97(23):1724–1733.

54. Kerbel RS, Kamen BA. The anti-angiogenic basis of metronomic chemotherapy. *Nature Reviews Cancer.* 2004;4(6):423–436.

55. Bello L, Carrabba G, Giussani C, et al. Low-dose chemotherapy combined with an antiangiogenic drug reduces human glioma growth in vivo. *Cancer Research.* 2001;61(20):7501–7506.

56. Stoll BR, Migliorini C, Kadambi A, et al. A mathematical model of the contribution of endothelial progenitor cells to angiogenesis in tumors: implications for antiangiogenic therapy. *Blood.* 2003;102(7):2555–2561.

57. Shannon C, Ashley S, Smith IE. Does timing of adjuvant chemotherapy for early breast cancer influence survival? *Journal of Clinical Oncology.* 2003;21(20):3792–3797.

58. Colleoni M, Bonetti M, Coates AS, et al. Early Start of Adjuvant Chemotherapy May Improve Treatment Outcome for Premenopausal Breast Cancer Patients with Tumors not Expressing Estrogen Receptors. *J Clin Oncol.* 2000;18(3):584.

59. Bellon JR, Come SE, Gelman RS, et al. Sequencing of chemotherapy and radiation therapy in early-stage breast cancer: updated results of a prospective randomized trial. *J Clin Oncol.* 2005;23:1934–1940.

60. Yarden Y, Sliwkowski MX. Untangling the ErbB signalling network. *Nature Reviews Molecular Cell Biology.* 2001;2(2):127–137.

61. Burstein HJ. The distinctive nature of HER2-positive breast cancers. [comment]. *New England Journal of Medicine.* 2005;353(16):1652–1654.

62. Slamon DJ, Clark GM, Wong SG, et al. Human breast cancer: correlation of relapse and survival with amplification of the HER-2/neu oncogene. *Science.* 1987;235(4785):177–182.

63. Romond EH, Perez EA, Bryant J, et al. Trastuzumab plus adjuvant chemotherapy for operable HER2-positive breast cancer. *New England Journal of Medicine.* 2005;353(16):1673–1684.

64. Gonzalez-Angulo AM, Hortobagyi GN, Esteva FJ. Adjuvant therapy with trastuzumab for HER-2/neu-positive breast cancer. *Oncologist.* 2006;11(8):857–867.

65. Wolff AC, Hammond MEH, Schwartz JN, et al. American Society of Clinical Oncology/College of American Pathologists guideline recommendations for human epidermal growth factor receptor 2 testing in breast cancer. *Journal of Clinical Oncology.* 2007;25(1):118–145.

66. Joensuu H, Kellokumpu-Lehtinen P-L, Bono P, et al. Adjuvant docetaxel or vinorelbine with or without trastuzumab for breast cancer. *New England Journal of Medicine.* 2006;354(8):809–820.

67. Piccart-Gebhart MJ, Procter M, Leyland-Jones B, et al. Trastuzumab after adjuvant chemotherapy in HER2-positive breast cancer. *N Engl J Med.* 2005;353:1659–1672.

68. Slamon D EWea. Phase III randomized trial comparing doxorubicin and cyclophosphamide followed by docetaxel, with doxorubicin and cyclophosphamide followed by docetaxel and trastuzumab, with docetaxel, carboplatin and trastuzumab in HER2 positive early breast cancer patients: BCIRG 006 study. *Breast Cancer Res Treat.* 2005;94(suppl 1):S5.

69. Smith I, Procter M, Gelber RD, et al. 2-year follow-up of trastuzumab after adjuvant chemotherapy in HER2-positive breast cancer: a randomised controlled trial. [see comment]. *Lancet.* 2007;369(9555):29–36.

70. Perez EA, Romond EH, Suman VJ, et al. Updated results of the combined analysis of NCCTG N9831 and NSABP B-31 adjuvant chemotherapy with/without trastuzumab in patients with HER2-positive breast cancer. *J Clin Oncol* (Meeting Abstracts) 2007;25(18 suppl):512.

71. Slamon D, Eiermann W, Robert N, et al. BCIRG 006: 2nd interim analysis phase III randomized trial comparing doxorubicin and cyclophosphamide followed by docetaxel (AC→T) with doxorubicin and cyclophosphamide followed by docetaxel and trastuzumab (AC→TH) with docetaxel, carboplatin and trastuzumab (TCH) in Her2neu positive early breast cancer patients. Paper presented at: 29th Annual San Antonio Breast Cancer Symposium; December 14-17, 2006; San Antonio, TX. Abstract 52. Available at: http://www.abstracts2view.com/sabcs06/view.php?nu=SABCS06L_78.

72. Burstein HJ, Harris LN, Gelman R, et al. Preoperative therapy with trastuzumab and paclitaxel followed by sequential adjuvant doxorubicin/cyclophosphamide for HER2 overexpressing stage II or III breast cancer: a pilot study. *J Clin Oncol.* 2003;21:46–53.

73. Carey LA, et al. Response to trastuzumab with paclitaxel immediately following 4AC as initial therapy for primary breast cancer. *Breast Cancer Res Treatment.* 2002;76 (Suppl 1)(109):Abstract 424.

74. Buzdar AU VV, Ibrahim N, et al. Prospective data of additional patients treated with neoadjuvant therapy treated with paclitaxel followed by FEC chemotherapy with trastuzumab in HER-2 positive operable breast cancer, and an update of initial study population. In: San Antonio Breast Cancer Symposium; December 2005; December 2005.

75. Hassett MJ, O'Malley AJ, Pakes JR, et al. Frequency and cost of chemotherapy-related serious adverse effects in a population sample of women with breast cancer. *Journal of the National Cancer Institute.* 2006;98(16):1108–1117.

76. Smith TJ, Khatcheressian J, Lyman GH, et al. 2006 update of recommendations for the use of white blood cell growth factors: an evidence-based clinical practice guideline. *Journal of Clinical Oncology.* 2006;24(19):3187–3205.

77. Demark-Wahnefried W, Winer EP, Rimer BK. Why women gain weight with adjuvant chemotherapy for breast cancer. *Journal of Clinical Oncology.* 1993;11(7):1418–1429.

78. Sadler IJ, Jacobsen PB. Progress in understanding fatigue associated with breast cancer treatment. *Cancer Invest.* 2001;19:723–731.

79. Holmberg L, Anderson H. HABITS (hormonal replacement therapy after breast cancer–is it safe?), a randomised comparison: trial stopped. *Lancet.* 2004;363(9407):453–455.

80. Grunfeld E, Dhesy-Thind S, Levine M. Steering Committee on Clinical Practice Guidelines for the Care and Treatment of Breast C. Clinical practice guidelines for the care and treatment of breast cancer: follow-up after treatment for breast cancer (summary of the 2005 update). *CMAJ Canadian Medical Association Journal.* 2005;172(10):1319–1320.

81. Parulekar WR, Day AG, Ottaway JA, et al. Incidence and prognostic impact of amenorrhea during adjuvant therapy in high-risk premenopausal breast cancer: analysis of a National Cancer Institute of Canada Clinical Trials Group Study–NCIC CTG MA.5. *Journal of Clinical Oncology.* 2005;23(25):6002–6008.

82. Curtis RE, Boice JD, Jr., Stovall M, et al. Risk of leukemia after chemotherapy and radiation treatment for breast cancer. *New England Journal of Medicine.* 1992;326(26):1745–1751.

83. Smith RE, Bryant J, DeCillis A, et al. National Surgical Adjuvant Breast and Bowel Project E. Acute myeloid leukemia and myelodysplastic syndrome after doxorubicin-cyclophosphamide adjuvant therapy for operable breast cancer: the National Surgical Adjuvant Breast and Bowel Project Experience. *Journal of Clinical Oncology.* 2003;21(7):1195–1204.

84. Pui CH, Relling MV. Topoisomerase II inhibitor-related acute myeloid leukaemia. *Br J Haematol.* 2000;109:13–23.

85. Von Hoff DD, Layard MW, Basa P, et al. Risk factors for doxorubicin-induced congestive heart failure. *Annals of Internal Medicine.* 1979;91(5):710–717.

86. Swain SM, Whaley FS, Ewer MS. Congestive heart failure in patients treated with doxorubicin: a retrospective analysis of three trials. *Cancer.* 2003;97(11):2869–2879.

87. Perez EA, Rodeheffer R. Clinical cardiac tolerability of trastuzumab. *Journal of Clinical Oncology.* 2004;22(2):322–329.

88. Vogel CL, Cobleigh MA, Tripathy D, et al. Efficacy and Safety of Trastuzumab as a Single Agent in First-Line Treatment of HER2-Overexpressing Metastatic Breast Cancer. *J Clin Oncol.* 2002;20(3):719–726.

89. Slamon DJ, Leyland-Jones B, Shak S, et al. Use of chemotherapy plus a monoclonal antibody against HER2 for metastatic breast cancer that overexpresses HER2. *New England Journal of Medicine.* 2001;344(11):783-792.

90. Seidman A, Hudis C, Pierri MK, et al. Cardiac Dysfunction in the Trastuzumab Clinical Trials Experience. *J Clin Oncol.* 2002;20(5):1215–1221.

91. Baselga J, Perez EA, Pienkowski T, et al. Adjuvant Trastuzumab: A Milestone in the Treatment of HER-2-Positive Early Breast Cancer. *Oncologist.* 2006;11(suppl_1):4–12.

92. Ewer MS, Vooletich MT, Durand J-B, et al. Reversibility of trastuzumab-related cardiotoxicity: new insights based on clinical course and response to medical treatment. *J Clin Oncol.* 2005;23:7820–7826.

93. Winer EP, Piccart-Gebhart MJ, Rugo HS. Management of HER-2 positive breast cancer. *American Society of Clinical Oncology.* 2006.

94. Early Breast Cancer Trialists' Collaborative Group. Systemic treatment of early breast cancer by hormonal, cytotoxic, or immune therapy: 133 randomised trials involving 31,000 recurrences and 24,000 deaths among 75,000 women. *The Lancet.* 1992; 339(8784):1–15.

95. Chan TW, Pollak M, Huynh H. Inhibition of insulin-like growth factor signaling pathways in mammary gland by pure anti-estrogen ICl 182,780. *Clinical Cancer Research.* 2001;7(8):2545–2554.

96. Gruvberger-Saal SK, Bendahl P-O, Saal LH, et al. Estrogen Receptor {beta} Expression Is Associated with Tamoxifen Response in ER{alpha}-Negative Breast Carcinoma. *Clin Cancer Res.* 2007;13(7):1987–1994.

97. Fisher B, Dignam J, Bryant J, et al. Five versus more than five years of tamoxifen for lymph node-negative breast cancer: updated findings from the National Surgical Adjuvant Breast and Bowel Project B-14 randomized trial. [see comment]. *Journal of the National Cancer Institute.* 2001;93(9):684–690.

98. Stewart HJ, Forrest AP, Everington D, et al. Randomised comparison of 5 years of adjuvant tamoxifen with continuous therapy for operable breast cancer. The Scottish Cancer Trials Breast Group. *British Journal of Cancer.* 1996;74(2):297–299.

99. Tormey DC, Gray R, Falkson HC. Postchemotherapy adjuvant tamoxifen therapy beyond five years in patients with lymph node-positive breast cancer. Eastern Cooperative Oncology Group. *J Natl Cancer Inst.* 1996;88:1828–1833.

100. Perez EA. Appraising adjuvant aromatase inhibitor therapy. *Oncologist.* 2006;11(10):1058–1069.

101. Bentzen SM, Skoczylas JZ, Overgaard M, et al. Radiotherapy-related lung fibrosis enhanced by tamoxifen. *Journal of the National Cancer Institute.* 1996;88(13):918–922.

102. Wazer DE, DiPetrillo T, Schmidt-Ullrich R, et al. Factors influencing cosmetic outcome and complication risk after conservative surgery and radiotherapy for early-stage breast carcinoma. *Journal of Clinical Oncology.* 1992;10(3):356–363.

103. Ahn PH, Vu HT, Lannin D, et al. Sequence of radiotherapy with tamoxifen in conservatively managed breast cancer does not affect local relapse rates. *Journal of Clinical Oncology.* 2005;23(1):17–23.

104. Harris EER, Christensen VJ, Hwang W-T, et al. Impact of concurrent versus sequential tamoxifen with radiation therapy in early-stage breast cancer patients undergoing breast conservation treatment. *Journal of Clinical Oncology.* 2005;23(1):11–16.

105. Castiglione-Gertsch M, O'Neill A, Price KN, et al. Adjuvant chemotherapy followed by goserelin versus either modality alone for premenopausal lymph node-negative breast cancer: a randomized trial. *J Natl Cancer Inst.* 2003;95(24):1833–1846.

106. Jakesz R, Hausmaninger H, Kubista E, et al. Randomized adjuvant trial of tamoxifen and goserelin versus cyclophosphamide, methotrexate, and fluorouracil: evidence for the superiority of treatment with endocrine blockade in premenopausal patients with hormone-responsive breast cancer–Austrian Breast and Colorectal Cancer Study Group Trial 5. *Journal of Clinical Oncology.* 2002;20(24):4621–4627.

107. Boccardo F, Rubagotti A, Amoroso D, et al. Cyclophosphamide, methotrexate, and fluorouracil versus tamoxifen plus ovarian suppression as adjuvant treatment of estrogen receptor-positive pre-/perimenopausal breast cancer patients: results of the Italian Breast Cancer Adjuvant Study Group 02 randomized trial. *Journal of Clinical Oncology.* 2000;18(14):2718–2727.

108. Suppression of Ovarian Function Trial (SOFT). A Phase III trial evaluating the role of ovarian function suppression (OFS) and the role of exemestane as adjuvant therapies for premenopausal women with endocrine-responsive breast cancer. Tamoxifen *versus* OFS + tamoxifen versus OFS + exemestane. BIG 2–02/IBCSG Trial 24–02. Available at International Breast Cancer Study Group (IBCSG website, http:/www.ibcsg,org).

109. Tamoxifen and Exemestane Trial (TEXT). A Phase III trial evaluating the role of exemestane plus GnRH analogue as adjuvant therapy for premenopausal women with endocrine-responsive breast cancer. Ovarian function suppression + tamoxifen *versus* ovarian function suppression + exemestane. BIG 3–02/IBCSG Trial 25–02. Available at International Breast Cancer Study Group (IBCSG website, http:/www.ibcsg,org.

110. Premenopausal Endocrine Responsive Chemotherapy Trial (PERCHE). A phase III trial evaluating the role of chemotherapy as adjuvant therapy for premenopausal women with endocrine-responsive breast cancer who receive endocrine therapy. http:/www.ibcsg,org. Accessed April 23, 2009.

111. Howell A, Cuzick J, Baum M, et al. Results of the ATAC (Arimidex, Tamoxifen, Alone or in Combination) trial after completion of 5 years' adjuvant treatment for breast cancer. *Lancet.* 2005;365(9453):60–62.

112. Dowsett M, Cuzick J, Wale C, et al. Retrospective analysis of time to recurrence in the ATAC trial according to hormone receptor status: an hypothesis-generating study. *Journal of Clinical Oncology.* 2005;23(30):7512–7517.

113. Thurlimann B, Keshaviah A, Coates AS, et al. A comparison of letrozole and tamoxifen in postmenopausal women with early breast cancer. *New England Journal of Medicine.* 2005;353(26):2747–2757.

114. Coates AS, Keshaviah A, Thurlimann B, et al. Five Years of Letrozole Compared With Tamoxifen As Initial Adjuvant Therapy for Postmenopausal Women With Endocrine-Responsive Early Breast Cancer: Update of Study BIG 1-98. *J Clin Oncol.* 2007;25(5):486–492.

115. Coombes RC, Hall E, Gibson LJ, et al. A randomized trial of exemestane after two to three years of tamoxifen therapy in postmenopausal women with primary breast cancer. *N Engl J Med.* 2004;350:1081–1092.

116. Boccardo F, Rubagotti A, Puntoni M, et al. Switching to Anastrozole Versus Continued Tamoxifen Treatment of Early Breast Cancer: Preliminary Results of the Italian Tamoxifen Anastrozole Trial. *J Clin Oncol.* 2005;23(22):5138–5147.

117. Kaufmann M, Jonat W, Hilfrich J, et al. Survival benefit of switching to anastrozole after 2 years' treatment with tamoxifen versus continued tamoxifen therapy: The ARNO 95 study. *J Clin Oncol* (Meeting Abstracts) 2006;24(18 suppl):547.

118. Coombes RC, Paridaens R, Jassem J, et al. First mature analysis of the Intergroup Exemestane Study. *J Clin Oncol* (Meeting Abstracts) 2006;24(18 suppl):LBA527.

119. Goss PE, Ingle JN, Martino S, et al. A randomized trial of letrozole in postmenopausal women after five years of tamoxifen therapy for early-stage breast cancer. *New England Journal of Medicine.* 2003;349(19):1793–1802.

120. Ingle JN, Tu D, Pater JL, et al. Duration of letrozole treatment and outcomes in the placebo-controlled NCIC CTG MA.17 extended adjuvant therapy trial. *Breast Cancer Res Treat.* 2006;99(3):295–300.

121. Perez EA, Josse RG, Pritchard KI, et al. Effect of letrozole versus placebo on bone mineral density in women with primary breast cancer completing 5 or more years of adjuvant tamoxifen: a companion study to NCIC CTG MA.17. *Journal of Clinical Oncology.* 2006;24(22):3629–3635.

122. Ravdin PM, Siminoff LA, Davis GJ, et al. Computer program to assist in making decisions about adjuvant therapy for women with early breast cancer. *J Clin Oncol.* 2001;19:980–991.

123. Olivotto IA, Bajdik CD, Ravdin PM, et al. Population-based validation of the prognostic model ADJUVANT! for early breast cancer. *Journal of Clinical Oncology.* 2005;23(12):2716–2725.

124. Lundin J, Lundin M, Isola J, et al. A web-based system for individualised survival estimation in breast cancer. *BMJ* 2003; 326(7379):29.

125. Geyer CE, Forster J, Lindquist D, et al. Lapatinib plus capecitabine for HER2-positive advanced breast cancer. *New England Journal of Medicine.* 2006;355(26):2733–2743.

126. Lin NU, Carey LA, Liu MC, et al. Phase II trial of lapatinib for brain metastases in patients with human epidermal growth factor receptor 2-positive breast cancer. *J Clin Oncol.* 2008;26:1993–1999.

127. Roy V, Perez EA. New therapies in the treatment of breast cancer. *Seminars in Oncology.* 2006;33(3 Suppl 9):S3–S8.

128. Miller KD, Chap LI, Holmes FA, et al. Randomized phase III trial of capecitabine compared with bevacizumab plus capecitabine in patients with previously treated metastatic breast cancer. *Journal of Clinical Oncology.* 2005;23(4):792–799.

129. Miller K, Wang M, Gralow J, et al. Paclitaxel plus bevacizumab versus paclitaxel alone for metastatic breast cancer. *N Engl J Med.* 2007;357: 2666–2676.

130. NCCN Clinical Practice Guidelines in Oncology. *Breast Cancer* V.2.2008. Available at www.nccn.org.

131. Goldhirsch A, Wood WC, Gelber RD, et al.; 10th St. Gallen conference. Progress and promise: highlights of the international expert consensus on the primary therapy of early breast cancer 2007. *Ann Oncol.* 2007;18:1133–1144.

132. American Society of Clinical Oncology Technology Assessment on the Use of Aromatase Inhibitors As Adjuvant Therapy for Postmenopausal Women With Hormone Receptor-Positive Breast Cancer: Status Report 2004. Available at www.asco.org.

COMMENTARY
Mary E. Cianfrocca and William J. Gradishar

Dr. Perez and colleagues provide an excellent overview of adjuvant therapy for early-stage breast cancer, covering prognostic/predictive factors, decision-making tools, as well as treatment options using chemotherapy, endocrine therapy, and trastuzumab. As the authors point out, the widespread application of adjuvant therapy has contributed to the reduction in breast cancer-related deaths in the United States (1). Some of the largest advances in adjuvant therapy, in terms of mortality reductions, have been in endocrine therapy for estrogen receptor (ER)-positive women (2). The most recent Early Breast Cancer Trialists' Collaborative Group (EBCTCG) overview analysis demonstrated that 5 years of adjuvant tamoxifen reduced the annual death rate by 31% among ER-positive women regardless of age. Approximately 75% of postmenopausal and 50% of premenopausal breast cancers are ER-positive, leading to a large percentage of breast cancer patients able to benefit from advances in endocrine therapy.

In postmenopausal women, the use of aromatase inhibitors (AIs) has become standard practice. The American Society of Clinical Oncology Technology Assessment Panel in 2004 concluded that optimal adjuvant endocrine therapy for a postmenopausal, ER-positive woman should include an AI either as initial therapy or after a period of tamoxifen treatment (3). The panel left open the questions of optimal AI (three are commercially available in the United States) as well as the optimal treatment regimen. As a survival benefit has been observed in trials of 2 to 3 years of tamoxifen followed by 2 to 3 years of an AI (4–6), 5 years of tamoxifen for postmenopausal women is no longer considered to be the optimal strategy. It is currently unknown, though, whether 5 years of an AI is superior to 2 to 3 years of tamoxifen followed by 2 to 3 years of an AI. Although several theoretical models examining the optimal therapy sequence (AI upfront vs. tamoxifen followed by an AI) have been proposed, their validity in clinical decision making remains uncertain (7,8). The Breast International Group (BIG) 1-98 trial will hopefully answer the question of optimal sequencing in a prospective fashion as the trial randomized postmenopausal women with ER-positive breast cancer to one of four arms: 5 years of tamoxifen; 5 years of letrozole; 2 years of tamoxifen followed by 3 years of letrozole; or 2 years of letrozole followed by 3 years of tamoxifen (9).

For premenopausal women, 5 years of tamoxifen remains the standard adjuvant therapy recommendation. A significant issue in these women, however, is tamoxifen metabolism. Tamoxifen undergoes extensive primary and secondary metabolism, and data suggest that a specific tamoxifen metabolite, 4-hydroxy-N-desmethyl tamoxifen (endoxifen) contributes significantly to the anticancer effect of this agent (10). Endoxifen is primarily formed by the CYP2D6-mediated oxidation of N-desmethyl-tamoxifen (11). Women who either possess genetic variants leading to low or absent CYP2D6 activity or who receive concomitant medications that inhibit CYP2D6 activity have significantly lower levels of endoxifen (12). Goetz et al. (13) recently demonstrated that women with the CYP2D6*4/*4 genotype have a lower incidence of hot flashes and a higher risk of disease relapse, suggesting that variations in tamoxifen metabolism have clinical implications.

The role of AIs in premenopausal women is investigational and being explored in multiple trials as discussed by Dr. Perez and colleagues. The usefulness of ovarian suppression (OS) is also an area of active investigation. Numerous trials have addressed the role of OS as a substitute for cytotoxic chemotherapy; however, interpretation of these trials is hampered by multiple factors, including mixed populations of ER-positive and

ER-negative patients, lack of tamoxifen in the chemotherapy arms, lack of an anthracycline in the majority of the trials, and lack of a taxane in all of the trials. The general interpretation of these trials is that combined endocrine therapy with OS and tamoxifen is likely comparable to chemotherapy with cyclophosphamide, methotrexate, and 5-fluorouracil (CMF) (14–21).

As Dr. Perez and colleagues noted, a portion of the benefit of adjuvant chemotherapy in premenopausal women has been attributed to its common side effect of ovarian failure. Chemotherapy may lead to a temporary or permanent cessation of ovarian function. Resumption of menses after chemotherapy may occur after a prolonged period of time, even after 2 to 3 years of amenorrhea (22). Very young women are less likely than older premenopausal women to develop permanent amenorrhea as a consequence of adjuvant chemotherapy (23). In a recent analysis of 166 patients ≤40 years of age treated with anthracycline and taxane-based chemotherapy, 15% developed long-term amenorrhea (≥12 months) and 85% resumed menstruation (24). Furthermore, data suggest that very young (age <35), ER-positive women primarily treated with chemotherapy have a statistically significantly higher risk of relapse than older premenopausal patients, while younger and older premenopausal, ER-negative patients had similar outcomes (25). For women <35 years of age who did not have chemotherapy-induced amenorrhea, 10-year disease-free survival (DFS) was 23% compared with 38% for those with amenorrhea. These observations are hypothesis-generating and suggest that young premenopausal women with ER-positive disease who fail to develop complete ovarian failure after chemotherapy may potentially benefit from OS. This hypothesis has been examined in multiple trials. However, these trials had diverse entry criteria with some allowing ER-negative or unknown tumors as well as differing chemotherapy regimens.

The International Breast Cancer Study Group (IBCSG) Trial VIII randomized 1,063 pre- or perimenopausal, node-negative women to one of three regimens: goserelin every 28 days for 24 months, six cycles of CMF, or six cycles of CMF followed by goserelin every 28 days for 18 months (15). Goserelin (Zoladex) is an injectable gonadotropin-releasing hormone (GnRH) agonist that produces ovarian suppression (26). Among patients aged ≥40 years, more than 90% were amenorrheic by the end of CMF therapy. In contrast, for the women aged ≤39 years, chemotherapy led to amenorrhea in only 50% by the end of CMF therapy, and among the patients in this age group not randomized to goserelin, menses resumed in approximately 15%. Overall, for patients with ER-positive disease, there was a trend toward improvement in 5-year DFS with CMF followed by goserelin compared with CMF alone (86% vs. 81%; confidence interval = 82%-91%). The benefit of the sequential regimen increased as the median age of the patient subpopulation decreased below 43 years of age. Although the goserelin-alone group had a marked improvement or less deterioration in quality of life (QOL) measures over the first 6 months compared with CMF-treated patients, QOL was similar for CMF alone and CMF followed by goserelin (27).

The Intergroup trial 0101/ECOG5188 led by the Eastern Cooperative Oncology Group randomized 1,504 premenopausal, node-positive women to three arms: cyclophosphamide, doxorubicin, and 5-fluorouracil (CAF) alone, CAF

plus 5 years of monthly goserelin, or CAF plus 5 years of tamoxifen and monthly goserelin (28). Unfortunately, there was no arm of CAF plus tamoxifen without goserelin. A significant benefit was seen for the addition of tamoxifen to CAF plus goserelin but not for the addition of goserelin alone to CAF. In an exploratory subset analysis, however, a possible trend for benefit for goserelin after CAF was observed in women younger than 40 years of age (9-year DFS of 55% vs. 48%).

The ZIPP (Zoladex in Premenopausal Patients) was a four-arm trial using a 2 × 2 factorial design to compare 2 years of therapy with tamoxifen, goserelin, or tamoxifen plus goserelin. An event-free and overall survival benefit was observed in the goserelin arms that was less pronounced in patients treated with tamoxifen or chemotherapy (28).

However, not all trials have shown a benefit for OS after chemotherapy. The Adjuvant Breast Cancer (ABC) Ovarian Ablation or Suppression Trial randomized 2,144 pre- or perimenopausal women with early-stage breast cancer receiving 5 years of tamoxifen with or without chemotherapy to ovarian ablation versus no ovarian ablation (29). There was no significant benefit for ovarian ablation even in the subgroup of women younger than 40 years of age.

OS is not without potential toxicities, which may include weight gain, sexual dysfunction, and hot flashes. Although some physicians and patients perceive OS as being associated with less toxicity than chemotherapy, this is not necessarily the case. The Danish Breast Cancer Cooperative Group (DBCG) trial 89-B randomized premenopausal, ER-positive women with early-stage breast cancer to nine cycles of CMF versus oophorectomy (30). A subgroup of 317 patients was invited to participate in a longitudinal QOL study with assessments at 1, 3, 5, 9, 15, and 24 months after randomization. After 2 years, 75% had completed all six questionnaires. Overall, while the chemotherapy-treated patients reported more symptoms at the first three time points, there were few differences between the two groups at later assessments. During treatment, chemotherapy patients reported a larger detrimental effect on cognitive functioning, social function, and global health status/QOL than patients who underwent oophorectomy. Some symptoms such as weight gain and anticipatory nausea persisted after chemotherapy was completed. The women who underwent oophorectomy, on the other hand, reported more pronounced hot flashes and sweats during the first 9 months after randomization. For some QOL aspects such as physical function, role function, emotional function, anxiety, work, and sexual functioning, there was no difference between the two groups.

At present, OS should not be routinely used either as a substitute for, or in addition to, adjuvant chemotherapy. Multiple clinical trials, including the Suppression of Ovarian Function Trial (SOFT) as well as the Tamoxifen and Exemestane Trial (TEXT) address the issue of adjuvant OS and will hopefully clarify the potential role of this modality for premenopausal women.

REFERENCES

1. Berry DA, Cronin KA, Plevritis SK, et al. Effect of screening and adjuvant therapy on mortality from breast cancer. *N Engl J Med.* 2005;353:1784–1792.

2. Effects of chemotherapy and hormonal therapy for early breast cancer on recurrence and 15-year survival: an overview of the randomized trials. *Lancet.* 2005;365:1687–1717.

3. Winer E, Hudis C, Burstein HJ, et al. American Society of Clinical Oncology technology assessment on the use of aromatase inhibitors as adjuvant therapy for postmenopausal women with hormone receptor-positive breast cancer: status report 2004. *J Clin Oncol.* 2004;23:619–629.

4. Coombes RC, Paridaens R, Jassem J, et al. First mature analysis of the Intergroup Exemestane Study [abstract]. *J Clin Oncol.* 2006;24 (18 Suppl):527.

5. Kaufmann M, Jonat W, Hilfrich J, et al. Survival benefit of switching to anastrazole after 2 years of treatment with tamoxifen versus continued tamoxifen therapy: The ARNO 95 study [abstract]. *J Clin Oncol.* 2006;24(18 Suppl):547.

6. Jonat W, Gnanat M, Boccardo F, et al. Effectiveness of switching from adjuvant tamoxifen to anastrazole in postmenopausal women with hormone-sensitive early-stage breast cancer: a meta-analysis. *Lancet Oncol.* 2007;7:991–996.

7. Punglia RS, Kuntz KM, Winer EP, et al. Optimizing adjuvant endocrine therapy in postmenopausal women with early stage breast cancer: a decision analysis. *J Clin Oncol.* 2005;23:5178–5187.

8. Cuzick J, Howell A. Optimal timing of an aromatase inhibitor in the adjuvant treatment of postmenopausal hormone receptor-positive breast cancer [abstract 658]. *Proc Am Soc Clin Oncol.* 2005;23:43s.

9. Thurlimann B, Keshaviah A, Coates AS, et al. A comparison of letrozole and tamoxifen in postmenopausal women with early breast cancer. *N Engl J Med.* 2005;353:2747–2757.

10. Lim YC, Desta Z, Flockhart DA, et al. Endoxifen (4-hydroxy-N-desmethyl-tamoxifen) has ant-estrogenic effects in breast cancer cells with potency similar to 4-hydroxy-tamoxifen. *Cancer Chemother Pharmacol.* 2005;55:471–478.

11. Desta Z, Ward BA, Soukhova NV, et al. Comprehensive evaluation of tamoxifen sequential biotransformation by the human cytochrome P450 system in vitro: prominent roles for CYP3A and CYP2D6. *J Pharmacol Exp Ther.* 2004;310:1062–1075.

12. Jin Y, Desta Z, Stearns V, et al. CYP2D6 genotype, antidepressant use and tamoxifen metabolism during adjuvant breast cancer treatment. *J Natl Cancer Inst.* 2005;97:30–39.

13. Goetz MP, Rae JM, Suman VJ, et al. Pharmacogenetics of tamoxifen biotransformation is associated with clinical outcomes of efficacy and hot flashes. *J Clin Oncol.* 2005;23:9312.

14. Schmid P, Untch M, Wallweiner D, et al. Cyclophosphamide, methotrexate and fluorouracil (CMF) versus hormonal ablation with leuprolin acetate as adjuvant treatment of node-positive, premenopausal breast cancer patients: preliminary results of the TABLE study (Takeda adjuvant breast cancer study with leuprolin acetate). *Anticancer Res.* 2002;22:2325–2332.

15. Castiglione-Gertsch M, O'Neill A, Price KN, et al. Adjuvant chemotherapy followed by goserelin versus either modality alone for premenopausal lymph node-negative breast cancer: a randomized trial. *J Natl Cancer Inst.* 2003;95:1833–1846.

16. Thomson CS, Twelves CJ, Mallon EA, et al: Adjuvant ovarian ablation vs CMF chemotherapy in premenopausal breast cancer patients: trial update and impact of immunohistochemical assessment of ER status. *Breast.* 2002;11:419–429.

17. Scottish Cancer Trials Breast Group and ICRF Breast Unit, Guys Hospital London. Adjuvant ovarian ablation versus CMF chemotherapy in premenopausal women with pathologic stage II breast carcinoma: the Scottish trial. *Lancet.* 1993;341:1293–1298.

18. Ejlertsen B, Mouridsen HT, Jensen MB, et al: Similar efficacy of ovarian ablation versus cmf: results from a randomized comparison in premenopausal patients with node positive and hormone receptor positive breast cancer. *J Clin Oncol.* 2006;24:4956–4962.

19. Jakesz R, Hausmaninger H, Kubista E, et al: Randomized adjuvant trial of tamoxifen and goserelin versus cyclophosphamide, methotrexate, and fluorouracil: evidence for the superiority of treatment with endocrine blockade in premenopausal patients with hormone-responsive breast cancer—Austrian Breast and Colorectal Cancer Study Group trial 5. *J Clin Oncol.* 2002;20:4621–4627.

20. Boccardo F, Rubagotti A, Amoroso D, et al: Cyclophosphamide, methotrexate, and fluorouracil versus tamoxifen plus ovarian suppression as adjuvant treatment of estrogen receptor-positive preperimenopausal breast cancer patients: results of the Italian Breast Cancer Adjuvant Study Group 02 randomized trial. *J Clin Oncol.* 2000;18:2718–2727.

21. Roche H, Kerbrat P, Bonneterre J, et al: Complete hormonal blockade versus epirubicin-based chemotherapy in premenopausal, one to three node-positive, and hormone-receptor positive, early breast cancer patients: 7-year follow-up results of French Adjuvant Study Group 06 randomised trial. *Ann Oncol.* 2006;17:1221–1227.

22. Petrek JA, Naughton MJ, Case LD, et al. Incidence, time course, and determinants of menstrual bleeding after breast cancer treatment: a prospective study. *J Clin Oncol.* 2006;24:1045–1051.

23. Fornier MN, Modi S, Panageas KS, et al. Incidence of chemotherapy-induced, long-term amenorrhea in patients with breast carcinoma age 40 years and younger after adjuvant anthracycline and taxane. *Cancer.* 2005;104:1575–1579.

24. Goldhirsch A, Gelber RD, Yothers G, et al: Adjuvant therapy for very young women with breast cancer: need for tailored treatments. *J Natl Cancer Inst Monogr.* 2001;44:51.

25. Tan SH, Wolff AC. Luteinizing hormone-releasing hormone agonists in premenopausal hormone receptor-positive breast cancer. *Clin Breast Cancer.* 2007;7:455–464.

26. Bernhard J, Zahrieh D, Castiglione-Gertsch, et al. Adjuvant chemotherapy followed by goserelin compared with either modality alone: The impact in amenorrhea, hot flashes, and quality of life in premenopausal patients—The International Breast Cancer Study Group Trial VIII. *J Clin Oncol.* 2007;25:263–270.

27. Davidson NE, O'Neill AM, Vukov AM, et al. Chemoendocrine therapy for premenopausal women with axillary lymph node-positive, steroid hormone receptor-positive breast cancer: results from INT 0101 (E5188). *J Clin Oncol.* 2005;23:5973–5982.

28. Baum M, Hackshaw A, Houghton J, et al: Adjuvant goserelin in pre-menopausal patients with early breast cancer: results from the ZIPP study. *Eur J Cancer.* 2006;42:895–904.

29. The Adjuvant Breast Cancer Trials Collaborative Group. Ovarian ablation or suppression in premenopausal early breast cancer: results from the international adjuvant breast cancer ovarian ablation or suppression randomized trial. *J Natl Cancer Inst.* 2007;99:516–525.

30. Groenvold M, Fayers PM, Petersen MA, et al. Chemotherapy versus ovarian ablation as adjuvant therapy for breast cancer: impact on health-related quality of life in a randomized trial. *Breast Cancer Res Treat.* 2006;98:275–284.

21

Axillary Lymphadenectomy for Breast Cancer: Impact on Survival

Howard Silberman

Over the past century, the natural history of breast cancer has been formulated in three successive theoretical models (Table 21.1) (1,2). In the *Halstedian Model* (3) breast cancer is perceived as a disease that spreads exclusively via the lymphatic system. The primary tumor infiltrates adjacent lymphatic channels, thereby reaching regional lymph nodes from which systemic dissemination subsequently occurs by contiguous extension to distant sites. This concept logically led to the view that for a period of time, prior to systemic spread, breast cancer can be cured by regional surgical extirpation sufficiently extensive to encompass all of the potentially involved tissues, including the entire breast and its overlying skin, the underlying pectoral muscles, and all of the ipsilateral axillary lymph nodes—the *radical mastectomy* of Halsted (3) and Meyer (4). This approach was subsequently extended by Urban (5) to the "superradical" mastectomy, a procedure that also encompassed the internal mammary lymph nodes.

High rates of systemic failure despite satisfactory local control by surgical resection led to the *Systemic Model* of breast cancer spread. This paradigm, now widely adopted and promulgated primarily by Fisher and his associates (6–9), envisions two subtypes of breast cancer. One subtype is a local neoplasm with little propensity to spread distantly, whereas in the second subtype systemic dissemination is already present at the time of clinical diagnosis. In the first type, adequate local treatment to the breast is curative. In the second type, local therapy is seen as useful in dealing with the primary tumor and in controlling locoregional recurrence; but local treatment, no matter how radical, is deemed to have no impact on cure because distant disease, the determinant of survival, already exists at the time of diagnosis. The most important scientific support for this theoretical concept of breast cancer biology derives from work of Fisher et al. (8,9) under the auspices of the National Surgical Adjuvant Breast Project (NSABP). The major influence on therapy deriving from NSABP randomized trial B-04 is that axillary lymphadenectomy, heretofore regarded as an inherent component of the curative approach to breast cancer, in fact accords no improvement in the cure rate of breast cancer.

More recently, an intermediate theoretical model of breast cancer spread has emerged, the *Spectrum Model* (1,10), in which the disease is viewed as systemic in many *but not all cases*. In the latter group of patients, often with subclinical, image-detected disease, early diagnosis and effective regional treatment is deemed capable of improving survival because it is held that persistent disease, locally or *within draining lymph nodes,* may be the source of distant metastases (1,2).

It is widely accepted that axillary dissection is of value in preventing local recurrence of tumor in the axilla, in evaluating prognosis, and in influencing the decision for adjuvant therapy. The important, controversial clinical issue to be considered here is whether partial or complete axillary lymphadenectomy has a significant, clinically applicable impact on survival and quality of life in any subset of patients with invasive breast cancer. Resolution of this issue requires careful assessment of past and current data because the NSABP trial and its conclusions have been the subject of critical analysis (2,11) and, in addition, a wide range of new technological and scientific developments (such as new concepts in the biology of tumor dissemination; detection of microscopic, subclinical disease employing new or improved modalities of high-resolution breast imaging; sentinel node analysis; and immunohistochemical detection of nodal micrometastases) may have an impact on the worth of therapeutic lymphadenectomy in modern practice. Also necessary is a re-evaluation of the morbidity of axillary dissection in relation to any potential benefit.

Conceptually, removing axillary lymph nodes can effect survival only if the lymph nodes removed contain metastatic deposits, if these nodal metastases can be the source of distant disease, and if nodal involvement at least sometimes precedes *incurable* systemic dissemination. Therefore, in assessing the potential therapeutic value of axillary lymphadenectomy, the specific relevant issues to be considered include the following:

1. Can lymph node metastases spread to distant sites?
2. Are there problems or concerns in the conduct or in the interpretation of the NSABP trial (8,9) that are sufficient to weaken the strength of its conclusions or its applicability in current practice?
3. What are the data from other studies that may reasonably reflect on the value of treating axillary metastases?
4. Does *complete* axillary clearance, including level III lymph nodes, contribute to the benefit, if any, of lymphadenectomy?
5. What is the morbidity of axillary dissection in relation to any benefit observed?

DISSEMINATION OF AXILLARY METASTASES

Considerable evidence exists that metastases can, in fact, metastasize (12,13), and, further, that the microenvironment within

Table 21.1

Various Models of Breast Cancer Spread

Halsted	Systemic	Spectrum
Tumor spreads in an orderly manner based on mechanical considerations	There is no orderly pattern of tumor cell dissemination	In most patients, axillary nodal involvement precedes distant metastases
The positive lymph node is an indicator of tumor spread and is the instigator of distant metastases	The positive lymph node is an indicator of a host-tumor relationship that permits development of metastases, rather than the instigator of distant metastases	The positive lymph node is an indicator of a host-tumor relationship that is correlated with the subsequent appearance of distant disease
RLNs are barriers to passage of tumor cells	RLNs are ineffective as barriers to tumor cell spread	RLNs are ineffective as barriers to tumor spread, but involvement of RLNs is not always associated with distant metastases
The bloodstream is of little significance as a route of tumor dissemination	The bloodstream is of considerable importance in tumor dissemination	The bloodstream is of considerable importance in tumor dissemination
Operable breast cancer is a local-regional disease	Operable breast cancer is a systemic disease	Operable breast cancer is a systemic disease in many but not all cases
The extent and nuances of the operations are the dominant factors influencing a patient's outcome	Variations in local-regional therapy are unlikely to affect survival	Variations in local-regional therapy are unlikely to have a major influence on survival but are of significance in some patients

RLNs, regional lymph nodes.
From Hellman, Harris. In Harris et al. *Diseases of the breast*. Lippincott Williams & Wilkins, 2000;419.

lymph nodes appears suitable for dissemination of nodal metastases (14–16).

Zeidman and Buss (17) demonstrated in a rabbit model that lymph nodes initially formed an effective barrier to further spread of metastatic carcinoma, but metastases to more distant lymph nodes and viscera developed when nodal resection was delayed beyond a certain point.

In a series of experiments using parabiotic mice, Hoover and Ketcham (18) demonstrated that for several different tumor lines, including a mammary adenocarcinoma, tumor present only in lung metastases could spread from one animal to another when the primary tumor had been removed before joining the circulation of the metastases-bearing animal to that of its syngeneic counterpart.

Recent data have established that tumor progression is critically dependent on the ability of the tumor, through the process of angiogenesis, to induce a neovascular stroma (14,19,20). The small proportion of tumor cells that eventually acquire all of the requisite properties for dissemination must detach from the primary tumor, enter the circulation via vascular or lymphatic channels, embolize to the capillary bed of a receptive organ, proliferate, and establish a micrometastasis. Such microscopic deposits must then induce their own vascular stroma in order to grow and give rise to secondary metastases (i.e., metastasis of metastases) (13,21).

Several vascular endothelial growth factors (VEGFs) have been identified that regulate angiogenesis and, more recently, lymphangiogenesis (15,16,22–26), processes that appear essential for breast cancer progression (22). Two recently cloned members of the VEGF family, VEGF-C and VEGF-D, have been recognized as the major regulators of lymphangiogenesis. Overexpression of VEGF-C and VEGF-D by breast cancer cells evidently promotes peritumoral and possibly intratumoral growth and enlargement of lymphatic vessels, and such tumor lymphangiogenesis enhances metastases to lymph nodes (16,23,25).

In addition, VEGF-A, heretofore regarded as a blood vessel-specific growth factor, has now been shown to also act as a potent lymphangiogenesis factor that promotes lymphatic tumor spread. Tobler and Detmar (16) and Hirakawa and associates (27) found that VEGF-A-overexpressing primary tumors induce active proliferation of tumor-associated lymphatic vessels as well as tumor metastasis to the sentinel and more distant lymph nodes. Moreover, the lymphangiogenic activity of the tumor cells was maintained even after their metastasis to the draining sentinel lymph nodes.

Guidi and associates (14) assessed the extent of angiogenesis in primary tumors and axillary nodes containing metastases from patients with breast cancer. The primary tumor and the tumor-bearing lymph nodes were examined for the presence or absence of focal areas of relatively intense neovascularization (vascular "hot spots"), and a quantitative assessment of intratumoral microvessel density was performed. Patients who had increased neovascularization by these markers of angiogenesis in their axillary lymph node metastases (but not in the primary tumor) experienced a statistically significant decrease in overall- and disease-free survival.

Skobe et al. (25) have presented experimental evidence, based on an analysis of VEGF growth factors in human breast

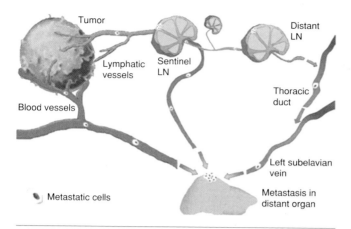

Figure 21.1 Model of malignant tumor cell dissemination. Several pathways can contribute to cancer cell dissemination. Metastatic cells enter the intra- or peritumoral lymphatic vessels and form metastases within the sentinel lymph node (LN). Further metastatic spread from the sentinel LN occurs to distant LNs and via the thoracic duct and the left subclavian vein to distant organs. Tumor cells may also spread directly to other organs via tumor-associated blood vessels or possibly via blood vessels within the metastatic LNs. (From Tobler NE, Detmar M. Tumor and lymph node lymphangiogenesis–impact on cancer metastasis. *J Leukoc Biol.* 2006;80:691–696, with permission.) (See color plates.)

cancers transplanted into nude mice, that tumor dissemination from metastatic lymph nodes can occur and does so via efferent lymphatics or through lymphatic-venous communications within the lymph node, and subsequently via the blood stream. Several studies in breast cancer patients show that VEGF-C levels around the primary tumor correlate with lymph node metastases and poor prognosis (23,26,28).

In an extensive review of the pathogenesis of metastatic dissemination and its relationship to lymphangiogenesis, Sleeman (15) concluded that the lymphatic system is highly amenable to the entry of metastasizing tumor cells and the formation of lymph node metastases, and, in addition, that these nodal metastases form a bridgehead for further metastatic spread.

The foregoing discussion supports the mechanism of tumor dissemination outlined by Tobler and Detmar (16), emphasizing the concept that nodal disease can be the source for distant metastases (Figure 21.1).

Thus, in the presence of the requisite microenvironment, it appears that lymph node metastases from human breast cancer can produce secondary metastatic deposits, evidently accounting for the adverse effect on survival observed by Guidi and associates (14) and others (23,28).

ANALYSIS OF NSABP PROTOCOL B-04

Between 1971 and 1974, Fisher and associates (8,9) enrolled patients in a prospective clinical trial to designed to compare the value of variations in locoregional treatment on the survival of patients with clinically evident, operable breast cancer. Patients judged to have clinically negative axillary nodes were randomly

assigned to be treated by radical mastectomy (n = 362), total mastectomy and regional irradiation (n = 352), or total mastectomy only (n = 365)

The impact of axillary lymphadenectomy was assessed by comparing outcome in the groups treated by radical mastectomy or total mastectomy only. At 10-year follow-up, the survival rate was 58% for the radical mastectomy group, compared with 54% for the total mastectomy-only group, a difference that was not statistically significant. At 25 years, the estimated disease-free survival was 19% in both groups. Among the 352 patients randomized to receive regional irradiation after total mastectomy, a significant reduction in local recurrence was observed, but there was no difference in survival compared with patients receiving total mastectomy alone.

These findings have led to the widely accepted conclusion that axillary lymphadenectomy (or nodal ablation by radiation) does not alter the incidence of systemic recurrence or patient survival, and, therefore, lymph node metastases are "indicators rather than instigators" of distant disease. The results of this trial are also offered as validating the *Systemic Model* of breast cancer spread (Table 21.1), wherein survival-determining systemic metastases are perceived as already present at the time of clinical diagnosis of the primary tumor and, therefore, locoregional therapy can have no impact on survival.

Critical reviews of this historic study suggest that a survival benefit attributable to axillary dissection may have been masked by several problematic clinical, pathologic, and statistical features of the protocol design (2,11,29):

1. Among the 365 patients assigned to receive total mastectomy only, 129 patients (35%) inadvertently had a limited axillary dissection, undoubtedly because of the anatomic interdigitation of breast tissue in the axillary tail with level I lymphoadipose tissue. In fact, up to 5 lymph nodes were removed in 23% of the patients; 6 to 10 nodes in 6%; and more than 10 nodes in 7%, including several patients with more than 20 nodes removed (29–31).

2. Despite a negative clinical examination, about 40% of the patients undergoing radical mastectomy had pathologically positive axillary nodes. Because patients were assigned in a statistically appropriate random manner to each of the treatment groups, the authors estimated that a similar percentage of the women in each arm of the study had axillary disease, therefore, including about 146 of the 365 patients in the mastectomy-only group. The trial protocol allowed for salvage surgery for postoperative axillary failure. At 25-year follow-up 68 patients (18.6%) in the mastectomy-only group developed clinically evident nodal metastases. This represents a 47% axillary relapse rate among the 146 patients estimated to have axillary metastases at the time of surgery. These patients were treated by delayed axillary dissection. Such delayed nodal relapse was not considered a treatment failure and was not included in the determination of disease-free survival (8,9). Moreover, the impact of the salvage lymphadenectomy on the survival of those patients remains unknown (2,11).

3. It is clear that axillary lymphadenectomy cannot improve the survival of patients free of nodal metastases, yet 60% of the patients in each arm of the study were estimated to be free of axillary disease. Consequently, only about 40% of the

patients, those who had axillary involvement, composed the true critical population to whom benefit could possibly accrue from axillary dissection. Taking this fact into account, and further, by estimating the likelihood of occult distant disease (which would preclude benefit from locoregional treatment) and considering the potential curative benefit of delayed salvage node dissection, Hellman and Harris (2) and Harris and Osteen (11) determined that only 9% of the total group could potentially benefit from initial axillary treatment. This analysis led the authors to conclude that the B-04 trial did not have the statistical power to prove or disprove the efficacy of axillary dissection because they calculated that approximately 1,000 patients in each arm would be required to have a 90% chance of detecting a 9% difference between two treatment arms in a clinical trial at a statistically significant level of $p = 0.05$.

4. Even if the conclusions of the B-04 trial were rigorously validated and true, new developments in diagnosis and treatment in the past 35 years, since the accrual of patients into that study, may alter the impact of axillary lymphadenectomy and unmask a survival benefit. Thus, patients entered into the B-04 trial had *clinically evident* primary tumors, measuring 3.3 to 3.7 cm in diameter. With current screening programs employing vastly improved, high-resolution imaging techniques, primary breast cancer is often diagnosed in a *preclinical*, even *microscopic*, phase in which regional lymph nodes may be involved *prior* to systemic dissemination. This concept, consistent with the *Spectrum Model* of breast cancer spread rather than the *Systemic Model* (Table 21.1), is supported by several lines of evidence. Modern mammographic screening of asymptomatic women, presumably resulting in earlier diagnoses, is associated with a decrease in breast cancer mortality of approximately 25% (see Chapter 16A) (2,32–34). If metastases always occur at the inception of breast cancer (*Systemic Model*) early detection could not be effective in preventing metastases or decreasing breast cancer mortality. Additional evidence supporting the *Spectrum Model* and, inferentially, the potential therapeutic benefit of axillary dissection, comes from the older literature wherein 26% to 50% of the long-term survivors of radical mastectomy alone had positive lymph nodes. Evidently, these surviving patients received effective regional treatment prior to systemic spread of their disease (31,35–38).

5. The advent of effective adjuvant chemotherapy is another advance that appears to alter the applicability of the B-04 data. Systemic occult metastases that were assumed to be survival-limiting in the population of patients studied in the NSABP trial, and which, therefore, precluded any benefit from lymphadenectomy, are now amenable to eradication by such adjuvant therapy (39,40). Current adjuvant chemotherapy regimens are evidently less effective against locoregional disease than systemic micrometastases (41), thereby raising the possibility of improving survival with regional ablative treatment even in patients with occult systemic disease. Support for this concept comes from reports of Overgaard et al. (42) and Ragaz and associates (43,44) and others (see later discussion).

6. In modern practice, sentinel lymph node analysis allows restriction of axillary lymphadenectomy only to those patients with a positive sentinel node and, therefore, at risk of having metastatic disease in the remaining, nonsentinel nodes. Evaluating the therapeutic efficacy of axillary dissection in patients with known axillary disease may well reveal a benefit masked in the B-04 series in which, as Harris and Osteen have pointed out (11), any favorable effect was diluted by including patients the majority of whom had no axillary metastases.

EFFECT OF RADIATION ON SURVIVAL AFTER LIMITED AXILLARY DISSECTION

Results have been published from two prospective, randomized trials designed to determine the worth of postoperative locoregional radiation therapy in patients with stage II and stage III breast cancer treated with modified radical mastectomy and adjuvant chemotherapy (42–44). A survival benefit was observed in the radiation arms of both studies. Although these findings might suggest that adjuvant radiation is routinely indicated after modified radical mastectomy for patients with high-risk breast cancer (41), such a conclusion is unfounded because very limited axillary dissections were performed in these trials, and the radiotherapy may have been only a surrogate for more adequate surgical dissection that would have removed residual axillary disease. Paradoxically, however, the results of radiation after *limited* axillary clearance derived from these trials provide important information reflecting on the worth of ablating axillary metastases.

In the Danish Breast Cancer Cooperative Group Trial (42), 1,708 premenopausal women who had undergone mastectomy for pathologic stage II or III breast cancer and who were to have adjuvant chemotherapy with cyclophosphamide, methotrexate, and fluorouracil (CMF) were randomly assigned to receive or not receive irradiation of the chest wall and regional lymph nodes. The axillary dissections performed were limited to level I and part of level II. A median of seven lymph nodes was removed; moreover, in 15% of the patients only zero to three nodes were retrieved and in 76% nine or fewer lymph nodes were removed. Axillary metastases were documented in 92% of the patients. Disease-free survival and overall survival at 10 years were significantly improved ($p <0.001$) in the cohort of patients receiving adjuvant radiation. In a subsequent analysis of overall failure pattern at 18-year follow-up, the Danish Breast Cancer Cooperative Group reported that a significant reduction in both locoregional recurrence and distant metastases was observed among patients receiving postmastectomy radiation. In the no-radiotherapy group, 45% of locoregional recurrences alone involved the axilla. The authors concluded that after locoregional recurrence, secondary dissemination to a distant site had occurred in a high number of patients (45).

Ragaz and associates (43,44) conducted a similar trial in Vancouver, British Columbia. Three hundred eighteen premenopausal women with node-positive breast cancer were randomly assigned, after modified radical mastectomy, to receive CMF chemotherapy plus radiotherapy or chemotherapy alone. Axillary dissection yielded a median of only 11 lymph nodes. Analysis of results at 20 years indicates that radiotherapy was associated with a significant improvement in overall survival (47% vs. 37%) and breast cancer-free survival (48% vs. 30%).

In addition, locoregional radiation significantly reduced both isolated locoregional recurrence (7% vs. 18%) and systemic recurrence (51% vs. 68%). Thus, systemic disease-free survival at 20 years was 48% in patients receiving radiation and 31% in the chemotherapy-only group ($p = 0.04$). The reduction in systemic recurrences associated with locoregional therapy observed in this trial also led these investigators to conclude that microscopic locoregional disease that survives both mastectomy and chemotherapy is the origin of subsequent systemic metastases.

Silberman and associates (46) analyzed the two trials in relation to their own experience. In 131 modified radical mastectomies performed in their series, a mean of 25 lymph nodes was removed in an operation designed to provide complete axillary clearance. These authors suggest that the radiotherapy employed in the Danish and British Columbia trials merely compensated for inadequate axillary surgery that resulted in a group of patients highly likely to have residual nodal disease (47). Thus, they believe that the results do not support the routine use of adjuvant postmastectomy radiotherapy when complete lymph node dissections are performed. Nevertheless, these two trials lend additional scientific support to the notion that obliteration of axillary metastases has a salutary effect on survival.

The addition of adjuvant chemotherapy in the Danish and British Columbia trials cannot account for the improvement in survival noted between the irradiated and nonirradiated groups, as the patients in both arms of the study received this therapy. Nevertheless, the *magnitude* of the potential survival benefit attributable to axillary treatment may well be enhanced by adjuvant chemotherapy because heretofore survival-limiting occult systemic micrometastases can now be cured in a significant proportion of patients who receive such systemic drug therapy. Regional treatment is required because current adjuvant chemotherapy regimens, although effective against systemic micrometastatic disease, appear to be less efficient in destroying microscopic locoregional disease among high-risk breast cancer patients (44,48).

OTHER STUDIES ASSESSING THE BENEFITS OF CONTROLLING LOCOREGIONAL DISEASE

The Early Breast Cancer Trialists' Collaborative Group (49) reported a meta-analysis of studies randomizing 8,500 women with node-positive disease to receive or not receive adjuvant locoregional radiation following mastectomy and "axillary clearance." A 17% reduction in local recurrence was observed in the radiation-treated group at 5 years. At 15 years the breast cancer mortality risk was modestly but significantly reduced in the radiation-treated group (54.7% vs. 60.1%). Among the node-negative patients, the reduction in local recurrence rate was statistically significant but very modest (6% vs. 2%); however, no significant reduction in 15-year breast cancer mortality accrued.

Gebski and associates (50) also concluded that in women with high-risk breast cancer, postmastectomy radiotherapy is associated with a reduction in locoregional recurrence and improved survival for up to 10 years. Their findings were based on a meta-analysis restricted to those randomized trials in which the study patients had received optimal and complete radiotherapy.

Whelan et al. (51) performed a meta-analysis of 18 randomized trials that involved 6,367 pre- and postmenopausal women, most of whom had positive nodes, and who were treated with modified radical mastectomy and systemic adjuvant treatment. Again, radiation therapy was associated with decreased locoregional recurrence and improved disease-free and overall survival.

OTHER STUDIES EXAMINING THE WORTH OF AXILLARY LYMPHADENECTOMY

Various additional studies examining the impact of axillary lymphadenectomy on survival have been published, but most, unfortunately, have method, design, or clinical features that tend to hinder definitive interpretation.

Orr (52) performed a meta-analysis of the results of trials published though 1998 in which standard treatment for breast cancer (mastectomy with axillary dissection or segmental mastectomy, breast radiation, and axillary dissection) was compared with standard treatment without axillary node dissection (Table 21.2) (9,53–62) Orr excluded from his analysis trials that referred to stage II patients only but included trials with mixtures of stage I and II patients. Six randomized controlled trials, consisting of nearly 3,000 patients and spanning 4 decades, were identified for inclusion in the meta-analysis. The trials included were those from Copenhagen (60,61), the South-East Scotland (SES) trial (54,56,62), the NSABP B-04 trial (results at 10 years) (9), Guy's Hospital in London (53,57–59), and the Institut Curie (55). All six trials, including two from Guy's Hospital, showed that prophylactic axillary node dissection improved survival, ranging from 4% to 16%, corresponding to a risk reduction of 7% to 46%. Combining the six trials showed an average survival benefit of 5.4% (95% confidence interval = 2.7-8.0, probability of survival benefit >99.5%). Adjusting for biases in the individual studies did not alter the conclusions, nor did subset analysis of stage I patients. The author concluded that axillary node dissection improves survival in women with operable breast cancer. However, he identified two important limitations of the analysis. First, few of the patients in the six trials had T1a tumors, so extrapolation of these results to this subset (and those with nonpalpable tumors) may be inappropriate. Second, essentially no patients in the six trials were treated with adjuvant therapy, as contrasted to current clinical practice, so that it is possible that the risk reduction seen in this meta-analysis may be altered in patients receiving adjuvant chemotherapy.

In an editorial critique of Orr's meta-analysis, Morrow (63) identified several additional limitations. The Guy's Hospital trials contributed 21% of the patients analyzed. These studies compared patients treated by radical mastectomy with those treated by wide local resection and a dose of breast irradiation deemed to be inadequate so that absence of axillary clearance may not have been the only factor contributing to the survival differences observed. Similarly, some patients included in the meta-analysis underwent extended radical mastectomies, with resection of internal mammary nodes.

Table 21.2

Meta-Analysis of Axillary Dissection (9,53–62)

Trial	Number of Patients	Follow-up (years)	Survival (%) Control	Survival (%) Treated	Difference) (%)	Reduction (%)	p-value
Copenhagen	425	10	46	50	4	7.4	NS
Guy's 1	370	10	43.6	51.6	8	14.2	NS
SES	498	10	51.5	61	9.5	19.6	0.04
B-04	727	10	54	58	4	8.7	NS
Guy's II	258	10	57	73	16	37.2	0.01
Curie	658	5	92.6	96.6	4	45.9	0.03

NS, not significant.
From *Orr, Ann Surg Oncol.* 1999;6:109.
The B-04 study authors reported survival of 19% in both the control and treated groups at 25 years' follow-up.

Finally, repeating the meta-analysis using the 25-year follow-up data from the NSABP B-04 trial may alter the findings as the survival rate in both arms of the study was 19%, eliminating the 4% benefit in favor of axillary dissection seen at 10 years (8).

AXILLARY RADIATION VERSUS AXILLARY DISSECTION

Between 1982 and 1987, Louis-Silvestre and associates (64) randomized 658 patients with breast tumors <3 cm in diameter and who were to be treated with segmental mastectomy and breast radiation to receive either axillary dissection (levels II and II) or axillary radiation. All patients had clinically negative axillae. At 15-year follow-up no difference in survival was observed, but axillary dissection was associated with a small but statistically significant decrease in the rate of axillary recurrence (1% vs. 3%). Twenty-one percent of the patients in the surgical group were node-positive.

In patients with clinically and image-negative axillae, the surgical approach to the axilla has the advantage that nodal ablation can be restricted to those with metastatic disease based on sentinel node analysis. An additional benefit of surgical treatment is that it provides tissue for histologic evaluation of the axillary contents and, therefore, accurate pathologic staging.

THE ARGUMENT FOR COMPLETE AXILLARY LYMPHADENECTOMY

In current practice, patients with invasive breast cancer who are known to have axillary disease preoperatively or who have a positive sentinel node at surgery, generally undergo an axillary dissection that encompasses the lymph nodes lateral to and deep to the pectoralis minor muscle (levels I and II), with the primary goal of achieving regional control and of providing staging information relevant to the decision for adjuvant therapy.

In contrast, for clinicians who perceive lymphadenectomy as potentially therapeutic, a strong case can be made for complete axillary clearance, including the apical lymph nodes medial to the pectoralis minor (level III nodes) and Rotter's interpectoral

nodes This recommendation is based on the fact that among patients with axillary metastases a significant proportion will harbor metastatic tumor in the apical nodes. In a report from the National Cancer Institute, Danforth and associates (65) analyzed the distribution of nodal metastases from breast cancer according to their anatomic location (Table 21.3). Among patients with axillary nodes found to be positive on pathologic examination but which were deemed negative on physical examination, 17% had level III metastases; among clinically and pathologically node-positive women, 45.9% had apical involvement. Overall, 27.7% of the 65 node-positive patients analyzed had level III nodal involvement.

In a review of published series (47,66–73), Moffat and associates (74) found that among women with pathologically involved axillary nodes, apical metastases were present in 16.4% to 58.1%, and up to 15% had involvement of Rotter's nodes (Table 21.4). Senofsky et al. (66) reported that when axillary metastases are present in level I and II lymph nodes, apical or Rotter's nodes are also involved in about one third of patients. Similarly, Veronesi and associates (75) found that the risk of level III metastases was 35% in women with tumors ≤2 cm in size when levels I and II were involved.

In a recent series of axillary dissections in 1,404 patients with positive sentinel nodes performed at Memorial Sloan-Kettering Cancer Center, 551 of the patients underwent dissection of level, I, II, and III nodes, at the discretion of the surgeon. Metastatic disease was found in level III nodes in 15.1% of the patients (76).

These data should logically lead surgeons who subscribe to the value of axillary clearance to perform a complete axillary lymphadenectomy in patients known to have axillary metastases based on clinical examination, preoperative needle biopsy, or sentinel node analysis. Surgeons still uncertain of the potential therapeutic value of nodal clearance would likely offer completely lymphadenectomy were it not for the prevailing fear of severe morbidity, primarily lymphedema, thought to accompany this procedure (77,78). In a review from the Mayo Clinic, Morrell and associates (79) assert that the incidence and severity of lymphedema correlate with the number of lymph nodes removed. Herd-Smith et al. (80) reported that, compared with patients with fewer than 20 lymph nodes removed, those who

Table 21.3

Distribution of Nodal Metastases in Patients with Pathologically Positive Nodes

Axillary Level	All Patients (%)	Clinically-node-negative Patients (%)	Clinically-node-positive Patients (%)
Na[a]	65	41	24
Level 1 only	20 (30.8)	15 (36.6)	5 (20.8)
Level II only	14 (21.5)	13 (31.7)	1 (4.2)
Level III only	2 (3.1)	1 (2.4)	1 (4.2)
Level 1, II	13 (20.0)	6 (14.6)	7 (29.2)
Level I, III	1 (1.5)	0 (0.0)	1 (4.2)
Level II, III	3 (4.6)	1 (2.4)	2 (8.3)
Level 1, II, III	12 (18.5)	5 (12.2)	7 (29.2)

[a] Number of patients with pathologically positive lymph nodes.
Modified after Danforth et al. *J Clin Oncol.* 1986;4:655–662.

had more than 30 nodes resected had only a borderline increased risk of lymphedema (hazard ratio = 1.64; 95% confidence interval: 0.99-2.74).

Many additional reports indicate that there is little increase in the incidence of lymphedema with extension of the surgical dissection to encompass the apical (level III) lymph nodes. In a review of collected series analyzing the incidence of lymphedema in relation to the extent of axillary dissection and the effect of concomitant axillary irradiation, Moffat and associates (74) at the University of Miami reported that lymphedema developed in 0% to 2.8% of patients undergoing axillary sampling procedures (81,82); in 2.7% to 7.4% of patients treated by partial (level I and II) axillary dissection (81–83); and in 3.1% to 8.0% of patients in whom complete axillary lymphadenectomy was performed

(66,84,85). Axillary irradiation alone was associated with an incidence of lymphedema of 2.1% to 8.3% (82,86–88). However, combined axillary dissection and irradiation (66,82,87–89) were synergistic in their effect on the development of lymphedema, resulting in a three- to sevenfold increase in incidence (Table 21.5) (66,81–89).

Veronesi et al. (85) reported an overall incidence of lymphedema of 5% following complete axillary clearance. Using a water-displacement technique to compare the volume of the two arms, Hoe et al. (90) determined that 7.6% of their patients developed lymphedema after full axillary dissection. Finally, in a study of lymphedema performed at the Memorial Sloan-Kettering Cancer Center, Werner and associates (91) reported that the level of node dissection was not statistically

Table 21.4

Incidence of Apical (Level III) and Rotter's (Interpectoral) Nodal Metastases in Patients with Pathologically Positive Nodes (47,66–73)

Reference	Number Cases	Number of pN+ Cases	Number with Apical Metastases (%)	Number with Rotter's Metastases (%)	Number with "Skip" Metastases[a] (%)
Senofsky et al.	278	92	24 (26.1)	14 (15,2)	5 (5.4)
Rosen et al.	933	429	104 (24.2)	1 (0.2)	2 (0.5)
Schwartz et al.	277	127	—	—	4 (3.1)
Pigott et al.	146	72[b]	30 (41.7)	—	3 (4.2)
Attiyeh et al.	—	105	61 (58.1)	—	12 (11.4)
Smith et al.	408	304	136 (44.7)	—	30 (9.9)
Veronesi et al.	—	539	102 (18.9)	—	2 (0.4)
Boova et al.	200	80	17 (21.3)	—	1 (1.3)
Cody et al.	500	134	—	13 (9.7)	—

Percentages in parentheses pertain to pN+ patients.
[a] For purposes of this discussion, "skip" metastases are defined as tumor in apical and/or Rotter's nodes in the absence of metastases in level I and II nodes.
[b] Seventy-two evaluable patients of 80 pN+ patients in this series.
Modified after Moffat et al. *J Surg Oncol.* 1992;51:8.

Table 21.5

Incidence of Lymphedema Following Treatment of the Axilla in Breast Cancer Patients (66,81–89)

	Number of Patients	Number with Lymphedema (%)	Follow-up
Axillary sampling			
Benson and Thorogood	463	13 (2.8)	2–7 years
Larson et al.	191[a]	12 (6.3)	45 months
Carabell et al.	84[a]	0 (0)	Minimum 1 year
Kissin et al.	17	0 (0)	Minimum 1 year
	22[a]	2 (9.1)	Minimum 1 year
Partial axillary lymphadenectomy			
Benson and Thorogood	497	25 (5.0)	2–7 years
Siegel et al.	259	7 (2.7)	27 months
Larson et al.	49[a]	18 (36.7)	45 months
Kissin et al.	94	7 (7.4)	Minimum 1 year
	47[a]	18 (38.3)	Minimum 1 year
Beadle et al.	109[a]	13 (11.9)	30 months
Total axillary lymphadenectomy			
Kissin et al.	50	4 (8.0)	5 years
Senofsky et al.	217	13 (6.0)	50 months
	61[a]	13 (21.3)	50 months
Veronesi et al.	352[b]	11 (3.1)	7 years
	349[c]	23 (6.6)	7 years
Radiotherapy only			
Delouche et al.	294	10 (3.4)	11 years
Larson et al.	235	10 (4.3)	45 months
Kissin et al.	12	1 (8.3)	Minimum 1 year
Beadle et al.	96	2 (2.1)	30 months

[a] These patients received postoperative adjuvant axillary radiotheraphy (XRT).
[b] Treated with conservative surgery, total axillary lymphadenectomy, and XRT.
[a] Treated by radical mastectomy.
Modified after Moffat et al. *J Surg Oncol* 1992;51:8.

related to the development of arm edema; the only factor that was significantly associated was obesity, manifest as a high body mass index. Moreover, the higher the body mass index, the greater was the frequency of lymphedema.

SUMMARY AND CONCLUSIONS

1. Breast cancer patients treated prior to the advent of modern, high-resolution, mammography and effective adjuvant chemotherapy often had large, palpable tumors. Such patients with nodal metastases were likely to have been unresponsive to locoregional treatment because of synchronous, survival-limiting systemic macro- or micrometastatic disease. The course of such patients is consistent with the *Systemic Model* of Fisher of breast cancer spread (6–9).

2. In modern practice, however, an increasing proportion of patients have tumors that are image-detected at the time of annual mammographic screening, nonpalpable, and often microscopic in size. These patients frequently are free of systemic disease at diagnosis or have micrometastatic systemic disease that is amenable to adjuvant chemotherapy. Such patients may have locoregional disease, including axillary metastases, which is survival-limiting if untreated because it may be the source of distant, systemic dissemination. Locoregional disease appears resistant to current chemotherapy regimens but can be successfully managed by locoregional therapy. Patients in this latter group have a course consistent with the *Spectrum Model* of Hellman (1,10) of breast cancer spread wherein locoregional therapy, including axillary lymphadenectomy, can improve survival.

3. Axillary surgery is preferable to axillary radiation because it can be restricted to patients known to have axillary disease (determined by preoperative biopsy or sentinel node analysis) and provides material for pathologic evaluation. Complete axillary lymphadenectomy has the advantage of clearing level III nodes that have a significant probability of harboring metastatic tumor when levels I and II are involved.

REFERENCES

1. Hellman S. The natural history of small breast cancers. *J Clin Oncol.* 1994;12:2229–2234.
2. Hellman S, Harris JR. Natural history of breast cancer. In: Harris JR, Lippman ME, Morrow M, et al., eds. *Diseases of the Breast*, 2nd ed. Philadelphia: Lippincott Williams & Wilkins; 2000:407–423.

3. Halsted W. The results of operations for the cure of cancer of the breast performed at the Johns Hopkins Hospital from June 1889 to January 1984. *Johns Hopkins Hosp Bull.* 1895;4:297.

4. Meyer W. An improved method of the radical operation for carcinoma of the breast. *Med Rec.* 1894;46:746.

5. Urban JA. Clinical experience and results of excision of the internal mammary lymph node chain in primary operable breast cancer. *Cancer.* 1959;12:14.

6. Fisher B. Breast cancer management: alternatives to radical mastectomy. *N Engl J Med.* 1979;310:326–328.

7. Fisher B. A commentary on the role of the surgeon in primary breast cancer. *Breast Cancer Res Treat.* 1981;1:17–26.

8. Fisher B, Jeong JH, Anderson S, et al. Twenty-five-year follow-up of a randomized trial comparing radical mastectomy, total mastectomy, and total mastectomy followed by irradiation. *N Engl J Med.* 2002;347:567–575.

9. Fisher B, Redmond C, Fisher ER, et al. Ten-year results of a randomized clinical trial comparing radical mastectomy and total mastectomy with or without radiation. *N Engl J Med.* 1985;312:674–681.

10. Hellman S, Harris J. The appropriate breast carcinoma paradigm. *Cancer Res.* 1987;2:339–342.

11. Harris JR, Osteen RT. Patients with early breast cancer benefit from effective axillary treatment. *Breast Cancer Res Treat.* 1985;5:17–21.

12. Fidler IJ. Molecular biology of cancer: invasion and metastasis. In: DeVita VT Jr, Hellman S, Rosenberg SA, eds. *Cancer: Principles & Practice of Oncology,* 5th ed. Philadelphia: Lippincott-Raven Publishers; 1997:135–152.

13. Fidler IJ. Seed and soil revisited: contribution of the organ microenvironment to cancer metastasis. *Surg Oncol Clin North Am.* 2001;10:257–269 .

14. Guidi AJ, Berry DA, Broadwater G, et al. Association of angiogenesis in lymph node metastases with outcome of breast cancer. *J Natl Cancer Inst.* 2000;92:486–492.

15. Sleeman J. The lymph node as a bridgehead in the metastatic dissemination of tumors. *Recent Results Cancer Res.* 2000;157:55–81.

16. Tobler NE, Detmar M. Tumor and lymph node lymphangiogenesis–impact on cancer metastasis. *J Leukoc Biol.* 2006;80:691–696.

17. Zeidman I, Buss JM. Experimental studies on the spread of cancer in the lymphatic system. I. Effectiveness of the lymph node as a barrier to the passage of embolic tumor cells. *Cancer Res.* 1954;14:403–405.

18. Hoover HC, Ketcham AS. Metastasis of metastases. *Am J Surg.* 1975;130:405–411.

19. Folkman J. What is the evidence that tumors are angiogenesis dependent? *J Natl Cancer Inst.* 1990;82:4–6.

20. Blood CH, Zetter BR. Tumor interactions with the vasculature: angiogenesis and tumor metastasis. *Biochem Biophys Acta.* 1990;1032:89–118.

21. Folkman J. Angiogenesis and breast cancer. *J Clin Oncol.* 1994;21:441–443.

22. Choi WW, Lewis MM, Lawson D, et al. Angiogenic and lymphangiogenic microvessel density in breast carcinoma: correlation with clinicopathologic parameters and VEGF-family gene expression. *Mod Pathol.* 2005;18:143–152.

23. Nakamura Y, Yasuoka H, Tsujimoto M, et al. Lymph vessel density correlates with nodal status, VEGF-C expression, and prognosis in breast cancer. *Breast Cancer Res Treat.* 2005;91:125–132.

24. Plate K. From angiogenesis to lymphangiogenesis. *Nat Med.* 2001;7:151–152.

25. Skobe M, Hawighorst T, Jackson DG, et al. Induction of tumor lymphangiogenesis by VEGF-C promotes breast cancer metastasis. *Nat Med.* 2001;7:192–198.

26. Thiele W, Sleeman JP. Tumor-induced lymphangiogenesis: a target for cancer therapy? *J Biotechnol.* 2006;124:224–241.

27. Hirakawa S, Kodama S, Kunstfeld R, et al. VEGF-A induces tumor and sentinel lymph node lymphangiogenesis and promotes lymphatic metastasis. *J Exp Med.* 2005;201:1089–1099.

28. Kinoshita J, Kitamura K, Kabashima A, et al. Clinical significance of vascular endothelial growth factor-C (VEGF-C) in breast cancer. *Breast Cancer Res Treat.* 2001;66:159–164.

29. Cody HS, III, Urban JA. The role of axillary dissection in managing patients with breast cancer: the case for complete axillary clearance. In: Wise L, Johnson H Jr., eds. *Breast Cancer: Controversies in Management.* Armonk, NY: Futura Publishing Company; 1994:69–176.

30. Fisher B, Wolmark N, Bauer M, et al. The accuracy of clinical nodal staging and of limited axillary dissection as a determinant of histologic nodal status in carcinoma of the breast. *Surg Gynecol Obstet.* 1981;152:765–772.

31. Kinne DW. Axillary clearance in opeable breast cancer: still a necessity? *Recent Results Cancer Res.* 1998;152:161–169.

32. Shapiro S. Determining the efficacy of breast cancer screening. *Cancer.* 1989;63:1873.

33. Tabar L, Fagerberg C, Duffy S, et al. Update of the Swedish two county program of mammographic screening for breast cancer. *Radiol Clin North Am.* 1992;30:187–210.

34. Wald N, Frost C, Cuckle H. Breast cancer screening: the current position. *BMJ.* 1991;302:845–846.

35. Adair F, Berg J, Joubert L, et al. Long term follow up of breast cancer patients: the 30 year report. *Cancer.* 1974;33:1145–1150.

36. Brinkley D, Haybrittle JL. The curability of breast cancer. *Lancet.* 1975;2:95–97.

37. Morrow M, Harris JR. Primary treatment of invasive breast cancer. In: Harris JR, Lippman ME, Morrow M, et al, eds. *Diseases of the Breast,* 2nd ed. Philadelphia: Lippincott Wilkins & Williams; 2000:515–560.

38. Rosen PP, Groshen S, Saigo PE, et al. A long-term follow-up study of survival in stage I (T1N0M0) and stage II (T1N1M0) breast carcinoma. *J Clin Oncol.* 1989;7:355–366.

39. Bonadonna G, Brusamolino E, Valagussa P, et al. Combination chemotherapy as an adjuvant treatment in operable breast cancer. *N Engl J Med.* 1976;294:405–410.

40. McCarthy NJ, Swain SM. Update on adjuvant chemotherapy for early breast cancer. *Oncology.* 2000;14:1267–1280.

41. Hellman S. Stopping metastases at their source. *N Engl J Med.* 1997;337:996–997.

42. Overgaard M, Hansen PS, Overgaard J, et al. Postoperative radiotherapy in high-risk premenopausal women with breast cancer who receive adjuvant chemotherapy. Danish Breast Cancer Cooperative Group 82b Trial. *N Engl J Med.* 1997;337:949–955.

43. Ragaz J, Jackson SM, Nhu L, et al. Adjuvant radiotherapy and chemotherapy in node-positive premenopausal women with breast cancer. *N Engl J Med.* 1997;337:956–962.

44. Ragaz J, Olivotto IA, Spinelli JJ, et al. Locoregional radiation therapy in patients with high-risk breast cancer receiving adjuvant chemotherapy: 20-year results of the British Columbia randomized trial. *J Natl Cancer Inst.* 2005;97:116–126.

45. Nielsen HM, Overgaard M, Grau C, et al. Study of failure pattern among high-risk breast cancer patients with or without postmastectomy radiotherapy in addition to adjuvant systemic therapy: long-term results from the Danish Breast Cancer Cooperative Group DBCG 82b and c randomized trials. *J Clin Oncol.* 2006;24:2268–2275.

46. Silberman AW, Sarna GP, Palmer D. Adjuvant radiation trials for high-risk breast cancer patients: adequacy of lymphadenectomy. *Ann Surg Oncol.* 2000;7:357–360.

47. Veronesi U, Rilke F, Luini A, et al. Distribution of axillary node metastases by level of invasion. An analysis of 539 cases. *Cancer.* 1987;59:682–687.

48. Harris J. Radiation therapy for invasive breast cancer: not just for local control. *J Clin Oncol.* 2005;23:1607–1608.

49. Clarke M, Collins R, Darby S, et al. Effects of radiotherapy and of differences in the extent of surgery for early breast cancer on local recurrence and 15-year survival: an overview of the randomised trials. *Lancet.* 2005;366:2087–2106.

50. Gebski V, Lagleva M, Keech A, et al. Survival effects of postmastectomy adjuvant radiation therapy using biologically equivalent doses: a clinical perspective. *J Natl Cancer Inst.* 2006;98:26–38.

51. Whelan TJ, Julian J, Wright J, et al. Does locoregional radiation therapy improve survival in breast cancer? A meta-analysis. *J Clin Oncol.* 2000;18:1220–1229.

52. Orr RK. The impact of prophylactic node dissection on breast cancer survival—a Bayesian meta-analysis. *Ann Surg Oncol.* 1999;6:109–116.

53. Atkins H, Hayward JL, Klugman DJ, et al. Treatment of early breast cancer: a report after ten years of a clinical trial. *Brit Med J.* 1972;2:423–429.

54. Bruce J. Operable cancer of the breast: a controlled clinical trial. *Cancer.* 1971;28:1443–1452.

55. Cabanes PA, Salmon RJ, Vilcoq JR, et al. Value of axillary dissection in addition to lumpectomy and radiotherapy in early breast cancer. *Lancet.* 1992;339:1245–1248.

56. Hamilton T, Langlands AO, Prescott RJ. The treatment of operable cancer of the breast: a clinical trial in the South-East region of Scotland. *Br J Surg.* 1974;61:758–761.

57. Hayward J, Caleffi M. The significance of local control in the primary treatment of breast cancer. *Arch Surg.* 1987;122:1244–1247.

58. Hayward JL. The Guy's trial of treatments of "early" breast cancer. *World J Surg.* 1977;1:314–316.

59. Hayward JL. The Guy's Hospital trials on breast conservation. In: Harris JR, Hellman S, Silen W, eds. *Conservative Management of Breast Cancer: New Surgical and Radiotherapeutic Techniques.* Philadelphia: JB Lippincott; 1983:77–90.

60. Johansen H, Kaae S, Schiodt T. Simple mastectomy with postoperative irradiation versus extended radical mastectomy in breast cancer: a twenty-five year follow-up of a randomized trial. *Acta Oncol.* 1990;29:709–715.

61. Kaae S, Johansen H. Does simple mastectomy followed by irradiation offer survival comparable to radical procedures? *Int J Radiation Oncol Biophys.* 1977;2:1163–1166.

62. Langlands AO, Prescott RJ, Hamilton T. A clinical trial in the management of operable cancer of the breast. *Br J Surg.* 1980;67:170–174.

63. Morrow M. A survival benefit from axillary dissection: was Halsted correct? *Ann Surg Oncol.* 1999;6:17–18.

64. Louis-Sylvestre C, Clough K, Asselain B, et al. Axillary treatment in conservative management of operable breast cancer: dissection or radiotherapy? Results of a randomized study with 15 years of follow-up. *J Clin Oncol.* Jan 1 2004;22(1):97–101.

65. Danforth DN, Findlay PA, McDonald HD, et al. Complete axillary lymph node dissection for stage I-II carcinoma of the breast. *J Clin Oncol.* 1986;4:655–662.

66. Senofsky GM, Moffat FL, Davis K, et al. Total axillary lymphadenectomy in the management of breast cancer. *Arch Surg.* 1991;126:1336–1342.

67. Rosen PP, Lesser ML, Kinne DW, Beattie EJ. Discontinuous or "skip" metastases in breast carcinoma. Analysis of 1228 axillary dissections. *Ann Surg.* 1983;197:276–283.

68. Schwartz GF, D'Ugo DM, Rosenberg AL. Extent of axillary dissection preceding irradiation for carcinoma of the breast. *Arch Surg.* 1986;121:1395–1398.

69. Pigott J, Nichols R, Maddox WA, et al. Metastases to the upper level of the axillary nodes in carcinoma of the breast and implications for nodal sampling procedures. *Surg Gynecol Obstet.* 1984;158:255–259.

70. Attiyeh FF, Jensen M, Huvos AG, et al. Axillary micrometastasis and macrometastasis in carcinoma of the breast. *Gynecol Obstet.* 1977;144:839–842.

71. Smith JA, Gamez-Araujo JJ, Gallager HS, et al. Carcinoma of the breast. Analysis of total lymph node involvement versus level of metastasis. *Cancer.* 1977;39:527–532.

72. Boova RS, Bonanni R, Rosato FE. Patterns of axillary node involvement in breast cancer. Predictability of level one dissection. *Ann Surg.* 1982;196:642–644.

73. Cody HS, III, Egeli RA, Urban JA. Rotter's node metastases. Therapeutic and prognostic considerations in early breast cancer. *Ann Surg.* 1984;199:266–270.

74. Moffat FL, Senofsky GM, Davis K, et al. Axillary node dissection for early breast cancer: some is good but all is better. *J Surg Oncol.* 1992;51:8–13.

75. Veronesi U, Luini A, Galimberti V, et al. Extent of metastatic axillary involvement in 1446 cases of breast cancer. *Eur J Surg Oncol.* 1990;16:127–133.

76. Naik AM, Park J, Dorn P, et al. Additional positive axillary nodes in 1404 breast cancer patients with a positive sentinel lymph node: Distribution by anatomic level. *Ann Surg Oncol.* 2006;13(Suppl):100.

77. Recht A, Houlihan MJ. Axillary lymph nodes and breast cancer: a review. *Cancer.* 1995;76:1491–1512.

78. Petrek JA, Lerner R. Lymphedema. In: Harris JR, Lippman ME, Morrow M, et al., eds. *Diseases of the Breast,* 2nd ed. Philadelphia: Lippincott Williams & Wilkins; 2000:1033–1040.

79. Morrell RM, Halyard MY, Schild SE, et al. Breast cancer-related lymphedema. *Mayo Clin Proc.* 2005;80:1480–1484.

80. Herd-Smith A, Russo A, Muraca MG, et al. Prognostic factors for lymphedema after primary treatment of breast carcinoma. *Cancer.* 2001;92:1783–1787.

81. Benson EA, Thorogood J. The effect of surgical technique on local recurrence rates following mastectomy. *Eur J Surg Oncol.* 1986;12:267–271.

82. Kissin MW, Querci della Rovere G, Easton D, et al. Risk of lymphedema following the treatment of breast cancer. *Br J Surg.* 1986;73:580–584.

83. Siegel BM, Mayzel KA, Love SM. Level I and II axillary dissection in the treatment of early-stage breast cancer. An analysis of 259 consecutive patients. *Arch Surg.* 1990;125:1144–1147.

84. Kissin MW, Thompson EM, Price AB, et al. The inadequacy of axillary sampling in breast cancer. *Lancet.* 1982;2:1210–1212.

85. Veronesi U, Saccozzi R, Del Vecchio M, et al. Comparing radical mastectomy with quadrantectomy, axillary dissection and radiotherapy in patients with small cancers of the breast. *N Engl J Med.* 1981;305:6–11.

86. Delouche G, Bachelot F, Premont M, et al. Conservation treatment of early breast cancer: long term results and complications. *Int J Radiation Oncol Biophys.* 1987;13:29–34.

87. Larson D, Weinstein M, Goldberg I, et al. Edema of the arm as a functionof the extent of axillary surgery in patients in stage I-II carcinoma of the breast treated with primary radiotherapy. *Int J Radiation Oncol Biophys.* 1986;12:1575–1582.

88. Beadle GF, Silver B, Botnick L, et al. Cosmetic results following primary radiation therapy for early breast cancer. *Cancer.* 1984;54:2911–2918.

89. Carabell SC, Richter MP, Bryan JH, et al. Radiation therapy as an alternative to mastectomy for breast cancer–the role of axillary sampling. *Int J Radiation Oncol Biophys.* 1981;7:31–32.

90. Hoe AL, Iven D, Royle GT, et al. Incidence of arm swelling following axillary clearance for breast cancer. *Br J Surg.* 1992;79:261–262.

91. Werner RS, McCormick B, Petrek JA, et al. Arm edema in conservatively managed breast cancer: obesity is a major predictive factor. *Radiology*. 1991;180:177–184.

COMMENTARY
Blake Cady

Dr. Silberman presents the potential therapeutic benefits of axillary dissection in breast cancer and describes an older concept of the controlling influence of regional nodal metastases on survival outcome. His review addresses breast cancer, but does not mention literature about regional node dissection in other primary cancers, which powerfully address the implication of regional nodal disease on outcome (1,2). Over 100 years ago, Halsted proposed that the lymphatic system was the primary route of breast cancer metastases: distant visceral disease resulted from direct or indirect lymphatic vessel connections between the breast, and its contained cancer, and the brain, lung, and liver. Local breast and regional nodal surgical options were paramount as they governed outcome by blocking lymphatic escape routes by cancer cells. This was the rationale for the Halsted radical mastectomy with radical axillary dissection. This Halstedian lymphatic dormant biological theory was nullified by randomized trials that revealed no survival benefit by regional axillary dissection in breast cancer, and in many other epithelial primary cancers by implication.

Fisher (3) proposed the subsequent "systemic from onset" biological theory from his many experiments in animals and the results of National Surgical Adjuvant Breast Project (NSABP) breast cancer randomized trials. Fisher determined that mortality depends on metastases to distant vital organs and the response to systemic treatment at an early micrometastatic stage. This obviated the effects of regional node metastases and the lymphatics, as breast cancer mortality was equivalent regardless of whether axillary dissection was performed. Local surgical treatment options did not determine survival outcome, and therapeutic priorities were systemic adjuvant treatments, either hormonal or chemotherapeutic. This systemic early hematogenous spread theory then dominated conceptual thinking in breast cancer treatment for the next 3 decades.

Hellman (4), after analyzing breast cancers at their earliest phases when discovered by mammographic screening, subsequently proposed a "spectrum" biological model. This biological theory, particularly defined in breast cancer by Hellman, was also apparent in gastric cancer in Japan, and colorectal and cervical cancers, other cancers favorably influenced by screening, indicates that the very earliest developing cancers modify their biological potential as they proceed in time and increase in size (5,6) Epithelial cancers originate in tiny foci with minimal virulence (5), and insignificant metastagenicity (6). As they grow in size and persist over time, the genetically abnormal original cancer cells evolve further with increasing genetic changes. Pathologic grade, initially low or better differentiated, dedifferentiates and evolves to higher grades or poorer differentiation as the cancers eventually become clinically detectable. Cancer prognosis is related to when the biologic progression to more aggressive behavior is interrupted by surgical removal. Widespread yearly mammographic screening results in breast cancers of 1 cm or less, and in the United States today the median diameter of all breast cancers, including patients with and without screening, is only 1.5 cm (7). The biological evolution of cancers detected by screening is interrupted early in their course and breast cancer mortality is very low. Increasing virulence (5) and metastagenicity (6) parallels the dedifferentiation that occurs with longer preclinical duration before becoming palpable. This proposed progression pattern is predominant but not universal in small cancers.

Two other biological varieties are recognized. A small subset of "systemic from origin" cancers may occur as a few even small breast cancers appear with poor differentiation and lymph vessel invasion or lymph node metastases and a poorer survival (8). Few breast cancer deaths occur with mammographically detected breast cancers <14 mm in size; however, three quarters of the infrequent deaths occur in the 14% of patients with such particular biological and mammographic features (9). Therefore, 86% of such small (≤14 mm) cancers display 20-year survival rates of over 97%. Contrariwise, some breast cancers apparently have no metastatic potential, with local growth potential only, even when large and clinically advanced. Patients reported by Halsted had a 15% long-term disease-free survival despite large size and an advanced presentation as an illustration of this small proportion of breast cancers without metastatic potential. T3 breast cancers without node metastases have a good long-term survival, even before the advent of adjuvant chemotherapy. These two minor categories within the "spectrum" model (i.e., 10% systemic from origin and 15% to 20% local growth potential only) leaves two-thirds to 75% conforming to the progressive type fitting the spectrum model of gradual progression to worse prognostic types as proposed by Hellman (4).

Randomized trials show no survival advantage for any variation of nodal resections or treatment in breast cancer (10). In other malignancies (melanoma and cancers of stomach, lung, esophagus, colon, and rectum), randomized trials comparing variations of nodal resections, or even just regional nodal observation, reveal no survival differences (1,2,10–13). Regional nodal removal increases staging accuracy and may result in stage shifting: the more nodes removed, the greater the stage accuracy, but no overall survival advantage occurs in randomized trials, except through the wider use of adjuvant therapies resulting from further discovery of node metastases.

Few 10-year survivors of breast, lung, colon and rectum, or stomach cancers had more than three node metastases at the time of initial resection (14). The American College of Surgeons' Gastric Cancer Report documented this very poor survival of patients with more than three node metastases present (15). Between 85% and 90% of all long-term survivors had either negative regional nodes or only one or two node metastases.

These many reports regarding the effects of regional nodal resections are manifestations of a comprehensive understanding of the anatomy, embryology, physiology, and function of the lymphatic system (16). The lymphatic system has only two original evolutionary purposes: to return interstitial fluid to the vascular space and nutrients from the digestive tract to the circulation. In later evolutionary development, collections of lymphocytes in lymph nodes interspersed in the lymphatic system developed for more sophisticated antigen recognition and humoral antibody and cytotoxic cells production to complete the functions of immunocompetence. Lymph nodes are not millipore filters but elaborate and ingenious organs for antigen recognition by lymphocytes. Labeled tumor cells injected into the nodal afferent lymphatic rapidly appear in efferent nodal lymphatics and the thoracic duct. If regional lymph nodes are destroyed by surgery, radiation therapy, parasitic infestation, or extensive metastases, regional edema is almost universal. Mammals, such as pigs, have numerous large regional lymph nodes because of constant exposure to environmental antigens (bacteria, parasites, viruses) but display no limb edema because lymph flow is not impeded by normal lymph nodes even if temporarily saturated with antigens that do not obstruct lymph flow, demonstrating that lymph nodes are porous, not millipore filters. A few cells detected by immunohistochemical staining of sentinel lymph nodes indicates the frequency of normal cells or cancer cells that are transiently detained but then may continue their passage without effecting distant metastases. Bone marrow metastatic cells detected by aspiration are an indicator for metastases risk, but in published data (17,18), they do not demonstrate the inevitability of metastases. As a matter of fact, over 80% of such patients survive metastases-free (18). In a meta-analysis of bone marrow aspiration studies (18) of patients with breast cancer, the prognostic effect of bone marrow cancer cells is identical to lymph node submicrometastases, indicating a similar prognostic effect for the risk of other distant vital organ metastatic disease. Thus, in themselves a few cells in bone marrow or lymph node are not a governing determination of survival, but only a prognostic indicator of the risk of clinical distant metastases.

Recent trials reported by Overgaard et al. (19,20) and Ragaz et al. (21) are different from previous trials by indicating a survival improvement by the addition of radiation to surgery in local surgical treatment of breast cancer after routine use of systemic therapy. Local recurrence after systemic adjuvant therapy, by definition, indicates chemoresistant or hormone-resistant cells. Previous trials not using systemic therapy revealed no survival advantage of local adjuvant radiotherapy (14). Neoadjuvant chemotherapy trials demonstrate this aspect of chemosensitivity (or resistance) because despite advanced clinical presentation of breast cancer with or without node metastases, and even inflammatory breast cancers, are cured in about 85% of cases if there is a complete pathologic response to primary chemotherapy (22). Such results display the chemosensitivity controlling influence on breast cancer survival regardless of the clinical stage of the primary presentation. These primary chemotherapy trials indicate the overriding importance of chemotherapy sensitivity in the survival of micrometastatic breast cancer.

Breast cancer survival is governed by the presence and growth or destruction of distant vital organ micrometastases: particular features of the primary cancer or regional nodal metastases are only general prognostic indicators. Cure in screen-detected small breast cancers is related to the absence of growth to a clinical distant metastasis, even though bone marrow or nodal micrometastases may be frequent. Breast cancer patients

never die of the local cancer, its recurrence, or regional nodal metastases or their recurrence, but only from distant vital organ clinical metastases. Because death does not result from axillary metastases or local disease, these manifestations of disease are indicators of outcome that is determined only by the distant clinical metastases that destroy some vital function: node metastases are statistically related to the likelihood of the controlling distant metastases but do not themselves cause death (1,2,10,16).

The biological explanation of the indicator function is displayed in animal research models demonstrating the cell and organ specificity of metastatic cancer (23). This is also demonstrated by distant vital organ oligometastatic disease, which can be cured by resection of liver metastases from colorectal carcinoma (24), and pulmonary metastases from sarcoma (25). Such cell and organ biological specificity applies to lymph node metastases in thyroid cancer (26) and islet cell cancers and carcinoid tumors (16). Brodt et al. (27) displayed unique cell and lymph node stroma characteristics that control lymph node metastases: a metastatic cell that progresses in a lymph node may have no capacity to grow in different organs. Liver metastases in colorectal cancer patients who survive long term following hepatic resection had huge quantities of circulating metastatic cells, but these cells apparently had no capacity to lodge and develop elsewhere. In differentiated thyroid cancer in young patients, lymph node metastases are present in 75% or more at regional node dissections, yet clinical distant metastases in lungs are uncommon (26) and the 20-year survival is over 98% disease-free. Apparently, cells that have the capacity to lodge and grow in cervical lymph nodes have no capacity to develop clinical metastases in other organs. On the other hand, sarcoma patients frequently develop lung metastases but seldom have regional nodal metastases; survival is determined only by lung metastases, not the uncommon nodal disease.

The indicator, but not governing, role of nodal metastases in breast cancer is emphasized by regional nodal recurrence; survival is better with longer disease-free intervals before regional recurrence. If lymph node metastases themselves had the capacity to cause vital organ distant metastases by further cell shedding, then the longer they were present (the longer the disease-free interval), the worse the survival should be because of longer periods of cell shedding, contrary to what is observed: longer disease-free intervals are associated with better survival. Lymph node recurrences and/or local recurrences may appear prior to, simultaneous with, or after distant metastases, or in isolation without distant metastases, in approximately equal proportions, yet a causative role of node metastases in survival can only be assumed if they recurred first, and later distant metastases appeared subsequently, which is the situation in only a minority of nodal recurrences (1,2,16). Indeed, when regional nodes are not surgically removed initially, but only at recurrence, the number of node metastases are the same and equivalent survival occurs, even though node metastases existed for long periods and were removed only late in disease evolution. Similar survival in initial prophylactic versus observation only, with later therapeutic nodal dissection when required that was demonstrated in breast cancer and melanoma trials, emphasizes this indicator function and clearly demonstrates the lack of any outcome- or survival-governing role of lymph node metastases.

Thus, a critical contemporary review of lymph node metastases and their surgery concludes that nodal metastases are indicators, not governors of outcome in breast cancer and all other cancer patients, with few exceptions. As a result, whether or not regional nodes are resected initially has no impact on survival. Dr. Silberman's chapter is of historical interest as its conclusions are not consistent with the contemporary literature or theory. Sentinel lymph node biopsy allows detection of nodal metastases for selection of adjuvant therapy and prognosis and can be performed under minimal anesthesia. Adjusting to this philosophy, even sentinel nodes in breast cancer that display metastases do not require subsequent axillary dissection, as demonstrated by recent articles (28–31); regional nodal recurrences are uncommon and survival is unaffected by such a policy of observation, only of proven metastatic disease, re-emphasizing the contemporary interpretation of this controversy.

REFERENCES

1. Gervasoni JE, Taneja C, Chung MA, et al. Biologic and clinical significance of lymphadenectomy. *Surg Clin North Am.* 2000;80:1631–1673.
2. Gervasoni JE Jr, Sbayi S, Cady B. The role of lymphadenectomy in the surgical treatment of solid tumors. An update on the clinical data. *Ann Surg Oncol.* 2007;14:2443–2462.
3. Fisher B. Laboratory and clinical research in breast cancer—a personal adventure: the David A. Karnovsky Memorial Lecture. *Cancer Res.* 1980;40:3863–3874.
4. Hellman S. Karnovsky Memorial Lecture. Natural history of small breast cancers. *J Clin Oncol.* 1994;12:2229–2234.
5. Heimann R, Ferguson D, Recant WM, et al. Breast cancer metastatic phenotype as predicted by histologic tumor markers. *Cancer J Sci Am.* 1997;3:224–229.
6. Heimann R, Hellman S. Aging, progression, and phenotype in breast cancer. *J Clin Oncol.* 1998;16:2686–2692.
7. Coburn, NG, Chung MA, Fulton J, et al. Decreased breast cancer size, stage and mortality in rhode island: an example of a well-screened population. *Cancer Control.* 2004;11:222–230.
8. Leitner SP, Swern AS, Weinberger D, et al. Predictors of recurrence for patients with small (one centimeter or less) localized breast cancer (T1a, NO, MO). *Cancer.* 1995;76:2266–2274.
9. Tabar L, Chen HH, Duffy S, et al. A novel method for prediction of long-term outcome of women with T1a, T1b, and 10-14 mm invasive breast cancers: a prospective study. *Lancet.* 2000;355:429–433.
10. Gervasoni JE, Taneja C, Chung MA, et al. Axillary dissection in the context of the biology of lymph node metastases. *Am J Surg.* 2000;180:278–283.
11. Balch CM, Soong SJ, Bartolucci AA, et al. Efficacy of elective regional lymph node dissection of 1 to 4 mm thick melanomas for patients 60 years and younger. *Ann Surg.* 1996; 224:255–263.
12. Bonenkamp JJ, Hermans J, Sasako M, et al. Extended lymph node dissection for gastric cancer. *N Engl J Med.* 1999;340:908–914.
13. Cuschieri A, Weeden S, Fielding J, et al. Patient survival after 0-1 and 0-2 resections for gastric cancer: long-term results of the MRC randomized surgical trial. *Br J Cancer.* 1999;79:1522–1530.
14. Cady B. Basic principles in surgical oncology. Presidential Address. *Arch Surg.* 1997;132:338–346.
15. Hundahl SA, Phillips Jl, Mench HR. The National Cancer Data Base Report on poor survival of U.S. gastric carcinoma patients treated with gastrectomy: fifth edition American Joint Committee on Cancer staging, proximal disease, and the "difference disease" hypothesis. *Cancer.* 2000;88:921–932.
16. Cady B. Regional lymph node metastases; a singular manifestation of the process of clinical metastases in cancer: contemporary animal research and clinical reports suggest unifying concepts. *Ann Surg Oncol.* 2007;14:1790–1800.
17. Diel IJ, Kaufmann M, Costa SO, et al. Micrometastatic breast cancer cells in bone marrow at primary surgery: prognostic value in comparison with nodal status. *J Natl Cancer Inst.* 1996;88:1652–1658.
18. Braun S, Vogl FD, Naume B, et al. A pooled analysis of bone marrow micrometastasis in breast cancer. *N Engl J Med.* 2005;353:793–802.
19. Overgaard M, Hansen PR, Overgaard J, et al. Postoperative radiotherapy in high-risk premenopausal women with breast cancer who receive adjuvant chemotherapy. *N Engl J Med.* 1997;337:949–955.
20. Overgaard M, Jensen MB, Overgaard J, et al. Postoperative radiotherapy in high-risk postmenopausal breast-cancer patients given adjuvant tamoxifen: Danish Breast Cancer Cooperative Group DBCG 82c randomised trial. *Lancet.* 1999;353:1641–1648.
21. Ragaz J, Jackson SM, Le N, et al. Adjuvant radiotherapy and chemotherapy in node-positive premenopausal women with breast cancer. *N Engl J Med.* 1997;337:956–962.
22. Buzdar AU, Ibrahim NK, Francis, D, et al. Significantly higher pathologic complete remission rate after neoadjuvant therapy with trastuzumab, paclitaxel, and epirubicin chemotherapy: results of a randomized trial in human epidermal growth factor receptor 2-positive operable breast cancer. *J Clin Oncol.* 2005;23:3376.
23. Chambers AF, Naumov GN, Varghese HJ, et al. Critical steps in hematogenous metastasis: an overview. *Surg Oncol Clin North Am.* 2001;10:243–255.
24. Cady B, Jenkins RL, Steele GO, et al. Surgical margin in hepatic resection for colorectal metastasis. *Ann Surg.* 1998;227:566–571.
25. Vezeridis MP, Moore R, Karakousis CP. Metastatic patterns in soft-tissue sarcomas. *Arch Surg.* 1983;118:915.
26. Cady B. Presidential address: beyond risk groups: a new look at differentiated thyroid cancer. *Surgery.* 1998;124:947–957.
27. Brodt P, Reich R, Moroz LA, et al. Differences in the repertoires of basement membrane degrading enzymes in two carcinoma sublines with distinct patterns of site-selective metastasis. *Biochem Biophys Acta.* 1992;77:1139.
28. Hwang RF, Gonzalez-Angulo AM, Yi M, et al. Low locoregional failure rates in selected breast cancer patients with tumor-positive sentinel lymph nodes who do not undergo completion axillary dissection. *Cancer.* 2007;119:723–730.
29. Naik AM, Fey J, Gemignani M, et al. The risk of axillary relapse after sentinel lymph node biopsy for breast cancer is comparable with that of axillary lymph node dissection. A Follow-up Study of 4008 Procedures. *Ann Surg.* 2004;240:68–77.
30. Guenther JM, Hansen NM, DiFronzo LA, et al. Axillary dissection is not required for all patients with breast cancer and positive sentinel nodes. *Arch Surg.* 2003;138:52–56.
31. Park J, Fey JV, Naik AM, et al. A declining rate of completion axillary dissection in sentinel lymph node-positive breast cancer patients is associated with the use of a multivariate nomogram. *Ann Surg.* 2007;245:462–468.

22

Sentinel Lymph Node Analysis in Breast Cancer: Indications, Techniques, and Results

Farin F. Amersi, Helen Mabry, and Armando E. Giuliano

Over the past 2 decades, evidence from randomized clinical trials has brought about major changes in the management of patients with breast cancer. Screening mammography, advances in adjuvant therapy, the implementation of breast-conservation surgery, and sentinel node biopsy (SNB) have had a substantial impact on the care of breast cancer patients. Intraoperative lymphatic mapping with SNB is becoming more widely accepted for regional lymph node staging in patients with early invasive breast cancer.

The presence of axillary lymph node metastases remains the most important predictor of overall recurrence and survival in patients with breast cancer (1–5). However, the value of axillary lymph node dissection (ALND) has been an area of controversy for many years as it has been widely viewed as a procedure for axillary staging and improving local control with no measurable survival benefit (6,7). Moreover, the decision to initiate adjuvant chemotherapy is no longer limited to patients with regional nodal involvement, but also depends on characteristics of the primary tumor including tumor size, histologic grade, histologic type, lymphovascular invasion, and receptor status.

ALND is associated with significant short- and long-term morbidity including increased risk of infection, pain, cosmetic deformity, and lymphedema, without providing any therapeutic benefit in node-negative patients (8–10). The appeal of SNB as an alternative to ALND for node-negative breast cancer patients is the ability to perform a smaller operation with less morbidity and complications, without compromising prognostic information.

To date, only one prospective randomized trial comparing SNB with ALND has been published, but several other large trials are pending (National Surgical Adjuvant Breast and Bowel Project [NSABP] B-32 and American College of Surgeons Oncology Group [ACOSOG] Z0010). Veronesi and colleagues (11) randomized patients with T1 tumors to either SNB followed by ALND or SNB alone. ALND was performed if the sentinel lymph node (SLN) contained metastases. A total of 516 patients were randomized. The incidence of SLN metastases was the same in both groups of patients. This suggested that SNB alone could predict axillary nodal metastases. Patients who received SNB only had less pain and better arm mobility. These patients developed no axillary recurrences and had the same short-term survival as the patients whose lymph nodes were tumor-free and treated with ALND. This study lacked the power to detect small differences in survival. The median follow-up was under

4 years (46 months). The false-negative rate of SNB was 8.8% (8 of 91 patients with node metastases were not identified) in the group undergoing complete ALND. The sensitivity was 91.2%, specificity was 100%, overall accuracy was 96.9%, and negative predictive value was 95.4%. This study used frozen section analysis of SLN and radioisotope only to locate the SLN.

NSABP B-32 is a prospective randomized trial designed to compare SNB with ALND in clinically node negative patients. A total of 5,611 patients were randomized from May 1999 to February 2004 when the trial was closed to accrual. This trial aims to compare disease-free survival, overall survival, and regional control of the axilla. There are 80 participating centers and 226 surgeons. The technical success rate for identifying the sentinel nodes was reported at 96.2% and there was a false-negative rate of 6.7% (12).

SENTINEL NODE BIOPSY INDICATIONS

SNB has become a powerful tool in staging of patients with early breast cancers. It significantly reduces the long-term risk of complications associated with ALND in node-negative patients. Moreover, most series report that patients with T1-T2 lesions have a 30% to 35% chance of metastases to axillary nodes (13–16). As the indications for adjuvant therapy have evolved over the last several years, SNB also provides a rational basis for identifying high-risk patients who can benefit from the use of systemic chemotherapy or hormonal therapy. SNB may provide local control if metastases were limited to the SLN. For patients with invasive tumors ≤1 cm the histopathologic status of the lymph nodes may be the deciding factor for or against adjuvant therapy.

Several consensus conferences such as American Society of Clinical Oncology (ASCO) Guidelines and Recommendations for Sentinel Lymph Node Biopsy in Early-stage Breast Cancer, Philadelphia Proceedings of the Consensus Conference on the Role of Sentinel Lymph Node Biopsy in Carcinoma of the Breast, April 19 to 22, 2001, and the 2005 International Consensus Conference on Image-detected Breast Cancer: State of the Art Diagnosis and Treatment have endorsed SNB as the preferred method for axillary staging of clinically node-negative patients with breast cancer (17–19). Nonetheless, SNB indications, techniques, and our understanding of the significance of the findings are still evolving. This chapter reviews the latest developments of SNB and future directions for its use.

HISTORY OF BREAST SENTINEL NODE BIOPSY

Morton and colleagues (20) developed lymphatic mapping and SNB for patients with early-stage melanoma. They defined the SLN as the first lymph node within the nodal basin to which the primary tumor drains. The SLN was localized by an intradermal injection with radiolabeled colloid or vital blue dye, or both together, and was highly predictive of the status of the remaining lymph nodes in that basin. This procedure was subsequently modified and applied to breast cancer by Giuliano et al. (21) in 1991. The initial experience that defined the technical aspects, and criteria for selecting patients for SNB, involved 172 patients with T1-T3 breast cancers, and included patients with or without palpable axillary adenopathy. Using a peritumoral injection of 5 mL of 1% isosulfan blue dye, the technique accurately predicted the tumor status of the axillary basin in 96% of these patients despite not having evolved the technique.

After the technique was optimized, the improvement in axillary staging by close histopathologic examination of sentinel nodes was prospectively evaluated in 162 patients with clinical T1N0 or T2NO breast cancer who underwent SNB followed by ALND compared with 134 patients who had ALND only (22). The SLNs were analyzed using both hematoxylin and eosin staining (H&E) and immunohistochemistry (IHC). This study demonstrated a significantly higher rate of detection of metastases in the group that had a SNB followed by completion ALND, than the group that had ALND only (42% vs. 29%), suggesting that a more focused examination of one or two SLNs by both H&E and IHC was more accurate than the histopathologic evaluation of the entire lymph node basin by H&E alone. Micrometastases were found in 3% of all ALND patients and 16% of all SNB patients because of the increased scrutiny of a smaller volume of tissue and the addition of IHC analysis. SNB provides the pathologist with the tissue most likely to contain metastases so that it can be the focus for intense study rather than the relatively large volume of tissue from ALND.

Other investigators validated the SNB technique in breast cancer. Albertini et al. (23) published the first use of both blue dye and filtered technetium-colloid for identifying the SLN, followed by completion ALND. Of the 62 patients in this study, the SLN was successfully identified in 92% of the patients with 100% specificity. Krag et al. (24) performed the first study using unfiltered technetium-colloid, and successfully identified the SLN in 18 of 22 patients (82%), with no false-negative cases. Veronesi et al. (25) performed SNB using a subdermal injection of technetium-99m (^{99m}Tc)-labeled human serum albumin and reported a 98% success rate in 160 of 163 patients, and accurately predicted the axillary status in 97% of the cases. These studies subsequently led to the first multicenter trial of 443 patients who had SLN dissection followed by ALND using radiotracer alone (26). Eleven surgeons from both academic and community programs successfully identified the SLN in 93% of the cases, with a false-negative rate of 11.4%. A similar multi-institutional study of 805 patients reported success with identifying the SLN using both a combination of radioactive colloid and blue dye (27). However, there were no statistically significant differences in the identification rate (92% vs. 89%), false-negative rate (1.6% vs. 8.7%), or the number of SLNs (2.2 vs. 2.0) removed between

the group that used blue dye versus a combination of blue dye and radiocolloid, respectively.

A meta-analysis of 11 published studies was performed with 912 patients that compared injection techniques with lymphoscintigraphy or blue dye or a combination of both in patients who had SLN dissection followed by ALND for in situ and invasive cancer (28). This study reported a significantly higher rate of identification if both radiocolloid and blue dye were used or radiocolloid alone compared with blue dye alone. Moreover, the SLN reflected the status of the axilla in 97% of the cases, with only a 5% false-negative rate reported. These studies demonstrate that the status of the SLN accurately predicts the status of the axillary nodal basin. The particular technique used is a matter of training and experience with verification of accuracy by ALND after SNB in the same patient.

SENTINEL NODE BIOPSY TRAINING

SNB can pose a technical challenge depending on the experience of the surgeon, pathologist, and the nuclear medicine radiologist. Cox et al. (29) reported on the need for adequate training and documentation of accuracy before performing lymphatic mapping and SLN biopsy. They studied the relationship between number of cases of SNB and the success rate of SLN identification. Sixteen surgeons performed lymphatic mapping in 2,255 breast cancer patients using a combination of blue dye and radiocolloid. They concluded that a learning curve exists to master the technique of SNB, with surgeons who perform more than six procedures per month identifying the SLN with 97% accuracy, whereas surgeons who performed three or less procedures per month had an average success rate of only 86%. Similar conclusions were also reached in the American College of Surgical Oncologist Group multicenter clinical trial for early-stage breast cancer, which examined individual surgeon's abilities to successfully identify the sentinel node (30). The authors found that surgeons who had accrued fewer than 50 patients in the study had a higher failure rate than those who accrued more.

TECHNICAL ASPECTS OF SLN BIOPSY

The SLN can be localized by either injection with radiolabeled colloid or vital blue or a combination of both. Lymphoscintigraphy is performed with ^{99m}Tc- labeled sulfur colloid. An advantage to the use of radiocolloid and lymphoscintigraphy is that it enables surgeons to identify drainage to areas away from the standard axillary nodal basin, including to supraclavicular, infraclavicular, and internal mammary nodes (Figure 22.1). Internal mammary draining nodes may be sampled or targeted for postoperative radiation (31–33).

Prior to surgery, patients are injected with the radiocolloid into the skin, subdermal, or peritumoral parenchyma of the breast (34). An injection of 0.5 mCi of filtered ^{99m}Tc sulfur colloid in a volume of 0.5 mL is standardly used. Imaging with a scintillation camera documents the drainage patterns through the lymphatics to the regional lymph nodes. Some surgeons do not use lymphoscintigraphy, but use the gamma probe to identify nodes intraoperatively. The location of the SLN is precisely marked on the skin, and a handheld gamma detection probe is

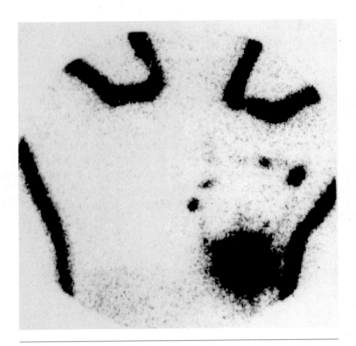

Figure 22.1 Lymphoscintigram demonstrating drainage to internal mammary nodes and axillary basin.

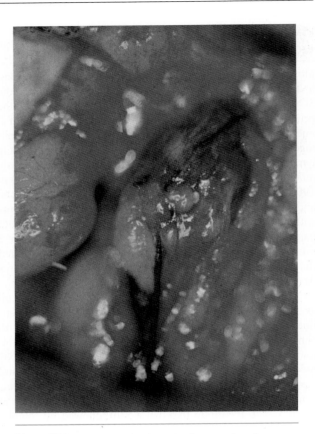

Figure 22.2 Intraoperative lymphatic mapping shows blue dye along the lymphatic channel into the sentinel node that is removed during sentinel lymph node dissection. (See color plates.)

used to identify the area of greatest activity in the axilla. This may help the surgeon in skin incision placement. Intraoperatively, the probe emits a signal that is used to guide the surgeon in identification of the sentinel node. Techniques vary; many surgeons believe that sentinel nodes should be removed until the baseline gamma probe signal is <10% of the highest signal value of a sentinel node; others remove only the node with the greatest signal.

Three to 5 mL of isosulfan blue dye (Lymphazurin 1%) injected subcutaneously or into the breast parenchyma surrounding the tumor will migrate to the sentinel node in approximately 5 minutes. Gentle massage of the breast tends to enhance migration. If the lesion has been excised, then the dye is injected into the breast parenchyma surrounding the cavity. If the lesion is not palpable, blue dye is injected into the parenchyma surrounding the area that has either been localized mammographically or through ultrasound guidance. A transverse incision is then made approximately 1 cm inferior to the hair-bearing area of the axilla, through the subcutaneous fat and clavipectoral fascia into the axillary fat pad. The SLN(s) is located by visual identification of a blue lymphatic tract or blue-stained node (Figure 22.2). If the SLN is not identified, regardless of technique, a full ALND should be performed. In addition, any additional palpable nodes that appear or feel clinically suspicious should be removed at the time of SNB.

Many factors contribute to the success of the procedure, including patient selection, injection technique, addition of massage, and timing of the incision. Older patients and patients with increased body mass index have been shown to have a decreased rate of SLN identification (35–38). The combination of blue dye and radioisotope enhances the ability to identify the SLN in all patient groups and may be especially helpful for sentinel node identification in obese or elderly patients.

Several investigators have studied which technique achieves the highest success rate in identifying the SLN with the lowest false-negative rate. A randomized trial by Morrow et al. (39) showed no significant difference in identifying the SLN when patients were randomized to either blue dye alone or the combination of blue dye and radiocolloid (86% vs. 88%, respectively) for surgeons learning the procedure. A significant predictor of SLN identification in this study was surgeon experience. Other studies confirm similar findings with either method (40–42).

The optimal injection technique continues to be debated. Several investigators, including the initial work by Giuliano et al. (21), have proposed that peritumoral intraparenchymal injection of blue dye or radiocolloid have a very low false-negative rate and have demonstrated 97% accuracy in identifying the SLN (Table 22.1). In addition, there is the advantage of not tattooing the skin using this technique compared with subdermal injections of blue dye. Other studies have proposed that subdermal injections yield similar identification rates as peritumoral injection (43,44). These authors conclude that, from a drainage standpoint, both techniques share similar lymphatic pathways. In a study by Vargas et al. (45), both radiocolloid and blue dye techniques identified SLNs with metastases with a concordance of 87%, with all patients in the study demonstrating successful uptake of radiocolloid and blue dye.

Subareolar injections of blue dye or radiotracer have been shown by some groups to be superior to peritumoral injections

Table 22.1

Injection Technique and Sentinel Lymph Node Identification

Study, Year (Ref.)	Patients	Site	(%) ID Rate
Linehan et al., 1999 (106)	200	IP vs. ID	92 vs. 100
Borgstein et al., 2000 (107)	210	ID vs. PT	100 vs. 100
Peley et al., 2004 (108)	100	SA vs. PT	99 vs. 100
Chagpar et al., 2004 (46)	3961	SA vs. PT	99 vs. 91
Lin et al., 2005 (109)	180	ID vs. PT	97 vs. 83
D'Eredita et al., 2006 (110)	195	SA vs. ID	95 vs. 100

ID, intradermal; IP, intraparenchymal; PT, peritumoral; SA, subareolar.

(46–48). Shimazu and colleagues (49) demonstrated a significantly higher success rate in identifying SLNs with subareolar injections of radioactive colloid when compared with peritumoral injection of blue dye (100% vs. 90%, respectively). These results support their hypothesis that the lymphatic drainage of the breast parenchyma and the subareolar plexus follow the same pathway to the SLN. Although many groups are proponents of peritumoral injections, there is considerable variation regarding the most appropriate technique for injection of blue dye or radiocolloid controversy, and individual experience and comfort with a particular technique is the most important factor in successful SNB. Cutaneous or subareolar injections rarely identify extra-axillary nodes.

The effect of gentle massage on the accuracy of SLN mapping remains controversial. Advocates of postinjection massage propose that the technique of massaging the breast encourages lymph flow and facilitates sentinel node detection (50).

In a study by Bass et al. (51), the addition of a 5-minute postinjection massage significantly improved the uptake of blue dye and radiocolloid by SLNs when compared with a control group of patients who did not receive a massage. Vigorous massage has never been definitively demonstrated to cause transportation of tumor cells into lymph nodes, but it appears to cause an increased incidence of benign epithelial cells in subcapsular sinuses of sentinel nodes, and may cause a false-positive finding of isolated tumor cells. In a study by Diaz et al. (52), a retrospective review of cytokeratin immunohistochemistry (CK-IHC)-positive cells in SLN of patients with intraductal carcinoma was performed. The authors found more CK-IHC–positive cells in SLN of patients who had received postinjection massage compared with SLN of patients without prior massage, and they concluded that pre-SLN biopsy breast massage may cause mechanical transport of epithelial cells to SLN. Other groups have also suggested that IHC-detected cells in SLNs of patients with breast cancer may represent mechanically displaced epithelial cells resulting from manipulation of the breast during mammography, breast biopsy, breast massage, or SLN biopsy (53–55). IHC employs monoclonal antibodies that are specific for epithelial cells, and are not tumor cell-specific, and it is possible that the CK-IHC–positive cells may represent mechanically displaced epithelial cells, and not tumor cells, which are unlikely to have clinical relevance. For now, there is no clear evidence that manipulation of the tumor with breast massage mechanically disrupts tumor cells, which may be transported into a SLN.

PATHOLOGICAL ANALYSIS OF THE SLN

Intraoperative Frozen Section of the SLN

Intraoperative analysis of SLNs is useful for rapidly identifying nodal metastases so that patients could undergo ALND during the same operation. The three methods for intraoperative analysis include gross inspection, imprint cytology, and frozen section. Brogi et al. (56) studied 305 SLNs from 133 patients with breast cancer. Each node underwent touch-preparation cytology and frozen section. Touch-preparation cytology and frozen section were fairly sensitive at detecting macrometastases (93% and 96%, respectively), but both had relatively poor sensitivity for detecting micrometastases (27% touch-preparation cytology and 27% frozen section). Turner et al. (57) also studied intraoperative analysis of SLNs from 278 patients with breast cancer comparing two-level frozen section combined with touch-preparation cytology to standard H&E-stained paraffin-embedded analysis. The two-level frozen section with touch-preparation cytology correctly identified 98% of all macrometastases, but only 28% of micrometastases, for an overall accuracy of 93%.

There is wide variation of frozen section protocols in different institutions in the United States and worldwide. Each institution must determine how best to analyze SLNs given the resources of their pathology departments. In most institutions permanent sections are more sensitive in detecting micrometastases than frozen sections. A frozen section to confirm metastases enables an ALND at the same operation and may be prudent to avoid a second operation; however, in most institutions intraoperative analyses are inadequate to reliably detect micrometastases.

Technique/Processing of SLN

Prior to SNB, staging of the axilla entailed the pathologist cutting one section of paraffin-embedded tissue from lymph nodes obtained from an ALND, and staining the sections with H&E. The process of examining multiple sections to detect micrometastatic

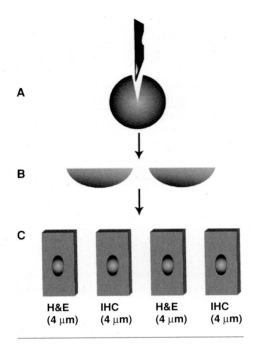

Figure 22.3 Technique of processing the sentinel lymph node (SLN) for histopathology. **(A)** Bisect SLN. **(B)** Section SLN. **(C)** Eight to 12 sections examined for immunohistochemistry (IHC) and hematoxylin and eosin (H&E) staining.

Table 22.2	
Indications for Sentinel Node Biopsy	
Approved Guidelines	Unapproved Indications
Prophylactic mastectomy	Prior axillary surgery
T1-T2 lesions	Pregnancy
Multicentric disease	T3-T4 lesions
Male breast cancer	Inflammatory breast cancer
Older patients	After neoadjuvant treatment
Obese patients	
DCIS	
Before neoadjuvant treatment	
Prior breast surgery	

DCIS, ductal carcinoma in situ.
Adapted from Lyman GH, Giuliano AE, Somerfield MR, et al. American Society of Clinical Oncology guideline recommendations for sentinel lymph node biopsy in early- stage breast cancer. *J Clin Oncol.* 2005;23:7703–7720.

disease can be time-consuming, arduous, and costly. SNB accurately predicts the histopathologic status of the axillary basin in breast cancer patients, allowing a more focused, less time-consuming, and more cost-effective analysis than ALND (11,58). The success of SNB depends in part on correct processing of the specimen after the SLN has been fixed briefly in 10% formalin. Because most tumor cells are found along the midplane and capsular sinus of the SLN, the node should be bisected through its length. The nodal tissue is then formalin-fixed, paraffin-embedded, and serially sectioned into at least 2- to 4-μm sections for H&E and IHC to identify micrometastases (Figure 22.3). IHC analysis requires the use of monoclonal antibodies specific for low- and intermediate-molecular-weight cytokeratins, which are present in cells of epithelial origin. This increases the sensitivity of detecting micrometastases. If the SLN does not demonstrate metastases by H&E or by IHC staining, the probability of metastases in a non-SLN from the same axillary basin is <1% in patients with small primary breast tumors and clinically nonpalpable axillary nodes (59). This analysis of SLN and nonsentinel nodes by the same technique was the first to confirm the SLN hypothesis.

INDICATIONS FOR SNB

SNB has improved the staging of breast cancer because it reliably predicts the status of the axilla with significantly less functional morbidity than an ALND. Although SNB has become well ac-

cepted in the staging and management of early-stage breast cancer patients, the role of SNB in the management of patients with ductal carcinoma in situ (DCIS), patients with previous breast and axillary surgery, clinically palpable axillary disease, neoadjuvant treatment, inflammatory breast cancer, and pregnancy-associated breast cancer, continues to be debated (Table 22.2).

PROPHYLACTIC MASTECTOMY

Indications for prophylactic mastectomy have become accepted for patients who have a strong family history of breast cancer, *BRCA1* and *BRCA2* gene mutation carriers, lobular carcinoma in situ, and for cosmesis or phobia of developing breast cancer in patients undergoing a contralateral mastectomy for breast cancer. In patients who have undergone a prophylactic mastectomy, the risk of finding an occult cancer has been reported to be about 5%; in addition, in patients with a history of breast cancer the risk of developing a contralateral breast cancer is about 1% per year (60,61). The feasibility of performing SNB is jeopardized in patients who choose to have a prophylactic mastectomy without axillary staging, and are subsequently found to have invasive cancer in the specimen; an ALND is then required to stage the axilla. If SNB is performed at the time of prophylactic mastectomy and the patient is found to have an invasive cancer with histologically negative SLNs, the morbidity associated with an ALND can be avoided. Dupont et al. (62) reported a series of 57 patients who underwent prophylactic mastectomy and SNB for lobular carcinoma in situ or were gene carriers of the *BRCA1* and *BRCA2* mutation, of whom two patients (3.5%) were found to have positive SLNs by IHC, in the absence of cancer in the mastectomy specimen. In addition, invasive breast cancer was found in two other patients with negative SLNs. As a result of these findings, 7% of the patients subsequently had a change in their surgical management. SNB may be offered to high-risk patients who choose to undergo prophylactic mastectomies.

PREVIOUS BREAST OR AXILLARY SURGERY

No large studies have reported success in identifying SLNs in patients who present with previous breast or axillary surgery. Many of the large trials excluded patients who had previous breast biopsies or previous axillary surgery (63–65). Of the limited studies available on SNB in patients who have had previous breast surgery, the data suggest that identifying the SLN can be achieved after previous breast biopsies, regardless of the size, location, or the length of time between the initial biopsy and the SLN procedure (66,67). In a retrospective review at the European Institute of Oncology, 543 patients were evaluated to determine the accuracy of SNB in patients who had previous breast biopsies (68). Lymphatic mapping identified the SLN in 99% of the patients. Based on clinical experience, a prior breast biopsy is not considered a contraindication to SLN.

Similarly, the effects of previous axillary operations on the accuracy of SNB have not been studied in large trials. The controversy surrounding the ability to successfully identify the SLN is due to disruption of lymphatic channels during surgery that can lead to aberrant lymphatic drainage patterns. A recent study was reported on the feasibility of performing a second SNB in a series of 18 patients who developed recurrences after breast conservation and SNB for early-stage breast cancer and who had negative SLNs at the time of their initial surgery (69). All patients underwent preoperative lymphoscintigraphy that demonstrated an SLN, and all patients had successful identification of the SLN intraoperatively, with an average of 1.3 SLNs removed. Two patients were found to have positive SLNs, requiring ALND. Of the 16 patients with negative SLNs, no recurrences were observed. In patients with prior axillary surgery, SNB may be offered and is best performed with both preoperative lymphoscintigraphy and blue dye for localization of SLN in unusual or nonaxillary locations.

DUCTAL CARCINOMA IN SITU

DCIS, by definition as a noninvasive lesion, does not have the ability to metastasize to regional lymph nodes. In theory, DCIS should not require SNB staging. However, because of sampling errors in about 20% of cases in which a core biopsy shows DCIS, invasive cancer will be found in the final specimen. Because of this, some surgeons will perform SNB for patients who have a core biopsy showing DCIS. Positive sentinel nodes have been reported in 0% to 13% of DCIS patients (70–75). Yen et al. (76) reviewed 398 patients diagnosed with DCIS on core biopsy and found that 20% had invasive disease on final pathology. On multivariate analysis, four independent risk factors for invasive disease were identified: age <55 (odds ratio [OR], 2.19; $p = 0.024$), diagnosis on a core biopsy (OR, 3.76; $p = 0.006$), mammographic size of DCIS >4 cm (OR, 2.92; $p = 0.001$), and high-grade DCIS (OR, 3.06; $p = 0.002$). Of these patients, 141

had SNB performed at the time of their initial operation. Seventy-three percent were diagnosed on core biopsy, 30% had invasive disease on final pathologic evaluation, and 10% (14/141) had SLN metastases. Of the 14 patients with positive nodes, 11 (79%) had invasive cancer found on their final pathology. Two of the 14 patients had metastases detected by IHC only. SNB should not be done after an excisional biopsy that shows DCIS only. If microinvasion is found, then SNB is indicated because these tumors have the ability to metastasize to axillary lymph nodes. SNB may be indicated in patients who have extensive DCIS requiring mastectomy. If invasive cancer is found on the final specimen, then postmastectomy SNB would be difficult. The patient would then require ALND. Further axillary surgery would be even more problematic if immediate reconstruction was completed, especially free flaps or flaps with transaxillary pedicles. For these reasons, SNB may be indicated for patients who require mastectomy for DCIS.

ASCO guidelines developed during a consensus conference in 2005 did not recommend routine use of SNB for breast-conserving DCIS treatment (17). If an invasive cancer is found, the patient can safely undergo SNB at another operation. Selective use of SNB is recommended in patients diagnosed with DCIS on core biopsy if there is a high risk of finding invasive disease. These may include patients undergoing mastectomy, palpable lesions, DCIS >40 mm, or high nuclear grade.

MULTICENTRIC LESIONS

Multicentric cancers found in different quadrants of the same breast occur in approximately 10% to 15% of patients. Multicentric tumors have been considered a contraindication to SNB; however, there is evidence that the entire breast may drain through the same afferent lymphatic channels to the same axillary sentinel node (Table 22.3) (77). In multiple small, nonrandomized studies SNB was performed with accuracy rates similar to patients with unifocal lesions (78,79). In a study by Goyal et al. (80), a mean number of 2.4 SLNs was found in 71 of 75 patients, with an identification rate of 94%. The SNB accurately predicted the status of the axilla in 96% of these patients. These results reflect similar outcomes in patients with unifocal invasive breast cancers. Most investigators report greater success using a combination of technetium sulfur colloid and blue dye. Some authors have suggested injecting radiocolloid at one site and blue dye at the tumor site.

CLINICALLY POSITIVE AXILLA

Most SNB studies have excluded patients with suspicious axillary lymph nodes. Determination of metastatic axillary disease by clinical examination is unreliable. The results of several series show a positive predictive value calculated as (true positive)/ (true positive + false positive) of 64% to 82%, a negative predictive value calculated as (true negative)/(true negative + false negative) of 50% to 63% and overall accuracy of 63% to 68% (81–84). Specht et al. (85) published a study of SNB in patients with clinically suspicious axillary nodes. Two experienced surgeons documented clinically suspicious axillary nodes in 106 patients preoperatively. The patients were

Table 22.3				
Sentinel Node Biopsy for Multicentric Disease				
Study, Year (Ref.)	Patients	No. of SLNs	% SLN ID Rate	% FN Rate
Shrenk and Wayand, 2001 (111)	19	1.9	100	0
Kumar et al., 2003 (75)	59	2.6	93	1.7
Tousimis et al., 2003 (76)	70	2.1	96	8
Goyal et al., 2004 (77)	842	2.4	94	8.8
Gentilini et al., 2006 (112)	42	1.36	100	2.3
Knauer et al., 2006 (113)	142	1.67	91	4

SLN, sentinel lymph node; ID, identification; FN, false-negative.

classified into two groups. The nodes of the first group were believed to be moderately suspicious and were described as "firm, shotty and more prominent that those on the contralateral side." Sixty-two patients were in this group. The nodes of the second group were thought to be "highly suspicious or unequivocally positive." Forty-four patients were in this group. All of these patients then underwent SNB. The positive predictive values of physical examination were 47% in the moderately suspicious group, 77% in the highly suspicious group, and 59% overall. The patients in the highly suspicious group had larger tumors (2.2 cm vs. 1.6 cm) and more lymphovascular invasion (41% vs. 32%). Both larger tumor size and lymphovascular invasion are known to correlate with a higher rate of axillary metastases. Overall, 41% of these patients with clinically involved nodes were node-negative and could be treated with SNB alone and spared ALND. This is some supportive evidence for use of SNB even in patients with a clinically involved axilla.

However, the more suspicious the axillary involvement, the more likely that the lymph nodes are truly involved. SNB is not recommended in patients with gross axillary disease. When performing SNB, any lymph node that is clinically suspicious for metastatic disease because of firm texture or enlarged size must be removed. These nodes are to be considered and evaluated as sentinel nodes even if they are not radioactive or blue. Some lymph nodes with large tumor deposits may have obstruction of the afferent lymphatics so that they cannot take up dye or radiocolloid. SNB may be attempted in patients with nodes clinically suspicious for metastatic disease; however, these patients, especially ones with large primary tumors or lymphovascular invasion, are likely to have nodal metastases and subsequently require ALND. However, there may be some patients with nodes clinically suspicious for metastatic disease who may be spared ALND, and SNB is worthwhile for them. ASCO guidelines recommended against performing SNB in patients with nodes clinically suspicious for metastases.

NEOADJUVANT CHEMOTHERAPY AND MANAGEMENT OF THE AXILLA

The use of neoadjuvant chemotherapy for patients with locally advanced breast cancer has received considerable attention over the last several years. The rationale for treating patients early with large operable tumors is reflected in many studies that demonstrate that systemic treatment downsized these large lesions, providing the alternative of breast conservation instead of mastectomy. Neoadjuvant chemotherapeutic regimens have led to axillary downstaging with a significant decrease in the number of palpable nodes after treatment (86,87). The use of SNB is being debated in patients who demonstrate a significant reduction in the number of nodes with metastatic disease, or who demonstrate a complete response. However, there is currently no evidence that ALND is not necessary even with a negative SLN after completion of neoadjuvant chemotherapy.

For patients with large lesions and clinically node-negative disease who are being considered for neoadjuvant chemotherapy, SNB is important in deciding which patients may need further therapy, including nodal radiation or ALND. Technical considerations including difficulty in identification of and retrieval of the SLN because of fat necrosis and fibrosis after neoadjuvant treatment can be avoided if the procedure is performed prior to the initiation of therapy (88–91).

The feasibility and accuracy of SNB after neoadjuvant treatment in patients who need axillary staging has also been debated. Many investigators have shown a high success rate in identifying SLNs with a low false-negative rate after neoadjuvant treatment (Table 22.4). The largest study demonstrating the feasibility and accuracy of SNB after neoadjuvant chemotherapy was conducted as part of the multicenter NSABP- B27 study (92). In this study, 428 patients were randomized to SNB with either lymphoscintigraphy, isosulfan blue dye, or a combination of both. The SLN was accurately identified in 85% of patients; however, the accuracy of identifying the SLN was significantly higher in the group that underwent SNB with radiocolloid, compared with blue dye or both, 90%, 77 %, and 88%, respectively. Of these patients, 323 went on to completion ALND. The SLN was the only involved node in 56% of patients with completion ALND. In addition, the authors demonstrated no difference in identifying the SLN based on tumor size or clinical status of the axilla. Although further studies with larger numbers and long-term follow-up are needed to fully evaluate the role of SNB after neoadjuvant treatment, there is supporting evidence that this technique is applicable in patients who demonstrate a complete clinical response. ASCO guidelines state that currently available data are not sufficient to recommend SNB or the appropriate timing related to preoperative chemotherapy, and the also expert panel

Table 22.4

Studies of Sentinel Node Biopsy After Neoadjuvant Chemotherapy

Study, Year (Ref.)	Tumor Stage	No. of Patients	% SLN ID Rate	% FN
Nason et al., 2000 (114)	2–3	15	87	33
Breslin et al., 2000 (115)	2–3	51	85	12
Fernandez et al., 2001 (116)	1–4	40	90	20
Haid et al., 2001 (117)	1–3	33	88	0
Julian et al., 2002 (118)	2–3	34	88	6
Miller et al., 2002 (119)	1–4	35	91	0
Piato et al., 2003 (120)	1–2	42	98	17
Jones et al., 2005 (121)	2–3	36	81	11
Mamounas et al., 2005 (92)	1–3	428	85	11
Tanaka et al., 2006 (122)	1–2	70	90	5

SLN, sentinel lymph node; ID, identification; FN, false-negative.

emphasizes that SNB should be performed only in patients with clinically negative axillary lymph nodes.

RECURRENT DISEASE/NEW PRIMARY BREAST CANCERS

Axillary staging of breast cancer with SNB is becoming more widely practiced and the dilemma of optimal treatment for new breast cancers or in-breast recurrences after previous ipsilateral SNB will arise. Although SNB has been successful in patients who have had previous biopsies, its role in patients who have had previous axillary surgery remains controversial. In patients who present with recurrent disease or a new primary, some investigators advocate a combination of both lymphatic mapping with radiocolloid and blue dye in identifying alternate lymphatic pathways such as internal mammary nodes or the contralateral axilla (93,94).

Port et al. (95) reported their experience with 32 patients who had prior axillary surgery for breast cancer and who developed in-breast recurrences. Of this group, the SLN was successfully identified in 75% of patients and there was a significant difference in the SLN identification rate if less than ten nodes had been removed during the previous axillary surgery compared with patients who had more than ten nodes removed (87% vs. 44%, respectively). The role of SNB in this group of patients remains to be established, and more data with larger numbers of patients are necessary to develop guidelines.

MALE BREAST CANCER

Breast cancer in men is uncommon, with approximately 1,600 new cases diagnosed each year according to the American Cancer Society. Although male patients usually present with larger tumors because of a delay in diagnosis, survival rates parallel women stage for stage (96). Men who develop breast cancer who undergo ALND are at similar risk of developing complications associated with this procedure. It seems logical that SNB could be used for men with breast cancer. In a study of 16 male

patients with T1 tumors, the SLN was successfully identified in 93% of patients (97). Although data are limited, the treatment and outcomes of men with breast cancer seem to be similar to women with breast cancer, and SNB may be offered to men with early breast cancer.

CONTRAINDICATIONS TO SNB: PREGNANCY-ASSOCIATED BREAST CANCER AND INFLAMMATORY BREAST CANCER

Pregnancy-associated breast cancer may have a delay in diagnosis because of lactation-associated changes of the breasts and difficulty in imaging pregnant patients. These patients may present with more advanced disease or metastatic disease. Breast conservation may be considered and radiation can be given postpartum without significant delay. Systemic chemotherapy can be administered after the first trimester of pregnancy. Hahn et al. (98) studied 57 pregnant women with breast cancer who received chemotherapy during pregnancy. All 57 women delivered live births. One child was born with Down syndrome and two have congenital anomalies including club foot and congenital bilateral ureteral reflux. The children appear to be healthy, but two have special educational needs. For patients who present with larger lesions, or present earlier in their pregnancy, modified radical mastectomy is commonly recommended. There are no studies that demonstrate the safety of lymphatic mapping during pregnancy. Blue dye should not be used in pregnant patients. A few studies have reported that the use of radiocolloid is considered safe because the fetal radiation exposure is likely to be minimal (99,100). Presently there is insufficient evidence for surgeons to recommend the use of SNB in pregnant patients with breast cancer. ASCO guidelines list pregnancy as a contraindication to SNB.

Inflammatory breast cancer represents one of the most aggressive forms of breast cancer. The diagnosis is based on the clinical presentation of diffuse inflammatory skin changes, with skin thickening, as well as histologic confirmation of dermal lymphatic invasion. The current management of inflammatory breast cancer includes neoadjuvant chemotherapy followed by modified radical mastectomy and postoperative radiation therapy. SNB is not recommended for patients with inflammatory breast cancer because of invasion and obstruction of dermal lymphatics by tumor cells.

AREAS OF CONTROVERSY

The accuracy of SNB depends on detailed histologic examination with serial sectioning of lymph nodes, as well as IHC to enhance detection of micrometastases, which may be missed on routine H&E staining. The definition of micrometastases has not always been consistent, and some reports have included isolated tumor cells. The American Joint Committee on Cancer divides lymph node metastases into those that measure ≤2 mm or >2 mm, and has now added the modifier (i+) for staging micrometastases found by IHC. For patients with micrometastases, additional nonsentinel node disease will be found in 8% to 35% (101).

The significance of isolated tumor cells (502 mm) as they relate to the risk of additional metastases in nonsentinel nodes, as well as prognosis, remains unclear. It has been suggested that SNB is adequate surgery for control of locoregional disease in patients with metastatic disease limited to isolated tumor cells. Chu et al. (102) studied 157 patients with T1-T2 breast cancers who had breast conservation and a SLN with metastatic disease, all of whom had completion ALND, and found that when the SLN contained micrometastases (≤2 mm), the rate of non-SLN involvement was only 7%, compared with 55% if the SLN contained macrometastases (>2 mm). A small number of patients with tumor-free SLNs may develop axillary recurrences due to the presence of undetected subclinical or occult disease. Clinically, nodal micrometastases can affect further treatment decisions by identifying high-risk patients who may be candidates for systemic therapy. The ACOSOG Z0010 trial was designed to determine the prognostic significance of micrometastases in SLN and bone marrow for patients with T1-2 N0 breast cancer. The goal of this study is to determine the significance, if any, of micrometastases detected by IHC on overall survival, disease-free survival, and axillary recurrence. The clinical relevance of micrometastases and isolated tumor cells is still not known. Studies designed to answer these questions are still pending. These studies include NSABP B-32 and (ACOSOG) Z0010. At the time of publication of the ASCO guidelines, this panel of experts recommended routine ALND for patients with micrometastases regardless of the method of detection.

FUTURE DIRECTION: MOLECULAR ANALYSIS OF SLN

Newer, more sensitive methods of detecting occult lymphatic metastases have been developed. The field of molecular oncology has identified multiple RNA and DNA markers that relate to cellular function, angiogenesis, invasion, metastases, and include tumor suppressor genes, oncogenes, tumor-associated antigens, transcription factors, and cellular mediators of apoptosis. Reverse transcriptase polymerase chain reaction (RT-PCR)

techniques detect tumor cells not only in tissue, but in lymph nodes, bone marrow, or blood. RT-PCR analysis of the SLN remains controversial because detection of tumor marker mRNA in histopathologically negative SLNs may result in the upstaging of some breast cancer patients, and the clinical significance of these findings are not known at this time. The significance of IHC-identified micrometastases is still subject to debate (103–105). Molecular techniques are limited by the specificity and sensitivity of markers and lack of standardization. Considerable work is still needed to develop clinically meaningful RT-PCR markers that are specific for breast cancer.

CONCLUSION

Since the early 1990s the development and wide acceptance of SNB has profoundly affected the management of breast cancer. The technique reliably stages the axilla with more accuracy and less morbidity than traditional ALND. SNB identifies node-positive patients who may need ALND for control of regional disease and identifies women at higher risk of recurrence. SNB has become an invaluable tool to clinicians to guide decisions regarding adjuvant treatment. Currently, the NSABP-32, a large multicenter randomized phase III clinical trial, aims to demonstrate that patients who have tumor-free SLN, with no further axillary surgery, will have the same outcomes, with less morbidity and better functional outcomes than those undergoing ALND, confirming the smaller randomized trial of Veronesi et al. (11).

Intense histopathologic assessment of the SLN has enhanced detection of clinically occult nodal metastases. The role of molecular technology in ultrastaging of the SLN remains to be established. Although some studies have demonstrated molecular evidence of SLN metastasis in patients with early-stage breast cancer, its clinical relevance has not been determined. Standardized protocols for histopathologic assessment, as well as treatment based on SLN status, are needed in order to determine the best prognostic and therapeutic interventions for patients with breast cancer.

REFERENCES

1. Carter CL, Allen C, Henson DE, et al. Relation of tumor size, lymph node status, and survival in 24,270 breast cancer cases. *Cancer.* 1989;63:181–187.
2. Beenken SW, Urist MM, Zhang Y, et al. Axillary lymph node status, but not tumor size predicts locoregional recurrence and overall survival after mastectomy for breast cancer. *Ann Surg.* 2003;237(5):732–738.
3. Kurtz JM, Kinkel K. Breast conservation in the 21st century. *Eur J Cancer.* 2000;36(15):1919–1924.
4. Huston TL, Simmons RM. Locally recurrent breast cancer after conservation therapy. *Am J Surg.* 2005;189(2):229–235.
5. Fortin A, Larochelle M, Laverdiere J, et al. Local failure is responsible for the decrease in survival for patients with breast cancer treated with conservative surgery and postoperative radiotherapy. *J Clin Oncol.* 1999;17(1):101–109.
6. Fisher B, Jeong H, Anderson S, et al. Twenty-five-year follow-up of a randomized trial comparing radical mastectomy, total mastectomy, and total mastectomy followed by irradiation. *N Engl J Med.* 2002;347(8):567–575.

7. Sosa JA, Diener-West M, Gusev V, et al. Association between extent of axillary lymph node dissection and survival in patients with stage I breast cancer. *Ann Surg Oncol.* 1998;5(2):140–149.

8. Schijven MP, Vingerhoets AJ, Rutten HJ et al. Comparison of morbidity between axillary lymph node dissection and sentinel node biopsy. *Eur J Surg Oncl.* 2003;29(4):341–350.

9. Burak WE, Hollenbeck ST, Zervos EE, et al. Sentinel lymph node biopsy results in less postoperative morbidity compared with axillary lymph node dissection for breast cancer. *Am J Surg.* 2002;183(1):23–27.

10. Swenson KK, Nissen MJ, Ceronsky C, et al. Comparison of side effects between sentinel lymph node and axillary lymph node dissection for breast cancer. *Ann Surg Oncol.* 2002;9:745–753.

11. Veronesi U, Paganelli G, Viale G, et al. A randomized comparison of sentinel node biopsy with routine axillary dissection in breast cancer. *N Engl J Med.* 2003;349(6):546–553.

12. Harlow SP, Krag D, Julian TB, et al. Prerandomization Surgical Training for the National Surgical Adjuvant Breast and Bowel Project (NSABP) B-32 Trial, a randomized phase III clinical trial to compare sentinel node resection to conventional axillary dissection in clinically node-negative breast cancer. *Ann Surg.* 2005;241(1):48–54.

13. Marrazzo A, Taormina P, David M, et al. The role of sentinel lymph node biopsy in the treatment of breast cancer. *Chir Ital.* 2006;58(3):299–304.

14. Pelosi E, Ala A, Bello E, et al. Impact of axillary nodal metastases on lymphatic mapping and sentinel lymph node identification rate in patients with early stage breast cancer. *Eur J Nucl Med Mol Imaging.* 2005;32(8):937–942.

15. Soni NK and Spillane AJ. Experience of sentinel node biopsy alone in early breast cancer without further axillary dissection in patients with negative sentinel node. *ANZ J Surg.* 2005;75(5):292–299.

16. Choi SH, Barsky SH, Chang HR. Clinicopathologic analysis of sentinel lymph node mapping in early breast cancer. *Breast J.* 2003;9(3):153–162.

17. Lyman GH, Giuliano AE, Somerfield MR, et al. American society of clinical oncology guideline recommendations for sentinel lymph node biopsy in early-stage breast cancer. *J Clin Oncol.* 2005;23(30):7703–7720.

18. Schwartz GF, Giuliano AE, Veronesi U, et al. Proceedings of the consensus conference on the role of sentinel lymph node biopsy in carcinoma of the breast, April 19-22, 2001, Philadelphia, Pennsylvania. *Cancer.* 2002;94:2542–2551.

19. Silverstein MJ, Lagios MD, Recht A, et al. Image-detected breast cancer: state of the art diagnosis and treatment. *J Am Coll Surg.* 2005;201(4):586–597.

20. Morton DL, Wen DR, Wong JH, et al. Technical details of intraoperative lymphatic mapping for early stage melanoma. *Arch Surg.* 1992;127(4):392–399.

21. Giuliano AE, Kirgan DM, Guenther JM, Morton DL. Lymphatic mapping and sentinel lymphadenectomy for breast cancer. *Ann Surg.* 1994;220(3):391–398.

22. Giuliano AE, Dale PS, Turner RR, et al. Improved axillary staging of breast cancer with sentinel lymphadenectomy. *Ann Surg.* 1995;222:394–401.

23. Albertini JJ, Lyman GH, Cox C, et al. Lymphatic mapping and sentinel node biopsy in the patient with breast cancer. *JAMA* 1996;276(22):1818–1822.

24. Krag DN, Weaver DL, Alex JC, et al. Surgical resection and radiolocalization of the sentinel node in breast cancer using gamma probe. *Surg Oncol.* 1993;2:335–340.

25. Veronesi U, Paganelli G, Galimberti V, et al. Sentinel-node biopsy to avoid axillary dissection in breast cancer with clinically negative lymph nodes. *Lancet.* 1997;349:1864–1867.

26. Krag D, Weaver D, Ashikaga T, et al. The sentinel node in breast cancer: a multicenter validation study. *N Engl J Med.* 1998;339(14):941–946.

27. McMasters KM, Wong SL, Tuttle TM, et al. Preoperative lymphoscintigraphy for breast cancer does not improve the ability to identify axillary sentinel lymph nodes. *Ann Surg.* 2000;231(5):724–731.

28. Miltenberg DM, Miller C, Karamlou TB, et al. Meta-analysis of sentinel lymph node biopsy in breast cancer. *J Surg Res.* 1999;84:138–142.

29. Cox CE, Salud CJ, Cantor A, et al. Learning curves for breast cancer sentinel lymph node mapping based on surgical volume analysis. *J Am Coll Surg.* 2001;193(6):593–600.

30. Posther KE, McCall LM, Blumencranz PW, et al. Sentinel node skills verification and surgeon performance: data from a multicenter clinical trial for early-stage breast cancer. *Ann Surg.* 2005;242(4):593–599; discussion 599–602.

31. Park C, Seid P, Morita E, et al. Internal mammary sentinel lymph node mapping for invasive breast cancer: implications for staging and treatment. *Breast J* 2005;11(1):29–33.

32. Farrus B, Vidal-Sicart S, Velasco M, et al. Incidence of internal mammary node metastases after a sentinel lymph node technique in breast cancer and its implication in the radiotherapy plan. *Int J Radiat Oncol Biol Phys.* 2004;60(3):715–721.

33. Estourgie SH, Nieweg OE, Olmos RA, et al. Lymphatic drainage patterns from the breast. *Ann Surg.* 2004;239(2):232–237.

34. Giuliano AE, Dale PS, Turner RR, et al. Improved axillary staging of breast cancer with sentinel lymphadenectomy. *Ann Surg.* 1995;222(3):394–401.

35. Sener SF, Winchester DJ, Brinkmann E, et al. Failure of sentinel lymph node mapping in patients with breast cancer. *J Am Coll Surg.* 2004;198(5):732–736.

36. Cox CE, Dupont E, Whitehead GF, et al. Age and body mass index may increase the chance of failure in sentinel lymph node biopsy for women with breast cancer. *Breast J* 2002;8(2):88–91.

37. Leppanen E, Leidenius M, Krogerus L, et al. The effect of patient and tumour characteristics on visualization of sentinel nodes after a single intratumoural injection of Tc 99m labelled human albumin colloid in breast cancer. *Eur J Surg Oncol.* 2002;28:821–826.

38. Derossis AM, Fey JV, Cody HS, et al. Obesity influences outcome of sentinel lymph node biopsy in early-stage breast cancer. *J Am Coll Surg.* 2003;197(6):896–901.

39. Morrow M, Rademaker AW, Bethke KP, et al. Learning sentinel node biopsy: results of a prospective randomized trial of two techniques. *Surgery.* 1999;126(4):714–720.

40. Reitsamer R, Peintinger F, Rettenbacher L, et al. Subareolar subcutaneous injection of blue dye versus peritumoral injection of technetium-labeled human albumin to identify sentinel lymph nodes in breast cancer patients. *World J Surg.* 2003;27(12):1291–1294.

41. Kern KA. Concordance and validation study of sentinel lymph node biopsy for breast cancer using subareolar injection of blue dye and technetium 99m sulfur colloid. *J Am Coll Surg.* 2002;195(4):467–475.

42. Cserni G, Rajtar M, Boross G, et al. Comparison of vital dye-guided lymphatic mapping and dye plus gamma probe-guided sentinel node biopsy in breast cancer. *World J Surg.* 2002;26(5):592–597.

43. Mateos JJ, Vidal-Sicart S, Zanon G, et al. Sentinel lymph node biopsy in breast cancer patients: subdermal versus peritumoural radiocolloid injection. *Nucl Med Commun.* 2001;22(1):17–24.

44. McMasters KM, Wong SL, Martin RC, et al. Dermal injection of radioactive colloid is superior to peritumoral injection for breast

cancer sentinel lymph node biopsy: results of a multiinstitutional study. *Ann Surg.* 2001;233(5):676–687.

45. Vargas HI, Tolmos J, Agbunag RV, et al. A validation trial of subdermal injection compared with intraparenchymal injection for sentinel lymph node biopsy in breast cancer. *Am Surg.* 2002;68: 87–91.

46. Chagpar A, Martin RC, Chao C, et al. Validation of subareolar and periareolar injection techniques for breast sentinel lymph node biopsy. *Arch Surg.* 2004;139(6):614–618.

47. Reitsamer R, Peintinger F, Rettenbacher L, et al. Subareolar subcutaneous injection of blue dye versus peritumoral injection of technetium-labeled human albumin to identify sentinel lymph nodes in breast cancer patients. *World J Surg.* 2003;27(12):1291–1294.

48. D'Eredita G, Ferrarese F, Cecere V, et al. Subareolar injection may be more accurate than other techniques for sentinel lymph node biopsy in breast cancer. *Ann Surg Oncol.* 2003;10(8):942–947.

49. Shimazu K, Tamaki Y, Taguchi T, et al. Comparison between periareolar and peritumoral injection of radiotracer for sentinel lymph node biopsy in patients with breast cancer. *Surgery.* 2002;131(3):277–286.

50. Haynes G, Garske D, Case D, et al. Effect of massage technique on sentinel lymph node mapping for cancer of the breast. *Am Surg.* 2003;69(6):520–522.

51. Bass SS, Cox CE, Salud CJ, et al. The effects of postinjection massage on the sensitivity of lymphatic mapping in breast cancer. *J Am Coll Surg.* 2001;192(1):9–16.

52. Diaz NM, Cox CE, Ebert M, et al. Benign mechanical transport of breast epithelial cells to sentinel lymph nodes. *Am J Surg Pathol.* 2004;28(12):1641–1645.

53. Rosser RJ. A point of view: Trauma is the cause of occult micrometastatic breast cancer in sentinel axillary lymph nodes. *Breast J.* 2000;6:209–212.

54. Hansen NM, Ye X, Grube BJ, et al. Manipulation of the primary breast tumor and the incidence of sentinel node metastases from invasive breast cancer. *Arch Surg.* 2004;139:634–640.

55. Turner RR, Giuliano AE. Does breast massage push tumor cells into sentinel nodes? *Am J Surg Pathol.* 2005;29(9):1254–1255.

56. Brogi E, Torres-Matundan E, Tan LK, et al. The results of frozen section, touch preparation, and cytological smear are comparable for intraoperative examination of sentinel lymph nodes: a study in 133 breast cancer patients. *Ann Surg Oncol.* 2005;12(2):173–180.

57. Turner RR, Hansen NM, Stern SL, et al. Intraoperative examination of the sentinel lymph node for breast carcinoma staging. *Am J Clin Pathol.* 1999;112(5):627–634.

58. McMasters KM, Tuttle TM, Carlson DJ, et al. Sentinel lymph node biopsy for breast cancer: a suitable alternative to routine axillary dissection in multi-institutional practice when optimal technique is used. *J Clin Oncol.* 2000;18(13):2560–2566.

59. Giuliano AE, Jones RC, Brennan M and Statman R. Sentinel lymphadenectomy in breast cancer. *J Clin Oncol.* 1997;15:2345–2350.

60. Hartmann LC, Schaid DJ, Woods JE, et al. Efficacy of bilateral prophylactic mastectomy in women with a family history of breast cancer. *N Engl J Med.* 1999;340(2):77–84.

61. Herrinton LJ, Barlow WE, Yu O, et al. Efficacy of prophylactic mastectomy in women with unilateral breast cancer: a cancer research network project. *J Clin Oncol.* 2005;23(19):4275–4286.

62. Dupont EL, Kuhn MA, McCann C, et al. The role of sentinel lymph node biopsy in women undergoing prophylactic mastectomy. *Am J Surg.* 2000;180:274–277.

63. Veronesi U, Galimberti V, Zurrida S, et al. Sentinel lymph node biopsy as an indicator for axillary dissection in early breast cancer. *Eur J Cancer.* 2001;37(4):454–458.

64. Viale G, Zurrida S, Mairoano E, et al. Predicting the status of axillary sentinel lymph nodes in 4351 patients with invasive breast carcinoma treated in a single institution. *Cancer.* 2005;103(3): 492–500.

65. Cox CE, Pendas S, Cox JM, et al. Guidelines for sentinel node biopsy and lymphatic mapping of patients with breast cancer. *Ann Surg.* 1998;227:645–653.

66. Heuts EM, van der ENT FW, Kengen RA, et al. Results of sentinel node biopsy not affected by previous excisional biopsy. *Eur J Surg Oncol.* 2006;32(3):278–281.

67. Dinan D, Cagle CE, Pettinga J. Lymphatic mapping and sentinel node biopsy in women with an ipsilateral second breast carcinoma and a history of breast and axillary surgery. *Am J Surg.* 2005;190(4):614–617.

68. Luini A, Galimberti V, Gatti G, et al. The sentinel lymph node biopsy after previous breast surgery: preliminary results on 543 patients treated at the European Institute of Technology. *Breast Cancer Res Treat.* 2005;89(2):159–163.

69. Intra M, Trifiro G, Viale G et al. Second biopsy of axillary sentinel lymph node for reappearing breast cancer after previous sentinel lymph node biopsy. *Ann Surg Oncol.* 2005;12(11):895–899.

70. Pendas S, Dauway E, Giuliano R, et al. Sentinel node biopsy in ductal carcinoma in-situ patients. *Ann Surg Oncol.* 2000;7(1):15–20.

71. Klauber-DeMoore N, Tan LK, Liberman L, et al. Sentinel Lymph Node Biopsy: Is It Indicated in Patients With High-Risk Ductal Carcinoma-In-Situ and Ductal Carcinoma-In-Situ With Microinvasion? *Ann Surg Oncol.* 2000;7(9):636–642.

72. Cox CE, Nguyen K, Gray RJ, et al. Importance of lymphatic mapping in ductal carcinoma in situ (DCIS): why map DCIS? *Am Surg.* 2001;67:513–519.

73. Kelly TA, Kim JA, Patrick R, et al. Axillary lymph node metastases in patients with a final diagnosis of ductal carcinoma in situ. *Am J Surg.* 2003;186(4):368–370.

74. Veronesi P, Intra M, Vento AR, et al. Sentinel lymph node biopsy for localized ductal carcinoma in situ? *Breast.* 2005;14(6):520–522.

75. Farkas EA, Stolier AJ, Teng SC, et al. An argument against routine sentinel node mapping for DCIS. *Am Surg.* 2004;70(1):13–17.

76. Yen TW, Hunt KK, Ross MI, et al. Predictors of invasive breast cancer in patients with an initial diagnosis of ductal carcinoma in situ: a guide to selective use of sentinel lymph node biopsy in management of ductal carcinoma in situ. *J Am Coll Surg.* 2005;200(4):516–526.

77. Jin Kim H, Heerdt AS, Cody HS, et al. Sentinel lymph node drainage in multicentric breast cancers. *Breast J.* 2002; 8(6):356–361.

78. Kumar R, Jana S, Heiba SI, et al. Retrospective analysis of sentinel node localization in multifocal, multicentric, palpable, or nonpalpable breast cancer. *J Nucl Med.* 2003;44(1):7–10.

79. Tousimis E, Van Zee KJ, Fey JV, et al. The accuracy of sentinel lymph node biopsy in multicentric and multifocal invasive breast cancers. *J Am Coll Surg.* 2003;197(4):529–535.

80. Goyal A, Newcombe RG, Mansel RE, et al. Sentinel lymph node biopsy in patients with multifocal breast cancer. *Eur J Surg Oncol.* 2004;30(5):475–479.

81. Cutler SJ, Axtell LM, Schottenfeld D, et al. Clinical assessment of lymph nodes in carcinoma of the breast. *Surg Gynelcol Obstet.* 1970;131:41–52.

82. Fisher B, Wolmark N, Banes M. The accuracy of clinical nodal staging and limited axillary dissection as a determinant of histologic nodal status in carcinoma of the breast. *Gynecol Obstet.* 1981;152:765–772.

83. De Freitas R Jr, Costa MV, Schneider SV, et al. Accuracy of ultrasound and clinical examination in the diagnosis of axillary lymph node metastases in breast cancer. *Eur J Surg Oncol.* 1991;17:240–244.

84. Vaidya JS, Vyas JJ, Thakur MH, et al. Role of ultrasound to detect axillary node involvement in operable breast cancer. *Eur J Surg Oncol.* 1996;22:140–143.

85. Specht MC, Fey JV, Borgen PI, et al. Is the clinically positive axilla in breast cancer really a contraindication to sentinel lymph node biopsy? *J Am Coll Surg.* 2005;200:10–14.

86. Vlastos G, Mirza NQ, Lenert JT, et al. The feasibility of minimally invasive surgery for stage IIA, IIB, and IIIA breast carcinoma patients after tumor downstaging with induction chemotherapy. *Cancer.* 2000;88(6):1417–1424.

87. Cance WG, Carey LA, Calvo BF, et al. Long-term outcome of neoadjuvant therapy for locally advanced breast carcinoma: effective clinical downstaging allows breast preservation and predicts outstanding local control and survival. *Ann Surg.* 2002;236(3): 295–302.

88. Kang SH, Kang JH, Choi EA, et al. Sentinel lymph node biopsy after neoadjuvant chemotherapy. *Breast Cancer.* 2004;11(3):233–241.

89. Patel NA, Piper G, Patel JA, et al. Accurate axillary nodal staging can be achieved after neoadjuvant therapy for locally advanced breast cancer. *Am Surg.* 2004;70:696–699.

90. Abrial C, Van Praagh I, Delva R, et al. Pathological and clinical response of a primary chemotherapy regimen combining Vinorelbine, Epirubicin, and Paclitaxel as neoadjuvant treatment in patients with operable breast cancer. *The Oncologist.* 2005;10(4): 242–249.

91. Rajan R, Esteva FJ, Symmans WF. Pathologic changes in breast cancer following neoadjuvant chemotherapy: implications for the assessment of response. *Clin Breast Cancer.* 2004;5(3):235–238.

92. Mamounas EP, Brown A, Anderson S, et al. Sentinel node biopsy after neoadjuvant chemotherapy in breast cancer: results from National Surgical Adjuvant Breast and Bowel Project Protocol B-27. *J Clin Oncol.* 2005;23(12):2694–2702.

93. Agarwal A, Heron DE, Sumkin J, et al. Contralateral uptake and metastases in sentinel lymph node mapping for recurrent breast cancer. *J Surg Oncol.* 2005;92(1):4–8.

94. Intra M, Trifiro G, Viale G, et al. Second biopsy of axillary sentinel lymph node for reappearing breast cancer after previous sentinel lymph node biopsy. *Ann Surg Oncol.* 2005;12(11):895–899.

95. Port ER, Fey J, Gemignani ML, et al. Reoperative sentinel lymph node biopsy: a new option for patients with primary or locally recurrent breast carcinoma. *J Am Coll Surg.* 2002;195(2):167–172.

96. Vetto J, Jun SY, Paduch D, et al. Stages at presentation, prognostic factors, and outcome of breast cancer in males. *Am J Surg.* 1999;177(5):379–383.

97. Port ER, Fey JV, Cody HS, Borgen PI. Sentinel lymph node biopsy in patients with male breast carcinoma. *Cancer.* 2001;91(2):319–323.

98. Hahn KM, Johnson PH, Gordon N, et al. Treatment of pregnant breast cancer patients and outcomes of children exposed to chemotherapy in utero. *Cancer.* 2006;107:1219–1226.

99. Morita ET, Chang J, Leong S. Principles and controversies in lymphoscintigraphy for breast carcinoma during pregnancy. *Surg Clin North Am.* 2000;80(6):1721–1737.

100. Gentilini O, Cremonesi M, Trifiro G, et al. Safety of sentinel node biopsy in pregnant patients with breast cancer. *Ann Oncol.* 2004;15(9):1348–1351.

101. McCready DR, Yong WS, Ng AK, et al. Influence of the new AJCC breast cancer staging system on sentinel lymph nodes positivity and false-negative rates. *J Natl Cancer Inst.* 2004;(96):873–875.

102. Chu KU, Turner RR, Hansen NM, et al. Do all patients with sentinel node metastasis from breast carcinoma need complete axillary node dissection? *Ann Surg.* 1999;229(4):536–541.

103. Klevasath MB, Bobrow LG, Pinder SE, et al. The value of immunohistochemistry in sentinel lymph node histopathology in breast cancer. *Br J Cancer.* 2005;92(12):2201–2205.

104. Chagpar A, Middleton LP, Sahin AA, et al. Clinical outcome of patients with lymph node-negative breast carcinoma who have sentinel lymph node micrometastases detected by immunohistochemistry. *Cancer.* 2005;15;103(8):1581–1586.

105. Sakorafas GH, Geraghty J, Pavlakis G. The clinical significance of axillary lymph node micrometastases in breast cancer. *Eur J Surg Oncol.* 2004;30(8):807–816.

106. Linehan DC, Hill AD, Akhurst T, et al. Intradermal radiocolloid and intraparenchymal blue dye injection optimize sentinel node identification in breast cancer patients. *Ann Surg Oncol.* 1999;6(5):450–445.

107. Borgstein PJ, Meijer S, Pijpers RJ, et al. Functional lymphatic anatomy for sentinel node biopsy in breast cancer: echoes from the past and the periareolar blue method. *Ann Surg.* 2000;232: 81–89.

108. Peley G, Sinkovics I, Toth J, et al. Subareolar injection of radioactive colloid for sentinel lymph node identification in breast cancer patients. *Am Surg.* 2004;70(7):625–629.

109. Lin KM, Patel TH, Ray A. et al. Intradermal radioisotope is superior to peritumoral blue dye or radioisotope in identifying breast cancer sentinel nodes. *J Am Coll Surg.* 2004;199(4):561–566.

110. D'Eredita G, Giardina C, Guerierri AM, et al. A further validation of subareolar injection technique for breast sentinel lymph node biopsy. *Ann Surg Oncol.* 2006;13(5):701–707.

111. Shrenk P, Wayand W. Sentinel-node biopsy in axillary lymphnode staging for patients with multicentric breast cancer. *Lancet.* 2001;357(9250):122–123.

112. Gentilini O, Trifiro G, Soteldo J, et al. Sentinel lymph node biopsy in multicentric breast cancer. The experience of the European Institute of Oncology. *Eur J Surg Oncol.* 2006;32(5):507–510.

113. Knauer M, Konstantinuik P, Haid A, et al. Multicentric breast cancer: a new indication for sentinel node biopsy–a multi-institutional validation study. *J Clin Oncol.* 2006;24(21):3374–3380.

114. Nason KS, Anderson BO, Byrd DR, et al. Increased false negative sentinel node biopsy rates after preoperative chemotherapy for invasive breast carcinoma. *Cancer.* 2000;89(11):2187–2194.

115. Breslin TM, Cohen L, Sahin A, et al. Sentinel lymph node biopsy is accurate after neoadjuvant chemotherapy for breast cancer. *J Clin Oncol.* 2000;18:3480–3486.

116. Fernandez A, Cortes M, Benito A, et al. Gamma probe sentinel node localization and biopsy in breast cancer patients treated with a neoadjuvant chemotherapy scheme. *Nucl Med Commun.* 2001;22(4):361–366.

117. Haid A, Tausch C, Lang A, et al. Is sentinel lymph node biopsy reliable and indicated after preoperative chemotherapy in patients with breast carcinoma? *Cancer.* 2001;92(5):1080–1084.

118. Julian TB, Dusi D, Wolmark N. Sentinel node biopsy after neoadjuvant chemotherapy for breast cancer. *Am J Surg.* 2002;184(4):315–317.

119. Miller AR, Thomason VE, Yeh IT, et al. Analysis of sentinel lymph node mapping with immediate pathologic review in patients receiving preoperative chemotherapy for breast carcinoma. *Ann Surg Oncol.* 2002;9(3):243–247.

120. Piato JR, Barros AC, Pincerato AM, et al. Sentinel lymph node biopsy in breast cancer after neoadjuvant chemotherapy. A pilot study. *Eur J Surg Oncol.* 2003;29(2):118–120.

121. Jones JL, Zabicki K, Christian RL, et al. A comparison of sentinel node biopsy before and after neoadjuvant chemotherapy: timing is important. *Am J Surg.* 2005;190(4):517–520.

122. Tanaka Y, Maeda H, Ogawa Y, et al. Sentinel node biopsy in breast cancer patients treated with neoadjuvant chemotherapy. *Oncol Rep.* 2006;15(4):927–931.

COMMENTARY 1
Michael S. Sabel

The sentinel lymph node (SLN) procedure has changed the landscape of breast surgery immeasurably, not only by greatly minimizing the morbidity associated with the surgical staging of breast cancer, but by improving our knowledge of the anatomy of the breast and axilla and the biology of breast cancer. However, no great advance comes without great controversy, and it is almost stunning how a procedure so beautifully simple in concept has led to such vigorous debate surrounding the most effective techniques and most appropriate application. It is expected that any new surgical procedure would prompt multiple articles confirming its efficacy, refining the technique and expanding its application, especially in breast disease, which commands such a prominent role in any surgeon's practice. The sheer volume of articles devoted to this topic, however, is somewhat overwhelming, especially given that the great majority of the literature is retrospective, single-institution data with a relative paucity of prospective, randomized data. This is likely a reflection of how rapidly the procedure was adopted, first by academic breast surgeons and shortly afterward by the community.

As we began to thoroughly examine the procedure, the answer to one question often led to many more questions. Can we inject the tracer subareolarly rather than peritumorally, and if so, what does this say about the embryologic development and lymphatic anatomy of the breast? If this works, then why should the procedure not be just as accurate for T3 lesions as T1 lesions, or multicentric cancers, for that matter? If we can perform SLN biopsy for very large lesions, how do we coordinate this with neoadjuvant chemotherapy? Should it be done only for invasive cancers? What about in situ cancer, or even prophylactic mastectomies?

Drs. Amersi, Mabry, and Giuliano do an excellent job of reviewing many of the questions that have arisen since the introduction of the SLN procedure, including those that have been settled and those that continue to cause debate both in the literature and at national meetings. The reader may walk away from this chapter choosing one side or the other for any particular controversy. However, the take-home message should be that for many of these debates, there is no right answer, no single approach or technique that should be universally applied. There are two primary reasons for this.

1. Unlike most surgical procedures, the successful SLN biopsy is dependent not only on the surgeon's skill and experience, but also on that of his or her colleagues in nuclear medicine and pathology. It is a true multidisciplinary procedure. Even a surgeon who has considerable experience in performing the procedure can have the results impacted by variations in lymphoscintigraphy and pathologic evaluation. It therefore becomes imperative not only for each institution to go through the proper learning curve, but also to periodically review its experience and identify areas for improvement. A thorough knowledge of an individual institution's level of expertise and limitations will help determine the best approach to many of these controversies.

2. Not only is the procedure multidisciplinary, but the management of breast cancer is multidisciplinary, and surgical staging will greatly impact both medical and radiation oncologists. It is therefore naïve to believe that there is one approach that should be used universally, whose advantages always trump its disadvantages. On the contrary, many of these questions should be discussed in a multidisciplinary setting, determining how the results may impact the choice of systemic agents, the fields for x-ray therapy, or even the most appropriate surveillance.

With these considerations in mind, we can examine many of these controversies from a different perspective and debate not "how should the surgeon do this" but rather "how will this impact the patient's complete treatment plan?"

BLUE DYE, RADIOACTIVE COLLOID, AND LYMPHOSCINTIGRAPHY

Whether to use blue dye alone, radioactive colloid alone, or the combination, is based on both surgeon preference and surgeon experience. There are several relative advantages and disadvantages to each approach. The use of blue dye only is much less expensive and greatly facilitates scheduling as there is no delay for the injection of the technetium-99m (^{99m}Tc) sulfur colloid or the lymphoscintigraphy to be performed. Surgeons experienced in blue dye-only SLN biopsy have a similar success rate and accuracy as those who used the combined technique. For surgeons trained with the combined technique, it may be difficult to shift to blue dye only, as the dissection is more delicate (taking care not to disrupt blue-stained lymphatics that may lead you to the SLN) and possibly more time-consuming. Even for experienced surgeons, the combined technique may be faster, and there is assuring comfort in identifying SLNs that are both blue and hot, particularly when different methods of injection are used. Therefore, in determining which approach is the right one, surgeons must consider their own experience and training. They must also look at their own practice and operating room (OR) availability, weighing the unavoidable delays in scheduling associated with nuclear medicine injection versus the added time in the OR that the blue dye-only technique may entail. In addition, the multidisciplinary team must ask itself how to approach the internal mammary (IM) lymph nodes.

One of the most significant areas of controversy in breast cancer surgery is that of the IM lymph nodes, a controversy that had essentially disappeared after the abandonment of the extended radical mastectomy but arose again with the introduction of lymphoscintigraphy. Whether to use radioactive colloid, how to inject it, and whether to obtain the lymphoscintigram, all hinge on the answer to this question, "If the lymphoscintigram shows drainage to the internal mammary chain, should these nodes be biopsied?" The answer to this question lies in two additional questions. One, what is the impact of leaving behind unrecognized disease in the IM nodes, and two, what impact would this information have on chemotherapy or radiation therapy? Neither of these questions is easily answered, and so this remains a central argument (Table 22C1.1).

If it is believed that there is no situation in which the surgeon would pursue an IM node because (a) the impact of residual disease is minimal and (b) adjuvant therapy would not be altered, then blue dye only is appropriate. Even for those surgeons who use radioactive colloid, lymphoscintigraphy provides little useful information and may be omitted (1). On the other hand, if it is believed that any drainage to the IM lymph nodes should be pursued, not only for adjuvant therapy decisions but also to reduce IM recurrences, then both the radioactive colloid and the lymphoscintigram are essential (2–4). In addition, the ^{99m}Tc sulfur colloid should be injected peritumorally, as the drainage to the IM nodes after other injection techniques is much less common.

Surgeons may also opt to pursue IM nodes selectively; for example, when there is no drainage to the axillary nodes or when

Table 22C1.1

Arguments Against and in Favor of Identifying Internal Mammary (IM) Sentinel Lymph Nodes (SLN)

Arguments in favor
- Regional control is important as IM recurrences are difficult to deal with.
- Rate of IM recurrences may be underestimated as some may be labeled as chest wall recurrences or sternal metastases.
- May impact adjuvant therapy decisions in the absence of axillary metastases.
- May upstage patients otherwise considered node-negative.
- May help determine whether IM node should receive radiation.
- Not technically complex with minimal risk.

Arguments against
- Many breast surgeons are not familiar with the procedure, which has a small risk of pneumothorax or injury to the intercostal vessels.
- Precludes the blue dye-only technique, or intradermal or periareolar injections for the radioactive colloid.
- It is rare to find metastases to the IM nodes, especially in absence of axillary nodes.
- It rarely impacts adjuvant therapy decisions as most node-negative patients are still offered chemotherapy.
- There are no data suggesting a survival benefit in identifying IM SLN.

the tumor size is associated with an equivocal indication for adjuvant chemotherapy (5,6). This is why it is imperative that surgeons not only ask themselves if they are comfortable with the IM node biopsy technique, but also how these results may impact their oncology colleagues. For example, how might this impact chemotherapy decisions? Does your radiation oncologist routinely include the IM nodes in the radiation fields, irradiate them for any node-positive patient (IM or axillary), irradiate them only when the lymphoscintigraphy shows drainage to the IM chain, or irradiate only when the IM nodes show documented metastases? This controversy highlights how multidisciplinary breast cancer treatment may impact the sentinel lymph node procedure.

SLN BIOPSY BEFORE OR AFTER NEOADJUVANT CHEMOTHERAPY

Another source of debate is what to do in the patient undergoing neoadjuvant chemotherapy. Prior to the widespread application of the SLN concept, there were very few drawbacks for patients undergoing preoperative chemotherapy in an attempt to downstage the primary tumor and allow for breast-conservation therapy. Currently, however, these women find themselves in a "catch-22." If they undergo mastectomy initially, they can have a SLN biopsy and avoid the morbidity of an axillary lymph node dissection (ALND) if they are SN node-negative. On the other hand, if they choose to receive neoadjuvant chemotherapy and then qualify for segmental mastectomy, they may be advised to undergo ALND as the accuracy of SLN biopsy after chemotherapy remains under study.

How to best incorporate SLN biopsy into the neoadjuvant paradigm became essential, and two approaches emerged (Table 22C1.2). Several surgeons argued for SLN biopsy prior to neoadjuvant chemotherapy (7–9). This avoided the issue surrounding the accuracy of SLN biopsy after chemotherapy and potentially provided information that might influence adjuvant therapy decisions. On the other hand, several institutions began trials of SLN biopsy after neoadjuvant chemotherapy, performed in conjunction with a completion ALND (10–13). Although the results vary, most of the data demonstrate a reasonable success rate and a false-negative rate of approximately 10% to 11% (14). This is only slightly higher than the false-negative rate of SLN biopsy overall, which is between 6% and 10%. However, the axillary recurrence rate after a negative SLN obtained *prior* to any chemotherapy is extremely low, whereas there are few data concerning the axillary recurrence rate after omitting ALND because the SLN is negative *after* chemotherapy. Until these data emerge, the impact of SLN biopsy after neoadjuvant chemotherapy is unclear.

Nonetheless, if one accepts now or in the future that SLN may be safely performed after chemotherapy, the controversy still exists. Proponents would argue that SLN biopsy after chemotherapy saves women who may have been node-positive prior to chemotherapy, but who have been converted to node negativity, from undergoing ALND. Knowing the nodal status after chemotherapy might be the most important prognostic information, as the nodal response rate might be the most important determinant of outcome. Proponents of SLN before chemotherapy might argue that knowing the true nodal status is more

Table 22C1.2

Arguments for and Against Sentinel Lymph Node (SLN) Biopsy Before or After Neoadjuvant Chemotherapy

	Following Neoadjuvant Chemotherapy	Before Neoadjuvant Chemotherapy
Pro	• Accuracy appears comparable to SLN biopsy in general. • Surgical sequence consistent with conventional neoadjuvant CTX regimens.	• More accurate staging of patients prior to initiating therapy. • Preferred by many medical and radiation oncologists. • More surgical experience with SLN biopsy in the pre-CTX setting. • Less concern about accuracy.
Con	• False-negative rates not yet optimized. • Range, 0%-40%. • Significant learning curve. • No data on axillary recurrence after negative SLN after neoadjuvant chemotherapy.	• Unnecessary ALNDs in patients with nodal disease limited to SLN or sterilized by chemotherapy. • Requires an additional surgical procedure

CTX, chemotherapy; ALND, axillary lymph node dissection.

important in determining which systemic agents (if any, given the emergence of the Oncotype DX assay) (Genomic Health, Redwood City, CA) or radiation fields should be used. Again, however, I would argue that it is naïve to believe that one universal approach is correct, as this is another example of why multidisciplinary management of breast cancer is so essential. Tumor board presentation of these patients, with input from medical and radiation oncologists, will identify some patients in whom SLN biopsy before chemotherapy may be preferable. These may include cases where the neoadjuvant regimen would change if the patient were known to be node-positive, if the radiation fields would be altered based on the pre-chemotherapy nodal status, or if the decision to offer postmastectomy radiation (should downstaging not occur) may change. On the other hand, there may be some patients in whom these decisions would not be altered by knowing the SLN node status, or where the post-chemotherapy nodal status might be more important. It is clear that not only is more research in this area needed, but that we have long passed the days of "one size fits all" in the multimodality treatment of breast cancer.

SLN BIOPSY FOR RECURRENT DISEASE OR A NEW PRIMARY CANCER

Another area addressed by Drs. Amersi, Mabry, and Giuliano is the role of SLN biopsy in the face of local recurrence or a new primary tumor. For patients who have undergone previous breast conservation and x-ray therapy and develop either a recurrence or new primary, mastectomy is the operation of choice with regard to the breast itself. In the past, patients previously treated for invasive cancer had all undergone an ALND. Today many patients with in-breast recurrences have their axillary lymph nodes intact, having previously had a negative SLN biopsy. The initial SLN studies were performed in patients with primary breast cancers; sentinel node techniques were discouraged in a previously operated axilla because of concerns regard-

ing altered drainage patterns and the resulting potential inaccuracy. As described in the chapter, more recent studies have clearly demonstrated the feasibility of sentinel node biopsy in patients with recurrent breast cancer.

For patients who had a negative SLN biopsy previously, intraoperative lymphatic mapping and SLN biopsy is reasonable, with ALND reserved for patients with demonstrated metastases. However, it must be remembered that patients with previous axillary surgery may have aberrant axillary drainage, including drainage to the IM, supraclavicular, or contralateral axilla, and the surgeon must be prepared to pursue the SLN in more unusual locations (15). A more difficult situation arises in the patient with a previous ALND. In this situation, the success rate of SLN biopsy is much lower and the incidence of aberrant axillary drainage much higher. Although intraoperative lymphatic mapping and SLN biopsy may still be attempted, the decision to proceed must be based on how the information will affect further treatment. Will the identification of nodal metastases, even in the face of an aberrant drainage pattern, help decide whether chemotherapy is recommended or accepted by the patient? Once again, the decision to restage the axilla is greatly facilitated by presentation of these patients in a multidisciplinary setting.

OTHER AREAS OF CONTROVERSY

Drs Amersi, Mabry, and Giuliano discuss several other areas of management that vary among surgeons, such as the best injection techniques (Table 22C1.3), the use of intraoperative pathologic examination (Table 22C1.4), or the use of SLN when there is a palpable lymph node. Again, there is no absolute right answer. Surgeons need to weigh the relative advantages and disadvantages, taking into account the resources they have available to them. For example, where to inject the ^{99m}Tc colloid sulfur may not be just an issue of surgeon preference but also a question of who is injecting the tracer? Intradermal or

Table 22C1.3

Relative Advantages and Disadvantages of Tracer Injection Site for Sentinel Lymph Node Biopsy in Breast Cancer

Site	Advantages	Disadvantages
Peritumoral (injected around the tumor or biopsy cavity)	• Conceptually the purest with the most experience. • Minimal "Blue Breast" • Nice correlation	• Requires knowledge of the tumor location for nonpalpable lesions. • Injection into cavity • ? Multiple tumors

Intradermal (injected in the skin over the tumor)	• Higher ID rate
	• Easier for nonpalpable
		• ? Multiple tumors
		• Blue tattooing of skin
		  ○ Necrosis with methylene blue
		  ○ Need to resect skin with mass
		• Requires knowledge of the tumor location for nonpalpable lesions.

Subareolar (injected in the subareolar plexus)	• Good for multiple tumors • Location of tumor irrelevant.	• "Blue Breast" ○ Not an issue for mastectomy • Low rate of internal mammary drainage
Periareolar (injected intradermally around the areola)	• Good for multiple tumors • Location of tumor irrelevant. • Highly accurate	• Tattooing of areola and breast ○ Not an issue for mastectomy • Low rate of internal mammary drainage

ID, identification.

peritumoral injections require knowledge of the tumor location in the breast. If a nuclear medicine specialist is being asked to perform the injection, will he or she be sufficiently skilled in interpreting the imaging to determine the tumor location in the case of nonpalpable lesions? If not, the surgeon may need to do the radioactive colloid injections. Although it is difficult to dispute the advantage to the patient of identifying a positive SLN intraoperatively so that an ALND may be performed at the same sitting, the feasibility of routine frozen section histology may depend on pathology resources. At busy academic centers, where multiple frozen sections are being requested simultaneously by other surgeons, routine intraoperative analysis of the SLN may not be reasonable. In addition, for breast surgeons, the additional time required to obtain frozen sections and the possibility that several patients on a given day may have positive SLNs thereby requiring conversion to complete axillary dissection could complicate OR scheduling and resources. Touch-preparation cytology may be preferable because it is a more rapid procedure, but interpretation requires the availability of an experienced cytopathologist.

The authors discuss the use of SLN biopsy in the face of a clinically palpable lymph node. It is clear that not all palpable adenopathy will represent metastases, and it would be unfortunate to perform an ALND for what in reality was a reactive lymph node. However, this situation may be avoided, and the use of SLN biopsy minimized, by the routine use of preoperative axillary

Table 22C1.4

Advantages and Disadvantages of Intraoperative Pathologic Analysis of the Sentinel Lymph Node in Breast Cancer

Analysis	Advantages	Disadvantages
None or highly selective	Minimal impact on scheduling Decreased time in OR Limit preop discussion of ALND	High number of patients returning to OR for ALND ? Cost ? Morbidity
Frozen section	Limit return to OR No false-positives	Adds 30 minutes per case Pathology resources False-negatives
Touch-preparation cytology	Limit return to OR Fast ? False-positive	Requires experienced cytopathologist Adds time to cases False-negatives

OR, operating room; ALND, axillary lymph node dissection.

Table 22C1.5

Sonographic Findings of Abnormal Lymph Nodes

- Enlarged diameter.
- Rounding of the normally ovoid shape.
- Markedly hypoechoic cortex.
- Right-to-left asymmetry.
- Cortical thickening.
- Eccentric hilar compression, indentation, displacement, or obliteration.
- Loss of echogenic outer capsule and angular margins.

ultrasound and ultrasound-guided fine-needle aspiration (FNA) biopsy of suspicious lymph nodes. Imaging of the axilla with ultrasound is rapidly becoming standard practice for preoperative axillary assessment in patients with biopsy-proven invasive cancers. The specificity of axillary ultrasound in identifying involved lymph nodes is between 87% and 95%, with a sensitivity from 50% to 70%. Abnormal lymph nodes are identified by either their size (a relatively weak sign) or a change in their morphology, which is significantly more useful in diagnosing metastasis (Table 22C1.5). Any abnormal lymph nodes identified on axillary ultrasound should undergo ultrasound-guided FNA to confirm the presence of metastases, which increases the specificity to nearly 100% in some studies (16–21). By working together with radiology, this approach can spare patients with FNA-proven regional disease the time and expense of SLN biopsy, proceeding directly to ALND at the time of their lumpectomy or mastectomy, as well as limit SLN biopsy in patients with palpable disease to those most likely to have a reactive lymph node.

It thus becomes obvious that successful lymphatic mapping and SLN biopsy are not associated exclusively with one particular approach, but that it is necessary that the procedures planned be consistent with the resources and treatment approaches of the institution in which they are to be performed. It is equally imperative that surgeons performing SLN biopsy periodically review their results in conjunction with nuclear medicine, pathology, radiology, medical oncology, and radiation oncology. Lower than expected success rates, higher than expected regional recurrence rates, or frequent disparities between the surgeon and the other members of the multidisciplinary team should prompt the surgeon to review and revise his or her technique.

THE FUTURE

Finally, the authors look toward the future and imagine the routine use of immunohistochemical staining or reverse transcriptase polymerase chain reaction in the evaluation of the SLN. If one looks only a little bit further into the future, one might imagine the abandonment of the SLN biopsy altogether. The prognostic benefit of SLN biopsy is still essential for adjuvant therapy decisions; however, the inadequacy of our current approach to staging is evidenced by the fact that only 10% of patients who are exposed to chemotherapy derive a benefit

(22,23). Although metastases to the lymph nodes is the most significant prognostic sign, 30% of node-negative patients will still relapse while up to 40% of node-positive patients will be alive at 10 years (24–26).

A more promising method of staging breast cancer patients may be to look at the tumor genome. DNA microarray analysis uses mRNA from fresh-frozen tissue to create double-stranded DNA. Using reverse transcription, amplified cRNA is labeled with fluorescent dye and hybridized to a panel of tens of thousands of genes on a chip. Computer-aided programs can then discern whether the gene is up-regulated or down-regulated within the cancer cells. Several groups have demonstrated the potential of microarray analysis in predicting outcome among breast cancer patients (27–31). This approach has already yielded a 21-gene assay that could predict the likelihood of distant recurrence among estrogen receptor-positive, node-negative breast cancer patients (32), and the benefit of adjuvant tamoxifen and chemotherapy (33,34). This represents the first step in moving from staging patients based on histopathologic features to staging patients based on genomic features. It is conceivable, however, that in the not-too-distant future, gene assays will be developed that can predict nodal involvement, or response to therapy regardless of tumor size or nodal status. When that time arrives, the need for SLN biopsy for staging purposes may disappear, and axillary lymph node dissection could become an obscure operation reserved for the unusual isolated axillary recurrence.

REFERENCES

1. Lawson LL, Sandler M, Martin W, et al. Preoperative lymphoscintigraphy and internal mammary sentinel lymph node biopsy do not enhance the accuracy of lymphatic mapping for breast cancer. *Am Surg.* 2004;70:1050–1055.
2. Plunkett TA, Correa I, Miles DW, Taylor-Papadimitriou J. Breast cancer and the immune system: opportunities and pitfalls. *J Mamm Gland Biol Neoplasia.* 2001;6:467–475.
3. Sugg SL, Ferguson DJ, Posner MC, et al. Should internal mammary nodes be sampled in the sentinel lymph node era? *Ann Surg Oncol.* 2000;7:188–192.
4. Purushotham AD, Cariati M. Internal mammary nodes and breast cancer. *Br J Surg.* 2005;92:131–132.
5. Bevilacqua JL, Gucciardo G, Cody HS 3rd, et al. A selection algorithm for internal mammary sentinel lymph node biopsy. *Eur J Surg Oncol.* 2002;28:603–614.
6. Park C, Seid P, Morita E, et al. Internal mammary sentinel lymph node mapping for invasive breast cancer: implications for staging and treatment. *Breast J.* 2005;11:29–33.
7. Sabel MS, Schott AF, Kleer CG, et al. Sentinel node biopsy prior to neoadjuvant chemotherapy. *Am J Surg.* 2003;186:102–105.
8. Jones JL, Zabicki K, Christian RL, et al. A comparison of sentinel node biopsy before and after neoadjuvant chemotherapy: timing is important. *Am J Surg.* 2005;190:517–520.
9. Schrenk P, Hochreiner G, Fridrik M, et al. Sentinel node biopsy performed before preoperative chemotherapy for axillary lymph node staging in breast cancer. *Breast J.* 2003;9:282–287.
10. Stearns V, Ewing CA, Slack R, et al. Sentinel lymphadenectomy after neoadjuvant chemotherapy for breast cancer may reliably represent the axilla except for inflammatory breast cancer. *Ann Surg Oncol.* 2002;9:235–242.
11. Kinoshita T, Takasugi M, Iwamoto E, et al. Sentinel lymph node biopsy examination for breast cancer patients with clinically

negative axillary lymph nodes after neoadjuvant chemotherapy. *Am J Surg.* 2006;191:225–229.

12. Seok Hyung K, Seok-Ki K, Youngmee K, et al. Decreased identification rate of sentinel lymph node after neoadjuvant chemotherapy. *World J Surg.* 2004;V28:1019–1024.

13. Mamounas EP, Brown A, Smith R, et al. Accuracy of sentinel node biopsy after neoadjuvant chemotherapy in breast cancer: updated results from NSABP B-27. *Proc Am Soc Clin Oncol.* 2002;21:140.

14. Xing Y, Foy M, Cox DD, et al. Meta-analysis of sentinel lymph node biopsy after preoperative chemotherapy in patients with breast cancer. *Br J Surg.* 2006;93:539–546.

15. Newman EL, Cimmino VM, Sabel MS, et al. Lymphatic mapping and sentinel lymph node biopsy for patients with local recurrence after breast-conservation therapy. *Ann Surg Oncol.* 2006;13:52–57.

16. van Rijk MC, Deurloo EE, Nieweg OE, et al. Ultrasonography and fine-needle aspiration cytology can spare breast cancer patients unnecessary sentinel lymph node biopsy. *Ann Surg Oncol.* 2006;13:31–35.

17. Khan A, Sabel MS, Nees A, et al. Comprehensive axillary evaluation in neoadjuvant chemotherapy patients with ultrasonography and sentinel lymph node biopsy. *Ann Surg Oncol.* 2005;12:697–704.

18. Lam WW YW, Chan YL, Stewart IE, et al. Detection of axillary lymph node metastases in breast carcinoma by technetium-99m sestamibi breast scintigraphy, ultrasound, and conventional mammography. *Eur J Nucl Med.* 1996;23:498–503.

19. Bonnema J van Geel AN, van Ooijen B, et al. Ultrasound-guided aspiration biopsy for detection of nonpalpable axillary node metastases in breast cancer patients: new diagnostic method. *World J Surg.* 1997;21:270–274.

20. Walsh JS, Dixon JM, Chetty U, Paterson D. Colour Doppler studies of axillary node metastasis in breast carcinoma. *Clin Radiol.* 1994;49:189–191.

21. Ciatto S, Brancato B, Risso G, et al. Accuracy of fine needle aspiration cytology (FNAC) of axillary lymph nodes as a triage test in breast cancer staging. Breast Cancer Res Treat.

22. Goldhirsch A, Glick JH, Gelber RD, et al. International consensus panel on the treatment of primary breast cancer. Seventh international conference on adjuvant therapy of primary breast cancer. *J Clin Oncol.* 2001;19:3817–3827.

23. Eifel P, Axelson JA, Costa J, et al. National Institutes of Health Consensus Development Conference Statement: adjuvant therapy for breast cancer, November 1-3, 2000. *J Natl Cancer Inst.* 2001;93:979–989.

24. Early breast cancer trialists collaborative group. Systemic treatment of early breast cancer by hormonal, cytotoxic or immune therapy. *Lancet.* 1992;339:1–15.

25. Fisher B, Redmond C, Dimitrov NV, et al. A randomized clinical trial evaluating sequential methotrexate and fluorouracil in the treatment of patients with node-negative breast cancer who have estrogen receptor negative tumors. *N Engl J Med.* 1989;320:473–478.

26. Mansour EG, Gray R, Shatila AH, et al. Survival advantage of adjuvant chemotherapy in high-risk node-negative breast cancer: ten year analysis—an intergroup study. *J Clin Oncol.* 1998;16:3486–3492.

27. van't Veer LJ, Dai H, van de Vijver MJ, et al. Gene expression profiling predicts clinical outcome of breast cancer. Nature 2002;415:530–536.

28. van de Vijver MJ, He YD, van't Veer LJ, et al. A gene-expression signature as a predictor of survival in breast cancer. *N Engl J Med.* 2002;347:1999–2009.

29. Ahr A, Karn T, Solbach C, et al. Identification of high risk breast-cancer patietns by gene expression profiling. *Lancet.* 2002;359:131–132.

30. West M, Blanchette C, Dressman H, et al. Predicting the clinical status of human breast cancer by using gene expression profiles. *Proc Natl Acad Sci U S A.* 2001;98:11462–11467.

31. Sorlie T, Perou CM, Tibshirani R, et al. Gene expression patterns of breast carcinomas distinguish tumor subclasses with clinical implications. *Proc Natl Acad Sci U S A.* 2001;98:10869–10874.

32. Paik S, Shak S, Tang G, et al. A multigene assay to predict recurrence of tamoxifen-treated, node-negative breast cancer. *N Engl J Med.* 2004;351:2817–2826.

33. Paik S, Shak S, Tang G, et al. Expression of the 21 genes in the Recurrence Score assay and prediction of clinical benefit from tamoxifen in NSABP study B-14 and chemotherapy in NSABP study B-20. Paper presented at: 27th Annual San Antonio Breast Cancer Symposium; 2004; San Antonio, TX. Abstract 24.

34. Paik S. Development and clinical utility of a 21-gene recurrence score prognostic assay in patients with early breast cancer treated with tamoxifen. *Oncologist.* 2007;12:631–635.

COMMENTARY 2
David Krag

The authors of Chapter 22 have provided a good and broad overview of the current status of sentinel node (SN) surgery for breast cancer. The editors of this book have requested that the commentary provide a different point of view or cover tangential issues. Given the experience of Dr. Giuliano's team and their coverage of the topic, there are few tangential issues to add. This commentary will provide some perspective on the rationale of the larger randomized trials comparing SN surgery with axillary node resection (ANR) and touch on the development of SN surgery.

RANDOMIZED TRIALS

As stated in the opening paragraph of the accompanying chapter, evidence from randomized trials has brought about major changes in the management of patients with breast cancer. Results from definitive clinical trials have consistently demonstrated that removing less breast tissue does not significantly reduce survival. Implementation of breast-conserving therapy became more widespread after completion of these trials. Indeed, a current measure of quality care for a surgeon is the fraction of patients receiving breast-conserving therapy versus mastectomy (1).

Although randomized trials have led to changes in how surgery of the breast is performed, changes in the management of lymph nodes by SN surgery has been implemented in the absence of randomized trials documenting survival or regional control equivalency. In fact, the frequency that patients are offered SN surgery has become a de facto quality measure for a surgical practice. Of the more than 2,500 articles published since 1993 exclusively on SNs in breast cancer, 47 articles describe practice patterns, 26 address training issues, and 25 articles describe SN practice guidelines. These latter 100 articles attest to the maturation of the procedural methods and the extensive implementation of the SN surgery technique in breast cancer. Adoption of SN surgery preceding results of randomized trials is different than the implementation of breast-conserving therapy, which largely occurred in reverse order.

As is true for surgical management of a variety of solid tumors, there are three main reasons to perform node surgery for breast cancer: improve survival, improve regional control, and provide staging information. ANR provides the most well-studied method of accomplishing these goals. The results of randomized trials available regarding the outcomes of ANR serve as a benchmark for SN surgery. A careful examination and analysis of six randomized trials of ANR versus observation (2–12) were performed by Orr (13). The most striking and compelling observation was that in every single trial, higher survival was observed in the group that had initial ANR. This includes the National Surgical Adjuvant Breast and Bowel Project (NSABP)-04 trial (9), which in the United States has been the reference standard. Given these findings, one might ask what data are available to justify the currently prevailing concept that there is no survival benefit from ANR? In combining the six trials, Orr (13) found that the average survival benefit favoring ANR versus observation was about 5.5%. It is this 5.5% difference that SN surgery needs to neutralize to demonstrate equivalent survival as ANR.

The magnitude of the survival advantage from ANR observed in randomized trials is important in analyzing the design of clinical trials comparing ANR with SN surgery (14). The maximum difference expected from ANR versus observation is in the range of 5.5%, so a trial of ANR versus SN surgery should at least be able to detect those differences. What reduction is survival would be considered acceptable in exchange for reduction in morbidity related to ANR? The answer should be as close to zero as possible. A clinical trial comparing ANR with SN surgery should be designed to detect as small a survival difference as possible. The NSABP B-32 trial (15) was designed to detect a survival difference of <2% between the two randomized arms.

REMOVAL OF VARIABLE NUMBER OF LYMPH NODES

Certainly removing any tissue, including SNs, that has no cancer should have no impact on cancer control. But how correct is the interpretation of the pathologist in declaring that a lymph node is free of cancer cells? When the pathologist says a case is node-negative, does that mean there are in fact no cancer cells present? The pathologist only samples a fraction of 1% of the node. Since at least 1948 it has been known that more aggressive analysis of lymph nodes in breast cancer cases will identify cancer cells in nodes that were initially determined to be negative (16). Many authors, including the authors of the accompanying chapter, have evaluated this issue related to SNs. They demonstrated considerable increase in frequency of cancer cell identification when more thorough analytical techniques are employed (17,18). This demonstrates that, especially for SNs, when the pathologist says there is no cancer, there

in fact often are cancer cells. The important conclusion is that conventional pathologic evaluation of nodes considerably underestimates the number of cases that have cancer cells in the nodes.

The main point for this discussion is that pathology reports indicating node-negative status describe a population in which a significant percent of cases in fact do have cancer cells present. What is not known is whether this is of clinical significance. If all the nodes are being removed as part of an ANR anyway, the issue of leaving nodes with residual cancer is irrelevant. If only a few nodes are being removed as part of a SN procedure, then many nodes with possible residual cancer cells will be left behind. Although this may have no impact on prognosis when a complete ANR is performed, what is the impact on survival or regional control when such nodes are left intact in the patient?

Resection of SNs falls somewhere between an ANR and observation relative to the amount of node tissue removed. It is a partial lymphadenectomy. In the absence of randomized trials evaluating the clinical outcomes of patients with variable number of nodes removed, retrospective analyses of large databases can provide suggestions of the outcomes. Based on the Surveillance Epidemiology and End Results (SEER) database a simple question was analyzed. In breast cancer patients who have had variable numbers of nodes removed, and the variation is in the number of pathologically negative nodes, is there a survival difference? In this data set, the answer to this question is yes. In some subsets of patients the difference is quite high (19). We found that among patients with one to three positive nodes, there is improved survival as more lymph nodes are removed. This is true even though the variable number of nodes removed are all pathologically negative (19). Although smaller differences were observed, a similar finding occurs with patients in which all of the lymph nodes were node-negative. These observations are not unique. The preponderance of data show very similar outcomes for a variety of cancers including colorectal cancer (20), malignant melanoma (21), and pancreatic cancer (22).

IMPLICATIONS FOR TECHNOLOGY TRANSFER

It is important to recognize that there is a long history leading to the SN procedures that are performed today. There are published reports related to the concept of the SN in almost every decade of the last century (23). This rich history, which predates 1990, includes dozens of articles describing SNs, blue dyes for lymphatic mapping, selective lymphadenectomy, and even a suggestion to alter our staging system to account for status of the SN (24). Advances in surgical technology are moving faster than the educational system can readily accommodate. How we adapt to these changes will set the stage for effectiveness at delivering quality care to our patients. It also impacts the initial training of residents and our own continuous training. The story behind SN surgery can be viewed critically as a dynamic example of how we incorporate and adapt new technology. Such an analysis will better guide our surgical community on how to incorporate new knowledge and track quality of care.

REFERENCES

1. McCahill LE, James TA. Measuring individual surgeon performance in breast cancer surgery. In: Proceedings of the Society of Surgical Oncology Meeting; March 16, 2007; Washington, DC.

2. Fisher B, Redmond C, Fisher ER, et al. Ten-year results of a randomized clinical trial comparing radical mastectomy and total mastectomy with or without radiation. *N Engl J Med.* 1985;312:674–681.

3. Atkins H, Hayward JL, Klugman DJ, et al. Treatment of early breast cancer: a report after ten years of a clinical trial. *Br Med J.* 1972;2:423–429.

4. Bruce J. Operable cancer of the breast: a controlled clinical trial. *Cancer.* 1971;28:1443–1452.

5. Hamilton T, Langlands AO, Prescott RJ. The treatment of operable cancer of the breast: a clinical trial in the South-East region of Scotland. *Br J Surg.* 1974;61:758–761.

6. Hayward J, Caleffi M. The significance of local control in the primary treatment of breast cancer. *Arch Surg.* 1987;122:1244–1247.

7. Hayward JL. The Guy's trial of treatments of "early" breast cancer. *World J Surg.* 1977;1:314–316.

8. Hayward JL. The Guy's Hospital trials on breast conservation. In: Harris JR, Hellman S, Silen W, eds. *Conservative Management of Breast Cancer: New Surgical and Radiotherapeutic Techniques.* Philadelphia: JB Lippincott; 1983:77–90.

9. Johansen H, Kaae S, Schiodt T. Simple mastectomy with postoperative irradiation versus extended radical mastectomy in breast cancer: a twenty-five year follow-up of a randomized trial. *Acta Oncol.* 1990;29:709–715.

10. Kaae S, Johansen H. Does simple mastectomy followed by irradiation offer survival comparable to radical procedures? *Int J Radiation Oncol Biophys.* 1977;2:1163–1166.

11. Langlands AO, Prescott RJ, Hamilton T. A clinical trial in the management of operable cancer of the breast. *Br J Surg.* 1980;67:170–174.

12. Cabanes PA, Salmon RJ, Vilcoq JR, et al. Value of axillary dissection in addition to lumpectomy and radiotherapy in early breast cancer. *Lancet.* 1992;339:1245–1248.

13. Orr RK. The impact of prophylactic axillary node dissection on breast cancer survival–a Bayesian meta-analysis. *Ann Surg Oncol* 1999;6:109–116.

14. Krag D, Ashikaga T. The design of trials comparing sentinel-node surgery and axillary resection. *N Engl J Med.* 2003;349:603–605.

15. Krag DN, Julian TB, Harlow SP, et al. NSABP-32: Phase III, randomized trial comparing axillary dissection with sentinel lymph node dissection: a description of the trial. *Ann Surg Oncol.* 2004;11(3 Suppl):208S–210S.

16. Saphir O, Amromin, G. Obscure axillary lymph-node metastasis in carcinoma of the breast. *Cancer.* 1948;1:238–241.

17. Dowlatshahi K, Fan M, Anderson JM, et al. Occult metastases in sentinel nodes of 200 patients with operable breast cancer. *Ann Surg Oncol.* 2001;8:675–681.

18. Bostick PJ, Huynh KT, Sarantou T, et al. Detection of metastases in sentinel lymph nodes of breast cancer patients by multiple-marker RT-PCR. *Int J Cancer.* 1998;79:645-651.

19. Krag DN, Single RM. Breast cancer survival according to number of nodes removed. *Ann Surg Oncol.* 2003;10:1152–1159.

20. Tepper JE, O'Connell MJ, Niedzwiecki D, et al. Impact of number of nodes retrieved on outcome in patients with rectal cancer. *J Clin Oncol.* 2001;19:157–163.

21. Chan AD, Essner R, Wanek LA, et al. Judging the therapeutic value of lymph node dissections for melanoma. *J Am Coll Surg.* 2000;191:16–22.

22. Schwarz RE, Smith DD. Extent of lymph node retrieval and pancreatic cancer survival: information from a large US population database. *Ann Surg Oncol.* 2006;13:1189–1200.

23. Krag DN. Minimal access surgery for staging regional lymph nodes: the sentinel-node concept. *Curr Probl Surg.* 1998;35:951–1016.

24. Cabanas RM. An approach for the treatment of penile carcinoma. *Cancer.* 1977;39:456–466.

23

Preoperative Chemotherapy for Locally Advanced and Inflammatory Breast Cancer

Cathie T. Chung

DEFINITIONS

Locally Advanced Breast Cancer

Locally advanced breast cancers (LABCs) are defined by several characteristics that comprise different TNM stage classifications for breast cancer, but exclude patients with distant metastatic disease. Generally, these tumors are considered primarily inoperable at time of initial presentation. Although there is no standard definition for LABC, these invasive breast cancers are usually defined by size >5 cm (T3) or primary cancers that involve the skin/chest wall (T4), independent of node (N) stage, and/or cancers that are associated with fixed/matted axillary lymph nodes (N2a) or internal mammary lymph nodes (N2b/N3b) (1). In addition, based on the most recent changes in the TNM staging system for breast cancer that were instituted in 2002, patients with ipsilateral supraclavicular lymph node involvement (now considered N3c as opposed to M1) are also categorized as having LABC (2). In support of the downstaging of patients with ipsilateral supraclavicular lymph node involvement from stage IV to stage IIIC disease, investigators at the University of Texas M.D. Anderson Cancer Center have shown that these patients have similar prognoses compared with patients with stage III breast cancer, if treated with curative intent (3). As shown in Table 23.1, features of LABC fall within stages IIIA, IIIB, and IIIC breast cancer, although in some series patients with stage IIB (T3N0) breast cancer have also been included as part of this group (1,4–6). In the advent of screening mammography, which has resulted in the increased detection of earlier stages of breast cancer, LABC consists of 5% to 15% of new breast cancers in the United States but about 40% to 60% of new breast cancers in nonindustrialized countries (7). Patients who present with LABC will often have locoregionally advanced disease due to delays in diagnosis or neglect (8).

Inflammatory Breast Cancer

Inflammatory breast cancer (IBC) is a subset of LABC, the clinical appearance of which was first described by Sir Charles Bell (9) in 1814 but then later described by Lee and Tannenbaum (10) in 1924, who introduced the term *inflammatory* to describe the striking clinical features of IBC. As both noninflammatory LABC and IBC were associated with poor prognoses, patients with these breast cancers were grouped together in older series of patients with LABC (11,12). More recently, however, IBC was found to have its own distinct clinical, pathologic, and molecular features (13,14) so that currently, IBC is distinguished from other stages of noninflammatory LABC.

IBC is a rapidly progressive form of invasive breast cancer, which more commonly involves ductal rather than lobular cancer. The distinguishing feature of IBC is that it is highly angioinvasive and aggressive (15). Despite recent advancements in treatment, median disease-free survival (DFS) for patients with IBC was reported to be <2.5 years (16). Moreover, compared with other subsets of noninflammatory LABC, IBC was found to be associated with younger age at diagnosis, increased rates of estrogen receptor-negative breast cancers, and cancers of poorer grade (14). Survival rates of patients with IBC were also found to be inferior, compared with those of patients with noninflammatory LABC (14,17). In the series of patients followed at The University of Texas M.D. Anderson Cancer Center (18), the median progression free survival was 24 months for patients with IBC, compared with 35 months for patients with stage III non-IBC. Similarly, overall survival (OS) was shorter for patients with IBC (42 months), compared with patients with stage III non-IBC (60 months). Updated trends in survival for women with breast cancer within nine SEER (The Surveillance, Epidemiology and End Results Program) registries have also been published (19) and show similar results. Using this database, median survival of women with IBC was 2.9 years and was statistically shorter, compared with median survivals of women with either noninflammatory LABC (6.4 years) or non-T4 breast cancers (>10 years). In the United States, IBC comprises about 1% to 6% of all breast cancers (20,21) but incidence rates for IBC were reported to have doubled between the periods 1975-1977 and 1990-1992 within SEER registries (17).

As its name implies, clinical signs of acute inflammation of the breast, which arise rapidly over time (weeks to months, as opposed to years), manifest the hallmarks of IBC. These cancers are highly dermatotropic, as evidenced by tumor emboli seen within dermal lymphatics by breast or skin biopsy (22), lending to clinical manifestations exhibited by erythema, fine dimpling (peau d'orange) of the skin, and warmth. Despite these pathologic findings, there are no unique histopathologic features of IBC because invasion of malignant cells within dermal lymphatics may also be seen in non-IBC and be absent in some patients with IBC who meet clinical criteria (15,16,23). As such, a diagnosis of IBC rests purely on physical examination and an appropriate clinical history.

Compared with noninflammatory LABC in which patients may present with history of a large palpable breast mass, a

Table 23.1

Classification of Locally Advanced Breast Cancer Based on the 6th Edition (2002) of the American Joint Committee on Cancer *Staging Manual for Primary Breast Cancer*

Stage IIIA: T0, N2, M0
    T1, N2, M0
    T2, N2, M0
    T3, N1, M0
    T3, N2, M0

Stage IIIB: T4, N0, M0
    T4, N1, M0
    T4, N2, M0

Stage IIIC: Any T, N3, M0

Primary tumor (T)

T1 = Tumor ≤2 cm in greatest dimension
T2 = Tumor >2 cm but ≤5 cm
T3 = Tumor >5 cm
T4 = Tumor of any size with direct extension to:
T4a = Chest wall, not including pectoralis muscle
T4b = Edema (including peau d'orange) or ulceration of the skin of the breast or satellite nodules confined to the same breast
T4c = Both T4a and T4b
T4d = Inflammatory carcinoma

Regional lymph nodes (N)

N0 = No regional lymph node metastasis
N1 = Metastasis to moveable ipsilateral axillary lymph node(s)
N2a = Metastasis to ipsilateral axillary lymph nodes fixed to one another (matted)
N2b = Metastasis only in clinically apparent ipsilateral internal mammary node(s) and in the absence of clinically evident axillary lymph node metastasis
N3a = Metastasis in ipsilateral infraclavicular lymph node(s)
N3b = Metastasis in ipsilateral internal mammary lymph nodes(s) and axillary lymph node(s)
N3c = Metastasis in ipsilateral supraclavicular lymph nodes(s)

Distant metastasis (M)

M0 = No distant metastasis

distinct breast mass is not appreciated in patients with IBC over 50% of the time (24,25). Instead, patients with IBC typically present with rapid onset of breast enlargement associated with diffuse induration (26) and skin features, as classically described by Haagensen (22). These skin features now define IBC and consist of warmth, erythema, and edema (peau d'orange), involving at least one third of the breast and the presence of a palpable ridge at the margin of induration. In the absence of lymph node involvement, patients with IBC are staged with IIIB disease (T4dN0). Physical examination of patients with IBC, however,

will more commonly detect palpable regional lymph nodes or matted axillary lymph nodes (23,25), rendering such patients with stage IIIB (T4dN1-2) or IIIC (T4dN3) disease. Primary IBC should be distinguished from secondary inflammatory changes that can arise in patients with neglected, noninflammatory LABC and patients who develop inflammatory changes of the chest wall after mastectomy (16,20,27). Because of the appearance of the breast, IBC is often misdiagnosed as infectious mastitis or abscess, leading to a delay in diagnosis (20).

TREATMENT OF LABC/IBC: HISTORICAL PERSPECTIVE

Although noninflammatory LABC and IBC are distinct disease entities, all patients with LABC present with similar treatment-related dilemmas and were historically treated with upfront radical mastectomy before the early 1980s. Haagenson and Stout (28) were among the first to carefully analyze their results of patients with LABC and defined clinical markers that, although not specific contraindications for radical mastectomy, were indicators of poor prognosis. These signs included ulceration and edema of the breast, fixation of the tumor to the chest wall, fixed axillary lymph nodes with tumor involvement, and supraclavicular lymph node involvement. Other poor prognostic features of LABC, which they described, included patients with satellite nodules in the skin overlying the breast and patients with skin involvement. In their series of 35 patients with these characteristics, at 5 years, local recurrence rate was 46% and only two patients were free of disease. These investigators thus developed criteria for breast cancer, which defined inoperability due to development of distant metastasis soon after mastectomy. Indeed, retrospective reviews of series of patients with LABC show that prior to the early 1980s, 5-year survival rates for patients with IBC treated with mastectomy alone ranged from 0% to 10%. Mean survival for these patients ranged from 12 to 32 months (20). For patients with noninflammatory LABC, 5-year survival rates ranged from 5% to 53% among different series of patients treated by surgery alone. The wider range in 5-year survival rates seen among these patients likely reflects heterogeneity in the classification of disease among patients, because nonuniform staging criteria were used at the time (29). Nevertheless, these earlier studies demonstrated the inadequacy of upfront mastectomy for patients with LABC, presumably because of the presence of undetected micrometastasis at time of presentation.

The role of radiotherapy in the primary treatment of patients with LABC has also been studied, either as single modality treatment or combined with surgery. For patients with IBC treated with radiotherapy alone prior to 1987, 5-year survival rates ranged from 0% to <10% and mean survival ranged from 4 to 29 months, results very similar to outcome with mastectomy alone. With the combination of radiation and mastectomy in the treatment of IBC, improvements in locoregional control were observed in some studies, compared with single-modality local therapy alone. However, 5-year survival rates for these patients still ranged from 0% to 20% and OS was no different, compared with either modality alone (20). Similarly, for patients with noninflammatory LABC, retrospective reviews of series of patients treated by radiation alone showed 5-year DFS rates to range from 16% to 28%, similar to results obtained from surgery alone. In addition, no survival advantage was seen by combining radiation and surgery (29).

COMBINED MODALITY TREATMENT WITH NEOADJUVANT CHEMOTHERAPY

Given the poor results of primary local therapy in the treatment of patients with LABC, the use of neoadjuvant (also known as induction, preoperative, or primary systemic) chemotherapy was first introduced in the 1970s (30) with the intent of converting unresectable tumors to tumors more amenable to local treatment by surgery or radiation. Advantages to this approach were conferred by early findings of the Oxford Overview, which have been updated and continue to show that systemic adjuvant polychemotherapy significantly reduces risks of breast cancer recurrence and death, presumably by eradicating micrometastatic disease in patients with early-stage breast cancer (31). These data paved the way for initiation of trials, which added systemic chemotherapy, before local therapies (surgery and/or radiation) for patients considered to have inoperable LABC. Although initial trials of neoadjuvant chemotherapy involved small numbers of patients with different durations of treatment and different entry criteria, most of these trials involved upfront use of an anthracycline, followed by local therapy and maintenance chemotherapy. Such strategies documented improvements of survival for patients with noninflammatory LABC and IBC, compared with historical controls treated with local therapy alone (20,29,32,33).

Few data exist from multi-institutional trials incorporating neoadjuvant chemotherapy in the treatment of patients with inoperable LABC. The CALGB (Cancer and Leukemia Group B), however, conducted an early trial involving 113 patients with stage III (T3 N1-2 and T4 N0-2) breast cancer who received three cycles of neoadjuvant CAFVP chemotherapy (cyclophosphamide, doxorubicin, 5-fluorouracil, vincristine, and prednisone), followed by randomization to either mastectomy (if determined to have operable disease) or radiation and continuation of CAFVP chemotherapy postoperatively for 2 years. Of these patients, 91 (81%) developed operable disease, and median OS for the mastectomy and radiation groups were no different at 39.3 and 39.0 months, respectively (34). These data indicated that high response rates could be achieved with chemotherapy and that impact on survival of patients with LABC rested on developments of better systemic treatments.

With these acknowledgments, the use of neoadjuvant chemotherapy as part of combined modality therapy with surgery and radiation was widely adopted for treatment of LABC (35,36). Indeed, clinical practice guidelines have been developed that commence with neoadjuvant chemotherapy in treatment algorithms for patients with LABC (37,38). Based primarily on data derived from small phase II clinical trials, single-institution case series, and limited data from randomized trials (39–41) of neoadjuvant chemotherapy for operable breast cancer (some of which incorporated patients with T3N0-1 disease),

---

Table 23.2

Theoretical Concepts Applied to the Use of Neoadjuvant Chemotherapy in the Treatment of Patients with Locally Advanced Breast Cancer

Advantages

- Earlier treatment of micrometastatic disease
- Potential to downstage breast and nodal disease to achieve operability/breast conservation
- Ability to monitor clinical tumor response to guide therapy and minimize toxicities from ineffective therapies
- Optimal drug delivery through an intact tumor vasculature
- Potential to use this paradigm to identify molecular markers of response or outcome by performing studies on pre- and posttreatment tumor tissue, which may lead to better therapies

Disadvantages

- Potential development of drug resistance early in the course of treatment
- Delay of local therapy, particularly in patients not responding to chemotherapy
- Inaccurate assessment of initial pathologic stage to refine estimates of prognosis or benefits from therapy

---

these guidelines established neoadjuvant chemotherapy as standard of care for the treatment of patients with LABC (35,36). Theoretical advantages and disadvantages of this approach, as opposed to standard treatment schemes of surgery followed by adjuvant chemotherapy for operable breast cancer, are shown in Table 23.2 and are subject to speculation. Given the foundation from which the strategy of neoadjuvant chemotherapy arose, however, it would no longer be feasible to conduct controlled randomized clinical trials of neoadjuvant chemotherapy versus adjuvant chemotherapy for patients with inoperable LABC, especially in Western countries where the prevalence of this disease is small.

However, a randomized trial performed in India with women defined as having operable, T4b N0-2M0 breast cancer, was reported (42). This trial involved 101 patients but excluded those who had either IBC, extensive edema of the arm or breast or axillary lymph nodes that were fixed to underlying structures. Patients were randomized to either of two arms: (A) three cycles of neoadjuvant chemotherapy (cyclophosphamide, epirubicin and 5-fluorouracil; CEF), followed by mastectomy and three additional cycles of the same chemotherapy, or (B) upfront mastectomy followed by six cycles of CEF chemotherapy in the adjuvant setting. All patients received radiation after completion of chemotherapy. With a median follow-up of 25 months, no significant difference was seen in DFS (61% and 76%, for the neoadjuvant and adjuvant groups, respectively) or OS (76% and 82% for the neoadjuvant and adjuvant groups, respectively), similar to other observations seen in randomized trials of neoadjuvant chemotherapy for operable breast cancer

(39,40). In the neoadjuvant group, however, significant shrinkage of the index tumor mass was achieved in 66% of patients, and among 41 patients who started with clinically palpable axillary lymph nodes, 32% achieved pathologically negative nodes. Although these effects of neoadjuvant chemotherapy were not shown to improve survival, the small number of patients and limited duration of follow-up limit interpretation of the data. Nevertheless, it was shown that the delay of surgery due to up-front chemotherapy was not detrimental. Thus, despite the lack of evidence from large, prospective, randomized trials of neoadjuvant chemotherapy in LABC, advantages of this approach out-weigh disadvantages.

LESSONS LEARNED FROM STUDIES ON COMBINED MODALITY THERAPY FOR LABC

Long-Term Outcome

Despite uniform acceptance of neoadjuvant chemotherapy as standard therapy for patients with LABC, there is no chemotherapy regimen, which has been established as the gold standard, and many basic questions remain unanswered (Table 23.3).

In this light, the design of optimal treatments for patients with LABC is still an evolving process but has been shaped

---

Table 23.3

Questions to Be Addressed in the Design of Neoadjuvant Clinical Trials for Patients with Locally Advanced Breast Cancer

- Optimal combination and number of non–cross-resistant drugs (anthracyclines ± taxanes or other agents)
- Optimal sequencing of drugs (concurrent versus sequential)
- Optimal duration of treatment (fixed number of preoperative cycles versus continuation of chemotherapy until maximal clinical response is achieved)
- Optimal scheduling of chemotherapy/dose density (daily, weekly, every 2 or 3 weeks)
- Optimal dose intensity
- Need for additional adjuvant chemotherapy after completion of local treatment (sandwich chemotherapy)
- Determination of best surrogate markers for long-term survival and prognosis
- Determination of molecular markers based on the biology of an individual's cancer to predict response and tailor use of optimal regimens
- Optimal incorporation of newer biologic agents (e.g., antiangiogenesis agents, signal transduction inhibitors of specific breast cancer growth pathways) to enhance response rates and prolong survival

---

by longitudinal single-institutional studies (11,32,33,43–46). Taken together, these studies show that a subset of patients with LABC are able to achieve long-term survival, reflecting the impact that multimodality therapy has had on changing the natural history of LABC. Compared with historical outcomes of patients with LABC prior to 1980, it is impressive that over the past 2 decades we have been able to attain 15-year survival rates of 20% to 28% for patients with IBC and 23% to 60% for patients with noninflammatory LABC. In addition, these studies established that although there is no uniformly favored neoadjuvant chemotherapy regimen, clearly anthracyclines were proven effective in achieving high clinical response rates (Tables 23.4 and 23.5). As such, these drugs have become standard in neoadjuvant chemotherapy regimens for both operable and inoperable breast cancers.

Surrogate Markers of Long-Term Survival after Preoperative Chemotherapy for LABC

For primary operable breast cancers, results from the National Surgical Adjuvant Breast and Bowel Project (NSABP) B-18 trial have now been reported after 9 years of follow-up (40). These results showed no difference in DFS (55% vs. 53% for the preoperative and postoperative chemotherapy groups, respectively; $p = 0.50$) or OS (69% vs. 70% for the preoperative and postoperative chemotherapy groups, respectively; $p = 0.80$), whether four cycles of doxorubicin/cyclophosphamide (AC) chemotherapy were given in the neoadjuvant or adjuvant setting. These findings were corroborated by a meta-analysis involving nine randomized trials that incorporated 3,946 patients with breast cancer who were treated with the same chemotherapy regimen, either preoperatively or postoperatively (39). Despite the lack of overall benefit in survival produced by trials of neoadjuvant chemotherapy, however, the NSABP B-18 trial clearly showed that among patients who received preoperative AC chemotherapy, improved outcomes could be seen in a small subset of patients who achieved a pathologic complete response (pCR). In this setting, pCR was defined as no residual invasive cancer within the breast at time of histologic examination, in which case OS was 85%, compared with 73% for patients who had residual invasive cancer within the primary breast specimen (pINV). Similarly, DFS was superior for patients who achieved a pCR (75%), compared to those with pINV (58%). These differences in outcome in favor of patients achieving a pCR were statistically significant and persisted after adjustment for other clinical variables, including tumor size prior to chemotherapy, lymph node status, and patient age (40).

Thus, current measures for judging the efficacy of preoperative chemotherapy regimens for treatment of breast cancer use rates of pCR as end points of study as these are considered surrogate markers of survival. Desired definitions for pCR, however, may vary (35). For example, in the series of 925 breast cancer patients who were treated with preoperative chemotherapy at M.D. Anderson Cancer Center and who had cytologically proven axillary lymph node metastasis prior to chemotherapy (N = 403), the status of the axillary lymph nodes after preoperative chemotherapy was a strong predictor of survival, regardless of whether residual disease remained within the primary breast specimen. At a median follow-up of 64 months, rates

Table 23.4

Long-term Outcome of Longitudinal Studies Using Combined Modality Therapy for Locally Advanced Breast Cancer

Institution	Study Interval	Number, Stage	Neoadjuvant CT	Median Follow-up		Survival	
NCI [11]	1980–1988	107, II 48, IIIA 46, IBC 13, IIIB, non-IBC	CAMF + HT	16.8 y		Median	15-y OS
					IIIA	12.2 y	50%
					IBC	3.8 y	20%
					IIIB, non-IBC	5.8 y	23%
U of Michigan (43)	1986–1993	89, IIIA, IIIB 40, IBC	CAMF + HT	4.5 y (0.9–8.2 y)		5-y DFS	OS
					IBC	38%	37%
					Non-IBC	50%	63%
U of North Carolina, Chapel Hill (44)	1992–1998	59, III 13, IBC	A, dose intense	70 mo		5-y OS	
					All patients	76%	
					IBC	67%	
Tenon Hospital, Paris, France (45)	1982–1998	120, no IBC	AVFC	140 mo		5-y OS = 81% 10-y OS = 67% 15-y OS = 60%	
U of Texas, M.D. Anderson Cancer Center (46)	1974–1993	178, All IBC	FAC ± VbP, 4 different protocols	45–215 mo		DFS, all groups 5 y = 32% 10 y = 28% 15 y = 28%	
U of Pennsylvania (32)	1983–1996	54, All IBC	CMF or CAF	5.1 y		5-y OS = 56% 10-y OS = 35%	
U of Florida, Gainesville (33)	1982–2001	61, All IBC	A based ± T	14 y		5-y OS = 45% 10-y OS = 28%	

CT, chemotherapy; NCI, National Cancer Institute; C, cyclophosphamide; A, anthracycline; M, methotrexate; F, fluorouracil; HT, hormonal therapy; OS, overall survival; IBC, inflammatory breast cancer; DFS, disease-free survival; V, vincristine or vindesine; Vb, vinblastine; P, prednisone; T, taxol.

of 5-year OS and relapse-free survival (RFS) were significantly better for the 22% of patients who achieved an axillary lymph node pCR, compared with those who had residual axillary lymph node metastases. In this situation, axillary lymph node pCR was defined by the eradication of residual axillary lymph node metastasis after preoperative chemotherapy, in which case 5-year OS and RFS rates were 93% and 87%, respectively. For those with residual axillary lymph node metastasis, 5-year OS and RFS rates were 72% and 60%, respectively, which was a statistically inferior outcome compared with those of patients who had achieved an axillary lymph node pCR ($p < 0.0001$) (6).

Outcomes of preoperative chemotherapy based on pathologic assessments of primary breast specimens and axillary lymph nodes have also been reported for LABC. In a study of 372 patients with LABC (none with IBC) who were treated in two prospective trials with four cycles of FAC (fluorouracil, Adriamycin, and cyclophosphamide) chemotherapy prior to breast surgery, 12% of patients achieved a pCR. In this instance, pCR was defined by the absence of residual invasive disease within the breast and axillary lymph nodes. At a median follow-up of 58 months, the 5-year OS and DFS rates were significantly better in the group that achieved a pCR, compared with the group

that had achieved less than a pCR (5-year OS and DFS rates = 89% and 87%, respectively for the pCR group vs. 64% and 58%, respectively, for the non-pCR group; $p < 0.01$). Factors more likely to be associated with a pCR included breast cancers that were estrogen receptor-negative and those that were smaller in size (5). Similar findings were reported in a retrospective review of 138 patients with LABC who were treated preoperatively with chemotherapy involving either CMF (cyclophosphamide, methotrexate, and fluorouracil) or Adriamycin for three or four cycles. In this series, 13% of patients had a pCR within the breast and 27% had a pCR within axillary lymph nodes. With a median follow-up of 52 months, both distant DFS and OS were significantly better for those who obtained a pCR within axillary lymph nodes, compared with those who had residual axillary lymph node metastasis. In the former group, rates of distant DFS and OS were 64% and 71%, respectively. These figures compared favorably with rates of distant DFS and OS of 41% and 54%, respectively, among those with one to nine positive residual axillary lymph nodes ($p = 0.03$) (47).

The poorer prognosis of patients with noninflammatory LABC and residual pathologic disease after preoperative chemotherapy was also shown in a smaller study of 52 patients.

Table 23.5

Long-term Local Control Rates in Patients with Locally Advanced Breast Cancer Treated with Neoadjuvant Chemotherapy

Ref. N	Number, Stage	Med F/Up	cRR	pCR	% LRR	Treatment Schemes
Shen et al. 2004 (12)	33, IIIB, IIIC (no IBC)	91 mo	85%	12%	15%	CT-BCT-CT-RT
Cance et al. 2002 (44)	62, IIIA, IIIB IBC = 13	70 mo	84%	15%	14%	CT-BCT-CT-RT (N = 22) CT-M-CT-RT (N = 40) (IBC not eligible for BCT)
Lerouge et al. 2004 (45)	120, IIIA,B,C (no IBC)	140 mo	58%	22%	M+RT = 4% BCT+RT = 23% RT only = 13%	CT-RT-M-RT-CT (N = 49) CT-RT-BCT+RT-CT (N = 32) CT-RT-RT-CT (N = 39)
Merajver et al. 1997 (43)	75, IIIA,B (IBC 40%)	4.5 y	97%	28%	M+RT = 13% RT only = 14%	CT-XRT-CT (N = 21) CT-M+RT-CT (N = 54)
Harris et al. 2003 (32)	54, IBC	5.1 y	73%	12%	8% at 5 yr 19% at 10 y	CT-RT-CT (N = 2) M-CT-RT-CT (N = 2) CT-M-RT-CT (N = 15) CT-RT-M-CT (N = 35)
Ueno et al. 1997 (46)	178, IBC	45-215 mo (4 protocols)	74%	NR	20%, all patients no difference among groups)	CT-RT-CT (N = 40) CT-M-CT-RT (N = 23) CT-M-CT-RT (N = 43) CT-M-CT-RT or CT-RT-M ± CT (N = 72)
Low et al. 2004 (11)	107 IIIA = 48 IBC = 46 IIIB, non-IBC = 13	16.8 y	IIIA: 50% IBC: 57% IIIB, non-IBC: 31%	29% 33% 23%	15% 28% 23%	CT+HT-M-RT-CT (N = 75) CT+HT-RT-CT (N = 32)
Liauw et al. 2004 (33)	61, IBC	14 y	91%	NR	22% (for patients who received tri-modality therapy)	CT-M-RT (N = 32) CT-RT-M (N = 10) CT-RT (N = 1) M-CT-RT (N = 12) M-RT-CT (N = 2) M-RT (N = 4)

cRR, clinical response rate after neoadjuvant chemotherapy; pCR, complete pathologic response of primary breast mass and axillary lymph nodes; LRR, locoregional recurrence; CT, chemotherapy; BCT, breast-conserving therapy; RT, radiation therapy; IBC, inflammatory breast cancer; M, mastectomy; HT, hormonal therapy; NR, not reported; y, years.

In this study in which patients received a median of three cycles of preoperative FAC chemotherapy, 12% achieved a pCR as defined by no residual disease within the breast and axillary lymph nodes. At a median follow-up of 34.5 months, no recurrences were seen among patients with a pCR. In those with residual pathologic disease after preoperative chemotherapy, inferior rates of 3-year DFS were correlated with increasing number of remaining pathologic lymph nodes (60% vs. 18% for those with one to three nodes and four to nine nodes, respectively; $p = .0003$) (48).

The influence of residual pathologic lymph nodes on outcome has also been studied in 175 patients with IBC (of whom 61 were known to have cytologically positive lymph nodes prior to treatment with neoadjuvant chemotherapy), using either FAC alone or FAC with taxane chemotherapy. In this study, 14 patients (23%) achieved an axillary lymph node pCR at the time

of surgery and 13 patients (21%) achieved a pCR involving both axillary lymph nodes and the primary breast specimen. With a median follow-up of 48 months, the median OS was 47.4 months. However, among patients who achieved an axillary lymph node pCR, OS rates at 5 years were statistically greater at 82.5%, compared to 37% ($p = 0.01$), in those who did not achieve an axillary lymph node pCR. Similarly, rates of RFS at 5 years were statistically greater in those who achieved an axillary lymph node pCR (78.6%) compared with those who did not (25%; $p = 0.0001$) (49).

Thus, patients with IBC can achieve similar rates of axillary lymph node pCR after preoperative chemotherapy as those with non-IBC. For these patients with IBC, prognosis after preoperative chemotherapy is exceptionally good. However, for patients with IBC who do not achieve an axillary lymph node pCR after primary systemic chemotherapy, survival is markedly shorter compared with patients with non-IBC. The introduction of better preoperative systemic therapies using newer combinations of chemotherapeutic agents or targeted biologic agents is needed in these instances. In this regard, several phase II trials of preoperative chemotherapy for LABC have been reported that have shown activity of chemotherapies including, cisplatin (50), carboplatin (51), vinorelbine (52), gemcitabine (53), and an analog of epothilone B (54).

Alternatively, another strategy that has been used to improve outcomes of patients with LABC who do not achieve pCR after primary systemic chemotherapy is to sandwich additional treatment with adjuvant chemotherapy, using non–cross-resistant drugs. Such a strategy is exemplified by a study that was performed among 193 patients with LABC. All enrolled patients were treated preoperatively with three cycles of chemotherapy using vincristine, doxorubicin, cyclophosphamide, and prednisone (VACP) and then stratified to different adjuvant chemotherapy regimens based on the volume of residual tumor found at the time of mastectomy. Patients with <1 cm^3 of residual tumor after preoperative VACP received five additional cycles of VACP postoperatively. However, patients with >1 cm^3 of residual tumor after preoperative VACP were randomized to receive either additional postoperative VACP or alternate chemotherapy with VbMF (vinblastine, methotrexate with leucovorin rescue, and fluorouracil). In this study, 12.2% of patients achieved a pCR within the breast (defined as no residual invasive cancer); with a median follow-up of 13.9 years, the median OS of this group of patients has not been reached. For those with <1cm^3 of residual disease at time of mastectomy, median OS was 163 months; for those with >1 cm^3 of residual disease at time of mastectomy, median OS was 68 months ($p = .002$). Among patients randomized to either VACP or VbMF as adjuvant chemotherapy, estimated 5-year OS was 47% in for the former group and 65% in the latter group ($p = .06$), suggesting a potential benefit of the incorporation of alternate non–cross-resistant adjuvant chemotherapy in patients with less than a pCR after primary systemic chemotherapy (55).

Thus, for patients with LABC treated with preoperative chemotherapy, the goals of primary systemic therapy are generally to achieve high pCR rates. However, even for these patients, the attainment of a pCR does not eliminate the risk of development of distant metastasis. For example, it was shown that the 10-year distant metastasis-free rate was 82% among 226 breast cancer patients who achieved a pCR after neoadjuvant chemotherapy. Among these patients, 36%, 27%, 23%, 12%, and 11% had stage II, IIIA, IIIB, IIIC disease, and IBC, respectively. Factors associated with development of distant metastasis after attainment of pCR included (a) combined clinical stage (clinical stages IIIB, IIIC, and IBC; hazard ratio [HR] = 4.24; 95% confidence interval [CI]: 1.96-9.18; p <0.0001), (b) identification of ten or less lymph nodes at time of surgery (HR = 2.94; 95% CI: 1.40-6.15; p = 0.004), and (c) premenopausal status (HR = 3.08; 95% CI: 1.25-7.59; p = .015). Freedom from distant metastasis at 10 years was 97% for patients with no factors, 88% for patients with one factor, 77% for patients with two factors, and 31% for patients with three factors (p <.0001) (56). Thus, premenopausal patients with LABC/IBC and suboptimal lymph node evaluation who achieve a pCR after

preoperative chemotherapy might also be candidates for investigational alternate adjuvant treatments.

Taxane Chemotherapy for LABC

In adjuvant chemotherapy for node-positive, early-stage breast cancer, the utility of the addition of taxane chemotherapy (either paclitaxel or docetaxel) to anthracycline-based regimens has been well documented in several large randomized trials. These trials generally have shown improvements in DFS and OS, whether anthracyclines and taxanes were given concurrently or sequentially (57–60). In neoadjuvant chemotherapy for operable breast cancers, the role of taxanes in clinical trials has been reviewed (61,62). One pivotal trial, however, was the NSABP B-27 trial as this was a large, randomized, phase III study involving 2,411 participants. In this trial, participants were randomized among three treatment arms, each combining simultaneous administration of chemotherapy and tamoxifen. In group 1, patients received four cycles of preoperative chemotherapy with Adriamycin and cyclophosphamide (AC) followed by surgery. In group 2, patients received four cycles of preoperative AC and four cycles of docetaxel, followed by surgery. In group 3, patients received four cycles of preoperative AC, followed by surgery and four cycles of docetaxel given in the adjuvant setting. At initial presentation of the data (63), the addition of preoperative docetaxel to AC (group 2) significantly increased the clinical complete response rate (40.1% vs. 63.6% for AC alone and AC followed by preoperative docetaxel, respectively; p <0.001) as defined by the absence of residual palpable tumor, both within the breast and axillary lymph nodes. With respect to pathologic response, the addition of preoperative docetaxel to AC also increased rates of pCR from 13.7% (for AC alone) to 26.1% (p <0.001), although it is debated whether this difference may have been due to imbalances in the total number of preoperative chemotherapy cycles among the three groups.

With the most recent updates of this trial at a median of 77.9 months of follow-up (41), no statistically significant differences in OS, DFS, or RFS were observed among the three groups. However, there was a nonsignificant trend toward improved DFS for groups 2 and 3 (5-year DFS = 71.1% and 70.0%, respectively) compared with group 1 (5-year DFS = 67.7%). In addition, there was a trend toward better RFS for group 2 (5-year RFS = 74%) compared with group 1 (5-year RFS = 69.6%, HR = 0.85; 95% CI L 0.71-1.02; p = 0.08). As would be predicted, DFS [HR = 0.45; p <0.0001] and OS (HR = 0.33; p <0.0001) were significantly better for patients who achieved a pCR (defined as no residual invasive cancer within the primary breast specimen) compared to patients who did not. Having achieved a pCR, however, the addition of docetaxel did not further improve survival.

Similarly, in a review of all patients at M.D. Anderson Cancer Center who were treated with preoperative chemotherapy under five different protocols (6), higher pCR rates were observed among patients who received combined anthracycline/taxane-based regimens compared with those who received anthracycline-based regimens (29% vs. 19%, respectively; p = 0.03). However, as with the NSABP B-27 trial, no differences in OS were seen between groups. Taken together, these data provide evidence for a beneficial effect of the incorporation of taxanes into preoperative chemotherapy regimens, principally because of the increased pCR rates. Although there has been no clear impact of preoperative taxanes on improving survival of patients who attain a pCR, this issue has yet to be resolved as the number of patients in these subsets are likely too small to be within the power of these studies to detect such a difference.

The role of taxanes as neoadjuvant chemotherapy for LABC, including IBC, has also been studied but largely in small, phase II trials (64–67). The Aberdeen study (68), however, was a phase III randomized trial for patients with large (>3 cm) or locally advanced (T3, T4, or N2) breast cancers. In this study, 162 patients received four cycles of preoperative chemotherapy with CVAP (cyclophosphamide, vincristine, doxorubicin, and prednisolone), after which patients who had a clinical response (either partial or complete) were randomized to either four additional cycles of preoperative CVAP or four cycles of preoperative docetaxel. All patients who had no clinical response to four initial cycles of preoperative CVAP received four cycles of preoperative docetaxel (nonrandomized). Among randomized participants who completed all eight cycles of preoperative chemotherapy, pCR rates (defined as no invasive tumor within the primary breast specimen) were higher in the group that received sequential docetaxel compared with the group that received CVAP alone (34% vs. 16%, respectively; $p = 0.04$). Clinical response rates (both complete and partial) were similarly greater in the sequential docetaxel group than in the CVAP-alone group (94% vs. 66%, respectively; $p = 0.001$). On examination of the axillary lymph nodes, however, no difference was seen between groups, with 33% and 38% of patients in the CVAP and sequential docetaxel groups, respectively, having residual axillary lymph node metastases. In patients who had no initial response to CVAP, the crossover to docetaxel resulted in a clinical response rate (complete and partial) of 55%, with 2% achieving a pCR. With respect to survival, at a median follow-up of 38 months, DFS (90% vs. 77% for the sequential docetaxel and CVAP-alone groups, respectively; $p = 0.03$) and 3-year survival (97% vs. 84% for the sequential docetaxel and CVAP groups, respectively; $p = 0.05$) were significantly improved with the incorporation of docetaxel (69). Thus, these data show that the incorporation of non–cross-resistant drugs to anthracycline-based neoadjuvant chemotherapy regimens can improve pCR and survival rates for patients with LABC. In addition, because all patients in this study received the same total number of preoperative chemotherapy cycles (as opposed to participants who enrolled in the NSABP B-27 trial), these data would support enhanced effects of taxanes because of their intrinsic biologic activities in breast cancer, including induction of apoptosis (64).

Targeted Preoperative Regimens for *HER2*- Positive LABC

The *HER2* gene, which encodes the growth factor receptor *HER2*, is amplified in 25% to 30% of all breast cancers and portends a worse prognosis (70). With the development of trastuzumab (a recombinant monoclonal antibody targeted against *HER2*), systemic treatments for *HER2*-positive breast cancers have been influenced by the beneficial effects of combining trastuzumab with chemotherapy. For patients with metastatic breast cancer, the impact of trastuzumab in improving response rates, time to progression, and survival, when combined with either AC chemotherapy or paclitaxel, was demonstrated in a pivotal phase III randomized trial (71). More recently, several large random-

ized clinical trials have also demonstrated superior DFS and OS when trastuzumab was added to adjuvant chemotherapy for patients with early-stage breast cancer (72–74).

In this setting, the utility of incorporating trastuzumab into preoperative chemotherapy regimens for patients with breast cancer has also been evaluated in several clinical trials. In a study of 42 patients, which included patients with stage II to IIIA breast cancer (no IBC allowed), patients were randomized to four cycles of preoperative paclitaxel followed by four cycles of preoperative FEC (fluorouracil, epirubicin, and cyclophosphamide), either in the absence or presence of weekly concurrent trastuzumab. Although the primary objective of this study was to demonstrate a 20% improvement of pCR rate with the addition of trastuzumab to chemotherapy (planned sample size was 164 patients), the study was closed early by the Data Monitoring Committee when the superiority of trastuzumab became evident after 34 patients had completed treatment. At that time, pCR rates were 25% and 66.7% for the chemotherapy-only and chemotherapy plus trastuzumab groups, respectively ($p = 0.02$). No data were provided on survival, but this was not a predetermined end point of the study (75). The very high pCR rate achieved in this study with the addition of trastuzumab to preoperative chemotherapy is supported by a phase II study involving 33 patients with stage II/III, noninflammatory, *HER2*-positive, operable breast cancers. In this study, patients were treated with trastuzumab combined with docetaxel for six cycles prior to surgery. A clinical response rate was observed in 96% of patients, with 73% achieving a complete clinical response and 47% achieving a pCR (as defined by absence of tumor seen in both the breast and lymph nodes) (76).

In another study designed to examine the cellular response to preoperative trastuzumab, 35 patients with LABC were treated with weekly trastuzumab alone for 3 weeks, followed by weekly trastuzumab with docetaxel for 12 weeks and then surgery. Serial core biopsies were taken at baseline and within the first 3 weeks of treatment with trastuzumab. Immunohistochemical studies were then applied to these core biopsy specimens to identify markers of cell cycle activity, proliferation, apoptosis, and survival (e.g., Ki-67, p27, phosphorylated MAPK, and phosphorylated Akt). Early tumor regression was seen after only 3 weeks of trastuzumab alone, with 23% of patients having achieved a partial clinical response. Of those who were found to have a clinical response, biomarker studies done on serial core biopsy specimens demonstrated a 35% increase in apoptosis (77). These trials in conjunction with preliminary reports of other neoadjuvant trials incorporating trastuzumab with combination chemotherapy (51,78) exemplify the synergistic effects that can be achieved by the identification and targeting of select molecular pathways that drive the growth of certain breast cancers. With the many new monoclonal antibodies and growth factor tyrosine kinase inhibitors currently under development, preoperative treatments for LABC and IBC will continue to improve and hopefully will also have an impact on survival.

LOCOREGIONAL CONTROL OF DISEASE

Inflammatory Breast Cancer

The rewards of neoadjuvant chemotherapy in LABC have spawned new dilemmas in that, with prolongation of survival of patients, locoregional control of disease emerges as an important consideration in the comprehensive care of patients. In this regard, for patients with IBC who achieve a response after neoadjuvant chemotherapy, mastectomy followed by radiation would be considered standard of care based on the long-term follow-up of studies shown in Table 23.5. It is noted, however, that a subset of 40 patients with IBC treated on one of the early protocols (protocol A) developed at the M.D. Anderson Cancer Center (46) received induction chemotherapy with FAC followed by radiation alone and adjuvant chemotherapy. In this group of patients, locoregional recurrence (LRR) rate was 18%, which was no different from that of other patients who were treated with mastectomy on protocols B (26%), C (14%), and D (22%). Protocols B and C followed the same treatment scheme with induction chemotherapy, followed by mastectomy, adjuvant chemotherapy, and radiotherapy but involved two different chemotherapy regimens, either FAC alone (protocol B) or FACVP (protocol C). In protocol D, patients received induction chemotherapy with FAVCP and then, depending on response, either proceeded to mastectomy, adjuvant chemotherapy and radiation (in the case of complete or partial response), or further treatment with alternate non–cross-resistant chemotherapy (MV), followed by radiation, mastectomy (if feasible), and adjuvant chemotherapy (in the case of less than a partial response or progression of disease after initial FAVCP chemotherapy). Although the numbers of patients enrolled in each of these protocols were small (40, 23, 43, and 72 patients enrolled in protocols A, B, C, and D, respectively), these data suggest that some patients with IBC may achieve good local control with radiation and without mastectomy.

At the National Cancer Institute in Bethesda, Maryland (11), a different approach was used to treat patients with LABC, but outcome with respect to overall rate of LRR for patients with IBC was similar, compared with data obtained at the M.D. Anderson Cancer Center (Table 23.5). In this series that consisted of patients with IBC and noninflammatory LABC, patients received induction therapy with combination chemotherapy and hormonal therapy (hormonal synchronization), and in instances in which residual disease was detected, patients then proceeded to mastectomy, radiation, and further adjuvant chemotherapy. For patients who were noted to have a complete clinical response, multiple incisional biopsies were performed to document pathologic response, and in this instance, patients received radiation alone followed by adjuvant chemotherapy. Although not statistically significant, it was determined that for patients with IBC, a higher local recurrence rate was seen in patients who achieved a pathologic response and received radiation alone (40%), compared with patients who had residual disease and proceeded to mastectomy and radiation (23%). Limitations of this study exist because the methods used to determine pathologic response might not have been accurate. As such, higher rates of local relapse in the group of patients who were treated by radiation alone may have resulted from undetected residual disease after neoadjuvant chemotherapy.

In compiling the multiple studies using combined modality therapy, it would appear that for patients with IBC, mastectomy and radiation are the most effective treatments to minimize local recurrences, but even so, rates of LRR are about 20%. None of the studies shown in Table 23.5 omitted radiation but a few omitted mastectomy, indicating that for some highly selected patients

with IBC who respond to chemotherapy, radiation alone may provide good local control. As yet, there are no data on the safety of lumpectomy/segmental resection for patients with IBC after neoadjuvant chemotherapy, regardless of response to treatment.

Noninflammatory Locally Advanced Breast Cancer

For patients with noninflammatory LABC, standard local therapy also has been with mastectomy and radiation. However, as opposed to operable breast cancer for which consensus guidelines have been established for postmastectomy radiation based on accurate assessment of initial pathologic stage (79,80), no such guidelines have been created for inoperable LABC. Thus, for these patients, uncertainty exists as to whether recommendations for postmastectomy radiation should be based on initial clinical stage or final pathologic stage at completion of neoadjuvant chemotherapy.

To address this concern, a retrospective review was conducted of 150 patients derived from five clinical trials (total study population = 883) of neoadjuvant chemotherapy at the M.D. Anderson Cancer Center (81). Among these patients, 55% had stage III disease, 43% had stage II disease, and 1% had stage I disease. All patients had non-IBC and received neoadjuvant chemotherapy (mostly anthracycline-based), followed by mastectomy and adjuvant chemotherapy in 92% of cases. As postmastectomy radiation was not specified in these protocols, none of these 150 patients received radiation. With a median follow-up of 4.1 years, the LRR rate was 27% at both 5 and 10 years. As would be expected, factors associated with increased risk of LRR included increasing clinical stage with 5-year rates of LRR being 5%, 16%, 17%, 50%, and 79% for stages IIA, IIB, IIIA, IIIB, and IIIC breast cancer, respectively. LRR rates, however, were also associated with increased extent of pathologic disease seen within the breast and axillary lymph nodes. For example, the 5-year rate of LRR was 10% for pathologic T1 tumors without nodal involvement but 20% with node involvement. By combining both clinical and pathologic staging information, 5-year rates of LRR for clinical T1-2 tumors were 5% when associated with no pathologic lymph nodes but 13% when associated with positive pathologic lymph nodes. For clinical T3-4 tumors, 5-year rates of LRR were 34% when associated with no pathologic lymph nodes and 36% when associated with positive pathologic lymph nodes. For the 10% of patients who achieved a complete pathologic response (defined as no residual invasive or in situ disease in the breast and lymph nodes), the 5-year rate of LRR was 15%, which was not statistically different from that of patients who had pathologic residual disease (28%). Taken together, these data indicate that recommendations for postmastectomy radiation after neoadjuvant chemotherapy should take into account initial clinical stage because patients may still be at relatively high risk for LRR despite successful downstaging of disease. In support of this recommendation, a follow-up study was done by the same group of investigators at the M.D. Anderson Cancer Center (82) in which the outcome of 134 patients from the cohort previously described was compared with that of 542 patients from the original study population who received postmastectomy radiation after neoadjuvant chemotherapy.

This follow-up study showed that irradiated patients had lower rates of LRR (10-year LRR rate = 11%), compared with nonirradiated patients (10-year LRR rate = 22%). In addition, radiation reduced rates of LRR for patients with greater than clinical stage IIB disease, tumors that were >2 cm based on pathologic size, or who had four or more pathologic lymph nodes. Radiation also significantly reduced the rate of LRR for patients who had clinical stage III disease but achieved a pathologic complete response (10-year rate of LRR = 33 and 3% for patients without and with radiation, respectively). As such, it would appear that all or nearly all patients with LABC who undergo mastectomy after neoadjuvant chemotherapy would be candidates for radiation, regardless of pathologic stage at completion of chemotherapy. Risk of LRR after postmastectomy radiation is low, with 5- and 10-year rates of LRR reported to be 9% and 11%, respectively. In multivariate analysis, factors that were independently associated with LRR after postmastectomy radiation were skin/nipple involvement, supraclavicular lymph node involvement, extracapsular extension, and estrogen receptor-negative disease (82).

Although mastectomy has been standard of care after neoadjuvant chemotherapy for patients with LABC, evidence now exists that shows that for some patients, reasonable local control rates can also be achieved with breast conservation, including excision with radiation or radiation alone (Table 23.5). It should be noted that unlike the large randomized trials comparing mastectomy versus lumpectomy for patients with operable breast cancer (83), the trials of breast conservation for patients with LABC were not randomized and, in fact, only highly selected patients were deemed eligible for this procedure. In the French series of patients (45), patients were eligible for breast conservation if tumors reduced in size to ≤3 cm after neoadjuvant chemotherapy, in which case patients proceeded to wide local excision and radiation rather than mastectomy plus radiation. For patients who had no residual palpable disease after neoadjuvant chemotherapy, local radiation alone was administered. Ten-year DFS was comparable among groups (63%, 51%, and 66% for the mastectomy plus radiation, excision plus radiation, and radiation alone groups, respectively). However, the 10-year local failure rate was lower in the mastectomy plus radiation group (4%), compared with the group that underwent excision plus radiation (23%) or radiation alone (13%).

In the series of patients from the University of North Carolina, Chapel Hill (44), non-IBC patients were eligible for breast-conserving therapy if tumors reduced in size to ≤4 cm after neoadjuvant chemotherapy and an acceptable cosmetic effect could be achieved. For these patients, the 5-year OS rate was 96%, whereas for non-IBC patients who underwent mastectomy the rate was 51%. In this instance, differences in survival between the non-IBC patients who underwent either mastectomy or breast conservation presumably reflect differences in responsiveness to chemotherapy so that patients who underwent breast preservation had a better outcome because of chemosensitive disease. Local recurrence rates, however, were similar between groups and were 10% and 16% for the breast conservation and mastectomy groups, respectively.

Taken together, it would appear that no standard recommendation can be made with regard to breast conservation for patients with non-inflammatory LABC and that this decision needs to be made on an individual basis. Nevertheless, for a subset of patients who respond to induction chemotherapy, breast preservation may be an option because although it may be associated with a higher local recurrence rate, compared with mastectomy it does not appear to be associated with inferior survival.

FUTURE DIRECTIONS

Systemic treatments for patients with LABC, including IBC, have evolved over time based on better understanding of the natural history of this disease, as influenced by both anatomy and biology. In this regard, we have identified a subset of patients with invasive breast cancer who benefit from preoperative chemotherapy based on anatomic features such as size of tumor, extent of lymph node involvement, and morphologic appearance of the breast and overlying skin. On a deeper level, an understanding of the biology of these cancers has led to refinements in treatment strategies so that, for example, the identification of the importance of amplification of the *HER2* gene in some cases of LABC has led to more tailored treatments associated with higher pCR rates. For IBC, this is particularly relevant as these cancers are more likely to be *HER2*-positive. Other candidate genes that may lead to novel treatment strategies for IBC include the *RhoC GTPase* oncogene, a member of the Ras superfamily of GTP-binding proteins, which is overexpressed in IBC and shown to regulate breast cancer cell migration, invasion, and angiogenesis (84,85). The *WISP3* gene (an insulinlike growth factor0binding, protein-related protein), on the other hand, is more often underexpressed in IBC, conferring the potential for breast cancer progression by loss of tumor suppressor activity (86). As such, future strategies for treatment of IBC will be directed toward continued efforts to inhibit or restore the function of select target genes.

On a more sophisticated level, the development of treatment strategies for LABC/IBC has now gone beyond the boundaries of anatomy and biology to approach the molecular level. In this light, analyses of gene expression arrays have identified distinct molecular signatures for IBC (13,87), and several studies have correlated molecular signatures of LABC with responsiveness to neoadjuvant chemotherapy. The evolution of these types of studies will refine and identify predictors of response, thereby enabling better selection of therapies for individual patients (88–91). Thus, over the past 25 years, significant improvements have been achieved for treatment of patients with LABC/IBC and the prediction would be that, with more advanced treatments, the natural history of this disease will change, leading to better prognoses and outcomes for these patients.

REFERENCES

1. Giordano SH. Update on locally advanced breast cancer. *Oncologist*. 2003;8:521–530.
2. Singletary SE, Allred C, Ashley P, et al. Revision of the American Joint Committee on Cancer staging system for breast cancer. *J Clin Oncol*. 2002;20:3628–3636.
3. Brito RA, Valero V, Buzdar AU, et al. Long-term results of combined modality therapy for locally advanced breast cancer with ipsilateral supraclavicular metastases: the University of Texas M.D. Anderson Cancer Center Experience. *J Clin Oncol*. 2001;19:628–633.
4. Sikov WM. Locally advanced breast cancer. *Curr Treat Options Oncol*. 2000;3:228–238.

5. Kuerer HM, Newman LA, Smith TL, et al. Clinical course of breast cancer patients with complete pathologic primary tumor and axillary lymph node response to doxorubicin-based neoadjuvant chemotherapy. *J Clin Oncol.* 1999;17:460–469.

6. Hennessy BT, Hortobagyi GN, Rouzier R, et al. Outcome after pathologic complete eradication of cytologically proven breast cancer axillary node metastases following primary chemotherapy. *J Clin Oncol.* 2005;23:9304–9311.

7. Esteva FJ, Hortobagyi GN. Locally advanced breast cancer. *Hematol/Oncol Clin North Am.* 1999;13:457–472.

8. Ahern V, Brennan M, Ung O, et al. Locally advanced and inflammatory breast cancer. *Aust Fam Physician.* 2005;34:1027–1032.

9. Bell C. *A System of Operative Surgery.* Hartford, CT: Hale and Hosner, 1814.

10. Lee BJ, Tannenbaum NE. Inflammatory carcinoma of the breast: a report of twenty eight cases for the breast clinic of Memorial Hospital. *Surg Gynecol Obstet.* 1924;39:580–595.

11. Low JA, Berman AW, Steinberg SM, et al. Long-term follow-up for locally advanced and inflammatory breast cancer patients treated with multimodality therapy. *J Clin Oncol.* 2004;22:4067–4074.

12. Shen J, Valero V, Buchholz TA, et al. Effective local control and long-term survival in patients with T4 locally advanced breast cancer treated with breast conservation therapy. *Ann Surg Oncol.* 2004;11:854–860.

13. Bertucci F, Finetti P, Rougemont J, et al. Gene expression profiling for molecular characterization of inflammatory breast cancer and prediction of response to chemotherapy. *Cancer Res.* 2004;64:8558–8565.

14. Anderson WF, Chu KC, Chang S. Inflammatory breast carcinoma and non-inflammatory locally advanced breast carcinoma: distinct clinicopathologic entities? *J Clin Oncol.* 2003;21:2254–2259.

15. Cariati M, Bennett-Britton TM, Pinder SE, et al. Inflammatory breast cancer. *Surg Oncol.* 2005;14:133–143.

16. Kleer CG, Van Golen KL, Merajver SD. Molecular biology of breast cancer metastasis. Inflammatory breast cancer: clinical syndrome and molecular determinants. *Breast Cancer Res.* 2000;2:423–429.

17. Chang S, Parker SL, Pham T, et al. Inflammatory breast cancer incidence and survival. The Surveillance, Epidemiology and End Results Program of the National Cancer Institute, 1975–1992. *Cancer.* 1998;82:2366–2372.

18. Cristofanilli M, Buzdar AU, Hortobagyi GN. Update on inflammatory breast cancer. *Oncologist.* 2003;8:141–148.

19. Hance KW, Anderson WF, Devesa SS, et al. Trends in inflammatory breast carcinoma incidence and survival: the Surveillance, Epidemiology and End Results Program at the National Cancer Institute. *J Natl Cancer Inst.* 2005;97:966–975.

20. Jaiyesimi IA, Buzdar AU, Hortobagyi G. Inflammatory breast cancer: a review. *J Clin Oncol.* 1992;10:1014–1024.

21. Wingo PA, Jamison PM, Young JL, et al. Population-based statistics for women diagnosed with inflammatory breast cancer (United States). *Cancer Causes Control.* 2004;15:321–328.

22. Haagensen C. *Diseases of the Breast.* Philadelphia: Saunders, 1971.

23. Merajver SD, Sabel MS. Inflammatory breast cancer. In: Harris JR, Lippman ME, Morrow M, et al., eds. *Diseases of the Breast,* 3rd ed. Philadelphia: Lippincott Williams & Wilkins; 2004;971–982.

24. Tardivon AA, Viala J, Corvellec Rudelli A, et al. Mammographic patterns of inflammatory breast carcinoma: a retrospective study of 92 cases. *Eur J Radiol.* 1997;24:124–130.

25. Giordano SH, Hortobagyi GN. Inflammatory breast cancer. Clinical progress and the main problems that must be addressed. *Breast Cancer Res.* 2003;5:284–288.

26. Taylor G, Meltzer A. Inflammatory carcinoma of the breast. *Am J Cancer.* 1938;33:33–49.

27. Lerebours F, Bieche I, Lidereau R. Update on inflammatory breast cancer. *Breast Cancer Res.* 2005;7:52–58.

28. Haagensen C, Stout A. Carcinoma of the breast II: criteria of operability. *Ann Surg.* 1943;118:859–868.

29. Hunt KK, Ames FC, Singletary SE, et al. Locally advanced noninflammatory breast cancer. *Surg Clin North Am.* 1996;76:393–410.

30. De Lena M, Zucali R, Viganotti G, et al. Combined chemotherapy-radiotherapy approach in locally advanced (T3b-T4) breast cancer. *Cancer Chemother Pharmacol.* 1978;1:53–59.

31. Early Breast Cancer Trialists' Collaborative Group (EBCTCG). Effects of chemotherapy and hormonal therapy for early breast cancer on recurrence and 15-year survival: an overview of randomized trials. *Lancet.* 2005;365:1687–1717.

32. Harris EE, Schultz D, Bertsch H, et al. Ten-year outcome after combined modality therapy for inflammatory breast cancer. *Int J Radiat Oncol Biol Phys.* 2003;55:1200–1208.

33. Liauw SL, Benda RK, Morris CG, et al. Inflammatory breast carcinoma: outcomes with trimodality therapy for nonmetastatic disease. *Cancer.* 2004;100:920–928.

34. Perloff M, Lesnick GJ, Korzon A, et al. Combination chemotherapy with mastectomy or radiation for stage III breast carcinoma. A Cancer and Leukemia Group B study. *J Clin Oncol.* 1988;6:261–269.

35. Kaufmann M, Hortobagyi GN, Goldhirsch A, et al. Recommendations from an international expert panel on the use of neoadjuvant (primary) systemic treatment of operable breast cancer: an update. *J Clin Oncol.* 2006;24:1940–1949.

36. Wolff AC, Davidson NE. Preoperative therapy in breast cancer: lessons learned from the treatment of locally advanced disease. *Oncologist.* 2002;7:239–245.

37. Shenkier T, Weir L, Levine M, et al. Steering Committee on Clinical Practice Guidelines for the Care and Treatment of Breast Cancer. Clinical practice guidelines for the care and treatment of breast cancer: 15. Treatment for women with stage III or locally advanced breast cancer. *CMAJ.* 2004;170:983–994.

38. NCCN practice guidelines in oncology. V.2.2006 www.nccn.org. Accessed November 10, 2006.

39. Mauri D, Pavlidis N, Ioannidis JP. Neoadjuvant versus adjuvant systemic treatment in breast cancer: a meta-analysis. *J Natl Cancer Inst.* 2005;97:188–194.

40. Wolmark N, Wang J, Mamounas E, et al. Preoperative chemotherapy in patients with operable breast cancer: nine-year results from the National Surgical Adjuvant Breast and Bowel Project B-18. *J Natl Cancer Inst Monogr.* 2001;30:96–102.

41. Bear HD, Anderson S, Smith RE, et al. Sequential preoperative or postoperative docetaxel added to preoperative doxorubicin plus cyclophosphamide for operable breast cancer: National Surgical Adjuvant Breast and Bowel Project Protocol B-27. *J Clin Oncol.* 2006;24:2019–2027.

42. Deo SV, Bhutani M, Shukla N, et al. Randomized trial comparing neo-adjuvant versus adjuvant chemotherapy in operable locally advanced breast cancer (T4bN0-2 MO). *J Surg Oncol.* 2003;84:192–197.

43. Merajver SD, Weber BL, Cody R, et al. Breast conservation and prolonged chemotherapy for locally advanced breast cancer: the University of Michigan experience. *J Clin Oncol.* 1997;15:2873–2881.

44. Cance WG, Carey LA, Calvo BF, et al. Long-term outcome of neoadjuvant therapy for locally advanced breast carcinoma: effective clinical downstaging allows breast preservation and predicts outstanding local control and survival. *Ann Surg.* 2002;236:295–303.

45. Lerouge D, Touboul E, Lefranc J-P, et al. Combined chemotherapy and preoperative irradiation for locally advanced noninflammatory breast cancer: updated results in a series of 120 patients. *Int J Radiat Biol Phys.* 2004;59:1062–1073.

46. Ueno NT, Buzdar AU, Singletary SE, et al. Combined-modality treatment of inflammatory breast carcinoma: twenty years of experience at M.D. Anderson Cancer Center. *Cancer Chemoth Pharmacol.* 1997;40:321–329.

47. Gajdos C, Tartter PI, Estabrook A, et al. Relationship of clinical and pathologic response to neoadjuvant chemotherapy and outcome of locally advanced breast cancer. *J Surg Oncol.* 2002;80:4–11.

48. Yildirim E, Semerci E, Berberoglu U. The analysis of prognostic factors in stage III-B non-inflammatory breast cancer. *Eur J Surg Oncol.* 2000;26:34–38.

49. Hennessy BT, Gonzalez-Angulo AM, Hortobagyi GN, et al. Disease-free and overall survival after pathologic complete disease remission of cytologically proven inflammatory breast carcinoma axillary lymph node metastases after primary systemic chemotherapy. *Cancer.* 2006;106:1000–1006.

50. Ezzat AA, Ibrahim EM, Ajarim DS, et al. High complete pathological response in locally advanced breast cancer using paclitaxel and cisplatin. *Breast Cancer Res Treat.* 2000;62:237–244.

51. Mehta RS, Schubbert T, Hsiang D, et al. High pathologic complete remission rates with paclitaxel and carboplatin ± trastuzumab (TC±H) following dose dense doxorubicin and cyclophosphamide (AC) supported by GM-CSF in breast cancer-a phase II study. *Breast Cancer Res Treat.* 2005;94(Suppl 1):S225.

52. Limentani SA, Brufsky AM, Erban JK, et al. Phase II study of neoadjuvant docetaxel/vinorelbine followed by surgery and adjuvant doxorubicin/ cyclophosphamide in women with stage II/III breast cancer. *Clin Breast Cancer.* 2006;6:511–517.

53. Sanchez-Rovira P, Anton A, Barnadas A, et al. Biweekly gemcitabine, doxorubicin and paclitaxel (GAT) regimen as neoadjuvant chemotherapy in locally advanced stage IIb-III breast cancer patients: interim results from the 2002-01 GEICAM study. *Breast Cancer Res Treat.* 2004;88(Suppl 1):S107.

54. Low JA, Wedam SB, Lee JJ, et al. Phase II clinical trial of Ixabepilone (BMS-247550), an epothilone B analog in metastatic and locally advanced breast cancer. *J Clin Oncol.* 2005;23:2726–2734.

55. Thomas E, Holmes FA, Smith TL, et al. The use of alternate, non-cross resistant adjuvant chemotherapy on the basis of pathologic response to a neoadjuvant doxorubicin-based regimen in women with operable breast cancer: long-term results from a prospective randomized trial. *J Clin Oncol.* 2004;22:2294–2302.

56. Gonzalez-Angulo AM, McGuire SE, Buchholz TA, et al. Factors predictive of distant metastases in patients with breast cancer who have a pathologic complete response after neoadjuvant chemotherapy. *J Clin Oncol.* 2005;23:7098–7104.

57. Martin M, Pienkowski T, Mackey J, et al. Adjuvant docetaxel for node-positive breast cancer. *N Engl J Med.* 2005;352:2302–2313.

58. Henderson IC, Berry DA, Demetri GD, et al. Improved outcomes from adding sequential paclitaxel but not from escalating doxorubicin dose in an adjuvant chemotherapy regimen for patients with node-positive primary breast cancer. *J Clin Oncol.* 2003;21:976–983.

59. Mamounas EP, Bryant J, Lembersky B, et al. Paclitaxel after doxorubicin plus cyclophosphphamide as adjuvant chemotherapy for node-positive breast cancer: results from NSABP B-28. *J Clin Oncol.* 2005;23:3686–3696.

60. Roché H, Fumoleau P, Spielmann M, et al. 6 cycles of FEC100 vs 3FEC100 followed by 3 cycles of docetaxel for node-positive breast cancer patients: analysis at 5 years of the adjuvant PACS 01 trial. *Breast Cancer Res Treat.* 2004;88(Suppl 1):S16.

61. Trudeau M, Sinclair SE, Clemons M. Neoadjuvant taxanes in the treatment of non-metastatic breast cancer: a systematic review. *Cancer Treatment Rev.* 2005;31:283–302.

62. Estévez LG, Gradishar WJ. Evidence-based use of neoadjuvant taxane in operable and inoperable breast cancer. *Clinical Cancer Res.* 2004;10:3249–3261.

63. Bear HD, Anderson S, Brown A, et al. The effect on tumor response of adding sequential preoperative docetaxel to preoperative doxorubicin and cyclophosphamide: preliminary results from the National Surgical Adjuvant Breast and Bowel Project Protocol B-27. *J Clin Oncol.* 2003;21:4165–4174.

64. Than Y-L, Gomez LF, Mohsin S, et al. Clinical response to neoadjuvant docetaxel predicts improved outcome in patients with large locally advanced breast cancers. *Breast Cancer Res Treat.* 2005;94:279–284.

65. Gogas H, Papadimitriou C, Kalofonos HP, et al. Neoadjuvant chemotherapy with a combination of pegylated liposomal doxorubicin (Caelyx) and paclitaxel in locally advanced breast cancer: a phase II study by the Hellenic Cooperative Oncology Group. *Ann Oncol.* 2002;13:1737–1742.

66. de Matteis A, Nuzzo F, D'Aiuto G, et al. Docetaxel plus epidoxorubicin as neoadjuvant treatment in patients with large operable or locally advanced carcinoma of the breast. *Cancer.* 2002; 94:895–901.

67. Espinosa E, Morales S, Borrega P, et al. Docetaxel and high dose epirubicin as neoadjuvant chemotherapy in locally advanced breast cancer. *Cancer Chemother Pharmacol.* 2004;54:546–552.

68. Smith IC, Heys SD, Hutcheon AW, et al. Neoadjuvant chemotherapy in breast cancer: significantly enhanced response with docetaxel. *J Clin Oncol.* 2002;20:1456–1466.

69. Hutcheon AW, Heys SD, Sarkar TK, and the Aberdeen Breast Group. Neoadjuvant docetaxel in locally advanced breast cancer. *Breast Cancer Res Treat.* 2003;79(Suppl 1):S19–24.

70. Vogel CL, Cobleigh MA, Tripathy D, et al. Efficacy and safety of trastuzumab as a single agent in first line treatment of HER2-overexpressing metastatic breast cancer. *J Clin Oncol.* 2002;20:719–726.

71. Slamon DJ, Leyland-Jones B, Shak S, et al. Use of chemotherapy plus a monoclonal antibody against HER2 for metastatic breast cancer that overexpresses HER2. *N Engl J Med.* 2001;344:783–792.

72. Romond EH, Perez EA, Bryant J, et al. Trastuzumab plus adjuvant chemotherapy for operable HER2-positive breast cancer. *N Engl J Med.* 2005;353:1673–1684.

73. Piccart-Gebhart MJ, Procter M, Leyland-Jones B, et al. Trastuzumab after adjuvant chemotherapy in HER2-positive breast cancer. *N Engl J Med.* 2005;353:1659–1672.

74. Joensuu H, Kellokumpu-Lehtinen PL, Bono P, et al. Adjuvant docetaxel or vinorelbine with or without trastuzumab for breast cancer. *N Engl J Med.* 2006:354:809–820.

75. Buzdar AU, Ibrahim NK, Francis D, et al. Significantly higher pathologic complete remission rate after neoadjuvant therapy with trastuzumab, paclitaxel, and epirubicin chemotherapy: results of a randomized trial in human epidermal growth factor receptor 2-positive operable breast cancer. *J Clin Oncol.* 2005;23:3676–3685.

76. Coudert BP, Arnould L, Moreau L, et al. Preoperative systemic (neoadjuvant) therapy with trastuzumab and docetaxel for HER2 overexpressing stage II or III breast cancer: results of a multicenter phase II trial. *Ann Oncol.* 2006;17:409–414.

77. Mohsin SK, Weiss HL, Gutierrez MC, et al. Neoadjuvant trastuzumab induces apoptosis in primary breast cancers. *J Clin Oncol.* 2005;23:2460–2468.

78. Coudert B, Largillier R, Chollet P, et al. Pathological complete response with neoadjuvant docetaxel, carboplatin and trastuzumab in HER2-positive locally advanced breast cancer on behalf of the GETNA Group. *Breast Cancer Res Treat.* 2005;94(Suppl 1):S223.

79. Recht A, Edge SB, Solin LJ, et al. Postmastectomy radiotherapy: guidelines of the American Society of Clinical Oncology. *J Clin Oncol.* 2001;19:1539–1569.

80. Pierce LJ. Treatment guidelines and techniques in delivery of postmastectomy radiotherapy in management of operable breast cancer. *J Natl Cancer Inst Monogr.* 2001;30:117–124.

81. Buchholz TA, Tucker SL, Masullo L, et al. Predictors of local-regional recurrence after neoadjuvant chemotherapy and mastectomy without radiation. *J Clin Oncol.* 2002;20:17–23.

82. Huang EH, Tucker SL, Strom EA, et al. Postmastectomy radiation improves local-regional control and survival for selected patients with locally advanced breast cancer treated with neoadjuvant chemotherapy and mastectomy. *J Clin Oncol.* 2004;22:4691–4699.

83. Fisher B, Anderson S, Bryant J, et al. Twenty-year follow-up of a randomized trial comparing total mastectomy, lumpectomy, and lumpectomy plus irradiation for the treatment of invasive breast cancer. *N Engl J Med.* 2002;347:1233–1241.

84. van Golen KL. Relationship between growth factor signaling and motility in aggressive cancers. *Breast Cancer Res.* 2003;5:174–179.

85. van Golen KL, Bao LW, Pan Q, et al. Mitogen activated protein kinase pathway is involved in RhoC GTPase-induced motility, invasion and angiogenesis in inflammatory breast cancer. *Clin Exp Metastasis.* 2002;19:301–311.

86. Kleer CG, Zhang Y, Pan Q, et al. WISP3 and RhoC guanosine triphosphatase cooperate in the development of inflammatory breast cancer. *Breast Cancer Res.* 2004;6:R110–115.

87. Van Laere S, Van der Auwera I, Van den Eynden GG, et al. Distinct molecular signature of inflammatory breast cancer by cDNA microarray analysis. *Breast Cancer Res Treat.* 2005;93:237–246.

88. Dressman HK, Hans C, Bild A, et al. Gene expression profiles of multiple breast cancer phenotypes and response to neoadjuvant chemotherapy. *Clin Cancer Res.* 2006;12:819–826.

89. Hannemann J, Oosterkamp HM, Bosch CA, et al. Changes in gene expression associated with response to neoadjuvant chemotherapy in breast cancer. *J Clin Oncol.* 2005;23:3331–3342.

90. Chang JC, Wooten EC, Tsimelzon A, et al. Patterns of resistance and incomplete response to docetaxel by gene expression profiling in breast cancer patients. *J Clin Oncol.* 2005;23:1167–1177.

91. Gianni L, Zambetti M, Clark K, et al. Gene expression profiles in paraffin-embedded core biopsy tissue predict response to chemotherapy in women with locally advanced breast cancer. *J Clin Oncol.* 2005;23:7265–7277.

COMMENTARY
Kevin R. Fox

Discussions of the preoperative or neoadjuvant therapy of breast cancer are challenging. The literature on the subject of neoadjuvant therapy is vast but scattershot, with the majority of publications, with few exceptions, representing discussions of nonrandomized observations in relatively small numbers of patients. Dr. Chung's foregoing chapter on this difficult subject is a remarkably concise and painstaking effort to make sense of this difficult subject. The following comments will emphasize the issues of applying preoperative chemotherapy in the context of day-to-day clinical practice, focusing on the utility of preoperative chemotherapy as a product of a limited literature, and the use of legitimate clinical evidence derived from this literature.

We must keep in mind that the overwhelming bulk of the medical literature on the treatment of potentially "curable" breast cancers, most of which are "operable," follows a traditional algorithm of "surgery first," establishment of recurrence risk using accepted prognostic factors, and administration of a variety of therapies, including systemic chemotherapy, hormonal therapy, and more recently, targeted immunotherapy in an effort to enhance curability. Dozens of clinical trials, involving tens of thousands of patients, have led to complex but widely accepted care standards using this traditional algorithm. The literature on preoperative chemotherapy affords us no such body of evidence.

As Dr. Chung's discussion of this subject begins, appropriately, with an examination of the history of preoperative chemotherapy, readers should remember that the basic tenets of this therapeutic approach began in the 1960s and 1970s in a subset of patients that represented then, and represent now, a minority of the patients we see day-to-day. Patients with truly "inoperable" cancers of the breast, and patients with "inflammatory" breast cancers, will always constitute a small portion of any oncology practice. The ability of systemic chemotherapy to bring about clinical responses, to enhance the operability of these patients, and to improve the natural history of their breast cancers, thus improving survival, is unquestioned. As one reads on, the discussion gravitates away from this subset of patients and to the more recent literature, at least some of which is composed of large, thoughtfully designed, randomized clinical trials. In these clinical trials a variety of critical questions are asked, and occasionally answered, but these findings are largely confined to patients whose breast cancers were considered operable at the time of presentation.

If you follow the exhaustive time line of Dr. Chung's chapter, a remarkable similarity between inoperable and operable patients appears. Regardless of the size of the trial, or the presence or absence of randomization, or the state of "operability" of the patient at the time of initiation of therapy, there appear to be a few universal truths: first, the majority of patients will respond to chemotherapy, particularly if the chemotherapy is anthracycline-based. Second, when the patient reaches the point of definitive surgery, the complete disappearance of all evidence of invasive cancer is rather unusual. And third, if the patient is so fortunate to have complete resolution of all evidence of invasive cancer, then her prognosis seems to be quite good, relative to her counterparts who do not enjoy such a robust pathologic response.

Beyond this, relatively little can really be said about the subject. Perhaps it is best, then, to begin a more detailed discussion of the topic by asking the question, "What do we really know about the utility of preoperative chemotherapy in patients with breast cancer?" and just as critically, "What don't we know?" If we consider both inoperable and operable patients as a collective group of potentially curable candidates for preoperative chemotherapy, then the "facts," as they stand now, are as follows.

1. Most patients, if given anthracycline-based chemotherapy, will have a clinical response to treatment.
2. Most patients, having then undergone surgery, will not have complete pathologic eradication of their breast cancers.

3. Patients who attain pathologic complete responses have a better long-term prognosis than those who do not.
4. Patients who receive preoperative chemotherapy will probably have a reduction in the number of positive nodes in the axilla.
5. Inoperable patients will often achieve an operable state.
6. Operable patients will occasionally become candidates for breast conservation when they were originally considered not to be so.
7. The overall survival of these patients does not differ whether they received their chemotherapy preoperatively or postoperatively.

That, for all intents and purposes, is the extent of our relative certainty about the subject, and begs an equivalent list of statements regarding the deficiencies in our knowledge base:

1. The optimum chemotherapy regimen for preoperative application has not been defined.
2. The incorporation of hormonal therapy, whether alone or in conjunction with chemotherapy for hormone-receptor positive populations, has not been defined.
3. The use of trastuzumab in the preoperative treatment strategy for patients whose breast cancers overexpress *HER2* has not been defined, despite encouraging data.
4. The pathologic complete response rate, while predicting a better outcome for patients receiving a given chemotherapeutic regimen, has not been shown to be a "surrogate" predictor of overall survival when different chemotherapy regimens are compared in randomized trials.
5. The role of the sentinel node procedure in the management of patients receiving preoperative chemotherapy has not been defined.
6. By foregoing complete surgical treatment and staging until after chemotherapy is completed, precise predictions of local recurrence and systemic risk is compromised.
7. The need for, or selection of, postoperative therapy in patients who have residual disease in the breast following preoperative chemotherapy is completely uncertain.

It is best, perhaps, to take a critical look at what we have learned thus far from clinical trials to date. Fortunately, for the sake of discussion, the number of clinical trials—by virtue of their size, randomization, follow-up, and ease of interpretation—is rather small, and these pivotal trials will be discussed in more detail.

NATIONAL SURGICAL ADJUVANT BREAST AND BOWEL PROJECT (NSABP) CLINICAL TRIAL B-18.

This clinical trial, in all of its published forms (1–3), stands as the benchmark study from which the basic tenets of preoperative therapy have been derived, and stands as the foundation for most of the subsequently completed clinical trials worthy of discussion. This trial, notable above all for its simplicity of design and hypothesis, was the first randomized trial of legitimate size to examine the simple question of whether the preoperative application of a standard chemotherapy regimen (cyclophosphamide

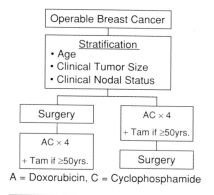

Figure 23C.1. *National Surgical Adjuvant Breast and Bowel Project* B-18 schema. Tam, tamoxifen; A, doxorubicin; C, cyclophosphamide.

and doxorubicin) conferred any advantage over the same regimen administered postoperatively (Figure 23C.1). This clinical trial randomized 1,523 patients who had in common (a) palpable breast cancer at presentation, (b) diagnosis rendered by needle aspiration or core biopsy only, (c) clinical tumor stage from T1 to T3, and (d) clinical N0 or N1 disease at presentation. The results of this clinical trial are now well known, with over 9 years of follow-up. These results are summarized in Table 23C.1. The disease free-survival and overall survival between the groups did not differ. In patients receiving preoperative chemotherapy, 80% showed a clinical response in the breast, while 36% had a complete clinical response. Of the patients who enjoyed a complete clinical response, 26%, in turn had a complete pathologic response in the breast.

Two additional and very relevant lessons were learned from this clinical trial. As surgeons were required to "propose" their intended operation (mastectomy vs. breast-conservation procedure) based on clinical findings prior to randomization, the number of breast-conservation procedures actually performed could be compared with the proposed number. These data are summarized in Table 23C.2. In patients receiving preoperative chemotherapy, the rate of lumpectomy rose from 60% (proposed) to 67% (performed), while in the group undergoing surgery first, the rate of lumpectomy fell from 66% (proposed) to 60% (performed). This improvement in breast-conservation rate was most striking in patients with tumors >5 cm at presentation, wherein the rate of "proposed" versus "performed"

Table 23C.1

Results of NSABP Trial B-18 at Nine Years of Follow-up

	Preop. Chemotherapy	Postop. Chemotherapy	p
Disease-free survival	55%	53%	0.50
Overall survival	69%	70%	0.80

Table 23C.2		
NSABP B-18 Proposed Versus Performed Rates of Breast Conservation Surgery (BCS)		
	Proposed BCS	Performed BCS
Preoperative chemotherapy	60%	67%
Postoperative chemotherapy	66%	60%

breast-conservation procedures rose from 8% to 22% after pre-operative chemotherapy. Although the enhancement of breast-conservation rates may be the most enduring lesson learned from this clinical trial, there has remained an obvious concern that the rates of ipsilateral breast tumor recurrence in patients treated with breast conservation, who were originally not considered as candidates for such an approach, might be excessively high. The rates for ipsilateral breast tumor recurrence were indeed higher for the preoperative versus postoperative treatment groups at a median follow-up of 9 years (10.7% vs. 7.6%, respectively), but this difference was not statistically significant.

The second critical observation from this clinical trial corroborated clinical impressions from many older, smaller, and nonrandomized trials. In the patients assigned to receive preoperative chemotherapy, there was a striking difference in overall, disease-free, and relapse-free survival when patients were divided into groups that had achieved a pathologic complete response (pCR) versus those who did not (pINV). The figures at 9 years of follow-up are included in Table 23C.3.

This observation, which is encouraging enough, applies to only a small proportion of the entire group of patients receiving chemotherapy (fewer than 15%) and leaves us with a large group of women with either clinical or pathologic residual disease in the breast for which outcomes are clearly worse, but for whom effective treatment strategies have yet to be developed.

This clinical trial has been criticized on two principle grounds. First, patients under the age of 50 were not required to take tamoxifen if their cancers were hormone receptor-positive, in keeping with the standards of the time. This problem has been remedied in all subsequently designed clinical trials of this nature. Second, it has been argued that the chemotherapy regimen

using doxorubicin and cyclophosphamide might not be the optimum regimen for the postoperative (and therefore preoperative) therapy of all breast cancer patients, and that a chemotherapy regimen including a taxane component might be a more representative standard. This particular issue was addressed in the next clinical trial under discussion, NSABP trial B-27.

NSABP TRIAL B-27

By the mid 1990s, the effectiveness of the taxanes, paclitaxel and docetaxel, as therapies for metastatic breast cancer was readily apparent, and by the late 1990s, the value of these same compounds as additions to anthracycline-based postoperative adjuvant therapies had been widely accepted in the United States (4,5). Clinical trial B-27 (6,7) (Figure 23C.2) was designed to incorporate docetaxel into the treatment scheme. In this trial, 2,411 women, whose presentation and selection criteria were identical to the criteria set forth in clinical trial B-18, were randomized to one of three treatment arms. All patients received four cycles of preoperative AC (doxorubicin and cyclophosphamide). One group (AC-S) went on to surgery at that point, and received no further chemotherapy. The second group (AC-T-S) received four cycles of docetaxel (T) after AC, then proceeded to surgery. The third group (AC-S-T) underwent surgery after four cycles of AC, then received four cycles of postoperative docetaxel regardless of the pathologic findings.

A list of selected outcomes, with a median follow-up of approximately 6.5 years, is shown in Table 23C.4. The addition of docetaxel to the preoperative treatment regimen virtually doubled the rate of pathologic complete response. Although there was a definite trend in the reduction of locoregional recurrences (and a statistically significant reduction in local recurrences only) in patients receiving docetaxel preoperatively, the other outcomes, with respect to overall survival and number of patients developing distant metastases, did not differ. Therefore, the rate of pCR failed to act as a "surrogate" marker for overall survival in this study. However, two other observations deserve mention, as shown in Table 23C.5. Regardless of treatment, the achievement

Table 23C.3		
NSABP B-18 Rates of Overall Survival and Disease-Free Survival at Nine Years Follow-up According to Pathological Response in Patients Receiving Preoperative Chemotherapy		
	pCR	pINV
Disease-free survival	75%	58%
Overall survival	85%	73%

pCR, no evidence of invasive carcinoma at surgery
pINV, residual invasive carcinoma at surgery

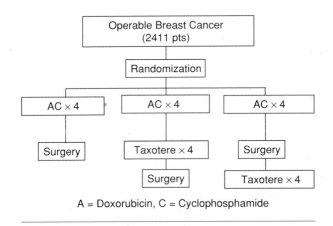

Figure 23C.2. *National Surgical Adjuvant Breast and Bowel Project B-27 schema. A, doxorubicin; C, cyclophosphamide.*

Table 23C.4

NSABP B-27: Outcomes at Six and One-half Years of Median Follow-up

	AC-Surgery	AC-T-Surgery	AC-surgery-T
Total number of patients	802	803	799
All local recurrences (%)	68 (8.5%)	38 (4.7%)*	44 (5.5%)*
Ipsilat. breast recurrences (%)	32 (4.0%)	19 (2.4%)	21 (2.6%)
Metastases	134 (16.7%)	132 (16.7%)	127 (15.9%)
5-Year DFS/OS (%)	67.7%/80.4%	71.1%/80.6%	70%/78.6%

A, doxorubicin, C, cyclophosphamide, D, docetaxel
*p, .003 compared with AC-surgery arm

of a pCR, either by AC alone (in groups AC-S and AC-S-T) or by AC-T (group AC-T-S) predicted a better overall and disease-free survival when compared with the majority of patients who failed to achieve a pCR. Second, as shown in Table 23C.6, the rate of proposed versus performed breast-conservation procedures rose in all groups, but the addition of docetaxel preoperatively did not improve the breast-conservation rate overall.

Why did this trial fail to show a survival advantage for patients receiving docetaxel? Two explanations come quickly to mind, although there may be others. First, in any large clinical trial, a significant proportion of patients will be estrogen receptor-positive, and in trial B-27, over 1,000 patients were known to be so. The worth of the taxanes in reducing the risk of metastatic disease in clinical trials of postoperative therapy in patients with hormone receptor-positive breast cancer has been brought into question recently (8). Table 23C.7 illustrates the pCR rates by estrogen receptor status. The reduced impact of preoperative chemotherapy in producing pCR rates is demonstrated here, as the patients who were known to be estrogen receptor-positive, while enjoying a higher pCR rate with the addition of preoperative docetaxel, had an overall markedly reduced overall rate of this particular outcome.

In theory, the addition of docetaxel in general is of little overall importance in this subset of patients, in whom adjuvant hormonal therapy is of equal or greater value than adjuvant systemic chemotherapy. Second, we must consider the overall risk of recurrence and death for the entire group of patients under study. By enrolling patients onto a clinical trial of preoperative therapy without knowledge of the pathologic status of the axillary lymph

nodes, clinical trials such as this one will treat an uncertain number of "node-negative" patients. In fact, clinical trial B-18 showed that of the patients treated on the "postoperative" chemotherapy arm, that is, patients who were identified as candidates for the clinical trial and then underwent surgery after randomization, fully 43% were identified as pathologically node-negative before any chemotherapy was initiated. One can hypothesize that in clinical trial B-27, if a significant number of these patients were pathologically node-negative at entry, then the ability to demonstrate an improved outcome with docetaxel would be very difficult to demonstrate statistically, as this group of patients is at an inherently lower risk of recurrence and death overall.

Nonetheless, clinical trial B-27 will remain a landmark study in the evolving clinical science of preoperative chemotherapy, and serves as a natural springboard for the proposed clinical trials that represent the next generation of studies of preoperative chemotherapy to be discussed in the following section.

THE ROLE OF PREOPERATIVE TRASTUZUMAB

In patients whose breast cancers overexpress *HER2*, the worth of postoperative trastuzumab in reducing the risk of recurrence, and perhaps even death from breast cancer, is now well known, and the administration of up to 1 year of trastuzumab, in addition to chemotherapy, is now an accepted practice standard (9–12). The incorporation of trastuzumab into the preoperative treatment of patients remains an active research question, and

Table 23C.5

NSABP B-27 Outcomes Based on Pathological Response at the Time of Surgery, Regardless of Treatment Given

	pCR*	non-pCR	p
n	410	1899	
DFS	81.5%	64.5%	<.0001
OS	92%	77.9%	<.0001

*pCR defined as no evidence of invasive cancer at surgery

Table 23C.6

Patients Undergoing Breast Conservation Surgery in NSABP B-27 Bases on Preoperative Chemotherapy Regimen

	n	Proposed	Performed
AC-surgery−+/−T	1606	48.4%	61.6%*
AC-T-surgery	805	50.8%	63.7%

A, doxorubicin, C, cyclophosphamide, T, docetaxel
*p, .33

Table 23C.7

Pathological Complete Response Rates in NSABP B-27 Bases on Estrogen Receptor (ER) Status and Preoperative Chemotherapy Regimen

	ER-negative	ER-positive	ER-unknown
Number of patients	738	1038	510
AC-surgery −+/−T*	13.6%	5.7%	31.6%
AC-T-surgery*	22.8%	14.1%	50.8%

A, doxorubicin, C, cyclophosphamide, T, docetaxel
*p <0024 for all comparisons of AC-surgery +/−T to AC-surgery-T

whether this should be done in a clinical practice setting is uncertain. However, preliminary evidence from one clinical trial suggests that preoperative trastuzumab may have a profound impact on the subsequent operative findings if it is administered in conjunction with preoperative chemotherapy.

As discussed by Dr. Chung, only one report of a randomized trial is available for review, and this trial was unfortunately suspended because of the robust nature of the pathologic findings. In the M.D. Anderson Cancer Center trial, a clinical study of preoperative chemotherapy (Figure 23C.3) enrolled 42 patients with *HER2* overexpressing breast cancers to receive preoperative chemotherapy with four cycles of paclitaxel, followed by four cycles of cyclophosphamide, fluorouracil, and epirubicin (FEC), with or without the concurrent administration of 24 weeks of weekly trastuzumab (13). Most of these patients had lesions that were clinically staged as T1-3, N0-1 as in the previously discussed NSABP trials. All patients underwent definitive surgery after the completion of the previously mentioned treatment, and

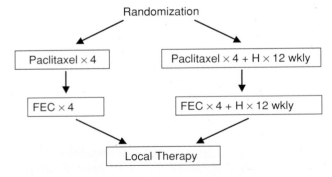

Operable Breast Cancer Her–2 +

Randomization

Paclitaxel × 4

Paclitaxel × 4 + H × 12 wkly

FEC × 4

FEC × 4 + H × 12 wkly

Local Therapy

F = fluorouracil, E = epirubicin, C = cyclophosphamide,
H = trastuzuamab; patients received endocrine therapy if HR+

Figure 23C.3. M.D. Anderson Cancer Center trial of preoperative chemotherapy with or without trastuzumab (H) in patients with *HER2* overexpressing breast cancer. Patients received endocring therapy if they were *HER2*-positive. F, fluorouracil; E, epirubicin; C, cyclophosphamide.

at the time of surgery, the pCR rate was an astonishing 66.7% in the group receiving preoperative trastuzumab, as opposed to 25% in the patients who did not. Although this study was stopped because of this marked difference in pathologic outcomes, the same investigators have reported on a subsequent supplementary group of patients treated presumptively with the chemotherapy/trastuzumab combination (14), reporting a pCR rate of 54.5% in 22 additional patients treated in this manner.

It is unknown if the inclusion of trastuzumab should now become a routine part of clinical practice in the preoperative treatment scheme of patients with *HER2* overexpressing breast cancers. Two uncertainties remain: if part of the goal of preoperative trastuzumab is to alter the surgical prospects of the patient who is inoperable, or to improve the likelihood of a breast-conserving operation in a patient who at presentation is not considered a candidate for breast conservation, the M.D. Anderson Cancer Center trial is not able to provide information regarding the likelihood of success. Second, this clinical trial was designed to coadminister trastuzumab with an anthracycline-based regimen (FEC) for a 12-week period. Although no excess cardiac toxicity was reported as a result of this strategy, the coadministration of trastuzumab with anthracyclines in not routinely recommended, and cannot be recommended outside a clinical trial. Whether or not the practitioner should choose to incorporate trastuzumab into the preoperative treatment scheme remains an unresolved issue; if this choice is made in a non–clinical trial setting, then we must acknowledge our obligation to extend the trastuzumab therapy beyond the point of surgery for the balance of 1 calendar year of total trastuzumab therapy.

TAILORING POSTOPERATIVE THERAPY AFTER "INSUFFICIENT" PREOPERATIVE THERAPY

Perhaps the most vexing problem for medical oncologists who choose to administer preoperative chemotherapy is confronting the patient who completes a prescribed course of preoperative therapy, undergoes an operation, and has residual disease in the breast. This scenario is the rule, rather than the exception, as the majority of patients fail to achieve a pCR. Furthermore, both clinical trials of the NSABP, as previously outlined, and numerous other studies of varying size, have emphasized the fact that patients failing to achieve a pCR have a significantly greater risk of recurrence and death. It is fully understandable that the medical oncologist, on confronting such a patient, feels obligated to recommend additional therapy; however, the existing literature provides us with absolutely no guidance as to what to do. Only three clinical trials of have been designed to examine "non–cross-resistant" therapy in a randomized fashion in patients who failed to respond "adequately" to an initial chemotherapy regimen, and none of these clinical trials can be said to demonstrate, conclusively, the real advantages of doing so. Two of these trials, one of which was conducted at the M.D. Anderson Cancer Center in the late 1980s, which is hampered by the absence of taxane therapy in the treatment scheme (15), and the other, known as the "Aberdeen" trial (16), are discussed by Dr. Chung. Although both trials suggest that a patient who responds inadequately (based on pathologic determination in the M.D. Anderson Cancer Center trial, and based on clinical determination in the Aberdeen trial) might better be served by prescribing a different chemotherapy than the one given initially, each trial is relatively small, and the true benefits of such a strategy remain unproven.

The largest clinical trial designed to evaluate the worth of non–cross-resistant therapy in poor chemotherapy responders is the German "GEPARTRIO" trial, the schema of which is shown in Figure 23C.4. This clinical trial, which has been published in preliminary form (17) and subsequently updated (18), has now treated over 2,000 patients, and although no information is available on the rates of recurrence and death in these patients, there are facets of this study that deserve mention.

The clinical design of the GEPARTRIO trial is quite straightforward. Eligible patients (those with T2-4, N0-3 lesions), who could be perceived as either operable or inoperable, all received two cycles of "TAC" chemotherapy (docetaxel, doxorubicin, and cyclophosphamide). If the patients failed to show a >50% reduction in tumor size (by ultrasound examination), they were defined as showing "low chemosensitivity," and were randomized to continue with the same chemotherapy regimen (TAC) for four additional cycles, or to receive a novel, non–cross-resistant regimen of vinorelbine and capecitabine (NX). Patients who showed, on the other hand, more than a 50% reduction in tumor size, were deemed "high chemosensitivity" patients, and were randomized to receive either four or six additional cycles of TAC. Following the completion of the assigned chemotherapy, all patients underwent surgery.

Thus far, two lessons have been learned from this clinical trial. First, the low chemosensitivity patients, after completing their prescribed therapy and before undergoing surgery, were re-evaluated by ultrasound. Table 23C.8 shows the percentage of patients achieving a "sonographic response" in the low chemosensitivity group. There was no particular advan-

Table 23C.8

Final Sonographic Response Rate for "Low Chemosensitivity" Patients After Completion of all Chemotherapy

Chemotherapy regimen	NX	TAC
Sonographic responses	63.5%	60%

N, vinorelbine, X, capecitabine, T, docetaxel, A, doxorubicin, C, cyclophosphamide

Difference not statistically significant in 627 patients.

tage, at least sonographically, in switching to the non–cross-resistant NX regimen. The second lesson is illustrated in Table 23C.9. The ultimate pCR rate for the low chemosensitivity and high chemosensitivity patients, all of whom have undergone surgery, is shown. Clearly, a greater initial clinical response to TAC chemotherapy predicted for a better pathologic result, but the low chemosensitivity patients had a poor overall pCR rate regardless of the chemotherapy regimen administered.

Although data on recurrence and survival of the patients in this enormous clinical trial are awaited, the information to date serves as yet another cautionary note: the appropriate chemotherapeutic strategy for patients who do not respond well to initial preoperative chemotherapy simply is not known.

LESSONS FOR CLINICAL PRACTICE AND PROSPECTS FOR FURTHER RESEARCH

The practicing oncologist, on confronting a patient in whom preoperative therapy is a consideration, must take seriously

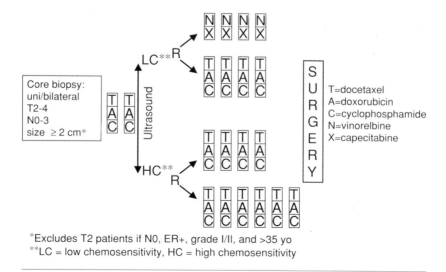

*Excludes T2 patients if N0, ER+, grade I/II, and >35 yo
**LC = low chemosensitivity, HC = high chemosensitivity

Figure 23C.4. The GEPARTRIO trial of preoperative chemotherapy based on clinical response. *Excludes patients with T2 lesions if N0, estrogen receptor-positive, grade 1/2, and >35 years old. **LC, low chemosensitivity; HC, high chemosensitivity. R, T, docetaxel; A, doxorubicin; C, cyclophosphamide; N, vinorelbine; X, capecitabine.

Table 23C.9

Clinical Outcomes in the GEPARTRIO Trial Based on Response to Initial Chemotherapy

	Low Chemosensitivity	High Chemosensitivity
CR by palpation	14%	47%
CR by ultrasound	10%	31%
Pathological CR	5.6%	25.2%
Mastectomy rate	71.5%	59.3%

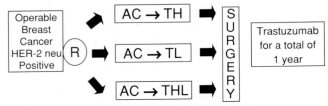

A = doxorubicin, C = cyclophosphamide, T = paclitaxel, H = trastuzumab, L = lapatinib

Figure 23C.5. Proposed trial *National Surgical Adjuvant Breast and Bowel Project* B-41 for patients with operable, *HER2* overexpressing, breast cancer. R, randomization; A, doxorubicin; C, cyclophosphamide; T, paclitaxel; H, trastuzumab; L, lapatinib.

the limitations of our current knowledge base, and make the best treatment decision based on those things that preoperative chemotherapy can accomplish. Preoperative chemotherapy can, in effect, accomplish only two legitimate clinical goals, and can accomplish them simultaneously. First, and perhaps foremost, it can alter the surgical prospects for the patient by rendering the inoperable patient operable, or rendering the operable patient a candidate for breast-conserving therapy when, at presentation, she was not thought to be such a candidate. Second, preoperative therapy can and will improve the patient's chances of long-term freedom from recurrence and likelihood of cure, just as conventional postoperative therapy would. With these two goals in mind, it is incumbent on the practitioner to devise the entire chemotherapeutic strategy at the outset, determining which regimen will result in the best long-term outcome for the patient, and administering the preselected chemotherapy regimen while hoping, at the same time, to achieve the intended surgical goal. With this in mind, perhaps the optimum preoperative chemotherapy regimen should "mirror" the treatment regimen that would be given had the patient been given postoperative therapy instead. Although it can be argued that preoperative chemotherapy also affords us the chance to evaluate the effectiveness of a given regimen, we are sorely lacking in the knowledge as to what to do if the patient proves to be even partially resistant to this strategy. Modifying the chemotherapy regimen "midstream" for a patient who responds less than exuberantly is dangerous territory, and proper clinical decisions simply cannot be made based on our available data.

This commentary by no means diminishes the field of preoperative chemotherapy as a valuable research tool. However, the most enduring lessons from research in preoperative therapy can only be achieved through the design and implementation of large, randomized clinical trials. Two of the clinical trials that have been either proposed or activated by the NSABP are shown in Figures 23C.5 and 23C.6. The first clinical trial, designated B-41, is intended for patients with operable, *HER2* overexpressing breast cancers. All patients will receive a full course of preoperative chemotherapy with doxorubicin, cyclophosphamide, and paclitaxel, and all patients will receive the balance of 1 year of trastuzumab postoperatively. However, the randomization will affect the patient's preoperative treatment strategy, wherein one third of the patients will receive trastuzumab concurrently with the taxane, one-third will receive the newer targeted therapy lapatinib, and one-third will receive

a combination of both trastuzumab and lapatinib. This clinical trial thus takes into account the potential benefits of preoperative *HER2-targeted* therapy, but ensures that all patients will also receive an adequate course of postoperative trastuzumab to ensure an optimum outcome for all patients enrolled. The second clinical trial, designated B-40 and currently enrolling patients, is directed at non-*HER2* expressing patients and is more complex. Patients will be randomized to receive one of three preoperative chemotherapy regimens, all of which employ doxorubicin, cyclophosphamide, and docetaxel, but will add preoperative gemcitabine or capecitabine in two of the patient groups. Patients will also be randomized to receive, or not receive, the antiangiogenic compound bevacizumab both during preoperative chemotherapy and after definitive surgery.

Clearly, preoperative chemotherapy has its place, although a limited place, in the standard treatment of patients with operable breast cancer, and a much more easily defined place in patients deemed inoperable at presentation. A significant number of questions remain as to the optimum chemotherapeutic approach in these patients, but accumulating evidence from current, completed clinical trials, and trials yet to be completed

HER-2 negative breast cancer by core biopsy, palpable mass ≥2.0 cm, Randomized to one of six preoperative chemotherapy regimens

| T × 4 → AC × 4→ Surgery | TX × 4→ AC × 4→ Surgery | TG × 4→ AC × 4→ Surgery | TB × 4 → ACB × 2→ AC × 2 → Surgery → B × 10 | TXB × 4→ ACB × 2→ AC × 2 → Surgery→ B × 10 | TGB × 4→ ACB × 2→ AC × 2 → Surgery → B × 10 |

T = docetaxel, X = capecitabine, G = gemcitabine, A = doxorubicin, C = cyclophosphamide, B = bevacizumab
Patients randomized to receive preoperative bevacizumab will also receive ten postoperative doses of bevacizumab

Figure 23C.6. *National Surgical Adjuvant Breast and Bowel Project* clinical trial B-40 of preoperative therapy for patients with operable, *HER2*-negative breast cancer. Patients randomized to receive preoperative bevacizumab (B) will also receive ten postoperative doses of B. T, docetaxel; A, doxorubicin; C, cyclophosphamide; X, capecitabine; G, gemcitabine.

will clarify some, if not all, of these uncertainties in the next several years. The current status of preoperative chemotherapy is nicely summarized by a recent international expert panel, and perhaps a proper concluding statement can be taken from their recommendations on "NST" (neoadjuvant systemic therapy) (19):

> First, the disease-free survival and overall survival are equivalent in patients treated with the same adjuvant or neoadjuvant regimen. However, NST has the clinical advantage of improving the surgical options (e.g., more breast conserving procedures). Second, it has been demonstrated that the response to NST is a predictor of long-term outcome. Indeed, pCR is strongly associated with improved disease-free and overall survival. However, it has not been proven that increasing pCR rates with more active regimens improves overall survival ... So far, the optimal regimen has not been defined ... It seems clear that NST has not been exploited to the fullest, and as more is known about operable breast cancer—its biology and treatment—and about NST, the closer we will come to achieving this aim.

REFERENCES

1. Fisher B, Brown A, Mamounas E, et al. Effect of preoperative chemotherapy on local-regional disease in women with operable breast cancer: findings from National Surgical Adjuvant Breast and Bowel Project B-18. *J Clin Oncol.* 1997;15:2483–2493.
2. Fisher B, Bryant J, Wolmark N, et al. Effect of preoperative chemotherapy on the outcome of women with operable breast cancer. *J Clin Oncol.* 1998;16:2672–2685.
3. Wolmark N, Wang J, Mamounas E, et al. Preoperative chemotherapy in patients with operable breast cancer: nine-year results from National Surgical Adjuvant Breast and Bowel Project B-18. *J Natl Cancer Inst Monogr.* 2001;30:96–102.
4. Henderson I, Berry D, Demetri G, et al. Improved outcomes from adding sequential paclitaxel but not from escalating doxorubicin dose in an adjuvant chemotherapy regimen for patients with node-positive breast cancer. *J Clin Oncol.* 2003;21:976–983.
5. Martin M., Pienkowski T., Mackey J, et al. Adjuvant docetaxel for node-positive breast cancer. *N Engl J Med.* 2005;352:2302–2313.
6. Bear H, Anderson S, Brown A, et al. The effect on tumor response of adding sequential preoperative docetaxel to preoperative doxorubicin and cyclophosphamide: preliminary results from National Surgical Adjuvant Breast and Bowel Project protocol B-27. *J Clin Oncol.* 2003;21:4165–4174.
7. Bear H, Anderson S, Smith R, et al. Sequential preoperative or postoperative docetaxel added to preoperative doxorubicin plus cyclophosphamide for operable breast cancer: National Surgical Adjuvant Breast and Bowel Project protocol B-27. *J Clin Oncol.* 2006;24:2019–2027.
8. Berry D, Cirrincione C, Henderson IC, et al. Estrogen-receptor status and outcomes of modern chemotherapy for patients with node-positive breast cancer. *JAMA.* 2006;295:1658–1667.
9. Romond E, Perez E, Bryant J, et al. Trastuzumab plus adjuvant chemotherapy for operable HER-2 positive breast cancer. *N Engl J Med.* 2005;353:1673–1684.
10. Piccart-Gebhart M, Procter M, Leyland-Jones B, et al. Trastuzumab after adjuvant chemotherapy in HER-2 positive breast cancer. *N Engl J Med.* 2005;353:1659–1672.
11. Joensuu H, Kellokumpu-Lehtinen P, Bono P, et al. Adjuvant docetaxel or vinorelbine with or without trastuzumab for breast cancer. *N Engl J Med.* 2006;354:809–820.
12. Slamon D, Eiermann W, Robert N, et al. Phase III randomized trial comparing doxorubicin and cyclophosphamide followed by docetaxel (AC-T) with doxorubicin and cyclophosphamide followed by docetaxel and trastuzumab (AC-TH) with docetaxel, carboplatin and trastuzumab (TCH) in HER2 positive early breast cancer patients: BCIRG 006 study. *Breast Can Res Treat.* 2005;94(Supp 1):S5.
13. Buzdar A, Ibrahim N, Francis D, et al. Significantly higher pathologic complete remission rate after neoadjuvant therapy with trastuzumab, paclitaxel, and epirubicin chemotherapy: results of a randomized trial in human epidermal growth factor receptor-2 positive operable breast cancer. *J Clin Oncol.* 2005;23:3676–3685.
14. Buzdar A, Valero V, Ibrahim N, et al. Prospective data of additional patients treated with neoadjuvant therapy with paclitaxel followed by FEC chemotherapy with trastuzumab in HER-2 positive operable breast cancer, and an update of initial study population. *Breast Cancer Res Treat.* 2005;94(Suppl):S223.
15. Thomas E, Holmes F, Smith T, et al. The use of alternate, non-cross-resistant adjuvant chemotherapy on the basis of pathological response to a neoadjuvant doxorubicin-based regimen in women with operable breast cancer: long-term results from a prospective randomized trial. *J Clin Oncol.* 2004;22:2294–2302.
16. Smith I, Heys S, Hutcheon A, et al. Neoadjuvant chemotherapy in breast cancer: significantly enhanced response with docetaxel. *J Clin Oncol.* 2002;20:1456–1466.
17. von Minckwitz G, Blohmer J-U, Raab G, et al. In vivo chemosensitivity-adapted preoperative chemotherapy in patients with early-stage breast cancer: the GEPARTRIO pilot study. *Ann Oncol.* 2005;16:56–63.
18. von Minckwitz G, Kuemmel S, duBois A, et al. Individualized treatment strategies according to in-vivo chemosensitivity assessed by response after 2 cycles of neoadjuvant chemotherapy. Final results of the Gepartrio study of German Breast Group. *Breast Cancer Res Treat.* 2006;100(Suppl 1):558.
19. Kaufmann M, Hortobagyi G, Goldhirsch A, et al. Recommendations from an international expert panel on the use of neoadjuvant (primary) systemic treatment of operable breast cancer: an update. *J Clin Oncol.* 2006;24:1940–1946.

24

Evolution of Elective Lymph Node Dissection for Cutaneous Malignant Melanoma

Daniel F. Roses

The ablation of clinically occult regional nodal metastases to improve survival has been the focus of the longest standing controversy in the surgical management of cutaneous malignant melanoma. Throughout the second half of the last century, studies purportedly demonstrating a survival advantage for patients having elective regional lymph node dissections were countered by studies purportedly demonstrating that they might be more appropriately reserved only for those patients whose nodes became clinically palpable. Uncertainty on this issue led to varied practices among major institutions with broad experience in the treatment of malignant melanoma (1). This controversy was heightened by a dramatic rise in the incidence of malignant melanoma as reported by the Surveillance, Epidemiology and End Results (SEER) program initiated in 1973 (2). This documentation coincided with the uniform microstaging of primary lesions, and the SEER data also demonstrated a markedly increased percentage of patients with lesions diagnosed early in their evolution and with favorable outcomes (2). Such patients had a predictably lower incidence of regional lymph node metastases, further stimulating a significantly more critical and selective approach to the surgical management of regional lymph nodes.

The recent introduction and broad acceptance of selective sentinel lymphadenectomy has clearly changed the intensity of debate on the appropriateness of surgery for regional lymph nodes, but the therapeutic impact of any elective surgical approach to the nodal drainage site of a primary melanoma continues to spark controversy. What is clear is that sentinel lymphadenectomy has recast the fundamental issue of the role regional lymph node metastases have in the natural history of melanoma with far greater sensitivity. What might have been previously undetected micrometastases by traditional pathologic assessment of nodal dissection specimens are now being increasingly detected by advanced immunohistochemical and biotechnologic techniques applied to multiply sectioned sentinel nodes. This has largely deflated, if not eliminated, the validity of studies of elective lymph node dissections from prior eras and has necessitated an entire reassessment of the issue. This review of the evolution of surgical approaches to regional nodes in patients with cutaneous malignant melanoma will consider the sources of controversy and the recent experience directed at making surgery more selective and consistent with a broader biologic understanding of the disease.

EVOLUTION OF ELECTIVE REGIONAL LYMPH NODE DISSECTION FOR CUTANEOUS MELANOMA

The concept that regional lymph nodes provide an early barrier to systemic dissemination was empirically embraced as early as the 18th century. It was granted scientific legitimacy in the 19th century by the development of microscopic pathology. Like breast cancer, melanoma provided an accessible neoplasm for study in that era. Discussing breast cancer in his seminal volume *Cellular Pathology*, Virchow (3) in 1858 stated that axillary lymph nodes served as a temporary barrier and provided a period of protection from the further spread of disease, eventually becoming an independent source for further dissemination. In 1892, this concept was applied to the treatment of melanoma by H. L. Snow (4), who proposed wide excision and elective lymph node dissection before nodal metastases became palpable as essential to curing the disease. He emphasized that the initial spread of melanoma was always to the regional lymph nodes, echoing the contemporary approach to breast cancer then being forcefully advocated by W. S. Handley in Great Britain and W. S. Halsted in the United States. Snow wrote of regional nodal metastases from melanoma:

> Eventually they pass beyond such "traps" into the blood current; then death with multiple visceral metastases ensues. Palpable enlargement of these glands is unfortunately but a late symptom of deposit therein; by the time it occurs there is almost always implication of deeper organs or tissues . . . We further see the paramount importance of securing, whenever possible, the perfect eradication of those lymph glands which will necessarily be first infected; before enlargement takes place radical removal of such organs in the axilla, groin, surface regions of the neck . . . is a safe and easy measure which, under the conditions indicated, should never be neglected.

This view was endorsed in 1903 by Frederick Eve (5), who, in reviewing the experience at the London Hospital, found regional lymph node involvement to be present in the great majority of cases, whether palpable or not.

The most influential advocate of the surgical treatment of melanoma based on a presumed orderly pattern of lymphatic permeation was Handley (6). He extended his conceptualization of the natural history of breast cancer to melanoma in two Hunterian lectures published in 1907 in *Lancet*. Handley asserted that the "growth of tendril-like cylinders of cells along the finer lymphatics that surround the primary growth" was the major mechanism of metastasis from melanoma, and that "embolic spread by way of the blood stream is a later event, dependent on the infiltration and invasion of the veins and arteries from concomitant permeated lymphatics" (6). Curiously, his specific point of reference for these dictates on the pattern of dissemination was an autopsy study of a single patient who had died with widely disseminated metastatic melanoma.

Handley advocated that the surgical treatment of a primary malignant melanoma should be its excision with a margin of skin by "what is judged by present standards to be a safe and practicable distance" (6). He also advised excising the deep fascia and even a portion of muscle subjacent to the lesion as well as the regional lymph nodes as part of the first operation. If two regional drainage basins were involved, he advocated dissection of both. Handley's contemporary, J. H. Pringle (7), further elaborated on the surgical treatment of malignant melanoma in an article the following year advising that the operation be extended beyond the local skin, subcutaneous tissue, and fascia by an en bloc resection of the areas of "lymphatic permeation" between the primary neoplasm and the regional lymph nodes. Inherent in all of these surgical approaches was the concept that permeation of malignant melanocytes through regional lymphatic channels to regional lymph nodes might serve to seed further local or distant metastases, a concept reinforced by the development and wide acceptance of contemporaneous en bloc radical resections for a variety of other solid neoplasms, particularly breast cancer. Melanoma presented a particular challenge to this concept of lymphatic permeation because the regional nodal groups were often at a significantly discontinuous anatomic site from the primary lesions.

The concept of lymphatic permeation was accepted with little challenge. Beginning in the 1930s, however, increasing evidence that cancer cells were rarely observed in lymphatic channels extending from the primary site to regional lymph nodes and that cancer cells could bypass lymph nodes and extend from lymphatics to blood vessels began to slowly erode the concept of contiguous lymphatic permeation and even orderly tumor embolization (8–11). The underlying biologic premise of elective regional lymph node dissection for many solid malignant neoplasms, including melanoma, began to be met with skepticism. Increasingly, tumor cells proliferating in regional lymph nodes became viewed as biologically selected and, rather than being initiators, were viewed as a reflection of more widespread tumor dissemination. For some patients, it was hypothesized, micrometastatic disease in lymph nodes might even be destined for tumor destruction rather than tumor proliferation, and its presence could even provide an advantageous immunologic interface between tumor and host. The growing recognition of the heterogeneity of tumor cells within a given neoplasm and their varied metastatic potential, and even predilection for specific metastatic locations, further challenged the concept of an orderly progression of disease whereby regional lymph nodes served as the first metastatic site (12).

Perhaps the most important and easily definable stimulus to the reassessment of surgical therapy for melanoma was microstaging of the primary lesion, initially enunciated and validated by Clark (13). His histopathologic studies made clear that the potential for metastatic spread was related to the level of invasion of the melanoma from its origin in the epidermis. This concept was refined by Breslow (14), who related prognosis to the thickness of the lesion as precisely measured by an ocular micrometer from the top of the granular zone of the epidermis to the base of the neoplasm. Thickness soon supplanted level of invasion as the major prognostic variable in the histologic staging of cutaneous melanoma, to which was also added ulceration as a dominant adverse determinant of survival.

Such precise assessment of prognosis from the histopathologic evaluation of the primary lesion made clear that, at least for —thin" nonulcerated melanomas (generally <1.0 mm in thickness), elective regional lymph node dissection was unlikely to have an impact on survival (15–19). In a study of 119 patients from New York University with stage I primary cutaneous malignant melanoma undergoing regional lymph node dissection, each of the lymph nodes in the dissection specimen was evaluated by serial sections, and micrometastases were correlated with primary tumor thickness. None of the patients with lesions <1.0 mm in thickness had nodal micrometastases (18). Data from major centers, as reported by such investigators as Balch et al. (19) and Essner and Morton (20), correlated thickness with nodal micrometastases and survival, and made clear that microstaging of the primary lesion was essential in considering whether elective lymph node dissection provided a survival benefit.

MORBIDITY OF LYMPH NODE DISSECTION

Any assessment of the benefits of elective lymph node dissection for melanoma had to consider the potential morbidity of such procedures. Until an improvement in survival could be demonstrated, the potential morbidity of such procedures would have heightened significance. With the introduction of more limited sentinel lymphadenectomy, as will be discussed, morbidity has been largely eliminated and the controversy shifted to the need for further ablation of the entire nodal drainage sites proven to contain microscopic sentinel node metastases.

Complication rates for regional lymph node dissections approaching or even exceeding 50% have been reported (21,22). Such high rates resulted from stringent criteria for defining morbidity, and varied depending on such patient characteristics as age, obesity (23), and, most importantly, the specific nodal dissections considered (24–26). Most reported complications associated with elective lymph node dissections were in the early postoperative period and related to wound infection, flap necrosis, seroma, and temporary nerve dysfunction (27–34).

Many reports on complications also combined elective dissections of nonpalpable nodes with therapeutic dissections for palpable disease, the latter having a greater potential for local complications. Even prior biopsy of a palpable lymph node could negatively affect a subsequent lymph node dissection (35). Coit et al. (36) found that other factors increasing the risk of complications in patients undergoing either groin or axillary dissection included obesity, age older than 60 years, and a history of smoking, hypertension, or diabetes. Multiple risk factors were found to be additive in predisposing to complications. Less definable and difficult to assess was the experience of the surgeon and the impact of appropriate and careful surgical technique in decreasing morbidity.

Certainly the greatest source of long-term morbidity has been persistent extremity lymphedema after axillary or inguinal node dissection. In the axilla, this was infrequent, with a reported incidence of ≤2% in most series (23,26,37), although a rate of 10% was reported (24). A lack of comparable objective criteria may have been responsible for such variations. Groin dissections, however, had more predictable rates of significant edema, particularly when deep iliac and obturator dissections were performed along with superficial inguinal dissections (22,24,38). Urist and associates (23) reported that 26% of patients experienced leg edema for 6 months or longer following dissection of inguinal nodes, but that 8% suffered significant functional deficit. Usually, edema was confined to the thigh (23,26,32) and was relatively asymptomatic; however, up to 10% of patients had long-term edema that impaired function (23,26). Edema occurred less frequently in patients undergoing groin dissection for primary melanoma of the trunk rather than extremities, as scars from wide excisions on the lower extremity could further impair lymphatic flow. Prophylactic measures such as elastic stockings and elevation (24,39) could decrease the incidence, but the effect of these measures was difficult to define.

Long-term numbness or paresthesias might result from the division of cutaneous sensory nerves such as branches of the femoral nerve, the lateral cutaneous nerve in the groin, the intercostobrachial in the axilla, and the rich distribution of sensory nerves in the head and neck. Popliteal node dissections, rarely performed electively but therapeutically performed for occasional instances of popliteal node involvement, require careful preservation of the sciatic nerve, and tibial and common peroneal nerves, but may result in denervation of the sensory medial and lateral sural cutaneous nerves (40). Even as elective radical neck dissection was supplanted by selective and modified procedures that preserved the spinal accessory nerve, any dissection of the posterior cervical triangle risked limitation in shoulder mobility. The facial nerve and its branches were at risk in superficial parotid resections for melanomas with drainage pathways to the preauricular nodes or to submandibular or facial nodes in the vicinity of the marginal mandibular nerve. In the head and neck region in particular, even limited dissections having no definable functional morbidity were associated with potential cosmetic morbidity.

Clearly, arguments against elective lymph node dissection that cited such morbidity had to be countered with evidence of their therapeutic efficacy. Citing a low rate of morbidity in an effort to contain a potentially lethal neoplasm as justification for elective lymph node dissection alone without such evidence became unacceptable. Whether elective node dissection offered patients a survival advantage was first assessed in retrospective analyses and then, more importantly, in prospective trials.

RETROSPECTIVE STUDIES OF ELECTIVE LYMPH NODE DISSECTION

The justification for elective lymph node dissection prior to microstaging was primarily derived from comparing the survival of patients with micrometastases in elective regional lymphadenectomy specimens with those having therapeutic lymph node dissection for clinically palpable disease. By this criteria, Pack et al. (41) in 1952, reported a 27% improvement in 5-year survival for patients having elective regional lymphadenectomy. Several studies since, including some in which patients' primary lesions were microstaged, reported a comparable improvement in survival (42–47) for patients with proven nodal micrometastases in elective regional lymphadenectomy specimens compared with those with clinically palpable metastases having therapeutic lymph node dissections (Table 24.1). The inference of such analyses was that micrometastatic nodal disease, for a significant subset of patients, was a harbinger of clinically palpable disease which, if allowed to progress, would lead to further disease progression. Even allowing for lack of optimal assessment of identifiable prognostic factors, most importantly thickness (Breslow) (42,47–55), such retrospective analyses were flawed by comparison of what may be biologically different patient populations, those with micrometastases versus those with macrometastases, and compromised the validity of any conclusions. Even if there were no biologic dissimilarity, a lead-time bias favoring the micrometastatic group would require prolonged follow-up and close matching for other prognostic variables to make comparisons meaningful. This was not achievable in such retrospective studies.

Table 24.1

Survival of Patients with Regional Node Metastases on Pathological Examination in Relation to Clinical Status of Regional Nodes (42–47)

Source	Lone-term Survival		
	CS-I (%)	CS-II (%)	Difference (%)
McNeer and Das Gupta (1964)	52	19	33
Cohen et al. (1977)	55	38	17
Das Gupta (1977)	69	20[a]	49
Balch et al. (1981)	48	24	24
Gallery et at. (1982)	48	36	12
Roses et al. (1985)	44	20	24
Average	53	26	27

CS-I = clinical stage I: regional lymph nodes not palpable or suspicious.
CS-II = clinical stage II: regional lymph nodes enlarged by palpation and suspicious for metastases.
All data are for 5-year survival rates, except in Cohen et al., which are 10-year results.
[a] Patients with Clark's levels III and IV.
From Morton, et al. (101)

One means of overcoming the inherent flaws in such retrospective studies was to perform multivariate analyses, comparing large groups of patients without clinically palpable nodes, who either did or did not have elective regional lymphadenectomy, matched by available prognostic indicators. The most significant study in this regard came from a combined series from the University of Alabama and the Melanoma Unit in Sydney, Australia, as reported by Balch et al. (16). The major prognostic determinants of survival were tumor thickness and ulceration. Reports of their experiences (16,49–51), as well as those from more limited series (52,53), supported a survival benefit for elective lymph node dissection for those patients with a primary tumor between 0.76 mm and 4.0 mm in thickness ("intermediate thickness"). At 8 years, the survival advantage for patients who had elective lymph node dissections with a primary lesion between 1.5 mm and 4.0 mm in thickness was sustained in rates as high as 20% to 40% (1,16,49,53). The benefit was more modest for patients with a primary tumor between 0.76 mm and 1.5 mm in thickness. The apparent failure of elective regional lymphadenectomy to improve survival for patients with a thicker primary tumor in those studies was attributed to the probable high frequency of occult distant metastases already present at the time of initial surgical treatment. In contrast, the great majority of patients with a thin primary tumor would accrue no survival advantage from elective regional lymphadenectomy because of a very low incidence of both occult nodal and distant metastases.

Other retrospective analyses demonstrated thickness to be a significant prognostic determinant even for patients with nodal micrometastases (46,56,57). In a review from New York University of the prognostic relevance of the extent of nodal metastases, lesion thickness, level of invasion, site of lesion, satellitosis, age, and sex for 213 consecutive patients with regional nodal metastases (157 with clinically negative/histologically positive disease and 56 with clinically positive/histologically positive disease), the difference in survival between patients with clinically negative/histologically positive nodes and clinically positive/histologically positive nodes was apparent throughout the follow-up period, as had been observed by others (47). In particular, a 10-year survival rate of 65% was achieved for the clinically negative patients having primary lesions of <2.0 mm in thickness, while it was 19% for patients having primary lesions of ≥5.0 mm in thickness. Balch and associates (58) were further able to show ulceration to be the only adverse tumor-related determinant in their node-positive patients.

In 1991, Morton and associates (59) at the John Wayne Cancer Institute (Santa Monica, CA) reviewed their experience with 1,134 melanoma patients with nodal metastases. Elective regional lymphadenectomy was performed in patients with primary lesions thicker than 0.65 mm. Although univariate analysis indicated that the number of involved nodes, gender, primary site (extremity versus trunk), and depth of inversion was prognostically significant, as with previous studies, survival rates at 5 and 10 years were significantly better for those patients who underwent elective regional lymphadenectomy with occult metastases than for those undergoing therapeutic regional lymphadenectomy for clinically evident disease. Likewise, a retrospective review of 3,616 patients from 9 centers in Germany demonstrated a 5-year survival advantage of 20% for male patients with axial and acral melanomas with thicknesses of 1.5 to 4.5 mm and a 5% to 10% advantage for women with melanomas with thicknesses of 2.5 to 5.0 mm who had elective lymph node dissections (60).

Despite such large retrospective studies, many employing multivariate analyses to adjust for multiple prognostic determinants, and supporting the efficacy of elective lymph node dissection, other retrospective studies reached different conclusions. Elder and associates (61) reviewed their experience with 72 patients who had a minimum of 5 years of follow-up and reported statistically equivalent survival at both 5 and 10 years for patients having wide excision alone or wide excision with elective lymphadenectomy. Binder and associates (62) and Bagley and associates (63) similarly found equivalent 5-year survival in a review of 168 patients having wide excision alone and 147 patients having wide excision and elective lymphadenectomy. A review of the Duke University Melanoma Clinic experience with 910 patients having wide excision and elective lymphadenectomy and 2,023 patients having wide excision alone failed to demonstrate a survival difference at 5 and 10 years (64). Equivalent survival was demonstrated as well when these groups were analyzed by increasing Breslow thickness range (0.75 to 1.50 mm, 1.51 to 2.99 mm, and 3.0 to 3.99 mm). This experience was further analyzed in a review of 4,682 patients by Singluff and associates (54), which again failed to demonstrate an advantage to elective lymphadenectomy. A large review from the Sydney Melanoma Unit (which had previously reported a survival advantage for elective lymphadenectomy for intermediate-thickness melanoma) of 1,278 patients with melanomas of the trunk or limbs exceeding 1.5 mm thickness, treated from 1960 to 1991, also failed to demonstrate a survival advantage for patients having elective lymphadenectomy (55). This study excluded patients referred after definitive local treatment elsewhere, as inclusion of patients whose first evidence of failure was regional and who were then referred to the Sydney Melanoma Unit, may have created a selection bias favoring elective lymphadenectomy in the earlier analyses.

Whereas the largest reported experience had been with melanomas of the trunk and limbs, more limited experience with melanomas of the head and neck added to the controversy. In a series of 206 patients with head and neck melanomas from New York University (65), 90 of whom had regional lymph node dissections, the dominant prognostic determinant was the presence of nodal metastases, but a survival advantage could not be demonstrated for clinically occult compared with palpable disease. A report by Belli and associates (66) on their experience with 93 patients with regional node metastases from melanomas in the head and neck region reached a similar conclusion. O'Brien and associates (67) reporting from the Sydney Melanoma Unit, noted that an improvement in survival could be seen for patients who had elective lymph node dissection with lesions in the 1.5- to 3.9-mm thickness range using a univariate analysis, but the benefit was lost in a multivariate analysis that adjusted for prognostic variables.

Of note in the New York University study on head and neck melanoma was the pattern of metastases, affecting lymph nodes adjacent to the primary melanoma site and extending beyond that site in some instances but never skipping over the initial draining nodal depot. This suggested a predictable anatomic progression of regional nodal metastases. Radical and modified radical neck dissections were abandoned, and more limited dissections to include the nodal group adjacent or subjacent to the anatomic site of the primary lesion were adopted.

In looking at retrospective analyses from that era, it is apparent that divergent conclusions were often reached, and certainly a definitive case for elective node dissection had not been made. Although patients with nodal metastases were a heterogeneous group, there did emerge the suggestion that any benefit of elective lymph node dissection would probably be for those patients with "intermediate-thickness" lesions. This emerging hypothesis was compelling enough to justify its evaluation in more stringently controlled prospective trials. Notably, while some prospective trials had already been initiated before the universal application of microstaging criteria, microstaging now provided a framework for structuring prospective trials of elective lymph node dissection.

PROSPECTIVE, RANDOMIZED STUDIES OF ELECTIVE LYMPH NODE DISSECTION

Even before microstaging had become standardized for prognostic assessment, two prospective, randomized trials had been conducted to address the issue of whether elective lymph node dissection provided a survival advantage. In both, patients with malignant melanomas of the extremities were randomized to either wide excision alone or wide excision and elective lymph node dissection. Both studies failed to show a statistically significant benefit to elective lymphadenectomy. The earlier of these two studies, performed at the Mayo Clinic between 1971 and 1976, as reported by Sim and associates (68), randomized 171 patients with extremity melanomas to wide excision alone (reserving lymph node dissection only if nodes became clinically positive), to wide excision and immediate elective lymph node dissection, or to elective lymph node dissection 1 to 3 months after wide excision. A second larger multicenter study of melanomas on the distal two thirds of the extremities in Europe, under the auspices of the World Health Organization (WHO), as reported by Veronesi and associates (69), had two randomization arms: wide excision and elective lymph node dissection, or wide excision alone, reserving lymph node dissection if the nodes became clinically positive. As both trials were initiated before the microstaging systems of Clark and Breslow had been widely adopted, patients were not prospectively stratified for those variables. The WHO study had a predominance of lesions in women, a group with a more demonstrably favorable gender-specific survival for distal extremity lesions. Furthermore, ulceration was not a stratification criterion.

In these studies, 5-year survival was not statistically different in any treatment group. In the WHO study, survival in patients with occult microscopic disease who had elective lymph node dissection was not significantly different from survival for those who had wide excisions alone, for whom therapeutic node dissection was reserved if clinically positive nodes developed during observation (36.8% vs. 30.2%). These studies became the most frequently cited to counter proponents of elective lymph node dissection.

Reservations about the Mayo and WHO studies were amplified by publication of the data of Balch and associates (16) demonstrating a survival advantage for patients with intermediate-thickness melanoma having elective lymph node dissections. It was noted that the percentage of patients with melanomas that were microstaged and in the 1.5- to 4.0-mm thickness range in the WHO study was only 34%. These were the patients for whom the greatest potential benefit from elective lymph node dissection might be realized. Furthermore, there was a 5-year survival difference in the WHO study, although not statistically significant, for patients with melanomas of 1.6- to 4.5-mm thickness, favoring wide excision and elective lymph node dissection compared with wide excision alone (78.5% vs. 69.7%). The possibility existed that, with much larger numbers of patients with malignant melanomas in this intermediate-thickness range, a statistically significant benefit for elective lymph node dissection might have been demonstrated. Furthermore, 21% of patients with melanomas of 1.5 to 4.0 mm in thickness were found to have metastases in the elective node dissections, while 56% of patients in this thickness range treated by wide excision alone developed clinical nodal metastases treated by subsequent therapeutic dissections (70,71). This raised the possibility that occult nodal disease may have been pathologically undetected in elective node dissection specimens presumed to be negative for metastases.

Because subgroups of patients may have benefited from elective lymph node dissection, Cascinelli and associates (72) re-evaluated survival 15 years after the original publication of the WHO study, according to prognostic criteria: sex, tumor thickness, Clark levels III and IV, and ulceration. No significant survival differences were noted in any of these subgroups. Of the entire group of 286 patients who had wide excision alone, 75 (26%) went on to develop nodal metastases requiring regional node dissection; survival in this group at 10 years was not statistically different from survival in the 54 patients who had been randomized to have elective lymphadenectomy and in whom nodal micrometastases had been diagnosed histologically in the lymph node dissection specimens. To assess a possible survival advantage for patients with intermediate tumor thickness, a multivariate analysis was performed on the subgroup of 185 melanoma patients with primary tumor thicknesses between 1.5 and 4.0 mm, and this also failed to show a benefit for elective lymph node dissection (73). Ulceration of the melanoma, as defined by histologic rather than clinical evaluation, was the only prognostic variable along with thickness that had an impact on survival. Other factors, including initial surgical treatment (wide local excision with or without elective lymph node dissection as noted), sex, age, and maximal tumor diameter, failed to correlate with survival.

Because the first WHO trial was limited to lesions on the extremities and was initiated before the widespread adoption of microstaging by thickness, and before the availability of retrospective data on the potential value of elective node dissection for intermediate-thickness lesions, another trial was initiated for melanomas thicker than 1.5 mm located on the trunk. Patients were randomized to receive wide excision alone or wide excision and elective lymph node dissection (74). Of the 252 patients entered in the study, 21% having nodal dissections were found to have micrometastases, while 26% in the wide excision group developed clinically detectable regional nodal metastases during follow-up. The overall survival of the two groups of patients was statistically equivalent. Survival according to type of treatment was also evaluated in two subgroups of patients: those with tumor thickness between 1.5 and 4.0 mm, and those with tumor thickness >4.0 mm. An observed difference in the intermediate-thickness subgroup favoring the elective lymph node dissection group was statistically significant ($p = 0.03$). There was no difference for lesions >4.0 mm in thickness. In an analysis at 8 years of follow-up, patients with micrometastases in elective lymph node dissection specimens had a 5-year survival rate of 48.2%, versus 26.6% for patients having a delayed dissection when clinically palpable nodal metastases were detected ($p = 0.04$) (75,76).

To specifically evaluate elective lymph node dissection for intermediate-thickness melanomas (1.0 to 4.0 mm), an Intergroup Melanoma Surgical Trial was initiated and directed by Balch et al. (77,78) and supported by the National Cancer Institute. Also included in the study was an assessment of differing margins of excision around the primary lesion, the other surgical issue in the treatment of melanoma requiring prospective analysis. After randomization to either 2.0 cm or 4.0 cm margins of excision, patients with melanomas of the trunk or proximal extremities were randomized to have or not to have elective lymph node dissection. Patients with head and neck and distal extremity melanomas were also included if a 2.0-cm margin excision could be achieved and then also randomized to have or not have an elective lymph node dissection. Patients were stratified according to: (a) melanoma thickness (1.0 to 2.0 mm, 2.0 to 3.0 mm, 3.0 to 4.0 mm), (b) location of the primary melanoma (proximal extremity vs. trunk, or distal extremity vs. head and neck), and (c) ulceration of the epidermis overlying the melanoma on microscopic sections.

The Intergroup Melanoma Surgical Trial prerandomized 786 patients, of whom 740 were eligible and evaluable for study. The average follow-up when reported in 1996 was 7.4 years. Adverse prognostic indicators were greater tumor thickness, ulceration, site of the primary melanoma on the trunk, and patient age, most significantly over 60 years. There was no statistically significant difference between patients having or not having elective lymph node dissection at 10 years (77% vs. 73%; $p = 0.12$). However, subset analysis did demonstrate a survival advantage for elective lymph node dissection for patients with nonulcerated melanomas (84% vs. 77%; $p = 0.03$), with a tumor thickness of 1.0 to 2.0 mm (86% vs. 80%; $p = 0.03$). For patients 60 years of age or younger, the advantage was even more significant ($p = 0.0006$) (Figure 24.1).

This was the first prospectively randomized study designed to assess whether a survival advantage could be demonstrated for elective lymph node dissection in specific subsets of patients. The improvement demonstrated for patients with nonulcerated lesions of 1.0 to 2.0 mm in thickness lesions lent some support to the traditional hypothesis that there might be a time interval in the progression of melanoma during which ablation of regional lymph nodes for patients with occult nodal disease but a low risk of systemic disease might prevent the further dissemination of disease. However, the low incidence of nodal micrometastases in the elective node dissection specimens for patients with melanomas 1.0 to 2.0 mm thick (5%) compared

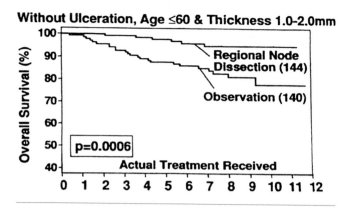

Figure 24.1 Effect of elective regional lymph node dissection in patients ≤60 years old with lesions 1.0 to 2.0 mm in thickness and without ulceration. This was the subset of patients in the Intergroup Melanoma Trial in which the most significant improvement in survival was observed. (From Balch CM, Soong S-J, Bertolucci AA, et al. Efficacy of an elective regional lymph node dissection of 1.0 to 4.0 mm-thick melanomas for patients 60 years of age and younger. *Ann Surg.* 1996; 224:255–266.)

with patients having wide excision alone who subsequently developed clinical node metastases (13%) further highlighted the potential inadequacy of pathologic analyses based on random sampling of limited sections from a specimen in which multiple nodes were grossly dissected (79).

ELECTIVE "SELECTIVE" REGIONAL LYMPHADENECTOMY

If elective lymph node dissection does provide subsets of patients with a survival advantage, it should be most compellingly demonstrated in those proven to have nodal micrometastases. As noted, these patients would also be those who would not have evolving metastases at other sites. As most patients with intermediate-thickness melanomas have a reported incidence of nodal metastases in elective lymph node dissection specimens no greater than 25%, and if those with nodal metastases who also harbored occult systemic disease were eliminated, the potential advantage of elective nodal dissection would be limited to even fewer patients. If only those patients who had micrometastases to regional lymph nodes could be accurately and reliably identified, studies might then be designed to focus with statistical magnitude on the fundamental biologic significance of whether the ablation of nodal micrometastases does, in fact, affect survival. This became realized by the introduction of sentinel lymphadenectomy, clearly a major advance in refining the surgical treatment of malignant melanoma. Sentinel lymphadenectomy was made possible by the confluence of advances in nuclear imaging and lymphatic mapping and, most importantly, histopathology.

Lymphatic Mapping

The understanding of cutaneous lymphatic drainage for most of the 20th century was grounded in the classic 19th-century studies of Sappey (80), in which the lymphatics were mapped by cutaneous injections of red oxide of mercury. Sappey's elegant illustrations provided a detailed delineation of lymphatic anatomy and suggested a uniform pattern of lymphatic drainage to regional nodes (81). His studies were adapted by surgeons to delineate the nodal drainage sites for the dissemination of malignant melanoma, a cutaneous neoplasm with a propensity for dermal lymphatic invasion. However, clinical experience demonstrated that central locations on the trunk and the head and neck were not always predictable, and might even drain to multiple nodal sites. Nuclear lymphatic mapping techniques were therefore adopted to determine the direction of nodal drainage from these ambiguous areas.

Several investigators contributed to the development of nuclear lymphatic mapping. Sherman and Ter-Pogossian (82) used radioactive colloidal gold (^{198}Au) to demonstrate cutaneous lymphatic flow, following which Fee and associates (83) applied this technique for the determination of lymphatic pathways from specific cutaneous melanoma sites. Because of the high radiation exposure from ^{198}Au, other tracers for lymphoscintigraphy were evaluated, among which were technetium-99m (^{99m}Tc)-labeled sulfur colloid (84), ^{99m}Tc-labeled antimony sulfide, and ^{99m}Tc-labeled human serum albumin (85). Lymphoscintigraphy required that the skin surrounding the primary melanoma site be injected with radiocolloid intradermally with care taken to raising a wheal to insure intradermal entry of radiocolloid into the dermal lymphatics. Images were then obtained at approximately 15-to 20-minute intervals. Lymphatic mapping revealed that, whereas nodal drainage pathways from the extremities were invariably directed to the ipsilateral axilla or groin, for distal extremity lesions they might be uncommonly directed to epitrochlear or popliteal nodes as well. Most importantly, several studies confirmed that drainage pathways from primary lesions on the trunk and the head and neck were less predictable.

Before lymphoscintigraphy, surgeons had relied on guidelines originally derived from the studies of Sappey, which had established a dividing line on the trunk from the second lumbar vertebra to the umbilicus, drainage above going to the ipsilateral axilla, and below to the ipsilateral groin. The exceptions were zones surrounding this dividing line in which drainage could be to either or both the axilla and groin, and in the midline, for a distance of 2.5 cm, where drainage could be contralateral or bidirectional. In a study by Norman and associates (86), it was noted that up to 59% of elective regional lymphadenectomies determined by such guidelines might have resulted in the ablation of the wrong nodal group or a failure to dissect one of multiple nodal groups to which the truncal melanoma drained. Other studies have confirmed that as many as 50% of melanoma sites will drain to multiple lymphatic basins or have pathways that are not predictable by Sappey's studies (87–94). For head and neck sites, Wanebo and associates (89) reported that the predictability of cutaneous lymphatic flow may be less certain than believed by strict anatomic criteria. This was also substantiated by other reports demonstrating a discordance of one-third from lymphoscintigraphic findings and anatomically predicted pathways (90–94). In a study from the Moffitt Cancer Center (Tampa, FL) of 212 patients who were candidates for elective lymph node dissection and had preoperative lymphoscintigraphy, the discordance rate in the head and neck for lymphoscinti-

graphic pattern compared to predicted anatomic pathways was 63%, while for truncal lesions, the discordance rate was 32%. Lymphoscintigraphy changed the plan of operative intervention in 47%, with 19% having a basin dissected that would not have been predicted by traditional criteria, and 28% did not have a dissection because of failure of the lymphoscintigram to indicate a predominant drainage basin from a constellation of multiple sites (95).

A formidable experience with 1,759 melanoma patients having lymphoscintigraphy, as reported by Thompson and associates (96), has provided a particularly compelling confirmation of the importance of precisely delineating the pattern of lymphatic flow from cutaneous sites, which they found to not infrequently differ from classic teaching. Lymphoscintigraphy showed 1,089 patients to have drainage to 1 nodal field, 491 to 2 nodal fields, 134 to 3 nodal fields, and 6 to 5 nodal fields. In many instances, the pathways were at variance with traditional precepts including interval nodes outside drainage basins as well as contralateral nodal sites. An initial drainage pattern to interval nodes was confirmed by Summer and associates (97) to occur in as many as 5% of melanoma patients. Such studies clearly weakened the assumptions derived from studies on elective node dissection in which lymphoscintigraphy was not used in the planning of surgery, particularly for large numbers of patients having truncal and head and neck melanomas. In a report from the Sydney Melanoma Unit, de Wilt et al. (98) reported a discordance rate of 31.6% for 362 patients with head and neck melanomas between sentinel nodes identified by lymphoscintigraphy compared with locations that would have been clinically predicted. It should be noted that of the prospective trials of elective lymph node dissection, only the Intergroup Melanoma Trial required lymphoscintigraphy to identify the nodal basin(s) at risk for truncal melanomas.

Sentinel Lymphadenectomy

Lymphoscintigraphy demonstrated the feasibility of applying lymphatic mapping for surgical planning. A logical extension was the hypothesis that within the specific lymph node drainage basin, the initial site(s) of lymph node metastases might also be identified. If this was achievable then surgery could be precisely directed, the frequency of complete regional lymph node dissection significantly limited, and, most importantly, the study of clinically occult lymph node metastases and any advantage resulting from their removal greatly enhanced. For this to be achieved, techniques for intraoperative lymphatic mapping were required.

Investigations by Kinmonth (99), using patent blue V dye to demonstrate the regional lymphatics in preparation for lymphangiography, established that agent as well suited for intraoperative lymphatic mapping. Investigators at the John Wayne Cancer Institute (100) compared patent blue V, methylene blue, isosulfan blue, and Evans blue dyes in cats to determine the optimal agent. Patent blue V and isosulfan blue were demonstrated to be the most consistent and useful. They then proceeded to apply lymphatic mapping clinically in melanoma patients. In a landmark report by Morton and associates (101), patent blue V or isosulfan blue was injected intradermally at the primary melanoma site in 223 consecutive patients as a means of mapping the sentinel node(s). By "sentinel" was meant the node or nodes that drained the specific cutaneous sites and were presumed to be the initial potential repository of a regional nodal micrometastasis. The technique was found to be effective for sites draining to the neck, axilla, and groin. A standardized technique was used in conjunction with preoperative lymphoscintigraphy, successfully enabling blue-stained nodes along with their blue-stained afferent lymphatics to be identified. To test the hypothesis that metastases from a specific site would preferentially affect a draining sentinel node or nodes, the incidence of micrometastases in the sentinel node was correlated with the remaining nodes in a completed lymph node dissection specimen. In the reports on their initial 4-year experience, sentinel nodes were successfully identified in 194 of 237 (82%) patients who also had a completion regional lymph node dissection. Micrometastases were demonstrated in 47 (18%) of 259 sentinel nodes. Nonsentinel nodes were the sole site of metastases in only two (0.06%) of 3079 nonsentinel nodes from the 194 lymphadenectomy specimens from patients who had identifiable sentinel nodes. This clearly supported the predictability of sentinel nodes being the initial site of occult microscopic nodal metastases. It confirmed that the lymphatic drainage of primary melanoma sites could be traced to sentinel nodes and that the absence of metastases in these nodes accurately reflected the absence of metastases in the remaining nodal basin.

The introduction of sentinel lymphadenectomy using blue dye extended the experience gained with lymphoscintigraphy into the operating room. Preoperative lymphoscintigraphy was employed for planning of the specific nodal sites for surgery. Injection or reinjection prior to surgery was also employed by several investigators using a gamma-probe in the operating room as the primary means of identifying the sentinel node(s) that had concentrated the radioisotope. Alex and associates (102) first reported on this technique using a handheld gamma-probe alone without blue dye. A report by Krag and associates (103) followed. Thereafter, several investigators applied this approach in conjunction with the dye technique, further directing the site of incision, refining the dissection, and augmenting identification of the sentinel nodes (104–110). The radioisotope, most commonly filtered ^{99m}Tc sulfur colloid, was injected intradermally around the melanoma biopsy site at least 1 hour prior to surgery, allowing the sentinel node to concentrate the radioisotope, which was then readily identified using a gamma-probe. Optimally, the radioactive counts in the harvested bed would be <10% of the ex vivo counts of the harvested node(s). Although concordance between radioactive node(s) and blue node(s) was expected, it was argued that persistence of significant radioactivity might then direct the surgeon to additional sentinel node(s) that may not have concentrated the dye.

Successful sentinel node identification has been verified in several large series from numerous centers, most confirming the optimal efficacy of a combined technique with gamma-probe identification complementing the visual identification of blue-stained nodes. Although a blue-stained sentinel node with an afferent blue-stained lymphatic clearly became the standard for positive identification, in a robust axilla or in many areas of the head and neck, tracing blue lymphatic channels could be difficult and was facilitated by the use of radioisotopes. Conversely, where the sentinel node(s) was subjacent or directly adjacent to the primary melanoma site, and "shine through" of radioactivity might have compromised the specificity of radioisotopic identification, the blue dye technique remained essential. Morton and associates (111) have further demonstrated a differential concentration of dye and isotope in a specific segment of a sentinel node using carbon dye as a mapping adjunct, suggesting that these specific agents are indeed trapped in a specific segment of the node, and this segment corresponds to the site of micrometastasis.

Morton and associates (112) also validated that intraoperative lymphatic mapping with sentinel lymphadenectomy can be successfully learned and applied. In a Multicenter Selective Lymphadenectomy Trial Group study, 551 patients accrued from 16 international centers were compared to 584 patients from the organizing group at the John Wayne Cancer Institute. In both groups, blue dye plus radiocolloid was more successful (99.1%) than blue dye alone (95.2%; $p = 0.014$). Most importantly, after a learning phase of 30 cases in which a completion lymph node dissection was performed, an accuracy rate of 93.3% for sentinel node identification was achieved by the participating centers compared with 95.3% for the John Wayne Cancer Institute, with a comparable incidence of nodal metastases after adjusting for risk factors. A review of the reported experience with lymphatic mapping and sentinel lymphadenectomy from ten clinical trials (113) using dye or radioisotopes or a combination, has further confirmed a sentinel node identification rate of 82% to 100%, with micrometastasis detected in 15% to 26% of patients.

It was recognized that a sentinel node evaluated as negative for micrometastatic disease does not abrogate the need for further clinical surveillance of the regional nodal basin from which it has been harvested. The John Wayne Cancer Institute reported a 4.8% incidence of same-basin recurrence at a median follow-up of 45 months (112). However, recurrences were as likely to represent pathologic failure to identify micrometastasis as technical errors leading to a misidentification of the true sentinel node(s) (113,114). As institutional validation of the capability of both the surgical team and the quality of nuclear imaging was evident, the necessity of detailed nodal histopathology became equally apparent.

Histopathology of Regional Lymph Nodes

As early as 1958, Lane and associates (115) demonstrated that the survival rate for patients with melanoma and metastatic nodal involvement was highest for those with a single microscopic focus within a lymph node and that, whereas regional lymph nodes might be pronounced normal after thorough but routine pathologic examination, serial sections of the same nodes often demonstrated the presence of microscopic melanoma. In the study of regional node micrometastases at New York University, trisecting each node and step-sectioning each segment led to a detection of micrometastases in 28% of patients with melanomas 1.0 to 2.0 mm in thickness and in 50% of patients with melanoma >4.0 mm in thickness (18). Although routine hematoxylin and eosin (H&E) staining could identify most nodal micrometastases and was traditionally the basis of assessing trials of elective regional lymphadenectomy, the identification and ability to immunohistochemically stain for melanoma markers significantly added to the sensitivity of detecting nodal disease. The opportunity to study a single sentinel node, compared to an entire regional nodal group, now provided pathologists the means to not only prepare additional sections but to readily apply such advanced staining techniques as well. It is now clearly recognized that failure to serially section and, most importantly, use immunohistochemical staining of sentinel nodes may be responsible for understaging nodal pathology. Gershenwald and associates (114) reported on ten first recurrences in a previously mapped nodal basin from which a sentinel node had been negative by H&E staining from a series of 243 sentinel lymphadenectomies. Re-evaluation by immunohistochemical staining of the sentinel node revealed previously undetected metastases in seven patients.

The optimal immunohistochemical staining technique, or combination of techniques, has not been defined. Immunohistochemical staining with antibody to S-100 protein has demonstrated its presence in primary and metastatic melanoma cells, as well as in normal melanocytes and non-melanocytic cell types, including neurons, pituicytes, Langerhans' cells, dendritic cells, and macrophages. Anti-S-100 antibody staining was first used as an adjunct in the diagnosis of histologically ambiguous primary melanomas, including amelanotic and desmoplastic lesions, and then for diagnosing histopathologically undifferentiated metastatic melanomas, particularly in the absence of a definable primary lesion. Anti-S-100 antibody staining is quite sensitive, with 90% of primary and metastatic lesions being positive, including clinically occult foci of metastatic melanoma in lymph nodes (116,117). Therefore, S100 protein is routinely used as a screening melanocytic marker. Although S100 staining of lymph nodes can detect greater numbers of metastases than H&E alone (29% vs. 10%), as reported by Cochran and associates (117), benign nerve cells within lymph nodes, as well as cells of neuroectodermal origin may be stained as well.

Staining with the monoclonal antibody HMB-45 directed against the protein gp100 present in premelanosomes improves the specificity of identifying metastases. gp100 is present in the functional component of melanocytic nevi and primary and metastatic melanoma cells (118,119). Goscin et al. (120) have indicated, however, that it may have a sensitivity of only 50% for micrometastatic melanoma in lymph nodes. Other investigators have also confirmed that the intensity and uniformity of staining may be variable and inadequate to identify all metastases (121–123). Staining for the antigen Melan-A, a product of the *MART-1* gene and present in melanocytes, may have the advantage of both the specificity of HMB-45 but with greater sensitivity (124,125). A variety of immunohistochemical stains for other markers have been, and are being, investigated. These include tyrosinase, an enzyme required for the hydroxylation of tyrosine as the initial step in melanogenesis (126), microphthalmic transcription factor necessary for the development of melanocytes (127), and NKI/C3, an antibody to the 25-110 kD glycoprotein found in the inner membrane of cytoplasmic vesicles of melanocytes (128). Busam and associates (129) have recently reported on PNL2, a monoclonal antibody that shows immunoreactivity against melanocytes and melanocytic-derived tumors and demonstrated high sensitivity for metastatic melanoma (87%). The sensitivity of PNL2 appears similar to that of HMB-45. However, this marker may prove to be of value for HMB-45–negative cases. The optimal marker or combination of markers identifiable by immunohistochemical staining has not yet been defined.

The traditional argument that even those patients without histologically documented nodal metastases in elective regional lymphadenectomy specimens may, in fact, harbor micrometastases that are undetected by standard pathologic sectioning and H&E staining is supported by the experience since sentinel lymphadenectomy was introduced. Experience with sentinel node histopathology has confirmed the early observations of Cochran and colleagues (130,131), who reported that the rate of detecting micrometastases rose 14% in regional lymph nodes examined by immunohistochemical techniques, as compared with routine staining methods. Spanknebel and associates (132) have reported on the use of immunohistochemical-enhanced pathology in the study of 95 sentinel lymph nodes harvested from 39 patients assessed by H&E, S100 protein, and HMB-45 stains at 50-mcm intervals for 20 levels or until the sentinel lymph node was exhausted. Metastatic melanoma was discovered in nodes from 20 of the 39 patients. No single method detected all the metastases with S100 staining having the highest yield (86%), followed by HMB-45 (81%) and H&E (52%). All 20 levels were required to identify 100% of the micrometastases, 17 levels resulted in the positive identification of 95% of nodes, 15 levels resulted in 90% positive identification, 10 levels in 75%, and 3 levels in 42%. The authors concluded that sentinel node positivity could be increased to 71% by performing three levels of 250-mcm intervals, each level being composed of a set of three sections stained with H&E, S-100 protein, and HMB-45, respectively. Clearly, the refinement of surgical sentinel lymphadenectomy must be matched by meticulous pathologic technique in both sectioning and staining. Nevertheless, the inherent limitations of nodal sectioning and even immunohistochemical staining has led to the application of a reverse transcriptase-polymerase chain reaction (RT-PCR) assay, which allows the amplification and detection of the messenger RNA of melanoma specific markers.

RT-PCR has the capability of detecting submicroscopic disease, even isolated malignant cells, with great sensitivity, and is being studied to even further upstage the identification of nodal metastases (133–135). Reintgen and associates (136) reported on the use of this assay for evaluating the lymph nodes of 29 patients with intermediate-thickness melanoma. Standard pathologic staining was compared with RT-PCR. Eleven (38%) were pathologically positive and 19 (66%) were RT-PCR–positive. In a study by Goydos and associates (137), the sentinel nodes of 50 patients were evaluated after sectioning along their long axes, one half of the node by H&E and immunohistochemical staining "when appropriate" and the other half frozen in liquid nitrogen for RT-PCR. Ten patients had micrometastases detected by routine histopathology, and an additional three patients had micrometastases identified by RT–PCR. The sensitivity of this assay is clearly increased compared to previous techniques.

The prognostic significance of RT–PCR-detected tumor-positive nodes that are otherwise undetectable by other histopathologic techniques has not been defined, and is being assessed in more long-term follow-up. Bostick and associates (138) reported a significant correlation of recurrence from a group of 72 patients, whose sentinel nodes demonstrated expression using a multiple mRNA marker RT–PCR despite being negative by immunohistochemical staining. Morton and associates (111) have demonstrated that the assay may be effectively augmented by the use of carbon identification of potential preferential intranodal sites of metastases as previously cited. Twenty-five of 166 patients (16%) studied had nodal metastases found only in nodal areas containing carbon particles. As carbon particles remained in the nodes, from which dye may have dissipated, they could be readily identified by the pathologist. In 162 patients with negative findings on immunohistochemical staining, 49 (30%) were positive when nodes were re-evaluated by a multimarker RT–PCR assay, and these patients had a significantly higher risk of recurrence and decreased survival than patients who had negative findings by both immunohistochemical staining and the multiple mRNA marker assay. Significant increased recurrence and decreased survival has also been reported by Li and associates (139) for patients with disease detected by RT–PCR but whose sentinel nodes were histologically negative, while contrary data has been presented by Kammula and associates (140) showing no difference in survival for patients with RT–PCR positivity or negativity if the sentinel nodes were histologically negative. Although molecular upstaging of sentinel lymph nodes may provide important information for prognosis, the use of single molecular or varying panels of markers presently makes interpreting the benefits of RT-PCR difficult. As the method for RT-PCR becomes more standardized and specificity improves, this approach to the molecular staging of metastatic melanoma and its impact on prognosis and therapy may become more sensitive and reliable.

Molecular assays of sentinel nodes may allow further stratification of patients who previously would have been considered node-negative into more favorable groups if RT–PCR–negative and higher risk groups if RT–PCR–positive. Clearly, the introduction of lymphatic mapping, sentinel lymphadenectomy, and refinement in the histologic and biochemical detection of nodal micrometastases has recast the issue of the benefits of elective nodal dissection. It has also reinvigorated precepts favoring nodal metastases as initial sites of metastatic disease and potential instigators of further metachronous dissemination.

SENTINEL LYMPHADENECTOMY TRIALS

The development of intraoperative lymphatic mapping and sentinel lymphadenectomy with immunohistochemical staining made clear the inherent flaws in previous trials that had broadly assessed the value of lymph node dissection for all patients, even when stratified by specified thickness. Morton (141) and colleagues at the John Wayne Cancer Institute accordingly organized the Multicenter Selective Lymphadenectomy Trial (MSLT) with other institutions having a documented breadth of experience in the treatment of cutaneous malignant melanoma. Patients with a clinically localized primary cutaneous melanoma with a Breslow thickness of ≥1 mm or Clark level IV or V regardless of Breslow level were randomly assigned to either wide excision and postoperative observation of regional lymph nodes with lymphadenectomy if nodal relapse occurred, or to wide excision and sentinel node biopsy with immediate lymphadenectomy if nodal micrometastases were detected on biopsy. The trial

provided the opportunity to evaluate the efficacy of the elective ablation of nodal micrometastases using lymphatic mapping to determine the nodal sites and specific nodes at greatest risk and selecting only those patients with micrometastases diagnosed by enhanced histopathology of sentinel nodes for complete lymph node dissection. Even before completion of this first prospective trial, sentinel lymphadenectomy had found broad acceptance as a staging procedure, independent of its possible inherent therapeutic value (142).

Enrollment in the MSLT trial was closed in March 2002 after the accrual of over 2,000 patients. In addition to validating the technique and its reproducibility in the centers participating in the trial (143), an interim analysis examined the morbidity and accuracy of lymphatic mapping and sentinel lymphadenectomy for detection of sentinel nodal metastases (144). In 1,191 patients treated with sentinel lymphadenectomy, the rate of sentinel node identification was 95.3%, with a nodal recurrence rate in a tumor-negative dissected nodal basis of 5.2% after an initial case volume of 25 cases had been completed at each center. Morbidity of sentinel lymphadenectomy was predictably low (10.1%), complications increasing to 37.2% with the addition of a completion lymph node dissection. Almost all were related to early wound problems. This analysis further confirmed the accuracy and reproducibility of the technique.

The results from the third interim analysis of the trial were published in September 2006 (145). Among 1,269 patients with an intermediate-thickness primary melanoma (1.2 to 3.5 mm), the mean ($\pm$SE) estimated 5-year disease-free survival rate for the population was 78.3% $\pm$ 1.6% in the biopsy group and 73.1% $\pm$ 2.1% in the observation group (hazard ratio for death, 0.74; 95% confidence interval [CI]: 0.59$^-$0.93; $p = 0.009$). Five-year melanoma-specific survival rates were similar in the two groups (87.1% $\pm$ 1.3% and 86.6% $\pm$ 1.6%, respectively). In the biopsy group, the presence of metastases in the sentinel node was the most important prognostic factor; the 5-year survival rate was 72.3% $\pm$ 4.6% among patients with tumor-positive sentinel nodes and 90.2% $\pm$ 1.3% among those with tumor-negative sentinel nodes (hazard ratio for death, 2.48; 95% CI: 1.54-3.98; p <0.001). The incidence of sentinel node micrometastases was 16.0% (122 of 764 patients), and the rate of nodal relapse in the observation group was 15.6% (78 of 500 patients). The corresponding mean number of tumor-involved nodes was 1.4 in the biopsy group and 3.3 in the observation group (p <0.001), indicating disease progression during observation. Among patients with nodal metastases, the 5-year survival rate was higher among those who underwent immediate lymphadenectomy than among those in whom lymphadenectomy was delayed (72.3% $\pm$ 4.6% vs. 52.4% $\pm$ 5.9%; hazard ratio for death, 0.51; 95% CI: 0.32-0.81; $p = 0.004$).

Sentinel lymphadenectomy has become a standard of practice in the surgical management of primary cutaneous melanoma. Discussion has now focused on the indications for the procedure based on tumor thickness, location, and patient age among other clinical and histopathologic variables. Of these, tumor thickness has particular significance because, while the risk of metastases is predictably low for lesions <1.0 mm in thickness, an ever-increasing majority of patients are diagnosed with melanomas in this thickness range. Reported rates of nodal metastases for lesions <1.0 mm is no greater than 7% and no greater than 3% for lesions <0.75 mm (146–149). However, the increasing sensitivity of detecting sentinel nodal metastases coupled with the low morbidity of the procedure may well lower the threshold of indications based on thickness.

Another compelling issue is the appropriateness of completion regional lymphadenectomy for those patients demonstrated to have a sentinel nodal metastasis. It has been well established that the great majority of patients with a sentinel nodal micrometastasis will have no additional regional nodal metastases in nonsentinel lymph nodes in the completion nodal dissection specimen (150–157). Although the value of many series is limited by the routine histologic assessment of nonsentinel nodes compared with the detailed immunohistochemical assessment of sentinel nodes, the low yield of additional nonsentinel node metastases supports the hypothesis that sentinel nodes may concentrate and limit the further lymphatic dissemination of melanoma. In this sense, they may be true sentinels or guardians. Indeed, the combination of primary tumor thickness and the extent of microscopic sentinel node metastases may increasingly be viewed as indicators of possible additional nodal involvement. Morton and associates (111) demonstrated that metastases from melanomas of 1.01 to 2.00 mm in thickness were more likely to only be in the sentinel nodes, whereas thicker lesions ≥2.01 mm were more likely to involve additional lymph nodes as well as metastasize to distant sites. Cochran and associates (158,159) have further suggested that the tumor area relative to the nodal area may provide a particularly strong indicator of the likelihood of nonsentinel nodal metastases. They noted that 65.4% of patients in whom metastatic melanoma occupied >4% of the sentinel node had nonsentinel nodal metastases compared with 3.1% in whom the tumor occupied <4% of the sentinel node.

Observations on tumor thickness and nodal metastatic burden may be viewed as supporting a temporal relationship whereby a sentinel node concentrates tumor cells for a time, before further growth and more widespread dissemination (111). Certainly, limiting surgery to sentinel lymphadenectomy alone for a majority of patients with a demonstrated micrometastasis would even more fully realize the potential of the procedure to optimize any prognostic and therapeutic advantage, while further limiting the morbidity of a complete regional node dissection. Trials have been initiated to assess this issue. A Multicenter Sunbelt Melanoma Trial randomizes patients with melanoma of at least 1.0 mm in thickness, in whom sentinel lymph nodes were negative by immunohistochemical staining but positive on RT-PCR, to undergo either observation, completion lymph node dissection, or completion lymph node dissection with adjuvant interferon-α-2b therapy. A second Multicenter Selection Lymphadenectomy Trial (MSLT-II) randomizes patients with proven sentinel nodal metastases to either completion regional nodal dissection or observation.

SENTINEL LYMPHADENECTOMY IN THE ASSESSMENT OF PROGNOSIS AND ADJUVANT THERAPY

The prognostic assessment of a primary cutaneous malignant melanoma has been more precisely defined than any other solid malignant neoplasm. Tumor thickness and ulceration are

well established as the most significant variables in this regard. Within any thickness range, the presence or absence of regional lymph node metastases becomes an even more powerful predictor (160). A report from the Stanford University Medical Center on their experience with sentinel lymphadenectomy over a 7-year period demonstrated a 46% recurrence rate for patients having sentinel nodal metastases compared with 14% for those without (p <0.001) (161). Recurrence rates were more significant for tumors >2 mm in thickness with 53% having sentinel nodal metastases recurring compared with 24% if sentinel nodes were negative. The Sydney Melanoma Unit (162) also reported a 5-year survival rate of 56% for patients who were sentinel node-positive compared with 90% for patients who were sentinel node-negative. Several other studies have confirmed the dominance of lymph node status independent of tumor thickness and ulceration, and among patients with thick melanomas (163–171). Although the prognostic assessment by histologic examination of lymph nodes has been advanced as a major reason to perform elective regional lymphadenectomies, the increased pathologic sensitivity and decreased morbidity of sentinel lymphadenectomy have provided a more compelling incentive to stage the regional nodal basin. Furthermore the prognostic variability for patients with nodal metastases can be more specifically defined.

In an analysis of the prognostic impact of clinical versus pathologic nodal staging among 5,345 patients in the American Joint Committee on Cancer database, Balch et al. (169) reported that patients with clinically evident nodal disease (N+) had diminished 5-year survival rates compared with patients initially clinically staged as having no evidence of nodal metastases (N–) but who were subsequently staged pathologically positive after either sentinel node biopsy or elective regional node dissection. These survival differences were statistically significant among all T substages except T4b (>4.0 mm with ulceration) (Table 24.2). In addition, a 5-year survival rate of 69% was noted for those with only one sentinel node with a micrometastasis and a non-ulcerated melanoma compared to 13% for those having an ulcerated melanoma, palpable nodal disease and more than three nodes with histologic metastases (168,169).

Whether sentinel lymphadenectomy is appropriate for patients with thin melanomas (≤1.0 mm), and certainly stage 1A (≤0.75 mm), is controversial and at the present time unresolved in view of the low rate of nodal metastases (172). The status of the sentinel lymph node has clearly emerged as an essential prognostic variable for almost all patients without palpable nodal disease. Reports of large experiences from both the M.D. Anderson Cancer Center and the Moffitt Cancer Center have confirmed the presence or absence of sentinel node metastases to be the most dominant prognostic indicator for both disease-free and disease-specific survival (109). As a result, sentinel lymph node pathology has become essential for defining patients at high risk of recurrence and to structure trials for evaluating the efficacy of systemic adjuvant strategies.

Efforts to alter the progression of disease for high-risk patients with adjuvant systemic therapies have been ongoing for more than 3 decades, involving a variety of chemotherapeutic and immunotherapeutic approaches. The earliest efforts showing the promise of prolonging survival used a nonspecific immunostimulant, *Bacillus Calmette-Guérin* (BCG). A survival advantage was not sustained when randomized trials were

Table 24.2

Clinical vs. Pathologic Nodal Staging. Five-Year Survival Rates of Patients with Clinically Negative (N-) Nodal Metastases who were Pathologically Staged After Regional Lymph Node Dissection or Sentinel Lymphadenectomy Compared to Patients with Clinically Positive Nodes (N+)

T stage	Path Nodes (N)	5-Year, Survival % ± S.E.	P-value*
T1a	N − (n = 379)	94 ± 2.0	0.0035
	N + (n = 15)	64 ± 17.7	
T1b	N − (n = 319)	90 ± 2.5	0.0039
	N + (n = 18)	76 ± 14.9	
T2a	N − (n = 1480)	94 ± 0.8	<0.0001
	N + (n = 150)	73 ± 5.6	
T2b	N − (n = 408)	83 ± 2.3	<0.0001
	N + (n = 62)	56 ± 8.8	
T3a	N − (n = 808)	86 ± 1.6	<0.0001
	N + (n = 177)	59 ± 6.0	
T3b	N − (n = 639)	72 ± 2.1	<0.0001
	N + (n = 176)	49 ± 4.5	
T4a	N − (n = 203)	75 ± 3.9	0.0116
	N + (n = 66)	61 ± 7.4	
T4b	N − (n = 330)	53 ± 3.1	0.2403
	N + (n = 116)	44 ± 5.5	

*The p-value based on the comparison of survival curves using the log rank test.
Adapted from Balch, et al. (169)

conducted (173), an experience that was repeated with levamisole (174,175) and transfer factor (176). Results with *Corynebacterium parvum*, when compared with BCG in patients with resected regional node metastases, showed a prolongation in disease-free interval, although a statistically significant improvement in survival could not be demonstrated (177). Likewise, randomized adjuvant chemotherapy trials using single agents, most commonly dacarbazine, as well as combination or chemoimmunotherapy regimens, have failed to demonstrate a benefit in high-risk patients to date (178,179). Nonspecific active immunotherapeutic treatments have given way to efforts at active specific immunotherapy, most commonly with a variety of vaccines using irradiated melanoma cells, shed antigens from melanoma cells maintained in cell culture, peptides, gangliosides, or cell lysates, as well as autologous and allogeneic whole cells often in conjunction with other immunologic adjuvants as well as dendritic cells, initially evaluated in patients with systemic disease (180–187). Data from randomized trials to date in node-positive patients have failed to demonstrate an improvement in survival (188–192). In a trial reported by Sondak and associates (193) (SW06-9035) using an allogeneic melanoma cell lysate vaccine, a subset of patients positive for human leukemic antigen (HLA-A2 and/or HLA-C3) had a significant 5-year survival benefit of 93% in the treatment group

compared with 74% for patients in the nontreatment group ($p = 0.009$), although overall survival for treated or nontreated patients showed no statistical difference in survival. A study based on HLA-A2 or HLA-C3 has been proposed.

Initial trials using interferon-α in patients with advanced melanoma have demonstrated partial or complete responses in approximately 15% to 20% (194). In keeping with other immunotherapy regimens, patients free of disease but at high risk of recurrence have been the focus of efforts to improve survival using interferon-α. The Eastern Cooperative Oncology Group (ECOG) conducted a randomized, controlled study (Trial 1684) of 1 year of high-dose interferon-α-2b ($n = 143$) versus observation ($n = 137$), which generated great interest. As reported by Kirkwood and associates (195), a statistically significant prolongation of relapse-free and overall survival for treated patients was observed. At 5 years, the estimated survival in the treated group was 46%, compared with 37% in the untreated group. The survival benefit was greatest in node-positive patients. Hepatoxicity was noted, with two patients dying of this complication early in the study. A WHO study of 444 patients, with resected node-positive patients randomized to receive low-dose interferon-α-2a versus observation, failed to demonstrate an advantage in disease-free or overall survival (196). Other studies of interferon-α-2a (179–182), using different dosages and schedules, also failed to show a statistically significant advantage in disease-free or overall survival (197–199). A confirmatory trial by ECOG (1690), which also assessed possibly less toxic doses of interferon, failed to show a survival improvement for high-dose or low-dose interferon compared with the untreated patients (200–201). In an updated analysis, however, a trend toward recurrence-free survival was reported for the high-dose interferon group (202). The Sunbelt Melanoma Trial randomizes patients with melanomas ≥ 1.0 mm thick and histologically negative but RT-PCR–positive sentinel lymph nodes to observation or completion lymph node dissection. For patients with histologically positive sentinel node(s), a completion lymph node dissection is performed. If found to have no additional positive nodes, they are randomly assigned to observation and 1 month of high-dose adjuvant interferon-α followed by 1 year of subcutaneous injections. If there are additional positive nodes or extracapsular extension of the single positive node, they all receive adjuvant interferon.

Although effective adjuvant therapy for high-risk melanoma patients continues to elude investigators, it is also clear that sentinel lymphadenectomy has become an essential means of stratifying ongoing and future trials, providing vital prognostic information with limited morbidity. Efforts to reproducibly enlist the ability of the immune system to destroy melanoma cells have been elusive, but the study of sentinel nodal metastases may further enhance our understanding of the mechanisms of immune recognition and reactivity. This may prove to be the greatest benefit of sentinel lymphadenectomy.

CONCLUSION

Sentinel lymphadenectomy requires not only refined techniques in surgery, but in nuclear imaging and histopathology as well. Sentinel lymphadenectomy has clearly been adopted with an enthusiasm not dissimilar to that of elective lymph node dissection a century earlier. This procedure has dramatically altered the surgical approach to malignant melanoma, and evidence is emerging that ablating micrometastases has a salutary impact on the natural history of the disease. The study of this issue continues with approaches of far greater sensitivity and specificity than previously.

Sentinel node identification is a reproducible and validated technique. It would appear that, with some exceptions, the performance of an elective lymph node dissection without a properly performed sentinel lymphadenectomy to confirm the presence of regional nodal micrometastases is no longer appropriate. Indeed, whether completion regional node dissection is required for all patients with proven sentinel node metastases remains to be tested. Conversely, it has even been provocatively suggested that protein resonance spectroscopy of nodal fine-needle aspiration biopsy samples might replace surgical sentinel node biopsy in the future (203).

One hundred years after Handley (6) embraced lymphatic permeation as the basis for the surgical treatment of malignant melanoma, it is sobering and challenging to consider that despite a century of progress toward understanding the biology, improving the diagnostic accuracy, and refining the prognostic assessment of malignant melanomas, the pathophysiology of lymph node metastases remains to be elucidated. However, we may be on the threshold of understanding host-tumor interaction within the specific nodal site targeted by a primary melanoma and even the molecular characteristics of a micrometastasis that might allow further proliferation at systemic sites. Genetic profiling of primary melanomas and nodal metastases may well improve our understanding of the progression of metastatic disease and certainly direct the application and even the development of unique biologic treatments (204,205). For now, an ever more precise identification of nodal tumor pathology should guide the need for further surgery and, far more importantly, the use and evaluation of adjuvant systemic therapies.

REFERENCES

1. McCarthy WH, Shaw HM, Cascinelli N, et al. Elective lymph node dissection for melanoma: two perspectives. *World J Surg.* 1992;16:203–213.
2. Surveillance, Epidemiology and End Results (SEER) Program. Public-use data (1973-2000), National Cancer Institute, DC-CPS, Surveillance Research Program, Cancer Statistics Branch. Released April 2004. Based on the November 2003 submission. http://www.seer.cancer.gov/publicdata. Accessed in 2006.
3. Virchow R. *Cellular Pathology.* Chance F, trans. London: J. Churchill; 1860:187.
4. Snow HL. Melanotic cancerous disease. *Lancet.* 1892;2:872–874.
5. Eve F. A lecture on melanoma. *The Practitioner.* 1903;70:165–174.
6. Handley WS. The pathology of melanotic growths in relation to their operative treatment: lectures I & II. *Lancet.* 1907; 1:927–35, 996–1003.
7. Pringle JH. A method of operation in cases of melanotic tumours of the skin. *Edinburgh Med J.* 1908.
8. Gray, JH. The relationship of lymphatic vessels to the spread of cancer. *Br J Surg.* 1938, 2b; 462–495.
9. Engell, HC. Cancer cells in the circulating blood. *Acta Chir Scand Suppl.* 1955;201:1–79.
10. Fister, B, Fisher, ER. The interrelationship of hematogenous and lymphatic tumor cell dissemination. *Surg Gynecol Obstet* 1966; 122:791.
11. Edwards JM, Kinmouth JB. Lymphovenous shunts in man. *British Med J* 1969;4:579–584.
12. Weiss L. Site-associated differences in cancer cell populations. *Clin Exp Metastasis.* 1991;9:193–197.
13. Clark WH, From L, Bernardino EH, Mihm MC. The histogenesis and biologic behavior of primary human malignant melanomas of the skin. *Cancer Res* 1969;29:705–727.
14. Breslow A. Thickness, cross-sectional areas, and depth of invasion in the prognosis of cutaneous melanoma. *Ann Surg.* 1970;172: 902–908.
15. Balch CM, Soong SJ, Murad TM, et al. A multifactorial analysis of melanoma. II: Prognostic factors in patients with stage I (localized) melanoma. *Ann Surg.* 1979;86:343–351.
16. Balch CM, Soong SJ, Milton GW, et al. A comparison of prognostic factors and surgical results in 1,786 patients with localized (stage I) melanoma treated in Alabama, USA, and New South Wales, Australia. *Ann Surg.* 1982;196:677–684.
17. Balch CM, Milton GW, Cascinelli N, Sim FH. Elective lymph node dissection: pros and cons. In: Balch CM, Houghton AN, Milton GW, et al., eds. *Cutaneous melanoma,* 2nd ed. Philadelphia: JB Lippincott, 1992;345–366.
18. Roses DF, Harris MN, Hidalgo D, et al. Correlation of the thickness of melanoma and regional lymph node metastases. *Arch Surg.* 1982;117:921–925.
19. Balch CM, Murad TM, Soong S, et al. Tumor thickness as a guide to surgical management of clinical stage I melanoma patients. *Cancer.* 1979;43:883–888.
20. Essner R, Morton DL. Elective lymph node dissection. In: Lejeune FJ, Chaudhar AK, DasGupta TK, eds. *Malignant melanoma.* New York: McGraw-Hill, Inc., 1994;207.
21. Polk HC Jr, Bland KI. Routine elective lymph node dissection in melanoma: unnecessary treatment? In: O'Connell TX, ed. *Surgical oncology: controversies in cancer treatment.* Boston: GK Hall, 1981;122–136.
22. McCarthy JG, Haagenson CD, Herter FP. The role of groin dissection in the management of melanoma of the lower extremity. *Ann Surg.* 1972;179:156–159.
23. Urist MM, Maddox WA, Kennedy JE, et al. Patient risk factors and surgical morbidity after regional lymphadenectomy in 204 melanoma patients. *Cancer.* 1983;51:2152–156.
24. Ingvar C, Erichsen C, Johnsson P. Morbidity following prophylactic and therapeutic lymph node dissection: a comparison. *Tumori.* 1984;70:529–533.
25. Bowsher WG, Taylor BA, Hughes LE. Morbidity, mortality, and local recurrence following regional node dissection for melanoma. *Br J Surg.* 1986;73:906–908.
26. Holmes EC, Moseley HS, Morton DL, et al. A rational approach to the surgical management of melanomav. *Ann Surg.* 1977;186:481–490.
27. Karakousis CP, Goumas W, Rao U, Driscoll DI. Axillary node dissection in malignant melanoma. *Am J Surg.* 1991;162:202–207.
28. Gumport SL, Harris MN. Results of regional lymph node dissection for melanoma. *Ann Surg.* 1974;179:105–108.
29. Coit DG, Brennan MF. Extent of lymph node dissection in melanoma of the trunk or lower extremity. *Arch Surg.* 1989;124: 162–166.
30. Baas PC, Koops HS, Hoekstra JH, et al. Groin dissection in the treatment of lower extremity melanoma, short-term and long-term morbidity. *Arch Surg.* 1992;127:281–286.
31. Finck SJ, Giuliano AE, Mann BD, Morton DL. Results of ilioinguinal dissection for stage II melanoma. *Ann Surg.* 1982;196:180–186.

32. Karakousis CP, Heiser MA, Moore RH. Lymphedema after groin dissection. *Am J Surg.* 1983;145:205–208.

33. Karakousis CP, Driscoll DL, Rose B, et al. Groin dissection in malignant melanoma. *Ann Surg Oncol.* 1994;1:271–277.

34. Shaw JHF, Rumball EM, Complications and local recurrence following lymphadenectomy. *Br J Surg.* 1990;77:760–764.

35. Shaw JH, Koea J. Morbidity of lymphadenectomy for melanoma. *Surg Oncol Clin North Am.* 1992;1(2):195–203.

36. Coit DG, Peters M, Brennan MF. A prospective randomized trial of perioperative Cefazolin treatment in axillary and groin dissection. *Arch Surg.* 1991;126:1366–1369.

37. Silberman AW. Malignant melanoma: practical considerations concerning regional lymph node dissection. *Ann Surg.* 1987;206:206–209.

38. Karakousis CP, Emrich LJ, Rao U. Groin dissection in malignant melanoma. *Am J Surg.* 1985;152:491–495.

39. Harris MN, Gump SL, Berman IR, et al. Ilio-inguinal lymph node dissection for melanoma. *Surg Gynecol Obstet.* 1973;136:33–39.

40. Karakousis, CP. The technique of popliteal lymph node dissection. *Surg Gynecol Obstet.* 1980;181:420–423.

41. Pack GT, Gerber DM, Scharnagel IM. End results in the treatment of malignant melanoma. A report of 1190 cases. *Ann Surg.* 1952;136:905–911.

42. Balch CM, Soong S, Murad TM, et al. Multifactorial analysis of melanoma. III: prognostic factors in patients with regional lymph node metastases (stage II). *Ann Surg.* 1981;193:377–388.

43. McNeer G, Das Gupta TK. Prognosis in malignant melanoma. *Surgery.* 1964;56:512–518.

44. Cohen MH, Ketcham AS, Felix EL, et al. Prognostic factors in patients undergoing lymphadenectomy for malignant melanoma. *Ann Surg.* 1977;186:635–642.

45. Das Gupta TK. Results of treatment of 269 patients with primary cutaneous melanoma: a five-year prospective study. *Ann Surg.* 1977;186:201–209.

46. Callery C, Cochran AJ, Roe DJ, et al. Factors prognostic for survival in patients with malignant melanoma spread in the regional lymph nodes. *Ann Surg.* 1982;196:69–75.

47. Roses DF, Provet JA Harris MN, Gumport SL, Dubin N. Prognosis of patients with pathologic stage II cutaneous malignant melanoma. *Ann Surg.* 1985;201:103–107.

48. Wanebo JH Fortner JG, Woodruff J, et al. Selection of the optimum surgical treatment of stage I melanoma by depth of microinvasion: use of the combined microstage technique (Clark-Breslow). *Ann Surg.* 1975;182:302–315.

49. Balch CM, Murad TQ, Soong S, et al. Tumor thickness as a guide to surgical management of clinical stage I melanoma patients. *Cancer.* 1979;43:883–888.

50. Milton GW, Shaw HM, McCarthy WH, et al. Prophylactic lymph node dissection in clinical stage I cutaneous melanoma: results of surgical treatment in 1319 patients. *Br J Surg.* 1982;69:108–111.

51. McCarthy WH, Shaw HM, Milton GW. Efficacy of elective lymph node dissection in 2,347 patients with clinical stage I malignant melanoma. *Surg Gynecol Obstet.* 1985;161:575–580.

52. Biess B, Broker EB, Drepper H, et al. Should elective lymph node dissection be used for treatment of primary melanoma? *J Cancer Res Clin Oncol.* 1989;115:470–473.

53. Reintgen DC, Cox EB, McCarty KS, et al. Efficacy of elective lymph node dissection in patients with intermediate thickness primary melanoma. *Ann Surg.* 1983;198:379–385.

54. Singluff EL, Stidham KR, Ricci WM, et al. Surgical management of regional lymph nodes in patients with melanoma. Experience with 4,682 patients. *Ann Surg.* 1994;219:120–130.

55. Coates AS, Ingvar CI, Petersen-Schaefer K, et al. Elective lymph node dissection in patients with primary melanoma of the trunk and limbs treated at the Sydney Melanoma Unit from 1960 to 1991. *J Am Coll Surg.* 1995;180:402–409.

56. Day CL, Sober SJ, Lew RA, et al. Malignant melanoma patients with positive nodes and relatively good prognosis: microstaging retains prognostic significance in clinical stage I patients with metastases to regional nodes. *Cancer.* 1981;47:955–962.

57. Slingluff CL, Vollmer R, Seigler HF. Stage II malignant melanoma: presentation of a prognostic model and an assessment of specific active immunotherapy in 1273 patients. *Surg Oncol.* 1988;39:139–147.

58. Balch CM, Soong SJ, Murad TM, et al. A multifactorial analysis of melanoma. III. Prognostic factors in patients with lymph node metastases (stage II). *Ann Surg.* 1981;193:377–385.

59. Morton DL, Wanek L, Nizze JA, et al. Improved long-term survival after lymphadenectomy of melanoma metastatic to regional nodes; analysis of prognostic factors in 1134 patients from the John Wayne Cancer Clinic. *Ann Surg.* 1991;214:491–499.

60. Drepper H, Kohler CO, Bastian B, et al. Benefit of elective lymph node dissection in subgroups of melanoma patients. *Cancer.* 1993;72:741–749.

61. Elder DE, Guerry D, VanHorn M, et al. The role of lymph node dissection for clinical stage I malignant melanoma of intermediate thickness (1.51-3.99 mm). *Cancer.* 1985;56:413–418.

62. Binder M, Pehamberger H, Steiner A, et al.Elective regional node dissection in malignant melanoma. *Eur J Cancer.* 1990;26:871–873.

63. Bagley FH, Cady B, Lee A, et al. Changes in clinical presentation and management of malignant melanoma. *Cancer.* 1981;47:2126–2134.

64. Crowley NJ. The case against elective lymphadenectomy. *Surg Oncol Clin North Am.* 1992;1(2):223–246.

65. Roses DF, Harris MN, Grunberger I, et al. Selective surgical management of cutaneous melanoma of the head and neck. *Ann Surg.* 1980;192:629–632.

66. Belli F, Nova M, Santinami M, et al. Management of nodal metastases from head and neck melanoma. *J Surg Oncol.* 1989;42:47–53.

67. O'Brien CJ, Gianoutsos MP, Morgan MJ. Neck dissection for cutaneous malignant melanoma. *World J Surg.* 1992;16:222–226.

68. Sim FH, Taylor WF, Ivins JC, et al. A prospective randomized study of the efficacy of routine prophylactic lymphadenectomy in management of malignant melanoma: preliminary results. *Cancer.* 1978;41:946–956.

69. Veronesi U, Adamus J, Bandierra DC, et al. Inefficacy of immediate node dissection on stage I melanoma of the limbs. *N Engl J Med.* 1977;297:627–630.

70. Veronesi U, Adamus J, Bandiera DC, et al. Delayed regional lymph node dissection in stage I melanoma of the skin of the lower extremities. *Cancer.* 1982;49:2420.

71. Veronesi U, Adamus J, Bandiera DC, et al. Stage I melanoma of the limbs: Immediate versus delayed node dissection. *Tumori.* 1980;66:373.

72. Cascinelli N, Santinami M, Belli I. The case against elective lymph node dissection. *World J Surg.* 1992;16:206–213.

73. Cascinelli N. The role of clinical trials in assessing optimal treatment of cutaneous melanoma not extending beyond the regional nodes. *Eur J Surg Oncol.* 1996;22:123–135.

74. Cascinelli N, Morabito A, Santinami M, et al. Immediate or delayed dissection of regional nodes in patients with melanoma of the trunk: a randomized trial. *Lancet.* 1998;351:783–796.

75. Balch CM, Cascinelli N, Sim FH, et al. Elective lymph node dissection: results of prospective randomized surgical trials. In: Balch CM et al., eds. *Cutaneous melanoma,* 3rd ed. St Louis, MO: Quality Medical Publishing Inc., 1998;209–225.

76. Cascinelli N, Morabito A, Santinami M, MacKie RM, Belli F. Immediate or delayed dissection of regional lymph nodes in patients with melanoma of the trunk. *Lancet.* 1998;351:793–796.

77. Balch CM, Soong S-J, Bertolucci AA, et al. Efficacy of an elective regional lymph node dissection of 1.0 to 4.0 mm-thick melanomas for patients 60 years of age and younger. *Ann Surg.* 1996;224:255–266.

78. Balch CM, Soong S-H, Ross MI, et al. Long-term results of a multi-institutional randomized trial comparing prognostic factors and surgical results for intermediate thickness melanomas (1.0 to 4.0 mm). *Ann Surg Oncol.* 2000;7:87–97.

79. Balch C. Randomized surgical trials involving elective node dissection for melanoma. *Advances in Surgery.* 1999;32:255–270.

80. Sappey MPC. *Injection preparation et conservation des vaisseaux lymphatiques.* Thèse pour le doctorate en medecine, N. 241. Paris Rignoux Imprimeur de la faculte de Medecine, Paris, 1843.

81. Sappey MPC. *Anatomie, Physiologie, Pathologie des Vaisseux Lymphotiques Consideres Chez L'Home et les Vertebres.* Paris: A. DeLahaye and E. Lecrosnier; 1874.

82. Sherman A, Ter-Pogossian M. Lymph node concentration of radioactive colloid gold following interstitial injection. *Cancer.* 1953;6:1238–1240.

83. Fee HJ, Robinson DS, Sample WF, Graham LS, Holmes EC, Morton DL. The determination of lymph shed by colloidal gold scanning patients with malignant melanoma: a preliminary study. *Surgery.* 1978;84:626–632.

84. Sullivan DC, Croker BP Jr, Harris CC, Deery P, Seigler HF. Lymphoscintigraphy in malignant melanoma: ^{99m}Tc-antinomy sulfur colloid. *Am J Roentgenol.* 1981;137:847–851.

85. Lamki LM, Haynie TP, Balch CM, et al. Lymphoscintigraphy in the surgical management of patients with truncal melanoma: comparison of Tc human serum albumin (abstract). *J Nucl Med.* 1989;30:844.

86. Norman J, Cruse CW, Espinosa C, et al. Redefinition of cutaneous lymphatic drainage with the use of lymphoscintigraphy for malignant melanoma. *Am J Surg.* 1991;162:432–437.

87. Lamki LM, Logic JR. Defining lymphatic drainage patterns with cutaneous lymphoscintigraphy. In Balch CM, Houghton AN, Milton GW, et al. eds. *Cutaneous melanoma,* 2nd ed. Philadelphia: JB Lippincott, 1992;367–375.

88. Reintgen DS, Cruse CW, Wells K, et al. The orderly progression of melanoma nodal metastases. *Ann Surg.* 1994;220:759–767.

89. Wanebo HJ, Harpole D, Teates CD. Radionuclide lymphoscintigraphy with technetium ^{99m} antimony sulfide colloid to identify lymphatic drainage of cutaneous melanoma at ambiguous sites in the head and neck and trunk. *Cancer.* 1985;55:1403–1413.

90. Uren RF, Howman-Giles RB, Shaw HM, et al. Lymphoscintigraphy in high risk melanoma of the trunk: predicting draining node groups, defining lymphatic channels, and locating the sentinel node. *J Nucl Med.* 1993;34:1435–1440.

91. Berman DG, Norman J, Cruse CW, et al. Lymphoscintigraphy in malignant melanoma. *Ann Plast Surg.* 1992;28L:29–32.

92. Berger DH, Feig B, Podoloff D, et al. Lymphoscintigraphy as a predictor of lymphatic drainage from cutaneous melanoma. *Ann Surg Oncol.* 1997;4:247–251.

93. Wells RE, Cruse CW, Daniels S, et al. The use of lymphoscintigraphy in melanoma of the head and neck. *Plast Reconstr Surg.* 1994;93:757–761.

94. O'Brien CJ, Uren RF, Thompson JF, et al. Prediction of potential metastatic sites in cutaneous head and neck melanoma using lymphoscintigraphy. *Am J Surg.* 1995;170:461–466.

95. Reintgen DS, Rapaport DP, Tanabe K, et al. Lymphatic mapping and sentinel lymphadenectomy. In Balch CM et al., eds. *Cutaneous melanoma.* St Louis, MO: Quality Medical Publishing Inc., 1998;227–244.

96. Thompson JF, Uren RF, Shaw HM, et al. Location of sentinel lymph nodes in patients with cutaneous melanoma; new insights into lymphatic anatomy. *J Am Coll Surg.* 1999;189:195–206.

97. Sumner WE, Ross MI, Mansfield PF, et al. Implications of lymphatic drainage to unusual sentinel lymph node sites in patients with primary cutaneous melanoma. *Cancer.* 2002;95:354–360.

98. DeWilt J, Thompson JF, Uren RF, et al. Correlation between preoperative lymphoscintigraphy and metastatic nodal disease sites in 362 patients with cutaneous melanomas of the head and neck. *Ann Surg.* 2004;239:544–552.

99. Kinmonth JB. *The Lymphatics: Diseases, Lymphography, and Surgery.* Baltimore: Williams & Wilkins; 1972.

100. Wong JH, Cagle LH, Morton DL. Lymphatic drainage of skin to a sentinel lymph node in a feline model. *Ann Surg.* 1991;214:637–641.

101. Morton DL, Wen D-R, Wong JH, et al. Technical details of intraoperative lymphatic mapping for early stage melanoma. *Arch Surg.* 1992;127:392–399.

102. Alex JC, Weaver DL, Fairbank JJ, et al. Gamma-probe-guided lymph node localization in malignant melanoma. *Surg Oncol.* 1993;2:303–308.

103. Krag DN, Meijer ST, Weaver DL, et al. Minimal-access surgery for staging of malignant melanoma. *Arch Surg.* 1995;130:654–658.

104. Albertini JJ, Cruse CW, Rapaport D, et al. Intraoperative radiolymphoscintigraphy improves sentinel lymph node identification for patients with melanoma. *Ann Surg.* 1996;223:217–224.

105. Leong SP, Steinmetz I, Habib FA, et al. Optimal selective sentinel lymph node dissection in primary malignant melanoma. *Arch Surg.* 1997;132:666–673.

106. Thompson JF, McCarthy WH, Bosch CM, et al. Sentinel lymph node status as an indicator of the presence of metastatic melanoma in regional lymph nodes. *Melanoma Res.* 1995;5:255–260.

107. Lingam MK, Mackie RM, McKay AJ. Intraoperative identification of sentinel lymph node in patients with malignant melanoma. *Br J Cancer.* 1997;75:1505–1508.

108. Bostick P, Essner R, Glass E, et al. Comparison of blue dye and probe-assisted intraoperative lymphatic mapping in melanoma to identify sentinel nodes in 100 lymphatic basins. *Arch Surg.* 1999;134:43–49.

109. Gershenwald JE, Thompson W, Mansfield PF, et al. Multi-institutional melanoma lymphatic mapping experience: the prognostic value of sentinel lymph node status in 612 stage I or II melanoma patients. *J Clin Oncol.* 1999;17:976–983.

110. Haddad FF, Costello D, Reintgen DS. Radio guided surgery for melanoma. *Surg Onc Cl N Amer.* 1999;8:413–426.

111. Morton DL, Hoon DSB, Cochran AJ, et al. Lymphatic mapping and sentinel lymphadenectomy for early-stage melanoma: therapeutic utility and implications of nodal microanatomy and molecular staging for improving the accuracy of detection of nodal micrometastases. *Ann Surg.* 2003;238:538–550.

112. Morton DL, Thompson JF, Essner R, et al. Validation of the accuracy of intraoperative lymphatic mapping and sentinel lymphadenectomy for early stage melanoma: a multicenter trial. *Ann Surg.* 1999;23:453–465.

113. Morton DL, Chan AD. Current status of intraoperative lymphatic mapping and sentinel lymphadenectomy for melanoma: is it standard of care? *J Am Coll Surg.* 1999;189:214–223.

114. Gershenwald JE, Colome MI, Lee JE, et al. Patterns of recurrence following a negative sentinel lymph node biopsy in 243 patients with stage I or II melanoma. *J Clin Oncol.* 1998;16:2253–2260.

115. Lane N, Lattes R, Malm J. Clinico-pathological correlation in a series of 117 malignant melanomas of the skin of adults. *Cancer.* 1958;11:1025–1043.

116. Ordonez NG, Ji XL, Hickey RC. Comparison of HMB-45 monoclonal antibody and S-100 protein in the immunohistochemical diagnosis of melanoma. *Am J Clin Pathol.* 1988;12:612–618.

117. Cochran AJ, Lu HF, Li PX, et al. S-100 protein remains a practical marker for melanocytic and other tumours. *Melanoma Res.* 1993;3:325–330.

118. Wick MR, Swanson PE. Recognition of malignant melanoma by monoclonal antibody HMB-45: an immunohistochemical study of 200 paraffin-embedded cutaneous tumors. *J Cutan Pathol.* 1988;15:201–207.

119. Fernando SS, Johnson S, Bate J. Immunohistochemical analysis of cutaneous malignant melanoma: comparison of S-100 protein, HMB-45 monoclonal antibody and NKI/C3 monoclonal antibody. *Pathology.* 1994;26:16–19.

120. Goscin C, Glass F, Messina JL. Pathologic examination of the sentinel lymph node in melanoma. *Surg Oncol Clin North Am.* 1999;8:427–434.

121. Clarkson KS, Surdgess I, Molyneux A. The usefulness of tyrosinase in the immunohistochemical assessment of melanocytic lesions: a comparison of the novel T311 antibody (antityrosinase) with S-100, HMB-45, and A103 (anti-melan-A). *J Clin Pathol.* 2001;54:196–200.

122. Cochran AJ, Essner R, Rose D, Glass E. Principles of sentinel lymph node identification: background and clinical implications. *Langenbecks Arch Surg.* 2000;385:252–260.

123. Mahmood MN, Lee MW, Linden MD, Nathanson SD, Hornyak TJ, Zarbo RJ. Diagnostic value of HMB-45 and anti-melan A staining of sentinel lymph nodes with isolated positive cells. *Mod Pathol.* 2002;15:1288–1293.

124. Jungbluth AA, Busam KJ, Gerald WL, Stockert E, Coplan KA, Iversen K, et al. A103: an anti-melan-A monoclonal antibody for the detection of malignant melanoma in paraffin-embedded tissues. *Am J Surg Pathol.* 1998;22:595–602.

125. Blessing K, Sanders D, Grant J. Comparison of immunohistochemical staining of the novel antibody melan-A with S100 protein and HMB-45 in malignant melanoma and melanoma variants. *Histopathology.* 1998;32:139–146.

126. Kaufmann O, Koch S, Burghardt J, et al. Tyrosinase, Melan-A and KBA62 as markers for the immunohistochemical identification of metastatic amelanotic melanomas on paraffin sections. *Mod Pathol.* 1998;11:740–746.

127. Miettinen M, Fernandez M, Franssila K, et al. Microphthalmia transcription factor in immunohistochemical diagnosis of metastatic melanoma: comparison with four other melanoma markers. *Am J Surg Pathol.* 2001;25:205–211.

128. Yu LL, Flotte TJ, Tanabe KK, et al. Detection of microscopic melanoma metastases in sentinel lymph nodes. *Cancer.* 1999;86:617–627.

129. Busam KJ, Kucukgol D, Sato E, et al. Immunohistochemical analysis of novel monoclonal antibody PNL2 and comparison with other melanocyte differentiation markers. *Am J Surg Pathol.* 2005;29:400–406.

130. Cochran AJ, Wen D-R, Herschman HR. Occult melanoma in lymph nodes detected by anti-serum to S-100 protein. *Int J Cancer.* 1984;34:159–163.

131. Cochran AJ, Wen D-R, Morton DL. Occult tumor cells in the lymph nodes of patients with pathological stage I malignant melanoma. *Am J Surg Pathol.* 1988;12:612–618.

132. Spanknebel K, Coit DG, Bieligk SE, et al. Characterization of micrometastatic disease in melanoma sentinel lymph nodes by enhanced pathology: recommendations for standardizing pathologic analysis. *Am J Surg Pathol.* 2005;29:305–317.

133. Wang X, Heller R, VanVoorhis N, et al. Detection of submicroscopic lymph node metastases with polymerase chain reaction in patients with malignant melanoma. *Ann Surg.* 1994;220:786–774.

134. Sarantou T, Chi DD, Garrison DA, et al. Melanoma associated antigens as messenger RNA detection markers for melanoma. *Cancer Res.* 1997;57:1371–1376.

135. Kuo CT, Bostick PJ, Irie RF, et al. Assessment of messenger RNA of $\beta 14 \rightarrow$ N-acetylgalactosaminyl-transferase as a molecular marker for metastatic melanoma. *Clin Cancer Res.* 1998;4:411–418.

136. Reintgen D, Albertini J, Miliotes G, et al. The accurate staging and modern-day treatment of malignant melanoma. *Cancer Res Therapy Control.* 1995;4:183–197.

137. Goydes JS, Ravikumar TS, Germino FJ, et al. Minimally invasive staging in patients with melanoma: sentinel lymphadenectomy and detection of the melanoma-specific proteins MART-1 and tyrosinase by reverse transcriptase polymerase chain. *J Am Coll Surg.* 1998;187:182–190.

138. Bostick PJ, Morton DL, Turner RR, et al. Prognostic significance of occult metastases detected by sentinel lymphadenectomy and reverse transcriptase-polymerase chain reaction in early-stage melanoma patients. *J Clin Oncol.* 1999;17:3238–3244.

139. Li W, Stall A, Shivers SC, et al. Clinical relevance of molecular staging for melanoma: a comparison of RT-PCR and immunohistochemistry staining in sentinel lymph nodes of patients with melanoma. *Ann Surg.* 2000;231:795–803.

140. Kammula US, Ghossein R, Bhattacharya S, Coit DG. Serial follow-up and the prognostic significance of reverse transcriptase-polymerase chain reaction: staged sentinel lymph nodes from melanoma patients. *J Clin Oncol.* 2004;22:3989–3996.

141. Morton DL. Sentinel lymphadenectomy for patients with clinical stage I melanoma. *J Surg Oncol.* 1997;66:267–269.

142. Gershenwald J, Thompson W, Mansfield P, et al. Multi-institutional melanoma lymphatic mapping experience: the prognostic value of sentinel lymph node status in 612 stage I or II melanoma patients. *J Clin Oncol.* 1999;17:976–983.

143. Morton DL, Thompson JF, Eisner JR, et al. Validation of the accuracy of intraoperative lymphatic mapping and sentinel lymphadenectomy for early stage melanoma: a multicenter trial. *Ann Surg.* 1998;230:453–465.

144. Morton DL, Cochran AJ, Thompson JF, et al. Sentinel node biopsy for early stage melanoma: accuracy and morbidity in MSLT-I, an International Multicenter Trial. *Ann Surg.* 2005;242:302–313.

145. Morton DL, Thompson JF, Cochran AJ, et al. Sentinel-node biopsy or nodal observation in melanoma. *N Engl J Med.* 2006;355:1307–1317.

146. Bleicher RJ, Essner R, Foshag LJ, et al. Role of sentinel lymphadenectomy in thin invasive cutaneous melanomas. *J Clin Oncol.* 2003;21:1326–1331.

147. Jacobs IA, Chang CK, DasGupta TK, Salti GI. Role of sentinel node biopsy in patients with thin (<1 mm) primary melanoma. *Ann Surg Oncol.* 2003;10:558–561.

148. Bedrosian I, Faries MB, Guerry DT, et al. Incidence of sentinel node metastasis in patients with thin primary melanoma (< or = 1 mm) with vertical growth phase. *Ann Surg Oncol.* 2000;7:262–267.

149. Karakousis GC, Gimosty PA, Botbyl JD, et al. Predictors of regional nodal disease in patients with thin melanomas. *Ann Surg Oncol.* 2006;13:533–541.

150. McMasters KM, Wong SL, Edwards MJ, et al. Frequency of non-sentinel lymph node metastasis in melanoma. *Ann Surg Oncol.* 2002;9:137–141.

151. Reeves ME, Delgado R, Busam KJ, et al. Prediction of nonsentinel lymph node status in melanoma. *Ann Surg Oncol.* 2003;10:27–31.

152. Wagner JD, Gordon MS, Chuang TY, et al. Predicting sentinel and residual lymph node basin disease after sentinel lymph node biopsy for melanoma. *Cancer.* 2000;89:453–462.

153. Elias N, Tanabe KK, Sober AJ, et al. Is completion lymphadenectomy after a positive sentinel lymph node biopsy for cutaneous melanoma always necessary? *Arch Surg.* 2004;139:400–405.

154. Sabel MS, Griffith K, Sondale VK, et al. Predictors of nonsentinel lymph node positivity in patients with a positive sentinel lymph node for melanoma. *J Amer Coll Surg.* 2005;201:39–47.

155. Joseph E, Brobeil A, Glass F, et al. Results of complete lymph node dissection in 83 melanoma patients with positive sentinel nodes. *Ann Surg Oncol.* 1998;5:119–125.

156. Clary BM, Brady MS, Lewis JJ, Coit DG. Sentinel lymph node biopsy in the management of patients with primary cutaneous melanoma: review of a large single-institutional experience with an emphasis on recurrence. *Ann Surg.* 2001;233:250–258.

157. Wagner JD, Gordon MS, Chuang T-Y, et al. Predicting sentinel and residual lymph node basin disease after sentinel lymph node biopsy for melanoma. *Cancer.* 2000;89:453–462.

158. Cochran AJ, Wen D-R, Huang R-R, et al. Prediction of metastatic melanoma in nonsentinel nodes and clinical outcome based on the primary melanoma and the sentinel node. *Mod Pathol.* 2004;17:747–755.

159. Cochran AJ, Roberts A, Wen D-R, et al. Optimized assessment of sentinel lymph nodes for metastatic melanoma: implications for regional surgery and overall treatment planning. *Ann Surg Oncol.* 2004;12:1565–1615.

160. Coit DG. Prognostic factors in patients with melanoma to regional lymph nodes. *Surg Oncol Clin North Am.* 1992;1:281–295.

161. Berk DR, Johnson DL, Uzieblo A, Kiernan M, Swetler SM. Sentinel lymph node biopsy for cutaneous melanoma. The Stanford Experience, 1997-2004. *Arch Dermatol.* 2005;141:1016–1022.

162. Yee VS, Thompson JF, McKinnon JG, et al. Outcome in 846 cutaneous melanoma patients from single center after a negative sentinel node biopsy. *Ann Surg Oncol.* 2005;12:429–439.

163. Alaia TA, Gershenwald JE. Management of early stage cutaneous melanoma. *Curr Prob Surg.* 2005;42:457–534.

164. Ferrone CR, Panageas KS, Busam K, Brady MS, Coit DG. Multivariate prognostic model for patients with thick cutaneous melanoma: importance of sentinel lymph node status. *Ann Surg Oncol.* 2002;9:637–645.

165. McMasters KM, Sondak V, Lotze M, Ross M. Recent advances in melanoma staging and therapy. *Ann Surg Oncol.* 1999;6:467–475.

166. Zettersten E, Shaikh L, Ramirez R, Kashani-Sabet M. Prognostic factors in primary cutaneous melanoma. *Ann Surg Oncol.* 1999;83:61–75.

167. Thompson J. The Sydney Melanoma Unit experience of sentinel lymphadenectomy for melanoma. *Ann Surg Oncol.* 2001;8:445–478.

168. Balch C, Soong S, Gershenwald J, Thompson J, et al. Prognostic factor analysis of 17,600 melanoma patients: validation of the American Joint Committee on Cancer melanoma staging system. *J Clin Oncol.* 2001;19:3622–3634.

169. Balch C, Buzaid AC, Soong SJ, et al. Final version of the AJCC staging system for cutaneous melanoma. *J Clin Oncol.* 2001;19:3635–3648.

170. Gershenwald JE, Mansfield P, Lee J, et al. Role for lymphatic mapping and sentinel lymph node biopsy in patients with thick (> or = 4 mm) primary melanoma. *Ann Surg Oncol.* 2000;7:160–165.

171. Thompson JF, Shaw H. The prognosis of patients with thick primary melanomas: is regional lymph node status relevant and does removing positive regional nodes influence outcome? *Ann Surg Oncol.* 2002;9:719–722.

172. Vaquerano J, Kraybill WG, Driscoll DL, et al. American Joint Committee on Cancer Clinical Stage as a selection criterion for sentinel lymph node biopsy in thin melanoma. *Ann Surg Oncol.* 2006;13:198–204.

173. Morton DL, Holmes EC, Eilber FR, et al. Adjuvant immunotherapy of malignant melanoma: results of a randomized trial in patients with lymph node metastases. In Terry WD, Rosenberg SA, eds. *Immunotherapy of human cancer.* Amsterdam: Elsevier North Holland, 1982;245–249.

174. Quirt IC, Shelley WE, Paters JL, et al. Improved survival in patients with poor-prognosis malignant melanoma treated with adjuvant levamisole: a phase III study by the National Cancer Institute of Canada Clinical Trials Group. *J Clin Oncol.* 1991;9:729–735.

175. Spitler LE. A randomized trial of levamisole versus placebo as adjuvant therapy in malignant melanoma. *J Clin Oncol.* 1991;9:736–740.

176. Miller LL, Spitler LE, Allen RE, et al. A randomized double-blind, placebo-controlled trial of transfer factor as adjuvant therapy for malignant melanoma. *Cancer.* 1988;61:1543–1549.

177. Lipton A, Harvey HA, Balch CM, et al. *Corynebacterium parvum* versus Bacille Calmette-Guérin adjuvant immunotherapy of stage II malignant melanoma. *J Clin Oncol.* 1991;9:1151–1156.

178. Karakousis CP, Didolkar MS, Lopez R, et al. Chemoimmunotherapy (DTIC and *Corynebacterium parvum*) as adjuvant treatment in malignant melanoma. *Cancer Treat Rep.* 1979;63:1739–1743.

179. Cuningham TJ, Schoenfeld D, Nathanson L, et al. A controlled ECOG study of adjuvant therapy with BCG or BCG plus DTIC in patients with stage I and II malignant melanoma. In Terry WD, Rosenberg SA, eds. *Immunotherapy of human cancer.* Amsterdam: Elsevier North Holland, 1982;271–277.

180. Bystryn J, Zeleniuch-Jacquotte A, Oratz R, et al. Double-blind trial of a polyvalent, shed-antigen melanoma vaccine. *Clin Cancer Res.* 2001;7:1882–1887.

181. Rosenberg S, Yang J, Schwartzentruber D, et al. Immunologic and therapeutic evaluation fo a synthetic peptide vaccine for the treatment of patients with metastatic melanoma. *Nat Med.* 1998;4(3):321–327.

182. Salgaller M, Marincola F, Cormier J, et al. Immunization against epitopes in the human melanoma antigen gp100 following patient immunization with synthetic peptides. *Cancer Res.* 1996;56(20):4749–4757.

183. Ravindranath M, Morton D, Irie R. An epitope common to gangliosides O-acetyl-GD3 and GD3 recognized by antibodies in melanoma patients after active specific immunotherapy. *Cancer Res.* 1989;49(14):3891–3897.

184. Wallack M, Scoggin S, Sivanandham M. Active specific immunotherapy with vaccinia melanoma oncolysate. *Mt Sinai J Med.* 1992;59(3):227–233.

185. Nestle F, Alijagic S, Gilliet M, et al. Vaccination of melanoma patients with peptide or tumor lysate-pulsed dendritic cells. *Nat Med.* 1998;4(3):269–270.

186. Bedrosian I, Mick R, Xu S, et al. Intradnodal administration of peptide-pulsed mature dendritic cell vaccines results in superior CD8+ T-cell function in melanoma patients. *J Clin Oncol.* 2003;21:3826–3835.

187. Farles MB, Morton DL. Melanoma: Is immunotherapy of benefit? *Advances in Surgery.* 2003;37:139–162.

188. Verma S, Quirt I, McCready D, et al. Systematic review of systemic adjuvant therapy for patients at high risk for recurrent melanoma. *Cancer.* 2006;106:1431–1442.

189. Wallack MK, Sivanandham M, Balch CM, et al. Surgical adjuvant active specific immunotherapy for patients with Stage III

melanoma: the final analysis of data from a Phase III, randomized, double-blind, multicenter vaccinia melanoma oncolysate trial. *J Am Coll Surg.* 1998;187:69–77.

190. Livingston PO, Wong GY, Adluri S, et al. Improved survival in Stage III melanoma patients with GM2 antibodies: a randomized trail of adjuvant vaccination with GM2 ganglioside. *J Clin Oncol.* 1994;12:1036–1044.

191. Bystryn JC, Zeleniuch-Jacquotte A, Oratz R, Shapiro RL, Harris MN, Roses DF. Double-blind trial of a polyvalent shed-antigen, melanoma vaccine. *Clin Cancer Res.* 2001;7:1882–1887.

192. Hersey P, Coates AS, McCarthy WH, et al. Adjuvant immunotherapy of patients with high-risk melanoma using vaccinia viral lysates of melanoma: results of a randomized trial. *J Clin Oncol.* 2002;20:4181–4190.

193. Sondak VK, Liu PY, Tuthill RJ, et al. Adjuvant immunotherapy of resected, intermediate-thickness, node-negative melanoma with an allogeneic tumor vaccine: overall results of a randomized trial of the Southwest Oncology Group. *J Clin Oncol.* 2002;20:2058–2066.

194. Kirkwood JM, Agarwala S. Systemic cytotoxic and biologic therapy of melanoma. *PPO Updates.* 1993;7:1–16.

195. Kirkwood JM, Strawdrerman MH, Ernstoff MS, et al. Interferon alpha-2b adjuvant therapy of high-risk resected cutaneous melanoma: the Eastern Cooperative Oncology Group Trial 5T 1684. *J Clin Oncol.* 1996;14:7–17.

196. Cascinelli N. Evaluation of efficacy of adjuvant IFN-α-2a in melanoma patients with regional node metastases. *Proc Am Soc Clin Oncol.* 1995;14:410 (abstract).

197. Grob J, Dreno B, Delauney M, et al. Results of the French multicenter trial on adjuvant therapy with interferon-α-2a in resected primary melanoma (1.5 mm). *Proc Am Soc Clin Oncol.* 1996;15:437.

198. Pehamberger H, Soyer P, Steiner A, et al. Adjuvant interferon α-2a treatment in resected primary cutaneous melanoma. *Melanoma Res.* 1997;7(Suppl. 1):531.

199. Creagan E, Dalton R, Ahmann D, et al. Randomized, surgical adjuvant clinical trial of recombinant interferon α-2a in selected patients with malignant melanoma. *J Clin Oncol.* 1999;13:2776–2783.

200. Kirkwood JM, Ibrahim JG, Sondak VK, et al. High- and low-dose interferon alfa-2b in high-risk melanoma: first analysis of Intergroup Trial E1690/S9111/C9190. *J Clin Oncol.* 2000;18:2444–2458.

201. Kirkwood J, Ibrahim J, Sondak V, et al. Role of high-dose IFN in high-risk melanoma: preliminary results of the E1690/S9111/C9190 U.S. Intergroup Postoperative Adjuvant Trial of high- and low-dose IFNα-2b (HDI and LDI) in resected high-risk primary or regionally lymph node metastatic melanoma in relation to 10-year updated results of E1684. Symposium on Advances in Biology and Treatment of Cutaneous Melanoma, November 7, 1998, Boston.

202. Kirkwood J, Manola J, Ibrahim J, et al. A pooled analysis of Eastern Cooperative Oncology Group and Intergroup trials of adjuvant high-dose interferon for melanoma. *Clin Cancer Res.* 2004;10:1670–1677.

203. Stretch JR, Somorjai R, Bourne R, et al. Melanoma metastases in regional lymph nodes are accurately detected by proton magnetic resonance spectroscopy of fine-needle aspirate biopsy samples. *Ann Surg Onc.* 2005;12:943–949.

204. Carr KM, Bittner M, Trent JM. Gene expression profiling in human cutaneous melanoma. *Oncogene.* 2003;22:3076–3080.

205. Baldi A, Santini D, DeLuca A, Paggi M. cDNA array technology in melanoma: an overview. *J Cell Physiol.* 2003;196:219–223.

COMMENTARY

Lisa K. Jacobs, Julie R. Lange, and Charles M. Balch

The chapter by Dr. Daniel Roses is a comprehensive, lucid, and scholarly treatise on the evaluation and management of the regional lymph nodal basins in patients with melanoma. It is well referenced and has a particularly good section on the history of lymphadenectomy and lymph node metastases.

We agree with Dr. Roses on his surgical recommendations, including his conclusion that the use of elective lymph node dissection has been completely supplanted by the more accurate and "selective" method of lymphatic mapping and sentinel node excision. In a national study, the number of patients diagnosed with stage III melanoma increased by over 55% between 1998 and 2001, and this corresponded to a 53% increase in the number of sentinel node biopsies performed (1).

A therapeutic completion lymphadenectomy should be performed as a standard of care in the approximately 20% of patients with histologically demonstrated metastases in the sentinel lymph node (SLN) inasmuch as there is a 15% to 24% probability that other (nonsentinel) lymph nodes will also contain occult micrometastases (2,3). In a recent report by Scheri and colleagues (4), even patients with isolated tumor cells (nests of metastatic cells <0.2 mm) in the sentinel nodes had a significantly higher risk of melanoma-specific death than those with tumor-negative SLNs, and they had a 12% likelihood of having nonsentinel node metastasis. The authors suggest that patients with micrometastases and isolated tumor cells should be considered for completion lymphadenectomy. Other series have not detected nonsentinel nodal metastases when the volume of sentinel node metastases is <0.2 mm or <0.1 mm in diameter (5,6).

Indeed, the use of SLN biopsy has dramatically changed the current surgical management of melanoma, and it offers many significant benefits to our patients. Initially described by Morton et al. (7), sentinel lymphadenectomy is a highly accurate, minimally invasive method of identifying those primary melanoma patients who may have clinically occult nodal metastases. The majority of patients have node-negative disease and can be safely treated without completion dissection as they have a low-to-intermediate risk for future metastases. Unless participating in a clinical trial, patients with a positive sentinel node biopsy should undergo a completion lymphadenectomy and can be considered for adjuvant therapy if deemed appropriate. The concept of the sentinel node is now well established and should be used in those melanoma patients in whom the information obtained will be useful for staging and treatment planning.

In this commentary, we provide some additional perspective to Dr. Roses' comprehensive chapter by framing our discussion on the clinical management of the regional node basin in a model of surgical decision making.

GOALS AND RATIONALE FOR LYMPH NODE SURGERY IN MELANOMA

There are three major goals of cancer surgery: staging, cure, and palliation. Identifying and then excising metastatic melanoma in the regional lymph nodes is one of the few surgical situations in which all three goals would potentially apply. However, even in a noncurative, palliative situation, surgery often provides the most effective treatment for relieving or preventing disabling symptoms from bulky regional disease despite metastatic growth in a distant vital organ.

Decisions regarding node dissection for clinically occult disease are more rational today because of improved staging techniques and the technology associated with intraoperative lymphatic mapping and sentinel lymphadenectomy. Microstaging of a primary melanoma with the combined use of tumor thickness and ulceration now can provide accurate statistical probability of a patient having clinically occult nodal metastases. The incidence of nodal metastases is related to the thickness of the primary melanoma (8,9). In patients with lesions <0.76 mm thick, the likelihood of finding a positive sentinel node is minimal. For melanomas 0.76 to 1 mm thick, the probability of finding a metastatic sentinel node is 5% to 6%. For melanomas 1.1 to 1.5 mm thick, the chance is 7% to 8%. For melanomas 1.5 to 4.0 mm thick, the figure is 18% to 19%, and for melanomas 4 mm or thicker, the risk of sentinel node disease is 29% to 34% (8).

Over the past few years, there has been a worldwide validation of the staging accuracy and reproducibility of intraoperative lymphatic mapping and sentinel lymphadenectomy (10–14). This surgical technique has provided the surgeon with a precise tool that, when properly used, can stage for the presence or absence of a metastatic tumor down to a threshold of 10^5 to 10^6 cells with an accuracy of 95%. In fact, the technique has proved so reproducible and valuable as a staging procedure that the American Joint Committee on Cancer (AJCC) Melanoma Committee and the National Comprehensive Cancer Network guidelines have recommended that patients with T2, T3, and T4 melanomas be considered for sentinel lymphadenectomy to guide clinical decision making and for staging prior to entry into a melanoma clinical trial. The overall yield of finding occult nodal metastases averages about 20% and increases as melanomas become thicker or have features of a poorly differentiated tumor, such as ulceration or increased mitotic rate (2,9,15,16). Even patients with T1b melanomas (i.e., those melanomas <1.0 mm thickness with either ulceration of the surface or a Clark level IV depth) can be considered for the sentinel node procedure because the incidence of nodal metastases is approximately 10% to 14% (13,15,17).

SURGICAL DECISION MAKING: DO THE BENEFITS OUTWEIGH THE RISKS?

Surgeons treating melanoma patients make a sequence of decisions as they select from an array of therapeutic options concerning the management regional lymph nodes that are either clinically negative but might harbor micrometastases, or are clinically suspicious for nodal metastases. After an appropriate eval-

uation and staging, a treatment plan must be formulated that takes into consideration the critical question, "Do the potential benefits of surgery outweigh the potential risks?" The first decision is whether to recommend lymphatic mapping followed by a sentinel node excision with a careful pathologic evaluation of the resected node(s). A second decision is whether to perform a completion lymphadenectomy in patients with a positive sentinel node, especially if the tumor volume within the node is small.

In considering a recommendation for SLN analysis in patients with clinically negative (N0) nodes, the elements of decision making on the "benefits" side include:

1. Achieving one or more of the three goals of cancer surgery, that is:
   a. Diagnosis/staging of metastases
   b. Regional disease control, and/or
   c. Increased survival rates
2. Discerning the features of nodal metastases that predict the risk of distant metastases such as the number of nodal metastases and extracapsular invasion, and
3. "Quality of life" issues as perceived by the patient.

The elements of decision making on the "risk" side include:

1. The morbidity of a sentinel node procedure and, if necessary, a completion lymphadenectomy (e.g., wound complications, lymphedema, numbness)
2. Patient comorbidity risk factors (e.g., obesity, older age)
3. Risk of not performing a lymphadenectomy that may increase the probability of future regional recurrence
4. Risk of not receiving adjuvant systemic therapy with occult metastatic lymph nodes

Understanding the risks of morbidity when making operative decisions is important. We believe the estimates summarized in Dr. Roses' chapter overstate the morbidity in current practice. The risk/benefit analysis must also include the risk of the SLN procedure and the future risk to the patient if a clinically palpable nodal recurrence occurs. Serious postsurgical complications of sentinel node biopsy are uncommon. Estimates of morbidity rates in several series range from 5% to 20%, and are mainly confined to transient wound complications (12,18–21). After sentinel node biopsy, some patients have a self-limited lymphocele at the site of node excision. The risk of lymphocele can be minimized by ligating or clipping all lymphatic channels encountered during the sentinel node resection. If a lymphocele is large or painful, a simple office aspiration should provide adequate management. Small, asymptomatic lymphoceles can be observed and usually resolve spontaneously. Mild lymphedema has been reported in patients after sentinel node biopsy of the axilla and the inguinal area. However, the incidence is low, and the swelling usually subsides over time. It has been suggested that performing a sentinel node procedure might increase the incidence of in-transit or intralymphatic metastases, but a careful analysis of available data has shown convincingly that this concern is not valid (22,23).

Complete lymphadenectomy for regionally metastatic melanoma carries a risk of seroma, sensory loss, and lymphedema. A few patients have a seroma or prolonged drain output. Lymphedema is the most feared common complication of lymph node dissection and can occur after axillary or inguinal lymphadenectomy. However, the risk of lymphedema is low, and most cases are mild to moderate and controllable with diligent care.

The morbidity after an inguinal lymphadenectomy is higher than that associated with an axillary or cervical lymphadenectomy. In the older literature, morbidity rates of 50% were quoted, resulting in a reluctance to perform this operation, especially by surgeons who encounter this situation infrequently. More recent publications report a much lower rate of significant wound complications and lymphedema (24,25). Important data that emphasize the benefit of applying sentinel node technology in detecting clinically occult inguinal disease come from Sabel et al. (24) at the University of Michigan. These authors compared the pathology results and morbidity among 132 patients who underwent completion inguinal lymphadenectomy after a metastatic sentinel node was identified with the morbidity experienced by 80 patients who underwent inguinal lymphadenectomy for clinically palpable disease. Age, gender, and body mass index were similar in both groups. Overall, there was a 19% incidence of significant wound complications. The complication rate following lymphadenectomy was significantly higher among patients with clinically evident nodal disease compared with those who had a dissection for micrometastasis in a sentinel node (28% vs. 14%; $p = 0.02$). Lymphedema occurred in 41% of patients who presented with clinical disease and in 24% in those with clinically occult disease ($p = 0.02$). These results demonstrate that management of inguinal nodal disease when it is clinically occult is associated with reduced morbidity compared with management when the disease is clinically apparent (24).

INDICATIONS FOR LYMPHATIC MAPPING AND SENTINEL NODE EXCISION

Sentinel lymphadenectomy is a highly accurate, minimally invasive method of identifying those primary melanoma patients who may have clinically occult nodal metastases (14). Indeed, it is the most accurate, reproducible and cost-effective test available today for detecting regional node micrometastases. At Johns Hopkins, we recommend this procedure for patients when (a) the yield or incidence of clinically occult nodal metastases is 5% or greater, (b) the information gained will be used in subsequent treatment decisions (including completion lymphadenectomy), and (c) the morbidity of the procedure is low. In general, we recommend lymphatic mapping and sentinel node biopsy for patients with T1b, T2, T3, or T4 lesions.

Preoperative lymphoscintigraphy is vital to the success of sentinel node biopsy. Radioisotope and blue dye are the two commonly used tracers, and many groups use both. With truncal or head and neck primary lesions, drainage often occurs to more than one nodal basin, and it is important to retrieve the sentinel node(s) from each nodal basin in which a sentinel node is identified (8,26). Preoperative lymphoscintigraphy facilitates the identification of sentinel nodes that lie outside traditional nodal basins or at unexpected sites. Sentinel nodes have occasionally been identified at popliteal and epitrochlear sites and in

the triangular intramuscular space in the back, at the supraclavicular fossa, and at internal mammary and paravertebral sites.

PATHOLOGIC EXAMINATION OF SENTINEL LYMPH NODES

The sentinel node should be placed in formalin for permanent fixation. Frozen section analysis is discouraged because it inevitably wastes nodal tissue that might contain micrometastases and, moreover, it is difficult to reliably identify melanoma metastases by frozen section. Thus, it is preferable to save the entire lymph node intact for permanent processing. Multiple sections should be prepared for routine and immunohistochemical staining (e.g., HMB-45, S100, Melan-A) to search for micrometastases. Immunohistochemical staining increases the node-positive rate by 10% to 12% compared with staining with hematoxylin and eosin alone (27,28). In a series of 243 patients with histologically negative sentinel nodes, eight of the ten patients (4.1% of the total group) who subsequently relapsed in the previously mapped nodal basin were found to have occult disease in the original sentinel node on retrospective re-evaluation with serial sectioning or immunohistochemical staining (26). Finally, we agree with Dr. Roses that the prognostic significance of molecular markers of metastases by reverse transcriptase-polymerase chain reaction methods has still not been defined, and thus molecular markers should not be used in routine clinical practice.

RESULTS OF THE MULTICENTER SELECTIVE LYMPHADENECTOMY TRAIL (MSLT) I

Dr. Roses has nicely summarized this seminal randomized surgical trial comparing SLN biopsy and nodal observation conducted by Dr. Donald Morton and colleagues (29). The SLN procedure was performed by scores of surgeons practicing in three continents with only a 3.4% false-negative rate and minimum morbidity. They demonstrated that the sentinel node biopsy provides important prognostic information and identifies patients with nodal metastases whose survival can be prolonged by lymphadenectomy (29). Importantly, this is the first randomized trial to directly assess the staging value of SLN biopsy and confirms the importance of detecting clinically occult (i.e., microscopic) metastases as a staging tool and as a predictor of survival outcome. It conclusively showed that nodal metastases could be detected by SN analysis a median of 16 months earlier compared with the "watch and wait" approach in the 20% of patients who had nodal metastases. In the SLN biopsy arm, the SLN status was the most significant predictor of survival in a multifactorial analysis. These results confirm other analyses specifically examining the prognostic significance of SLN biopsy (30). The AJCC Melanoma Database analysis (30) of more than 16,000 melanoma patients demonstrated that the presence of nodal micrometastases was such a strong predictor of survival that it has been included among the elements of the melanoma TNM classification.

In the MSLT I trial, the nodal observation group had multiple follow-up examinations before nodal metastases became clinically detectable and a radical lymphadenectomy performed. In this group, there were a larger mean number of metastatic lymph nodes (3.3 metastatic lymph nodes vs. 1.4 in the SLN group). The implications for this higher number of nodal metastases are important. First, the regional recurrence rates significantly increase as the number of metastases increase in a nodal basin, and reach about a 20% regional failure rate after standard lymphadenectomy for patients with four or more metastatic nodes (compared with <5% in patients with a single metastatic node) (29). In many melanoma centers, patients with multiple, grossly detectable nodal metastases (i.e., stage IIIB and IIIC) receive adjuvant radiation therapy to the nodal basin (28), and would more likely receive adjuvant high-dose interferon (31). In contrast, patients with one or two micrometastases (stage IIIA) would not be considered for adjuvant radiation therapy but would be candidates for other systemic treatments, especially in clinical trials, such as melanoma vaccine trials, in lieu of high-dose interferon.

The survival rates in the two randomized groups were comparable. However, among patients with nodal metastases, 16% in each group, the 5-year survival rate was superior in the cohort of patients undergoing early surgical intervention as directed by the SLN biopsy (72% vs. 52%; $p = 0.004$) (29). Although this result was a secondary issue in the study, it was a clearly stated secondary outcome objective in the design of the trial. The dilutional effect on overall survival rates by the 84% of patients who never had nodal metastases will make it difficult to demonstrate a survival advantage of the group undergoing SLN biopsy. It would also be difficult—perhaps even impossible—to have a different design of a randomized trial to address this issue, as the presence or absence of nodal metastases is only known retrospectively after either the SLN procedure or after close clinical examination of the regional nodal basin by palpation or ultrasound. The assessment of long-term survival rates is still ongoing; the results so far demonstrate that disease-free survival rates are improved in the SLN group compared to the nodal observation group, although the melanoma-specific mortality rates are essentially the same.

RATIONALE FOR COMPLETION NODE DISSECTION FOR MICROSCOPICALLY POSITIVE REGIONAL NODES

The rationale for a completion node dissection is to determine how many nodes are positive, to provide regional control of disease, and to give the patient an opportunity for improved survival. If the patient already has distant microscopic metastases, removing regional nodal metastases should usually be avoided because a survival benefit is unlikely. Results from the Intergroup Melanoma Surgical Trial demonstrate that prognostic factors (especially tumor thickness and ulceration) can prospectively identify a subset melanoma patients who are at a high risk for occult regional metastases and yet at a low risk for having occult distant metastases, so that surgical excision of their regional lymph nodes is justified with the aim of achieving a therapeutic benefit (32). The window of time for which early surgical intervention halts the further dissemination of melanoma metastases from regional to distant sites might be estimated at 16 months, which is the average relapse time for patients who had a primary excision and nodal observation, and whose original nodal micrometastases evolved into clinically detectable disease.

There is also a very compelling rationale for pathologic staging of the regional lymph nodes for patients prior to entry into adjuvant systemic therapy trials. Differences in 2- and 5-year survival rates for patients with and without clinically occult nodal metastases can vary by as much as 20% to 25%. Indeed, some of the problems in interpreting and comparing past clinical trials of melanoma patients has been the inability to fully account for the pathologic differences in nodal status in a heterogeneous group of T3 and T4 patients, some of whom had pathologic assessment of their regional nodes while others had only clinical assessment.

REGIONALLY METASTATIC MELANOMA: PREDICTING RECURRENCE AND SURVIVAL

The features of a primary melanoma and nodal metastases can be accurately used to categorize patients into homogeneous subgroups based on metastatic risk. These predictive or prognostic parameters are also indispensable in multidisciplinary treatment planning and are essential in design, analysis, and comparability of clinical trials.

In patients with metastatic regional metastases, the stage grouping for pathologic stage III melanoma uses four major determinants of outcome:

1. The number of metastatic lymph nodes;
2. The tumor burden, either microscopic (i.e., clinically occult and detected pathologically by sentinel node biopsy or elective lymphadenectomy) or macroscopic (i.e., clinically apparent by physical or radiologic examination and verified pathologically);
3. Ulceration of the primary melanoma; and
4. Satellite or in-transit metastases (30,33).

The presence of one to three microscopic (i.e., clinically occult) nodal metastases (N1a and N2a) identified after sentinel or elective lymphadenectomy in patients with a nonulcerated primary melanoma (T1-4a) is associated with a 5-year survival of 63% to 69%. Patients with one to three microscopic (clinically occult) metastatic nodes (N2a) arising from an ulcerated primary melanoma (T1-4b) are equivalent prognostically to patients with one to three macroscopic metastatic nodes (N1b and N2b) arising from a nonulcerated primary melanoma (T1-4a) and are grouped together as pathologic stage IIIB. All patients with four or more macroscopically positive nodes (N3) or those with any nodal disease in the presence of satellite or in-transit metastases are at especially high risk for systemic metastases and are grouped as pathologic stage IIIC (30).

UNCERTAINTY IN THE VALUE OF LYMPHADENECTOMY FOR MICROSCOPIC NODAL DISEASE

As Dr. Roses stated, the value of routine dissection for patients with microscopically positive nodes has been questioned (34).

There are now two prospective clinical trials ongoing to determine the magnitude of any benefit in this population, especially those patients with truly microscopic metastases in the sentinel node, a circumstance associated with a lower probability of having adjacent nonsentinel nodes involved with metastases. We support these studies and have activated the MSLT II trial at our own institution. We believe that participation in these studies is critically important. The widespread use of elective node dissection as practiced decades ago has been replaced by lymphatic mapping, sentinel node biopsy, and "selective" lymphenectomy as the result of numerous studies supporting the accuracy and clinical value of sentinel node biopsy in providing prognostic information. Completion dissection for patients with demonstrated regional metastases remains the standard of care today, but there may be defined cohorts of patients that might be spared this additional procedure and its attendant morbidity. On the other hand, we have an obligation as physicians to prove that we can provide more conservative treatment safely and this can only be done using the clinical trials process.

SUMMARY AND RECOMMENDATIONS

Management of the regional lymph node basin in patients with melanoma has been one of the most controversial surgical management issues for over 30 years. Fortunately, advances in our understanding of prognosis, clinical trials, and sentinel node technology now enable surgeons to better stage melanoma patients and recommend a treatment plan that is more precisely and individually tailored to the biology and natural history of their disease presentation. Currently, most melanoma experts recommend lymphatic mapping and sentinel lymphadenectomy as a staging procedure for patients with clinical stage I or II melanoma if their primary tumor is at least 1 mm thick, or, if thinner, when the melanoma is ulcerated, or is Clark level IV or V (i.e. T1bN0M0). The morbidity of the procedure is low and the staging information gained is valuable. Patients found to be node-positive are then classified as having pathologic stage III melanoma and should undergo a therapeutic lymphadenectomy of that nodal basin and should be considered for systemic adjuvant therapy. The concept of the sentinel node is now well established and should be applied to all melanoma patients in whom the information is likely to be useful for staging and treatment planning. Furthermore, the routine use of sentinel node biopsy in the appropriate patients will allow for more accurate stratification of patients entering trials of adjuvant systemic therapies.

Despite recent advances, there is still much research to be done, especially in the area of molecular staging, assessment of the value of completion node dissection, and effective adjuvant systemic therapy. Progress in these areas is paramount to improving cure rates for this increasingly common cancer.

REFERENCES

1. Cormier JN, Xing Y, Ding M, et al. Population-based assessment of surgical treatment trends for patients with melanoma in the era of sentinel lymph node biopsy. *J Clin Oncol.* 2005;23:6054–6062.
2. Essner R, Scheri R, Kavanagh M, et al. Surgical management of the groin lymph nodes in melanoma in the era of sentinel lymph node dissection. Arch Surg. 2006;141:877–82; discussion 882–884.
3. Sabel MS, Griffith K, Sondak VK, et al. Predictors of nonsentinel lymph node positivity in patients with a positive sentinel node for melanoma. *J Am Coll Surg.* 2005;201:37–47.
4. Scheri RP, Essner R, Turner RR, et al. Isolated tumor cells in the sentinel node affect long-term prognosis of patients with melanoma. *Ann Surg Oncol.* 2007;14:2861–2866.
5. Govindarajan A, Ghazarian DM, McCready DR, et al. Histological features of melanoma sentinel lymph node metastases associated with status of the completion lymphadenectomy and rate of subsequent relapse. *Ann Surg Oncol.* 2007;14:906–912.
6. van Akkooi AC, de Wilt JH, Verhoef C, et al. Clinical relevance of melanoma micrometastases (<0.1 mm) in sentinel nodes: are these nodes to be considered negative? *Ann Oncol.* 2006;17:1578–1585.
7. Morton DL, Wen DR, Wong JH, et al. Technical details of intraoperative lymphatic mapping for early stage melanoma. *Arch Surg.* 1992;127:392–399.
8. Gershenwald JE, Thompson W, Mansfield PF, et al. Multi-institutional melanoma lymphatic mapping experience: the prognostic value of sentinel lymph node status in 612 stage I or II melanoma patients. *J Clin Oncol.* 1999;17:976–983.
9. Sondak VK, Taylor JM, Sabel MS, et al. Mitotic rate and younger age are predictors of sentinel lymph node positivity: lessons learned from the generation of a probabilistic model. *Ann Surg Oncol.* 2004;11:247–258.
10. Thompson JF, Uren RF, Shaw HM, et al. Location of sentinel lymph nodes in patients with cutaneous melanoma: new insights into lymphatic anatomy. *J Am Coll Surg.* 1999;189:195–204.
11. Morton DL, Thompson JF, Essner R, et al. Validation of the accuracy of intraoperative lymphatic mapping and sentinel lymphadenectomy for early-stage melanoma: a multicenter trial. Multicenter Selective Lymphadenectomy Trial Group. *Ann Surg.* 1999;230:453–465.
12. Morton DL, Cochran AJ, Thompson JF, et al. Sentinel node biopsy for early-stage melanoma: accuracy and morbidity in MSLT-I, an international multicenter trial. *Ann Surg.* 2005;242:302–313.
13. Karakousis GC, Gimotty PA, Botbyl JD, et al. Predictors of regional nodal disease in patients with thin melanomas. *Ann Surg Oncol.* 2006;13:533–541.
14. Balch CM, Cascinelli N. Sentinel-node biopsy in melanoma. *N Engl J Med.* 2006;355:1370–1371.
15. Vaquerano J, Kraybill WG, Driscoll DL, et al. American Joint Committee on Cancer clinical stage as a selection criterion for sentinel lymph node biopsy in thin melanoma. *Ann Surg Oncol.* 2006;13:198–204.
16. Paek SC, Griffith KA, Johnson TM, et al. The impact of factors beyond Breslow depth on predicting sentinel lymph node positivity in melanoma. *Cancer.* 2007;109:100–108.
17. Rousseau DL Jr, Ross MI, Johnson MM, et al. Revised American Joint Committee on Cancer staging criteria accurately predict sentinel lymph node positivity in clinically node-negative melanoma patients. *Ann Surg Oncol.* 2003;10:569–574.
18. Wrightson WR, Wong SL, Edwards MJ, et al. Complications associated with sentinel lymph node biopsy for melanoma. *Ann Surg Oncol.* 2003;10:676–680.
19. de Vries M, Vonkeman WG, van Ginkel RJ, et al. Morbidity after axillary sentinel lymph node biopsy in patients with cutaneous melanoma. *Eur J Surg Oncol.* 2005;31:778–783.
20. Wasserberg N, Tulchinsky H, Schachter J, et al. Sentinel-lymph-node biopsy (SLNB) for melanoma is not complication-free. *Eur J Surg Oncol.* 2004;30:851–856.
21. de Vries M, Vonkeman WG, van Ginkel RJ, et al. Morbidity after inguinal sentinel lymph node biopsy and completion lymph node dissection in patients with cutaneous melanoma. *Eur J Surg Oncol.* 2006;32:785–789.

22. van Poll D, Thompson JF, Colman MH, et al. A sentinel node biopsy does not increase the incidence of in-transit metastasis in patients with primary cutaneous melanoma. *Ann Surg Oncol.* 2005;12:597–608.

23. Pawlik TM, Ross MI, Johnson MM, et al. Predictors and natural history of in-transit melanoma after sentinel lymphadenectomy. *Ann Surg Oncol.* 2005;12:587–596.

24. Sabel MS, Griffith KA, Arora A, et al. Inguinal node dissection for melanoma in the era of sentinel lymph node biopsy. *Surgery.* 2007;141:728–735.

25. van Akkooi AC, Bouwhuis MG, van Geel AN, et al. Morbidity and prognosis after therapeutic lymph node dissections for malignant melanoma. *Eur J Surg Oncol.* 2007;33:102–108.

26. Gershenwald JE, Colome MI, Lee JE, et al. Patterns of recurrence following a negative sentinel lymph node biopsy in 243 patients with stage I or II melanoma. *J Clin Oncol.* 1998;16:2253–2260.

27. Cochran AJ, Essner R, Rose DM, et al. Principles of sentinel lymph node identification: background and clinical implications. *Langenbecks Arch Surg.* 2000;385:252–260.

28. Burmeister BH, Mark Smithers B, Burmeister E, et al. A prospective phase II study of adjuvant postoperative radiation therapy following nodal surgery in malignant melanoma-Trans Tasman Radiation Oncology Group (TROG) Study 96.06. *Radiother Oncol.* 2006;81:136–142.

29. Morton DL, Thompson JF, Cochran AJ, et al. Sentinel-node biopsy or nodal observation in melanoma. *N Engl J Med.* 2006;355:1307–1317.

30. Balch CM, Soong SJ, Gershenwald JE, et al. Prognostic factors analysis of 17,600 melanoma patients: validation of the American Joint Committee on Cancer melanoma staging system. *J Clin Oncol.* 2001;19:3622–3634.

31. Kirkwood JM, Manola J, Ibrahim J, et al. A pooled analysis of eastern cooperative oncology group and intergroup trials of adjuvant high-dose interferon for melanoma. *Clin Cancer Res.* 2004;10:1670–1677.

32. Balch CM, Soong S, Ross MI, et al. Long-term results of a multi-institutional randomized trial comparing prognostic factors and surgical results for intermediate thickness melanomas (1.0 to 4.0 mm). Intergroup Melanoma Surgical Trial. *Ann Surg Oncol.* 2000;7:87–97.

33. Balch CM, Buzaid AC, Soong SJ, et al. Final version of the American Joint Committee on Cancer staging system for cutaneous melanoma. *J Clin Oncol.* 2001;19:3635–3648.

34. Wong SL, Morton DL, Thompson JF, et al. Melanoma patients with positive sentinel nodes who did not undergo completion lymphadenectomy: a multi-institutional study. *Ann Surg Oncol.* 2006;13:809–816.

25

Adjuvant Therapy for Melanoma:
Review of Published Data and Studies in Progress

Omid Hamid, Vernon K. Sondak, and Jeffrey S. Weber

The search for effective adjuvant therapy of melanoma over the last 20 years has resulted in the testing of a broad variety of therapeutic agents. Until recently, there was little evidence in any randomized trial to suggest survival benefit for any adjuvant therapy. The demonstration of activity for adjuvant high-dose interferon alfa (IFN-α) in cooperative group trial EST 1684 resulted in approval by the United States Food and Drug Administration (FDA) in 1995, but the melanoma landscape was surrounded by controversy since the E1690/Southwest Oncology Group (SWOG) 9111 trial results became available and failed to confirm those results. The recent Eastern Cooperative Oncology Group (ECOG) 1694/SWOG 9512 data have restored IFN's place as a standard against which other adjuvant treatments may be measured. In this chapter, we review all the randomized adjuvant trials conducted to date in melanoma, discuss pertinent studies, and offer recommendations for the adjuvant treatment of melanoma patients with various stages of disease (Table 25.1) who have been rendered clinically disease-free by surgery.

BACKGROUND

Because of our limited success in treating metastatic melanoma, with no single agent having more than a 20% response rate, and the high failure rates associated with surgical therapy for locally and regionally advanced disease, the search for effective adjuvant therapy of melanoma has generated intense interest. Few of the available cytotoxic chemotherapeutic agents have had more than limited efficacy against advanced disease, with response rates of no more than 15% to 20% for dacarbazine, cisplatin, vinblastine, paclitaxel, and temozolomide, indicating that single chemotherapy agents are unlikely to manifest activity as adjuvant therapy. That fact, combined with the assessment that melanoma was an immunogenic tumor susceptible to attack by the host's immune system, resulted in the testing of a remarkably broad spectrum of therapeutic agents, many of which have no applications in treatment for other forms of cancer. The adjuvant therapy trials that were performed were often flawed and always greatly underpowered to detect a significant difference in survival between the arms. Not surprisingly, then, past reviews of the status of adjuvant therapy of melanoma have been little more than litanies of negative results. Occasionally, post·hoc (data-derived) subset analyses appeared promising in one or another trial, but the lack of a compelling rationale for the efficacy of the therapy in the particular subset analyzed usually resulted in insufficient enthusiasm for further testing. The individual practitioner has had little motivation to treat melanoma patients with adjuvant therapy, despite the high risk of and lack of effective therapy for recurrent disease.

This situation changed after approval by the FDA of IFN-α-2b for the postsurgical adjuvant therapy of high-risk melanoma in late 1995, followed shortly thereafter by publication of the results of the clinical trial that resulted in this approval (1). High-dose IFN-α-2b became the standard of care and was used by many oncologists in the community. Yet the trial that showed benefit for IFN-α-2b, the ECOG trial EST1684, suffered from many of the same ailments that plagued previous adjuvant therapy trials (2,3). Unfortunately, the results of the confirmatory trial, E1690/SWOG 9111, did not reproduce the original positive results of the earlier trial, throwing the field back into confusion. That situation has been clarified by the recent data from the ECOG 1694/SWOG 9512 trial, which terminated early after the data suggested that relapse-free and overall survival (OS) were improved with high-dose IFN-α-2b.

Time and the maturation of several additional completed trials will further clarify the role of high-dose IFN-α-2b adjuvant therapy. Unfortunately for the field, the results of two recently completed randomized phase III vaccine trials have negated 20 years of work on allogenic cellular vaccines as adjuvant therapy. But the melanoma landscape has already been permanently changed, and adjuvant therapy research in this disease is in the process of a paradigm shift. The challenge now is to build on the successful model of large randomized well-powered phase III trials with appropriate control arms using new knowledge on antigen-specific immune responses to melanoma gained by basic immunologists over the last 5 to 10 years. Doing so in a rational manner, including adding more specific immune therapies to established IFN-α-2b will require improvements in several areas: increased understanding of the mechanisms of action of the available therapeutic agents (in particular, allowing the rational design of combination therapies), better ability to prognosticate an individual's risk of recurrence (allowing the appropriate inclusion or exclusion of patients from protocol or non-protocol therapy), and a commitment to design and conduct clinical trials that possess sufficient statistical power to detect therapeutically meaningful differences. The intent of this review chapter is to briefly but critically analyze the many adjuvant therapy trials conducted to date, including those in progress and those closed to accrual but awaiting maturation of the results, and describe briefly new and earlier phase trials of antigen-specific vaccines that may revolutionize the field. We hope to highlight the

Table 25.1

TMN Staging System for Melanoma

DEFINITIONS

Primary Tumor (T)

TX	Primary tumor cannot be assessed (e.g., shave biopsy or regressed melanoma)
T0	No evidence of primary tumor
Tis	Melanoma *in situ*
T1	Melanoma ≤1.0 mm with or without ulceration
T1a	Melanoma ≤1.0 mm in thickness and level II or III, no ulceration
T1b	Melanoma ≤1.0 mm in thickness and level IV or V or with ulceration
T2	Melanoma 1.01–2.0 mm in thickness with or without ulceration
T2a	Melanoma 1.01–2.0 mm in thickness, no ulceration
T2b	Melanoma 1.01–2.0 mm in thickness, with ulceration
T3	Melanoma 2.01–4 mm in thickness with or without ulceration
T3a	Melanoma 2.01–4.0 mm in thickness, no ulceration
T3b	Melanoma 2.01–4.0 mm in thickness, with ulceration
T4	Melanoma greater than 4.0 mm in thickness with or without ulceration
T4a	Melanoma >4.0 mm in thickness, no ulceration
T4b	Melanoma >4.0 mm in thickness, with ulceration

Regional Lymph Nodes (N)

NX	Regional lymph nodes cannot be assessed
N0	No regional lymph node metastasis
N1	Metastasis in one lymph node
N1a	Clinically occult (microscopic) metastasis
N1b	Clinically apparent (macroscopic) metastasis
N2	Metastasis in 2 to 3 regional nodes or intralymphatic regional metastasis without nodal metastasis
N2a	Clinically occult (microscopic) metastasis
N2b	Clinically apparent (macroscopic) metastasis
N2c	Satellite or in-transit metastasis without nodal metastasis
N3	Metastasis in four or more regional nodes, or matted metastatic nodes, or in-transit metastasis or satellite(s) with metastasis in regional node(s)

Distant Metastasis (M)

MX	Distant metastasis cannot be assessed
M0	No distant metastasis
M1	Distant metastasis
M1a	Metastasis to skin, subcutaneous tissues, or distant lymph nodes
M1b	Metastasis to lung
M1c	Metastasis to all other visceral sites or distant metastasis at any site associated with an elevated serum lactic dehydrogenase (LDH)

PATHOLOGIC STAGE GROUPING

Stage 0	Tis	N0	M0
Stage IA	T1a	N0	M0
Stage IB	T1b	N0	M0
	T2a	N0	M0
Stage IIA	T2b	N0	M0
	T3a	N0	M0
Stage IIB	T3b	N0	M0
	T4a	N0	M0
Stage IIC	T4b	N0	M0
Stage IIIA	T1–4a	N1a	M0
	T1–4a	N2a	M0
Stage IIIB	T1-4b	N1a	M0
	T1–4b	N2a	M0
	T1–4a	N1b	M0
	T1–4a	N2b	M0
	T1–4a/b	N2c	M0
Stage IIIC	T1–4b	N1b	M0
	T1–4b	N2b	M0
	Any T	N3	M0
Stage IV	Any T	Any N	M1

CLINICAL STAGE GROUPING

Stage 0	Tis	N0	M0
Stage IA	T1a	N0	M0
Stage IB	T1b	N0	M0
	T2a	N0	M0
Stage IIA	T2b	N0	M0
	T3a	N0	M0
Stage IIB	T3b	N0	M0
	T4a	N0	M0
Stage IIC	T4b	N0	M0
Stage III	Any T	N1	M0
	Any T	N2	M0
	Any T	N3	M0
Stage IV	Any T	Any N	M1

From the AJCC Cancer Staging Manual. 6th edition. New York: Springer-Verlag, 2002.

challenges for clinicians and clinical researchers alike for adjuvant therapy of melanoma in the new millennium.

OVERVIEW OF METHODOLOGIC PROBLEMS IN MELANOMA ADJUVANT TRIALS

Virtually all of the adjuvant therapy trials reported to date have suffered from one or more basic methodologic problems that limit the degree of confidence that can be placed in their results.

Inadequate Statistical Power

Without an adequate sample size, a clinical trial will have very little power to detect a *clinically* significant difference as statistically significant. Most of the randomized, controlled trials of adjuvant therapy conducted in melanoma have had fewer than 250 patients per arm. To put this into perspective, a 5% increase in 5-year survival for patients with melanoma metastatic to the regional lymph nodes (which would translate to at least 400 to 500 additional 5-year survivors in this country annually) would require over 1,250 patients per arm for a two-arm trial with 80% power to detect that difference. Most of the largest randomized trials completed in melanoma to date have had 700 to 800 patients total, and some of these have been multiarm trials. Multiarm trials with smaller patient groups will have lower statistical power than two-arm trials of the same total size, because of the need to account for multiple comparisons.

Improper or Imbalanced Control Group

The results of a randomized controlled trial are only as good as the control group used. Historic controls are clearly inappropriate in melanoma adjuvant trials, and have led to recognizable and predictable errors (4). Even consecutive series from a single institution or investigator are poor controls: the thoroughness with which patients are evaluated for metastatic disease has increased over the years (including widespread use of sentinel node biopsies combined with immunohistochemical techniques to evaluate regional nodal metastases, magnetic resonance imaging scanning to screen for CNS metastases, and positron emission tomography scanning for the sensitive detection of occult metastases), resulting in stage migration and improved survival within stages in the absence of effective therapy. In randomized trials, the need for use of a placebo has never fully been addressed (5). Very few melanoma adjuvant trials have used a placebo control, which often presents a difficult decision for participating patients. Some studies have not used a no-treatment control of any kind, relying instead on allegedly inactive agents such as the vaccinia viral oncolysate trial in which vaccinia virus alone was used as the control, and the two Canvaxin trials, which used Bacille Calmette-Guérin (BCG) plus placebo as the control arm. When the study result is negative, the question of unrecognized activity of the control group arises and can obscure the results (6).

However, one of the biggest problems encountered in randomized controlled trials of adjuvant therapy of melanoma to date has been a known or potential imbalance of recognized prognostic factors between the treatment and control arms. For example, in the EST1684 trial of adjuvant high-dose IFN-α, there was a known imbalance between the treatment and control arms for the presence of ulceration in the primary tumor (favoring the control arm) for patients in the stratum with pT4N0M0 disease (thick primary, pathologically negative nodes). This limited the ability to generalize the positive results of this trial from node-positive patients to high-risk node-negative patients. But even more importantly, one of the primary prognostic factors for node-positive patients—the number of tumor-involved nodes—was not recognized at the time this study was designed (1). Hence, it was unknown whether the treatment and control arms were balanced with respect to that crucial factor. The use of randomization does not guarantee that the two groups are equivalent in this regard; rather, it allows us to conclude that there is only a 5% or lesser chance that the two groups are sufficiently imbalanced to result in the erroneous conclusion that IFN-α-2b is active when in fact it is not.

Heterogeneous Risk Groups

Compounding the problems inherent in trials with small sample sizes and potentially imbalanced risk factors is the inclusion of heterogeneous groups of at-risk patients in many of the adjuvant trials conducted to date. Current thinking, based in part on the existing TNM system for melanoma, would stratify patients into four risk categories as follows: low risk (stage I), primary tumor <2.0 mm with negative nodes; intermediate risk (stage IIA), primary tumor 2.0 to 4.0 mm with negative nodes; high risk (stages IIB/C and III), primary tumor >4.0 mm with or without ulceration with negative nodes or any primary tumor with positive nodes, satellitosis, or in-transit metastases; and very high-risk (stage IV), resected metastatic melanoma beyond the regional nodes. Patients with noncutaneous primaries, multiple (more than ten) positive nodes or gross extracapsular extension appear to be at higher risk than the average "high-risk" patient, but precisely where they should fit into this classification scheme remains to be defined. The updated staging criteria developed in 2001 now include such factors as ulceration of the primary lesion, which portends a worse prognosis for early-stage disease and sentinel node positivity by immunohistochemical staining only, which suggests a better outcome for patients with stage III disease. The new staging criteria will completely change the accrual patterns to future adjuvant trials and render the use of historic controls impossible to interpret.

Lack of Active Agents

Perhaps no problem has posed a greater problem in devising melanoma clinical trials than the lack of effective agents. No available single agent has a >20% objective response rate against measurable metastatic disease, and combination therapy has not yet been established to be superior to single agents. Dacarbazine and IFNα2b are two of the active single agents in metastatic disease, and have been evaluated in several adjuvant therapy trials. Vinblastine, cisplatin, paclitaxel, and temozolomide have 10% to 15% single-agent activity and are unlikely to be evaluated in randomized adjuvant therapy trials. Several trials have been published suggesting that combination therapy either with dacarbazine, cisplatin, biscloronitrosomea (BCNU), and tamoxifen or dacarbazine plus IFN-α has no survival advantage over dacarbazine alone in the treatment of metastatic disease (7). Most of the other agents that have been investigated in the adjuvant setting have either no or minimal activity against metastatic disease. It has often been postulated, but never substantiated, that agents lacking activity against metastatic disease (particularly immunotherapeutic agents) could still prove efficacious in the adjuvant setting. Unfortunately, the mechanisms of action of these agents are poorly understood. When trials with these agents have yielded negative results, there has rarely been sufficient biologic information obtained to conclude whether the agent or agents actually achieved the desired surrogate or biologic effect. This has perpetuated the uncertainty regarding the adjuvant use of immunomodulatory agents, leaving few new leads on which to build.

Variable or Inadequate Follow-up

Although patients with stage IV (disseminated) melanoma generally have short median survival duration in the range of 7 to 9 months, patients with earlier-stage disease can have long disease-free intervals prior to relapse or recurrence. For this reason, an adequate length of patient follow-up to ensure that enough "events" (relapse or death from disease) occur is critical in adjuvant therapy trials. There are instances of melanoma trials that were initially reported as positive only to be reanalyzed later and re-reported as negative (8,9).

The methodologic problems previously described are present to some extent in virtually every trial reported to date. They make comparisons of trials difficult, even when the trials allegedly study similar interventions, and they preclude lending serious weight to the results of subset analyses. In the sections that follow, we provide an overview of the adjuvant trials conducted in melanoma to date, focusing on randomized, controlled trials that incorporate a no-treatment control arm, but also discussing new developments in antigen-specific therapy in detail. Generally, only the overall results of comparisons between the treatment arm and the control arm for disease-free survival (DFS) and survival are presented. Results of multiarm trials are considered separately for each treatment arm, recognizing that appropriate statistical adjustments for multiple comparisons may or more likely may not have been made. The reader is referred to the specified reference for more details about a particular trial.

NONSPECIFIC IMMUNOSTIMULANTS

Bacille Calmette-Guérin

Morton (10) demonstrated that intralesional injection of viable BCG organisms could lead to the regression of intradermal metastases of melanoma, a local therapy that still has clinical use today. Even more significantly, uninjected lesions occasionally regressed. This suggested that the human immune system could be primed to destroy distant melanoma and stimulated the conduct of clinical trials using BCG in the adjuvant setting. Although several nonrandomized trials using historic controls and two small randomized trials of intralesional or intralymphatic BCG showed a statistically significant benefit in favor of BCG (10,11), a number of other randomized trials failed to substantiate this benefit (12–21). Virtually all of these trials were small and employed heterogeneous populations of patients at intermediate and high risk of recurrence. A small randomized trial employing the methanol extracted residue of BCG was performed, and no beneficial effect of treatment was found (21).

Corynebacterium Parvum

Corynebacterium parvum is another micro-organism that nonspecifically stimulates the human immune system, and has been used as an adjuvant in murine antitumor vaccination studies. It has an advantage compared with BCG in that viable organisms are not required for adjuvant efficacy. Based on data from murine studies, adjuvant treatment with *C. parvum* has been compared with untreated controls in two studies, neither of which demonstrated a significant overall benefit for the therapy (22,23). *Corynebacterium parvum* was also compared directly with BCG (without an untreated control group) in two adjuvant trials. Lipton et al. (24) found a statistically significant DFS advantage for the subgroup of patients with positive nodes who were treated with *C. parvum*, but no such advantage for node-negative patients. Balch et al. (25) conducted a slightly larger trial and found a nonsignificant increase in median survival in favor of the BCG-treated patients. *Corynebacterium parvum* has never found widespread adoption as a therapeutic agent in melanoma or any other malignancy.

Levamisole

Levamisole is an antihelminthic agent for which various immunomodulatory properties have been reported (i). Four randomized, controlled trials of levamisole in melanoma have been conducted. In three of the four, no benefit for levamisole therapy was identified (5,27). In one study, a significant increase in 5-year survival was seen in favor of levamisole. This significance of this difference disappeared, however, in multivariate analysis, raising the possibility of an imbalance of prognostic factors rather than a true treatment effect (26).

Other Nonspecific Immunostimulants

Transfer factor, an extract of disrupted leukocytes thought to transfer delayed-type hypersensitivity and act as a nonspecific immunostimulant (28), was tested in two small randomized, controlled trials in melanoma without evidence of efficacy (29,30). Transfer factor has never found widespread adoption as a therapeutic agent in melanoma or any other malignancy. Isoprinosine, a mixture of inosine, acedoben, and dimepranol with putative immunostimulatory properties, has been tested in the adjuvant therapy of melanoma in several small randomized trials (31,32). A suggestion of improved DFS seen in one study was not confirmed in the other. A single small study of the thymic factor thymostimuline suggested a short-term advantage in disease-free and OS in favor of the treated group (33), but two other studies did not (34,35).

In conclusion, in the absence of a solid scientific rationale, the empiric use of nonspecific immunostimulants would not seem to be worth pursuing in the adjuvant therapy of melanoma.

ACTIVE SPECIFIC IMMUNOTHERAPY

Unlike the nonspecific immunostimulants previously described, active specific immunotherapy is mediated by vaccine reagents that elicit a specific host immune response to known or unknown tumor-associated antigens. To date, only a limited number of melanoma-associated antigens have been defined, and peptide or whole antigen vaccines have been developed for only a few of these, which will be discussed later. Few vaccine trials have been conducted that included as part of the study appropriate immune monitoring to verify that the desired immunologic surrogate end point had been achieved. The lack of no-treatment control arms has also complicated the interpretation of several studies.

Autologous Tumor Vaccines

Because few melanoma-associated antigens have been defined, and those few may not be present or may not be sufficiently immunogenic in a given individual to mediate tumor regression (i.e., a "tumor regression antigen"), a number of investigators have worked with autologous cellular tumor vaccines. This approach theoretically ensures that all biologically relevant antigens are available for presentation to the immune system. Of course, this approach is limited to individuals with sufficient tumor to prepare a vaccine, is predicated on tumor regression antigens being present at a sufficiently high concentration on the tumor cell surface with neither antigen down-modulation nor active suppression being present, and presumes that antigens on tumor cells are capable of presentation to immune cells. This has restricted melanoma adjuvant trials to patients with bulky nodal or resectable distant metastatic disease. Such patients have a poor overall prognosis and are likely to have significant residual tumor burden and tumor-related immune suppression, making them less than ideal candidates for any immunotherapeutic approach. Even then, only enough tumor is usually obtained to provide for a limited number of vaccinations. Furthermore, the technical complexities inherent in harvesting tumor and preparing a vaccine have, to date, precluded multi-institutional trials to formally test the efficacy of autologous tumor vaccines. Two small randomized trials (15 and 31 patients, respectively) comparing irradiated or neuraminidase-treated autologous tumor cells plus BCG to a control group found that the treatment group appeared to fare no better or perhaps even worse than the control group (36–38). In addition, a somewhat larger randomized, controlled trial of adjuvant therapy with autologous tumor cells plus BCG in renal cell carcinoma failed to show any evidence of benefit for vaccine treatment (39). A large compilation has been published that describes a total of 214 patients with stage III resected melanoma after lymphadenectomy and received multiple intradermal injections of an autologous, dinitrophenol-modified melanoma cell vaccine mixed with BCG. Four vaccine dosage schedules all included low-dose cyclophosphamide. Median survival was 44 months for this cohort of stage IIIB/IIIC patients. Survival and relapse correlated with delayed-type hypersensitivity (DTH) reactivity to modified and native tumor cells (40). These survival data are comparable with the control arms of prior IFN trials, as well as the control arm of the randomized Canvaxin trial described later, and in the absence of randomized data are difficult to interpret. Nonetheless, single-institution studies incorporating historic controls (41), as well as the potential of genetically modifying tumor cells to render them more immunogenic (42), continue to stimulate interest in this approach.

Allogenic Tumor Cell Vaccines

Specific immunotherapy has been evaluated as a therapy for melanoma for many years. Given the existence of spontaneous clinical remissions, the prognostic significance of lymphocytic infiltration in the primary lesion, and demonstrated objective tumor response with cytokines such as IFN and interleukin (IL)-2, investigators have explored vaccines as an immunologic approach to adjuvant therapy for melanoma (43). Allogeneic tumor cell vaccines, generally prepared from cultured cell lines or lysates, offer several important advantages over autologous vaccines: they are readily available, even for patients who lack sufficient tumor to produce an autologous tumor cell vaccine, and can be standardized, preserved, and distributed in a manner akin to any other pharmacologic or therapeutic agent, with specific potency tests and release criteria. This property allows for the use of multiple vaccinations over months or years and facilitates the performance of large-scale, multi-institutional clinical trials. The majority of trials that have been completed to date, however, have been small, single institution studies. None of these trials demonstrated an unequivocal benefit for immunotherapy with allogenic tumor cells administered in conjunction with BCG when compared with an untreated (44) or a BCG-treated control group (45).

Considerable uncertainty remains as to the optimal immunologic adjuvant to use in conjunction with an allogenic tumor cell vaccine, but there is reason to suspect that BCG may not be ideal (46,47). Also controversial is the role of immunomodulators given concomitantly with vaccination, most notably cyclophosphamide. Two randomized studies have been conducted in which allogenic melanoma vaccines were administered without or with cyclophosphamide given for 3 days prior to vaccination. The results of these studies have been conflicting, with one suggesting no detectable difference (48) and one suggesting a decrease in suppressor cell activity and augmented antibody response (49).

The SWOG has completed a large (>600 patients) randomized trial comparing an allogenic melanoma cell lysate (Melacine) coadministered with detoxified endotoxin/mycobacterial cell wall skeleton (DETOX), given without cyclophosphamide, to an untreated control group in patients with intermediate-thickness, node-negative melanoma (S9035). After a median follow-up of 4.1 years, 95 events, defined as recurrences or deaths, occurred among 300 eligible patients randomized to the vaccine versus 106 events among 300 eligible patients randomized to observation. When the entire randomized population of 689 patients was considered, there were 103 events among 346 patients randomized to the vaccine compared with 125 events among 343 patients assigned to observation. Tissue type played an important role in outcome; vaccine was more likely to be effective in patients who were A2-positive or C3-positive. With 553 of 689 (80%) patients serotyped for HLA class I antigens, a striking benefit of vaccine in terms of DFS was shown among those patients who expressed two or more of the five antigens; HLA-A2, -A28, -B44, -B45, and -C3 (referred to as M5). This effect was based predominantly on HLA-A2 and HLA-C3 expression. The HLA analyses were prospectively planned and were multivariate, adjusted for tumor thickness, site, ulceration, gender, and nodal staging method. Updated analysis with 15 months of additional follow-up (median, 5.6 years) also examined OS. Overall, there was no longer a significant advantage of vaccine treatment on outcome for the patient population as a whole (eligible or all randomized). However, among patients with two or more of M5, vaccine patients had a better DFS ($p = 0.0002$) and improved OS ($p = 0.001$). Among patients expressing HLA-A2 and/or HLA-C3, vaccine patients had a better DFS ($p = 0.004$) and improved OS ($p = 0.003$). This analysis further supports the association of HLA class I antigens with a benefit from Melacine (50).

Canvaxin, a polyvalent cell vaccine composed of a combination of allogenic cell lines, entered randomized phase III testing based on promising phase II data in resected stage II, III, and IV melanoma (51). Previously, in a single arm trial (52), Canvaxin was administered to 77 patients with resected high-risk stage IV melanoma, and correlates of relapse-free and OS were assessed. There was a significant correlation between OS and development of immunoglobulin (Ig) M antibodies directed against TA-90, a recently characterized tumor-associated glycoprotein on melanomas. In this analysis, TA-90 IgM levels correlated more strongly with outcome than DTH to the vaccine components, suggesting that TA-90 antibodies might be a new prognostic marker for patients with resected high-risk melanoma.

Unfortunately, recent presentation of data from interim analysis of separate randomized phase III trials comparing

Canvaxin with BCG to placebo with BCG in resected melanoma stage III and stage IV disease failed to show any progression-free or OS advantage (53). The median OS for resected stage IV patients who received Canvaxin was 31.5 months, and 38.7 months for patients who received placebo. The 5-year OS rate was 39.6% for patients receiving Canvaxin and 44.9% for patients who received placebo. The median and 5-year DFS for patients who received Canvaxin was 8.3 months and 27.4% versus 7.2 months and 20.9%, in the control arm. None of these results were statistically significantly different. For the trial of patients with resected stage III disease, in an interim analysis, the 5-year survival rate was 59.1% for patients taking Canvaxin and 67.7% for patients receiving placebo. Although Canvaxin did not show any survival advantage at 5 years, and in fact appeared to have an inferior survival rate to placebo plus BCG, the median survival in resected stage III (>5.75 years) and stage IV melanoma (38 months) in the placebo arm has established a contemporary standard for future clinical trials (53).

Viral Oncolysates

The allogenic vaccine trials previously cited incorporated an immunologic adjuvant to generate a sufficient local immune response so that priming of an immune response to tumor-associated antigens could occur. An alternative approach to allogenic vaccination involves the use of a virus to lyse the tumor cells prior to inoculation. In theory, the admixture of viral and tumor proteins should provoke an intense nonspecific immune response that would lead to recognition and rejection of tumor cells by the host. A pilot study of melanoma patients treated with Newcastle disease virus lysates of either autologous or allogenic tumor cells for 5 years suggested an improved survival compared with historic controls (54). This observation prompted two larger randomized trials using vaccinia viral lysates of allogenic tumor. One trial incorporated a control arm in which patients were treated with vaccinia virus alone, without tumor cells (6). The other trial used a no-treatment control arm (55). Both studies demonstrated no evidence of benefit for the vaccinia oncolysate treatment. Although it is possible that a small immunomodulatory effect of vaccinia virus by itself could have obscured the beneficial effect of the viral oncolysate in one trial, the negative results of the other trial suggest that this is not the case. The results of these two randomized trials, in such marked contrast to the beneficial effect seemingly found in a nonrandomized trial (6,55), emphasizes yet again the perils of relying on historic nonrandomized control groups in evaluating melanoma therapy (4).

DEFINED ANTIGEN VACCINES

In the last decade, a number of antigens present on melanoma cells that could potentially serve as targets for the human immune response have been identified and defined. Although all of these antigens may not be present on every tumor cell, as the number of defined antigens increases, the likelihood increases that at least one relevant antigenic target can be identified for every patient's melanoma. Still lacking, however, but in the process of development are reliable and reproducible methods for immunizing humans against each of these defined antigens, and

only one randomized clinical trial using a defined antigen vaccine has been completed to date (56).

Gangliosides

Gangliosides are a group of related glycolipids present on melanoma cells and some nonneoplastic cells (particularly neural tissues and granulocytes) (57–59). Ganglioside GD3, for example, is distributed widely on melanocytes, nevi, and practically all melanomas, as well as some normal tissues, and naturally occurring anti-GD3 antibodies are rare. Administration of a monoclonal antibody to GD3 (in conjunction with macrophage-colony stimulating factor) resulted in objective regressions of melanoma metastases (60). Ganglioside GM2 is expressed on a large percentage of melanoma tumors, is rarely detected on normal tissues, and about 5% of melanoma patients have naturally occurring anti-GM2 antibodies. Patients with antiganglioside antibodies (whether spontaneously occurring or secondary to therapy) appear to have a better prognosis than those without antibodies (61,62). Livingston et al. (61) conducted a small randomized trial comparing BCG with treatment with BCG plus purified GM2 ganglioside as adjuvant therapy for patients with node-positive melanoma. There was no significant survival difference between the two treatment arms. Interpretation was hampered by the small size of the trial and the fact that there was an imbalance between the two arms with respect to the number of patients with pre-existing anti-GM2 antibodies. Since the completion of that study, the investigators have focused on ways to increase the humoral response to GM2 vaccination. By conjugating the GM2 to the xenogeneic protein keyhole limpet hemocyanin and replacing the BCG with the saponin-derived adjuvant QS-21, they were able to achieve high levels of IgG and IgM anti-GM2 antibodies in a very high percentage of patients (56).

Another technique for stimulating an immune response to nonprotein antigens such as gangliosides is by administration of anti-idiotype antibodies. These "anti-antibodies" are antibodies raised against antiganglioside antibodies so that the variable regions of the antibody are essentially mirror images of the ganglioside itself, only composed of protein (63). When an immune response occurs to this mirror-image protein, it is also cross-reactive against the original antigen (64). To date, anti-idiotype antibodies have been produced against GD2 and GD3; these antibodies have undergone phase I and II testing and have been shown to be capable of generating high titers of anti-GD3 antibodies in patients with metastatic and resected melanoma. In a phase II trial in 47 patients with metastatic melanoma who received an anti-idiotype antibody with QS-21 adjuvant (65), anti-anti-idiotype or Ab3 was documented in 40 of 47 patients. One complete responder and 18 stable patients were noted. The same investigators went on to immunize 44 patients without evidence of disease after resection, and 42 patients developed high-titer Ab3. The anti-idiotype antibodies have not yet been subjected to testing in randomized trials (66,67).

HLA-Restricted Melanoma-Associated Antigenic Peptides

It is now recognized that T cells recognize antigenic peptides in an HLA-restricted manner, meaning that a given peptide must be presented to the T cell in the antigen-binding groove of that particular HLA molecule in order to stimulate an immune response (68,69). From a practical standpoint, this means that even if a tumor possesses a known tumor-regression antigen, the patient's HLA type will determine whether or not individual epitope peptides encoded by that antigen can be recognized. At present, a number of HLA-restricted melanoma-associated antigenic peptides have been defined, and vaccines are being constructed and tested in appropriate patients (70). Initial experiments with the HLA-A1 restricted MAGE-3 peptide EVDPIGHLY given in aqueous solution at low (100 to 300 mcg per injection) doses to 12 patients with metastatic melanoma indicated that 6 were able to complete 3 injections at monthly intervals, and 3 of the 6 had objective clinical responses (71). Surprisingly, no evidence of boosted T-cell immunity against MAGE-3 was detected in the peripheral blood.

The MART-1 27-35 and 26-35, tyrosinase 1-9 and 368-376, as well as several gp100 peptides (280-288 and 457-467) have been tested alone and in combination in patients with metastatic or resected melanoma. Jaeger and colleagues (72) immunized six metastatic melanoma patients intradermally with multiple peptides from MART-1, gp100, and tyrosinase in aqueous solution at 100 mcg each weekly for four immunizations. When granulocyte-macrophage colony-stimulating factor was injected at 75 mcg per dose subcutaneously as an adjuvant for 3 days prior to and 2 days after immunization with multiple antigen peptides, significant boosting of immune reactivity was seen compared with vaccination with peptides alone. Three of six patients showed increased immune reactivity to tyrosinase peptide 1-9, and one had increased reactivity to MART-1 26-35. In three evaluable patients, three objective clinical responses were seen, including two partial regressions in involved lymph nodal, cutaneous and liver lesions, and one complete regression in a patient with subcutaneous disease.

Cebon and colleagues (73) immunized patients with metastatic melanoma using intradermally administered MART-1 26-35 peptide with IL-12 in increasing doses given either subcutaneously or intravenously. The main toxicity of IL-12 by either route was flulike symptoms. Of the first 15 patients, one complete response, one partial response, and one mixed response, were noted. Immune assays for T-cell generation included DTH, which was seen in patients with or without IL-12. Positive cytotoxic T-lymphocyte (CTL) assays were seen in patients with evidence of clinical benefit, but not in patients without regression.

A number of small pilot studies have been conducted in which patients with metastatic melanoma received multiple subcutaneous injections of a single peptide emulsified with incomplete Freund's adjuvant (IFA) at 3-week intervals. MART-1 27-35, gp100 209-217, 154-162, and 280-288 have been used in these trials (74,75). In one study, escalating doses of the gp100 209 (ITDQVPSFY), 280 (YLEPGPVTA), or 154 (KTWGQYWQV) peptides at doses from 1 to 10 mg were administered subcutaneously every 3 weeks with IFA (76). Immune assays were performed using the previously mentioned "native" peptides for antigenic stimulation and substituted 209-2M (IMDQVPFSY) and 280-9V (YLEPGPVTV) peptides. Ninety percent to 100% of patients had strong evidence of boosted immune reactivity postvaccination as shown by an assay in which release of gamma IFN from peripheral blood mononuclear cells (PBMCs) restimulated 1 to 3 times in the presence of IL-2 and peptide antigen was measured by enzyme-linked immunosor-

bent assay. Seven of seven patients had boosted gp100 reactivity postvaccine after only one restimulation with the 209-2M peptide, and five of six patients were boosted with one restimulation with the 280-9V peptide. Higher release of cytokine was seen after four immunizations rather than two in most patients, and a greater level of reactivity was observed when substituted peptides were used in assays contrast with native peptides. Boosted cytokine release was shown to correlate with cytolytic responses. When tumor cell lines expressing the correct MHC restriction element and antigen were used as a stimulator in cytokine release assays, lower levels of cytokine were observed compared with T2 cells pulsed with the relevant peptide, suggesting that peptide density on the target was important for recognition by effector cells in PBMC. Objective partial and complete remissions were uncommon, with 1 of 20 patients having a complete regression. No clear correlation was observed between the level of immune response and the rare clinical responses, so no statement about clinical benefit could be made.

In a second study of escalating doses of the MART-1 27-35 peptide administered subcutaneously every 3 weeks with IFA, 15 of 16 patients had evidence of boosting of immunity directed against the native MART-1 27-35 peptide, with increased reactivity after 4 compared with fewer vaccinations (77). No objective clinical responses were seen. In an adjuvant study, 25 melanoma patients with high-risk resected stage III/IV disease were treated with increasing doses of the MART-1 27-35 peptide emulsified with IFA every 3 weeks subcutaneously (78). Ten of 22 patients had evidence of boosted immunity by cytokine release assays, and a correlation was observed between the absolute level of gamma IFN released after multiple restimulations of peptide-pulsed patient PBMCs postvaccination and time to relapse, with a *p* value of 0.003. The correlation of immune reactivity with time to relapse suggests that a positive response to peptide vaccination may incur clinical benefit.

The anchor amino acids that form hydrogen bonds between epitope peptides and class I MHC molecules can be modified to strengthen their binding, resulting in greater immunogenicity in vitro and in vivo. When such heteroclytic peptides derived from gp100 were used to restimulate PBMCs from patients with metastatic melanoma immunized with a wild type gp100 peptide, immune reactivity was detected with greater frequency and sensitivity (77). Patients immunized with the heteroclytic gp100 peptide demonstrated a higher level of immune reactivity compared with the wild type peptide. The MART-1 27-35 peptide has been shown to be "naturally" processed and is immunodominant. However, the MART-1 26-35 peptide has been shown to be a better MHC binder and more immunogenic in vitro (79), and was more effective at the detection and quantitation of MART-1–specific CTL in a flow cytometry assay when used for the generation of MHC/peptide tetramers (80). Heteroclytic gp100 peptides combined with IFA have been used to immunize patients with metastatic melanoma, and >90% of the patients in one vaccine study had evidence of boosted immunity detected after one restimulation in vitro, suggesting that the substituted peptide was more immunogenic than natural peptide in vivo (81). When the same substituted gp100 peptide was injected and followed within several days by high-dose intravenous IL-2, surprisingly no detectable augmented immune response was observed, but 13 of 31 patients had an antitumor response, including 12 partial responses and 1 complete response for an overall response rate of 42%, significantly greater than rates observed with IL-2 alone (15% to 20%) (81).

The utility of a peptide vaccination added to high-dose IL-2 as an "adjuvant" is being explored in two ongoing multicenter randomized trials. At our institution, the heteroclytic gp100 209-217 (210M) and tyrosinase 368-376 (370D) peptides emulsified in IFA with or without IL-12 as an adjuvant were examined in a randomized phase II trial in patients with high-risk resected stage III/IV melanoma in which immune response is one end point and time to relapse is the clinical end point, suggesting that multiple melanoma peptides injected simultaneously with adjuvant result in boosted immunity to both antigens in virtually all patients with resected high-risk melanoma. Whether IL-12 administration results in augmented skin test reactivity or increased antigen-specific immune responses measured by cytokine release or tetramer assays awaits a more detailed analysis. Thirty-four of 40 patients developed a positive skin test response to the gp100 peptide but none to tyrosinase. The data suggested that a significant proportion of patients with resected melanoma mounted antigen-specific immune response against a peptide vaccine and indicated that IL-12 may increase the immune response, supporting further development of IL-12 as a vaccine adjuvant (82).

IL-12, an immune stimulating cytokine, has also been subsequently tested with alum as an adjuvant in patients with stage IIB/III and IV resected melanoma receiving a multipeptide vaccine. Higher doses of IL-12 with alum induced a higher rate of immune response and prolonged time to recurrence in patients receiving a peptide vaccine. In that trial, time to recurrence was associated with immune response, supporting further development of IL-12 with alum as a vaccine adjuvant (83).

Slingluff et al. (84) have found that vaccination with multiple peptides in an emulsion of granulocyte-macrophage colony-stimulating factor in adjuvant was immunogenic, and that vaccination with the same peptides pulsed onto monocyte-derived immature dendritic cells was only weakly immunogenic. These data support continued investigation of vaccination with peptides administered in granulocyte-macrophage colony-stimulating factor as adjuvant. Another recent phase II trial was performed to assess the value of IL-2 as a systemic adjuvant to augment T-cell immune responses to a peptide vaccine in patients with stage IV melanoma. Patients receiving IL-2 prior to peptide dosing showed paradoxically diminished magnitude and frequency of cytotoxic T-lymphocyte responses to these peptides (85). It is difficult to define the best approach for future vaccine development, given the discouraging results from recent cellular vaccine trials. Only through continued clinical investigation of immune activation and suppression mechanisms in cancer can we hope to define promising adjuvants and vaccines.

MISCELLANEOUS AGENTS: HORMONES, COUMARIN, AND RETINOIDS

A small randomized, controlled trial using the progestational agent megestrol acetate (Megace) was conducted that demonstrated a trend for improved survival in favor of the treated group (86). Although this difference failed to achieve statistical significance, it prompted a larger-scale evaluation by the North Central Cancer Treatment Group in which adjuvant therapy with megestrol acetate oral suspension administered at a dose of 160 mg twice a day for 2 years was not found to be effective in prolonging progression-free survival or OS in patients with surgically resected, locally advanced melanoma. On the theory that differentiation agents might be useful in the adjuvant setting, several studies have compared retinoic acid or 13-cis-retinoic acid to observation (87,88). One additional trial compared BCG plus retinoic acid with BCG alone (80). All of these studies failed to demonstrate a benefit for the adjuvant use of retinoids. A study with 27 patients and using the anticoagulant coumarin (from which Coumadin is derived) revealed an increased DFS in the treated group (89).

SINGLE-AGENT CYTOTOXIC CHEMOTHERAPY

Single agents with recognized but modest activity against advanced disease include dacarbazine (DTIC), the nitrosoureas (carmustine [BCNU], lomustine [CCNU], and semustine [methyl-CCNU]), the vinca alkaloids (vincristine, vinblastine, and vindesine), cisplatin, paclitaxel, and bleomycin (90). Single-agent therapy with dacarbazine results in objective responses in about 18% to 22% of patients with measurable metastatic disease. Response durations are generally short, and durable complete responses are quite uncommon. Despite this modest activity, DTIC has been rather extensively evaluated in the adjuvant setting (91). These trials have provided no evidence that DTIC has significant efficacy as a postsurgical adjuvant. One multiarm trial incorporated single agent methyl-CCNU in one treatment arm. There was a nonsignificant trend in favor of the chemotherapy arm (92), but significant renal toxicity and the risk of treatment-induced myelodysplasia mitigated against further evaluation of this agent in the adjuvant setting.

MULTIAGENT CYTOTOXIC CHEMOTHERAPY

Multiagent chemotherapy has never been definitively documented to be superior to single-agent therapy when used for metastatic melanoma. A definitive phase III trial was performed under the auspices of the Eastern Cooperative Oncology Group (ECOG) to compare DTIC alone with the Dartmouth regimen of BCNU, CDDP, DTIC, and tamoxifen (7). There were 240 patients randomized to the trial, in which median survival for DTIC was 6.3 months compared with 7.7 months for the combination. There were no significant differences between the two groups in survival or response rate, suggesting that the Dartmouth regimen should no longer be used in the routine treatment of patients with metastatic melanoma. By default, DTIC remains the standard of care to which new experimental chemotherapies should be compared. Nonetheless, several adjuvant therapy trials have been conducted in which chemotherapy was combined with immunotherapy or where multiple cytotoxic agents were employed.

Adjuvant Chemoimmunotherapy

Several small trials have explored postoperative adjuvant therapy with DTIC plus BCG, with or without a no-treatment arm (93–96). DTIC plus BCG does not appear to have any efficacy in the adjuvant setting, hardly surprising in view of the lack of activity of the individual agents and the absence of any suggestion of synergy between them. DTIC with or without cyclophosphamide plus *C. parvum* also failed to prove to be superior to *C. parvum* alone (97) or to a no-treatment control group (98). BCG with or without *C. parvum* has been combined with DTIC-based multiagent chemotherapy in a few studies, all without a no-treatment control arm (99–102). No suggestion of benefit for chemoimmunotherapy was seen in these studies. Finally, a small randomized trial of DTIC plus IFN revealed no evidence of benefit compared with a no-treatment control group (103).

Adjuvant Biochemotherapy

The clinical benefit for adjuvant therapy with high-dose IFN (HDI) is currently hotly debated. Unfortunately, all other investigational options have failed to show significant clinical benefit as measured by consistent relapse-free or OS benefit. Given the improved response rates with biochemotherapy (BC) in the metastatic setting (104), this regimen was evaluated in a phase III randomized trial of adjuvant BC versus IFN-α-2b in resected stage III patients with high risk for melanoma recurrence. The primary end points were OS and relapse-free survival. In an interim analysis presented at the American Society for Clinical Oncology meeting in Atlanta in 2006, there were no significant differences in both relapse-free survival and OS between HDI and BC groups (105). Although there may be multiple reasons presented for the failure to see a difference, the complexity of this regimen and the inpatient therapy associated with BC render it difficult to give in the community setting. Further investigation with BC in the adjuvant setting may need to incorporate maintenance therapy. This approach has been noted to have a better median survival in metastatic melanoma in comparison to historic controls.

Adjuvant Multiagent Cytotoxic Therapy

Multiagent cytotoxic chemotherapy without immunotherapy has received relatively little attention in the postoperative adjuvant setting. Karakousis and Blumenson (106) found no benefit for the combination of DTIC and estramustine in a small, three-arm study comparing multiagent chemotherapy or BCG to a no-treatment control group. Four two-arm, randomized controlled trials of multiagent chemotherapy have been done. A trial using BCNU, dactinomycin, and vincristine (107), and a small trial of DTIC, CCNU, and vincristine (108) both suggested a benefit for multiagent chemotherapy, while two other trials did not (109). Interestingly, no adjuvant trials have been performed to date with cisplatin-containing combinations, although recent data previously discussed in which a combination chemotherapy regimen failed to demonstrate a survival advantage over single-agent dacarbazine render any such adjuvant trials premature.

Preoperative (Neoadjuvant) Chemoimmunotherapy

Preoperative chemotherapy has become commonplace in the treatment of some tumor types, but has not found widespread application in melanoma. Nonetheless, patients with bulky nodal disease, resectable metastatic disease, and noncutaneous primary melanomas (such as anorectal melanomas) would be logical candidates for a preoperative approach aimed at shrinking the tumor and assessing in vivo chemosensitivity. A number of recent nonrandomized phase II studies have revealed high response rates (40% to 65%) in patients with metastatic melanoma to chemoimmunotherapy regimens with cisplatin, Velban, dacarbazine, IL-2, and IFN-α (110,111). A similar regimen including cisplatin, vinblastine, and DTIC administered concurrently with IL-2 and IFN-α (112) has shown a 44% response rate used preoperatively, suggesting a possible role for this neoadjuvant approach. Patients who are candidates for this type of therapy, however, are also candidates for autologous tumor vaccines as well as postoperative IFN-α on cooperative group trials. Thus, the precise role of preoperative chemoimmunotherapy will need to be defined in a prospective, randomized relative to these other approaches.

Intensive Chemotherapy with Autologous Bone Marrow Support

A limited experience has been accumulated with autologous marrow support following intensive chemotherapy for metastatic melanoma. Although intensive chemotherapy for metastatic melanoma has not found widespread use, one small randomized trial was conducted in patients with multiple involved lymph nodes (113). No advantage for the treatment group was found. Of interest was the high frequency of local/regional recurrence in this study, doubtless reflective of the high regional disease burden of eligible patients.

INTERFERONS AND OTHER CYTOKINES

Although their precise antitumor effects remain poorly understood, no agents have been more intensively studied in melanoma than the interferons. This has resulted in multiple adjuvant trials involving these agents. Other cytokines, such as the interleukins and tumor necrosis factor-α, have also undergone detailed evaluations, but as yet have received limited attention in the adjuvant setting.

Interferon Gamma

The immunologic activities of IFN-γ have been extensively characterized, including studies in melanoma patients (114–117). These studies provided a compelling rationale for the use of IFN-γ in the adjuvant treatment of melanoma (118). A randomized trial of the SWOG, however, failed to indicate any benefit for adjuvant treatment with an immunologically active dose of IFN-γ in patients at intermediate and high risk of recurrence (119). The results of this trial were disclosed early because of a suggestion that the treatment arm actually fared worse than the control arm (120), prompting the National Cancer Institute of

Canada to close its adjuvant therapy trial comparing levamisole and IFN-γ. A total of 89 patients were entered onto this study when it was closed; there was no apparent difference in DFS or OS between the two groups (121). From 1988 to 1996, a total of 830 patients were randomized in the European Organization for Research and Treatment of Cancer Melanoma Group (EORTC-MG) prospective, randomized phase III adjuvant trial to evaluate the efficacy and toxicity of low dose recombinant IFN-α-2b (rIFN-alpha2b) (1 MU) or recombinant IFN-γ (rIFN-gamma) (0.2 mg), both given subcutaneously, every other day, for 12 months in comparison with an untreated control group. The German Cancer Society (DKG) added a fourth arm with Iscador M, a popular mistletoe extract. High-risk stage II patients (lesions of thickness >3 mm) and stage III patients (those with positive lymph nodes) without distant metastasis were treated until their first progression or death. At median follow-up of 8.2 years, a total of 537 relapses and 475 deaths were reported. At 8 years, the disease-free interval rate was 32.4% and the OS rate was 40.0%. In terms of OS, the corresponding estimates for the three treatment comparisons were: IFN-alpha2b, 0.96 (95% confidence interval [CI]: 0.76–1.21); rIFN-gamma, 0.87 (95% CI: 0.69–1.10); and Iscador M 1.21 (95% CI: 0.84–1.75). There was no clinical benefit for adjuvant treatment with low-dose rIFN-alpha2b or rIFN-gamma or with Iscador M in high-risk melanoma patients. Given the long list of favorable immunologic effects associated with IFN-γ, the lack of efficacy is difficult to explain but should prompt a rethinking of the widely held tenet that immunologic agents that lack activity in metastatic disease are appropriate candidates for evaluation in the adjuvant setting (122).

Interferon Alfa

Unlike IFN-γ, IFN-α does possess a significant degree of activity against metastatic melanoma (123), in addition to a broad range of immunologic effects (124). These properties have prompted a number of studies of IFN-α in the adjuvant setting. These trials have employed varying doses, routes of administration, durations of therapy, and risk groups, making comparisons all but impossible. Nonetheless, on closer inspection some patterns have emerged.

One nonrandomized trial evaluated a low-dose IFN-α regimen (2 to 3 MU subcutaneously twice or thrice weekly) administered for 20 months to patients at intermediate risk of recurrence. This study suggested an early increase in DFS compared with historic controls who disappeared once therapy was stopped (125). Whether this represented a true biologic effect of IFN therapy or not is impossible to determine in a nonrandomized trial, but this observation has nonetheless prompted concerns about the duration of IFN treatment in the adjuvant setting. The World Health Organization looked at a similar low-dose regimen (3 MU subcutaneously thrice weekly) administered for 3 years to patients with positive nodes in a randomized trial that has been showed no benefit in terms of either relapse-free or OS compared to observation (126,127). Several interim analyses had been published or presented, initially with a suggestion of significant benefit (128) and later without (129). The mature results of this trial do not indicate a prolongation of survival for patients with stage III resected disease, nor do they shed light onto whether there is indeed a "rebound" effect after IFN treatment is discontinued.

A different approach was taken by Creagan et al. (130) and the North Central Cancer Treatment Group in a randomized trial of patients at intermediate and high risk of recurrence. In this study, patients on the treatment arm received a 3-month course of high-dose (20 MU/m^2) IFN-α2a administered intramuscularly. Overall, there was no significant difference in outcome between the treatment and control arms. Patients in the high-risk group (involved nodes), however, had an increased DFS (40% vs. 30% alive and well at 5 years) that reached statistical significance when adjusted for prognostic factors. OS was also better in the node-positive patients who received IFN-α2a (47% vs. 39% alive at 5 years), but not significantly so. No benefit was detected for the node-negative patients on this trial. The relatively small size of the study (262 patients overall, 160 node-positive patients) severely limited the power to detect a significant treatment effect, and makes any conclusions about subset effects tenuous at best, but suggested that higher doses of IFN may be beneficial.

Like Creagan et al. (130), Kirkwood et al. (1) chose to employ a very high dose of IFN, this time IFN-α2b, but for a longer interval (1 year), in a randomized controlled trial for ECOG. Both node-positive and high-risk node-negative (T4N0M0) patients were included; the majority of patients had relapsed in the regional nodes after prior wide excision. The regimen involved an initial "induction" phase of 20 MU/m^2 intravenously 5 days a week for 4 weeks and was followed by a "maintenance" phase of 10 MU/m^2 subcutaneously 3 days a week for 11 months. This regimen was deliberately chosen to be at or near the maximally tolerated dose, and indeed was quite toxic. Treatment was reduced or discontinued in over half the patients, and there were two treatment-related deaths. The overall results, however, were positive: patients randomized to receive IFN-α2b had a significant 33% improvement in DFS and a 27% improvement in OS compared with the control group. There was no evidence of an increased relapse rate after the IFN-α2b treatment ended, indeed the results demonstrated a plateau of increased long-term survival. One observation was similar to the NCCTG trial: the beneficial effect was confined to node-positive patients. Indeed, in the small subset of node-negative patients (accounting for about 11% of the 280 total patients), the group randomized to receive IFN-α2b actually fared worse. The small size of this subset, and the presence of an imbalance between the treatment and control arms in the percentage of patients with ulcerated primaries, makes it impossible to determine whether there is truly a difference in the response of node-positive and node-negative patients to IFN treatment. Despite the lack of a mature confirmatory trial, the FDA approved the use of adjuvant high-dose IFN-α2b for melanoma patients who are 18 years or older and free of disease "at high risk of recurrence" in December 1995. That the results of a quality-adjusted time without symptoms or toxicity (Q-TWiST) analysis, confirmed the benefit of IFN-α2b therapy even after accounting for its significant toxicity (131) and also played a role in the FDA decision. This analysis was done retrospectively, without prospective collection of quality of life data from participants in the original ECOG trial, but still provides a basis for assuring patients that the significant toxicity of therapy appears justified. One additional reservation must be stated regarding the ECOG trial: patients were not evaluated for a recognized prognostic factor, the number of positive lymph nodes. Hence, it is possible that there was an unrecognized imbalance between the treatment and control groups of node-positive patients that could have influenced the outcome (2).

A confirmatory study was conducted as an ECOG-coordinated Intergroup trial, with accrual completed in June 1995. Patients were grouped prior to randomization into eight strata based on American Joint Committee on Cancer stage of disease at randomization and by number of involved lymph nodes (0, 1, 2 to 3, and ≥4). They were then randomized within each stratum to treatment with high-dose IFNα-2b (HDI) for 1 year, low-dose IFN-α-2b (LDI) for 2 years, or observation. HDI was similar to ECOG 1684 and LDI was 3 MIU/day subcutaneously 3 times a week (132). In E1690, data were gathered from 642 patients from February 1991 to June 1, 1995, and the analyzed database was current to September 1998. The initial analysis was performed at a median follow-up of 52 months (4.3 years). In contrast to E1684, patients with T4 (Breslow depth >4 mm) primary lesions and no clinical evidence of lymph node metastasis (T4cN0) were not required to undergo lymphadenectomy based on the absence of any survival benefit associated with elective lymph node dissection in four randomized trials. The demographics of E1690 differ from those of E1694 in the distribution of patients with pN1 and cN1 lesions, and a higher proportion of patients with recurrent nodal disease. At 52 months of follow-up, the median relapse-free survival in patients treated with HDI was 2.4 years, compared with 1.6 years for patients in the observation arm (7). In the HDI group, the estimated 5-year relapse-free survival was 44% compared with 35% in the observation arm ($p_2 = 0.054$; $p = 0.025$) in the intention-to-treat (ITT) analysis, a 28% greater risk of recurrence for the observation group compared with the HDI group; however, the difference in relapse-free survival between the HDI and observation groups was not statistically significant. Treatment with LDI was associated with a somewhat smaller relapse-free survival benefit than HDI when compared with observation, but did not reach statistical significance.

Interestingly, interstudy improvement for the control arm was seen with a p value <0.001, suggesting that therapy in general, staging criteria, and supportive care had improved since the 1980s. Relapse-free survival time was clearly prolonged as in the prior E1684 study, but the time from relapse to death in the control arm significantly increased, resulting in no survival difference. The explanation for this has been debated with no clear-cut answer, but it was intriguing that patients who relapsed on the observation arm were more commonly treated with HDI or chemobiotherapy than patients on the treatment arms, which may account for the improvement in survival between the two studies.

The third in a series of IFN adjuvant trials was ECOG 1694/SWOG 9512 in which 774 patients were allocated randomly to receive the EST 1684 1-year regimen of IFN or 96 weeks of a vaccine called GM2-KLH/QS-21 (GMK), which generates antiganglioside antibodies, in patients with resected stage IIB-III melanoma. The trial was stopped prematurely by the data safety monitoring board because relapse-free survival in the IFN arm was clearly superior to that in the vaccine arm in a planned interim analysis. Among the total of 774 eligible patients, 151

of 389 patients treated with GMK (39%) and 98 of 385 patients treated with IFN-α-2b (25%) experienced relapse. The hazard ratio for relapse for patients treated with IFN-α-2b decreased by nearly 50% compared with those treated with GMK in both the analysis of all eligible patients and the ITT analysis (p <0.0015). OS was also greater in the IFN-α-2b group, with 52 deaths compared with 81 deaths in the GMK group. There was a 52% increase in the hazard of death for eligible patients treated with GMK compared with those treated with IFN-α-2b, again in both the analysis of all eligible patients and the ITT analysis (p <0.023). Median relapse-free survival was 22.5 months for the GMK group, but was not reached in the IFN-α-2b group. Median OS was not reached in either arm. The estimated 2-year relapse-free survival rates for the IFN-α-2b and GMK groups were 62% and 49%, respectively, and the respective estimated 2-year OS rates for the IFN-α-2b and GMK groups were 78% and 73% (133).

On review, 2-year relapse-free survival rates in the HDI groups from the analyses of the eligible populations in trials E1684, E1690, and E1694 indicates that relapse-free survival improved with each successive trial (48%, 52%, and 62%, respectively). This can be attributed to differences in the study populations. Trials E1690 and E1694 had a higher proportion of node-negative patients (25% and 23%, respectively) compared with E1684 (11%) and a smaller percentage of patients with recurrent disease (51% and 36%, respectively) compared with E1684 (61%). Another major difference among the trials is the subset of patients who gained the greatest relapse-free survival benefit. In E1694, the greatest benefit was observed in node-negative patients. In E1684, the greatest relapse-free survival benefit was derived by patients with one positive lymph node, and in E1690, patients with two to three positive nodes derived the greatest relapse-free survival benefit, suggesting that relapse-free survival benefit may be independent of disease stage. This improvement was similar for OS. OS rates were 63%, 71%, and 77%, respectively, in the E1684, E1690 and E1694 trials.

Wheatley et al. (134) recently reviewed 14 comparisons of IFN alfa in 12 randomized, controlled clinical trials in a recent meta-analysis. Four studies evaluated HDI or IFN-α-2a, with or without vaccine therapy, compared with observation. These were the ECOG 1684 trial, Intergroup E-1690 trial (which also evaluated LDI), and the North Central Cancer Treatment Group and ECOG 2696 trials. Analyses of data from the four studies of HDI demonstrated a 26% reduction in the risk of recurrence when compared with control, a two-sided p value of 0.00009. When the high-dose arms of the three ECOG/Intergroup trials were examined, mortality was reduced by 15%, a two-sided p value of 0.06. The EORTC 18952 trial compared intermediate-dose IFN-α-2b and observation for 1- and 2-year study periods. Six studies compared LDI or IFN-α-2b with observation: the WHO-16 trial, the low-dose arm of the Intergroup E-1690 trial, and the United Kingdom Coordinating Committee on Cancer Research Adjuvant in Melanoma (AIM), French Centre de Génétique Moléculaire (CGM), Austrian Malignant Melanoma Cooperative Group (MMCG), and Scottish Melanoma Group (MG) trials. Very low doses of IFN-α-2b were compared with observation in the EORTC 18871 and DKG-80 trials. Significant trend for dose-dependent effect on recurrence-free survival with increasing doses of IFN-α was seen ($p = 0.02$) (134).

High-dose IFN is the standard of care in patients with resected stage III melanoma against which other regimens should be measured. Updated results from E1694 for OS continue to support a benefit for HDI. However, these data must be interpreted cautiously in light of a recent review of the long-term data from the EST 1684 and 1690 trials. At a median follow-up of 12.6 years, the survival benefit previously seen in that trial was lost, although there remained a significant difference in relapse-free survival with $p = 0.006$ (135). In contrast, an encouraging note stems from a recent multicenter pilot study through ECOG in which patients were randomly assigned to receive HDI for 1 year or IFN plus a GM2 vaccine (136). The results of this trial indicated that no diminution in antibody responses to the vaccine was seen with concurrent HDI, suggesting that as new vaccine strategies are developed, they may be added to the existing standard IFN-α regimen with a reasonable chance that the vaccine-induced immune response will not be diminished.

Confounding Factors

Intergroup trial E1690 demonstrated that HDI therapy was associated with a relapse-free survival advantage. Neither HDI nor LDI therapy demonstrated a benefit for OS compared with observation in this study; however, salvage of regional recurrences with IFN-α–containing regimens may have confounded the survival analysis. Relapse occurred in 114 patients in the HDI group and 121 in the observation group. Similar proportions of patients in each group received chemotherapy, surgery, radiation therapy, or no treatment at relapse. However, the proportion of patients in the observation group that received an IFN-α–containing salvage regimen (31%) was significantly larger than that in the HDI group (15%; $p = 0.003$). Twice as many patients in the observation group as in the HDI group (21% vs. 10%) received HDI therapy (i.e., 10 MIU/m^2 subcutaneously three times a week [TIW]) at relapse. Similarly, a greater proportion of patients in the observation group than in the HDI group (17% vs. 6%) were treated with a biochemotherapy regimen ($p = 0.013$). There were no substantial differences between the HDI and observation groups in the proportion of patients who received an IL-2–containing regimen either as single-agent or combination therapy. A Kaplan-Meier estimate of OS for subgroups of patients in the HDI and observation groups demonstrated that an IFN-α–containing salvage regimen provided a postrelapse survival advantage for patients in the observation group. Compared with the median survival of 0.8 years for the 83 patients in the observation group who relapsed, median survival was 2.2 years for the 23 patients who were treated with an IFN-α–containing postrelapse regimen ($p = 0.0024$). The hazard ratio for this comparison was 2.13 (95% CI: 1.29-3.53). The assumption in this analysis is that patients in the observation group who received IFN-α–containing salvage therapy were clinically comparable at relapse to those who did not. A Cox regression analysis was performed to determine whether prognostic factors such as age, sex, performance status, ulceration, disease stage, and number of positive nodes at randomization differed between patients in the observation group who did or did not receive IFN-α–containing salvage therapy. After adjusting for these variables, only salvage therapy with an IFN-α–containing regimen had a meaningful effect on survival, with a hazard ratio of 2.14. Furthermore, the median time from randomization to initial relapse for the 38 patients in the observation group who received IFN-α–containing salvage therapy was 0.9 years, not substantially different from the median relapse-free survival of 0.5 years for the 83 patients who relapsed but did not receive IFN-α.

These data suggest that IFN-α–containing salvage therapy may account for the prolonged postrelapse survival of the 38 patients in the observation group who received it. Indeed, 17 of these patients received adjuvant IFN-α therapy for resectable regional relapse that was indistinguishable from the setting in which the original E1684 trial tested the role of IFN-α. For patients in the HDI group who relapse, however, there was no apparent survival advantage associated with IFN-α–containing salvage therapy; however, the number of patients in the HDI arm who received IFN-α–containing therapy postrelapse was small (n = 17) (136). These data may suggest that IFN could be used up front as an adjuvant therapy or delayed until nodal relapse with equal utility.

The assumption in this analysis is that patients in the observation group who received IFN-α–containing salvage therapy were clinically comparable at relapse to those who did not. A Cox regression analysis was performed to determine whether prognostic factors such as age, sex, performance status, ulceration, disease stage, and number of positive nodes at randomization differed between patients in the observation group who did or did not receive IFN-α–containing salvage therapy. After adjusting for these variables, only salvage therapy with an IFN-α–containing regimen had a meaningful effect on survival, with a hazard ratio of 2.14. Furthermore, the median time from randomization to initial relapse for the 38 patients in the observation group who received IFN-α–containing salvage therapy was 0.9 years, not substantially different from the median relapse-free survival of 0.5 years for the 83 patients who relapsed but did not receive IFN-α. These data suggest that IFN-α–containing salvage therapy may account for the prolonged postrelapse survival of the 38 patients in the observation group who received it. Indeed, 17 of these patients received adjuvant IFN-α therapy for resectable regional relapse that was indistinguishable from the setting in which the original E1684 trial tested the role of IFN-α.

NeoAdjuvant Interferon Therapy

A subset of patients may benefit from briefer IFN regimens after resection of high-risk melanoma, but that group has not yet been defined. Because of the significant morbidity associated with adjuvant HDI therapy, the role for neoadjuvant IFN therapy in melanoma has expanded in an effort to identify subgroups that would benefit from continued maintenance therapy. Moschos et al. (137) treated 20 patients with stages IIIB and IIIC disease with a month of HDI using the EST 1684 regimen. In that group of patients, biopsy samples were informative for 17, with 55% demonstrating an objective clinical response and 15% with a complete pathologic response. At a median follow-up of 18.5 months (range, 7 to 50 months) ten patients had no evidence of recurrent disease. Clinical responders had significantly greater increases in immune response. Although encouraging, this trial was underpowered to define the role of clinical response at 4 weeks as a surrogate marker for OS.

IFN-α has also been investigated at lower dosages as part of a neoadjuvant biochemotherapy regimen for patients with stage III melanoma with clinical response rates of approximately 40% and pathologic response in 10% of patients (138,139). In a trial of 92 patients with stage III melanoma, the overall response rate was 26% (140). The toxicity of the biochemotherapy regimen was high but manageable. At a median follow-up of 40.4 months, relapse-free survival and OS were 64% and 78%, respectively. There was a lower relapse rate and improved survival for patients with a positive sentinel lymph node compared with patients with clinically detected lymph nodes, although this difference did not reach statistical significance. An Intergroup trial (SWOG trial 0008) currently is evaluating a similar regimen of three postoperative courses of biochemotherapy versus HDI in patients with resected stage III disease and two or more positive nodes. It is hoped that this trial will clarify the role of a biochemotherapy regimen as adjuvant therapy in stage III melanoma.

Low-Dose Interferon

A number of randomized, controlled studies have evaluated lower doses of IFN-α-2b (LDI) for intermediate- and high-risk resected melanoma. LDI administered for 2 to 3 years had no effect in high-risk melanoma, induced a transient delay in relapse for intermediate-risk melanoma, and provided no survival benefit in intermediate and high-risk disease (141–144). The negative results of these trials of LDI were confirmed in the AIM HIGH trial; the largest single randomized controlled study of LDI published to date (145). The EORTC trial 18952 tested "intermediate" doses of IFN-α-2b given for 1 or 2 years. At 3 years' median follow-up, there was neither an OS nor relapse-free survival benefit for the two intermediate dosages of 5 MU 3 times per week (5 MU/m^2) and 10 MU 3 times per week administered subcutaneously, both for 2 years (145). These trials confirm the importance of initial high-dose therapy and put into question the lower dose maintenance portion of therapy, which is now standard.

Interleukin 2 and Other Cytokines

Besides IFN-α, IL-2 is the only other cytokine that has documented efficacy in advanced disease, an indication for which it was approved by the FDA. Unfortunately, significant toxicity has precluded evaluation of this agent in the adjuvant setting. The National Cancer Institute attempted to conduct an adjuvant trial of high-dose IL-2 in patients at extremely high risk of recurrence (ten or more involved lymph nodes), but even in this poor prognosis group the severe toxicity of treatment led to premature closure of the study. There are currently insufficient data to justify the use of other cytokines in the systemic adjuvant therapy of melanoma patients.

CTLA-4 INHIBITION AND T-CELL ACTIVATION

CTL antigen-4 (CTLA-4) is a molecule on T cells thought to be of primary importance in maintaining immune homeostasis and the induction of tolerance to self-antigens (146). Its effects are mediated through inhibitory T-cell signaling and blockade of the CD28-B7 costimulatory pathway. Knockout of the *CTLA-4* gene in mice leads to a lymphoproliferative syndrome and subsequent lymphocytic tissue infiltration and destruction. Ipilimumab (MDX-010), a human anti-CTLA-4 antibody shown to have clinical activity in melanoma and renal cancer, is associated with inflammatory-type adverse events termed *immune breakthrough events* (IBEs) (147–149). When given to patients with metastatic melanoma MDX-010 has approximately a 15% response rate with prolonged remissions. Work in mice showed that CTLA-4 abrogation with an antibody can augment immunity to a vaccine and cause regression of established tumors. In trials of MDX-010 with a peptide vaccine combined with adjuvant Montanide ISA 51, Sanderson et al. (150) have shown both immune responses and the occurrence of IBEs. The occurrence of IBEs is associated with prolonged time to relapse in patients with resected high-risk melanoma receiving MDX-010, and patients with certain CTLA-4 polymorphisms can have a higher rate of IBEs and lower chance of recurrence. Prolonged remissions have been observed with MDX-010 (151). A similar anti-CLA-4 antibody from Pfizer, Tremelimumab, has also shown antitumor responses in melanoma that are associated with IBEs (152). Phase II trials of CTLA-4 antibodies alone or with vaccine are ongoing as adjuvant therapy in pilot trials of patients with high risk melanoma.

REGIONAL ADJUVANT THERAPY

Not all adjuvant therapy needs be administered systemically; regional treatments have also been extensively evaluated in melanoma. Elective lymph node dissection can be considered an "adjuvant" to wide excision of the primary tumor; the results of clinical trials evaluating node dissections are discussed elsewhere in this book. The two other techniques for increasing regional control that have been evaluated in melanoma include external-beam radiation therapy and hyperthermic isolation limb perfusion.

External-Beam Radiation Therapy

Radiation therapy has traditionally had a very limited role in the management of melanoma, primarily confined to treatment of central nervous system metastases (153). There is reason to suspect, however, that adjuvant treatment with radiation can decrease recurrence after lymph node dissection (154). Surprisingly, only one small randomized trial of adjuvant radiotherapy has been completed in cutaneous melanoma, and this yielded a negative result (155). This study used conventional radiation fractions and a treatment break, both currently thought to be suboptimal for melanoma. A small nonrandomized phase II study of adjuvant radiation therapy delivered in large fractions to patients with lymph nodal melanoma in the neck suggested a very favorable survival and time to relapse compared with historic controls. Based on these promising phase II data, the Radiation Therapy Oncology Group initiated a randomized trial of postoperative irradiation using larger treatment fractions in patients undergoing neck dissections for melanoma. Accrual to this trial has been poor, however, and the approval of IFN-α as adjuvant therapy further jeopardized its success, resulting in the trial being modified to include IFN-α treatment for all randomized patients. Accrual to the trial has been suspended. Nonetheless, it remains clear that patients with multiple lymph nodes involved with melanoma are at great risk of regional and distant recurrence, especially with extranodal extension. Such patients could potentially benefit from an integrated strategy involving both IFN and radiotherapy. Preliminary studies are necessary to define the optimal scheduling of these two modalities, but if these can be conducted, a randomized trial comparing IFN alone with IFN plus radiation for melanoma patients with multiple involved nodes would seem to be worthwhile. Adjuvant radiation therapy is also being evaluated in the management of ocular melanoma, in a multicenter collaborative trial (156).

Hyperthermic Isolation Limb Perfusion

Extremity isolation limb perfusion is conducted as a surgical procedure under general anesthesia, by cannulating the main artery and vein to the arm or leg and diverting the blood flow in that extremity through a cardiac surgery bypass oxygenation apparatus. Tourniquets are applied to effectively isolate the entire limb from the systemic circulation, and antineoplastic agents are then introduced into the bypass circuit, perfusing the limb but not the systemic circulation. The temperature of the perfusate can be adjusted, and most perfusions are carried out at elevated temperatures (39°C to 41.5°C). The most commonly used drug for perfusion has been melphalan (157), but cisplatin, dactinomycin, and most recently tumor necrosis factor-α with or without IFN-γ (158) have also been used. Although hyperthermic isolation limb perfusion with any of these agents induces a high rate of objective remissions in patients with measurable cutaneous ("in transit") metastases, response durations are typically short and these patients generally succumb to distant disease regardless of whether or not local control is achieved.

Isolation limb perfusion has been evaluated in the adjuvant setting, with the goal of reducing in transit recurrences. Trial design has been hampered by the difficulty in defining a patient population at high enough risk of cutaneous recurrence who do not also have a prohibitively high risk of developing distant metastases. Several suggestive retrospective reviews led to two small randomized trials, which showed evidence of an overall or DFS benefit for adjuvant isolation limb perfusion with melphalan (159,160). This prompted a large randomized international, Intergroup trial of adjuvant limb perfusion (over 700 patients). Final results revealed no evidence of a survival or DFS benefit for melphalan perfusion (161). Hence, once again retrospective studies and small randomized trials suggested a benefit that was not confirmed in a well-designed, appropriately powered randomized study. Given the technical complexity, risks, and lack of demonstrated benefit of this adjuvant therapy, its further routine use as adjuvant therapy for patients with resected in-transit limb melanoma should not be considered. Whether the availability of new perfusion therapies such as tumor necrosis factor-α will lead to a rethinking of this position remains to be seen. If so, any future adjuvant trials should probably be confined to patients with primary tumors at very high risk of local/regional recurrence (i.e., thick primaries with ulceration, satellitosis, or extensive angiolymphatic spread and/or patients with completely resected local or in-transit recurrences).

SUMMARY AND FUTURE CONSIDERATIONS

Who is an appropriate candidate for systemic adjuvant therapy?

Metastatic malignant melanoma remains a highly lethal disease; hence, the prevention of its development is a clinical priority. Of the myriad of agents tested over the years, IFN-α-2b was the only one to gain FDA approval on the basis of a survival advantage, albeit in a single but well-designed phase III randomized trial. A confirmatory trial (ECOG 1690/SWOG9111) did not confirm this benefit, but ECOG 1694 study suggests that it must be considered to be a standard treatment for patients for whom adjuvant therapy is prescribed. But what should patients do who have indeterminate and high risk of disease recurrence?

- *Resected stage III melanoma:* Otherwise healthy patients should be offered entry to randomized clinical trials comparing new approaches to adjuvant therapy such as vaccines or other biologics with or without HDI. These patients should be given a clear understanding of the relapse-free and OS benefit and toxicity of therapy. A discussion of the results of the Q-TWiST analysis of the E1684 trial, the developments in the confirmatory three-arm trial, as well as the prematurely halted ECOG 1694/SWOG 9512 trial is often a helpful exercise in allowing prospective patients to weigh the toxic costs of therapy against the possible gains in freedom from relapse and OS. Patients with multiple (ten or more) involved lymph nodes, extracapsular invasion, or other risk factors for regional recurrence should also be considered for concomitant adjuvant external-beam radiation with large fractions. Substantive questions remain about the use and proper scheduling of adjuvant radiation that are worthy of a large-scale clinical trial. If patients are to receive HDI, one common practice is to initiate radiation therapy in these patients after the completion of the 1 month of intravenous IFNα-2b concomitant with the start of subcutaneous therapy. Patients with bulky nodal disease should be strongly considered for investigations of neoadjuvant chemoimmunotherapy or combination therapy with tumor vaccines.

- *Resected stage IV melanoma:* Resection of isolated melanoma metastases remains the best option for curative treatment of metastatic melanoma in those few individuals amenable to this therapy. It should be offered to eligible patients whenever possible. Referral of these patients to treatment centers where aggressive surgery and investigational protocols are available is advocated. These patients should be strongly considered for investigations of adjuvant chemoimmunotherapy or novel combination therapy or phase II peptide or antigen-specific vaccine trials. Off protocol, adjuvant therapy with two to three cycles of chemoimmunotherapy or the use of HDI if administered with careful informed consent is acceptable, given the extremely high risk of relapse in this patient population.

- *Resected stage IIB melanoma:* Patients with thick ($\geq$4.0 mm) primary tumors, especially if ulcerated, and clinically or pathologically negative lymph nodes ideally should be considered for participation in clinical trials assessing vaccines and other biologic therapies. This approach is justified by the high risk of recurrence combined with the equivocal benefit for

IFNα-2b in this subgroup. Given the high risk of occult nodal involvement in these patients, lymphatic mapping and selective lymph node dissection should be employed when possible, and patients with pathologically positive nodes treated as outlined for stage III patients, as there was a benefit for IFN-α seen in this subgroup in the most recently completed EST 1694 trial.

- *Resected stage IIA melanoma:* Patients with intermediate-thickness primary tumors and clinically or pathologically negative lymph nodes are not candidates for adjuvant therapy with the 1-year regimen of HDI, but are at sufficient risk of relapse to justify participation in clinical trials incorporating a no-treatment control. Experimental approaches appropriate for this group might include brief HDI regimens as is being tested by ECOG, and defined antigens such as peptides, vector, or protein approaches. Given the moderate risk of occult nodal involvement in patients with intermediate thickness primary melanomas, lymphatic mapping and selective lymph node dissection is indicated for those patients. Morton et al. (162) recently reported that earlier detection of nodal positivity by sentinel node analysis leading to immediate lymphadenectomy in patients with lesions 1.2 to 3.5 mm in thickness was associated with prolonged survival compared with similar patients randomized to postoperative observation and delayed lymphadenectomy at the time of nodal relapse. Such patients determined to have pathologically positive nodes sentinel nodes would then receive adjuvant therapy as outlined for stage III patients

- *Resected stage I melanoma:* Patients with thin primary tumors and clinically negative lymph nodes are not candidates for adjuvant therapy, and if the primary tumor is <1 mm, they have insufficient risk of occult nodal involvement to justify lymphatic mapping and selective lymph node dissection unless the lesion is ulcerated. Such patients are at high enough risk for the development of second primary melanomas (and nonmelanoma skin cancers) to justify participation in experimental trials aimed at melanoma prevention, a fertile field of future research.

- *Resected no-cutaneous melanoma:* The use of adjuvant therapy in mucosal and choroidal melanomas must still be considered purely investigational, and should therefore ideally take place in the context of randomized controlled phase III or pilot phase II trials. Because many patients with mucosal melanomas—and some patients with choroidal melanomas—are at very high risk of local/regional and distant recurrence, multicenter and cooperative group trials addressing multimodality therapy in these diseases should be developed. An increased understanding of the biologic and therapeutic differences (if any) between cutaneous and noncutaneous melanomas would certainly facilitate the design and conduct of such trials.

REFERENCES

1. Kirkwood JM, Strawderman MH, Ernstoff MS, et al. Interferon alfa-2b adjuvant therapy of high-risk resected cutaneous melanoma: the Eastern Cooperative Oncology Group trial EST 1684. *J Clin Oncol.* 1996;14:7–17.

2. Balch CM, Buzaid AC. Finally, a successful adjuvant therapy for high-risk melanoma. *J Clin Oncol.* 1996;14:1–3.

3. Nathanson L. Interferon adjuvant therapy of melanoma. *Cancer.* 1996;78:944–947.

4. Balch CM. How patient referral bias can confuse interpretation of clinical results: elective lymph node dissections at the Sydney Melanoma Unit. *J Am Coll Surg.* 1995;180:490–492.

5. Spitler LE. A randomized trial of levamisole versus placebo as adjuvant therapy in malignant melanoma. *J Clin Oncol.* 1991;9:736–740.

6. Wallack MK, Sivanandham M, Balch CM, et al. A phase III randomized, double-blind, multiinstitutional trial of vaccinia melanoma oncolysate—active specific immunotherapy for patients with stage II melanoma. *Cancer.* 1995;75:34–42.

7. Saxman SB, Meyers ML, Chapman PB, et al. A phase III multicenter randomized trial of DTIC, Cisplatin, BCNU and Tamoxifen versus DTIC alone in patients with metastatic melanoma. In: Proceedings of the American Society of Clinical Oncology; May 17–19, 1999; San Diego, CA. Abstract 2068.

8. Stevenson HC, Green I, Hamilton JM, et al. Levamisole: known effects on the immune system, clinical results, and future applications to the treatment of cancer. *J Clin Oncol.* 1991;9:2052–2066.

9. Loutfi A, Shakr A, Jerry M, et al. Double blind randomized prospective trial of levamisole/placebo in stage I cutaneous malignant melanoma. *Clin Invest Med.* 1987;10:325–328.

10. Morton DL. Immunological studies with human neoplasms. *J Reticuloendothelial Soc.* 1971;10:137–146.

11. Pinsky CM, Hirshaut Y, Oettgen HF. Treatment of malignant melanoma by intratumoral injections of BCG NCI Monographs. 1973;39:255.

12. Mastrangelo MJ, Sulit HL, Prehn LM. Intralesional BCG in the treatment of metastatic malignant melanoma. *Cancer.* 1976;37:684.

13. Morton DL, Eilber FR, Holmes EC, et al. BCG immunotherapy of malignant melanoma: Summary of a seven year experience. *Annals of Surgery.* 1974;180:635–650.

14. Gutterman JU, Mcbride C, Freireich EJ, et al. Active immunotherapy with BCG for recurrent malignant melanoma. *Lancet.* 1973;I:1208–1213.

15. Paterson AH, Wilans DJ, Jerry LM, et al. Adjuvant BCG immunotherapy for malignant melanoma. *Can Med Assoc J.* 1984;131:744.

16. Czarnetzki BM, Macher E, Suciu S, et al. Long-term adjuvant immunotherapy in stage I high risk malignant melanoma, comparing two BCG preparations versus non-treatment in a randomised multicentre study (EORTC Protocol 18781). *European Journal of Cancer.* 1993;29A(9):1237–1242.

17. Paterson AH, Willans DJ, Jerry LM, et al. Adjuvant BCG immunotherapy for malignant melanoma. *CMAJ.* 1984;131(7):744–748.

18. Silver HK, Ibrahim EM, Evers JA, et al. Adjuvant BCG immunotherapy for stage I and II malignant melanoma. *CMAJ.* 1983;128(11):1291–1295.

19. Byrne MJ, Van Hazel G, Reynolds PM, et al. Adjuvant immunotherapy with BCG in stage II malignant melanoma. *J Surg Oncol.* 1983;23:114–116.

20. Cochran AJ, Buyse ME, Lejeune FJ, et al. Adjuvant reactivity predicts survival in patients with "high-risk" primary malignant melanoma treated with systemic BCG. EORTC Malignant Melanoma Cooperative Group Writing Committee. *International Journal of Cancer.* 1981;28(5):543–550.

21. O'Connor TP, Labandter HP, Hiles RW, et al. A clinical trial of BCG immunotherapy as an adjunct to surgery in the treatment

of primary malignant melanoma. *British Journal of Plastic Surgery.* 1978;31(4):317–322.

22. Christie GH, Bomford R. Mechanisms of macrophage activation by Corynebacterium parvum I. In vitro experiments. *Cell Immunol.* 1975;17:150–159.

23. Lipton A, Harvey HA, Lawrence B, et al Corynebacterium parvum versus BCG adjuvant immunotherapy in human malignant melanoma. *Cancer.* 1983;51:57–66.

24. Lipton A, Harvey HA, Balch CM, et al. Corynebacterium parvum versus Bacille Calmette-Guerin adjuvant immunotherapy of stage II malignant melanoma. *J Clin Oncol.* 1991;9:1151–1158.

25. Balch CM, Smalley RV, Bartolucci AA, et al. A randomized prospective clinical trial of adjuvant C. parvum immunotherapy in 260 patients with clinically localized melanoma (stage I): prognostic factors analysis and preliminary results of immunotherapy. *Cancer.* 1982;49:1079–1086.

26. Lejeune FJ, Macher E, Kleeberg U, et al. An assessment of DTIC versus levamisole or placebo in the treatment of high risk stage I patients after surgical removal of a primary melanoma of the skin: a phase III adjuvant study. EORTC protocol 18761. *Eur J Cancer Clin Oncol.* 1988;24:S81–S90.

27. Loutfi A, Shakr A, Jerry M, et al. Double blind randomized prospective trial of levamisole/placebo in stage I cutaneous malignant melanoma. *Clin Invest Med.* 1987;10:325–328.

28. Lawrence HS. The transfer in humans of delayed skin sensitivity to streptococcal M substance and to tuberculin with disrupted leucocytes. *J Clin Invest.* 1955;34:219–230.

29. Bukowski RM, Deodhar S, Hewlett JS, et al. Randomized controlled trial of transfer factor in stage II malignant melanoma. *Cancer.* 1983;51:269–272.

30. Miller LL, Spitler LE, Allen RE, et al. A randomized, double-blind, placebo-controlled trial of transfer factor as adjuvant therapy for melanoma. *Cancer.* 1988;61:1543–1549.

31. Martinez J, Miller L, Allen R, et al. A randomized trial of isoprinosine as surgical adjuvant therapy of melanoma: final report. *Proc Am Assoc Cancer Res.* 1990;31:203.

32. Khayat D, Pompidou A, Soubrane C, et al. Results of two successive randomized prospective studies of nonspecific adjuvant immunotherapy of thin malignant melanoma. *Fourth International Congress on Anti-cancer Chemotherapy.* Paris, France, 1993:118.

33. Azizi E, Brenner HJ, Shoham J. Postsurgical adjuvant treatment of malignant melanoma patients by the thymic factor thymostimulin. *Arzneimittel Forschung.* 1984;34:1043–1046.

34. Bernengo MG, Doveil GC, Lisa F, et al. The immunological profile of melanoma and the role of adjuvant thymostimulin immunotherapy in stage I patients. *Thymic Factor Therapy: Serono Symp Publ.* 1984;16:329–339.

35. Norris RW, Byrom NA, Nagvekar NM, et al. Thymostimulin plus surgery in the treatment of primary truncal malignant melanoma: preliminary results of a U.K. multi-centre clinical trial. *Thymic Factor Therapy: Serono Symp Publ.* 1984;16:341–348.

36. McIllmurray MB, Embleton MJ, Reeves WG, et al. Controlled trial of active immunotherapy in management of stage IIB malignant melanoma. *Br Med J.* 1977;1(6060):540–542.

37. McIllmurray MB, Reeves WG, Langman MJS, et al. Active immunotherapy in melanoma [letter]. *Br Med J.* 1978;1(6112):579.

38. Aranha GV, McKhann CF, Grage TB, et al. Adjuvant immunotherapy of malignant melanoma. *Cancer.* 1979;43:1297–1303.

39. Galligioni E, Quaia M, Merlo A, et al. Adjuvant immunotherapy treatment of renal carcinoma patients with autologous tumor cells and Bacillus Calmette-Guèrin. Five-year results of a prospective randomized study. *Cancer.* 1996;77:2560–2566.

40. Berd D, Sato T, Maguire HC Jr, et al. Immunopharmacologic analysis of an autologous, hapten-modified human melanoma vaccine. *J Clin Oncol.* 2004;22(3):403–415.

41. McCulloch PB, Dent PB, Blajchman M, et al. Recurrent malignant melanoma: effect of adjuvant immunotherapy on survival. *Can Med Assoc J.* 1977;117:33–36.

42. Dranoff G, Jaffee E, Lazenby A, et al. Vaccination with irradiated tumor cells engineered to secrete murine granulocyte-macrophage colony stimulating factor stimulates potent, specific, and long-lasting anti-tumor immunity. *Proc Natl Acad Sci U S A.* 1993;90:3539–33543.

43. Sosman JA, Ashani T, Weeraratna S, et al. When Will Melanoma Vaccines Be Proven Effective? *J Clin Oncol.* 2004:387–389.

44. Morton DL. Adjuvant immunotherapy of malignant melanoma: status of clinical trials at UCLA. *Int J Immunother.* 1986;2:31–36.

45. Hedley DW, McElwain TJ, Currie GA. Specific active immunotherapy does not prolong survival in surgically treated patients with stage IIB melanoma and may promote early recurrence. *Br J Cancer.* 1978;37:491–496.

46. Schultz N, Oratz R, Chen D, et al. Effect of DETOX as an adjuvant for melanoma vaccine. *Vaccine.* 1995;13:503–508.

47. Helling F, Zhang A, Shang A, et al. GM2-KLH conjugate vaccine: increased immunogenicity in melanoma patients after administration with immunological adjuvant QS-21. *Cancer Res.* 1995;55:2783–2788.

48. Oratz R, Dugan M, Roses DF, et al. Lack of effect of cyclophosphamide on the immunogenicity of a melanoma antigen vaccine. *Cancer Res.* 1991;51:3643–3647.

49. Hoon DSB, Foshag LJ, Nizze AS, et al. Suppressor cell activity in a randomized trial of patients receiving active specific immunotherapy with melanoma cell vaccine and low dosages of cyclophosphamide. *Cancer Res.* 1990;50:5358–5364.

50. Sosman JA, Unger JM, Liu PY, et al. Adjuvant immunotherapy of resected, intermediate-thickness node-negative melanoma with an allogeneic tumor vaccine. Impact of HLA class I antigen expression on outcome. *J Clin Oncol.* 2002;20:2067–2075.

51. Morton DL, Hseuh EC, Essner R, et al. Prolonged survival of patients receiving active immunotherapy with Canvaxin therapeutic polyvalent vaccine after complete resection of melanoma metastatic to regional lymph nodes. *Ann Surg.* 2002:438–448.

52. Hsueh EC, Gupta RK, Qi, K, et al. Correlation of specific immune responses with survival in melanoma patients with distant metastases receiving ployvalent melanoma cell vaccine. *J Clin Oncol.* 1998;16(9):2913–2920.

53. Data from Society for Surgical Oncology Annual meeting 2006. San Diego, CA.

54. Cassel WA, Murray DR, Phillips HS. A phase II study on the postsurgical management of stage II malignant melanoma with a Newcastle disease virus oncolysate. *Cancer* 1983;52:856–860.

55. Hersey P, Coates P, McCarthy WH. Active immunotherapy following surgical removal of high risk melanoma: present status and future prospects. *SBT93: Society for Biological Therapy.* In: Proceedings from the 8th Annual Scientific Meeting; November 10–14, 1993; Nashville, TN. Abstract 432.

56. Livingston PO, Wong GYC, Adluri S, et al. Improved survival in stage III melanoma patients with GM2 antibodies: a randomized trial of adjuvant vaccination with GM2 ganglioside. *J Clin Oncol.* 1994;12:1036–1044.

57. Hersey P. Ganglioside antigens in tissue sections of skin, naevi, and melanoma: implications for treatment of melanoma. *Cancer Treat Res.* 1991;54:137–151.

58. Hamilton WB, Helling F, Lloyd KO, et al. Ganglioside expression on human malignant melanoma assessed by quantitative immune thin-layer chromatography. *Int J Cancer.* 1993;53:566–573.

59. Tai T, Cahan LD, Tsuchida T, et al. Immunogenicity of melanoma-associated gangliosides in cancer patients. *Int J Cancer.* 1985;35:607–612.

60. Minasian LM, Yao TJ, Steffens TA, et al. A phase I study of anti-GD3 ganglioside monoclonal antibody R24 and recombinant human macrophage-colony stimulating factor in patients with metastatic melanoma. *Cancer.* 1995;75:2251–2257.

61. Livingston PO, Ritter G, Srivastava P, et al. Characterization of IgG and IgM antibodies induced in melanoma patients by immunization with purified GM2 ganglioside. *Cancer Res.* 1989;49:7045–7050.

62. Takahashi T, Chang C, Morton DL, et al. IgM antibodies to ganglioside GM3 and GD3 induced by active immunization correlated with survival in melanoma patients. *Proc Am Assoc Cancer Res.* 1995;36:485.

63. Chatterjee MB, Foon KA, Köhler H. Idiotypic antibody immunotherapy of cancer. *Cancer Immunol Immunother.* 1994;38:75–82.

64. Mittelman A, Wang X, Matsumoto K, et al. Antiantiidiotypic response and clinical course of the disease in patients with malignant melanoma immunized with mouse antiidiotypic monoclonal antibody MK2-23. *Hybridoma.* 1995;14:175–181.

65. Foon KA, Lutzky J, Hutchins L, et al. Clinical and immune responses in melanoma patients immunized with an anti-idiotype (ID) antibody mimicking GD2. In: Proceedings of the American Society of Clinical Oncology; May 17–19, 1999; San Diego, CA. Abstract 1672.

66. Saleh MN, Stapleton JD, Khazaeli MB, et al. Generation of a human anti-idiotypic antibody that mimics the GD2 antigen. *J Immunol.* 1993;151:3390–3398.

67. McCaffery M, Yao TJ, Williams L, et al. Immunization of melanoma patients with BEC2 anti-idiotypic monoclonal antibody that mimics GD3 ganglioside: enhanced immunogenicity when combined with adjuvant. *Clin Cancer Res.* 1996;2:679–686.

68. Townsend ARM, Gotch RM, Davey J. Cytotoxic cells recognize fragments of the influenza nucleoprotein. *Cell.* 1985;42:457–467.

69. Townsend ARM, Rothbard J, Gotch FM, et al. The epitopes of influenza nucleoprotein recognized by cytotoxic T lymphocytes can be defined with short synthetic peptides. *Cell.* 1986;44:959–968.

70. Robbins PF, Kawakami Y. Human tumor antigens recognized by T cells. *Curr Opin Immunol.* 1996;8:628–636.

71. Marchand M, et al. Tumor regression responses in melanoma patients treated with a peptide encoded by MAGE-3. *Int J Cancer.* 1995;63:883–885.

72. Jaeger E, Ringhoffer M, Dienes HP, et al. Granulocyte macrophage colony stimulating factor enhances immune responses to melanoma associated peptides in vivo. *Int J Cancer.* 1997;67:54–62.

73. Cebon JS, Jaeger E, Gibbs P, et al. Phase I studies of immunization with Melan-A and IL-12 in HLA-A2 positive patients with stage III and IV metastatic melanoma. In: Proceedings of the American Society of Clinical Oncology; May 17–19, 1999; San Diego, CA. Abstract 1671.

74. Salgaller MM, Marincola FM, Cormier JN, et al. Immunization against epitopes in the human melanoma antigen gp100 following patient immunization with synthetic peptides. *Cancer Res.* 1996;56:4749–4757.

75. Salgaller ML, Afshar A, Marincola FM, et al. Recognition of multiple epitopes of the human melanoma antigen gp100 by peripheral blood lymphocytes stimulated in vitro with synthetic peptides. *Cancer Res.* 1995;55:4972–4977.

76. Cormier JN, Salgaller ML, Prevette T, et al. Enhancement of cellular immunity in melanoma patients immunized with a peptide from MART-1/Melan A. *Cancer Journal From Scientific American.* 1997;3:37–44.

77. Parkhurst MR, Salgaller ML, Southwood S, et al. Improved induction of melanoma reactive CTL with peptides from melanoma antigen gp100 modified at HLA-A0201 binding residues. *J Immunology.* 1996;157:2536–2548.

78. Wang F, Bade E, Kuniyoshi C, et al. Phase I trial of a MART-1 peptide vaccine with Incomplete Freund's Adjuvant for resected high-risk melanoma. *Clin Cancer Res.* 1999;5(10):2756–2765.

79. Valmori D, Fonteneau JF, Lizana CM, et al. Enhanced generation of specific tumor-reactive CTL in vitro by selected Melan-A/MART-1 immunodominant peptide analogues. *J Immunol.* 1998;160:1750–1758.

80. Romero P, Dunbar PR, Valmori D, et al. Ex vivo staining of metastatic lymph nodes by class I major histocompatibility complex tetramers reveals high numbers of antigen-experienced tumor specific cytolytic T lymphocytes. *J Exp Med.* 1998;188:1641–1650.

81. Rosenberg SA, Yang JC, Schwartzentruber DJ, et al. Immunologic and therapeutic evaluation of a synthetic peptide vaccine for the treatment of patients with metastatic melanoma. *Nature Medicine.* 1998;4:321–327.

82. Lee P, Wang F, Kuniyoshi J, et al. Effects of interleukin-12 on the immune response to a multipeptide vaccine for resected metastatic melanoma. *J Clin Oncol.* 2001;19:3836–3847.

83. Weber J, Hamid O, Lee PP, et al. Randomized phase II trial of melanoma peptides with Montanide ISA 51 and different doses of IL-12 with Alum for resected stages IIC/III and IV melanoma. In: Proceedings of the American Society of Clinical Oncology; May 13–17, 2005; Orlando, FL. Abstract 2506.

84. Slingluff CL, Petroni GR, Yamshchikov GV, et al. Clinical and immunologic results of a randomized phase II trial of vaccination using four melanoma peptides either administered in granulocyte macrophage colony-stimulating factor in adjuvant or pulsed on dendritic cells. *J Clin Oncol.* 2003;21:4016–4026.

85. Slingluff CL Jr, Petroni GR, Yamshchikov GV, et al. Immunologic and clinical outcomes of vaccination with a multiepitope melanoma peptide vaccine plus low-dose interleukin-2 administered either concurrently or on a delayed schedule. *J Clin Oncol.* 2004;22:4474–4485.

86. Creagan ET, Ingle JN, Schutt AJ, et al. A prospective, randomized controlled trial of megestrol acetate among high-risk patients with resected malignant melanoma. *Am J Clin Oncol.* 1989;12:152–155.

87. Meyskens FL Jr, Liu PY, Tuthill RJ, et al. Randomized trial of vitamin A versus observation as adjuvant therapy in high risk primary malignant melanoma: a Southwest Oncology Group study. *J Clin Oncol.* 1994;12:2060–2065.

88. Lotan R, Hendrix MJC, Lippman SM. Retinoids in the management of melanoma. In: Marks R ed. *Retinoids in Cutaneous Malignancy.* Blackwell Scientific, London. 1991:133.

89. Meyskens FL Jr, Booth AE, Goff P, et al. Randomized trial of BCG ± vitamin A for stages I and II cutaneous malignant melanoma. In: Salmon SE, ed. *Adjuvant Therapy of Cancer* 5th ed. New York: Grune & Stratton; 1987:665–682.

90. Thornes RD, Daly L, Lynch G, et al. Treatment with coumarin to prevent or delay recurrence of malignant melanoma. *J Cancer Res Clin Oncol.* 1994;120:S32–S34.

91. Houghton AN, Legha S, Bajorin DF. Chemotherapy for metastatic melanoma. In: Balch CM, Houghton AN, Milton GW, et al. eds. *Cutaneous Melanoma* 2nd ed. J.B. Lippincott, Philadelphia. 1992:498.

92. Hill GJ II, Moss SE, Golomb FM, et al. DTIC and combination therapy for melanoma: III. DTIC (NSC 45388) Surgical Adjuvant Study COG protocol 7040. *Cancer.* 1981;47:2556–2562.

93. Quirt IC, DeBoer G, Kersey PA, et al. Randomized controlled trial of adjuvant chemoimmunotherapy with DTIC and BCG after complete excision of primary melanoma with a poor prognosis or melanoma metastases. *Can Med Assoc J.* 1983;128:929–933.

94. Wood WC, Cosimi AB, Carey RW, et al. Randomized trial of adjuvant therapy for "high-risk" primary malignant melanoma. *Surgery*. 1978;83:677–681.

95. Knost JA, Reynolds V, Greco FA, et al. Adjuvant chemoimmunotherapy stage I/II malignant melanoma. *J Surg Oncol*. 1982;19:165–170.

96. Sterchi JM, Wells HB, Case LD, et al. A randomized trial of adjuvant chemotherapy and immunotherapy in stage I and II cutaneous melanoma: an interim report. *Cancer* 1985;55:707–712.

97. Castel T, Estapé J, Viñolas N, et al. Adjuvant treatment in stage I and II malignant melanoma: a randomized trial between chemoimmunotherapy and immunotherapy. *Dermatologica*. 1991;183:25–30.

98. Balch CM, Murray D, Presant C, et al. Ineffectiveness of adjuvant chemotherapy using DTIC and cyclophosphamide in patients with resectable metastatic melanoma. *Surgery*. 1984;95:454–459.

99. Karakousis CP, Didolkar MS, Lopez R, et al. Chemoimmunotherapy (DTIC and *Corynebacterium parvum*) as adjuvant treatment in malignant melanoma. *Cancer Treat Rep*. 1979;63:1739–1743.

100. Banzet P, Jacquillat C, Civatte J, et al. Adjuvant chemotherapy in the management of primary malignant melanoma. *Cancer*. 1978;41:1240–1248.

101. Quagliana J, Tranum B, Neidhardt J, et al. Adjuvant chemotherapy with BCNU, Hydrea and DTIC (BHD) with or without immunotherapy (BCG) in high risk melanoma patients: a SWOG study. *Proc Am Assoc Cancer Res*. 1980;21:399.

102. Misset JL, Delgado M, De Vassal F, et al. Immunotherapy or chemoimmunotherapy as adjuvant treatment for malignant melanoma: a G.I.F. trial. In: Salmon SE, Jones SE eds. *Adjuvant Therapy of Cancer III*. Grune & Stratton, New York. 1981:225.

103. Kerin MJ, Gillen P, Monson JRT, et al. Results of a prospective randomized trial using DTIC and interferon as adjuvant therapy for stage I malignant melanoma. *Eur J Surg Oncol*. 1995;21:548–550.

104. Kim KB, Legha SS, Gonzalez R, et al. A phase III randomized trial of adjuvant biochemotherapy (BC) versus interferon-α-2b (IFN) in patients (pts) with high risk for melanoma recurrence. In: *J Clin Oncol* 2006 ASCO Annual Meeting Proceedings (Post-Meeting Edition). Vol 24, No. 18S (June 20 Suppl): Abstract 185.

105. O'Day S, Atkins M, Weber J, et al. A phase II multi-center trial of maintenance biotherapy (MBT) after induction concurrent biochemotherapy (BCT) for patients (Pts) with metastatic melanoma (MM). *J Clin Oncol*. 2005;23:7503.

106. Karakousis C, Blumenson L. Adjuvant chemotherapy with a nitrosourea-based protocol in advanced malignant melanoma. *Eur J Cancer*. 1993;29A:1831–1835.

107. Hansson J, Ringborg U, Lagerlof B, et al. Adjuvant chemotherapy of malignant melanoma. A pilot study. *Am J Clin Oncol*. 1985;8:47–50.

108. Jacquillat C, Banzet P, Civatte J, et al. Adjuvant chemotherapy or chemoimmunotherapy in the management of primary malignant melanoma of level III, IV, or V. *Recent Results Cancer Res*. 1979;68:346–358.

109. Tranum BL, Dixon D, Quagliana J, et al. Lack of benefit of adjunctive chemotherapy in stage I malignant melanoma: a Southwest Oncology Group Study. *Cancer Treat Rep*. 1987;71:643–644.

110. Richards J, Mehta N, Ramming K, et al. Sequential chemoimmunotherapy in the treatment of metastatic melanoma. *J Clin Oncol*. 1992;10:1338–1346.

111. Legha SW, Ring S, Eton O, et al. Development of a biochemotherapy regimen with concurrent administration of cisplatin, vinblastine, dacarbazine, interferon alfa and interleukin-2 for patients with metastatic melanoma. *J Clin Oncol*. 1998;16:1752–1759.

112. Buzaid AC, Legha S, Bedikian A, et al. Neoadjuvant biochemotherapy in melanoma patients (pts) with local regional metastases (LRM). In: Proceedings of the American Society of Clinical Oncology; May 18–21, 1996; Phildelphia, PA. Abstract.

113. Meisenberg BR, Ross M, Vredenburgh JJ, et al. Randomized trial of high-dose chemotherapy with autologous bone marrow support as adjuvant therapy for high-risk, multi-node-positive malignant melanoma. *J Natl Cancer Inst*. 1993;85:1080–1085.

114. Herlyn M, Guerry D, Koprowski H. Recombinant interferon gamma induces changes in expression and shedding of antigens associated with normal human melanocytes, nevus cells, and primary and metastatic melanoma cells. *J Immunol*. 1985;134:4226–4230.

115. Kurzrock R, Rosenblum MG, Sherwin SA, et al. Pharmacokinetics, single-dose tolerance and biological activity of recombinant gamma interferon in cancer patients. *Cancer Res*. 1985;45:2866–2872.

116. Maluish AE, Urba WJ, Longo DL, et al. The determination of an immunologically active dose of interferon-gamma in patients with melanoma. *J Clin Oncol*. 1988;6:434–445.

117. Schiller JH, Pugh M, Kirkwood JM, et al. Eastern Cooperative Group trial of interferon gamma in metastatic melanoma: an innovative study design. *Clin Cancer Res*. 1996;2:29–36.

118. Jaffe HS, Herberman RB. Rationale for recombinant human interferon-gamma adjuvant immunotherapy for cancer. *J Natl Cancer Inst*. 1988;80:616–618.

119. Meyskens FL Jr, Kopecky K, Taylor CW, et al. Randomized trial of adjuvant human interferon gamma versus observation in high-risk cutaneous melanoma. *J Natl Cancer Inst* 1995;87:1710–1713.

120. Meyskens FL Jr, Kopecky K, Samson M, et al. Recombinant human interferon gamma: adverse effects in high-risk stage I and II cutaneous malignant melanoma [letter]. *J Natl Cancer Inst*. 1990;82:1071.

121. Osoba D, Zee B, Sadura A, et al. Measurement of quality of life in an adjuvant trial of gamma interferon versus levamisole in malignant melanoma. In: Salmon SE ed. *Adjuvant Therapy of Cancer VII*. J.B. Lippincott, Philadelphia, Pennsylvania. 1993:412.

122. Kleeberg UR, Suciu S, Brocker EB, et al. Final results of the EORTC 18871/DKG 80–1 randomised phase III trial. rIFN-alpha2b versus rIFN-gamma versus ISCADOR M versus observation after surgery in melanoma patients with either high-risk primary (thickness >3 mm) or regional lymph node metastasis. *Eur J Cancer*. 2004;40:390–402.

123. Parkinson DR, Houghton AN, Hersey P, et al. Biologic therapy for melanoma. In: Balch CM, Houghton AN, Milton GW, et al. eds. *Cutaneous Melanoma* (2nd ed). J.B. Lippincott, Philadelphia. 1992:522.

124. Leffer LM, Dinarello CA, Herberman RB, et al. Biologic properties of recombinant alpha-interferons: 40th anniversary of the discovery of interferons. *Cancer Res*. 1998;58(12):2489–2499.

125. Kokoschka EM, Trautinger F, Knobler RM, et al. Long-term adjuvant therapy of high-risk malignant melanoma with interferon α2b. *J Invest Dermatol*. 1990;95:S193–S197.

126. Rusciani L, Petralgia S, Alotto M, et al. Postsurgical adjuvant therapy for melanoma: evaluation of a 3-year randomized trial with recombinant interferon-alpha after3 aqnd 5 years of follow-up. *Cancer*. 1997;79:2354–2360.

127. Cascinelli N. Evaluation of efficacy of adjuvant rIFN 2A in melanoma patients with regional node metastases. In: Proceedings of the American Society of Clinical Oncology; May 21–23, 1995; Los Angeles, CA. Abstract.

128. Cascinelli N, Bufalino R, Morabito A, et al. Results of an adjuvant interferon study in the WHO melanoma programme. *Lancet*. 1994;343:913–914.

129. Caraceni A, Gangeri L, Martini C, et al. Neurotoxicity of interferon-alpha in melanoma therapy: results from a randomized, controlled trial. *Cancer.* 1998;83(3):482–489.

130. Creagan ET, Dalton RJ, Ahmann DL, et al. Randomized, surgical adjuvant clinical trial of recombinant interferon alfa-2a in selected patients with malignant melanoma. *J Clin Oncol.* 1995;13:2776–2783.

131. Cole BF, Gelber RD, Kirkwood JM, et al. Quality-of-life—adjusted survival analysis of interferon alfa-2b adjuvant treatment of high-risk resected cutaneous melanoma: an Eastern Cooperative Oncology Group study. *J Clin Oncol.* 1996;14:2666–2673.

132. Kirkwood JM, Ibrahim J, Sondak V, et al. High- and low-dose in high-risk melanoma: first analysis of the intergroup trial E1690/S9111/C9190. *J Clin Oncol.* 2000;18(12):2444–2458.

133. Kirkwood JM, Ibrahim JG, Sosman JA, et al. High-dose interferon alfa-2b significantly prolongs relapse-free and overall survival compared with the GM2-KLH/QS-21 vaccine in patients with resected stage IIB-III melanoma: results of intergroup trial E1694/S9512/C509801. *J Clin Oncol.* 2001;19:2370–2380.

134. Wheatley K, Ives N, Hancock B, et al. Does adjuvant interferon-alpha for high-risk melanoma provide a worthwhile benefit? A meta-analysis of the randomised trials. *Cancer Treat Rev.* 2003;29:241–252.

135. Kirkwood JM, Manola J, Ibrahim J, et al. for the Eastern Cooperative Oncology Group. A pooled analysis of eastern cooperative oncology group and intergroup trials of adjuvant high-dose interferon for melanoma. *Clin Cancer Res.* 2004;10:1670–1677.

136. Kirkwood JM, Ibrahim J, Lawson JH, et al. High dose interferon alfa-2b does not diminish antibody response to GM2 vaccination in patients with resected melanoma: Results of the multicenter Eastern Cooperative Oncology Group phase II trial E2696. 2001;19(5):1430–1436.

137. Moschos SJ, Edington HD, Land SR, et al. Neoadjuvant treatment of regional stage IIIB melanoma with high-dose interferon alfa-2b induces objective tumor regression in association with modulation of tumor infiltrating host cellular immune responses. *J Clin Oncol.* 2006;24:3164–3171.

138. Buzaid AC, Colome M, Bedikian A, et al. Phase II study of neoadjuvant concurrent biochemotherapy in melanoma patients with local-regional metastases. *Melanoma Res.* 1998;8:549–556.

139. Gibbs P, Anderson C, Pearlman N, et al. A phase II study of neoadjuvant biochemotherapy for stage III melanoma. *Cancer.* 2002;94:470–476.

140. Lewis KD, Robinson WA, McCarter M, et al. Phase II multicenter study of neoadjuvant biochemotherapy for patients with stage III malignant melanoma. *J Clin Oncol.* 2006;24:3157–3163.

141. Cascinelli N, Belli F, MacKie RM, et al. Effect of long-term adjuvant therapy with interferon alpha-2a in patients with regional node metastases from cutaneous melanoma: A randomized trial. *Lancet.* 2001;358:866–869.

142. Eggermont AMM, Kleeberg UR, Ruiter DJ, et al. The European Organization for Research and Treatment of Cancer Melanoma Group trial experience with more than 2000 Patients, evaluating adjuvant therapy treatment with low or intermediate doses of interferon alpha-2b. In: Perry GM, ed. Alexandria, VA: American Society of Clinical Oncology; 2001:88–93.

143. Cameron DA, Cornbleet MC, Mackie RM, et al. Adjuvant interferon alpha 2b in high risk melanoma: The Scottish study. *Br J Cancer.* 2001;84:1146–1149.

144. Kirkwood JM, Ibrahim JG, Sondak VK, et al. High- and low-dose interferon alfa-2b in high-risk melanoma: First analysis of Intergroup trial E1690/S9111/C9190. *J Clin Oncol.* 2000;18:2444–2458.

145. Moschos SJ, Kirkwood JM, Konstantinopoulos PA. Present status and future prospects for adjuvant therapy of melanoma: time to build upon the foundation of high-dose interferon alfa-2b. *J Clin Oncol.* 2004;22:11–14.

146. Egen JG, Kuhns MS, Allison JP. CTLA-4: new insights into its biological function and use in tumor immunotherapy. *Nat Immunol.* 2002;3(7):611–618.

147. Hodi FS, Mihm MC, Soiffer RJ, et al. Biologic activity of cytotoxic T lymphocyte-associated antigen 4 antibody blockade in previously vaccinated metastatic melanoma and ovarian carcinoma patients. *Proc Natl Acad Sci U S A.* 2003;100(8):4712–4717.

148. Korman A, Yellin M, Keler T. Tumor immunotherapy: pre-clinical and clinical activity of CTLA-4 antibodies. *Curr Opin Invest Drugs.* 2005;6:582–591.

149. Phan GQ, Yang JC, Sherry RM, et al. Cancer regression and autoimmunity induced by cytotoxic T lymphocyte-associated antigen 4 blockade in patients with metastatic melanoma. *Proc Natl Acad Sci U S A.* 2003;100:8372–8377.

150. Sanderson K, Scotland R, Lee P, et al. Autoimmunity in a phase I trial of a fully human anti-cytotoxic T-lymphocyte antigen-4 monoclonal antibody with multiple melanoma peptides and Montanide ISA 51 for patients with resected stages III and IV melanoma. *Clin Oncol.* 2005;23(4):741–750.

151. Attia P, Phan GQ, Maker AV, et al. Autoimmunity correlates with tumor regression in patients with metastatic melanoma treated with anti-cytotoxic T-lymphocyte antigen-4. *J Clin Oncol.* 2005;23(25):6043–6053.

152. Ribas A, Camacho LH, Lopez-Berestein G, et al. Antitumor activity in melanoma and anti-self responses in a phase I trial with the anti-cytotoxic T lymphocyte-associated antigen 4 monoclonal antibody CP-675,206. *J Clin Oncol.* 2005;23(35):8968–8977.

153. Schmidt-Ullrich RK, Johnson CR. Role of radiotherapy and hyperthermia in the management of malignant melanoma. *Semin Surg Oncol.* 1996;12:407–415.

154. Ang KK, Peters LJ, Weber RS, et al. Postoperative radiotherapy for cutaneous melanoma of the head and neck region. *Int J Radiat Oncol Biol Phys.* 1994;30:795–798.

155. Creagan ET, Cupps RE, Ivins JC, et al. Adjuvant radiation therapy in the treatment of regional nodal metastases from malignant melanoma: a randomized prospective study. *Cancer.* 1978;42:2206–2210.

156. Kirkwood JM, Earle JD, Fine SL, et al. Five-year progress report: the Collaborative Ocular Melanoma Study. In: Proceedings of the American Society of Clinical Oncology; 1992.

157. Cumberlin R, De Moss E, Lassus M, et al. Isolation perfusion for malignant melanoma of the extremity: a review. *J Clin Oncol.* 1985;3:1022–1031.

158. Lienard D, Ewalenko P, Delmotte JJ, et al. High-dose recombinant tumor necrosis factor alpha in combination with interferon gamma and melphalan in isolation perfusion of the limbs for melanoma and sarcoma. *J Clin Oncol.* 1992;10:52–60.

159. Ghussen F, Krüger I, Smalley RV, et al. Hyperthermic perfusion with chemotherapy for melanoma of the extremities. *World J Surg.* 1989;13:598–602.

160. Hafström L, Rudenstam CM, Blomquist E, et al. Regional hyperthermic perfusion with melphalan after surgery for recurrent malignant melanoma of the extremities. *J Clin Oncol.* 1991;9:2091–2094.

161. Lejeune FJ, Vaglini M, Schraffordt-Koops H, et al. A randomized trial on prophylactic isolation perfusion for Stage I high-risk (i.e., greater than 1.5-mm thickness) malignant melanoma of the limbs. An interim report. *Special International Columbus Meeting on Surgical Oncology.* Genoa, Italy, 1992:75.

162. Morton DL, Thompson JF, Cochran AJ, et al. Sentinel-node biopsy or nodal observation in melanoma. *N Engl J Med.* 2006;355:1307–1317.

COMMENTARY
Lilah F. Morris and James S. Economou

Despite decades of research, metastatic melanoma is almost uniformly fatal, with an average life expectancy of 6 to 9 months. Less than 20% of patients will respond to any therapy. Although complete surgical excision is the foundation of melanoma treatment, surgery has a very limited role in metastatic disease. Traditional chemotherapies have minimal efficacy, and they never provide long-term control of disease.

Immune-based therapies are the only treatment modalities that have the potential to offer long-term survival in some patients with widely metastatic disease. Interleukin (IL)-2 and interferon therapy are the only two Food and Drug Administration–approved immunotherapies for melanoma. Their role in treatment of melanoma was well described in Chapter 25.

Many vaccine-based therapies—including whole tumor cell, peptide, ganglioside, DNA, viral, and dendritic cell-based treatments—have been studied in metastatic disease. However, vaccine trials have had limited success. A recent review of over 1,300 vaccine treatments found a 3.3% objective response rate (1). Despite the low response rate, the majority of responders achieved long-term control of their disease. This demonstrated that manipulation of the immune system could be an effective therapeutic modality in the treatment of metastatic melanoma. Here we focus on current knowledge in adoptive immunotherapy.

ADOPTIVE TRANSFER THERAPY FOR METASTATIC MELANOMA

Adoptive immunotherapy involves the transfer of tumor-specific T cells into a tumor-bearing host, with the goal of tumor regression. The cellular arm of the immunologic cascade—the recognition, proliferation, and activation of cytotoxic CD8+ T lymphocytes (CTLs)—is required for effective cancer immunotherapy. Tumor-associated antigens (TAAs), or short peptides expressed on the surface of most human cancers and presented by major histocompatibility complexes (MHCs), are recognized by a corresponding CTL T-cell receptor (TCR). Successful adoptive immunotherapy requires sufficient numbers of tumor-reactive T cells, avid recognition of the cognate antigen by the TCR, trafficking and infiltration of T cells into tumor sites, and activation of T cells that are able to kill tumors.

The major obstacle with initial attempts at adoptive transfer therapy was the ability to generate sufficient numbers of autologous immune cells with antitumor activity. Adoptive cell transfer methods were pioneered in humans in the early 1980s, when autologous antitumor lymphocytes were derived from incubation of peripheral blood mononuclear cells with IL-2, generating lymphocytes that preferentially lysed tumor cells, but not normal cells. Termed *lymphokine-activated killer* (LAK) cells, these cells were characterized as a distinct subset of lymphocytes, without B- or T-cell surface markers, and different from natural killer cells and cytotoxic T lymphocytes. A major study of this approach reported a 30% response rate, with 8 of 106 patients having complete regression of all tumor (2). Limitations of this method were the large numbers of tumor-reactive cells required to induce cancer regression ($3 \times 10^{10} - 3 \times 10^{11}$), the toxic effects of high-dose IL-2, and lack of confirmation of these response rates.

While human trials of LAK/IL-2 therapy were underway, a preclinical immunotherapy model using tumor-infiltrating lymphocytes (TILs) was introduced. Tumors were harvested from mice, digested in DNase and collagenase, and cultured with IL-2. Within 2 weeks, a 100-fold expansion of the original number of TILs was observed, with nearly complete destruction of tumor cells. Adoptive transfer of expanded TILs was 50 to 100 times more potent in antitumor activity than LAK cell adoptive transfer (3). Promising responses from an initial clinical trial were seen in patients with melanoma and renal cell carcinoma who were administered autologous expanded TILs and IL-2 (objective tumor responses of 23% and 29%, respectively, lasting 3 to 14 months) (4). However, further studies of this method were limited by the TIL inability specifically to traffic to tumor sites (5).

In order to improve adoptive immunotherapy, researchers began to study other endogenous factors that may influence persistence, activation, and tumor trafficking of adoptively transferred cells. A major breakthrough came with the discovery that the effects of adoptive transfer therapy are more pronounced if the host immune system is depleted. Preconditioning, with either total-body radiation or chemotherapy, depletes "cytokine sinks," or competition from endogenous cells for cytokines that activate tumor-reactive T cells (6). In addition, elimination of the suppressor activity of CD4+/CD25+/foxp3+ regulatory T cells, and improved function of antigen-presenting cells, may increase antitumor immune response (6,7). In fact, clinical trials of TIL adoptive immunotherapy after lymphodepletion in patients with metastatic melanoma refractory to other therapies demonstrated 46% to 51% objective clinical response (8,9).

Despite promising responses from TIL adoptive immunotherapy, this treatment modality is limited to patients who have resectable tumor and whose TILs can be harvested. The advantage of clonally expanding a patient's autologous tumor-reactive T cells is that the TAA of interest need not be identified. Despite the ability to produce large numbers of cells via ex vivo clonal expansion, there is an inverse relationship between in vitro effector function and in vivo antitumor efficacy. CD8+ cells in a late effector phase of terminal differentiation are 100 times less effective in antitumor activity than T cells in an early effector stage (10). In addition to appropriate effector function, clonally expanded antitumor T cells need to survive in circulation in order to control tumor growth. Phase I studies in metastatic melanoma using ex vivo clonal expansion of antigen-specific CD8+ T cells have been limited by the short persistence of the adoptively transferred cells (8,11).

Several common TAAs have been identified in melanoma, including gp100, tyrosinase, MART-1, and tyrosinase-related protein-2. With the identification of these TAAs, more focus was placed on the interaction between the specific CD8+ TCR and its cognate tumor antigen. For instance, in order to obtain more tumor-specific CTLs, a recent phase I trial clonally expanded patients' CTL in the presence of Melan-A-pulsed dendritic cells.

This small trial had a 27% antitumor response rate (12). Normally, CTLs that bear a TCR recognizing common melanoma antigens exist, but their normal frequency in the body is low (<0.001% of the T-cell repertoire) and their binding affinities are weak. Innovative preclinical models have demonstrated methods to overcome both of these obstacles.

To better study these issues, several groups developed transgenic mice with a model TCR recognizing a TAA. Pmel-1 transgenic mice express the alpha and beta chains of a TCR that recognize the MHC class I-restricted epitope corresponding to amino acids 25-33 on gp100, a melanoma antigen present in both human melanoma and in B16, a spontaneous murine melanoma (13). Despite pmel-1 mice having >95% of their CD8+ T cells express the TCR-recognizing gp100, B16 melanoma grows progressively in these mice. Thus, this model proved that the presence of CTL recognizing a specific melanoma antigen is necessary, but not sufficient, to eradicate large, established tumors.

In order to understand more completely why the mere presence of tumor antigen-specific CTLs does not mediate tumor regression, several modified adoptive cell transfer experiments using the pmel-1 model were performed. Lymphodepleting preconditioning regimens of chemotherapy or total body radiation that deplete endogenous competitive or suppressor immune cells greatly enhance adoptive cell transfer therapy. Recent preclinical work suggests that more profound, myeloablative preconditioning regimens, similar to those administered prior to bone marrow transplantation, delivered along with bone marrow, render adoptive transfer more effective (14). Studies to understand this effect are underway. In addition, antigen-specific vaccination, combined with administration of high-dose IL-2, are necessary in this model to break T-cell functional tolerance (13).

The pmel-1 model has illustrated that in adoptive transfer strategies, both high precursor frequency of tumor-reactive T cells and efficient recognition and binding between the TCR and its cognate antigen are necessary to eradicate established tumor. Translation of this adoptive transfer strategy into humans has focused on cloning a specific TAA-recognizing TCR into a viral vector, then ex vivo activating and transducing autologous human peripheral blood mononuclear cells, bone marrow, or stem cells.

Proof of principle for antitumor efficacy using murine hematopoietic stem cells (HSCs) virally transduced with a TCR-recognizing tumor antigen used the xenoantigen ovalbumin (15). Murine TCRs specific for ovalbumin presented in the context of MHC class I or class II (called MOT-1 and MOT-2, respectively) were cloned and virally transduced into HSCs. After mice were immunized with transduced HSCs, subcutaneous E.G7 tumors (a murine lymphoma, EL.4, genetically modified to express the ovalbumin antigen) were implanted. Tumor growth was completely suppressed long term in 50% of mice, while the other half experienced short-term tumor growth suppression.

The genes encoding the CD8+ TCR specific for several TAAs have been cloned from patients who had near-complete responses to immune therapy. Recent efforts have attempted to introduce these TCRs, via a viral vector, into peripheral blood lymphocytes of patients with advanced cancers. A promising study from the National Cancer Institute in patients with metastatic melanoma demonstrated durable (>20 months) disease regression in 2 of 17 patients whose peripheral blood lymphocytes were transduced with a retrovirus expressing the MART-1 TCR and adoptively transferred after lymphodepleting preconditioning regimens (16). As in other trials of immune therapies for metastatic melanoma, all of these patients had been refractory to prior therapy with IL-2.

Despite the low response rate in this trial, it serves as proof of principle of the efficacy of adoptive immunotherapy using a virally transduced, cloned TCR. This trial also brings to light several important issues that will determine the future direction of adoptive immunotherapy. Although patients in this trial were lymphodepleted prior to adoptive transfer, myeloablative preconditioning might promote more robust expansion and activation of adoptively transferred cells, as has been demonstrated in preclinical animal models (14). If more profound preconditioning regimens promote in vivo expansion of adoptively transferred cells, this will obviate the need for prolonged ex vivo expansion of these cells. Adoptively transferred cells exposed to less ex vivo expansion should be more effective with an early effector, rather than an exhausted memory, phenotype (10). Modifying cloned TCRs to have higher affinity for their cognate antigen should improve tumor antigen recognition and tumor lysis.

Finally, patients in this trial received adoptive transfer of both CD4+ and CD8+ T cells transduced with the MART-1 TCR. However, the function of CD4+ cells with an MHC class I-restricted TCR on their surface has not been studied. Although CD4+ cells provide help to tumor antigen-specific CD8+ T cells, little is known about the role of tumor antigen-specific CD4+ T cells. It is possible that the help CD4+ cells provide CD8+ CTLs is abrogated by tumor antigen-specific CD4+ cells with a regulatory phenotype.

Although many questions remain, adoptive transfer therapy for metastatic melanoma is a promising area of study. Further clinical trials will help refine adoptive transfer strategies, and ultimately may provide the potential for cure in this otherwise fatal disease.

REFERENCES

1. Rosenberg S, Yang JC, Restifo NP. Cancer immunotherapy: moving beyond current vaccines. *Nat Med.* 2004;10:909–915.
2. Rosenberg S, Lotze MT, Muul LM, et al. A progress report on the treatment of 157 patients with advanced cancer using lymphokine-activated killer cells and interleukin-2 or high-dose interleukin-2 alone. *N Engl J Med.* 1987;316:889–897.
3. Rosenberg S, Spiess P, Lafreniere R. A new approach to the adoptive immunotherapy of cancer with tumor-infiltrating lymphocytes. *Science.* 1986;233:1318–1321.
4. Kradin R, Kurnick JT, Lazarus DS, et al. Tumour-infiltrating lymphocytes and interleukin-2 in treatment of advanced cancer. *Lancet.* 1989;1:577–580.
5. Economou J, Belldegrun AS, Glaspy J, et al. In vivo trafficking of adoptively transferred interleukin-2 expanded tumor-infiltrating lymphocytes and peripheral blood lymphocytes. Results of a double gene marking trial. *J Clin Invest.* 1996;97:515–521.
6. Klebanoff C, Khong HT, Antony PA, et al. Sinks, suppressors and antigen presenters: how lymphodepletion enhances T cell-mediated tumor immunotherapy. *Trends Immunol.* 2005;26:111–117.

7. North R. Cyclophosphamide-facilitated adoptive immunotherapy of an established tumor depends on elimination of tumor-induced suppressor T cells. *J Exp Med.* 1982;155:1063–1074.

8. Dudley M, Wunderlich JR, Yang JC, et al. A phase I study of non-myeloablative chemotherapy and adoptive transfer of autologous tumor antigen-specific T lymphocytes in patients with metastatic melanoma. *J Immunother.* 2002;25:243–251.

9. Dudley M, Wunderlich JR, Yang JC, et al. Adoptive cell transfer therapy following non-myeloablative but lymphodepleting chemotherapy for the treatment of patients with refractory metastatic melanoma. *J Clin Oncol.* 2005;23:2346–2357.

10. Gattinoni L, Klebanoff CA, Palmer DC, et al. Acquisition of full effector function in vitro paradoxically impairs the in vivo antitumor efficacy of adoptively transferred CD8+ T cells. *J Clin Invest.* 2005;115:1616–1626.

11. Yee C, Thompson JA, Byrd D, et al. Adoptive T cell therapy using antigen-specific CD8+ T cell clones for the treatment of patients with metastatic melanoma: in vivo persistence, migration, and antitumor effect of transferred T cells. *Proc Natl Acad Sci U S A.* 2002;99:16168–16173.

12. Mackensen A, Meidenbauer N, Vogl S, et al. Phase I study of adoptive T-cell therapy using antigen-specific CD8+ T cells for the treatment of patients with metastatic melanoma. J Clin Oncol. 2006;24:5060–5069.

13. Overwijk W, Theoret MR, Finkelstein SE. Tumor regression and autoimmunity after reversal of a functionally tolerant state of self-reactive CD8+ T cells. *J Exp Med.* 2003;198:569–580.

14. Wrzesinski C, Paulos CM, Gattinoni L, et al. Hematopoietic stem cells promote the expansion and function of adoptively transferred antitumor CD8 T cells. *J Clin Invest.* 2007;117:492–501.

15. Yang L, Baltimore D. Long-term in vivo provision of antigen-specific T cell immunity by programming hematopoietic stem cells. *Proc Natl Acad Sci U S A.*. 2005;102:4518–4523.

16. Morgan R, Dudley ME, Wunderlich JR, et al. Cancer regression in patients after transfer of genetically engineered lymphocytes. *Science.* 2006;314:126–129.

26

Melanoma: Surgical Approach to Metastatic Disease

James M. McLoughlin, Jonathan S. Zager, Andrew S. Sloan, and Vernon K. Sondak

Metastatic melanoma can present with a wide variety of symptoms and in almost any organ system in the body. Most patients with metastatic melanoma have disease that is too extensive to resect or that is unresectable by virtue of its location. Even patients with regional metastases (i.e., in-transit disease) or with isolated, potentially resectable distant metastases most often harbor microscopic metastases that preclude long-term disease control by surgery. Nonetheless, numerous retrospective studies and some prospective trials have demonstrated better-than-expected survival rates in metastatic melanoma patients undergoing complete surgical resection. Moreover, advances in imaging technologies as well as improvements in surgical techniques and perioperative care raise the prospect that patients with truly isolated metastatic disease can be identified and safely subjected to surgery. A surgical approach requires an understanding of the disease process, adequate imaging, and careful patient selection.

More than any other factor, the inherent biology of the tumor determines the ultimate outcome. Reported survival rates for patients with metastatic melanoma vary widely, and it has long been recognized that patients selected for more aggressive treatments tend to be those who would have lived longer even in the absence of therapy. Retrospective reports have noted that a long disease-free interval from primary diagnosis to the diagnosis of metastases, fewer metastatic lesions, and limited numbers of organ systems involved by disease all identify patients that are more likely to have prolonged survival after surgical intervention, but also after systemic therapies as well (1–4). Although it is likely that someday high-throughput techniques for gene expression analysis will reliably identify patients who will benefit from surgical intervention as well as those who will not, for now, clinical predictors must be used in the selection of patients with metastatic melanoma for surgery.

THE NATURAL HISTORY OF DISTANT METASTATIC MELANOMA

Long-term survival after an intervention may be as much a reflection of the natural history of the disease as a result of the intervention itself (4,5). The underlying expectation of a uniformly poor outcome in the absence of surgery may influence the surgeon to choose a surgical approach that may not actually alter the disease outcome. Conversely, an inappropriately pessimistic view of the likelihood of a good outcome after surgery may lead to the addition of untested adjunctive therapies, with any good outcomes subsequently attributed to the nonsurgical therapy. There is a distinct lack of clinical trials that evaluate patients with a clinically and radiographically resectable lesion randomized to nonsurgical versus surgical therapy, and we are only beginning to gain insights from prospective trials of surgery alone or with postoperative adjuvant therapy. The literature is replete, however, with retrospective studies, analyses of prospectively acquired databases, and a multitude of case reports attesting to the potential value of surgical treatment of metastatic melanoma in properly selected cases (1–3,5–9). We will present data from studies that may help clarify a baseline against which surgical interventions can be compared in hopes of shedding light on whether or not a resection would make a difference in an individual with metastatic melanoma.

The Surveillance Epidemiology and End Results (SEER) database represents 71,842 patients with melanoma, treated or not, from 17 sites throughout the United States during the period of 1999 to 2005 (10). In this database, patients are classified only as having localized, regional, or distant disease. The 1,957 patients with distant disease in this database had an approximately 15% survival at f5 years (Table 26.1). It is not known what percentage of patients had surgery as primary treatment for their metastatic disease, but it likely was a small minority. The database of the American Joint Committee on Cancer (AJCC), as described by Balch et al. (11), is composed of data from 17,600 patients treated within a clinical trial context or at institutions with prospective databases. In the 2002 AJCC staging system (Table 26.2), patients with distant metastatic melanoma are subclassified based on sites of disease (skin/soft tissue and nodes vs. lung vs. other visceral sites) and serum lactate dehydrogenase level (LDH). Patients with M1a disease have only skin, soft-tissue, or nodal metastases and a normal LDH, and have the best 5-year survival (18.8%) (Table 26.1). Patients with non-pulmonary visceral metastases or an elevated serum LDH (M1c) constitute the majority of patients with metastatic disease in the AJCC database, and these patients had a 5-year survival of only 9.5%. As with the SEER database, few patients were likely to have had surgery as primary treatment for their metastatic disease. Chang et al. (12) identified 823 patients in the National Cancer Data Base with a diagnosis of stage IV melanoma, and reported an overall 5-year survival of 17.9% (Table 26.1). Patients in this database were categorized based on therapy received. Even in the absence of any treatment, 15.9% of patients survived beyond 5 years (12). Patients who received surgery, with or without adjuvant radiation therapy, as treatment for their

Table 26.1

Five-Year Survival of Patients with Distant Metastatic Melanoma in Large Databases

Ref.	Database	Total No. of Patients in Database	No. of Patients with Distant Metastatic Melanoma	5-Year Survival for Patients with Distant Metastatic Melanoma (%)
SEER (10)	SEER	48,923	1,957	15.3
Balch et al. (11)	AJCC	17,600	M1a-179	18.8
			M1b-186	6.7
			M1c-793	9.5
Chang et al. (12)	National Cancer Database	84,836	823	17.9

SEER, Surveillance Epidemiology and End Results; AJCC, American Joint Committee on Cancer.

Table 26.2

American Joint Committee on Cancer Staging System for Melanoma

T1a	Tumor $\leq$ 1.0 mm thick, and ulceration absent, and Clark Level II or III
T1b	Tumor $\leq$ 1.0 mm thick and ulceration present or Clark Level IV or V
T2a	Tumor 1.01–2.0 mm thick and ulceration absent
T2b	Tumor 1.01–2.0 mm thick and ulceration present
T3a	Tumor 2.01–4.0 mm thick and ulceration absent
T3b	Tumor 2.01–4.0 mm thick and ulceration present
T4a	Tumor >4.0 mm thick and ulceration absent
T4b	Tumor >4.0 mm thick and ulceration present
N1a	Micrometastasis in one regional lymph node
N1b	Macrometastasis in one regional lymph node
N2a	Micrometastasis in two or three regional lymph nodes
N2b	Macrometastasis in two or three regional lymph nodes
N2c	In-transit metastasis(es) or satellite(s) without metastatic lymph nodes
N3	Four or more regional lymph nodes, or matted metastatic lymph nodes, or in-transit metastasis(es) or satellite(s) with lymph node(s)
M1a	Metastasis in skin, subcutaneous tissue, or nonregional lymph nodes and normal serum LDH level
M1b	Lung metastasis and normal serum LDH level
M1c	All other visceral metastasis and normal serum LDH level
	Any distant metastasis and elevated serum LDH level

	Pathologic Stage			Clinical Stage		
Stage	T	N	M	T	N	M
Stage IA	T1a	N0	M0	T1a	N0	M0
Stage IB	T1b or T2a	N0	M0	T1b or T2a	N0	M0
Stage IIA	T2b or T3a	N0	M0	T2b or T3a	N0	M0
Stage IIB	T3b or T4a	N0	M0	T3b or T4a	N0	M0
Stage IIC	T4b	N0	M0	T4b	N0	M0
Stage III				Any T	N1–N3	M0
Stage IIIA	T1-4a	N1a or N2a	M0			
Stage IIIB	T1-4b	N1a or N2a	M0			
Stage IIIC	T1-4b	N1b or N2b	M0			
	Any T	N3	M0			
Stage IV	Any T	Any N	Any M1	Any T	Any N	Any M1

From Greene FL, Page DL, Balch CM, et al. (eds). *AJCC Cancer Staging Manual*, 6th edition. New York: Springer-Verlag; 2002.

Table 26.3

Five-Year Survival of Patients with In-Transit or Regionally Metastatic Melanoma

Ref.	Database	Total No. of Patients in Database	No. of Patients with In-Transit or Regional Melanoma	5-Year Survival for Patients with Regionally Metastatic Melanoma (%)
SEER (10)	SEER	48,923	5,871—regional	64.9
Balch et al. (11)	AJCC	17,600	Stage IIIB (all patients)—543	53
			Stage IIIC (in-transit with nodes)—396	26.7
Chang et al. (12)	National Cancer Database	84,836	1,251—Stage III	49.0

AJCC, American Joint Committee on Cancer.

distant metastatic disease had a 5-year survival of 20.3%. Institutional database reports have also described long-term survival for metastatic melanoma patients who were both surgically and nonsurgically treated (13,14). These results highlight the observation that, although the median survival for stage IV melanoma is poor, some patients with distant disease will survive 5 years and even beyond.

NATURAL HISTORY OF IN-TRANSIT MELANOMA

The SEER data (10) indicate a 5-year survival of 61.9% for patients with regional spread of their melanoma (stage III). Chang et al. (12) report a 49% 5-year survival of all stage III cutaneous melanomas (Table 26.3). The outcome for patients with stage III melanoma varies widely based on a number of clinicopathologic factors. Survival for stage III melanoma patients is impacted by the number of nodes involved with metastatic tumor and by whether the nodal metastases are detected when clinically occult (during elective node dissection or sentinel node biopsy of clinically negative nodes) or clinically overt (identified by palpation or imaging studies). Interestingly, even after the development of nodal metastases, ulceration of the primary tumor retains independent prognostic significance. Thus, in the AJCC database (11), the 5-year survival for the group of stage III patients in the most favorable prognostic category (one microscopically involved lymph node from a nonulcerated primary tumor) was 63%, as opposed to 17% for the group in the least favorable category (clinically evident involvement of four or more nodes from an ulcerated primary tumor).

Stage III melanoma status also encompasses patients with cutaneous and subcutaneous metastases that develop in the dermal or subdermal lymphatics between the primary tumor site and the regional lymph node basin(s), termed *in-transit metastases*. Some classification schemes have arbitrarily distinguished satellite lesions from in-transit metastases based on their distance from the primary tumor: satellites are defined as occurring within 2 cm of the original primary, whereas in-transit metastases are more than 2 cm from the original lesion. The prognosis for both in-transit and satellite lesions are similar, however, and in the cur-

rent AJCC staging system, in-transit and satellite lesions are combined (Table 26.2). Satellite and/or in-transit metastases have been reported to develop in 4% to 7% of patients with cutaneous melanoma. They are most common in patients with thick, ulcerated primary tumors, and somewhat more common in patients with lower extremity rather than upper extremity primaries.

In the AJCC guidelines, in-transit or satellite disease is classified as N2c if it occurs in the absence of nodal involvement, and as N3 if any nodes are involved. Five-year survival for patients with stage IIIB cancer with N2c disease can be as high as 46% with no ulceration and 24% with ulceration of the primary lesion. Patients with stage IIIC disease, which includes N3 disease, have a 27% 5-year survival with or without ulceration of the primary lesion. Clearly, in-transit and satellite disease should be considered as manifestations of regional lymphatic involvement and treated aggressively, as long-term survivors are not uncommon.

SYSTEMIC THERAPY FOR METASTATIC MELANOMA

When considering a surgical intervention, the tumor's response to medical therapy should also be understood. A multitude of systemic options are available for treating advanced melanoma. Long-term survival has been reported in small numbers of patients treated with immunotherapy or cytotoxic chemotherapy, either as single-agent therapy or in combination regimens (14–16). Khan et al. (17) evaluated 212 patients treated by a variety of medical approaches. A significantly improved survival was noted in a small subset of patients who had objective responses to any type of systemic therapy (18 patients in all, or 8.5%) as opposed to those who did not respond ($p = .0001$) (Figure 26.1). This result may partly reflect an inherent difference in tumor biology in addition to the effect from therapy. Adjuvant treatment for patients with melanoma who have been resected free of clinically evident disease has been extensively tested. Therapies investigated have ranged from immunotherapy (18) to vaccines (19), chemotherapy (14), and radiation (20,21). The advantages of adjuvant therapy have been small and their impact on overall survival is debatable (18,19). Nonetheless, both high-dose

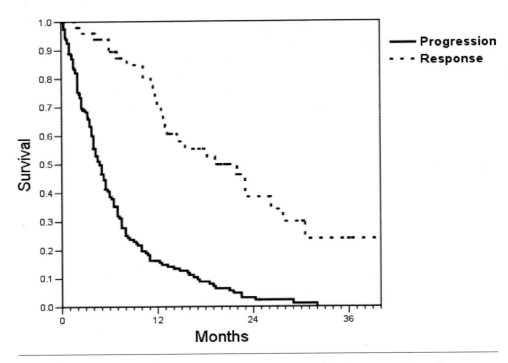

Figure 26.1 Survival for metastatic melanoma patients treated with systemic chemotherapy, comparing patients with progressive disease and patients with a response to treatment. $P = 0.0001$. (Khan et al)[17] Reproduced with permission.

interferon and postoperative radiation are employed to variable degrees in patients at high risk of recurrence after surgery. Neither therapy, however, reliably controls unresectable or gross residual melanoma after incomplete resection.

Using the multicenter published databases as a baseline, it is then useful to compare reported results after surgery for patients with metastatic melanoma. In Table 26.4, multiple studies are highlighted to emphasize the variability associated with published reports. In aggregate, the studies that report data about excisions achieving microscopically clear margins of resection (R0 resection) strongly support the interpretation that surgical intervention impacts survival only when all grossly evident disease can be removed. The data suggest that the actual location of metastasis may not be as important as the ability to achieve complete removal of all disease. To maximize the chances for complete resection of metastatic disease, all patients being considered for surgery should have a thorough preoperative evaluation including appropriate imaging studies.

PREOPERATIVE ASSESSMENT

To select patients with regional or distant metastatic melanoma who have the potential to benefit from surgery, the preoperative evaluation focuses on understanding the patient's risk for complications and thoroughly assessing the extent of the melanoma. A thorough history and physical examination should be performed, looking particularly for signs and symptoms that may reflect metastatic disease in sites where imaging studies have low sensitivity, such as the small bowel. Patients should be questioned for weight loss, nausea, emesis, headaches, melena, hemoptysis, night sweats, or any new or changing symptoms.

Physical examination is highly sensitive for evaluating the skin and subcutaneous tissue for metastases, less sensitive for lymph node metastases, and very insensitive for lung, visceral, and central nervous system metastases. Determining the appropriate radiologic evaluation is controversial because of a lack of reliable studies. Routine preoperative imaging in stage I, II, and IIIA melanoma patients is unproductive and has an unacceptably high rate of false-positive findings (22–27). For patients with stage IIIB/C and stage IV melanoma being considered for surgical treatment, however, the rate of identification of clinically occult metastases is high enough to justify the risk of encountering false-positive findings. Prospective data are surprisingly limited, but the available evidence supports brain magnetic resonance imaging (MRI), chest, abdominal and pelvic computed tomography (CT), and whole-body positron emission tomography (PET) scanning as worthwhile in the preoperative evaluation of stage IIIB/C and IV melanoma patients (28,29).

Although not an absolute contraindication to surgery for extracerebral metastases, the presence of brain metastases generally leads to a decision not to operate on such a patient until and unless the central nervous system (CNS) disease can also be controlled. Hence, routine preoperative evaluation of the CNS is justified (30). Gadolinium-enhanced MRI is the most sensitive test for detecting brain metastases from melanoma and should be routinely employed. CT is an alternative in patients with a contraindication to MRI. PET scans can be used for the brain, but standard ^{18}F-fluorodeoxyglucose (^{18}F-FDG) PET is an insensitive test for identifying brain metastases because of the brain's high baseline glucose utilization.

For the remainder of the body, the ^{18}F-FDG PET scan has emerged as a useful and sensitive study to identify unsuspected

Table 26.4

Results of Resection for Patients with Metastatic Melanoma from Institutional Series

Author	Year	N	Location	MDFS	MOS	5-yr
Pawlik et al[62]	2006	40	Liver	Ocular: 8.3 mo	29.4 mo	20.5%
				Cutaneous: 4.7 mo	23.6 mo	0%
Essner et al[80]	2004	1,574	GI tract	—	36.7	28%
Wood et al[13]	2001	60	Abdominal organs	R_0: 15 mo (1–47)	27.6 mo (1–112)	24%
				R_2: 0	8.4 mo	0%
Rose et al[81]	2001	24	Liver	R_0: 12 mo	28 mo (2–147)	29%
				R_2: 0	4 mo	0%
Gutman et al[86]	2001	35	GI tract	R_0: —	17 mo	0%
Leo et al[6]	2000	282	Lung	—	19 mo	22%
Ollila et al[82]	1999	211	All sites	R_0: 8 mo (0.6–91)	18.2 mo	20%
				R_2: 0	—	7%
				Observation: 0	—	2.1%
Haigh et al[57]	1999	27	Adrenal	R_0: 12 mo	18.6 mo (1–67)	10%
				R_2: 0	7.7 mo (1–61)	—
Agrawal et al[85]	1999	68	GI tract	—	8.2 mo	18%
Eton et al[87]	1998	57	All sites	—	10 mo	5%
Ollila et al[1]	1996	69	GI Tract	R_0: —	48.9 mo	41%
				R_2: —	5.4 mo	—
				Observation: —	5.7 mo	—
Barth et al[84]	1995	1521	All Sites	M1a: —	12.5 mo	14%
				M1b: —	8.3 mo	4%
				M1c: —	4.4 mo	3%
Tafra et al[52]	1995	106	Lung	—	18 mo	27%
Wong et al[83]	1993	144	All Sites	—	—	20%

MDFS, median disease free survival; MOS, median overall survival; R, resection status.

metastatic lesions. Glucose is readily concentrated in melanoma; however, the PET scan does have limitations. As with all imaging studies, the sensitivity of PET scans for detecting tumors <1 cm in size diminishes. Because PET is a purely functional study, anatomic localization can be problematic. To improve the anatomic localization, PET is often combined with a CT scan to produce a study referred to as a PET/CT fusion. However, hypermetabolic areas on PET with no corresponding CT abnormality are commonly encountered, and can be difficult if not impossible to categorize as true- or false-positive findings. The development of handheld probes capable of detecting ^{18}F-FDG intraoperatively may help overcome this problem in the future (31).

Several prospective trials have evaluated PET in the preoperative setting. Brady et al. (29) studied 103 patients imaged for preoperative evaluation of stage IIC, III, and IV melanoma. They concluded that PET is better than CT in identifying distant disease, but the combination of the two studies is more accurate than each individually. The scan findings of additional disease impacted surgical decision making in their series, but false-positive and indeterminate findings were common. In 36 of 103 patients, findings on imaging resulted in management changes. Of these 36 patients, 34 had a change in their management by findings either exclusively seen on PET or seen on both PET and CT, whereas only 2 had a change in management based on CT findings in the absence of a PET abnormality. Ultimately, 19 of 36 patients had their planned surgery canceled because of the extent of disease discovered by the imaging studies.

False-positive findings, however, were not uncommon. Among the 59 patients undergoing both CT and PET, 5 had false-positive findings and 10 had false-negative results. False-negative results were defined those as having a normal PET and developing a metastasis within the following 4 months. Fuster et al. (28) retrospectively evaluated PET scans in patients with known metastatic melanoma as a surveillance tool compared with standard screening techniques including physical examination, CT scans, MRI, ultrasound, liver function blood tests, and plain x-rays. They concluded that PET scanning alone was more accurate overall than all other standard screening techniques combined. The false-negative rate for lung lesions was 12 of 89 with an overall sensitivity of 57% (Table 26.5).

As previously noted, studies suggest that patients with stage I and II disease derive little benefit from routine preoperative imaging because of high false-positive rates and a low yield of true positive findings (22–27). However, in preparing to operate

Table 26.5

Comparison of Positron Emission Tomography and Other Imaging Modalities in Patients with Melanoma

Author	Year	Role		TP	FP	TN	FN
Brady (29) N = 103	2005	Preoperative staging	CT:	48%	5%	95%	52%
			PET:	68%	8%	92%	32%
			PET/CT:	77%	8%	92%	23%
Reinhardt (88) N = 250	2006	Correlation with clinical staging	CT:	78.8%	15.7%	–	–
			PET:	92.8%	4.3%	–	–
			PET/CT:	97.2%	1.2%	–	–
Fuster (29) N = 101	2004	Screening for pulmonary recurrence	PET:	68%	16%	12%	5%
			CT:	51%	26%	2%	22%

TP, true positive; FP, false positive; TN, true negative; FN, false negative; PE, Physical Exam; LFT, liver function tests.

on patients with in-transit metastases or stage IV disease, PET combined with CT imaging can identify clinically significant disease that changes the management algorithm in a substantial number of patients, justifying the risk of encountering false-positive findings.

In the workup for in-transit disease, the presence of concomitant lymph node metastasis affects the surgical approach. Therefore, preoperative evaluation of the lymph node basin is an important consideration. Even though PET and CT can both identify nodal metastases, particularly those larger than a centimeter, ultrasound of the nodal basin has emerged as a more sensitive test that can also be used to provide localization if a needle biopsy is required (32,33).

A chest x-ray is often used in the preoperative evaluation in patients with stage III and stage IV disease. CT has a much higher sensitivity for small pulmonary metastases, including metastases below the threshold for detection by PET, but also identifies a large number of tiny and indeterminate lesions (23,28). Blood tests are notoriously insensitive and nonspecific in metastatic melanoma patients, and no highly accurate melanoma-specific serologic markers exist. Mild elevations of serum LDH are very nonspecific, but marked elevations usually indicate widespread disease (11,23). Nonetheless, a patient with otherwise resectable stage III or IV melanoma should not be denied resection on the basis of LDH elevation alone.

TREATMENT ALGORITHMS

In-Transit Disease

When treating in-transit disease, surgery should be attempted first if anatomically possible with the goal of a complete resection. Attention should also be directed to the lymph node basin, as survival is worse if lymph node metastasis is present (11,34–36). Surgical approaches to in-transit disease are based on the feasibility of resection as well as minimizing morbidity. We propose an algorithmic approach to treating in-transit disease (Figure 26.2). Once the preoperative workup has been performed to exclude the presence of systemic disease, patients with relatively few lesions can be treated with resection along with lymph node

dissection if nodal basins are found to be positive. A skin graft may be needed for closure, and consideration should be given to radiating the region of in-transit disease to minimize local recurrence (20,21). A histologically negative margin is a sufficient goal when resecting in-transit metastases; unlike resection for a primary tumor, no predetermined margin of normal tissue is established. After an initial resection of in-transit metastases, further recurrence in the same extremity is commonplace. Dong et al. (37) reviewed 648 patients with recurrent melanoma in a locoregional distribution. Fifty-five of those surgically treated experienced a second relapse within 2 years, and by 5 years, 82% percent had a local recurrence. When recurrence is limited to one or a few nodules, repeat resection is an appropriate approach. Frequent recurrences after surgery, radiation, and systemic therapy or recurrences presenting with a larger numbers of lesions may require an alternative approach. Local treatments such as intralesional therapy or laser therapy (38,39) have been used but have not had the same local control success as isolated limb infusion or isolated limb perfusion (40–49).

If surgery cannot achieve a complete resection of all in-transit metastases, patients have a choice of regional or systemic treatment approaches. A trial of systemic therapy is not unreasonable given the high risk of eventual development of distant metastases in patients with in-transit disease, particularly with prior or concomitant nodal involvement. Patients with very bulky or symptomatic in-transit metastases are more likely to obtain relief from a regional chemotherapy approach. Currently, regional chemotherapy is administered by either hyperthermic isolated limb perfusion (40,41) or by the minimally invasive technique of isolated limb infusion (42–45).

The limb perfusion technique involves the surgical isolation and cannulation of the inflow and outflow vessels of an extremity from the remainder of the body. A heart-lung bypass machine is connected to the cannulae and high concentrations of a therapeutic agent at hyperthermic temperatures are perfused through the limb for an hour or more. Melphalan (L-phenylalanine mustard) is the perfusion drug of choice in the United States. Tumor necrosis factor-α has also been used in the United States and in Europe, but has not shown significant benefit compared with melphalan in randomized trials (41), and

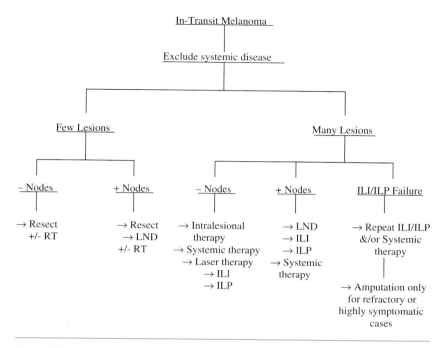

Figure 26.2 Algorithm of treatment options for in-transit melanoma. RT, radiation therapy; ILI, isolated limb infusion; ILP, isolated limb perfusion; LND, lymph node dissection; → Treatment Options.

is not available for use in the United States. Side effects in the perfused limb can range from mild erythema to extensive epidermolysis. Deep tissue damage can require fasciotomies or urgent amputations. If tumor necrosis factor-α is used, great care must be exercised to prevent leakage of the cytokine into the systemic circulation, which can induce a severe systemic inflammatory response that can be life-threatening (40,41,46,47). Randomized trials of limb perfusion in the adjuvant setting, after resection of an intermediate- or high-risk primary melanoma, have failed to demonstrate a survival benefit and the significant toxicity of limb perfusion cannot be justified in the adjuvant setting (48). However, in the therapeutic setting overall response rates up to 90% have been reported, and long-term survival is not uncommon (41,43,44).

Isolated limb infusion, generally using melphalan plus dactinomycin (actinomycin D), is a less invasive form of regional chemotherapy using radiologically placed cannulae and tourniquet occlusion to isolate the limb (42,45,49). It is an option for some patients who would be poor candidates for limb perfusion because of medical comorbidities, extremity edema, or circulatory problems, or because of extensive prior surgeries hindering access to the vessels. It may also be more appropriate for patients undergoing palliative regional therapy in the presence of documented distant metastasis. Isolated limb infusion has been shown in small studies in the United States (49) as well as from the Sydney Melanoma Unit (43,44) to provide durable regional disease-free control rates that are comparable to those historically reported for limb perfusion. It has not, however, been prospectively compared with limb perfusion in patients who are good candidates for both procedures. In our algorithm, we consider performing isolated limb infusion prior to using isolated limb perfusion because of the less severe side effect profile

of isolated limb infusion. We would consider repeating isolated limb infusion one or more times prior to proceeding to isolated limb perfusion.

Multiple individual lesions can be treated at one time by intralesional therapy. Little is known of the long-term efficacy of this approach, however. Intralesional therapy with bacille Calmette-Guérin, granulocyte-macrophage colony-stimulating factor (GM-CSF), interleukin 2 or other cytokines has also been employed in anecdotal cases or small series of patients (50). Injected lesions frequently regress, and occasional regressions of noninjected lesions have been observed, but the long-term control rate is far below that seen with limb perfusion or infusion. Nonetheless, intralesional therapy remains an option for patients with significant comorbidities that would preclude limb infusion or perfusion, and for those with recurrences after perfusion. Ongoing investigations of intralesional gene therapy offer the hope that techniques can be developed that would have a high likelihood of leading to regression of uninjected lesions and even protection against subsequent metastatic disease with minimal toxicity (51).

Pulmonary Metastases

The lungs are the most common visceral site of metastasis in melanoma. Between 12% and 36% of patients with metastatic melanoma will develop one or more pulmonary metastases. If a metastatic lesion is truly isolated to the lung, pulmonary resection is an acceptable treatment. Several studies have reported a median survival rate between 10 and 28 months and a 5-year survival of 6% to 27% (6,52–56). Even in the presence of multiple nodules, some patients will benefit from resection as long as a complete resection can be performed. The advent

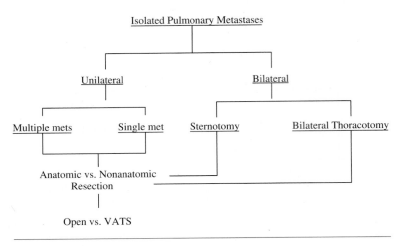

Figure 26.3 Algorithm for treating isolated pulmonary metastases. VATS, video-assisted thoracic surgery; met, metastasis.

of video-assisted thoracotomy has increased the interest in resecting metastases of all types, including melanoma, although precisely how much advantage this approach provides is a matter of debate. Wedge resections are the appropriate procedure for most melanoma metastases; lobectomies should be rare and pneumonectomy is almost never indicated (52). In our algorithm, surgical resection is considered when no other evidence of systemic disease is identified. Little has been documented about the proper approach to bilateral metastases, but a sternotomy would be an acceptable initial approach (52) (Figure 26.3).

Abdominal Metastases

The abdomen is a common site of metastasis in melanoma, but only splenic, adrenal, and gastrointestinal metastases are commonly approached surgically. Of all patients with melanoma, 1.5% to 4.4% will develop symptomatic metastasis to the gastrointestinal tract. Typical symptoms, when present, include pain, gastrointestinal bleeding, anemia, obstruction, weight loss, and a palpable mass. In the evaluation of metastases to abdominal organs, surgery should be considered if all disease can be removed. The ability to resect all disease has consistently proven to be the most important factor in prolonging survival. Ollila et al. (1) reviewed 124 patients evaluated for melanoma metastatic to the gastrointestinal tract. Of the 124 patients, 69 patients underwent surgical resection. Forty-six of the patients were treated for cure and had a 48.9-month median survival. Twenty-three patients were treated for palliation of symptoms and had a 5.4-month median survival. The remaining 55 patients treated nonoperatively had a 5.7-month overall survival.

Metastases to the gastrointestinal tract may present with bleeding or obstruction, conditions often requiring surgical intervention for palliation. In bleeding patients, the source of hemorrhage is often difficult to identify at surgery, and the patient is found to have multiple intestinal lesions, which even if not currently symptomatic can be anticipated to produce symptoms in the near future. Therefore, palliation may require resection of multiple loops of bowel or, in the case of obstruction, an intestinal bypass to achieve symptomatic relief. In contrast to

the survival benefit associated with curative surgery in which all known metastatic disease is removed, several studies, including the previously mentioned study by Ollila et al. (1), have demonstrated that palliative surgery does not prolong survival; in fact, in some studies the survival is worse than with a nonoperative approach. Nevertheless, symptomatic relief can be achieved in carefully selected patients operated on by experienced surgical teams.

Metastases to the adrenal gland may occasionally be the only site of disease. Several studies have demonstrated prolonged survival in resected patients when no other site of disease was encountered (57–60). If technically feasible, a laparoscopic adrenalectomy can be performed as long as negative margins can be achieved. Laparoscopy has the advantage of evaluating the abdomen for intra-abdominal metastases that can be missed on preoperative imaging. Many times the adrenal metastases are locally invasive or incite an inflammatory response that necessitates an open approach to safely achieve negative margins. Bilateral adrenal metastases do occur and can be resected laparoscopically. Adrenal preservation may be considered, but long-term steroid replacement would be preferred to leaving a positive margin (Figure 26.4). Haigh et al. (57) demonstrated that survival was significantly longer when adrenal metastases were treated for cure rather than for palliation. The median survival was 25.7 months for the curative group, 9.9 months for the palliative group, and 7.7 months for those patients treated nonoperatively. Metastases to the spleen should also be considered for resection if no other evidence of disease is identified. Laparoscopic and open procedures have been described, and either approach is satisfactory if complete tumor excision can be accomplished (61).

Metastases to the liver often present with multiple lesions or disease in unresectable locations. However, in the select patients who have resectable disease, surgery may be considered. Intraoperative ultrasound is very useful to identify additional lesions not seen preoperatively. Surgical resection can be performed with an anatomic or nonanatomic approach and may require the addition of radiofrequency ablation to achieve negative margins. Ablative techniques can be used as a sole treatment

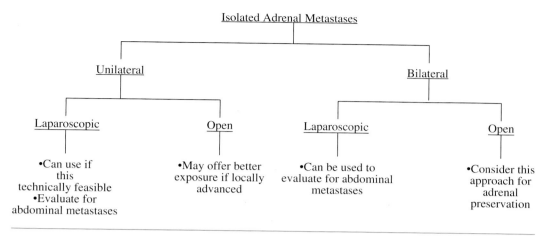

Figure 26.4 Algorithm for treating isolated metastases to the adrenal gland.

method as well (Figure 26.5). Overall, the outcomes tend to be poor. Pawlik et al. (62) demonstrated a median survival of 23.6 months in 24 patients with cutaneous melanoma metastatic to the liver, with no patient surviving longer than 45 months. It remains unclear why the outcomes for resection of apparently isolated liver metastases seem so much worse than for other isolated visceral melanoma metastases, but at present liver resection should be employed for the treatment of metastatic melanoma only in highly selected cases, if at all, and only after a thorough search for other intra- and extrahepatic disease. Hepatic arterial chemoembolization is an alternative therapy to resection. Sharma et al. (69), demonstrated improved survival in select patients with isolated, metastatic melanoma to the liver. Further investigation is still needed to determine the role and efficacy of chemoembolization as current data is very limited.

Brain Metastases

Brain metastases are common in patients with melanoma, which is the third most common cause of brain metastases. The incidence of clinically relevant brain metastases in patients with melanoma has been as high as 10% to 19% in patients with regional (stage III) disease and 18% to 26% in patients with stage IV

disease, and the prevalence at autopsy is 49% to 75% (63). Factors associated with brain metastases in melanoma are male gender, mucosal or head and neck or trunk primaries, and deep or ulcerated lesions (64). Melanoma brain metastases are frequently symptomatic because of hemorrhage or seizure, with the clinical manifestations of individual cases related to the precise anatomic location of the metastases.

The treatment of melanoma brain metastases remains controversial. There are few randomized trials on management of melanoma brain metastases and thus no definitive management paradigm. At present, treatment is typically determined by the size and location of the lesions, the clinical and neurologic condition of the patient, and the wishes of the patient and family.

Most chemotherapeutic agents do not penetrate the blood–brain barrier well enough to achieve therapeutic intracranial concentrations. Although temozolomide penetrates the brain well, efficacy is limited (65). Whether or not temozolomide will ultimately have a role in conjunction with whole-brain or localized radiation remains to be seen. Melanoma is relatively radio-resistant, and whole-brain radiotherapy (WBRT) alone has limited efficacy, with median survival of 2 to 4 months (66,67).

Prospective randomized trials have established that surgical resection combined with WBRT is the definitive treatment

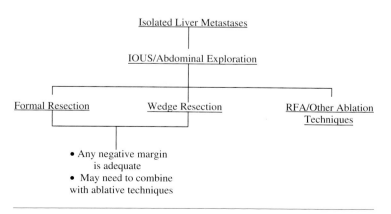

Figure 26.5 Algorithm for treating isolated liver metastases.
IOUS, intraoperative ultrasound; RFA, radiofrequency ablation.

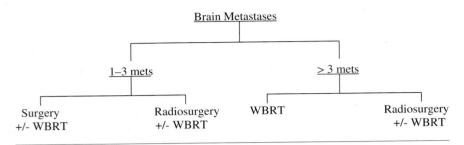

Figure 26.6 Algorithm for treating brain metastases. WBRT, whole-brain radiation therapy.

for single cortical brain metastases from solid tumors (68,69). However, few melanoma patients were represented in these trials, and the propensity for multiple brain metastases in patients with melanoma as well as the failure of melanoma to respond to typical doses of radiation (30 Gray total in 10 fractions of 2 Gray each) limit the applicability of these results to the management of patients with melanoma brain metastases. In melanoma patients with a one to three superficial metastases amenable to resection, surgery with or without WBRT is associated with median survival of 8 to 11 months (66,67). Improved outcome is associated with good prognostic indicators including Karnofsky performance status >70%, controlled primary, age <65 years, and no evidence of extracranial systemic metastases (66,70).

Recently, investigators have demonstrated the efficacy of stereotactic radiosurgery (SRS) for patients with brain metastases. Radiosurgery employs a multidisciplinary approach to treatment and allows multiple intracranial lesions to be treated simultaneously in an outpatient setting. Important limitations to radiosurgery include limited efficacy for tumors >3.5 cm in maximal diameter and a delayed treatment effect (typically 6 to 12 weeks), which does not necessarily lead to tumor shrinkage, making it ineffective in relieving mass effect. The neurosurgeon and the radiation oncologist review the images in order to identify the metastatic lesion or lesions and the structures at risk (such as the optic nerve and chiasm, and brainstem). Working at a computerized SRS planning station, the size, location, and shape of the radiation beam are determined as well as the dose to the target lesion and surrounding brain. An immobilizing frame or mask is placed on the patient prior to treatment, after which the linear accelerator moves about the patient's head to deliver the previously calculated, precisely shaped beams of radiation to the tumor with minimal dose to the surrounding normal brain. Because of the noninvasive fixation devices now employed, the stereotactic radiation can be delivered in one to five fractions to optimize tumor control while minimizing risk to the surrounding normal brain. Typically, however, 15 to 24 Gray is delivered in a single dose, which is an order of magnitude greater than the dose commonly used in WBRT. A recent Radiation Therapy Oncology Group prospective, randomized trial demonstrated SRS combined with WBRT improved survival in solid tumor patients with one to three lesions compared with WBRT alone (71). Again, however, few melanoma patients were represented in this study. A smaller phase II study of SRS sponsored by the Eastern Cooperative Oncology Group and the Southwest Oncology Group for patients with one to three brain metastasis, of whom more than one-third had melanoma, demonstrated a median survival of approximately 6 months after SRS alone (72). Other retrospective studies of SRS combined with WBRT have demonstrated survival of 7 to 8 months (73,74). A more recent retrospective study of patients with five metastasis or fewer treated with SRS demonstrated median survival of 11.1 months and found that WBRT did not improve survival (84). Median survival of up to 28 months has been reported in selected patients with good prognostic indicators (age <60, Karnofsky performance status ≥90, and with stable extracranial disease) (75). An ongoing prospective, randomized phase III trial sponsored by the American College of Surgeons Oncology Group and the North Central Cancer Treatment Group will evaluate SRS with or without WBRT to address this issue in the next few years (Figure 26.6).

Unknown Primary

Patients occasionally present with distant metastases of melanoma from unknown primary sites. In such cases, the patient evaluation requires a thorough history of any lesions that may have been removed, even if the pathology was unknown or presumed to be benign. Furthermore, a thorough skin examination from the scalp to between the toes should be performed, with attention paid to areas of depigmentation that could represent a regressed primary site. In some cases, illumination with a Wood's lamp (ultraviolet or "black" light) can highlight depigmented areas of skin. Although some have speculated that metastatic melanoma from an "unknown primary" actually represents primary visceral or nodal melanoma arising in noncutaneous melanocytes, the literature suggests that the survival of patients with unknown primary melanomas is equivalent to that for patients with known primary tumors and similar clinicopathologic features. Accordingly, we treat unknown primary melanoma patients in exactly the same fashion as patients with a known primary. The one exception to this rule is the isolated finding of a single dermal or subcutaneous nodule of melanoma with no epidermal component. Such lesions are frequently classified by the pathologist as "metastatic melanoma," but the biologic behavior is much more in keeping with a primary melanoma. It is likely that most cases represent a traumatized primary tumor that has lost its epidermal component, although some cases may represent melanoma arising in deep dermal or subcutaneous melanocytes without overlying epidermal involvement. We employ identical surgical margins and use sentinel node mapping in these cases exactly as we would for a typical cutaneous primary melanoma of similar thickness (76,77).

ADJUVANT THERAPY AFTER RESECTION OF METASTATIC MELANOMA

No prospective randomized trials to date have shown a relapse-free or survival advantage for patients with resected metastatic melanoma (either in-transit disease or distant metastases) treated with adjuvant systemic immunotherapy or chemotherapy. High-dose interferon given for 1 year is the accepted standard adjuvant therapy for patients with "high-risk" melanoma metastatic to the regional nodes, but such therapy has never been adequately tested in patients with resected in-transit or distant metastatic melanoma. Nonetheless, because of its role in other high-risk situations, patients with resected metastatic melanoma who have not been treated with interferon should at least be informed about this therapy, and if they are appropriate candidates, referred for evaluation by a medical oncologist. Adjuvant therapy with GM-CSF has been widely employed because of a single, nonrandomized phase II trial that involved patients with resected stage IV disease and showed improved survival compared with a historical control cohort (78). However, it is clear that the historical control cohort chosen was from an earlier era than the patients in the trial, and likely had a markedly inferior prognosis based on advances in imaging and patient selection. Nonetheless, this phase II trial led to the performance of a cooperative-group phase III trial (E4697) evaluating the role of GM-CSF as well as a peptide vaccine in patients with resected stage III and IV melanoma (79). This trial recently completed accrual of approximately 800 patients and should provide definitive evidence regarding the role, if any, of GM-CSF and vaccines in the adjuvant therapy of resected metastatic melanoma.

"Debulking" or cytoreductive surgery is sometimes performed in metastatic malignancies of various types, with the underlying rationale being to reduce the tumor burden to a level at which systemic therapies can become effective. This strategy has proven valuable in ovarian cancer, but to date has never shown to be of any value in melanoma. There are simply no available systemic therapies for melanoma that work any better with "limited residual disease" than they do with more extensive residual disease. Except within a carefully designed clinical trial, metastatic melanoma patients who cannot be resected to a disease-free state should not undergo surgery, except in very limited situations where palliation—not cytoreduction—is the therapeutic intent.

SUMMARY

In the treatment of metastatic melanoma, complete surgical extirpation of disease is the best option for cure. However, the art of surgery relies on the ability to determine which patient will benefit from intervention. Evaluation requires a thorough history and physical examination and staging studies, including a PET/CT scan, an MRI of the brain, and an LDH level. The literature is limited in what can be proven with scientifically sound and reproducible data. However, what is evident is that a select group of patients will have their disease process altered by an appropriate and aggressive surgical intervention.

REFERENCES

1. Ollila DW, Essner R, Wanek LA, et al. Surgical resection for melanoma metastatic to the gastrointestinal tract. *Arch Surg.* 1996; 131:975–979.
2. Balch CM, Soong SJ, Murad TM, et al. A multifactorial analysis of melanoma. IV. Prognostic factors in 200 melanoma patients with distant metastases (stage III). *J Clin Oncol.* 1983;1:126–134.
3. Karakousis CP, Temple DF, Moore R, et al. Prognostic parameters in recurrent malignant melanoma. *Cancer.* 1983;52:575–579.
4. Flaherty LE, Liu PY, Unger J, et al. Comparison of patient characteristics and outcome between a single-institution phase II trial and a cooperative-group phase II trial with identical eligibility in metastatic melanoma. *Am J Clin Oncol.* 1997;20:600–604.
5. Ollila DW, Stern SL, Morton DL. Tumor doubling time: a selection factor for pulmonary resection of metastatic melanoma. *J Surg Oncol.* 1998;69:206–211.
6. Leo F, Cagini L, Rocmans P, et al. Lung metastases from melanoma: when is surgical treatment warranted? *Br J Cancer.* 2000;83:569–572.
7. Wong SL, Coit DG. Role of surgery in patients with stage IV melanoma. *Curr Opin Oncol.* 2004;16:155–160.
8. Ollila DW, Caudle AS. Surgical management of distant metastases. *Surg Oncol Clin North Am.* 2006;15:385–398.
9. Allen PJ, Coit DG. The surgical management of metastatic melanoma. *Ann Surg Oncol.* 2002;9:762–770.
10. SEER Cancer Statistics Review. 1996-2002.
11. Balch CM, Buzaid AC, Soong SJ, et al. Final version of the American Joint Committee on Cancer staging system for cutaneous melanoma. *J Clin Oncol.* 2001;19:3635–3648.
12. Chang AE, Karnell LH, Menck HR. The National Cancer Data Base report on cutaneous and noncutaneous melanoma: a summary of 84,836 cases from the past decade. The American College of Surgeons Commission on Cancer and the American Cancer Society. *Cancer.* 1998;83:1664–1678.
13. Wood TF, DiFronzo LA, Rose DM, et al. Does complete resection of melanoma metastatic to solid intra-abdominal organs improve survival? *Ann Surg Oncol.* 2001;8:658–662.
14. Vuoristo MS, Hahka-Kemppinen M, Parvinen LM, et al. Randomized trial of dacarbazine versus bleomycin, vincristine, lomustine and dacarbazine (BOLD) chemotherapy combined with natural or recombinant interferon-alpha in patients with advanced melanoma. *Melanoma Res.* 2005;15:291–296.
15. Rosenberg SA, Yang JC, Topalian SL, et al. Treatment of 283 consecutive patients with metastatic melanoma or renal cell cancer using high-dose bolus interleukin 2. *JAMA.* 1994;271:907–913.
16. Eton O, Legha SS, Bedikian AY, et al. Sequential biochemotherapy versus chemotherapy for metastatic melanoma: results from a phase III randomized trial. *J Clin Oncol.* 2002;20:2045–2052.
17. Khan MA, Andrews S, Ismail-Khan R, et al. Overall and progression-free survival in metastatic melanoma: analysis of a single-institution database. *Cancer Control.* 2006;13:211–217.
18. Verma S, Quirt I, McCready D, et al. Systematic review of systemic adjuvant therapy for patients at high risk for recurrent melanoma. *Cancer.* 2006;106:1431–1442.
19. Tagawa ST, Cheung E, Banta W, et al. Survival analysis after resection of metastatic disease followed by peptide vaccines in patients with Stage IV melanoma. *Cancer.* 2006;106:1353–1357.

20. Ballo MT, Ross MI, Cormier JN, et al. Combined-modality therapy for patients with regional nodal metastases from melanoma. *Int J Radiat Oncol Biol Phys.* 2006;64:106–113.

21. Ballo MT, Ang KK. Radiotherapy for cutaneous malignant melanoma: rationale and indications. *Oncology (Williston Park).* 2004;18:99–107.

22. Garbe C, Paul A, Kohler-Spath H, et al. Prospective evaluation of a follow-up schedule in cutaneous melanoma patients: recommendations for an effective follow-up strategy. *J Clin Oncol.* 2003;21:520–529.

23. Wang TS, Johnson TM, Cascade PN, et al. Evaluation of staging chest radiographs and serum lactate dehydrogenase for localized melanoma. *J Am Acad Dermatol.* 2004;51:399–405.

24. Wagner JD, Schauwecker D, Davidson D, et al. Inefficacy of F-18 fluorodeoxy-D-glucose-positron emission tomography scans for initial evaluation in early-stage cutaneous melanoma. *Cancer.* 2005;104:570–579.

25. Longo MI, Lazaro P, Bueno C, et al. Fluorodeoxyglucose-positron emission tomography imaging versus sentinel node biopsy in the primary staging of melanoma patients. *Dermatol Surg.* 2003;29:245–248.

26. Hafner J, Schmid MH, Kempf W, et al. Baseline staging in cutaneous malignant melanoma. *Br J Dermatol.* 2004;150:677–686.

27. Fink AM, Holle-Robatsch S, Herzog N, et al. Positron emission tomography is not useful in detecting metastasis in the sentinel lymph node in patients with primary malignant melanoma stage I and II. *Melanoma Res.* 2004;14:141–145.

28. Fuster D, Chiang S, Johnson G, et al. Is ^{18}F-FDG PET more accurate than standard diagnostic procedures in the detection of suspected recurrent melanoma? *J Nucl Med.* 2004;45:1323–1327.

29. Brady MS, Akhurst T, Spanknebel K, et al. Utility of preoperative ^{18}F-fluorodeoxyglucose-positron emission tomography scanning in high-risk melanoma patients. *Ann Surg Oncol.* 2006;13:525–532.

30. Fogarty GB, Tartaguia C. The utility of magnetic resonance imaging in the detection of brain metastases in the staging of cutaneous melanoma. *Clin Oncol (R Coll Radiol).* 2006;18:360–362.

31. Gulec SA, Daghighian F, Essner R. PET-Probe: Evaluation of technical performance and clinical utility of a handheld high-energy gamma probe in oncologic surgery. *Ann Surg Oncol.* 2006 (e-pub).

32. Kahle B, Hoffend J, Wacker J, et al. Preoperative ultrasonographic identification of the sentinel lymph node in patients with malignant melanoma. *Cancer.* 2003;97:1947–1954.

33. Blum A, Schmid-Wendtner MH, Mauss-Kiefer V, et al. Ultrasound mapping of lymph node and subcutaneous metastases in patients with cutaneous melanoma: results of a prospective multicenter study. *Dermatology.* 2006;212:47–52.

34. Kretschmer L, Beckmann I, Thoms KM, et al. Factors predicting the risk of in-transit recurrence after sentinel lymphonodectomy in patients with cutaneous malignant melanoma. *Ann Surg Oncol.* 2006;13:1105–1112.

35. Kang JC, Wanek LA, Essner R, et al. Sentinel lymphadenectomy does not increase the incidence of in-transit metastases in primary melanoma. *J Clin Oncol.* 2005;23:4764–4670.

36. Chao C, Wong SL, Ross MI, et al. Patterns of early recurrence after sentinel lymph node biopsy for melanoma. *Am J Surg.* 2002;184:520–524.

37. Dong XD, Tyler D, Johnson JL, et al. Analysis of prognosis and disease progression after local recurrence of melanoma. *Cancer.* 2000;88:1063–1071.

38. Hayes AJ, Clark MA, Harries M, et al. Management of in-transit metastases from cutaneous malignant melanoma. *Br J Surg.* 2004;91:673–682.

39. Gibson SC, Byrne DS, McKay AJ. Ten-year experience of carbon dioxide laser ablation as treatment for cutaneous recurrence of malignant melanoma. *Br J Surg.* 2004;91:893–895.

40. Grunhagen DJ, Brunstein F, Graveland WJ, et al. One hundred consecutive isolated limb perfusions with TNF-alpha and melphalan in melanoma patients with multiple in-transit metastases. *Ann Surg.* 2004;240:939–947.

41. Cornett WR, McCall LM, Petersen RP, et al. Randomized multicenter trial of hyperthermic isolated limb perfusion with melphalan alone compared with melphalan plus tumor necrosis factor: American College of Surgeons Oncology Group Trial Z0020. *J Clin Oncol.* 2006;24:4196–4201.

42. Thompson JF, Kam PC. Isolated limb infusion for melanoma: a simple but effective alternative to isolated limb perfusion. *J Surg Oncol.* 2004;88:1–3.

43. Lindner P, Thompson JF, De Wilt JH, et al. Double isolated limb infusion with cytotoxic agents for recurrent and metastatic limb melanoma. *Eur J Surg Oncol.* 2004;30:433–439.

44. Lindner P, Doubrovsky A, Kam PC, et al. Prognostic factors after isolated limb infusion with cytotoxic agents for melanoma. *Ann Surg Oncol.* 2002;9:127–136.

45. Bonenkamp JJ, Thompson JF, de Wilt JH, et al. Isolated limb infusion with fotemustine after dacarbazine chemosensitisation for inoperable loco-regional melanoma recurrence. *Eur J Surg Oncol.* 2004;30:1107–1112.

46. Vrouenraets BC, Kroon BB, Ogilvie AC, et al. Absence of severe systemic toxicity after leakage-controlled isolated limb perfusion with tumor necrosis factor-alpha and melphalan. *Ann Surg Oncol.* 1999;6:405–412.

47. Vrouenraets BC, Hart GA, Eggermont AM, et al. Relation between limb toxicity and treatment outcomes after isolated limb perfusion for recurrent melanoma. *J Am Coll Surg.* 1999;188:522–530.

48. Koops HS, Vaglini M, Suciu S, et al. Prophylactic isolated limb perfusion for localized, high-risk limb melanoma: results of a multicenter randomized phase III trial. European Organization for Research and Treatment of Cancer Malignant Melanoma Cooperative Group Protocol 18832, the World Health Organization Melanoma Program Trial 15, and the North American Perfusion Group Southwest Oncology Group-8593. *J Clin Oncol.* 1998;16:2906–2912.

49. Zager JS, Gershenwald J, Aldrink J, et al. Isolated limb infusion for locally recurrent and in-transit extremity melanoma: a combined institutional initial experience. *Ann Surg Oncol.* 2006;13:84.

50. Morton DL, Eilber FR, Holmes EC, et al. BCG immunotherapy of malignant melanoma: summary of a seven-year experience. *Ann Surg.* 1974;180:635–643.

51. Heller L, Merkler K, Westover J, et al. Evaluation of toxicity following electrically mediated interleukin-12 gene delivery in a B16 mouse melanoma model. *Clin Cancer Res.* 2006;12:3177–3183.

52. Tafra L, Dale PS, Wanek LA, et al. Resection and adjuvant immunotherapy for melanoma metastatic to the lung and thorax. *J Thorac Cardiovasc Surg.* 1995;110:119–128.

53. Karp NS, Boyd A, DePan HJ, et al. Thoracotomy for metastatic malignant melanoma of the lung. *Surgery.* 1990;107:256–261.

54. Karakousis CP, Velez A, Driscoll DL, et al. Metastasectomy in malignant melanoma. *Surgery.* 1994;115:295–302.

55. Harpole DH Jr, Johnson CM, Wolfe WG, et al. Analysis of 945 cases of pulmonary metastatic melanoma. *J Thorac Cardiovasc Surg.* 1992;103:743–748.

56. Gorenstein LA, Putnam JB, Natarajan G, et al. Improved survival after resection of pulmonary metastases from malignant melanoma. *Ann Thorac Surg.* 1991;52:204–210.

57. Haigh PI, Essner R, Wardlaw JC, et al. Long-term survival after complete resection of melanoma metastatic to the adrenal gland. *Ann Surg Oncol.* 1999;6:633–639.

58. Branum GD, Epstein RE, Leight GS, et al. The role of resection in the management of melanoma metastatic to the adrenal gland. *Surgery.* 1991;109:127–131.

59. Lo CY, van Heerden JA, Soreide JA, et al. Adrenalectomy for metastatic disease to the adrenal glands. *Br J Surg.* 1996;83:528–531.

60. Kim SH, Brennan MF, Russo P, et al. The role of surgery in the treatment of clinically isolated adrenal metastasis. *Cancer.* 1998;82:389–394.

61. de Wilt JH, McCarthy WH, Thompson JF. Surgical treatment of splenic metastases in patients with melanoma. *J Am Coll Surg.* 2003; 197:38–43.

62. Pawlik TM, Zorzi D, Abdalla EK, et al. Hepatic resection for metastatic melanoma: distinct patterns of recurrence and prognosis for ocular versus cutaneous disease. *Ann Surg Oncol.* 2006;13:712–720.

63. Barnholtz-Sloan JS, Sloan AE, Davis FG, et al. Incidence proportions of brain metastases in patients diagnosed (1973 to 2001) in the Metropolitan Detroit Cancer Surveillance System. *J Clin Oncol.* 2004;22:2865–2872.

64. Sampson JH, Carter JH Jr, Friedman AH, et al. Demographics, prognosis, and therapy in 702 patients with brain metastases from malignant melanoma. *J Neurosurg.* 1998;88:11–20.

65. Margolin K, Atkins B, Thompson A, et al. Temozolomide and whole brain irradiation in melanoma metastatic to the brain: a phase II trial of the Cytokine Working Group. *J Cancer Res Clin Oncol.* 2002; 128:214–218.

66. Broadbent AM, Hruby G, Tin MM, et al. Survival following whole brain radiation treatment for cerebral metastases: an audit of 474 patients. *Radiother Oncol.* 2004;71:259–265.

67. Fife KM, Colman MH, Stevens GN, et al. Determinants of outcome in melanoma patients with cerebral metastases. *J Clin Oncol.* 2004;22:1293–1300.

68. Patchell RA, Tibbs PA, Walsh JW, et al. A randomized trial of surgery in the treatment of single metastases to the brain. *N Engl J Med.* 1990; 322:494–500.

69. Patchell RA, Tibbs PA, Regine WF, et al. Postoperative radiotherapy in the treatment of single metastases to the brain: a randomized trial. *JAMA.* 1998;280:1485–1489.

70. Harrison BE, Johnson JL, Clough RW, et al. Selection of patients with melanoma brain metastases for aggressive treatment. *Am J Clin Oncol.* 2003;26:354–357.

71. Andrews DW, Scott CB, Sperduto PW, et al. Whole brain radiation therapy with or without stereotactic radiosurgery boost for patients with one to three brain metastases: phase III results of the RTOG 9508 randomised trial. *Lancet.* 2004;363:1665–1672.

72. Manon R, O'Neill A, Knisely J, et al. Phase II trial of radiosurgery for one to three newly diagnosed brain metastases from renal cell carcinoma, melanoma, and sarcoma: an Eastern Cooperative Oncology Group study (E 6397). *J Clin Oncol.* 2005;23:8870–8876.

73. Lavine SD, Petrovich Z, Cohen-Gadol AA, et al. Gamma knife radiosurgery for metastatic melanoma: an analysis of survival, outcome, and complications. *Neurosurgery.* 1999;44:59–64.

74. Mori Y, Kondziolka D, Flickinger JC, et al. Stereotactic radiosurgery for cerebral metastatic melanoma: factors affecting local disease control and survival. *Int J Radiat Oncol Biol Phys.* 1998;42:581–589.

75. Hasegawa T, Kondziolka D, Flickinger JC, et al. Brain metastases treated with radiosurgery alone: an alternative to whole brain radiotherapy? *Neurosurgery.* 2003;52:1318–1326.

76. Norman J, Cruse CW, Wells KE, et al. Metastatic melanoma with an unknown primary. *Ann Plast Surg.* 1992;28:81–84.

77. de Wilt JH, Farmer SE, Scolyer RA, et al. Isolated melanoma in the lung where there is no known primary site: metastatic disease or primary lung tumour? *Melanoma Res.* 2005;15:531–537.

78. Spitler LE, Grossbard RL, Ernstoff MS, et al. Adjuvant therapy of stage III and IV malignant melanoma using granulocyte-macrophage colony-stimulating factor. *J Clin Oncol.* 2000;18:1614–1621.

79. Lawson DH. Choices in adjuvant therapy of melanoma. *Cancer Control.* 2005;12:236–241.

80. Essner R, Lee JH, Wanek LA, et al. Contemporary surgical treatment of advanced-stage melanoma. *Arch Surg.* 2004;139:961–966.

81. Rose DM, Essner R, Hughes TM, et al. Surgical resection for metastatic melanoma to the liver: the John Wayne Cancer Institute and Sydney Melanoma Unit experience. *Arch Surg.* 2001;136:950–955.

82. Ollila DW, Hsueh EC, Stern SL, et al. Metastasectomy for recurrent stage IV melanoma. *J Surg Oncol.* 1999;71:209–213.

83. Wong JH, Skinner KA, Kim KA, et al. The role of surgery in the treatment of nonregionally recurrent melanoma. *Surgery.* 1993;113: 389–394.

84. Barth A, Wanek LA, Morton DL. Prognostic factors in 1,521 melanoma patients with distant metastases. *J Am Coll Surg.* 1995; 181:193–201.

85. Agrawal S, Yao TJ, Coit DG. Surgery for melanoma metastatic to the gastrointestinal tract. *Ann Surg Oncol.* 1999;6:336–344.

86. Gutman H, Hess KR, Kokotsakis JA, et al. Surgery for abdominal metastases of cutaneous melanoma. *World J Surg.* 2001;25:750–758.

87. Eton O, Legha SS, Moon TE, et al. Prognostic factors for survival of patients treated systemically for disseminated melanoma. *J Clin Oncol.* 1998;16:1103–1111.

88. Reinhardt MJ, Joe AY, Jaeger U, et al. Diagnostic performance of whole body dual modality 18F-FDG PET/CT imaging for N- and M-staging of malignant melanoma: experience with 250 consecutive patients. *J Clin Oncol.* 2006;24:1178–1187.

COMMENTARY
Richard Essner

Melanoma, once an uncommon disease, has become a major health concern in the United States and abroad. An estimated 62,480 Americans developed melanoma in 2008 and more than 8,400 will succumb to the disease (1). Melanoma is now the fifth most common cancer in men and sixth most common in women in the United States. It continues to be an increasing health concern, in part because of the young age of the patients, and the disproportionate amount of lost productivity compared with other malignancies.

The surgical management of melanoma has evolved over the last 150 years as more is known about its biology and natural history. Surgical resection is the mainstay of treatment of the primary lesion. Early approaches to melanoma were wide excision with 5-cm margins and complete removal of all the regional lymph nodes. For most melanomas, wide excisions employing only 1- to 2-cm margins and the regional lymph nodes are evaluated by sentinel node dissection, a minimally invasive alternative to the conventional management of the regional lymph node basin.

The staging of metastatic melanoma has been improved by more sensitive and specific computed tomography (CT) scans, magnetic resonance imaging (MRI), and whole-body positron emission tomography with ^{18}F-fluorodeoxyglucose (PET), which accurately determine the extent of metastatic disease (2). Improvements in patient risk assessment, support medications, and intensive care management have diminished the morbidity and mortality of treatment.

NATURAL HISTORY

Once melanoma has spread to distant sites, the median survival is estimated to be 7 to 8 months and overall survival is <5%, with few long-term survivors. This poor prognosis has remained unchanged for the last 50 years and reflects the continued inadequacy of therapy for metastatic melanoma (3). Nonsurgical approaches continue to be unsatisfactory, and developments in chemotherapy and biotherapy have not kept pace with those for breast, colon, and other solid-tumor malignances. In part, this likely relates to the relatively low incidence of metastatic melanoma so that few medical centers in the United States or abroad have a large enough population of such patients to evaluate alternative therapeutic strategies in single institutional or even multi-institutional randomized trials. Moreover, conventional chemotherapy is toxic and expensive, and even the addition of interleukin-2 (Proleukin) has only enhanced partial response rates with little effect on survival. Newer drugs such as sorafenib (Bay43-9006) and anti-CTLA-4 antibodies have demonstrated mixed responses in melanoma (4). Neither drug has been approved by the Food and Drug Administration for melanoma.

The prognosis of metastatic melanoma also depends on the site of disease and number of lesions. Balch and associates (5) examined the American Committee on Cancer database and demonstrated that 5-year survival rates are highest for involvement of skin and subcutaneous tissue and decrease progressively for involvement of distant lymph nodes, gastrointestinal tract, and lung, bone, liver, and brain.

The number of organ sites containing metastases also is important, with median survival of 7 months for patients with a single site of disease as compared with only 2 to 4 months for patients with two or more metastatic sites. The disease-free interval before development of distant metastases is also important. The median survival for patients who progress from regional to distant metastases is 5.6 months if prior disease-free interval is <18 months, as compared with 8 months if disease-free interval exceeds 18 months (6,7).

The association between disease-free interval and survival reflects the biological characteristics of the tumor and, in particular, its growth rate and doubling time, factors that if known would influence the decision for resection of the metastatic lesion. The complex interaction between host and tumor can be estimated by determining the tumor doubling time (TDT) (8,9). TDT for pulmonary lesions can be calculated by comparing measurements from at least two chest x-rays with both posterior/anterior and lateral views (9). In a study of patients with pulmonary metastases, Ollila et al. (9) reviewed the outcome of 45 patients with calculated TDTs who underwent resection

of the pulmonary lesions. When TDT was <60 days, median survival was 16.0 months and 5-year survival rate was zero; when TDT was ≥60 days, median survival was 29.2 months (log-rank test; significant at p <0.0001) and 5-year survival rate was 20.7% (6 of 29; p <0.0001). The authors concluded that TDT is the most significant preoperative prognostic factor for patients undergoing pulmonary resection of metastatic melanoma. If TDT is <60 days, they recommended a preoperative neoadjuvant regimen of chemotherapy and biologic therapy and, further, that pulmonary metastasectomy should not be attempted if TDT cannot be increased to ≥60 days by the systemic treatment.

Assessing growth rates for metastases at other sites is more difficult, especially trying to determine tumor volume based on PET, CT, or MRI. An alternative approach, "watch and wait," calls for a period of clinical observation (often weeks or months) that may provide important information on tumor growth rates and the possibility of subclinical metastases becoming evident at other sites that may preclude benefit from surgery. On the other hand, such a delay in resection could be associated with progression of disease and potentially deterioration in performance status, making subsequent surgery more difficult or even contraindicated In cases in which TDT can be determined, it seems reasonable to wait for this calculation to confirm eligibility for surgery and avoid resection in patients who are unlikely to benefit.

RATIONALE FOR RESECTION

Surgical resection remains the single most effective therapy for metastatic melanoma. Surgery can be effective in part because most patients with metastatic disease will have tumor limited to one or just a few sites. The most common first sites of metastases include the lung, followed by the skin, lymph nodes, brain, liver, and gastrointestinal tract (3).

Despite the fact that surgical resection may be technically possible in many patients, the surgeon's role is often limited to complete resection of a solitary visceral metastasis or surgery for palliation of symptomatic disease due to bleeding, bowel obstruction, neurologic symptoms, or pain (10). Many of these patients are seen initially by a medical oncologist who initiates treatment with chemotherapy or biotherapy. Unfortunately, in many cases surgical consultation is not sought until there is no longer a role for resection. Given the absence of effective biologic and chemotherapy agents for systemic metastases, all patients with metastatic disease should be evaluated by both medical and surgical oncologists to create a treatment plan.

There are a variety of theoretical reasons for considering resection of metastases. Reducing the tumor burden may allow the patient to overcome immunosuppressive substances produced by the tumor (i.e., interleukin-10, transforming growth factor-beta) and decrease the amount of specific tumor-enhancing agents such as vascular endothelial growth factor that could be produced by metastases (11–14). Although metastatic deposits of melanoma ≥2 cm in size are difficult to completely destroy with systemic therapy, these tumors often can be readily removed by surgery. We have found that most patients with metastatic melanoma have only one to three sites of initial synchronous metastases, many of which can be controlled by resection alone (3,15). Improvements in sophisticated imaging techniques such as CT, MRI, and PET can better differentiate between single and multiple metastatic sites, allowing for better preoperative planning and eliminating those individuals who are not eligible for resection. Long-term survival after resection of all clinically evident metastatic disease may be a function of the loss of immunosuppressive and growth enhancing agents from the tumor microenvironment, and these changes may slow the growth of other subclinical occult metastases. In addition, a number of studies have demonstrated that patients can successfully undergo resection of multiple asynchronous metastases (16). Finally, if surgical resection is not successful, these patients often remain candidates for systemic therapy; on the other hand, patients who fail initial treatment systemic therapy often will have lost the opportunity for surgical resection.

A patient's candidacy for surgery depends on the site, disease status, and duration of anticipated survival. If survival is estimated at weeks or a few months, then surgical resection may not be warranted. However, a patient with a long disease-free interval after treatment of primary disease or a patient with very slow-growing metastatic disease or those who respond well to systemic therapy may be eligible for resection. Older patients with significant comorbid conditions, such as cardiopulmonary disease, diabetes, or poor pulmonary performance, probably are not good candidates for surgery. Certainly, the risk of perioperative morbidity should be weighed against the potential benefits of surgery and nonsurgical therapy. The same considerations apply to patients who need surgery for palliation of bleeding or obstruction, although the goals of surgical resection and the anticipated long-term follow-up are different. Potential candidates for palliative resection must be evaluated by a surgeon.

SUMMARY

The surgical management of melanoma has evolved over the last 150 years. Changes in our approach to early-stage disease have resulted in decreasing margins of resection and a minimally invasive technique of evaluating the regional lymph nodes. Surgery for metastatic melanoma has also been improved through the development of better radiographic staging modalities and perioperative patient care.

Surgical resection generally has not been popular for initial treatment of metastatic disease because surgery is considered a local therapy and is thought to have little effect on the growth of disseminated disease. Most early studies of surgical resection of melonoma focused on palliation of symptoms only. Theoretical data suggest that removal of macroscopic disease may hinder development of microscopic metastases (17). Unlike chemotherapy or biotherapy, complete resection rapidly renders a patient disease-free usually with a short recovery period and minimal morbidity. With chemotherapy, the response to treatment is based on changes of tumor appearance on radiographic imaging. These findings can be misleading, whereas resection with clear surgical margins can control metastases with a high rate of success. Patients whose metastases are completely resected can experience long periods of disease-free and occasionally long-term survival regardless of the site of the disease and number of metastases.

REFERENCES

1. Jemal A, Siegel R, Ward E, et al. Cancer statistics, 2008. *CA Cancer J Clin*. 2008;58:71–96.
2. Schwimmer J, Essner R, Patel A, et al. A review of the literature for whole-body FDG PET in the management of patients with melanoma. *Q J Nucl Med*. 2000;44:153–167.
3. Barth A, Wanek LA, Morton DL. Prognostic factors in 1,521 melanoma patients with distant metastases. *J Am Coll Surg*. 1995; 181:193–201.
4. Atkins MB. Cytokine-based therapy and biochemotherapy for advanced melanoma. *Clin Cancer Res*. 2006;12:2353S–2358S.
5. Balch CM, Soong S-J, Gershenwald JE, et al. Prognostic factors analysis of 17,600 melanoma patients: validation of the American Joint Committee on Cancer Melanoma staging system. *J Clin Oncol*. 2001;19:3622–3634.
6. Lee ML, Tomsu K, Von Eschen KB. Duration of survival for disseminated malignant melanoma: results of a meta-analysis. *Melanoma Res*. 2000;10:81–92.
7. Balch CM, Soong S-J, Murad TM, et al. A multifactorial analysis of melanoma IV. Prognostic factors in 200 melanoma patients with distant metastases (stage III). *J Clin Oncol*. 1983;1: 126–134.
8. Joseph WL, Morton DL, Adkins PC. Prognostic significance of tumor doubling time in evaluating operability in pulmonary metastatic disease. *J Thorac Cardiovasc Surg*. 1971;61:23–32.
9. Ollila DW, Stern SL, Morton DL. Tumor doubling time: a selection factor for pulmonary resection of metastatic melanoma. *J Surg Oncol*. 1998;69: 206–211.
10. Ollila DW, Essner R, Wanek LA, et al. Surgical resection for melanoma metastatic to the gastrointestinal tract. *Arch Surg*. 1996; 131:975–979.
11. Dadras SS, Lange-Asschendfeldt B, Velasco P, et al. Tumor lymphangiogenesis predicts melanoma metastasis to sentinel lymph nodes. *Mod Pathol*. 2005;18:1232–1242.
12. Hendrix MJ, Seftor EA, Kirschmann DA, et al. Remodeling of the microenvironment by aggressive melanoma tumor cells. *Ann N Y Acad Sci*. 2003;995:151–161.
13. Bergers G, Benjamin LE. Tumorigenesis and the angiogenic switch. *Nat Rev Cancer*. 2003;3:401–410.
14. Avradopoulous K, Mehta S, Blackinton D, et al. Interleukin-10 as a possible mediator of immunosuppressive effect in patients with squamous cell carcinoma of the head and neck. *Ann Surg Oncol*. 1997;4:184–190.
15. Essner R, Lee JH, Wanek LA, et al. Contemporary surgical treatment of advanced-stage melanoma. *Arch Surg*. 2004;139:961–966.
16. Ollila DW, Hsueh EC, Stern SL, et al. Metastasectomy for recurrent stage IV melanoma. *J Surg Oncol*. 1999;71:209–213.
17. Chakraborty NJ, Twardzik DR, Sivanandham MT, et al. Autologous melanoma-induced activation of regulatory T cells that suppress cytotoxic response. *J Immunol*. 1990;145:2359–2364.

27

Soft-Tissue Sarcomas

Chapter 27A
Management of Soft-Tissue Sarcomas of the Extremity

James F. Huth

Soft-tissue sarcomas are a heterogeneous group of cancers that arise from tissue of mesenchymal origin. There are many histologically distinct tumors that fall under this general category, and these tumors can arise from any of a variety of connective tissues within the body. According to data collected by the American Cancer Society (1), these tumors comprise approximately 1% of adult malignancies, but 7% to 10% of malignancies in children. Of the 8,300 cases diagnosed yearly in the United States, 50% of the cases will arise in the extremity, followed by 20% of cases that occur in the retroperitoneum. The disease occurs in all age groups, and there is no significant difference in occurrence based on gender. This is a challenging group of malignant neoplasms with approximately 50% of the patients diagnosed with sarcoma eventually succumbing to the disease.

Treatment strategies have changed dramatically over the past 25 years. Current therapies have focused on improving outcomes in three major areas of concern: (a) improving survival, (b) decreasing local recurrence rates, and (c) improving quality of life. Decisions regarding therapy depend on a number of factors, including location of the primary tumor and the pathologic staging of the disease.

ETIOLOGY

There are a number of factors known to increase the risk for development of sarcomas, but in most patients there is no identifiable agent responsible for the development of the tumor. Certain syndromes are associated with development of connective tissue tumors, such as Gardner syndrome. Specific genetic mutations have also been implicated such as the *RB1* genes associated with retinoblastoma and osteosarcoma. Patients with neurofibromatosis have been found to have abnormalities on chromosome 17 (NF-1) and chromosome 22 (NF-2), and these patients are at increased risk of developing neurofibrosarcoma. The *p53* gene has been associated with distinct familial cancer syndromes including the Li-Fraumeni syndrome (2), a rare inherited disorder characterized by high risk for the development of sarcomas of bone and soft tissue, breast, and other tumors. As the distribu-

tion of the *p53* gene mutations becomes better understood, it is clear that this tumor suppressor gene is critical in cell regulation and its mutation is associated with a wide variety of human tumors (3).

Exposure to radiation can result in the development of sarcomas, as evidenced by the increased incidence of this disease in individuals who have industrial exposure (4) or received radiation treatment for childhood and adult tumors (5). It was initially hypothesized that orthovoltage (low kilovoltage) radiation of at least 2,000 cGy was required to induce tumors, whereas megavoltage and high doses (>4,000 cGy) would decrease the rate of carcinogenesis. Children appear to be more susceptible, and there appears to be a dose-response curve with a relative risk of 0.6 in those receiving <1,000 cGy (i.e., no increased risk when compared with the general population) to 38.3 in those receiving >6,000 cGy (6). Of the radiation-induced sarcomas, approximately 70% are malignant fibrous histiocytoma. The latency period is 7 to 25 years and the tumors are associated with a poor long-term prognosis. Laskin et al. (7) reported a 26% 5-year survival in a series of 53 patients who developed sarcomas after receiving radiation therapy for other conditions.

Chemical agents have also been found to be causative agents in the development of sarcomas. 3-Methyl cholanthrene causes soft tissue sarcomas in laboratory animals, and Thorotrast and vinyl chloride have been thought to be causative agents for development of hepatic angiosarcomas in humans (8). Agent Orange, a dioxin-containing herbicide used in the Vietnam War, has been implicated as a causative agent for sarcomas developing in veterans who were exposed. Follow-up studies have been inconclusive (9,10). Individuals infected with the human immunodeficiency virus are at increased risk for the development of Kaposi sarcoma.

DIAGNOSIS AND STAGING

Soft-tissue sarcomas most commonly present as a painless mass. In many cases, patients do not immediately seek medical attention, and when they do, the mass is attributed to a hematoma or "pulled muscle." When the mass fails to resolve after several weeks' duration, further diagnostic possibilities are entertained. Important elements of the history include duration of the presence of the mass, any history of trauma, any change in size or consistency over time, associated pain, paresthesias, and any of the risk factors previously described. In general, a biopsy should be performed on any soft-tissue mass that is symptomatic or enlarging, any new mass that persists for >4 weeks, or any soft-tissue mass that is >5 cm in diameter.

A number of modalities are available for obtaining tissue including fine-needle aspiration, core needle biopsy (CNB), incisional biopsy, and excisional biopsy. Because most soft-tissue masses are larger that 2 cm, CNB is the best initial procedure, providing that the reviewing pathologist is experienced and confident with this technique. Use of CNB read by an experienced pathologist provides sufficient material 93% of the time, and is 95% accurate in making the appropriate diagnosis (11). If the diagnosis cannot be made by CNB, then an open biopsy is indicated. Care must be taken with an open biopsy to avoid dissemination of tumor cells and the location of the incision must take into account the incision required for radical excision of a subsequently diagnosed malignant tumor. Tumors <5 cm may be biopsied with an excision if the tumor is superficial and not adjacent to major neurovascular structures. One wants to be sure that a re-excision in fresh tissue planes can be performed should the diagnosis turn out to be malignant. For larger lesions, an incisional biopsy is most appropriate. Care should be taken to place the incision in an appropriate place for inclusion in a larger incision when definitive surgery is performed. No skin flaps should be raised at the time of the incisional biopsy, and there should be meticulous attention to hemostasis to avoid a hematoma that could disseminate tumor cells through adjacent tissue planes. On the extremity, incisions should be made along the long axis of the limb in order to obtain adequate proximal and distal control of the neurovascular bundle at the time of definitive excision of the tumor.

Preoperative imaging is an important part of the evaluation of a patient with a sarcoma of the extremity. Magnetic resonance imaging (MRI) has supplanted other imaging modalities in the evaluation of these patients. This is because of the unparalleled soft-tissue contrast, tissue specificity, and multiplanar capabilities of MRI. Imaging routinely includes axial pre- and post-contrast T1-weighted images and T-2 weighted images and stir sequences. Coronal T1-weighted images are used for localization and for three-dimensional measurement of tumors. Contrast enhancement is also important for detecting and characterizing areas of vascularity and necrosis. Special techniques can also be used for evaluating proximity to neurovascular structures, a distinct advantage of MRI in evaluation of extremity tumors. Specific patterns on MRI can be very useful in limiting the differential diagnosis of mass lesions of the extremity (12). Although MRI, like any imaging modality, does not provide histologic information regarding whether a tumor is benign or malignant, certain diagnoses may be strongly suspected by MRI characteristics. These diagnoses include lipoma, liposarcoma, benign vascular lesions such as hemangioma, arteriovenous malformation, and pseudoaneurysm, hemosiderin-laden lesions such as pigmented villonodular synovitis, fibromatosis, subacute hematoma, and ganglion cyst. Thus a close working relationship between surgeon and radiologist is required in order to obtain the optimum MRI evaluation in each individual case. In addition to imaging at the local site, a chest computed tomography scan is a useful screening tool to evaluate for pulmonary metastases.

A great deal of prognostic information can be gained by a thorough histopathologic evaluation of soft-tissue tumors. These tumors are given a histologic classification based on the type of tissue that they form, not the site of origination. For the extremity tumors, the most common histologic type is malignant fibrous

Table 27A.1

Grading of Sarcomas

Low-Grade Sarcoma	High-Grade Sarcoma
Well differentiated Normal nuclear/ cytoplasmic ratio	Poorly differentiated High nuclear/cytoplasmic ratio
Hypocellular	Hypercellular
Hypovascular	Hypervascular
Much stroma	Minimal stroma
Minimal necrosis	Much necrosis
<5 mitoses/high power field	>5 mitoses/high power field

histiocytoma, followed by liposarcoma, synovial sarcoma, fibrosarcoma, leiomyosarcoma, and malignant peripheral nerve tumor. However, the histologic classification is not the primary determinant of prognosis, and pathologists may enhance the histopathologic diagnosis by knowing the clinical presentation, size, and site of the tumor, and age of the patient. The three most important components required for accurate assessment of the malignant potential of a sort tissue sarcoma are (a) histologic grade of the tumor, (b) the size of the tumor, and (c) the depth of the tumor relative to the fascia of the underlying muscle. Histologic grade, the primary determinant of pathologic stage, is based on the various criteria outlined in Table 27A.1.

Tumor stage is determined by a combination of grading criteria as well as by the size and location of the tumor. Table 27A.2 is a scheme of staging based on the report of the 2002 American Joint Committee on Cancer (13). This is a TNM system, in which the T classification is determined by tumor size and tumor location criteria. T1 tumors are <5 cm, and T2 tumors are >5 cm. The "a" subtype indicates a tumor that is superficial to the muscle fascia for extremity tumors, while the "b" subtype is a tumor that invades the fascia or is beneath it. The grade of the tumor is not designated by a T rating. Histopathologic tumor grade is the primary determinant of stage, with variations based on size and location. A tumor that is low grade, small, and superficial is designated as stage I, but a tumor of the same size and location that is poorly differentiated would be designated stage II. High-grade tumors that are large and deep receive a stage III designation.

SURGICAL THERAPY

Simple excision of soft-tissue sarcomas of the extremity resulted in an unacceptable high rate of local recurrence (14,15). This resulted in a change is therapy to amputation or compartment resection in an effort to improve local control rates, but local failure still occurred in 20% to 30% of cases (16). Over the past 3 decades, significant advances have been made with respect to multimodality treatment of this disease, achieving local control rates of 95% and an amputation rate of <10%.

Of historical interest is the use of the compartment excision. This was a limb-sparing technique that was limited to tumors occupying a single muscle compartment and not extending

Table 27A.2

Staging of Extremity Soft-Tissue Sarcomas

T Staging (Primary Tumor)

TX	Primary tumor cannot be assessed
T0	No evidence of primary tumor
T1	Tumor ≤5 cm greatest dimension
T1a	superficial tumor
T1b	deep tumor
T2	Tumor >5 cm
T2a	Superficial tumor
T2b	Deep tumor

Histologic Grade

GX	Grade cannot be assessed
G1	Well differentiated
G2	Moderately differentiated
G3	Poorly differentiated

Group Staging

Stage I

T1a	N0	M0	G1
T1b	N0	M0	G1
T2a	N0	M0	G1
T2b	N0	M0	G1

Stage II

T1a	N0	M0	G2,3
T1b	N0	M0	G2,3
T2a	N0	M0	G2,3

Stage III

T2b	N0	M0	G2,3

Stage IV

T1,2	N1	M0	G1,2,3
T1,2	N0	M1	G1,2,3

N Staging (Regional lymph nodes)

NX	Nodes cannot be assessed
N0	No nodal metastases
N1	Regional node metastases

M Staging (Distant Metastases)

MX	Distant metastases cannot be assessed
M0	No distant metastases
M1	Distant metastases

From American Joint Committee on Cancer. AJCC Cancer Staging Manual, 6th ed. New York: Springer-Verlag, 2002.

through the enveloping fascia. The entire muscle and investing fascia were removed from origin to insertion. Because the extent of the muscle was usually far greater along its long axis than the extent of the tumor, this technique involved opening large tissue planes in order to remove the entire muscle.

In 1982, Rosenberg and associates (17) at the National Cancer Institute reported the results of a randomized trial comparing amputation versus limb-sparing surgery combined with radiation therapy for the treatment of extremity soft-tissue sarcomas. In the limb-sparing group, wide local excision was followed by 5,000 cGy to the entire anatomic areas with a boost to 6,000 to 7,000 cGy to the tumor bed. Although there were four local recurrences (14.8%) compared with no local recurrences in the amputation group, there was no difference in disease-free survival or overall survival between the two groups. A multivariate analysis showed that the only correlate of local recurrence was the final margin of resection. Numerous other studies have also been conducted combining radiation and surgery. These studies have combined either preoperative radiotherapy (18) or postoperative radiotherapy (19) with extremity-sparing surgery, or trials

have included preoperative chemotherapy combined with radiation therapy in the treatment regimen with excellent results (20).

Brennan (21) at Memorial Sloan-Kettering Cancer Center described a management strategy using excision and postoperative brachytherapy. A prospective trial from Memorial Sloan-Kettering Cancer Center included patients with extremity or superficial soft-tissue sarcomas of the trunk. Eighty-six patients were randomized to receive limb-sparing surgery alone, and 78 patients received limb-sparing surgery plus brachytherapy. The brachytherapy was conducted using iridium 192 afterloading catheters that delivered 4,500 cGy over 4 to 6 days. The median follow-up for this study was 76 months. The 5-year actuarial survival was 82% in the brachytherapy group compared with 69% in the surgery-only group. This beneficial effect was noted only in patients with high-grade tumors.

A study at the National Cancer Institute randomized extremity soft-tissue sarcoma patients to limb-sparing surgery alone versus limb-sparing surgery plus external-beam irradiation (22). The radiation was delivered in 180-cGy fractions to a total dose of 4,500cGy to a wide field, followed by an 1,800 cGy boost to the tumor bed. After a median follow-up of 115 months, 17 of the 71 patients in the surgery-only arm had local failure compared with 1 of 70 failures in the radiation therapy arm.

Eilber and colleagues (23) at the University of California at Los Angeles have had extensive experience with the use of neoadjuvant chemotherapy and radiation therapy in the treatment of extremity soft-tissue sarcomas. The concept was to give preoperative therapy before extensive surgical resection. The theoretical advantages of this approach were that (a) chemotherapy and radiation are given to the tumor with undisturbed tissue planes and therefore better blood supply, (b) preoperative treatment provides an in vitro evaluation of the clinical response of the tumor to chemotherapy and radiation, and (c) the reduction in tumor size and clarification of the tumor pseudocapsule allow for more adequate excision of the primary tumor. They conducted a series of trials looking at intra-arterial Adriamycin followed by varying doses of external-beam radiation therapy. The radiation therapy was given over a short time course (10 days) at high fraction 175 to 350 cGy per fraction. Ultimately, it appeared that a total fraction of 2,800 cGy in 10 fractions resulted in a local control rate of >90% with a 27% local wound complication rate and an amputation rate of 4.5%. Eventually, the intra-arterial Adriamycin was replaced with systemic therapy, including Adriamycin and ifosfamide yielding similar results.

Other approaches to the in situ treatment of extremity sarcomas prior to resection are being evaluated. Because of success seen in the treatment of in-transit melanoma of the extremity, there has been an interest in the use of isolated limb perfusion (24). In European trials using tumor necrosis factor in combination with interferon, doxorubicin, or melphalan, complete response rates of 18% to 60% have been achieved in small series of patients with limb salvage achieved in 63% to 90% of patients. These preliminary results await the completion of larger multi-institutional trials for verification of efficacy and evaluation of toxicity.

Most patients with high-grade soft-tissue sarcomas of the extremity receive either preoperative or postoperative radiation therapy. Pollack et al. (25) have suggested that the degree of oxygenation within the tumor and its surrounding tissue bed has direct consequences regarding the chance of achieving local control. Therefore, they suggest that the tumor status at the time of presentation should dictate the timing of radiotherapy. They reviewed the cases of 128 patients given preoperative radiotherapy (median dose, 5,000 cGy) to 165 patients who received postoperative radiotherapy (median dose, 6,400 cGy). Local control rates were similar between the two groups (82% for preoperative vs. 81% for postoperative). However, the status of the disease at the time of presentation was an important determinant of outcome. In patients who presented with gross disease that was being treated for the first time, preoperative therapy resulted in an 88% local control rate at 10 years compared with 67% local control for patients treated with postoperative therapy. Another set of patients were those who presented for treatment after an excision biopsy elsewhere (i.e., no gross residual disease). Those who were treated with immediate re-excision followed by postoperative radiation had a local control rate of 91% at 10 years, compared with a 72% local control rate at 10 years for those receiving preoperative radiation therapy ($p = 0.02$).

ADJUVANT CHEMOTHERAPY

Despite the excellent results that can be achieved with local control and limb-sparing surgery, approximately 40% of patients with extremity sarcoma eventually die from metastatic disease. Numerous combinations of drugs have been studied with varying results (26). Bramwell and associates (27) reported on a randomized trial comparing cyclophosphamide, doxorubicin, and dacarbazine (CYVADIC) with no adjuvant therapy in 317 patients. After a median follow-up of 80 months, the chemotherapy group had a lower relapse-free survival of 56% versus 43% ($p = 0.007$), but overall survival was similar between the two groups (63% vs. 56%; $p = 0.64$). A trial by European Organisation for Research and Treatment of Cancer (28) randomized patients between doxorubicin alone versus CYVADIC versus doxorubicin and ifosfamide. No statistically significant differences were found in terms of overall survival (52 weeks vs. 51 weeks) between the groups. All adjuvant chemotherapy studies have suffered from small numbers of patients entered into the trials. The Sarcoma Meta-analysis Collaboration tried to circumvent this problem by performing a meta-analysis of adjuvant chemotherapy for soft-tissue sarcomas (29). The study analyzed the data from 158 patients enrolled in 14 trials of doxorubicin-based adjuvant chemotherapy with a median follow-up of 9.4 years. They calculated a benefit from chemotherapy of 6% for local relapse-free interval (hazard ratio, 0.73), 10% for distant relapse-free (hazard ratio, 0.70), and 10% for recurrence-free survival (hazard ratio, 0.75). For overall survival, the hazard ratio of 0.89 was not significant. Although this study is subject to the pitfalls of meta-analysis, it is based on a large number of patients. On subset analysis, patients with extremity sarcoma had an absolute survival benefit of 7% at 10 years. Several randomized trials are currently underway in an attempt to further delineate the role of adjuvant chemotherapy in the treatment of this disease.

Clearly there is a need for well-conducted clinical trials regarding the use of adjuvant chemotherapy for extremity sarcomas. It is important to clearly define risk factors for development of metastatic disease so that the patient can be properly stratified in these trials. Staging systems incorporate tumor grade, size, and location, which are the three factors most commonly associated with distant recurrence in this disease. However, several other factors may play a role. Failure to achieve a histologically negative margin at the time of resection of an extremity sarcoma has been found to correlate with survival (30,31). Similarly, local recurrence has been associated with distant relapse (32). Pathologic response to preoperative therapy has been shown to correlate with survival in patients with extremity sarcomas. Eilber et al. (33) examined the extent of pathologic necrosis in 496 patients with high-grade extremity sarcomas. Patients who had >95% necrosis after treatment with neoadjuvant chemotherapy were less likely to develop local recurrence and had better survival than patients who did not have this type of pathologic response to therapy. Henshaw et al. (34) had similar results using doxorubicin, intra-arterial cisplatin, and ifosfamide prior to surgery. Patients achieving a response with >95% tumor necrosis has a superior disease-free survival (88% vs. 77%) and overall survival (74% vs. 65%) than patients who did not achieve this response. Wendtner et al. (35) had similar findings in patients with retroperitoneal or visceral soft-tissue sarcomas. Forty patients with large, high-grade, locally advanced tumors were treated with neoadjuvant chemotherapy and hyperthermia. The 15 patients who demonstrated a radiographic or pathologic response had a significant improvement in 5-year survival (60% vs. 10%).

Thus, there appear to be a number of prognostic variables that may impact prognosis and influence the decision whether to recommend adjuvant chemotherapy for the patient with a soft-tissue sarcoma of the extremity. Grobmyer and Brennan (36) have developed a nomogram that incorporates the major prognostic factors that are used to assess the 12-year sarcoma-specific death of patients with extremity tumors. This nomogram is based on tumor size, grade, histology, depth of tumor, and patient age. However, the treatment-related variables previously discussed are not included in the nomogram, which may limit its usefulness in light of these recent advances.

FUTURE CONSIDERATIONS

There have been many advances in knowledge regarding the molecular basis of malignancy. This involves mutations in tumor promoter and tumor suppressor genes. For instance, gastrointestinal stromal tumors (GIST) have been shown to be the result of a mutation in the growth factor receptor c-Kit (37), a tyrosine kinase receptor. A mutation of this gene results in constitutive phosphorylation and dysregulation of its downstream signaling pathway. STI-571 (Gleevec) is a tyrosine kinase inhibiter directed at c-Kit. It was found that 89% of symptomatic patients with GIST had an improvement in symptoms when treated with STI-57 (38–40). New trials are underway including American College of Surgeons Oncology Group (ACOSOG) 9000, "A phase II study of adjuvant STI571 (Gleevec) therapy in patients following completely resected high-risk primary gastrointestinal stromal tumor (GIST)" and Radiation Therapy Oncology Group Trial S-0132, "A phase II study of neoadjuvant/adjuvant STI571 in patients with primary or recurrent respectable malignant GIST." The use of tyrosine kinase inhibitors and similar compounds represents an important new concept in the treatment of sarcomas and other tumors. It will be exciting to observe the clinical relevance of other molecularly targeted drugs and the efficacy of antiangiogenic therapy in the treatment of these tumors.

REFERENCES

1. Jemal A, Thomas A, Murray T, et al. Cancer Statistics, 2002. *CA Cancer J Clin.* 2002;52:23–47.
2. Birch JM, Hartley AL, Tricker KJ, et al. Prevalence and diversity of constitutional mutations in the p53 gene among 21 Li-Fraumeni families. *Cancer Res.* 1994;54:1298–1304.
3. Toguchida J, Yamaguchi T, Dayton SH, et al. Prevalence and spectrum of germline mutations of the p53 gene among patients with sarcoma. *N Engl J Med.* 1992;326:1350–1352.
4. Martland HS, Humphries RE. Osteogenic sarcoma in dial painters using luminous paint. *Arch Pathol.* 1929;7:406–417.
5. Robinson E, Neugut AL, Wylie P. Review: clinical aspects of post-irradiation sarcomas. *J Natl Cancer Inst.* 1988;80:233–240.
6. Tucker MA, D'Angio GJ, Boice JD, et al. For the Late Effects Study Group. Bone sarcomas linked to radiotherapy and chemotherapy in children. *N Engl J Med.* 1987;317:588–593.
7. Laskin WB, Silverman, TA, Enzinger, FM. Post-radiation soft tissue sarcomas. An analysis of 53 cases. *Cancer.* 1988;62:2230–2240.
8. Lloyd JW. Angiosarcoma of the liver of vinyl chloride/polyvinyl chloride production worker. *J Occup Med.* 1975;17:222–224.
9. Collins JJ, Strauss ME, Levinskas GJ, et al. The mortality experience of workers exposed to 2,3,7,8-tetrachlorobenzo-p-dioxine in a trichlorophenol process accident. *Epidemiology.* 1993;4:7–13.
10. Suruda AJ, Ward EM, Fingerhut MA. Identification of soft tissue sarcoma deaths in cohorts exposed to dioxin and to chlorinated naphthalenes. *Epidemiology.* 1995;48:539–544.
11. Heslin MJ, Lewis JJ, Woodruff JM, et al. Core needle biopsy for diagnosis of extremity soft tissue sarcoma. *Ann Surg Oncol.* 1997;4:425–431.
12. Fenstermacher MJ. Imaging evaluation of patients with soft tissue sarcoma. *Surg Oncol Clin North Am.* 2003;12:305–322.
13. American Joint Committee on Cancer. *AJCC Cancer Staging Manual,* 6th ed. New York: Springer-Verlag; 2005.
14. Alho A, Alvegard, TA, Berlin O, et al. Surgical margin in soft tissue sarcoma: the Scandinavian Sarcoma Group experience. *Acta Orthop Scand.* 1989;60:687–692.
15. Cantin J, McNeer GP, Chu FC, et al. The problem of local recurrence after treatment of soft tissue sarcoma. *Ann Surg.* 1968;168:47–53.
16. Rosenberg, SA, Glatstein EJ. Perspectives on the role of surgery and radiation therapy in the treatment of soft tissue sarcomas of the extremities. *Semin Oncol.* 1981;8:190–200.
17. Rosenberg, SA, Tepper, J, Glatstein E, et al. The treatment of soft tissue sarcomas of the extremities: prospective randomized evaluations of (1) limb–sparing surgery plus radiation therapy compared with amputation and (2) the role of adjuvant chemotherapy. *Ann Surg.* 1982;196:305–315.
18. Suit, HD, Poppe KH, Mankin HJ et al. Preoperative radiation therapy for sarcoma of soft tissue. *Cancer.* 1981;47:2269–2274.
19. Lindberg RD, Martin RG, Romsdahl MD, et al. Conservative surgery and postoperative radiotherapy in 300 adults with soft tissue sarcomas. *Cancer.* 1982;47:2391–2397.
20. Eilber FR, Morton DL, Eckardt J, et al. Limb salvage for skeletal and soft tissue sarcomas: multidisciplinary preoperative therapy. *Cancer.* 1984;53:2579–2584.
21. Brennan MF. Management of extremity of soft-tissue sarcomas. *Am J Surg.* 1989;158:71–78.
22. Yang JC, Chang AE, Baker AR, et al. Randomized prospective study of the benefit of adjuvant radiation therapy in the treatment of soft tissue sarcomas of the extremity. *J Clin Oncol.* 1998;16:197–203.
23. Eilber FR, Eckardt, GR, Yao SF, et al. Neoadjuvant chemotherapy and radiation therapy in the multidisciplinary management of soft tissue sarcomas of the extremity. *Surg Oncol Clin North Am.* 1993;2:511–520.
24. Eggermont AMM. Isolated limb perfusion in the management of locally advanced extremity soft tissue sarcoma. *Surg Clin North Am.* 2003;12:469–483.
25. Pollack A, Zagars GK, Goswitz MS, et al. Preoperative radiotherapy in the treatment of soft tissue sarcomas: a matter of presentation. *Int J Radiat Oncol Biol Phys.* 1998;42:563–572.
26. McCarter MD, Jaques DP, Brennan MF. Randomized clinical trials in soft tissue sarcoma. *Surg Oncol Clin North Am.* 2002;11:11–23.
27. Bramwell V, Rouesse J, Steward W, et al. Adjuvant CYVADIC chemotherapy for adult soft tissue sarcoma-reduced local recurrence but no improvement in survival: a study of the European Organization for Research and Treatment of Cancer Soft Tissue and Bone Sarcoma group. *J Clin Oncol.* 1994;12:1137–1149.
28. Santoro A, Tursz T, Mouridsen H, et al. Doxorubicin versus CYVADIC versus doxorubicin plus ifosfamide in first-line treatment of advanced soft tissue sarcomas: a randomized study of the

European Organization for Research and Treatment of Cancer Soft Tissue and Bone Sarcoma Group. *J Clin Oncol.* 1995;13:1537–1545.

29. Sarcoma Meta-analysis Collaboration. Adjuvant chemotherapy for localized respectable soft-tissue sarcoma of adults: meta-analysis of individual data. *Lancet.* 1997;350:1647–1654.

30. Tanabe KK, Pollock RE, Ellis LM, et al. Influence of surgical margins on outcome in patients with preoperatively irradiated extremity soft tissue sarcomas. *Cancer.* 1994;73:1652–1659.

31. Stojadinovic A, Leung DH, Hoos A, et al. Analysis of the prognostic significance of microscopic margins in 2.084 localized primary adult soft tissue sarcomas. *Ann Surg.* 2002;235:424–434.

32. Pisters PW, Leung DH, Woodruff J, et al. Analysis of prognostic factors in 1,041 patients with localized soft tissue sarcomas of the extremities. *J Clin Oncol.* 1996;14:1679–1689.

33. Eilber FR, Rosen G, Eckardt J, et al. Treatment-induced pathologic necrosis: a predictor of local recurrence and survival in patients receiving neoadjuvant therapy for high-grade extremity soft tissue sarcomas. *J Clin Oncol.* 2001;19:3202–3209.

34. Henshaw RM, Priebat D, Perry D, et al. Induction chemotherapy for high grade extremity soft tissue sarcomas: histologic response and correlation of tumor necrosis to long term disease free and overall patient survival. In: Proceedings of the American Society of Clinical Oncology. 2000;19:553a. Abstract 2177.

35. Wendtner CM, Abdel-Rahman S, Ktych M, et al. Response to neoadjuvant chemotherapy combined with regional hyperthermia predicts long-term survival for adult patients with retroperitoneal and visceral high-risk soft tissue sarcomas. *J Clin Oncol.* 2002;20:3156–3164.

36. Grobmyer SR, Brennan MF. Predictive variable detailing the recurrence rate of soft tissue sarcomas. *Curr Opin Oncol.* 2003;15:319–326.

37. Sarlomo-Rikala M, Kovatich AJ, Barusevicius A, et al. CD117: a sensitive marker for gastrointestinal stromal tumors that is more specific than CD 34. *Mod Pathol.* 1998;11:728–734.

38. Blanke CD, von Mehren M, Joensuu H, et al Evaluation of the safety and efficacy of an oral molecularly-targeted therapy, STI571, in patients with unresectable or metastatic gastrointestinal stromal tumors (GIST) expressing C-KIT (CD117). In: Proceedings of the American Society of Clinical Oncology. 2001:20:1a.

39. Van Oosterom AT, Judson I, Verweij J, et al. STI571, an active drug in metastatic gastrointestinal stromal tumors (GIST), An EORTC phase I study [abstract 2]. *Proc Am Soc Clin Oncol* 2110;20:1a.

40. Joensuu H, Roberts, PJ, Sarlomo-Rikala M, et al. Effect of the tyrosine kinase inhibitor STI571 in a patient with a metastatic gastrointestinal stromal tumor. *N Engl J Med.* 2001;344:1042–1046.

COMMENTARY

Frederick R. Eilber and Fritz C. Eilber

The chapter by Dr. James Huth presents an excellent review of the current management of extremity soft-tissue sarcomas. This clearly is a very rare disease with few institutions and/or individuals having the critical volume of experience to appropriately treat patients with these tumors. Soft-tissue sarcomas are a heterogeneous group of connective tissue malignancies with over 50 different histologic subtypes, an annual incidence of only about 8,000 cases, and a disease-specific mortality of up to 50% (1,2). As such, these tumors represent rare high-risk malignancies that are difficult to diagnose and treat. Effective treatment of soft-tissue sarcomas requires careful preoperative planning by an experienced multidisciplinary team of physicians. This necessitates the collaborative effort of a number of different specialties and should include surgical oncology, orthopaedic oncology, medical oncology, radiation therapy, pathology, and radiology. In our weekly sarcoma conference at the University of California at Los Angeles, at which about 1,000 cases are discussed per year, the importance of this multidisciplinary preoperative treatment planning is clearly evident. Simply having the pathology slides reviewed by one of our experienced sarcoma pathologist results in a change in the histologic diagnosis in approximately 10% of the cases. Additional input from all members of the team results in prompt treatment planning and presents an opportunity to enroll patients in protocol-driven therapy.

Although Dr. Huth's chapter is well organized and extremely well written, we believe several points require elaboration.

DIAGNOSIS

Any painless mass larger than 2 cm that is deep to the subcutaneous tissue, immobile, and firm should be considered to be a sarcoma until proven otherwise. In the presence of any of these clinical features, cross-sectional imaging and tissue diagnosis are essential in guiding further treatment. Cross-sectional imaging with either computerized tomography (CT) or magnetic resonance imaging provides anatomic information necessary to guide potential surgical resection. CT-guided core biopsy is the best method to obtain an accurate tissue diagnosis (3,4). CT guidance allows for precise tissue sampling, and core biopsy allows for adequate tissue collection for histologic diagnosis. In the rare case that CT-guided core biopsy is unable to provide an adequate histologic diagnosis, an open biopsy can be performed. Unfortunately it is not uncommon to see a series of errors that can place a potentially curable patient into a limb- and/or life-threatening situation. An example would be the excision of a presumed thigh lipoma (no preoperative imaging or tissue diagnosis) through a transverse incision with the development of a postoperative hematoma.

LOCAL CONTROL

A positive margin is a significant independent adverse prognostic factor for local recurrence and should be re-resected whenever possible (5,6). Patients referred to a specialty center after undergoing resection of a primary extremity tumor at another institution require re-imaging and re-resection of the surgical site (7,8). It is very difficult to determine the exact extent of the initial surgery and there is often a limited pathologic assessment of the tumor/margins, making it difficult to determine if there is residual disease. Finally, re-resection has been shown to provide an improved survival (8).

One of the principal mistakes in treating soft-tissue sarcomas is to underestimate significance of a local recurrence. Not only are patients who develop a local recurrence at an increased risk of developing a subsequent local recurrences, but the ability to resect recurrent disease is significantly less than for patients with primary disease (5). For patients with locally recurrent extremity lesions, this translates into a significantly higher amputation rate. Regardless of the site, the development of a local recurrence is a significant factor associated with decreased survival (5,6). A patient who develops a large local recurrence in a short interval indicates a biologically aggressive tumor with a high tumor-specific mortality, and such patients should be treated with neoadjuvant systemic therapy (9).

The best treatment of a local recurrent disease is preventing it. This necessitates aggressive surgical treatment of the primary disease as adjuvant therapies cannot compensate for inadequate surgery. It is a morbid and lethal misconception for patients who receive suboptimal treatment of their primary disease to think that they can be referred to a specialty center when and if a recurrence develops.

NEOADJUVANT/ADJUVANT THERAPY

In general, patients who have low-grade soft-tissue sarcomas are treated with surgery alone. Low-grade tumors that are very large or recurrent should be considered for treatment with adjuvant radiation therapy. Patients with high-grade tumors (>5 cm) are treated with surgery, radiation therapy, and chemotherapy (neoadjuvantly or adjuvantly). Based on a series of studies, ifosfamide-based chemotherapy appears to be the most effective current systemic treatment. In patients with high-risk (high-grade, large, deep) primary extremity soft-tissue sarcomas, treatment with ifosfamide-based chemotherapy was associated with an improved disease-specific survival compared with patients who revived no chemotherapy (10–16). It has been our experience that neoadjuvant high-dose ifosfamide, doxorubicin, and radiation has been most effective (11). However, this is a very toxic and difficult regimen to administer and should only be given by medical oncologists and radiation therapists experienced in the management of sarcomas, ideally in the setting of a specific protocol.

Although soft-tissue sarcomas have historically been lumped together, the importance of identifying histology-specific chemotherapy is becoming increasingly important in the current era in which soft-tissue sarcomas are being classified and treated based on their molecular and genetic characteristics. In our experience, ifosfamide-based chemotherapy is most effective in treating patients with synovial sarcomas, malignant fibrous histiocytoma (now called *myxofibrosarcoma*), and pleomorphic or dedifferentiated liposarcomas (12,13,16). Patients with malignant peripheral nerve sheath tumors and angiosarcoma have a typically poor response to this treatment. Patients who have no response are those with extraosseous chondrosarcoma and epithelioid sarcoma. Gemcitabine and Taxotere, initially described for leiomyosarcoma of the uterus, have shown efficacy in soft-tissue sarcomas (17). This regimen is less toxic than high-dose ifosfamide and appears particularly effective for nonuterine leiomyosarcomas. Finally, as touched on by Dr. Huth, the success of the tyrosine kinase inhibitor STI571 (Gleevec) in treating patients with gastrointestinal stromal sarcomas is likely a glimpse of the future when molecularly target treatments will be employed.

In summary, we believe this an excellent chapter that can provide the general guidelines for diagnosis and treatment of soft-tissue sarcoma. Because these are rare, high-risk malignancies that are difficult to diagnose and treat, they should be managed by an experienced multidisciplinary team of physicians. Local control is critical and the best opportunity to render a patient disease-free is in the setting of the primary tumor. Management of primary disease requires aggressive multimodality, histology-specific treatment.

REFERENCES

1. Kattan MW, Leung DH, Brennan MF. Postoperative nomogram for 12-year sarcoma-specific death. *J Clin Oncol.* 2002;20:791–796.
2. Eilber FC, Brennan MF, Eilber FR, et al. Validation of the postoperative nomogram for 12-year sarcoma-specific death. *Cancer.* 2004;15;101:2270–2275.
3. Heslin MJ, Lewis JJ, Woodruff JM, et al. Core needle biopsy for diagnosis of extremity soft tissue sarcoma. *Ann Surg Oncol.* 1997;4:425–431.
4. Yao L, Nelson SD, Seeger LL, et al. Primary musculoskeletal neoplasms: effectiveness of core-needle biopsy. *Radiology.* 1999;212:682–686.
5. Eilber FC, Rosen G, Nelson SD, et al. High-grade extremity soft tissue sarcomas: factors predictive of local recurrence and its effect on morbidity and mortality. *Ann Surg.* 2003;237:218–226.
6. Lewis JJ, Leung D, Heslin M, et al. Association of local recurrence with subsequent survival in extremity soft tissue sarcoma. *J Clin Oncol.* 1997;15:646–652.
7. Giuliano AE, Eilber FR. The rationale for planned reoperation after unplanned total excision of soft-tissue sarcomas. *J Clin Oncol.* 1985;3:1344–1348.
8. Lewis JJ, Leung D, Espat J, et al. Effect of reresection in extremity soft tissue sarcoma. *Ann Surg.* 2000;231:655–663.
9. Eilber FC, Brennan MF, Riedel E, et al. Prognostic factors for survival in patients with locally recurrent extremity soft tissue sarcomas. *Ann Surg Oncol.* 2005;12:228–236.
10. Frustaci S, Gherlinzoni F, De Paoli A, et al. Adjuvant chemotherapy for adult soft tissue sarcomas of the extremities and girdles: results of the Italian randomized cooperative trial. *J Clin Oncol.* 2001;19:1238–1247.
11. Eilber FC, Rosen G, Eckardt J, et al. Treatment induced pathologic necrosis: a predictor of local recurrence and survival in patients receiving neoadjuvant therapy for high grade extremity soft tissue sarcomas. *J Clin Oncol.* 2001;19:3203–3209.
12. Eilber FC, Brennan MF, Eilber FR, et al. Chemotherapy is associated with improved survival in patients with primary extremity synovial sarcoma. *Ann Surg.* 2007;245:105–113.
13. Eilber FC, Eilber FR, Eckardt J, et al. The impact of chemotherapy on the survival of patients with high-grade primary extremity liposarcoma. *Ann Surg.* 2004;101:686–695.
14. DeLaney TF, Spiro IJ, Suit HD, et al. Neoadjuvant chemotherapy and radiotherapy for large extremity soft-tissue sarcomas. *Int J Radiat Oncol Biol Phys.* 2003;56:1117–1127.
15. Grobmyer SR, Maki RG, Demetri GD, et al. Neo-adjuvant chemotherapy for primary high-grade extremity soft tissue sarcoma. *Ann Oncol.* 2004;15:1667–1672.
16. Eilber FC, Tap WD, Nelson SD, et al. Advances in chemotherapy for patients with extremity soft tissue sarcoma. *Orthop Clin North Am.* 2006;37:15–22.
17. Hensley ML, Maki R, Venkatraman E, et al. Gemcitabine and docetaxel in patients with unresectable leiomyosarcoma: results of a phase II trial. *J Clin Oncol.* 2002;20:2824–2831.

Chapter 27B
Soft-Tissue Sarcomas of the Retroperitoneum

James R. Ouellette, Farin F. Amersi, David V. Cossman, and Allan W. Silberman

Retroperitoneal sarcomas are rare, insidious tumors accounting for approximately 0.1% of all malignancies and <15% of adult soft-tissue sarcomas (1). Like soft-tissue sarcomas of the extremities, they are a varied group of malignancies arising from mesenchymal tissue (2). A review from Memorial Sloan-Kettering Cancer Center analyzing 500 patients with retroperitoneal sarcomas showed liposarcoma (41%) and leiomyosarcoma (27%) to be the most common histologic subtypes (3) (Table 27B.1). Early symptoms of retroperitoneal sarcomas are usually vague, as the loose areolar tissue of the retroperitoneal space allows the tumor to expand relatively easily in several directions except into the posterior musculature. Consequently, these tumors are often quite large when symptoms first occur and a diagnosis is established. The most frequent clinical presentation is weight loss and abdominal pain and/or a palpable abdominal or flank mass, but nonspecific symptoms such as nausea, vomiting, and back pain are not unusual. More subtle presentations include neurologic symptoms from pressure or invasion of nerves, like the femoral, genitofemoral, or obturator nerve, or lower extremity swelling or edema from encroachment on the inferior vena cava (IVC) or iliac veins. These more subtle signs and symptoms often cause delays in diagnosis because the diagnostic evaluation is directed to neurologic or vascular studies of the lower extremity, while the abdomen and retroperitoneum are not initially considered.

Although the pathologic subtypes and histologic grade of retroperitoneal sarcomas are similar to those of the extremity soft-tissue sarcomas, management is more complex because of the difficult location in the retroperitoneum and the proximity of surrounding vital structures (4). In addition, the use of multimodality therapy, particularly radiation therapy, commonly used in extremity sarcomas is more difficult to deliver in the patient with a retroperitoneal sarcoma because of the large fields involved and the presence of radiation-sensitive normal tissues like bowel, liver, kidney, bladder, and spinal cord (5). Chemotherapy, like radiation therapy, is also commonly used in extremity sarcomas; however, its efficacy in retroperitoneal sarcomas remains unproven (6). Surgery remains the mainstay of treatment; however, considerable expertise is required for a successful outcome. A clear pathologic margin is the goal of surgery, but this often requires multiple organs to be removed, including major vascular structures.

DIAGNOSIS

As previously noted, the initial presentation of a patient with a retroperitoneal sarcoma is most commonly an asymptomatic abdominal mass. Pain is present in 40% to 60% of patients (7). Hassan et al. (8) reviewed the Mayo Clinic experience and found that 61% of patients present with multiple signs and symptoms, specifically pain (57%), abdominal mass (36%), distention (25%), nonspecific gastrointestinal complaints (26%), and weight loss (29%).

Computed tomography (CT) is the single most useful diagnostic procedure in the preoperative evaluation of patients with retroperitoneal masses. In addition to demonstrating the size and consistency of the tumor and its relationship to, and possible displacement of, adjacent retroperitoneal structures, CT-directed biopsies, either fine-needle aspirates or needle core biopsies, can lead to a tissue diagnosis that can be helpful in treatment planning and consideration of neoadjuvant therapy. Moreover, preoperative CT-guided biopsies will sometimes establish a diagnosis of a nonsarcomatous retroperitoneal malignancy, which may be more appropriately treated with nonsurgical therapy. This group can include lymphomas, germ cell tumors, or other primary tumors extending into the retroperitoneum (colon, renal, adrenal, pancreatic) (9). Biopsy is discouraged by some if, based on imaging, a tumor is believed to be a sarcoma, because of the concern for needle track seeding and implantation. Therefore, unless the treatment course will be altered, biopsy should be considered carefully and in concert with the surgeon (10).

Magnetic resonance imaging (MRI) scans are increasingly being obtained preoperatively and can add information regarding tumor heterogeneity and vascular involvement. However, in

Table 27B.1

Histologic Subtypes of Soft-Tissue Extremity and Retroperitoneal Sarcomas

Extremity (Adapted from ref. 2)		Retroperitoneal (Adapted from ref. 3)	
Site	%	Site	%
Malignant fibrous histiocytoma	28	Liposarcoma	41
Liposarcoma	15	Leiomyosarcoma	27
Leiomyosarcoma	12	Other	14
Synovial sarcoma	10	Malignant fibrous histiocytoma	7
Malignant peripheral nerve sheath tumors	6	Fibrosarcoma	6
Rhabdomyosarcoma	5	Hemangiopericytoma	3
Other	≤3	Malignant peripheral nerve sheath tumors	3

this cost-cutting environment, it is difficult to justify both CT and MRI unless a specific question—for instance, patency of the portal vein or superior mesenteric vein—is being evaluated. The ability to perform magnetic resonance angiography has almost eliminated the need for angiography in evaluation of these lesions. Barium studies, intravenous pyelography, and arteriography, although still occasionally used in the preoperative evaluation of the patient with a retroperitoneal mass, have assumed much less importance since the introduction of CT and MRI.

The diagnosis of a retroperitoneal sarcoma should prompt a minimum of a chest and liver CT scan searching for distant metastatic disease. This knowledge may modify the treatment plan, or at least the treatment order. No known serum markers are available for the evaluation of a sarcoma; however, markers for germ cell tumors may be measured if this is part of the differential diagnosis.

STAGING

Patients with retroperitoneal sarcomas have been staged using the American Joint Committee on Cancer (AJCC) staging system (Table 27B.2) (11). This system uses the TNM classification to describe solid tumors. Unfortunately, this system has been

Table 27B.2

American Joint Committee on Cancer Staging System

Category	Definition
Tumor status (primary)	
T0	No evidence of primary tumor
T1	Tumor ≤5 cm (T1a, superficial; T1b, deep)
T2	Tumor >5 cm (T2a, superficial; T2b, deep)
Lymph node status	
N0	No regional node involvement
N1	Regional node metastasis
Metastasis	
M0	No metastasis
M1	Distant metastasis
Stage grouping	
IA	T1a, N0, M0 (low grade)
	T1b, N0, M0 (low grade)
IB	T2a, N0, M0 (low grade)
	T2b, N0, M0 (low grade)
IIA	T1a, N0, M0 (high grade)
	T1b, N0, M0 (high grade)
IIB	T2a, N0, M0 (high grade)
III	T2b, N0, M0 (high grade)
IV	Any T, N1, M0 (any grade)
	Any T, any N, M1 (any grade)

Data derived from American Joint Committee on Cancer. *AJCC Cancer Staging Manual*, 6th ed. New York: American Joint Committee on Cancer; 2002:193–197.

Table 27B.3

The Dutch/Memorial Sloan-Kettering Cancer Center Classification System

Classification Stage	Definition
I	Low grade, complete resection, no metastases
II	High grade, complete resection, no metastases
III	Any grade, incomplete resection, no metastases
IV	Any grade, any resection, distant metastases

Data derived from van Dalen T, Hennipman A, Van Coevorden F, et al. Evaluation of a clinically applicable post-surgical classification system for primary retroperitoneal soft-tissue sarcoma. *Ann Surg Oncol*. 2004;11: 483–490.

designed and validated for use with soft-tissue sarcomas of the extremities, not retroperitoneal sarcomas, which are all deep and usually >5 cm. Thus, the category T2b, N0, M0 (stage IB) would be the minimum stage of a retroperitoneal sarcoma with no possibility of a stage II (A or B) tumor. The histologic grade of the tumor becomes the major determinant of stage.

A recently proposed classification system for retroperitoneal sarcomas was developed in concert by the Dutch Soft Tissue Sarcoma Group and the Sarcoma Disease Management Team at Memorial Sloan-Kettering Cancer Center (Table 27B.3) (12). This system relies on the postresection characteristics of the tumor, namely macroscopic total resection, histologic grade, and distant metastases. Microscopic margins are difficult to reliably state because of the size of these lesions, so they were not included in the staging system. This resulted in a more even distribution of patients than the AJCC system.

SURGICAL TREATMENT

The treatment of retroperitoneal sarcomas is simply stated, but often difficult to achieve: complete removal of the tumor with clear surgical margins. As in other solid tumors, it is clear that the first surgical attempt at tumor removal is the best chance to cure the patient. In the analysis by Lewis et al. (3) of 500 patients with retroperitoneal sarcomas, those presenting with primary disease had an 83% resection rate with a median survival of 72 months. Those patients presenting with a local recurrence had a resection rate of 52% with a median survival of 28 months. Other authors have reported anywhere between 65% and 78% resectability rates for first-attempt retroperitoneal sarcomas, with resectability dropping to approximately 55% to 57% for recurrences (3,13).

We recently analyzed outcomes in our single-center experience with 44 patients who underwent resection for a retroperitoneal sarcoma, and assessed the impact on patient outcomes of factors such as gender, histology, and grade of the primary tumor, resection of a primary lesion or recurrent disease, tumor size, tumor location, vascular involvement, status

Table 27B.4

Clinical and Pathologic Features of Patients with Retroperitoneal Sarcomas

Variable Data	
Total number of patients:	44
Age: Mean/median (years)	61.8/62.3
Female/male	23/21
Primary/recurrent	27/17
Tumor Histology	**No. (%) of Patients**
Liposarcoma	19(44.0)
Leiomyosarcoma	11(25.0)
Malignant peripheral nerve sheath tumors	5(11)
Malignant fibrous histiocytoma	2(5)
Other	7(16)
Tumor Grade	**No. (%) of Patients**
Low	7(16)
Intermediate	14(3%)
High	23(52)
Mean tumor size	**16.9 cm**
Tumor Location	**No. (%) of Patients 51 (81%)**
Right retroperitoneal	14(33)
Left retroperitoneal	17(40)
Pelvic	6(14)
Mid abdomen	6(14)

of the surgical margins, neoadjuvant treatment, as well as either adjuvant chemotherapy and/or radiation (14). Over the 20-year study period, 27 patients (61.3%) had resection of the primary lesion, and 17 (38.6%) presented with resection for recurrent disease (Table 27B.4). Complete surgical resection (R0 or R1) was achieved in 79.1% of the patients, of whom 26 (59%) had clear surgical margins. At a median follow-up of 4.2 years, overall 1-, 3-, and 5-year survival was 87%, 53%, and 39%, respectively, for the patients who underwent resection of their primary disease; however, survival for patients was lower for those who underwent resection for recurrent disease, with overall 1-, 3-, and 5-year survival rates of 69%, 38%, and 19%, respectively. We performed univariate analysis on this group of patients, looking at factors that predict outcome. Only 2 of the 12 variables studied significantly affected survival. Tumor grade and tumor size with lesions >15 cm were found to be significant predictors of overall survival. Of the variables found to affect recurrence, only tumor size and vascular involvement were found to be statistically significant.

Complete surgical resection is the goal in all patients explored for resection. The first surgical attempt of a left-sided retroperitoneal sarcoma may involve resection of diaphragm, stomach, pancreas, spleen, adrenal, kidney and ureter, small bowel, colon, pelvic organs, and vascular structures, with or without grafting (Figure 27B.1). Removal of a right-sided retroperitoneal sarcoma may also involve resection of liver, biliary tract, and duodenum (Figure 27B.2). The MRI shown in Figure 27B.1 is from a patient presenting to our group who previously underwent two attempts at resection for a left-sided, well-differentiated liposarcoma in which no organs were removed at either previous operation. Seventy percent distal pancreatectomy, splenectomy, adrenalectomy, ureteronephrectomy, small bowel resection, and left hemicolectomy were required to achieve complete resection. Similarly, a pelvic sarcoma may require removal of pelvic organs or extension into the groin or scrotum for complete removal. These can be formidable, time-consuming operations and should be done at institutions at which there is both experience and interest in the problem. There can be no hesitation to resect involved organs; moreover, bowel and kidney will often approximate the tumor mass, but not be directly invaded. These organs should be resected to provide adequate margin.

Our strategy for the safe, surgical removal of retroperitoneal sarcomas can be outlined as follows:

1. Preoperative evaluation: A thorough assessment of the patient's cardiopulmonary function and renal function must be performed. A renal scan is obtained to establish the function of the *contralateral* kidney in case a nephrectomy is being considered. In cases in which ureteral involvement may be an issue, cystoscopy with ureteral catheter insertion can be helpful in identifying a displaced ureter. A formal bowel preparation is mandatory as small bowel and colon resections are commonly required. If major vascular structures are involved, particularly at the aortoiliac bifurcation, it should be anticipated from the outset that blood products may be required; in addition, consideration should be given to cell-saver technology.

2. Incision: The choice of incision should depend on the location of the tumor and the organs potentially involved. Often the exact choice of incision is not made until the patient is positioned on the operating table and the tumor palpated with the patient in a relaxed state. Most tumors can be approached through a midline incision, a midline incision with a T-transverse extension, a bilateral subcostal incision with or without a T-midline extension (chevron), or a thoracoabdominal incision. Exposure is the key to both safety and success.

3. Intraoperative considerations: Once the abdomen is opened, an exploration is done to determine resectability and to determine which organs may have to be sacrificed. This exploration is often difficult because of the massive size of some of these tumors and the reluctance to "burn a bridge" before the decision to proceed is made. Not uncommonly, either the left or right colon and its mesentery are draped over the tumor. Transecting the bowel above and below the tumor often helps in further defining the situation and allowing the surgical team to begin to develop the posterior dissection plane. We dissect the tumor from all directions in an attempt to isolate the point of retroperitoneal fixation, which is often muscular (psoas, iliacus, paravertebral, diaphragm), but, as previously noted, multiple organs can be adherent to the tumor and require resection. Resection of contiguous organs en bloc

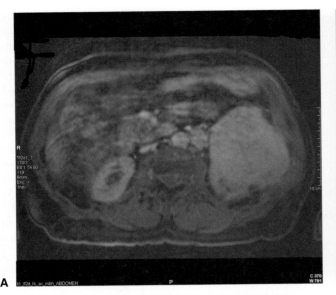

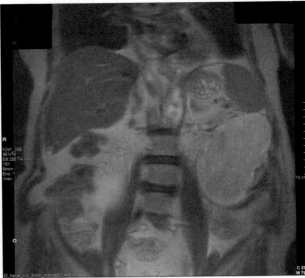

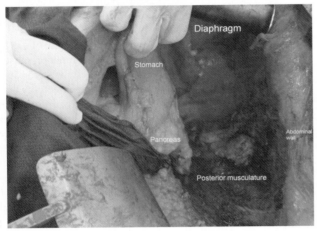

Figure 27B.1. (**A**) A Magnetic resonance imaging scan demonstrating large, recurrent left-sided retroperitoneal liposarcoma possibly invading the left kidney and spleen. (**B**) Coronal view of anatomic relationship with stomach and spleen. (**C**) Resection required removal of retroperitoneal musculature along with spleen, left kidney, left adrenal, left colon, distal pancreas, and partial gastrectomy. A large defect is left between the diaphragm superiorly and the pelvis inferiorly.

with tumor is required in 63% to 83% of patients, with over 50% necessitating more than one organ resection (3,8,13).

Although the kidney is commonly resected because of location and proximity to tumor, it must be noted that invasion is uncommon. Jaques et al. (13) noted that of the 30 nephrectomies performed in their series, only 2 kidneys were involved on pathologic examination. Our experience has been similar. In addition, the colon, another commonly resected organ, is often not involved directly by tumor; however, the colonic mesentery frequently is draped over the tumor and thus requires resection.

Resectability, as defined by most current studies, consists of complete removal of all macroscopic disease (R0, R1 resections). R0 indicates that the margins are free, both grossly and microscopically; R1 indicates gross removal, but microscopic involvement. Because of the size of most retroperitoneal sarcomas, evaluation of microscopic margins becomes impractical. Distant metastatic disease, peritoneal sarcomatosis, extensive vascular involvement, mesenteric root involvement, and neural (spinal cord) invasion are clear signs of unresectability (9,13). Barring these issues, most of these tumors can be grossly removed. Although complete resection rates

(R0 and R1) are between 59% and 95% depending on the study, local recurrence rates remain between 23% and 49%, even from groups well versed in the care of these tumors (3,8,13,15–17).

4. Major vascular involvement: Major vascular involvement has often been cited as a criterion for unresectability; however, several groups, including our own, have successfully resected retroperitoneal sarcomas with incontinuity arterial resections necessitating bypass grafting, including extra-anatomic reconstructions (18). If major vascular involvement is anticipated, magnetic resonance imaging, CT angiography, or conventional arteriography is important in planning reconstruction. Contrast imaging confirms that the target vessel is suitable for bypass and is in continuity with the distal vascular bed. This is especially important in patients who have had prior procedures in the groin, have extensive arteriosclerotic occlusive disease, or have had prior radiation therapy to the operative field. Absence of femoral pulses is an indication for conventional dye arteriography. Because venous reconstruction is optional, preoperative venous assessment is adequately performed with contrast-enhanced cross-sectional, and sagittal imaging to evaluate venous invasion by tumor.

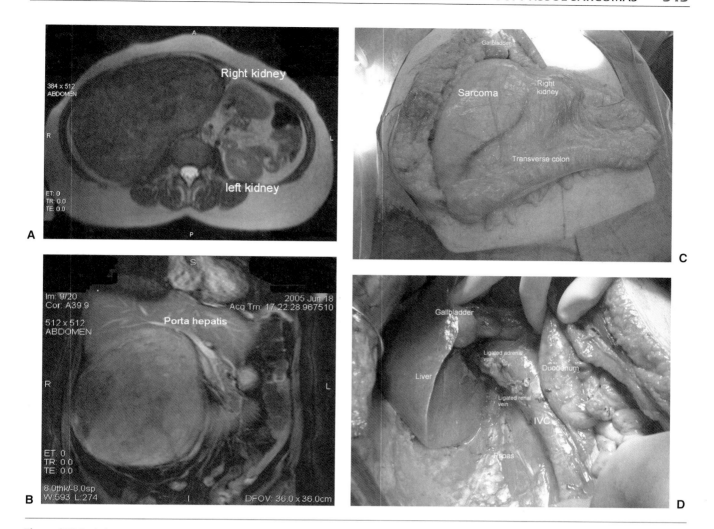

Figure 27B.2. (**A**) A computed tomography scan demonstrating right-sided retroperitoneal liposarcoma displacing right kidney anteriorly to the left of midline. (**B**) Tumor mass pushing on right lobe of liver with possible invasion and displacement of portal structures. (**C**) Resection of mass required right hemicolectomy and right ureteronephrectomy along with portions of retroperitoneal musculature. The liver was uninvolved. (**D**) The resection bed shows a normal liver capsule, the inferior vena cava (IVC), and duodenal margin.

Extra-anatomic reconstructions, such as axillofemoral and/or femoral-femoral bypass grafts, are useful ways of keeping prosthetic grafts and anastomoses out of the main surgical field when there has been bowel spillage, leakage of potentially contaminated urine from the ureter or bladder, or when the tumor itself is necrotic and bacterial contamination cannot be immediately ruled out. In addition, the surgical team must be prepared to use venovenous bypass techniques or even total circulatory arrest with profound hypothermia in certain situations (18,19).

In studies addressing major vascular resection (20–22), major venous ligation has often resulted in transient, severe, lower extremity edema. However, this rarely leads to persistent venous stasis and edema. This is regardless of whether the major vein (IVC or iliac/femoral vein) was patent at the time of surgery. Venous collaterals appear to form quickly and resolve severe lower extremity edema within 6 to 8 weeks. Although the infrarenal IVC can frequently be ligated with-

out long-term consequence, this may not be the case in an irradiated field. According to Matsushita and colleagues (23), resection of the iliac or femoral veins is sometimes more likely to result in chronic venous disease. Of the ten patients in their study, none had venous reconstruction and no patients had complications resulting in limb loss because of venous ligation. If venous reconstruction is used, autologous vein or a prosthetic graft may be placed as interposition conduits. In addition, an arteriovenous fistula may be temporarily added to increase blood flow through the graft. Grotemeyer et al. (24) described six patients with invasion of tumor into the IVC. After tumor resection, the involved IVC segments were replaced by polytetrafluoroethylene (PTFE) grafts to restore IVC continuity. In three patients, an adjunctive arteriovenous (AV) fistula was constructed between the femoral artery and the femoral vein. Graft patency after a mean follow-up of 30.2 months (range, 1 to 79) was 83.3%. The only graft occlusion occurred in a patient without an AV fistula. There were no

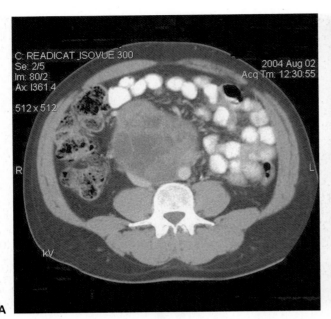 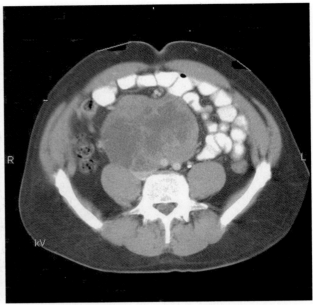

Figure 27B.3. (**A**) A computed tomography scan demonstrating a large pelvic/retroperitoneal sarcoma completely encasing the aorta and vena cava at the level of the bifurcation. (**B**) Distally, the internal and external iliac vessels were also involved. Resection was performed en bloc with right colon, right kidney, and aortocaval bifurcation. Reconstruction of the aorta was performed, and the infrarenal inferior vena cava was oversewn (not shown).

perioperative deaths and no major complications requiring reoperation. The authors suggest that in patients with tumor involvement of the IVC, the clinical outcome depends heavily on the vascular surgical co-procedure. After resection of the IVC, a PTFE graft is recommended in combination with an AV fistula. Anticoagulation is recommended for 3 months, followed by ligation of the AV fistula.

A recent case of ours highlights the problem of major vascular involvement (Figure 27B.3). The patient presented with a poorly differentiated pelvic sarcoma that completely encased the aorta and vena cava at aortoiliac/IVC bifurcation. He initially was treated with neoadjuvant chemotherapy, but despite the development of extensive tumor necrosis, there was no tumor shrinkage or change in vascular invasion. The tumor was resected en bloc with the right colon, right kidney, distal aorta, and vena cava. Reconstruction with an aortobifemoral graft was completed. The vena cava was ligated below the renal veins and no reconstruction was attempted. Massive scrotal and lower extremity swelling resolved within 6 weeks.

RADIATION THERAPY

Radiotherapy has been extensively studied in the treatment of soft-tissue sarcomas of the extremity (25–31). The goal of adjuvant or neoadjuvant radiation therapy is to achieve local control without resorting to amputation (limb-salvage therapy). Adverse prognostic factors affecting local recurrence after limb-salvage therapy include positive microscopic margins, a prior local recurrence, radiotherapy dose and field size, histologic grade, and histologic subtype (30,32–34).

With the use of multimodality therapy, local control with limb salvage is no longer the main issue with extremity sarcomas. Instead, the main focus has become the prevention and treatment of distant metastatic disease, primarily to the lung. This is in contradistinction to retroperitoneal sarcomas for which patients usually die from locally recurrent disease. In the study by Lewis et a. (3), 75% of their patients with primary retroperitoneal disease died in the *absence* of distant disease. The use of postoperative radiation in the adjuvant setting certainly makes theoretical sense; however, a survival advantage using radiation has been difficult to prove. High-grade histology, large size, and close or positive margins (35) are often reasons given to proceed with radiation; however, problems with large fields and damage to normal organs often makes this a more idealistic rather than realistic choice of therapy. Fein and colleagues (36) evaluated 21 patients retrospectively who were treated with surgical resection followed by radiation at a mean dose of 54 Gy. However, only one patient had negative microscopic margins. The 2-year local control and overall survival rates were 72% and 69%, respectively. There appeared to be some improvement in local control with doses >52.2 Gy. Tzeng and colleagues (37) studied preoperative radiation with selective dose escalation to the margin at risk in 16 patients with biopsy-proven retroperitoneal sarcomas. This included 45 Gy in 25 fractions to the entire tumor plus a boost dose of 57.5 Gy to the volume predicted as high risk for positive surgical margins. Fourteen of 16 patients (88%) underwent complete macroscopic resection. With a median follow-up of 28 months, there were only two local recurrences.

Intraoperative radiation therapy (IORT) has also been investigated. Sindelar et al. (38) evaluated 35 patients and found that using 20 Gy IORT followed by 35 to 40 Gy of external-beam radiation (EBRT) resulted in a 60% local control rate as compared with 20% in the surgery plus EBRT alone group. This small study did have a somewhat higher local recurrence rate than those seen by other investigators. However, no improvement in survival was found. In fact, the surgery plus IORT plus EBRT group had a 45-month median survival compared with the surgery plus EBRT group, whose survival was 52 months. A more recent report from Dziewirski et al. (5) used intraoperative brachytherapy (IOBRT) with and without EBRT in a group of 70 patients. After intraoperative evaluation and resection, only 46 patients were eligible for IOBRT. Half of these patients also received EBRT. This regimen resulted in an 88% 3-year local recurrence-free survival in the group treated with adjuvant EBRT, and only 58% in the IOBRT group, with no overall survival advantage. This led the authors to conclude that EBRT remains a necessary element of treatment for local control.

A phase 1 trial using preoperative doxorubicin with EBRT, followed by surgery and IORT was evaluated at M.D. Anderson Cancer Center. The goal was to evaluate the feasibility of the technique and toxicity of the regimen. A dose-escalation technique was used for EBRT ranging from 18 to 50.4 Gy based on reversible toxicity. Thirty-one of 35 patients completed the initial chemoradiation regimen without the need for hospitalization. Only 29 patients proceeded to laparotomy and 26 underwent either an R0 or R1 resection, with 22 patients receiving the IORT dose. No complications were attributable to IORT alone, but one patient developed ureteral strictures after the complete regimen that was thought to represent a cumulative effect of EBRT and IORT in addition to operative dissection (39).

CHEMOTHERAPY

Patients with high-grade retroperitoneal sarcomas and/or close surgical margins are often considered for postoperative adjuvant chemotherapy in addition to radiation therapy even though a survival advantage has not been clearly demonstrated. Glenn and associates (40) performed the only prospective trial and studied 37 patients with postoperative chemotherapy and radiation. There appeared to be an improvement in locoregional control, but no survival advantage; however, because of the small sample size and multiple arms in the study, it was difficult to draw any firm conclusions.

Meric and associates (6,41) from M.D. Anderson Cancer Center reviewed the morbidity of neoadjuvant chemotherapy in 108 patients with retroperitoneal sarcomas. The most common morbidities were wound complications. They concluded that neoadjuvant therapy did not increase morbidity, but did not address effectiveness. The radiographic response to neoadjuvant chemotherapy was a predictor of local control and survival in soft tissue sarcoma of both extremity and retroperitoneal types (6).

Wendtner et al. (42) added regional hyperthermia to neoadjuvant chemotherapy in an effort to further improve response. The authors selected a cohort of 58 patients who were all deemed unlikely to have an R0 resection, that is, they were considered unresectable. Forty-five of those patients had previous surgical resection or radiation prior to inclusion in the study. The overall response rate was 13%. Thirty patients went on to resection, but

28 developed progression, died, or refused surgery. Complete resection was achieved in eight patients (27%). This represents a cumbersome, but potentially useful therapeutic regimen that needs further study.

POSTTREATMENT REGIMEN

There is no well-defined follow-up regimen for patients with retroperitoneal sarcomas, although proposed schedules are published by the National Comprehensive Cancer Network (43). Because most recurrences occur in the first 2 years after resection, a combination of physical examination and imaging should be done more frequently during this time (44). Early detection of recurrences may allow for more effective treatment, especially if surgical intervention is required. Unfortunately, no proof currently exists to show an overall survival benefit to early detection with imaging. Clear evidence will continue to be difficult to obtain because of the overall low incidence of retroperitoneal sarcoma; however, we continue with intensive surveillance and aggressive treatment of recurrence and certain cases of metastatic disease.

FUTURE DIRECTIONS

There is a clear need for improvement in the treatment of patients with soft-tissue sarcomas, both retroperitoneal and non-retroperitoneal. Aggressive surgical therapy remains the mainstay of treatment for retroperitoneal sarcomas as local recurrence is the most common cause of death; however, improved radiation techniques and more effective systemic therapies will be needed to achieve long-term success in these patients. Recently, targeted molecular therapies have been found to be effective against certain types of tumors. For example, imatinib (Gleevec), a protein tyrosine kinase inhibitor, has been successfully used in patients with advanced and metastatic gastrointestinal stromal tumors with responses up to 60% (45,46). The role of imatinib in the adjuvant and neoadjuvant setting of resectable lesions is currently under investigation, but no data are yet available.

Some subtypes of soft-tissue sarcomas have identifiable molecular targets. Dermatofibrosarcoma and giant cell fibrosarcoma both express a fusion protein caused by translocation of the collagen type I alpha 1(*COLIA1*) and platelet-derived growth factor beta-chain (*PDGFB*) genes. The resultant protein is considered a functional PDGFB. Because imatinib inhibits the receptor of *PDGFB*, it may be effective against these histologic subtypes (47,48). Synovial cell sarcoma can express epidermal growth factor receptors and may therefore respond to epidermal growth factor-receptor inhibitors such as gefitinib (Iressa) (49).

Vascular endothelial growth factor (VEGF) has also been shown to be present in certain soft-tissue sarcomas and has been proposed as a tumor marker (50). Because bevacizumab (Avastin), a VEGF neutralizing antibody, has been successful in treating other tumors, it may also have activity against sarcomas that express this receptor. Although no results are available, the European Organisation for Research and Treatment of Cancer is developing clinical studies of VEGF receptor antagonists. We await further studies and results with these newer modalities.

REFERENCES

1. Clark JA, Tepper JE. Role of radiation therapy in retroperitoneal sarcomas. *Oncology (Williston Park)*. 1996;10:1867–1874.

2. American Cancer Society. *Cancer Facts and Figures 2006*. Atlanta, GA: American Cancer Society; 2006.

3. Lewis JJ, Leung D, Woodruff JM, et al. Retroperitoneal soft-tissue sarcoma: analysis of 500 patients treated and followed at a single institution. *Ann Surg*. 1998;228:355–365.

4. Clark MA, Fisher C, Judson I, et al. Soft-tissue sarcomas in adults. *N Engl J Med*. 2005;353:701–711.

5. Dziewirski W, Rutkowski P, Nowecki ZI, et al. Surgery combined with intraoperative brachytherapy in the treatment of retroperitoneal sarcomas. *Ann Surg Oncol*. 2006;13:245–252.

6. Meric, F, Hess KR, Varma DG, et al. Radiographic response to neoadjuvant chemotherapy is a predictor of local control and survival in soft tissue sarcomas. *Cancer*. 2002;95:1120–1126.

7. Alvarenga JC, Ball AB, Fisher C, et al. Limitations of surgery in the treatment of retroperitoneal sarcoma. *Br J Surg*. 1991;78:912–916.

8. Hassan, I, Park SZ, Donohue JH, et al. Operative management of primary retroperitoneal sarcomas: a reappraisal of an institutional experience. *Ann Surg*. 2004;239:244–250.

9. Feig BW. Retroperitoneal sarcomas. *Surg Oncol Clin North Am*. 2003;12:369–377.

10. Clark MA, Thomas JM. Port site recurrence after laparoscopy for staging of retroperitoneal sarcoma. *Surg Laparosc Endosc Percutan Tech*. 2003;13:290–291.

11. American Joint Committee on Cancer. *AJCC Cancer Staging Manual*, 6th ed. New York: American Joint Committee on Cancer; 2002: 193–197.

12. van Dalen T, Hennipman A, Van Coevorden F, et al. Evaluation of a clinically applicable post-surgical classification system for primary retroperitoneal soft-tissue sarcoma. *Ann Surg Oncol*. 2004;11:483–490.

13. Jaques, DP, Coit, DG, Hadju, SI, et al. Management of primary and recurrent soft-tissue sarcoma of the retroperitoneum. *Ann Surg*. 1990;212:51–59.

14. Ouellette JR, Amersi FF, Alban R, et al. Surgical resection for retroperitoneal sarcomas: analysis of factors determining outcome [abstract P284]. *Ann Surg Oncol*. 2007;14:118.

15. Karakousis CP, Gerstenbluth R, Kontzoglou K, et al. Retroperitoneal sarcomas and their management. *Arch Surg*. 1995;130:1104–1109.

16. Stoeckle E, Coindre JM, Bonvalot S, et al. Prognostic factors in retroperitoneal sarcoma: a multivariate analysis of a series of 165 patients of the French Cancer Center Federation Sarcoma Group. *Cancer*. 2001;92:359–368.

17. Gronchi A, Casali PG, Fiore M, et al. Retroperitoneal soft tissue sarcomas: patterns of recurrence in 167 patients treated at a single institution. *Cancer*. 2004;100:2448–2455.

18. Ouellette JR, Cossman DV, Sibert KS, et al. Tumors at the aortoiliac/inferior vena cava bifurcation: pre-operative, anesthetic, and intra-operative considerations. *Am Surg*. 2007;73:440–446.

19. McCready, RA, Fehrenbacher, JW, Divelbiss JL, et al. Surgical resection of a large recurrent pelvic arteriovenous malformation using deep hypothermic circulatory arrest. *J Vasc Surg*. 2004;39:1348–1350.

20. Hollenbeck ST, Grobmyer SR, Kent KC, et al. Surgical treatment and outcomes of patients with primary inferior vena cava leiomyosarcoma. *J Am Coll Surg*. 2003;197:575–579.

21. Sarkar R, Eilber FR, Gelabert HA, et al. Prosthetic replacement of the inferior vena cava for malignancy. *J Vasc Surg*. 1998;28:75–83.

22. Hardwigsen J, Baque P, Crespy B, et al. Resection of the inferior vena cava for neoplasms with or without prosthetic replacement: a 14-patient series. *Ann Surg*. 2001;233:242–249.

23. Matsushita M, Kuzuya A, Mano N, et al. Sequelae after limb-sparing surgery with major vascular resection for tumor of the lower extremity. *J Vasc Surg*. 2001;33:694–699.

24. Grotemeyer D, Pillny M, Luther B, et al. Reconstruction of the inferior vena cava for extended resection of malignant tumors. *Chirurg*. 2003;74:547–553.

25. Rosenberg SA, Tepper J, Glatstein E, et al. The treatment of soft-tissue sarcomas of the extremities: prospective randomized evaluations of (1) limb-sparing surgery plus radiation therapy compared with amputation and (2) the role of adjuvant chemotherapy. *Ann Surg*. 1982;196:305–315.

26. Tepper JE, Suit HD. Radiation therapy alone for sarcoma of soft tissue. *Cancer*. 1985;56:475–479.

27. Tanabe KK, Pollock RE, Ellis LM, et al. Influence of surgical margins on outcome in patients with preoperatively irradiated extremity soft tissue sarcomas. *Cancer*. 1994;73:1652–1659.

28. Pisters PW, Harrison LB, Leung DH, et al. Long-term results of a prospective randomized trial of adjuvant brachytherapy in soft tissue sarcoma. *J Clin Oncol*. 1996;14:859–868.

29. Yang JC, Chang AE, Baker AR, et al. Randomized prospective study of the benefit of adjuvant radiation therapy in the treatment of soft tissue sarcomas of the extremity. *J Clin Oncol*. 1998;16:197–203.

30. Pollack A, Zagars GK, Goswitz MS, et al. Preoperative vs. postoperative radiotherapy in the treatment of soft tissue sarcomas: a matter of presentation. *Int J Radiat Oncol Biol Phys*. 1998;42:563–572.

31. Harrison LB, Franzese F, Gaynor JJ, et al. Long-term results of a prospective randomized trial of adjuvant brachytherapy in the management of completely resected soft tissue sarcomas of the extremity and superficial trunk. *Int J Radiat Oncol Biol Phys*. 1993;27:259–265.

32. Keus RB, Rutgers EJ, Ho GH, et al. A limb-sparing therapy of extremity soft tissue sarcomas: treatment outcome and long-term functional results. *Eur J Cancer*. 1994;30A:1459–1463.

33. Mundt AJ, Awan A, Sibley GS, et al. Conservative surgery and adjuvant radiation therapy in the management of adult soft tissue sarcoma of the extremities: clinical and radiobiological results. *Int J Radiat Oncol Biol Phys*. 1995;32:977–985.

34. Dinges S, Budach V, Budach W, et al. Local recurrences of soft tissue sarcomas in adults: a retrospective analysis of prognostic factors in 102 cases after surgery and radiation therapy. *Eur J Cancer*. 1994;30A:1636–1642.

35. Heslin MJ, Lewis JJ, Nadler E, et al. Prognostic factors associated with long-term survival for retroperitoneal sarcoma: implications for management. *J Clin Oncol*. 1997;158:2832–2839.

36. Fein DA, Corn BW, Lanciano RM, et al. Management of retroperitoneal sarcomas: does dose escalation impact on local control? *Int J Radiat Oncol Biol Phys*. 1995;31:129–134.

37. Tzeng CWD, Fiveash JB, Popple RA, et al. Preoperative radiation therapy with selective dose escalation to the margin at risk for retroperitoneal sarcoma. *Cancer*. 2006;107:371–379.

38. Sindelar WF, Kinsella TJ, Chen PW, et al. Intraoperative radiotherapy in retroperitoneal sarcomas. Final results of a prospective, randomized, clinical trial. *Arch Surg*. 1993;128:402–410.

39. Pisters PW, Ballo MT, Fenstermacher M, et al. Phase I trial of preoperative concurrent doxorubicin and radiation therapy, surgical resection, and intraoperative electron-beam radiation therapy for patients with localized retroperitoneal sarcoma. *J Clin Oncol*. 2003;21:3092–3097.

40. Glenn, J, Sindelar WF, Kinsella T, et al. Results of multimodality therapy of resectable soft-tissue sarcomas of the retroperitoneum. *Surgery*. 1985;97:316–325.

41. Meric, F, Milas M, Hunt KK, et al. Impact of neoadjuvant chemotherapy on postoperative morbidity in soft tissue sarcomas. *J Clin Oncol*. 2000;18:3378–3383.

42. Wendtner CM, Abdel-Rahman S, Krych M, et al. Response to neoadjuvant chemotherapy combined with regional hyperthermia predicts long-term survival for adult patients with retroperitoneal and visceral high-risk soft tissue sarcomas. *J Clin Oncol.* 2002;20:3156–3164.

43. National Comprehensive Cancer Network (NCCN). Clinical practice guidelines in oncology, soft tissue sarcoma 2006:1–48. www.nccn.org.

44. Stojadinovic A, Leung DH, Allen P, et al. Primary adult soft tissue sarcoma: time-dependent influence of prognostic variables. *J Clin Oncol.* 2002;20:4344–4352.

45. Hirota S, Isozaki K, Moriyama Y, et al. Gain-of-function mutations of c-kit in human gastrointestinal stromal tumors. *Science.* 1998;279:577–580.

46. Demetri GD, von Mehren M, Blanke CD, et al. Efficacy and safety of imatinib mesylate in advanced gastrointestinal stromal tumors. *N Engl J Med.* 2002;347:472–480.

47. Shimizu A, O'Brien KP, Sjoblom T, et al. The dermatofibrosarcoma protuberans-associated collagen type Ialpha1/platelet-derived growth factor (PDGF) B-chain fusion gene generates a transforming protein that is processed to functional PDGF-BB. *Cancer Res.* 1999;59:3719–3723.

48. Maki RG, Awan RA, Dixon RH, et al. Differential sensitivity to imatinib of 2 patients with metastatic sarcoma arising from dermatofibrosarcoma protuberans. *Int J Cancer.* 2002;100:623–626.

49. Nielsen TO, Hsu FD, O'Connell JX, et al. Tissue microarray validation of epidermal growth factor receptor and SALL2 in synovial sarcoma with comparison to tumors of similar histology. *Am J Pathol.* 2003;163:1449–1456.

50. Hayes AJ, Mostyn-Jones A, Koban MU, et al. Serum vascular endothelial growth factor as a tumour marker in soft tissue sarcoma. *Br J Surg.* 2004;91:242–247.

COMMENTARY
Murray F. Brennan

The authors of Chapter 27B present a comprehensive overview of the management of retroperitoneum sarcomas. The commonest histopathology, as they rightly point out, is liposarcoma. At Memorial Sloan-Kettering Cancer Center, we have been most unsatisfied with the benefits of fine-needle biopsy, particularly in well-differentiated fatty lesions. These can usually be clearly identified on the preoperative computed tomography scan and so biopsy is rarely necessary. However, the authors are correct

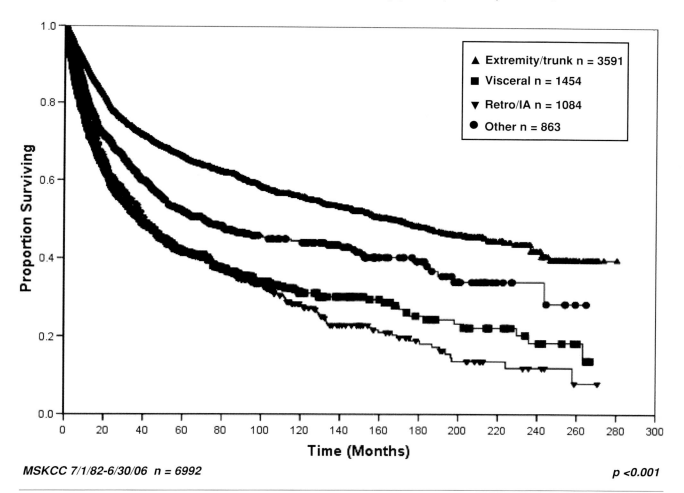

Figure 27B.C1 Overall survival by site for patients with soft-tissue sarcoma. Memorial Sloan-Kettering Cancer Center (MSKCC) 7/1/82 to 6/30/06.

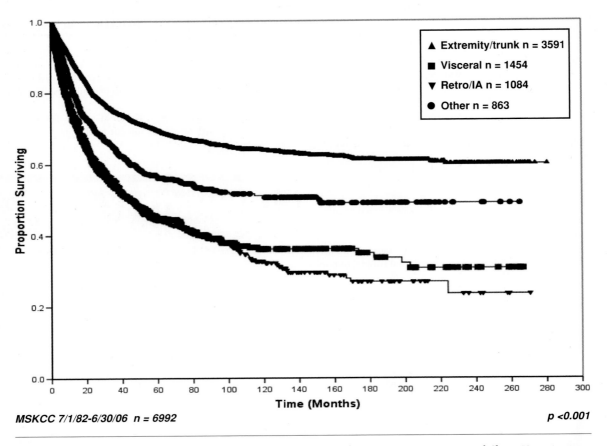

Figure 27B.C 2 Disease-specific survival by site for patients with soft-tissue sarcoma. Memorial Sloan-Kettering Cancer Center (MSKCC) 7/1/82 to 6/30/06.

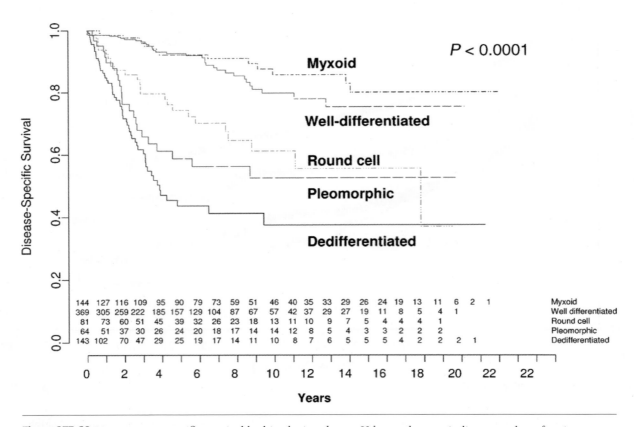

Figure 27B.C 3 Liposarcoma-specific survival by histologic subtype. Values at bottom indicate number of patients at risk. (From Moore DK, Kattan MW, Antonescu CR, et al. Subtype specific prognostic nomogram for patients with primary liposarcoma of the retroperitoneum, extremity or trunk. *Ann Surg.* 2006;244:381–391, with permission.)

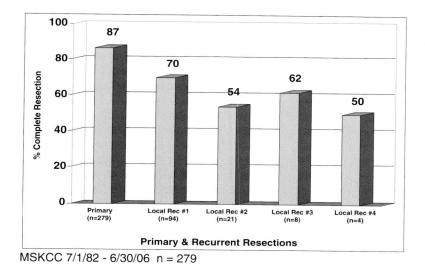

MSKCC 7/1/82 - 6/30/06 n = 279

Figure 27B.C 4 Percentage of complete resections for primary and recurrent (Rec) retroperitoneal soft-tissue sarcoma. Memorial Sloan-Kettering Cancer Center (MSKCC) 7/1/82 to 6/30/06.

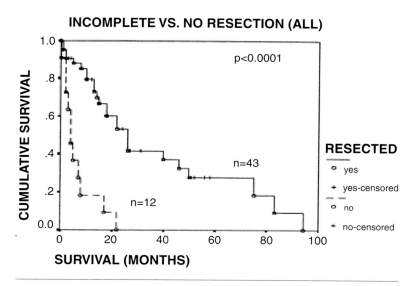

Figure 27B.C 5 Disease-specific survival comparing incomplete resection versus exploration and biopsy alone for patients with retroperitoneal liposarcoma. (From Shibata D, Lewis JJ, Leung DH, et al. Is there a role for incomplete resection in the management of retroperitoneal liposarcomas? *J Am Coll Surg*. 2001;193:373–379, with permission.)

that when there is the potential for a germ cell tumor or a lymphoma, then tissue core biopsy is a reasonable first approach. In the absence of that suspected pathology, unless neoadjuvant therapy is considered, which in my opinion should only be in a clinical trial situation, we proceed directly to operation.

The techniques of operation are well outlined. Appropriate emphasis is made on the fact that more extended operations beyond complete gross resection do not translate into a survival benefit (1). In addition, it is surprisingly rare to have true parenchymal invasion of the kidney by low-grade liposarcoma, which occurs in <10% of all patients, even those in whom the tumor completely encompasses the kidney (2). Resection of the kidney is often required because of the inability to have a complete gross resection and maintain adequate access to the vascular hilum. Patients should be made aware that the pathology may return without true parenchymal invasion of the kidney, but to obtain a complete resection, the kidney may need to be sacrificed. Conversely, when there is minimal involvement of the kidney, particularly in the reoperative situation when the contralateral kidney is gone, then the simple expedient of taking the kidney capsule can often render a complete gross resection without sacrifice of renal mass.

Major vascular involvement is well described; we are less enthusiastic about the major arterial resection described, as once major arterial involvement occurs, the lesion is usually sufficiently extensive that a complete gross resection cannot be obtained even with arterial reconstruction. Vena cava involvement often by primary leiomyosarcoma is well described, and the importance, in our opinion, of not performing complicated reconstructive processes that are rarely successful is emphasized (3). The vena cava can readily be ligated and resected, and with diligent attention to support hose, long-term peripheral edema can be completely avoided. A simple technique for repairing a partial resection of the inferior vena cava, in which the defect is large but only involves part of the inferior vena cava, is the use of a peritoneal fascial patch (4).

The authors rightfully describe the outcome, and an update of long-term survival in our prospectively followed database is appended (Figure 27.C1). Disease-specific survival by site with over 6,000 cases is shown in Figure 27B.C2. Prognosis is well defined by these two slides emphasizing the important point made by the authors that local recurrence is a factor in disease-specific survival for retroperitoneal sarcomas in contradistinction to systemic disease, which is the usual cause of death in visceral and extremity lesions. The evaluation of prognosis can now be done in general with defined sarcoma nomograms (5). As the authors point out, retroperitoneal lesions are all large and usually deep, and so the precision of this definition for the retroperitoneal lesion has been questioned. More recently we have provided a nomogram for liposarcoma, the most common histopathology (6). This gives a more accurate picture of the expected outcome based on the histology. Future nomograms directed at site-specific changes are likely to be of similar value (Figure 27B.C3).

The authors do not address the difficult problem of recurrence. Given the natural history of this disease, the majority of patients have recurrence. We have previously shown that approximately 80% of patients can undergo a first resection that is complete. However, with increasing subsequent resections, the likelihood of complete resection progressively diminishes (Figure 27B.C4).

Historically, we have always thought that only complete resection translates into a survival benefit, but it now appears clear with increasing numbers that, at least in liposarcoma (6), complete resections done for palliation can translate into an association with improved long-term survival (Figure 27B.C5) (7).

REFERENCES

1. Bevilacqua RG, Rogatko A, Hajdu SI, et al. Prognostic factors in primary retroperitoneal soft tissue sarcoma. *Arch Surg*. 1991;126:328–334.
2. Russo P, Kim Y, Ravindran S, et al. Nephrectomy during operative management of retroperitoneal sarcoma. *Ann Surg Oncol*. 1997;4:421–424.
3. Hollenbeck ST, Grobmyer SR, Kent KC, et al. Surgical treatment and outcome of patients with primary inferior vena cava leiomyosarcoma. *J Am Coll Surg*. 2003;197:575–579.
4. Suzman MS, Smith A, Brennan MF. Fascio-peritoneal patch repair of the IVC: A workhorse in search of work? *J Am Col Surg*. 2000;191:218–220.
5. Kattan MW, Leung DH, Brennan MF. Postoperative nomogram for 12-year sarcoma-specific death. *J Clin Oncol*. 2002;20:791–796.
6. Dalal KM, Kattan MW, Antonescu CR, et al. Subtype specific prognostic nomogram for patients with primary liposarcoma of the retroperitoneum, extremity or trunk. *Ann Surg*. 2006;244:381–391.
7. Shibata D, Lewis JJ, Leung D, et al. Is there a role for incomplete resection in the management of retroperitoneal liposarcomas? *J Am Coll Surg*. 2001;193:373–379.

Chapter 27C
Experience with Cryosurgery in the Management of Soft-Tissue Sarcomas

Lawrence R. Menendez, Yuri Falkinstein, and Elke R. Ahlmann

The treatment of soft-tissue sarcomas remains controversial, but there is general agreement that local control of the tumor is essential in order to achieve a cure. The mainstay of treatment, therefore, has been wide surgical excision, and in the case of extremity lesions, limb-sparing resection or amputation. In order to reduce the risk of local recurrence, radiation therapy has also been extensively used as a surgical adjuvant in the treatment of these tumors. The combination of surgery and radiation therapy has been generally effective in treating low-grade sarcomas, but results have been less satisfactory with high-grade lesions. Consequently, patients with high-grade soft-tissue sarcomas are often treated with adjunctive systemic chemotherapy and radiotherapy in the adjuvant or neoadjuvant setting in an attempt to improve local control and increase patient survival (see Chapter 29).

There are problems inherent with each of these treatment modalities. Obtaining wide surgical margins requires a plane of resection through normal tissue to eliminate any satellite lesions in the reactive zone of the tumor. Resections to assure tumor-free margins may result in major functional deficits and cosmetic deformities and, in addition, are sometimes difficult to achieve, especially when the tumor is adjacent to major neurovascular structures. In limb-salvage procedures surgical margins are sometimes very narrow and the plane of resection between the tumor and the adjacent vital structures may actually be through the reactive zone of the tumor. The resulting "marginal" margin may leave satellite lesions behind. Radiation therapy is also associated with significant risk and morbidity, including, for example, epidermolysis, fibrosis, stiffness, delayed wound healing, wound infection, radionecrosis of bone, degenerative arthritis, peripheral neuropathy, and the development of radiation-induced sarcomas (1–4). The morbidity of systemic chemotherapy in the treatment of cancer is well recognized and the efficacy of this modality in the treatment of soft-tissue sarcomas is controversial (5–7). Additionally, these adjuvants are often contraindicated in certain groups of patients, including elderly patients, those with multiple medical conditions, those who have previously been treated with the maximum allowable dose of radiation or chemotherapy, and those with tumors that are unresponsive to these modalities. In the past, such patients had no option other than to undergo surgical resection without prior treatment of their tumors. Cryoablation may be a viable option for these patients to reduce the tumor burden and make limb-salvage a surgical possibility.

PRINCIPLES OF CRYOABLATION

Cryosurgical ablation is a therapeutic method of treating neoplastic disease by freezing the malignant tissue in situ in order to cause devitalization (8). Cryosurgery generally requires special instrumentation to produce freezing of tissue. Successful cryosurgery requires that the same volume of tissue must be frozen as would have been excised had the tumor been treated with conventional wide resection alone. Thus, the amount of tissue surrounding the tumor that is devitalized cryosurgically must extend past the reactive zone of a tumor and into surrounding normal tissue to produce a margin sufficiently wide to encompass and thereby destroy any existing satellite lesions. This is the same principle of care that is applied when performing a curative en bloc surgical resection of a malignant tumor.

The literature contains many reports detailing the development of cryosurgery The use of freezing techniques in the treatment of malignancies began in the mid-19th century when iced saline solutions were used to treat advanced carcinomas of the breast and cervix (8). In the early 20th century, cryosurgery was used to treat various skin diseases (8). Modern cryosurgery made a significant breakthrough in 1961 with the development of an automated cryosurgical apparatus using liquid nitrogen (9).

Cryosurgery is most useful in easily accessible areas of the body, but recent advances in technology now make it possible to treat tumors that are deep and relatively inaccessible. Cryoprobe transducers can provide a controllable and predictable area of necrosis, and their use is now the preferred method of cryosurgery in many situations. In addition, dramatic advances in imaging technology, especially the development of computer-enhanced, real-time intraoperative ultrasonography, have allowed the safe and precise monitoring of deep-seated visceral lesions that cannot be completely visualized.

Benign and malignant tumors in many parts of the body, including bone, have been treated with cryosurgical techniques (10–61). Cryoablation is now a recognized approach to the treatment of various malignant tumors, including carcinoma of the skin (13,31–33), tumors of the eye (34–38), carcinomas of the oral cavity (39,40), carcinoma of the liver, both primary and metastatic (41–46), carcinoma of the vulva, vagina, and uterus (47,48), carcinoma of the prostate (10,14,49–52), and primary bone tumors (53–61). To date, however, soft-tissue sarcomas have not been treated extensively with this modality, although these tumors are present in relatively accessible locations.

PATHOPHYSIOLOGY OF CRYOABLATION

Cryosurgical techniques for the treatment of neoplastic disease is based on the concept of tumor destruction by the sequence of rapid freezing, slow thawing, and the immediate repetition of the freeze-thaw cycle (62,63). The coldest temperature reached in tissue has been demonstrated to be the most important determinant in causing cell necrosis (64). All living tissue subjected to a temperature of $-20°C$ or below for 1 minute or longer will undergo necrosis (65). However, most authorities recommend a treatment goal of at least $-40°C$ for 1 minute or more in all areas of the tumor to ensure cell necrosis and thereby minimize the risk of local recurrence (8,65). The damaging effects on cellular integrity result from severe cold as well as from the process of freezing and thawing. Hypothermia deprives cells of the energy required to drive cellular processes, resulting in both metabolic uncoupling and compromised integrity of cell membranes and organelles. Tissue freezing results in both extracellular and intracellular propagation of pure water without electrolytes and proteins. The osmotic gradient that develops draws water from the intracellular spaces, leading to cell shrinkage and membrane damage (66). The shearing forces from ice crystals are mechanically disruptive to organelles and cell membrane. Rapid freezing additionally maximizes cellular energy depletion (8).

The thawing process also disrupts cellular integrity by creating osmotic gradients and mechanical shearing forces thus destroying any remain reactive cells.

In the early phases of warming, small ice crystals recrystallize into larger ones that produce destructive shearing activity. As warming progresses, melting occurs and intact cells become exposed to a hypotonic environment. These new osmotic forces cause volume expansion and bursting of the cells. In contrast to the rate of freezing, a slow thaw is associated with optimal cellular damage. Thrombosis and tissue obliteration of tissue microvasculature also occur throughout the entire cryodestructive process, and thus contribute to tissue anoxia and hypoxic cell death (8,66,67).

The probability of achieving total cell necrosis increases with two freeze-thaw cycles (8). Although there is some debate as to the necessity of more than one freeze-thaw cycle in clinical practice, most surgeons performing cryoablation of malignant tumors perform two freeze-thaw cycles to assure maximal tissue destruction (8). In many cases, the initial freeze is followed by a slow passive thaw, and the second freeze is followed by a relatively active thaw.

The effects of freezing are nonselective, meaning that normal and malignant tissues are destroyed equally. An exception to this is the muscular wall of large arteries, which have been shown to be relatively impervious to the effects of freezing (68–71). Blood flow through these vessels acts like a heat sink and prevents freezing of the entire arterial wall. For this reason, a tourniquet should not be used when performing a cryosurgical ablation of an extremity sarcoma. These large vessels will show no evidence of thrombosis or wall damage after thawing (68–71). The close proximity of major vessels to a sarcoma therefore should not be a contraindication to performing cryoablation; however, care should still be taken to protect and retract vascular structures as far as possible from the tumor bed to prevent unnecessary freezing.

Another exception to the nonselective effects of freezing involves peripheral nerves. Peripheral nerve palsies were documented after cryosurgical treatment of bone tumors (55,60). Peripheral nerves that are frozen develop a neuropraxia and cease to function initially but this has been found to resolve 3 and 12 months after the initial insult (55,60,72). Peripheral nerve palsies associated with cryosurgery appear to be transient, and there have been no reported cases of permanent nerve dysfunction (55,60,72,73). In fact, intraoperative intercostal nerve freezing often has been used to prevent postthoracotomy pain, and this surgically induced neurapraxia was also found to be transient (74). This may be because of the unusual histology of peripheral nerves, which demonstrate long axons extending great distances from centrally located nuclei.

After cryoablation, the necrotic tissue is often allowed to resorb. The time required for resorption depends to some degree on the stoma. Thus, cellular tissue resorbs more rapidly than tissues with abundant fibrous stroma, such as connective tissue (8).

Cryosurgical ablation can be performed with use of either liquid nitrogen or gaseous argon, and multiple devices can be used, ranging from expensive automated instruments to simple, handheld devices that are nothing more than modified Thermos bottles or funnels. The type of apparatus chosen for use depends on the nature of the area of disease. Currently, the surgeon has the option of using liquid nitrogen in one of several ways. Liquid nitrogen can be poured or sprayed directly onto the tissues or it can be applied via a closed system with a cryoprobe so that the liquid nitrogen is never released on or into the tissue. Gaseous argon is available only using the cryoprobe system. We currently have been using a cryoprobe system that uses argon gas, which has the advantage of freezing faster and being colder than liquid nitrogen and enables the achievement of temperatures as low as −186°C. The major disadvantages of the spray or pour techniques are related to the difficulty in controlling runoff of the liquid nitrogen onto normal tissues during treatment. In addition, there is a risk of insufflation of tissue with associated nitrogen embolism if the spray technique is used.

The cryoprobe technique provides a controllable and predictable area of necrosis and is now the preferred method of cryosurgery in many situations, especially in large, bulky lesions in which a greater depth of freezing is required. During the freezing process, the white, frosted appearance of frozen tissue gradually extends away from the probe. When the freezing has encompassed a satisfactory volume of tissue, the process is stopped, the tissue is allowed to thaw, and the freeze-thaw cycle is repeated.

There are a variety of cryoprobe systems available that vary in size and the dimension of the freeze zone created. The systems also vary in the number of probes that can be accommodated simultaneously. Thus, it is important that the surgeon choose the appropriate cryoprobe in order to rationally plan a safe and effective cryosurgical procedure.

Ultrasound is routinely used during the cryoablation of hepatic and prostate tumors and other deep-seated visceral lesions (41). The freezing interfaces visualized as an advancing hyperechoic hemispheric rim with complete posterior or acoustic shadowing. As the ice ball expands, the hyperechoic rim increases in size, as does the area of acoustic shadowing (41). On the video monitor, the area of ice ball appears as a black mass lined by a white rim. Ultrasound monitoring is important for reasons of both efficacy and safety. The temperature at the periphery of

the cryolesion visualized on the ultrasound may only be 0°C to −10°C. There is a 10°C/mm to 20°C/mm decrease in the temperature from the outer rim of the ice ball toward the center (42). Because a freezing temperature of −40°C is required to assure tissue necrosis, there is a small rim of frozen tissue inward from the ice ball's edge that may contain viable cells. Thus, as with traditional surgical resection, a margin of normal tissue surrounding the neoplasm is also frozen in order to assure adequate treatment. Consequently, the surgeon should strive whenever possible to extend the ice ball beyond the tumor margin into normal tissue for a distance of 5 to 10 mm (41). Ultrasound monitoring of the freezing process can thus allow the surgeon to freeze the tumor while preventing undue freezing and necrosis of surrounding normal tissue. Freezing time varies, depending on the size of the tumor. It can range from 5 to 20 minutes or longer, depending on the size of the lesion. In a passive thaw, the ice ball is allowed to defrost at room temperature. In an active thaw, heated gaseous nitrogen or helium at approximately 60°C is pumped into the probe to help accelerate the thawing process.

While performing cryoablation, care should be taken to isolate the tissue to be frozen from any surrounding vital structures if possible. Surgical packs and Gelfoam® (Upjohn Co., Kalamazoo, Michigan) can also be used to help with isolation. The outer portion of the probe and the delivery line should also be isolated from critical structures.

CRYOSURGERY OF MUSCULOSKELETAL SOFT-TISSUE SARCOMAS: EXPERIENCE AT THE UNIVERSITY OF SOUTHERN CALIFORNIA

We previously reported the results of a phase 1 study demonstrating the safety and feasibility of cryoablation of soft-tissue extremity sarcomas (75). We have now completed a further study in which we have evaluated the oncologic and functional results of patients treated by this method (76). In this retrospective analysis, we reviewed the records of 38 patients with a biopsy-proven primary musculoskeletal soft-tissue sarcoma treated with cryoablation followed by immediate surgical resection. None of the patients had prior treatment with neoadjuvant chemotherapy or radiation. The study included 20 male and 18 female patients with an average age of 59 years (range, 28 to 92 years). The minimum follow-up was 6 months (average, 37 months; range, 6 to 98 months). All living patients had a minimum of 24 months of follow-up. Patients who died of disease before reaching 24 months of follow-up were also included in the study.

Locations of the tumors were the thigh (13), leg (4), forearm (3), chest wall (3), buttocks (3), pelvis (3), shoulder (1), arm (1), and hand (1). Diagnoses included malignant fibrous histiocytoma (16), myxoid liposarcoma (6), extraskeletal chondrosarcoma (5), leiomyosarcoma (3), synovial cell sarcoma (3), malignant Schwannoma (2), epithelioid sarcoma (1), and fibrosarcoma (1).

The lesion and a cuff of normal tissue around it were exposed through a longitudinal incision over the tumor. Neurovascular structures not in direct continuity with the pseudocapsule of the tumor were mobilized and retracted. After taking care to adequately protect the surrounding soft tissues, neurovascular structures, and skin, cryosurgical ablation commenced. Ultrasonography of the lesion was performed using 5-MHz or 7.5-MHz intraoperative transducers (3535 Ultrasound Scanning System, B-K Medical Systems, Wilmington, Massachusetts) to assist with strategic placement of the cryoprobes. Probes 3, 8, or 10 mm in diameter were inserted sequentially into the lesion at the discretion of the surgeon, depending on which cryosystem was used. The initial five cases were performed using the Cryotech LCS 3000 system (Candela Laser Corporation, Wayland, Massachusetts), and the ensuing seven cases were performed with the CMS AccuProbe 450 cryosurgical system (Cryomedical Sciences, Inc., Rockville, Maryland). Both systems circulate gaseous nitrogen through the cryoprobes to effect freezing of tissue. Since 2001 the authors have been using the CRY-Ocare system (Endocare Inc., Irvine, California), which uses argon gas and therefore has the advantage of freezing faster and colder than liquid nitrogen to achieve temperatures as low as $-186°C$.

For all cryoablative procedures, the probes were placed to ensure a complete freeze of the tumor as well as a minimum 10-mm cuff of normal tissue. Intralesional temperatures of $-160°C$ were maintained for 15 minutes with constant monitoring using thermocouples. The freeze cycle was also monitored with ultrasonography by visualizing the freezing interface as an advancing hyperechoic hemispheric rim with complete acoustic shadowing. The ice ball was extended 10 mm beyond the tumor margin into normal tissue in an attempt to freeze satellite lesions that may have been present in the reactive zone of the tumor. Once the ice ball reached the appropriate size, the tumor was allowed to slowly thaw by circulating helium gas through the probes and maintaining a temperature of $0°C$ for 5 minutes. The cycle was then repeated for a total of two cycles of fast-freeze/slow-thaw. Warm distilled water was then used to aid with thawing of the ice ball that encompassed the tumor, as well as to enhance the tumoricidal effect. At the end of the second thawing cycle, the probes were removed and the holes left by the cryoprobes were packed with Gelfoam. Wide resection of the tumor was then performed, often necessitating the use of osteotomes to resect the frozen tissue. The cryoablation was considered successful at the time of surgery in each of the 38 patients inasmuch as the ice ball appeared to encompass the entirety of the tumor and a wide surrounding margin. Overall, the entire cryoablative process added approximately 60 minutes to the procedure.

Histologic evaluation of permanent specimens revealed that 16 of the 38 patients (42%) had evidence of near-complete ($\geq$95%) tumor necrosis, and 11 of these (29%) had complete (100%) histologic necrosis. However, the majority of specimens revealed <95% necrosis. In 58% of cases, cryoablation was not effective in achieving complete devitalization of tumor tissue. The percent necrosis for these 22 cases was 90% (3), 80% (4), 70% (1), 50% (4), 40% (3), 30% (1), 20% (2), 10% (2), and 5% (2). In all cases the viable tissue seen in the resected tumor was only at the periphery or rim, indicating that there was inadequate freezing and the ice ball did not encompass the entire tumor. Six of these patients had relatively large tumors with a volume >1,000 cm^3 (mean,

1,894 cm^3). In these cases only a 1- to 2-cm rim of viable tumor remained at the periphery. All tumors were resected with a clear margin of 10 mm between the surgical margin and evidence of tumor. With the numbers available, we found no difference in percent tumor necrosis for those tumors <1,000 cm^3 and >1,000 cm^3, indicating there should be no contraindication to treating large tumors with cryoablative techniques. We observed no bias toward a certain grade of tumor, demonstrating either an entirely favorable or unfavorable amount of tumor necrosis.

No differences were detected in the recurrence rate in those patients with complete freezing of the tumor indicated by evidence of >95% necrosis from the rate in patients with <95% necrosis. The *recurrence-free survival* was 87% at both 2 and 5 years for patients with >95% necrosis, and 87% and 72%, respectively, for those with <95% necrosis based on Kaplan-Meier survivorship analysis. Local tumor recurrence occurred in three patients with an average time from surgical resection to the development of local recurrence of 16 months (range, 5 to 37 months). All tumors were malignant fibrous histiocytomas, and all demonstrated <95% necrosis. Tumor necrosis for these patients was an average of 50% (range, 10% to 50%), and average tumor volume was 3,132 cm^3 (range, 956.3 to 6,300 cm^3). All patients were treated with re-excision and adjuvant cryoablation and were free of disease at the time of this writing.

Kaplan-Meier survivorship curves with 95% confidence intervals show that patients with adequate freezing indicated by more than 95% histologic necrosis had a greater ($p = 0.006$) *overall survival* than those patients who had less-than-optimal tumor freezing. The 2-year and 5-year survivorships are 94% and 86%, respectively, for patients with >95% necrosis. For patients with <95% necrosis, survival was 53% at 2 years and 34% at 5 years.

Similarly, patients with adequate freezing had a greater ($p = 0.021$) *disease-free survival* than those patients who had less than optimal tumor freezing. Patients with >95% necrosis had a disease-free survival of 85% at 2 and 5 years, respectively. Patients with <95% necrosis had 60% and 50% 2- and 5-year disease-free survival, respectively.

The most common complication associated with the procedure was the development of serous wound drainage and seroma occurring in 8 patients (21%). This complication is seen frequently with cryoablative procedures because of both the resulting liquefaction of residual frozen tissue as well as the large volumetric defect created as a result of resection. The average tumor volume resected in the patients who developed seromas was 1,369 cm^3 (range, 16.5 to 6,800 cm^3). None of the patients with serous drainage or seromas became infected. The wound drainage subsided within 6 weeks (range, 2 to 6 weeks). In six patients, seromas resolved after aspiration performed between 1 and 4 weeks postoperatively. Two patients with large seromas that recurred after aspiration required surgical evacuation. No patients in this study required soft-tissue coverage with muscle flaps.

Peripheral nerve palsies occurred in five patients (13%), all of whom had their respective nerves deliberately frozen, as we believed mobilizing the nerves from their respective locations in close proximity to the tumor would potentially contaminate the surgical margin. There were three palsies of the sciatic nerve and one of the posterior tibial nerve, which occurred after resection of tumors of the posterior compartment of the thigh. The remaining patient developed palsies of both the radial and ulnar nerves after resection of a tumor from the arm. All five cases initially had complete motor and sensory neurapraxias but demonstrated complete recovery of function, two within 1 week of cryoablation, two within 3 months, and the remaining patient within 6 months.

Superficial wound infections that resolved after a course of oral antibiotics occurred in three patients. No cases of deep wound infection, deep venous thrombosis, pulmonary embolism, or skin slough occurred in this study.

Postoperatively, patients achieved good-to-excellent postoperative function corresponding to 87% of baseline function. The patients with poorer postoperative function were those who had experienced nerve palsies and, therefore, had prolonged recovery time. All patients in this study were able to return to activities of daily living and occupation-related activities.

The differences in overall survival and disease-free survival we found based on the amount of histologic necrosis emphasize the importance of complete freezing of the tumor. The fact that only 42% of tumors had either complete or near-complete necrosis highlights the technical difficulty of the cryoablation procedure. Of the patients with <95% necrosis, five were treated with the Cryotech LCS 3000 and seven with the CMS Accu-Probe 450 system. Both commercially available models of probes were designed for treatment of liver, prostate, and uterine tumors and can accommodate only a maximum of five probes simultaneously.

When freezing large, bulky tumors, five probes are sometimes inadequate. In such cases, the tumor must be frozen in sections, which may not be ideal. The CRYOcare system that we presently use can accommodate up to eight probes simultaneously, and thus a greater volume of tumor can be frozen at one time. In this study, all cases without favorable histologic responses to cryoablation can be explained by inadequate freezing. The resected tissue specimens showed pockets of viable tumor or interspersed viable cells throughout the tumor margins. The cells at the center of the tumor that were adequately frozen became necrotic, as expected, while at the periphery some viable cells remained because the tumors were not completely frozen at their margins. Of the 14 patients with <50% necrosis, eight of these cases were performed early in our experience with this technique.

The lack of complete necrosis can be attributed to several factors, including poor intraoperative imaging and the initial lack of use of thermocouples to monitor temperature. Early in our experience the propagating ice ball often could not be well visualized. We have not encountered this problem with the current use of more technologically advanced ultrasound transducers and have been able to more easily assess propagation of the ice ball to encompass the entirety of the tumor. Another problem we initially encountered was the inability to accurately assess the temperature of the tumor in all dimensions during propagation of the ice ball. We have since used thermocouples to monitor the temperature at the periphery of the ice ball and have been able to assure an adequate margin of devitalized tissue at the periphery of the tumor. We recommend the placement of multiple thermocouples at the expected margin of later resection to assure a temperature of at least −40°C for more than 1 minute.

THE ROLE OF CRYOABLATION IN THE TREATMENT OF SOFT-TISSUE SARCOMAS

Our experience at the University of Southern California indicates that cryoablation is a safe, technically feasible, and effective adjunctive treatment for musculoskeletal soft-tissue sarcomas (75,76). Cryosurgical ablation, however, should not be used in lieu of conventional treatment techniques, but may be an effective surgical adjuvant in improving oncologic outcome in certain groups of patients. It can be employed in conjunction with surgery, chemotherapy, and radiotherapy. Our current indications for the use of cryosurgery in the treatment of soft-tissue sarcomas include elderly patients and those with multiple medical conditions who are unable to tolerate chemotherapy, those who have previously been treated with the maximum allowable dose of radiation or chemotherapy, and those with tumors that are unresponsive to these modalities.

The major complications associated with this technique are those involving peripheral nerves. Although some patients do develop neurapraxia after direct exposure of the peripheral nerves to cryodestructive procedures, none has been permanent, indicating that the neurapraxia resulting from cryoablation is transient in nature.

No instances of thrombosis of major vessels in patients with cryoablation of extremity sarcomas have been reported. The major problem with vital structures is concern with peripheral nerves, blood vessels, and in certain instances bone. Isolating these structures when possible can minimize the morbidity of the procedure. When the location of these structures in relationship to the tumor makes mobilization and isolation impossible, both peripheral nerves and blood vessels can be safely included in the freeze zone without sustaining permanent damage.

At present, there are several inherent problems with the cryoablation of soft-tissue sarcomas. Of greatest concern is the quality of intraoperative imaging with ultrasound. If the tumor and propagating ice ball are not adequately visualized, a portion of the tumor may not be adequately frozen. Lack of 100% tumor necrosis is secondary to inadequate freezing, which, in our experience, is the result of poor intraoperative imaging. The importance of achieving ≥95% tumor necrosis was demonstrated in our study, in which patients with ≥95% necrosis had a significantly increased overall survivorship and disease-free survivorship. Further technical advances must be made in order to solve the problem with inadequate imaging. If imaging is satisfactory, complete tumor necrosis should and can be realized.

There are also concerns regarding the potential for local contamination when the cryoprobes are inserted. In order to minimize this risk, the tissues should be meticulously protected with surgical packing before the probes are inserted. The tracts created by the probes should also be plugged with Gelfoam immediately on their removal, while the tissue is still frozen and there is little or no bleeding.

REFERENCES

1. Kuklo TR, Temple HT, Owens BD, et al. Preoperative versus postoperative radiation therapy for soft-tissue sarcomas. *Am J Orthop.* 2005;34:75–80.

2. Livi L, Santoni R, Paiar F, et al. Late treatment-related complications in 214 patients with extremity soft-tissue sarcoma treated by surgery and postoperative radiation therapy. *Am J Surg.* 2006;191:230–234.

3. Paulino AC. Late effects of radiotherapy for pediatric extremity sarcomas. *Int J Radiat Oncol Biol Phys.* 2004;60(1):265–274.

4. Zagars GK, Ballo MT, Pisters PW, et al. Preoperative vs. postoperative radiation therapy for soft tissue sarcoma: a retrospective comparative evaluation of disease outcome. *Int J Radiat Oncol Biol Phys.* 2003;56:482–488.

5. Cormier JN, Huang X, Xing Y, et al. Cohort analysis of patients with localized, high-risk, extremity soft tissue sarcoma treated at two cancer centers: chemotherapy-associated outcomes. *J Clin Oncol.* 2004;22:4567–4574.

6. Grobmyer SR, Maki RG, Demetri GD, et al. Neo-adjuvant chemotherapy for primary high-grade extremity soft tissue sarcoma. *Ann Oncol.* 2004;15:1667–1672.

7. Eilber FC, Eilber FR, Eckardt J, et al. The impact of chemotherapy on the survival of patients with high-grade primary extremity liposarcoma. *Ann Surg.* 2004;240:686–695.

8. Gage AA. Cryosurgery in the treatment of cancer. *Surg Gynecol Obstet.* 1992;174:73–92.

9. Cooper IS, Lee ASJ. Cryostatic congelation: a system for producing a limited, controlled region of cooling or freezing of biologic tissue. *J Nerv Ment Dis.* 1961;133:259–263.

10. Gonder MJ, Soanes WA, Smith V. Experimental prostate cryosurgery. *Invest Urol.* 1964;1:610–619.

11. Rand RW, Rashe Am, Paglia DE, et al. Stereotactic cryo-hypophysectomy. *JAMA.* 1964;189:255–259.

12. Gage AA, Keopf S, Wehrle D, et al. Cryotherapy for cancer of the lip and oral cavity. *Cancer.* 1965;18:1649–1651.

13. Zacarian S, Adham M. Cryotherapy of cutaneous malignancy. *Cryobiology.* 1966;2:212–218.

14. Gonder MJ, Soanes WA, Shulman S. Cryosurgical treatment of the prostate. *Invest Urol.* 1966;3:372–378.

15. Barton R. Cryosurgical treatment of nasopharyngeal neoplasms. *Am Surg.* 1966;32:744–747.

16. Hill C. Preliminary report on cryosurgery in otolaryngology. *Laryngoscope.* 1966;76:109–111.

17. Kaplan J, Kaplan I. Cryogenic electrocoagulation and spontaneous necrosis of a bladder neoplasm: a preliminary comparative study. *J Urol* 1966;95:531–535.

18. Jordan W, Walker D, Miller G, et al. Cryotherapy of benign and neoplastic tumors of the prostate. *Surg Gynecol Obstet.* 1967;25:1265–1268.

19. Lincoff H, McLean J, Long R. The cryosurgical treatment of intraocular tumors. *Am J Ophthalmol.* 1967;63:389–399.

20. Crisp WE, Asadourian L, Ramberber W. Application of cryosurgery to gynecologic malignancy. *Obstet Gynecol.* 1967;30:668–673.

21. Blackwood J, Moore FT, Pace WG. Cryotherapy for malignant tumors. *Cryobiology.* 1967;4:33–38.

22. Ostergard D, Townsend DE. Malignant melanoma of the female urethra treated by cryotherapy with radical vulvectomy and anterior exenteration. *Obstet Gynecol.* 1968;31:75–82.

23. Dowd J, Flint L, Zinman L, et al. Experiences with cryosurgery of the prostate in the poor-risk patient. *Surg Clin North Am.* 1968;48:627–632.

24. Gage AA. Cryotherapy for inoperable cancer. *Dis Colon Rectum.* 1968;2:36–44.

25. Torre D. Cutaneous cryosurgery. *J Cryosurg.* 1968;1:202–209.

26. Beggs JH. Cryotherapy as a palliative maneuver. *JAMA.* 1968;207:1570–1572.

27. Marcove RC, Miller TR. Treatment of primary and metastatic bone tumors by cryosurgery. *JAMA.* 1969;207:1890–1894.

28. Crisp WE. The use of cryosurgery in cancer of the uterine cervix. *Int Surg.* 1969;52:451–454.

29. Gage A. Cryosurgery for cancer—an evaluation. *Cryobiology.* 1969;5:241–249.

30. Miller D, Metzner D. Cryosurgery for tumors of the head and neck. *Trans Am Acad Ophthalmol Otolaryngol.* 1969;73:300–309.

31. Lubritz RR. Cryosurgery management of multiple skin carcinomas. *J Dermatol Surg Oncol.* 1977;3:414–416.

32. Kuflik EG. Cryosurgery for multiple basal-cell carcinomas on the nose: a case report. *J Dermatol Surg Oncol* 1984;10:16–18.

33. Graham G, Clark L. Statistical analysis in cryosurgery of skin cancer. *Clin Dermatol.* 1990;8:101–107.

34. Abramson D, Lisman R. Cryopexy of a choroidal melanoma. *Ann Ophthalmol.* 1979;11:1418–1421.

35. Fraunfelder FT, Boozman FW, Wilson RS, et al. No-touch technique for intraocular malignant melanomas. *Arch Ophthalmol.* 1977;95:1616–1620.

36. Wilson RS, Fraunfelder FT. Circum-tumor cryoenucleation: a new no-touch technique for the prevention of metastatic seeding of intraocular cancer. *Int Congr Ser.* 1979;2:1870–1873.

37. Lazar M, Geyer O, Rosen N, et al. A transconjunctival cryosurgical approach for intraorbital tumors. *Aust NZ J Ophthalmol.* 1985;13:417–420.

38. Hurwitz JJ, Mishkin SK. The value of cryoprobe-assisted removal of orbital tumors. *Ophthalmic Surg.* 1988;19:94–97.

39. Weaver A, Smith D. Cryosurgery for head and neck cancer. *Am J Surg.* 1974;128:466–470.

40. Smith D, Weaver A. Cryosurgery for oral cancer—a six-year retrospective study. *J Oral Surg.* 1976;34:245–248.

41. Kane RA. Ultrasound-guided hepatic cryosurgery for tumor ablation. *Semin Intervent Radiol.* 1993;10:132–142.

42. Ravikumar TS, Steel G Jr, Kane R, et al. Experimental and clinical observations on hepatic cryosurgery for colorectal metastases. *Cancer Res.* 1991;51:6323–6327.

43. Zhov XD, Tang ZY, Yu YQ, et al. Clinical evaluation of cryosurgery in the treatment of primary liver cancer. Report of 60 cases. *Cancer.* 1988;61:1889–1892.

44. Ravikumar TS, Kane R, Cady B, et al. A 5-year study of cryosurgery in the treatment of liver tumors. *Arch Surg.* 1991;126:1520–1524.

45. Polk W, Fong Y, Kerpeh M, et al. A technique for the use of cryosurgery to assist hepatic resection. *J Am Coll Surg.* 1995;180:171–176.

46. Steele G Jr. Cryoablation in hepatic surgery. *Sem Liver Dis.* 1994;14:120–125.

47. Wright VC, Davies EM. The conservative management of cervical intraepithelial neoplasia: the use of cryosurgery and the carbon dioxide laser. *Br J Obstet Gynaecol.* 1981;88:663–668.

48. Goncalves J. Cryovulvectomy—A new surgical technique for advanced cancer. *Skin Cancer.* 1986;1:17–31.

49. Bonney WW, Fallon B, Gerber WL. Cryosurgery in prostatic cancer: survival. *Urology.* 1982;19:37–42.

50. Bonney WW, Fallon B, Gerber WL. Cryosurgery in prostatic cancer: elimination of local lesion. *Urology.* 1982;22:8–15.

51. Gursel E, Roberts M, Veenema R. Regression of prostatic cancer following sequential cryotherapy to the prostate. *J Urol.* 1972;108:928–932.

52. Eltahir K, Rietrich F. Clinical observations on tumor immunity in urologic cryosurgery. *Z Urol Nephrol.* 1976;69:135–140.

53. Bickels J, Meller I, Schmookler BM, et al. The role and biology of cryosurgery in the treatment of bone tumors. A review. *Acta Orthop Scand.* 1999;70:308–315.

54. Gage A, Erikson R. Cryotherapy and curettage for bone tumors. *J Cryosurg.* 1968;1:60–66.

55. Marcove RC, Weis LD, Vaghaiwalla MR, et al. Cryosurgery in the treatment of giant cell tumors of bone. A report of 52 consecutive cases. *Cancer.* 1978;41:957–969.

56. Jacobs PA, Clemency RE Jr. The closed cryosurgical treatment of giant cell tumor. *Clin Orthop Rel Res.* 1985;192:149–158.

57. Marcove R, Stovel P, Huvos A, et al. The use of cryosurgery in the treatment of low and medium chondrosarcoma. *Clin Orthop Rel Res.* 1977;122:147–156.

58. Malawer MM, Bickels J, Meller I, et al. Cryosurgery in the treatment of giant cell tumor. A long-term follow-up study. *Clin Orthop Rel Res.* 1999;(359):176–188.

59. Malawer MM, Dunham W. Cryosurgery and acrylic cementation as surgical adjuncts in the treatment of aggressive (benign) bone tumors. Analysis of 25 patients below the age of 21. *Clin Orthop Rel Res.* 1991;(262):42–57.

60. Marcove RC, Lyden JP, Huvos AG, et al. Giant cell tumors treated with cryosurgery. *J Bone Joint Surg Am.* 1973;55:1633–1644.

61. Schreuder HWB, Pruszczynski M, Veth RPH, et al. Treatment of benign and low-grade malignant intramedullary chondroid tumors with curettage and cryosurgery. *Eur J Surg Oncol.* 1998;24:120–126.

62. Gage AA. Probe cryosurgery. In: Epstein E, Epstein E Jr, eds. *Skin Surgery.* Philadelphia: WB Saunders; 1987:465–479.

63. Gage AA, Torre D. Cryosurgery. In: Webster J. *Encyclopedia of Medical Devices and Instrumentation.* New York: Wiley and Sons; 1988:893–908.

64. Gage A. What temperature is lethal for cells. *J Dermatol Surg Oncol.* 1979;5:459–461.

65. Cooper IS. Cryosurgery for cancer. *Fed Proc.* 1965;24:5237–5240.

66. Reite C. Mechanical forces as a cause of cellular damage by freezing and thawing. *Biol Bull.* 1966;131:197–203.

67. Mazur P. Physical and chemical factors underlying cell injury in cryosurgical freezing. In: Rand RW, Rinfret AP, Von Leder H, eds. *Cryosurgery.* Springfield, IL: Charles C Thomas; 1968, 32–51.

68. Cooper IS, Samma K, Wisniewska K. Effects of freezing in major arteries. *Stroke.* 1971;2:471–482.

69. Gage AM, Montes M, Gage AA. Freezing the canine thoracic aorta in situ. *J Surg Res.* 1979;27:331–340.

70. Bowers WD Jr, Hubbard RW, Daum RC, et al. Ultrastructural studies on muscle cells and vascular endothelium immediately after freeze-thaw injury. *Cryobiology.* 1973:10:9–21.

71. Giampapa VC, Oh C, Aufses AH. The vascular effect of cold injury. *Cryobiology.* 1981;1:49–54.

72. Miles TS, Hribar D. Recovery of function after cryosurgical lesions of peripheral nerves in rats. *Neurosci Lett.* 1981;24:285–288.

73. Myers RR, Powell HC, Hechman HM, et al. Biophysical and pathological effects of cryogenic nerve lesion. *Ann Neurol.* 1981;10:478–485.

74. Nelson KM, Vincent RG, Bourke RS, et al. Intraoperative intercostal nerve freezing to prevent post-thoracotomy pain. *Ann Thorac Surg.* 1974;18:280–285.

75. Menendez LR, Tan MS, Kiyabu MT, et al. Cryosurgical ablation of soft tissue sarcomas: a phase I trial of feasibility and safety. *Cancer.* 1999; 86:50–57.

76. Ahlmann ER, Falkinstein Y, Fedenko AN, et al. Cryoablation and resection influences patient survival for soft tissue sarcomas: impact on survivor ship and local recurrence. *Clin Orthop Relat Res.* 2007;459: 174–181.

COMMENTARY
Dror Robinson

HISTORICAL REVIEW

Cryosurgery in orthopaedic oncology is entering its fifth decade, and as expected at this venerable age, appears mature and well established. However, evolution of this modality still continues with efforts to develop more precise methods of tissue ablation with resultant feasibility to modify the type of surgery required from wide and radical resections into marginal and even intralesional procedures.

Treating bone tumors by cryosurgery began in the mid-1960s in the United States using direct instillation of liquid nitrogen (1). To a certain extent, this method decreased the recurrence rate of bone tumors and reduced the requirement for amputation. The major drawbacks were the danger of potentially deadly embolic events, originally thought to be due to nitrogen emboli, as well as unpredictable tissue freezing. (2). The pathogenesis of these embolic events during surgery has not been thoroughly elucidated. It is known that embolic events, thought to be due to venous air embolism, occur during hip arthroplasty in approximately 5% of patients (3). During hip arthroplasty, Spiess et al. (3) reported that all embolic events producing hemodynamic changes were detected by precordial Doppler ultrasound, but the incidence of increased end-tidal nitrogen and carbon dioxide was low, as was the incidence of air in central venous catheter aspirations. These latter findings led to the hypothesis that many of the embolic events actually may be due to bone marrow extravasation rather than gas embolism. Kropfl et al. (4) found that during conventional reamed femoral nailing, the incidence of bone marrow extravasation correlated with the rise in intramedullary pressure. In an experimental study in rats and rabbits, de Vries and associates (5) found that cryosurgery of intact bone resulted in increased intramedullary pressure that could cause bone marrow extravasation, resulting in embolization of bone marrow particles into extraosseous veins with resulting occlusion of pulmonary vasculature. The authors theorized that the increased intramedullary pressure was due to edema in the medullary cavity caused by cryosurgical damage to cell membranes.

A method to circumvent the danger of using liquid nitrogen in vivo is the option of ex vivo freezing. This involves temporary excision of the affected part of the bone, freezing it outside the body in liquid nitrogen and then retransplanting it. This method has the drawback that liquid nitrogen makes the bone very brittle. Transplantation may be followed by breakage of the bone due to fatigue fracture or even splitting of the bone during insertion of the osteosynthesis materials.

In 1980, Kerschbaumer and associates (6) developed a closed system of cryosurgery, allowing controlled freezing without exposure of living tissues to liquid nitrogen. This system eliminated the problem gas embolism and reduced the risk of inadvertent soft-tissue damage. In their studies, the authors concluded that the safest way of freezing bone selectively without exposure of the soft tissues to unnecessary risks is by intramedullary freezing, as contrasted to periosteal freezing.

A further advance was made during the 1990s when an argon-based system developed for prostate cryosurgery was applied to the treatment of musculoskeletal tumors. This system allows real-time monitoring of tissue temperatures in the surrounding soft tissue as well as ensuring adequate freezing of the tumor bed (7). The argon-based system, which uses argon gas and therefore has the advantage of freezing faster and colder than liquid nitrogen, achieves temperatures down to −186°C. In previous studies, my colleagues and I have shown that a minimum of two freezing cycles is necessary in order to achieve cellular necrosis of chondrosarcomas in situ (8). This therapy has revolutionized the treatment of low-grade chondrosarcomas, and instead of mutilating bone resections, it is possible to perform intralesional resection with similar clinical results (9).

As they describe in the accompanying chapter, Dr. Menendez and colleagues at the University of Southern California (10) have reported similar results in soft-tissue sarcomas, wherein about 50% of cases demonstrated >95% necrosis histologically following cryoablation.

MECHANISM OF CRYOABLATION

As the University of Southern California authors point out, with the exception of the muscular wall of large arteries and nerve tissue, the effects of freezing are nonselective; normal and malignant tissues are destroyed equally (11).

Although major blood vessels are relatively protected during cryosurgery, microvascular damage appears to be the mechanism leading to tissue damage in most tissues. Endothelial cells lining the vessel wall are thought to be the initial target of freezing. There is mounting evidence that the endothelium may play an important role in cryosurgical treatments by acting to locally foster thrombi in the microvasculature of various tissues after freezing. It was found that the initial cell shape change was mainly controlled by water dehydration, dependent on the cooling rate, resulting in the shrinkage of cells in the direction normal to the free surface. Quantitative analysis showed that the freezing-induced dehydration greatly enhanced the cell surface stresses, especially in the axial direction. This could be one of the major causes of the final breaking of the cell junction and cell detachment (12).

Another mechanism of cell damage is related to intracellular ice formation (IIF). IIF was found to occur at lower temperatures (18°C) in many cell types than would be expected, and the phenomenon is particularly important at cooling rates ≥25°C/min (13).

Thus it appears that the minimal temperature of the ice ball formed should be about −20°C to ensure tissue damage due to IIF. In addition, rapid freezing appears of importance and thus the use of multiple probes is indicated.

A third mechanism of cell death associated with cryosurgery is apoptosis or gene-regulated cell death (14). Apoptosis is additive with both the direct ice-related cell damage that occurs during the operative freeze-thaw intervals and coagulative necrosis that occurs over days posttreatment.

Subfreezing temperatures, when sequentially applied with low-dose chemotherapy, may provide improved cancer cell death in the freeze zone periphery due to apoptosis. Apoptotic cells exhibit nonrandom DNA cleavage, blebbing of the membranes, phospholipid inversion in the membranes, and caspase activation in the cells. Once in an apoptotic state, not all cells will eventually die. Less-damaged cells can repair themselves and survive, therefore requiring further injury to complete the lethal effect. Thus, it appears that cryosurgery when used in combination with cytotoxic chemical and physical agents designed to initiate apoptosis, will have clinical benefit.

RECOMMENDED PROTOCOL FOR MUSCULOSKELETAL ONCOLOGY

Repetitive freeze-thaw cycles have been reported to improve therapeutic outcomes at warmer subfreezing temperatures (−20° to −40°C). Temperatures must be achieved at a safe margin (positive margin) around a tumor, which in hepatic tumors, for example, is commonly accepted to be 1 cm beyond the edge of the lesion. This margin is often accepted in musculoskeletal oncology as well. Baust and Maiwand (15) state that the cryosurgeon should aim for a temperature of −25°C in the periphery of the abnormal tissue. As mentioned previously, a minimum of two freeze-thaw cycles is necessary to achieve cell necrosis rates of >95% in chondrosarcomas (8). In a study of renal cell carcinoma, complete loss of cell viability was evident at temperatures of −25°C and colder. Extended freeze hold times over 5 minutes and passive thawing rates resulted in more extensive cell damage. Additionally, a double freeze-thaw cycle significantly increased cell death compared with a single cycle (16).

In conclusion, it appears that the ice ball should extend to at least 1 cm from the edge of the lesion, that two or more freeze-thaw cycles should be used, that the minimal hold time is 5 minutes, and that the temperature at the margins should be lower than −25°C. Slow thawing is preferred to rapid one.

FUTURE PROSPECTS

The most exciting recent developments in the field of musculoskeletal cryoablation are related to pain relief and closed image-guided treatment of bone metastasis. The techniques were initially developed for the treatment of prostate and renal cancer. They are based on the insertion of a thin probe under image guidance and then monitoring of the ice ball formation and isotherms within its borders (17). The same technique has been successfully employed in bone metastasis (18). External-beam radiation therapy is the current standard of care for cancer patients who present with localized bone pain, but 20% to 30% of patients treated with this modality do not experience pain relief and, unfortunately, few further options exist for these patients. High-temperature treatment using radiofrequency ablation and low-temperature treatment using cryoablation therapy are most commonly used. Complete ablation of metastatic lesions is not readily achieved with radiofrequency ablation because the zone of ablation can only be estimated. In contrast, with cryosurgery, the zone of ablation can be visualized on computed tomography scanning as a low-attenuation area corresponding to the ice ball or by ultrasound, as previously described. Cryoablation also allows the simultaneous use of multiple cryoprobes, which allows complete ablation of large lesions (up to approximately 8-cm diameter) in a single session (18).

In conclusion, it appears that cryosurgery is a safe and reliable modality in the treatment of both soft-tissue and bone lesions. The cryosurgical treatment of soft-tissue tumors is currently reserved as a modality adjunctive to surgical resection in malignant tumors. However, further research is necessary to determine whether benign lesions could be treated with minimally invasive methods using only image-guided cryoablation.

The use of cryoablation is indicated in both benign aggressive and malignant bone lesions as an adjunct to surgical resection, making it possible to employ intralesional resection in at least some malignant primary bone tumors without compromising oncologic results. The most promising field that is expected to rapidly expand over the next few years is the palliative treatment of bone metastasis.

REFERENCES

1. Marcove RC, Miller TR. Treatment of primary and metastatic bone tumors by cryosurgery. *JAMA.* 1969;207:1890–1894.
2. Schreuder HW, van Beem HB, Veth RP. Venous gas embolism during cryosurgery for bone tumors. *J Surg Oncol.* 1995;60:196–200.
3. Spiess BD, Sloan MS, McCarthy RJ, et al. The incidence of venous air embolism during total hip arthroplasty. *J Clin Anesth.* 1988;1:25–30.
4. Kropfl A, Berger U, Neureiter H, et al. Intramedularry pressure and bone marrow fat intravasation in unreamed femoral nailing. *J Trauma.* 1997;42:946–954.
5. de Vries J, Oosterhuis JW, Oldhoff J. Bone marrow embolism following cryosurgery of bone: an experimental study. *J Surg Res.* 1989;46:200–206.
6. Kerschbaumer F, Russe W, Weiser G, et al. Cryolesions of bone. An experimental study. Part I: examinations in technique of controlled cryolesion in bone. *Arch Orthop Trauma Surg.* 1980;96:5–9.
7. Rehman J, Landman J, Lee D, et al. Needle-based ablation of renal parenchyma using microwave, cryoablation, impedance- and temperature-based monopolar and bipolar radiofrequency, and liquid and gel chemoablation: laboratory studies and review of the literature. *J Endourol.* 2004;18:83–104.
8. Robinson D, Yassin M, Nevo Z. Cryotherapy of musculoskeletal tumors–from basic science to clinical results. *Technol Cancer Res Treat.* 2004;3:371–375.
9. Ahlmann ER, Menendez LR, Fedenko AN, et al. Influence of cryosurgery on treatment outcome of low-grade chondrosarcoma. *Clin Orthop Relat Res.* 2006;451:201–207.
10. Ahlmann ER, Falkinstein Y, Fedenko AN, et al. Cryoablation and resection influences patient survival for soft tissue sarcomas: impact on survivorship and local recurrence. *Clin Orthop Relat Res.* 2007;459:174–181.
11. Bowers WD Jr, Hubbard RW, Daum RC, et al. Ultrastructural studies on muscle cells and vascular endothelium immediately after freeze-thaw injury. *Cryobiology.* 1973;10:9–21.
12. Zhang A, Xu LX, Sandison GA, et al. Morphological study of endothelial cells during freezing. *Phys Med Biol.* 2006;51:6047–6060.
13. Berrada MS, Bischof JC. Evaluation of freezing effects on human microvascular-endothelial cells (HMEC). *Cryo Lett.* 2001;22:353–366.
14. Baust JG, Gage AA, Clarke D, et al. Cryosurgery—a putative approach to molecular-based optimization. *Cryobiology.* 2004;48:190–204.
15. Baust J, Maiwand MO. Fundamental aspects of cryosurgery. *Cryosurgery.* 2002;6:6–8.
16. Clarke DM, Robilotto AT, Rhee E, et al. Cryoablation of renal cancer: variables involved in freezing-induced cell death. *Technol Cancer Res Treat.* 2007;6:69–79.
17. Maybody M, Solomon SB. Image-guided percutaneous cryoablation of renal tumors. *Tech Vasc Interv Radiol.* 2007;10:140–148.
18. Callstrom MR, Charboneau JW Image-guided palliation of painful metastases using percutaneous ablation. *Tech Vasc Interv Radiol.* 2007;10:120–131.

28

Diagnosis and Treatment of Malignant Tumors of Bone

Earl Brien and James R. Ouellette

Malignant tumors of the bone mirror soft-tissue sarcomas in their complexity. An understanding of the basic biology and pathology of bone tumors is essential for appropriate treatment planning. In this chapter, we review the unique biological behavior of bone sarcomas. This provides the basis for their staging, resection, and the use of appropriate neoadjuvant or adjuvant treatment modalities.

OSTEOSARCOMA

Intramedullary, high-grade osteosarcoma is the most common malignant bone tumor of childhood. Malignant cells that produce osteoid define an osteosarcoma. The distal femur, proximal tibia, and proximal humerus are the most frequent sites of involvement. It is most commonly seen in the second decade of life with a second peak in the sixth decade usually seen as a secondary sarcoma. Patients will often present with a painful mass. Approximately 4% of tumors about the knee will be misdiagnosed initially as athletic injuries. Arthroscopy is the most common procedure performed in such patients (1). Radiographs frequently reveal a blastic, intramedullary lesion with an associated density in the soft tissues. The differential diagnosis includes infection, lymphoma, and osteoblastoma. Telangiectatic osteosarcoma is characterized radiographically by a lytic, destructive lesion of bone. This will often appear similar to a giant cell tumor, Ewing sarcoma, or infection.

Imaging Studies

Plain radiographs are best in diagnosing bone tumors. Many benign tumors can be diagnosed without ordering additional studies (2). If a malignant tumor is suspected, magnetic resonance imaging (MRI) of long bones best demonstrates intramedullary and soft-tissue tumor extension. Total-body bone scan is important to determine additional osseous lesions. Computed axial tomography (CAT) scan of the chest may be done after confirmation of malignancy to determine the presence of lung metastases. MRI should be done after chemotherapy has been administered and prior to definitive surgery to evaluate response and confirm your surgical plans based on the initial MRI. This should include the entire involved bone to evaluate skip metastasis. Serial plain radiographs of the extremity and chest are performed in 3-month intervals for the first 2 years. CAT

scan of the chest is performed every 6 months, providing chest x-rays are normal. These recommendations may be modified, particularly if patients are being actively treated for metastatic disease.

Osteosarcoma may be subcategorized by location or histologic variants. Osteosarcomas about the surface of the bone are most commonly parosteal or periosteal osteosarcomas. Parosteal osteosarcoma is low grade and is commonly found pasted to the posterior surface of the femur. Low-grade, intramedullary osteosarcoma (Figure 28.1) has similar histologic features as fibrous dysplasia, but also requires wide excision as opposed to curettage, grafting, and internal fixation, which is typically performed with fibrous dysplasia. The low-grade osteosarcoma may have only subtle anaplasia and lacks mitotic activity. Periosteal osteosarcoma may mimic malignant cartilaginous tumors microscopically. It is important to differentiate periosteal osteosarcoma from low- to intermediate-grade chondrosarcoma because periosteal osteosarcoma will have a better response to chemotherapy. Radiographically, it commonly has a "sunburst" appearance and is also considered a periosteal or juxtacortical lesion.

The majority of osteosarcomas are high-grade and intramedullary (Figure 28.2). However, exceptions include high-grade surface osteosarcomas. The histologic variations are far more complex than defining osteosarcoma by location. Osteosarcoma is the great mimicker histologically of numerous benign tumors such as giant cell tumor, aneurysmal bone cyst (telangiectatic osteosarcoma), chondroblastoma, osteoblastoma, and early fracture callous. Unfortunately, the histologic differences between these lesions and osteosarcoma may be subtle, and without an experienced pathologist, radiologist, and clinician, grave diagnostic errors may occur.

Surgical Staging

Three critical factors are evaluated with surgical staging: grade, compartment, and metastases. The grade (low or high) of the tumor determines if the lesion is stage I or II. Whether the tumor is intra- or extracompartmental is designated by *a* or *b*. The presence of metastatic disease, regardless of grade or compartment status, is stage III. The typical osteosarcoma patient at presentation has stage IIb lesion. This means that it is a high-grade lesion that is extracompartmental without evidence of gross disease in the lung (3,4). We know from historic data that nearly

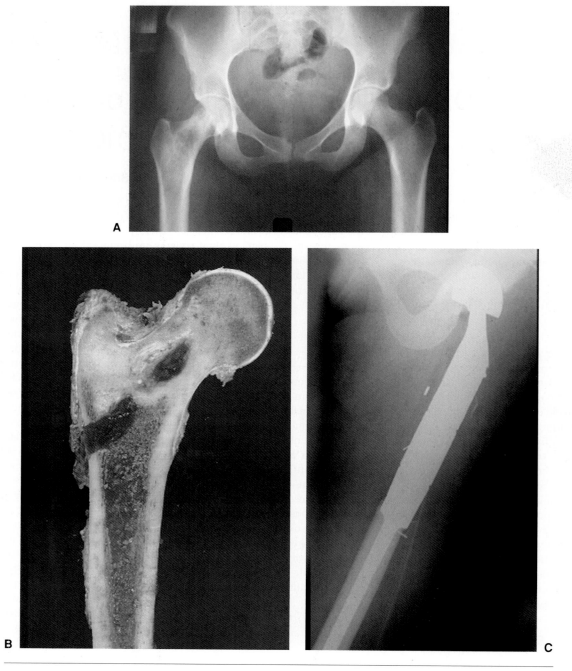

Figure 28.1 Intramedullary proximal femoral osteosarcoma. This figure represents a 22-year-old woman diagnosed with low-grade, intramedullary proximal femoral osteosarcoma. This was originally diagnosed as fibrous dysplasia at an outside institution; however, progressive pain and an abnormal radiograph (**A**) led to repeat biopsy, which showed subtle anaplasia, characteristic of low-grade osteosarcoma. Proximal femoral resection (**B**) and proximal femoral resection was treated with hemiarthorplaty (**C**). This provides immediate stabilization of the proximal femur to the acetabulum and reduces the risk of dislocation often resulting from a loss of the stabilizing hip abductor forces perioperatively.

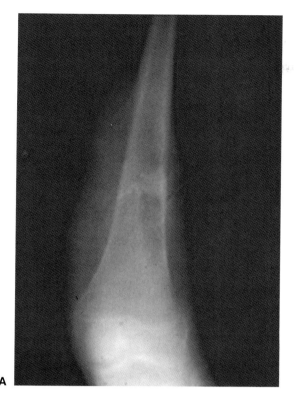

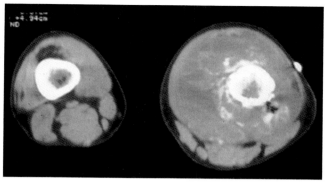

Figure 28.2 High-grade osteosarcoma of the distal femur. This figure represents a classic osteogenic sarcoma of the distal femur treated with wide excision and endoprosthetic reconstruction with a modular rotating hinged knee. Although there was a large, soft-tissue component (**A**), the tumor responded nicely to chemotherapy. Tumor response is determined by pain relief and reduction in soft-tissue mass. Monthly evaluation of thigh circumference at the biopsy site is adequate to determine tumor response. Magnetic resonance imaging (MRI) should be performed prior to definitive surgery to evaluate extent of disease in both bone and soft tissues (**B**). However, we use tumor resection measurements from original MRI to avoid intraoperative contamination.

90% of patients with osteosarcoma present with microscopic metastatic disease.

Treatment

Biopsy should be planned to limit contamination and allow for excision of the biopsy site to be best incorporated with the definitive surgery. In the extremities, a longitudinal incision is most easily excised and reduces soft-tissue contamination. Incisions through the muscle belly may provide better hemostasis and avoid neurovascular contamination. The capsule should be reapproximated, often over gel foam, to achieve hemostasis. For scapula and pelvic tumors, the incision is placed in line with the planned excision. Biopsy should provide the pathologist with adequate tissue while limiting the risk of pathologic fracture and significant contamination. Drains are generally avoided with biopsies. Mankin et al. (5,6) have published several articles regarding the hazards of biopsy in patients with malignant primary bone tumors. Non–weight bearing should be considered to further reduce the risk of fracture prior to definitive treatment of long bones. Percutaneous core biopsy is an alternative to open biopsy and may reduce contamination. In some cases, particularly cystic lesions like telangiectatic osteosarcoma, open biopsy should be considered because percutaneous biopsy may not be adequate. External central lines in the young (<10 years of age) and implanted catheters are placed either at the time of biopsy, if diagnosis can be confirmed on frozen section, or after definitive diagnosis is made.

Treatment for classic high-grade osteosarcoma is preoperative combination chemotherapy (Adriamycin, methotrexate, iphosphamide, and/or cisplatinum). Bacci et al. (7,8) and Ferrari et al. (9) reviewed 510 consecutive patients with high-grade os-

teosarcoma of the extremity and found that four drug regimens and telangiectatic tumors each correlated with an improved prognosis. Most patients can receive limb-salvage surgery, and this includes en bloc excision and reconstruction. Reconstructive surgery includes endoprosthesis, composite (endoprosthesis plus allograft), or allograft alone. Intra-articular excision (cutting through the joint to remove the diseased bone) is the standard approach to limb-salvage surgery. However, Dr. Brien has had many cases in the past 15 years in which such an excision would have resulted in contamination and subsequent local recurrence. This inevitably would lead to amputation of the extremity. Initially, local fascial flaps are developed, the nerve and blood vessels are identified and dissected from the tumor, and resection of the bone is approximately 3 to 5 cm from the proximal extent of the tumor. In cases in which the tumor has a large soft-tissue extension and is in close proximity of the joint, one should strongly consider extra-articular excision and reconstruction. The capsule and its adjacent structures about the knee and shoulder do not act as a barrier to soft-tissue spread. Despite a more aggressive surgical approach, patients have excellent function postoperatively.

Bickels et al. (10) reviewed 110 reconstructions of distal femoral replacements with nearly 8-year follow-up and identified a 5.4% infection rate, 5.4% recurrence rate, and 10.8% loosening rate. The authors' preferred method depends on the site and extent of tumor. Endoprosthesis with a rotating hinge knee is ideal for distal femoral resections. We prefer a similar approach for proximal tibial resections; however, a gastrocnemius flap should be used to further support the patellar tendon reconstruction. There are recent data supporting composite reconstruction with proximal femoral replacement; however, with careful reconstruction of the hip abductors with Mersilene tape and fiber wire, hip abduction can be restored. For osteosarcoma of the proximal humerus, in which intra-articular resection can be performed, composite reconstruction may have benefit for shoulder abduction similar to the hip. However, when performing composite reconstruction, one should be cognizant of the difficulty of getting an excellent fit distally with adequate stem size and length. Diaphyseal sarcomas are best managed by intercalary allograft (11). Rigid fixation is essential and best achieved by spanning the entire allograft with either a plate or intramedullary rod and further stabilizing the host allograft junction with derotation plates. We have preferred double-plating technique in the past; however, with the current locking plates, one may consider intramedullary nailing in conjunction with derotating locking plates at junctional sites.

The most common complication of intercalary allograft is nonunion, which ranges between 10% and 20% at each host/allograft site. Autograft should be considered at the initial surgery or subsequent surgery. Osteosarcoma in the pediatric group can be treated with an expandable prosthesis. This does not require reopening the incision to provide additional growth. Lengthening can be achieved by an external cuff that works through an electromagnetic field and allows a spring-loaded device to increase the length of the prosthesis. Early data on this technique have been published from several centers regarding pediatric limb reconstruction (12–15).

Amputation is considered in patients with vascular involvement, pathologic fracture where significant contamination has occurred, and in a patient whose tumor has responded poorly to chemotherapy. However, >90% of patients with osteosarcoma will have limb-salvage surgery as opposed to amputation. Several studies have been published comparing functional outcome of patients having amputation versus limb salvage for high-grade bone sarcomas (16,17). Bone transport has also been considered in such cases (18). Vascular bypass has been used in cases in which the blood vessels have been encased by tumor and when patients have refused amputation.

Lung metastasis is not uncommon and CT scan of the chest is used to evaluate and monitor disease. Early recognition of lung lesions is imperative. Patients who respond well to chemotherapy and have fewer than four lung nodules have an excellent prognosis. Immunotherapy, such as interferon, should be considered in patients with poor chemotherapy response or in patients who have had lung recurrence despite chemotherapy and surgery.

It should be noted that for low-grade, intramedullary, and parosteal osteosarcoma, treatment is surgery alone, consisting of wide excision followed by limb reconstruction. Wide excision with clear margins is essential to avoid local recurrence and later progression into a high-grade osteosarcoma. We strongly favor en bloc excision for low-grade osteosarcoma of the distal femur as opposed to partial excision of the femur and stabilization with bone strut. This unique tumor is nearly always cured with wide excision; however, if there is incomplete resection of the tumor, local recurrence follows. Amputation should be considered because these tumors will often step up in grade and lead to systemic disease and late death.

CHONDROSARCOMA

Primary chondrosarcoma is the most common tumor of flat bones in skeletally mature patients (Figure 28.3). Fifth decade is peak age. Night pain is an early presentation and is often followed by a painful mass. Low-grade intramedullary chondrosarcoma may be a primary or secondary neoplasm. Secondary low-grade chondrosarcomas arise from either enchondromas or osteochondromas. Intramedullary chondrosarcoma must be diagnosed histologically in conjunction with plain radiographs. Cytology in cartilaginous tumors is variable. Many benign cartilaginous tumors may look more cytologically ominous than the low-grade chondrosarcoma. Intramedullary, low-grade chondrosarcoma should be histologically evaluated on low power. Mirra et al. (19) were able to distinguish low-grade chondrosarcoma from enchondroma by describing four histologic features characteristic of chondrosarcoma. These histologic features include the chondrosarcoma permeation pattern, invasion

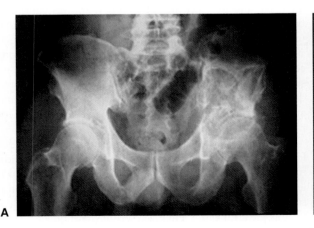
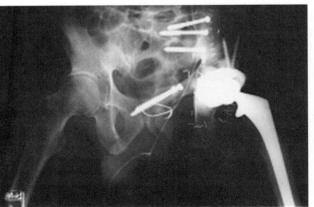

Figure 28.3 Chondrosarcoma of the pelvis. A 57-year-old man with chondrosarcoma of the pelvis (**A**) was treated with pelvic allograft and total hip replacement (**B**). Allograft has a high failure and infection rate. Other reconstruction includes saddle prosthesis or extended girdlestone excision. Pelvic excisions and reconstruction are some of the most challenging cases in orthopaedic oncology. Many articles have been written specifically on this topic (22–24).

of the Haversian canal, marrow with bands of fibrosis, and extraosseous involvement. Radiographic features of chondrosarcoma include mixed lytic/blastic lesion, cortical thickening, overall enlargement of the bone, and soft-tissue extension. Chondrosarcoma may arise from osteochondroma as well. Osteochondroma of the pelvis and scapula are the most common sites of malignant degeneration. Osteochondroma is best evaluated by MRI, which reveals a cartilaginous cap of ≥2 cm. Infrequently, bursal fluid can mimic an enlarged cap and may require biopsy. Biopsy should be performed to evaluate the cap and must be orientated from superficial to deep. If a biopsy is given to the pathologist who shaves the cap, it may appear to have a thickened cap of cartilage. This would be misleading and most likely lead to an incorrect diagnosis. One should consider removing osteochondromas about the pelvis and scapula, particularly if their growth cannot be monitored clinically, because delay in diagnosing malignant degeneration may occur and a high-grade, dedifferentiated sarcoma may develop from such low-grade sarcomas.

Low-grade chondrosarcoma commonly occurs in the fourth and fifth decades of life. Again, this may be either primary or secondary. For a diagnosis to be made of secondary chondrosarcoma, either radiographs or histology must reveal a primary benign cartilaginous lesion. Lesions such as synovial chondromatosis and juxtacortical chondroma are often misdiagnosed as chondrosarcoma because of the cytologic features. The average age of dedifferentiated chondrosarcoma occurs approximately 10 to 15 years later than the low-grade chondrosarcoma (sixth decade is most common) (20). These patients require aggressive chemotherapy and wide excision. Prognosis is poorer than other high-grade malignant bone tumors, most likely because of patients' inability to tolerate high-dose chemotherapy.

Clear cell chondrosarcoma is a rare variant of chondrosarcoma. Radiographically, the lesion extends to the subchondral surface and is termed *epiphyseal*. Histologically, clear cartilaginous cells are seen. Osteoid production is common and may mimic osteosarcoma; however, osteoblastic rimming is usually present, indicating reactive bone production (21). Cells of the clear cell chondrosarcoma may have to be distinguished from melanoma and clear cell carcinoma. Wide excision without chemotherapy is recommended. Chondrosarcoma is insensitive to both radiation and chemotherapy.

Extraskeletal myxoid chondrosarcoma is another rare variant of chondrosarcoma. This tumor is unique because it may present as multiple lesions. It can arise from either the bones or soft tissue. Surgical excision is recommended and close observation of the entire body with positron emission tomography or bone scan should be performed.

CHORDOMA

Chordoma is a malignant disease of the neuroectoderm and involves the midline from the spheno-occipital region to the tip of the coccyx. The most common location is the sacrum (Figure 28.4). It is a low-to-intermediate grade tumor characterized histologically by physaliphorous cells that, if not completely removed, will recur and spread hematogenously to the lungs. It must be differentiated from the benign, giant notochordal hamartoma described by Mirra and Brien (25). Giant notochordal hamartoma has physaliphorous cells, as seen in chordoma, but these lack the invasive and aggressive features that its malignant counterpart demonstrates. Chordoma nearly always has an associated soft-tissue mass unlike giant notochordal hamartoma. Radiographic differential diagnosis includes metastatic disease, osteosarcoma, chondrosarcoma, and giant cell tumor. Treatment for notochordal hamartoma is observation, unlike the necessary wide excision for chordoma. Instability of the lower spine occurs if >50% of the sacral ala is removed. Bowel, bladder, and erectile function may be maintained if one side of S2 and S3 nerve roots can be preserved. Radiation therapy may reduce the risk of local recurrence; however, chordoma is not exquisitely radiosensitive. Standard chemotherapy has not been successful; however, current trials are underway using TOR (target of rapamycin) inhibition or imatinib (Gleevec) with early positive results.

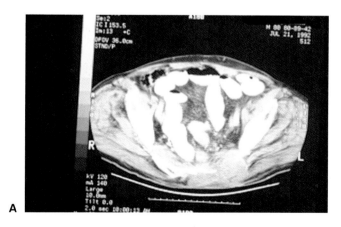

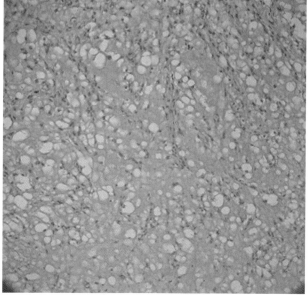

Figure 28.4 Chordoma. (**A**) A destructive mass of the sacrum with soft-tissue extension can be seen on computed tomography (CT) scan. Calcifications may be seen on plain radiographs or CT scan as well. (**B**) Cells are bubbly and clear and often form chords.

ROUND CELL TUMORS

Ewing Sarcoma

Ewing sarcoma is a rare, aggressive round cell tumor. It most commonly presents in the flat bones of skeletally immature patients as a primary bone lesion extending into the soft tissues. Most patients present with metastatic disease to the lung. Histologically, the round cells of a Ewing sarcoma must be distinguished from other round cell malignancies and infection. Ewing cells stain positive for CD99 and OK 13. Immunostains can distinguish Ewing sarcoma from lymphoma, neuroblastoma, round cell osteosarcomas, rhabdomyosarcoma, and other lesions characterized by round cells. Radiologic differential diagnosis may include eosinophilic granuloma, infection, and round cell osteosarcoma. Treatment includes chemotherapy, radiation, and wide excision. These lesions often involve patients in their first and second decades and may require unique reconstructions for limb salvage (26). Although these tumors are highly responsive to chemotherapy and radiation therapy, survival rates vary between 45% and 75%. Proximal lesions (spine, pelvis, and shoulder) have a worse prognosis. Metastatic disease to distant sites other than the lung is more common in Ewing sarcoma than osteosarcoma. Close monitoring for such lesions should be performed.

Lymphoma

Lymphoma of bone is a rare round cell bone tumor that is characterized by either lytic or blastic changes. Similar to Ewing sarcoma, lymphoma has a propensity for the diaphysis of long bones, but also may be seen in the spine. The blastic process seen in the spine has been described as "ivory vertebrae" (Figure

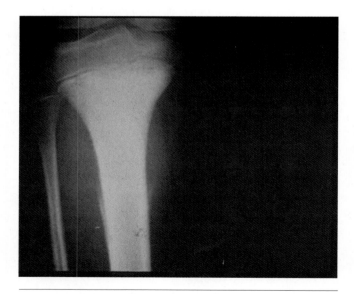

Figure 28.5 Lymphoma of bone. This figure represents a classic case of lymphoma of bone in a 14-year-old male patient. Bone has characteristic features of "ivory" and must be distinguished from chronic sclerosing osteomyelitis of Garre, Ribbings disease, and other sclerosing lesions of bone. Also seen radiographically is subtle elevation of periosteum laterally about the tibia.

28.5). Histology and cytology must distinguish this tumor from other round cell tumors, particularly Ewing sarcoma, because treatment includes radiation and chemotherapy alone. Prognosis is excellent (>90%).

Neuroblastoma (Metastatic)

Similar to lymphoma and Ewing sarcoma, metastatic neuroblastoma is a round cell tumor. It is not surgically treated but managed with chemotherapy and radiation therapy. Neuroblastoma should be strongly considered in patients younger than 5 years old with a round cell malignancy. They usually present as multifocal lesions and may be mistaken for infection or eosinophilic granuloma clinically. Special stains are again useful in distinguishing these lesions from other round cell tumors.

Plasmacytoma/Multiple Myeloma

Myeloma is the most common primary malignancy of bone. It usually presents as multiple lesions but occasionally is seen in an isolated bone (plasmacytoma). It is characterized radiographically as a lytic, sometimes expansile, lesion with an associated soft-tissue mass. Histologically, malignant plasma cells (round cells with eccentric nuclei and abundant cytoplasm) can distinguish it from other round cell tumors and infection. Treatment includes chemotherapy, radiation therapy, and surgical stabilization of the bone. In cases in which it is isolated to a single bone, we have treated plasmacytoma as a primary bone tumor with wide excision after chemoradiation. Although this is commonly a systemic disease, survival varies from months to years depending on the response to chemotherapy. New drug therapies such as bortezomib (Velcade), thalidomide, and others have lengthened survival times. Studies evaluating Cox-2 inhibitors such as celecoxib (Celebrex) in the treatment of multiple myeloma are also underway.

MALIGNANT FIBROUS HISTIOCYTOMA

Malignant fibrous histiocytoma (MFH) is a common soft-tissue sarcoma; however, it may also present as a primary malignancy of bone. It is characterized histologically by malignant cells in a storiform pattern. Fibrosarcoma is also a rare bone tumor and can be distinguished histologically from MFH by its "herring bone" pattern. MFH is most common in skeletally mature patients and presents as a lytic, destructive bone lesion. It may also occur often as a secondary tumor. Previously radiated bone and Paget disease are the most common pre-existing diseases seen with MFH. Differential diagnosis includes metastatic disease, osteosarcoma, and lymphoma. Giant cell tumors may be seen as a secondary lesion of Paget disease and may have a similar aggressive appearance as malignancy, but are managed with corticosteroids (27).

Treatment of high-grade MFH includes chemotherapy and wide excision. Some would also consider radiation therapy. Prognosis is poor, with <50% survival rates. Prognosis is poorer in these patients because such patients are usually older and often have comorbidities that may prohibit high-dose chemotherapy. However, younger patients with such histologic variants probably behave in a similar manner to their age-matched cohort.

Secondary Sarcomas: Postradiation and Bone Infarct

Postradiation sarcoma was initially described by Cahan et al. (28) in 1948. Inclusion criteria were patients who received radiation therapy with the tumor developing within the radiation field after several years. Osteosarcoma and MFH are the most common sarcomas arising from prior radiation treatment. Postradiation sarcomas can occur in previously normal bone or bones with prior tumors such as giant cell tumor of bone. Similarly, bone infarct may lead to secondary sarcomas. A similar case was described by Bahk (29) and associates in a report of a case of osteochondritis dissecans associated with an incipient high-grade sarcoma.

ADAMANTINOMA

Adamantinoma is a rare malignant tumor nearly always involving the tibia (Figure 28.6). It must be distinguished from another

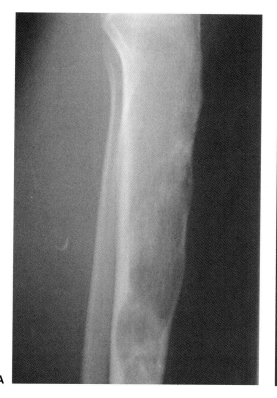

A

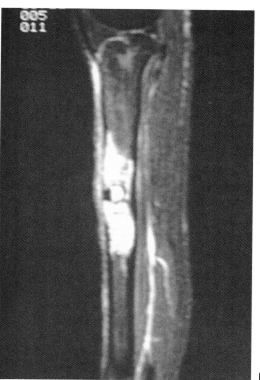

B

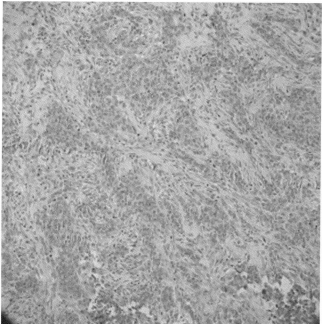

C

Figure 28.6 Adamantinoma. A 19-year-old woman presented with a lytic lesion of the tibia (**A**). There is no bowing of the bone, and magnetic resonance imaging (**B**) reveals a soft-tissue mass associated with intramedullary signal abnormality. Biopsy revealed numerous nests of epithelial cells consistent with adamantinoma (**C**).

rare, but benign, bone tumor called osteofibrous dysplasia. Both have a strong predilection for the tibia. Osteofibrous dysplasia usually presents in childhood, presents with progressive bowing of the tibia, and has a smooth border about its periphery radiologically. Adamantinoma usually occurs in skeletally mature patients (third to fourth decades). Radiographically, adamantinoma may reveal a "shark bite" lesion of the tibia; however, it may have similar features to osteofibrous dysplasia. There may be histologic overlap between these two entities as well, yet the adamantinoma has nests or clusters of epithelial cells that are keratin-positive.

Treatment is surgery alone, and systemic disease is less common than in high-grade sarcomas. Adamantinoma commonly involves the diaphysis of bone, and intercalary allograft may be required. However, this unique tumor does have a predilection for lymphatic spread, and popliteal and inguinal lymph nodes need to be evaluated clinically. Without metastatic disease at presentation, prognosis is excellent.

ANGIOSARCOMA

Angiosarcoma is a rare disease of bone and soft parts that affects adults. Aggressive local spread characterizes the disease. Bone involvement may be diffuse and may not only involve the entire limb, but lymph node involvement is not uncommon. Radiographically, it must be distinguished from metastatic disease or multiple myeloma. Histologically, malignant endothelial cells are readily seen and may shed into the lumen of the blood vessel. Metastatic disease is common and prognosis is guarded. We have yet to observe an angiosarcoma in childhood. Cellular hemangiomas may appear quite ominous and if a diagnosis is made of angiosarcoma, expert pathologic consultation is recommended. Surgical ablation is required and amputation is more common than limb salvage for this tumor.

BENIGN TUMORS MIMICKING MALIGNANT TUMORS

Benign aggressive bone tumors may mimic sarcomas. The most aggressive benign tumors include giant cell tumor, aneurysmal bone cyst, and chondroblastoma. Radiographically, these lesions can demonstrate significant bone loss. Such tumors may require surgical excision similar to sarcomas.

BONE METASTASES

Currently, patients are surviving longer with metastatic disease because of improved systemic therapy and radiation therapy. Patients often receive radiation therapy for bone metastases. The most common spread of disease to bone is the spine, ribs, and pelvis/hip. Such lesions often require stabilization with internal fixation. In patients with metastatic renal cell carcinoma (RCC) to bone, local bone recurrence is common. Les et al. (30) found that 53% of patients treated with intralesional procedures for metastatic RCC required reoperation. Only 3% of patients treated with en bloc excision required repeat surgery. A more aggressive surgical approach should be considered in patients with RCC metastasis.

Despite the use of long-acting bone-strengthening medications (bisphosphonates), fractures may not heal, and hardware failure is becoming more prevalent because of longer survival. Such cases often require limb-salvage surgery similar to primary sarcomas because bone healing cannot be achieved. In patients with an isolated renal cell metastasis or an isolated bone metastasis stable for >3 years after initial treatment, one should consider wide resection of these lesions if the patient is free from other metastatic disease (31).

REFERENCES

1. Muscolo DL, Ayerza MA, Makino A, et al. Tumors about the knee misdiagnosed as athletic injuries. *J Bone Joint Surg Am.* 2002;85:1209–1214.
2. Aboulafia AJ, Levin AM, Blum J. Preferential evaluation of patients with suspected bone and soft tissue tumors. *Clin Orthop.* 2002;397:83–88.
3. Enneking WF, Spanier SS, Goodman MA. A system for the surgical staging of musculoskeletal sarcoma. *Clin Orthop.* 1980;153:106–120.
4. Nelson TE, Enneking WF. Staging of bone and soft-tissue sarcomas revisited. In: Stauffer RN, ed. *Advances in Operative Orthopedics.* Vol 2. St. Louis, MO: Mosby Year-Book; 1994:379–391.
5. Mankin HJ, Lange TA, Spanier SS. The hazards of biopsy in patients with malignant primary bone and soft-tissue tumors. *J Bone Joint Surg Am.* 1982;64:1121–1127.
6. Mankin HJ, Mankin CJ, Simon MA. The hazards of biopsy, revisited: Members of the Musculoskeletal Tumor Society. *J Bone Joint Surg Am.* 1996;78:656–663.
7. Bacci G, Ferrarri S, Bertoni F, et al. Histologic response of high-grade nonmetastatic osteosarcoma of the extremity to chemotherapy. *Clin Orthop.* 2001;386:186–196.
8. Bacci G, Longhi A, Fagioli F, et al. Adjuvant and neoadjuvant chemotherapy for osteosarcoma of the extremities: 27 year experience at Rizzoli Institute, Italy [published online ahead of print November 17, 2005]. *Eur J Cancer.* 2005;41:2836–2845.
9. Ferrari S, Smeland S, Mercuri M, et al. Italian and Scandinavian Sarcoma Groups. Neoadjuvant chemotherapy with high-dose Ifosfamide, high-dose methotrexate, cisplatin, and doxorubicin for patients with localized osteosarcoma of the extremity: a joint study by the Italian and Scandinavian Sarcoma Groups [published online ahead of print October 24, 2005]. *J Clin Oncol.* 2005;23:8845–8852.
10. Bickels J, Wittig JC, Kollender Y, et al. Distal femoral resection with endoprosthetic reconstruction. *Clin Orthop.* 2002;400:225–235.
11. Chang DW, Weber KL. Use of a vascularized fibula bone flap and intercalary allograft for diaphyseal reconstruction after resection of primary extremity bone sarcomas. *Plast Reconstr Surg.* 2005;116:1918–1925.
12. Gupta A, Meswania J, Pollock R, et al. Non-invasive distal femoral expandable endoprosthesis for limb-salvage surgery in paediatric tumours. *J Bone Joint Surg Br.* 2006;88:649–654.
13. Weisstein JS, Goldsby RE, O'Donnell RJ. Oncologic approaches to pediatric limb preservation. *J Am Acad Orthop Surg.* 2005;13:544–554.
14. Wilkins RM, Camozzi AB, Gitelis SB. Reconstruction options for pediatric bone tumors about the knee. *J Knee Surg.* 2005;18:305–309.
15. Gitelis S, Neel MD, Wilkins RM, et al. The use of a closed expandable prosthesis for pediatric sarcomas. *Chir Organi Mov.* 2003;88:327–333.

16. Simon MA, Aschliman MA, Thomas N, et al. Limb-salvage treatment versus amputation for osteosarcoma of the distal end of the femur. 1986. *J Bone Joint Surg Am.* 2005;87:2822.

17. Pardasaney PK, Sullivan PE, Portney LG, et al. Advantage of limb salvage over amputation for proximal lower extremity tumors. *Clin Orthop Relat Res.* 2006;444:201–208.

18. Ehrhart N. Longitudinal bone transport for treatment of primary bone tumors in dogs: technique description and outcome in 9 dogs. *Vet Surg.* 2005;34:24–34.

19. Mirra JM, Gold R, Downs J, et al. Aner histologic approach to the differentiation of enchondroma from chondrosarcoma of bones. A clinico-pathologic analysis of 51 cases *Clin Orthop.* 1985;210: 214–237.

20. Brien E, Mirra J, Kerr R. Pathogenesis of cartilagenous tumors, intramedullary tumors. *Skel Radiol.* 1997;26:325–353.

21. Brien E, Mirra JM, Ippolito V. Clear cell chondrosarcoma with elevated alkaline phosphatase. Skel Radiol. 1996;25:770–774.

22. Aydinli U, Ozturk C, Yalcinkaya U, et al. Limb-sparing surgery for primary malignant tumours of the pelvis. *Acta Orthop Belg.* 2004;70:417–422.

23. Donati D, El Ghoneimy A, Bertoni F, et al. Surgical treatment and outcome of conventional pelvic chondrosarcoma. *J Bone Joint Surg Br.* 2005;87:1527–1530.

24. Hoffmann C, Gosheger G, Gebert C, et al. Functional results and quality of life after treatment of pelvic sarcomas involving the acetabulum. *J Bone Joint Surg Am.* 2006;88:575–582.

25. Mirra J, Brien E. Giant notochordal hamartoma of intraosseous origin: a newly reported benign entity to be distinguished from chordoma. Report of two cases. *Skel Radiol.* 2001;30:698–709.

26. Mankin HJ, Gebhardt MC, Tomford WW. The use of frozen cadaveric allografts in the management of patients with bone tumors of the extremities. *Orthop Clin North Am.* 1987;18:275–289.

27. Jacobs TP, Michelsen J, Polay JS, et al. Giant cell tumor in Paget's disease of bone. *Cancer.* 1979;44:742–747.

28. Cahan WG, Woodard HQ, Higinbotham NL, et al. Sarcoma arising in irradiated bone. Report of eleven cases. *Cancer.* 1948;1:3–29.

29. Bahk W, Brien E, Mirra J. Osteosarcoma associated with osteochondritis dissecans. A case report and review of the literature. *J Bone Joint Surg Am.* 1997;79:1849–1853.

30. Les KA, Nicholas RW, Rougraff B, et al. Local progression after operative treatment of metastatic kidney cancer. *Clin Orthop.* 2001;390:206–211.

31. Jung ST, Ghert MA, Harrelson JM, et al. Treatment of osseous metastases in patients with renal cell carcinoma. *Clin Orthop.* 2003;409:223–231.

COMMENTARY
J. Sybil Biermann and Laurence H. Baker

Drs. Brien and Ouellette present a comprehensive treatise on the diagnosis and management of bone tumors, including a discussion of the most common types of bone tumors, the importance of staging and biopsy, the treatment with multiagent chemotherapy, and methods of bone reconstruction. They go on to detail various types and subtypes of bone sarcoma with description of the ages, locations, and pathology of specific subtypes.

However, a most important aspect of contemporary management of bone tumors, while briefly mentioned, is *not*, in our opinion, sufficiently underscored in this work—the vital importance of multidisciplinary management of bone tumors, and the value of treatment of sarcomas in centers, both to optimize individual patient outcome and to further advance the understanding of these rare diseases.

Sarcomas in general and bone sarcoma in particular are rare diseases. The American Cancer Society estimates that in 2009 there will be 2,570 new cases of bone sarcoma and 10,660 new cases of soft tissue sarcoma in the United States, in contrast to 219,440 new lung cancers and 192,280 new cases of prostate cancer (1). Because of the rarity of sarcomas, clinicians in the community usually have less familiarity with the diagnosis, treatment, prognosis, and overall management than with other more commonly occurring tumors. Not only are sarcomas much less common, but they are also much more heterogeneous than the common epithelial cancers.

Furthermore, evidence is accruing that suggests that this lack of familiarity has implications for patient outcome. In a rigorous analysis of over 4,000 sarcoma patients, Gutierrez (2) has shown a significantly improved outcome for patients treated in high-volume sarcoma centers compared with those treated at lower-volume centers, with significantly longer median survival times and lower amputation rates.

Drs. Brien and Ouellette briefly mention the hazards of biopsy in musculoskeletal tumors, citing Mankin et al. (3). In 1982, they reviewed a series of 329 patients contributed by members of the Musculoskeletal Tumor Society (MSTS). These data represented a case series of unselected, newly diagnosed patients with malignant primary bone or soft-tissue tumors. In this series, the authors found that the optimum treatment plan was altered as a result of biopsy problems (poor placement, poor technique, or other) in 18% of patients. An amputation was performed in 4.5%, which would have been unnecessary had the biopsy been optimized! Ten years later similar data were once again collected and published by the MSTS (4). In this second series, comprising 597 patients, the rate of diagnostic error was still 18%, with a rate of 3% unnecessary amputations related to poor biopsy technique. Although errors can and do occur in any institution, errors, complications, and changes in the course and outcome were 2 to 12 times greater when the biopsy was done in a referring institution instead of a treatment center.

In soft-tissue sarcoma, the problem is likely even worse, in part because of the multiple surgical disciplines (e.g., general surgery, gynecology, otolaryngology, orthopaedics) who service this population (5). Looking at a series of nearly 6,000 sarcomas in the United States, Lawrence et al. (6) found that nearly half the sarcomas were biopsied by excision, rather than the preferred needle or incisional biopsy. This leads to wider re-excisions, difficulty ascertaining the exact location of the initial tumor when planning postoperative radiation therapy, and perhaps missed opportunities for neoadjuvant chemotherapy.

Improvement in survival rates for osteosarcoma and Ewing sarcoma began by collaboration between orthopaedic surgeons and pediatric or medical oncologists. Prior to 1970, bone sarcomas were typically managed by amputation by orthopaedic surgeons, resulting in very poor survival (7). Orthopaedic surgeons at the time began working with implant manufacturers to create custom-made implants to facilitate limb salvage in this unfortunate group of patients. However, fabrication times were lengthy and local progression of disease during the manufacture of the implant often made the final product unusable. Turning to their pediatric and medical oncology colleagues for help, with the goal of chemotherapy to delay the progression of the local disease during this unavoidable interval, led to a surprising result. Not only was disease progression reduced, but also a survival benefit was noted for those patients receiving chemotherapy. Furthermore, at the time of resection an avenue was created for the evaluation of efficacy of chemotherapy as a predictive test for survival (8).

For the next 30 years, successive improvements in longevity of patients with bone sarcomas have followed this pattern. Gradual improvements in survival have resulted from successive, usually randomized controlled studies of bone sarcoma patients, both in osteosarcoma and later in Ewing sarcoma, performed primarily in large-volume centers where the expertise to perform full-dose chemotherapy with growth factor support, sophisticated limb-sparing surgery, and detailed pathologic analysis of the specimens are present. In fact, early studies were clouded by the inclusion of a variety of pathologic variants of osteosarcoma; their increasing recognition by pathology experts has markedly improved the precision with which these clinical studies can be performed.

Pretreatment referral is often necessary to establish correct diagnosis. Increasingly, the diagnosis and treatment planning for sarcomas depends not only upon light microscopic diagnosis but also on cytogenetic or molecular testing, usually only available in referral centers (9). For example, the prognosis of synovial sarcoma has been shown to rest in the exact region of translocation (10). This has significant import for the categorization of patients in clinical trials and anticipated outcomes. However, partly because of financial and technical constraints, molecular testing for sarcomas is rarely available in low-volume centers.

An illustrative model of the importance of centralization of bone sarcoma in studying and providing optimal patient care comes from Italy, where the majority of osteosarcomas in the country are treated at the Rizzoli Institute in Bologna. Investigators have treated and studied an impressive series of 1,126 patients with extremity nonmetastatic high-grade osteosarcoma over a 27-year period (in this country with a 2007 population of 58 million) and have sufficient power in their data to show conclusively that the two most important predictors of outcome are adequate surgical margins and histologic response to preoperative chemotherapy (11).

Changing health care initiatives, health maintenance organizations, and economic realities currently challenge the system of centralized care of these patients as well as the frequent desire for patients and their families to be treated as close to home as possible. However, not only is care for individual patients likely to be associated with an improved outcome, but also advancement of the field in general is reliant on enrollment of these patients with rare diseases on clinical trials in centers equipped to perform them.

Recent guidelines published by the National Comprehensive Cancer Center Network (12) provide recommendations that patients with suspected primary bone malignancy be referred *prior to biopsy and treatment* to an appropriate center where integration of care among multiple specialists (orthopaedic oncology, medical oncology, pediatric oncology pathology, radiation oncology, and diagnostic radiology) can be present. A high index of suspicion for primary bone malignancy is necessary for community practitioners who, depending on their practice, may encounter only one such lesion every several years. Familiarity with the vagaries of biopsy, staging, and treatment clearly is not expected, and the best service one may do for the patient in this situation is to promptly refer to a fully staffed bone tumor center prior to any intervention.

REFERENCE

1. Jemal A, Siegel R, Ward E, et al. Cancer statistics, 2009. *CA Cancer J Clin*. 2009. Published online May 27, 2009. Doi:10.3322/caaa.20006.
2. Gutierrez J. Should soft tissue sarcomas be treated at high-volume centers? *Ann Surg*. 2007;245:952–958.
3. Mankin HJ, Lange TA, Spanier SS. The hazards of biopsy in patients with malignant primary bone and soft-tissue tumors. *J Bone Joint Surg Am*. 1982;64:1121–1127.
4. Mankin HJ, Mankin CJ, Simon MA. The hazards of the biopsy, revisited. Members of the Musculoskeletal Tumor Society. *J Bone Joint Surg Am*. 1996;78:656–663.
5. Biermann JS, Baker LH. The future of sarcoma treatment. *Semin Oncol*. 1997;24:592–597.
6. Lawrence W Jr, Donegan WL, Natarajan N, et al. Adult soft tissue sarcomas. A pattern of care survey of the American College of Surgeons. *Ann Surg*. 1987;205:349–359.
7. Marcove RC, Miké V, Hajek JV, et al. Osteogenic sarcoma under the age of twenty-one. A review of one hundred and forty-five operative cases. *J Bone Joint Surg Am*. 1970;52:411–423.
8. Rosen G, Marcove RC, Caparros B, et al. Primary osteogenic sarcoma: the rationale for preoperative chemotherapy and delayed surgery. *Cancer*. 1979;43:2163–2177.
9. Lazar A, Abruzzo LV, Pollock RE, et al. Molecular diagnosis of sarcomas: chromosomal translocations in sarcomas. *Arch Pathol Lab Med*. 2006;130:1199–1207.
10. Kawai A, Woodruff J, Healey JH, et al. SYT-SSX gene fusion as a determinant of morphology and prognosis in synovial sarcoma. *N Engl J Med*. 1998;338:153–160.
11. Bacci G, Forni C, Longhi A, et al. Local recurrence and local control of non-metastatic osteosarcoma of the extremities: a 27-year experience in a single institution. *J Surg Oncol*. 2007;96:118–123.
12. NCCN Clinical Practice Guidelines in Oncology. *J Natl Compr Canc Netw*. 2007;5:420–437.

29

Chemotherapy for Soft-Tissue Sarcomas

Charles A. Forscher

Surgery is the main treatment modality for the management of soft-tissue sarcomas, but radiation therapy and chemotherapy are often used as adjunctive treatments. Chemotherapy is routinely employed when treating the common childhood soft-tissue sarcoma, rhabdomyosarcoma, and is the standard of care for bone tumors such as osteosarcoma and Ewing sarcoma. However, the role of chemotherapy for adult soft-tissue sarcomas remains controversial. The reasons for this disparity are not fully understood. Trials of chemotherapy in adults often include many different sarcoma subtypes with differing sensitivities to chemotherapy, adults may have comorbid illnesses making delivery of chemotherapy more difficult, and there may be other as yet unrecognized factors to account for the purported difference between the activity of chemotherapy for soft-tissue sarcomas in adults as compared with bone tumors and soft-tissue sarcomas in children.

SINGLE AGENTS AND COMBINATIONS FOR ADVANCED DISEASE

The most active single drugs for treating soft-tissue sarcomas are doxorubicin and ifosfamide. Doxorubicin was first used in the 1970s and overall response rates between 13% and 34% have been reported, with a complete response rate of 6% (1–3). A dose-response relationship exists with higher response rates observed at doses of 75 mg/m^2 compared to doses of 50 mg/m^2 when given every 3 weeks (4). Cardiomyopathy is the major dose-limiting toxicity of doxorubicin, with an incidence approaching 30% at cumulative doses above 550 mg/m^2 (5–7). Cardiotoxicity may be lessened by continuous-infusion administration as opposed to bolus dosing. In addition, the use of agents such as dexrazoxane may reduce the risk of developing cardiotoxicity (8,9) without compromising the activity of the drug. It is not clear whether analogues of doxorubicin, such as epirubicin, have less potential for inducing cardiac damage.

Ifosfamide, an analogue of cyclophosphamide, is also active in treating soft-tissue sarcomas. When compared with cyclophosphamide, it is more active with less myelosuppression, producing a response rate of 18% compared with 7.5% for cyclophosphamide in the setting of advanced disease (10). When given at doses ranging from 5 to 14 g/m^2, it has yielded responses in the range of 12% to 38% and demonstrated responsiveness in patients with progressive disease after doxorubicin, suggesting a lack of cross-resistance between the two compounds. It can be given as a short 1-hour bolus or as a continuous infusion over 24 hours. Higher doses can be divided over multiple-day

regimens. The drug must be administered with mesna (sodium 2-mercaptothanesulfonate), which acts as a bladder protectant, to prevent hemorrhagic cystitis induced by acrolein, a biologically inactive metabolite. Other toxicities can include central nervous system effects such as lethargy and confusion and renal effects such as azotemia and acquired Fanconi syndrome (11). With the advent of infusion pumps, multiple-day administration of ifosfamide is no longer limited to the inpatient setting but can be safely done on an outpatient basis. Longer infusions of ifosfamide at a lower dose of 1 g/m^2 for 14 to 21 days have shown activity even in those who have progressed on ifosfamide given at lower dose and on shorter schedules (12). Whether this benefit was due to the higher cumulative dose or the prolonged schedule of administration is not clear.

Dacarbazine (DTIC) has a response rate of 17% when used as a single agent in the sarcomas (13). It is usually given at a dose of 1 g/m^2 over 4 to 5 days. Dose-limiting toxicity is emesis, which may be diminished if the drug is given as a continuous infusion.

Cyclophosphamide, cisplatin, mitomycin, vincristine, actinomycin D, bleomycin, etoposide, and methotrexate have all been evaluated as single agents for soft-tissue sarcomas, with response rates in the 10% to 15% range. More recently, gemcitabine has been evaluated with response rates in the 3% to 18% range (14–16). Docetaxel has also been studied with response rates ranging from 0% to 21%. Interestingly, the same cooperative group, European Organisation for Research and Treatment of Cancer (EORTC), reported results of an initial trial with a 21% response rate and a follow-up comparison trial with doxorubicin in which no responses were seen in the docetaxel arm (17,18). Thus, a drug with consistent response rate over 20% in soft-tissue sarcomas has not been found in over 15 years.

Given the limited activity of single chemotherapeutic agents in the sarcomas and following the example of other solid tumors such as breast cancer, it seemed logical to test the activity of combinations of drugs in the sarcomas. However, unlike some other solid tumors, the superiority of combination chemotherapy over single agents for sarcomas is much less clear. Studies combining doxorubicin with DTIC have generally shown higher response rates for the combination compared with single-agent doxorubicin but have not shown an impact on overall survival. In addition, the combination regimens have been associated with increased toxicity (19,20). The addition of either vincristine or cyclophosphamide to doxorubicin-DTIC yielded no advantage for the three-drug combination (21,22). And a study comparing doxorubicin alone to combinations of doxorubicin with cyclophosphamide and vincristine or cyclophosphamide with actinomycin D and vincristine found single-agent doxorubicin to be the most active and least toxic regimen (23).

Ifosfamide has been added to doxorubicin for the treatment of advanced sarcomas (24,25). Again, the benefit for combination chemotherapy has proved elusive. Despite initial reports suggesting higher response rates for combinations incorporating ifosfamide, the EORTC trial comparing doxorubicin with ifosfamide and doxorubicin versus CYVADIC (cyclophosphamide, vincristine, doxorubicin, and dacarbazine) showed similar response rates for the three regimens. In addition, remission duration and overall survival were not statistically different among the regimens. Single-agent doxorubicin was associated with less myelosuppression. The EORTC concluded that single-agent doxorubicin remains the standard against which other regimens should be compared (26). One possible explanation for the failure of the combinations to improve on the activity of single-agent doxorubicin is that the dose of doxorubicin was decreased from 75 to 50 mg/m^2 when combined with ifosfamide. A subsequent EORTC study tried to eliminate this factor by comparing a standard dose combination of ifosfamide and doxorubicin (5 g/m^2 with 50 mg/m^2) with a high-dose regimen (5 g/m^2 with 75 mg/m^2) with growth factor support (27). No statistically significant difference was seen between the two arms in terms of response rate, 21% for the standard dose arm versus 23.3% for the augmented arm. However, the progression-free survival was significantly longer for the intensive regimen, with a median time to progression of 19 weeks in the conventional arm versus 29 weeks for the intensified arm. Overall survival was not different between the two arms.

Higher doses of ifosfamide in combination with doxorubicin have produced higher response rates in a single-institution trial from M.D. Anderson Cancer Center. Ifosfamide at a dose of 10 g /m^2 given over 4 to 5 days with doxorubicin at doses between 75 and 90 mg/m^2 given over 3 days yielded an overall response rate of 64% (3 complete responses and 18 partial responses in 33 patients). Increased toxicity was observed in the more intensive regimen, but the authors concluded this approach was appropriate in selected patients (28).

Another trial of high-dose ifosfamide and doxorubicin with growth factor support from the Swiss Group for Clinical Research evaluated 33 patients (with 20 soft-tissue sarcomas, 11 gynecologic sarcomas, and 2 bone sarcomas) (29). Doses of ifosfamide ranged between 10 and 12 g/m^2. Doses of doxorubicin began at 50 mg/m^2 and escalated to 90 mg/m^2. Thirty-one patients were evaluable, with an overall response rate of 55%, 4 (13%) complete responses, and 13 (42%) partial responses. Median survival was 2 years, with 25% survival at 3 years. The authors thought the dose level of ifosfamide at 10 g/m^2 and doxorubicin at 90 mg/m^2 with growth factor support (granulocyte-macrophage colony-stimulating factor [GM-CSF]) was manageable and recommended it for further study.

Despite their relatively low response rates as single agents, the combination of gemcitabine and docetaxel has recently shown activity in advanced sarcomas. Initially used in uterine leiomyosarcomas with a reported response rate of 53% (3 complete responses and 15 partial responses in 34 patients) in the setting of unresectable or recurrent disease, this combination has produced an overall response rate of 43% (5 complete and 10 partial responses in 35 patients) in a study with a variety of different soft-tissue sarcomas (30,31). The factors that account for the improvement in activity for this combination are not clear, but the sequencing of the drugs, gemcitabine before docetaxel, and the more prolonged infusion time of gemcitabine, 90 minutes, may play a role. Additional studies with this regimen are in progress, which should help determine the proper role for this combination. This combination appears to be less active in leiomyosarcoma originating from other sites, such as the gastrointestinal tract.

Currently, either single-agent chemotherapy or multiagent chemotherapy can be considered appropriate for the treatment of patients with advanced sarcomas. More aggressive regimens may be used in younger patients or in those in whom a better response might allow for a surgical option for resection. Those with poor performance status may be considered candidates for treatment with single agents, possibly at lower doses, or supportive care. Whether single agents or combinations are employed, median survival in advanced sarcoma remains in the range of 12 months (32).

ADJUVANT CHEMOTHERAPY

Although local failure rates for extremity sarcomas have decreased to the range of 5% to 10% with modern surgical techniques, 40% to 60% of patients with high-grade sarcomas still develop metastatic disease and die within 5 years from diagnosis. Despite the relatively low response rates for the drugs and regimens available, adjuvant chemotherapy has been tried in the soft-tissue sarcomas. There are now multiple randomized trials of the use of chemotherapy in the adjuvant setting for soft-tissue sarcomas. All the studies include doxorubicin either alone or in combination. Some of these studies were limited to patients with extremity sarcoma, others included sarcomas at other sites such as the abdomen, retroperitoneum, and the head and neck, and some trials have evaluated uterine sarcomas.

The National Cancer Institute conducted several sequential trials of adjuvant chemotherapy for high-grade sarcomas and included substantial numbers of patients with extremity lesions (33–35). The first trial used doxorubicin at 50 mg/m^2 with cyclophosphamide at 500 mg/m^2 given in escalating doses. When the cumulative dose of doxorubicin reached 500 to 550 mg/m^2, high-dose methotrexate was substituted for an additional six cycles. The subsequent trial eliminated the methotrexate and capped the cumulative dose of doxorubicin at 350 mg/m^2. The first reports of the initial trial showed a disease-free and overall survival benefit for the patients with extremity lesions who received chemotherapy. However, with additional follow-up, disease-free survival remained improved, but overall survival was no longer better to a statistically significant level. This may have been partly due to a 14% incidence of doxorubicin-associated cardiomyopathy. The later trial with lower cumulative dose doxorubicin produced disease-free survival and overall survival rates similar to those seen with the higher-dose regimen.

Studies from M.D. Anderson Cancer Center randomized patients between observation and chemotherapy with cyclophosphamide, doxorubicin, vincristine, and actinomycin D along with local radiation at 6,500 cGy (VACAR) (36,37). Initial findings suggested inferior disease-free and overall survival rates for the chemotherapy-treated group. However, more mature data with a median follow-up of 10 years revealed improved disease-free survival and a trend toward improved overall survival in the chemotherapy arm.

The Rizzoli Institute in Italy reported a benefit from the use of doxorubicin given at 75 mg/m^2 for six cycles compared with observation in patients with high-grade extremity lesions (38). Some patients received preoperative chemotherapy with doxorubicin and radiation followed by surgery, and were then randomized to observation versus an additional four cycles of doxorubicin. The other patients, who were deemed not suitable for conservative surgery, underwent amputation and then underwent randomization. Disease-free survival was 73% for the chemotherapy arm and 43% for the observation arm (p <0.02). Overall survival rates were 91% and 70% (p <0.05), respectively. However, an update of this study with longer follow-up failed to show a continued benefit in disease-free and overall survival in the chemotherapy arm (39).

The Gynecologic Oncology Group evaluated the use of doxorubicin in the adjuvant setting for resected uterine sarcomas at a dose of 60 mg/m^2 versus observation (40). There was no difference in disease-free survival, and overall survival was not statistically significantly improved: 73 months for the treated group and 55 months for the control group.

The Eastern Cooperative Oncology Group (41), the Intergroup (Southwest Oncology Group, Cancer and Leukemia Group B and the Eastern Cooperative Oncology Group) (42–44), and a group of Boston hospitals (Dana-Farber Cancer Institute and Massachusetts General Hospital) conducted studies of doxorubicin at doses ranging from 70 to 90 mg/m^2 and found no significant differences between chemotherapy and control groups.

A study of the Scandinavian Sarcoma Group (45), using a somewhat lower dose of doxorubicin, 60 mg/m^2, given for nine cycles also found no advantage for the chemotherapy arm.

Another doxorubicin trial from the University of California at Los Angeles (UCLA) used preoperative local radiation therapy with intra-arterial doxorubicin for all patients with a postoperative randomization to additional intravenous doxorubicin or observation. No benefit was found for the postoperative chemotherapy (46).

Two studies using the CYVADIC regimen have been reported. A large study with over 400 patients from the EORTC found no significant differences in disease-free or overall survival between the treatment and control groups (47). However, a smaller study from the Foundation Bergonie in France with 59 patients found both a disease-free and overall survival benefit for the chemotherapy arm (disease-free survival: 65% vs. 37% and overall survival 83% vs. 43%), which was statistically significant (48).

The Mayo Clinic used regimens of vincristine, cyclophosphamide, and actinomycin D alternating with vincristine, doxorubicin, and dacarbazine and found no difference in overall survival between the groups (49). They did observe a decrease in the incidence of pulmonary metastasis in the chemotherapy group.

The Italian Sarcoma Study Group evaluated the combination of ifosfamide and epirubicin versus observation for extremity sarcomas. Initial reports showed a significant improvement in disease-free survival for the chemotherapy-treated group (72% vs. 55%, p <0.002), which led to early closure of the trial (50).

However, with longer follow-up, the differences between the two groups have narrowed (51). Although overall survival continues to be better for the chemotherapy, the benefit in disease-free and overall survival is no longer statistically significant.

A more recent trial from Brodowicz and colleagues (52) used an intensive combination of ifosfamide, doxorubicin, and dacarbazine given every 2 weeks with growth factor support. Disease-free survival was improved in the chemotherapy group compared with control (77% vs. 57%), but this was not statistically significant, perhaps owing to the small sample size of the study, 59 patients. Both the chemotherapy and control groups in the study have overall survival rates above 80%, but the follow-up for this study is relatively short.

Given the small size of many of these studies, several attempts at meta-analyses of data from many of these studies have been performed. Antman et al. (53) pooled the data from the Boston, Eastern Cooperative Oncology Group, and Intergroup studies and found no difference in overall survival between the chemotherapy and control groups with 10-year follow-up (53). Zalupski et al. (54) performed a meta-analysis for patients with extremity sarcomas and found a benefit in overall survival (71% to 81%) and disease-free survival (68% to 53%) for the chemotherapy group. Both these differences were statistically significant. A larger meta-analysis reported by Tierney et al. (55) pooled data from over 1,500 patients and observed improved survival at both 2 and 5 years for the chemotherapy-treated patients. The largest meta-analysis, including 1,568 patients, was published by the Sarcoma Meta-analysis Collaboration (56). Overall survival was improved with chemotherapy from 50% to 54% but this was not statistically significant. However, disease-free survival was improved from 45% to 55%, which was statistically significant, and perhaps somewhat surprisingly, local disease-free survival was better for those treated with chemotherapy. When the extremity sarcoma patients were analyzed separately, overall survival was increased by 7%, which was statistically significant.

Thus, a small, but real, benefit appears to exist for adjuvant chemotherapy for extremity soft-tissue sarcomas. Any advantage for adjuvant chemotherapy in the management of soft-tissue sarcomas arising at other sites is less clear based on the data from the meta-analyses.

NEOADJUVANT TRIALS

Following the experience with preoperative chemotherapy for osteosarcoma, several centers initiated regimens with chemotherapy and radiation given preoperatively for soft-tissue sarcomas. The potential advantages for preoperative treatment are several-fold. Early institution of chemotherapy may allow for less drastic surgery, possibly allowing for an increased possibility for limb preservation. Preoperative chemotherapy can serve as an "in vivo" test of chemosensitivity, can allow for the early treatment of any micrometastatic disease, and can suggest the need for a change in treatment if no objective response is observed. The latter can potentially spare patients the administration of inactive but toxic treatments. Favorable response to preoperative treatment may serve as a prognostic tool to guide subsequent chemotherapy. Preoperative radiation can be given when tissue planes are undisturbed and the target is well defined, and it is often possible to deliver preoperative radiation in a shorter period of time compared with postoperative external-beam radiation. The drawbacks to preoperative treatment are that it delays definitive surgery, may increase local complications, and may not be active against the tumor.

The study mentioned in the previous section from UCLA was one of several studies done there to evaluate preoperative treatment for extremity soft-tissue sarcomas (57). The initial study of 77 patients used intra-arterial doxorubicin at a dose of 30 mg/day for 3 days with radiation at a dose of 35 cGy. Local recurrence occurred in 7 patients (9%); wound complications were seen in 27 patients (35%). Median pathologic necrosis in the tumor specimens was 70%, with complete pathologic necrosis seen in 9 patients (11.7%).

In the follow-up study, the dose of radiation was reduced to 17.5 cGy. Although wound complications were decreased, the local recurrence rate rose to 15%, median necrosis decreased to 45%, and the pathologic complete response rate fell to 3.5%.

The subsequent UCLA study increased the dose of radiation to 28 cGy and compared intravenous doxorubicin with intra-arterial doxorubicin. The local recurrence rate was 9%, median tumor necrosis was 60%, and the complete pathologic response rate was 6.3%. There were no differences based on the route of doxorubicin administration.

As there appeared to be no advantage for intra-arterial doxorubicin, the fourth UCLA regimen used intravenous doxorubicin and cisplatin with radiation at 28 cGy. Median tumor necrosis was 70%, with complete pathologic response seen in 10.9% of patients.

The fifth UCLA study added ifosfamide to doxorubicin/cisplatin with radiation at 28 cGy. Two cycles of ifosfamide were given at doses ranging from 14 to 18 g/m^2 followed by one cycle of doxorubicin/cisplatin at doses of 60 to 75 mg/m^2 and 100/120 mg/m^2, respectively. Of 44 patients, there was only one local recurrence, median tumor necrosis was 95%, and complete pathologic necrosis was observed in 17 patients (39%). Eilber and colleagues (58) concluded that ifosfamide had a major impact on the rate of pathologic necrosis observed after preoperative treatment, as this was the highest rate of pathologic necrosis of any of their tested regimens.

Overall survival at 5 years was 77% for the ifosfamide-treated group and 64% for all the prior regimens, and this benefit persisted at 10 years, 71% versus 58% (p <0.03). Treatment-induced pathologic necrosis was an independent predictor of both local recurrence and overall survival. All patients in these studies received preoperative chemotherapy and radiation without a control arm.

Mack and colleagues (59) in Canada treated 75 patients with extremity or truncal sarcomas on a modified Eilber (UCLA) regimen of doxorubicin at 30 mg/day (fixed dose) for 3 days with sequential radiation, 300 cGy/day for 10 days. The majority of the tumors (66%) were >5 cm and 71% were grade II/III. Of 67 patients with negative margins at the time of surgery, the local control rate was 97% at 5 years with an overall survival rate of 63%. Minor wound complications were seen in eight patients (10.6%) and reoperation was necessary in three patients. The authors concluded that this regimen allowed for excellent local control. Again, all patients received treatment with both chemotherapy and radiation.

Additional evaluation of preoperative radiation with sensitizing doxorubicin was reported by Wanebo and colleagues (60) in a study initiated by the Southeastern Cancer Study Group and maintained in three institutions. Sixty-six patients were randomized between two dose levels of radiation, 30 to 35 Gy in 10 fractions or 46 Gy in 23 to 25 fractions with intra-arterial doxorubicin at 30 mg/day for 3 days. Postoperative radiation was given to 31 patients. Wound complications were observed in 41% of the patients. Overall survival and disease-free survival at 5 years were 59% and 49%, respectively. Limb salvage surgery was possible in 60 patients. The authors thought this approach permitted excellent immediate local control and reasonable long-term local control but that distant metastases remained a challenge.

Levine and colleagues (61) also examined the use of preoperative doxorubicin with concomitant radiation. They treated 55 patients with intra-arterial doxorubicin at 10 mg/m^2/day for 10 days with 25 Gy radiation. The majority of tumors were stage T2 (41 patients); 7 patients had low-grade tumors. Initial limb-preserving surgery was possible in 47 patients (87%). Complications secondary to treatment occurred in 26% of patients. Overall survival at 5 years was 69% and disease-free survival was 51%. Because of complications, the long-term limb salvage rate was 81% This trial also concluded that intra-arterial doxorubicin was associated with significant morbidity, but the investigators thought the approach was justified.

The M.D. Anderson Cancer Center has performed several trials of preoperative treatment. One series, first reported in 1997, summarized the experience with doxorubicin-based chemotherapy in 76 patients with stage IIIB tumors (62). Patients received doxorubicin and dacarbazine (ADIC), cyclophosphamide and ADIC (CYADIC), or other doxorubicin-based regimens. Objective radiologic responses were observed in 27% of patients (complete response in 9%, partial response in 19%). The 5-year actuarial rates for local relapse-free survival (LRFS), distant metastasis-free survival (DMFS), disease-free survival, and overall survival were 83%, 52%, 46%, and 59%, respectively. There were no significant differences in the survival rates between responding and nonresponding patients, and the rates appeared comparable to those achieved with postoperative chemotherapy.

Another trial from M.D. Anderson Cancer Center studied 27 patients with intermediate- and high-grade extremity sarcomas using continuous-infusion intravenous doxorubicin with radiation given in 25 2-Gy fractions (63). The doxorubicin was given as an initial bolus of 4 mg/m^2 followed by a continuous infusion at doses ranging from 12.5 to 20.0 mg/m^2/wk. The maximum tolerated dose for the combined approach was 17.5 mg/m^2. Twenty-two patients were treated at the 17.5 mg/m^2 dose level, and 11 had ≥90% tumor necrosis at the time of surgery with 2 complete responses, which the authors thought was encouraging.

The Mayo Clinic has also studied preoperative treatment for extremity soft-tissue sarcomas (64). Their regimen included ifosfamide, doxorubicin, mitomycin, and cisplatin given intravenously for two cycles followed by 5 weeks of radiation (4,500 cGy). During the radiation, a third cycle of chemotherapy was given at reduced dose for three additional cycles. Patients received sargramostim (GM-CSF) support. Additional radiation was given to a total of 5,500 to 6,500 cGy by either intraoperative electron beam, brachytherapy, or external beam. Kaplan-Meier estimated 5-year survival was approximately 80%, and 2-year estimated metastasis-free survival was 85%.

Gortzak and colleagues (65) reported a phase 2 study from the EORTC and the National Cancer Institute of Canada using ifosfamide (5 g/m^2 over 24 hours) and Doxorubicin (50 mg/m^2) both given intravenously for three cycles versus immediate surgery for high-risk soft-tissue sarcomas. These included tumors ≥8 cm of any grade, grade II/III tumors <8 cm, or grade II/III tumors that were locally recurrent or had recent surgery with inadequate margins. There were 134 patients, 67 in each arm. The limb preservation rate was 88%. The 5-year estimated disease-free survival was 52% for the no-chemotherapy arm and 56% for the chemotherapy arm ($p = 0.3548$). The 5-year overall survival was 64% and 65%, for each arm, respectively. This study was not powered to draw conclusions on benefit, but it seemed unlikely that major benefits would accrue from the use of this dose and schedule. Based on these results and slow accrual, a planned phase 3 trial was not performed.

However, a retrospective analysis of ifosfamide and doxorubicin given prior to surgery compared with surgery alone reported by Grobmeyer and colleagues (66) found a benefit in disease-specific survival for those receiving chemotherapy. There were 74 patients in the chemotherapy group and 282 in the control group. The 3-year disease-specific survival for extremity tumors >10 cm was 62% for the control group and 83% for the treated group. This group (those whose tumors were >10 cm) appeared to derive the greatest benefit from the neoadjuvant approach.

Two trials of neoadjuvant MAID (mesna, doxorubicin, ifosfamide, and dacarbazine) chemotherapy with radiation have been reported. Ifosfamide was given at 2 g/m^2/day for 3 days, doxorubicin was given at 20/mg/m^2/day for 3 days, and dacarbazine was given at 250 mg/m^2 for 4 days. There were three courses of preoperative chemotherapy with two cycles of interdigitated radiation therapy each at 22 Gy. Three additional cycles of MAID were given postoperatively with 16 Gy radiation for positive margins. Forty-eight patients with large (>8 cm) high-grade tumors were treated in the initial study and compared with historical controls (67). The 5-year rates for actuarial local control, freedom from distant metastases, disease-free survival, and overall survival were 92% and 86%, 75% and 44%, 70% and 42%, and 87% and 58% for the MAID and control groups, respectively. The rates for improvement in freedom from distant metastases, disease-free survival, and overall survival were all statistically significant.

On the basis of this initial trial, the Radiation Therapy Oncology Group conducted a follow-up phase 2 trial with this treatment in 66 patients (68). Sixty-four patients were analyzed, 61 underwent surgery, with 5 patients requiring amputation. Disease-free survival at 3 years was estimated at 56.6%, with an estimated 64.5% distant disease-free survival, and an estimated 75.1% overall survival. Fifty-three patients (83%) experienced grade IV toxicity, with grade V toxicity in 3 patients. These results are similar to the first trial and demonstrated the ability to deliver combined modality chemotherapy and radiation in a multi-institutional setting.

A provocative trial from Henshaw and colleagues (69) tested the use of induction chemotherapy without radiation in high-grade soft-tissue sarcomas. Thirty-three patients were studied and all received both preoperative and postoperative chemotherapy. Two different regimens were employed. The first group (n = 18) was treated for two cycles with intravenous doxorubicin at 60 mg/m^2 over 72 hours following intra-arterial cisplatin at 120 mg/m^2 over 2 hours. The second group (n = 15) received an initial cycle with ifosfamide at 2.25 g/m^2 day for 4 days with intravenous doxorubicin at 75 mg/m^2 as a continuous intravenous infusion over 72 hours followed by filgrastim support. Cycles 2 and 3 also included doxorubicin at the same dose as cycle 1, with intra-arterial cisplatin at 120 mg/m^2 over 4 hours. Postoperatively, the group 1 patients received four additional cycles of doxorubicin at 60 mg/m^2 and cisplatin at 120 mg/m^2. Those in group 2 received three cycles of ifosfamide at 2.25 g/m^2 for 4 days with intravenous doxorubicin at 75 mg/m^2 over 72 hours.

Histologic response was evaluable for 29 patients. Tumor necrosis ranged from 50% to 100% with a median value of 95%, with 22 of 29 patients having estimated tumor necrosis of ≥90%. Two patients developed local recurrence, one of whom was reported alive after repeat resection and external-beam radiation. The other patient died of metastatic disease without developing further local involvement. Thus, the limb-salvage rate was 94%. Kaplan-Meier estimated relapse-free and overall survival was 80% and 88%. Limb preservation was possible in 31 patients, with 2 patients requiring primary amputation. Although this study was small, the rate of local control was quite good, and this raises the issue as to whether radiation treatment is necessary for the management of all high-grade extremity sarcomas.

It is not clear what accounts for the differences in the results from these trials. Sarcomas are a heterogenous group of tumors, and it is possible that some studies included an excess of relatively resistant sarcoma subtypes (e.g., leiomyosarcoma). Some of these trials used only doxorubicin, and some studies gave only preoperative treatment without postoperative chemotherapy. Many, but not all, of the studies that produced improved results with chemotherapy included ifosfamide. Most studies included radiation, but the study by Henshaw et al. (69) produced excellent results in terms of local control without radiation therapy. Preoperative chemotherapy with (or possibly without) radiation may be considered in the management of large, high-grade soft-tissue sarcomas of the extremity. The definitive trial to address this issue is yet to be performed.

Hybrid Studies

Two recent studies have tried to address some of these questions. A cohort analysis of patients with high-risk extremity sarcomas was reported from M.D. Anderson Cancer Center and Memorial Sloan-Kettering Cancer Center (70). There were 674 patients analyzed, with half receiving local therapy only and the other half receiving local therapy along with doxorubicin-based chemotherapy. All patients had primary stage III extremity sarcomas. Some patients (214, 64%) received preoperative chemotherapy, and 122 (36%) received postoperative chemotherapy. Most patients received doxorubicin either alone or in combination with dacarbazine or cyclophosphamide. A smaller group of patients received ifosfamide either alone or in combination. It is not clear how many patients received both doxorubicin and ifosfamide. Although attempts were made to account for known prognostic variables, the study was not randomized. A benefit for chemotherapy in terms of disease-specific survival existed only during the first year after treatment. Beyond 1 year, those in the no-chemotherapy control group had superior disease-specific survival. In fact, local control rates, specifically local relapse-free interval and local disease-free survival, also favored the no-chemotherapy control group after the first year. The authors concluded that the benefits of chemotherapy are time-dependent and fade after the first year following treatment.

Another cohort analysis was confined to extremity liposarcomas (71). It again included patients from Memorial Sloan-Kettering Cancer Center but this time they were grouped with patients from UCLA. There were 245 patients included, again in a nonrandomized assessment. Patients received either no chemotherapy (99, 40%), doxorubicin-based chemotherapy (83, 34%), or ifosfamide-based chemotherapy (63, 26%). The majority of those treated with ifosfamide were from UCLA. Some patients received only adjuvant chemotherapy and some received both preoperative and adjuvant chemotherapy. Those who received doxorubicin-based chemotherapy had a 5-year disease-specific survival of 64% (confidence interval [CI] 53%–74%) compared with 56% (CI 51%–79%) for the no-chemotherapy group (log-rank $p = 0.28$). However, those treated with ifosfamide-based chemotherapy had a 5-year disease-specific survival of 92% (CI 84%–100%) compared with 65% (50%–76%) for the no-chemotherapy group (CI 51%–79%), which was statistically significant (log rank $p = 0.0003$). Rates for local control were similar among the groups. In this study, the benefit for chemotherapy did not vary with time and remained significant at 5 years. Patients whose tumors were between 5 and 10 cm and those whose tumors had myxoid/round cell histology also fared better.

What accounts for the differing conclusions from these two studies? One explanation is that ifosfamide does make a difference in extremity sarcomas, or at least in extremity liposarcomas. Another explanation is that both these studies are nonrandomized, and although large by the standards of sarcoma studies, still relatively small. Thus, the definitive determination of the value of chemotherapy in the soft-tissue sarcomas in the adjuvant/neoadjuvant setting remains unresolved.

REFERENCES

1. Blum RH. An overview of studies of Adriamycin (NSC-123127) in the United States. *Cancer Chemother Rep.*1975;6:247–251.
2. O'Bryan RM, Luce JK, Talley RW, et al. Phase II Evaluation of Adriamycin in human neoplasis. *Cancer.* 1973;32:1–8.
3. Benjamin RS, Wiernik PH, Bachur NR. Adriamycin: A new effective agent in the therapy of disseminated sarcomas. *Med Pediatr Oncol.* 1975;1:63–76.
4. O'Bryan RM, Baker LH, Gottlieb JE, et al. Dose-response evaluation of Adriamycin in human neoplasia. *Cancer.* 1977;39:1940–1948.
5. Henderson IC, Frei E. Adriamycin cardiotoxicity. *Am Heart J.* 1980;99:671–674.
6. Lefrak EA, Pitha J, Rosenheim S, et al. A clinico-pathologic analysis of Adriamycin cardiotoxicity. *Cancer.* 1973;32:302–314.
7. Unverferth DV, Magorien RD, Leier CV, et al. Doxorubicin cardiotoxicity. *Cancer Treat Rev.* 1982;9:149–164.
8. Wexler LH, Andrich MP, Venzon D. Randomized trial of the cardioprotective agent ICRF-187 in pediatric sarcoma patients treated with doxorubicin. *J Clin Oncol.* 1996;14(2):362–372.
9. Seymour L, Bramwell V, Moran LA. Use of Dexrazoxane as a cardio protector in patients receiving doxorubicin or epirubicin chemotherapy for the treatment of cancer. *Cancer Prev. Control.* 1999;3(2):145–159.
10. Bramwell VH, Mouridsen HT, Santoro A, et al. Cyclophosphamide versus ifosfamide. Final report of a randomized phase II trial in adult soft tissue sarcomas. *Eur J Cancer Clin Oncol.* 1987;3:311–321.
11. Zalupski M, Baker LH Ifosfamide. *J Natl Cancer Inst.* 1988;80:556–566.
12. Frustaci S, Comandone A, Bearz A,, et al. Efficacy and tolerability of an ifosfamide continuous infusion (IFO-CI) in soft tissue sarcoma patients. *Proc Am Soc Clin Oncol.* 1998;17A1993 (abstract).
13. Gottlieb JA, Benjamin RS, Baker LH, et al. The role of DTIC(NSC-45388) in the chemotherapy of sarcomas. *Cancer Treat Rep.* 1976;60:199–293.
14. Von Burton G, Rankin C, Zalupski MM, et al. Phase II trial of gemcitabine as first line chemotherapy in patients with metastatic or unresectable soft tissue sarcoma. *Am J Clin Oncol.* 2006;29:59–61.
15. Svancarova L, Blay JY, Judson IR, et al. Gemcitabine in advanced adult soft-tissue sarcomas. A phase II study of the EORTC Soft Tissue and Bone Sarcoma Group. *Eur J Cancer.* 2002;38:556–559.
16. Patel SR, Gandhi V, Jenkins J, et al. Phase II clinical investigation of gemcitabine in advanced soft tissue sarcomas and window evaluation of dose rate on gemcitabine triphosphate accumulation. *J Clin Oncol.* 2000;19(5):3483–3489.
17. Verweij J, Catimel G, Sulkes A, et al. Phase II studies of docetaxel in the treatment of various solid tumors. EORTC Early Clinical Trials Group and the EORTC Soft Tissue and Bone Sarcoma Group. *Eur J Cancer.* 1995;31A(Suppl 4):21–24.
18. Verweij J, Lee DM, Ruka W, et al. Randomized phase II study of docetaxel versus doxorubicin in first and second-line chemotherapy for locally advanced or metastatic soft tissue sarcoma in adults: a study of the European organization for research and treatment of cancer soft tissue and bone sarcoma group. *J Clin Oncol.* 2000;18(10):2081–2086.
19. Gottlieb JA, Baker LH, Quagliana JM, et al. Chemotherapy of sarcomas with a combination of Adriamycin and demethyl triazeno imidazole carboxamide. *Cancer.* 1972;30:1632–1638.
20. Borden EC, Amato D, Rosenbaum C, et al. Randomized comparison of three Adriamycin regimens for metastatic soft tissue sarcomas. *J Clin Oncol.* 1987;5:40–850.
21. Gottlieb JA, Baker LH, O'bryan RM, et al. Adriamycin (NSC-123127) used alone or in combination for soft tissue and bony sarcomas. *Cancer Chemother Rep.* 1975;6:271–282.
22. Baker LH, Frank J, Fine G, et al. Combination chemotherapy using Adriamycin, DTIC, cyclophophamide and actinomycin D in advanced soft tissue sarcomas: A randomized comparative trial. A phase III, Southwest Oncology Group Study (7613). *J Clin Oncol.* 1987;5:851–861.
23. Schoenfeld D, Rosenbaum C, Horton J, et al. A comparison of Adriamycin versus vincristine, and Adriamycin and cyclophosphamide versus vincristine, actinomycin D and cyclophosphamide for advanced sarcoma. *Cancer.* 1982;50:2757–2762.
24. Elias AD, Antman KH. Doxorubicin, ifosfamide, and dacarbazine (AID) with mesna uroprotection for advance untreated sarcoma: a phase I study. *Cancer Treat Rep.* 1986;70:827–833.
25. Loehrer PJ Sr, Sledge GW Jr, Nicaise C, et al. Ifosfamide plus doxorubicin in metastatic adult sarcomas: A multi-institutional phase II trial. *J Clin Oncol.* 1989;7:1655–1659.

26. Santoro A, Tursz T, Mouridsen H, et al. Doxorubicin versus CYVADIC versus doxorubicin plus ifosfamide in first-line treatment of advanced soft tissue sarcomas: a randomized study of the European Organization for Research and Treatment of Cancer Soft Tissue and Bone Sarcoma Group. *J Clin Oncol.* 1995;13(7): 1537–1545.

27. LeCesne A, Judson I, Crowther D, et al. Randomized phase III study comparing conventional-dose doxorubicin plus ifosfamide versus high-dose ifosfamide plus recombinant human granulocyte-macrophage colony-stimulating factor in advanced soft tissue sarcomas: A trial of the European Organization for Research and Treatment of Cancer/Soft Tissue and Bone Sarcoma Group. *J Clin Oncol.* 2000;18(14):2676–2684.

28. Patel SR, Vadhan-RAj S, Burgess MA, et al. Results of two consecutive trials of dose-intensive chemotherapy with doxorubicin and ifosfamide in patients with sarcomas. *Am J Clin Oncol.* 1998;21(3):317–321.

29. Leyvraz S, Bacchi M, Cerny T, et al. Phase I multicenter study of combined high-dose ifosfamide and doxorubicin in the treatment of advanced sarcomas. Swiss Group for Clinical Research(SAKK). *Ann Oncol.* 1998;9(8):877–884.

30. Hensley ML, Maki R, Venkatraman E, et al. Gemcitabine and docetaxel in patients with unresectable leiomyosarcoma: results of a phase II trial. *J Clin Oncol.* 2002;20(12):2824–2831.

31. Leu KM, Ostruska LJ, Shewach D, et al. Laboratory and clinical evidence of synergistic cytotoxicity of sequential treatment with gemcitabine followed by docetaxel in the treatment of sarcoma. *J Clin Oncol.* 2004;22(9):1706–1712.

32. Van Glabbeke M, van Oosterum AT, Oosterhuis JW, et al. Prognostic factors for the outcome of chemotherapy in advanced soft tissue sarcomas: an analysis of 2,185 patients treated with anthracycline containing first-line regimens—an European Organization for Research and Treatment of Cancer Soft Tissue and Bone Sarcoma Study Group. *J Clin Oncol.* 1999;17(1):150–157.

33. Rosenberg SA, Tepper J, Glatstein E, et al. Prospective randomized evaluation of adjuvant chemotherapy in adults with soft tissue sarcomas of the extremities. *Cancer.* 1982;52:424–434.

34. Potter DA, Kinsella T, Glatstein E, et al. High grade soft tissue sarcomas of the extremities. *Cancer.* 1986;58:190–205.

35. Chang AE, Kinsella T, Glatstein E, et al. Adjuvant chemotherapy for patients with high-grade soft-tissue sarcomas of the extremity. *J Clin Oncol.* 1998;6:1491–1500.

36. Lindberg R, Murphy W, Benjamin R, et al. Adjuvant chemotherapy in the treatment of primary soft tissue sarcomas. A preliminary report. Management of Primary Bone and Soft Tissue Tumors. Chicago: Year Book Medical Publishers; 1997;343–352.

37. Benjamin RS, Terjanian TO, Fenoglio GL, et al. The importance of combination chemotherapy for adjuvant treatment of high-risk patients with soft-tissue sarcomas of the extremities. In: Salmon S, ed. *Adjuvant Therapy of Cancer V.* Orlando: Grune and Stratton; 1987:735–744.

38. Gherlinzoni F, Bacci G, Picci P, et al. A randomized trial for the treatment of high-grade soft-tissue sarcomas of the extremities: Preliminary observations. *J Clin Oncol.* 1986;5:552–558.

39. Gherlinzoni F, Picci P, Bacci G, et al. Late results of a randomized trial for the treatment of soft tissue sarcomas (STS) of the extremities in adult patients. *Proc Am Soc Clin Onol.* 1993;12:a1633.

40. Omura GA, Blessing JA, Major F, et al. A randomized clinical trial of adjuvant adriamycin in uterine sarcomas: a Gynecologic Oncology Group study. *J Clin Oncol.* 1985;3(9):1240–1245.

41. Lerner, HJ, Damato DA, Savlov ED, et al. Eastern Cooperative Oncology Group: A comparison of adjuvant doxorubicin and observation for patients with localized soft tissue sarcoma. *J Clin Oncol.* 1987;5:613–617.

42. Antman K, Amato D, Pilepich M, et al. A preliminary analysis of a randomized intergroup (SWOG, ECOG, CALGB, NCOG) trial of adjuvant doxorubicin for soft tissue sarcomas. In Salmon S (ed) Adjuvant therapy of Cancer V. Orlando Grune and Stratton 1987:725–734.

43. Antman K, Suit H, Amato D, et al. Preliminary results of a randomized trial of adjuvant doxorubicin for sarcomas: Lack of apparent difference between treatment groups. *J Clin Oncol.* 1984;2: 601–608.

44. Antman K, Amato D, Lerner H, et al. Adjuvant doxorubicin for sarcomas: Data from the ECOG and MGH/DFCI studies. *Cancer Treat Symp.* 1985;3:109–115.

45. Alvegard TA Adjuvant chemotherapy with Adriamycin in high grade malignant soft tissue sarcoma—a Scandinavian randomized study. *Proc Am Soc Clin Oncol.* 1986;5:a485.

46. Eilber FR, Giuliano AE, Huth JF et al. Postoperative adjuvant chemotherapy (Adriamycin) in high grade soft tissue sarcoma: A randomized prospective clinical trial. In: Salmon S, ed. *Adjuvant Therapy of Cancer V.* Orlando: Grune and Stratton; 1987: 719–724.

47. Bramwell V, Rouesse J, Steward W, et al. European experience of adjuvant chemotherapy for soft tissue sarcoma: Interim report of a randomized trial of CyVADIC versus control. In: Ryan J, Baker L, eds. *Recent Concepts in Sarcoma Treatment.* The Netherlands: Kluwer Academic; 1988:157–164.

48. Ravaud A, Bui NB, Coindre JM, et al. Adjuvant chemotherapy with CyVADIC in high risk soft tissue sarcoma: a randomized prospective clinical trial. In: Salmon SE, ed. *Adjuvant Therapy of Cancer VI.* Philadelphia: WB Saunders; 1990:556.

49. Edmonson JH, Fleming TR, Ivins JC, et al. Randomized study of systemic chemotherapy following complete excision of nonosseous sarcomas. *J Clin Oncol.* 1984;2:1390–1396.

50. Frustaci S, Gherlinzoni F, De Paoli A, et al. Adjuvant chemotherapy for adult soft tissue sarcomas of the extremities and girdles: results of the Italian randomized cooperative trial. *J Clin Oncol.* 2001;19(5)1238–1247.

51. Frustaci S, De Paoli A, Bidoli E, et al. Ifosfamide in the adjuvant therapy of soft tissue sarcomas. *Oncology.* 2003;(Suppl 2):80–84.

52. Brodowicz T, Schwameis E, Widder J, et al. Intensified adjuvant IFADICchemotherapy for adult soft tissue sarcoma. A prospective randomized feasibility trial. *Sarcoma.* 2000;4:151.

53. Antman K, Ryan I, Borden E, et al. Pooled results from three randomized adjuvant studies of doxorubicin versus observation in soft tissue sarcomas: 10 year results and review of the literature. In: Salmon SE, ed. *Adjuvant Therapy of Cancer,* 6th ed. Philadelphia: WB Saunders; 1990:529.

54. Zalupski MM, Ryan JR, Hussein ME, et al. Defining the role of adjuvant chemotherapy for patients with soft tissue sarcomas of the extremities. In: Salmon SE, ed. *Adjuvant Therapy of Cancer,* 7th ed. Philadelphia: JB Lippincott; 1993:385.

55. Tierney JF, Mosseri V, Stewart LA, et al. Adjuvant chemotherapy for soft-tissue sarcoma: Review and meta-analysis of the published results of randomized clinical trials. *Br J Cancer.* 1995;72: 469–475.

56. Sarcoma Meta-Analysis Collaboration: Adjuvant chemotherapy for localized respectable soft-tissue sarcoma of adults: Meta-analysis of individual data. *Lancet.* 1997;350:1647–1654.

57. Eilber FR, Eckardt J, Yao L, et al. Neoadjuvant chemotherapy in the multidisciplinary management of soft tissue sarcomas of the extremity. *Surg Oncol Clin North Am.* 1993;2(6):511–520.

58. Eilber FC, Rosen G, Eckardt J et al. Treatment-induced pathologic necrosis: a predictor of local recurrence and survival in patients receiving neoadjuvant therapy for high-grade extremity soft tissue sarcomas. *J Clin Oncol.* 2001;19(13):3203–3209.

59. Mack LA, Crowe PJ, Yang JL et al. Preoperative chemoradiotherapy (modified Eilber protocol) provides maximum local control and minimal morbidity in patients with soft tissue sarcoma. *Ann Surg Oncol.* 2005;12(8):646–653.

60. Wanebo HJ, Temple WJ, Popp MB, et al. Preoperative regional therapy for extremity sarcoma. A tricenter update. *Cancer.* 1995;75(9):2299–2306.

61. Levine EA, Trippon M, Das Gupta TK. Preoperative multimodality treatment for soft tissue sarcomas. *Cancer.* 1993;71(11):3685–3689.

62. Pisters PW, Patel SR, Varma DG, et al. Preoperative chemotherapy for stage IIIB extremity soft tissue sarcoma: long-term results from a single institution. *J Clin Oncol.* 1997;15(12):3481–3487.

63. Pisters PW, Patel SR, Prieto VG, et al. Phase I trial of preoperative doxorubicin-based concurrent chemoradiation and surgical resection for localized extremity and body wall soft tissue sarcomas. *J Clin Oncol.* 2004;22(16):3375–3380.

64. Edmonson JH, Petersen IA, Shives TC, et al. Chemotherapy, irradiation and surgery for function-preserving therapy of primary extremity soft tissue sarcomas: initial treatment with ifosfamide, mitomycin, doxorubicin and cisplatin plus granulocyte macrophage-colony-stimulating factor. *Cancer.* 2002;94(3):786–792.

65. Gortzak E, Azzarelli A, Buesa J, et al. A randomised phase II study on neo-adjuvant chemotherapy for "high-risk" adult soft-tissue sarcoma. *Eur J Cancer.* 2001;37(9)1096–1103.

66. Grobmeyer SR, Maki RG, Demetri GD, et al. Neo-adjuvant chemotherapy for primary high-grade extremity soft tissue sarcoma. *Ann Oncol.* 2004;15(11):1667–1672.

67. DeLaney TF, Spiro IJ, Suit HD et al. Neoadjuvant chemotherapy and radiotherapy for large extremity soft-tissue sarcomas. *Int J Rad Onc Biol Phy.* 2003;56(4):1117–1127.

68. Kraybill WG, Harris J, Spiro IJ, et al. Phase II study of neoadjuvant chemotherapy and radiation therapy in the management of high-risk, high-grade, soft tissue sarcomas of the extremities and body wall: Radiation Therapy Oncology Group Trial 9514. *J Clin Oncol.* 2006;24(4):619–625.

69. Henshaw RM, Priebat DA, Perry DJ, et al. Survival after induction chemotherapy and surgical resection for high-grade soft tissue sarcoma. Is radiation necessary? *Ann Surg Oncol.* 2001;8:484–495.

70. Cormier JN, Huang X, Xing Y, et al. Cohort analysis of patients with localized, high-risk, extremity soft tissue sarcoma treated at two cancer centers: Chemotherapy-associated outcomes. *J Clin Oncol.* 2004;22(22):456745–74.

71. Eilber FC, Eilber FR, Eckardt J, et al. The impact of chemotherapy on the survival of patients with high-grade primary extremity liposarcoma. *Ann Surg.* 2004;240(4):686–697.

COMMENTARY
Karen Antman

The author had no commercial relationships with manufacturers of products or providers of services discussed in this chapter. Most drugs discussed in this chapter do not have Food and Drug Administration approval for use in the treatment of sarcoma.

In his excellent review of the chemotherapy literature for soft tissue sarcomas, Dr. Charles Forscher outlines the current evidence base for treatment decision making for adults with these neoplasms. In his chapter, he comments on the outcomes for children versus adults with sarcomas and reviews adjuvant treatment and combined modality therapies as well as chemotherapy for advanced disease.

Dr. Forscher has detailed the modest activity of the available drug regimens and the conflicting results of the few relatively small cooperative group randomized studies as well as many retrospective small single-institution studies. Whereas cooperative studies in other tumors comprise thousands of patients, the largest sarcoma studies include several hundred patients and even the meta-analyses include only just over 1,000 patients. Thus, using standard criteria for levels of evidence, few treatment decisions for adults with soft-tissue sarcoma are based on the most reliable (level one) evidence, that is, several large randomized trials with consistent results.

WHY DO WE HAVE CONFLICTING EVIDENCE FOR MANAGEMENT DECISIONS IN ADULTS WITH SOFT-TISSUE SARCOMAS?

The Number of Sarcoma Patients Is Not the Problem

Why do we lack reliable level-one evidence based on multiple large randomized trials in adult sarcomas? The intuitive answer is that sarcomas are uncommon and thus adequately sized studies cannot be done. However, larger collaborative studies in less common malignancies, for example, Hodgkin disease, testis cancer, and even rare sarcomas, such as gastrointestinal stromal tumors (GISTs), and rhabdomyosarcomas in children, have provided the basis for steady progress in disease treatments and improved outcomes. The estimated number of newly diagnosed sarcomas in the United States in 2008, 12,770 (Table 29C.1), comprises <1% of the 1,437,180 newly diagnosed malignancies in the United States and about 15% of pediatric malignancies (1). However, there are even fewer cases of Hodgkin disease and testis cancer in the United States, and yet many more randomized studies in connection with these diseases have been published.

Table 29C.1

Sarcomas: Incidence and Mortality Data in the United States for 2008

| Sarcoma | Cases | | | Deaths |
	Males	Females	Total	Total
Soft-tissue sarcoma	5,720	4,670	10,390	3,680
Sarcomas of bones and joints	1,270	1,110	2,380	1,470
Total sarcomas	6,990	5,780	12,770	5,150

Data are from ref. 1. American Cancer Society. Cancer Facts & Figures 2008. Atlanta: American Cancer Society; 2008.

In fact, sarcomas actually are more common than these statistics suggest. Visceral sarcomas, coded as gastrointestinal, urinary, or gynecologic malignancies, are not included in these statistics. Furthermore, because sarcomas are difficult to diagnose by inexperienced pathologists, they are underdiagnosed. The actual incidence of sarcoma is probably about double these estimates.

The overall survival rate of patients with sarcoma in the United States is also helpful to appropriately interpret the data in the clinical trials described in Dr. Forscher's chapter. The 5-year relative survival rates (comparing the survival of the cancer patients with that of the general population) for 1996-2003 from the 17 Surveillance Epidemiology and End Results (SEER) geographic areas was 66% overall for soft-tissue sarcomas and 70% for sarcomas of bone and joints (1).

Lack of a Consolidated United States Sarcoma Study Group

Why have studies succeeded in even less common sarcomas such as GISTs and in childhood rhabdomyosarcomas? The impact of organizations committed to accrual of all children with these rare malignancies, studied in an orderly sequence of clinical trials in the United States (the Children's Cancer Study Group) and in Europe, cannot be underestimated.

In the United States, most children with cancer are referred to centers and entered onto clinical trials. In contrast, only 3% to 5% of adults with cancer participate in clinical trials. Cooperative groups are not funded to handle large number of patients and data.

In the past, cooperative groups in the United States facilitated accrual of patients into studies of uncommon tumors. As studies became larger and more expensive, cooperative groups increasingly have focused on hematologic malignancies and the most common solid tumors (breast, lung, colon, and prostate); therefore, fewer resources remain for the study of uncommon solid tumors.

Finally, accrual of patients with sarcoma has been divided over the several cooperative groups in the United States. In comparison, the European Organisation for Research and Treatment of Cancer (EORTC) supports a single committed sarcoma group, which has provided the majority of recent randomized sarcoma study results.

Regulatory Costs to Keep Studies Open for Uncommon Cancers Have Increased Significantly

The cost of opening a study was considerably lower at the time sarcoma studies flourished. Regulatory agencies did not require regular review and annual reapprovals of each open study at an institution, and thus institutions could afford to open and maintain studies onto which they projected few if any accruals. Today, annual renewal of clinical protocols costs thousands of dollars per year per study, and thus institutions cannot afford to keep open studies in diseases for the few patients seen at any given institution. One solution to this problem is referral of sarcoma patients to a few regional sarcoma centers with active studies.

TREATMENT OF SOFT-TISSUE SARCOMAS

Comparison of Sensitivity of Childhood and Adult Sarcomas

Rhabdomyosarcomas and Ewing sarcomas in children are exquisitely sensitive to cytotoxic chemotherapy, whereas fibrosarcomas, liposarcomas, and leiomyosarcomas in adults have low response rates to drugs tested to date. Children with rhabdomyosarcoma are generally treated with multiagent chemotherapy in regimens combining vincristine, actinomycin, and either cyclophosphamide or ifosfamide (2,3). Doxorubicin-based regimens are often used in adults (4). Chemotherapy is followed by resection of residual rhabdomyosarcoma and radiation therapy. Lymph node metastases are more common than in other adult sarcomas. Although children with metastatic disease are sometimes cured, adults have a poor prognosis despite often excellent responses to primary aggressive chemotherapy (5).

Dr. Forscher comments on the differences in the sensitivity of soft-tissue sarcomas in adults versus those in children and attributes the poorer progress in sarcomas in adults to combining sarcoma histologic variants, to comorbid diseases in adults that limit treatment options, and to "unrecognized factors."

Certainly, differences in cytogenetics and molecular signatures and in intrinsic sensitivity to agents currently available are major factors. Cytogenetics and molecular signatures of sarcomas that are common in adults vary substantially from those of childhood sarcomas. Combining adult sarcomas of different histologies into a single trial can dilute the data and thereby obscure the recognition of activity in a single histologic variant. Separate studies of each of the various sarcoma histologies would require a national accrual base.

New Therapeutic Agents

The identification of active new agents provides a powerful impetus for funding pivotal studies. Certainly the activity of imatinib in GISTs resulted in rapid accrual in what was previously thought to be a small subset of soft-tissue sarcomas. Because of the lack of organized sarcoma studies in the United States, many new agents are never evaluated in adult sarcomas.

Dr. Forscher observes that ifosfamide, evaluated in the 1980s, is the most recently identified active agent for adult soft-tissue sarcomas. In fact, the last moderately sized randomized trials of soft-tissue sarcoma in the United States were studies of doxorubicin-based chemotherapy with or without the addition of ifosfamide. These trials were begun in the late 1980s collaboratively by the Southwest Oncology Group and the Cancer and Leukemia Group B (6), and separately by the Eastern Cooperative Oncology Group (7). Both of these studies documented an increased response rate for the ifosfamide-containing arm. However, the European EORTC trial showed no difference (8).

The differences between the two positive American studies (6,7) compared with the negative EORTC study (8) may have been due to a difference in the ifosfamide administration schedule. Based on the pharmacokinetic data suggesting saturation of the enzyme that activates the prodrug, the United States studies called for providing the ifosfamide dose over several days, whereas the EORTC study delivered ifosfamide over a single day. A subsequent EORTC study used the same dose and schedule of ifosfamide (5 g/m^2 over 24 hours), versus 3 g/m^2 per day, administered over 4 hours on 3 consecutive days, every 3 weeks. Of 103 patients receiving first-line treatment, the 1-day schedule yielded five partial responses (response rate 10%), versus 12 (25%) for the 3-day schedule (9). Because the study changed both dose and schedule, the components contributing to the difference cannot be separated, but the minimal activity on the 1-day schedule may explain the discrepancy between the American and European results. One randomized study conducted in the United States that compared two ifosfamide doses (6 g/m^2 vs. 12 g/m^2) showed no dose effect for ifosfamide (10).

Special Considerations in Adjuvant Chemotherapy

Adjuvant chemotherapy as the standard of care for rhabdomyosarcomas, osteosarcomas, and Ewing sarcomas was established in studies that included only single histologies. Adjuvant chemotherapy remains controversial for other adult soft-tissue sarcomas. Most sarcoma centers do not recommend adjuvant therapy for low-grade lesions (given their low probability of metastatic spread) or for high-grade lesions smaller than 5 cm, because of their excellent prognosis.

Several of the meta-analyses reviewed in the chapter summarized only published data. However, one meta-analysis considered the computerized databases of 1,568 individual patients from all randomized doxorubicin-based adjuvant trials in patients with sarcoma. Adjuvant chemotherapy improved local and distant recurrence-free survival (hazard ratios, 0.73 and 0.70; $p = 0.016$ and 0.0003, respectively). However, the group receiving chemotherapy had a nonsignificant 4% survival advantage (hazard ratio, 0.89; $p = 0.12$) (11). Adjuvant trials of doxorubicin and ifosfamide regimens produce conflicting results (12,13). Because surgical resection of local recurrences and even pulmonary metastases can be curative (see following discussion), disease-free survival is less meaningful than overall survival as a primary endpoint.

Therapy for Advanced Soft-Tissue Sarcomas
Surgical Resection

Resection of subpleural metastases in carefully selected patients provides disease-free survival in about 20% of patients (14–17). Patients with fewer than three to five nodules, a tumor doubling time of more than 20 days, and a disease-free interval longer than 12 months have a better prognosis. A randomized study of a combined-modality approach (chemotherapy and resection) versus surgery alone has yet to be published.

Single-Agent Chemotherapy

Single-agent chemotherapy is generally chosen for palliation, particularly in older patients and in those with lower-grade lesions. Doxorubicin, the most active single agent in soft-tissue sarcomas, has a response rate of 15% to 35%. Doxorubicin at 60 to 70 mg/m^2 every 3 weeks produced significantly higher response rates than dose rates of 50 mg/m^2 or less in randomized trials (18–20).

Dacarbazine has a single-agent response rate of about 16% for most adult sarcomas and response rates of up to 44% when used in combination with doxorubicin for leiomyosarcomas. Nausea and flulike symptoms are significantly diminished by continuous-infusion administration (21–23).

Ifosfamide, a cyclophosphamide analogue, is effective against sarcoma alone or in combination with doxorubicin, but requires mesna coadministration to prevent bladder injury (6,24).

Combination Chemotherapy

Combination chemotherapy may be used (a) if a response would facilitate curative resection of a primary lesion and (b) for palliation of unresectable or metastatic sarcoma, particularly for patients aged younger than 50 years with high-grade lesions. A combination of doxorubicin and ifosfamide produces response rates of 17% to 25% (6,7). The median survival of patients with unresectable or metastatic sarcoma is 12 months, with no significant chemotherapy impact on median survival. (No effect on survival would be expected given a response rate considerably below 50%.) A new regimen of gemcitabine and Taxotere appears active (25), but has not been compared in a randomized study against doxorubicin and ifosfamide-based chemotherapy.

Treatment of Special Histologic Variants of Soft-Tissue Sarcoma

Management of GISTs, mesotheliomas, rhabdomyosarcomas, and Kaposi sarcoma (KS) differ from that of the classic adult soft-tissue sarcomas. Rhabdomyosarcomas, GISTs, and KS are considerably more sensitive to currently available agents than the classic sarcomas.

Kaposi Sarcoma

Four variants of KS have been identified: classic, transplant-associated, lymphadenopathic, and acquired immunodeficiency syndrome (AIDS)-associated. Over 95% of KS lesions, regardless of clinical subtype are human herpes virus 8 (HHV8)-associated. HHV8 and Epstein-Barr virus, both gamma herpesviruses, cause tumors, particularly lymphoproliferative disorders and lymphomas. HHV8 infection rates are low in Europe, the United States, and Asia, intermediate around the Mediterranean, and >50% in some Central African locations such as Uganda, Zambia, and South Africa (26). HHV8 rates parallel the global incidence of KS.

The classic KS variant presents most commonly in elderly men of Mediterranean origin as multiple purple skin lesions of the lower legs that progress over time to nodules and plaques. Transplant-associated KS develops, predominantly in men, an average of 16 months after organ transplant, particularly if the organ donor or recipient is of Mediterranean origin. Lymphadenopathic KS, an aggressive variant often in young children, is endemic in parts of Africa (27).

The most aggressive variant, human immunodeficiency virus (HIV)-associated KS, presents as cutaneous or oral mucosal lesions or adenopathy. HIV-associated KS lesions often begin on the face, trunk, or arms. Men who acquire HIV by sexual contact with men develop KS more commonly than those who acquire AIDS after intravenous drug use. Lesions of the classic variant of KS generally respond to resection, radiotherapy, or interferon alfa, or low-dose vinblastine or doxorubicin.

Adjusting the dose of immunosuppression therapy may control transplantation-associated KS. Doxorubicin, vinblastine, or paclitaxel, as single-agents or in combination, are used for advanced or visceral disease. Interferon alfa is usually used as a single agent (27–30). Responses in HIV-associated KS are shorter than in classic KS.

REFERENCE

1. American Cancer Society. Cancer Facts & Figures 2008. Atlanta: American Cancer Society; 2008.

2. Lager JJ, Lyden ER, Anderson JR, et al. Pooled analysis of phase II window studies in children with contemporary high-risk metastatic rhabdomyosarcoma: a report from the Soft Tissue Sarcoma Committee of the Children's Oncology Group. *J Clin Oncol.* 2006;24:3415–3422.

3. Crist WM, Anderson JR, Meza JL, et al. Intergroup rhabdomyosarcoma study-IV: results for patients with nonmetastatic disease. *J Clin Oncol.* 2001;19:3091–3102.

4. Antman K, Crowley J, Balcerzak SP, et al. A Southwest Oncology Group and Cancer and Leukemia Group B phase II study of doxorubicin, dacarbazine, ifosfamide, and mesna in adults with advanced osteosarcoma, Ewing's sarcoma, and rhabdomyosarcoma. *Cancer.* 1998;82:1288–1295.

5. Joshi D, Anderson JR, Paidas C, et al. Age is an independent prognostic factor in rhabdomyosarcoma: a report from the Soft Tissue Sarcoma Committee of the Children's Oncology Group. *Pediatr Blood Cancer.* 2004;42:64–73.

6. Antman K, Crowley J, Balcerzak SP, et al. An Intergroup phase III randomized study of doxorubicin and dacarbazine with or without ifosfamide and mesna in advanced tissue and bone sarcomas. *J Clin Oncol.* 1993;11:1276–1285.

7. Edmonson JH, Ryan L, Blum RH, et al. Randomized comparison of doxorubicin alone vs ifosfamide and doxorubicin or mitomycin, doxorubicin, cisplatin against advanced soft tissue sarcomas. *J Clin Oncol.* 1993;11:1269–1275.

8. Santoro A, Tursz T, Mouridsen H, et al. Doxorubicin versus CYVADIC versus doxorubicin plus ifosfamide in first-line treatment of advanced soft tissue sarcomas: a randomized study of the European Organization for Research and Treatment of Cancer Soft Tissue and Bone Sarcoma Group. *J Clin Oncol.* 1995;13:1537–1545.

9. van Oosterom AT, Mouridsen HT, Nielsen OS, et al. Results of randomised studies of the EORTC Soft Tissue and Bone Sarcoma Group (STBSG) with two different ifosfamide regimens in first- and second-line chemotherapy in advanced soft tissue sarcoma patients. *Eur J Cancer.* 2002;38:2397–2406.

10. Worden FP, Taylor JM, Biermann JS, et al. Randomized phase II evaluation of 6 g/m2 of ifosfamide plus doxorubicin and granulocyte colony-stimulating factor (G-CSF) compared with 12 g/m^2 of ifosfamide plus doxorubicin and G-CSF in the treatment of poor-prognosis soft tissue sarcoma. *J Clin Oncol.* 2005;23:105–112.

11. Tierney JF. A meta-analysis using individual patient data from randomised clinical trials of adjuvant chemotherapy for soft tissue sarcomas [abstract 2024]. *J Clin Oncol.* 1996;14:1751.

12. Frustaci S, Gherlinzoni F, De Paoli A, et al. Adjuvant chemotherapy for adult soft tissue sarcomas of the extremities and girdles: results of the Italian randomized cooperative trial. *J Clin Oncol.* 2001;19:1238–1247.

13. Gortzak E, Azzarelli A, Buesa J, et al. A randomised phase II study on neo-adjuvant chemotherapy for "high-risk" adult soft-tissue sarcoma. *Eur J Cancer.* 2001;37:1096–1103.

14. Chao C, Goldberg M. Surgical treatment of metastatic pulmonary soft-tissue sarcoma. *Oncology (Williston Park).* 2000;14:835–847.

15. Porter GA, Cantor SB, Walsh GL, et al. Cost-effectiveness of pulmonary resection and systemic chemotherapy in the management of metastatic soft tissue sarcoma: a combined analysis from the University of Texas M. D. Anderson and Memorial Sloan-Kettering Cancer Centers. *J Thorac Cardiovasc Surg.* 2004;127:1366–1372.

16. Temple LK, Brennan MF. The role of pulmonary metastasectomy in soft tissue sarcoma. *Semin Thorac Cardiovasc Surg.* 2002;14:35–44.

17. Weiser MR, Downey RJ, Leung DH, et al. Repeat resection of pulmonary metastases in patients with soft-tissue sarcoma. *J Am Coll Surg.* 2000;191:184–191.

18. Bodey GP, Rodriguez V, Murphy WK, et al. Protected environment-prophylactic antibiotic program for malignant sarcoma: randomized trial during remission induction chemotherapy. *Cancer.* 1981;47:2422–2429.

19. Pinedo HM, Branwell VHC, Mouridsen HT, et al. CYVADIC in advanced soft tissue sarcoma: a randomized study comparing two schedules. A study of the EORTC Soft Tissue and Bone Sarcoma Group. *Cancer.* 1984;53:1825–1832.

20. Schoenfeld D, Rosenbaum C, Horton J, et al. A comparison of Adriamycin versus vincristine and Adriamycin, and cyclophosphamide for advanced sarcoma. *Cancer.* 1982;50:2757–2762.

21. Benjamin RS, Gottlieb JA, Baker LH. CYVADIC vs CYVADACT-A randomized trial of cyclophosphamide, vincristine and Adriamycin, plus either dacarbazine or actinomycin D in metastatic sarcomas. *Proc Annu Meet Am Assoc Cancer Res.* 1976;17:256.

22. Borden EC, Amato D, Enterline HT, et al. Randomized comparison of Adriamycin regimens for treatment of metastatic soft tissue sarcomas. *J Clin Oncol.* 1987;5:840–850.

23. Zalupski M, Metch B, Balcerzak S, et al. Phase III comparison of doxorubicin and dacarbazine given by bolus versus infusion in patients with soft-tissue sarcomas: a Southwest Oncology Group Study. *J Natl Cancer Inst.* 1991;83:926–932.

24. Bramwell V, Mouridsen HT, Santoro A, et al. Cyclophosphamide vs ifosfamide: Final report of a randomized phase II trial in adult soft tissue sarcoma. *Eur J Cancer Clin Oncol.* 1987;23:311–321.

25. Maki RG, Wathen JK, Patel SR, et al. Randomized phase II study of gemcitabine and docetaxel compared with gemcitabine alone in patients with metastatic soft tissue sarcomas: results of sarcoma alliance for research through collaboration study 002 [corrected]. *J Clin Oncol.* 2007;25:2755–2763.

26. Serraino D, Toma L, Andreoni M, et al. A seroprevalence study of human herpesvirus type 8 (HHV8) in eastern and Central Africa and in the Mediterranean area. *Eur J Epidemiol.* 2001;17:871–876.

27. Antman K, Chang Y. Kaposi's sarcoma. *N Engl J Med.* 2000;342:1027–1038.

28. Krown SE, Li P, Von Roenn JH, et al. Efficacy of low-dose interferon with antiretroviral therapy in Kaposi's sarcoma: a randomized phase II AIDS clinical trials group study. *J Interferon Cytokine Res.* 2002;22:295–303.

29. Ramirez-Amador V, Esquivel-Pedraza L, Lozada-Nur F, et al. Intralesional vinblastine vs. 3% sodium tetradecyl sulfate for the treatment of oral Kaposi's sarcoma. A double blind, randomized clinical trial. *Oral Oncol.* 2002;38:460–467.

30. Stallone G, Schena A, Infante B, et al. Sirolimus for Kaposi's sarcoma in renal-transplant recipients. *N Engl J Med.* 2005;352:1317–1323.

30

The Pathogenesis of Esophageal Carcinoma

Parakrama Chandrasoma

Carcinoma of the esophagus is caused by a genetic change or series of changes that gives the proliferating cells of the esophagus the growth characteristics that are recognized by their phenotypic expression. The carcinoma cells develop a growth advantage over the neighboring noncancer cells, which cause them to appear as mass lesions. Carcinoma cells can be differentiated from their benign counterparts by the fact that they have new capabilities such as invasiveness and metastasis.

This chapter will concentrate on the pathogenesis of esophageal carcinoma in terms of how the normal cells are converted into cells that have the potential of cancer. There is much unknown about this process. When this process is understood, it will be described in a few sentences that detail a series of genetic events with the phenotypic result of each of them. At this time, the best we can do is make deductions from observed phenotypic abnormalities.

The genetic changes of cancer in the esophagus require that the actively proliferating pool of cells in the esophageal epithelium interact with a carcinogenic agent. The proliferating pool of cells in the esophageal epithelium is derived from the stem cells that constantly divide to renew the epithelial cells that are continually lost from the surface (1). Renewal requires multiplication and differentiation of the stem cell into the surface cell, which is usually a terminally differentiated, nonmitotic cell.

THE ESOPHAGEAL STEM CELL

The stem cells in the esophagus are derived from the embryonic foregut endoderm (2). During fetal life, the stem cell shows multiple lines of differentiation (2,3). In the first trimester, the esophageal epithelium consists of a primitive stratified columnar epithelium. This is replaced in the second trimester by a pseudostratified ciliated columnar epithelium. Beginning in the 22nd week of gestation, the stem cell acquires a genetic signal that causes it to differentiate into stratified squamous epithelium. This progressively replaces the ciliated pseudostratified columnar epithelium, beginning in the midpart of the esophagus and extending in both directions. In late fetal life, squamous epithelium lines much of the esophagus except for small areas at the proximal and distal ends, which are lined by a nonciliated columnar epithelium that is associated with mucosal mucous glands. This small area of fetal columnar epithelium is located above the gastroesophageal junction; the epithelium at the gastroesophageal junction and in the stomach is gastric oxyntic mucosa from early fetal life (4). When epithelial development is completed, the entire esophagus is lined by squamous epithe-

lium to the gastroesophageal junction, where it transitions into gastric oxyntic mucosa (5).

After development, therefore, the esophageal stem cell differentiates into squamous epithelium throughout the esophagus. The genetic signal that drives the stem cell to squamous differentiation is unknown. All the fetal genetic signals that caused the stem cell to differentiate into various types of columnar epithelia have been suppressed.

The esophageal stem cell is located in the basal layer of the stratified squamous epithelium. Its continuous division produces a pool of proliferating cells that can be recognized in histologic sections stained for Ki-67, which identifies an antigen in the nucleus that is active in proliferating cells only (Figure 30.1). In the normal esophageal squamous epithelium, the proliferating cell pool is restricted to one to two cell layers above the basal layer. The more superficial cells are nonmitotic Ki-67 cells that are terminally differentiated keratinocytes (5).

The stratified squamous epithelium is eminently suited to the only function of the esophagus, which is to transmit a bolus of food from the pharynx to the stomach. It presents an impermeable surface that prevents entry of luminal molecules into the epithelium by virtue of the tight cell junctions between keratinocytes (6). The normal loss of surface cells by the abrasion of swallowing is effectively replaced from below. The mucosa is lubricated by the mucous secretion of the esophageal submucosal glands that drain through the mucosa to the surface by ducts. The stem cells and the proliferating pool of cells are sequestered in the deeper region of the stratified epithelium and do not normally come into contact with luminal molecules.

PATHOGENESIS OF SQUAMOUS CARCINOMA

Squamous carcinoma of the esophagus is a carcinoma that arises in the cells of the proliferating pool that have the normal squamous differentiating genetic signal. With neoplastic transformation, the cells retain their differentiation toward keratinocytes.

The pathogenesis of squamous carcinoma is largely unknown except for the fact that it is not significantly associated with gastroesophageal reflux disease (7). The carcinogen is therefore either a blood-borne carcinogen that reaches the esophageal stem cell or one that is present in the lumen either normally or during the act of swallowing. The likelihood that a luminal antigen is responsible for squamous carcinoma is low. The only normal secretion of the esophagus is limited

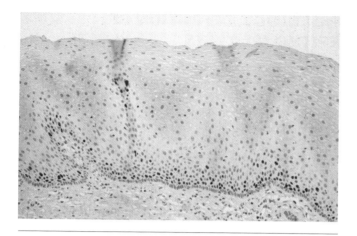

Figure 30.1 Stratified squamous epithelium of the esophagus, stained by immunoperoxidase technique for Ki-67, showing the proliferating pool of cells limited to the suprabasal region.

to that of the mucous glands. Swallowing includes saliva and food. The esophagus rapidly propels luminal contents during swallowing, where a primary peristaltic wave develops in the pharynx and passes down the entire esophagus, pushing the bolus down into the stomach with the synchronized relaxation of the lower esophageal sphincter. The collection of any luminal material apart from swallowing is believed to evoke a secondary peristaltic wave, which similarly clears the esophagus and keeps its lumen empty. The time available for a luminal carcinogen to act is extremely small. When this is coupled with the fact that the normal squamous epithelium presents an impermeable barrier to the entry of luminal molecules, it is unlikely that any luminal carcinogen can come into contact with the proliferating cells that are sequestered in the basal region of the epithelium.

Most squamous carcinomas occur in patients without a preexisting esophageal disease and the etiology of this usual squamous carcinoma of the esophagus is unknown; no specific carcinogen has been identified. In the United States, the incidence is around 2 per 100,000 population (8). The incidence is much higher, in the 50 to 200 per 100,000 range in a large Asian belt ranging from the eastern edge of the Caspian Sea to northern China along the ancient Silk Route (9). The reason for this distribution is not known, although many food factors such as the contamination of food by the fungus *Geotrichum candidum* (10)[10] and viruses have been suggested. A recent study from Linxian, China, showed that human papillomas virus infection was not associated with esophageal carcinoma (11).

In the United States, squamous carcinoma of the esophagus is associated with male sex, low socioeconomic status, alcoholism, and smoking and is more common in African Americans than whites. Patients with a history of lye-induced esophageal injury (12), tylosis palmaris (13), and Plummer-Vinson syndrome have a high risk of future squamous carcinoma; those with achalasia of the cardia have a slightly increased risk, with an incidence of 3.4 per 1,000 patients (14). Patients with head and neck cancer have an increased tendency to develop squamous carcinoma of the esophagus (15). An area of high incidence in

coastal South Carolina has been associated a particular type of moonshine liquor (16).

Esophageal squamous carcinoma involves the entire esophagus with a tendency to have the highest incidence in the middle third. The tumor generally does not manifest clinically until dysplasia occurs, usually at an advanced stage. In countries where the incidence of gastroesophageal carcinoma is sufficiently high for screening, early esophageal squamous carcinomas are detected and treated at a curable stage. Early screening includes balloon cytology, used in high-risk areas of China (17), and upper endoscopy with Lugol's iodine staining in China and Japan (18). The finding of an early squamous carcinoma of the esophagus is rare in the United States at the present time.

The incidence trends of esophageal squamous carcinoma in the United States have shown an encouraging decline over the past 3 decades but this has not occurred in high-risk countries. In the United States, the incidence declined from 31 per million in 1973-1975 to 19 per million in 2001 (8). The reason for this decline in incidence is unknown. Improved food supply with a decrease in the use of preservatives, which generate potentially carcinogenic nitric acid metabolites, is suggested as a possible reason for the decline in the United States.

PATHOGENESIS OF ADENOCARCINOMA OF ESOPHAGUS

Adenocarcinoma of the esophagus is increasing in epidemic fashion in the United States, Western Europe, Canada, Australia, and New Zealand. In the United States, the incidence increased approximately sixfold from 3.8 per million in 1973-1975 to 23.3 per million in 2001 (8). The mortality from esophageal adenocarcinoma has paralleled this incidence increase, increasing from 2 per million in 1975 to 15 per million in 2001 (8). The number of patients in the United States with adenocarcinoma of the esophagus exceeded the number with squamous carcinoma in the mid-1990s (19).

After epithelial development has been completed at or soon after birth, no part of the esophagus is normally lined by columnar epithelium. This was not always an accepted fact; in fact, some physicians still believe there exists a phantom normal columnar epithelium. Adenocarcinoma in the esophagus arises after the normal squamous epithelium has undergone columnar metaplasia to form the columnar-lined esophagus.

COLUMNAR-LINED ESOPHAGUS

Columnar-lined esophagus is the precursor lesion of adenocarcinoma of the esophagus. Controversy surrounds the definition of the entity and this must be addressed in order to accurately identify all patients who are at risk for adenocarcinoma. Ninety percent of esophageal adenocarcinoma is diagnosed too late in its course to prevent death (20). The overall mortality in adenocarcinoma of the esophagus is over 80% (21). The mortality is much lower in patients who develop adenocarcinoma while under surveillance for Barrett's esophagus (22).

The present definitions of the early stages of reflux disease and the practice guidelines that are based on these definitions ignore a large number of persons at risk. This results from a failure of understanding of the pathogenesis of gastroesophageal reflux disease (5). It is therefore worthwhile to attempt to recognize the early changes with the hope that this will permit more effective prevention of reflux-induced adenocarcinoma in the future.

Original Description of the Columnar-Lined Esophagus

Allison and Johnstone (23) first described columnar-lined esophagus in 1953. Before this, the accepted viewpoint was that the esophagus ended at the squamocolumnar junction. When the squamocolumnar junction was displaced proximally in patients with columnar-lined esophagus, this definition resulted in the columnar-lined esophagus being called an *intrathoracic tubular stomach* (24). In 1953, Allison and Johnstone (23) proved that in some patients, there was a columnar-lined esophagus interposed between the stomach and the proximally displaced squamocolumnar junction.

The first description of the columnar-lined esophagus was well nigh perfect (23). In the description of the pathology of one of their specimens, Dr. D. H. Collins describes the method they used: "The oesophagus was separated with a knife from the stomach along the line of the peritoneal reflection. A vertical slice was then made through the centre of the reconstituted specimen, i.e., up the posterior wall, and three vertically contiguous blocks were prepared" (23). Histology carried out on this vertical slice showed: "The stomach below the anatomical junction with the oesophagus is lined by gastric mucosa of fundal type. . . . Cardiac glands and cardiac gastric mucosa do not appear until 0.6 cm up the anatomical oesophagus. . . . The rather villous type of cardiac mucosa, its lack of depth, and a diffuse fibrosis of the submucosa in the zone for 2 to 4 cm above the stomach orifice, suggest healing of previous shallow ulcerations." Allison and Johnstone (23) identify the esophageal characteristics of the columnar-lined segment between the squamocolumnar junction and the true gastroesophageal junction as follows: ". . . it has no peritoneal covering, that the musculature is that of the normal oesophagus, that there may be islands of squamous epithelium within it, that there are no oxyntic cells in the mucosa, and that in addition to gastric glands there are present typical oesophageal mucous glands."

To Allison and Johnstone (23), the entity was clearly definable as extending from the squamocolumnar junction proximally to the gastroesophageal junction distally. It was also clearly definable by histology because of the fact that normal gastric oxyntic mucosa was present at the gastroesophageal junction and the columnar-lined esophagus was lined by epithelia that we today call cardiac and oxyntocardiac mucosa that were readily differentiated from gastric oxyntic mucosa under the microscope. Their argument was so persuasive that Norman Barrett (25) reversed his viewpoint that this structure was a tubular stomach, reversed his definition of the esophagus as "that part of the foregut lined by squamous epithelium" and, in a classic article of 1957, coined the term *columnar-lined esophagus* that still bears his name. There is considerable injustice that Barrett's name is applied to an entity so perfectly described by Allison and Johnstone.

HISTOLOGIC DEFINITION OF EPITHELIAL TYPES

There are five basic epithelia that line the entire esophagus and the entire stomach to the point where pyloric antral mucosa arises in the distal stomach (5,26,27). These are stratified squamous epithelium and four types of columnar epithelia. All types of columnar epithelia have a surface and foveolar epithelium consisting of mucous cells. The four types of columnar epithelia are defined as follows: (a) gastric oxyntic mucosa, which contains straight tubular glands containing parietal cells and no mucous cells; (b) cardiac mucosa, which is composed of mucous cells without any parietal cells or goblet cells; (c) oxyntocardiac mucosa, which has glands composed of mucous and parietal cells; and (d) cardiac mucosa with intestinal metaplasia characterized by the presence of goblet cells. Other cell types may be found in these columnar epithelia: chief cells, Paneth cells, neuroendocrine cells, and pancreatic cells; these do not affect the basic classification of the four epithelial types.

Anatomic Location of Different Columnar Epithelia

Two of these epithelial types are universally present, usually lining a large surface area. The esophagus is lined by squamous epithelium and most of the proximal stomach is lined by gastric oxyntic mucosa. The majority of people have one, two, or three types of the other three columnar epithelia interposed between the gastric oxyntic mucosa and esophageal squamous epithelium (28).

Whenever a validated definition of the gastroesophageal junction such as the peritoneal reflection used by Allison and Johnstone (23), the epithelium at and distal to the junction is gastric oxyntic mucosa. De Hertogh et al. (4), in a recent study of fetal autopsy specimens, showed that the epithelium at and distal to the angle of His is gastric oxyntic mucosa. By these two validated definitions of the gastroesophageal junction, the other three columnar epithelial types are proximal to the junction and therefore represent columnar-lined esophagus. They are not found in the stomach.

What was absolutely clear in 1953 is in total confusion today. Over the years, physicians have introduced and used unvalidated definitions of the gastroesophageal junction brought on by the need to identify the junction endoscopically. The peritoneal reflection is neither visible at endoscopy nor demonstrable by biopsy.

In 1961, Hayward (29), in a highly influential article that was not accompanied by any data, introduced end of the tubular esophagus as the definition of the gastroesophageal junction: "The oesophagus is defined as the tube conducting food from the throat to the stomach and all of this tube is regarded as the oesophagus, irrespective of its lining." The intent of this statement was to confirm Allison and Johnstone's definition of the columnar-lined esophagus and debunk the concept of a tubular stomach. The unintended consequence was that the esophagus became equivalent to a tube and therefore ended at the distal end of the tube. The end of the tubular esophagus is still used as the definition of the gastroesophageal junction. In 2000, the Association of Directors of Anatomic and Surgical Pathology recommended that a horizontal line be drawn at the point where the tubular esophagus became the saccular stomach to define the junction (30). This is the standard of practice in the pathologic dissection of esophagogastrectomy specimens.

In patients who have a hiatal hernia, the demarcation of the end of the tubular esophagus is frequently not clear. The esophagus, rather than having a sharp angle of His, tapers gradually into the stomach like the neck of a bottle of chardonnay. In 1987, McClave et al. (31) described the proximal limit of the gastric rugal folds as a reliably definable endoscopic landmark. Over the years, this landmark has become accepted almost universally as the endoscopic gastroesophageal junction.

When the gastroesophageal junction is defined as either the end of the tubular esophagus or the proximal limit of the rugal folds, cardiac mucosa with and without intestinal metaplasia and oxyntocardiac mucosa straddle the junction and are partly in the esophagus and partly in the stomach. Because the columnar epithelia that line columnar-lined esophagus are identical microscopically to those in the "normal gastric cardia" distal to these definitions of the gastroesophageal junction, histologic examination no longer has the ability to diagnose columnar lined esophagus.

It is clear that there is a discrepancy between the original description by Allison and Johnstone and the present definitions. In a recent study (32), Chandrasoma et al. tested the present definitions of the gastroesophageal junction. They selected ten esophagectomy specimens that satisfied the following criteria (Figure 30.2): (a) they had a clearly demarcated junction

between the end of the tubular esophagus and the saccular structure distal to this; (b) the "gastric" rugal folds came all the way to the end of the tubular esophagus; and (c) the gastric oxyntic mucosa near the distal resection margin was without inflammation or *Helicobacter pylori* infection. Following the method of Allison and Johnstone (23), they separated the esophagus from the stomach at the line of the end of the tubular esophagus, which was the same as the line of the proximal limit of the rugal folds in these selected specimens. The entire circumference of the area distal to the end of the tubular esophagus was cut in with vertical sections, permitting mapping of the columnar epithelial types. Cardiac mucosa with and without intestinal metaplasia and oxyntocardiac mucosa extended 0.31 to 2.06 cm distal to the end of the tubular esophagus in these ten specimens, at which point the epithelium became gastric oxyntic mucosa (Figure 30.3). They correlated the presence of submucosal glands in these full-thickness sections and showed that submucosal glands were found within 0.5 cm proximal to the proximal limit of gastric oxyntic mucosa. Submucosal glands were never found under gastric oxyntic mucosa.

Submucosal glands are found in the esophagus and not in the stomach. Johns (3), in an extensive embryologic study of the esophagus, showed that these deep glands develop in the esophagus after fetal life and after the surface epithelium has developed into squamous epithelium. They do not develop in relation to fetal columnar epithelium in either the esophagus or the stomach.

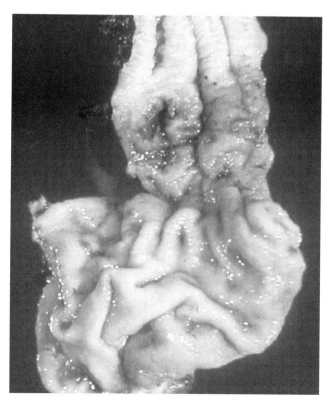

Figure 30.2 Esophagectomy specimen. A columnar-lined esophagus and adenocarcinoma are present in the tubular esophagus. There is a sharp line where the tubular esophagus ends. The rugal folds come all the way up to the end of the tubular esophagus.

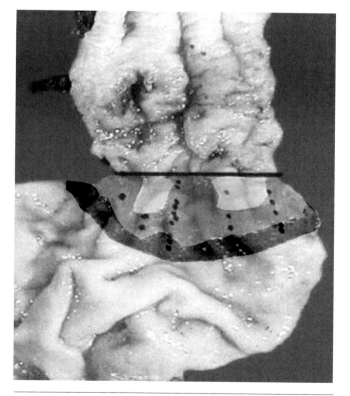

Figure 30.3 Mapping of epithelial types (yellow = cardiac mucosa with intestinal metaplasia; green = cardiac mucosa; pink = oxyntocardiac mucosa) and submucosal esophageal glands (black dots) in the proximal part of the saccular organ of specimen shown in Figure 30.2. (See color plates.)

We concluded that the data in our study prove that a variable part of the saccular organ distal to the end of the tubular esophagus and the proximal limit of the rugal folds is anatomically esophageal by the presence of submucosal glands. We suggested the term *dilated end-stage esophagus* to this area of esophagus. When the true gastroesophageal junction is defined as the proximal limit of gastric oxyntic mucosa, the dilated end-stage esophagus is accurately defined by the fact that the epithelium lining it consists of cardiac mucosa with and without intestinal metaplasia and oxyntocardiac mucosa.

Our study confirms the finding of Allison and Johnstone (23) that the epithelial lining at and distal to the true gastroesophageal junction (the peritoneal reflection) is gastric oxyntic mucosa. The dilated end-stage esophagus defined by our study shows several of the features that Allison and Johnstone used in 1953 to convince Norman Barrett that what he was calling a tubular stomach was actually esophagus. These include the presence of esophageal submucosal glands and a columnar lining other than gastric oxyntic mucosa. We did not find squamous islands in this region, but these have been reported to be present up to 3 cm distal to the proximal limit of rugal folds in 3% of endoscopies (33).

In a similar study of esophagectomy specimens, Sarbia et al. (34) reported the presence of cardiac and oxyntocardiac mucosa up to a maximum of 2.8 cm distal to the end of the tubular esophagus. In 25% of these cases, submucosal glands were present in this region. Jain et al. (35) showed the presence of cardiac mucosa in a biopsy taken 2 cm distal to the proximal limit of rugal folds in 3% of patients.

In all of these studies, the dilated end-stage esophagus has a limit of 3 cm distal to the end of the tubular esophagus. This is the approximate maximum length of the abdominal part of the normal lower esophageal sphincter (36). It is well known that gastroesophageal reflux disease is associated with a progressive loss of the lower esophageal sphincter, even in the early stages of the disease (37). Loss of sphincter tone in the abdominal esophagus is theoretically capable of causing dilatation of this part of the damaged esophagus, explaining both the dilatation and the maximal observed extent of the dilated end-stage esophagus.

DEFINITION OF COLUMNAR-LINED AND BARRETT'S ESOPHAGUS

Although the existence of columnar-lined esophagus was known since the early 20th century, the medical community throughout history has had an inexplicable need to underestimate its importance. Initially, by declaring that the esophagus ended at the squamocolumnar junction, the very existence of the columnar-lined esophagus was denied; it was called a tubular stomach (24). When Allison and Johnstone (23) defined the entity in 1953, both they and Barrett (25) initially regarded it as a relatively harmless congenital anomaly.

By the end of 1950s, it had become recognized that columnar-lined esophagus was not congenital; rather, it was caused by gastroesophageal reflux. In 1961, Hayward (29) wrote: "When the normal sphincteric and valvular mechanism in the lower oesophagus and oesophago-gastric junction, i.e., what I call the cardia, fails, ... reflux from the stomach occurs and acid and pepsin reach the squamous epithelium and begin to

digest it.... the destroyed epithelium may re-form, often with leucoplakia, or junctional (= cardiac) epithelium, usually not very healthy-looking, may replace it.... With repetition over a long period the metaplastic junctional (= cardiac) epithelium may creep higher and higher until it reaches the level of the arch of the aorta."

When columnar-lined esophagus was recognized as an acquired disease resulting from gastroesophageal reflux, it became necessary to define it by endoscopic criteria. Hayward (29), in his influential 1961article, declared without any supporting data, that "the lower centimetre or two of this tube (the esophagus) is normally lined by columnar epithelium, previously called cardiac and regarded as gastric, but in this paper called junctional and regarded as oesophageal. Thus the view that the oesophagus is lined only by squamous epithelium is rejected." He also stated that this "junctional" or "cardiac" columnar epithelium that lines the distal esophagus "extends a little way into the stomach" and "it must lie, as it does, astride the gastro-oesophageal junction partly in the oesophagus and partly in the stomach" (29). By this edict, cardiac mucosa moved into the stomach below the gastroesophageal junction.

The finding by Allison and Johnstone (23) that the columnar-lined esophagus ended at the true peritoneal reflection and gastric oxyntic mucosa was now modified without any evidence to justify it. The columnar-lined esophagus that Allison and Johnstone had described was effectively divided into three segments by Hayward (29): (a) "normal" cardiac mucosa lining the proximal stomach distal to the end of the tubular esophagus; (b) cardiac mucosa "normally" lining the distal 2 cm of the tubular esophagus; and (c) columnar-lined esophagus, recognized as abnormal only when it exceeded the 2 cm defined as normal by Hayward's edict.

This led to an incorrect practice at endoscopy wherein patients with <2 cm (this was actually increased to 3 cm for no good reason) of columnar lining in the esophagus were considered normal and not subject to biopsy till the mid-1990s. This practice resulted in only the most severely affected patients falling within the definition of an abnormal columnar-lined esophagus. In a screening study of 961 persons, Rex et al. (38) showed that only 12 of 65 (18.5%) persons with Barrett's esophagus by the present definition had columnar-lined esophagus exceeding 3 cm in length. Fifty-three patients with short-segment Barrett's esophagus would have been ignored between 1961 and 1994. The definition of the time made Barrett's esophagus a rare entity.

In the 1980s, evidence emerged that only patients with intestinal metaplasia in the columnar-lined esophagus were at risk for developing reflux-associated esophageal adenocarcinoma (39,40). This caused the definitions to change. The term *Barrett's esophagus* was now restricted to patients who had intestinal metaplasia in a biopsy and the intent of making the diagnosis of Barrett's esophagus became to identify risk of future adenocarcinoma. Columnar-lined esophagus without intestinal metaplasia was ignored and the fact that this was a manifestation of gastroesophageal reflux disease was lost.

Spechler et al. (41), in 1994, showed that when biopsies are taken from the 2 cm segment of "normal" columnar epithelium in the distal esophagus, 18% of patients had intestinal metaplasia. When, over the next few years, this was shown to be a significant risk for adenocarcinoma of the esophagus, short-segment Barrett's esophagus was recognized. Two elements are necessary to make a diagnosis of short-segment Barrett's esophagus: (a) a columnar-lined segment of esophagus must be seen at endoscopy above the proximal limit of the rugal folds; and (b) intestinal metaplasia must be present in a biopsy taken from this abnormal area.

These data caused a significant change in clinical practice (42). Biopsies were taken in any patient who had a visible columnar-lined esophagus. When the biopsies showed intestinal metaplasia, a diagnosis of Barrett's esophagus was made. In the screening study of Rex et al. (38), 164 of the 961 patients were found to have a visible columnar-lined esophagus measuring between 0.5 and 3 cm. Of these, 53 had intestinal metaplasia and therefore short-segment Barrett's esophagus. The prevalence of Barrett's esophagus increased more than fourfold by these new definitional criteria.

We presently recognize the following groups of patients who have columnar epithelia other than gastric oxyntic mucosa between the squamocolumnar junction and the proximal limit of gastric oxyntic epithelium: (a) *Patients with long-segment Barrett's esophagus* who have intestinal metaplasia in columnar-lined esophagus extending to >2 cm above the end of the tubular esophagus. (b) *Patients with >3 cm of columnar-lined esophagus without intestinal metaplasia*; this group is rare but does not fit into any presently recognized disease entity. In Europe, there is still a tendency for patients with >3 cm of columnar-lined esophagus to be diagnosed as having Barrett's esophagus even when they do not have intestinal metaplasia (7). (c) *Patients with short-segment Barrett's esophagus* who have intestinal metaplasia with a visible columnar-lined esophagus <2 cm long. (d) *Patients who have no intestinal metaplasia in a biopsy from a visible segment of columnar-lined esophagus*. These patients are ignored; they do not fit into any recognized disease entity. (e) *Patients without an endoscopically visible columnar-lined esophagus*. The present practice guidelines are to not biopsy these normal people, even when they have symptoms of reflux. If biopsies are taken distal to the endoscopic gastroesophageal junction, these patients have extremely varied histologic features. Most patients will have oxyntocardiac mucosa; some will have cardiac mucosa and a significant number will have intestinal metaplasia in cardiac mucosa. In the study by Chandrasoma et al. (43), 40% of patients in this category had neither intestinal nor cardiac mucosa, and 15% had intestinal metaplasia. Patients who have intestinal metaplasia in a biopsy distal to the endoscopic gastroesophageal junction are presently diagnosed as having "intestinal metaplasia of the gastric cardia."

It must be recognized that by the criteria of Allison and Johnstone (23) and the study by Chandrasoma et al. and Sarbia et al. (32,34), the true gastroesophageal junction is always lined by gastric oxyntic mucosa and may be as much as 2.8 cm distal to the presently recognized endoscopic definition of the gastroesophageal junction. This means that all patients who have a normal endoscopic appearance who have cardiac mucosa with and without intestinal metaplasia and oxyntocardiac mucosa in a biopsy distal to the endoscopic junction have microscopic columnar-lined esophagus in a reflux-damaged dilated end-stage esophagus that is presently mislabeled as stomach. The patients within this group who have intestinal metaplasia are at risk for esophageal adenocarcinoma. These patients are missed by present definitions and practice guidelines. The similarity to the mistake that resulted in short-segment Barrett's esophagus being missed for 35 years is eerie.

ESTABLISHING NORMALCY

The important question about columnar-lined esophagus is: What it normal? How much columnar epithelium, if any, normally exists between the normal squamous lining of the esophagus and the gastric oxyntic mucosa that normally lines the stomach? If such columnar epithelium normally exists, is it in the stomach or the esophagus? Histology textbooks still state that the distal 1 to 2 cm of the esophagus and the proximal 1 to 2 cm of the stomach are normally lined by cardiac mucosa (44,45).

The first autopsy study that was undertaken in an attempt to define normalcy was the study by Chandrasoma et al. (28). Although ultimately published in 2000, this study was referred to in many earlier articles because of the difficulty that was encountered getting it accepted (46,47). In the prospective part of this study, in which 18 specimens from patients who had died without any evidence of esophageal disease during life were completely examined, we showed that cardiac mucosa was absent in 10 (56%), the extent of cardiac mucosa was 0 to 2.75 mm, oxyntocardiac mucosa was present in all patients although it was absent from some part of the circumference in 9 (50%), and the maximum extent of combined cardiac and oxyntocardiac mucosa found separating squamous epithelium from gastric oxyntic mucosa was 8.05 mm. Only 4 (22%) of these 18 patients had a maximum combined cardiac and oxyntocardiac mucosal length exceeding 5 mm.

The results of the normal autopsy study should be compared with our study of esophagectomy specimens in patients undergoing resection for esophageal disease (32). The two patients with squamous carcinoma had a total separation of squamous from gastric oxyntic mucosa of 3.1 and 4.3 mm, which is similar to the autopsy population, reflecting the fact that squamous carcinoma has no known association with reflux disease. The eight patients with esophageal adenocarcinoma had a separation of squamous from gastric oxyntic mucosa ranging from 11.5 to 70.5 mm; this includes the columnar-lined segment in the tubular esophagus as well as the dilated end-stage esophagus.

These studies show that the separation of squamous from gastric oxyntic mucosa is very close to zero in normal persons and increases dramatically with reflux disease. In extreme cases, nonoxyntic columnar epithelia line almost the entire tubular esophagus and extend to 3 cm distal to the end of the tubular esophagus. We take this as strong evidence to suggest that all columnar epithelia other than gastric oxyntic mucosa are abnormal in this region and represent reflux-induced metaplasia of the esophageal squamous epithelium (5,27).

This concept is not yet accepted. The main objection to it is that oxyntocardiac mucosa is universally present at the junction, albeit in very small amounts. Most authorities now accept that cardiac mucosa may be absent, although they cling to the fact that a small amount (<4 mm) should be acceptable as normal (48), despite considerable proof that this is not correct (5,27).

Irrespective of whether a minute amount of cardiac and oxyntocardiac mucosa is universally present or not, it is likely that it is abnormal rather than normal. If gastroesophageal reflux is tested in the normal population by placing a pH or impedance probe in the lower esophagus, virtually everyone in the population will have episodes of reflux (49). An abnormal 24-hour pH study demands an exposure of the distal esophagus to a pH

>4.5% (or 64 minutes) of a 24-hour period (49). It is very likely that very small amounts of cardiac and oxyntocardiac mucosa found in most people is a reflection of this near-universal reflux. Universality does not equate to normalcy; otherwise we are in danger of regarding atherosclerosis of the abdominal aorta to be normal in adult males in the United States.

SIGNIFICANCE OF COLUMNAR EPITHELIA

There has never been any argument that columnar-lined esophagus is the result of a metaplastic change in the squamous epithelium of the esophagus resulting from damage caused by gastroesophageal reflux. Csendes et al. (50) demonstrated that the length of the columnar-lined esophagus directly correlated with the severity of reflux. Chandrasoma et al. compared a series of patients with measured biopsies taken from columnar-lined esophagus and showed that patients who had >2 cm of columnar-lined esophagus had a highly significantly greater severity of reflux as quantitated by a 24-hour pH study than patients with <2 cm of columnar-lined esophagus (26).

This correlation between severity of reflux has been shown to exist with very small lengths of cardiac and oxyntocardiac mucosa separating the squamous epithelium from gastric oxyntic mucosa. Oberg et al. (37), in a study of biopsies taken from endoscopically normal patients, showed that patients who had either cardiac or oxyntocardiac mucosa in their biopsies had a higher acid exposure in 24-hour pH tests and a significantly greater likelihood of abnormalities of the lower esophageal sphincter than patients who did not have these mucosal types in their biopsies. Glickman et al. (51), in a study of pediatric patients, many of whom had clinical reflux disease, showed that patients who had >1 mm of cardiac mucosa in their biopsy specimen had a greater likelihood of having symptoms of reflux than patients with <1 mm of cardiac mucosa. It is to be stressed that even patients with <1 mm of cardiac mucosa in this study had evidence of reflux disease, although at a lower frequency than those with longer segments of cardiac mucosa.

It appears clear from these studies that the presence of any cardiac or oxyntocardiac mucosa between the squamocolumnar junction and gastric oxyntic mucosa is associated with and caused by gastroesophageal reflux. The only normal epithelia in this region are squamous (esophageal) and gastric oxyntic. In the absolutely normal person, who is difficult to find in the population because of the almost universal prevalence of gastroesophageal reflux, the esophageal squamous epithelium transitions at the gastroesophageal junction into gastric oxyntic mucosa (28). Cardiac mucosa with and without intestinal metaplasia and oxyntocardiac mucosa are metaplastic esophageal epithelia and always represent columnar-lined esophagus.

Recognition of these facts permits a rational histology-based diagnosis of reflux disease that can define the presence of reflux and its severity. There are four gradations of disease severity: (a) no reflux: patients with only squamous epithelium and gastric oxyntic mucosa; (b) mild reflux: patients who are endoscopically normal but have epithelia denoting columnar-lined esophagus in biopsies taken distal to the squamocolumnar junction and proximal to the true gastroesophageal junction (proximal limit

of gastric oxyntic mucosa); (c) moderate reflux: patients with visible columnar-lined esophagus <2 cm long; and (d) severe reflux: patients with >2 cm of columnar-lined esophagus. In all these groups, the presence of intestinal metaplasia in cardiac mucosa represents Barrett's esophagus. Although the four groups are classified according to severity of reflux disease, the presence of intestinal metaplasia indicates increased risk of cancer, irrespective of risk. The combination of the two results in a new classification of gastroesophageal reflux disease (Table 30.1) (5,27).

Table 30.1

Classification of Gastroesophageal Reflux Disease Based on Risk of Adenocarcinoma of the Esophagus[a]

Grade zero: No risk of adenocarcinoma (55%–65%)

Definition: No cardiac mucosa or intestinal metaplasia in any biopsy.
Subgroups:
Group 0a: Normal: Only squamous epithelium and gastric oxyntic mucosa
Group 0b: Compensated reflux: Oxyntocardiac mucosa as the only epithelium in the metaplastic columnar esophagus.

Grade 1: Reflux disease (30%–45%)

Definition: Cardiac mucosa (reflux carditis) present; oxyntocardiac mucosa also present in most cases.
Subgroups:
Group 1a: Mild reflux disease: Cardiac mucosa length <1 cm. Endoscopy normal.
Group 1b: Moderate reflux disease: Cardiac mucosa and oxyntocardiac mucosa length = 1–2 cm.
Group 1c: Severe reflux disease: Cardiac mucosa and oxyntocardiac mucosa length >2 cm.

Grade 2: Barrett's esophagus (5%–15%)

Definition: Intestinal metaplasia (goblet cells) present in cardiac mucosa; nonintestinalized cardiac mucosa and oxyntocardiac mucosa also present in most cases.
Subgroups:
Group 2a: Barrett's esophagus in reflux disease limited to dilated end-stage esophagus (microscopic Barrett's esophagus): Endoscopy normal.
Group 2b: Short-segment Barrett's esophagus: Endoscopy shows a columnar-lined esophagus <2 cm long.
Group 2c: Long-segment Barrett's esophagus: Endoscopy shows a columnar-lined esophagus >2 cm long.

Grade 3: Neoplastic Barrett's esophagus

Definition: Dysplasia or adenocarcinoma present.
Subgroups:
Group 3a: Low-grade dysplasia.
Group 3b: High-grade dysplasia.
Group 3c: Adenocarcinoma.

[a] The percentage of the population within each group is in parentheses.

RECLASSIFICATION OF ADENOCARCINOMA OF THE GASTRIC CARDIA

Present pathologic classification of adenocarcinomas in this region is based on the gastroesophageal junction being defined as the end of the tubular esophagus. A tumor with its epicenter above this line is esophageal and below this line is gastric. Tumors that involve the junctional region are classified under the gastric cardia code in the International Classification of Diseases.

The error associated with the present definition of the gastroesophageal junction raises the possibility that tumors presently classified as adenocarcinoma of the gastric cardia are truly adenocarcinomas of the esophagus. In a study of 36 adenocarcinomas classified by present criteria as tumors of the gastric cardia, we mapped the epithelium at the epicenter and distal edge of the tumor and showed that only 16 had gastric oxyntic mucosa at the distal edge, indicating that 20 of these tumors were entirely within the esophagus if the proximal limit of gastric oxyntic mucosa was the gastroesophageal junction (27). Of the remaining 16 patients, the epithelium at the epicenter of the tumor was not gastric oxyntic in any patient, indicating that >50% of these tumors were esophageal. We suggested that most adenocarcinomas of the gastric cardia are in reality adenocarcinomas of the distal esophagus occurring in the dilated end-stage esophagus presently misclassified as gastric cardia.

This would explain the epidemiologic anomalies where the increasing incidence curve of adenocarcinoma of the gastric cardia has largely paralleled that of adenocarcinoma of the esophagus and the increased risk of adenocarcinoma of the gastric cardia in patients with symptomatic gastroesophageal reflux disease.

The correction of this error will result in a doubling of the present incidence of reflux-induced adenocarcinoma because adenocarcinoma of the gastric cardia has a numerical incidence that is equal to or greater than that of esophageal adenocarcinoma. Correct delineation of risk of cancer in reflux disease drives all calculations of cost-effectiveness of proposed preventive measures.

THE REFLUX-ADENOCARCINOMA SEQUENCE

The pathogenesis of esophageal adenocarcinoma passes through three stages: (a) columnar metaplasia of the squamous-lined esophagus to produce the columnar-lined esophagus; (b) intestinal metaplasia, which is Barrett's esophagus; and (c) carcinogenesis, which occurs in the intestinal metaplastic type of columnar lined esophagus.

Columnar Metaplasia of Esophageal Squamous Epithelium

The normal squamous epithelium is impermeable to luminal molecules (6). The primary effect of acid reflux is to cause damage that increases the permeability of the epithelium. Tobey et al. (6,52) showed that acid damage of squamous epithelium causes separation of the keratinocytes ("dilated intercellular spaces") and permits the passage of molecules up to 20 kD in size into the epithelium. As the degree of damage increases, larger molecules gain access to increasing depths of the epithelium. Acid reflux is the key that opens the permeability lock of normal squamous epithelium.

The entry of complex molecules in the refluxate permits the interaction between receptors in the proliferating cells and molecules in the refluxate. An unknown molecular-cell interaction must cause a switch in the genetic signal of these proliferating cells that causes them to change the differentiation from squamous to columnar. This is the genetic and molecular basis of columnar metaplasia of the esophagus. The fact that this change is extremely common suggests that the molecule responsible is ubiquitous in the gastric refluxate. The exact nature of the genetic switch involved is unknown.

Columnar metaplasia leads to the replacement of stratified squamous to a simple columnar epithelium composed of a flat layer of columnar mucous cells. This quickly invaginates and organizes itself into a complex columnar epithelium composed of surface and foveolar columnar cells and glands composed of mucous cells. This is cardiac mucosa.

The fact that cardiac mucosa is the first epithelium to arise from columnar metaplasia of squamous epithelium is shown by two sets of data. First, reflux-induced columnar metaplasia of the esophagus in children consists largely of cardiac mucosa without intestinal metaplasia (53). Second, patients who have had esophagogastrectomy with a gastric pullup have been shown to develop cardiac mucosa above the anastomotic line as the first evidence of postoperative columnar metaplasia (54–56). This is followed, often several months or years later, by the occurrence of intestinal metaplasia in some patients.

Intestinal Metaplasia in Cardiac Mucosa

The occurrence of intestinal metaplasia in cardiac mucosa is the definitive criterion for the diagnosis of Barrett's esophagus in a patient with columnar-lined esophagus. There is evidence that activation of *CDX* genes is associated with intestinal metaplasia in cardiac mucosa (57,58). *CDX* genes are normally expressed in the small and large intestine, but suppressed in the normal esophagus.

The likelihood of intestinal metaplasia increases as the length of columnar-lined esophagus increases. In our mapping study (43), intestinal metaplasia had a prevalence of 15% when the columnar epithelial length was <1 cm; 70% at 1 to 2 cm; 90% at 3 to 4 cm; and 100% when the columnar lined segment reached 5 cm. In patients who develop intestinal metaplasia, the goblet cells are most likely to occur and are most prevalent in the most proximal part of the columnar-lined segment (59).

The fact that intestinal metaplasia is invariably present when the columnar epithelial length reaches 5 cm suggests that the molecule that causes intestinal metaplasia is invariably present in gastric refluxate. The distribution of intestinal metaplasia in the most proximal zone of the columnar-lined esophagus suggests the possibility that this is a pH-related event.

In patients who have no reflux, the pH of the esophagus is neutral to the end of the lower esophageal sphincter, at which point there is a sudden change in pH to normal gastric pH, which is normally 1 to 3. When reflux occurs, the acid gastric

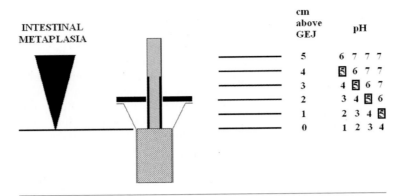

Figure 30.4 The effect of pH in the pathogenesis of intestinal metaplasia in cardiac mucosa. Four different baseline gastric pHs (1–4) are shown to the right. With different reflux volumes, there is a varying time exposure and gradient of increasing alkalinity to the normal pH of 7 in the esophagus. If intestinal metaplasia is favored by a pH of 5 (highlighted in a box), the maximal tendency to intestinal metaplasia of cardiac mucosa will occur most proximally where the highest volume reflux has the appropriate pH. GEJ, gastroesophageal junction.

juice decreases the esophageal pH, displacing proximally the point at which neutrality is reached. This sets up a pH gradient from the normal 1 to 3 at the gastroesophageal junction to 7 at the point in the esophagus either above the column of refluxate or where the refluxed acid is neutralized. The exact pH gradient in the esophagus and the time of exposure of the cell to refluxate depends on the volume and frequency of reflux.

Cardiac metaplasia of the esophagus must exist for intestinal metaplasia to occur. The length of cardiac mucosa in different people is a function of the cumulative effect of reflux damage in that patient. The fact that intestinal metaplasia is most prevalent in long segments of columnar-lined esophagus and occurs in the most proximal region suggests that intestinal metaplasia occurs in the region of the greatest degree of alkalinity (27) (Figure 30.4). The fact that intestinal metaplasia is less likely to occur in the distal regions of a columnar-lined segment suggests that the lower pH (more acid) environment of the more distal region inhibits intestinal metaplasia.

If it is true that the occurrence of intestinal metaplasia is induced by alkalinity, it would follow that acid-suppressive drugs would promote intestinal metaplasia in columnar-lined esophagus. The inevitable and desired result of acid suppression is to increase baseline gastric pH. This is the reason why symptoms of reflux are controlled and erosive esophagitis heals with acid suppression. However, an unwanted effect of this would be the promotion of intestinal metaplasia in cardiac mucosa. This would explain the historic increase in the prevalence of intestinal metaplasia over the past 5 decades.

Carcinogenesis in Barrett's Esophagus

The induction of carcinoma in Barrett's esophagus depends on an unknown sequence of irreversible genetic mutations. The target cells for carcinogens are limited to proliferative cells in columnar-lined epithelium that is marked by the presence of intestinal metaplasia. It is as if the genetic switch that causes the

esophageal cell to differentiate into goblet cells makes it receptive to carcinogenic molecules.

Esophageal adenocarcinoma has the characteristic of a tumor caused by the effect of a luminal molecule associated with gastroesophageal reflux. The carcinogen involved is unknown but must reside in the gastric juice. There is a significant body of evidence that suggests that bile acid metabolites are implicated in the genesis of esophageal adenocarcinoma (60–63). The entry of bile into the stomach by duodenogastric reflux is a very common phenomenon in humans. In a patient with normal gastric acidity in the 1 to 3 pH range, bile acids precipitate into harmless insoluble molecules. At a pH above 6, the bile acids remain in an ionized form that precludes their entry into cells. Between a pH of 3 and 6, the bile acids and their metabolites are converted to un-ionized soluble molecules that can penetrate cell membranes and enter epithelial cells (64). Bile acid metabolites have been shown to have capability in entering epithelial cells and binding with cellular receptors in esophageal progenitor cells to activate many different metabolic pathways in experimental models using cell lines. Jaiswal et al. (61,62) showed that the conjugated bile salt glycochenodeoxycholic acid was highly effective in activating genetic pathways in a Barrett adenocarcinoma cell line and a nonneoplastic Barrett cell line. These pathways are known to promote cell proliferation and inhibit apoptosis.

Acid suppression, particularly when it is uncontrolled as in most patients who take these medications, both over-the-counter and prescribed, has the effect of increasing gastric pH into the critical 3 to 6 pH range, where it promotes the generation of carcinogenic molecules from the endogenous bile acids when these are present in the stomach.

The genetic changes of carcinogenesis occur in the esophagus when there is an interaction of sufficient duration between the target cell and the carcinogen. The two factors involved operate in diametrically opposite locations: (a) intestinal metaplasia, which contains the target cells, tend to occur maximally in the more proximal part of the columnar-lined esophagus, whatever

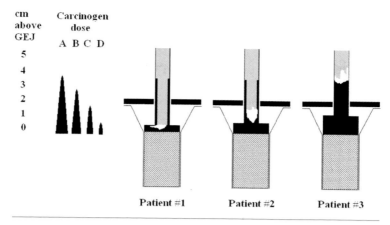

Figure 30.5 Interplay between different carcinogen doses (A–D) and the level of intestinal metaplasia in the esophagus. Carcinogenesis will not occur unless a sufficient carcinogenic dose reaches an area where there is intestinal metaplasia. In patient 1 (very short-segment Barrett's esophagus limited to the dilated end-stage esophagus), carcinogenesis is possible in all four dose levels A–D. In patient 2, carcinogenesis will occur only in dose levels A, B, and C; it will not occur in the lowest level D. Patient 3 is at risk of cancer only with the highest carcinogen dose environment (A) because it is only at this level that carcinogenic effect reaches the area of intestinal metaplasia proximally in the esophagus. Lowering the level at which intestinal metaplasia is present in the esophagus increases carcinogen interaction in all patients. GEJ, gastroesophageal junction.

its length, and (b) the carcinogen dose is always maximal in the stomach and declines as it moves up the esophagus at a rate that depends on the severity of reflux (Figure 30.5). The fact that esophageal adenocarcinomas tend to occur in the more distal region of a long segment of Barrett's esophagus provides support for the concept that the carcinogen milieu is highest in the distal esophagus. Delivery of an adequate carcinogen dose to target cells will be enhanced by anything that promotes intestinal metaplasia in the more distal regions of the columnar-lined segment. If the previous suggestion that the generation of intestinal metaplasia in cardiac mucosa is promoted by increasing alkalinity of gastric juice, a theoretical basis exists for acid-suppressive drugs promoting cancer (Figure 30.6).

There is, in fact, evidence that the use of acid-suppressive drugs promote esophageal adenocarcinoma. In the landmark study that established the association between symptomatic reflux and adenocarcinoma of the esophagus and gastric cardia, Lagergren et al. (7) report: *"We compared the risk of esophageal adenocarcinoma among persons who used medication for symptoms of reflux at least five years before the interview with that among symptomatic persons who did not use such medication. The odds ratio was 3.0 (95 percent confidence interval, 2.0 to 4.6) without adjustment for the severity of symptoms and 2.9 (95 percent confidence interval, 1.9 to 4.6) with this adjustment."* There are no contrary data that prove that acid-suppressive drug use either decreases or does not increase the risk of cancer. Most studies show a trend that suggest that acid-suppressive drugs may promote cancer but do not have the statistical power to prove this.

It is not difficult to understand why acid-suppressive drugs can theoretically promote carcinogenesis. Acid suppression does not prevent reflux; it simply removes the acid from the reflux-ate (65). Reflux continues unabated; the esophageal epithelium is exposed to all the molecules in the refluxate except acid. Because columnar-lined esophagus is probably generated relatively early in life, the use of acid-suppressive drugs, by increasing the tendency to intestinal metaplasia in columnar-lined esophagus and increasing the carcinogenicity of bile acid derivatives, would theoretically be expected to promote cancer.

CLINICAL MANAGEMENT IMPLICATIONS

The management of gastroesophageal reflux disease at the present time is almost entirely based on controlling symptoms and healing erosive esophagitis with acid-suppressive drugs. The entire population is encouraged to do this. The government, by permitting the most powerful acid-suppressive agents to be sold over-the-counter without prescription, has permitted the pharmaceutical companies that produce these drugs to directly market to the consumer and create an impression that these are miracle drugs that can cure reflux disease. "Pop a purple pill and eat whatever you want without the penalty of acid reflux" is the mantra that comes over the television airways.

Although this may have been appropriate in the days when the penalty of reflux disease was pain, erosions, and strictures, it is certainly not appropriate today. Reflux disease has reared a new ugly head—adenocarcinoma—and the medical community has done nothing to alter its course in how this disease is managed. We still look at reflux disease as a disease that causes heartburn and erosions and not as a disease that causes the death by reflux-induced adenocarcinoma of approximately 14,000

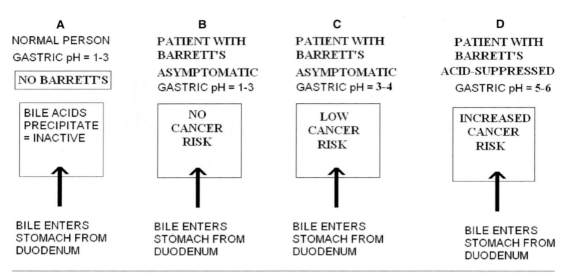

Figure 30.6 The effect of gastric pH on bile acids. Carcinogenic molecules are produced from bile acids at intermediate levels of gastric pH. Note that bile acids are derived from duodenogastric reflux; entry of bile acids is inevitably associated with alkalinization of gastric juice (B). This natural alkalinization is enhanced in patients receiving acid-suppressive drugs (C), shown as increasing carcinogenicity.

Americans per year. We do nothing to find most of these people before they present with advanced cancer. By treating reflux disease at all stages with acid suppression only, we subscribe to the naïve and incorrect notion that every manifestation of reflux disease, including cancer, is caused by the acid in the reflux. In fact, while the acid may cause all the pain and the strictures, it may actually protect against the development of intestinal metaplasia in columnar-lined esophagus and carcinogenesis in intestinal metaplasia. Acid suppression, while curing the symptoms, may promote intestinal metaplasia and cancer. It is important to understand that there need not be proof of this to consider the use of acid-suppressive drugs unsafe. The burden is not to prove that acid-suppressive drugs cause cancer; rather, the burden is to prove that they do not cause cancer by the people producing them and using them.

Antireflux surgery is the alternate form of treatment of gastroesophageal reflux disease. At present, this is most commonly a laparoscopic Nissen fundoplication. Antireflux surgery is a highly effective method of controlling the most severe of reflux symptoms and curing erosive reflux disease (66,67). It is at least as effective as acid-suppressive drugs. Unlike acid-suppressive drugs, a successful fundoplication creates a new valve at the gastroesophageal junction and effectively prevents gastroesophageal reflux (68). Not only is the exposure of the esophagus to acid prevented, but also the exposure of the esophagus to every other molecule in the refluxate (Figure 30.7). If the surgery is successful, the progression of reflux disease must stop if this is a disease that is produced by luminal molecules.

The only downside to antireflux surgery is the fact that it is a surgical procedure, albeit laparoscopic and associated with a short hospital stay, that there is a failure rate of approximately 20% at the present time, and that there are complications such as dysphagia. Surgery results in a front-end cost, but it has been shown in European studies that the lifetime cost is actually reduced because 80% of patients do not require lifelong acid-suppressive drug treatment (69,70).

At the present time, antireflux surgery is used only when medical treatment has failed or when the disease is severe and complicated. Although the frequency of antireflux procedures has increased, the total number of patients treated in this manner still remains relatively small. In this milieu, it is impossible to find data that prove that antireflux surgery has a protective effect against cancer. In the absence of proof, the statement is made that there is no evidence to support the use of antireflux surgery as a cancer-preventive treatment in patients with reflux. This is a classic catch-22 argument. Even if large-scale randomized clinical trials were undertaken today, the low incidence of adenocarcinoma and the slow rate of development of adenocarcinoma in reflux disease would mean that the statistical power to provide proof will take many years. During this time, all that the medical community is doing is continuing the present treatment with acid-suppressive drugs, which has a known theoretical and demonstrated risk of promoting cancer and which has been associated with a sixfold increase in incidence over the past 30 years. Parrilla et al. (68), in a well-designed randomized clinical trial, have shown that even with a small number of patients followed over a relatively short time, there is at least a suggestion, if not proof, that successful antireflux surgery decreases the progression of intestinal metaplasia to increasing dysplasia and cancer. We have shown that reversal of intestinal metaplasia frequently occurs in columnar-lined esophagus after antireflux surgery.

The combination of the abject failure of present acid-suppressive drug regimens in preventing reflux-induced cancer and the availability of a surgical procedure that theoretically prevents disease progression and has been demonstrated in small studies to practically decrease the risk of adenocarcinoma should result in a dramatic and immediate shift of the treatment of gastroesophageal reflux disease from medical acid suppression to antireflux surgery. As the number of patients so treated increases, it is likely that the expertise will increase, the number of complications will decrease, and the failure rate will decrease. When this is coupled with the fact that the cost of treatment is less

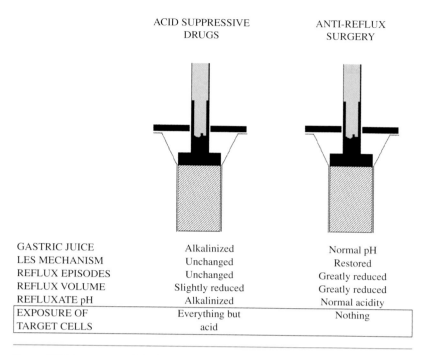

Figure 30.7 Depiction of the fundamental difference between the effect of acid-suppressive drug therapy and antireflux surgery. Acid-suppressive drugs simply change acid reflux to non–acid reflux of similar volume. The target cells in the esophagus continue to be bombarded by all refluxate molecules except H^+. Antireflux surgery eradicates all reflux when it is successful. LES, lower esophageal sphincter.

than lifelong acid suppression, there is no argument that antireflux surgery is the clear first-line treatment of choice at least in the symptomatic patient with gastroesophageal reflux disease. The expectation of a greatly increased use of antireflux surgery is a reversal of the trend of increasing adenocarcinoma of the esophagus.

REFERENCES

1. Karam SM. Lineage commitment and maturation of epithelial cells in the gut. *Front Biosci.* 1999;4:286–298.
2. Liebermann-Meffert D, Duranceau A, et al. Anatomy and embryology. In: Orringer MB, Heitmiller R, eds. *The Esophagus.* Vol 1. Zudeima GD, Yeo CJ. *Shackelford's Surgery of the Alimentary Tract.* 5th ed. Philadelphia: WB Saunders; 2002:3–39.
3. Johns BAE. Developmental changes in the oesophageal epithelium in man. *J Anat.* 1952;86:431–442.
4. De Hertogh G, Van Eyken P, Ectors N, et al. On the existence and location of cardiac mucosa; an autopsy study in embryos, fetuses, and infants. *Gut.* 2003;52:791–796.
5. Chandrasoma P. Controversies of the cardiac mucosa and Barrett's esophagus. *Histopathology.* 2005;46:361–373.
6. Tobey NA, Hosseini SS, Argore CM, et al. Dilated intercellular spaces and shunt permeability in non-erosive acid-damaged esophageal epithelium. *Am J Gastroenterol.* 2004;99:13–22.
7. Lagergren J, Bergstrom R, Lindgren A, et al. Symptomatic gastroesophageal reflux as a risk factor for esophageal adenocarcinoma. *N Engl J Med.* 1999;340:825–831.
8. Pohl H, Welch HG. The role of overdiagnosis and reclassification in the marked increase of esophageal adenocarcinoma incidence. *J Natl Cancer Inst.* 2005;97:142–146.
9. Kirby TJ, Rice TW. The epidemiology of esophageal cancer: The changing face of a disease. *Chest Surg Clin North Am.* 1994;4:217–225.
10. Chang F, Syrjanen S, Wang L, et al. Infectious agents in the etiology of esophageal cancer. *Gastroenterology.* 1992;103:1336–1348.
11. Gao GF, Roth MJ, Wei WQ, et al. No association between HPV infection and the neoplastic progression of esophageal squamous cell carcinoma: Result from a cross-sectional study in a high-risk region of China. *Int J Cancer.* 2006;119:1354–1359.
12. Isolauri J, Markkula H. Lye ingestion and carcinoma of the esophagus. *Acta Chir Scand.* 1989;155:269–271.
13. Harper PS, Harper RM, Howel-Evans AW. Carcinoma of the esophagus with tylosis. *QJ Med.* 1970;39:317–333.
14. Peracchia A, Segalin A, Bardini R, et al. Esophageal carcinoma and achalasia: Prevalence, incidence and results of treatment. *Hepatogastroenterology.* 1991;38:514–516.
15. Matsumoto M, Natsugoe S, Okumura H, et al. Clinicopathological and biological characteristics of esophageal squamous cell carcinoma associated with head and neck cancer. *Oncology.* 2004;67:98–102
16. Brown LM, Blot WJ, Schuman SH, et al. Environmental factors and high risk of esophageal cancer among men in coastal South Carolina. *J Natl Cancer Inst.* 1988;80:1620–1625.
17. Wang LD, Yang HH, Fan ZM, et al. Cytological screening and 15 years' follow-up (1986-2001) for early esophageal squamous cell carcinoma and precancerous lesions in a high-risk population in

Anyang County, Henan Province, Northern China. *Cancer Detect Prev.* 2005;29:317–322.

18. Katagiri A, Kaneko K, Konishi K, et al. Lugol staining pattern in background epithelium of patients with esophageal squamous cell carcinoma. *Hepatogastroenterology.* 2004;51:713–717.

19. Devesa SS, Blot WJ, Fraumeni JF. Changing patterns in the incidence of esophageal and gastric carcinoma in the United States. *Cancer* 1998;83:2049–2053.

20. Dulai GS, Guha S, Kahn KL, et al. Preoperative prevalence of Barrett's esophagus in esophageal adenocarcinoma: a systematic review. *Gastroenterology.* 2002;122:26–33.

21. Spechler SJ. Barrett's esophagus. *N Engl J Med.* 2002;346:836–842.

22. Peters JH, Clark GWB, Ireland AP, et al. Outcome of adenocarcinoma arising in Barrett's esophagus in endoscopically surveyed and nonsurveyed patients. *J Thorac Cardiovasc Surg.* 1994;108:813–821.

23. Allison PR, Johnstone AS. The oesophagus lined with gastric mucous membrane. *Thorax.* 1953;8:87–101.

24. Barrett NR. Chronic peptic ulcer of the oesophagus and "oesophagitis." *Br J Surg.* 1950;38:175–182.

25. Barrett NR. The lower esophagus lined by columnar epithelium. *Surgery.* 1957;41:881–894.

26. Chandrasoma PT, Lokuhetty DM, DeMeester, TR, et al. Definition of histopathologic changes in gastroesophageal reflux disease. *Am J. Surg Pathol.* 2000;24:344–351.

27. Chandrasoma PT, DeMeester TR. *GERD: From Reflux to Esophageal Adenocarcinoma.* San Diego: Academic Press; 2006.

28. Chandrasoma PT, Der R, Ma Y, et al. Histology of the gastroesophageal junction: an autopsy study. *Am J Surg Pathol.* 2000;24:402–409.

29. Hayward J. The lower end of the oesophagus. *Thorax.* 1961;16:36–41.

30. Association of Directors of Anatomic and Surgical Pathology. Recommendations for reporting of resected esophageal adenocarcinomas. *Am J Surg Pathol.* 2000;31:1188–1190.

31. McClave SA, Boyce HW Jr, Gottfried MR. Early diagnosis of columnar lined esophagus: A new endoscopic diagnostic criterion. *Gastrointest Endosc.* 1987;33:413–416.

32. Chandrasoma P, Makarewicz K, Wickramasinghe K, et al. A proposal for a new validated histologic definition of the gastroesophageal junction. *Human Pathol.* 2006;37:40–47.

33. Fass R, Sampliner RE. Extension of squamous epithelium into the proximal stomach: a newly recognized mucosal abnormality.*Endoscopy.* 2000;32:27–32.

34. Sarbia M, Donner A, Gabbert HE. Histopathology of the gastroesophageal junction. A study on 36 operation specimens. *Am J Surg Pathol.* 2002;26:1207–1212.

35. Jain R. Aquino D, Harford WV, et al. Cardiac epithelium is found infrequently in the gastric cardia [abstract]. *Gastroenterology.* 1998;114:A160.

36. DeMeester TR, Peters JH, Bremner CG, et al. Biology of gastroesophageal reflux disease: pathophysiology relating to medical and surgical treatment. *Annu Rev Med.* 1999;50:469–506.

37. Oberg S, Peters JH, DeMeester TR, et al. Inflammation and specialized intestinal metaplasia of cardiac mucosa is a manifestation of gastroesophageal reflux disease. *Ann Surg.* 1997;226:522–532.

38. Rex DK, Cummings OW, Shaw M, et al. Screening for Barrett's esophagus in colonoscopy patients with and without heartburn. *Gastroenterology.* 2003;125:1670–1677.

39. Haggitt RC, Dean PJ. Adenocarcinoma in Barrett's epithelium. In: Spechler SJ, Goyal RK, eds. *Barrett's Esophagus: Pathophysiology, Diagnosis and Management.* New York: Elsevier Science Publishing; 1985:153–166.

40. Reid BJ, Weinstein WM. Barrett's and adenocarcinoma. *Annu Rev Med.* 1987;38:477–492.

41. Spechler SJ, Zeroogian JM, Antonioli DA, et al. Prevalence of metaplasia at the gastroesophageal junction. *Lancet.* 1994;344:1533–1536.

42. Sampliner RE. Practice guidelines on the diagnosis, surveillance, and therapy of Barrett's esophagus. *Am J Gastroenterol.* 1998;93:1028–1031.

43. Chandrasoma PT, Der R, Ma Y, et al. Histologic Classification of Patients Based on Mapping Biopsies of the Gastroesophageal Junction. *Am J Surg Pathol.* 2003;27:929–936.

44. De Nardi FG, Riddell RH. Esophagus. In: Sternberg SS, ed. *Histology for Pathologists,* 2nd edition. Philadelphia: Lippincott-Raven Publishers; 1997:461–480.

45. Owen DA. Stomach. In: Sternberg SS, ed. *Histology for Pathologists,* 2nd edition. Philadelphia Lippincott-Raven Publishers; 1997:481–493.

46. Chandrasoma P. Pathophysiology of Barrett's esophagus. *Semin Thoracic Cardiovasc Surg.* 1997;9:270–278.

47. Chandrasoma P. Non-neoplastic diseases of the esophagus. In: Chandrasoma P. *Gastrointestinal Pathology.* Stamford, CT: Appleton & Lange; 1999:9–36.

48. Odze RD. Unraveling the mystery of the gastroesophageal junction: a pathologist's perspective. *Am J Gastroenterol.* 2005;100:1853–1867.

49. Jamieson JR, Stein HJ, DeMeester TR, et al. Ambulatory 24-hour esophageal pH monitoring: normal values, optimal thresholds, specificity, sensitivity, and reproducibility. *Am J Gastroenterol.* 1992;87:1102–1111.

50. Csendes A, Maluenda F, Braghetto I, et al. Location of the lower esophageal sphincter and the squamocolumnar mucosal junction in 109 healthy controls and 778 patients with different degrees of endoscopic esophagitis. *Gut.* 1993;34:21–27.

51. Glickman JN, Fox V, Antonioli DA, et al. Morphology of the cardia and significance of carditis in pediatric patients. *Am J Surg Pathol.* 2002;26:1032–1039.

52. Tobey NA, Carson JL, Alkiek RA, et al. Dilated intercellular spaces: a morphological feature of acid reflux-damaged human esophageal epithelium. *Gastroenterology.* 1996;111:1200–1205.

53. Hassall E. Barrett's esophagus: new definitions and approaches in children. *J Pediatiatr Gastroenterol Nutr.* 1993;16:345–364.

54. Dresner SM, Griffin SM, Wayman J, et al. Human model of duodenogastro-oesophageal reflux in the development of Barrett's metaplasia. *Br J Surg.* 2003;90:1120–1128.

55. Lord R, Wickramasinghe K, Johansson JJ, et al. Cardiac mucosa in the remnant esophagus after esophagectomy is an acquired epithelium with Barrett's-like features. *Surgery.* 2004;136:633–640.

56. Oberg S, Johansson J, Wenner J, et al. Metaplastic columnar mucosa in the cervical esophagus after esophagectomy. *Ann Surg.* 2002;235:338–345.

57. Silberg DG, Furth EE, Taylor JK, et al. CDX1 protein expression in normal, metaplastic, and neoplastic human alimentary tract epithelium. *Gastroenterology.* 1997;113:478–486.

58. Phillips RW, Frierson HF, Moskaluk CA. Cdx2 as a marker of epithelial differentiation in the esophagus. *Am J Surg Pathol.* 2003;27:1442–1447.

59. Chandrasoma PT, Der R, Dalton P, etal. Distribution and significance of epithelial types in columnar lined esophagus. *Am J Surg Pathol.* 2001;25:1188–1193.

60. Nehra D. Howell P, Williams CP, et al. Toxic bile acids in gastro-oesophageal reflux disease: influence of gastric acidity. *Gut.* 1999;44:598–602.

61. Jaiswal K, Tello V, Lopez-Guzman C, et al. Bile salt exposure causes phosphtidyl-inositol-3-kinase-mediated proliferation in a Barrett's adenocarcinoma cell line. *Surgery.* 2004;136:160–168.

62. Jaiswal K, Lopez-Guzman C, Souza RF, et al. Bile salt exposure increases proliferation through p38 and ERK-MAPK pathways in non-neoplastic Barrett's cell line. *Am J Physiol Gastrointest Liver Physiol.* 2006;290:G335–342.

63. Stamp DH. Bile acids aided by acid suppression therapy may be associated with the development of esophageal cancers in Westernized societies. *Med Hypothesis.* 2002;59:398–405.

64. Kauer WK, Stein HJ. Bile reflux in the constellation of gastroesophageal reflux disease. *Thorac Surg Clin.* 2005;15:335–340.

65. Tamhankar AP, Peters JH, Portale G, et al. Omeprazole does not reduce gastroesophageal reflux: new insights using multichannel intraluminal impedance technology. *J Gastrointest Surg.* 2004;8: 890–898.

66. Eubanks TR, Omelanczuk P, Richards C, et al. Outcomes of laparoscopic antireflux procedures. *Am J Surg.* 2000;179:391–395.

67. Lundell L, Miettinen P, Myrvold HE, et al. Continued (5-year) followup of a randomized clinical study comparing antireflux surgery and omeprazole in gastroesophageal reflux disease. *J Am Coll Surg.* 2001;192:172–179.

68. Parrilla P, deHaro LFM, Ortiz A, et al. Long term results of a randomized prospective study comparing medical and surgical treatment of Barrett's esophagus. *Ann Surg.* 2003;237:291–298.

69. Van Den Boom G, Go PM, Hameeteman W, et al. Cost effectiveness of medical versus surgical treatment in patients with severe or refractory gastroesophageal reflux disease in the Netherlands. *Scand J Gastroenterol.* 1996;31:1–9.

70. Viljakka M, Nevalainen J, Isolauri J. Lifetime costs of surgical versus medical treatment of severe gastro-oesophageal reflux disease in Finland. *Scand J Gastroenterol.* 1997;32:766–772.

COMMENTARY
Hanlin L. Wang

Esophageal carcinogenesis is a complex, multistep process that apparently involves different etiopathogenetic mechanisms in different types of carcinoma. For both adenocarcinoma and squamous cell carcinoma, a dysplasia-carcinoma sequence has been well established. Dysplasia of the lining epithelium of the esophagus, either squamous or columnar, is not only the most important precursor for cancer development but also the most important morphologic marker for early cancer detection (1,2). In the case of adenocarcinoma, the occurrence of dysplasia is preceded by a metaplastic process known as *Barrett's esophagus* in which stratified squamous epithelium is replaced by specialized columnar epithelium containing goblet cells (incomplete and complete intestinal metaplasia).

As an authority in gastrointestinal pathology, Dr. Chandrasoma contributes a considerable and provocative discussion in the preceding chapter on the perplexing subject of esophageal carcinogenesis that continues to brew exciting clinical and scientific research interest. Instead of following his chapter in a point-to-point fashion, several controversial topics are selected for further discussion in this commentary.

THE CONTROVERSY OF THE GASTROESOPHAGEAL JUNCTION

It is difficult to believe that we are still unsure of where the esophagus ends and where the stomach begins in the era of molecular medicine. Undoubtedly, an explicit definition of the gastroesophageal junction (GEJ) is of practical importance for the diagnosis and management of Barrett's esophagus. It is apparent that Dr. Chandrasoma holds a strong belief that the true stomach begins with pure oxyntic mucosa. Any other types of columnar-lined mucosa detected in the GEJ region between squamous and oxyntic mucosa are abnormal and represent reflux-induced metaplasia of the esophageal squamous epithelium. Therefore, the so-called gastric cardia is not a legitimate part of the stomach but rather a saccular dilatation of the distal esophagus lined by metaplastic columnar epithelium (dilated end-stage esophagus).

As Dr. Chandrasoma pointed out in his chapter, this concept has not yet gained popularity in the community. In current practice, the proximal limit of the gastric folds has been widely accepted as the best endoscopic landmark of the GEJ. In fact, all 18 participants of the 2003 American Gastroenterological Association Barrett's Esophagus Workshop unanimously endorsed this practice, although recognizing that there are scant data to validate it (3). By this definition, the gastric cardia does exist. Studies on populations with a very low risk of gastroesophageal reflux disease (GERD), such as neonates, infants, and children, support the notion that the existence of the cardia is the result of normal embryonic development of the stomach and does not necessarily represent evidence of a metaplastic response to reflux. In addition, as summarized in a recent review article by Odze (4), these studies consistently demonstrate that the cardia is extremely short (<0.4 cm), and consists of either pure mucous glands (cardiac mucosa) or mixed mucous and oxyntic glands (oxyntocardiac mucosa). Given the fact that these types of mucosa are also present in the gastric antrum and antral-body transitional region, it is difficult to accept the concept that the stomach has to begin with pure oxyntic mucosa. The same argument can also be made that pure oxyntic glands detected in the cardiac region in a subset of individuals, mainly adults, may actually result from a metaplastic process possibly secondary to GERD. In fact, it is not unusual to detect pure oxyntic mucosa in biopsies from the distal portion of the tubular esophagus with endoscopic evidence of columnar-lined esophagus.

The dilated end-stage esophagus theory appears to explain the epidemiologic data of increasing incidence of adenocarcinoma of the gastric cardia while a concomitant decrease in the prevalence of gastric cancer is observed. However, it is difficult to imagine that such a narrow region (<0.4 cm) has such a great potential for cancer development. Apparently, the confusing definitions of cardiac carcinoma are at least partially responsible. The assignment of tumor location in this region (including the cardia, GEJ, and distal esophagus) is arbitrary many times because tumor invasion has destroyed the anatomic landmark and/or histologic evidence of mucosal origin (5). For instance, an adenocarcinoma originally arising in an ultrashort Barrett's esophagus may be considered cardiac if the tumor invades into the stomach with the epicenter located in the proximal region of the gastric folds. Tumor cells may also replace intestinal metaplasia of the esophageal mucosa such that the background of Barrett's esophagus cannot be demonstrated.

Nevertheless, a variable degree of chronic inflammation is almost always present in biopsies from the gastric cardia (or dilated end-stage esophagus). Intestinal metaplasia is also a frequent histologic finding. The biologic significance of intestinal metaplasia in this region is unknown but it may serve as a predisposing condition for cancer development similar to Barrett's esophagus. What may be different from Barrett's esophagus, however, is that intestinal metaplasia in this region may not always be the result of GERD. Studies have shown that *Helicobacter pylori* infection is another cause of intestinal metaplasia in the cardia, as it is in the remaining part of the stomach. This columnar-to-columnar metaplasia of the gastric cardia may have a natural history and carcinogenic potential different from GERD-induced squamous-to-columnar metaplasia of the esophagus (4).

The current working definition of Barrett's esophagus is the endoscopic recognition of proximal displacement of the squamocolumnar junction relative to the GEJ (the proximal limit of gastric folds) with histologic evidence of intestinal metaplasia (3). With the dilated end-stage esophagus concept, the GEJ is not an endoscopically recognizable landmark. Rather, it is located in the proximal portion of the gastric folds and can be recognized only under a microscope. This apparently poses a challenge to endoscopists because the dilated end-stage esophagus is grossly indistinguishable from the remaining part of the stomach.

MULTISTEP CARCINOGENESIS IN BARRETT'S ESOPHAGUS

There has been no doubt that esophageal adenocarcinoma is causally associated with GERD. It remains elusive, however, why many patients with severe recurrent reflux esophagitis never develop Barrett's esophagus and why only a very small proportion of the patients with established Barrett's esophagus progress to dysplasia and finally carcinoma. Genetic predisposition thus serves a critical role, yet the genetic factors that determine the susceptibility or a "Barrett gene" have not been discovered.

The reflux-metaplasia-dysplasia-carcinoma sequence starts with the detrimental effects of acid, bile, gastric, and pancreatic enzymes in the refluxate (6–9). The cytokines and chemokines released by damaged epithelial cells attract inflammatory cells that produce additional inflammatory mediators, including reactive oxygen species, to further cause cell injury and DNA damage. The development of intestinal metaplasia is thought to be an adaptive response mediated by direct exposure of esophageal stem cells to the abnormal reflux environment and activation of genes that are involved in intestinal differentiation. One of the important genes, *CDX2*, which is a transcription factor exclusively expressed in intestinal epithelium under normal circumstances, has been shown to be activated in inflamed esophageal mucosa even before morphologic transformation (10,11). Activation of *CDX2* expression has been suggested to be responsible for the transcription of other intestinal-specific genes such as *MUC2* (6).

Intestinal metaplasia appears to confer cells a higher proliferative potential and a lower apoptotic activity when compared

with other types of columnar metaplasia (9). A repeated injury and healing process may lead to the selection of a cell clone with critical genetic or epigenetic alterations in specific genes and subsequent clonal expansion because of its growth advantage. One of the candidate genes in this regard is the tumor suppressor *p16* that has been shown to be frequently inactivated, mainly through promoter hypermethylation, at the stage of metaplasia (8,12). There is evidence to suggest that *p16* inactivation is not only necessary for clonal selection and expansion, but also provides a genetic background for the loss of function of another important tumor suppressor gene *p53* via either mutations or loss of heterozygosity (8,13). Because *p53* serves a pivotal role in the cell-cycle control and genomic stability, loss of *p53* function has been thought to be one of the most critical and earliest genetic events in the progression to dysplasia and carcinoma (8,14).

The molecular alterations briefly described here are just a few examples observed along the reflux-metaplasia-dysplasia-carcinoma sequence. Numerous studies have convincingly shown that neoplastic progression in Barrett's esophagus involves a series of molecular abnormalities resulting from the complex interplay between refluxate and mucosal response. In brief, the important alterations include aberrant expression of growth factors and their receptors, activation of proto-oncogenes, inactivation of tumor suppressors, deregulation of cell-cycle control, induction of angiogenesis, and alteration of cell-adhesion mechanisms. A detailed discussion of these molecular abnormalities is beyond the scope of this commentary; interested readers are referred to recent comprehensive reviews for further reading (6,8,15–18).

CONCEPTS OF CANCER PREVENTION IN BARRETT'S ESOPHAGUS

The logic of cancer prevention in Barrett's esophagus seems straightforward: reflux causes cancer, blocking reflux blocks cancer development. However, the effectiveness of two currently available options of intervention, acid-suppression therapy and antireflux surgery, has not been well demonstrated. It is also unclear from the current literature exactly what roles acid, bile, and other elements in the refluxate serve during carcinogenesis, although accumulating evidence suggests bile acids are likely the most important carcinogens (19,20).

Effective acid suppression by proton pump inhibitors (PPIs) has been shown to inhibit cell proliferation and promote differentiation in Barrett mucosa (21). A recent retrospective study by El-Serag and colleagues (22) showed that the use of PPIs was independently associated with reduced incidence of dysplasia in patients with Barrett's esophagus in comparison with those receiving no therapy or treated with H_2-receptor antagonists, which are less-effective acid suppressors. This study also showed that among those taking PPIs, a longer duration of use was associated with less frequent occurrence of dysplasia. These data thus suggest that long-term effective acid suppression may halt or slow the progression of Barrett metaplasia to dysplasia.

Chronic acid suppression has potential drawbacks, however (15,20,23). For example, achlorhydria is a known risk factor for gastric cancer. Secondary elevation of serum gastrin levels may stimulate cell proliferation in Barrett mucosa. Acid suppression may also lead to bacterial overgrowth, which facilitates the production of carcinogens. Furthermore, acid suppression may render bile acids more carcinogenic, as discussed by Dr. Chandrasoma in the preceding chapter. From that perspective, gastric acid appears to protect Barrett's esophagus from neoplastic transformation despite its detrimental effect on the cells. Aggressive acid suppression may thus actually promote esophageal carcinogenesis (15,24).

In contrast to acid-suppression therapy that selectively inhibits gastric acid secretion, antireflux surgery is scientifically more appealing as it is aimed at correcting the fundamental defect that causes reflux. However, the currently available clinical data have not convincingly demonstrated that antireflux surgery is more advantageous in cancer prevention in patients with Barrett's esophagus (3,23). A large population-based retrospective cohort study conducted in Sweden failed to show a reduction in the incidence of esophageal and cardiac adenocarcinomas in GERD patients after antireflux surgery (25). The study by Spechler and colleagues (26) specifically compared the long-term outcomes of medical and surgical therapies for GERD patients in a randomized trial. In this study, 4 of 165 patients (2.4%) in the medical group and 1 of 82 (1.2%) in the surgical group developed esophageal adenocarcinoma during 10 to 13 years of follow-up. The difference between these two treatment groups was not statistically significant. However, as the authors acknowledged, this study did not have sufficient statistical power to detect small differences, given such a low incidence of the tumor. In a more recent study coauthored by Dr. Spechler, the incidence of esophageal adenocarcinoma in 946 patients who received antireflux surgery was 0.072% during a mean follow-up time of 11.8 years, whereas the incidence in 1,892 age-matched, medically treated GERD patients was 0.04% during a mean follow-up time of 10.6 years (27). These data thus emphasize that there is insufficient evidence to support the contention that antireflux surgery reduces the risk of cancer development in GERD patients. In addition, a meta-analysis of 34 studies including 754 surgically treated and 918 medically treated patients with Barrett's esophagus showed no significant protective effect of antireflux surgery on cancer development (28). Despite the intrinsic defect of these comparative studies that the patients who underwent surgical procedures usually had more severe diseases and thus might have a higher cancer risk, these observations have led to the recommendation by authorities that antireflux surgery should not be advised for the treatment of GERD with the expectation that it will prevent esophageal adenocarcinoma (3,24,29).

The possibility exists that the molecular alterations triggering the progression of the metaplasia-dysplasia-carcinoma sequence may have already occurred in some individuals such that normalization of the luminal milieu after the critical point, either by acid suppression or antireflux surgery, may not be able to stop the cellular events that eventuate in neoplastic transformation. In this regard, chemoprevention using aspirin and other nonsteroidal anti-inflammatory drugs has shown promise for reducing cancer risk in patients with Barrett's esophagus (30,31). Instead of blocking the entry of potential carcinogens into the esophagus, nonsteroidal anti-inflammatory drugs presumably intervene in the inflammatory response at the early stage of carcinogenesis by selectively inhibiting a cellular process, the activity of cyclooxygenases that mediate the production of prostaglandins.

ROLE OF HUMAN PAPILLOMAVIRUS IN ESOPHAGEAL SQUAMOUS CARCINOGENESIS

A causal association of human papillomavirus (HPV) with esophageal squamous carcinogenesis was first suggested by Syrjänen (32) 25 years ago, but whether HPV infection is indeed a risk factor as for cervical and anal cancers is still the subject of continuing debate. In reviewing a number of studies published between 1982 and 2001, Syrjänen (32) concluded that HPV appeared to play an important role in esophageal squamous carcinogenesis. Of the several thousands of carcinomas analyzed, the average HPV detection rate was 23% by in situ hybridization and 15% by polymerase chain reaction, but the detection rates were highly variable among different studies, ranging from 0% to up to 70%. It is apparent that many technical factors contribute to this considerable variation, such as different methods and different types of specimens used for HPV detection by different investigators. However, there appears to be a trend for a higher HPV detection rate in geographic regions with a higher incidence of esophageal squamous cell carcinoma. If this observation holds true, it would suggest that the underlying etiologies of esophageal squamous carcinogenesis differ among geographic areas and that HPV plays a more significant role in areas with a higher prevalence of the disease (32,33). This would potentially, at least in part, explain the wide geographic variation in incidence of esophageal squamous cell carcinoma. The data reported in a number of recent studies appear to substantiate this explanation (34–39).

In tumors harboring HPV, high-risk types 16 and 18 are most commonly detected. It has been well established that the E6 and E7 oncoproteins of these high-risk HPVs mediate their oncogenic effects by functional inactivation of two important cellular tumor suppressors $p53$ and Rb through physical protein-protein interactions and accelerated protein degradation. It is puzzling, however, that some of the HPV-positive squamous cell carcinomas of the esophagus simultaneously harbor $p53$ gene mutations (32), while these two events are typically mutually exclusive in cervical and anal cancers.

Despite the continuing debate, it appears reasonable to believe that HPV infection is one of the many risk factors responsible for a fraction of esophageal squamous cell carcinoma. With the advent of HPV vaccines, it would be interesting to see if there will be a reduction in the incidence of this disease in the future generations in prevalent regions.

REFERENCES

1. Casson AG, Williams L, Guernsey DL. Epidemiology and molecular biology of Barrett's esophagus. *Semin Thorac Cardiovasc Surg.* 2005;17:284–291.
2. Dry SM, Lewin KJ. Esophageal squamous dysplasia. *Semin Diagn Pathol.* 2002;19:2–11.

3. Sharma P, McQuaid K, Dent J, et al. A critical review of the diagnosis and management of Barrett's esophagus: the AGA Chicago Workshop. *Gastroenterology.* 2004;127:310–330.

4. Odze RD. Unraveling the mystery of the gastroesophageal junction: a pathologist's perspective. *Am J Gastroenterol.* 2005;100:1853–1867.

5. Dent J. Pathogenesis and classification of cancer around the gastroesophageal junction—not so different in Japan. *Am J Gastroenterol.* 2006;101:934–936.

6. Bax DA, Siersema PD, Van Vliet AH, et al. Molecular alterations during development of esophageal adenocarcinoma. *J Surg Oncol.* 2005;92:89–98.

7. Guillem PG. How to make a Barrett's esophagus: pathophysiology of columnar metaplasia of the esophagus. *Dig Dis Sci.* 2005;50:415–424.

8. Maley CC. Multistage carcinogenesis in Barrett's esophagus. *Cancer Lett.* 2007;245:22–32.

9. Turcotte S, Duranceau A. Gastroesophageal reflux and cancer. *Thorac Surg Clin.* 2005;15:341–352.

10. Eda A, Osawa H, Satoh K, et al. Aberrant expression of CDX2 in Barrett's epithelium and inflammatory esophageal mucosa.*J Gastroenterol.* 2003;38:14–22.

11. Moons LM, Bax DA, Kuipers EJ, et al. The homeodomain protein CDX2 is an early marker of Barrett's oesophagus. *J Clin Pathol.* 2004;57:1063–1068.

12. Bian YS, Osterheld MC, Fontolliet C, et al. p16 inactivation by methylation of the CDKN2A promoter occurs early during neoplastic progression in Barrett's esophagus. *Gastroenterology.* 2002;122:1113–21.

13. Maley CC, Galipeau PC, Li X, et al. Selectively advantageous mutations and hitchhikers in neoplasms: p16 lesions are selected in Barrett's esophagus. *Cancer Res.* 2004; 64:3414–3427.

14. Merola E, Claudio PP, Giordano A. p53 and the malignant progression of Barrett's esophagus. *J Cell Physiol.* 2006;206:574–577.

15. Atherfold PA, Jankowski JA. Molecular biology of Barrett's cancer. *Best Pract Res Clin Gastroenterol.* 2006;20:813–827.

16. Koppert LB, Wijnhoven BP, van Dekken H, et al. The molecular biology of esophageal adenocarcinoma. *J Surg Oncol.* 2005;92:169–190.

17. Spechler SJ. Barrett's esophagus: a molecular perspective.*Curr Gastroenterol Rep.* 2005;7:177–181.

18. Tannapfel A. Molecular findings in Barrett's epithelium. *Dig Dis.* 2004;22:126–133.

19. Bernstein H, Bernstein C, Payne CM, et al. Bile acids as carcinogens in human gastrointestinal cancers. *Mutat Res.* 2005;589:47–65.

20. Sital RR, Kusters JG, De Rooij FW, et al. Bile acids and Barrett's oesophagus: a sine qua non or coincidence? *Scand J Gastroenterol.* 2006;41(Suppl 243):11–17.

21. Jankowski JA, Anderson M. Management of oesophageal adenocarcinoma—control of acid, bile and inflammation in intervention strategies for Barrett's oesophagus. *Aliment Pharmacol Ther.* 2004;20 (Suppl 5):71–80.

22. El-Serag HB, Aguirre TV, Davis S, et al. Proton pump inhibitors are associated with reduced incidence of dysplasia in Barrett's esophagus. *Am J Gastroenterol.* 2004;99:1877–1883.

23. Souza RF, Spechler SJ. Concepts in the prevention of adenocarcinoma of the distal esophagus and proximal stomach. *CA Cancer J Clin.* 2005;55:334–351.

24. Stamp DH. Bile acids aided by acid suppression therapy may be associated with the development of esophageal cancers in westernized societies. *Med Hypotheses.* 2006;66:154–157.

25. Ye W, Chow WH, Lagergren J, et al. Risk of adenocarcinomas of the esophagus and gastric cardia in patients with gastroesophageal reflux diseases and after antireflux surgery. *Gastroenterology.* 2001;121:1286–1293.

26. Spechler SJ, Lee E, Ahnen D, et al. Long-term outcome of medical and surgical therapies for gastroesophageal reflux disease: follow-up of a randomized controlled trial. *JAMA.* 2001;285:2331–2338.

27. Tran T, Spechler SJ, Richardson P, et al. Fundoplication and the risk of esophageal cancer in gastroesophageal reflux disease: a Veterans Affairs cohort study. *Am J Gastroenterol.* 2005;100:1002–1008.

28. Corey KE, Schmitz SM, Shaheen NJ. Does a surgical antireflux procedure decrease the incidence of esophageal adenocarcinoma in Barrett's esophagus? A meta-analysis. *Am J Gastroenterol.* 2003;98:2390–2394.

29. Shaheen NJ. Does fundoplication change the risk of esophageal cancer in the setting of GERD? *Am J Gastroenterol.* 2005;100:1009–1011.

30. Corley DA, Kerlikowske K, Verma R, et al. Protective association of aspirin/NSAIDs and esophageal cancer: a systematic review and meta-analysis. *Gastroenterology.* 2003;124:47–56.

31. Vaughan TL, Dong LM, Blount PL, et al. Non-steroidal anti-inflammatory drugs and risk of neoplastic progression in Barrett's oesophagus: a prospective study. *Lancet Oncol.* 2005;6:945–952.

32. Syrjänen KJ. HPV infections and oesophageal cancer. *J Clin Pathol.* 2002;55:721–728.

33. Sur M, Cooper K. The role of the human papilloma virus in esophageal cancer. *Pathology.* 1998;30:348–354.

34. Shen ZY, Hu SP, Lu LC, et al. Detection of human papillomavirus in esophageal carcinoma. *J Med Virol.* 2002;68:412–416.

35. Zhou XB, Guo M, Quan LP, et al. Detection of human papillomavirus in Chinese esophageal squamous cell carcinoma and its adjacent normal epithelium. *World J Gastroenterol.* 2003;9:1170–1173.

36. Farhadi M, Tahmasebi Z, Merat S, et al. Human papillomavirus in squamous cell carcinoma of esophagus in a high-risk population. *World J Gastroenterol.* 2005;11:1200–1203.

37. Katiyar S, Hedau S, Jain N, et al. p53 gene mutation and human papillomavirus (HPV) infection in esophageal carcinoma from three different endemic geographic regions of India. *Cancer Lett.* 2005;218:69–79.

38. Yao PF, Li GC, Li J, Xia HS, et al. Evidence of human papilloma virus infection and its epidemiology in esophageal squamous cell carcinoma. *World J Gastroenterol.* 2006;12:1352–1355.

39. Souto Damin AP, Guedes Frazzon AP, de Carvalho Damin D, et al. Detection of human papillomavirus DNA in squamous cell carcinoma of the esophagus by auto-nested PCR. *Dis Esophagus.* 2006;19:64–68.

31

Surgical Management of Cancer of the Esophagus

Seth A. Spector and Alan S. Livingstone

Despite improvements in rates of resectability and periop-erative mortality, cancer of the esophagus remains among the solid tumors most resistant to a consistently successful ther-apeutic approach. Esophageal cancer is relatively uncommon in the United States. The American Cancer Society estimated that 16,470 men and women (12,970 men and 3,500 women) were diagnosed with cancer of the esophagus in 2008, and 14,280 (11,250 men and 3,030 women) died of the disease in the same year (1). The overall 5-year relative survival rate for patients di-agnosed between 1996 and 2003 was estimated to be 16% (18% for white patients and 11% for African Americans). These esti-mates represent significant improvements (*p* <0.05) compared to the comparable survival rates among patients diagnosed be-tween 1975 and 1977 (5% for all races, 6% for whites, and 3% for African Americans) (1). These modest advances in out-come appear to be associated with an increased understanding of pathogenesis, advances in techniques allowing earlier diag-nosis, and possibly extended surgery for invasive disease and combined multimodal therapy.

Based on Surveillance, Epidemiology, and End-Results (SEER) data published in 2009, 23% of cases of invasive can-cer of the esophagus currently are diagnosed while the cancer is still confined to the primary site (localized stage); 30% are diagnosed after the cancer has spread to regional lymph nodes or directly beyond the primary site; 32% are diagnosed after the cancer has already metastasized (distant stage); and for the remaining 15%, the staging information is unknown. The corre-sponding 5-year relative survival rates are: 37.1% for localized; 18.5% for regional; 3.1% for distant; and 11.7% for unstaged disease (2).

PATHOLOGY AND EPIDEMIOLOGY

There is a dichotomy in the presentation of this disease both in the histology (adenocarcinoma vs. squamous cell carcinoma) and in its geographic distribution. Squamous cell carcinoma is the predominant histologic type in the cervical esophagus and in the upper and middle thirds of the thoracic esophagus. Most of these lesions arise in the middle third of the esophagus. Ade-nocarcinoma is the predominate histology in the distal third of the esophagus, where it most commonly occurs, often associated with Barrett's esophagus (3).

Worldwide, squamous cell is the commonest histologic type, but the incidence appears to be declining, possibly due to a reduction in smoking and alcohol intake and increased consumption of fresh fruits and vegetables (4). Squamous cell carcinoma is relatively uncommon outside Asia but is among the leading causes of cancer death in central and Southeast Asia. High incidence areas for squamous carcinoma include Turkey, Iran, the southern republics of the former Soviet Union, north-ern China, southern coast of China, southern Thailand, and the mountainous regions of Japan (3,5,6). Interestingly, Fernan-des et al. (7) reported that between 1968 and 2002, there was a progressive and statistically significant decrease in the inci-dence of squamous cell cancer in Singapore and a trend to an increase in adenocarcinoma. The authors attributed the decline in squamous cancer to the known decrease in frequency of smok-ing in Singapore. They suggested that the apparent increase in adenocarcinoma may be due to rise in the frequency of reflux esophagitis and obesity. A decreased incidence of the disease has also been observed in Hong Kong. This trend appears to be correlated with decreased consumption of alcohol and tobacco and increased intake of fresh rather than preserved foods (8). In the United States, the overall incidence of squamous cell cancer has remained stable, but has increased among African American men (5). High incidence areas in the Untied States include the low country of the Carolinas and in major metropolitan cen-ters such as Los Angeles, New York, Detroit, and Washington, D.C. (5).

In the Western world, the incidence of adenocarcinoma of the esophagus and esophagogastric junction has increased dra-matically. A sixfold increase in incidence was observed in the United States between 1975 and 2001 (9). Devesa et al. (10) reported that throughout the 1990s, the incidence of adeno-carcinoma surpassed that of squamous cell carcinoma in North America. Bollschweiler et al. (11) studied the demographic vari-ation in the incidence of esophageal adenocarcinoma among white men in North America, Europe, and Australia. The esti-mated incidence for the year 2000 was highest in Great Britain (5.0 to 8.7 cases per 100,000 population) and in Australia (4.8 cases per 100,000 population) followed by the Netherlands (4.4 cases per 100,000 population), the United States (3.7 cases per 100,000 population), and Denmark (2.8 cases per 100,000 pop-ulation). Low rates (<1.0 cases per 100,000 population) were found in Eastern Europe. The largest changes in incidence were reported in the southern European countries, with an estimated average increase of 30% per year; in Australia, with an average increase of 23.5% per year; and in the United States, with an average increase of 20.6% per year. The rates of increase ranged from 8.7% to 17.5% on average in Northern Europe, Central Europe, and the United Kingdom. In contrast, at most there was only a minor rise in incidence in Eastern Europe.

SCREENING AND SURVEILLANCE

In squamous cell carcinoma for which there are no common associated precancerous lesions or markers, mass screening programs, such as are practiced in China and other highly endemic areas, are not practical in the United States or other low-risk countries (12). Screening, however, may be advisable in patients with various uncommon conditions that have been associated with the development of squamous cancer, such as tylosis, Plummer-Vinson (Paterson Kelly) syndrome, caustic injury to the esophagus, achalasia, and prior aerodigestive tract malignancy (3).

In contrast, for patients at risk for adenocarcinoma, in whom progression from dysplasia to invasion may be observed over time, surveillance programs may be beneficial with the goal of earlier diagnosis and improved outcome. The Practice Parameters Committee of the American College of Gastroenterology recommends in their 2008 updated guidelines (13) that patients with Barrett's esophagus without evidence of dysplasia be followed with endoscopy at 3-year intervals. The presence of low-grade dysplasia warrants follow-up endoscopy within 6 months to ensure that no higher grade of dysplasia is present. If none is found, yearly surveillance endoscopy with biopsy is recommended until no dysplasia is observed on two annual examinations. Thereafter periodic surveillance is recommended, with no specific interval suggested. Pathologically confirmed high-grade dysplasia calls for surgical intervention or intensive endoscopic surveillance, with endoscopic examinations every 3 months. The latter recommendation by the Committee is controversial. Many authorities recommend some form of ablation, with esophagectomy regarded as the gold standard in the management of high-grade dysplasia (14,15).

Endoscopic surveillance consists of four-quadrant biopsies at intervals of 2 cm in addition to biopsies of any suggestive lesions. In patients with high-grade dysplasia undergoing surveillance, biopsies at 1-cm intervals are recommended (16). Methods under investigation to enhance the yield of surveillance protocols include chromoendoscopy, high-magnification endoscopy, optical coherence tomography, fluorescence endoscopy, and narrow band imaging (15,17).

Despite recommended protocols for surveillance, the efficacy of serial endoscopic biopsies is unestablished inasmuch as there is no convincing data demonstrating that surveillance prevents cancer or improves life expectancy (3,18).

CLINICAL PRESENTATION

Patients with early-stage disease are usually asymptomatic. Patients with early-stage adenocarcinoma are commonly identified in the course of evaluation of gastrointestinal reflux disease or as a result of surveillance of Barrett's esophagus. Significant symptoms generally reflect locally advanced or metastatic disease. Dysphagia, first to solids and then liquids, and weight loss are the commonest presenting symptoms. Other symptoms may in-

clude heartburn, vomiting or regurgitation, odynophagia, chest pain, recurrent cough as a result of aspiration or direct tracheal involvement, and hoarseness reflecting recurrent laryngeal nerve involvement (19,20).

DIAGNOSIS AND CLINICAL STAGING

Esophagogastroscopy, the mainstay of diagnosis, defines the location and extent of the lesion, and endoscopic biopsies combined with cytologic brushings are highly accurate in confirming the diagnosis (3). Endoscopy may also provide some information regarding the stage of disease as large circumferential tumors are more often than not transmural, and 80% of these will have lymph node involvement (21). Barium swallow, an important diagnostic test in the past, has been largely replaced by the endoscopic examination. Bronchoscopy is indicated for patients with tumors of the middle and upper thirds of the esophagus to assess the possibility of tracheal involvement.

Once the diagnosis of cancer is established, additional evaluation is necessary to determine the stage of the disease, including the extent of the tumor (T stage), the status of regional lymph nodes (N stage), and the presence or absence of metastatic disease (M stage) (Table 31.1). Computed tomography (CT) of the chest, abdomen, and pelvis with oral and intravenous contrast is usually the initial test ordered to assess the presence and extent of systemic disease, such as metastatic disease of the lungs, liver, and adrenal glands, and peritoneal carcinomatosis. CT scanning is less accurate in assessing the T stage and nodal involvement although the images may reveal thickening of the esophagus or a mass effect and lymphadenopathy. Combined CT-positron emission tomography imaging appears to improve the accuracy of noninvasive staging, especially for the detection of distant metastases (22).

Endoscopic ultrasound (EUS) is a key modality in assessing the depth of invasion (T stage) and the presence of adjacent involved lymph nodes (N stage), but the procedure is highly operator- and instrument-dependent. EUS can differentiate intramural from transmural disease, but its ability to distinguish mucosal from submucosal, and submucosal from intramuscular is limited. Miniprobe high-frequency (20 MHz) sonographic catheters that can be passed through the standard endoscope are more accurate in making these differentiations. Murata et al. (23) claimed that they could achieve a 94% accuracy in defining differences between mucosal and submucosal tumors. The accuracy is also dependent on the part of the esophagus bearing the tumor. The tubular esophagus is much easier to assess than the area of the gastroesophageal junction. May et al. (24) reported 91% accuracy in the tubular esophagus but only 14% with lesions limited exclusively to the gastroesophageal junction.

EUS is also used to assess nodal status. The reported accuracy of EUS in determining pathologic adenopathy ranges from 50% to 80% (25,26). The accuracy of nodal staging has been enhanced by the use of apparatus that allows the performance of ultrasound-guided endoscopic fine-needle aspiration biopsies (EUS-FNA). In comparing EUS-FNA with EUS alone for lymph node staging, Vazquez-Sequeiros and associates (27) found that

Table 31.1

American Joint Committee on Cancer Staging of Esophageal Cancer

Tx: tumor cannot be assessed	Nx: regional nodes cannot be assessed	Mx: metastases cannot be assessed
T0: no evidence of tumor	N0: no regional lymph node metastases	M0: no distant metastases
Tis: carcinoma in situ	N1: regional Lymph node metastases present	M1: distant metastases present
T1: tumor invades lamina propria or submucosa	—	M1a: positive celiac nodes with a lower thoracic tumor or positive cervical nodes with an upper third tumor
T2: tumor invades muscularis propria	—	M1b: other distant metastases in an upper or lower third tumor
T3: Tumor invades adventitia	—	—
T4: Tumor invades adjacent structures	—	—

Stage 0	Tis N0 M0
Stage 1	T1 N0 M0
Stage 2A	T2-3 N0 M0
Stage 2B	T1-2 N1 M0
Stage 3	T3 N1 M0 or T4 N0-1 M0
Stage 4	Any T, any N M1
Stage 4a	Any T, any N M1a
Stage 4b	Any T, any N M1b

Data derived from the *AJCC Cancer Staging Manual.* 6th ed. New York: Springer-Verlag; 2002:91–98.

EUS-FNA was more sensitive, 93% versus 63% ($p = 0.01$) and more accurate, 93% versus 70% ($p = 0.02$).

HISTORY OF ESOPHAGEAL SURGERY

Law and Wong (20) have briefly outlined the history of esophageal surgery. In 1877, Czerny was the first surgeon to successfully resect a cervical esophageal cancer. In 1913, Torek (28) performed the first successful transthoracic resection. The high mortality rates associated with transthoracic resection at that time led to the development of the transhiatal approach to esophagectomy, which was introduced by Denk in 1913, refined by Turner in 1931, and popularized by Orringer (29–36) during the last 25 years.

During the early experience with esophagectomy, the proximal and distal ends after resection were brought out subcutaneously and connected by external plastic tubes, skin tubes, or flaps. In 1933, Ohsawa (37) reported the first use of the stomach for reconstruction of the resected esophagus, a technique he employed in 18 patients in Japan. In 1946, Lewis (38) described his two-stage approach to esophageal resection, employing a right thoracotomy and a separate laparotomy. This technique remains widely employed in current practice. In 1976, McKeown (39) suggested a three-stage operation, with an incision in the neck through which the anastomosis was created to avoid the severe consequences of an intrathoracic anastomotic leak. In 1982 and 1994, Akiyama and Tsurumaru (40,41) described their technique of esophagectomy with preservation of the vagus nerve.

Swanstrom and Hansen (42) reported an early experience with laparoscopic total esophagectomy in 1997.

MANAGEMENT OF PREMALIGNANT CONDITIONS AND EARLY CARCINOMA

The management of Barrett's esophagus with high-grade dysplasia and superficial cancers of the esophagus is controversial. An array of therapeutic options have been studied, including photodynamic therapy (PDT), endoscopic mucosal resection (EMR), radiofrequency ablation, argon beam plasma coagulation (43), and esophagectomy with or without vagal-sparing.

The selection of therapy is influenced by various epidemiologic studies that are often inconsistent in their conclusions. Important factors to be considered in recommending management include the following:

1. Barrett's esophagus is considered a premalignant condition that is thought to carry a 30- to 125-fold increased risk of cancer compared with an age-matched population (15,18).
2. The cumulative incidence of progression from high-grade dysplasia to esophageal cancer ranges from 16% to 59% in various studies over a 5- to 8-year period of surveillance (15,44–46).
3. It has been widely published that 30% to 50% of patients undergoing esophagectomy for a preoperative diagnosis of high-grade dysplasia are found to have an occult invasive carcinoma in the resected specimen (3,14). In contrast, in

a review of the literature, Konda et al. (47) selected the records of 213 patients who had undergone an esophagectomy for high-grade dysplasia in which an occult lesion was found and in which the pathologist specified the occult lesion as either intramucosal cancer (noninvasive, T1a lesion) or submucosal disease (invasive, T1b lesion) (48). The authors determined that only 12.7% of the patients really had invasive disease, whereas 28.2% had an intramucosal carcinoma.

4. In the absence of an endoscopic abnormality, occult adeno-carcinomas found in patients with pre-resection biopsies re-vealing only high-grade dysplasia generally are confined to the mucosa and are associated with nodal metastases in <5% of patients (14). However, an endoscopically visible lesion within the Barrett's mucosa, which on biopsy reveals adeno-carcinoma, cannot be assumed to be confined to the mucosa, no matter how small. Such lesions may penetrate into the submucosa, where the risk of nodal disease is at least 25% (14,47).

5. The depth of invasive of small visible lesions may be diffi-cult to determine preoperatively, even with endoscopic ul-trasound. Some authorities believe that endoscopic mucosal resection is the only accurate method to determine the depth of invasion of small visible lesions (14).

Photodynamic Therapy

This locally ablative therapy employs a photosensitizing drug, such as sodium porfimer, which is preferentially retained in neoplastic tissue. When the drug is endoscopically exposed to light of the proper wavelength, an oxidative photochemical re-action is generated which results in destruction of the diseased mucosa (15). PDT has been employed in the management of Barrett's esophagus with high-grade dysplasia and early carci-noma. About half of the patients treated for high-grade dyspla-sia experience complete ablation of all of the Barrett's changes in addition to ablation of the area of high-grade dysplasia (49,50). Strictures complicate this therapy in up to half of treated pa-tients (15,49). In addition, in areas of apparent squamous re-epithelialization, patches of subsquamous intestinal metaplasia of uncertain biological significance have been found (15).

Overholt et al. (49) treated 103 patients with Barrett's esophagus with high-grade dysplasia, low-grade dysplasia, or early carcinoma with PDT supplemented by focal contact neodymium:yttrium-aluminium-garnet(Nd:YAG) laser pho-toablation and acid-suppressive therapy with the proton pump inhibitor, omeprazole. In their intention-to-treat analysis of the 103 patients, the success rate for controlling low-grade dyspla-sia, high-grade dysplasia, and early cancer was 92.9%, 77.5%, and 44.4%, respectively. There was also a significant reduction in the length of Barrett's mucosa. Three of 65 patients (4.6%) with high-grade dysplasia developed subsquamous adenocarcinoma. Subsquamous, nondysplastic, metaplastic epithelium was found in four patients (4.9%). Strictures occurred in 18% with one session of PDT, and 50% with two treatments, 30% overall. The authors concluded that PDT with supplemental Nd:YAG pho-toablation and continuous treatment with omeprazole reduces the length of Barrett's mucosa, eliminates high-grade dysplasia, and, by comparison with historical data, may reduce the ex-pected frequency of carcinoma.

Subsequently, Overholt and associates (51) conducted a multi-institutional randomized trial comparing PDT plus omeprazole with omeprazole alone in the management of Barrett's esophagus with high-grade dysplasia. At 5 years of follow-up, the combined therapy was associated with a signifi-cantly greater rate of eliminating high-grade dysplasia (77% vs. 39%; p <0.0001) and a reduced incidence of progression to cancer (15% vs. 29%; $p = 0.027$).

The University of Pittsburgh experience (15) with PDT in-cludes 50 high-risk patients with either high-grade dysplasia or localized cancer. At a mean follow-up period of 28.1 months, 16 patients (32%) were alive and free of disease, 30% were alive with residual or recurrent disease, and 38% had died with re-current disease. The overall survival at 36 months was 31%. Strictures occurred in 42% of the patients. The intent-to-treat success rate was 38% in high-grade dysplasia and 30% in cases of focal carcinomas.

In a retrospective study from the Mayo Clinic (52), the long-term survival of 129 patients with high-grade dysplasia treated with PDT was compared with that observed among 70 patients treated with transhiatal or transthoracic esophagectomy. Overall mortality in the PDT group was 9% (11/129) and in the surgery group was 8.5% (6/70) over a median follow-up period of 59 ± 2.7 months for the PDT group and 61 ± 5.8 months for the surgery group. Overall survival was similar between the two groups (Wilcoxon test = 0.0924; $p = 0.76$). The treatment modality was not determined to be a significant predictor of mortality on multivariate analysis. The authors concluded that in this single-center, retrospective study the overall survival at 5 years of patients with high-grade dysplasia treated with PDT appears to be comparable to that of patients treated with esopha-gectomy.

In a subsequent pilot study from the Mayo Clinic (44) biomarkers that have been associated with progression of neo-plasia in Barrett's esophagus were measured in a group of patients with high-grade dysplasia or mucosal cancer who were treated with PDT. The biomarkers that were assessed included loss of 9p21 (site of the $p16$ gene) and 17p13.1 (site of the $p53$ gene) loci; gains of the 8q24 (*c-myc*), 17q (*HER2/neu*), and 20q13 loci; and multiple gains. The elimination of dysplasia with PDT was generally associated with loss of the biomarkers. However, 25% of the patients who responded to the ablative therapy had per-sistence of one or more of the biomarkers, and a third of these patients developed recurrent high-grade dysplasia. None of the patients with assays negative for the biomarkers had recurrence over a median follow-up period of 22 months.

Endoscopic Mucosal Resection

EMR has been employed in the management of nodular or focal high-grade dysplasia or early carcinomas. Ell et al. (53) reported the outcome in 100 consecutive patients undergoing EMR in the management of early adenocarcinomas arising in Barrett's metaplasia. No major complications occurred. Complete local remission was achieved in 99 of the 100 patients after 1.9 months (range, 1 to 18 months) and a maximum of three resections. Within a short mean follow-up period of 36.7 months, recurrent or metachronous carcinomas were found in 11% of the patients, but successful repeat treatment with endoscopic resection was possible in all of these cases. The calculated 5-year survival rate was 98%.

In order to avoid recurrent or metachronous lesions, Lopes and associates (54) performed circumferential EMR in 41 patients with Barrett's high-grade dysplasia, in 23 of whom early cancers were detected on endoscopic ultrasound. The aim of the technique was to remove not only the neoplastic lesion but also the remaining Barrett's epithelium. During a mean follow-up of 31.6 months, Barrett's epithelium was completely replaced by squamous epithelium in 31 (75.6%) cases. Despite the circumferential technique, Barrett's epithelium recurred in ten (24.4%) patients and recurrent or metachronous early cancer was detected in five (12.2%), all but one of whom were treated again by EMR; the fifth patient was referred to surgery.

Larghi et al. (55) at the University of Chicago also employed EMR to achieve complete Barrett's eradication in the treatment of patients with high-grade dysplasia or intramucosal adenocarcinoma. Twenty-four patients underwent a total of 44 EMR sessions. After a median follow-up of 28 months (range, 15 to 51 months), persistent endoscopic and histologic eradication of Barrett's esophagus was demonstrated in 21 patients (87.5%). In two patients, Barrett's epithelium was detected beneath the neosquamous epithelium 3 months after completion of the resection. In the remaining patient, intramucosal adenocarcinoma was found in a nodule seen and removed by EMR at 12-month surveillance endoscopy.

In another approach to reduce the incidence of recurrence or metachronous lesions, Buttar and associates (56) treated 17 patients with superficial adenocarcinomas with EMR followed by PDT. No new or recurrent cancers developed in 16 (94%) of the patients receiving the combined therapy, although residual Barrett's was present in 47%.

In Japan, Shimizu at al. (57) performed an extended EMR in 26 consecutive patients with squamous cell esophageal carcinoma invading the muscularis mucosa or submucosa. In this prospective, but nonrandomized, study the results were compared with those observed in a control group of 44 consecutive patients with esophageal carcinoma invading the muscularis mucosae or upper third of the submucosa and no preoperative evidence of lymph node metastasis who underwent esophagectomy during the same period. Overall survival rates at 5 years in the extended endoscopic mucosal resection group and surgical resection group were 77.4% and 84.5%, respectively. There was no significant difference between survival distributions. Cause-specific survival rates at 5 years in extended endoscopic mucosal resection and surgical resection groups were 95.0% and 93.5%, respectively. Survival curves for the groups were similar.

In contradistinction to other endoscopic ablative techniques, EMR excises a disc of esophageal wall down to the muscularis propria, thereby providing a specimen for histologic review that includes both mucosa and submucosa. To assess the staging accuracy of EMR, Maish and DeMeester (58) treated seven patients with small, visible adenocarcinomas with EMR followed by esophagectomy. Pathologic examination of the resected esophagus confirmed that EMR had accurately determined the depth of tumor invasion in all seven cases. However, in two of the seven patients (29%) an additional cancer was found in the resected specimen that had not been detected preoperatively despite multiple endoscopies. The authors concluded that

EMR is a valuable staging procedure that can identify patients with lesions confined to the mucosa that have a low risk of nodal involvement and therefore for whom there is no need to perform lymphadenectomy at the time of esophagectomy.

Radiofrequency Ablation

Several studies (59–62) have indicated the safety and efficacy of radiofrequency ablation using the HALO 360 (BARRX Medical, Sunnyvale, CA), endoscopic balloon-based ablation device. The data indicate that this technique can reliably ablate residual dysplastic Barrett's esophagus after endoscopic mucosal resection of an intramucosal cancer, or as the sole therapy for patients with high-grade dysplasia in the absence of a visible lesion or ulcer.

In 2009, Shaheen and associates (62) reported the results of a multicenter, sham-controlled trial in which 127 patients with dysplastic Barrett's esophagus were randomly assigned in a 2:1 ratio to receive either radiofrequency ablation (ablation group) or a sham procedure (control group). Primary outcomes at 12 months included the complete eradication of dysplasia and intestinal metaplasia. Among the patients with low-grade dysplasia, complete eradication of dysplasia occurred in 90.5% of those in the ablation group, as compared with 22.7% of those in the control group (p <0.001). Among the patients with high-grade dysplasia, complete eradication occurred in 81.0% of those in the ablation group, as compared with 19.0% of those in the control group (p<0.001). Overall, 77.4% of patients in the ablation group had complete eradication of intestinal metaplasia, as compared with 2.3% of those in the control group (p<0.001). Patients in the ablation group had less disease progression (3.6% vs. 16.3%, p = 0.03) and fewer cancers (1.2% vs. 9.3%, p = 0.045).

Esophagectomy

Total esophagectomy eliminates all of the Barrett's metaplasia, interrupts the potential progression of high-grade dysplasia to adenocarcinoma, removes any intramucosal cancers, and precludes the development of recurrent and metachronous esophageal lesions that may occur with the endoscopic ablative techniques previously described. However, there has been reluctance to offer esophagectomy for high-grade dysplasia and intramucosal cancers because of the magnitude of the procedure and its potential associated morbidity. Because of the extremely low incidence of nodal involvement with intramucosal lesions, several authorities (14,63,64) recommend esophagectomy without systematic lymphadenectomy as the gold standard against which other, less aggressive treatment should be compared. Their argument is supported by data purporting to show significantly less morbidity with this operation compared with that associated with radical en bloc esophagectomy.

Williams et al. (64) at the University of Rochester retrospectively reviewed their experience with esophagectomy in the management of 35 patients with biopsy-proven high-grade dysplasia. Thirty-three patients (94.3%) underwent an esophagectomy via a transhiatal approach and two (5.7%) through a combined laparotomy and right thoracotomy. Of those patients undergoing transhiatal esophagectomy (THE), four (12.1%) were completed using a vagal-sparing technique. All but one patient underwent a cervical incision with cervical esophagogastric anastomosis, regardless of approach. A single patient underwent esophagogastric anastomosis performed in the high intra-thoracic position. All patients, except those undergoing vagal-sparing esophagectomy, underwent either pyloromyotomy or pyloroplasty for gastric drainage. Thirty-day perioperative and in-hospital mortality was zero. Complications occurred in 13 of 35 patients (37%) including 3 patients with pneumonia and 3 with self-limited anastomotic leaks. Foregut symptoms improved in all patients except complaints of dysphagia and choking. Dysphagia and choking, however, were mild, occurring less often than once per month in 83% (10/12) of these patients. Three patients developed symptoms that occurred daily. Of these patients, one had chest pain and one had epigastric pain. Both described these symptoms as short-lasting and occurring at meals. One patient experienced daily dysphagia. Two thirds (23/34) of patients were taking antacid medications for symptoms of heartburn or regurgitation, all with good relief. Most patients (82%) required at least one postoperative dilation for dysphagia. Patient satisfaction was high (97%), with almost all patients stating they would choose surgery again if given the choice. Medium-term survival was excellent, approaching 100% at nearly 3-years of follow-up.

At the University of Southern California (USC), the decision for esophagectomy or an attempt at esophageal preservation for patients with high-grade dysplasia and intramucosal adenocarcinoma is based on the extent and severity of the mucosal disease and the functional status of the esophagus and associated pathophysiologic abnormalities (14,63,64). In general, patients with short-segment Barrett's and normal esophageal body function with a small or moderate-sized hiatal hernia are considered ideal potential candidates for esophageal preservation. If a visible lesion is present in these patients, they undergo endoscopic mucosal resection of the lesion, and if it is completely excised and confined to the mucosa on pathologic review of the specimen, the residual Barrett's is treated with radiofrequency ablation. The patients are maintained on high-dose proton pump inhibitor medication and have surveillance endoscopy with biopsies every 3 months for a year to confirm complete elimination of all Barrett's esophagus. After a year of negative biopsies (no Barrett's esophagus or cancer) patients are considered for antireflux surgery to eliminate reflux and potentially reduce the likelihood of recurrent Barrett's esophagus.

In contrast, patients who are considered poor candidates for esophageal preservation by the USC group are those that present with high-grade dysplasia or an intramucosal adenocarcinoma and have severe reflux symptoms or dysphagia, long-segment Barrett's esophagus with a large, fixed hiatal hernia and poor esophageal body motility. These patients, who do not require lymphadenectomy, are treated with a vagal-sparing esophagectomy. Vagal-sparing esophagectomy is also undertaken for patients with multiple lesions within long-segment Barrett's esophagus or lesions with positive lateral margins after endoscopic mucosal resection.

A vagal-sparing esophagectomy is carried out through an abdominal and left neck approach, either via laparotomy or as a laparoscopic procedure. A highly selective vagotomy is then performed along the lesser curvature of the stomach from the crow's foot up to the gastroesophageal junction. A formal abdominal lymphadenectomy is not part of this procedure inasmuch as preservation of the vagal branches along the lesser curvature

of the stomach precludes a lymph node dissection around the left gastric vessels. Gastrointestinal continuity is restored with a gastric pullup. No pyloroplasty procedure is required because the antral innervation is preserved.

The vagal-sparing technique is preferred by surgeons at USC in view of their findings in a retrospective comparison of experience at USC with en bloc, transhiatal, and vagal-sparing esophagectomies for high-grade dysplasia and intramucosal carcinoma (14,63,64). The study revealed equivalent oncologic outcome among the procedures; however, the vagal-sparing procedure was associated with a reduced incidence of postvagotomy symptoms and less weight loss postoperatively compared with transhiatal or en bloc resections. In addition, they found that perioperative morbidity including infectious, respiratory, and anastomotic complications were all reduced in patients who had the vagal-sparing procedure.

SURGICAL MANAGEMENT OF INVASIVE DISEASE

Esophagectomy is the mainstay of treatment for localized, resectable carcinoma of the esophagus, either as the sole therapy or as the key component in multimodality treatment. Approaches to esophageal resection for cancer in current practice are outlined in Table 31.2. The main controversial aspects in surgical management relate to the optimal technique of esophagectomy, transthoracic or transhiatal, and the extent of lymphadenectomy. Proponents of the transhiatal approach emphasize the shorter operative procedure, fewer pulmonary complications, longer proximal margins of resection, and a cervical rather than an intrathoracic anastomosis, where the risk of significant sepsis after leak is much less. Advocates of the transthoracic approach discuss the benefits of dissection under direct vision and an extended lymphadenectomy to more adequately stage the disease and provide local control. Two small randomized trials showed similar morbidity and mortality and survival rates between the two approaches (65,66).

Rindani et al. (67) reviewed 44 series published between 1986 and 1996 reporting the results of THE or transthoracic resection using the Ivor Lewis approach. There were 2,675 patients who underwent THE and 2,808 who had a thoracotomy. There were no differences in morbidity between the two groups with respect to pulmonary or cardiac complications or survival at 5 years. The authors calculated that in order to demonstrate a significant difference in morbidity or long-term survival between the two techniques, 3,100 patients would be required in each arm of a prospective, randomized trial.

Transhiatal Esophagectomy

In 2007, Orringer et al. (32), at the University of Michigan, reported the results of 30 years of experience in the performance of 2,007 THE procedures, including 1,063 procedures performed between 1976 and 1998 (group I) and 944 from 1998 to 2006 (group II). The procedure was undertaken for cancer in 1,525 of the patients. Following removal of the esophagus from the posterior mediastinum, the stomach was used as the esophageal substitute in 97% of the cases. The stomach was advanced through the original esophageal bed in the posterior mediastinum into

Table 31.2

Approaches to Esophageal Resection for Cancer

Transhiatal esophagectomy
  Laparotomy and cervical approach
  Peritumoral or two-field lymph node dissection
  En bloc resection feasible for distal esophageal tumors
  Cervical anastomosis

Transthoracic
  Ivor Lewis two-stage technique (38)
    Right thoracotomy and laparotomy
    Peritumoral or two-field lymph node dissection
    En bloc resection feasible for middle or distal thoracic tumors
  McKeown three-stage technique (39)
    Right thoracotomy, laparotomy, cervical approach
    Peritumoral, two-field or three-field lymph node dissection
    En bloc resection feasible for middle or distal thoracic tumors
    Cervical anastomosis

Left thoracotomy
  Left thoracotomy with or without cervical approach
  Peritumoral lymph node dissection
  Intrathoracic or cervical anastomosis

Left thoracoabdominal
  Left thoracoabdominal approach
  Peritumoral or two-field lymph node dissection
  Intrathoracic anastomosis

Minimally invasive techniques
  Laparoscopic and thoracoscopic approaches
  Robotically assisted approach

Modified after Posner MC, Minsky BD, Ilson DH. Cancer of the esophagus. In: DeVita VT Jr, Lawrence TS, Rosenberg SA, eds. *Cancer Principles and Practice of Oncology.* 8th ed. Philadelphia: Lippincott Williams & Wilkins; 2008:993–1043.

the neck where cervical esophagogastric anastomosis was performed. In recent years the anastomosis was performed in a stapled side-to-side fashion. The adoption of this refinement in technique has resulted in the reduction in the incidence of anastomotic leak and subsequent stricture formation. A pyloromyotomy was routinely performed. Accessible subcarinal, paraesophageal, gastrohepatic ligament, and celiac axis lymph nodes were routinely sampled in patients with esophageal carcinoma, but an *en bloc* wide resection of the esophagus and adjacent regional lymph nodes was not performed.

In comparing the earlier experience of the Michigan group with this operation (group I) and their more recent experience (group II), significant improvements (p <0.001) were observed in overall hospital mortality (4% vs. 1%); mean blood loss (677 vs. 368 mL); the rate of anastomotic leak (14% vs. 9%); and the frequency of hospital discharge within 10 days (52% vs. 78%). Major complications remained infrequent: wound infection/dehiscence, 3%; atelectasis/pneumonia, 2%; and intratho-

racic hemorrhage, recurrent laryngeal nerve paralysis, chylothorax, and tracheal laceration, <1% each. A 3% hospital mortality rate was observed among the 1,525 patients undergoing esophagectomy for cancer. The improvements over time were attributed to technical refinements in the performance of the procedure, a strict protocol of perioperative management, and the high-volume experience at the University of Michigan.

The overall 5-year survival for patients with cancer was 29%. Significant differences in 5-year survival were observed depending on (a) the site of the tumor, with midesophageal tumors having the worst prognosis (p <0.0001; Figure 31.1); (b) the histologic type (adenocarcinoma, 31% vs. squamous, 23%; p <0.0001), and (c) the stage of disease (stage 0 and I significantly longer than more advanced stages; p <0.0001 (Table 31.3). Among 583 cancer patients who received neoadjuvant chemoradiation, 121 (21%) had complete pathologic responses. These complete responders had a significantly better 5-year survival rate (58%) than those with residual disease (22%) (p <0.0001).

Transthoracic Esophagectomy with Extended Lymphadenectomy

The benefit of systematically removing lymph nodes at the time of esophagectomy remains controversial. Various studies consider patient outcome in relation to the total number of lymph nodes removed, the number of metastatic nodes found, the ratio of metastatic to total nodes retrieved, and the survival benefit of a formal en bloc lymphadenectomy with resection to include the abdominal and mediastinal lymph nodes (two-field dissection) or extended further to include the cervical lymph node basin (three-field dissection).

Schwarz and Smith (68) reviewed the records of 5,620 patients with adenocarcinoma (57% of cases) and squamous cell carcinoma (43%) extracted from the SEER 1973–2003 database. Relationships between the number of lymph nodes examined and overall survival were analyzed. On multivariate analysis, total lymph node count (or negative lymph node count, respectively) was an independent prognostic variable, aside from age, race, resection status, radiation, T category, N category (all at p <0.0001), and M category (p = 0.0003). Higher total lymph node count (>30) and negative lymph node count (>15) categories were associated with best overall survival and lowest 90-day mortality (p <0.0001). The numeric lymph node effect on overall survival was independent from nodal status or histology. The authors concluded that greater total and negative lymph node counts are associated with longer survival from cancer of the esophagus. Although they were unable to define the mechanism for these findings, the authors contend that the results were not due solely to stage migration.

In a study of a subset of 972 node-negative patients extracted from the SEER database, Greenstein et al. (69) found that disease-specific survival rates increased with a higher number of negative lymph nodes. The 5-year disease-specific survival rate was 55% among patients with 10 or fewer negative lymph nodes, compared with 66% and 75%, respectively, for those with 11 to 17 negative lymph nodes and 18 or more negative lymph nodes. The number of negative lymph nodes was found to be significantly associated with survival in analyses

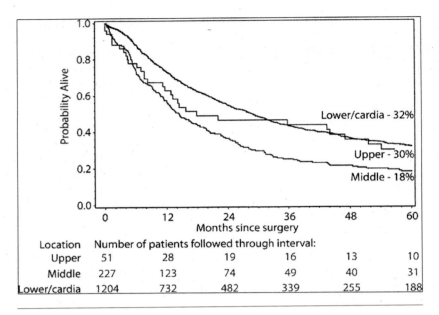

Figure 31.1 Site-dependent Kaplan-Meier survival curves in patients undergoing transhiatal esophagectomy for carcinoma of the intrathoracic esophagus and cardia. Differences in survival were significantly different (*p* <0.0001). (From Orringer MB, Marshall B, Chang AC, et al. Two thousand transhiatal esophagectomies: changing trends, lessons learned. *Ann Surg.* 2007;246:363–374.)

stratified by tumor status. On multivariate regression controlling for age, race/ethnicity, sex, histology, tumor status, and postoperative radiotherapy, a higher number of negative lymph nodes was found to be independently associated with higher disease-specific survival. The authors concluded that for determining accurate stage and prognosis, and for postoperative treatment planning, patients undergoing surgical resection for esophageal cancer should have at least 18 lymph nodes removed.

Table 31.3

Kaplan-Meir Survival after Transhiatal Esophagectomy by Tumor Stage

TNM Stage	No. Patients	Survival (%, 95% CI)	
		2 Yr	5 Yr
0	154	80.8 (73.0–86.5)	58.8 (49.1–67.3)
1	279	85.5 (80.0–89.7)	65.1 (56.5–72.5)
IIA	310	53.7 (47.5–59.6)	27.8 (22.2–33.7)
IIB	171	50.6 (42.3–58.3)	29.5 (21.8–37.5)
III	469	31.7 (27.4–36.2)	11.1 (8.2–14.5)
IVA	44	17.3 (7.7–30.1)	9.9 (3.2–21.2)
IVB	45	7.0 (1.8–17.2)	0
Unstaged	2	—	—

CI, confidence interval.
From Orringer MB, Marshall B, Chang AC, et al. Two thousand transhiatal esophagectomies: changing trends, lessons learned. *Ann Surg.* 2007;246:363–374.

Transthoracic en bloc esophagectomy has been studied extensively by DeMeester and his colleagues at USC. In 2001, the USC group (70) published an analysis of a series of 100 consecutive patients with potentially curable esophageal adenocarcinoma treated by en bloc resection, including a systematic abdominal and mediastinal lymph node dissection. None of the patients received neoadjuvant radiation or chemotherapy. The two-field en bloc procedure was performed through an initial right thoracotomy followed by a midline laparotomy. In all patients the proximal anastomosis was performed through an incision in the left neck. The thoracic dissection included removal of the azygos vein with its associated nodes, the thoracic duct, and the low paratracheal, subcarinal, paraesophageal, and parahiatal nodes in continuity with the resected esophagus. The block of tissue removed was bounded laterally on each side by the excised mediastinal pleura, anteriorly by the pericardium and membranous trachea, and posteriorly by the aorta and vertebral bodies. The abdominal dissection included removal of the lymph nodes along the hepatic artery and portal vein from the porta hepatis to the celiac trunk, around the celiac trunk, and along the left gastric artery and lesser curvature of the stomach. In addition, all the retroperitoneal tissue cephalad to the hepatic artery was removed, including the tissue that lies over the inferior vena cava and the right crus of the diaphragm. On the left side, the tissues and lymph nodes surrounding the splenic artery and the tissue overlying the adrenal gland and left crus of the diaphragm were removed. In 62 patients the spleen and the lymph nodes along the splenic artery and in the splenic hilum were also removed. In 72 patients gastrointestinal continuity was reestablished by the use of an isoperistaltic colon interposition based on the left colic artery. In these patients, the abdominal dissection also included the removal of the proximal two thirds of the stomach, the omentum, and the lymph nodes along the proximal two thirds of the greater curvature of the stomach. In 28 patients the esophageal reconstruction was done by creating a gastric tube after a wide resection of the gastric cardia down to the fourth vein on the lesser curvature of the stomach. The use of the stomach for reconstruction was based on the size of the primary tumor, the degree to which it involved the proximal stomach, and the presence of intrinsic colonic disease (e.g., polyps, diverticula) or variations in vascular supply that precluded the use of the colon.

The overall actuarial survival rate at 5 years was 52%. Survival rates by American Joint Commission on Cancer staging system were stage 1 (n = 26), 94%; stage a (n = 11), 65%; stage 2b (n = 13), 65%; stage 3 (n = 32), 23%; and stage 4 (n = 18), 27%. The perioperative mortality rate was 6%. The median number of lymph nodes removed per patient was 48. No nodal recurrences were detected within the surgical field; there was one anastomotic recurrence. Six patients developed recurrences beyond the limits of the two-field dissection in cervical and/or superior mediastinal nodes.

Survival in this series of patients was inversely related to tumor depth, the presence of nodal metastases, the number of nodal metastases per patient, and the ratio of involved nodes to the total number of nodes removed. Tumor invasion of the muscularis propria or deeper was associated with lymph node involvement in 75% to 85% of patients, with up to 45% having more than four involved nodes, of which 30% to 40% were distant in location and 23% to 27% involved celiac nodes. The authors believe that these findings support their recommendation for transthoracic en bloc esophagectomy in patients with invasive disease. However, adjuvant chemotherapy is recommended in the presence of more than four metastatic nodes or a lymph node ratio of >10% as these findings identify a subset of patients with ≥80% risk of developing systemic metastases. In the authors' experience, surgical resection alone is unlikely to be curative in these patients.

In 2004, the USC group published a study (71) in which they compared the survival of patients with T3 N1 adenocarcinoma of the distal esophagus who were treated either by THE (22 patients) or transthoracic en bloc esophagectomy (27 patients). This was a retrospective case-control study between nonrandomized patients with similarly sized transmural tumors and lymph node metastases and the following matched criteria: tumors of similar location, more than 20 lymph nodes in the surgical specimen, R0 resection, no previous chemotherapy or radiation therapy, and follow-up until death or for a minimum of 5 years. The number of nodes harvested was greater with en bloc esophagectomy than with THE (median, 52 vs. 29 [range, 21 to 85 vs. 20 to 60]; p <0.001). The median number of involved nodes was similar with en bloc esophagectomy and THE (median, 5 vs. 7 [range, 1 to 19 vs. 1 to 16]). However, the only two independent factors that affected survival in a Cox proportional hazards analysis were the number of involved lymph nodes ($p = 0.01$) and the type of resection($p = 0.03$). Patients who underwent en bloc esophagectomy had an overall survival benefit over those who underwent THE ($p = 0.01$). However, the survival benefit of en bloc esophagectomy was limited to patients with eight or fewer nodes (p <0.001), with no difference in outcome seen between the two procedures when nine or more nodes were

involved ($p = 0.96$). The authors contend that the method of their study removed the effect of inaccurate preoperative staging and minimized the effect of postoperative stage migration because all patients had N1 disease. Inaccurate staging and stage migration are factors that have often confounded the interpretation of other published comparative studies. The authors hypothesize that the improved survival after transthoracic en bloc esophagectomy observed in the present study was because of more complete removal of local-regional nodes that harbored occult, micrometastatic disease.

In 2008, the USC group (72) reported that the improved outcome that they observed with en bloc esophagectomy was sustained even among patients who had received neoadjuvant therapy. Among 58 patients who had received neoadjuvant therapy, 40 had an en bloc resection and 18 had a THE. A complete pathologic response occurred in 17 (29.3%) of 58 patients. Overall survival at 5 years and survival in patients with residual disease after neoadjuvant therapy was significantly better with an en bloc resection (overall survival: 51% for en bloc resection and 22% for transhiatal resection [$p = 0.04$]; survival with residual disease: 48% for en bloc resection and 9% for transhiatal resection [$p = 0.02$]). Survival in patients with complete pathologic response tended to be better after an en bloc resection (en bloc, 70%; transhiatal, 43%; $p = 0.3$).

In view of reports indicating involvement of cervical lymph nodes in as many as one third of patients with esophageal carcinoma of either cell type (73,74), Akiyama et al. (75) in Japan, performed a series of operations in which they extended the en bloc lymphadenectomy to include an extensive thoracocervical node dissection (three-field dissection). In a retrospective review of their results among 717 patients who had undergone an R0 resection, the authors reported a 5-year survival rate of 55% in patients in whom the more extensive node dissection was performed compared to the 38.3% rate observed after a two-field dissection ($p = 0.0013$).

Altorki et al. (76) from Cornell University published the results of a prospective observational study of esophagectomy with three-field lymphadenectomy performed in 80 patients. Hospital mortality rate was only 4%, but significant morbidity was observed. Minor complications occurred in 15% of patients; however, major complications developed in 31%, including recurrent laryngeal nerve injury in 9%. Metastases to the recurrent laryngeal and/or deep cervical nodes occurred in 36% of patients irrespective of cell type (adenocarcinoma, 37%; squamous, 34%) or location within the esophagus (lower third, 32%; middle third, 60%). Although the frequency of cervicothoracic nodal disease was independent of cell type or tumor location within the esophagus, the frequency of such nodal metastases was influenced by the nodal status within the abdomen and/or mediastinum. Forty-three percent of patients with node-positive disease in the abdomen and/or mediastinum also had nodal metastases in the cervicothoracic region. In contrast, among patients with node-negative disease in the abdomen and mediastinum, only 13% had isolated metastases in the cervicothoracic nodes. Overall 5-year and disease-free survival rates were 51% and 46%, respectively. The 5-year survival rate for node-negative patients was 88%; that for those with nodal metastases was 33%. The 5-year survival rate in patients with positive cervical nodes was 25% (squamous, 40%; adenocarcinoma, 15%).

In this series, 32% of the patients were upstaged, primarily from stage III to stage IV, resulting in an improvement in stage-specific survival. In contrast to the authors' previously reported 34% 5-year survival in stage III patients following two-field en bloc resection (77), stage III survival was 53% in their current report. This apparent improvement in outcome was at least partly due to stage migration, as stage III patients in this series represented a more homogeneous group. To determine whether the three-field procedure results in a survival benefit for patients with stage IV disease, the authors call for a randomized controlled trial comparing the two approaches to lymph node management.

The value of a three-field dissection is apparently limited inasmuch as isolated postoperative recurrences in the third-field of nodal clearance after a two-field dissection are uncommon. Thus, Law et al. (78) and Dresner et al. (79) reported isolated cervical relapses in only 4% and 6%, respectively, of patients undergoing curative esophagectomy, and Hagen et al. (70) observed an isolated cervical and/or superior mediastinal nodal recurrence in only 6% of their patients at USC. In addition, any potential benefit must be weighed against the significant morbidity of the procedure reported even in experienced hands (76).

At the University of Miami we believe that excellent local control can be achieved without formal lymphadenectomy. We conducted a phase 2 trial to evaluate neoadjuvant and adjuvant combination chemotherapy for patients with T3N1 esophageal adenocarcinoma (80). Thirty of 33 enrolled patients underwent esophagectomy either by the transhiatal approach (24 patients) or the Ivor Lewis approach (six patients) without radical lymphadenectomy. With a median follow-up of over 50 months, only one patient had local recurrence. We contend that survival of patients with widely invasive disease or nodal disease depends on control of systemic disease and little can be achieved with extended local treatment to improve outcome.

Minimally Invasive Esophagectomy

Various centers have evaluated the feasibility of a minimally invasive approach to esophagectomy for patients with cancer. Luketich et al. (81) from the University of Pittsburgh reported their experience with a laparoscopic transhiatal approach combined with a right video-assisted thoracoscopic approach to mobilize the intrathoracic esophagus and facilitate a more complete node dissection. Continuity was restored with a cervical esophagogastrostomy. The procedure was attempted in 222 patients and successfully completed in 206; 16 patients (7.2%) required nonemergent conversion to an open procedure. Indications for the operation included 47 patients with high-grade dysplasia and 175 for cancer. Operative mortality was 1.4%; the median hospital stay was 7 days (range, 3 to 75). Kaplan-Meir survival rates at 40 months were approximately 95% for patients with high-grade dysplasia or carcinoma in situ and 70%, 20%, and 25% for stage I, II, and III disease, respectively. Employing a similar combined approach, Nguyen et al. (82) reported the results in 38 cancer patients. Operative mortality was 4.3%. The mean number of lymph nodes retrieved was 10.3. Three-year survival was 57%. Avital et al. (83) performed a laparoscopic THE in 19 cancer patients with an operative mortality of 4.5%. Lymphadenectomy yielded an average of 14.3 nodes. At a mean follow-up of 30 months, overall survival was 61%.

Early experience with robotically assisted laparoscopic THE was reported by Galvani and associates (84) at the University of Illinois. There was no perioperative mortality among 18 patients treated for esophageal adenocarcinoma. Mean operative time was 267 minutes with an estimated blood loss of 54 mL. The surgical specimen yielded an average of 14 lymph nodes per patient. At a mean follow-up period of 22 months, 11 patients (61%) remained disease-free. Kernstine et al. (85) have described a technique of completely robotic esophagectomy with three-field lymphadenectomy. Among eight patients so treated, there was no perioperative mortality. The extended lymphadenectomy yielded a mean of 25 lymph nodes.

TECHNICAL CONSIDERATIONS IN THE PERFORMANCE OF ESOPHAGECTOMY

Methods of Reconstruction

At the University of Miami, we believe that the preferred method of reconstruction after esophagectomy is the use of tubularized stomach drawn through the posterior mediastinum. The posterior mediastinum provides a more direct and shorter route that enables the gastric conduit to easily reach the neck or the esophagus at a level above the azygos vein and is associated with better gastric emptying. We occasionally use the alternative retrosternal route, especially if there is significant locoregional disease in the posterior mediastinum that may require further therapy, such as radiation. The retrosternal route, however, has limitations inasmuch as boluses of food may not progress easily across the thoracic inlet. Therefore, when we use this route for reconstruction, we usually remove the manubrium and medial part of the clavicle with an oscillating saw in order to increase the width of this space. The tubularized stomach is the preferable conduit for reconstruction because it has a well-defined and consistent blood supply and generally is of sufficient length to reach most areas, thereby allowing reconstruction with a single anastomosis.

In preparing the gastric conduit, the stomach and proximal duodenum need to be fully mobilized while preserving the right gastroepiploic artery. Preservation of this vessel is especially important if the conduit must reach the neck. If there is concern about the adequacy of the blood supply, the left gastric can be preserved, but this would necessitate an Ivor Lewis approach with an anastomosis in the right chest. If the stomach is not available or is unsuitable because of tumor involvement or inadequate length, the colon can be used for reconstruction. The potential use of the colon for reconstruction must be anticipated preoperatively as the vascular supply to the colon must be assessed with mesenteric angiography; colonoscopy is required to identify any unforeseen disease; and mechanical bowel preparation is necessary. Preferably, the left colon is used to construct an interposition graft, basing the blood supply on the ascending branch of the left colic or on the left branch of the middle colic. The colon is then brought up to the neck in an antiperistaltic manner. It is critical to determine that the colon graft is not twisted and that its length is appropriately measured. The colonic segment will elongate over time, which may produce a redundancy that impairs the passage of food. On the other hand, a benefit of reconstruction with the colon is a reduced incidence of leak and stricture.

Gastric Outlet Procedures

Because most esophagectomies involve a bilateral vagotomy, the advisability of performing a pyloric drainage procedure, such as pyloroplasty, pyloromyotomy or pyloromyectomy, to assure adequate gastric emptying must be considered. Most surgeons perform a pyloromyotomy or pyloroplasty to avoid gastric stasis and the possibility of aspiration pneumonia that may accompany a functional gastric outlet obstruction. Others (86), however, omit an emptying procedure claiming that symptomatic delay in gastric emptying only affects about 20% of patients, which, when it occurs, can be treated with prokinetic agents or balloon dilatation of the pylorus. In addition, omitting an emptying procedure avoids complications with which it may be associated, such as the dumping syndrome and bile reflux affecting the residual esophagus. Urschel and associates (87) performed a meta-analysis of nine randomized controlled trials that included 553 patients; the study was designed to compare the effect of pyloric drainage versus no drainage on patient outcomes. Early outcomes assessed by the meta-analysis included operative mortality, esophagogastric anastomotic leaks, pulmonary morbidity, pyloric drainage complications, fatal pulmonary aspiration, and gastric outlet obstruction. Late outcomes included gastric emptying (scintigraphic studies), bile reflux, food intake and nutritional status, and obstructive foregut symptoms. The results based on this small number of patients indicated that pyloric drainage procedures reduce the occurrence of early postoperative gastric outlet obstruction after esophagectomy with gastric reconstruction, but they have little effect on other early and late patient outcomes.

Anastomotic Leaks

Anastomotic leaks are uncommon in modern practice, occurring in about 6% to 9% of patients with either cervical or thoracic anastomoses (32,87–89). Many leaks are asymptomatic and are identified on routine contrast imaging. Symptomatic patients may present with a wide spectrum of clinical manifestations, which range from mild to severe.

Asymptomatic leaks in the neck discovered only on an x-ray contrast study require little specific treatment. Usually a delay of oral intake, especially solids, for a few days will suffice. In the presence of a minor, well-contained leak, ortal intake is withheld and antibiotics and parenteral nutrition are considered. Lerut et al. (89) prescribe somatostatin to diminish the volume of gastric secretion and a proton pump inhibitor to neutralize gastric acid secretion. Symptomatic leakage in the neck is generally associated with local inflammation, seroma, hematoma, or fistulous drainage of saliva or air. In a series of 2,007 THE procedures, Orringer et al. (32) encountered 232 cervical esophagogastric anastomotic leaks. All but 15 of the leaks were managed successfully in the short term by opening the neck wound at the bedside and local wound packing until healing by secondary intent occurred. Gastric tip necrosis necessitating takedown of the intrathoracic stomach and a cervical esophagostomy occurred in 15 patients.

Intrathoracic anastomotic leaks may be asymptomatic or may present with a wide array of clinical manifestations ranging from mild to severe and including circulatory collapse and multiorgan system failure. The severity of presentation largely depends on whether pleural space contamination and gastric necrosis occur. Among 761 patients who had undergone an esophagectomy with intrathoracic anastomosis at the Mayo Clinic (88) 48 patients (6.3%) developed an anastomotic leak. The esophageal leak was asymptomatic in 31.9% of the patients. Signs and symptoms were present in the remaining 68.1% and included pleural effusion in 27 patients, leukocytosis in 25 patients, shortness of breath in 19 patients, fever in 16 patients, chest pain in 8 patients, hypotension in 6 patients, atrial dysrhythmias in 6 patients, bilious drainage from the chest tube in 6 patients, hydropneumothorax in 6 patients, vomiting in 4 patients, subcutaneous emphysema in 4 patients, and renal failure in 2 patients.

Forty-five patients (95.7%) underwent diagnostic evaluation that included oral contrast examination in 37 patients (78.7%), CT of the chest with oral contrast in 23 patients (48.9%), and both in 15 patients (31.9%). Esophageal contrast examination demonstrated the leak in 42 (93.3%) of the 45 patients, although the initial contrast swallow failed to document the leak in nearly half of the patients. The leak was limited to the mediastinum in 28 patients (62.2%). Twenty-four of these mediastinal leaks were localized and considered contained; the remaining four were diffuse and therefore considered noncontained. The leak extended into the pleural space in 14 patients (33.3%) and involved the right pleural cavity in 12 patients, the left pleural cavity in one patient, and both cavities in one patient; all were considered noncontained. Overall, contrast examination revealed that the leak was contained in 24 patients and noncontained in 18 patients.

Surgical intervention was undertaken for symptomatic, noncontained intrathoracic leaks and for those leaks for which conservative management had failed. Twenty-seven patients (57.4%) were managed nonoperatively. Twenty patients (42.6%) required surgical intervention that included primary anastomotic repair in 14 patients, reinforcement of the anastomosis with viable tissue in 6 patients, and esophageal diversion in 2 patients. A single reoperation was done in 15 patients, and 5 patients required two reoperations. The mortality rate was 8.5%.

HEALTH-RELATED QUALITY OF LIFE AFTER SURGERY FOR CANCER OF THE ESOPHAGUS

Parameswaran and associates (90) reviewed randomized trials and longitudinal and cross-sectional studies that assessed health-related quality of life (HRQL) after esophagectomy with multidimensional, validated questionnaires. At a minimum, HRQL measures capture physical, psychological (including emotional and cognitive), and social functioning as well as assessing global quality of life. The study revealed that patients experience a global deterioration in almost all aspects of HRQL immediately after surgery, irrespective of the approach (i.e., open transthoracic or THE), from which it takes approximately 9 to 12 months to return to baseline values. Emotional functions, however, remained stable or even improved after surgery. In addition, dysphagia scores generally improve after surgery; however, relief of dysphagia is often replaced with other symptoms such as loss of appetite, change in taste, nausea, and diarrhea. The authors also found that surgical technique and perioperative outcomes seemed to influence HRQL. Patients who had a cervical esophagogastric anastomosis seemed to have better physical and social functions and fewer problems with insomnia and vomiting after surgery compared with those with an intrathoracic anastomosis, whereas patients who had a pyloroplasty had fewer problems with psychosocial functions, indigestion, and dysphagia. Postoperative complications like anastomotic leaks, sepsis, and cardiopulmonary complications adversely affected HRQL. Patients who subsequently developed recurrence of tumor or who died within 2 years after surgery seemed to have worse HRQL compared with those who remained disease-free. The authors recommend that methods be developed to provide patients with HRQL data as part of the preoperative informed consent process inasmuch as such data may have an impact on surgical decision making.

REFERENCES

1. Jemal A, Siegel R, Ward E, et al. Cancer statistics, 2008. *CA Cancer J Clin.* 2008;58:71–96.
2. Surveillance Epidemiology and End Results (SEER) Cancer of the Esophagus. 2009. Available at http://seer.cancer.gov/. Accessed June 13, 2009.
3. Posner MC, Minsky BD, Ilson DH. Cancer of the esophagus. In: DeVita VT Jr, Lawrence TS, Rosenberg SA, eds. *Cancer Principles and Practice of Oncology,* 8th ed. Philadelphia: Lippincott Williams & Wilkins; 2008:993–1043.
4. Brown LM, Devesa SS. Epidemiologic trends in esophageal and gastric cancer in the United States. *Surg Oncol Clin North Am.* 2002; 11:235–256.
5. Altorki NK. Carcinoma of the esophagus. In: Bland KI, Daly JM, Karakousis CP, eds. *Surgical Oncology: Contemporary Principles and Practice.* New York: McGraw-Hill; 2001:609–622.
6. Henteleff H, Casson AG. Epidemiology of malignant neoplasms. In: Pearson FG, Cooper JD, Deslauriers J, Ginsberg RJ, et al., eds. *Esophageal Surgery,* 2nd ed. New York: Churchill Livingstone; 2002:668–676.
7. Fernandes ML, Seow A, Chan YH, et al. Opposing trends in incidence of esophageal squamous cell carcinoma and adenocarcinoma in a multi-ethnic Asian country. *Am J Gastroenterol.* 2006;101:1430–1436.
8. Tse LA, Yu IT, Mang OW. Time trends of esophageal cancer in Hong Kong: age, period and birth cohort analyses. *Int J Cancer.* 2007;120:853–858.
9. Pohl H, Welch HG. The role of overdiagnosis and reclassification in the marked increase of esophageal adenocarcinoma incidence. *J Natl Cancer Inst.* 2005;97:142–146.
10. Devesa SS, Blot WJ, Fraumeni JF Jr. Changing patterns in the incidence of esophageal and gastric carcinoma in the United States. *Cancer.* 1998;83:2049–2053.
11. Bollschweiler E, Wolfgarten E, Gutschow C, et al. Demographic variations in the rising incidence of esophageal adenocarcinoma in white males. *Cancer.* 2001;92:549–555.
12. Jacob P, Kahrilas PJ, Desai T, et al. Natural history and significance of esophageal squamous cell dysplasia. *Cancer.* 1990;65:2731–2739.
13. Wang KK, Sampliner RE. Undated guidelines 2008 for the diagnosis, surveillance, and therapy of Barrett's esophagus. *Am J Gastroenterol.* 2008;103:788–797.
14. DeMeester SR. New options for the therapy of Barrett's high-grade dysplasia and intramucosal adenocarcinoma: endoscopic mucosal resection and ablation versus vagal-sparing esophagectomy. *Ann Thorac Surg.* 2008;85:S747–750.
15. Schuchert MJ, Luketich JD. Barrett's esophagus-emerging concepts and controversies. *J Surg Oncol.* 2007;95:185–189.
16. Reid BJ, Blount PL, Feng Z, et al. Optimizing endoscopic biopsy detection of early cancers in Barrett's high-grade dysplasia. *Am J Gastroenterol.* 2000;95:3089–3096.
17. Wilson BC. Detection and treatment of dysplasia in Barrett's esophagus: a pivotal challenge in translating biophotonics from bench to bedside. *J Biomed Opt.* 2007;12:051401.
18. Yousef F, Cardwell C, Cantwell MM, et al. The incidence of esophageal cancer and high-grade dysplasia in Barrett's esophagus: a systematic review and meta-analysis. *Am J Epidemiol.* 2008;168: 237–249.
19. Finley RJ. Adenocarcinoma of the esophagus and esophagogastric junction. In: Pearson FG, Cooper JD, Deslauriers J, et al., eds. *Esophageal Surgery,* 2nd ed. New York: Churchill-Livingstone; 2002: 724–734.
20. Law SYK, Wong J. Management of squamous cell carcinoma of the esophagus. In: Pearson FG, Cooper JD, Deslauriers J, et al., eds. *Esophageal Surgery,* 2nd ed. New York: Churchill-Livingstone; 2002: 705–724.
21. Nigro JJ, DeMeester SR, Hagen JA, et al. Node status in transmural esophageal adenocarcinoma and outcome after en bloc esophagectomy. *J Thorac Cardiovasc Surg.* 1999;117:960–968.
22. Plukker JT, van Westreenen HL. Staging in oesophageal cancer. *Best Pract Res Clin Gastroenterol.* 2006;20:877–891.
23. Murata Y, Suzuki S, Ohta M, et al. Small ultrasonic probes for determination of the depth of superficial esophageal cancer. *Gastrointest Endosc.* 1996;44:23–28.
24. May A, Gunter E, Roth F, et al. Accuracy of staging in early oesophageal cancer using high resolution endoscopy and high resolution endosonography: a comparative, prospective, and blinded trial. *Gut.* 2004;53:634–640.
25. Botet JF, Lightdale CJ, Zauber AG, et al. Preoperative staging of esophageal cancer: comparison of endoscopic US and dynamic CT. *Radiology.* 1991;181:419–425.
26. Nishimaki T, Tanaka O, Ando N, et al. Evaluation of the accuracy of preoperative staging in thoracic esophageal cancer. *Ann Thorac Surg.* 1999;68:2059–2064.
27. Vazquez-Sequeiros E, Norton ID, Clain JE, et al. Impact of EUS-guided fine-needle aspiration on lymph node staging in patients with esophageal carcinoma. *Gastrointest Endosc.* 2001;53:751–757.
28. Torek F. The first successful case of resection of the thoracic portion of the esophagus for carcinoma. *Surg Gynecol Obstet.* 1913;16: 614–617.
29. Orringer MB. Technical aids in performing transhiatal esophagectomy without thoracotomy. *Ann Thorac Surg.* 1984;38:128–132.
30. Orringer MB. Transhiatal esophagectomy without thoracotomy for carcinoma of the thoracic esophagus. *Ann Surg.* 1984;200:282–288.
31. Orringer MB. Current status of transhiatal esophagectomy. *Adv Surg.* 2000;34:193–236.
32. Orringer MB, Marshall B, Chang AC, et al. Two thousand transhiatal esophagectomies: changing trends, lessons learned. *Ann Surg.* 2007;246:363–374.
33. Orringer MB, Marshall B, Iannettoni MD. Transhiatal esophagectomy: clinical experience and refinements. *Ann Surg.* 1999;230: 392–403.
34. Orringer MB, Marshall B, Iannettoni MD. Eliminating the cervical esophagogastric anastomotic leak with a side-to-side stapled anastomosis. *J Thorac Cardiovasc Surg.* 2000;119:277–288.
35. Orringer MB, Marshall B, Iannettoni MD. Transhiatal esophagectomy for treatment of benign and malignant esophageal disease. *World J Surg.* 2001;25:196–203.
36. Van den Broek WT, Makay O, Berends FJ, et al. Laparoscopically assisted transhiatal resection for malignancies of the distal esophagus. *Surg Endosc.* 2004;18:812–817.

37. Ohsawa T. Esophageal surgery. *J Jpn Surg Soc.* 1933;34:950–1318.

38. Lewis I. The surgical treatment of carcinoma of the oesophagus with special reference to a new operation for growths of the middle third. *Br J Surg.* 1946;34:18–31.

39. McKeown KC. Total three-stage oesophagectomy for cancer of the oesophagus. *Br J Surg.* 1976;63:259–262.

40. Akiyama H, Tsurumaru M, Kawamura T, Ono Y. Esophageal stripping with preservation of the vagus nerve. *Int Surg.* 1982;67:125–128.

41. Akiyama H, Tsurumaru M, Ono Y, et al. Esophagectomy without thoracotomy with vagal preservation. *J Am Coll Surg.* 1994;178:83–85.

42. Swanstrom LL, Hansen P. Laparoscopic total esophagectomy. *Arch Surg.* 1997;132:943–949.

43. Attwood SE, Lewis CJ, Caplin S, et al. Argon beam plasma coagulation as therapy for high-grade dysplasia in Barrett's esophagus. *Clin Gastroenterol Hepatol.* 2003;1:258–263.

44. Prasad GA, Wang KK, Halling KC, et al. Correlation of histology with biomarker status after photodynamic therapy in Barrett's esophagus. *Cancer.* 2008;113:470–476.

45. Schnell TG, Sontag SJ, Chejfec G, et al. Long-term nonsurgical management of Barrett's esophagus with high-grade dysplasia. *Gastroenterology.* 2001;120:1607–1619.

46. Weston AP, Sharma P, Topalovski M, et al. Long-term follow-up of Barrett's high-grade dysplasia. *Am J Gastroenterol.* 2000;95:1888–1893.

47. Konda VJ, Ross AS, Ferguson MK, et al. Is the risk of concomitant invasive esophageal cancer in high-grade dysplasia in Barrett's esophagus overestimated? *Clin Gastroenterol Hepatol.* 2008;6:159–164.

48. Liu L, Hofstetter WL, Rashid A, et al. Significance of the depth of tumor invasion and lymph node metastasis in superficially invasive (T1) esophageal adenocarcinoma. *Am J Surg Pathol.* 2005;29:1079–1085.

49. Overholt BF, Panjehpour M, Halberg DL. Photodynamic therapy for Barrett's esophagus with dysplasia and/or early stage carcinoma: long-term results. *Gastrointest Endosc.* 2003;58:183–188.

50. Wang KK. Current status of photodynamic therapy of Barrett's esophagus. *Gastrointest Endosc.* 1999;49(3 Pt 2):S20–23.

51. Overholt BF, Wang KK, Burdick JS, et al. Five-year efficacy and safety of photodynamic therapy with Photofrin in Barrett's high-grade dysplasia. *Gastrointest Endosc.* 2007;66:460–468.

52. Prasad GA, Wang KK, Buttar NS, et al. Long-term survival following endoscopic and surgical treatment of high-grade dysplasia in Barrett's esophagus. *Gastroenterology.* 2007;132:1226–1233.

53. Ell C, May A, Pech O, et al. Curative endoscopic resection of early esophageal adenocarcinomas (Barrett's cancer). *Gastrointest Endosc.* 2007;65:3–10.

54. Lopes CV, Hela M, Pesenti C, et al. Circumferential endoscopic resection of Barrett's esophagus with high-grade dysplasia or early adenocarcinoma. *Surg Endosc.* 2007;21:820–824.

55. Larghi A, Lightdale CJ, Ross AS, et al. Long-term follow-up of complete Barrett's eradication endoscopic mucosal resection (CBE-EMR) for the treatment of high grade dysplasia and intramucosal carcinoma. *Endoscopy.* 2007;39:1086–1091.

56. Buttar NS, Wang KK, Lutzke LS, et al. Combined endoscopic mucosal resection and photodynamic therapy for esophageal neoplasia within Barrett's esophagus. *Gastrointest Endosc.* 2001;54:682–688.

57. Shimizu Y, Tsukagoshi H, Fujita M, et al. Long-term outcome after endoscopic mucosal resection in patients with esophageal squamous cell carcinoma invading the muscularis mucosae or deeper. *Gastrointest Endosc.* 2002;56:387–390.

58. Maish MS, DeMeester SR. Endoscopic mucosal resection as a staging technique to determine the depth of invasion of esophageal adenocarcinoma. *Ann Thorac Surg.* 2004;78:1777–1782.

59. Gondrie JJ, Pouw RE, Sondermeijer CM, et al. Effective treatment of early Barrett's neoplasia with stepwise circumferential and focal ablation using the HALO system. *Endoscopy.* 2008;40:370–379.

60. Sharma VK, Wang KK, Overholt BF, et al. Balloon-based, circumferential, endoscopic radiofrequency ablation of Barrett's esophagus: 1-year follow-up of 100 patients. *Gastrointest Endosc.* 2007;65:185–195.

61. Smith CD, Bejarano PA, Melvin WS, et al. Endoscopic ablation of intestinal metaplasia containing high-grade dysplasia in esophagectomy patients using a balloon-based ablation system. *Surg Endosc.* 2007;21:560–569.

62. Shaheen NJ, Sharma P, Overholt BF. Radiofrequency ablation in Barrett's esophagus with dysplasia. *N Engl J Med.* 2009;360:2277–2288.

63. Peyre CG, DeMeester SR, Rizzetto C, et al. Vagal-sparing esophagectomy: the ideal operation for intramucosal adenocarcinoma and barrett with high-grade dysplasia. *Ann Surg.* 2007;246:665–674.

64. Williams VA, Watson TJ, Herbella FA, et al. Esophagectomy for high grade dysplasia is safe, curative, and results in good alimentary outcome. *J Gastrointest Surg.* 2007;11:1589–1597.

65. Chu KM, Law SY, Fok M, et al. A prospective randomized comparison of transhiatal and transthoracic resection for lower-third esophageal carcinoma. *Am J Surg.* 1997;174:320–324.

66. Goldminc M, Maddern G, Le Prise E, et al. Oesophagectomy by a transhiatal approach or thoracotomy: a prospective randomized trial. *Br J Surg.* 1993;80:367–370.

67. Rindani R, Martin CJ, Cox MR. Transhiatal versus Ivor-Lewis oesophagectomy: is there a difference? *Aust N Z J Surg.* 1999;69:187–194.

68. Schwarz RE, Smith DD. Clinical impact of lymphadenectomy extent in resectable esophageal cancer. *J Gastrointest Surg.* 2007;11:1384–1394.

69. Greenstein AJ, Litle VR, Swanson SJ, et al. Effect of the number of lymph nodes sampled on postoperative survival of lymph node-negative esophageal cancer. *Cancer.* 2008;112:1239–1246.

70. Hagen JA, DeMeester SR, Peters JH, et al. Curative resection for esophageal adenocarcinoma: analysis of 100 en bloc esophagectomies. *Ann Surg.* 2001;234:520–531.

71. Johansson J, DeMeester TR, Hagen JA, et al. En bloc vs transhiatal esophagectomy for stage T3 N1 adenocarcinoma of the distal esophagus. *Arch Surg.* 2004;139:627–633.

72. Rizzetto C, DeMeester SR, Hagen JA, et al. En bloc esophagectomy reduces local recurrence and improves survival compared with transhiatal resection after neoadjuvant therapy for esophageal adenocarcinoma. *J Thorac Cardiovasc Surg.* 2008;135:1228–1236.

73. Isono K, Ochiai T, Okuyama K, et al. The treatment of lymph node metastasis from esophageal cancer by extensive lymphadenectomy. *Jpn J Surg.* 1990;20:151–157.

74. Kato H, Watanabe H, Tachimori Y, et al. Evaluation of neck lymph node dissection for thoracic esophageal carcinoma. *Ann Thorac Surg.* 1991;51:931–935.

75. Akiyama H, Tsurumaru M, Udagawa H, et al. Radical lymph node dissection for cancer of the thoracic esophagus. *Ann Surg.* 1994;220:364–373.

76. Altorki N, Kent M, Ferrara C, et al. Three-field lymph node dissection for squamous cell and adenocarcinoma of the esophagus. *Ann Surg.* 2002;236:177–183.

77. Altorki NK, Girardi L, Skinner DB. En bloc esophagectomy improves survival for stage III esophageal cancer. *J Thorac Cardiovasc Surg.* 1997;114:948–956.

78. Law SY, Fok M, Wong J. Pattern of recurrence after oesophageal resection for cancer: clinical implications. *Br J Surg.* 1996;83:107–111.

79. Dresner SM, Griffin SM. Pattern of recurrence following radical oesophagectomy with two-field lymphadenectomy. *Br J Surg.* 2000;87:1426–1433.

80. Ardalan B, Spector SA, Livingstone AS, et al. Neoadjuvant, surgery and adjuvant chemotherapy without radiation for esophageal cancer. *Jpn J Clin Oncol.* 2007;37:590–596.

81. Luketich JD, Alvelo-Rivera M, Buenaventura PO, et al. Minimally invasive esophagectomy: outcomes in 222 patients. *Ann Surg.* 2003; 238:486–495.

82. Nguyen NT, Roberts P, Follette DM, et al. Thoracoscopic and laparoscopic esophagectomy for benign and malignant disease: lessons learned from 46 consecutive procedures. *J Am Coll Surg.* 2003; 197:902–913.

83. Avital S, Zundel N, Szomstein S, et al. Laparoscopic transhiatal esophagectomy for esophageal cancer. *Am J Surg.* 2005;190: 69–74.

84. Galvani CA, Gorodner MV, Moser F, et al. Robotically assisted laparoscopic transhiatal esophagectomy. *Surg Endosc.* 2008;22:188–195.

85. Kernstine KH, DeArmond DT, Shamoun DM, Campos JH. The first series of completely robotic esophagectomies with three-field lymphadenectomy: initial experience. *Surg Endosc.* 2007;21:2285–2292.

86. Velanovich V. Esophagogastrectomy without pyloroplasty. *Dis Esophagus.* 2003;16:243–245.

87. Urschel JD, Blewett CJ, Young JE, et al. Pyloric drainage (pyloroplasty) or no drainage in gastric reconstruction after esophagectomy: a meta-analysis of randomized controlled trials. *Dig Surg.* 2002;19:160–164.

88. Crestanello JA, Deschamps C, Cassivi SD, et al. Selective management of intrathoracic anastomotic leak after esophagectomy. *J Thorac Cardiovasc Surg.* 2005;129:254–260.

89. Lerut T, Coosemans W, Decker G, et al. Anastomotic complications after esophagectomy. *Dig Surg.* 2002;19:92–98.

90. Parameswaran R, McNair A, Avery KN, et al. The role of health-related quality of life outcomes in clinical decision making in surgery for esophageal cancer: a systematic review. *Ann Surg Oncol.* 2008;15:2372–2379.

COMMENTARY
Mitchell C. Posner

Chapter 31, "Surgical Management of Cancer of the Esophagus," provides a broad overview of the challenges inherent in present-day management of patients with esophageal cancer. At a time when greater emphasis has been appropriately placed on the multidisciplinary treatment of patients with solid tumors while surgery has inappropriately been viewed by many experts as a modality of less significance, three areas or issues deserve further attention:

1. The extent of surgical resection and its impact on outcome,
2. Surgeon/hospital volume and its relationship to adequate performance of esophagectomy, and
3. The role of surgery in the era of multimodality therapy of cancer of the esophagus.

I would like to address these issues separately, but the reader should be well aware that these areas are all interrelated in the ultimate goal of providing both high-quality and consistent care for the patient with esophageal cancer.

EXTENT OF SURGICAL RESECTION

There is no issue that engenders more debate among experts than the optimal surgical approach to a patient with esophageal cancer. The controversy can be distilled down to whether a more extended resection through a transthoracic approach provides superior oncologic outcome to a resection with more limited morbidity and mortality via a transhiatal approach.

There have been two large meta-analyses (1,2) using collective reviews of numerous individual studies comparing transhiatal esophagectomy with transthoracic esophagectomy. Most of the studies included in these meta-analyses were retrospective in nature and were not consistent with respect to the surgical technique used and what therapy in addition to surgery was delivered. The meta-analysis by Rindani et al. (1) involved almost 5,500 patients from 44 published series over a decade beginning in 1986. Drs. Spector and Livingstone correctly point out that there were no differences in overall perioperative morbidity between the two surgical approaches. However, transhiatal esophagectomy was associated with a higher incidence of certain complications: anastomotic leak, anastomotic stricture, and recurrent laryngeal nerve injury. Importantly, postoperative mortality was substantially higher in the transthoracic esophagectomy group (9.5%) than in the transhiatal group (6.3%). Overall 5-year survival was equivalent. The second large meta-analysis, not mentioned in the chapter, involved over 7,500 patients gleaned from 50 studies over a 9-year period beginning in 1990 (2). Transthoracic esophagectomy was associated with a statistically significant higher risk of pulmonary complications. Transhiatal esophagectomy was associated with a statistically significant higher rate of anastomotic leaks. Again, postoperative mortality was significantly higher in the transthoracic group, but 5-year survival was no different between the transthoracic and transhiatal esophagectomy cohorts.

Until recently, these meta-analyses and other retrospective reviews were the only data available to help guide practitioners with regard to the relative merits of transthoracic versus transhiatal esophagectomy. However, in 2002 Hulscher et al. (3) provided level I evidence regarding this controversial issue in an article published in the *New England Journal of Medicine*. Two hundred twenty patients were randomly assigned to either transthoracic or transhiatal esophagectomy. Patients undergoing transthoracic esophagectomy were statistically more likely to develop postoperative pulmonary complications and prolonged intensive care unit and hospital stay. Although transthoracic esophagectomy was associated with a higher perioperative morbidity rate, there was no significant increase in hospital mortality between the two groups. Importantly, there were no statistically significant differences in median disease-free or overall survival between the two surgical approaches at a median follow-up of almost 5 years. Furthermore, rates of local regional and distant recurrence were the same between the two treatment arms. These data suggest that oncologic outcome is not substantially influenced by the surgical approach to esophagectomy and that either procedure is associated with acceptable morbidity and mortality in the hands of experienced surgeons.

SURGEON/HOSPITAL VOLUME AND ESOPHAGECTOMY

Common sense would dictate that better outcomes on a more consistent basis would be achieved the more frequently a surgical procedure is performed by an individual or at an institution. This is borne out by increasing evidence that patients who undergo complex oncologic resections at high-volume hospitals by experienced high-volume surgeons have significantly lower rates of perioperative morbidity and mortality (4–6). Postoperative morbidity and operative mortality following esophagectomy has been consistently demonstrated to be strongly associated with hospital/surgeon volume, and that relationship is one of the strongest among all complex cancer operations (4–6). Furthermore, a recent analysis of the National Surveillance Epidemiology and End Results–Medicare-linked database (7) suggests that not only is short-term outcome following esophagectomy influenced by hospital/surgeon volume but long-term survival is also volume-dependent. The probability of surviving 5 years following esophagectomy in high-volume hospitals was 34%, whereas 5-year survival probability in low-volume hospitals was only 17%. This 17% absolute difference in 5-year survival following esophagectomy between high- and low-volume hospitals was the highest among all cancer resections surveyed. The volume-dependent discrepancy in 5-year survival could not be attributed to differences in the delivery of adjuvant therapy. Therefore, not only are short-term procedure-related outcomes associated with surgical experience, but long-term oncologic outcomes may also be driven by surgeons in centers where esophageal resection is frequently performed. The basis for this improved survival has not been defined and requires further investigation.

ROLE OF SURGERY IN THE MULTIMODALITY THERAPY ERA

Relative 5-year survival rates for patients with esophageal cancer have improved over the 3 most recent successive decades beginning in the 1970s (8). Although the reason for this trend is surely multifactorial, this improvement in survival corresponds with the widespread acceptance and use of a multimodality treatment approach to esophageal cancer. This has led some investigators to examine the value of surgery in combined modality treatment regimens and others to suggest a diminished role for resection in the modern management of esophageal cancer. The former premise is based on hypothesis-driven scientific testing of surgery in the context of clinical trials and is appropriate. However, the latter subjective conclusion is at best premature and at worst irrational and has the potential to compromise delivery of treatment that offers the best opportunity for long-term survival. In an attempt to address this issue, as alluded to by Drs. Spector and Livingstone, squamous cell carcinoma and adenocarcinoma of the esophagus are distinct entities and should be considered as such when defining optimal therapy.

A recent report (9) updating the results of a multicenter trial conducted in the United States and designed to assess the value of preoperative chemotherapy plus surgery versus surgery alone provides some insight regarding the worth of achieving local control via surgery. Although there was no difference in disease-free or overall survival among those patients randomized to receive either chemotherapy plus surgery or surgery alone, only patients who underwent a resection resulting in microscopically negative margins (R0 resection) had a substantial chance of surviving disease-free over a long period. Thus, those patients who underwent such a complete, margin-negative resection had a 3-year survival of 39%, while those patients undergoing an R1 resection (microscopically positive margins) had a 3-year survival of 12%. Those patients with grossly positive margins (R2 resection) or who underwent no resection at all had an equivalent 3-year survival of only 4%. Of importance is the additional finding that there was no significant difference in the median survival among patients undergoing a R1 or R2 resection or no resection at all. Of the 467 patients registered for the study, there were equivalent numbers of those patients with squamous cell carcinoma and adenocarcinoma of the esophagus. These data strongly suggest that residual microscopic or gross tumor is associated with poor outcome and that a proper oncologically sound esophagectomy is an important component of a long-term disease-free state.

One question that might be asked is whether the addition of radiation therapy to the preoperative chemotherapy regimen is sufficient to provide adequate local control and, therefore, render surgery an unnecessary requirement for appropriate combined modality therapy. Results from the Radiation Therapy Oncology Group 85-01 trial (10) that randomized patients to definitive chemoradiotherapy versus radiation therapy alone (without surgery in either arm) suggests that a substantial number of patients will have residual disease following chemoradiotherapy. In this trial almost 50% of patients developed local failure as a first sign of failure following chemoradiotherapy. One can speculate that the addition of surgery to this regimen would have improved local control and potentially improved survival. Further evidence to support this contention can be found in the results of a phase 2 trial my colleagues and I conducted in which almost 60% of actual (not actuarial) 5-year survivors had residual tumor identified in their esophagectomy specimen following preoperative chemoradiotherapy (11). One can conclude that it is unlikely that patients who have residual tumor following chemoradiotherapy and do not have that disease resected would be counted among the long-term survivors. However, only level I evidence in the form of outcome results from phase 3 trials would provide scientific proof of the value of resection, or for that matter any other therapeutic intervention.

Two randomized trials began to address the role of surgery following chemoradiotherapy in patients with squamous cell carcinoma of the esophagus. A trial in France (FFCD9102) randomized 259 patients who had a partial response to chemoradiotherapy to either surgery or additional chemoradiotherapy (12). There was no significant difference in either 2-year survival or median survival in patients undergoing surgery versus those treated with chemoradiotherapy alone. Likewise, the German Oesophageal Cancer Study Group randomized 172 patients with esophageal squamous cell carcinoma to preoperative chemoradiotherapy plus surgery versus chemoradiotherapy alone (13). Although there was a decrease in 2-year local failure in those patients randomized to the surgical arm, there was no significant difference in 3-year survival between the preoperative chemotherapy followed by surgery versus chemoradiotherapy alone arms. Therefore, it could be reasonably argued that the addition of surgery to an effective regimen of chemoradiotherapy in patients with squamous cell carcinoma of the esophagus is of unproven value. In patients with squamous cell carcinoma, local control achieved with either radiation or surgery may, in fact, be equivalent and proper selection of treatment modalities will require further study.

No such level I evidence exists regarding the utility of resection in patients with adenocarcinoma of the esophagus, by far the more common histology identified in patients in the United States. In contradistinction to squamous cell esophageal carcinoma, the more pressing issue for patients with esophageal adenocarcinoma is the controversy regarding the value of preoperative combined modality therapy, not the worth of esophagectomy. Based on numerous phase 2 trials and five phase 3 trials (14–18) that compared concurrent preoperative chemoradiotherapy followed by surgery with surgery alone, it is not clear that preoperative chemoradiotherapy can be declared as standard of care. What has been documented is that the majority of patients are downstaged with preoperative chemoradiotherapy, and for those patients who have a substantial response (complete pathologic response or major partial response defined by residual microscopic disease in the resected specimen) to preoperative chemoradiotherapy there is a survival advantage. Surgery appears to be a critical component of combined modality therapy to eliminate residual disease following chemoradiotherapy leading to improved local regional and improved long-term survival. However, failure at a distant site is common and is the most frequent cause of death.

Although definitive proof of the benefit of preoperative chemoradiotherapy in the treatment of patients with esophageal cancer is lacking, the combined-modality approach has been adopted in most centers in the United States and is by far the most frequent therapeutic option offered to patients with cancer of the esophagus. A recent meta-analysis reported that preoperative chemoradiotherapy improved 3-year survival by 13% over surgery alone with similar improvement identified in patients with both squamous cell carcinoma and adenocarcinoma histology (19). Although the role of surgery has been questioned, there is little controversy that select patients benefit from esophageal resection, and in other patients surgery provides no additional advantage. Patients who have complete pathologic response to combined chemoradiotherapy probably gain little from undergoing esophagectomy, considering the substantial morbidity and mortality associated with the procedure. On the other hand, it is counterintuitive that patients with residual disease following preoperative combined-modality treatment would not benefit from eradicating that residual disease with resection to give them the best opportunity for a long-term disease-free state.

The challenge that confronts those interested in this disease is to be able to accurately stratify patients, either through advanced imaging and/or molecular genetic technology, to tailor therapy including surgery to individual patients that would provide optimal outcome. Surgeons should be among those investigators leading the way toward this goal.

REFERENCES

1. Rindani R, Martin CJ, Cox MR. Transhiatal versus Ivor-Lewis oesophagectomy: is there a difference? *Aust N Z J Surg.* 1999;69:187–194.
2. Hulscher JB, Tijssen JG, Obertop H, et al. Transthoracic versus transhiatal resection for carcinoma of the esophagus: a meta-analysis. *Ann Thorac Surg.* 2001;72:306–313.
3. Hulscher JB, van Sandick JW, de Boer AG, et al. Extended transthoracic resection compared with limited transhiatal resection for adenocarcinoma of the esophagus. *N Engl J Med.* 2002;347:1662–1669.
4. Birkmeyer JD, Siewers AE, Finlayson EVA, et al. Hospital volume and surgical mortality in the United States. *N Engl J Med.* 2002;346:1128–1137.
5. Begg CB, Cramer LD, Hoskins WJ, et al. Impact of hospital volume on operative mortality for major cancer surgery. *JAMA.* 1998;280:1747–1751.
6. Killeen SD, O'Sullivan MJ, Coffey JC, et al. Provider volume and outcomes for oncological procedures. *Br J Surg.* 2005;92:389–402.
7. Birkmeyer JD, Sun MS, Wong SL, et al. Hospital volume and late survival after cancer surgery. *Ann Surg.* 2007;245:777–783.
8. Jemal A, Siegel R, Ward E, et al. Cancer Statistics 2007. *CA Cancer J Clin.* 2007;57:43–66.
9. Kelsen DP, Winter KA, Gunderson LL, et al. Long-term results of RTOG Trial 8911 (USA Intergroup 113): A random assignment trial comparison of chemotherapy followed by surgery compared with surgery alone for esophageal cancer. *J Clin Oncol.* 2007;25:3719–3725.
10. Al-Sarraf M, Martz K, Herskovic A, et al. Progress report of combined chemoradiotherapy versus radiotherapy alone in patients with esophageal cancer: An intergroup study. *J Clin Oncol.* 1997;15:277–284.
11. Posner MC, Gooding WE, Lew JI, et al. Complete 5-year follow-up of a prospective phase II trial of preoperative chemoradiotherapy for esophageal cancer. *Surgery.* 2001;130:620-628.
12. Bedenne L, Michel P, Bouche O, et al. Chemoradiation followed by surgery compared to chemoradiation alone in squamous cancer of the esophagus: FFCD 9102. *J Clin Oncol.* 2007;25:1160–1168.
13. Stahl M, Stuschke M, Lehmann N, et al. Chemoradiation with and without surgery in patients with locally advanced squamous cell carcinoma of the esophagus. *J Clin Oncol.* 2005;23:2310–2317.
14. Urba SG, Orringer MB, Turrisi A, et al. Randomized trial of preoperative chemoradiation versus surgery alone in patients with locoregional esophageal carcinoma. *J Clin Oncol.* 2001;19:305–313.
15. Bosset JF, Gignoux M, Triboulet JP, et al. Chemoradiotherapy followed by surgery compared with surgery alone in squamous cell cancer of the esophagus. *New Engl J Med.* 1997;337:161–167.
16. Walsh TN, Noonan N, Hollywood D, et al. A comparison of multimodal therapy and surgery for esophageal adenocarcinoma. *New Engl J Med.* 1996;335:462–467.
17. Burmeister BH, Smithers BM, Gebski V, et al Surgery alone versus chemoradiotherapy followed by surgery for resectable cancer of the oesophagus: a randomised controlled phase III trial. *Lancet Oncol.* 2005;6:659–668.
18. Tepper J, Krasna M, Niedzwiecki D, et al. Phase III trial of trimodality therapy with cisplatin, fluorouracil, radiotherapy, and surgery compared with surgery alone for esophageal cancer: CALGB 9781. *J Clin Oncol.* 2008;26(7):1086–1092.
19. Gebski V, Burmeister B, Smithers BM, et al. Survival benefits from neoadjuvant chemoradiotherapy or chemotherapy in oesophageal carcinoma: a meta-analysis. *Lancet Oncol.* 2007;8:226–234.

32

Neoadjuvant Therapy for Esophageal Cancer

Lawrence Leichman and Cynthia Gail Leichman

NEOADJUVANT CANCER THERAPY

A working definition of neoadjuvant treatment of solid tumors, its goals, and a brief survey of its application in other solid tumors will lay the foundation for this chapter regarding neoadjuvant therapy for patients with esophageal cancer.

Neoadjuvant cancer therapy is an additional treatment administered prior to so-called established or standard therapy with the primary goals of increasing overall survival (OS) and improving the cure rate. Other objectives for neoadjuvant therapy include improved local tumor control, increased time to recurrence, less radical surgery, including organ-sparing procedures, and, by using degree of response as guide, designing optimal future treatment for an individual patient (1).

At diagnosis, regardless of histology, most locally advanced solid tumors (stage III) have clinically occult distant metastases, and a lesser number of early-stage tumors (stages I and II) will also have occult distant metastases. Thus, systemic treatment of microscopic distant metastases without delaying postoperative healing and rehabilitation is a scientifically sound strategy. Employing a local treatment such as radiation prior to surgery makes it possible to eradicate tumor cells sterilizing the periphery of the surgical margins. This will decrease both local and distant metastases and, in anal cancers, rectal cancers, and laryngeal cancers, maintains cure rates while sparing organ function and integrity (2). Whether a preoperative treatment plan uses systemic chemotherapy or radiation therapy, or both, patients are generally treated early in their clinical course, before the necessity of recovery and rehabilitation following surgery but without the benefit of surgical staging.

Chemotherapy prior to surgery and radiation is now frequently administered to patients with locally advanced breast cancer (3), advanced transitional cell bladder cancer (4), and advanced squamous cell tumors of the head and neck and uterine cervical tumors (5,6). In many centers, chemotherapy plus radiation prior to surgery is now the preferred method for treatment of rectal cancer (7). Although some studies have found improved local control of solid tumors with preoperative chemotherapy and radiation (8), it has been more difficult to prove that such therapy results in significantly fewer metastases. Furthermore, there is no evidence from randomized clinical trials that neoadjuvant treatments lead to superior survival compared with postoperative adjuvant treatments. Without such evidence, the question may be raised as to how did neoadjuvant therapy gain the favor of surgeons, radiation therapists, and medical oncologists? The most compelling and most oft-cited reasons include (a) downstaging, (b) organ preservation, (c) improved local control, and (d) an early systemic attack on tumors with a strong propensity for early distant dissemination. Also, investigators have assumed (with little hard evidence) that effective therapy for the primary tumor means effective therapy for distant metastases and, by corollary, have used response or lack thereof to neoadjuvant chemotherapy to guide decisions regarding appropriate postoperative therapy. Neoadjuvant treatment of solid tumors has offered numerous insights into the molecular and genetic factors that make a primary tumor sensitive or resistant to chemotherapy and/or radiation.

Among the most consistent observations regarding neoadjuvant treatments, from small phase 2 to large phase 3 randomized trials, is that patients obtaining a complete pathologic response (pCR) after neoadjuvant therapy (or a near pCR) have the greatest chance for prolonged survival and the greatest opportunity to be cured (9–11). Therefore, pCR has become the most important early end point for clinicians and their patients. In current phase 2 and phase 3 trials, pCR is frequently used as surrogate end point for OS.

ESOPHAGEAL CANCER DEMOGRAPHICS

Esophageal cancer is a highly lethal tumor of the upper gastrointestinal tract. Although relatively uncommon in terms of incidence, it is the seventh leading cause of cancer death in the United States; worldwide it is the sixth leading cause of cancer death (12). It is estimated that in 2009, 16,470 individuals (12,940 men and 3,530 women will develop cancer of the esophagus and then it will be 14,530 deaths from this disease (13) in 2009 (13). The overwhelming number of these deaths will be from tumor that has disseminated beyond the esophagus, to bone, liver, lungs, lymph nodes, and brain. Although 90% of esophageal cancers can be histologically classified as squamous cell carcinoma and adenocarcinoma, with distinct epidemiologic characteristics, after factoring in stage, survival does not favor one histologic type over the other. Progress has been made in the understanding of environmental and molecular factors leading to esophageal squamous cell carcinomas and adenocarcinomas, but this has not been matched by similar advances in therapeutic choices or outcome. Once diagnosed, *all* patients presenting with esophageal cancer have an OS of approximately 15%. Even in publications reporting patients treated with intent to cure, the published 5-year survival rates for patients with esophageal cancer are generally <30% (14).

Esophageal cancer incidence increases with age. Although patients who are reported in clinical trial data are generally younger, the median age at diagnosis of esophageal cancer is 69 years; the median age at death for this patient population is 70 years. The ratio of men to women diagnosed with esophageal cancer in the United States is greater than 4:1 (7.8/100,000 and 1.8/100,000, respectively). The prevalence of esophageal cancer is greater in the African American population (10.5/100,000 for men and 3.0/100,000 for women) than in the white population in the United States. Moreover, in comparison to the white population in the United States, the African American population has a higher death rate from esophageal cancer (15). For esophageal cancers, the overall 5-year relative survival rate determined by the Surveillance, Epidemiology, and End Results (SEER) cancer registries of the National Cancer Institute (NCI) from 17 geographic areas in the United States is 15.6%. For African American men and women, who have a higher incidence of squamous cell tumors of the esophagus, the overall 5-year survival rates are 10.8% and 11.8%, respectively. In comparison, the 5-year relative survival rates for white men and women are 16.2% and 16.8%, respectively (2).

Over the past 2 decades, in the United States the incidence of esophageal adenocarcinoma for men and women has increased over 400% and 300%, respectively (16). The reasons for the rapidly increasing incidence of esophageal adenocarcinoma are not well understood, but current theories point to lifestyle changes that increase chronic reflux esophagitis inducing Barrett esophagus, the frequently visible premalignant condition leading to adenocarcinoma of the esophagus (17,18). Although the majority of esophageal cancer patients in recently reported trials from the United States have adenocarcinoma, in parts of the United States and Western Europe heavy smoking, alcohol consumption, and a relatively low consumption of raw fruits and vegetables contribute to diagnosis of squamous cell histology for over 50% of newly diagnosed esophageal cancers (16).

STAGING ESOPHAGEAL CANCER

TNM

Currently, definitive staging for esophageal cancer takes place after surgery. Thus, definitive postoperative staging for esophageal cancer is done with collaboration of the surgeon and the pathologist. Nevertheless, in a tumor for which preoperative treatment is a strong consideration, clinical staging is essential. Indeed, an understanding of esophageal cancer staging and its relationship to outcome is essential to the appropriate application of neoadjuvant therapy for esophageal cancer patients. The current American Joint Committee on Cancer (AJCC) staging system for esophageal cancer classifies a primary tumor (T) depth of invasion into mucosa only as Tis or carcinoma in situ; when the primary tumor invasion is up to, but not through the submucosa it is T1; invasion up to but not through muscularis propria is T2; transmural invasion of the primary tumor into periesophageal tissues is T3; and invasion of the primary tumor into adjacent structures is T4. Each T-category has been shown to be an independent variable for survival after surgery. However, metastatic cancer to regional lymph node (N status) from

a primary esophageal cancer is more closely related to OS than the depth of primary tumor invasion (T status). Of course, the probability that any individual esophageal cancer patient will have a metastatic lymph node becomes greater with each increment in T stage (19). In the current AJCC staging system, lymph node involvement is designated only as N0 or N1. However, as in other tumors of the gastrointestinal tract, the number of involved lymph nodes appears to have such critical role in long-term survival that an N2 designation has been suggested for patients with five or more cancer-involved lymph nodes (20). Distant cancer metastases are designated with an M status. As a few patients exhibit long-term survival when celiac nodes are involved, there is controversy regarding the utility of denoting an M1a classification when these lymph nodes are involved for a primary tumor in the distal esophagus or gastroesophageal junction (GEJ). Metastatic esophageal cancer beyond celiac lymph nodes is designated M1b. At this time, TNM staging and stage grouping (see following discussion) for squamous cell carcinomas and adenocarcinomas of the esophagus are identical. Table 32.1 outlines the current TNM system for esophageal cancer; Table 32.2 shows the stage grouping for esophageal cancer.

Table 32.1

TNM System for Cancer of the Esophagus

Primary Tumor (T)

TX	Primary tumor cannot be assessed
T0	No evidence of primary tumor
Tis	Carcinoma in situ
T1	Tumor invades lumina propria or submucosa
T2	Tumor invades muscularis propria
T3	Tumor invades adventitia
T4	Tumor invades adjacent structures

Regional Lymph Nodes (N)

NX	Cannot asses lymph node status
N0	No metastases to regional lymph nodes
N1	Metastases to regional lymph nodes

Distant Metastases (M)

MX	Cannot assess distant metastases
M0	No distant metastases
M1	Distant metastasis

Tumors of the lower thoracic esophagus
M1a Metastases in celiac lymph nodes
M1b Other distant metastases

Tumors of the midthoracic esophagus
M1a Not applicable
M1b Nonregional lymph nodes and/or distant metastases

Tumors of the upper thoracic esophagus
M1a Metastases to cervical lymph nodes
M1b Other distant metastases

Table 32.2

Stage Grouping for Cancer of the Esophagus

Stage Groupings	TNM Classification		
0	Tis and/ or T0	N0	M0
I	T1	N0	M0
IIA	T2	N0	M0
	T3	N0	
IIB	T1	N1	M0
	T2	N1	*
III	T3	N1	M0
	T4	N any	
IV	T any	N any	M1
IVA	T any	N any	M1a
IVB	T any	N any	M1b

Preoperative, Noninvasive Staging

The AJCC and the International Union Against Cancer make no distinction between pathologic stage and clinical stage for esophageal cancer. Moreover, neither has a current designation for patients treated with preoperative or neoadjuvant radiation or chemotherapy and radiation (CRT). In the postoperative staging systems for esophageal cancer, the effort is a collaborative process between the surgeon and pathologist. However, when standard curative treatment specifies two potentially difficult treatment programs, major surgery or CRT-accurate noninvasive staging is needed.

The most readily available clinical staging tools such as physical examination, routine blood studies, barium swallow, and chest radiographs will not suffice to accurately stage most patients with esophageal cancer. Realistically, blood and serum determinations will document a patient's overall fitness by noting values of total protein, serum albumin, and renal and liver function. These studies and the patient's blood count are not direct staging procedures for patients with esophageal cancer. Physical examination may demonstrate metastatic cancer, but few patients present with such physical findings. Barium studies have largely been replaced with flexible endoscopy and oral contrast used for computerized tomography (CT) scans.

Currently, CT scans, endoscopic ultrasonography (EUS), and positron emission tomography (PET) scans have established roles in the pretreatment evaluation of patients with esophageal malignancies. No doubt, these "modern," noninvasive staging technologies, whether analyzed individually or in aggregate, accurately characterize most esophageal cancers prior to surgery. However, even when all three of these modalities are used together, inaccuracies are found for primary tumor, nodal metastases, and distant metastases in 21%, 18%, and 36% of patients, respectively (21,22).

Endoscopic Ultrasonography

Unless the primary esophageal mass prohibits passage of the endoscope, EUS is generally considered the best method for ac-

curately identifying T stage and local lymph node metastases. At the usual ultrasound frequencies of 7.5 or 12 MHz, EUS will accurately image structures up to 5 cm from the esophageal wall. Higher frequencies allow for greater detail at less distance from the esophagus (23). In general, operators attempt to identify five layers through the esophageal wall: a boundary echo and superficial mucosa, the mucosa and muscularis mucosa, the submucosa, the muscularis mucosa, and the adventitia. Experienced operators can use EUS to biopsy suspicious, visible lymph nodes outside the esophageal wall (24). Lymph nodes considered likely candidates for metastatic cancer by CT scans are >0.8 cm. Similar size criteria are used by EUS operators. In addition, suspicious lymph nodes by EUS are uniformly hypoechoic, well set off from surrounding fat, and well rounded. Reviews of EUS accuracy suggest that EUS T-stage assessment correlates with surgical pathology findings at a rate of 80% to 85%. Although nodal accuracy by EUS is less precise (75%) than T stage, EUS is more accurate in correctly predicting positive and negative lymph nodes than either CT or PET scans (25). However, when CT is combined with EUS, the published staging accuracies have been in the range of 62% to 90% (26).

Computerized Tomography/Magnetic Resonance Imaging

After the primary tumor is evaluated and diagnosed by esophageal-gastric endoscopy and EUS, body imaging studies such as CT or magnetic resonance imaging (MRI) scans of chest, abdomen, and pelvis are generally performed to evaluate an esophageal mass and to detect proximal and distant lymph node metastases and metastatic cancer. Other than the expertise of local radiologists, there is no reason to recommend one type of imaging over another. However, CT scans are widely available in the United States and are most often used in the clinical staging of esophageal cancers. Because most patients in the United States present with advanced T stage and with positive lymph nodes (stages IIA, IIB, and III), CT scans are most often used to detect distant metastatic cancer to other organs or lymph nodes. Bulky esophageal tumors and lymph nodes at ≥1 cm diameter can readily be identified by CT scans (27).

Positron Emission Tomography Scans

[18]F-fluoro-deoxy-D-glucose (FDG)-PET scanning using is approved by Medicare for the preoperative staging of esophageal cancers (28). As a "metabolic" study, relying on differences between tumor cell metabolism and normal cell metabolism, PET is generally complementary to cross-sectional imaging studies such as CT or MRI scans. PET scans are generally more reliable in picking out positive regional lymph nodes than CT scans, but not as accurate or reliable as EUS in determining regional nodal involvement (29). Although there have been investigations into the role of PET scans in determining immediate response to therapy (30,31), PET scans currently are most useful for detecting metastases unidentified by other imaging modalities, with an accuracy of 80% (32), for detecting unsuspected second primary tumors (especially lung tumors) and for improving interpretation of "lesions" seen by CT scanning. Regardless of the degree of certainty noted by the PET scan interpretation, the impact of a positive PET scan distant from regional lymph nodes has such a

profound bearing on the on the patient's treatment and prognosis that it remains incumbent on physicians evaluating esophageal cancer patients to obtain histologic proof of incurability.

Clinical Workup

Fortunately, there are an increasing number of patients who have very early esophageal adenocarcinomas that are now being found because of the relationship between esophageal reflux symptoms and carcinoma. If confirmed by EUS, further staging of patients suspected of harboring an in situ (Tis) adenocarcinoma of the esophagus by whole-body imaging with CT or MRI scans plus PET scans cancer is not necessary. Although only about 10% of patients with T1 lesions confirmed by EUS have positive lymph nodes at operation, some clinicians still require a full workup with CT and PET before deciding on definitive therapy for patients with clinically staged as T1N0M0. Thus, in practice, regardless of symptoms, any patient with an invasive cancer found by endoscopic evaluation should receive an evaluation by CT scan prior to making a decision regarding definitive therapy. For patients found to have invasive cancer of the esophagus without a definable mass by CT or MRI scans, EUS should be done to determine the depth of invasion of the primary tumor and to assess regional lymph nodes.

If clinically fit for definitive surgery, patients with T1N0 lesions who are not upstaged by PET scan should proceed to surgery. Patients with EUS-defined T2 esophageal primary tumors lesions need further evaluation by CT scans and PET scans. If, in the opinion of the evaluating clinicians, a patient has stage I cancer (T1N0M0), there is no value in current systemic or local therapy prior to surgery. Current NCI-sponsored clinical phase 2 trials for neoadjuvant CRT for esophageal cancers include patients with clinical stages IIA, IIB, and III. In the ongoing Southwest Oncology Group (SWOG) Trial S0356, eligibility is limited to those patients with clinical stages IIA, IIB, and IIIB; patients must have a negative PET scan before enrolling in the SWOG trial.

NEOADJUVANT THERAPY FOR ESOPHAGEAL CANCER

The need for upgrading the standard of care for patients with esophageal cancer was clearly and effectively stated, perhaps understated, by two articles in the *British Journal of Surgery* in summer of 1980, which demonstrated the dismal results of either standard of care, surgery, or radiation. In these reports, Earlam and Cunha-Melo (33,34) compiled a survey of the medical literature that described over 18,000 patients. They found the 5-year survival of patients with esophageal cancer who were treated with radiation as the only modality was 6%. Surprisingly, those patients treated with surgery alone fared even less well, with a 5-year survival of 4%. Moreover, they concluded that "... oesophageal resection for squamous cell carcinoma has the highest operative mortality of any routinely performed surgical procedure today" (1,2). Although these authors did not specifically call for a new approach to curing esophageal cancer, these articles helped pave the way for new clinical research in esophageal cancer.

Neoadjuvant Radiation Therapy

Neoadjuvant radiation, as a single modality prior to surgery, has been generally unsuccessful in improving OS for patients with esophageal cancer. However, a brief review of radiation prior to surgery does indicate that experienced surgeons can safely operate on patients after external-beam radiation and that a trend toward improved survival can be found with radiation prior to surgery.

There have been randomized trials comparing radiation alone with radiation prior to surgery in which patients received doses of external-beam radiation between 4,000 and 5,500 cGy. In general, these trials showed no differences in the R0 resection rates, local failure, and OS (35). A recent meta-analysis of these trials reviewed 1,147 patients with a median follow-up of 9 years. The authors of the meta-analysis found the hazard ratio (HR) of 0.89 (95% confidence interval [CI]: 0.78–1.01). Furthermore, meta-analysis found that radiation prior to surgery reduces the risk of death by 11%, with a 3% and 4% absolute survival benefit at 2 and 5 years, respectively ($p = 0.062$). The authors of the meta-analysis note that it is plausible that if they had a patient base of over 2,000 with which to work, preoperative radiation prior to surgery may have reached statistical significance (36). Nevertheless, as it has become increasing clear that invasive tumors of the esophagus disseminate beyond surgical and radiation fields relatively early in their development (28,37,38), new randomized trials testing radiation as single modality prior to surgery versus surgery alone are unlikely to be undertaken.

Neoadjuvant Chemotherapy

For esophageal cancer, a tumor that tends to early distant dissemination, a strategy to kill occult microscopic cancer is needed. Although single-agent response rates of various chemotherapeutic agents against esophageal cancers (adenocarcinomas or squamous cell carcinomas) are modest, there are enough agents with response rates reported between 15% and 30% (39) that clinical trials have been designed using combinations of these agents prior to surgery. More recently, newer analogues of cisplatin and 5-fluorouracil (5-FU), oxaliplatin, and capecitabine, respectively, have been tested in combination without data on single-agent activity data. Comparing and interpreting trials that have used systemic chemotherapy is challenging because investigators have tended to "lump" patients for whom response of the primary esophageal tumor is the primary objective of the trial with patients for whom response of a measurable metastatic deposit is the primary objective. In general, those with measurable primary cancers will have a higher performance status than those with measurable metastatic liver or lung lesions. The patients for whom response of the primary tumor is the main goal can have clinically meaningful symptomatic relief without significant change in tumor size. Furthermore, the molecular parameters that will determine a tumor's resistance or response are not necessarily the same in the primary tumor and metastatic lesions. In general, response rates reported for chemotherapy in the neoadjuvant setting tend to be greater than those reported in the setting of disseminated cancer. For example, single-agent 5-FU and single-agent cisplatin administered in a neoadjuvant clinical trial have reported responses rates of 85% and 72%, respectively (40,41). The same drugs administered to those with

Table 32.3

Systemic Chemotherapeutic Agents and Response Rates Against Disseminated Esophageal and/or Gastroesophageal Junction Cancers

Systemic Agent/s (Ref.)	No. of Patients	Response Rate (%)	Histology
5-Fluorouracil (5-FU) (40)	26	16	S
Cisplatin (44)	222	23	S
Paclitaxel (45)	51	32	S & A
Docetaxel (46)	22	18	A
Irinotecan (47)	43	14	A
Cisplatin/5-FU (48,49)	94	34	S
Irinotecan/cisplatin (50)	39	36	S & A
Docetaxel/cisplatin (51)	14	43	A
Docetaxel/cisplatin/5-FU (51)	22	59	A
Oxaliplatin/capecitabine (52)	43	35	A
Docetaxel/capecitabine (53)	44	39	A

S, squamous cell cancer; A, adenocarcinoma.

metastatic esophageal cancer have reported response rates of 16% and 21%, respectively (42,43). Currently, there are little data to suggest that particular systemic agents or combinations have more or less activity on squamous cell esophageal cancers versus adenocarcinomas of the esophagus. Table 32.3 summarizes the most frequently used systemic treatments against disseminated esophageal and gastroesophageal junction (GEJ) cancers (40,44–53).

The value of preoperative chemotherapy without radiation for patients with esophageal and GEJ tumors remains uncertain and controversial (54–60). For most oncologists in North America, the question of administering chemotherapy prior to surgery appeared to be settled with the publication of the North American Intergroup trial 0013. In this randomized clinical trial, 467 patients were randomized to receive three cycles of preoperative chemotherapy with cisplatin and infusion 5-FU prior to surgery. If patients appeared to respond to therapy, postoperative treatment with the same drugs was to be continued. If the patient had less than an R0 resection, that is, microscopic positive margins or gross tumor at the margins, then radiation was allowed after surgery. Of the eligible patients, 51% had adenocarcinoma, 44% had squamous cell carcinoma, and 5% had epithelial esophageal cancers that could not be histologically characterized. The final report in 1998 indicated no improvement in survival for the patients who received neoadjuvant chemotherapy (54).

In 2002, the British Medical Research Council (MRC) reported a far larger phase 3 randomized trial in which patients with esophageal cancer (adenocarcinomas or squamous cell cancers) were randomized to receive either chemotherapy prior to surgery or surgery alone (57). In the MRC trial, 802 patients were randomized to receive either two cycles of cisplatin and infusion 5-FU prior to esophagectomy versus esophagectomy without prior chemotherapy. In the MRC trial, 66% of the enrolled patients had adenocarcinoma and 31% had squamous cell carcinomas. Approximately 9% of the patients in the MRC trial received some external-beam radiation prior to surgery. OS was

statistically significantly better for the patients who received preoperative chemotherapy (HR, 0.79; 95% CI: 67–93; $p = 0.004$). Few experts in this field have been able to explain the reason for contradictory results in trials that seemed, on the surface, to be similar in design and eligibility criteria. Is less "up front" chemotherapy better (favoring MRC)? Did postoperative systemic chemotherapy have a negative impact on survival for patients treated in the North American Intergroup? Are esophageal adenocarcinomas (more in the MRC trial) more sensitive to cisplatin and 5-FU than squamous cell esophageal carcinomas? Did the 9% of patients in the MRC trial who received preoperative radiation contribute to improved survival? Did all these factors combine to make the MRC trial positive? Although these questions remain unanswered, the standard of care in Great Britain for patients with potentially curable esophageal cancers is chemotherapy prior to surgery. Even with further analysis, it is not likely that the reasons for the very different results of the North American Intergroup and the MRC trials will be fully understood. Unfortunately, such an understanding could significantly contribute to the design of future clinical trials for patients with esophageal cancer.

After the MRC trial results were published, Malthaner et al. (58) conducted a meta-analysis of phase 3 randomized trials to determine whether preoperative chemotherapy improves survival for esophageal cancer patients. The review included 11 phase 3 trials in which 2,019 patients with potentially resectable esophageal cancer (any histology) were randomized to chemotherapy prior to surgery versus surgery alone. Cancers of the cervical esophagus were excluded. In eight of the trials, in which 1,729 patients were studied, sufficient details were provided to allow inclusion in a meta-analysis for the primary outcome of survival. The authors reviewed survival on a yearly basis. The meta-analysis by these authors and others (56) published prior to MRC results found no improvement in survival for esophageal cancer patients treated with preoperative chemotherapy. In the most recent meta-analysis (58), it was found that the rate of R0 resections was not influenced by preoperative chemotherapy and that chemotherapy did not influence operative complications. Although the ability to determine recurrence patterns was limited, this analysis reported that chemotherapy decreased local recurrences by 19% (not statistically significant). The mortality rate prior to surgery for patients receiving chemotherapy was 2.5% (not statistically significant). Only 3% of patients treated with chemotherapy achieved a pCR. At 1- and 2-year follow-ups, no differences in survival were noted. However, at the 3-year interval, the risk ratios found a 21% increase in survival in favor of the patients who received preoperative chemotherapy (relative risk [RR], 1.21; 95% CI: 0.88–1.68; $p = 0.68$). At the 5-year follow-up mark, OS survival significantly favored those patients who received chemotherapy. These patients had 44% improvement in survival (RR, 1.44; 95% CI: 1.05–1.97; $p = 0.02$). Three of the trials in this analysis attempted to give chemotherapy postoperatively. Of note, if these trials are excluded from the review, the advantage for preoperative chemotherapy becomes statistically significant at 4 years (RR, 1.49; 95% CI: 1.14–1.96; $p = 0.004$) and stronger at 5 years (RR, 1.71; 95% CI = 1.35– 2.15) (57). The MRC trial had the strongest impact on the findings of the most recent meta-analysis, but the authors also noted that two randomized trials, published in 1997 (59) and 2001 (60), had matured and showed a survival advantage for patients receiving chemotherapy.

It is unlikely that the findings of the recent meta-analysis regarding the modest survival from chemotherapy at 5 years will influence the practice in the United States for those charged with the care of patients with potentially resectable esophageal cancer. The meta-analysis examined clinical trials results, not primary data from each trial. Indeed, the authors suggest that this type of detailed analysis needs to be undertaken in the future (60). Although most trials in the meta-analysis treated patients with a combination of cisplatin and 5-FU, doses differed, length of treatments differed, and the populations and their histologies were heterogeneous. The very low pCR rate of 3% will also have a negative influence on those who believe that pCR, or near pCR, is essential for effective neoadjuvant therapy for esophageal cancer.

Neoadjuvant Chemotherapy and Radiation

Concern about postoperative wound healing and misunderstandings regarding the propensity of most solid tumors to spread systemically held back combining preoperative radiation with concomitant chemotherapy. However, in developing a neoadjuvant CRT program for squamous cell cancer tumors of the anal canal, Nigro and colleagues (61) at Wayne State University (WSU) demonstrated that radical surgery (abdominoperineal resection [APR] or Miles procedure) was safe. 5-FU and mitomycin C were used with 30 Gy of external-beam radiation. Although the systemic therapy (5-FU and mitomycin C) were initially thought to act as "radiation sensitizers," both agents are effective cytotoxics against systemic metastases from anal and rectal cancers. The methods and results of the WSU anal cancer program were informative for much current thinking about CRT prior to surgery for patients with solid tumors. The WSU investigators performed posttreatment biopsies for all patients and found that those without tumor in the posttreatment biopsies of the anal canal did not have cancer in the APR specimen. They

recognized that their patients without cancer in the anal biopsies prior to APR had a very different prognosis from those with residual cancer: (a) those without cancer were likely to be cured, and the corollary, those with cancer tumor were not likely to be cured even after radical surgery; (b) for those with cancer in the biopsies, systemic chemotherapy was ineffective at eradicating microscopic disease as distant recurrences appeared within 2 years of operation; and (c) sparing the rectum for those without cancer in the posttreatment biopsies did not alter the excellent outcome for those patients (62). The elimination of the microscopically visible primary anal cancer (pCR) indicated that the chemotherapy was effective in treating microscopic metastatic cancer (63). The thesis that pCR of the primary tumor is the key to prognosis after neoadjuvant CRT, while most robust in the treatment of anal cancer, has held up very well in other solid tumors, especially cancer of the esophagus.

Using the same schedule of 5-FU, mitomycin C, and external-beam radiation developed by Nigro et al. (61) for anal cancers, Franklin and colleagues (64) reported the rate of surgical resections, surgical complications after therapy, the toxicities, and the pCR rate for patients with squamous cell cancers of the esophagus. The published results showed that the treatment was relatively effective but because of bone marrow suppression, the potential for pulmonary toxicity (in a group of patients with long-term smoking histories) and the fact that a new drug cisplatin had synergy of platinum with 5-FU and radiation, cisplatin in combination with infusion-5-FU soon supplanted mitomycin C in testing neoadjuvant combined-modality treatment for esophageal cancers. The first published trial using this new combination enrolled patients with squamous cell tumors. Although operative mortality because of pulmonary failure was significant, median survival for the whole group was 18.6 months, with a long-term survivorship (and the potential for cure) reported for the 21% who had a pCR (65). Since then, more than 75 reports of nonrandomized single or multi-institutional trials using the backbone of cisplatin and 5-FU with minor variations of external-beam radiation prior to prior surgery have been published. Despite more sophisticated preoperative staging and the entry of more and more patients with adenocarcinomas into the treatment milieu, pCR rates remain between 20% and 33%, with median survivals reported between 16 and 30 months. Indeed, the best results are in the single-institution trials in which patient selection is determined by a multidisciplinary team well versed in preoperative CRT.

Randomized Clinical Trials
Neoadjuvant CRT versus Surgery Alone

Six prospectively randomized clinical trials comparing neoadjuvant CRT prior to surgery against surgery alone have been published in peer-reviewed articles. The six randomized controlled trials include a total of 764 patients. None of the trials used EUS or PET scanning in their preoperative or clinical staging. Although each trial used cisplatin in the chemotherapy combinations, four used cisplatin and 5-FU, one used cisplatin alone, and one added vinblastine to cisplatin and 5-FU. External-beam radiation doses ranged between 24 and 51.7 Gy in varying fractions (Table 32.4). The combined pCR rate for patients on these trials was 21%.

Table 32.4

Randomized Clinical Trials Testing Neoadjuvant Chemotherapy and Radiation Therapy (CRT) Prior to Surgery Against Surgery Alone

Ref.	No. CRT + S/Surg	SCC/Adeno	No. Surgery/ No. Randomized	Xrt Fx Daily Dose (Gy)	Xrt Total Dose (Gy)	Chemo
Nygaard et al. (67)	53/50	100/0	44/53, 45/50	1.75	41.1	CDDP Bleo
Apinop et al. (69)	35/30	100/0	26/35, 39/45	2	33.6	CDDP 5-FU
Le Prise et al. (74)	41/45	100/0	33/41, 39/45	2	24	CDDP 5-FU
Walsh et al. (70)	58/55	0/100	39/58, 52/55	2.67	50.7	CDDP 5-FU
Bosset et al. (68)	151/146	100/0	94/151, 97/146	3.7	50/.7	CDDP
Urba et al. (66)	50/50	75/25	34/50, 42/50	1.5×2	51.7	CDDP 5-FU Vbl

CRT+ S/Surg, chemoradiotherapy plus surgery versus surgery alone; SCC, squamous cell cancer; Adeno, adenocarcinoma; XRT, radiation therapy; Fx, fraction/day; Chemo, chemotherapy; CDDP, cisplatin; Bleo, bleomycin; 5-FU, 5-fluorouracil; Vbl, vinblastine.

With the exception of one trial (66), all surgery was done by transthoracic resection. Only two of the six trials were multi-institutional (67,68); the largest trial evaluated 269 patients (68) and the smallest evaluated 69 patients (69). No trial included stage I patients. Walsh and colleagues (70) restricted entry to patients with adenocarcinoma; Urba et al. (66) allowed entry patients with both adenocarcinomas and squamous cell carcinomas; the other four trials included only esophageal squamous cell carcinomas.

Although the effect of neoadjuvant CRT trended toward improved survival for several trials and showed no difference for others, only Walsh et al. (70) found a statistically significant improvement of survival for chemotherapy and radiation prior to surgery. Although the trial by Walsh and colleagues has been criticized because patients randomized to surgery alone had a median survival of 12 months, the median survival of 17 months for the patients treated preoperatively with CRT was also less than usually reported (71).

Meta-Analyses of Randomized Clinical Trials

With the heterogeneity of the esophageal neoadjuvant randomized clinical trials and the small number of patients in each trial, several meta-analyses have been undertaken and published. Each meta-analysis reviewed the results of individual trials, but not the records of individual patients within the trials. As expected, the meta-analyses themselves were somewhat heterogeneous in their scope.

In their meta-analysis, Fiorica et al. (72) found the pooled estimate of the treatment effect was statistically significant in improving survival (odds ratio [OR], 0.53; 95% CI: 0.31–0.92). However, if either of the trials that included patients with adenocarcinoma were excluded, the effect of preoperative CRT lost statistical significance. In reviewing surgical complications, they found adverse postoperative events in 39% of patients who received neoadjuvant CRT, compared with 34% of those who had surgery without preoperative CRT (not statistically significant). Although not statistically significant, postoperative mortality trended upward as the dose of radiation increased.

Kaklamanos et al. (73) conducted their meta-analysis using data from 11 randomized clinical trials in which chemotherapy and/or CRT was administered prior to surgery versus surgery alone. Five of the trials analyzed by Kaklamanos et al. have not yet been published in a peer-reviewed journal. This meta-analysis found 2-year survival ranging from 23% to 46% with CRT prior to surgery versus 13% to 41% with surgery alone, with a net gain in survival of 6.4% favoring preoperative CRT. This trend was not statistically significant ($p = 0.86$).

Urschel and Vasan (75) reviewed the six trials in Table 32.4 (66–70,74) and an additional three trials for which only abstract data, not peer-reviewed data, were available. Their analysis included 1,116 patients. At 2 years, Urschel and Vasan found no significant survival advantage in their comparison of preoperative CRT versus surgery alone. At 3 years, if the data were restricted to those trials for which chemotherapy and radiation were concurrently administered, 3-year survival strongly favored neoadjuvant CRT (OR, 0.45; 95% CI: 0.26–0.79; $p = 0.005$). Rates of regional recurrence favored neoadjuvant CRT (OR, 0.38; 95% CI: 0.23–0.63; $p = 0.0002$). However, they found no treatment effect on the rates of distant metastases. In this report, a nonsignificant trend toward increased operative mortality for CRT was found (OR, 1.72; 95% CI: 0.96–3.07; $p = 0.07$).

In their meta-analysis Greer et al. (76) attempted to extend the time for survival analysis for the six randomized trials to 5 years. However, only three of the trials reported 5-year survival data; thus, extrapolations were made for the three trials reporting 3-year survival data. Five of the six trials individually reported small, nonstatistically significant improvements in long-term survival for patients who were treated with preoperative CRT.

Similarly, the meta-analysis summary measure of survival indicated the RR of death was 0.86 for the CRT followed by surgery compared with surgery alone (95% CI: 0.74–1.01; $p = 0.07$).

Patterns of Care

A patterns of care study funded by the NCI found that between 1992 and 1994, there was a dramatic rise in the utilization of CRT either alone or prior to surgery for esophageal cancer patients in the United States (77). A second, follow-up study conducted between 1996 and 1999 found further evidence for the increasing use of neoadjuvant CRT prior to surgery (78). In a patterns of care study published in 2005, the authors reviewed the outcome for 11,340 esophageal cancer patients (76.9% male, 48.7% squamous cell cancers; median age, 64), 6,398 (56.4%) were treated with chemotherapy and radiation, 3,758 (32%) were treated with CRT prior to surgery, and 1,229 (10.8%) were treated with radiation therapy alone or radiation prior to surgery. The univariate analysis used by these authors to evaluate factors predictive for survival in esophageal cancer patients with clinical stages II and III found that the treatment approach predicted statistically significant differences in the risk of death. Patients treated with neoadjuvant chemotherapy prior to surgery had a 0.53 HR for survival ($p = 0.0001$). In the multivariate analysis, patients treated with CRT prior to surgery maintained an HR for death of 0.52 ($p = 0.0001$) (79).

The failure of Cancer Leukemia Group B C9781 (which also was an NCI Intergroup Trial) to complete enrollment clearly reflects the patterns of care studies. In this trial patients were randomized to surgery alone versus two cycles of preoperative cisplatin and 5-FU with concomitant external-beam radiation. After several years of poor accrual, the trial was closed with only 59 eligible patients entered. However, an abstract of this aborted trial was presented in a plenary session of the 2006 meeting of the American Society of Clinical Oncology. The authors reported a highly statistically significant benefit in OS for the patients randomized to preoperative CRT ($n = 29$) (80). Commentary on this trial suggested that preoperative CRT could now join surgery alone and chemotherapy and radiation as an acceptable potentially curable definitive therapy for patients with esophageal cancer.

Summary of Neoadjuvant CRT

Aside from the opportunity to treat all esophageal cancer patients presenting without clinical evidence of distant metastases, the common threads among preoperative CRT reports for esophageal cancer patients are high overall response rates, lower stages than expected (downstaging) if surgery were being performed alone, and a clear association between long-term survival with pCR or near pCR rates (81). With the exclusion of esophageal cancer patients who would not need preoperative downstaging or would not likely benefit from any form of adjuvant therapy (those patients with in situ and stage I tumors), regardless of preneoadjuvant staging, survival after preoperative CRT survival depends on the posttherapy stage. Because many more patients will undergo potentially curative surgery if treated by CRT, the improvement of survival by downstaging has undoubtedly had a major role in determining the overall popularity

Table 32.5

Patient and Tumor Characteristics of 593 Patients with Esophageal Cancer Treated at the M.D. Anderson Cancer Center Between 1985 and 2003

	Surgery Only n = 354	CRT ⇒ Surgery n = 239	p Value
Gender			0.02
Male	289 (82%)	206 (86%)	
Female	65 (18%)	33 (14%)	
Clinical Stage			<0.01
0	3 (1%) (in situ)	0 (0%)	
I	43 (12%)	0 (0%)	
IIA/B	264 (75%)	139 (58%)	
III	38 (11%)	87 (36%)	
IV	6 (2%)	13 (5%)	
Pathologic Stage			<0.01
0	0 (0%)	69 (28%)	
I	72 (20%)	25 (10%)	
IIA/B	107 (30%)	84 (35%)	
III	139 (39%)	46 (19%)	
IV	36 (10%)	15 (6%)	

CRT, chemotherapy and radiation.
Adapted from Swisher SG, Hofstetter W, Wu TT, et al. Proposed revision of the esophageal cancer staging system to accommodate pathologic response (pP) following preoperative chemoradiation (CRT). *Ann Surg.* 2005;241:810–820.

of CRT prior to surgery. Table 32.5, adapted from Swisher et al. (81) shows these data.

Swisher and his colleagues (81) also found that after CRT the pTNM cancer-specific survival for patients with stages II and III was similar to those who underwent surgery without CRT ($p = 0.98$). Table 32.6 outlines these data. These results are similar to those of other retrospective reviews that have indicated an association between pathologic response to preoperative CRT and survival (82,83). They also illustrate major points regarding esophageal cancer patients undergoing CRT prior to surgery: (a) Unlike anal canal tumors in which a pCR is tantamount to cure, approximately 40% of esophageal patients with stage 0 pathology on surgical resection after CRT will relapse and die of their cancer. (b) Although those patients downstaged to stage 0 have the best 5-year survival rates, for those downstaged to stages I and II 5-year survivals are found in approximately 47% and 35%, respectively.

CURRENT RESEARCH STRATEGIES AND TRENDS

Current strategies by single institutions and NCI-sponsored cooperative oncology groups to improve survival for patients with

Table 32.6

Impact of Chemotherapy and Radiation Therapy (CRT) on Pathologic TNM and Stage-Specific Survival

Pathologic Stage (at Surgical Resection)	Surgery Only (n = 354) Median (mo), 3y, 5y	CRT ⇒ Surgery (n = 239) Median (mo), 3y, 5y	p Value
0	—	133.2, 69%, 58%	—
I	162.8, 85%, 82%	52.6, 63%, 47%	0.01
IIA/B	41.2, 51%, 39%	39.6, 54%, 35%	0.85
III	14.9, 17%, 7%	13.3, 21%, 5%	0.78
IV	11.4, 17%, 17%	13.6, 13%, 13%	0.72

Adapted from Swisher SG, Hofstetter W, Wu TT, et al. Proposed revision of the esophageal cancer staging system to accommodate pathologic response following preoperative chemoradiation (CRT). *Ann Surg.* 2005;241:810–820.

locally advanced esophageal cancer are appropriately focused on increasing the percent of esophageal cancer patients achieving a stage 0 (pCR) status following neoadjuvant CRT. pCR rates of 35% to 45% will undoubtedly lead to improved OS for esophageal cancer patients with locally advanced (stages II and III) tumors. To accomplish this, most new investigational treatment protocols feature innovative chemotherapeutic regimens. However, there are some important issues regarding surgery and radiation that still need clinical testing.

Surgery

Surgical results for esophageal cancer have improved in recent decades. Operative mortality is now expected to be <5%. Although debate continues as to the best operative procedure, the progress in survival and mortality is more likely a product of better patient selection and improved postoperative care rather than the chosen procedure (84,85). The transthoracic esophagectomy is performed most often in the Western world. In this operation, the surgeon performs an en bloc resection with two-field lymphadenectomy. An Ivor-Lewis approach is a form of transthoracic esophagectomy (TTE) that uses laparotomy for gastric mobilization with resultant anastomosis in the upper thorax via a right thoracotomy. Using the en bloc esophagectomy, DeMeester (86) has reported a local recurrence of only 1% in 100 consecutive patients with adenocarcinoma of the distal esophagus. Japanese surgeons have advocated a three-field lymphadenectomy that extends the lymph node dissection to include the cervical and upper thoracic region. As the majority of esophageal cancer patients treated in Japan have squamous cell cancers, this operation is appropriate (87). A transhiatal esophagectomy (THE) uses cervical and abdominal incisions to construct a cervical anastomosis. Advocates of the THE cite few pulmonary complications because they can avoid a thoracotomy, a shorter operative time, decreased incidence of gastric reflux, and improved operative morbidity. Of course, the number of lymph nodes removed by

the THE is limited, causing some patients undergoing THE to be understaged. A Dutch surgical trial randomized patients with adenocarcinoma of the esophagus or gastric cardia between TTE and THE. As expected, more lymph nodes were dissected by the TTE procedure but a lower morbidity was seen in the patients undergoing THE. Although median survival, disease-free survival, and quality-adjusted survival were not statistically different between the two groups, there appeared to be a trend toward improved 5-year survival favoring the group who received TTE (88).

As systemic therapy should be targeted appropriately, surgery must be individualized as well. Patients with esophageal cancer limited to the mucosa or submucosa may not need radical operations. On the other hand, patients with invasive cancers will need a true cancer operation. Currently, esophageal surgeons make those types of decisions based on tumor position, previous treatments, and body habitus to decide whether the patient should have an anastomosis in the chest or neck or the choice of conduit (stomach, colon, or jejunum) (89). Whether the operative procedure should be modified in the face of effective neoadjuvant CRT remains an answered question.

Preoperative CRT requires an expert team. The initial evaluation of the patient with esophageal cancer for neoadjuvant therapy has to include all members of the team. No team member is more important than the surgeon who must agree that the patient's clinical stage, overall performance status, and general health status will allow an attempt at esophageal resection with intent to cure. Data regarding surgical results clearly indicate that the best outcomes from surgery are found when patients are operated on by an expert team with a high-volume practice (90). At this time, there are no published data regarding the importance of the operative team's experience in a patient who received neoadjuvant CRT. No doubt, a surgical team with experience operating in a field that has been irradiated and giving postoperative care to patients who have had cytotoxic CRT will improve outcomes.

Radiation Therapy

At the outset of preoperative CRT for esophageal cancer, recommendations regarding radiation field size suggested that margins should be at approximately 5 cm above and below the primary lesion (91). Using these parameters, the marginal failure rate may be as high as 15% to 25% (92). A recent Radiation Therapy Oncology Group trial demonstrated that increasing the dose of external-beam radiation with preoperative chemotherapy results in unacceptable toxicity (93). Advances in shaping of the irradiated field and changes in fractionation schema will probably be more effective than increasing radiation total dose. Although it is now standard of care to include major nodal areas at risk in the radiation field, there has been little clinical research on the utility of including lymph nodes within the celiac axis. As celiac lymph nodes are at risk for patients with adenocarcinomas of the GEJ, and increasing the radiation field to include them will increase toxicity, routine inclusion of these lymph nodes is a relevant question for clinical investigators. Whether radioprotective agents such as amifostine will allow increased external-beam radiation doses to be administered with less toxicity is currently being studied (94).

Systemic Treatment

Cisplatin and 5-FU in combination with external-beam radiation will produce symptomatic improvement for the majority of patients treated. Using current, noninvasive staging techniques to choose the best possible group of patients, it is still unlikely that this combination will produce more than a 25% pCR rate or a median survival >2 years. In the hands of experienced surgeons who are familiar with operating on patients who have received CRT, it appears that operative mortality is not substantially increased when compared with surgery without preoperative CRT (95).

New Agents

Taxanes (paclitaxel and docetaxel), the camptothecin analogue, irinotecan, the platinum analogue, oxaliplatin, and the fluoropyrimidine analogue, capecitabine, have been introduced into therapeutic trials for esophageal cancer patients. In an effort to maximize chemotherapy intensity and exposure to non-cross-resistant agents, investigators also have used combination chemotherapy as the initial treatment, followed by chemotherapy and radiation, followed by surgery. A report by Ajani and colleagues (51) of a prospectively randomized trial for patients with advanced GEJ and gastric cancers showed that adding docetaxel to 5-FU and cisplatin produced a higher response and a statistically improved survival. Ilson (50) and colleagues have developed a safe dose and schedule of the combination irinotecan and cisplatin for patients with metastatic or unresectable esophageal cancer (squamous cell and adenocarcinomas). In a multicenter phase 2 trial, this combination had a confirmed 36% response rate.

Recently, induction chemotherapy prior to neoadjuvant CRT has been tested by several groups. Pisani et al. (96) reported on locally advanced esophageal cancer in 47 patients with adenocarcinomas and squamous cell carcinomas treated with docetaxel and cisplatin prior to protracted-infusion 5-FU and 40 Gy of external-beam radiation. Thirty-nine patients (83%) had an R0 resection. Although no patient died in the hospital following surgery, two patients died within 2 months of surgery. Fourteen patients (29%) had a pCR. Ajani et al. (97) have used four systemic agents in their preoperative therapy of tumors of the esophagus and GEJ. This clinical protocol administered two 6-week cycles of irinotecan and cisplatin followed by paclitaxel and 5-FU given concomitantly with 45 Gy of external-beam radiation followed by surgery. Although 63% and 84% had clinical stage T3 and N1, respectively, 39 of 43 patients (92%) underwent an R0 resection (5% postoperative mortality). In this cohort, 11 patients (28%) had a pCR and an additional 16 patients (37%) had <10% viable tumor in the resected specimen. The median survival for all patients treated was 22 months (97). In an attempt to maximize dose and minimize toxicity of a platinum analogue, Khushalani and colleagues (98) tested oxaliplatin and protracted infusion 5-FU with 50.5 Gy of external-beam radiation. Although this trial was designed as a phase 1 to find the best possible dose of oxaliplatin, and included stage IV patients, 38% of the patients who underwent esophagectomy had T0N0M0 lesions. Some of these strategies are currently being tested in the multi-institutional settings of the NCI-funded cooperative oncology groups. The key objective of these trials is to safely raise the pCR rate above the threshold 25%.

Chemotherapy and Radiation without Surgery

With the publication of the Radiation Therapy Oncology Group trial noting a statistically significant survival for patients who received 5-FU and cisplatin with concomitant radiation versus radiation alone, chemotherapy and radiation has been defined as acceptable definitive, potentially curative therapy for patients with either squamous cell carcinoma or adenocarcinoma of the esophagus (99,100). Updated results of this trial at 5 and 10 years have shown a median survival of 14 months for patients who received CRT versus 9.3 months for patients treated with radiation alone. At 5 years, 27% of the 61 patients who were treated with CRT were alive; of the 62 patients randomized to receive radiation alone, none were alive beyond 3 years (p <0.001) (101). At 10 years, the OS for the combined-modality group was 21% (102). The Eastern Cancer Oncology Group reported their prospectively randomized study in which 119 patients were randomized to receive 5-FU and mitomycin C with radiation versus radiation alone. Although the investigators found that chemotherapy and radiation improved median survival from 9 months to 15 months (p = 0.04), they did not find an improvement in 5-year survival in their two groups. Because an estimated 50% of the patients enrolled in the Eastern Cancer Oncology Group trial received subsequent surgery, these results had only a modest impact on clinical practice (103). In a meta-analysis considering 11 randomized prospective trials comparing CRT against radiation alone, the authors concluded that combined-modality therapy is statistically superior to radiation alone. The HR for OS was 0.73 (95% CI: 0.64–0.84) in favor of the combined-modality therapy. However, the absolute benefit for the combination of radiation and chemotherapy is only a modest 9% (104).

The Role of Surgery in Combined-Modality Treatments of Esophageal Cancer

Posttreatment biopsies of the esophagus prior to surgery do not indicate which patients will have no tumor in the resected esophagus. Because the risk of leaving microscopic tumor in the esophagus has such an important role in the patient's ultimate prognosis, it is unlikely that PET scanning will be able to determine which patients will have a pCR at surgery. There have been very few trials comparing a surgical versus nonoperative curative approach to esophageal cancer. However, a recent report by Stahl and colleagues (105) from Germany details the results of a trial conducted in Germany for 172 patients age 70 years or less with T3N0-1M0 squamous cell esophageal cancers. In this trial, patients were randomized to receive either three courses of induction chemotherapy with etoposide, 5-FU, and cisplatin followed by cisplatin and etoposide administered concomitantly with 4,000 cGy of external-beam radiation followed by transthoracic esophagectomy or the same induction chemotherapy and chemotherapy and radiation with the addition of further radiation to at least 6,500 cGy without surgery. Eighty-six patients were randomized in each arm of this trial. With a median observation time of 6 years, the following was noted: two toxic deaths from chemotherapy were found in both arms of the study; no patient treated definitively with CRT died within 30 days of completing treatment, whereas 7 of patients in the surgical group died within 30 days of the operation; median survival was 16.4 months for the group taken to surgery and 14.9 months for the group definitively treated with CRT. At 3 years, the survival curves spread in favor of the group that had surgery, but the differences were not statistically significant. The group who underwent surgery had significantly fewer local recurrences. Of the 172 patients randomized, 131 had their induction chemotherapy response analyzed by an outside panel: 44 patients had an objective response to chemotherapy; 87 did not respond. At 3 years 58% of those undergoing surgery were alive compared with 55% of those treated definitively without surgery. Although nonresponders to CRT had a median survival of <1 year, nonresponders who could still undergo an R0 resection had a 32% 3-year survival (105).

An abstract from a French group reported preliminary results for patients with esophageal squamous cell and adenocarcinomas (T3-4, N0-1, M0) treated with two cycles of cisplatin and 5-FU sandwiched between external-beam radiation. Responding patients were then randomized to surgery alone or further CRT. Median survival for the randomized group was 17.7 months for those undergoing surgery versus 19.3 months for those treated definitively with CRT (106).

Despite these provocative results, the arguments for surgery for most patients after CRT remain strong. With current therapy, the pCR rate is generally under 30%. Following CRT, none of our current noninvasive studies accurately predict patients with who will have pCR (107,108). For patients with adenocarcinoma of the esophagus, successful CRT does not apparently eradicate Barrett esophagus. In a study by Theisen et al. (109), Barrett mucosa was unmasked and later documented by biopsy or histologic assessment in 18 of 20 patients who did not have Barrett esophagus identified prior to CRT. If the Barrett esophagus remains, the patient is at risk for a second primary esophageal adenocarcinoma, and endoscopic surveillance for these patients becomes a life-long project unless the esophagus is removed. The pCR is clearly a surrogate for survival and can place a new regimen into the forefront of clinical trials. Thus the efficacy of new systemic and radiation treatments for esophageal cancer patients can best be measured by complete surgical extirpation of the esophagus. Clearly, it would be a major improvement toward individualizing patient care if investigators could determine if patients destined to be cured by CRT prior to surgery are the same or different from patients destined to be cured by CRT without surgery.

MOLECULAR TARGETS FOR ESOPHAGEAL CANCER

Information regarding the importance of molecular profiling in esophagus cancer falls into three categories: oncogenic progression, prognosis, and prediction. With the knowledge that Barrett esophagus is the precursor lesion for the development of adenocarcinoma of the esophagus, research has been focused on molecular changes that inform for progression into the malig-

nant phenotype. Prognostic genetic changes within the tumor will indicate which patients are likely to fare better or more poorly regardless of the treatment. Predictive gene analyses are directed toward examination of molecular parameters within the tumor or host for genes known to be active in specific drug metabolism or radiation repair pathways. At times, molecular changes and their translation into the clinical arena may overlap, such that clinical intervention for prevention may equally apply in disease treatment.

Oncogenic Progression and Prognosis

Investigative methods may use analysis of specific genes or gene groups based on preclinical leads, or may involve genome studies of esophageal cancers looking for clusters of genes that are overexpressed, deleted, or mutated. As most of the advanced technology for performing these analyses occurred in the time when esophageal cancer treatment was moving toward neoadjuvant therapy, there are few studies with purely prognostic information from surgery-only series. Recently published data from investigations in the areas of cancer progression and prognosis are summarized in the following section.

Investigators at the University of Washington have focused on the role of the tumor suppressor genes *p53* and *p16* in the development of esophageal adenocarcinoma using mapped interval biopsies (2 cm apart) in a cohort of patients with Barrett esophagus enrolled in a surveillance program. They have reported loss of heterozygosity in the chromosomes harboring these genes, aneuploid and tetraploid populations, as identified by flow cytometry lead to progression to the malignant phenotype (110,111). Additionally, promoter hypermethylation of the *p16* gene predicts for such progression and, as demonstrated more recently by Maley et al. (112), the area over which theses clonal expansion occur impacts risk of cancer development.

Vallbohmer et al. (113) examined expression levels of *COX-2*, *VEGF*, and *EGFR* in 91 tissue samples from patients with Barrett esophagus and adenocarcinoma. Gene selection was made on the basis of available targeted agents against these gene functions. Their findings suggest a stepwise increase in expression of *COX2* and *VEGF* over the progression from normal to metaplasia to cancer. Earlier studies from this group demonstrated that increased expression of bFGF occurred even earlier than increases in *VEGF* expression (114). These results indicate that trials of early intervention, using currently available inhibitors of *COX2* and *VEGF* might be valuable in the areas of cancer prevention and cancer therapy.

Using methods of comparative genomic hybridization and serial analysis of gene expression, investigators from Finland (115) and the Netherlands (116) have identified a number of chromosomal regions with clustering of overexpressed genes from esophageal adenocarcinomas. Some of these genes have known functions in the development and progression of cancer (growth factors, protease inhibitors, and proliferation markers); the functions of others have yet to be defined as to their relevance in the malignant process. Nonetheless, identification of these overexpressions gives us tools for sorting among esophageal cancers for prognosis, and identifies potential targets for therapeutic indications.

Specific epigenetic changes leading to cancer development may provide a clue as to tissue of origin. As systemic treatments become more sophisticated, this will be clinically relevant to treatment decisions for adenocarcinomas of the lower esophagus versus those originating in the stomach. Schildhaus et al. (117) examined hypermethylation of the promoter region, which causes gene silencing, of five genes known to have tumor suppressor activity: $p16^{INK4a}$, E-cadherin, O^6-MGMT, DAPK, and FHIT. In addition to determining the site of origin, differences in these gene activities may identify cancers that might be more sensitive to specific classes of drugs (e.g., alkylators). As methylation is a target of drug development; further elaboration of these patterns in individual tumors may direct where these new agents should most appropriately be evaluated in future clinical trials.

Table 32.7 summarizes the studies previously noted as well as prognostic studies of Fas overexpression by Chan et al. (118) and lysosomal enzyme activity by Altorjay et al. (119).

Analysis of Predictive Gene Expression

Investigations into combinations of specific genes involved in the metabolic or known resistance pathways of commonly used treatment modalities are becoming more relevant as systemic therapeutic options have widened. As discussed earlier in this

Table 32.7

Investigations of Molecular Correlates of Malignant Genotype and Prognosis

Molecular Parameter/ Method	No. of Patients/ Histology	Treatment	Correlative Data	Ref.
Gene array—(HLA) high-level amplifications—associated genes	14 Adeno-GEJ: 11 male, 3 female. Fresh-frozen tissue	None	Characterization of 11 HLA; most up-regulated at 7q = hepatocyte growth factor (HGF)	Van Dekken et al. (116)
Gene expression: CGH, SAGE	18 Adeno-GEJ/xenograft fresh-frozen tissue	None	DNA amplification regions associated with gene overexpression and chromosome location	Koon et al. (115)
p16, p53; flow cytometry, DNA amplification and mutation analysis; LOH analysis; promoter methylation	267 Barrett metaplasia; interval mapped biopsy; fresh tissue	None	Size (area) of clonal expansion of p53 and p16 LOH predicts for development of cancer	Maley et al. (112)
VEGF; bFGF; fresh-frozen tissue; RT-PCR, IHC	77 Adeno: 16 metaplasia, 11 dysplasia, 15 carcinoma, 35 normal mucosa	None	Increased levels of both in cancer vs. normal or premalignant; bFGF up-regulated more in dysplasia	Lord et al. (114)
COX-2, VEGF, EGFR/ fresh-frozen, RT-PCR	75 Adeno: 44 adeno, 15 metaplasia, 16 normal	None	Progression of expression of COX-2 and VEGF but not EGFR in the metaplasia-dysplasia-carcinoma sequence	Vallbohmer et al. (113)
Promotor hypermethylation: fresh tissue; PCR, IHC	29 Adeno: 10 esophagus (Barretts), 7 prox gastric, 12 GEJ	None	5 genes; distribution of silencing by location; implications: field defect, apoptosis, drug sensitivity	Schildhaus et al. (117)
Fas overexpression; IHC	58 Squamous, paired normal tissue	Surgery	High Fas correlates with better survival	Chan et al. (118)
Lysosomal enzyme activity	47: 29 Adeno, 18 squamous	Surgery	Specific and relative activities re: path type and normal tissue; correlate with survival in adeno	Altorjay et al. (119)

Adeno, adenocarcinoma; GEJ, gastroesophageal junction; CGH, comparative genomic hybridization; SAGE, serial analysis of gene expression; LOH, loss of heterozygosity; RT-PCR, reverse transcription polymerase chain reaction; IHC, immunohistochemical.

chapter, the most common trimodality therapy for initial treatment of esophagus is a 5FU-cisplatin–based chemotherapy with external-beam radiation followed by surgical resection. Genes involved in anabolism and catabolism of these drugs, as well as cell repair, have thus been examined in esophageal tumor tissue. Trials have been designed to examine pretreatment and posttreatment gene expression to assess if initial levels or changes over the course of therapy can provide a predictive profile for survival for complete pathologic response, the only outcome consistently associated with improved survival.

Prospective trials of tissue acquisition in conjunction with protocol therapy were conducted by investigators at Roswell Park Cancer Institute (120) and at the University of Southern California (121). These trials demonstrated declining levels of the genes of interest between pretreatment biopsies and posttreatment tissue. In the Roswell trial, decline in thymidylate synthetase (*TS*), the target enzyme for 5-FU activity, was associated with survival in early analysis (but lost statistical significance later); decline in expression of *XPA*, a gene involved in nucleotide excision repair and thus resistance to platinum compounds, correlated with survival in late analysis. In the University of Southern California trial, although all gene expressions declined over the course of therapy, only the decline in expression level of epidermal growth factor receptor (EGFR), which has been associated with resistance to radiation, significantly correlated with response to therapy.

Retrospective trials examining similar groupings of gene expressions have been published by investigators at Duke University (122,123) and Munich, Germany (124). Harpole et al. (123) correlated pretreatment gene expression with cancer-free survival. Low initial gene expression of the multidrug resistance gene, *MDR* and *GSTπ1*, both of which are associated with platinum resistance, and *TS* were correlated with improved cancer-free survival independently of other clinical factors. Multivariate analysis demonstrated worsening of cancer-free survival with the addition of each overexpressing gene. Joshi et al. (122) examined pretreatment biopsies for gene expression levels of *TS1*, glutathione S-transferase (*GSTP1*), and the DNA repair gene *ERCC1*. They demonstrated an inverse relationship of *TS1* expression with response to neoadjuvant therapy, decreased cancer-specific survival with high expression levels of all three genes, and increased risk of cancer recurrence with high *TS1* and *ERCC1* levels. The German study demonstrated association of initially high levels of methylenetetrahydrofolate reductase (*MTHFR*, associated with 5-FU activation) and *MDR1* with response as the primary outcome.

Using a different method, Wu et al. (125) demonstrated genetic polymorphisms of *MTHFR* and *MDR* that were associated with reduced recurrence risk and improved survival, as well as a variant allele of the nucleoside repair gene *XRCC1*, which is associated with the absence of pCR and poor survival. Liao et al. (126) examined a polymorphism for the *TS* gene and found a nonsignificant trend for higher local-regional control for the patient cohort with the 6bp/6bp polymorphism at the 3′ UTR (untranslated region).

A number of the genes that have not previously been reported to be predictive of response to current standard 5-FU, platinum, and radiation-based regimens have been shown to change over the course of neoadjuvant therapy and to correlate with better or poorer prognosis. Although a larger database is needed, selecting treatments based on the most favorable gene profile available for chemotherapy and radiation response, and by further subselecting for gene expression predictive of response to available targeted agents, response benefit for specific agents will be maximized.

Although the inducible *COX-2* gene has been shown to be associated with carcinogenesis through increase in angiogenesis and suppression of apoptosis in response to a number of tumor-promoting factors, several groups have evaluated its role in resistance to neoadjuvant treatment of esophageal cancer. Xi et al. (127) demonstrated variable expression *COX-2* across therapy, with high posttreatment levels associated with minor response and poor prognosis. Sivula et al. (128) confirmed that high levels of *COX-2* in the esophageal cancer postchemotherapy had a negative effect on outcome. In a proof-of-principle study, Tuynman et al. (129) demonstrated down-regulation of *COX-2* expression with 4 weeks of celecoxib therapy in a small number of patients with esophageal adenocarcinoma. Thus, with further elucidation of the impact of initial expression of *COX-2* on outcome, rationale exists for studying the incorporation of *COX-2* inhibitor in neoadjuvant treatment strategies.

Up-regulation of *NFκB*, a transcription factor associated with promoting cancer progression by blunting of apoptosis and promotion of multidrug resistance, has been investigated in esophageal carcinoma by Abdel-Latif et al. (130,131). High initial expression of *NFκB* was inversely associated with major or complete pathologic response. Furthermore, the cytokines expressed when *NFκB* is activated were down-regulated in patients who had a pCR with CRT prior to surgery. A number of agents that block *NFκB* activity have been tested clinically in other malignancies and these may have a future role in combined-modality therapy of esophagus cancer.

Overexpression of the genes *c-erbB-1* (*EGFR, HER1*) and *c-erbB-2* (*HER2/neu*) has been associated with poor outcome in a number of cancers. Several agents directed toward modulation of these genes are currently in use in clinical practice in breast, lung, colon, and head and neck cancers. In head and neck cancer, definitive therapy with cetuximab administered concurrently with radiation produced a longer survival time than radiation alone (132). The addition of trastuzumab to chemotherapy in the adjuvant treatment of breast cancer that overexpresses *HER2/neu* improves survival beyond that achieved with chemotherapy alone (133). Schneider et al. (121) demonstrated reduction of expression levels of both of these genes during the course of therapy and demonstrated an association between this change in the *EGFR* gene and histologic grade of regression. However, in pretreatment esophageal cancer specimens, Miyazono et al. (134) dichotomized *c-erbB-1* and *c-erbB-2* gene expression levels and demonstrated that low expression levels of *c-erbB-2* (but not *c-erbB-1*) correlated with major histopathologic response to CRT. The *EGFR* inhibitor cetuximab is currently being evaluated in phase 2 cooperative group and single-institution trials for patients with disseminated esophageal cancer, and results from this approach are awaited. The differing signals from these studies may also suggest a role for investigating some of the newer monoclonal antibodies and multitarget tyrosine kinase inhibitors in order to inactivate both pathways. These reports are summarized in Table 32.8 (120–135).

Table 32.8

Investigations of Molecular Correlates of Treatment Response

Molecular Parameter/ Method	No. of Patients/ Histology	Treatment	Correlative Data	Ref.
TS, DPD, ERCC-1, γGCS, γGT, GSH, MRP-2/ fresh-frozen, RT-PCR	38: 32 adeno, 4 squamous	5-FU/oxaliplatin XRT, surgery; serial biopsy	XPA, TS correlate with survival in a time-dependent fashion; TS, γGCS, ERCC-1 decline over Tx	Leichman et al. (120)
TS, DPD, ERCC-1, GST-π, EGFR, and Her2/neu/ paraffin, RT-PCR	24: 7 Adeno, 17 squamous	5-FU/CDDP; XRT; surgery serial bx	TS, DPD, ERCC-1, GST-π, EGFR, decline over Tx; Δ of EGFR correlates with survival	Schneider et al. (121)
TS1, GSTP1, ERCC1; paraffin, RT-PCR	99: 70 Adeno, 29 squamous	5-FU/CDDP; XRT; surgery	High expression *TS1* = poor Tx response; high expression all 3 genes = poor survival; high *TS1*, ERCC1 = high recurrence risk	Joshi et al. (122)
TS, GST-π 1, metallothionen (MT), P-gp (MDR)/ paraffin, IHC	118: 82 Adeno, 36 squamous	5-FU/CDDP; XRT; surgery	Low expression of *TS, GST-π*, and P-gp correlate with improved DFS	Harpole et al. (123)
Polymorphisms: *MTHFR, TS, MDR1, GSTP1, NER, XRCC-1*/paraffin, RT-PCR	210:174 Adeno, 36 squamous	5-FU/CDDP/taxanes; XRT; surgery	Variant alleles *MTHFR* and *MDR1* improve survival with 5-FU/CDDP; Variant *XRCC1* decreases pCR and survival	Wu et al. (125)
Polymorphism: *3'-UTR (TS gene)*/paraffin, RT-PCR	146: Adeno	5-FU/CDDP; XRT; surgery	Trend to association of 6bp/6bp genotype and improved locoregional control	Liao et al. (126)
TS, TP, DPD, MTHFR, MAP7, ELF3, ERCC-1, ERCC-4 HER2/neu, GADD-45; caldesmon/paraffin, RT-PCR	38 Adeno	5-FU/CDDP; surgery	*MTHFR, MRP1*, Caldesmon and *ERCC4* expression associate with response	Langer et al. (124)
P53, p21, Ki67/paraffin, IHC	30 Adeno	5-FU/LV/IFNα; 5-FU/MTX; or carboplatin/ epirubicin/etoposide; surgery	No correlation with response; *p53+* → *p53−*; *p21−* → *p21+* = better survival	Heeren et al. (135)
COX-2, MET, VEGF/MTT, Western blot, IHC, RT-PCR	27 Adeno: 12 treated, 15 control	Celecoxib (4 weeks); surgery	*Cox-2, MET*, and VEGF decreased in Tx group vs. control	Tuynman et al. (129)
COX-2/fresh-frozen, IHC, RT-PCR	52: 20 Adeno, 32 squamous	5-FU/CDDP; XRT; surgery; serial biopsy	High *COX-2* expression post-Tx correlates with poor outcome	Xi et al. (127)
COX-2/paraffin, IHC	117 Squamous	CDDP/etoposide & surgery (n = 36); surgery (n = 81); only postop specimen	*COX-2* expression not correlated with response; low expression = poor outcome with neoadjuvant Tx	Sivula et al. (128)
c-erbB-1, c-erbB-2/ fresh-frozen, RT-PCR	36: 13 Adeno, 23 squamous	5-FU/CDDP; XRT; Surgery	Low *c-erbB-2* expression correlates with response; no correlation *c-erbB-1*	Miyazono et al. (134)

(Continued)

Table 32.8

Investigations of Molecular Correlates of Treatment Response (*Continued*)

Molecular Parameter/ Method	No. of Patients/ Histology	Treatment	Correlative Data	Ref.
NF-κB, RelA, IκB-α/ fresh-frozen (n = 30), paraffin (n = 97); electrophoresis, IHC	30 Adeno, (fresh-frozen): 15 Barretts, 10 Barretts adjacent adeno, 30 adeno CA	5-FU/CDDP; XRT (n = 58); surgery (n = 39)	*NFκB* expression inverse correlate with response, survival	Abdel-Latif et al. (131)
NF-κB, IL-1β, IL-8; electrophoresis, ELISA	20 Adeno: 10 NF-κB, 10 cytokine; pre- and post-TX analysis	5FU/CDDP; XRT; surgery	Decline in NF-κB IL-1β, IL-8 correlates with pCR	Abdel-Latif et al. (130)

RT-PCR, reverse transcription polymerase chain reaction; Adeno, adenocarcinoma; 5-FU, 5-fluorouracil; XRT, radiation therapy; Tx, treatment; CDDP, cisplatin; IHC, immunohistochemical; DFS, disease-free survival; pCR, complete pathological response; LV, IFNα, interferon alfa; MTX, methotrexate; MTT, ELISA, enzyme-linked immunosorbent assay.

CONCLUSIONS

Neoadjuvant therapy for locally advanced esophageal cancer has a niche as a new standard of care. Nevertheless, because current esophageal preoperative treatments are inadequate for most patients, a standard neoadjuvant therapy remains to be defined. Outside a clinical trial, cisplatin combinations with fluoropyrimidines or taxanes or topoisomerase I inhibitors such as irinotecan are reasonable treatment strategies for systemic therapy in combination with radiation. Clinical trials testing new agents and new ways of administering systemic and regional treatments are necessary. Patients should be encouraged to seek these well-designed, institutional review board-approved trials.

Clinicians and patients must appreciate that the addition of local and systemic therapy to surgery adds a small but detectable increase morbidity and mortality. Only patients with clinical stage II and stage III esophageal tumors should be included in current combined-modality neoadjuvant programs. Preoperative therapy should be given by experienced medical and radiation oncologists, and surgery should be performed only by a team experienced in operating on patients pretreated by radiation and chemotherapy. A strong team approach toward this group of patients is mandatory to bring the maximum number of patients to a favorable outcome.

It is clear that progress has been made in identifying new targets for systemic therapy. Learning to combine new specifically designed targeted agents with current agents that already have targets in their metabolic pathways or in the DNA repair pathways will require innovative translational research for patients with esophageal cancer. However, retrospective analyses have already identified a variety of genes involved in the cancer developmental pathway as well as those that could segregate these cancers on the basis of response and survival. These analyses need to be extended to larger populations in order to provide a more robust database. Furthermore, where the data are currently most robust, trials must be designed in which patients will be selected for specific treatments on the basis of their tumor's molecular profile. Only with this type of proof of principle will we be able to move forward with design and selection of cancer treatments based not on histology and anatomy, but on relevant molecular biologic behavior.

REFERENCES

1. Thomas E, Holmes FA, Smith TL, et al. The use of alternate, non-cross-resistant adjuvant chemotherapy on the basis of pathologic response to a neoadjuvant doxorubicin-based regimen in women with operable breast cancer: long term results from a prospective randomized trial. *J Clin Oncol.* 2004;22:2294–2302.

2. Chau I, Brown G, Cunningham D, et al. Neoadjuvant capecitabine and oxaliplatin followed by synchronous chemoradiation and total mesorectal excision in magnetic resonance imaging-defined poor-risk rectal cancer. *J Clin Oncol.* 2006;24:668–674.

3. Chen AM, Meric-Bernstam F, Hunt KK, et al. Breast conservation after neoadjuvant chemotherapy: The M.D. Anderson Cancer Center Experience. *J Clin Oncol.* 2004;22:2303–2312.

4. Vogelzang NJ. Neoadjuvant MVAC: The long and winding road is getting shorter and straighter. (ed) *J Clin Oncol.* 2001;20:4003–4004.

5. Harari PM. Why has induction chemotherapy for advanced had and neck cancer become a United States community standard of practice? *J Clin Oncol.* 1997;15:2050–2055.

6. Benedetti-Panici P, Greggi S, Colombo A, et al. Neoadjuvant chemotherapy and radical surgery versus exclusive radiotherapy in locally advanced squamous cell cervical cancer: Results from the Italian multicenter randomized study. *J Clin Oncol.* 2002;20:179–188.

7. Tepper JE, Goldberg RM, et al. An embarrassment of riches: Neoadjuvant therapy of rectal cancer. (ed) *J Clin Oncol.* 2005;23:1399–1341.

8. Adelstein DJ, LeBlanc M. Does induction chemotherapy have a role in the management of locoregionally advanced squamous cell head and neck cancer? *J Clin Oncol.* 2006;24: 2624–2628.

9. O'Connell MJ. Combined modality therapy for rectal cancer (ed). *J Clin Oncol.* 2005;23;5450–5451.

10. Ring A, Webb A, Ashley S, et al. Is surgery necessary after complete remission following neoadjuvant chemotherapy for early breast cancer. *J Clin Oncol.* 2003;21:4540–4545.

11. Chireac LR, Swisher SG, Ajani JA, et al. Posttherapy pathologic stage predicts survival in patient with esophageal carcinoma receiving preoperative chemoradiation. *Cancer.* 2005;103:1347–1355.

12. Ries LAG, Eisner MP, Kosary C, et al. eds. SEER cancer statistics review 1973–1999. Bethesda Md.: National Cancer Institute 2002.

13. Jernal A, Murray T, Ward E, et al. Cancer statistics, 2005. *CA Cancer J Clin.* 2005. Published online:doi:10.3322/caac.20006.

14. Edwards BK, Brown ML, Wingo PA et al. Annual report to the nation on the status of cancer, 1975–2002, featuring population-based trends in cancer treatment. *J Natl Cancer Inst.* 2005;97:1407–1427.

15. Miller JAG, Rege RV, Ko, CY, et al. Health care access and poverty do not explain the higher esophageal cancer mortality in African Americans. *Am J Surg.* 2004;188:22–26.

16. Brown LM, Devesa SS. Epidemiologic trends in esophageal and gastric cancer in the United States. *Surg Oncol Clin N Am.* 2002;11:235–256.

17. Lagergren J, Berstrom R, Lindgren A, et al. Symptomatic gastroesophageal reflux as a risk factor for esophageal adenocarcinoma. *N Engl J Med.* 1999;340:825–831.

18. Wijnhoven BP, Tilanus HW, Dinjens WN. Molecular biology of Barrett's adenocarcinoma. *Ann Surg.* 2001;233:322–337.

19. Rice TW, Zuccaro G Jr, Adelstein DJ, et al. Esophageal carcinoma: depth of tumor invasion is predictive of regional lymph node status. *Ann Thorac Surg.* 1998;65:787–792.

20. Korst RJ, Rusch VW, Venkatraman E, et al. Proposed revision of the staging classification for esophageal cancer. *J Thorac Cardiovasc Surg.* 1998;115:660–669. discussion 669–670.

21. Flamen P, Lerut A, Cutsem E, et al. Utility of positron emission tomography for the staging of patients with potentially operable esophageal carcinoma. *J Clin Oncol.* 2000;18:3202–3210.

22. Wallace MB, Nietert PJ, Earle C, et al. An analysis of multiple staging management strategies for carcinoma of the esophagus: computed tomography, endoscopic ultrasound, positron emission tomography, and throacoscopy/laparasocopy. *Ann Thorac Surg.* 2002;74:1026–1032.

23. Rosch T: Endosonographic staging of esophageal cancer: A review of literature results. *Ganstrointest Endosc Clin N Am.* 1995;5:537–547.

24. Fockens P, VAndenBrande J, vanDjullemenH, et al. Endosonographic T-staging of esophageal carcinoma: *A learning curve Gastrointest Endosc.* 1996;44:58–62.

25. Dancygier H, Lightdale CJ (eds): Endoscopic Sonography in Gastroenterology. Stuttgart, Germany, Thieme, 1999.

26. Abdalla EK, Pisters PWT. Staging and preoperative evaluation of upper gastrointestinal malignancies. *Seminars in Oncology,* 31, No. 2004;4:513–514.

27. Lightdale CJ: Esophageal cancer: Practice Guidelines *Am J Gastroenterol.* 1999;94:20–29.

28. Lightdale C. Positron emission tomography: another useful test for staging esophageal cancer. *J Clin Oncol.* 2000;18:3199–3201.

29. Meltzer C Luketich JD, Friedman D, et al. Whole-body FDG positron emission tomographic imaging for staging esophageal cancer comparison with computed tomography. *Clin Nucl Med.* 2000;25:882–887.

30. Weber WA, Ott K, Becker K, et al. Prediction of response to preoperative chemotherapy in adenocarcinomas of the esophagogas-

tric junction by metabolic imaging. *J Clin Oncol.* 2001;19:3058–3065.

31. Downey RJ, Akhurst T, Ilson D, et al. Whole body 28FDG-PET and the response of esophageal cancer to induction therapy: results of a preoperative trial. *J Clin Oncol.* 2003;21:428–432.

32. Luketich JD, Schauer PER, Meltzer CC, et al. The role of positron emission tomography in staging esophageal cancer. *Ann Thorac Surg.* 1997;64:765–769.

33. Earlam R, Cunha-Melo JR. Oesophageal squamous cell carcinoma: I. A critical review of surgery. *Br J Surg.* 1980;67:381–390.

34. Earlam R, Cunha-Melo JR. Oesophageal squamous cell carcinoma: II. A critical view of radiotherapy. *Br J Surg.* 1980;67:457–461.

35. Denittis AS. Esophagus. In *Principles and Practice of Radiation Oncology,* (4th ed). Lippicott Williams & Wilkins, Philadelphia, 2004.

36. Arnott SJ, Duncan W, Gignoux M, et al. Preoperative radiotherapy in esophageal carcinoma: A meta-analysis using individual patient data (esophageal cancer collaborative group). *Int J. Radiat Oncol Biol Phys.* 1998;41:579–582.

37. Montravade R, Ladd T, Briele H, et al. Carcinoma of the esophagus: sites of failure. *Int J Radiat Oncol Biol Phys.* 1982;8:1897–1902.

38. Hosch SB, Stoecklein NH, Pichlmeier U, et al. Esophageal cancer: the model of lymphatic tumor cell spread and its prognostic significance. *J Clin Oncol.* 2001;19:1970–1975.

39. Shah MA, Schartz GK. Treatment of metastatic esophagus and gastric cancer. *Semin Oncol.* 2004;21:574–587.

40. Lokich J, Shea M, Chaffey J, et al. Sequential infusional 5-fluorouracil followed by concomitant radiation for tumors of the esophagus and gastroesophageal junction. *Cancer.* 1987;60:275–279.

41. Miller JI, McIntyre B, Hatcher CR. Combined treatment approach in surgical management of carcinoma of the esophagus: a preliminary report. *Ann Thorac Surg.* 1985;40:289–293.

42. Ezdinli EZ, Gelber R, Desai DV, et al. Chemotherapy of advanced carcinoma of the esophagus: Eastern Cooperative Oncology Group. *Cancer.* 1980;46:2149–2153.

43. Panettiere F, Leichman L, Tilchen E, et al. Chemotherapy for advanced epidermoid carcinoma of the esophagus with single agent cisplatin: a final report on Southwest Oncology Group study. *Cancer Treat Rep.* 1984;68:1023–1024.

44. Enzinger P, Ilson DH, Kelsen D. Chemotherapy in esophageal cancer. *Semin Oncol.* 1999;26 (suppl 15):12–20.

45. Ajani JA, Ilson DH, Daugherty K, et al. Activity of taxol in patients with squamous cell carcinoma of he esophagus. *J Natl Cancer Inst.* 1994;86:1086–1091.

46. Heath EI, Urba S, Marshall J, et al. Phase II trial of docetaxel chemotherapy in patients with incurable adenocarcinomas of the esophagus. *Invest New Drugs.* 2002;20:95–99.

47. Ensinger PC, Kulke MH, Clark JW, et al. A phase II trial of irinotecan in patients with previously untreated advanced esophageal and gastric adenocarcinoma. *Dig Dis Sci.* 2005;50:2218–2223.

48. Hayashi K, Ando N, Watanabe H, et al. Phase II evaluation of protracted infusion of cisplatin and 5-fluorouracil in advanced squamous cell carcinoma of the esophagus: A Japan Esophageal Oncology Group (JEOG) trial (JCOG 9407). *Jpn J Clin Oncol.* 2001;31:419–423.

49. Bleiberg H, Conroy T, Paillot B, et al. Randomized phase II study of cisplatin and 5-fluorouracil versus cisplatin alone in advanced squamous cell oesophageal cancer. *Eur J Cancer.* 1997;33:1216–1220.

50. Ilson DH. Phase II trial of weekly irinotecan/cisplatin in advanced esophageal cancer. *Oncology (Williston Park).* 2004;18: (14 Suppl) 22–25.

51. Ajani JA, Fodor MB, Tjulandin SA, et al. Phase II multi-institutional trial of docetaxel plus cisplatin with or without fluorouracil in patient with untreated, advanced gastric or gastroesophageal adenocarcinoma. *J Clin Oncol.* 2005;23:5660–5667.

52. Jatoi A, Murphy BR, Foster NR, et al. Oxaliplatin and capecitabine in patients with metastatic adenocarcinoma of the esophagus, gastroesophageal junction and gastric cardia: a phase II study from the North Central Cancer Treatment Group. *Ann Oncol.* 2006;17:29–34.

53. Giordano KF, Jatoi A, Stella PJ, et al. Docetaxel and capecitabine in patients with metastatic adenocarcinoma of the stomach and gastroesophageal junction: a phase II study from the North Central Cancer Treatment Group. *Ann Oncol.* 2006;17:652–656.

54. Kelsen DP, Ginsberg R, Pajak TF, et al. Chemotherapy followed by surgery compared with surgery alone for localized esophagus cancer. *N Engl J Med.* 1998;339:1979–1984.

55. Malthaner R, Fenlon D. Preoperative chemotherapy for respectable thoracic esophageal cancer (Cochrane Review) in: *Cochrane Database Syst Rev,* 2001;1–1.

56. Urschel JD, Vasan H, Blewett CJ. A meta-analysis of randomized controlled trials that compared neoadjuvant chemotherapy and surgery to surgery alone for respectable esophageal cancer. *Am J Surg.* 2002;183:274–279.

57. Medical Research Council Oesophageal Cancer Working Group. Surgical resection with or without preoperative chemotherapy in oesophageal cancer: a randomised controlled trial. *Lancet.* 2002;359:1727–1733.

58. Malthaner RA, Collin S, Fenlon D, Rhopes S. Preoperative chemotherapy for resectable thoracic esophageal cancer. *Cochrane Database Syst Rev.* 2006;3:CD001556.

59. Kok TC, vLanschot J, Siersema PD, et al. Neoadjuvant chemotherapy in operable esophageal squamous cell cancer: a final report of a phase III multicenter randomized controlled trial. *Proc Am Soc Clin Oncol.* 1997;16:277a. Abstract 984.

60. Wang C, Ding T, Cheng L. A randomized clinical study of preoperative chemotherapy for esophageal carcinoma. *Zhonghua Zhong Liu Za Zhi.* 2001;23:254–255.

61. Nigro ND, Vaitkevicius VK, Considine B Jr. Combined therapy for cancer of the anal canal: a preliminary report. *Dis Colon Rectum.* 1974;17:354–356. *Dis Colon Rectum* 1974;36:709–711.

62. Nigro ND, Vaitkeviceus VK, Herskovic AM, et al. Preservation of function in the treatment of cancer of the anus. *Important Adv Oncol.* 1989;161–177.

63. Leichman L, Nigro N, Vaitkevicius VK, et al. Cancer of the anal canal: a model for pre-operative adjuvant combined modality therapy. *Am J Med.* 1985;78:211–215.

64. Franklin R, Steiger Z, Vaishampayan G, et al. Combined modality therapy for esophageal squamous cell carcinoma. *Cancer.* 1983;51:1062–1071.

65. Leichman L, Steiger Z, Seydel HG, et al. Pre-operative Chemotherapy and Radiation Therapy for Patients with Cancer of the Esophagus: A Potentially Curative Approach. *J Clin Oncol.* 1984;2(2):75–79.

66. Urba SG, Orringer MB, Turrisi DA, et al. Randomized trial of preoperative chemoradiation versus surgery alone in patients with locoregional esophageal cancer. *J Clin Oncol.* 2001;19:305–313.

67. Nygaard K, Hagen S, Hansen HS, et al. Preoperative radiotherapy prolongs survival in operable oesophageal carcinoma: a randomized multicenter study of preoperative radiotherapy and chemotherapy. *World J Surg.* 1992;16:1104–1109.

68. Bosset JF, Gignoux M, Triboulet JP, et al. Chemoradiotherapy followed by surgery compared with surgery alone in squamous cell cancer of the esophagus. *N Engl J Med.* 1997;337:161–167.

69. Apinop C, Puttisak P, Preecha N, et al. A prospective study of combined therapy in oesophageal cancer. *Hepatogastroenterology.* 1994;41:391–393.

70. Walsh TN, Noonan N, Hollywood D, et al. Comparison of multimodal therapy and surgery for oesophageal adenocarcinoma. *N Engl J Med.* 1996;335:462–467.

71. Walsh TN, Grennell M, Mansoor S, et al. Neoadjuvant treatment of advanced stage esophageal adenocarcinoma increases survival. *Dis Esophagus.* 2002;15:121–124.

72. Fiorica F, Di Bona D, Schepis F, et al. Preoperative chemoradiotherapy for oesophageal cancer: systematic review and met-analysis. *Gut.* 2004;53:925–930.

73. Kaklamanos IG, Walker GR, Ferry K, et al. Neoadjuvant treatment for respectable cancer of the esophagus and gastroesophageal junction: a meta-analysis of randomized clinical trials. *Ann Surg Oncol.* 2003;10:754–761.

74. Le Prise E, Etienne PL, Meuniere B, et al. A randomized study of chemotherapy, radiation therapy, and surgery versus surgery for localized squamous cell carcinoma of the esophagus. *Cancer.* 1994;73:1779–1784.

75. Urschel JD, Vasan H. A meta-analysis of randomized controlled trials that compared neoadjuvant chemoradiation and surgery to surgery alone for respectable esophageal cancer. *Am J Surg.* 2003;185:538–543.

76. Greer SE, Goodney PP, Sutton JE, et al. Neoadjuvant chemoradiotherapy for esophageal carcinoma: A meta-analysis. *Surgery.* 2005;137:172–177.

77. Coia LR, Minsky BD, John MJ, et al. The evaluation and treatment of patients receiving radiation therapy for carcinoma of the esophagus: Results of the 1992, 1994 Patterns of Care Study. *Cancer.* 1999;85:2499–2505.

78. Suntharalingam M, Moughan J, Coia LR, et al. The national practice for patients receiving radiation therapy for carcinoma of the esophagus: Results of the 1996-1999 Patterns of Care Study. *Int J Radiat Oncol Biol Phys.* 2003;56:981–987.

79. Suntharalingam M, Moughan J, Coia LR, et al. Outcome results of the 1996-1999 Patterns of Care Survey of the National Practice for Patients Receiving Radiation Therapy for Carcinoma of the Esophagus. *J Clin Oncol.* 2005;23:2325–2331.

80. Tepper JE, Krasna M, Niedzwiecki D, et al. Superiority of trimodality therapy to surgery alone in esophageal cancer : results of CALGB 9781. *Proc Am Soc Clin Oncol.* 2006;24:4012 (abstr).

81. Swisher SG, Hofstetter W, Wu TT, et al. Proposed revision of the esophageal cancer staging system to accommodate pathologic response (pP) following preoperative chemoradiation (CRT). *Ann Surg.* 2005;241:810–820.

82. Mandard AM, Dalibard F, Mandard JC, et al. Pathologic assessment of tumor regression afer preoperative chemotherapy of esophageal carcinoma. *Cancer.* 1994;73:2680–2686.

83. Schneider PM, Baldr SE, Metzger R, et al. Histomorphologic tumor regression and lymph node metastases determine prognosis following neoadjuvant radiochemotherapy for esophageal cancer: implications for response classification. *Ann Surg.* 2005;242:684–692.

84. Urschel JD, Vasan H. A meta-analysis of randomized controlled trials that compared neoadjuvant chemoradiation and surgery to surgery alone for respectable esophageal cancer. *Am J Surg.* 2003;185:538–543.

85. Whooley BP, Law S, Murphy SC, et al. Analysis of reduced death and complication rates after esophageal resection. *Ann Surg.* 2001;233:338–344.

86. DeMeester SR. Adenocarcinoma of the esophagus and cardia: A review of the disease and its treatment. *Annals of Surgical Oncology.* 2006;13:12–30.

87. Ando N, Ozawa S, Kitagawa Y, et al. Improvement in the results of surgical treatment of advanced squamous esophageal carcinoma during 15 consecutive years. *Ann Surg.* 2000;232:225–232.

88. Hulscher JBF, Van Sandick JW, De Boer A GEM, et al. Extended transthoracic resection compared with limited transhiatal resection for adenocarcinoma of the esophagus. *N Engl J Med.* 2002;347:1662–1669.

89. Bolton JS, Teng S. Transthoracic or transhiatal esophagectomy for cancer of the esophagus: does it matter? *Surg Oncol Clin North Am.* 2002;11:365–375.

90. Chang AC, Birkmeyer JD. The volume-performance relationship in esophagectomy. *Thorac Surg Clin.* 2006;16:87–94.

91. Pearson JG. The value of radiotherapy in the management of esophageal cancer. *AJR Am J Roentagenol.* 1977;105:500–513.

92. Herskovic A, Leichman L, Lattin P, et al. Chemo/radiation with and without surgery in the thoracic esophagus: the Wayne State experience. *Int J Radiat Oncol Biol Phys.* 1988;15:655–662.

93. Minsky BD, Pajak TF, Ginsberg RJ, et al. INT 0123 (Radiation Therapy Oncology Group 94-05) phase III trial of combined modality therapy for esophageal cancer: High-dose versus standard-dose radiation therapy. *J Clin Oncol.* 2002;20:1167–1174, (comment).

94. Gunderson LL, Haddock Mg, Braich T, et al. Chemoradiation for Esophageal Cancer. In: *American Society for Clinical Oncology 2003 Educational Book.* Alexandria, VA: American Society for Clinical Oncology; 2003:441–449.

95. Kelsen DP, Multimodality therapy of local regional esophageal cancer. *Semin Oncol.* 2005;32 (suppl 9) S6–S10.

96. Pasini F, de Manzoni G, Pedrzzani C, et al. High pathological response rate in locally advanced esophageal cancer after neoadjuvant combined modality therapy: dose finding of a weekly chemotherapy schedule with protracted infusion of 5-fluorouracil and dose escalation of cisplatin, docetaxel and concurrent radiotherapy. *Ann Oncol.* 2005;16:1133–1139.

97. Ajani JA, Walsh G, Komaki R, et al. Preoperative induction of CPT-11 and cisplatin chemotherapy followed by chemoradiation in patients with locoregional carcinoma of the esophagus or gastroesophageal junction. *Cancer.* 2004;100:2347–2354.

98. Khushalani NI, Leichman CG, Proulx G, et al. Oxaliplatin in combination with protracted-infusion 5-fluorouracil and radiation: Report of a clinical trial for patients with esophageal cancer. *J Clin Oncol.* 2002;20:2844–2850.

99. Herskovic A, Martz K, Al Sarraf M, et al. Combined chemotherapy and radiotherapy compared with radiotherapy alone in patients with cancer of the esophagus. *N Engl J Med.* 1992;326:1593–1598.

100. Haller DG. Treatments for esophageal cancer. (ed) *N Engl J Med.* 1992;326:629–631.

101. Al Sarraf M, Martz A, Herskovic A, et al. Progress report of combined chemoradiotherapy versus radiotherapy alone in patients with esophageal cancer: An Intergroup Study. *J Clin Oncol.* 1997;15:277–284.

102. Cooper JS, Guo MD, Herskovic A, et al. Chemotherapy of locally advanced esophageal cancer: long term follow-up of a prospective randomized trial (RTOG 85-01). *JAMA.* 1999;281:1623–1627.

103. Smith TJ, Ryan LM, Douglass HO, et al. Combined chemoradiotherapy vs. radiotherapy alone for early stage esophagus squamous cell carcinoma of the esophagus. *In J Radiat Oncol Biol Phys.* 1998;42:269–276.

104. Wong R, Malthaner R. Combine chemotherapy and radiotherapy (without surgery) compared with radiotherapy alone in localized carcinoma of the esophagus (Review). The Cochrane Collaboration. *The Cochrane Library Issue.* 2006;2.

105. Stahl M, Stuschke M, Lehmann N, et al. Chemoradiation with and without surgery in patients with locally advanced squamous cell carcinoma of the esophagus. *J Clin Oncol.* 2005;23:2310–2317.

106. Bedenne L, Michel P, Bouche O, et al. Randomized phase III trial in locally advanced esophageal cancer: radiochemotherapy followed by surgery versus radiochemotherapy alone (FCD 9102). *Proc Am Soc Clin Oncol.* 2002;21:130a, (abstr 519).

107. Westerterp M, van Westreenen HL, Reitsma JB, et al. Esophageal Cancer: CT endoscopic US and FDG PET for assessment of response to neoadjuvant therapy—systematic review. *Radiology.* 2005;236:841–851.

108. Yang Q, Cleary KR, Yao JC, et al. Significance of postchemoradiation biopsy in predicting residual esophageal carcinoma in the surgical specimen. *Diseases of the Esophagus.* 2004;17:38–43.

109. Theisen J, Stein HJ, Dittler HJ, et al. Preoperative chemotherapy unmasks underlying Barrett's mucosa in patient with adenocarcinoma of the distal esophagus. *Surg. Endosc.* 2002;16:671–673.

110. Galipeau PC, Prevo LJ, Sanchez CA, et al. Clonal expansion and loss of heterozygosity at chromosomes 9p and 17p in pre-malignant esophageal (Barrett's) tissue. *J Natl Cancer Inst.* 1999;91:2087–2095.

111. Barrett MT, Pritchard D, Palanca-Wessels C, et al. Molecular phenotype of spontaneously arising 4N (G2-tetraploid) intermediates of neoplastic progression in Barrett's esophagus. *Cancer Res.* 2003;63:4211–4217.

112. Maley CC, Galipeau PC, Xiaohong L, et al. J. The combination of genetic instability and clonal expansion predicts progression to esophageal adenocarcinoma. *Cancer Res.* 2004;64:7629–7633.

113. Vallbohmer D, Peters JH, Kuramochi H, et al. Molecular determinants in targeted therapy for esophageal adenocarcinoma. *Arch Surg.* 2006;141:476–482.

114. Lord, R VN, Park JM, Wickramasinghe K, et al. Vascular endothelial growth factor and basic fibroblast growth factor expression in esophageal adenocarcinoma and Barrett esophagus. *J Thorac Cardiovasc Surg* 2003;125:246–253.

115. Koon N, Zaika A, Moskaluk C, et al. Clustering of Molecular Alterations in Gastroesophageal Carcinomas. *Neoplasia* 2004;6:143–149.

116. Van Dekken H, Vissers K, Tilanus HW, et al. Genomic array and expression analysis of frequent high-level amplifications in adenocarcinomas of the gastro-esophageal junction. *Cancer Genetics and Cytogenetics* 2006;166:157–162.

117. Schildhaus HU, Krockel I, Lippert H, et al. Promoter hypermethylation of p16^{INK4a}, E-cadherin, O^6-MGMT, DAPK and FHIT in adenocarcinomas of the esophagus, esophagogastric junction and proximal stomach. *International Journal of Oncology* 2005;26:1493–1500.

118. Chan KW, Lee PY, Lam AK, et al. Clinical relevance of *Fas* expression in oesophageal squamous cell carcinoma. *J Clin Path.* 2006;59:101–104.

119. Altorjay A, Paal , Sohar N, et al. Significance and prognostic value of lysosomal enzyme activities measured in surgically operate adenocarcinomas of the gastroesophageal junction and squamous cell carcinomas of the lower third of esophagus. *World J Gastroenterology.* 2005;11:5751–5756.

120. Leichman L, Lawrence D, Clark K, et al. Expression of genes related to Oxaliplatin and 5-Fluorouracil activities in endoscopic biopsies of primary esophageal cancer in patients receiving Oxaliplatin, 5-Flourouracil and radiation: characterization and exploratory analysis with survival. *J Chemother.* 2006;18:514–524.

121. Schneider S, Uchida K, Brabender J, et al. Downregulation of TS, DPD, ERCC1, GST-Pi, EGFR, and HER2 gene expression after neoadjuvant three-modality treatment in patients with esophageal cancer. *J Am Coll Surg.* 2005;200:336–344.

122. Joshi M-B M, Shirota Y, Danenberg KD, et al. High gene expression of *TS1, GSTP1,* and *ERCC1* are risk factors for survival in patients treated with trimodality therapy for esophageal cancer. *Clin Cancer Res.* 2005;11:2215–2221.

123. Harpole DH Jr., Moore MB, Herndon JE II, et al. The prognostic value of molecular marker analysis in patients treated with tri-modality therapy for esophageal cancer. *Clinical Cancer Research.* 2001;7:562–569.

124. Langer R, Specht K, Becker K, et al. Association of pretherapeutic expression of chemotherapy-related genes with response to neoadjuvant chemotherapy in Barrett Carcinoma. *Clinical Cancer Research.* 2005;11:7462–7469.

125. Wu X, Gu J, Wu TT, et al. Genetic variations in radiation and chemotherapy drug action pathways predict clinical outcomes in esophageal cancer. *Journal of Clinical Oncology.* 2006;24:3789–3798.

126. Liao Z, Liu H, Swisher SG, et al. Polymorphism at the 3'-UTR of the thymidylate synthase gene: a potential predictor for outcomes in Caucasian patients with esophageal adenocarcinoma treated with pre-operative chemoradiation. *Int J Radiat Oncol Biol Phys.* 2006;64:700–708.

127. Xi H, Baldus SE, Warnecke-Eberz U, et al. High Cyclooxygenase-2 expression following neoadjuvant radiochemotherapy is associated with minor histopathologic response and poor prognosis in esophageal cancer. *Clinical Cancer Research.* 2005;11:8341–8347.

128. Sivula A, Buskens CJ, van Rees BP, et al. Prognostic role of cyclooxygenase-2 in neoadjuvant-treated patients with squamous cell carcinoma of the esophagus. *Int J Cancer.* 2005;116:903–908.

129. Tuynman JB, Buskens C, Kemper K, et al. Neoadjuvant Selective COX-2 inhibition down-regulates important oncogenic pathways in patients with esophageal adenocarcinoma. *Annals of Surgery.* 2005;242:840–850.

130. Abdel-Latif MMM, O'Riordan JM, Ravi N, et al. NF-κB activation in esophageal adenocarcinoma. *Annals of Surgery.* 2004;239:491–500.

131. Abdel-Latif MMM, O'Riordan JM, Ravi N, et al. Activated nuclear factor-kappa B and cytokine profiles in the esophagus parallel tumor regression following neoadjuvant chemoradiotherapy. *Diseases of the Esophagus.* 2005;18:246–252.

132. Bonner JA, Harari PM, Giralt J, et al. Radiotherapy plus cetuximab for squamous-cell carcinoma of the head and neck. *N Engl J Med.* 2006;354:567–578.

133. Romond EH, Perez EA, Bryant J, et al. Trastuzumab plus adjuvant chemotherapy for operable HER2-positive breast cancer. *N Engl J Med.* 2005;353:1673–1684.

134. Miyazono F, Metzger R, Warnecke-Eberz U, et al. Quantitative c-erbB-2 but not c-erbB-1 mRNA expression is a promising marker to predict minor histopathologic response to neoadjuvant radiochemotherapy in oesophageal cancer. *Br J Cancer.* 2004;91:666–672.

135. Heeren PA, Kloppenberg FW, Hollema H, et al. Predictive effect of p53 and p21 alteration on chemotherapy response and survival in locally advanced adenocarcinoma of the esophagus. *Anticancer Res.* 2004;24:2579–2583.

COMMENTARY
Bach Ardalan and Olga Kozyreva

The management of patients with esophageal carcinoma presents some of the greatest challenges currently faced by physicians. Despite current staging modalities and aggressive strategies, esophageal carcinoma remains a fatal disease. The direction of its future treatment is uncertain.

Approximately 50% of these patients present with locoregional disease, for which the optimal therapy is unclear. Options include primary surgery, definitive chemoradiation, neoadjuvant chemoradiation or chemotherapy, adjuvant chemotherapy, adjuvant radiation, or adjuvant chemoradiation. Although surgical therapy may be curative in the early stages of esophageal carcinoma, 5-year survival rarely exceeds 30% for regionally advanced cases—a number closely matched by definitive chemoradiation trials (1). Despite potentially curative surgical resection, 30% to 40% of patients with locally advanced esophageal carcinoma will suffer from local and/or systemic relapse within 24 months after surgery and ultimately die from their disease. A reason for such an early tumor relapse in these patients is the presence of clinically undetectable micrometastatic disease at the time of diagnosis. Only 50% to 60% of the resectable patients who underwent surgery with curative intent had a R0 resection or microscopically margin-negative surgery. In addition, 70% to 80% of all resected surgical specimens harbored lymph node metastases (2,3). Many recent studies have shown the presence of occult metastases in lymph nodes from patients with esophageal cancer staged as pathologically node-negative (4–11). These studies indicate that 1% to 17% of histologically negative lymph nodes and 11% to 50% of pathologically node-negative patients (p_{N0}) have nodal metastases that are missed by routine pathologic evaluation (4,6,7,9). Interestingly, studies confirm the presence of micrometastases in rib marrow in 75% to 88% of esophageal cancer patients undergoing curative surgery (12,13). The prognostic relevance of isolated tumor cells in the bone marrow is still a matter of controversy. Several studies support the hypothesis that minimal residual disease or isolated tumor cells in the bone marrow of cancer patients can be regarded as the precursor of clinically manifested distant metastases.

ADJUVANT THERAPY FOR ESOPHAGEAL CANCER

The Leichmans have provided a very scholarly and comprehensive discussion of the status of neoadjuvant therapy. Here we focus on the available information evaluating postoperative adjuvant therapy. The intent of adjuvant therapy is to eradicate micrometastatic residual disease following curative resection of a primary tumor with the goal to improve overall survival. The benefit of adjuvant chemotherapy for high-risk colon cancer, early breast carcinoma, and non-small cell lung cancer is well established (14–16).

Although "adjuvant therapy," strictly defined, implies the absence of any detectable residual disease after surgical resection, in the study of esophageal cancer some of the "adjuvant" trials include patients with known residual disease after a resection intended to cure.

Adjuvant Radiation

The advantage of adjuvant radiation therapy in contrast to preoperative radiation is that the intraoperative and histopathologic findings guide the treatment. Thus it is possible to deliver radiation to areas at high risk for recurrence in accurately staged patients. The disadvantages of postoperative therapy include the presence of the radiation-sensitive esophageal substitute and wider fields of radiation in the postoperative patient.

Table 32C.1

Characteristics of Randomized Clinical Trials in which Surgery and Postoperative Radiation were Compared with Surgery Alone

Series	Year	S+RT N	S N	Radiation Dose	Median Survival S+RT vs. S (mo)	3-Year Survival S+RT vs. S (%)	5-Year Survival S+RT vs. S (%)	Local Recurrence Rate S+RT vs. S (%)
Fok et al. (17)	1993	65	65	49–52 Gy/14–15 fr	8.7 vs. 15.2	16 vs. 21		15 vs. 31
Zieren et al. (19)	1995	33	35	45–55 Gy/25 fr	14 vs. 13	22 vs. 20		45 vs. 54
Ténière et al. (18)	1991	102	119	55.8 Gy/31 fr	18 vs. 18	27 vs. 29	21 vs. 19	70 vs. 85
Kasai et al. (21)	1978	52	59	60 Gy	26 vs. 14	—	—	—
Xiao et al. (20)	2003	220	275	50–60 Gy/25–30 fr	36 vs. 26	51 vs. 44	41 vs. 37	19.8 vs. 44.9
Total		472	553					

S, surgery; RT, radiotherapy; N, number of patients randomized; fr, fractions; boost of 0 to 10 Gy.

The role of postoperative radiation was evaluated in five randomized prospective trials (17–21). The study's characteristics and results are summarized in Table 32C.1. Although all studies specified the absence of distant metastases as an inclusion criterion, Zieren et al. (19) and Teniere et al. (18) included patients with M1 disease (celiac node involvement). Three of five studies conducted in Asia (Hong Kong, Japan, and China) were performed in patients with squamous cell carcinomas. The trial end points were toxicity, local recurrence, and overall survival. The quality of life was assessed in only one trial (19). Radiotherapy was delivered within 6 weeks after surgery in the trials by Fok et al. (17), Zieren et al. (19), and Xiao et al. (20), but in the trial by Teniere et al. (18), radiation therapy began within 3 months. The radiotherapy doses in these trials were higher than in the preoperative series. Fok et al. (17) used a hypofractionated schedule with three fractions per week for a total dose that depended on margin status between 49 and 52.5 Gy. Zieren et al. (19) delivered 45 to 55 Gy in 25 fractions with a boost of 0 to 10 Gy. Teniere et al. (18) delivered a total of 55.8 Gy in 31 fractions. The dose of radiation in the study by Xiao et al. (20) was 50 to 60 Gy in 25 to 30 fractions delivered over 5 to 6 weeks. The toxicity reported by Fok et al. (17) was significant. The upper gastrointestinal ulceration and bleeding in 24 of 65 patients in the treatment group resulted in five deaths, perhaps owing to the hypofractionated (3.5 Gy) method used. In the 33 patients receiving radiation, Zieren et al. (19) reported only mild toxicity. Their results indicate more rapid recovery of quality of life with surgery alone compared with postoperative radiotherapy.

In summary, two of these trials (18,19) have shown that radiation therapy did not improve survival. The local control was significantly better in postoperative radiotherapy groups in three trials (17–19). Two studies indicated that for those patients who did not have lymph nodal metastases, the prophylactic postoperative radiation therapy improved survival when patients underwent a curative resection (20,21). The trial by Fok et al. (17) reported a shorter survival with the postoperative radiotherapy group compared with surgery.

Although investigators cannot recommend the use of routine postoperative radiotherapy outside the clinical trial setting, it may be effective for the individuals at high risk for local recurrence and for patients with known microscopic or gross residual tumor after surgery. In clinical trials, investigators continue to evaluate postoperative radiation therapy.

Postoperative Chemotherapy and Surgery versus Surgery Alone

In three randomized controlled trials, surgery and postoperative chemotherapy were compared with surgery alone (22–24). All three trials used cisplatin-based regimens. Ando et al. (23), in their early trial, randomized 205 patients to receive two cycles of postoperative cisplatin and vindesine or surgery alone. Pouliquin et al. (22) randomized 120 patients to receive six to eight cycles of postoperative cisplatin and 5-fluorouracil (5-FU) or no treatment. In the latest study, Ando et al. (24) randomized 242 patients based on the patients' lymph node status to either receive two cycles of cisplatin and 5-FU or surgery alone. After 5 years of follow-up, the survival rates of the two arms in each study were nearly identical. The study characteristics and results are summarized in Table 32C.2.

In addition, in each of the groups stratified for complete versus incomplete resection, Pouliquin et al. (22) found that the addition of postoperative chemotherapy had no impact on survival. The toxicity levels were significant in two trials. Investigators did not provide operative mortality in either study; however, in two of the studies, there were four postoperative deaths attributed to the toxicity of chemotherapy. In one study, investigators assessed the quality of life and concluded that the duration of improved dysphagia was similar for both groups (22). However, in the latest study, Ando et al. (24) demonstrated that postoperative adjuvant chemotherapy with cisplatin and fluorouracil is better able to prevent relapse in patients with esophageal cancer than surgery alone. Risk reduction by postoperative chemotherapy was remarkable in the subgroup with lymph node metastasis.

Although these trials included only patients with squamous cell histology, and some resections were palliative in nature, the data demonstrate that the use of postoperative chemotherapy for esophageal carcinoma cannot be recommended outside the clinical trial setting.

Table 32C.2

Characteristics of Randomized Clinical Trials of Surgery Plus Postoperative Chemotherapy versus Surgery Alone

Series	Year	CT+S N	S	Chemotherapy Regimen	CT-Associated Mortality CT+S (%)	Median Survival (mo) CT+S	S	Survival Rate (%) 1-yr CT+S vs. S	2-yr	3-yr	4-yr	5-yr	Grade III/IV Toxicity CT+S (%)
Ando et al. (23)	1997	105	100	Cisplatin 70 mg/m² + vindesine 3 mg/m² × (2 cycles)	4 (4)	57	47	90 vs. 90	67 vs. 67	58 vs. 54	58 vs. 48	48 vs. 45	29
Pouliquen et al. (22)	1996	52	68	Cisplatin 100 mg/m² + 5-FU (6–8 cycles)	4 (8)	13	14	83 vs. 70	34 vs. 44	32 vs. 32	18 vs. 20	17 vs. 12	29
Ando et al. (24)	2003	120	122	Cisplatin 80 mg/m² + 5-FU (2 cycles)	NA	Not reached	84	93 vs. 90	75 vs. 75	68 vs. 66	66 vs. 58	52 vs. 61	NA
Total		277	290										

CT, chemotherapy; S, surgery; N, number of patients randomized; 5-FU, 5-fluorouracil; NA, not applicable.

633

Postoperative Chemoradiotherapy

Concurrent chemoradiotherapy has been shown to be superior to radiation therapy alone in patients with localized carcinoma of the esophagus (25–27). In the prospective combined phase 1 and 2 trial conducted by Nishimura et al. (28), the role of concurrent chemoradiation in an adjuvant setting was evaluated. The study enrolled 16 patients with postoperative locoregional recurrence of esophageal cancer, and two patients with incompletely resected esophageal cancer. Patients received two cycles of continuous infusion of 5-FU 250 to 300 mg/m^2 on days 1 to 14, cisplatin 10 mg/m^2 on days 1 to 5 and 8 to 12, and a concurrent radiotherapy dose of 30 Gy in 15 fractions over 3 weeks. Thirteen (72%) patients completed the chemotherapy-radiation therapy (CT-RT) protocol; complete response was observed in 40% (4/10) of patients without prior chemotherapy. The 2-year survival rate was 19%, with a median survival time of 9.5 months. Toxicity in this study was significant, although no treatment-related death was reported.

Postoperative Immunotherapy With Radiotherapy or Chemoradiation

One Japanese trial evaluated protein-bound polysaccharide K (PSK) as an adjunct to postoperative RT or chemoradiation (CRT) in resected esophageal cancer. PSK, obtained from basidiomycetes, is a biological response modifier also known to suppress metastasis and inhibit tumor invasion (29,30). This trial involved 174 patients with squamous cell carcinoma who underwent esophagectomy and then were randomly assigned to four treatment groups. The 3-year survival rates for RT, RT + PSK, CRT, and CRT + PSK were 43.3%, 45.5%, 33.5%, and 44.3%, respectively. There was no significant difference in survival rates when RT and RT + PSK were compared or when CRT and CRT + PSK were compared (30). In the eligible patients, multivariate regression analysis indicated that postoperative therapy with or without PSK was the most significant prognostic factor. Study results also indicate that PSK may have a beneficial effect on esophageal carcinoma when given in combination with CT + RT.

Postoperative Chemotherapy versus Postoperative Radiotherapy

One randomized trial evaluated postoperative chemotherapy versus postoperative radiotherapy following curative esophagectomy (31). Patients received cisplatin and vindesine (n = 126) or radiotherapy at a dose of 50 Gy (n = 127). The median survival was 38 months for both groups. At 3 years, no difference in the survival rate was detected (52% for chemotherapy vs. 51% for radiotherapy at 3 years; log-rank $p = 0.806$). The toxicity was more significant among patients randomized to chemotherapy compared with the RT group. In this trial, the quality of life was not assessed.

Preoperative and Postoperative Chemotherapy and Surgery versus Surgery Alone

Two randomized trials evaluated preoperative and postoperative chemotherapy to surgery alone (32,33). On analysis, neither Roth et al. (32), using a now outdated combination of cisplatin, vindesine, and bleomycin, nor the largest North American trial, reported by Kelsen et al. (33), using cisplatin and 5-FU, detected a statistically significant difference in overall survival. There was no significant difference in the risk of death detected with preoperative and postoperative chemotherapy and surgery compared with surgery alone.

Combined Preoperative and Postoperative Chemotherapy Without Radiation (University of Miami Experience)

At the University of Miami we enrolled 33 patients over a 6-year period in a phase 2 trial to evaluate neoadjuvant and adjuvant combination chemotherapy without RT for stage III, resectable, esophageal adenocarcinoma (34). All patients were staged with computed axial tomography scans and endoscopic ultrasounds prior to enrollment. The CT cycles included cisplatin, taxol, Fluorodeoxyuridine (FUDR), and leucovorin. The chemotherapy was given for 16 weeks prior to surgery, followed by adjuvant chemotherapy for patients whose pathology at the time of surgery demonstrated microscopic disease. Overall toxicities were acceptable and 30 patients demonstrated clinical response, with ten patients showing no gross pathologic disease. The Kaplan-Meier estimates of overall survival at 1, 3, and 5 years were 73% (95% confidence interval [CI]: 58%-88%), 52% (95% CI: 34%-69%), and 29% (95% CI: 13%-45%), respectively. Median survival was 42 months (95% CI: 14-52 months) (Figure 32C.1). Ten patients are alive after a median follow up of 73 months (range, 45 to 89 months). Twenty-nine patients were eligible for adjuvant chemotherapy. Fourteen patients did not receive the therapy; 15 patients received at least one cycle. Comparison of the 29 patients eligible for adjuvant chemotherapy showed a survival benefit when at least one cycle of adjuvant therapy was given ($p = 0.040$). Survival for the 15 patients who received at least one cycle of adjuvant chemotherapy was 54 months as compared with 23 months for those who did not (Figure 32C.2). We found that this regimen of combination chemotherapy for locally advanced esophageal adenocarcinoma was safe and comparable with those regimens that contain radiation. In this cohort, local recurrence was seen in only one patient. To avoid local complications of surgery, omission of radiation may allow for a more aggressive chemotherapy. In addition, we have shown a significant survival benefit in resected patients who have received adjuvant therapy after complete surgical resection. This study needs to be confirmed in a larger phase 2 or in a randomized phase 3 trial.

CONCLUSIONS

The recent interest in developing improvements in diagnosis and treatment of esophageal carcinoma has yet to define the optimal therapy for this difficult disease. Squamous cell carcinoma of the esophagus has historically presented difficulties in management. The recent rise in esophageal adenocarcinomas has further complicated the treatment. As with any other malignancy, the most advantageous treatment of patients with esophageal carcinoma depends on accurate staging. Currently, definitive staging for esophageal cancer takes place after surgery. Many techniques exist for improving diagnostic accuracy before

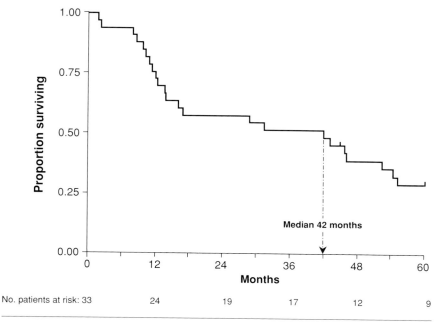

Figure 32C.1 Kaplan-Meier survival curve for 33 patients with stage III, resectable esophageal adenocarcinoma treated with combined preoperative and postoperative chemotherapy without radiation at the University of Miami. (From Ardalan B, Spector SA, Livingstone AS, et al. Neoadjuvant, surgery and adjuvant chemotherapy without radiation for esophageal cancer. *Jpn J Clin Oncol.* 2007;37:590–596, with permission.)

surgery, but a single method has not demonstrated significant advantages over the others. Even when computed tomography, endoscopic ultrasound, and positron emission tomography are used together to evaluate the primary tumor, nodal and distant metastases, the sensitivity, specificity, and accuracy of these methods may vary (35–39). Selecting the best method for tumor staging has proven controversial, as well as choosing the

superior resection technique. Various resection techniques offer advantageous alternatives, but one particular method has not demonstrated superiority in diminishing perioperative risk and improving survival.

Developments in neoadjuvant and adjuvant therapies have also led to mixed conclusions. Single-modality therapies of surgery, chemotherapy, or radiation alone have not verified

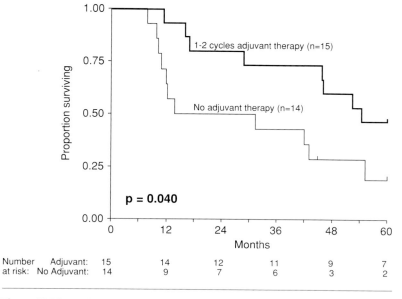

Figure 32C.2 Kaplan-Meier estimates of survival according to whether or not patient received adjuvant chemotherapy for stage III, resectable esophageal adenocarcinoma. (From Ardalan B, Spector SA, Livingstone AS, et al. Neoadjuvant, surgery and adjuvant chemotherapy without radiation for esophageal cancer. *Jpn J Clin Oncol.* 2007;37:590–596, with permission.)

improved survival rates for esophageal carcinoma. Preoperative radiotherapy has not shown overall superiority to surgery alone (40–42), even though one trial has illustrated an improvement in locoregional failure rate in the preoperative radiation group (40). Although some trials have shown improvements for recurrence rates with postoperative radiation, no survival benefit has been confirmed (17–19). Roth et al. (32), Law et al. (43), Kok et al. (44), and Clark (45) have illustrated advantageous median survival rates after preoperative chemotherapy. On the basis of the overall data, preoperative and postoperative chemotherapy studies have not shown conclusive results.

Efforts to combine preoperative chemoradiation and surgery have not illustrated any benefit to surgery alone (46). However, it may improve resectability and locoregional control. This combination has been widely associated with severe toxicity, but improved toxicity profiles have recently been shown with newer agents and advanced radiation planning technique. The only positive study supporting neoadjuvant chemoradiation is the study by Walsh et al. (47), although the poor outcome in the surgical arm received criticism. Current use of camptothecins and taxanes in combination with radiotherapy has shown the potential to improve survival rates.

In early adjuvant trials between 1978 and 1995, most patients were *clinically* staged. Endoscopic ultrasound, or ^{18}F-fluoro-deoxy-D-glucose positron emission tomography, scans were unavailable at that time, thus preventing accurate staging of these patients. Squamous cell carcinoma was the most prevalent histology at that time. Thus, most clinical trials had few patients with a histologic diagnosis of adenocarcinoma. Although patients with adenocarcinoma were included in some trials, they were not separated from those diagnosed with squamous cell carcinoma. Early studies did not consistently find that they responded differently to chemotherapy or radiation. Later in larger European series (with over 1,000 consecutive esophagectomies) investigators described adenocarcinoma as a "favorable" predictor for long-term survival, as compared with squamous histology (48). In addition, the pattern of lymphatic metastases of esophageal adenocarcinoma appears to differ from that of squamous cell esophageal carcinoma.

In face of the dramatic shifting to adenocarcinoma in Western countries, interpretation of the adjuvant therapy trials is very difficult and confusing. Based on these facts, new trials are necessary to reevaluate the role of adjuvant therapy. Currently, the treatment of resectable esophageal cancer differs in the United States and Europe. The United States standard is preoperative, neoadjuvant chemoradiation, whereas the European standard is chemotherapy alone, followed by surgery (48). Addition of radiation therapy in the United States trials has not significantly reduced the rate of local recurrence as compared with the European trials. Moreover, the addition of radiation therapy in the United States trials could significantly hamper the administration of optimal chemotherapy. The radiation therapy has increased the incidence of surgically resected complete pathologic response in the United States trials. It is questionable whether the local tumor response, as the result of radiation therapy, would translate into improved overall survivorship. In the European trial, without the administration of radiation, the result is comparable to the survivorship in the United States trials (49). Therefore, it seems clear that

investigators need to address esophageal carcinoma as a systemic disease. Our European colleagues are planning to add new chemotherapeutic or biologic agents to the original platform of cisplatin and 5-FU. The United States investigators are planning to include new chemotherapeutic and biologic agents in the original platform of chemoradiation with the understanding that radiation therapy should continue to be a major part of therapy.

Although our study is small and nonrandomized, it provokes certain questions (34). Without radiation therapy, only one local recurrence occurred in 33 patients. Based on our findings, we conclude that the safest optimal therapy excludes radiation therapy. Deletion of radiation therapy has allowed us to offer more intensive neoadjuvant therapy to our patients as compared with European investigators who used more modest chemotherapy regimens. Another point of deviation between our study and that of the European investigators is the use of adjuvant therapy. It is very interesting and intriguing that in our study, those patients who received adjuvant chemotherapy overall experienced a superior survival (34). We consider this an important point, which we hope European investigators will use to conduct larger and statistically powered studies.

Interest in adjuvant trails for adenocarcinoma of the esophagus is ongoing. Currently, there are several trials evaluating the role of adjuvant therapy. One trial is a phase 3 study of adjuvant chemoradiation after resection in patients with gastric or gastroesophageal carcinomas (National Cancer Institute protocol ID NCT00052910). The second is a phase 2 nonrandomized trial of sunitinib (Sutent), a new oral multikinase inhibitor, following chemotherapy, radiation, and surgery (National Cancer Institute protocol ID NCT00400114). The details of these trials are available at the Web site of the National Cancer Institute (50). The Japanese Cooperative Oncology Group is currently performing a randomized trial comparing preoperative chemotherapy with postoperative chemotherapy.

The overall management of esophageal carcinoma has become quite complex. Interpretation of the randomized trials is difficult because of the heterogeneous treatments—surgical technique, chemotherapy, and radiation dosages. The poor prognosis of esophageal carcinoma demands attention to new chemotherapeutic and biologic agents, radiation schedules, and surgical techniques. Toward this end, positive steps forward are studies that demonstrate a moderate success in detecting molecular markers that may predict treatment response. (nitrotyrosine, *PTEN* tumor suppressor gene, *p53*, thymidine phosphorylase, and thymidylate synthase) (51–55). Although this will impact the treatment regimen in the future, progress in the management of esophageal carcinoma will remain slow and incremental. All clinicians are encouraged to enter patients in clinical trials to improve the therapy of esophageal cancer.

REFERENCES

1. Cooper JS, Guo MD, Herskovic A, et al. Chemoradiotherapy of locally advanced esophageal cancer: long-term follow-up of a prospective randomized trial (RTOG 85-01). Radiation Therapy Oncology Group. *JAMA.* 1999;281:1623–1627.
2. Izbicki JR, Hosch SB, Pichlmeier U, et al. Prognostic value of immunohistochemically identifiable tumor cells in lymph nodes of

patients with completely resected esophageal cancer. *N Engl J Med.* 1997;337:1188–1194.

3. Matsumoto M, Natsugoe S, Nakashima S, et al. Clinical significance of lymph node micrometastasis of p_{N0} esophageal squamous cell carcinoma. *Cancer Lett.* 2000;153:189–197.

4. Bonavina L, Ferrero S, Midolo V, et al. Lymph node micrometastases in patients with adenocarcinoma of the esophagogastric junction. *J Gastrointest Surg.* 1999;3:468–476.

5. Nakamura T, Ide H, Eguchi R, et al. Clinical implications of lymph node micrometastasis in patients with histologically node-negative (p_{N0}) esophageal carcinoma. *J Surg Oncol.* 2002;79:224–229.

6. Komukai S, Nishimaki T, Watanabe H, et al. Significance of immunohistochemically demonstrated micrometastases to lymph nodes in esophageal cancer with histologically negative nodes. *Surgery.* 2000;127:40–46.

7. Vazquez-Sequeiros E, Wang L, Burgart L, et al. Occult lymph node metastases as a predictor of tumor relapse in patients with node-negative esophageal carcinoma. *Gastroenterology.* 2002;122:1815–1821.

8. Kijima F, Natsugoe S, Takao S, et al. Detection and clinical significance of lymph node micrometastasis determined by reverse transcription-polymerase chain reaction in patients with esophageal carcinoma. *Oncology.* 2000;58:38–44.

9. Godfrey TE, Raja S, Finkelstein SD, et al. Prognostic value of quantitative reverse transcription-polymerase chain reaction in lymph node-negative esophageal cancer patients. *Clin Cancer Res.* 2001;7:4041–4048.

10. Kassis ES, Nguyen N, Shriver SP, et al. Detection of occult lymph node metastases in esophageal cancer by minimally invasive staging combined with molecular diagnostic techniques. *JSLS.* 1998;2:331–336.

11. Luketich JD, Kassis ES, Shriver SP, et al. Detection of micrometastases in histologically negative lymph nodes in esophageal cancer. *Ann Thorac Surg.* 1998;66:1715–1718.

12. O'sullivan GC, Sheehan D, Clarke A, et al. Micrometastases in esophagogastric cancer: high detection rate in resected rib segments. *Gastroenterology.* 1999;116:543–548.

13. Noguchi T, Shibata T, Fumoto S, et al. Detection of disseminated cancer cells in rib marrow of patients with esophageal cancer. *Oncol Rep.* 2003;10:623–627.

14. NIH consensus conference. Adjuvant therapy for patients with colon and rectal cancer. *JAMA.* 1990;264:1444–1450.

15. Gill S, Loprinzi CL, Sargent DJ, et al. Pooled analysis of fluorouracil-based adjuvant therapy for stage II and III colon cancer: who benefits and by how much? *J Clin Oncol.* 2004;22:1797–1806.

16. Douillard J, Rosell R, Delena M, et al. ANITA: phase III adjuvant vinorelbine and cisplatin versus observation in completely resected (stage I-III) non-small cell lung cancer patients: final results after 70-month median follow-up. *J Clin Oncol.* 2005;23(Suppl 16S):624s.

17. Fok M, Sham JS, Choy D, et al. Postoperative radiotherapy for carcinoma of the esophagus: a prospective, randomized controlled study. *Surgery.* 1993;113:138–147.

18. P. Teniere J-M, Fingerhut HA, Fagniez PL. Postoperative radiation therapy does not increase survival after curative resection for squamous cell carcinoma of the middle and lower esophagus as shown by a multicenter controlled trial *Surg Gynecol Obstet.* 1991;173:123–130.

19. Zieren HU, Müller JM, Jacobi CA, et al. Adjuvant postoperative radiation therapy after curative resection of squamous cell carcinoma of the thoracic esophagus: a prospective randomized study *World J Surg.* 1995;19:444–449.

20. Xiao ZF, Yang ZY, Liang J, et al. Value of radiotherapy after radical surgery for esophageal carcinoma: a report of 495 patients. *Ann Thorac Surg.* 2003;75:331–336.

21. Kasai M, Mori S, Watanabe T. Follow-up results after resection of thoracic esophageal carcinoma. *World J Surg.* 1978;2:543–551.

22. Pouliquen X, Levard H, Hay JM, et al. 5-Fluorouracil and cisplatin therapy after palliative surgical resection of squamous cell carcinoma of the esophagus. A multicenter randomized trial. French Associations for Surgical Research. *Ann Surg.* 1996;223:127–133.

23. Ando N, Iizuka T, Kakegawa T, et al. A randomized trial of surgery with and without chemotherapy for localized squamous carcinoma of the thoracic esophagus: the Japan Clinical Oncology Group Study. *J Thorac Cardiovasc Surg.* 1997;114:205–209.

24. Ando N, Iizuka T, Ide H, et al. A randomized trial of surgery alone vs surgery plus postoperative chemotherapy with cisplatin and 5-fluorouracil for localized squamous carcinoma of the thoracic esophagus: The Japan Clinical Oncology Group Study (JCOG 9204). *J Clin Oncol.* 2003;21:4592–4596.

25. Herskovic A, Martz K, Al-Sarraf M, et al. Combined chemotherapy and radiotherapy compared with radiotherapy alone in patients with cancer of the esophagus. *N Engl J Med.* 1992;326:1593–1598.

26. Al-Sarraf M, Martz K, Herskovic A, et al. Progress report of combined chemoradiotherapy versus radiotherapy alone in patients with esophageal cancer: an Intergroup study. *J Clin Oncol.* 1997;15:277–284.

27. Smith TJ, Ryan LM, Douglass HO Jr, et al. Combined chemoradiotherapy vs. radiotherapy alone for early stage squamous cell carcinoma of the esophagus: a study of the Eastern Cooperative Oncology Group. *Int J Radiat Oncol Biol Phys.* 1998;42:269–276.

28. Nishimura Y, Koike R, Nakamatsu K, et al. Concurrent chemoradiotherapy with protracted infusion of 5-FU and cisplatin for postoperative recurrent or residual esophageal cancer. *Jpn J Clin Oncol.* 2003;33:341–345.

29. Kobayashi et al., PSK as a chemopreventive agent. *Cancer Epidemiol Biomarkers Prev.* 1993;2:271–276.

30. Ogoshi K, Satou H, Isono K, et al. Immunotherapy for esophageal cancer. A randomized trial in combination with radiotherapy and radiochemotherapy. Cooperative Study Group for Esophageal Cancer in Japan. *Am J Clin Oncol.* 1995;18:216–222.

31. Iizuka T, for the Japanese Esophageal Oncology Group. A comparison of chemotherapy and radiotherapy as adjuvant treatment to surgery for esophageal carcinoma. Japanese Esophageal Oncology Group. *Chest.* 1993;104:203–207.

32. Roth JA, Pass HI, Flanagan MM, et al. Randomized clinical trial of preoperative and postoperative adjuvant chemotherapy with cisplatin, vindesine, and bleomycin for carcinoma of the esophagus. *J Thorac Cardiovasc Surg.* 1988;96:242–248.

33. Kelsen DP, Ginsberg R, Pajak TF, et al. Chemotherapy followed by surgery compared with surgery alone for localized esophageal cancer. *N Engl J Med.* 1998;339:1979–1984.

34. Ardalan B, Spector SA, Livingstone AS, et al. Neoadjuvant, surgery and adjuvant chemotherapy without radiation for esophageal cancer. *Jpn J Clin Oncol.* 2007;37:590–596.

35. Kobori O, Kirihara Y, Kosaka N, et al. Positron emission tomography of esophageal carcinoma using (11)C-choline and (18)F-fluorodeoxyglucose: a novel method of preoperative lymph node staging. *Cancer.* 1999;86:1638–1648.

36. Buenaventura P, Luketich JD. Surgical staging of esophageal cancer. *Chest Surg Clin North Am.* 2000;10:487–497.

37. Block MI, Patterson GA, Sundaresan RS, et al. Improvement in staging of esophageal cancer with the addition of positron emission tomography. *Ann Thorac Surg.* 1997;64:770–776.

38. Rice TW. Clinical staging of esophageal carcinoma: CT, EUS, and PET. *Chest Surg Clin North Am.* 2000;10:471–485.

39. Kim K, Park SJ, Kim BT, et al. Evaluation of lymph node metastases in squamous cell carcinoma of the esophagus with positron emission tomography. *Ann Thorac Surg.* 2001; 71:290–294.

40. Gignoux M, Roussel A, Paillot B, et al. The value of preoperative radiotherapy in esophageal cancer: results of the study of the EORTC. *World J Surg.* 1987;110:426–432.

41. Launois B, Delarue D, Campion JP, et al. Preoperative radiotherapy for carcinoma of the esophagus. *Surg Gynecol Obstet.* 1981;153:690–692.

42. Arnott SJ, Duncan W, Kerr GR, et al. Low dose preoperative radiotherapy for carcinoma of the oesophagus: results of a randomized clinical trial. *Radiother Oncol.* 1992;24:108–113.

43. Law S, Fok M, Chow S, et al. Preoperative chemotherapy versus surgical therapy alone for squamous cell carcinoma of the esophagus: a prospective randomized trial. *J Thorac Cardiovasc Surg.* 1997;114:210–217.

44. Kok TC, van Lanscho J, Siersema PD, et al. Neoadjuvant chemotherapy in operable esophageal squamous cell cancer: final report of a phase III multicenter randomized controlled trial. *Proc Am Soc Clin Oncol.* 1997;16:277 (Abstract).

45. Clark, P. Surgical resection with or without preoperative chemotherapy in oesophageal cancer: an updated analysis of a randomized controlled trial conducted by UK medical research Council Upper Alimentary Tract Cancer Group. *Proc Am Soc Clin Oncol.* 2001;20:126(Abstract).

46. Urba SG, Orringer MB, Turrisi A, et al. Randomized trial of preoperative chemoradiation versus surgery alone in patients with locoregional esophageal carcinoma. *J Clin Oncol.* 2001;19:305–313.

47. Walsh TN, Noonan N, Hollywood D, et al. A comparison of multimodal therapy and surgery for esophageal adenocarcinoma. *N Engl J Med.* 1996;335:462–467.

48. Schneider BJ, Urba SG. Preoperative chemoradiation for the treatment of locoregional esophageal cancer: the standard of care? *Semin Radiat Oncol.* 2007;17:45–52.

49. Ross P, Nicolson M, Cunningham D, et al. Prospective randomized trial comparing mitomycin, cisplatin, and protracted venous-infusion fluorouracil (PVI 5-FU) with epirubicin, cisplatin, and PVI 5-FU in advanced esophagogastric cancer. *J Clin Oncol.* 2002;20:1996–2004.

50. National Cancer Institute. http://clinicaltrials.gov. Accessed June 16, 2009.

51. Siewert J, Stein H, Feith M, et al. Histologic tumor type is an independent prognostic parameter in esophageal cancer: lessons from over 1000 consecutive resections at a single center in the western world. *Ann Surg.* 2001;234:360–369.

52. Tachibana M, Shibakita M, Ohno S, et al. Expression and prognostic significance of PTEN product protein in patients with esophageal squamous cell carcinoma. *Cancer.* 2002;94:1955–1960.

53. Shimada H, Takeda A, Shiratori T, et al. Prognostic significance of serum thymidine phosphorylase concentration in esophageal squamous cell carcinoma. *Cancer.* 2002;94:1947–1954.

54. Kato H, Miyazaki T, Yoshikawa M, et al. Expression of nitrotyrosine is associated with angiogenesis in esophageal squamous cell carcinoma. *Anticancer Res.* 2001;21:3323–3329.

55. Aloia TA, Harpole DH Jr, Reed CE, et al. Tumor marker expression is predictive of survival in patients with esophageal cancer. *Ann Thorac Surg.* 2001;72:859–866.

33

Cancer of the Stomach: Surgical Management

Bruce E. Stabile and Brian R. Smith

Worldwide, gastric cancer is second only to carcinoma of the lung as the leading cause of death from malignancy (1). The great majority of cancers arising in the stomach are adenocarcinomas, with lymphomas and malignant gastrointestinal stromal tumors and carcinoids together constituting <10% of the total. Although these much less common tumors are often amenable to successful management by operative resection or other means, the adenocarcinomas are particularly aggressive and surgeons remain frustrated by their inability to reliably cure them after more than 125 years of trying. This long experience has made it clear that simple removal of the adenocarcinoma-bearing stomach is inadequate therapy for the majority of patients and that a better understanding of the pathogenesis and progression of the malignant process is sorely needed.

The role of radical gastrectomy combined with an aggressive regional lymphadenectomy for adenocarcinoma remains controversial despite several randomized clinical trials that have largely failed to support its validity. Adjuvant therapies of various types and combinations have also historically been ineffective in prolonging life or improving its quality. Nonetheless, outcome data are emerging that might be cause for reassessment of the roles of both aggressive surgery and adjuvant therapy in selected patient groups. There are, in fact, reasons for optimism about a disease that historically has elicited only nihilism from physicians in Westernized countries. Most importantly, new insights into the etiology of gastric adenocarcinoma hold promise for opportunities to actually prevent this widespread and highly lethal tumor. Specifically, the consensus within the scientific community that the bacterium *Helicobacter pylori* plays a central role in most human gastric oncogenesis presents possibilities for both infection prevention and eradication that might be expected to effectively abort the development of the majority of gastric cancers (2,3).

GASTRIC ADENOCARCINOMA

Because of its continued high prevalence in densely populated underdeveloped countries, adenocarcinoma of the stomach persists as the number two cause of cancer mortality globally, with approximately 650,000 deaths per year (1). Westernized countries that have attained high overall standards of living tend to have relatively lower mortality rates. In the United States, gastric adenocarcinoma is only the 13th most common cause of cancer deaths, with only about 12,000 per year (4). The annual death rate in the United States is a mere 5 per 100,000 compared to 90 per 100,000 in Japan (5). This low figure does not represent a low-case mortality rate but rather a low disease prevalence.

The recorded incidence of gastric cancer has been falling in the United States for over 70 years, most likely due in large part to a decrease in the incidence of *H. pylori* infection (6). Improvements in public sanitation, personal hygiene, and general living conditions over the past century have been responsible for reductions in infection rates, particularly among children (7,8). Notably, however, the beginning of the decline of gastric cancer in the United States antedated the introduction of antibiotics by a number of years. More recently, the immigration of large numbers of Hispanic, Middle Eastern, and Pacific Rim peoples appears to be responsible for a leveling-off of the decline in some regions of the country (9).

Regardless of geographic locale or frequency of disease, the risk for development of gastric adenocarcinoma increases with age and the disease afflicts men nearly twice as often as women (Figure 33.1) (5). There are also significant ethnic predilections, and both African American men and women have almost double the incidence of their white American counterparts. Despite the observed overall decline in distal (noncardia) gastric cancer in most Westernized countries, a paradoxic sharp rise in proximal (cardia) cancers has recently been noted (4). In fact, recent United States data indicate that adenocarcinoma of the gastric cardia is rising at a faster rate than any other cancer except for the closely related adenocarcinoma of the distal esophagus (10).

HISTOLOGIC CLASSIFICATION

The now widely accepted classification system first described by Laurén (11) has greatly simplified the histologic evaluation of gastric adenocarcinoma and has provided a sound basis for understanding its development. The more common intestinal type cancers are typically located distally in the stomach, are well differentiated, and form glandular structures reminiscent of colonic carcinoma. The cells are polarized, mucus-containing, cohesive, and are found in a histologic setting of chronic atrophic gastritis with associated intestinal metaplasia and dysplasia (12). Intestinal type of tumors are most frequently located in antral mucosa and tend to be localized rather than extensively infiltrating. The less common diffuse type of cancers are poorly differentiated and tend to spread widely through the submucosa in the form of linitis plastica. The tumors usually arise in a field of chronic gastritis but without accompanying atrophy or metaplasia. They often afflict younger patients, may be familial, and are more frequently found in the proximal stomach. The cells are highly pleomorphic, poorly cohesive, and do not form glandular structures. They frequently assume a signet ring configuration and are postulated to arise de novo from stem cells located in the

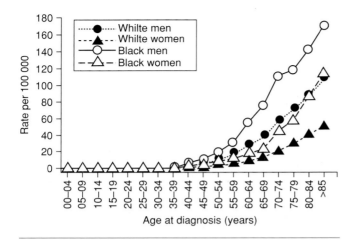

Figure 33.1 United States incidence rates for gastric cancer by age and ethnicity. (From Hohenberger P, Gretschel S. Gastric cancer. *Lancet*. 2003;362:305–312, with permission.)

proliferative zone at the neck regions of gastric glands (13). Diffuse-type tumor histology implies a more aggressive malignant behavior and a worse prognosis. Tumors with mixed glandular and diffuse histologic features are not uncommon and expression of the intestinal phenotype may be a time-dependent event (14).

ETIOLOGY

Both genetic and environmental factors interact in complex ways to culminate in gastric carcinogenesis (Table 33.1). Although much data in both areas are available, the integration of etiologic information remains minimal at this time. The diffuse type of gastric cancer may be the more genetically determined type based on its similar incidence in men and women, its greater frequency in younger patients, and its association with blood group A (15). There is also familial clustering that confers a two- to three-fold increased risk among first-degree relatives. Gastric cancer is known to have a high incidence in inherited syndromes such as familial adenomatous polyposis, Gardner syndrome, hereditary nonpolyposis colon cancer, and Peutz-Jeghers syndrome. At least two molecular phenotypes are associated with distinct genomic destabilization pathways (16). One manifests high-level microsatellite instability and the other manifests chromosomal and intrachromosomal instability. High-level microsatellite instability has been found in 17% to 59% of gastric cancers in Western populations. Such tumors harbor mutations in the coding and noncoding regions of a variety of cancer-related genes. Interestingly, the presence of *H. pylori*-induced chronic gastritis adjacent to gastric cancer is positively correlated with microsatellite instability-phenotypic tumors.

Polymorphisms at the interleukin-1β and N-acetyl cystine 1 genes have been demonstrated to be consistently associated with gastric cancer (16). The interleukin-1β polymorphism has also been noted to be involved with the hypochlorhydria associated with *H. pylori* infection (17). Such host genetic factors thus appear to be linked significantly to the development of gastric cancer in infected individuals. Polymorphisms of numerous

Table 33.1

Genetic and Environmental Factors Associated with Gastric Adenocarcinoma

Genetic	Environmental
Familial tumor syndromes	*Helicobacter pylori* infection
Familial adenomatous	Tobacco smoking
polyposis	Vitamin C deficiency
Gardner syndrome	Low dietary fruits/vegetables
Hereditary nonpolyposis	High dietary
colon cancer	Salt
Peutz-Jeghers syndrome	Fat
Blood group A	Nitrates
Genetic abnormalities	Polycyclic hydrocarbons
Interleukin-1β	
N-acetyl cystine 1	
Adenomatous polyposis	
coli	
E-cadherin	
β-catenin	
Cyclin E	
TGF-βIIR	
p53	
BAX	
K-ras	
bcl-2	
c-met	

TGF, transforming growth factor.

proinflammatory cytokine gene clusters, including several additional interleukins and tumor necrosis factor, appear to confer a twofold or greater increase in the risk of noncardia gastric cancer. Mutations of the *p53* gene, loss of heterozygosity, and abnormal protein expression are all well described in gastric cancer, with the majority of tumors containing one or more mutations and loss of heterozygosity (18). The mechanism of *p53* tumor suppressor dysfunction and telomerase reactivation appears to lead to gastric cancer in conjunction with an *H. pylori*-induced decrease in apoptosis combined with enhanced cellular proliferation (19). The *p53* mutation and its associated gastric metaplasia and dysplasia may derive from significantly increased mucosal free radical levels that accompany *H. pylori* infection (20).

The diffuse type of gastric cancer represents only 5% to 10% of all cases and may depend on an autosomal dominant, incomplete penetrance pattern of inheritance (21). Germ line mutations of the gene that encodes the epithelial cell adhesion molecule E-cadherin have been identified in a number of families with high prevalences of gastric cancer. These instances may represent the small minority of cases that develop exclusive of *H. pylori* infection or other known external factors. Histologic examination of prophylactic gastrectomy specimens from such family members reveal minute intramucosal foci of diffuse-type adenocarcinoma in the complete absence of any epithelial inflammation or metaplasia.

Environmental exposures of various types appear to be dominant in the development of the intestinal type of gastric cancer. This is evidenced by demographic clustering, the dramatic

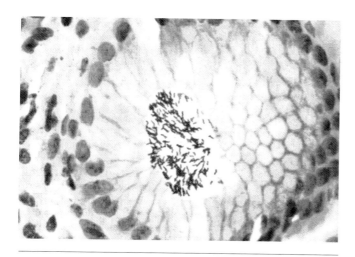

Figure 33.2 Photomicrograph of antral biopsy (×1000) prepared with Genta stain and showing a gastric pit filled with *Helicobacter pylori*. (From Genta RM, Graham DY. *Helicobacter pylori* in a gastric pit. *N Engl J Med.* 1996;335:250, with permission.)

decline in the incidence of the disease in developed countries, and its association with low socioeconomic status, diet, tobacco smoking, and, most importantly, *H. pylori* infection (22). Although a myriad of environmental factors are known to impact the development of gastric cancer, over the past 2 decades it has become evident that *H. pylori* infection is the single most important external determinant of the disease (Figure 33.2). The prevalence of infection is highest in areas of the world where gastric cancer is particularly common. Best estimates suggest that infection plays an important causative role in substantially greater than half of all gastric adenocarcinomas (23). In a recent

prospective study of 1,526 Japanese persons followed for a mean of nearly 8 years, all of the 36 (2.9%) newly diagnosed gastric cancers occurred in infected individuals and none developed in uninfected individuals (Figure 33.3) (24). This longitudinal study dramatically supports an association between *H. pylori* infection and the development of gastric cancer, and reinforces the findings of an earlier meta-analysis that demonstrated an odds ratio of 2.3 in favor of an association between *H. pylori* infection and gastric cancer (25).

The growing consensus that *H. pylori* plays a highly important etiologic role in gastric carcinogenesis has been fortified by a better understanding of serum antibody assays and mucosal biopsies in the diagnosis of the infection. Earlier studies attempting to associate *H. pylori* infection and gastric cancer were flawed by false-negative antibody and biopsy results (5,24). This was due to a lack of understanding of the phenomenon of spontaneous resolution of infection that occurs with the development of severe mucosal atrophy that renders the local environment unsuitable to the organism (26). The infection therefore resolves by the time the cancer is diagnosed but only after having set in motion an irreversible sequence of events that inevitably culminates in cancer development. The point in the pathologic sequence from *H. pylori*-induced gastritis to carcinoma at which inevitability occurs remains unknown, but recent evidence suggests that eradication of the infection must be effected early in the progression if cancer is to be prevented. A randomized clinical trial of *H. pylori* eradication demonstrated a 37% relative decrease in cancer incidence after a mean of 7.5 years of follow-up among patients treated for infection compared with those given placebo (2). Although the difference was not significant, a subgroup analysis of those infected patients without precancerous lesions of the gastric mucosa at study entry did demonstrate a significant reduction among treated patients (Figure 33.4). In fact, no patient in the eradication group developed cancer,

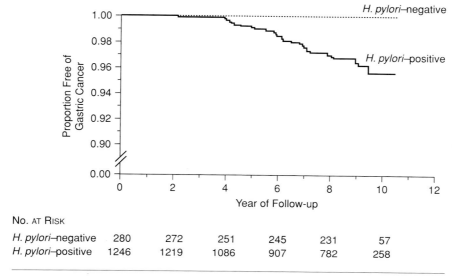

No. AT RISK						
H. pylori–negative	280	272	251	245	231	57
H. pylori–positive	1246	1219	1086	907	782	258

Figure 33.3 Proportions of *Helicobacter pylori*-positive and *H. pylori*-negative patients who remained free of gastric cancer over time. Uninfected individuals were significantly unaffected compared with infected individuals. (From Uemura N, Okamoto S, Yamamoto S, et al. *Helicobacter pylori* infection and the development of gastric cancer. *N Engl J Med.* 2001;345:784–789, with permission.)

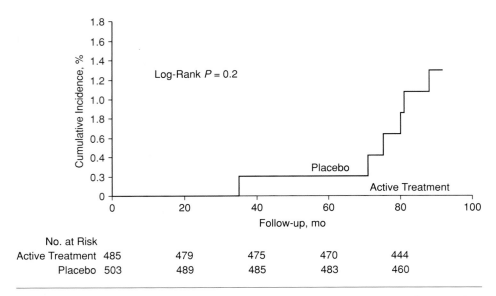

Figure 33.4 Cumulative incidence of gastric adenocarcinoma among patients infected with *Helicobacter pylori* but without precancerous mucosal changes on initial biopsy and who had been randomized to antibiotic treatment of the infection or to placebo. During an 8-year follow-up, no actively treated patients developed gastric cancer. (From Wong BC-Y, Lam SK, Wong WM, et al. *Helicobacter pylori* eradication to prevent gastric cancer in a high-risk region of China: a randomized controlled trial. *JAMA.* 2004;291:187–194.)

strongly supporting the hypothesis that *H. pylori* infection is the dominant cause of gastric adenocarcinoma (2).

A large amount of epidemiologic evidence indicates that the acquisition of *H. pylori* infection is greatest in early childhood, particularly before the age of 5 years (27). Transmission is believed to be oral-oral or fecal-oral and most commonly between siblings or parent and child. Host susceptibility is an additional important factor for infection, with highest concordance between monozygotic twins. It appears that both genetically determined susceptibility to *H. pylori* infection and gastric cancer plus actual infection in early life are important risk factors for the prolonged process of gastric carcinogenesis.

Although more than half of the world's population is infected with *H. pylori,* only about half of infected individuals progress to any degree along the preneoplastic histologic sequence toward gastric cancer and <2% develop overt malignancy (12). In addition to host genetic susceptibility factors, the pathogenicity of the particular infecting *H. pylori* strain is also a critically important determinant of cancer development. The most important identified virulence factor that can be produced by the bacterium is derived from a gene known as cytotoxin-associated gene A (*cagA*) (28). The gene product, the CagA protein, is injected by the bacterium into gastric epithelial cells by an associated gene-encoded type IV secretion system that involves a molecular "syringe" mechanism (29). Inside the host cell, the CagA protein causes tyrosine phosphorylation and subsequent dephosphorylation of cellular proteins, inductions of interleukins, expression of several proto-oncogenes, and a growth factor-like effect that promotes cellular proliferation (23). CagA-positive *H. pylori* infection is associated with a more intense gastritis than CagA-negative infection and it appears that this more severe inflammation increases the risk of gastric cancer

over the long term (30). A number of studies have indicated that CagA seropositivity substantially raises the odds ratio for cancer compared with CagA seronegative but *H. pylori* seropositive subjects (31,32). Furthermore, the CagA protein found in East Asian *H. pylori* strains exhibits a greater binding affinity for host cell tyrosine phosphatase compared to that found in Western CagA-positive strains, suggesting a mechanism for the observed greater virulence of East Asian strains (33).

The other much investigated *H. pylori* virulence factor is the protein produced by the vacuolating-associated cytotoxin A (*vacA*) gene (34). This is a bacterial exotoxin that induces endosomal vacuolization of epithelial cells (35). VacA is known to be synergistic with CagA and several other gene products in causing intestinal metaplasia of gastric mucosal cells. In sum, these virulence factors confer on *H. pylori* a substantial capacity for not only promoting enduring infection and chronic pangastritis but also a progressive destruction of the gastric mucosa that leads to atrophy, metaplasia, dysplasia, and ultimately, adenocarcinoma (Figure 33.5). The apparent glaring exception to this sequencing is adenocarcinoma of the gastric cardia, for which *H. pylori* has consistently been found not to be a risk factor (15,25,36).

As early as 1994 the weight of epidemiologic evidence supported a causal relationship between *H. pylori* infection and gastric adenocarcinoma, resulting in the categorization of the bacterium as a type I carcinogen by both the International Agency for Research on Cancer and the World Health Organization (23). A 2001 analysis of 12 case-control studies conducted by the Helicobacter and Cancer Collaborative Group reviewed 1,228 noncardia gastric cancer patients and reverified the association between *H. pylori* infection and gastric cancer (Figure 33.6) (37).

Over the past decade, there has been demonstration in a number of animal models of the carcinogenic role of *H. pylori* in

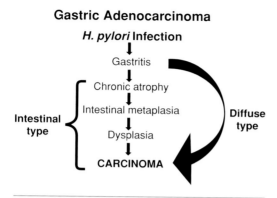

Gastric Adenocarcinoma

Figure 33.5 The progression from gastritis to carcinoma as a consequence of *Helicobacter pylori* infection. Development of intestinal-type carcinoma typically includes all stages of the sequence from chronic atrophic gastritis through carcinoma, and the diffuse type may arise from gastritis in the absence of any intermediate stage.

the development of severe gastritis, intestinal metaplasia, dysplasia, and adenocarcinoma. Gastric inoculation of the bacterium into Mongolian gerbils resulted in the development of intestinal-type adenocarcinoma in 37% of experimental animals but none of the control animals at 62 weeks (38). Even more universal development of gastric carcinoma in response to *H. pylori* in-

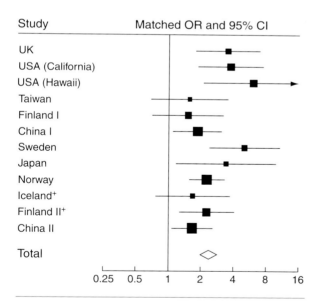

Figure 33.6 Matched odds ratios (OR) and 95% confidence intervals (CI) for the association between *Helicobacter pylori* infection and gastric carcinoma. Square size is proportional to study size from among 12 studies. +, unpublished data, per the original citation. (From the Helicobacter and Cancer Collaborative Group. Gastric cancer and *Helicobacter pylori*: a combined analysis of 12 case control studies nested within prospective cohorts. *Gut.* 2001;49:347–353, with permission.)

fection has been demonstrated in a transgenic hypergastrinemic mouse model, although only in male animals (39,40). Thus, the totality of evidence that *H. pylori* causes gastric adenocarcinoma is overwhelmingly strong (22). The relationship holds true for both intestinal and diffuse histologic types and for all gastric locations with the exception of the gastric cardia.

A number of noninfectious cofactors important to the pathogenesis of gastric adenocarcinoma have been known for a long time. Important among these are exposure of the gastric mucosa to high levels of nitrates, alcohol, and a variety of organic toxins associated with tobacco smoking (1,32). Cigarette smoking, in particular, has been found to have synergistic promotion of gastric intestinal metaplasia in conjunction with *H. pylori* infection (41). The mechanism appears to be through augmented duodenogastric reflux with increased pH and bile acid concentrations in the stomach.

The association between gastric cancer and the lack of intake of fresh vegetables and fruits appears to be related to vitamin C deficiency, a condition known to be exacerbated by *H. pylori* infection and its reduction of luminal secretion and systemic bioavailability of the vitamin (42). Although the decline in gastric cancer in industrialized countries may be attributed to a falling prevalence of *H. pylori* infection, it may also be attributed to the availability of fresh produce through modern refrigeration (1). Safe and reliable food preservation has been accompanied by a decreased requirement for salting, pickling, spicing, and smoking, all of which have been implicated in gastric carcinogenesis (5,18,32). However, there exists no prospective proof of the relationship between diet and gastric cancer.

DIAGNOSIS

Because of its aggressive biologic nature, cure of gastric adenocarcinoma is possible only if the disease is discovered at an early stage. The incidence of the disease is low in the United States and most Westernized countries, so aggressive screening is not cost-effective and generally not practiced. The key to early diagnosis is recognition of the alarm symptoms and signs that suggest gastric cancer rather than benign dyspeptic conditions. These alarm symptoms and signs include anorexia, early satiety, weight loss, fatigue, emesis or hematemesis, melena, anemia, and a palpable abdominal mass. Dyspeptic pain unresponsive to standard antisecretory therapy also suggests the possibility of cancer and should prompt early esophagogastroduodenoscopy. Failure to endoscopically examine the patient with atypical pain or some alarm symptom or sign is the single most correctable cause of delayed diagnosis of gastric cancer.

Whenever gastric cancer is suspected, the diagnostic procedure of choice is flexible fiberoptic esophagogastroduodenoscopy. Multiple biopsies of any gastric mucosal abnormality, ulceration, or mass lesion are always indicated and have a diagnostic accuracy of >95% for malignancy (1,43). Barium upper gastrointestinal radiographic studies are no longer routinely performed for diagnosis. Early gastric cancer and sessile nonbulky tumors are easily missed and radiographic discrimination between benign and malignant gastric ulcers is relatively poor. Because any mucosal abnormality identified on upper gastrointestinal series requires endoscopic biopsy for definitive diagnosis, the radiographic study is inherently redundant and not cost-effective.

STAGING

Accurate preoperative and intraoperative disease staging are essential to the successful surgical management of gastric cancer. The TNM staging system is outlined in Table 33.2. Technologic advances in tumor imaging have allowed refinement of treatment algorithms designed to improve cure rates and minimize unnecessary interventions. Computed tomography (CT), and to a lesser extent, magnetic resonance (MR) scans, have been the mainstays for detection of distant metastases (M staging) involving the liver, lungs, and ovaries. CT and MR have not been particularly useful in defining nonbulky peritoneal or omental (also M staging) and lymph nodal metastases (N staging). An even greater deficiency of both CT and MR has been assessment of the depth of gastric wall penetration by the primary tumor

(T staging). These problems have been addressed to a substantial degree by the application of endoscopic ultrasonography (EUS) and laparoscopy to the staging process. With regard to T staging, the accuracy of EUS has been in the range of 80% to 90%, compared with only 20% to 30% for CT scanning (44). Similarly, for N staging, the figures have been 70% to 80% compared with 30% to 40% for EUS and CT, respectively (45). Lymph nodes as small as 4 mm have been imaged by EUS (46). Small-volume malignant ascites and occult left lobe liver metastases not appreciated by CT or MR have also been detected by EUS. Furthermore, EUS-guided fine-needle aspiration (FNA) has been successfully employed to obtain cytologic confirmation of malignant cells in lymph nodes, liver, and ascitic fluid, thereby avoiding nontherapeutic laparotomy in selected patients with incurable disease (47). The high degree of concordance between

---

Table 33.2

TNM Staging System for Stomach Cancer

DEFINITIONS

Primary Tumor (T)

TX	Primary tumor cannot be assessed
T0	No evidence of primary tumor
Tis	Carcinoma *in situ*: intraepithelial tumor without invasion of the lamina propria
T1	Tumor invades lamina propria or submucosa
T2	Tumor invades muscularis propria or subserosa
T2a	Tumor invades muscularis propria
T2b	Tumor invades subserosa
T3	Tumor penetrates serosa (visceral peritoneum) without invasion of adjacent structures
T4	Tumor invades adjacent structures

Regional Lymph Nodes (N)

NX	Regional lymph nodes(s) cannot be assessed
N0	No regional lymph node metastasis
N1	Metastasis in 1 to 6 regional lymph nodes
N2	Metastasis in 7 to 15 regional lymph nodes
N3	Metastasis in more than 15 regional lymph nodes

Distant Metastasis (M)

MX	Distant metastasis cannot be assessed
M0	No distant metastasis
M1	Distant metastasis

Histologic Grade (G)

GX	Grade cannot be assessed
G1	Well differentiated
G2	Moderately differentiated
G3	Poorly differentiated
G4	Undifferentiated

Residual Tumor (R)

RX	Presence of residual tumor cannot be assessed
R0	No residual tumor
R1	Microscopic residual tumor
R2	Macroscopic residual tumor

Stage Grouping

0	Tis	N0	M0
IA	T1	N0	M0
IB	T1	N1	M0
	T2a/b	N0	M0
II	T1	N2	M0
	T2a/b	N1	M0
	T3	N0	M0
IIIA	T2a/b	N2	M0
	T3	N1	M0
	T4	N0	M0
IIIB	T3	N2	M0
IV	T4	N1-3	M0
	T1-3	N3	M0
	Any T	Any N	M1

Adapted from *AJCC Cancer Staging Manual*, 6th ed. New York: Springer-Verlag; 2002:105–106.

preoperative EUS staging and the pathologic staging of gastric cancer has also allowed accurate prediction of postoperative recurrence risk (48).

There currently exists no indirect imaging modality capable of detecting occult metastatic peritoneal tumor metastases. As a result, their discovery has typically been made only at the time of exploratory laparotomy undertaken for planned curative gastric resection. Laparoscopy prior to laparotomy permits minimally invasive direct visualization and biopsy of metastatic deposits for frozen section histologic examination together with aspiration of small-volume ascites or peritoneal lavage for immediate cytologic evaluation (49). Laparoscopic ultrasonography (LUS) can further enhance tumor staging by detection of small (<1 cm) liver metastases and nonresectable distant nodal metas-

tases (49,50). The accuracy of staging of laparoscopy has been found to be as high as 99% for occult hepatic metastases, 94% for peritoneal metastases, but only 65% for nodal metastases (49). Clinical experience suggests that laparoscopic staging can alter the clinical stage in nearly one third of patients (50,51). The combined modalities of EUS with fine-needle aspiration and laparoscopy with LUS have proven efficacy in the more precise staging of gastric cancer and their use in the preoperative staging sequence has become common at many centers. Their inclusion in management algorithms for gastric cancer has allowed for reductions in nontherapeutic laparotomy rates as well as overall perioperative mortality from the elimination of the excessive mortality associated with nontherapeutic laparotomy (Figure 33.7) (9,52,53).

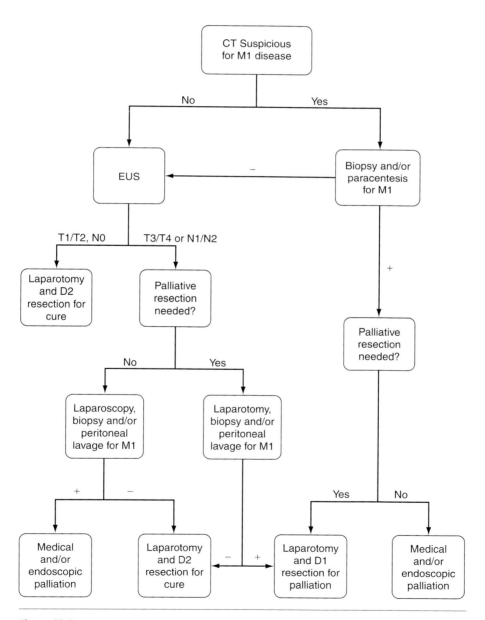

Figure 33.7 Algorithm for management of gastric adenocarcinoma with computed tomography scan suspicious for metastatic (M1) disease. CT, computed tomography; EUS, endoscopic ultrasound.

Recent experience with preoperative EUS in the diagnosis of small-volume ascites has verified the concept that occult ascites is an important predictive factor for the presence of occult peritoneal metastases in gastric cancer patients (54). Even in the absence of definable ascites, laparoscopic peritoneal lavage that detects the presence of free peritoneal tumor cells portends the subsequent manifestation of peritoneal carcinomatosis and contraindicates attempted curative gastric resection (55,56). Among 371 patients without evidence of peritoneal metastases at laparoscopy, 6% had positive lavage cytology that was associated exclusively with T3 and T4 primary tumors and was associated with a median survival of only 15 months (57). Thus detection of either occult ascites or free peritoneal tumor cells strongly suggests peritoneal tumor spread and argues for palliative medical or surgical interventions only.

EXTENT OF GASTRIC RESECTION

Surgeons have been successfully performing gastrectomy for the past 125 years and surgical resection remains the only proven curative therapy for invasive gastric adenocarcinoma. Over the course of the second half of the last century, considerable debate surrounded the issue of the extent of gastrectomy required to confer the maximal potential for long-term survival in the absence of excessive perioperative morbidity and mortality. Based on a number of retrospective experiences, a high subtotal (85%) distal gastrectomy was considered by most to be equal to total gastrectomy as a curative operation for antral and midbody gastric cancers, provided an adequate negative surgical margin could be achieved (58,59). Large tumors of the midstomach or fundus were agreed to require total gastrectomy. Cancers localized to the gastric cardia have usually been managed by total gastrectomy with limited intra-abdominal or transhiatal resection of the distal esophagus to achieve a negative margin (60). Cardia tumors with extension into the distal esophagus have required transmediastinal or thoracoabdominal esophagogastrectomy.

The most persistent controversy regarding extent of gastrectomy has been over tumors situated in the distal half of the stomach. In a French multicenter randomized trial of 169 patients that compared subtotal and total gastrectomy, there were no statistically significant differences in perioperative morbidity, mortality, or 5-year survival rates (48% in both groups) related to the extent of resection (61). A similar but larger and more recent randomized trial conducted by the Italian Gastrointestinal Tumor Study Group involved 622 patients allocated to subtotal gastrectomy or total gastrectomy (62). Both procedures included aggressive regional lymphadenectomies. The 5-year survival probabilities were similar, 65% after subtotal and 62% after total gastrectomy. Furthermore, a quality of life assessment using multiple patient symptom and satisfaction indices has shown significantly better outcomes 1 year after subtotal gastrectomy compared with total gastrectomy (63). With equal perioperative and long-term survival rates, and superior quality of life following subtotal gastrectomy, its place as the procedure of choice for distal cancers has been convincingly established. However, for any partial gastrectomy to be as curative as total gastrectomy, a proximal tumor-free margin of 6 cm confirmed by frozen section examination must be assured (62).

For tumors of the gastric cardia not extending into the esophagus, the large prospective Multicenter German Gastric Cancer Study database largely established the primacy of transabdominal total gastrectomy with limited distal esophagectomy as the preferred operation over more extensive transmediastinal or thoracoabdominal esophagogastrectomy (60,64). Perioperative mortality after procedures that included extended esophagectomy was 5.6% versus only 1.9% after total gastrectomy (64). Long-term survival was not increased by extended esophageal resection but rather depended on inclusion of an en bloc regional lymphadenectomy and achievement of a complete (R0) tumor resection. Furthermore, a United States single-institution study found a threefold increase in perioperative morbidity following major esophagectomy as compared with total gastrectomy, and no 5-year survival differences (65). A very recently presented randomized trial from Japan compared the left thoracoabdominal approach with the abdominal and transhiatal approach for gastric cardia cancer extending <3 cm into the esophagus (66). Among 167 patients treated, the 5-year survival rates were 36% and 49%, respectively. Pulmonary function and quality of life measures also favored the abdominal approach. Certainly for tumors ascending >3 cm into the esophagus, transmediastinal or thoracoabdominal esophagectomy is virtually mandatory. In most instances in which cure is intended, an en bloc lymphadenectomy should be included, as the 5-year survival is twice that of less extensive resection (67–69). Therefore, when the esophagus is significantly invaded, a transthoracic approach may be superior as it affords a more anatomic and complete cancer resection.

EXTENT OF LYMPHADENECTOMY

The lymphatic drainage of the stomach is multidirectional and involves a wide network of anastomosing lymphatic channels. As a result, the lymph node metastases associated with gastric adenocarcinoma are somewhat unpredictable and not uncommonly include skip metastases (70). This fact combined with the recognized aggressiveness of gastric adenocarcinoma led to the concept of surgical clearance of second-level (regional) lymph nodes in addition to the first-level (perigastric) lymph nodes as an optimal oncologic lymphadenectomy for the disease (Figure 33.8). The more extensive second-level (D2) lymphadenectomy (Figure 33.9) has been rigorously compared to the more conservative first-level (D1) lymphadenectomy in both retrospective and several prospective trials, yet controversy persists regarding the ideal approach (71–73).

Despite an extensive Japanese literature supporting aggressive D2 lymph node dissection, the majority of American and European surgeons have been reluctant to embrace the operation (22,73). There have been a number of cogent reasons for this reluctance. These have included (a) the usually advanced stage of disease at diagnosis, (b) the lack of scientifically valid data in support of the putative benefit attending aggressive node dissection, (c) concerns over the reported higher morbidity and mortality of D2, and (d) a lack of familiarity and experience with the operative technique of D2 dissection. With the overall decline in training experience with gastrectomy and the absence of randomized trial results in support of D2, there has been little

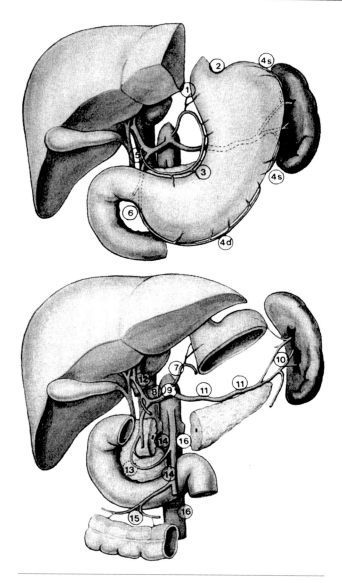

Figure 33.8 Gastric lymph node levels and stations. First-level nodes include stations 1 through 6 (*top figure*), most or all of which are removed by a D1 lymphadenectomy. Second-level nodes include stations 7 through 12 (*bottom figure*), most or all of which are removed in addition to first-level nodes by a D2 lymphadenectomy. Third-level nodes include stations 13 through 16 (*bottom figure*), which are rarely removed with curative intent. (From Hartgrink HH, van de Velde CJH, Putter H, et al. Extended lymph node dissection for gastric cancer: who may benefit? Final results of the randomized Dutch Gastric Cancer Group Trial. *J Clin Oncol.* 2004;22:2069–2077, with permission.)

compelling reason for Western surgeons to adopt the procedure. Nevertheless, critical examination of completed randomized trials, awareness of the early results from newer trials of superior design and conduct, and use of modern techniques that allow earlier diagnosis and more accurate preoperative staging, challenge the notion that D2 dissection should be discounted as having any therapeutic advantage.

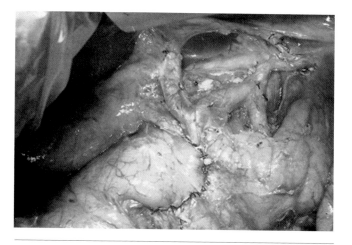

Figure 33.9 Operative field following total gastrectomy and D2 lymphadenectomy for adenocarcinoma showing skeletonized celiac, common and proper hepatic, and proximal splenic, left gastric, and gastroduodenal arteries superior to the closed duodenal stump and pancreas.

Of the several randomized controlled trials examining aggressive D2 lymphadenectomy in comparison to limited D1 lymphadenectomy and having mature data, only the British Medical Research Council Gastric Cancer Surgical Trial and the Dutch Gastric Cancer Trial have had sample sizes large enough to provide any potential for meaningful results (74–80). Unfortunately, both of these trials were flawed by design and performance problems as evidenced by inclusion of patients beyond any reasonable possibility of surgical cure and unacceptably high perioperative morbidity and mortality rates (76,78,79). In both trials the perioperative mortality and morbidity rates for D2 gastrectomy were greater than 10% and 40%, respectively (Table 33.3). The poor short-term outcomes likely reflect the unfamiliarity of many participating surgeons with the technique of D2 dissection and the inclusion of pancreaticosplenectomy in a large number of cases. Routine inclusion of pancreaticosplenectomy has not been shown to enhance long-term survival after radical gastrectomy (76,81). However, resection of the distal pancreas and spleen do increase the rates of anastomotic dehiscence, fistulization, and

Table 33.3

Results of British and Dutch Randomized Clinical Trials Comparing D1 and D2 Lymphadenectomies for Gastric Adenocarcinoma

Trial	Operation	Operative Mortality (%)	Operative Morbidity (%)	5-Year Survival (%)
British	D1	6	28	35
	D2	13	46	33
Dutch	D1	4	25	45
	D2	10	43	47

Table 33.4

Stage-Stratified 11-Year Survival Rates from the Dutch Randomized Clinical Trial Comparing D1 and D2 Lymphadenectomies for Gastric Adenocarcinoma

Stage	D1 (%)	D2 (%)	p Value
IA	60	58	0.84
IB	47	44	0.65
II	23	37	0.10
IIIA	4	22	0.38
IIIB	0	10	0.55
IV	0	3	0.19
ALL	30	35	0.53

mortality (76). Furthermore, adequate lymphadenectomy along the splenic artery can be accomplished without the inclusion of pancreaticosplenectomy (81).

Although the perioperative morbidity and mortality results from the British and Dutch trials were very similar, the 5-year survival figures were not (77,79). The survival rate differences for D1 versus D2 operations were statistically insignificant in both trials, but survival rates in the Dutch trial were 10% higher after D1 and 14% higher after D2 gastrectomy compared with the British trial (77,79). Stage stratification data recently provided by the Dutch trial also contain definite trends for increased 11-year survival for patients with stage II and stage IIIA cancer treated with D2 lymphadenectomy (Table 33.4) (80). Substantially enhanced survival was specifically noted for patients with N2 nodal involvement after D2 (Table 33.5). The insignificant nature of these stratified data simply may be the result of inadequate sample sizes (type 2 statistical error). This argument and the likely superiority of extensive lymphadenectomy for midstage (II and IIIA) gastric cancer is fortified by the nonrandomized but prospective data derived from the Multicenter German Gastric Cancer Study (82). This trial included 1,654

patients and documented a highly statistically significant increase in long-term survival among patients with stage II disease treated by D2 lymphadenectomy (Figure 33.10). Importantly, this was accomplished without any increase in perioperative morbidity or mortality attending the more extensive dissection.

A recent Italian Gastric Cancer Study Group randomized trial has further corroborated the safety of D2 lymphadenectomy (83). D2 dissection was performed without pancreaticosplenectomy and accomplished with a perioperative morbidity rate of only 16%, and with no mortality. Long-term survival data from this trial are not yet available. Nevertheless, the results from the prospective German trial and the randomized Italian trial clearly indicate the safety of D2 lymphadenectomy without pancreaticosplenectomy (82,83). The long-term survival data provided by the German trial, along with supporting trends from the Dutch randomized trial, strongly suggest efficacy of D2 dissection for midstage gastric cancer (80,82).

Aside from the survival advantage that well may be provided by D2 lymphadenectomy, a recent study has verified the concept that only D2 lymphadenectomy can provide a sufficient number of lymph nodes for accurate pathologic staging of gastric adenocarcinoma (84). The American Joint Commission on Cancer in 1997 established a guideline of 15 lymph nodes as the minimal number for adequate pathologic staging of the disease. The validity of the revised staging system as the most accurate prognostic indicator for gastric cancer has subsequently been well established (85). A direct comparison of D1 versus D2 has highlighted the inadequacy of the former as a cancer staging operation. Whereas the mean and median members of lymph nodes harvested by D1 lymphadenectomy were only 12.4 and 12, respectively, D2 lymphadenectomy yielded 25.2 and 22 lymph nodes, respectively (84). Only 20% of D1 operations provided the necessary 15 or greater lymph nodes, and this was accomplished by 86% of D2 operations. Morbidity and mortality rates associated with D2 lymphadenectomy were again no greater than that of D1 lymphadenectomy. In addition to its likely therapeutic superiority, it would appear that D2 lymphadenectomy should be performed in most instances in which gastrectomy is performed with curative intent in order to provide accurate pathologic staging and appropriate postoperative adjuvant therapy planning.

Table 33.5

Nodal Stage-Stratified 11-Year Survival Rates from the Dutch Randomized Trial Comparing D1 and D2 Lymphadenectomies for Gastric Adenocarcinoma

Nodal Stage	D1 (%)	D2 (%)	p Value
N0	52	51	0.93
N1	20	30	0.46
N2	0	21	0.08
N3	0	0	0.30
Negative	52	51	0.93
Positive	13	23	0.28

ADJACENT ORGAN RESECTION

The results provided by several randomized controlled trials have clearly demonstrated the inappropriateness of resection of adjacent organs (spleen, pancreas) not directly involved by the cancer (76,78,86). Combined with data from several thousand retrospectively studied patients, there has been no evidence of enhanced long-term survival deriving from routine adjacent organ removal. In addition, pancreaticosplenectomy significantly increases the rates of postoperative pancreatic fistula, abscess, and anastomotic leakage (87,88). These results do not, however, contraindicate organ resections in instances in which the tumor extends to adjacent organs in patients who are otherwise potentially curable (89). En bloc resection of such T4 primary tumors is appropriate only for patients without grossly apparent lymph node or other metastatic disease. As T4 tumors

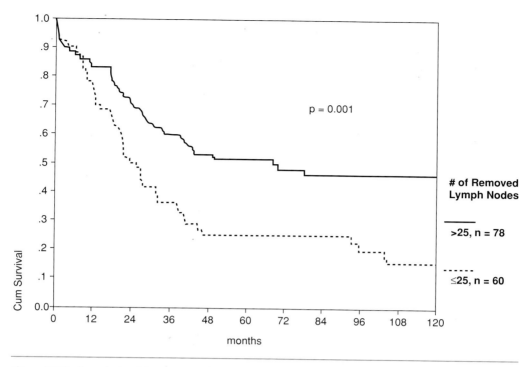

Figure 33.10 Cumulative (Cum) survival in patients after gastrectomy for stage II (T2N1) adenocarcinoma. Removal of ≤25 nodes was considered a D1 lymphadenectomy and >25 nodes was considered a D2 lymphadenectomy. (From Siewert JR, Bottcher K, Stein HJ, et al. Relevant prognostic factors in gastric cancer: ten-year results of the German Gastric Cancer Study. *Ann Surg.* 1998;228:449–461, with permission.)

accompanied by nodal metastases are classified as stage IV disease by the American Joint Commission on Cancer, aggressive en bloc resections are accompanied by poor risk-benefit ratios and should be avoided. In a series of 353 patients with T4 gastric cancers who underwent gastrectomy and en bloc adjacent organ resection, the perioperative mortality rate was 14%, and those with positive lymph nodes had a 5-year survival of only 15% (90). Nevertheless, nonmetastatic primary tumors directly invading the distal pancreas or spleen, left lateral segment of the liver, transverse colon or mesocolon, greater or lesser omenta, or diaphragmatic crura are appropriate for en bloc radical resection in selected cases. For distal gastric cancers invading the head of the pancreas, a somewhat more conservative approach is advisable. Because of the added morbidity and mortality associated with pancreaticoduodenectomy (Whipple procedure), it should be reserved only for the highly selected younger patient who is staged preoperatively and intraoperatively to have a very favorable T4N0M0 antral gastric tumor.

In most instances, the biology and stage of the tumor are the most important prognostic factors in gastric cancer. Therefore, the surgeon's ability to affect the course of the disease is inherently limited. Optimal surgical care is required to maximize the relatively small therapeutic opportunity. Adequate margins of resection, aggressive regional lymphadenectomy for midstage tumors, minimization of operative blood loss, and a secure restorative anastomosis are the critical elements within the surgeon's

control that must be achieved in order to serve the patient's best interests.

RECONSTRUCTION AFTER GASTRECTOMY

Limited distal gastrectomy (antrectomy) for small prepyloric and pyloric channel carcinomas offers the option of either Billroth I gastroduodenostomy or Billroth II gastrojejunostomy for reconnection of the gastrointestinal tract. Conventional wisdom has held that the latter procedure is preferable because it tends to provide greater margins of resection and removal of a greater number of juxtapyloric lymph nodes. It may also reduce the likelihood of late anastomotic obstruction secondary to local tumor recurrence. There are little reliable data to support the superiority of one or the other procedure. Nevertheless, a single randomized controlled trial comparing Billroth I with Billroth II anastomotic techniques in patients with antral cancers demonstrated no significant differences in perioperative morbidity or mortality, margins of resections, numbers of the lymph nodes removed, anastomotic strictures, frequencies of digestive complaints, or long-term survival (91). There were, however, more anastomotic fistulas and a trend toward more local tumor recurrences at the hepatoduodenal ligament after the Billroth I operation. It would appear that the Billroth I is an acceptable reconstruction for early-stage antral cancers without gross nodal involvement wherein distal gastrectomy with wide margins and a low probability of local reoccurrence can be anticipated. However, in the absence of any well-demonstrated disadvantage of Billroth II gastrojejunostomy, it continues to be the reconstruction of choice for most distal cancers in view of its demonstrated safety and ease of construction. The Roux-en-Y variant of the Billroth II has been advocated by some because of its prevention of bile reflux gastritis and esophagitis (92). Two problems, namely the Roux stasis syndrome and the development of late stomal ulceration when vagotomy is omitted, combine to discourage the application of this more complicated construction in most instances (93,94).

Provided that a 6-cm proximal margin can be assured, there is no demonstrated disadvantage of subtotal gastrectomy compared with total gastrectomy for resectable gastric cancers not involving the cardia, fundus, or proximal corpus (62). For proximal tumors not requiring extensive esophagectomy, total gastrectomy is the operation of choice (60). Proximal gastrectomy with esophagoantral reconstruction has been used in the past but is associated with a high incidence of severe and debilitating alkaline reflux esophagitis and is no longer recommended (64). Therefore, the appropriateness of total gastrectomy for any proximal or bulky midstomach cancer is well established and can be accomplished with minimal perioperative morbidity and mortality (60). However, controversy continues to abound regarding the efficacies of various reconstruction techniques after total gastrectomy. Over the past century more than 50 operations for intestinal reconstruction following total gastrectomy have been described (95). The majority of these have been designed to prevent bile reflux esophagitis, prevent dumping syndrome, provide a substitute food intake reservoir, maintain duodenal food passage, or some combination thereof. Achieving these ends has been believed to be important in maintaining optimal nutritional status and quality of life among long-term survivors.

Simple end-to-side loop esophagojejunostomy is an unacceptable reconstruction because it inevitably leads to severe bile reflux esophagitis and fails to provide any advantages other than ease and speed of construction (96). Some form of Roux-en-Y esophagojejunostomy, with or without a food reservoir pouch, has proved safe and durable for most patients (97). The Roux-en-Y limb procedure reliably eliminates alkaline reflux provided the length of jejunum between the esophagojejunal and distal jejunojejunal anastomosis is a minimum of 40 cm.

Consensus regarding the efficacy of jejunal reservoir pouch reconstruction after total gastrectomy has not been achieved (98,99). The complexity of the respective physiologic consequences of simple Roux-en-Y esophagojejunostomy compared with the myriad of jejunal pouch configurations, combined with the lack of adequately powered randomized trials, makes analysis of this issue extremely problematic. The findings of retrospective studies have clearly failed to demonstrate any superiority of the more complicated pouch reconstructions over simple Roux-en-Y anastomosis (93,98). Similarly, a review of the small number of modern prospective controlled trials of various reconstructive operations offers no clear direction because of small sample sizes and insignificant differences between groups (97,98). Detailed analysis of the long-term nutritional consequences of pouch reconstruction has failed to demonstrate any sustained, objectively assessed advantage. Long-term dietary support ap-

pears to be a more important determinant of chronic nutritional health than is the use of a pouch reservoir (100,101). Similarly, preservation of duodenal food passage by use of a jejunal interposition graft between the distal esophagus and proximal duodenum, with or without pouch reservoir construction, has not been demonstrated to confer any clinical advantage with regard to gastrointestinal function or patient satisfaction (97,99). Until such time as a randomized trial of sufficient size clearly demonstrates some advantage to more complex intestinal reconstruction, standard Roux-en-Y end-to-side esophagojejunostomy combined with diligent and sustained nutritional guidance can be considered an entirely acceptable procedure following total gastrectomy for gastric cancer.

MINIMALLY INVASIVE SURGERY

Laparoscopy and LUS are now well-established staging techniques that complement preoperative procedures such as CT and EUS (49–51). In combination, these techniques are extremely useful in selecting appropriate patients who may benefit from radical gastrectomy with curative intent. However, staging laparoscopy is superfluous and is not indicated in patients with incurable but resectable gastric cancers who would benefit from palliative gastrectomy to alleviate bleeding, obstruction, or severe pain. Neither is laparoscopy useful in incurable patients with bleeding or obstruction that can be managed with such newer endoscopic techniques as argon beam photocoagulation, laser ablation, or luminal stenting (102,103). On the other hand, laparoscopy and LUS to rule occult distant metastases (M1) prior to embarking on laparotomy and planned curative gastrectomy represent reliable techniques that provide accurate assessment of stage and resectability, and thus the opportunity to avoid unnecessary laparotomy when surgical palliation is not needed (52,53). Staging laparoscopy has been demonstrated to increase resectability rates and decrease nontherapeutic laparotomy rates and lengths of hospital stay in patients with unresectable tumors (104,105). Proper patient selection based on clinical status and preoperative assessment with CT and EUS are clearly required for the cost-effective application of staging laparoscopy and LUS.

Over the past 15 years laparoscopic resection has been used with increasing frequency for both early (T1) and, more recently, advanced (>T1) tumors (106,107). The early experience was largely confined to laparoscopic wedge resection of small cancers confined to the gastric mucosa. As technical advances have allowed for endoscopic mucosal resection of these very early gastric cancers, the need for laparoscopic wedge resection has declined (108). Nevertheless, the technical success and patient satisfaction afforded by laparoscopic resection has served as an impetus for the development and application of laparoscopic gastrectomy with lymph node dissection for more advanced-stage tumors (109). Most particularly, laparoscopy-assisted distal gastrectomy is now accepted in Japan as a valid alternative to traditional open distal gastrectomy for the treatment of early gastric cancer, even in cases with some risk of lymph node metastases (107). Over the past several years, both distal and total gastrectomy with D2 lymphadenectomy have been pursued with at least short-term success by a number of surgeons from around the world (109–111). A recently reported randomized controlled trial comparing laparoscopy-assisted distal gastrectomy with open distal gastrectomy in 59 patients found no significant differences in numbers of lymph nodes resected, operative morbidity or mortality rates, 5-year overall, or disease-free survival rates (112). Both the laparoscopic and open subtotal gastrectomies included D2 lymphadenectomies for advanced gastric cancers. There was reduced blood loss, shorter time to resumption of oral intake, and earlier hospital discharge in the laparoscopic group. Clearly, a substantial learning curve is required to achieve mastery and safe performance of laparoscopic subtotal gastrectomy with D2 lymphadenectomy. Regionalization of laparoscopic resection for advanced gastric cancer will likely occur in the future if the procedure becomes widely accepted based on verification of the efficacy of D2 lymphadenectomy and of its laparoscopic application.

Because extended lymphadenectomy performed laparoscopically is inherently difficult and tedious, the most appropriate and well-established indication for laparoscopic gastric resection remains early gastric cancer (107). By definition, these tumors penetrate into the mucosa or submucosa only, and only the latter tumors have lymphatic access and thus the potential for lymph node metastasis. Tumors staged as T1N0 by CT and EUS have a low likelihood of requiring lymphadenectomy and therefore are theoretically ideal for laparoscopic resection. In order to optimize selection of patients for laparoscopic resection without lymphadenectomy, the concept of sentinel lymph node identification and biopsy has recently been promulgated (106,113). Over the past several years, experience at multiple centers (primarily Japanese) encompassing several hundreds of patients and employing both radioisotope labeled colloid and dye-guided methods indicates that detection rates of sentinel nodes generally range between 95% and 100% with sensitivity for positive lymph nodes averaging between 85% and 100% (106). Some 5% to 10% of sentinel nodes in gastric cancer patients are located in the second-level nodal compartment rather than the perigastric nodal compartment (106). The important anatomic information derived from sentinel lymph node mapping is currently being used in a few centers to determine the extent of operative radicality (113,114). For sentinel lymph nodes found to be positive by frozen section histologic examination, a laparoscopic or open radical gastrectomy with D2 lymphadenectomy is performed. Alternatively, a negative sentinel node biopsy provides a rationale for a wedge resection, segmental resection, or limited proximal or distal gastrectomy with lymphadenectomy limited to the one to several sentinel nodes identified (Figure 33.11). In this manner, sentinel lymph node biopsy may provide an opportunity for a paradigm shift for the surgical management of early gastric cancer.

Laparoscopic endoluminal gastric surgery represents a new minimally invasive operative modality that combines the use of laparoscopic transgastric instrumentation with endoscopic guidance. The inflated stomach provides an adequate working space for laparoscopic maneuvering using standard instrumentation (Figure 33.12). Nearly 260 resections of early gastric cancers confined to the mucosa and a variety of benign lesions have been accomplished with good results over the past 15 years by Japanese surgeons (115). The technique is demanding and its place in the surgical armamentarium for gastric cancer remains to be determined.

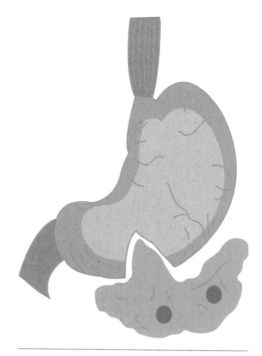

Figure 33.11 Wedge resection of the stomach with adjacent sentinel node basin lymphadenectomy appropriate for small, early gastric cancer with negative sentinel lymph node biopsy. (From Kitagawa Y, Fujii H, Kumai K, et al. Recent advances in sentinel node navigation for gastric cancer: a paradigm shift of surgical management. *J Surg Oncol.* 2005;90:147–152, with permission.)

PALLIATIVE SURGERY

The role of palliative operation for adenocarcinoma of the stomach has diminished considerably in recent years. Improved preoperative staging through refinements in CT, EUS, and laparoscopy have substantially reduced the frequency of laparotomy for locally unresectable primary tumors and limited but incurable metastatic disease. Acutely bleeding incurable tumors are now being managed with various endoscopic methods to achieve hemostasis, including electrocautery, laser, or argon beam photocoagulation (102,103). Patients with gastric inlet or outlet obstruction are obtaining satisfactory re-establishment of luminal patency by means of laser ablation or expandable metallic endoscopic stent placement. Stenting, in particular, has provided patency adequate for oral food intake in 85% to 97% of cases with an average uninterrupted duration of function of 5 to 6 months (102,103). Furthermore, nonoperative approaches to obstruction in incurable patients allow institution of palliative chemotherapy much sooner than after surgical resection or bypass.

Palliative surgical resection remains an effective strategy for patients with technically resectable but incurable tumors who suffer from bleeding, obstruction, or severe pain not manageable by endoscopic or other nonoperative means. Patient

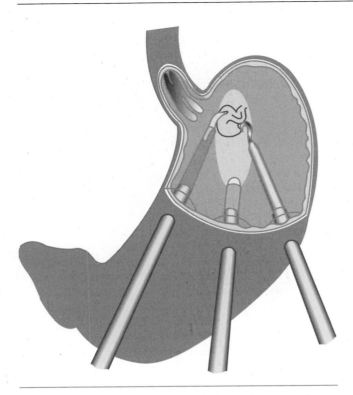

Figure 33.12 Laparoscopic intragastric mucosal resection for small, superficial, early gastric adenocarcinoma. (From Rosen MJ, Heniford BT. Endoluminal gastric surgery: the modern era of minimally invasive surgery. *Surg Clin North Am.* 2005;85:989–1007, with permission.)

selection is critically important and those with widely disseminated metastatic deposits, large-volume malignant ascites, severe nutritional deficits, advanced age, or poor functional status are generally not candidates for aggressive surgical intervention (116). Palliative gastric resection is often a formidable operation, particularly for very proximal or very distal bulky tumors. For the latter, a simple side-to-side gastrojejunostomy for proximal diversion of the food stream has been practiced frequently. However, gastric stasis has often precluded effective bypass of the obstructing lesion. In general, a limited distal gastrectomy provides better palliation than does proximal gastrojejunal bypass (117,118). Furthermore, the previously held notion that palliative total gastrectomy was too morbid an operation to be regularly applied has been well refuted and is clearly justified in selected patients (119,120). The operation affords not only symptom control, but also the potential elimination of severe complications (bleeding, perforation, and obstruction) caused by the primary tumor that shorten survival. Among a series of 53 patients who underwent palliative total gastrectomy, the mortality was an acceptable 8% and one-quarter survived 2 years or more, and the median survival was 19 months (119). The quality of life was judged to be good in 59% and poor in only 13%. Enhancement of the quality of life rather than prolongation of survival time per se should be the principal goal of palliative surgery. When operation is deemed appropriate as a palliative therapy and resection is not feasible, laparoscopic stapled side-

to-side gastrojejunostomy is now often preferred and can be accomplished with low morbidity and mortality. With the current panoply of minimally invasive techniques available, laparotomy for palliation of gastric cancer should rarely be the intervention of first choice.

GASTRIC LYMPHOMA

In contradistinction to gastric adenocarcinoma, gastric lymphoma is no longer primarily a surgical disease. With approximately 3,000 new cases of primary gastric lymphoma diagnosed in the United States each year, it ranks as the second most common malignancy of the stomach and accounts for 2% to 9% of the total (22,121). The tumor is the most common site of extranodal non-Hodgkin lymphoma and represents nearly half of all such cases. Unlike adenocarcinoma, gastric lymphoma afflicts men and women equally. It presents with symptoms similar to adenocarcinoma, mainly epigastric pain, anorexia, weight loss, and occasionally bleeding or perforation. Lymphoma B symptoms such as fever and night sweats are uncommon. Low-grade lesions often remain confined to the mucosa and submucosa and involve lymph nodes in only approximately 15% of cases. High-grade tumors tend to proliferate rapidly and spread to lymph nodes in >75% of cases (122).

Over the past 20 years, understanding of the etiology of gastric lymphoma has increased profoundly. Approximately 40% of all primary gastric lymphomas fall into the category of low-grade lymphoma and 98% of these are of the mucosa-associated lymphoid tissue (MALT) lymphoma type (123). In addition, one third of high-grade gastric lymphomas also contain some low-grade MALT component. In total, some 60% of all primary gastric lymphomas are characterized completely or in part by low-grade MALT histopathology. The tumors are of extranodal B-cell origin. They typically demonstrate a dense lymphoid cell infiltration of the gastric mucosa that ultimately destroys and replaces normal gastric glands. Most MALT lesions are biologically indolent, while high-grade tumors are typically aggressive. It is not clear whether the pure high-grade lymphomas arise from low-grade lesions that are subsequently obliterated or develop de novo as high-grade tumors (124).

What has become clear in recent years is the central role of *H. pylori* infection in the pathogenesis of MALT lymphomas (125). The organism has been found in 92% to 98% of stomachs resected for MALT lymphoma (126,127). A carefully conducted case-control study has shown that *H. pylori* gastritis long antedates development of the tumor and represents a pre-MALT lymphoma condition (128). CagA and other *H. pylori* virulence factors appear to initiate an inflammatory response that includes specific T cells that express a number of cytokines capable of inducing B-cell proliferation within gastric mucosa that is normally devoid of lymphoid tissue (129). An initial reactive oligoclonal and finally a monoclonal lymphoproliferative malignant transformation occurs that culminates after a number of years with a MALT lymphoma (130). It has been postulated that the lower grades of chronic gastritis caused by some *H. pylori* favor the development of MALT lymphoma compared with other *H. pylori*-induced disease states, including adenocarcinoma (131). Thus, specific antigens elaborated by relatively weak strains of *H. pylori* may be central to the pathogenesis of MALT lymphomas (132). Alterations in the *p53* suppressor gene may also be involved, as partial inactivation may lead to low-grade tumors while complete inactivation may promote high-grade lymphoma development (133).

Of central importance in the understanding of the etiologic role of *H. pylori* in gastric MALT lymphoma is the observation that eradication of the infection has led to complete tumor regression. More than 20 clinical series comprising 708 patients have now documented complete remission rates ranging from 35% to 100% (22). In the most recent and largest study to date, a complete response rate of 81% and a partial response of 9% were documented following a 2-week course of therapy directed against *H. pylori* among 120 patients with unequivocal low-grade MALT lymphomas (134). Only 10% had no tumor response to the antibiotic regimen. Subsequently, there were 9 recurrences among 97 patients with initial complete remissions. Some caution regarding the accuracy of diagnosis of complete remission based on endoscopic biopsy material is warranted, however. In some instances, residual tumor may be evident only in the deeper layers of the gastric wall, and the characteristic lymphoepithelial lesions of MALT lymphoma may not be evident following *H. pylori* eradication. The persistence of monoclonal B cells in the mucosa of nearly half of patients otherwise thought to be in complete remission emphasizes the unproven and still experimental nature of *H. pylori* eradication as a sole treatment modality (134).

A recent literature review indicates that the success of eradication is tumor stage-dependent (124). When lymph node involvement is present, complete responses are likely rare. Lymphomas penetrating beyond the submucosa have responded poorly in most instances (135,136). Clearly, the long-term efficacy of the unique antibacterial therapeutic strategy for MALT lymphoma must await long-term follow-up results. Nevertheless, with the introduction of therapy directed against *H. pylori* as a potentially curative treatment for low-grade MALT gastric lymphoma, the enthusiasm for resection has substantially declined. If the early success rates observed with *H. pylori* eradication are sustained over the long term, gastrectomy will rightfully be eliminated as a primary treatment consideration for localized MALT lymphomas.

Previously, surgical resection also played a prominent role in the treatment of non-MALT gastric lymphomas (137). Localized lymphomas of all types have long been effectively managed by partial or total gastrectomy, either as sole therapy or together with radiation therapy or combination radiation and chemotherapy. The validity of surgical resection was based on 5-year survival rates that routinely exceeded 90% (124,138). Nevertheless, the perioperative morbidity and mortality associated with major gastrectomy has long argued for alternative, safer therapies that could deliver comparable long-term disease-free outcomes. Both radiation and chemotherapy as primary modalities have provided very acceptable therapeutic results for localized MALT and non-MALT lymphomas of the stomach and have largely replaced gastrectomy, except in instances of exigent hemorrhage or perforation (124). In a series of 51 patients treated with the median radiation dose of 30 Gy, complete remission was achieved in 89% of patients after 4 years of follow-up (139). Comparable results have been obtained with chemotherapy alone and in combination with radiation therapy, and with both modalities combined with surgery (123). Specifically, the outcomes among the 185 patients treated in the prospective German Multicenter Study demonstrated equal effectiveness of radiation alone and gastrectomy followed by radiation for stage I tumors (123). When chemotherapy is used, the combination of cyclophosphamide, vincristine, and prednisolone (COP) is usually preferred.

The same equivalent efficacies of chemoradiation alone and gastrectomy followed by chemoradiation have been found for high-grade lymphomas as well. Overall 5-year survival rates in the German study were 84% and 82%, respectively, and significant toxicity from chemotherapy and/or radiation therapy was distinctly uncommon (123). The chemotherapeutic regimen for aggressive lesions typically has included cyclophosphamide, doxorubicin, vincristine, and prednisolone (CHOP). Importantly, with radiation and/or chemotherapy as primary treatment, concerns regarding the complications of gastric perforation and bleeding have not materialized, with rates of only approximately 2% (123). Recently, the anti-CD20 monoclonal antibody rituximab has been used both alone and in combination with chemotherapy, with promising results (140).

Surgical resection is no longer the primary treatment of choice for localized gastric lymphoma. Radiation therapy and chemotherapy either alone or in combination have achieved comparably good results without the morbidity and mortality associated with gastrectomy. As most low-grade lymphomas are of MALT derivation, and most of these are associated with *H. pylori* infection, eradication of the organism has become first-line therapy because of the high rates of remission achieved. For patients failing *H. pylori* eradication, and for early lymphoma not associated with *H. pylori*, chemotherapy or radiotherapy alone is as effective as gastrectomy. Elimination of surgery as primary treatment has the advantage of eliminating any delay in initiating systemic therapy. Operative intervention should no longer be considered a primary treatment and should be reserved for tumor-related complications such as perforation, major hemorrhage, or persistent disease confined to the stomach.

REFERENCES

1. Fuchs CS, Mayer RJ. Gastric carcinoma. *N Engl J Med.* 1995;333: 32–41.
2. Wong BCY, Lam SK, Wong WM, et al. *Helicobacter pylori* eradication to prevent gastric cancer in a high-risk region of China: a randomized controlled trial. *JAMA.* 2004;291:187–194.
3. Del Giudice G, Covacci A, Telford JL, et al. The design of vaccines against *Helicobacter pylori* and their development. *Annu Rev Immunol.* 2001;19:523–563.
4. Jemal A, Tiwari RC, Murray T, et al. Cancer statistics, 2004. *CA Cancer J Clin* 2004;54:8–29.
5. Hohenberger P, Gretschel S. Gastric cancer. *Lancet.* 2003;362:305–315.
6. Sipponen P. *Helicobacter pylori:* a cohort phenomenon. *Am J Surg Pathol.* 1995;19(Suppl 1):S30–S36.
7. Moss SF, Sood S. *Helicobacter pylori. Curr Opin Infect Dis.* 2003;16: 445–451.

8. Roosendaal R, Kuipers EJ, Buitenwerf J, et al. *Helicobacter pylori* and the birth cohort effect: evidence of a continuous decrease of infection rates in childhood. *Am J Gastroenterol.* 1997;92:1480–1482.

9. Smith BR, Stabile BE. Gastric adenocarcinoma: reduction of perioperative mortality by avoidance of nontherapeutic laparotomy. *J Gastrointest Surg.* 2007;11:127–132.

10. Kubo A, Corley DA. Marked regional variation in adenocarcinomas of the esophagus and the gastric cardia in the United States. *Cancer.* 2002;95:2096–2102.

11. Laurén P. The two histological main types of gastric carcinoma: diffuse and so-called intestinal-type carcinoma. An attempt at a histo-clinical classification. *Acta Pathol Microbiol Scand.* 1965;64:31–49.

12. Correa P. Human gastric carcinogenesis: a multistep and multifactorial process: first American Cancer Society Award Lecture on Cancer Epidemiology and Prevention. *Cancer Res.* 1992;52:6735–6740.

13. Hattori T. Development of adenocarcinomas in the stomach. *Cancer.* 1986;57:1528–1534.

14. Bamba M, Sugihara H, Kushima R, et al. Time-dependent expression of intestinal phenotype in signet ring cell carcinomas of the human stomach. *Vichows Arch.* 2001;438:49–56.

15. Imrie C, Rowland M, Bourke B, et al. Is *Helicobacter pylori* infection in childhood a risk factor for gastric cancer? *Pediatrics.* 2001;107:373–380.

16. Gonzalez CA, Sala N, Capella G. Genetic susceptibility and gastric cancer risk. *Int J Cancer.* 2002;100:249–260.

17. Machado JC, Figueiredo C, Canedo P, et al. A proinflammatory genetic profile increases the risk for chronic atrophic gastritis and gastric carcinoma. *Gastroenterology.* 2003;125:364–371.

18. Nardone G, Morgner A. *Helicobacter pylori* and gastric malignancies. *Helicobacter.* 2003;8(Suppl 1):44–52.

19. Lan J, Xiong YY, Lin YX, et al. *Helicobacter pylori* infection generated gastric cancer through p53-Rb tumor-suppressor system mutation and telomerase reactivation. *World J Gastroenterol.* 2003;9:54–58.

20. Morgan C, Jenkins GJ, Ashton T, et al. Detection of p53 mutations in precancerous gastric tissue. *Br J Cancer.* 2003;89:1314–1319.

21. La Vecchia C, Negri E, Franceschi S, et al. Family history and the risk of stomach and colorectal cancer. *Cancer.* 1992;70:50–55.

22. Stabile BE, Smith BR, Weeks DL. *Helicobacter pylori* infection and surgical disease—Part II. *Curr Prob Surg.* 2005;42:791–862.

23. Suerbaum S, Michetti P. *Helicobacter pylori* infection. *N Engl J Med.* 2002;347:1175–1186.

24. Uemura N, Okamoto S, Yamamoto S, et al. *Helicobacter pylori* infection and the development of gastric cancer. *N Engl J Med.* 2001;345:784–789.

25. Huang JQ, Sridhar S, Chen Y, et al. Meta-analysis of the relationship between *Helicobacter pylori* seropositivity and gastric cancer. *Gastroenterology.* 1998;114:1169–1179.

26. Sipponen P, Kosunen TU, Valle J, et al. *Helicobacter pylori* infection and chronic gastritis in gastric cancer. *J Clin Pathol.* 1992;45:319–323.

27. Go MF. Review article: natural history and epidemiology of *Helicobacter pylori* infection. *Aliment Pharmacol Ther.* 2002;16(Suppl 1):3–15.

28. Harris RA, Owens DK, Witherell H, et al. *Helicobacter pylori* and gastric cancer: what are the benefits of screening only for the CagA phenotype of *H. pylori*? *Helicobacter.* 1999;4:69–76.

29. Odenbreit S, Puls J, Sedlmaier B, et al. Translocation of *Helicobacter pylori* CagA into gastric epithelial cells by type IV secretion. *Science.* 2000;287:1497–1500.

30. Yamaoka Y, El-Zimaity HM, Gutierrez O, et al. Relationship between the cagA 3N repeat region of *Helicobacter pylori*, gastric histology, and susceptibility to low pH. *Gastroenterology.* 1999;117:342–349.

31. Huang JQ, Zheng GF, Sumanac K, et al. Meta-analysis of the relationship between cagA seropositivity and gastric cancer. *Gastroenterology.* 2003;125:1636–1644.

32. Machida-Montani A, Sasazuki S, Inoue M, et al. Association of *Helicobacter pylori* infection and environmental factors in non-cardia gastric cancer in Japan. *Gastric Cancer.* 2004;7:46–53.

33. Azuma T, Yamazaki S, Yamakawa A, et al. Association between diversity in the Src homology 2 domain-containing tyrosine phosphatase binding site of *Helicobacter pylori* CagA protein and gastric atrophy and cancer. *J Infect Dis.* 2004;189:820–827.

34. Leunk RD, Johnson PT, David BC, et al. Cytotoxic activity in broth-culture filtrates of *Campylobacter pylori*. *J Med Microbiol.* 1998;26:93–99.

35. Zambon CF, Navaglia F, Basso D, et al. *Helicobacter pylori* babA2, cagA and s1 vacA genes work synergistically in causing intestinal metaplasia. *J Clin Pathol.* 2003;56:287–291.

36. Kikuchi S. Epidemiology of *Helicobacter pylori* and gastric cancer. *Gastric Cancer.* 2002;5:6–15.

37. Helicobacter and Cancer Collaborative Group. Gastric cancer and *Helicobacter pylori*: a combined analysis of 12 case control studies nested within prospective cohorts. *Gut.* 2001;49:347–353.

38. Watanabe T, Tada M, Nagai H, et al. *Helicobacter pylori* infection induces gastric cancer in Mongolian gerbils. *Gastroenterology.* 1998;115:642–648.

39. Fox JG, Want TC, Rogers AB, et al. Host and microbial constituents influence *Helicobacter pylori*-induced cancer in a murine model of hypergastrinemia. *Gastroenterology.* 2003;124:1879–1890.

40. Fox JG, Rogers AB, Ihrig M, et al. *Helicobacter pylori*-associated gastric cancer in INS-GAS mice is gender specific. *Cancer Res.* 2003;63:942–950.

41. Nakamura M, Haruma K, Kamada T, et al. Cigarette smoking promotes atrophic gastritis in *Helicobacter pylori*-positive subjects. *Dig Dis Sci.* 2002;47:675–681.

42. Sobala GM, Schorah CJ, Shires S, et al. Effect of eradication of *Helicobacter pylori* on gastric juice ascorbic acid concentrations. *Gut.* 1993;34:1038–1041.

43. Gupta JP, Jain AK, Agrawal BK, et al. Gastroscopic cytology and biopsies in diagnosis of gastric malignancies. *J Surg Oncol.* 1983;22:62–64.

44. Pollack BJ, Chak A, Sivak MV Jr. Endoscopic ultrasonography. *Semin Oncol.* 1996;23:336–346.

45. Caletti G, Ferrari A, Brocchi E, et al. Accuracy of endoscopic ultrasonography in the diagnosis and staging of gastric cancer and lymphoma. *Surgery.* 1993;113:14–27.

46. Kuntz C, Herfarth C. Imaging diagnosis for staging of gastric cancer. *Semin Surg Oncol.* 1999;17:96–102.

47. Chang KJ, Katz KD, Durbin TE, et al. Endoscopic ultrasound-guided fine-needle aspiration. *Gastrointest Endosc.* 1994;40:694–699.

48. Smith JW, Brennan MF, Botet JF, et al. Preoperative endoscopic ultrasonography can predict the risk of recurrence after operation for gastric carcinoma. *J Clin Oncol.* 1993;11:2380–2385.

49. Stell DA, Carter CR, Steward I, et al. Prospective comparison of laparoscopy, ultrasonography and computed tomography in the staging of gastric cancer. *Br J Surg.* 1996;83:1260–1262.

50. Conlon KC, Karpeh MS. Laparoscopy and laparoscopic ultrasound in the staging of gastric cancer. *Semin Oncol.* 1996;23:347–351.

51. Burke EC, Karpeh MS, Conlon KC, et al. Laparoscopy in the management of gastric adenocarcinoma. *Ann Surg.* 1997;225:262–267.

52. Hulscher JB, Nieveen van Dijkum EJ, de Wit LT, et al. Laparoscopy and laparoscopic ultrasonography in staging carcinoma of the gastric cardia. *Eur J Surg.* 2000;166:862–865.

53. Yano M, Tsujinaka T, Shiozaki H, et al. Appraisal of treatment strategy by staging laparoscopy for locally advanced gastric cancer. *World J Surg.* 2000;24:1130–1136.

54. Lee YT, Ng EKW, Hung LCT, et al. Accuracy of endoscopic ultrasonography in diagnosing ascites and predicting peritoneal metastases in gastric cancer patients. *Gut.* 2005;54:1541–1545.

55. Bryan RT, Cruickshank NR, Needham SJ, et al. Laparoscopic peritoneal lavage in staging gastric and oesophageal cancer. *Eur J Surg Oncol.* 2001;27:291–297.

56. Ribeiro U Jr, Gama-Rodrigues JJ, Safatle-Ribeiro AV, et al. Prognostic significance of intraperitoneal free cancer cells obtained by laparoscopic peritoneal lavage in patients with gastric cancer. *J Gastrointest Surg.* 1998;2:244–249.

57. Bentrem D, Wilton A, Mazumdar M, et al. The value of peritoneal cytology as a preoperative predictor in patients with gastric carcinoma undergoing a curative resection. *Ann Surg Oncol.* 2005;12:347–353.

58. Dupont JB Jr, Lee JR, Bunton GR, et al. Adenocarcinoma of the stomach: review of 1,497 cases. *Cancer.* 1978;41:941–947.

59. Bozzetti F. Total versus subtotal gastrectomy in cancer of the distal stomach: facts and fantasy. *Eur J Surg Oncol.* 1992;18:572–579.

60. Siewert JR, Stein HJ, Sendler A, et al. Surgical resection for cancer of the cardia. *Semin Surg Oncol.* 1999;17:125–131.

61. Gouzi JL, Huguier M, Fogniez PL, et al. Total versus subtotal gastrectomy for adenocarcinoma of the gastric antrum. A French prospective controlled study. *Ann Surg.* 1989;209:162–166.

62. Bozzetti F, Marubini E, Bonfanti G, et al. Subtotal versus total gastrectomy for gastric cancer: five-year survival rates in a multicenter randomized Italian trial. Italian Gastrointestinal Tumor Study Group. *Ann Surg.* 1999;230:170–178.

63. Davies J, Johnston D, Sue-Ling H, et al. Total or subtotal gastrectomy for gastric carcinoma? A study of quality of life. *World J Surg.* 1998;22:1048–1055.

64. Siewert JR, Stein HJ. Adenocarcinoma of the gastroesophageal junction: classification, pathology and extent of resection. *Dis Esoph.* 1996;9:173–182.

65. Ito H, Clancy TE, Osteen RT, et al. Adenocarcinoma of the gastric cardia: what is the optimal surgical approach? *J Am Coll Surg.* 2004;199:880–886.

66. Sasako M, Yoshimura K, Sano T, et al. Morbidity and quality of life assessment in a phase III trial of surgical treatment for gastric cardia cancer comparing a left thoracoabdominal with abdominal and transhiatal approach. *Ann Surg.* (in press).

67. Hagen J, DeMeester S, Peters J, et al. Curative resection for esophageal adenocarcinoma: analysis of 100 en bloc esophagectomies. *Ann Surg.* 2001;234:520–531.

68. Altorki NMD, Skinner DMD. Should en bloc esophagectomy be the standard of care for esophageal carcinoma? *Ann Surg.* 2001;234:581–587.

69. Sihvo EI, Luostarinen ME, Salo JA. Fate of patients with adenocarcinoma of the esophagus and the esophagogastric junction: a population-based analysis. *Am J Gastroenterol.* 2004;99:419–424.

70. Kitagawa Y, Fujii H, Kumai K, et al. Recent advances in sentinel node navigation for gastric cancer: a paradigm shift of surgical management. *J Surg Oncol.* 2005;90:147–152.

71. Lim L, Michael M, Mann GB, et al. Adjuvant therapy in gastric cancer. *J Clin Oncol.* 2005;23:6220–6230.

72. Jansen EPM, Boot H, Verheij M, et al. Optimal locoregional treatment in gastric cancer. *J Clin Oncol.* 2005;23:4509–4517.

73. Swan R, Miner TJ. Current role of surgical therapy in gastric cancer. *World J Gastroenterol.* 2006;12:372–379.

74. Dent DM, Madden MV, Price SK. Randomized comparison of R1 and R2 gastrectomy for gastric carcinoma. *Br J Surg.* 1988;75:110–112.

75. Robertson CS, Chung SC, Woods SD, et al. A prospective randomized trial comparing R1 subtotal gastrectomy with R3 total gastrectomy for antral cancer. *Ann Surg.* 1994;220:176–182.

76. Cuschieri A, Fayers P, Fielding J, et al. Postoperative morbidity and mortality after D1 and D2 resections for gastric cancer: preliminary results of the MRC randomized controlled surgical trial. The Surgical Cooperative Group. *Lancet.* 1996;347:995–999.

77. Cuschieri A, Weeden S, Fielding J, et al. Patient survival after D1 and D2 resections for gastric cancer: long-term results of the MRC randomized surgical trial. Surgical Cooperative Group. *Br J Cancer.* 1999;79:1522–1530.

78. Bonenkamp JJ, Songun I, Hermans J, et al. Randomized comparison of morbidity after D1 and D2 dissection for gastric cancer in 996 Dutch patients. *Lancet.* 1995;345:745–748.

79. Bonenkamp JJ, Hermans J, Sasako M, et al. Extended lymph node dissection for gastric cancer. Dutch Gastric Cancer Group. *N Engl J Med.* 1999;340:908–914.

80. Hartgrink HH, van de Velde CJH, Bonenkamp JJ, et al. Extended lymph node dissection for gastric cancer: who may benefit? Final results of the randomized Dutch Gastric Cancer Group Trial. *J Clin Oncol.* 2004;22:2069–2077.

81. Kodera Y, Yamamura Y, Shimizu Y, et al. Lack of benefit of combined pancreaticosplenectomy in D2 resection for proximal-third gastric carcinoma. *World J Surg.* 1997;21:622–627.

82. Siewert JR, Bottcher K, Stein HJ, et al. Relevant prognostic factors in gastric cancer: ten-year results of the German Gastric Cancer Study. *Ann Surg.* 1998;228:449–461.

83. Degiuli M, Sasako M, Calgaro M, et al. Morbidity and mortality after D1 and D2 gastrectomy for cancer: interim analysis of the Italian Gastric Cancer Study Group randomized surgical trial. *Eur J Surg Oncol.* 2004;30:303–308.

84. Smith BR, Stabile BE. Aggressive D2 lymphadenectomy is required for accurate pathologic staging of gastric adenocarcinoma. *Am Surg.* (in press).

85. Wu CW, Hsieh MC, Lo SS, et al. Comparison of the UICC/AJCC 1992 and 1997 pN categories for gastric cancer patients after surgery. *Hepatogastroenterology.* 2001;48:279–284.

86. Csendes A, Burdiles P, Rojas J, et al. A prospective randomized study comparing D2 total gastrectomy versus D2 total gastrectomy plus splenectomy in 187 patients with gastric carcinoma. *Surgery.* 2002;131:401–407.

87. Kasakura Y, Fujii M, Mochizuki F, et al. Is there a benefit of pancreaticosplenectomy with gastrectomy for advanced gastric cancer? *Am J Surg.* 2000;179:237–242.

88. Otsuji E, Yamaguchi T, Sawai K, et al. Total gastrectomy with simultaneous pancreaticosplenectomy or splenectomy in patients with advanced gastric carcinoma. *Br J Cancer.* 1999; 79:1789–1793.

89. Martin RC 2nd, Jaques DP, Brennan MF, et al. Extended local resection for advanced gastric cancer: increased survival versus increased morbidity. *Ann Surg.* 2002;236:159–165.

90. Shchepotin IB, Chorny VA, Nauta RJ, et al. Extended surgical resection in T4 gastric cancer. *Am J Surg.* 1998;175:123–126.

91. Chareton B, Landen S, Manganas D, et al. Prospective randomized trial comparing Billroth I and Billroth II procedures for carcinoma of the gastric antrum. *J Am Coll Surg.* 1996;183:190–194.

92. Fukuhara K, Osugi H, Takada N, et al. Reconstructive procedure after distal gastrectomy for gastric cancer that best prevents duodenogastroesophageal reflux. *World J Surg.* 2002;26:1452–1457.

93. Gustavsson S, Ilstrup DM, Morrison P, et al. Roux-Y stasis syndrome after gastrectomy. *Am J Surg.* 1988;155:490–494.

94. Herrington JL, Scott HW, Sawyers JL. Experience with vagotomy-antrectomy and Roux-en-Y gastrojejunostomy in surgical treatment of duodenal, gastric and stomal ulcers. *Ann Surg.* 1984;199:590–596.

95. Lawrence W Jr. Reconstruction after total gastrectomy: what is preferred technique? *J Surg Oncol.* 1996;63:215–220.

96. Morrow D, Passaro E Jr. Alkaline reflux esophagitis after total gastrectomy. *Am J Surg.* 1976;132:287–291.

97. Lehnert T, Buhl K. Techniques of reconstruction after total gastrectomy for cancer. *Br J Surg.* 2004;91:528–539.

98. Espat NJ, Karpeh MS. Reconstruction following total gastrectomy: a review and summary of the randomized prospective clinical trials. *Surg Oncol.* 1999;7:65–69.

99. Nadrowski L. Is a distal jejunojejunal pouch nutritionally ideal in total gastrectomy? *Am J Surg.* 2003;185:349–353.

100. Braga M, Zuliani W, Foppa L, et al. Food intake and nutritional status after total gastrectomy: results of a nutritional follow-up. *Br J Surg.* 1988;75:477–480.

101. Bozzetti F, Bonfanti G, Castellani R, et al. Comparing reconstruction with Roux-en-Y to a pouch following total gastrectomy. *J Am Coll Surg.* 1996;183:243–248.

102. Nash CL, Gerdes H. Methods of palliation of esophageal and gastric cancer. *Surg Oncol Clin N Am.* 2002;11:459–483.

103. Adler DG, Baron TH. Endoscopic palliation of malignant gastric outlet obstruction using self-expanding metal stents: experience in 36 patients. *Am J Gastroenterol.* 2002;97:72–78.

104. Lehnert T, Rudek B, Kienle P, et al. Impact of diagnostic laparoscopy on the management of gastric cancer: prospective study 120 consecutive patients with primary gastric adenocarcinoma. *Br J Surg.* 2002;89:471–475.

105. Velanovich V. Staging laparoscopy in the management of intra-abdominal malignancies. *Surgery.* 1998:124:773–781.

106. Kitagawa Y, Kitano S, Kubota T, et al. Minimally invasive surgery for gastric cancer – toward a confluence of two major streams: a review. *Gastric Cancer.* 2005;8:103–110.

107. Kitano S, Shiraishi N. Minimally invasive surgery for gastric tumors. *Surg Clin N Am.* 2005;85:151–164.

108. Ono H, Kondo H, Gotoda T, et al. Endoscopic mucosal resection for treatment of early gastric cancer. *Gut.* 2001;48:225–229.

109. Etoh T, Shiraishi N, Kitano S. Laparoscopic gastrectomy for cancer. *Dig Dis.* 2005;23:113–118.

110. Adrales GL, Gandsas A, Mastrangelo MJ Jr, et al. An introduction to laparoscopic gastric resection. *Curr Surg.* 2003;60:385–389.

111. Noh SH, Hyung WJ, Cheong JH. Minimally invasive treatment for gastric cancer: approaches and selection process. *J Surg Oncol.* 2005;90:188–194.

112. Huscher CG, Mingoli A, Sgarzini G, et al. Laparoscopic versus open subtotal gastrectomy for distal gastric cancer: five-year results of a randomized prospective trial. *Ann Surg.* 2005;241:232–237.

113. Kitagawa Y, Fujii H, Kumai K, et al. Recent advances in sentinel node navigation for gastric cancer: a paradigm shift of surgical management. *J Surg Oncol.* 2005;90:147–152.

114. Isozaki H, Kimura T, Tanaka N, et al. An assessment of the feasibility of sentinel lymph node-guided surgery for gastric cancer. *Gastric Cancer.* 2004;7:149–153.

115. Rosen MJ, Heniford BT. Endoluminal gastric surgery: the modern era of minimally invasive surgery. *Surg Clin N Am.* 2005;85:989–1007.

116. Haugstvedt T. Benefit of resection in palliative surgery. *Dig Surg.* 1994;11:121–125.

117. Meijer S, De Bakker OJBG, Hoitsma HFW. Palliative resection in gastric cancer. *J Surg Oncol.* 1983;23:77–80.

118. Geoghegan JG, Keane TE, Rosenberg IL. Gastric cancer: the case for selective policy in surgical management. *J R Coll Surg Endinb.* 1993;38:208–212.

119. Monson JR, Donohue JH, Mc Ilrath DC, et al. Total gastrectomy for advanced cancer: a worthwhile palliative procedure. *Cancer.* 1991;68:1863–1868.

120. Miner TJ, Jaques DP, Karpeh MS, et al. Defining palliative surgery in patients receiving noncurative resections for gastric cancer. *J Am Coll Surg.* 2004;198:1013–1021.

121. Wayne JD, Bell RH Jr. Limited gastric resection. *Surg Clin N Am.* 2005;85:1009–1020.

122. Ko YH, Han JJ, Noh JH, et al. Lymph nodes in gastric B-cell lymphoma: pattern of involvement and early histological changes. *Histopathology.* 2002;40:497–504.

123. Koch P, del Valle F, Berdel WE, et al. Primary gastrointestinal non-Hodgkin's lymphoma: combined surgical and conservative or conservative management only in localized gastric lymphoma-results of the prospective German Multicenter Study GIT NHL 01/92. *J Clin Oncol.* 2001;19:3874–3883.

124. Yoon SS, Coit DG, Portlock CS, et al. The diminishing role of surgery in the treatment of gastric lymphoma. *Ann Surg.* 2004;240:28–37.

125. Lehours P, Ruskone-Fourmestraux A, Lavergne A, et al. Groupe d'Etude des Lymphomes Digestifs (GELD) for the Federation Francaise de Cancerologie Digestive (FFCD). Which test to use to detect *Helicobacter pylori* infection in patients with low-grade gastric mucosa-associated lymphoid tissue lymphoma? *Am J Gastroenterol.* 2003;98:291–295.

126. Wootherspoon AC, Ortiz-Hidalgo C, Falzon MR, et al. *Helicobacter pylori*-associated gastritis and primary B-cell gastric lymphoma. *Lancet.* 1991;338:1175–1176.

127. Eidt S, Stolte M, Fischer R. *Helicobacter pylori* gastritis and primary gastric non-Hodgkin's lymphomas. *J Clin Pathol.* 1994;47:436–439.

128. Parsonnet J, Hansen S, Rodriguez L, et al. *Helicobacter pylori* infection and gastric lymphoma. *N Engl J Med.* 1994;330:1267–1271.

129. Hussell T, Isaacson PG, Crabtree JE, et al. The response of cells from low-grade B-cell gastric lymphomas of mucosa-associated lymphoid tissue to *Helicobacter pylori.* *Lancet.* 1993;342:571–574.

130. Isaacson PG. Gastric MALT lymphoma: from concept to cure. *Ann Oncol.* 1999;10:637–645.

131. Meining A, Stolte M, Hatz R, et al. Differing degree and distribution of gastritis in *Helicobacter pylori*-associated diseases. *Virchows Arch.* 1997;431:11–15.

132. Qin Y, Greiner A, Trunk MJ, et al. Somatic hypermutation in low-grade mucosa-associated lymphoid tissue-type B-cell lymphoma. *Blood.* 1995;86:3528–3534.

133. Du M, Peng H, Singh N, et al. The accumulation of p53 abnormalities is associated with progression of mucosa-associated lymphoid tissue lymphoma. *Blood.* 1995;86:4587–4593.

134. Stolte M, Bayerdorffer E, Morgner A, et al. *Helicobacter* and gastric MALT lymphoma. *Gut.* 2002;50(Suppl 3):III19–III24.

135. Sackman M, Morgner A, Rudolph B, et al. Regression of gastric MALT lymphoma after eradication of *Helicobacter pylori* is predicted by endosonographic staging. MALT Lymphoma Study Group. *Gastroenterology.* 1997;113:1087–1090.

136. Nakamura S, Matsumoto T, Suekane H, et al. Predictive value of endoscopic ultrasonography for regression of gastric low-grade and high-grade MALT lymphomas after eradication of *Helicobacter pylori.* *Gut.* 2001;48:454–460.

137. Rosen CB, van Heerden JA, Martin JK Jr, et al. Is an aggressive surgical approach to the patient with gastric lymphoma warranted? *Ann Surg.* 1987;205:634–640.

138. Bartlett DL, Karpeh MS, Filippa DA, et al. Long-term follow-up after curative surgery for early gastric lymphoma. *Ann Surg.* 1996;223:53–62.

139. Yahalom J. MALT lymphomas: a radiation oncology viewpoint. *Ann Hematol.* 2001;80(Suppl 3):B100–B105.

140. Martinelli G, Laszlo D, Ferreri AJ, et al. Clinical activity of rituximab in gastric marginal zone non-Hodgkin's lymphoma resistant to or not eligible for anti-*Helicobacter pylori* therapy. *J Clin Oncol.* 2005;23:1979–1983.

COMMENTARY
Peter F. Crookes

On January 29, 1881, Theodor Billroth, Professor of Surgery at the Allgemeine Krankenhaus in Vienna, performed a distal gastrectomy for a stenosing antral tumor in a woman named Therese Heller. By February 4, 1881, he had written the report announcing the event. This was a landmark article, not because he was the first to perform a gastrectomy, but because his was the first patient to survive it. In Paris in 1879, Jules Pean had attempted the operation in similar circumstances but his patient died on the fifth postoperative day, most likely of sepsis consequent to an anastomotic leak. The following year, Ludwig Rydigyer also performed a gastrectomy in an older patient who died less than 24 hours later, probably from myocardial infarction. Billroth's initial success, although a major step forward, was very short-lived: the patient died of metastatic disease a few months later. However, the lessons from this early case—the primacy of surgery in the treatment of gastric cancer, the importance of technical skill, and the dismal results of incomplete excision—are with us today, over 120 years later. This brief commentary will attempt to place the review of Drs. Stabile and Smith in the context of the broad changes that have affected medical practice since Billroth's first partial success.

The current understanding of surgical techniques to which Billroth gave the initial impetus was fueled by the clinical problem of peptic ulcer disease, an extremely prevalent disease for which there was no effective medical treatment. In the days before H_2 receptor antagonists and proton pump inhibitors and an understanding of the role of *Helicobacter pylori*, surgery was the only effective measure to treat bleeding or perforated ulcers, or the stenosis that followed eventual healing. The technical capacity of surgeons to perform safe resections of the stomach rapidly developed in the first half of the 20th century. Later improvements in survival were the result of improved anesthesia and postoperative care, including the management of fluid and electrolyte disturbances, maintenance of nutrition, and the earlier detection and treatment of sepsis. Improved oncologic resections in Western centers rode on the back of these advances in surgery for benign disease of the stomach. In Southeast Asia, especially in Japan and later in Korea, the high incidence of gastric cancer was the dominant influence in the development of modern techniques of resection, and these techniques have, to some extent, influenced Western surgeons in specialized centers where the disease is commonly treated.

CONTINUING CONTROVERSIES

There are four major controversies that have continued to plague all surgeons interested in offering optimal therapy to their patients with gastric cancer: the extent of resection, the value of excision of adjacent organs, the extent of lymphadenectomy, and the value of adjuvant therapy. Clarity is beginning to emerge in the first two areas of controversy.

Extent of Resection

As Drs. Stabile and Smith point out in their chapter, there is abundant literature to support the use of subtotal rather than total gastrectomy in distal gastric cancer, because several studies have confirmed that it provides equivalent survival provided the proximal margin is adequate (1,2). Quality of life is also superior after subtotal gastrectomy, a fact that assumes greater importance if patients are destined to survive long term after gastrectomy (3). Thus, there is now broad agreement among surgeons that distal cancers involving only the antrum and not extending above the incisura angularis may be treated by subtotal gastrectomy with survival results comparable to total gastrectomy.

Excision of Adjacent Organs

Much cancer surgery had its roots in the Halsteadian concept of cancer spread, which emphasized direct extension rather than early systemic spread. In the proximal stomach, pathologic studies of patterns of lymph node spread pointed to the importance of spread to nodes along the splenic artery and the splenic hilum. It was believed that the only way to achieve a good cancer resection was to resect the spleen and tail of pancreas (4).

In the past 15 years, several large studies have shown convincingly that removal of the spleen has an independent negative effect on long-term survival, even after allowing for the fact that patients with concurrent splenectomy tend to have more advanced tumors. In addition, concurrent removal of the tail of the pancreas with the gastric specimen is responsible for the higher rate of subphrenic abscess, pancreatic fistula, and sepsis from anastomotic leakage.

Routine adjacent organ resection with a view to obtaining a wider oncologic margin must be distinguished from en bloc resection of adjacent organs invaded by a transmural tumor, in which leaving the adjacent organ behind would result in an incomplete tumor resection. Such an en bloc resection sometimes is necessary in transmural tumors of the greater curvature that invade the transverse mesocolon. Merely excising a disc of the mesocolon risks creating an ischemic segment of colon, and consequently a transverse colectomy may be required for an oncologically adequate gastrectomy. In very distal tumors invading the first portion of the duodenum, surgeons have occasionally attempted a concurrent pancreaticoduodenectomy, but the results of this procedure are especially poor. The combination of pancreatic resection with gastrectomy and extensive lymphadenectomy is hazardous because the stripping of the pancreatic capsule during the D2 dissection jeopardizes the pancreatic anastomosis. In these advanced tumors, although it may be necessary to resect adjacent organs merely to achieve an R0 resection, it must be recognized that the biology of the tumor is advanced and the prognosis is particularly poor.

Extent of Lymphadenectomy

The stimulus to study the worth of more extensive lymphadenectomy came from the careful histologic studies of Japanese surgeons, beginning over 50 years ago, as part of their national effort to improve survival from gastric cancer. During recent decades, investigators from Japanese centers consistently have reported survival and morbidity rates that are superior to those of most Western centers. The Japanese Research Society for Gastric Cancer has not enthusiastically endorsed the concept of randomized controlled trials on the grounds that their members can perform D2 lymph node dissections with extremely low mortality, there is no measurable difference in mortality or morbidity compared with less extensive node dissections; therefore, even if a D2 dissection confers only a tiny advantage, the patient should be offered that opportunity for benefit.

The potential explanations for this difference in perspective are complex, and go to the heart of what it means to be a surgeon. The assessment of the value of surgical therapy in any disease cannot be made in the same way as assessment of medical treatment. A defined dose of a given drug has the same effect regardless of who prescribes it. Multicenter studies comparing two different drugs can still have confidence that any differences in the outcome reflect actual differences in the studied drugs. This cannot be true for surgery. The recent emphasis on quality and publicly available outcome measures championed by Birkmeyer (5) serves only to emphasize the inherent differences between different surgeons and surgical centers. The importance of surgical technique and perioperative care may be difficult to quantify but is highly relevant to interpretation of the randomized controlled trials of D1 versus D2 gastrectomy.

Four such trials have been conducted but the long-term results of the most recent are still awaited. One early single-surgeon trial of 43 patients found no difference in outcome between D1 and D2 approaches, but the sample size was too small to detect any plausible difference (6). Two much larger, multicenter trials were the British Medical Research Council trial and the Dutch trial, in which 400 and 771 patients, respectively, were randomized to D1 or D2 dissections (7,8). Neither trial showed a survival advantage and both were characterized by excessive mortality and morbidity in the patients with extended lymphadenectomy. The Dutch trial had the benefit of a Japanese surgeon who demonstrated the technique of lymphadenectomy to the participating surgeons. Nevertheless, in both trials these extensive operations were performed by surgeons and in centers where familiarity with the procedure was low. Most of the morbidity and mortality appeared to be associated with the en bloc removal of the spleen and the tail of the pancreas mandated by the existing D2 protocol for middle and upper third tumors. The mortality of the more radical procedure (13% and 10%, respectively) would now be regarded as totally unacceptable. Further, the interpretation of the results is also obscured by two surgeon-related factors: noncompliance (performing a lesser resection than allocated) and contamination (performing

a more extensive resection than allocated). The net tendency of these two factors, affecting 50% to 80% of the specimens, was to lead to homogenization of the two groups. This would have the tendency to obscure any potential advantage of one procedure over the other.

The morbidity incurred in classic D2 resections for proximal tumors led Maruyama and associates (9) to develop a modification of the technique in which the extent of the lymphadenectomy is retained, including stations 10 and 11, but the pancreas and splenic vein are preserved.

A trial in north Italy using the Maruyama modification has recently been reported by Degiuli et al. (10). This trial has the advantage that one of the principal investigators was specifically trained in the technique of lymphadenectomy at the National Cancer Center Hospital in Tokyo, Japan. Because the potential benefit of a difficult procedure may be obscured by the effect of the learning curve, a failing that is likely to be amplified in multicenter studies, strict control of the training of the participating surgeons was necessary. The early postoperative results from this group are more promising and compare favorably with the results from large Japanese centers. The same investigators have now embarked on a randomized controlled trial using only those surgeons whose learning curve could be documented. Of 163 patients randomized so far, only one died in hospital (due to intraoperative stroke), an impressive operative mortality of 0.61% (11). The long-term results of this trial when published should finally demonstrate if extended lymphadenectomy offers a survival advantage without being offset by higher perioperative mortality.

Why has it been so difficult to demonstrate what seems on the surface to be such an intuitively straightforward question? The answer seems to lie in the difficulty of standardizing the minutiae of the surgical care. Surgeons are individualistic by nature, and extended lymphadenectomy is a difficult procedure to learn. It is estimated that the learning curve is approximately 3 years, and 15 to 25 procedures are required before mortality and morbidity reaches a plateau (12). In many of the multicenter surgical trials, the number of procedures performed by each participating surgeon was well below this figure, suggesting that operations of this nature should be restricted to high-volume centers where experience is concentrated.

Future directions of study in this area include the identification of the subgroups of patients most likely to benefit. There is already evidence that there may be little or no benefit to extended lymphadenectomy for early gastric cancer. It is also logical to suppose that very advanced tumors may also not benefit. The 10-year results of the German Gastric Cancer Study showed that although there was no benefit to extended lymphadenectomy for the population as a whole, patients with stage II cancer (T2N1 or T3N0 tumors) had a marked increase in survival, from 19.9% with a D1 dissection to 49.2% after a D2 dissection employing a further modification of the technique in which both the pancreas and the spleen were preserved (13). However, it is difficult to exclude the effect of stage migration in retrospective or nonrandomized studies. More extensive lymphadenectomy will inevitably result in patients being classified as a higher stage of disease, and will artificially improve the percentage survival for each stage. This phenomenon can only be truly circumvented by randomized trials.

If these more extensive resections prove to confer a survival benefit, future studies will focus on minimally invasive approaches to the problem. Although many reports of laparoscopic D2 resections are now in print, there seems little benefit to pursuing this area of investigation until the value of extended lymphadenectomy is established. Similarly, the identification of subgroups most likely to benefit will have to await larger studies than are currently available.

Adjuvant Therapy

Both chemotherapy and radiation therapy for gastric cancer have been extensively studied in the past decade. The application of these therapies to solid tumors in the hope of achieving the benefits observed in hematologic malignancies was partly fueled by the recognition of the poor results of surgical therapy alone. In addition, newer insights into cancer biology and the recognition that systemic spread may exist for long periods before it becomes clinically or radiographically evident have led to the concept that systemic therapy may offer a curative approach to such micrometastatic disease when provided in conjunction with surgical extirpation of the primary tumor. Different solid tumors have different proclivities to disseminate: it appears to happen very early for breast cancers, whereas cancers of the head and neck tend to remain locally advanced for prolonged periods before developing systemic disease. Gastric cancer appears to fall somewhere between these extremes. The concept is attractive: systemic chemotherapy should target cancer cells beyond the reach of local therapies, and radiation therapy should facilitate subsequent surgical resection or abolish any residual locoregional disease after operation. However, both these modalities have significant side effects and complications.

Chemotherapy

Postoperative, adjuvant chemotherapy has been extensively studied, and there are at least five meta-analyses of the available studies (14). In the most recent meta-analysis, 21 trials, 17 Western and 4 Asian, were reviewed. Only in the Asian studies was any benefit observed: no survival benefit was observed in the Western studies. The reported benefits were modest at best (15).

However, the combination of preoperative and postoperative chemotherapy in early trials showed sufficient promise to prompt a randomized study of perioperative chemotherapy with epirubicin, cisplatin, and fluorouracil, compared with a group of patients treated after surgery alone. This British Medical Research Council Adjuvant Gastric Cancer Infusional Chemotherapy (MAGIC) trial is the first major study to show a clear survival benefit. Two hundred fifty patients were randomized to the chemotherapy group, and 253 to surgery alone. After a mean of 47 months of follow-up, it was clear that the chemotherapy group had both superior overall survival (hazard ratio for death, 0.75) and disease-free survival (hazard ratio for progression, 0.66) (16). Encouraging though these results are, the study raises as many questions as it answers. It was notable that only 41.6% of the patients randomized to receive chemotherapy actually received all six cycles, and less than half of those who completed the preoperative cycles received any postoperative therapy. Whether the major benefit was produced by the preop-

erative or the postoperative cycles cannot be determined from this study. In addition, the gastric cancers were more heterogeneous than in many other studies as at least a quarter of both group were tumors of the gastroesophageal junction or lower esophagus. These doubts notwithstanding, the results are sufficiently encouraging to stimulate a new generation of studies, in the most current of which patients will be randomly assigned to receive perioperative chemotherapy with epirubicin, cisplatin, and capecitabine with or without the addition of bevacizumab (Avastin), an antivascular monoclonal antibody directed against vascular endothelial growth factor (17).

Radiation Therapy

Gastric cancer is relatively resistant to radiation therapy. The dose of radiation required to treat the tumor is toxic to nearby intestine and even the spinal cord (18). Administering radiation therapy after curative resection appeared to have no benefit (19).

Chemoradiation

A major step forward was noted when radiation and chemotherapy were combined. Not only is there the potential additive effect, but some chemotherapeutic agents act as radiosensitizers. The combination of radiation (45 Gy in 25 divided doses) and fluorouracil and leucovorin beginning 20 to 40 days after surgery was adopted by the Intergroup 0116 study and reported in 2001(20). This widely publicized study showed improved survival in the chemoradiation group at 3 years (50% vs. 41% for surgery alone). The median survival was 36 months for the chemoradiation group versus 27 months for surgery alone.

One of the major problems in this study is the variation in the surgical procedure performed. A subsequent analysis of 553 of the 556 patients showed that more than half of the patients had a minimal lymphadenectomy (D0). Only 10% of the patients in the trial underwent a D2 or greater dissection. Although the trial was not designed to study the effect of lymphadenectomy, it was noteworthy that patients with D0 dissection had a median survival of 27 months, compared with 29 months for D1 dissections and 48 months for D2 or greater dissections. This study raises concern that even in major academic centers, gastrectomy with few or even no resected lymph nodes is common, and that true R0 resections may be rarer than expected. In a subsequent article, the authors conceded that "surgical undertreatment seriously undermined survival" (21).

In this context, the beneficial effects of chemoradiation may to some extent make up for inadequate surgical excision. However, it must be weighed against the fact that a large percentage of the patients receiving chemoradiation developed what was described as a major toxic effect: 54% had hematologic toxicity, 33% had major gastrointestinal toxicity, and 3 (1%) died of causes directly related to the therapy. Widespread adoption of this protocol may therefore be premature.

CONCLUSION

Although it is generally accepted that treatment of gastric cancer may best take place in the context of a multidisciplinary team, the controversies surrounding the surgical component of the therapy continue to challenge surgeons. There is already pressure in the

United States to consider postoperative chemoradiation as so well established in the management of resectable gastric cancer that a surgeon failing to offer it may be criticized for falling below the standard of care. I believe this viewpoint to be misguided. The morbidity involved in administration of chemoradiation is substantial and its superiority over adequate surgery is far from established. It should not be forgotten that even in the 21st century, the best chance for survival in gastric cancer is to have an adequate excision. Lymphadenectomy in gastric cancer may be difficult to learn, but it seems destined to join the expanding pool of operations in which there is a clear link between volume and outcome. The patient is likely to be best served by referral to a specialist with the necessary training to perform the procedure safely and with the necessary institutional infrastructure to bring the patient safely through the postoperative recovery period.

REFERENCES

1. Gouzi JL, Huguier M, Fogniez PL, et al. Total versus subtotal gastrectomy for adenocarcinoma of the gastric antrum. A French prospective controlled study. *Ann Surg.* 1989;209:162–166.
2. Bozzetti F, Marubini E, Bonfanti G, et al. Subtotal versus total gastrectomy for gastric cancer: five-year survival rates in a multicenter randomized Italian trial. Italian Gastrointestinal Tumor Study Group. *Ann Surg.* 1989;230:170–178.
3. Davies J, Johnston D, Sue-Ling H, et al. Total or subtotal gastrectomy for gastric carcinoma? A study of quality of life. World J Surg. 1998;22:1048–1055.
4. The Japanese Research Society for Gastric Cancer. The general rules for gastric cancer study in surgery and pathology. *Jpn J Surg.* 1981;11:127–145.
5. Birkmeyer JD. Understanding surgeon performance and improving patient outcomes. *J Clin Oncol.* 2004;22:2765–2776.
6. Dent DM, Madden MV, Price SK. Randomized comparison of R1 and R2 gastrectomy for gastric carcinoma. *Br J Surg.* 1988;75:110–112.
7. Cuschieri A, Weeden A, Fielding J, et al. Patient survival after D_1 and D_2 resections for gastric cancer: long-term results of the MRC randomized surgical trial. *Br J Cancer.* 1999;79:1522–1530.
8. Hartgrink HH, van de Velde CJ, Putter H, et al. Extended lymph node dissection for gastric cancer: who may benefit? Final results of the randomized Dutch gastric cancer group trial. *J Clin Oncol.* 2004;22:2069–2077.
9. Maruyama K, Sasako M, Kinoshita T, et al. Pancreas-preserving total gastrectomy for proximal gastric cancer. *World J Surg.* 1995;19;532–536.
10. Degiuli M, Sasako M, Ponti A, et al. Morbidity and mortality after D2 gastrectomy for Gastric Cancer: results of the Italian Gastric Cancer Study Group prospective Multicenter Surgical study. *J Clin Oncol.* 1998;16:1–6.
11. Degiuli M, Calvi F. Survival of early gastric cancer in a specialized European center. Which lymphadenectomy is necessary? *World J Surg.* 2006;30:2193–2203.
12. Parikh D, Chagla L, Johnson M, et al. D2 gastrectomy: lessons from a prospective audit of the learning curve. *Br J Surg.* 1996;83:1595–1599.
13. Siewert JR, Bottcher K, Stein HJ, et al. Relevant prognostic factors in gastric cancer: ten-year results of the German Gastric Cancer Study. *Ann Surg.* 1998;228:449–461.
14. Ng K, Meyerhardt JA, Fuchs CS. Adjuvant and neoadjuvant approaches in gastric cancer. *Cancer J.* 2007;13:168–174.
15. Janunger KG, Hafstrom L, Glimelius B. Chemotherapy in gastric cancer: a review and updated meta-analysis. *Eur J Surg.* 2002;168:597–608.
16. Cunningham D, Allum WH, Stenning SP, et al. Perioperative chemotherapy versus surgery alone for resectable gastroesophageal cancer. *N Engl J Med.* 2006;355:11–20.
17. Chua YJ, Cunningham D. The UK NCRI MAGIC Trial of Perioperative Chemotherapy in resectable gastric cancer: implications for clinical practice. *Ann Surg Oncol.* 2007;14:2687–2690.
18. Moertel CG, Childs DS Jr, Reitemeyer RJ, et al. Combined 5-fluorouracil and supervoltage radiation therapy of locally unresectable gastrointestinal cancer. Lancet. 1969;2:865–867.
19. Hallissey MT, Dunn JA, Ward LC, et al. The second British Stomach Cancer Group trial of adjuvant radiotherapy or chemotherapy in resectable gastric cancer: five-year follow-up. *Lancet.* 1994;343:1309–1312.
20. Macdonald JS, Smalley SR, Benedetti J, et al. Chemoradiotherapy after surgery compared with surgery alone for adenocarcinoma of the stomach or gastroesophageal junction. *N Engl J Med.* 2001;345:725–730.
21. Hundahl SA, Macdonald JS, Benedetti J, et al. Surgical treatment variation in a prospective, randomized trial of chemoradiotherapy in gastric cancer: the effect of undertreatment. *Ann Surg Oncol.* 2002;9:278–286.

34

Gastric Cancer: Perioperative Adjunctive Therapy

Howard Silberman and Syma Iqbal

Gastric carcinoma, even when clinically localized, continues to resist curative surgical extirpation despite progressively more extensive operations, including subtotal gastrectomy, total gastrectomy, radical gastrectomy with splenectomy and distal pancreatectomy, and more recently, extended nodal dissections. Current efforts are now focused on designing and testing multimodal, perioperative strategies with the aim of achieving the same salutary effects observed with combined, multidisciplinary therapies employed in the treatment of other solid tumors, such as colon and rectal cancers, anal cancer, and breast cancer.

Systemic postoperative chemotherapy (adjuvant chemotherapy) and, to a lesser extent, preoperative chemotherapy (neoadjuvant chemotherapy) have been the adjunctive approaches most commonly studied. Although numerous phase 2 protocols have shown promise in improving survival, many such regimens have failed to withstand the rigors of randomized, controlled assessment while many others still await such confirmatory trials. Other therapeutic modalities currently under investigation in the clinic or in the laboratory include external-beam irradiation, often in combination with chemotherapy, intraoperative radiotherapy (IORT), hypothermia, intraperitoneal chemotherapy, immunotherapy, angiogenesis inhibitors, and blockers of oncogene function.

PRINCIPLES OF ADJUVANT AND NEOADJUVANT THERAPY

The scientific principles underlying current protocols for adjuvant and neoadjuvant chemotherapy in connection with the surgical management of various solid tumors derive substantially from the experimental work of Skipper [1], Skipper and Schabel [2], Norton and Simon [3], and Goldie and Coldman [4]. Based on quantitative chemotherapy studies, Skipper [1] and Skipper and Schabel [2] found that each dose of a chemotherapy agent kills a constant fraction of the tumor cell population, and between cycles of treatment the residual tumor cells resume proliferation ("fractional cell kill hypothesis"). They further found that most anticancer drugs have their greatest effect on actively proliferating cells. Because the rate of cell proliferation slows and the number of nonproliferating cells increases with growth of the tumor mass, chemotherapy is most effective when the tumor burden is lowest and cell proliferation is most active. Moreover, according to the Norton-Simon [3] hypothesis, the fractional cell kill of larger, slow-growing tumors is smaller than the fractional cell kill of smaller tumors.

The foregoing concepts are the basis for predicting a beneficial effect from adjuvant chemotherapy, defined as postoperative treatment for patients in whom tumor resection has rendered them free of any discernible disease and, therefore, any disease remaining is micrometastatic. In addition, based on the fractional cell kill hypothesis, it would be expected that the highest tolerable drug doses given at the shortest intervals possible would maximize the rate of cell kill [5].

It is thought that failure of chemotherapy primarily results from the presence of drug-resistant neoplastic stem cells that arise by mutation and that the drug-resistant phenotype is inherited and propagated [4,6]. Thus, as each tumor cell divides it has a certain probability, the mutation rate, of undergoing some type of hereditable change rendering it resistant to a given chemotherapeutic agent [4]. According to Goldie and Coldman [4], the probability of developing such drug resistance substantially increases as the tumor enlarges, a concept further contributing to the rationale for treatment in the adjuvant or minimal-disease setting. In addition, this mechanism of drug resistance is the basis for recommending multiagent protocols wherein a combination of non–cross-resistant drugs are administered with the aim of reducing the probability that any individual tumor cell will be resistant to all of the drugs in the combination [4].

A drawback of adjuvant therapy is that some patients will receive this aggressive therapy who, in fact, have no residual disease after surgical resection, and, therefore, no benefit from chemotherapy can accrue. In practice, patients with a given tumor are selected for adjuvant therapy based on the likelihood of relapse after surgery alone, determined from various features of the primary tumor, such as tumor size, depth of penetration, histologic grade, lymph node involvement, and extent of surgery.

In addition, any morbidity or otherwise slow recovery from major surgery may delay the start of systemic therapy, and in this setting, lower doses may be advisable to avoid intolerable toxicity. Finally, the major indicator of the effectiveness of a therapeutic chemotherapy program, the *complete remission rate* of measurable disease, is lost in the adjuvant setting because the primary tumor has already been removed. By necessity, the treatment protocol selected for individual patients is based on response rates observed in an entirely different population of patients: those with measurable residual disease of the same histologic type. In adjuvant programs, *relapse-free survival* or *disease-free survival* and *overall survival* are the major end points [7].

Neoadjuvant chemotherapy, systemic cytotoxic treatment given *prior* to surgical resection of the primary tumor, has several potential advantages compared with adjuvant therapy. Preoperative therapy may downstage the primary tumor, thereby facilitating surgical resection, and may sterilize microscopic marginal involvement. In addition, disseminated micrometastatic disease will be addressed weeks or even several months earlier than adjuvant therapy. Because tumor response to preoperative systemic treatment is measurable, neoadjuvant therapy serves as an in vivo chemosensitivity assay. A significant response indicates that the drug regimen is appropriate and, in addition, may be useful postoperatively. Lack of significant response indicates the need to choose another regimen or to proceed to surgery. Rapid progression of disease in the face of neoadjuvant therapy may identify a tumor so aggressive that a patient can be spared nontherapeutic surgery and its concomitant morbidity.

A disadvantage of neoadjuvant therapy is that it obscures accurate pathologic staging. In addition, surgical resection of the primary tumor is necessarily delayed and any undue toxicity further postpones operation with the possibility of disease progression in the interim.

REVIEW OF CLINICAL TRIALS IN GASTRIC CANCER

Adjuvant Systemic Chemotherapy

Adjuvant therapy of gastric cancer using an array of cytotoxic agents, administered singly or in combination, has been widely tested within the last 3 decades. Although chemotherapy alone following gastric resection has failed to consistently produce a clinically significant survival benefit among patients studied in the Western world (8,9), several randomized trials have reported positive results, but none so convincing as to establish the treatment protocol studied as standard of care (10–14).

In 1982, the Gastrointestinal Tumor Study Group (10) reported the results of a clinical trial in which 142 patients who had undergone curative gastric resection for adenocarcinoma were randomized to receive adjuvant methyl-CCNU and 5-fluorouracil (5-FU) or close observation only. After a median follow-up period of 4 years, a survival advantage appeared to be associated with the adjuvant therapy ($p < 0.03$). Median survival for the control patients was 33 months, whereas it was estimated to be in excess of 4 years in the treated group. Unfortunately, these favorable results were not confirmed in trials with the same agents subsequently reported from the Veterans Administration Surgical Oncology Group (15) and the Eastern Cooperative Oncology Group (16).

In 1991, Estape et al. (12) published the outcome of their randomized trial of adjuvant mitomycin C. Thirty-three patients received the drug and 37 patients were managed with surgery only. After 5 years of follow-up, the actuarial survival curve was statistically in favor of the adjuvant therapy ($p < 0.001$), a benefit that was sustained at 10 years ($p < 0.01$). Seventeen of 33 treated patients (52%) and 6 of 37 untreated patients (16%) were alive at 10 years. Patients with stage T3N0M0 disease benefited most. The most frequent site of relapse was the peritoneal cavity.

Neri et al. (13,14) studied the subset of resected patients with positive nodes. The experimental group received adjuvant epidoxorubicin, 5-FU, and leucovorin. At 3 years, 25% of treated patients but only 13% of control patients were alive. At that point, the median survival was 20.4 months versus 13.6 months in the treated and untreated groups, respectively, a statistically significant difference. In a follow-up report issued in 2001 after 5 years of follow-up (13), median survival time was 31 months versus 18 months in favor of the treated patients ($p < 0.01$).

Cirera et al. (11) assessed the efficacy of intravenous mitomycin in combination with oral tegafur in 148 patients with resected stage III disease. Analysis of this phase 3 trial after a median follow-up period of 37 months revealed that overall survival and disease-free survival were higher in the group of patients randomized to receive the chemotherapy ($p = 0.04$ for survival; $p = 0.01$ for disease-free survival). The overall 5-year survival rate and the 5-year disease-free survival rate were, respectively, 56% and 51% in the treatment group and 36% and 31% in the surgery-only control group.

In contrast to these studies reporting statistical benefit, modern adjuvant trials reported by Macdonald et al. (17) in 1995, Bajetta et al. (18) in 2002 and Chipponi et al. (19) in 2004 failed to demonstrate any favorable impact. Thus, in a phase 3 trial sponsored by the Southwest Oncology Group (17), 193 patients with resected stage I, II, or III disease were randomized to receive 1 year of 5-FU, doxorubicin, and mitomycin (FAM) or observation only. The two groups, accrued between 1978 and 1991, did not differ in disease-free survival ($p = 0.45$) or in overall survival ($p = 0.57$).

Similarly, in a randomized trial of 274 patients with locally advanced gastric cancer, the Italian Trials in Medical Oncology Group reported no significant survival difference with adjuvant etoposide, doxorubicin, and cisplatin followed by fluorouracil and folinic acid in comparison with surgery alone (18).

Chipponi et al. (19) compared treatment with adjuvant folinic acid, 5-FU, and cisplatinum with surgery only in a group of patients with positive nodes or serosal involvement, all of whom had undergone curative operations. The surgeons were free to perform D1 or D2 resections and any type of gastrectomy according to the site of the tumor. The 101 patients in the drug-treated group did not fare better than the 104 patients who had surgery alone. The 5-year survival rate was 39% in both groups.

The selected clinical trials described here serve to illustrate the heterogeneity of the patient populations studied, the wide array of drug protocols evaluated, the lack of uniformity in the extent of surgery, as well as the widely variable duration of observation and the inconsistent statistical and clinical results. Even the trials showing *statistical* benefit of adjuvant therapy were associated with disappointing *clinical* outcomes given the fact that in all adjuvant trials eligible patients are deemed to have been rendered free of disease by the surgical operation performed.

In an effort to resolve the inconclusive and conflicting results of the many randomized trials reported, data from these studies have been pooled and reanalyzed in seven published meta-analyses (9,20–25). In meta-analyses of randomized controlled studies, a combined or summary odds ratio and 95% confidence interval (CI) is calculated. An odds ratio with 95% CI of <1.0 is evidence of a statistically significant beneficial effect of the experimental treatment. An odds ratio of 1.0 indicates no effect of treatment, and a value >1.0 indicates a harmful effect.

Nakajima et al. (25) combined data from 1,177 patients entered into ten trials that were performed at the Cancer Institute Hospital in Tokyo. The pooled odds ratio was 0.63 with a 95% CI of 0.51-0.78, suggesting a survival benefit from the adjuvant chemotherapy employed, mitomycin C and/or 5-FU.

In 1993, Hermans et al. (26) published a meta-analysis of data from 2,096 patients evaluated in 11 randomized trials assessing the worth of primarily 5-FU–based adjuvant treatment versus surgery alone. The overall odds ratio of 0.88 with a 95% CI of 0.78-1.08 indicated that the postoperative drug therapy offered no significant survival benefit. However, the investigators (21) revised their conclusions the following year, based on the addition to their analysis of 318 patients from two relevant trials that had been inadvertently omitted. The new calculations, now based on 2,414 patients in 13 trials, yielded an odds ratio of 0.82 (95% CI: 0.68-0.98) indicating a statistically significant survival benefit. Nevertheless, the authors concluded that the evidence was insufficient to adopt such treatment as standard of care.

In 1999, Earle and Maroun (20) performed a meta-analysis of 13 trials into which 1,990 patients had been entered. Studies from Asian countries were excluded. The adjuvant treatment consisted of a 5-FU plus anthracycline-containing regimen in 6 of the 13 trials, and in 7 the regimens contained 5-FU and/or mitomycin C and/or a nitrosourea. The odds ratio was 0.80 (95% CI: 0.66-0.97), indicating that the adjuvant therapy appeared to confer a small survival benefit over surgery alone, but the results were of borderline statistical significance. In a subset analysis, the authors found that the beneficial effect appeared to be greater in node-positive patients, an observation consistent with that reported in the adjuvant treatment of patients with breast and colon cancer. The exclusion of Asian patients in this report, especially those from Japan, reflects the commonly held view that gastric cancer appears to behave more favorably in the Asian setting, possibly because of different biology, etiology, or surgical treatment.

In a report from Italy in 2000, Mari and associates (24) pooled data from 20 studies involving 3,658 patients comparing adjuvant postoperative chemotherapy with surgery alone. Three studies used single-agent chemotherapy, seven used a combination of 5-FU with an anthracycline, and ten a combination of 5-FU without anthracyclines. Chemotherapy reduced the risk of death by 18% (hazard ratio, 0.82, 95% CI: 0.75-0.89; p <0.001). The authors concluded that chemotherapy produces a small survival benefit in patients with curatively resected gastric cancer. They further stated, however, that taking into account the limitations of literature-based meta-analyses, adjuvant chemotherapy should still to be considered an investigational treatment.

In 2002, Janunger and associates (23) in Sweden published a meta-analysis of 21 trials in which 3,962 patients were randomized. A small but significant survival benefit for the treated patients was identified with an odds ratio of 0.84 (95% CI: 0.74-0.96). However, when Western and Asian studies were analyzed separately, no survival advantage was observed in the Western groups (odds ratio, 0.96; 95% CI: 0.83-1.12), and a benefit was

observed in the Asian trials (odds ratio, 0.58; 95% CI: 0.44-0.76), again emphasizing the apparent difference in the biology of gastric cancers arising in Western and Asian populations.

Panzini et al. (9) selected 17 trials for inclusion in a meta-analysis with a total of 3,118 patients. Similar to other meta-analyses, this 2002 report demonstrates a small but statistically significant advantage in survival with adjuvant chemotherapy (odds ratio, 0.72; 95% CI: 0.62-0.84).

In a meta-analysis published in December 2002, Hu et al. (22) pooled results from 14 English and Chinese language randomized trials involving 4,543 patients. A significant advantage was observed in favor of adjuvant therapy (odds ratio, 0.56; 95% CI: 0.40-0.79).

Thus, each of the seven meta-analyses reviewed here identifies an apparent statistical survival benefit associated with the administration of adjuvant chemotherapy after tumor resection compared with surgery alone. Nevertheless, for a variety of reasons, there is a general reluctance to conclude that chemotherapy should be routinely prescribed after curative gastric resection. For example, the favorable outcome observed in one of the seven analyses does not provide independent confirmation of the benefit observed in the others, as there is considerable overlap in the randomized trials selected for inclusion in the seven meta-analyses. In some of the studies, the favorable effect was of marginal statistical significance. In addition, when Asian patients are excluded from the analyses, the beneficial effect appears to be lost, again suggesting a biologic or epidemiologic variability in the disease between Asian and Western populations. Finally, Hu et al. (22) expressed the opinion that many of the randomized trials included in the various meta-analyses had methodologic flaws, thereby reducing the quality of the pooled data.

In a report published in 2007 by Sakuramoto and associates (27), and therefore subsequent to and consequently not included in the published meta-analyses, a salutary effect of adjuvant S-1 was described, again raising the hope of an effective adjuvant therapy. S-1 is an orally active combination of tegafur (a prodrug that is converted by cells to fluorouracil), gimeracil (an inhibitor of dihydropyrimidine dehydrogenase, which degrades fluorouracil), and oteracil (which inhibits the phosphorylation of fluorouracil in the gastrointestinal tract, thereby reducing the gastrointestinal toxic effects of fluorouracil). In the trial conducted by these investigators, 1,059 patients in Japan with stage II or III gastric cancer who underwent gastrectomy resulting in no residual tumor (R0 resection) with extended (D2) lymph node dissection were randomly assigned to undergo surgery followed by adjuvant therapy with S-1 or to undergo surgery only. In the S-1 group, administration of S-1 was started within 6 weeks after surgery and continued for 1 year. The trial was stopped on the recommendation of the independent data and safety monitoring committee because the first interim analysis, performed 1 year after enrollment was completed, showed that the S-1 group had a higher rate of overall survival than the surgery-only group ($p = 0.002$). Analysis of follow-up data showed that the 3-year overall survival rate was 80.1% in the S-1 group and 70.1% in the surgery-only group. The hazard ratio for death in the S-1 group, as compared with the surgery-only group, was 0.68 (95% CI: 0.52-0.87; $p = 0.003$). The authors concluded that S-1 is an effective adjuvant treatment, at least for East

Asian patients with locally advanced gastric cancer who have undergone curative surgery including a D2 lymphadenectomy.

Adjuvant Intraperitoneal Chemotherapy

The rationale for adjuvant intraperitoneal (IP) chemotherapy is based on the observation that the peritoneum is the site of first relapse in approximately 50% of patients following an apparently curative gastric resection (28). Several modern studies have been published evaluating the hypothesis that postresection IP chemotherapy will reduce intra-abdominal relapse and thereby improve survival compared with surgery alone.

In an attempt to prevent peritoneal recurrence, intraperitoneal hyperthermic chemoperfusion (IHCP) treatment with mitomycin C was combined with aggressive surgery by Fujimoto and associates (29) in Japan. Between March 1987 and December 1996, 141 gastric carcinoma patients with macroscopic serosal invasion were randomly allocated to one of two groups. Seventy-one patients underwent IHCP combined with surgery (IHCP group) and the remaining 70 patients underwent surgery alone (control group). IHCP was performed just after gastric resection and alimentary tract reconstruction under general anesthesia along with systemic hyperthermia. The authors found that the peritoneal recurrence rate in the IHCP group was significantly decreased ($p = 0.0000847$) compared with that in the control group. The 2-year, 4-year, and 8-year survival rates for the IHCP group were 88%, 76%, and 62%, respectively, whereas those for the control group were 77%, 58%, and 49%, respectively. The IHCP group thus enjoyed a significant survival benefit ($p = 0.0362$) compared with the control group.

From 1990 to 1995, Yu and associates (30) recruited a series of 248 Korean patients with biopsy-proven gastric cancer who were then randomized intraoperatively to receive early postoperative IP with mitomycin C on day 1 and 5-FU on postoperative days 2 through 5 (125 patients) versus surgery only (123 patients). Gastric resection plus early postoperative IP chemotherapy was associated with improved overall survival compared with surgery only (54% and 38%, respectively; $p = 0.0278$). There were statistically significant differences in patients with stage III (57% and 23%, respectively; $p = 0.0024$) and in those with stage IV (28% and 5%, respectively; $p = 0.0098$) gastric cancer. The improvement in survival rate was statistically significant for the subgroup of patients with gross serosal invasion (52% and 25%, respectively; $p = 0.0004$) and patients with lymph node metastasis (46% and 22%, respectively; $p = 0.0027$). These findings updated and confirmed these investigators' earlier work presented before the American Surgical Association in 1998 (31). The authors suggest that gross serosal invasion with or without frozen section evaluation of lymph nodes could be used as the major selection criterion for recommending early postoperative IP chemotherapy.

Korean investigators Kim and Bae (32) attempted to capitalize on in vitro observations that hyperthermia potentiates the effect of chemotherapeutic agents. Thus, a protocol was designed to evaluate the worth of IHCP in preventing and treating peritoneal metastasis after surgical resection of stomach cancer. In this trial, the authors studied 103 serosa-invasive gastric carcinoma patients who underwent surgical resection between 1990 and 1995. Fifty-two patients who underwent surgery plus IHCP were compared with 51 patients who underwent surgery only. IHCP was administered for 2 hours with an automatic IHCP device (closed-circuit system) just after surgical resection, with the patient under hypothermic general anesthesia (32.4°C to 34.0°C). The perfusate consisted of 1.5% peritoneal dialysis solution mixed with 10 mcg/mL of mitomycin C, warmed at an inflow temperature of over 44°C. The overall 5-year survival rate of the 103 patients was 29.97%. The 5-year survival rate was higher in the IHCP group than in the control group, at 32.7% and 27.1%, respectively, but this difference was not significant. However, among the 65 patients remaining with serosa-invasive gastric carcinoma after excluding those patients with stage IV disease, the 5-year survival was significantly higher ($p = 0.0379$) in the IHCP group than in the control group, at 58.6% and 44.4%, respectively.

In a similar study, Yonemura and associates (33) studied adjuvant IP chemotherapy with and without hyperthermia in patients with locally advanced disease. In this three-armed randomized trial, 139 Japanese patients with T2-4 gastric tumors underwent curative gastrectomy with extended lymphadenectomy. These patients were randomly allocated into the following three groups. Patients in the *CHPP* group received surgery plus chemohyperthermic peritoneal perfusion, and those in the *CNPP* group underwent surgery plus chemonormothermic peritoneal perfusion. The third, control, group underwent surgery alone. In the CHPP and CNPP groups, the peritoneal cavity was perfused using an extracorporeal circulation machine with 6 to 8 liters of saline containing 30 mg of mitomycin C and 300 mg of cisplatin and heated either to 42°C to 43°C or 37°C, respectively. Overall 5-year survival rates for the CHPP, CNPP, and surgery-alone groups were 61%, 43%, and 42%, respectively. In a subset analysis, patients with gastric cancer having serosal invasion or lymph node metastasis had a statistically significant improvement in survival when treated with chemohyperthermic peritoneal perfusion. However, chemonormothermic peritoneal perfusion had no survival benefit. By analyzing with the Cox proportional hazard model, chemohyperthermic peritoneal perfusion emerged as an independent prognostic factor for good survival. Surgery alone was associated with a threefold higher risk of death than chemohyperthermic peritoneal perfusion. The authors concluded that chemohyperthermic peritoneal perfusion with mitomycin C and cisplatin is indicated for patients with tumors infiltrating the serosal layer or node-positive disease.

The salutary effects of IP therapy in Asian patients in the reports previously cited were not confirmed in trials conducted in non-Asian patients. Sautner et al. (34) evaluated IP therapy with cisplatin. In this prospective randomized trial from the University of Vienna, 67 patients undergoing surgery for stage III and IV gastric cancer were randomized to one of two groups: 33 patients underwent adjuvant postoperative IP therapy with cisplatin, and 34 control subjects received no further treatment after surgical resection. Patients in the treatment group received a median of four IP therapy perfusions. The median disease-free survival was 12.7 months and 9.7 months in treated patients and controls, respectively ($p = 0.8$). After a median follow-up duration of 72 months, 54 patients (80%) had died of primary disease or related complications. The median survival for IP therapy patients was 17.3 months as compared with 16.0 months for controls ($p = 0.6$). Autopsies were performed on 12 (18%) of 54 patients who died, and showed tumor spread to the peritoneal cavity and/or to the liver, irrespective of the application of IP therapy. The authors concluded that adjuvant IP therapy with cisplatin is ineffective in patients with stage III and IV gastric cancer. The authors speculated that reasons for ineffectiveness of IP therapy may be the choice of an unsuitable chemotherapeutic agent, an inefficient method of administration, or a lack of sufficient drug penetration into the serosa or peritoneal metastasis.

In another report from Austria, the Austrian Working Group for Stomach Cancer (35) initiated a phase 3 trial assessing the worth of IP mitomycin for patients with tumors infiltrating the serosa. After radical gastric resection, 91 patients were randomized to the surgery-only control group or the experimental group, which received 50 mg of mitomycin bound to activated carbon particles intraperitoneally prior to closure of the surgical incision. Unfortunately, increased postoperative morbidity and mortality observed in the treated cohort with no apparent long-term survival benefit led the investigators to terminate further recruitment of patients.

Topuz and associates (36), in a series from Istanbul published in 2002, also described disappointing results with IP therapy. In this phase 2 trial, patients with stage II to III gastric cancer received a 2-liter IP solution of cisplatin, mitoxantrone, 5-FU, and folinic acid every 4 weeks for six cycles. Toxicity was limited, but after a median follow-up period of 23 months, survival rates appeared to be similar to those observed in patients previously treated with surgery alone.

In 2004, a meta-analysis evaluating IP chemotherapy in patients undergoing curative resection for locally advanced gastric cancer was published by Xu et al. (37). The analysis included 11 trials (2 from Austria, 4 from Japan, 4 from China, and one from Korea) involving 1,161 patients. The pooled odds ratio was 0.51 (95% CI: of 0.40-0.65), leading the authors to conclude that IP chemotherapy may confer a survival advantage, and further, that the combination of IP chemotherapy with hyperthermia or activated carbon particles may provide an additional benefit from the enhanced antitumor activity of the drugs employed.

Adjuvant Radiotherapy

In a prospective randomized trial conducted in the United Kingdom by Allum et al. (38) and Hallissey and associates (39), 153 patients with operable gastric cancer received postoperative radiotherapy and 145 patients were allocated to surgery only. Radiotherapy was given by parallel opposed anteroposterior/posteroanterior portals, including the splenic hilum on the left and the porta hepatis on the right. A midline dose of 4,500 Gy was given in 25 fractions over 35 days with the option of a further 500-Gy boost to a reduced field. After a minimum follow-up of 5 years, no survival advantage was observed in the treated group. The 5-year for surgery-alone was 20% and for surgery plus radiotherapy, only 12%.

Intraoperative radiotherapy (IORT) has been evaluated as an adjuvant modality that may improve survival by reducing locoregional relapse (40). Compared with external-beam radiotherapy, IORT allows the delivery of an increased radiation dose to the tumor bed while sparing exposure to surrounding structures. In 1993, investigators at the National Cancer Institute (41) reported the results of a prospectively randomized controlled

clinical trial comparing surgical resection and IORT with conventional therapy. Patients in the experimental group underwent gastrectomy after which IORT was administered to the gastric bed (20 Gy using 11 to 15 MeV electrons). Patients in the control group underwent gastrectomy alone for early-stage lesions confined to the stomach (stages I to II) or resection and postoperative external-beam radiotherapy to the upper abdomen (50 Gy using 6 to 10 mV photons) for advanced-stage lesions extending beyond the gastric wall (stages III to IV). One hundred patients were screened for the study, of whom 60 were randomized and underwent exploratory surgery. Nineteen patients were excluded intraoperatively because of unresectability or metastatic disease, leaving 41 patients in the study. Seven patients (17%) died of complications. The median survival for patients with tumors of all stages was 25 months for the IORT group and 21 months for the control group ($p = 0.99$). Locoregional disease failures occurred in 7 of 16 IORT patients (44%) and in 23 of 25 control patients (92%; $p < 0.001$). Complication rates were similar between IORT and control patients. Thus, IORT failed to afford a significant advantage over conventional therapy in overall survival, but IORT did significantly improve control of locoregional disease.

In another trial conducted by Abe and associates (42) patients were randomized to a surgery-only control group or to an experimental group to receive IORT. Again, no improvement in survival was observed between the two groups. However, there was a trend to improved survival in the subset of patients with serosal invasion and nodal disease beyond the perigastric (N1) echelon of lymph nodes.

Adjuvant Chemoradiation

Because of the apparent limited or inconsistent clinical effectiveness of adjuvant protocols providing chemotherapy only, on the one hand, and the demonstrated benefit of combined modality therapy with radiation and fluorinated pyrimidine in patients with known residual gastric and esophageal carcinoma on the other hand, a United States Intergroup Trial (SWOG-9008/INT0116) was initiated in 1991 to test whether the combination of 5-FU, leucovorin, and radiation after surgical resection would be of value to patients with resected gastric carcinoma (43,44). All patients entered into the trial had gastric surgery in which all detectable disease was excised and the margins of resection were microscopically free of tumor. The extent of regional lymphadenectomy was not standardized. A D0 lymphadenectomy (a partial N1 dissection) was performed in 54% of the patients; a D1 lymphadenectomy in 36%, and a D2 lymphadenectomy in 10%.

Of the 556 patients entered into the study, 281 were randomly allocated to the adjuvant chemoradiotherapy arm of the trial and 275 to the surgery-only arm. About two thirds of the patients in both arms had stage T3 or T4 tumors, and 85% had nodal metastases. The patients randomized to the adjuvant treatment group received 425 mg of fluorouracil per square meter of body surface area per day, plus 20 mg of leucovorin per square meter per day, for 5 days, followed by 4,500 cGy of radiation at 180 cGy per day, given 5 days per week for 5 weeks, with modified doses of fluorouracil and leucovorin on the first 4 and the last 3 days of radiotherapy. One month after the completion of radiotherapy, two 5-day cycles of fluorouracil (425 mg/m^2 per day) plus leucovorin (20 mg/m^2 per square meter per day) were given 1 month apart.

After a median follow-up period of 5 years, statistical analysis of the data indicated that disease-free and overall survival were significantly improved by this combined modality protocol with 5-FU, leucovorin, and radiation therapy. Median time to relapse was 30 months in the treatment arm versus 19 months in the control arm ($p < 0.001$; two-sided p value). Overall survival was also improved, with a median survival of 36 months in the treatment arm versus 27 months in the control arm ($p = 0.005$; two-sided p value). The 3-year overall survival rates were 50% in the chemoradiotherapy group and 41% in the surgery-only group. The corresponding 3-year rates for relapse-free survival were 48% and 31%, respectively. Toxicity associated with the adjuvant treatment included grade 3 toxic effects in 41% of the patients and grade 4 toxic effects in 32%. Three patients (1%) died from the adverse effects of the chemoradiation. The significant salutary effects observed led the authors to recommend that this combined-modality adjuvant treatment program be adopted as the standard of care for patients with high-risk, resectable gastric cancer.

In a critique of the study, Falcone (45) raised the question as to whether the benefit observed was simply compensation for the limited lymphadenectomy performed in most of the patients. This concern was based on data from the study that suggested that the survival benefit achieved appeared to have been derived primarily from improved local control rather than a reduction in the risk of distant metastases. The authors of the trial, however, thought this interpretation unlikely because no randomized trials conducted among non-Asian patients have proven a survival benefit attributable to extended lymphadenectomy (46,47). In another review of this Intergroup study, Hundahl and associates (48) obtained complete surgical information for the participants in the trial and calculated the Japanese Maruyama Index of Unresected Disease. These calculations led the authors to conclude that the surgical undertreatment observed in the trial adversely affected survival.

In another critique of the Intergroup trial, Leong (49) and Leong and associates (50) acknowledged the significant advantages achieved with the treatment protocol employed but expressed concerns about the considerable toxicity that occurred. They suggested that use of newer-generation cytotoxic agents and modern conformal techniques of radiation delivery may improve the outcome with less toxicity. Thus, these investigators designed a prospective phase 1 trial in which they evaluated the toxicity and feasibility of an alternative chemoradiation regimen. A total of 26 patients with adenocarcinoma of the stomach were treated with three-dimensional conformal radiation therapy to a dose of 45 Gy in 25 fractions with concurrent continuous infusional, rather than bolus, 5-FU. The majority of patients received epirubicin, cisplatin, and 5-FU as the systemic component given before and after concurrent chemoradiation. The overall rates of observed grade 3 and 4 toxicities were 38% and 15%, respectively. Gastrointestinal grade 3 toxicity was observed in 19% of patients, and hematologic grade 3 and 4 toxicities were observed in 23%. The authors concluded that their adjuvant regimen could be delivered safely and with acceptable toxicity, and, therefore, should be studied further.

Adjuvant Chemoimmunotherapy

The benefit of combined adjuvant chemotherapy and immunotherapy employing a streptococcal preparation, OK-432, in patients with curatively resected gastric cancer was assessed by Sakamoto and associates (51). These Japanese investigators conducted a meta-analysis of data derived from 1,522 patients enrolled in six randomized clinical trials. All six trials began between 1985 and 1993, and patients were followed for at least 3 years after surgery and enrollment of the last patient. In these trials, adjuvant chemotherapy, usually consisting of induction with mitomycin C plus long-term oral fluorinated pyrimidines, was compared with the same chemotherapy plus OK-432. OK-432 is a lyophilized preparation of a low virulence group A *Streptococcus pyogenes* (Su strain) of human origin that is inactivated by treatment with benzyl penicillin and heat. Administration of OK-432 has been reported to induce various cytokines, such as tumor necrosis factor-α, interferon-γ, interleukin (IL)-8, IL-12, granulocyte colony-stimulating factor, and granulocyte-macrophage colony-stimulating factor. OK-432 has also been shown to enhance cytotoxicity against autologous cells. The 3-year survival rate for all eligible patients in the six trials was 67.5% in the chemoimmunotherapy group versus 62.6% in the chemotherapy-only group. The 3-year overall survival odds ratio was 0.81 (95% CI: 0.65-0.99). The beneficial treatment effect was shown to be statistically significant ($p = 0.044$). The results of this meta-analysis were interpreted by the authors to suggest that chemoimmunotherapy after surgery with OK-432 can improve the survival of patients with successfully resected gastric cancer.

Neoadjuvant Therapy

Various preoperative treatment strategies have been studied with the goal of improving survival by downstaging the primary gastric tumor, thereby increasing the likelihood of achieving complete surgical resection with clear margins, and by controlling any micrometastatic disease.

Neoadjuvant Radiotherapy

In a randomized phase III study from China, 370 patients with apparently resectable adenocarcinoma of the gastric cardia were assigned to receive preoperative radiation therapy followed by surgery or surgery alone (52). The 10-year survival rate was higher in the radiotherapy group (20.26% vs. 13.3%; P = 0.009) as was the resection rate (89.5% vs. 79.4%, P < 0.01).

In another trial employing preoperative radiation (53), Skoropad and associates randomly assigned 78 patients to surgery alone or to an experimental regimen of preoperative radiation therapy (20 Gy), gastrectomy and intraoperative radiation therapy (20 Gy). No benefit was seen in patients with early stage disease, but a significant survival advantage was associated with the combined treatment in patients with node-positive disease (P = 0.04) or extragastric extension of the tumor (P = 0.042).

Neoadjuvant Chemotherapy

Investigators at New York University (54) studied the role of neoadjuvant CPT-11 (irinotecan) and cisplatin in downstaging locally advanced gastric cancer. Preoperative staging was performed with a combination of computed tomography scans, endoscopic ultrasonography and/or laparoscopy, and laparoscopic ultrasonography. Patients with locally advanced disease determined by preoperative clinical staging were eligible for entry. Neoadjuvant therapy consisted of two cycles of CPT-11 (75 mg/m^2) with cisplatin (25 mg/m^2) weekly 4 times every 6 weeks. This was followed by resection with D2 lymph node dissection. Twenty-two patients were entered into the study (four with T3N0 disease and 18 with T3N1 disease). Induction chemotherapy was well tolerated, with major toxicities being neutropenia and diarrhea. Two patients withdrew consent during the first cycle and were lost to follow-up. One patient progressed to stage IV disease during induction chemotherapy and did not undergo surgery. Nineteen patients underwent surgery. One patient had undetected stage IV disease (liver) and underwent a palliative R2 resection. Of the 18 remaining patients, 17 had curative R0 resections and one had a palliative R1 resection. A median of 21 lymph nodes (range, 1 to 121) were examined histologically. There was one postoperative death. Surgical morbidity did not appear to increase after the neoadjuvant regimen. Postoperative pathologic staging yielded 16% T3 lesions compared with 85% before treatment based on clinical staging; postoperative American Joint Committee on Cancer staging yielded 37% stage IIIA disease compared with 70% stage IIIA before treatment. The authors concluded that CPT-11-based neoadjuvant therapy downstages locally advanced gastric cancer.

In subsequent report from the same institution (55), the postoperative morbidity and mortality of the same neoadjuvant regimen was assessed. A total of 34 patients with locally advanced gastric cancer were placed on a phase 2 neoadjuvant chemotherapy protocol consisting of two cycles of CPT-11 (75 mg/m^2) with cisplatin (25 mg/m^2). Morbidity and mortality data were compared for these patients (CHEMO) versus 85 patients undergoing gastrectomy without neoadjuvant chemotherapy (SURG). Fifty-two percent of SURG patients had T3 or T4 tumors compared with 19% of CHEMO patients, consistent with tumor downstaging. The R0 resection rate was similar (80%). Morbidity was 41% in CHEMO patients and 39% in SURG patients. There were five postoperative deaths (4.4%), two in the CHEMO group and three in the SURG group ($p = $ NS). Thus, neoadjuvant chemotherapy with CPT-11 and cisplatin was not associated with increased postoperative morbidity compared with surgery alone.

Lowy and associates (56) at the University of Texas M.D. Anderson Cancer Center reported the results of three consecutive phase 2 trials using multiagent neoadjuvant chemotherapy to treat patients with potentially resectable gastric carcinoma. Among the 83 patients treated, 25 received etoposide, 5-FU, and cisplatin; 34 received etoposide, doxorubicin, and cisplatin; and 24 received 5-FU, alpha-interferon, and cisplatin. Patients remaining free of radiographic evidence of metastatic disease 4 to 6 weeks after completing the chemotherapy underwent a gastrectomy and a D2 lymphadenectomy with splenic preservation. A "curative" resection, defined as removal of all gross disease with negative pathologic margins, was achieved in 61 of the 83 patients studied. The clinical course of these 61 patients was correlated with the clinical and pathologic response to the preoperative drug therapy. There were 24 responders (39%) and 37 nonresponders (61%). A "responder" was defined as a patient in whom there was a >50% reduction in bidimensional tumor diameter on upper gastrointestinal series and computed tomography scan (clinical response) or in whom serial hematoxylin

and eosin-stained histologic sections revealed <10% viable tumor cells (pathologic response). Responders had an actuarial 5-year survival of 83% versus 31% for nonresponders (p <0.05). The median survival for nonresponders was 20 months, whereas the median survival for responders had not been reached at a median follow-up of 26 months. The authors cautioned that while these favorable results are encouraging, they must be interpreted carefully because they represent pooled data from three independent, nonrandomized prospective trials. For example, it is possible that the preoperative treatment served primarily to identify patients with biologically favorable tumors that would have been just as successfully treated with surgery alone.

Less encouraging results from the Netherlands were published in 2004 by Hartgrink and associates (57). These investigators performed a randomized trial comparing preoperative 5-FU, doxorubicin, and methotrexate (FAMTX) with surgery alone in order to evaluate the effect of this drug regimen on resectability and survival. A total of 59 patients with gastric cancer, excluding those with early (T1) tumors, were randomized to receive four courses of chemotherapy using FAMTX prior to surgery or to undergo surgery alone. Twenty-nine patients were allocated to the FAMTX regimen prior to surgery and 30 patients had surgery alone. Resectability rates were equal for both groups. A complete or partial response was achieved in 32% of the FAMTX group. With a median follow-up of 83 months, the median survival since randomization was 18 months in the FAMTX group versus 30 months in the surgery-alone group ($p = 0.17$). This trial, therefore, did not demonstrate a beneficial effect of preoperative FAMTX.

Neoadjuvant Chemoradiotherapy

Ajani and associates (58) designed a neoadjuvant protocol that called for the combination of preoperative drug therapy with preoperative radiotherapy. A multi-institutional study of the chemoradiotherapy regimen was then conducted to assess the R0 resection rate, the pathologic complete and partial response rates, and the safety and survival in patients with resectable gastric carcinoma. Patients with early-stage, T1N0, tumors or metastatic disease were excluded. Pretreatment staging was assessed by laparoscopy and endoscopic ultrasonography (EUS). Patients received up to two 28-day cycles of preoperative induction chemotherapy with fluorouracil, leucovorin, and cisplatin, followed by 45 Gy of radiation plus concurrent fluorouracil. Patients were then scheduled for surgery. Thirty-four patients were registered at three institutions. One ineligible patient was excluded. Most patients had disease staged T3N1 by EUS. Twenty-eight (85%) of 33 patients actually underwent surgery. The R0 resection rate was 70% and pathologic complete response rate was 30%. A pathologic partial response (<10% residual carcinoma in the primary) occurred in eight patients (24%). Comparison of the pretreatment T and N staging by EUS with the postoperative pathologic staging indicated that the neoadjuvant therapy was associated with significant downstaging (p <0.01). The median survival time for 33 patients was 33.7 months. Patients achieving a complete or partial pathologic response had a significantly longer median survival time (63.9 months) than those who did not (12.6 months; $p = 0.03$). There were two treatment-related deaths.

The authors concluded that their three-step strategy of preoperative induction chemotherapy followed by chemoradiotherapy and then surgery resulted in substantial pathologic responses that resulted in durable survival times. They thought that this preoperative regimen should next be compared with postoperative adjuvant chemoradiotherapy.

Combined Neoadjuvant and Adjuvant Therapy

Generally disappointing results achieved with preoperative or postoperative adjunctive therapy alone have led various investigators to test protocols providing therapy both before and after gastric resection.

Kelson and associates (59) identified a group of patients with apparently operable gastric cancer but at high risk for recurrence, based on staging with EUS. A cohort of such patients at the Memorial Sloan-Kettering Cancer Center was enrolled into a trial of combined preoperative neoadjuvant systemic chemotherapy and postoperative IP and systemic chemotherapy. In this phase 2 protocol, neoadjuvant therapy with FAMTX was given for three courses before planned laparotomy with the intention to perform curative resection. Postoperatively, IP cisplatin and 5-FU and intravenous 5-FU were administered to patients undergoing resection.

Fifty-six assessable patients were treated. Preoperative FAMTX therapy was tolerable, with the major toxicity being neutropenic fever. One treatment-related death was seen. Eighty-nine percent of patients underwent surgical exploration and 61% had potentially curative resections. There were two postoperative deaths. Comparison of pathologic tumor stage with EUS-predicted tumor stage showed apparent downstaging in 51% of patients. Postoperative IP chemotherapy was delivered to 75% of eligible patients. Toxicity was acceptable. There was no increase in operative morbidity or mortality compared with concurrent nonstudy patients undergoing a similar operative procedure and not receiving preoperative therapy. With a median follow-up time of 29 months, the median survival duration was 15.3 months. For patients who underwent potentially curative resections, the median survival duration was 31 months. Peritoneal failure was seen in 16% of patients.

The authors concluded that chemotherapy with the FAMTX regimen appears tolerable in patients with locally advanced gastric cancer, without an increase in operative morbidity or mortality. They further stated that IP therapy can be successfully delivered to most resected patients, and, with the protocol employed, the intra-abdominal failure pattern appears to be decreased compared with expected.

Crookes et al. (60) at the University of Southern California, employing a different combination of agents, also designed a protocol that called for preoperative systemic and postoperative IP chemotherapy. Fifty-nine patients who were deemed resectable for cure were entered into a clinical trial that called for two cycles of protracted infusion 5-FU with weekly leucovorin and cisplatin chemotherapy followed by surgery. Approximately 3 to 4 weeks after potentially curative surgery, patients were scheduled to receive two cycles of IP 5-fluoro-2′deoxyuridine and cisplatin.

Fifty-eight of the 59 patients studied (98%) received both cycles of systemic chemotherapy. Fifty-six patients (95%) underwent surgery: 40 patients (71%) had resections intended to

cure for stage 0 to IIIB disease, 15 patients (27%) had palliative surgery for stage IV gastric carcinoma, and one patient died intraoperatively without being staged. Two patients refused surgery, and the remaining patient died of progressive disease prior to surgery. Thirty-one of the 40 patients who underwent curative surgery completed both cycles of postoperative IP therapy; four patients received only one cycle. Three patients (5%) died secondary to treatment complications. There were two operative deaths, and one patient died of peritonitis associated with grade 4 granulocytopenia. Nine of the 40 patients (23%) whose carcinomas were resected for cure had recurrent carcinoma. With a median follow-up period exceeding 45 months, the calculated median survival for the 59 patients entered into the trial exceeded 4 years.

Thus, this combined pre- and postoperative regimen was found to be safe and appeared to decrease the gastric carcinoma recurrence rate, 23% here, in contrast to recurrence rates in the range of 60% to 70% in other reported prospective trials (8). Survival also appeared to be increased compared with historic controls.

Weese and associates (61) also conducted a trial of combined perioperative adjunctive therapy, in this case employing radiation as the postoperative adjuvant modality designed to reduce locoregional relapse. Variables evaluated included toxicity, response rate, locoregional control, and survival of a cohort of patients presenting with locally advanced disease. Patients with stage IIIA or early-stage IV gastric adenocarcinoma received neoadjuvant 5-FU, leucovorin, Adriamycin, and cisplatin, then underwent gastrectomy or esophagogastrectomy followed by IORT (1,000 cGY) to the gastric bed and postoperative radiation therapy. The authors reported that 9 of 15 patients (60%) with nodal metastases or transmural disease received IORT. There were two pathologically complete responses at the primary site. Eleven of 15 patients (73%) had tumor in perigastric lymph nodes; however, 9 of 15 patients (60%) had mucin-filled nodes without tumor cells. The treatment provided did not increase operative morbidity rates. Ten of 15 patients (67%) remained free of disease after a median follow-up period of 27 months (range, 6 to 60 months). Five patients died 13 to 41 months (median, 17 months) after diagnosis. The authors concluded that their program of multimodality pre- and postoperative therapy is safe, can downstage tumors, provides improved locoregional control, and appears to cause significant tumor regression that may result in long-term survival or cure.

In 2006, Cunningham and associates (62) reported the impressive beneficial effect of perioperative chemotherapy that was observed in the British Medical Research Council Adjuvant Gastric Infusional Chemotherapy (MAGIC) Trial. This trial was designed to assess whether the addition of a perioperative regimen of epirubicin, cisplatin, and infused fluorouracil to surgery improves outcomes among patients with potentially curable gastric cancer. The investigators randomly assigned 503 patients with resectable adenocarcinoma of the stomach (n = 372), esophagogastric junction (n = 58), or lower esophagus (n = 73) to either perioperative chemotherapy and surgery (250 patients) or surgery alone (253 patients).

Chemotherapy consisted of three preoperative and three postoperative cycles of intravenous epirubicin (50 mg/m² of body surface area) and cisplatin (60 mg/m²) on day 1, and a continuous intravenous infusion of fluorouracil (200 mg/m² per day) for 21 days. Surgery was scheduled to take place within 6 weeks after randomization in the surgery group and 3 to 6 weeks after completion of the third cycle of chemotherapy in the perioperative chemotherapy group. Postoperative chemotherapy was to be started 6 to 12 weeks after surgery. The primary end point was overall survival.

At the time of analysis, the median follow-up was 49 months in the perioperative-chemotherapy group and 47 months in the surgery group. Postoperative morbidity and mortality were similar in the two groups. As compared with the surgery group, the perioperative-chemotherapy group had a significantly higher likelihood of progression-free survival (hazard ratio for progression, 0.66; 95% CI: 0.53-0.81; p <0.001), and of overall survival (hazard ratio for death, 0.75; 95% CI: 0.60-0.93; p = 0.009). Five-year survival rates were 36.3% (95% CI: 29.5%–43.0%) among patients in the perioperative-chemotherapy group and 23.0% (95% CI: 16.6%–29.4%) among those in the surgery group. This estimated improvement of 13 percentage points in the five-year survival rate corresponds to a 25% reduction in the risk of death.

In addition, significant downstaging was observed. Thus, the median maximum diameter of resected tumors was smaller in the perioperative-chemotherapy group than in the surgery group (3 vs. 5 cm; p <0.001). This finding was thought to be consistent with tumor shrinkage in the chemotherapy group. Among all patients undergoing resection, there was a greater proportion of stage T1 and T2 tumors in the perioperative-chemotherapy group than in the surgery group (51.7% vs. 36.8%; p = 0.002 by the chi-square test for trend). Also, among patients with gastric cancer, there was a significant trend to less advanced nodal disease (i.e., N0 or N1) in the perioperative-chemotherapy group than in the surgery group (84.4% vs. 70.5%; p = 0.01 by the chi-square test for trend).

The authors point out that since the inception of the MAGIC trial, several new chemotherapy agents have become available. Currently, the oral fluoropyrimidine prodrug capecitabine and the nonnephrotoxic platinum compound oxaliplatin are being evaluated as substitutes for infused fluorouracil and cisplatin, respectively, in patients with previously untreated advanced esophagogastric cancer (63).

PRECLINICAL AND LABORATORY INVESTIGATIONS

Modulation of Tumoral Angiogenesis

Folkman (64,65) discovered that the growth of solid tumors and the formation of metastases depend on angiogenesis, manifest by the growth of new microvessels that converge on the tumor. The apparent effectiveness associated with the addition of the angiogenesis inhibitor bevacizumab (Avastin) to chemotherapy regimens in the management of colorectal, lung, and breast cancers (66) has led to investigations into the role of angiogenesis in gastric cancer and the possible therapeutic role of antiangiogenesis agents.

Erenoglu and associates (67) conducted a study to investigate the correlation between microvessel count (MVC), as a quantitative measure of angiogenesis, and various clinicopatho-

logic features in gastric carcinoma in order to evaluate the role of angiogenesis on the prognosis of gastric cancer and the rationale for testing adjuvant antiangiogenesis therapy. Fifty-seven patients who underwent surgical intervention for gastric carcinoma between 1993 and 1997 were reviewed retrospectively. The relationship between MVC and various clinicopathologic features was assessed. The effect of angiogenesis on overall survival and the role of MVC and other prognostic factors on distant metastases were assessed by multivariate analysis. Microvessels were outlined by antifactor VIII, which is a specific monoclonal antibody to factor VIII in vessel endothelial cells, and counted under light microscopy. There was no correlation between MVC and age or sex of the patient, duration of symptoms, or tumor size. However, proximally located, undifferentiated, diffuse type, serosal invasion-positive, lymph node invasion-positive, advanced stage, or distantly metastasized tumors had higher MVCs. Higher MVCs affected the overall survival adversely. Lymph node metastasis, serosal invasion, and MVC were found as independent prognostic factors affecting distant metastases. MVC was the sole factor affecting recurrent liver metastasis.

Maeda and associates (68) in Osaka, Japan, also observed a correlation between tumor angiogenic activity and progression of gastric carcinoma, again using immunohistochemical staining with antifactor VIII antibody. The MVC was determined in 124 specimens resected from patients with gastric carcinoma. Correlations between the MVC, various clinicopathologic factors, and prognosis were studied. The investigators found that the MVC increased with histologic stage and also was significantly higher in patients with lymph node metastases than in those without nodal disease. Moreover, in patients with a high MVC the prognosis was significantly poorer than in those with a low count. Multivariate analysis indicated that the MVC was an independent prognostic factor in patients with gastric cancer. Consistent with the report of Erenoglu et al. (67), these investigators found that the frequency of hepatic metastases was significantly increased in patients with a high MVC.

Thus, patients with a high MVC appear to be an appropriate population for the study of antiangiogenesis therapy. Several animal studies have demonstrated the effectiveness of angiogenesis inhibitors in reducing in the rate of tumor growth in gastric cancer models. Kanai and coworkers (69) studied the effect of the angiogenesis inhibitor TNP-470 on the progression of tumor growth in nude mice bearing orthotopically xenotransplanted human gastric cancers. The experimental data indicated that this agent not only slowed the growth of the primary tumor but was also effective in preventing liver metastases and peritoneal dissemination.

Using a similar experimental model, Teicher and associates (70) reported that treatment of nude mice with human gastric cancer xenografts with a protein kinase C (PKC) beta inhibitor resulted in a decrease in intratumoral microvessels and reduced tumor growth. These investigators also showed that the antitumor effect of gemcitabine was significantly enhanced when this cytotoxic agent was administered simultaneously with the PKC inhibitor.

In view of the apparent efficacy of bevacizumab in other solid tumors, Shah and colleagues (66) conducted a multicenter phase 2 trial to assess the safety and efficacy of the addition of bevacizumab to chemotherapy with irinotecan and cisplatin in the treatment of 47 patients with metastatic gastric or gastroesophageal junction adenocarcinoma. The authors concluded that bevacizumab can be safely given with chemotherapy in such patients, and they observed an apparent improvement is response rate, time to disease progression, and overall survival compared with historical controls.

Analysis of Molecular Markers

Evidence is emerging that analysis of various molecular markers may be a guide to identifying therapeutic agents apt to be effective in a given patient. For example, Ott and associates (71) evaluated microsatellite alterations and *p53* mutation status in biopsy material obtained from gastric tumors prior to any therapy. These investigators found that a high level of chromosomal instability defined a subset of patients who were more likely to benefit from cisplatin-based neoadjuvant chemotherapy. In contrast, in this study *p53* mutation status was not a useful marker for response prediction.

At the University of Southern California, investigators found that the gene expression of the enzyme thymidylate synthase (TS) within a gastric tumor had an inverse relationship to response and survival in patients receiving 5-FU-based chemotherapy (72). Thus, tumors that express low TS levels would be likely to benefit from 5-FU-based therapy, whereas limited preliminary data suggest that patients whose tumors express high TS levels may benefit from irinotecan (CPT-11) (73). The University of Southern California group also reported that the relative messenger ribonucleic acid (mRNA) level of the excision repair cross-complementing (*ERCC1*) gene was inversely associated with response and survival as an independent function of cisplatin efficacy (74).

Based on the observation that amplification or overexpression of the *erbB-2* oncogene, present in at least 20% of gastric cancers, is associated with an aggressive clinical course and poor prognosis, Kasprzyk and coworkers (75) evaluated the potential therapeutic effect of interfering with *erbB-2* function using monoclonal antibodies. In this study, the investigators demonstrated that a combination of two anti-*erbB-2*-specific antibodies inhibited the growth of human gastric tumor cells in vitro. This combination antibody therapy also inhibited the growth of human gastric tumor cell lines growing as xenografts in nude mice and was able to dramatically reduce established tumors.

Antisense Therapy

The concept underlying antisense therapy is that the effects of any particular gene might be blocked by administering a single-stranded oligodeoxynucleotide (ODN) with a sequence complementary to that of the gene's specific mRNA. By binding selectively to the mRNA, the antisense ODN would block its ability to synthesize protein and, consequently, would block the function of that particular gene (76). Kim and associates (77) studied antisense *bcl-2* in nude mice bearing tumors derived from xenotransplanted human cancer cells. The protein bcl-2 inhibits anticancer drug-induced apoptosis. Overexpression of *bcl-2* has been associated with drug resistance in various human malignancies, and overexpression has been observed in human gastric cancers. In this study, the antitumor effect of cisplatin and paclitaxel was significantly enhanced in the group of tumor-bearing mice that received these drugs in combination with antisense *bcl-2*.

CURRENT TREATMENT RECOMMENDATIONS AND STRATEGIES FOR THE FUTURE

Surgical resection remains the key component in the current treatment of gastric carcinoma; however, it is clear that improved outcome for patients even with apparently localized disease will depend not on more radical surgical extirpation (46,47) but on a coordinated, multidisciplinary effort engaging clinicians in surgical, medical, and radiation oncology, basic scientists, and medical statisticians.

At the present time, patients referred to the University of Southern California's Kenneth Norris Jr. Comprehensive Cancer Center with localized, resectable gastric cancer referred *prior* to surgical resection are offered the adjuvant chemoradiation program of postoperative 5-FU, leucovorin, and radiation that was shown effective in the United States Intergroup Trial (43,44) or the combined preoperative and postoperative regimen of epirubicin, cisplatin, and infusional 5-FU described in the British MAGIC trial (62). Patients referred *after* curative surgical resection are offered the postoperative chemoradiation regimen.

Further improvements in outcome await the results of various clinical trials now underway to test the safety and potential antitumor efficacy of new agents or, more likely, new combinations of agents and modalities in the optimal temporal relationship to the core surgical operation. Customizing chemotherapy based on the analysis of intratumoral molecular markers that correlate with drug efficacy needs to be pursued not only to identify the most appropriate therapy but also to avoid the toxicity of agents destined to be ineffective.

The new concept of targeted therapy, such as inhibition of tumor angiogenesis, is exciting based both on the original theoretical considerations of Folkman (64,65), favorable outcome in early clinical trials, and promising experience in the laboratory. It is hoped that bench research on antisense therapy, monoclonal antibodies, immunotherapy, and biologicals such as the interferons, interleukins, and vaccines will yield additional novel approaches to treatment, using agents administered alone or in combination with other therapies.

REFERENCES

1. Skipper HE. Laboratory models: some historical perspective. *Cancer Treat Rep.* 1986;70:3–7.
2. Skipper HE, Schabel FM Jr, Wilcox WS. Experimental evaluation of potential anticancer agents. Xiii. On the criteria and kinetics associated with "curability" of experimental leukemia. *Cancer Chemother Rep.* 1964;35:1–111.
3. Norton L, Simon R. The Norton-Simon hypothesis revisited. *Cancer Treat Rep.* 1986;70:163–169.
4. Goldie JH, Coldman AJ. A mathematic model for relating the drug sensitivity of tumors to their spontaneous mutation rate. *Cancer Treat Rep.* 1979;63:1727–1733.

5. Smith M, Chabner B. Systemic chemotherapy of solid tumors. In: Bland K, Daly J, Karakousis C, eds. *Surgical Oncology: Contemporary Principles & Practice.* New York: McGraw-Hill; 2001:147–158.

6. Carter S, Bakowski M, Hellmann K. *Chemotherapy of Cancer.* 3rd ed. New York: John Wiley & Sons; 1987.

7. Chu E, DeVita Jr VT. Principles of cancer management: chemotherapy. In: DeVita Jr VT, Hellman S, Rosenberg SA, eds. *Cancer: Principles & Practice of Oncology.* 6th ed. Philadelphia: Lippincott Williams & Wilkins; 2001:289–306.

8. Macdonald JS. Treatment of localized gastric cancer. *Semin Oncol.* 2004;31:566–573.

9. Panzini I, Gianni L, Fattori PP, et al. Adjuvant chemotherapy in gastric cancer: a meta-analysis of randomized trials and a comparison with previous meta-analyses. *Tumori.* 2002;88:21–27.

10. Controlled trial of adjuvant chemotherapy following curative resection for gastric cancer. The Gastrointestinal Tumor Study Group. *Cancer.* 1982;49:1116–1122.

11. Cirera L, Balil A, Batiste-Alentorn E, et al. Randomized clinical trial of adjuvant mitomycin plus tegafur in patients with resected stage III gastric cancer. *J Clin Oncol.* 1999;17:3810–3815.

12. Estape J, Grau JJ, Lcobendas F, et al. Mitomycin C as an adjuvant treatment to resected gastric cancer. A 10-year follow-up. *Ann Surg.* 1991;213:219–221.

13. Neri B, Cini G, Andreoli F, et al. Randomized trial of adjuvant chemotherapy versus control after curative resection for gastric cancer: 5-year follow-up. *Br J Cancer.* 2001;84:878–880.

14. Neri B, de Leonardis V, Romano S, et al. Adjuvant chemotherapy after gastric resection in node-positive cancer patients: a multicentre randomised study. *Br J Cancer.* 1996;73:549–552.

15. Higgins GA, Amadeo JH, Smith DE, et al. Efficacy of prolonged intermittent therapy with combined 5-FU and methyl-CCNU following resection for gastric carcinoma. A Veterans Administration Surgical Oncology, Group report. *Cancer.* 1983;52:1105–1112.

16. Engstrom PF, Lavin PT, Douglass HO Jr, et al. Postoperative adjuvant 5-fluorouracil plus methyl-CCNU therapy for gastric cancer patients. Eastern Cooperative Oncology Group study (EST 3275). *Cancer.* 1985;55:1868–1873.

17. Macdonald JS, Fleming TR, Peterson RF, et al. Adjuvant chemotherapy with 5-FU, adriamycin, and mitomycin-C (FAM) versus surgery alone for patients with locally advanced gastric adenocarcinoma: a Southwest Oncology Group study. *Ann Surg Oncol.* 1995;2:488–494.

18. Bajetta E, Buzzoni R, Mariani L, et al. Adjuvant chemotherapy in gastric cancer: 5-year results of a randomised study by the Italian Trials in Medical Oncology (ITMO) Group. *Ann Oncol.* 2002;13:299–307.

19. Chipponi J, Huguier M, Pezet D, et al. Randomized trial of adjuvant chemotherapy after curative resection for gastric cancer. *Am J Surg.* 2004;187:440–445.

20. Earle CC, Maroun JA. Adjuvant chemotherapy after curative resection for gastric cancer in non-Asian patients: revisiting a meta-analysis of randomised trials. *Eur J Cancer.* 1999;35:1059–1064.

21. Hermans J, Bonenkamp JJ. Meta-analysis of adjuvant chemotherapy in gastric cancer–in reply. *J Clin Oncol.* 1994;12:878–880.

22. Hu JK, Chen ZX, Zhou ZG, et al. Intravenous chemotherapy for resected gastric cancer: meta-analysis of randomized controlled trials. *World J Gastroenterol.* 2002;8:1023–1028.

23. Janunger KG, Hafstrom L, Glimelius B. Chemotherapy in gastric cancer: a review and updated meta-analysis. *Eur J Surg.* 2002;168:597–608.

24. Mari E, Floriani I, Tinazzi A, et al. Efficacy of adjuvant chemotherapy after curative resection for gastric cancer: a meta-analysis of published randomised trials. A study of the GISCAD (Gruppo Italiano per lo Studio dei Carcinomi dell'Apparato Digerente). *Ann Oncol.* 2000;11:837–843.

25. Nakajima T, Ota K, Ishihara S, et al. Meta-analysis of 10 postoperative adjuvant chemotherapies for gastric cancer in CIH. *Jpn J Cancer Chemother.* 1994;21:1800–1805.

26. Hermans J, Bonenkamp JJ, Boon MC, et al. Adjuvant therapy after curative resection for gastric cancer: meta-analysis of randomized trials. *J Clin Oncol.* 1993;11:1441–1447.

27. Sakuramoto S, Sasako M, Yamaguchi T, et al. Adjuvant chemotherapy for gastric cancer with S-1, an oral fluoropyrimidine. *N Engl J Med.* 2007;357:1810–1820.

28. Sugarbaker PH, Yu W, Yonemura Y. Gastrectomy, peritonectomy, and perioperative intraperitoneal chemotherapy: the evolution of treatment strategies for advanced gastric cancer. *Semin Surg Oncol.* 2003;21:233–248.

29. Fujimoto S, Takahashi M, Mutou T, et al. Successful intraperitoneal hyperthermic chemoperfusion for the prevention of postoperative peritoneal recurrence in patients with advanced gastric carcinoma. *Cancer.* 1999;85:529–534.

30. Yu W, Whang I, Chung HY, et al. Indications for early postoperative intraperitoneal chemotherapy of advanced gastric cancer: results of a prospective randomized trial. *World J Surg.* 2001;25:985–990.

31. Yu W, Whang I, Suh I, et al. Prospective randomized trial of early postoperative intraperitoneal chemotherapy as an adjuvant to resectable gastric cancer. *Ann Surg.* 1998;228:347–354.

32. Kim JY, Bae HS. A controlled clinical study of serosa-invasive gastric carcinoma patients who underwent surgery plus intraperitoneal hyperthermo-chemo-perfusion (IHCP). *Gastric Cancer.* 2001;4:27–33.

33. Yonemura Y, de Aretxabala X, Fujimura T, et al. Intraoperative chemohyperthermic peritoneal perfusion as an adjuvant to gastric cancer: final results of a randomized controlled study. *Hepatogastroenterology.* 2001;48:1776–1782.

34. Sautner T, Hofbauer F, Depisch D, et al. Adjuvant intraperitoneal cisplatin chemotherapy does not improve long-term survival after surgery for advanced gastric cancer. *J Clin Oncol.* 1994;12:970–974.

35. Rosen HR, Jatzko G, Repse S, et al. Adjuvant intraperitoneal chemotherapy with carbon-adsorbed mitomycin in patients with gastric cancer: results of a randomized multicenter trial of the Austrian Working Group for Surgical Oncology. *J Clin Oncol.* 1998;16:2733–2738.

36. Topuz E, Basaran M, Saip P, et al. Adjuvant intraperitoneal chemotherapy with cisplatinum, mitoxantrone, 5-fluorouracil, and calcium folinate in patients with gastric cancer: a phase II study. *Am J Clin Oncol.* 2002;25:619–624.

37. Xu DZ, Zhan YQ, Sun XW, et al. Meta-analysis of intraperitoneal chemotherapy for gastric cancer. *World J Gastroenterol.* 2004;10:2727–2730.

38. Allum WH, Hallissey MT, Ward LC, et al. A controlled, prospective, randomised trial of adjuvant chemotherapy or radiotherapy in resectable gastric cancer: interim report. British Stomach Cancer Group. *Br J Cancer.* 1989;60:739–744.

39. Hallissey MT, Dunn JA, Ward LC, et al. The second British Stomach Cancer Group trial of adjuvant radiotherapy or chemotherapy in resectable gastric cancer: five-year follow-up. *Lancet.* 1994;343:1309–1312.

40. Scaife CL, Calvo FA, Noyes RD. Intraoperative radiotherapy in the multimodality approach to gastric cancer. *Surg Oncol Clin North Am.* 2003;12:955–964.

41. Sindelar WF, Kinsella TJ, Tepper JE, et al. Randomized trial of intraoperative radiotherapy in carcinoma of the stomach. *Am J Surg.* 1993;165:178–187.

42. Abe M, Nishimura Y, Shibamoto Y. Intraoperative radiation therapy for gastric cancer. *World J Surg.* 1995;19:544–547.

43. Macdonald JS. Clinical overview: adjuvant therapy of gastrointestinal cancer. *Cancer Chemother Pharmacol.* 2004;54(Suppl 1):S4–11.

44. Macdonald JS, Smalley SR, Benedetti J, et al. Chemoradiotherapy after surgery compared with surgery alone for adenocarcinoma of the stomach or gastroesophageal junction. *N Engl J Med.* 2001;345:725–730.

45. Falcone A. Future strategies and adjuvant treatment of gastric cancer. *Ann Oncol.* 2003;14(Suppl 2):ii 45–47.

46. D'Angelica M, Gonen M, Brennan MF, et al. Patterns of initial recurrence in completely resected gastric adenocarcinoma. *Ann Surg.* 2004;240:808–816.

47. Hartgrink HH, van de Velde CJ, Putter H, et al. Extended lymph node dissection for gastric cancer: who may benefit? Final results of the randomized Dutch gastric cancer group trial. *J Clin Oncol.* 2004;22:2069–2077.

48. Hundahl SA, Macdonald JS, Benedetti J, et al. Surgical treatment variation in a prospective, randomized trial of chemoradiotherapy in gastric cancer: the effect of undertreatment. *Ann Surg Oncol.* 2002;9):278–286.

49. Leong T. Evolving role of chemoradiation in the adjuvant treatment of gastric cancer. *Expert Rev Anticancer Ther.* 2004;4:585–594.

50. Leong T, Michael M, Foo K, et al. Adjuvant and neoadjuvant therapy for gastric cancer using epirubicin/cisplatin/5-fluorouracil (ECF) and alternative regimens before and after chemoradiation. *Br J Cancer.* 2003;89:1433–1438.

51. Sakamoto J, Teramukai S, Nakazato H, et al. Efficacy of adjuvant immunochemotherapy with OK-432 for patients with curatively resected gastric cancer: a meta-analysis of centrally randomized controlled clinical trials. *J Immunother.* 2002;25:405–412.

52. Zhang ZX, Gu XZ, Yin WB, et al. Randomized clinical trial on the combination of preoperative irradiation and surgery in the treatment of adenocarcinoma of gastric cardia (AGC)–report on 370 patients. *Int J Radiat Oncol Biol Phys.* 1998;42:929–934.

53. Skoropad VY, Berdov BA, Mardynski YS, et al. A prospective, randomized trial of pre-operative and intraoperative radiotherapy versus surgery alone in resectable gastric cancer. *Eur J Surg Oncol.* 2000;26:773–779.

54. Newman E, Marcus SG, Potmesil M, et al. Neoadjuvant chemotherapy with CPT-11 and cisplatin downstages locally advanced gastric cancer. *J Gastrointest Surg.* 2002;6:212–223.

55. Marcus SG, Cohen D, Lin K, et al. Complications of gastrectomy following CPT-11-based neoadjuvant chemotherapy for gastric cancer. *J Gastrointest Surg.* 2003;7:1015–1023.

56. Lowy AM, Mansfield PF, Leach SD, et al. Response to neoadjuvant chemotherapy best predicts survival after curative resection of gastric cancer. *Ann Surg.* 1999;229:303–308.

57. Hartgrink HH, van de Velde CJ, Putter H, et al. Neo-adjuvant chemotherapy for operable gastric cancer: long term results of the Dutch randomised FAMTX trial. *Eur J Surg Oncol.* 2004;(30):643–649.

58. Ajani JA, Mansfield PF, Janjan N, et al. Multi-institutional trial of preoperative chemoradiotherapy in patients with potentially resectable gastric carcinoma. *J Clin Oncol.* 2004;22:2774–2780.

59. Kelsen D, Karpeh M, Schwartz G, et al. Neoadjuvant therapy of high-risk gastric cancer: a phase II trial of preoperative FAMTX and postoperative intraperitoneal fluorouracil-cisplatin plus intravenous fluorouracil. *J Clin Oncol.* 1996;14:1818–1828.

60. Crookes P, Leichman CG, Leichman L, et al. Systemic chemotherapy for gastric carcinoma followed by postoperative intraperitoneal therapy: a final report. *Cancer.* 1997;79:1767–1775.

61. Weese JL, Harbison SP, Stiller GD, et al. Neoadjuvant chemotherapy, radical resection with intraoperative radiation therapy (IORT): improved treatment for gastric adenocarcinoma. *Surgery.* 2000;128:564–571.

62. Cunningham D, Allum WH, Stenning SP, et al. Perioperative chemotherapy versus surgery alone for resectable gastroesophageal cancer. *N Engl J Med.* 2006;355:11–20.

63. Sumpter K, Harper-Wynne C, Cunningham D, et al. Report of two protocol planned interim analyses in a randomised multicentre phase III study comparing capecitabine with fluorouracil and oxaliplatin with cisplatin in patients with advanced oesophagogastric cancer receiving ECF. *Br J Cancer.* 2005;92:1976–1983.

64. Folkman J. What is the evidence that tumors are angiogenesis dependent? *J Natl Cancer Inst.* 1990;82:4–6.

65. Folkman J. Antiangiogenesis agents. In: DeVita V Jr, Hellman S, Rosenberg S, eds. *Principles and Practice of Oncology,* 6th ed. Philadelphia: Lippincott Williams and Wilkins; 2001:509–519.

66. Shah MA, Ramanathan RK, Ilson DH, et al. Multicenter phase II study of irinotecan, cisplatin, and bevacizumab in patients with metastatic gastric or gastroesophageal junction adenocarcinoma. *J Clin Oncol.* 2006;24:5201–5206.

67. Erenoglu C, Akin ML, Uluutku H, et al. Angiogenesis predicts poor prognosis in gastric carcinoma. *Dig Surg.* 2000;17:581–586.

68. Maeda K, Chung YS, Takatsuka S, et al. Tumor angiogenesis as a predictor of recurrence in gastric carcinoma. *J Clin Oncol.* 1995;13:477–481.

69. Kanai T, Konno H, Tanaka T, et al. Effect of angiogenesis inhibitor TNP-470 on the progression of human gastric cancer xenotransplanted into nude mice. *Int J Cancer.* 1997;71:838–841.

70. Teicher BA, Menon K, Alvarez E, et al. Antiangiogenic and antitumor effects of a protein kinase C beta inhibitor in human hepatocellular and gastric cancer xenografts. *In Vivo.* 2001;15:185–193.

71. Ott K, Vogelsang H, Mueller J, et al. Chromosomal instability rather than p53 mutation is associated with response to neoadjuvant cisplatin-based chemotherapy in gastric carcinoma. *Clin Cancer Res.* 2003;9:2307–2315.

72. Lenz HJ, Leichman CG, Danenberg KD, et al. Thymidylate synthase mRNA level in adenocarcinoma of the stomach: a predictor for primary tumor response and overall survival. *J Clin Oncol.* 1996;14:176–182.

73. Leichman CG. Thymidylate synthase as a predictor of response. *Oncology (Williston Park).* 1998;12(8 Suppl 6):43–47.

74. Metzger R, Leichman CG, Danenberg KD, et al. ERCC1 mRNA levels complement thymidylate synthase mRNA levels in predicting response and survival for gastric cancer patients receiving combination cisplatin and fluorouracil chemotherapy. *J Clin Oncol.* 1998;16:309–316.

75. Kasprzyk PG, Song SU, Di Fiore PP, et al. Therapy of an animal model of human gastric cancer using a combination of anti-erbB-2 monoclonal antibodies. *Cancer Res.* 1992;52:2771–2776.

76. Applebaum F. Targeted cancer therapy. In: Foley J, Vose J, Armitage J, eds. *Current Therapy in Cancer.* 2nd ed. Philadelphia: WB Saunders; 1999:523–33.

77. Kim R, Emi M, Tanabe K, et al. Preclinical evaluation of antisense bcl-2 as a chemosensitizer for patients with gastric carcinoma. *Cancer.* 2004;101:2177–2186.

COMMENTARY
John S. Macdonald

Drs. Silberman and Iqbal have provided an exhaustive and very timely review of approaches to adjunctive therapies to surgery in patients with resectable gastric adenocarcinomas. It is essential for clinicians to be aware of the applicable therapeutic strategies that may increase survival in patients with gastric cancers because these tumors will occur in over 900,000 people throughout the world each year (1).

Drs. Silberman and Iqbal delve into the clinical science of strategies employed over the last 30 years to increase the cure rate in patients with resectable gastric cancer. Not only do they provide a very complete cataloguing of what has been done, but they also give some insight into why clinical investigations in this area have very infrequently yielded compelling results. The authors also demonstrate how clinical trials might have been done better in patients with resectable stomach cancer.

There has been a plethora of approaches taken, including pre and postoperative chemotherapy and external-beam irradiation, and intraperitoneal chemotherapy with and without hyperthermia. Also, various schemes of immunotherapy have been evaluated. As noted by Drs. Silberman and Iqbal, all of these approaches were translated into clinical trials and had reasonable rationales that were potentially testable in well-designed clinical investigations. As also noted by the authors, most of these research concepts failed in clinical trials to produce any result that had an impacted on the standard of care in patients with resectable gastric cancer. Why was this the case? Were the ideas bad? Were the methods flawed? The fault, I am afraid, lies with us who do the clinical research and the methods we use, or in some cases, misuse. Many scientifically interesting concepts like intraperitoneal therapy, for example, were evaluated in relatively small phase 2 trials and never brought to adequate phase 3 evaluation. It is a fact that standards of care in medicine are almost universally changed only by level I evidence (2)—evidence that can only be derived from well-designed, well-powered, phase 3 clinical trials performed in carefully characterized patient populations. Unfortunately, the landscape of clinical research in gastric cancer is littered with phase 2 results that were never brought to phase 3 evaluation and with phase 3 trials that were underpowered to detect a clinically reasonable difference and therefore doomed to failure.

I also must add a word about meta-analysis. Drs. Silberman and Iqbal reference at least seven meta-analyses. The results of these meta-analyses almost always show benefit for the therapy under evaluation. With all these "statistically positive" data confronting clinicians, one must wonder why the therapies under evaluation were not adopted? One has to understand, as the authors do, that positive data derived from a meta-analysis are not of level I significance, but rather that a positive finding is an indication for conducting a prospective phase 3 clinical trial in order to generate level I data. The results of such a phase 3 trial may indeed have an impact on the standard of care. It should be reassuring to clinicians and their patients that positive results from meta-analyses have not been adopted as standards of care. A good example of the laudable caution of clinicians in regard to meta-analyses results is in the area of postoperative adjuvant chemotherapy (3,4). Essentially all the reported meta-analyses demonstrate benefit for postoperative chemotherapy, but clinicians have not accepted these data as clinically significant and still consider adjuvant chemotherapy to be investigational.

If we do not have adequate data to adopt all the "neat" approaches that Drs. Silberman and Iqbal describe, what do we know that may help patients with resectable stomach cancer? In the Western world, there are two studies that have altered the standard of care.

In 2006, Cunningham and colleagues (5) presented the results of the British Medical Research Council Adjuvant Gastric Cancer Infusional Chemotherapy (MAGIC) study. This was a well-designed and executed phase 3 trial evaluating the role of perioperative chemotherapy in the management of resectable gastric cancer. Patients with resectable gastric cancer were randomly allocated to a combination of chemotherapy and gastric resection or to gastric resection alone. The patients allocated to the chemotherapy and surgery treatment arm were to receive both pre- and postoperative therapy with three drugs: epirubicin, cisplatin, and 5-fluorouracil (ECF). The surgery-alone patients underwent curative intent gastectomy and received no adjuvant therapy. The major outcomes evaluated by Cunningham and colleagues (5) were progression-free and overall survival. The study enrolled 503 patients, with 250 receiving perioperative chemotherapy and 253 being treated with surgical resection alone. Analysis of the results provides convincing evidence of benefit from the use of ECF chemotherapy. Five-year overall survival was 36% for the chemotherapy-treated patients and 23% for the patients receiving surgical resection alone (log rank $p = 0.008$). This 13% improvement in survival corresponds with a 25% reduction in risk of death. Progression-free survival was also improved by chemotherapy with a log rank $p = 0.001$. In the chemotherapy/surgery/chemotherapy patients there were also encouraging trends in other outcomes such as decreased tumor size and reduction in the extent of nodal metastases. Toxicity of perioperative chemotherapy was manageable.

If perioperative chemotherapy with ECF improves survival, downstages tumors, and is reasonably safe, should it be considered a standard of care in the management of resectable gastric cancer? There are several aspects to this question. First, is ECF the "best" chemotherapy? Cunningham and colleagues (5) note that ECF is a chemotherapy program developed in the early 1990s (6) and that there are newer and less complex chemotherapy programs now available that are active in treating advanced gastric cancer (7,8). Are these more recently developed treatment programs better than ECF? The answer to this question is becoming available. The oral fluorinated pyrimidine, capecitabine, may be substituted for 5-flouorouracil in ECF-like regimens and it is highly likely that oxaliplatin will replace cisplatin in these regimens (8).

Although there undoubtedly will be debate among oncologists on which chemotherapy regimen is most appropriate in treating gastric cancer, a more important question is whether any sort of perioperative chemotherapy represents the best strategy to improve the cure rate in patients with resectable gastric adenocarcinoma. Part of the answer to this question hinges on when clinicians see cases of resectable gastric cancer. Although perioperative chemotherapy may be reasonable for patients seen prior to gastrectomy, patients who have already undergone gastric resection are not candidates for this treatment. It is common for patients with gastric cancer to be seen by oncologists after a gastrectomy with curative intent has been performed. Is there a standard of care for these patients? In 2001, data on a postoperative chemoradiation adjuvant therapy program were published (9). This study from the U.S. Intergroup Gastrointestinal Cancer Consortium, INT-0116, resulted in a postoperative chemoradiation treatment regimen being adopted as a standard of care for patients with resected gastric cancer. INT-0116 demonstrated that postoperative combined-modality therapy incorporating 5-fluorouracil and leucovorin chemotherapy along with external-beam radiation to the gastric resection site and the draining lymph node areas was beneficial for patients with resected gastric cancer. INT-0116 enrolled over 550 eligible patients. The patients on this study were randomly allocated to surgery alone or surgery followed by chemoradiation. These patients were generally at significant risk for relapse after gastric resection, with 85% of all patients having lymph node metastases and 65% having primary tumor invading completely through the gastric wall. The major outcomes analyzed were disease-free and overall survival. Chemoradiation significantly improved overall and disease-free survivals. Median survival increased from 27 to 36 months (log rank $p = 0.005$) for patients receiving the postoperative combined-modality therapy program, and disease-free survival was also improved from 19 to 30 months. This result was highly significant ($p < 0.001$). Updated results from INT-0116 with over 7 years of median follow-up indicated that the benefits for chemoradiation were maintained and did not deteriorate with increasing follow-up, and no significant long-term toxicity was observed (10).

The most important question for clinicians treating gastric cancer is how should MAGIC trial results and the INT-0116 data, or any of the approaches described by Drs. Silberman and Iqbal, influence the management of patients with resectable gastric cancer? Does perioperative chemotherapy represent such an advance in gastric cancer therapy that the standard of care must change? The MAGIC study, reported by Cunningham and colleagues (5), was well designed and well executed; therefore, clinicians may have confidence in the results of this phase 3 trial. The results provide solid evidence that perioperative therapy with ECF improves the outcome for patients with resectable gastric cancer identified before gastrectomy. Nevertheless, there are some concerns about the perioperative chemotherapy data reported by Chua and Cunningham (11). For example, will delaying surgery result in some patients not being able to undergo gastrectomy? Cunningham and colleagues (5) point out that 21 of 250 patients (8%) who were randomized to perioperative chemotherapy were unable to undergo resection and thus lost the opportunity for curative treatment. The major reason for being unable to undergo gastrectomy was disease progression. Would these patients have been able to undergo surgical resection of the primary neoplasm if they had not had operation delayed by up to 3 months for the administration of preoperative chemotherapy? One does not know, but a potential risk of perioperative therapy is losing the "window" for surgical resection.

Because patients on INT-0116 were identified postoperatively, there is no concern about loss of the opportunity for gastrectomy. However, in regard to postoperative chemoradiation, there are several concerns. One real concern germane to postoperative chemoradiation is the level of toxicity seen in the treatment arm of INT-0116. As noted by Drs. Silberman and Iqbal, over 90% of cases receiving postoperative chemoradiation develop grade 3 or 4 toxicities. Although this is a daunting statistic, it is important to understand that most of this toxicity was easily managed hematologic toxicity. There were only two definitely confirmed treatment-related toxic deaths, so there is no doubt that chemoradiation as delivered in INT-0116 can be given safely. Another significant factor in regard to INT-0116 is

the type of surgery performed in these patients. Only 10% of cases had a formal D2 dissection. Because 85% of all patients on the study had lymph node metastases, it is highly likely that many patients had unresected lymph node metastases. Does this mean that postoperative chemoradiation is effective because it controls unresected lymph node metastases? Would chemoradiation be unnecessary in a population of patients undergoing D2 dissection? The answer to this question can only be addressed by a phase 3 trial performed in a D2 dissection population. Such a trial has been initiated in Europe. What is known, without doubt, about postoperative chemoradiation is that this strategy is effective in the North American population treated on INT-0116.

So what is a clinician to do today with a patient with resectable or resected gastroesophageal cancer at high risk for relapse? Because adequate gastrectomy defined as a complete resection of the tumor with negative margins and containing at least 15 identifiable lymph nodes (a D2 resection) is important both for curative intent and adequate staging, the clinician should do all that he or she can to encourage this level of surgical care.

The results of the MAGIC perioperative chemotherapy study and the U.S. Intergroup study INT-0116 now give the clinician a choice of options (5,9–11). I believe that there is no "best" approach to adjunctive therapy in patients with resectable gastroesophageal cancer. Although there is no one best treatment, the good news is that now clinicians have effective options for patients with resected or potentially resectable tumors. Now just as postoperative chemoradiation is a proven treatment strategy for postgastrectomy patients, perioperative chemotherapy may be considered an appropriate option for patients with localized resectable gastric adenocarcinoma who have been identified preoperatively. The even better news, as described by Drs. Silberman and Iqbal, is that there is a great deal of active clinical and basic scientific effort occurring that should result in the future in continued improvements in outcome in patients with resectable stomach cancer.

REFERENCES

1. Parkin D, Bray F, Ferlay J, et al. Global Cancer Statistics, 2002. *CA Cancer J Clin.* 2005;55:74–108.
2. Locker GY, Hamilton S, Harris J, et al. ASCO 2006 update of recommendations for the use of tumor markers in gastrointestinal cancer. *J Clin Oncol.* 2006;24:5313–5327.
3. Hermans J, Bonenkamp JJ, Boon MC, et al. Adjuvant therapy after curative resection for gastric cancer: meta-analysis of randomized trials. *J Clin Oncol.* 1993;11:1441–1447.
4. Earle CC, Maroun JA. Adjuvant chemotherapy after curative resection for gastric cancer in non-Asian patients: revisiting a meta-analysis of randomized trials. *Eur J Cancer.* 1999;35:1059–1064.
5. Cunningham D, Allum WH, Stenning SP, et al. Perioperative chemotherapy versus surgery alone for resectable gastro-esophageal cancer. *N Engl J Med.* 2006;355:11–20.
6. Webb A, Cunningham D, Scarffe JH, et al. Randomized trial comparing epirubicin, cisplatin, and fluorouracil versus fluorouracil, doxorubicin, and methotrexate in advanced esophagogastric cancer. *J Clin Oncol.* 1997;15:261–267.
7. Sumpter K, Harper-Wynne C, Cunningham D, et al. Report of two protocol planned interim analyses in a randomized multicentre

phase III study comparing capecitabine with fluorouracil and oxaliplatin with cisplatin in patients with advanced esophagogastric cancer receiving ECF. *Br J Cancer.* 2005;92:1976–1983.

8. Cunningham D, Starling N, Rao S, et al. Capecitabine and oxaliplatin for advanced esophagogastric cancer. *N Engl J Med.* 2008;358:36–46.

9. Macdonald JS, Smalley SR, Benedetti J, et al. Chemoradiotherapy after surgery compared with surgery alone for adenocarcinoma of the stomach or gastroesophageal junction. *N Engl J Med.* 2001;345:725–730.

10. Macdonald JS. Role of postoperative chemoradiation in resected gastric cancer. *J Surg Oncol.* 2005;90:166–170.

11. Chua YJ, Cunningham D. The UK NCRI MAGIC trial of perioperative chemotherapy in resectable gastric cancer: implications for clinical practice [published online ahead of print July 27, 2007]. *Ann Surg Oncol.* 2007;14:2687–2690.

35

Cancer of the Pancreas: Surgical Management

Nicholas J. Zyromski, Attila Nakeeb, and Keith D. Lillemoe

Adenocarcinoma of the pancreas is one of the most lethal malignancies known to mankind. In 2009, it is estimated that 42,470 cases of pancreatic adenocarcinoma will be diagnosed in the United States, and 35,240 patients will die from the disease (1). The response of pancreatic cancer to chemotherapy and radiation therapy is poor, thus complete (R0) surgical resection offers the best hope for long-term survival. Unfortunately, only 15% to 20% of all patients with pancreatic cancer will have resectable disease at the time of diagnosis. Furthermore, patients with stage I pancreatic adenocarcinoma undergoing complete surgical resection, the best possible clinical scenario, still have a 5-year survival of only 15% to 20%. This is a striking contrast to the 80% to 90% 5-year survival generally realized by patients with other common epithelial tumors (such as breast and colon adenocarcinoma) of similar stage, and attests to the intrinsic biologic virulence of pancreatic adenocarcinoma.

Over the past 2 decades, major advances have been made in the operative and perioperative care of patients with pancreatic malignancy. These advances have translated directly to the dramatic decrease in perioperative mortality and acceptable postoperative complication rates currently reported from high-volume pancreatic surgical centers. This chapter reviews the pathology and diagnosis of pancreatic tumors, and principally focuses on the current surgical therapy of pancreatic adenocarcinoma, including both curative resection and palliation.

PATHOLOGY

Neoplasms of the pancreas are classified based on the cell type of origin, and can arise both from the exocrine (ductal epithelial, acinar, mesenchymal) and endocrine (islet) cells of the pancreas. Treatment of endocrine pancreatic neoplasms is reviewed in Chapter 42. Tumors arising from the exocrine pancreas are broadly classified as solid or cystic based on their gross appearance.

Solid Epithelial Tumors

Ductal Adenocarcinoma

It is of interest that although the pancreatic ductal epithelium comprises <10% of the pancreatic cell volume, ductal adenocarcinoma is by far the most common epithelial malignancy, accounting for at least 75% of all nonendocrine pancreatic malignancies. About 65% of ductal adenocarcinomas arise in the head of the pancreas, with 15% involving the body and tail, and 20% diffusely infiltrating the entire gland. Ductal adenocarcinoma of the pancreatic head frequently obstructs the intra-

pancreatic distal common bile duct, producing jaundice, and the main pancreatic duct, leading to a desmoplastic, fibrotic reaction and "obstructive chronic pancreatitis" (Figure 35.1). Ductal adenocarcinomas may invade locally into the duodenum, stomach, transverse colon, spleen, adrenal gland, or kidney. These malignancies also have a high frequency of microscopic infiltration into blood vessels, lymphatics, and the perineural sheath. Indeed, lymphovascular and perineural invasion have been shown to be independent prognostic factors of poor survival (2,3). At the time of resection, most ductal adenocarcinoma has invaded into local lymph nodes. As the disease progresses, distant metastases to the liver (80%), peritoneal cavity (60%), and lungs (50%) are common.

A large body of elegant experimental evidence has accumulated over the past decade suggesting that the development of pancreatic ductal adenocarcinoma follows a similar pattern to that observed in the colorectal adenoma to carcinoma sequence (4). Pancreatic intraepithelial neoplasias (PanINs) refer to proliferation of small pancreatic ducts, and are commonly observed in the resection specimens of patients with ductal adenocarcinoma (Figure 35.2). Molecular studies have shown that as PanINs progress, they accumulate the genetic changes similar to those commonly observed in pancreatic adenocarcinomas. Thus, PanINs are now widely accepted as "precursor" lesions to ductal adenocarcinoma.

Adenosquamous Carcinoma

Adenosquamous carcinoma is a rare variant of ductal adenocarcinoma that seems to arise more commonly in patients who have undergone chemoradiation therapy. The histology of adenosquamous carcinoma demonstrates both glandular and squamous cell differentiation. There is little difference in the clinical behavior of adenosquamous carcinoma compared with that of ductal adenocarcinoma.

Acinar Cell Carcinoma

Although acinar cells account for the bulk of the pancreatic parenchyma, true acinar cell carcinomas comprise only about 1% of all exocrine neoplasms. Histologically, the tumor cells resemble acinar cells, and may stain positive for trypsin, amylase, or lipase. Some patients may experience a clinical syndrome of polyarthralgia and peripheral fat necrosis related to tumor release of lipase. Grossly, these tumors are much larger than ductal adenocarcinomas, frequently >10 cm. The limited data available suggest that patients with acinar cell carcinomas may have a somewhat better prognosis than those with ductal adenocarcinomas.

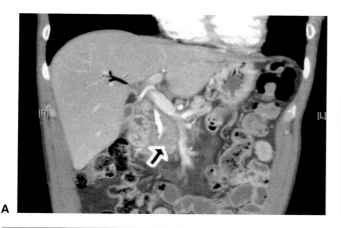
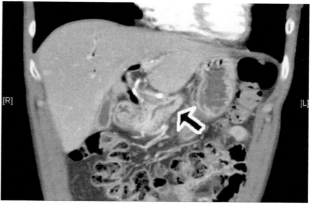

Figure 35.1 **(A)** Coronal computed tomography reconstruction demonstrating the relationship of a pancreatic head adenocarcinoma to the intrapancreatic bile duct (*arrow*); an endoscopically placed stent in the bile duct is white. Note the presence of pneumobilia in the right lobe of the liver. **(B)** Separate section of the patient depicted in **(A)** demonstrating dilated main pancreatic duct (*arrow*).

Pancreatoblastoma

Two thirds of pancreatoblastomas occur in children. These tumors demonstrate acinar as well as squamous cell differentiation. Similar to acinar cell carcinomas, pancreatoblastomas are also usually large, and may be associated with a slightly better clinical prognosis.

Cystic Epithelial Neoplasms

The majority of cystic lesions arising in the pancreas are benign pseudocysts related to a prior bout of pancreatitis. True cystic neoplasms of the pancreas are less common than solid epithelial neoplasms, and are generally categorized as serous or mucinous. In general, serous cystic neoplasms are thought of as benign, and mucinous cystic neoplasms are thought to have malignant potential. Many patients with cystic pancreatic neoplasms are asymptomatic and the lesion is only diagnosed incidentally by abdominal imaging performed for a separate indication. More

widespread use of cross-sectional abdominal imaging by computed tomography (CT) and magnetic resonance imaging (MRI) has contributed to an increased recognition of asymptomatic cystic pancreatic neoplasms. A recent study of over 24,000 abdominal CT and MRI scans demonstrated 168 unsuspected cystic pancreatic neoplasms in patients without a history of pancreatitis, for an estimated prevalence of 0.7% (5). The real malignant potential of mucinous cystic neoplasms combined with the occasional difficulty in differentiating between serous and mucinous cystic neoplasms frequently makes clinical management of these patients complex.

Serous Cystic Neoplasms

Histologically, serous cystic neoplasms (serous cystadenomas, SCAs) are usually composed of numerous small cysts, lined with a single layer of cuboidal cells and often demonstrating a central stellate scar. These morphologic features are often visible on

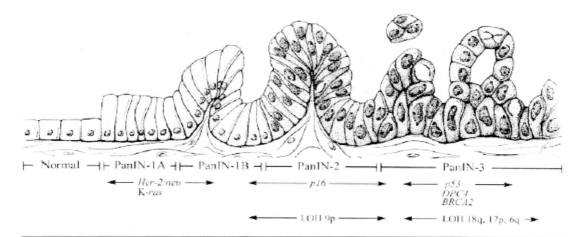

Figure 35.2 Schematic illustrating the progression of cellular dysplasia and accumulation of genetic defects in pancreatic ductal adenocarcinoma. PanIN, pancreatic intraepithelial neoplasia; LOH, loss of heterozygosity. (From Hruban RH, Goggins M, Parsons J, Kern SE. Progression model for pancreatic cancer. *Clin Cancer Res.* 2000;6:2969–2972, with permission.)

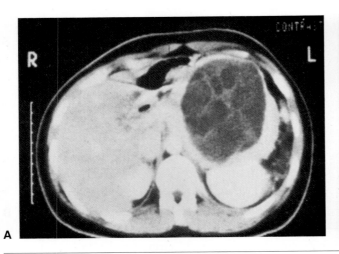 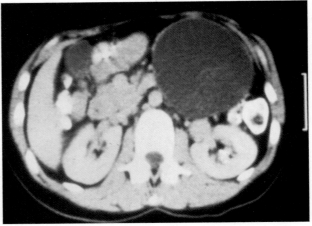

Figure 35.3 (A) Computed tomography (CT) demonstrating large serous cystadenoma with typical stellate scar. (B) CT of a large mucinous cystic neoplasm with typical smooth, unilocular appearance.

imaging studies (CT and MRI) and are helpful in differentiating SCAs from mucinous cystic lesions (Figure 35.3). Serous cystadenomas are more common in women [2:1], usually arise in the fifth or sixth decade of life, and are located more frequently in the body and tail of the pancreas. Most SCAs are benign; less than 10 cases of malignant serous cystadenocarcinoma have been reported in the literature (6). Most patients diagnosed with pancreatic SCA are asymptomatic, although the nonspecific abdominal symptoms of pain, nausea, dyspepsia, and vomiting may be present in 25% to 30% of patients, particularly those with large cysts.

Symptomatic patients with SCA should undergo surgical resection. Given the generally benign nature of these tumors, it is reasonable to observe patients with smaller, asymptomatic tumors with serial imaging. Recent data have documented an increased growth rate for SCAs >4 cm; therefore, resection should at least be discussed with younger, fit patients with larger tumors, even if they are asymptomatic (7). Resection of SCA should be conservative; a few authors advocate enucleation if technically possible (8).

Mucinous Cystic Neoplasms

Mucinous cystic neoplasms (MCNs) are composed of mucin-producing epithelial cells, most of which have an associated ovarian-type stroma of densely packed spindle cells (Figure 35.4). Similar to patients with SCA, most patients with MCN are female, in their 40s or 50s, and asymptomatic. Grossly, these tumors are predominantly macrocystic, although they may be multilocular or have adjacent cysts. MCNs generally do not communicate with the main pancreatic duct.

The major difference between SCA and MCN lies in the malignant potential of MCN. Two recent large series of MCN demonstrated invasive carcinoma in 36% and 29% of resected specimens (9,10). Therefore, *all* MCN must be considered malignant or premalignant, and resected whenever clinically feasible. The prognosis for patients with completely resected MCN without invasive carcinoma is excellent. In contrast, the prognosis of patients with invasive mucinous cystadenocarcinoma is grim,

with long-term survival rates paralleling those of patients with invasive ductal adenocarcinoma.

Intraductal Papillary Mucinous Neoplasms

Ohashi et al. (11) were the first to report the entity now known as intraductal papillary mucinous neoplasm (IPMN) as a "mucous secreting cancer of the pancreas" in the Japanese literature in 1982. For the next decade, little attention was paid to this report; however, over the subsequent 15 years, there has been a virtual explosion in the recognition of this tumor. IPMNs may arise from side branches or from the main pancreatic duct, and may be solitary or multifocal, occasionally involving the entire pancreatic ductal system. Similar to MCNs, IPMNs are considered to be premalignant lesions. Patients with IPMN may be asymptomatic or they may present with abdominal pain, pancreatitis, or biliary obstruction. The diagnosis of IPMN is suggested by the visualization of a cystic mass (or masses) on cross-sectional imaging,

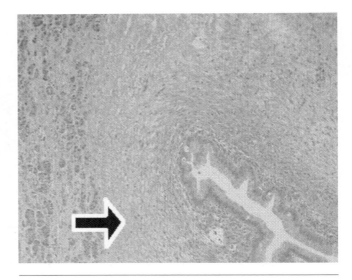

Figure 35.4 Micrograph of a pancreatic mucinous cystadenoma showing typical fibrous "ovarian stroma" (*arrow*).

or the finding of mucin extruding from a patulous "fish-mouth" papilla at the time of endoscopic retrograde cholangiopancreatography (ERCP). Cyst fluid obtained at the time of ERCP or endoscopic ultrasonography (EUS)-guided aspiration may help secure the diagnosis by positive cytology, presence of mucin, or elevation the tumor marker carcinoembryonic antigen to >200 ng/mL.

Despite the increasing number of patients with IPMN reported in the literature, long-term follow-up is lacking and the natural history of this disease remains unclear. Thus, the optimal surgical management of patients with IPMN remains controversial. Approximately 40% of patients with resected IPMN are found to have invasive carcinoma in the pathologic specimen, and the risk of developing invasive cancer is estimated to be 60% in patients who do not undergo surgical resection (12). The opportunity to resect a *premalignant* lesion and therefore *prevent* the development of pancreatic cancer must be carefully weighed against the risks of pancreatic surgery in an often elderly population with significant medical comorbidities. A recent consensus guideline recommends surgical resection of all IPMNs that involve the main pancreatic duct as well as side-branch lesions that are >3 cm in size (13). Clinical surveillance of patients after resection is important; magnetic resonance cholangiopancreatography (MRCP) is an extremely useful modality for surveillance of IPMN (Figure 35.5).

Solid and Cystic Neoplasms

Since its first description by Frantz (14) in 1959, this rare tumor has been reported in approximately 300 patients. Solid and cystic neoplasms generally develop in young females, and often grow to very large sizes (up to 20 cm) prior to diagnosis. Cytologically,

solid and cystic neoplasms are composed of both endocrine and exocrine components. Although generally considered a benign tumor, approximately one in six has been reported to metastasize, and thus aggressive surgical excision is indicated (15).

DIAGNOSIS AND CLINICAL STAGING

Early diagnosis of pancreatic cancer is challenging; the pancreas is inaccessible to clinical examination, and early symptoms such as vague abdominal discomfort, nausea, anorexia, and weight loss are nonspecific. Specific signs and symptoms of jaundice and epigastric/back pain arise only as the tumor enlarges and invades or obstructs adjacent structures. Indeed, it is not unusual for a patient with pancreatic cancer to be diagnosed within a few months of cholecystectomy performed for abdominal complaints due to presumed gallbladder disease.

Clinical Presentation

Jaundice is the most common physical finding in patients with pancreatic cancer, as most tumors arise in the head of the gland and obstruct the intrapancreatic portion of the common bile duct. The clinical finding of painless jaundice in an appropriate aged patient (fifth to sixth decade of life) must be considered pancreatic cancer until proven otherwise. The jaundice may be associated with darkening of the urine, acholic stools, and pruritus. Occasionally, hepatomegaly or an enlarged gallbladder (Courvoisier gallbladder) may be palpable on physical examination. Although less common, patients should also be examined for the presence of lymphadenopathy in the left supraclavicular (Virchow's node) and periumbilical (Sister Mary Joseph's node) distribution. Fine-needle aspiration biopsy of these nodes proves stage IV disease and allows treatment to be focused on palliation. Occasionally a "dropped metastasis" may be palpable on rectal examination (Blumer's shelf).

The pain associated with pancreatic cancer is typically epigastric and frequently radiates to the back. Pain may be caused by obstruction of the pancreatic duct or invasion of the tumor into the peripancreatic neural plexus. The presence of back pain in a patient with a known diagnosis of pancreatic cancer is ominous, and suggests presence of advanced disease. It is not uncommon for patients to complain of anorexia and weight loss.

In a small number of patients (10% to 15%), new-onset diabetes may be the first manifestation of pancreatic cancer. Similarly, patients may present with acute pancreatitis. It is important to keep pancreatic cancer in the differential diagnosis of acute pancreatitis, particularly for patients in their fifth to sixth decade without other obvious etiology (16).

Laboratory Findings

Patients whose tumor obstructs the bile duct typically have elevated levels of serum bilirubin and alkaline phosphecto. The transaminases may also be elevated, although usually to a lesser degree. It is important to measure coagulation parameters in patients with obstructive jaundice as impaired absorption of fat-soluble vitamins frequently leads to a prolonged prothrombin time. This is usually correctable by parenteral administration of vitamin K. Indices of nutritional status such as albumin, prealbumin, and transferrin are frequently low as a reflection of both

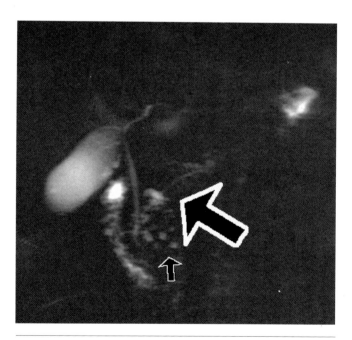

Figure 35.5 MRCP image of intraductal papillary mucinous neoplasm showing multifocal lesions. Numerous small lesions are visible in the head (*small arrow*) with a larger lesion at the genu (*large arrow*).

malabsorption and tumor cachexia. Serum levels of amylase and lipase are generally normal in patients with pancreatic cancer.

The tumor marker carbohydrate antigen 19-9 (CA19-9) is useful both for diagnosis and clinical follow-up of patients with pancreatic cancer. A CA19-9 value of >200 U/mL provides >95% accuracy for the diagnosis of pancreatic adenocarcinoma (17). Higher values are associated with larger tumors and metastatic disease, and thus are an indicator of unresectability and poor prognosis. This tumor marker is associated with the Lewis blood group, and so the 5% of the population who are Lewis blood group-negative are unable to produce CA19-9. It is also important to remember that CA19-9 levels may be spuriously elevated in the presence of jaundice. Serum levels of CA19-9 may be used to follow the response to adjuvant or neoadjuvant chemotherapy and radiation therapy, and are followed in the postoperative patient as an index of recurrent disease. Secondline adjuvant chemotherapy is often initiated on the basis of increasing CA19-9, even when recurrent or progressive disease can not be documented radiologically.

Radiologic Evaluation

A number of noninvasive radiologic tests are useful in the diagnosis of pancreatic cancer. These include transabdominal ultrasonography, CT, and MRI.

Transabdominal ultrasonography is rapid, inexpensive, and well tolerated by patients. In patients with tumors arising in the head of the pancreas, ultrasonography generally reveals a dilated intra- and extrahepatic biliary tree, and can identify the primary pancreatic tumor in up to 70% of patients. Transabdominal ultrasonography can also identify the presence of liver metastases, ascites, and enlarged peripancreatic nodes. Ultrasonography is highly operator-dependent, and the widespread availability of CT has limited the utility of ultrasonography as a principal modality for diagnosis and staging of pancreatic cancer.

Thin-slice, intravenous contrast-enhanced abdominal CT has become the imaging modality of choice for evaluation of patients with pancreatic cancer. Intravenous contrast is administered and the scanning sequence is timed to capture images in both arterial and portal venous phases ("pancreas protocol"). The primary pancreatic lesion appears as a focal, hypodense area within the pancreatic parenchyma. CT provides precise information about local extension of the tumor into vascular structures as well as the presence or absence of liver metastases and ascites (Figure 35.6). Using the specific, objective criteria of (a) absence of extrapancreatic disease, (b) a patent superior mesenteric-portal vein confluence, and (c) the absence of tumor invasion into the celiac axis or superior mesenteric artery, CT has been shown to predict resectability in up to 80% of patients (18). Despite advances in imaging techniques, the sensitivity of CT in detecting liver metastases <1cm in size and small peritoneal implants is still poor. CT allows image-directed biopsy; however, routine transabdominal biopsy of pancreatic lesions is discouraged and this modality should be reserved for highly selected situations.

MRI of the abdomen generally does not offer any advantages over CT in routine evaluation of patients with pancreatic cancer. Similar to CT, MRI provides cross-sectional imaging of the entire abdomen; however, MRI suffers from motion artifacts, lack of bowel opacification, and low spatial resolution. In addition, MRI is more costly than CT, and frequently more difficult for patients to tolerate. The one clear exception, however, lies in the evaluation of IMPNs. MRI and magnetic resonance cholangiopancreatography provide a reliable and reproducible method to evaluate IPMN, particularly in the case of patients being followed nonoperatively or those who require surveillance of the distal pancreatic remnant after pancreaticoduodenectomy (12).

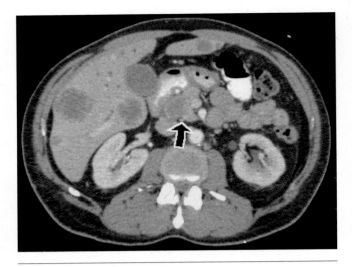

Figure 35.6 Computed tomography scan of a patient with pancreatic adenocarcinoma demonstrating the primary tumor in the head of the pancreas (*arrow*) and several large liver metastases.

Endoscopic Evaluation

ERCP and more recently EUS both play important roles in evaluating the patient with pancreatic adenocarcinoma. ERCP provides direct access to both the bile duct and the pancreatic duct. This offers the advantage of direct visualization of the duodenum, ampulla, and pancreatic and biliary ductal system with the capability of biopsy as necessary, as well as the opportunity to decompress the biliary tree in the patient with obstructive jaundice. The sensitivity of ERCP for diagnosing pancreatic cancer is >90%. The classic ERCP picture of a pancreatic head adenocarcinoma is that of the "double duct" sign (Figure 35.7).

Historically, ERCP (with biliary decompression) has been a routine step in the workup of patients with pancreatic cancer. A number of studies have demonstrated that preoperative biliary decompression is not mandatory in patients undergoing pancreatic resection (19,20). This, in combination with current advances in cross-sectional imaging techniques, has led to the current, more selective application of ERCP in the diagnosis of pancreatic cancer. Currently, ERCP is reserved for patients with obstructive jaundice in whom no pancreatic head mass is detected on CT, nonjaundiced patients with a pancreatic mass, and patients with chronic pancreatitis in whom development of malignancy is suspected either clinically or radiologically.

EUS of the pancreas (and upper gastrointestinal tract) has undergone tremendous advances over the past decade, and is now frequently applied in the workup of patients with pancreatic cancer. A recent review of the literature comparing EUS and CT in the evaluation of pancreatic cancer highlighted the accuracy of EUS in detecting pancreatic cancer, but concluded that

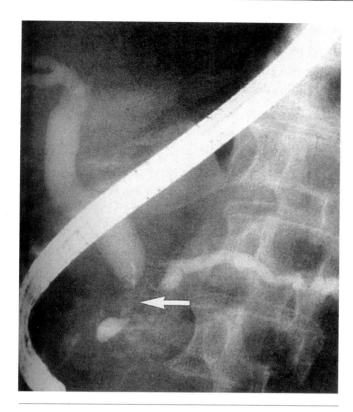

Figure 35.7 Endoscopic retrograde cholangiopancreatography demonstrating the "double duct" sign. The *arrow* shows the tumor obstructing both the bile duct (at 11 o'clock) and the pancreatic duct (at 3 o'clock).

these two tests are complementary (21). In performing EUS, a high-frequency ultrasound probe placed through an endoscope allows visualization of the pancreatic tumor, its relationship to adjacent vascular structures, reasonable views of the liver, and assessment for the presence of ascites. A major advantage of EUS lies in the capability for biopsy—either by fine needle or core needle—of the tumor, liver metastases, or ascites. EUS has also been shown to be more accurate than CT in assessing smaller pancreatic tumors (<3 cm). The major disadvantage of EUS is that the examination is technically challenging and operator-dependent. Although more endoscopists are becoming facile with the technical application of EUS, its current availability remains relatively limited.

RESECTION OF PANCREATIC CANCER

The pancreas has long been an organ that has defied surgical intervention. Walter Kausch (22) is credited for performance of the first pancreaticoduodenal resection, reported in 1912. The lead of Allan O. Whipple in the late 1930s, however, provided major impetus for surgeons to continue efforts at pancreatic resection, and his name remains synonymous with pancreaticoduodenectomy. In the 50 years following Whipple's landmark work, pancreatic surgery was plagued by extremely high morbidity, and mortality approaching 25%. These results combined with poor long-term survival from pancreatic cancer led some prominent American surgeons to call for a moratorium on pancreaticoduodenectomy as recently as the 1970s (23). Around this time,

reports of two series of pancreaticoduodenectomy performed without operative mortality encouraged surgeons to persist, and the past 3 decades have realized remarkable advances in pancreatic surgery (24,25). Pancreatic resection is now commonly performed, with high-volume centers routinely reporting mortality rates <4% (2,3,26).

The Role of Diagnostic Laparoscopy

Despite significant advances in radiology techniques, between 10% and 20% of patients with pancreatic cancer undergoing operative exploration with curative intent will be found to have unresectable disease, either because of undetected distant metastases or local invasion of adjacent major vascular structures. This has let to an increased interest in the use of laparoscopy as a specific staging tool (18,27). Staging laparoscopy can be performed with minimal morbidity, identifies patients (up to 20%) with radiologically undetected metastatic disease, and does not "burn any bridges" for subsequent resection in patients with localized disease (28). Proponents of routine laparoscopic staging in patients with pancreatic cancer argue that this modality spares a significant subset of patients from the morbidity associated with formal laparotomy, and allows earlier initiation of palliative therapy. The philosophy of routine staging laparoscopy is based on the view that palliation in unresectable patients can be achieved by nonoperative means. Our current practice is to offer staging laparoscopy selectively to patients with back pain, markedly elevated CA19-9, or a high clinical or radiologic suspicion of advanced disease.

The technique of staging laparoscopy starts with placement of four operating ports, one each at the umbilicus, epigastrium, and below the costal margin in the right and left midclavicular lines. The peritoneal cavity is systemically inspected in four quadrants, and suspicious peritoneal implants are biopsied. Some authors routinely send peritoneal washing for cytology: 200 mL of saline is irrigated and aspirated in the right and left upper quadrants and pelvis. The liver is systematically examined; use of intraoperative ultrasonography allows inspection of the deeper liver parenchyma and has been shown to increase the accuracy of laparoscopic staging. The transverse colon is elevated, and the root of the mesentery inspected for tumor invasion or enlarged lymph nodes around the middle colic vessels. The lesser sac is exposed by opening the pars flaccida, and the celiac axis and porta hepatis are evaluated. Enlarged celiac lymph nodes are biopsied. Finally, the primary tumor is evaluated. Ultrasound allows precise delineation of the tumor relationship to the adjacent organs and major vascular structures. Importantly, early concerns that staging laparoscopy would increase the incidence of abdominal wall ("port-site") metastases have not been borne out (29).

Proximal Pancreatic Resection (Pancreaticoduodenectomy)
Technique

Central venous and continuous arterial monitoring are routinely employed. Intravenous antibiotics should provide coverage of both skin and common biliary flora, particularly if preoperative biliary stenting has been used. Prophylaxis against venous thromboembolism, either with pneumatic compression cuffs or subcutaneous heparin derivatives, is begun preoperatively.

Either a midline or bilateral subcostal incision provides excellent exposure of the upper abdomen.

The first step in proximal pancreatic resection is a thorough abdominal exploration to exclude distant metastatic disease. The peritoneal surfaces and omentum are inspected and palpated, including those of the pelvis to exclude "dropped metastases." Suspicious nodules are biopsied for frozen section analysis. The transverse colon is elevated to inspect the root of the transverse mesocolon. Puckering of the transverse mesocolon by tumor should raise suspicion for major vascular involvement. The liver is palpated to detect small tumor implants that may not have been apparent on preoperative imaging. Use of intraoperative ultrasound allows more accurate appraisal of the deeper liver parenchyma, as well as providing important information about tumor relationship to the adjacent major vascular structures. The celiac axis is inspected for suspicious lymphadenopathy. Although metastatic disease in the celiac nodes suggests that the tumor has spread beyond the normal limits of resection, the presence of more localized tumor-bearing lymph nodes is not a contraindication to resection.

Having excluded distant metastases, the hepatic flexure of the colon is widely mobilized from the head of the pancreas. A generous Kocher maneuver is then performed to the level of the aorta. This allows the surgeon's left hand to be placed behind the head of the pancreas to evaluate the relationship of the tumor to the superior mesenteric vessels (Figure 35.8). Failure to identify a plane between the tumor and the superior mesenteric artery suggests direct involvement, and precludes complete resection. The superior mesenteric vein (SMV) is then exposed, and a plane is developed on the anterior surface of the SMV behind the neck of the pancreas. It is usually necessary to divide several small tributary veins to the SMV to complete this maneuver; care should be taken in dissecting these veins, as bleeding here can be troublesome. Should bleeding from these small veins be encountered, elevation of the pancreatic head ventrally with the surgeon's left hand is a helpful maneuver to slow hemorrhage and allow precise suture repair of the avulsed vessels and the superior mesenteric vein. Attention is then directed to the porta hepatis. The gallbladder is dissected from the liver bed and the cystic duct followed to the common bile duct. The common bile duct is encircled with a vessel loop and retracted laterally, exposing the portal vein. Early division of the bile duct in patients with jaundice in whom biliary bypass is planned may facilitate exposure. Dissection and ligation of the gastroduodenal artery also helps to expose the portal vein at the superior margin of the pancreas. Care should be exercised before dividing the gastroduodenal artery to ensure that this is not a replaced right hepatic artery, or in the rare case of celiac stenosis, that the blood supply of the hepatic artery does not depend solely on the superior mesenteric artery (30).

The anterior surface of the portal vein is dissected behind the pancreatic neck until this plane connects with the SMV dissection from below. At this point, the surgeon can be reasonably confident that resection will be technically possible. The bile

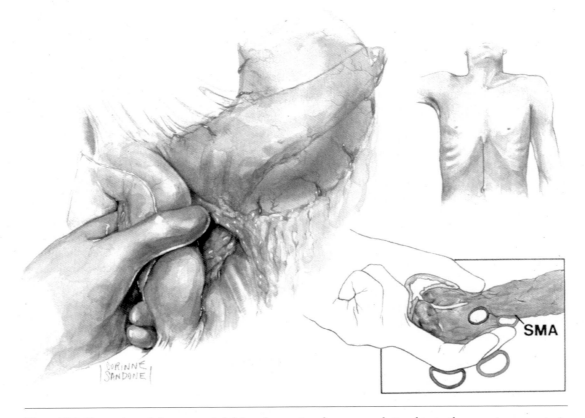

Figure 35.8 Illustration of the surgeon's left hand assessing the tumor relationship to the superior mesenteric vessels. SMA, superior mesenteric artery. (Adapted from Cameron JL, Sandone C. *Atlas of Gastrointestinal Surgery*, 2nd ed. Vol 1. Hamilton, Ontario: BC Decker, Inc., 2007:286.)

duct is divided and a circumferential biopsy sent for frozen section. If the pylorus-preserving modification of pancreaticoduo-denectomy is used, the duodenum is dissected from the head of the pancreas and divided approximately 2 cm distal to the pylorus. We routinely send a frozen section specimen from the duodenal margin. In the case of a classic Whipple operation, the stomach is divided to include approximately 40% of the stomach with the specimen. The neck of the pancreas is then divided, taking care to avoid injury to the underlying mesenteric vessels. A frozen section is sent of the pancreatic neck margin, marking the pancreatic duct with a suture for the pathologist. The transverse colon is elevated, and the jejunum divided approximately 10 cm distal to the ligament of Treitz. The mesentery of the proximal jejunum and distal duodenum is divided to the level of the uncinate process, at which point the specimen is rotated beneath the mesenteric vessels to the patient's right. Use of electrocoagulation devices such as the LigaSure (ValleyLab, Inc., Boulder, Colorado) or harmonic scalpel (Ethicon Endosurgery, Cincinnati, Ohio) has greatly facilitated this portion of the dissection (31).

The final step of the dissection involves transaction of the retroperitoneal soft-tissue margin. With the surgeon's left hand behind the head of the pancreas and rotating the specimen to the patient's right, the superior mesenteric artery is palpable, and the specimen is dissected flush with the right side of the superior mesenteric artery. The specimen, including head of the pancreas, duodenum (and distal stomach in the classic pancreaticoduo-denectomy), proximal jejunum, and gallbladder are now completely freed and can be removed from the operative field. The retroperitoneal soft-tissue margin is marked for the pathologist.

Reconstruction of enteric continuity begins with the pancreaticojejunostomy. The proximal jejunum is brought through the transverse mesocolon to lie adjacent to the pancreatic remnant with no tension. We favor an end-to-side, duct-to-mucosa pancreaticojejunostomy. This anastomosis is begun by placing a posterior layer of interrupted 3-0 sutures between the pancreatic capsule and jejunum. A small enterotomy is then made in the jejunum, and the pancreatic duct is sutured to the jejunal mucosa with 6-0 absorbable monofilament interrupted sutures. A short segment of pediatric feeding tube may be placed in the main pancreatic duct and used as a temporary stent, facilitating this portion of the anastomosis. The anastomosis is then completed with an anterior row of interrupted 3-0 sutures. In the case of a soft pancreas or small pancreatic duct, an alternate anastomosis may be constructed by extending the jejunotomy to equal the size of the pancreatic neck. A running anastomosis is then created, invaginating the neck of the pancreas 1 to 2 cm into the lumen of the jejunum. The biliary-enteric anastomosis is then created approximately 7 to 10 cm distal to the pancreaticojejunostomy in an end-to-side fashion with interrupted 5-0 absorbable sutures. T-tubes or transhepatic biliary stents are not routinely employed. The jejunum may be tacked to the hilar plate with laterally placed sutures to reduce tension. The final anastomosis is the duodeno-(gastro) jejunostomy, which is generally constructed in two layers and may be placed either in the retrocolic or antecolic position. Care should be taken to avoid excess redundancy of the jejunal limb. Figure 35.9 demonstrates the extent of resection and the final reconstruction after pancreaticoduodenectomy.

Extent of Resection

Whipple's description of pancreaticoduodenectomy included distal gastrectomy; this "classic" operation has been performed for decades. In the late 1970s, Traverso and Longmire (32)

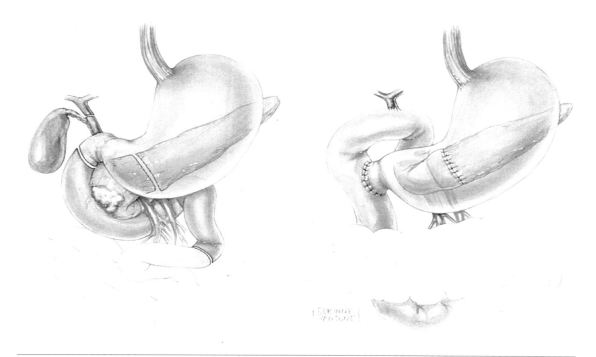

Figure 35.9 Diagram illustrating the extent of operative resection (**A**) and final reconstruction (**B**) after pancreaticoduodenectomy. (Adapted from Cameron JL, Sandone C. *Atlas of Gastrointestinal Surgery,* 2nd ed. Vol 1. Hamilton, Ontario: BC Decker, Inc.; 2007:302.)

popularized the concept of pylorus preservation. Preservation of the antral-pylorus complex offers the advantage of improved gastrointestinal function and the potential for reducing postgastrectomy complications, including marginal ulceration. In addition, the pylorus-preserving modification of pancreaticoduodenectomy is technically easier and less time-consuming than the classic Whipple procedure. The major concern with preserving the pylorus and proximal duodenum is the potential to compromise the proximal margin of resection. Clinical studies have indeed documented improved gastrointestinal function, while no difference in long-term survival has been seen when the two modifications are compared (33,34). Thus, the pylorus-preserving pancreaticoduodenectomy is widely employed.

Efforts to improve survival of patients with pancreatic cancer have led to the application of extended lymphadenectomy including complete dissection of celiac and periaortic nodes in conjunction with pancreaticoduodenectomy. Retrospective reports from the Japanese literature and one prospective Italian trial have suggested improved survival with extended retroperitoneal lymphadenectomy in pancreaticoduodenectomy (35,36). Unfortunately, these results have not been able to be reproduced in Western studies. Two recent large, prospective studies of pancreaticoduodenectomy with standard versus extended lymphadenectomy have been performed in the United States (37,38). Neither of these studies demonstrated a long-term survival advantage for patients undergoing extended lymphadenectomy. Additionally, both studies documented significantly increased morbidity rates, including pancreatic fistula and delayed gastric emptying, in patients undergoing extended lymphadenectomy. Therefore, most Western surgeons do not routinely apply extended lymphadenectomy to pancreaticoduodenectomy.

Extending resection for pancreatic cancer to include total pancreatectomy (with splenectomy) has been advocated by a few surgeons. The theoretical advantages of total pancreatectomy include elimination of multicentric disease and prevention of direct tumor spread to the distal pancreas. In addition, elimination of the pancreaticojejunostomy obviates the complication of pancreatic fistula, a major cause of morbidity and mortality after pancreatic resection. The major disadvantage of total pancreatectomy is the predictable development of endocrine dysfunction, which is often extremely difficult to control medically. To date, there is no evidence that total pancreatectomy reduces morbidity and mortality or improves long-term survival in patients with adenocarcinoma. Thus, this procedure should be reserved for the very select patients in whom a negative margin cannot be obtained on frozen section, or those with IPMN that involves the entire main pancreatic duct.

In 1973, Fortner (39) first described the concept of "regional pancreatectomy," which included resection of the superior mesenteric-portal vein confluence. For many years, vascular resection in conjunction with pancreatectomy was reserved for the situation in which vascular involvement by tumor was only appreciated after the pancreatic neck was divided (after the "point of no return" in the operation). Advances in technique and perioperative care have led to increasing use of elective superior mesenteric-portal vein resection by a number of centers (Table 35.1). It is now clear that vascular resection can be performed safely in conjunction with pancreatic resection, and while this has not been shown to confer any advantage in long-term survival, it does extend indications for resection.

Distal Pancreatectomy

Most patients with adenocarcinoma of the body and tail of the pancreas have metastatic disease at the time of clinical presentation. Of all patients with potentially resectable distal tumors (i.e., absence of liver metastasis and major vascular invasion on

Table 35.1

Select Reports of Vascular Resection With Pancreaticoduodenectomy

Ref.	First Author	Year	No. of Patients	Survival (months)	Mortality (%)
53	Sindelar	1989	20	12	20
25	Trede	1990	12	NR	0
54	Launois	1993	9	6	0
65	Harrison	1996	50	13	6
56	Roder	1996	22	8	0
57	Bold	1999	66	NR	2
58	Bachellier	2001	21	12	3
59	Van Geenen	2001	34	14	0
60	Howard	2003	13	13	8
61	Capussotti	2003	24	NR	0
62	Poon	2004	12	20	0
63	Jain	2005	48	40	6
64	Shimada	2006	86	14	1

NR, not reported.

good-quality abdominal CT), nearly 50% will be found to have occult metastasis at the time of diagnostic laparoscopy. Thus, surgical resection plays a more limited role in management of tumors of the pancreatic body and tail.

Technique

As with proximal resection, thorough abdominal exploration to rule out metastatic disease is the first step in distal resection. The liver, omentum, and peritoneal surfaces are closely inspected and suspicious nodules biopsied for frozen section. Particular attention should be directed to examination of the celiac axis, superior mesenteric artery, and aorta as tumors of the pancreatic neck and body frequently invade these vessels by direct extension. The lesser sac is widely opened by dividing the gastrocolic ligament from the right to left. Mobilization of the splenic flexure of the colon and avascular splenic ligaments exposes the inferior border of the pancreatic body and tail. The short gastric vessels are divided, and the stomach retracted superiorly, fully exposing the body and tail of the pancreas. The inferior border of the pancreas is dissected to the level of the SMV as it courses under the neck of the pancreas. If this vessel is free from tumor involvement, dissection proceeds. If possible, early control of the splenic artery and vein greatly facilitate subsequent dissection. The neck of the pancreas is divided, and the body and tail of the gland are elevated from the retroperitoneum and removed en bloc with the spleen.

Similar to pancreaticoduodenectomy, studies of extended lymphadenectomy with distal pancreatectomy have failed to demonstrate a survival advantage (40). Numerous techniques have been reported to control the proximal pancreatic neck; to date none has clearly demonstrated superiority in terms of reducing pancreatic fistula. Our preference is to directly suture ligate the pancreatic duct with nonabsorbable suture. A soft, closed-suction drain is routinely left in place at the cut edge of the pancreas.

Laparoscopic Distal Pancreatectomy

Since the mid 1990s, reports of laparoscopic distal pancreatectomy have accumulated. To date, these consist primarily of case reports and small, single-institution series (41). Laparoscopic distal pancreatectomy has principally been applied to patients with small islet cell tumors and cystic lesions. No data are currently available regarding long-term outcomes for laparoscopic resection of pancreatic adenocarcinoma. At present, therefore, laparoscopic distal pancreatectomy for adenocarcinoma should be restricted to experienced pancreatic surgeons in the context of an active clinical trial.

Outcomes After Pancreatic Resection

Perhaps the greatest surgical advance in pancreatic resection over the past 3 decades is the dramatic decrease in perioperative mortality. As recently as the 1970s, mortality after pancreatic resection approached 25% (23). Since the late 1980s, however, operative mortality has dropped substantially. Currently, high-volume centers routinely report perioperative mortality rates of 2% to 4% (2,3,26). In addition to advances in operative technique and perioperative care, this decrease in mortality can be directly linked to concentration of pancreatic surgery at high-volume centers with experienced pancreatic surgeons (65–67). Despite decreases in perioperative mortality, morbidity following pancreatic resection remains high, on the order of 30% to 40% even at high-volume centers. In addition to the general complications attending complex abdominal surgery, several complications are specific to pancreatic resection.

Pancreatic fistula continues to plague pancreatic surgeons, occurring in 5% to 15% of patients after pancreaticoduodenectomy and 5% to 30% after distal resection (2,26,40). A number of interventions to decrease rates of pancreatic fistula such as prophylactic administration of somatostatin analogues (42,43) and use of fibrin glue sealant on the pancreatic remnant (44) have been prospectively studied. Unfortunately, none have shown significant clinical benefit. Improvements in interventional radiology techniques have facilitated management of pancreatic fistula, and are likely a major reason for the observed decrease in mortality directly related to pancreatic fistula.

Delayed gastric emptying is a poorly understood phenomenon that occurs in 10% to 20% of patients undergoing pancreaticoduodenectomy. The motilin agonist erythromycin and prokinetic metoclopramide have both proved useful in treating this complication (45). Hemorrhage is a less common, but potentially lethal complication after pancreatic resection. Major hemorrhage frequently arises in the setting of pancreatic fistula, and is often related to pseudoaneurysm of the major visceral arteries. This complication is usually best managed by interventional radiology techniques (46).

Complete, margin-negative (R0) resection offers patients with pancreatic cancer the best possible chance for long-term survival. Historically, 5-year survival rates for patients undergoing pancreaticoduodenectomy were reported to be 5%. Recent studies have demonstrated increased survival rates of up to 17% at 5 years (2,3). It is worthwhile to note that the 5-year survival of patients undergoing pancreaticoduodenectomy for adenocarcinoma arising in the ampulla is substantially longer (39%) than for patients with adenocarcinoma arising in the head of the pancreas (3). Similarly, the outcome of patients with adenocarcinoma arising in the setting of IPMN appears to be somewhat more favorable. A recent large series from Johns Hopkins Hospital reported the median survival of 38 months for 90 patients with invasive cancer arising in IPMN as compared with 18 months for 1,175 patients with ductal adenocarcinoma without IPMN (47). The clinical outcome of patients undergoing distal pancreatectomy for adenocarcinoma mirrors that of patients undergoing pancreaticoduodenectomy, with 5-year survival rates of 12% to 17% (40). These dismal long-term outcomes reflect both the virulence of the tumor biology as well as failure of adjuvant chemoradiotherapy regimens to control micrometastatic disease.

PALLIATION

Despite the fact that the majority of patients with pancreatic adenocarcinoma are not candidates for complete surgical resection, surgical palliation remains a key consideration in providing optimal quality of life for patients with unresectable disease.

Palliation of pancreatic cancer has three major foci: providing relief of obstructive jaundice, gastric outlet obstruction, and pain.

Jaundice

Eighty percent of patients with adenocarcinoma of the pancreatic head will suffer from obstructive jaundice at some time during the course of their disease. If left untreated, jaundice results in malabsorption, cholestasis, progressive hepatic failure, and early death. In addition, the severe pruritus of obstructive jaundice can be debilitating and is extremely difficult to manage medically. Therefore, relief of obstructive jaundice is a critical component in palliation of unresectable pancreatic cancer. Patients with locally advanced unresectable pancreatic cancer have a life span of 6 to 18 months, and those with metastatic disease have a lifespan of 3 to 6 months. In the patient who is clearly unresectable, nonoperative (i.e., endoscopic or percutaneous radiologic) palliation of obstructive jaundice is indicated. Advances in endoscopic stent technology—specifically, the introduction of metallic biliary stents—has greatly improved the durability of these nonoperative approaches, and in most patients biliary obstruction is successfully managed without the need for surgery.

Surgical biliary bypass should be undertaken in all patients undergoing operative exploration with the intent of curative resection but found to be unresectable at the time of operation. Surgical biliary bypass may be performed by means of either choledochojejunostomy or cholecystojejunostomy. Choledochojejunostomy may be performed in a loop fashion (with Braun enteroenterostomy) or by Roux-en-Y bypass (Figure 35.10). Our preference is to bypass the biliary tree by means of Roux-en-Y choledochojejunostomy. This provides the advantage of removing a patent bilioenteric anastomosis from the alimentary stream, and avoids the 10% to 15% incidence of recur-

rent jaundice that occurs after cholecystojejunostomy. In patients with large tumors invading the porta hepatis or those with portal vein obstruction resulting in large periductal varices, cholecystojejunostomy is an acceptable alternative. In this case, the surgeon must demonstrate patency of the cystic duct, as well as ensure that the cystic duct enters the common bile duct at a suitable distance away from the tumor mass (ideally >2 cm). With improvements in laparoscopic techniques have come recent reports of palliative laparoscopic biliary bypass. To date, no prospective studies have compared the results of laparoscopic biliary bypass with either open biliary bypass or endoscopic stenting in the palliation of malignant biliary obstruction.

Gastric Outlet Obstruction

Gastric outlet obstruction may arise in the setting of both pancreatic head and body tumors. In all, approximately 20% of patients with pancreatic cancer will develop mechanical gastric outlet obstruction. The etiology of nausea and vomiting that is commonly seen in patients with pancreatic cancer is often more complex than a simple mechanical obstruction, and is likely related to neural invasion of the tumor with resultant dysmotility as well as malabsorption as a consequence of both biliary obstruction and pancreatic exocrine insufficiency. The indication for routine gastrojejunostomy in patients found to have unresectable disease at the time of exploration has historically been somewhat more controversial than that for biliary bypass. Two recent prospective, randomized studies have evaluated the role of prophylactic gastrojejunostomy in patients with periampullary cancer found to be unresectable at the time of operative exploration (48,49). Both demonstrated that performance of gastrojejunostomy in patients *without* preoperative symptoms of gastric outlet obstruction significantly reduced the incidence of subsequent gastric outlet obstruction as well as need for further intervention to treat this complication. Our practice, therefore, based on this level I evidence, is to routinely perform retrocolic, isoperistaltic gastrojejunostomy at the distal, dependent stomach in patients found to be unresectable at the time of exploration. Metallic stents have also been used to treat intestinal obstruction; this treatment is useful to treat gastric outlet obstruction in patients with advanced disease.

Pain

Virtually all patients with pancreatic cancer will develop pain related to their tumor. The pain of pancreatic cancer is likely related to neural invasion by the tumor and pancreatic ductal hypertension from tumor obstruction, but may also be related to biliary (and gallbladder) obstruction as well as gastrointestinal obstruction. Blockade of the celiac axis with chemical agents such as 50% ethanol or phenol has been shown to significantly improve pancreatic cancer pain, and in one prospective study to actually prolong the lifespan of patients with unresectable disease (50). Celiac neurolysis may be performed intraoperatively, percutaneously under CT guidance, or by EUS guidance (51,52). Intraoperative celiac blockade is performed by identifying the hepatic and splenic arteries as they arise from the celiac axis, and with the surgeon's left hand retracting these arteries caudally injecting 20 mL of 50% ethanol on each side of the aorta at the level of the celiac axis (Figure 35.11).

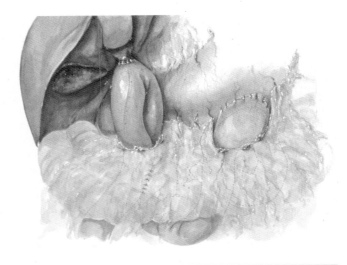

Figure 35.10 Illustration of completed palliative biliary bypass (in this case, loop hepaticojejunostomy with Braun enteroenterostomy) with concomitant retrocolic, isoperistaltic gastrojejunostomy. (Adapted from Cameron JL, Sandone C. *Atlas of Gastrointestinal Surgery,* 2nd ed. Vol 1. Hamilton, Ontario: BC Decker, Inc.; 2007:308.)

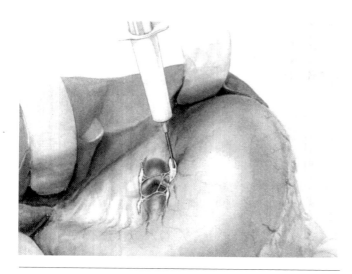

Figure 35.11 Diagram demonstrating intraoperative performance of celiac neurolysis. The hepatic artery and splenic artery are palpated and used to guide injection of 50% ethanol on either side of the aorta lateral to the celiac axis.

CONCLUSION

The surgeon continues to play a critical and central role in the management of patients with pancreatic cancer. Complete surgical resection currently offers patients with pancreatic cancer the best hope for long-term survival. In the patient with unresectable pancreatic cancer, surgical palliation by biliary bypass, gastrojejunostomy, and chemical celiac splanchnicectomy provides durable symptom relief. Refinements in operative technique and perioperative care have translated to dramatically decreased mortality after pancreatic surgery. Despite major surgical advances, long-term survival of patients with pancreatic cancer remains poor, which is a reflection of both the virulent tumor biology and the current lack of adequate adjuvant therapy. Surgeons must continue to lead research efforts in order to better understand the complex biology of this deadly disease (53–67).

REFERENCES

1. Jemal A, Siegel R, Ward E, et al. Cancer statistics, 2009. *CA Cancer J Clin.* Published online May 27, 2009. doi:10.3322 CAAC. 2006.
2. Sohn TA, Yeo CJ, Cameron JL, et al. Resected adenocarcinoma of the pancreas-616 patients: results, outcomes, and prognostic indicators. *J Gastrointest Surg.* 2000;4:567–579.
3. Cameron JL, Riall TS, Coleman J, et al. One thousand consecutive pancreaticoduodenectomies. *Ann Surg.* 2006;244:10–15.
4. Hruban RH, Goggins M, Parsons J, et al. Progression model for pancreatic cancer. *Clin Cancer Res.* 2000;6:2969–2972.
5. Spinelli KS, Fromwiller TE, Daniel RA, et al. Cystic pancreatic neoplasms: observe or operate. *Ann Surg.* 2004;239:651–657.
6. George DH, Murphy F, Michalski R, et al. Serous cystadenocarcinoma of the pancreas: a new entity? *Am J Surg Pathol.* 1989;13: 61–66.
7. Tseng JF, Warshaw AL, Sahani DV, et al. Serous cystadenoma of the pancreas: tumor growth rates and recommendations for treatment. *Ann Surg.* 2005;242:413–419.
8. Kiely JM, Nakeeb A, Komorowski RA, et al. Cystic pancreatic neoplasms: enucleate or resect? *J Gastrointest Surg.* 2003;7:890–897.
9. Zamboni G, Scarpa A, Bogina G, et al. Mucinous cystic tumors of the pancreas: clinicopathological features, prognosis, and relationship to other mucinous cystic tumors. *Am J Surg Pathol.* 1999;23:410–422.
10. Thompson LD, Becker RC, Przygodzki RM, et al. Mucinous cystic neoplasm (mucinous cystadenocarcinoma of low-grade malignant potential) of the pancreas: a clinicopathologic study of 130 cases. *Am J Surg Pathol.* 1999;23:1–16.
11. Ohashi K, Murakimi Y, Maruyama M, et al. Four cases of mucous secreting pancreatic cancer [in Japanese]. *Prog Dig Endosc.* 1982;20:348–351.
12. Schmidt CM, Lillemoe KD. IPMN-controversies in an "epidemic." *J Surg Oncol.* 2006;94:91–93.
13. Tanaka M, Chari S, Adsay V, et al. International consensus guidelines for management of intraductal papillary mucinous neoplasms and mucinous cystic neoplasms of the pancreas. *Pancreatology.* 2005;6:17–32.
14. Frantz VK. Tumors of the pancreas. In: *Atlas of Tumor Pathology,* section VII, fascicles 27 and 28. Washington, DC: Armed Forces Institute of Pathology; 1959.
15. Mao C, Guvendi M, Domenico DR, et al. Papillary cystic and solid tumors of the pancreas: a pancreatic embryonic tumor? Studies of three cases and cumulative review of the world's literature. *Surgery.* 1995;118:821–828.
16. Zyromski NJ, Haidenberg J, Sarr MG. Necrotizing pancreatitis caused by pancreatic ductal adenocarcinoma. *Pancreas.* 2001;22: 431–432.
17. Ritts RE, Pitt HA. CA 19-9 in pancreatic cancer. *Surg Oncol Clin North Am.* 1998;7:93–101.
18. Pisters PW, Lee JE, Vauthey JN, et al. Laparoscopy in the staging of pancreatic cancer. *Br J Surg.* 2001;88:325–337.
19. Pisters PW, Hudec WA, Hess KR, et al. Effect of preoperative biliary decompression on pancreaticoduodenectomy-associated morbidity in 300 consecutive patients. *Ann Surg.* 2001;234:47–55.
20. Martignoni ME, Wagner M, Krahenbuhl L, et al. Effect of preoperative biliary drainage on surgical outcome after pancreatoduodenectomy. *Am J Surg.* 2001;181:52–59.
21. Dewitt J, Devereaux BM, Lehman GA, et al. Comparison of endoscopic ultrasound and computed tomography for the preoperative evaluation of pancreatic cancer: a systematic review. *Clin Gastroenterol Hepatol.* 2006;4:717–725.
22. Kausch W. Das Carcinom der Papilla Duodeni und seine radikale Entfeinung. Beitrage zur Klinische Chirurgie 1912; 78: 439–486.
23. Crile G Jr. The advantages of bypass operations over radical pancreatoduodenectomy in the treatment of pancreatic carcinoma. *Surg Gynecol Obstet.* 1970;130:1049–1053.
24. Howard JM. Pancreatico-duodenectomy: forty-one consecutive Whipple resections without an operative mortality. *Ann Surg.* 1968;168:629–640.
25. Trede M, Schwall G, Saeger HD. Survival after pancreatoduodenectomy. 118 consecutive resections without an operative mortality. *Ann Surg.* 1990;211:447–458.
26. Schmidt CM, Powell ES, Yiannoutsos CT, et al. Pancreaticoduodenectomy: a 20-year experience in 516 patients. *Arch Surg.* 2004;139:718–725.
27. Conlon KC, Dougherty E, Klimstra DS, et al. The value of minimal access surgery in the staging of patients with potentially resectable peripancreatic malignancy. *Ann Surg.* 1996;223:134–140.
28. Vollmer CM, Drebin JA, Middleton WD, et al. Utility of staging laparoscopy in subsets of peripancreatic and biliary malignancies. *Ann Surg.* 2002;235:1–7.

29. Shoup M, Brennan MF, Karpeh MS, et al. Port site metastasis after diagnostic laparoscopy for upper gastrointestinal tract malignancies: an uncommon entity. *Ann Surg Oncol.* 2002;9:632–636.

30. Kurosaki I, Hatakeyama K, Nihei KE, et al. Celiac axis stenosis in pancreaticoduodenectomy. *J Hepatobiliary Pancreat Surg.* 2004;11:119–124.

31. Howard TJ, Mimms S. Use of a new sealing device to simplify jejunal resection during pancreaticoduodenectomy. *Am J Surg.* 2005;190:504–506.

32. Traverso LW, Longmire WP Jr. Preservation of the pylorus in pancreaticoduodenectomy. *Surg Gynecol Obstet,* 1978;146:959–962.

33. Kozuschek W, Reith HB, Waleczek H, et al. A comparison of long term results of the standard Whipple procedure and the pylorus preserving pancreatoduodenectomy. *J Am Coll Surg.* 1994;178:443–453.

34. Bell RH Jr. Pancreaticoduodenectomy with or without pylorus preservation have similar outcomes. *Cancer Treat Rev.* 2005;31:328–331.

35. Satake K, Nishiwaki H, Yokomatsu H, et al. Surgical curability and prognosis for standard versus extended resection for T1 carcinoma of the pancreas. *Surg Gynecol Obstet.* 1992;175:259–265.

36. Pedrazzoli S, DiCarlo V, Dionigi R, et al. Standard versus extended lymphadenectomy associated with pancreatoduodenectomy in the surgical treatment of adenocarcinoma of the head of the pancreas: a multicenter, prospective, randomized study. Lymphadenectomy Study Group. *Ann Surg.* 1998;228:508–517.

37. Yeo CJ, Cameron JL, Lillemoe KD, et al. Pancreaticoduodenectomy with or without distal gastrectomy and extended retroperitoneal lymphadenectomy for periampullary adenocarcinoma, part 2: randomized controlled trial evaluating survival, morbidity, and mortality. *Ann Surg.* 2002;236:355–366.

38. Farnell MB, Pearson RK, Sarr MG, et al. A prospective randomized trial comparing standard pancreatoduodenectomy with pancreatoduodenectomy with extended lymphadenectomy in resectable pancreatic head adenocarcinoma. *Surgery.* 2005;138:618–628.

39. Fortner JG. Regional resection of cancer of the pancreas: a new surgical approach. *Surgery.* 1973;73:307–320.

40. Strasberg SM, Drebin JA, Linehan D. Radical antegrade modular pancreatosplenectomy. *Surgery.* 2003;133:521–527.

41. Nakeeb A. The role of minimally invasive surgery for pancreatic pathology. *Adv Surg.* 2005;39:455–469.

42. Sarr MG. The potent somatostatin analogue vapreotide does not decrease pancreas-specific complications after elective pancreatectomy: a prospective, multicenter, double-blinded, randomized, placebo-controlled trial. *J Am Coll Surg.* 2003;196:556–564.

43. Yeo CJ, Cameron JL, Lillemoe KD, et al. Does prophylactic octreotide decrease the rates of pancreatic fistula and other complications after pancreaticoduodenectomy? Results of a prospective randomized placebo-controlled trial. *Ann Surg.* 2000;232:419–429.

44. Lillemoe KD, Cameron JL, Kim MP, et al. Does fibrin glue sealant decrease the rate of pancreatic fistula after pancreaticoduodenectomy? Results of a prospective randomized trial. *J Gastrointest Surg.* 2004;8:766–772.

45. Yeo CJ, Barry MK, Sauter PK, et al. Erythromycin accelerates gastric emptying after pancreaticoduodenectomy. A prospective, randomized, placebo-controlled trial. *Ann Surg.* 1993;218:229–237.

46. Zyromski, NJ, Viera, C, Stecker, M, et al. Improved outcomes in postoperative and pancreatitis-related visceral pseudoaneurysms. *J Gastrointest Surg.* 2007;11:50–55.

47. Winter JM, Cameron JL, Campbell KA, et al. 1423 pancreaticoduodenectomies for pancreatic cancer: a single-institution experience. *J Gastrointest Surg.* 2006;10:1199–1211.

48. Van Heek NT, De Castro SM, van Eijck CH, et al. The need for a prophylactic gastrojejunostomy for unresectable periampullary cancer: a prospective randomized multicenter trial with special focus on assessment of quality of life. *Ann Surg.* 2003;238:894–902.

49. Lillemoe KD, Cameron JL, Hardacre JM, et al. Is prophylactic gastrojejunostomy indicated for unresectable periampullary cancer? A prospective randomized trial. *Ann Surg.* 1999;230:322–328.

50. Lillemoe KD, Cameron JL, Kaufman HS, et al. Chemical splanchnicectomy in patients with unresectable pancreatic cancer. A prospective randomized trial. *Ann Surg.* 1993;217:447–455.

51. Wong GY, Schroeder DR, Carns PE, et al. Effect of neurolytic celiac plexus block on pain relief, quality of life, and survival in patients with unresectable pancreatic cancer: a randomized controlled trial. *JAMA.* 2004;291:1092–1099.

52. Cardenes HR, Chiorean EG, Dewitt J, et al. Locally advanced pancreatic cancer: current therapeutic approach. *Oncologist.* 2006;11:612–623.

53. Sindelar WF. Clinical experience with regional pancreatectomy for adenocarcinoma of the pancreas. *Arch Surg.* 1989;124:127–132.

54. Launois B, Franci J, Bardazoglou E, et al. Total pancreatectomy for ductal adenocarcinoma of the pancreas with special reference to resection of the portal vein and multicentric cancer. *World J Surg.* 1993;17:122–126.

55. Harrison LE, Klimstra DS, Brennan MF. Isolated portal vein involvement in pancreatic adenocarcinoma. A contraindication for resection? *Ann Surg.* 1996;224:342–347.

56. Roder JD, Stein HJ, Siewert JR. Carcinoma of the periampullary region: who benefits form portal vein resection? *Am J Surg.* 1996;171:170–174.

57. Bold RJ, Charnsangavej C, Cleary KR, et al. Major vascular resection as part of pancreaticoduodenectomy for cancer: radiologic, intraoperative, and pathologic analysis. *J Gastrointest Surg.* 1999;3:233–243.

58. Bachellier P, Nakano H, Oussoultzoglou PD, et al. Is pancreaticoduodenectomy with mesentericoportal venous resection safe and worthwhile? *Am J Surg.* 2001;182:120–129.

59. Van Geenen RC, ten Kate FJ, de Wit LT, et al. Segmental resection and wedge excision of the portal or superior mesenteric vein during pancreatoduodenectomy. *Surgery.* 2001;129:158–163.

60. Howard TJ, Villanustre N, Moore SA, et al. Efficacy of venous reconstruction in patients with adenocarcinoma of the pancreatic head. *J Gastrointest Surg.* 2003;7:1089–1095.

61. Capussotti L, Massucco P, Ribero D, et al. Extended lymphadenectomy and vein resection for pancreatic head cancer: outcomes and implications for therapy. *Arch Surg.* 2003;138:1316–1322.

62. Poon RT, Fan ST, Lo CM, et al. Pancreaticoduodenectomy with en bloc portal vein resection for pancreatic carcinoma with suspected portal vein involvement. *World J Surg.* 2004;28:602–608.

63. Jain S, Sacchi M, Vrachnos P, et al. Carcinoma of the pancreas with portal vein involvement: our experience with a modified technique of resection. *Hepatogastroenterology.* 2005;52:1596–1600.

64. Shimada K, Sano T, Sakamoto Y, et al. Clinical implications of combined portal vein resection as a palliative procedure in patients undergoing pancreaticoduodenectomy for pancreatic head carcinoma. *Ann Surg Oncol.* 2006;13:1569–1578.

65. Birkmeyer JD, Siewers AE, Finlayson EV, et al. Hospital volume and surgical mortality in the United States. *N Engl J Med.* 2002;346:1128–1137.

66. Fong Y, Gonene M, Rubin D, et al. Long-term survival is superior after resection for cancer in high-volume centers. *Ann Surg.* 2005;242:540–547.

67. Birkmeyer JD, Warshaw AL, Finlayson SRG, et al. Relationship between hospital volume and late survival after pancreaticoduodenectomy. *Surgery.* 1999;126:178–183.

Drs. Zyromski, Nakeeb, and Lillemoe have presented a very excellent and complete review of all aspects of pancreatic neoplasia based not only on extensive literature review but also on their own very extensive and impressive personal experience. This commentary is basically planned to emphasize some of their points by comparison and/or contrast or, at times, play the devil's advocate to stimulate additional thinking, perhaps in a new or different direction.

The major concern in pancreatic carcinoma is its basic biologic behavior. Article after article over many decades has shown that survival has not improved significantly, independent of progress in surgical and medical management. The majority of patients with pancreatic cancer are not resectable, and even among those patients who have their tumors resected only 10% to 20 % enjoy a 5-year survival. There is no substantial proof in any scientific report that earlier diagnosis, any type of screening, or more aggressive operations have produced any significant survivor benefit.

PATHOLOGY

The review of pathology by the authors is quite extensive and complete. I will address only the diagnosis of mucinous cystic neoplasms (MCNs). If there is unilocular cystic mass in the tail of the pancreas with no history of prior pancreatitis and a patient has no contraindications for surgery, then a presumptive diagnosis of MCN can be made and a distal pancreatectomy can be performed. However, with cystic mass present in the head, because of the increased morbidity and mortality associated with pancreaticoduodenectomy, a more extensive diagnostic workup may be indicated. This is usually accomplished by cyst aspiration. Although cytology may be part of the workup, I have not found this to be particularly helpful in recovering meaningful cells for diagnosis. Mucin should always be tested for in the aspirate as the presence of mucin indicates an MCN, whether premalignant or malignant. Carcinoembryonic antigen in the cyst fluid should also be measured routinely; however, I think a threshold of 400 ng/ml is better than the 200 ng/ml recommended in the chapter. It is important to balance the sensitivity versus the specificity; that is, the false-negatives versus the false-positives. Using the level of 400 ng/ml may mean a slight loss in sensitivity but a marked increase in specificity increasing the likelihood that the cyst is a significant MCN and should be resected. Because the purpose of the aspiration is to justify the need for pancreaticoduodenectomy, I think the use of the higher threshold may be more applicable.

PREOPERATIVE DIAGNOSIS AND MANAGEMENT

Most patients with surgically treatable disease have carcinoma in the head of the pancreas. Therefore, most patients present with

jaundice. In general, in patients with obstructive jaundice in the fifth decade or older, cancer should be the initial diagnosis until proven otherwise. This is especially true if they have no other reason to have jaundice, such as evidence of hepatitis, stones in the common duct, recent biliary operations with the possibility of iatrogenic duct stricture, or other diseases associated with bile duct stricture such as inflammatory bowel disease. The purpose of the preoperative workup is not so much to prove the diagnosis, which is already a given, but to determine which patients are unresectable because of liver metastases, extensive lymph node metastases, peritoneal carcinomatosis, and/or vascular invasion. By preoperative staging, patients who are clearly not resectable or curable by surgical means can avoid an unnecessary exploration.

The practical approach to the evaluation of patients with jaundice with a high suspicion of carcinoma follows:

1. *Helical (spiral) computerized tomography*. It should be emphasized that computerized tomography (CT) is not used so much to make a definite diagnosis of pancreatic cancer but rather to determine resectability. The problem with using the CT to make a definite diagnosis is the high rate of false-negative findings (approximately 20%). Often, the reason for a false-negative finding is a relatively small cancer in the head of the pancreas at the junction of the pancreatic and biliary duct that cannot be adequately imaged on the CT scan. However, these small lesions are often the earliest and most resectable; therefore, simply because the CT scan does not show such a definite pancreatic mass does not mean that the patients do not have cancer, especially a resectable cancer. The appearance of the double-duct sign—that is, a dilated bile duct and a dilated pancreatic duct—almost always indicates periampullary carcinoma, especially pancreatic cancer. The presence of a mass in the head of the pancreas may be helpful but is not 100% diagnostic because false-positive findings can be produced by pancreatic head pancreatitis, enlarged lymph nodes, other neoplasms, and so forth. Usually the CT scan will show intrahepatic and extrahepatic biliary dilatation that extends down to the pancreatic level. If it does, one can assume that this is due to either pancreatic cancer or another periampullary cancer and proceed accordingly. Obviously, if there is no extrahepatic biliary dilatation or if the dilatation extends only partially down the duct, other diagnoses should be suspected and substantiated with either endoscopic retrograde cholangiopancreatography (ERCP), percutaneous transhepatic cholangiography, or magnetic resonance cholangiopancreatography. Therefore, the CT is not used to make the diagnosis of pancreatic cancer but to establish evidence of unresectable disease.

2. *CA19-9*. CA19-9 should not be used a screening test in asymptomatic individuals because significantly sized lesions need to be present for the test to be positive. In addition, there are false-positive findings with other tumors producing elevations, such as upper gastrointestinal cancers, and colon cancers. Also there are no studies to prove that that using CA19-9 as a screening test improves patient outcomes. However, if the patient is jaundiced, an elevated CA19-9 may be helpful. Obviously, if the patient is jaundiced and has a significantly elevated CA19-9 (>200), the assumption is that the patient has malignancy as a cause be it pancreatic,

ampullary, or bile duct cancer. On the other hand, a negative test is of no particular help. Approximately 20% of patients with pancreatic cancer do not exhibit an elevated CA19-9 and therefore a negative test cannot exclude the diagnosis. On the other hand, there have been incidents of false-positive findings with CA19-9 in the setting of obstructive jaundice. Therefore, CA19-9 can be supportive to the clinical suspicions but should not be used alone. However, the test is easy to perform, inexpensive, noninvasive, and can be helpful in planning therapy and in early discussions with the patients.

3. *Laparoscopy.* I agree that laparoscopy should be performed only on selected individuals. Laparoscopy can be done on an individual with high suspicion of unresectable disease that has not been definitely proven on CT. This is especially true if one suspects carcinomatosis from the presence on CT of ascites or omental or mesentery thickening. Laparoscopy can be helpful in those patients with small liver metastases or peritoneal carcinomatosis but is not helpful in determining vascular involvement, retroperitoneal spread, and so forth. Therefore, laparoscopic examination is done on selective basis rather then as a routine.

4. *Endoscopic retrograde pancreatography.* I agree wholeheartedly that ERCP should not be done routinely. Reasons for this include the following:

   (a) The real purpose of preoperative testing is to determine resectability, and this is not possible with an ERCP.

   (b) There are potential complications of the ERCP, including cholangitis, perforations, and so forth.

   (c) The operation for ampullary, distal bile duct, or pancreatic cancer is exactly the same—that is, a pancreaticoduodenectomy—and a precise preoperative diagnosis is not needed to proceed in the proper fashion.

   (d) When an ERCP is performed, a stent is usually placed. This is done to help prevent cholangitis, which may be caused by the introduction of bacteria into the obstructed duct during ERCP. The preoperative placement of stents has not proven to be of significant benefit and may make the subsequent surgery more difficult by decreasing the diameter of the bile duct and causing periductal inflammation. Also, numerous reports have shown a higher rate of postoperative sepsis and infection when a preoperative ERCP stent was used.

   ERCP stenting, however, does have a place in certain circumstances: (a) When the patient is obviously not resectable as determined by CT scan or physical findings, a stent can produce palliation without the need for operation. (b) If the patient is currently not an operative candidate because of malnutrition, stenting may help decompress the liver and return the patient to operative status by improving the nutritional environment. (c) ERCP stenting may be helpful if surgery needs to be delayed by2 two weeks or longer because of the need for additional workup, treatment of comorbid conditions, or other reasons.

5. *Endoscopic ultrasonography.* Endoscopic ultrasonography is being increasing used, but there has been no proof that its routine use is beneficial in the management and outcome of these patients. Endoscopic ultrasound is used selectively when the clinical presentation and CT scans are not concordant or another diagnosis other than adenocarcinoma is suspected. In this case, endoscopic ultrasound may be helpful to make a correct diagnosis and lead to proper therapy.

OPERATIVE MANAGEMENT

After a helical CT scan that shows no evidence of unresectable disease, an operation is undertaken. The experienced surgeon then has to make the intraoperative decision that the patient has resectable periampullary or pancreatic cancer without a positive biopsy and then proceed with a pancreaticoduodenectomy (Whipple procedure). In a small percentage of cases, even with an experienced surgeon, a Whipple procedure will be performed for benign disease; that is, pancreatitis of the head. This is acceptable treatment for this diagnosis and avoids not treating a small resectable pancreatic cancer. Considerations in the operative approach include the following:

1. *Incision.* Although the authors state that either a midline incision or a bilateral subcostal, that is, transverse incision can be used equally, I much prefer the transverse incision, which gives better exposure to all aspects of the operation than the midline incision.

2. *Kocher maneuver.* I agree that an extensive Kocher maneuver should be the first step in the operative process after examining for resectability. This rules out invasion into the retroperitoneal structures and unresectability. In addition, a very extensive Kocher maneuver with rotation of the pancreas and duodenum forward places the retroperitoneal duodenum and pancreas into a much more anterior position, making all subsequent steps in the operation easier to perform. I do not think that examination of involvement of the superior mesenteric artery (SMA) during this maneuver adds anything to the finding of the CT scans done preoperatively. I have found this always to be a very difficult intraoperative assessment and have found that CT scans are much more accurate in making this determination.

3. *Pyloric sparing.* I agree with the authors that pyloric sparing is probably slightly preferable to the standard Whipple procedure with distal gastric resection. However, I think it is the surgeon's choice and the decision is to be based on the individual anatomic variation and the extent of disease seen at the time of operation. There has been little evidence to show that there is any significant survival benefit between the two procedures, and the difference in long-term nutritional effects between the two are not great.

4. *Variations in technique.* In general, I agree with the procedure that the authors have described in performing the Whipple procedure. However, I prefer certain variations.

   (a) It seems that the authors leave the gallbladder attached to the bile duct during the resection and remove it en bloc with the specimen. I find it very helpful for exposure purposes to remove the gallbladder early in the procedure.

   (b) Rather than first exposing the superior mesenteric vein (SMV) below the pancreas and proceeding upward, I think it is easier to start the dissection on the portal/SMV in the porta hepatis and proceeding downward toward the SMV, and then find and dissect SMV below the pancreas as the second step.

(c) I do not divide the bile duct early in the procedure but almost as my last step before removing the specimen. This is particularly so for patients who have ERCP stenting to decrease the amount of bile duct spillage and subsequent infection.

(d) The proximal bile duct and duodenum are, in my experience, not commonly involved with carcinoma, so these margins are not routinely sent for frozen section analysis. Although when not done as routine, obviously if there is any suspicious areas then they should be sent for frozen section analysis. However, the pancreatic margin is much more commonly affected, so a consideration can be given for routine frozen section examination.

(e) I free the jejunum distal to the ligament of Treitz and rotate it under the SMA and SMV to the right side prior to splitting the pancreas. I do this because this is not an irreversible step in the operation and this maneuver may show evidence of unresectability, and the operation can still be abandoned at the point. Secondly, I find that this maneuver increases the visibility and exposure for the pancreatic splitting and the rotated jejunum can be used as a handle to pull the specimen to the right and anteriorly, significantly aiding in the dissection of the SMV/portal vein and SMA.

5. *Pancreatic anastomosis.* The method of pancreatic anastomosis has always been controversial because one of the major complications of pancreaticoduodenectomy is pancreatic fluid leak and subsequent pancreatic fistula. Obviously, the pancreatic anastomosis can be handled in multiple fashions including end-to-end or end-to-side anastomoses or simply closing the head of the pancreas with the thoraco-abdominal (TA) stapling device or, especially in the case of a diabetic patient, a total pancreatectomy. Again, the technique used must be individually based on the training of the surgeon and any patient specifics, including consistency of the gland and size of the pancreatic duct. Although the authors routinely favor an end-to-side mucosa-to-mucosa pancreaticojejunostomy, I tend to favor invagination of the gland into the end of the jejunum. They also prefer this type of approach with the soft pancreas or a small duct, thinking that it is safer in these circumstances. However, if it is safer in these circumstances, I think that it is equally applicable when you have a firmer pancreas or a large duct. I tend to use the invagination procedure in most of my patients whether with dilated or normal duct. Again, our technique of invagination seems to be similar. The end of the pancreas is telescoped into the end of the pancreatic limb using a two-layer anastomosis with running 3–0 polypropylene suture externally and a running a 3–0 polyglactin suture internally. With this method, we have had a small percentage of leaks, well under 10%. All the anastomoses are drained by closed suction drainage because if there is a small leak it can be controlled by this drain. If there is no distal obstruction, a small fistula will close spontaneously. I have not in the recent past used any type of pancreatic stents as I have not seen the utility of their use and they may result in complications. The biliary jejunal anastomosis is done with a single layer of 4–0 running polyglactic suture. I agree

with the authors that a T-tube or biliary stent is not needed and is not used.

6. *Extended Whipple operation.* An extended Whipple procedure includes any combination of resection of the SMV and/or the SMA, total pancreatectomy, and/or extensive lymph node dissections outside the peripancreatic area. In general, I think these procedures are examples of the surgeon's wishful thinking captured in the quote from Alexander Pope, "Hope springs eternal." There is absolutely no evidence that any of these procedures increase survival significantly, and they certainly may increase the complication rate. As far as resecting vessels, there have been multiple studies showing that there is no real survival benefit resulting from this. The reason is that the patients generally fail with distant disease—that is, either liver or peritoneal metastases—and therefore removing the vessels does not have any impact on the occurrence of these metastases. Also, those patients who have vessel involvement have a poorer prognosis and a greater chance of having distant micrometastases than those patients whose vessels are not involved.

Not surprisingly, extensive lymph node dissections have not proven to have any benefit. Lymph node positivity, especially lymph node distance from the pancreas, is an indicator of systemic disease but not a determinant. The majority of patients do not fail locally in the lymph nodes but distantly in the liver and/or peritoneum. If the lymph nodes in the retroperitoneal, celiac, or para-aortic area are negative, then obviously the patient cannot benefit from having them removed. If they are positive, this is an indicator of distant disease and the patient is not benefited by their removal.

In general, major vessel resections are not part of the planned operation because of the limitations of it increasing survival for the patients. It may be able to be performed technically, but does it actually improve the outcome for the patients? This is severely in doubt. Occasionally during the operation, the anterior part of the SMV and portal vein is clear, but as you rotate the head of the pancreas to the right side and posteriorly it becomes obvious that the tumor involves the lateral or posterior portion of the vein. This usually occurs in a carcinoma in the uncinate process and is not discovered until after the pancreatic gland is split and the pancreas is rotated. At this point, one must proceed with the Whipple procedure out of necessity. A partial or complete resection of the portal vein can be performed to complete the Whipple procedure with no expectation that the cure rate is increased by this maneuver. On the other hand, one is occasionally confronted with a young, otherwise healthy patient who has involvement of the SMV or portal vein determined preoperatively. This patient wants to have the most aggressive therapy and understands the limitations. At the same time, you wish to avoid unnecessary and potentially dangerous procedure with the patient. In these very specific incidences, I have pretreated the patient with chemoradiation to the area of the pancreatic head. This may allow downsizing of the tumor but more importantly leaves one a window of approximately 3 months to re-evaluate the patient for metastatic disease before proceeding with the extended Whipple procedure. In this way, the patient with the potentially better biological outcome, that is, the patient who has not developed metastases during this waiting period, is selected. That said, there is no good evidence even with this approach that we have changed significantly the outcome in these patients.

7. *Distal pancreatectomy.* I agree with the authors that resectability, and more importantly cure, is very limited for pancreatic adenocarcinoma in the body and tail. This is probably a combination of the aggressive biological activity of these tumors and late presentation due to of lack of significant symptoms until an advanced stage is reached. Although adenocarcinoma of the pancreas occurring in the distal pancreas can be occasionally resected, distal pancreatectomy is usually done for other neoplasms such as MCN, either adenoma or cyst adenocarcinoma of the distal pancreas. My approach to distal pancreatectomy differs slightly from that of the authors. I do not proceed first to the SMV or along the inferior board of the pancreas. After determining respectability, I believe the easiest way to resect the distal pancreas is to swing both the spleen and tail of the pancreas forward and expose the posterior portion of the pancreas where the splenic artery, splenic vein, and its confluence with SMV lay, and thus increase the exposure. Transaction of the pancreas is done with a TA stapler. Although the pancreatic resection margin is routinely drained, we have not had any significant problem with pancreatic fistulas as long as there is no proximal obstruction in the pancreatic duct.

OUTCOMES AFTER PANCREATIC RESECTION

I agree with the authors that a pancreatic fistula is one of the more significant complications of the Whipple procedure and also agree that the use of octreotide, fibrin glue, and other approaches have not been of any particular benefit. I think a proper anastomosis with adequate drainage prevents most of these leaks and controls the few that do occur without significant complications.

Gastric outlet obstruction still occurs in 10% to 15% of the patients, lasting from a few days to many weeks. Although this is not a serious complication, it can be extremely upsetting for the patients during its resolution. Although I do not have good data to support my approaches, I generally start metoclopramide prophylactically the day after surgery and use gastrografin on the third or fourth day therapeutically before starting feeding. The gastrografin seems to stimulate gastric emptying by increasing peristalsis, by reducing edema in anastomoses by its osmotic effect, and by being a mucolytic agent.

Palliative Treatment

It must be realized that most of our efforts in treating patients with pancreatic cancer presently are in reality palliative. The majority of Whipple procedures that we perform, even those we think are curative, actually turn out to be merely palliative because there is distant microscopic disease of which we are not aware. This is the reason that even extensive surgery still shows a 5-year survival rate that does not exceed 20%. Therefore, at least 80% of pancreatectomies for pancreatic carcinoma are, in fact, palliative. However, I do not recommend an obvi-

ously purposeful palliative Whipple procedure when patients have obvious distance disease in the liver, peritoneal metastases, and so forth. This can expose patients to excessive morbidity to produce palliative results that can be obtained easily by simple bypass procedures.

In patients with obviously unresectable disease determined preoperatively, palliation should be attempted nonoperatively. This can generally be performed with a stent placed by ERCP for resolution of the jaundice. As far as gastric outlet obstruction is concerned, this is in general not as common a problem as bile duct obstruction. However, when it does occur, again a nonoperative approach should be tried to decrease morbidity to the patients. We have had increasing success with endoscopic dilation and stenting of the obstruction to produce adequate palliation.

Although most palliative attempts should be done nonoperatively, there is the occasion in which we are operating on the patient and then find that the tumor is unresectable. Palliation therefore should be undertaken during the operative procedure. Although the objectives of the palliation, that is, the treatment of the obstructive jaundice and the prevention of gastric outlet obstruction are the same, I have different approaches than the authors:

1. Unless there are signs of impending gastric outlet obstruction, I do not routinely perform a gastrojejunostomy. There are potential complications both short term and long term of the gastrojejunostomy, especially when no obstruction is actually present. In addition, it has been our experience that only a small percentage of patients (10%) develop gastric outlet obstruction before they die (1). Therefore, 90% of patients never need a bypass. In those patients who do develop an obstruction, this can generally be treated nonoperatively with the previously mentioned endoscopic stent.

2. Obviously, when unresectability is confirmed intraoperatively, bile duct obstruction should be treated operatively. However, I differ with the authors for their preference of doing a choledochojejunostomy or a cholecystojejunostomy. In general, I think that a cholecystojejunostomy is a very poor form of biliary drainage and does not have long durability. I also favor a cholecystoduodenostomy over a Roux-en-Y choledochojejunostomy because it is simpler and easier to perform; more physiologic, delivering bile back into the duodenum; and if subsequent obstruction occurs, it is easier to access by ERCP and stenting (2).

FUTURE TREATMENT

Perioperative adjunctive therapies are discussed in detail in Chapter 36. It is in this area where emphasis needs to be placed. There is some evidence that there is a minor impact of adjuvant chemoradiation after a Whipple procedure, although the effect is not marked and almost all of the patients fail outside the radiated area.

Over the past several years, performing extensive preoperative workup, especially with helical CT scans, has decreased the amount of unnecessary operations. This has increased the rate of successful resections and has saved many patients from needless surgery. More sensitive preoperative evaluation is certainly a significant move forward, allowing us to be as selective as we can in the care of our patients. Also, I think more experience and better preoperative staging have perhaps decreased the absolute number of Whipple procedures that are performed, and have slightly increased the percentage of the patients who have had 5-year survival after this operation. However, it may not have increased the absolute number of patients surviving 5 years, but simply the percentage. In the years ahead, I think we should continue to try to devise new methods of assessment, such as positron emission tomography and molecular markers, to select even more accurately those patients who have truly local disease and who can, therefore, benefit from pancreaticoduodenectomy.

The authors have stated that there have been extensive strides over the past years in the operative care of the patients with pancreatic cancer, with significant decreases in both the mortality and the morbidity of the operation. I agree; however, these apparent advances have not been matched by a significant increase in the surgical cure of these patients. I think all of us, as surgeons, need to come to a better understanding of the biology of pancreatic cancer. We have to understand that by the time patients are seen, most already have distance disease and cannot be cured by a pancreaticoduodenectomy or even bigger and supposedly better operations such as extensive lymph node dissections, vascular resections, and so forth. We must respond to the biology of the disease and understand that this is usually a systemic disease when first seen and that effective adjuvant therapy needs to be developed to significantly change the survival outcomes for patients with pancreatic carcinoma. Only with the development of effective adjuvant treatments will we see any significant and meaningful increase in the survival of our patients with pancreatic cancer.

REFERENCES

1. DiFronzo LA, Cymerman J, Egar S, et al. Non resectable pancreatic carcinoma: correlating length of survival with choice of palliative bypass. *Am Surg.* 1999;65:955–958.
2. DiFronzo LA, Egar S, O'Connell TX. Choledochoduodenostomy for palliation in unresectable pancreatic cancer. *Arch Surg.* 1998;133: 820–825.

36

Cancer of the Pancreas: Adjuvant and Neoadjuvant Therapy

David J. Park and Heinz-Josef Lenz

Cancer of the pancreas continues to pose a formidable clinical challenge with limited effective management options. Although it accounts for only 2% of malignancies in men and women in the United States, it is the fourth leading cause of cancer-related death (1).

Since first described in 1935 by Whipple et al. (2), pancreaticoduodenectomy has remained the principal surgical procedure for radical "curative" resection for most localized cancers of involving the head of the pancreas. However, depending on its location and extent, removal of tumor by distal pancreatectomy or total pancreatectomy may be required. Over the years, the "Whipple" procedure has undergone various modifications and standardization that have led to a decrease in perioperative morbidity and mortality. In experienced hands the perioperative mortality rate now approaches 1% to 2% (3).

Unfortunately, only about 10% to 15% of patients diagnosed with pancreatic cancer are eligible to undergo radical curative resection, mainly because of advanced disease at presentation. Even after a curative resection, only 5% to 20% of patients are expected to be alive in 5 years, because of relapse of disease (4). Most recurrences after curative resection are local or hepatic. Sperti and associates (5) analyzed 78 patients who underwent curative resection for pancreatic cancer and found that 97% of recurrences were either local (78%) or hepatic (61.5%). Ninety-five percent of the recurrences were diagnosed within 24 months following surgery. This group of patients had a median disease-free survival of 8 months, and a 5-year survival rate of 3%. Westerdahl et al. (6) reviewed the course of 74 patients who died within 6 months of curative surgery with recurrent disease. Local recurrence and hepatic metastases were present in 64 and 68 patients, respectively.

The poor results associated with radical surgery, the only potentially curative treatment now available, underscores the urgent need for effective perioperative therapy that can eradicate micrometastatic disease. Adjuvant and neoadjuvant strategies have used chemotherapy, radiation, or a combination of these two modalities. The inherent chemo- and radioresistant properties of pancreatic tumors have made this a challenging endeavor. Progress has been characterized by small, incremental gains compared with the more rapid advances achieved in other gastrointestinal malignancies, such as colon and rectal cancer.

In this chapter, we provide a review of the worldwide experience with adjuvant and neoadjuvant strategies (chemotherapy, external-beam radiotherapy, and combination of chemotherapy and radiotherapy) for localized pancreatic cancer. Locally advanced, apparently unresectable pancreatic cancer, is also considered because the line between resectability and unresectability is sometimes unclear. Intraoperative radiotherapy is a management modality undergoing study in a limited number of centers and is discussed briefly here.

ADJUVANT THERAPY: CHEMOTHERAPY AND CHEMORADIATION

Several randomized controlled trials of adjuvant treatment following curative resection of pancreatic cancer have been reported (7–11) (Table 36.1). In the United States, data supporting multimodality therapy come from a relatively small phase 3 evaluation of postoperative adjuvant chemoradiation conducted by the Gastrointestinal Tumor Study Group (GITSG) and published in 1985 (7). The study regimen consisted of two courses of radiotherapy, each 20 Gy, combined with bolus injections of 5-fluorouracil (5-FU; 500 mg/m^2 for 3 days), followed by weekly 5-FU for 2 years or until recurrence occurred. This trial was closed early because of poor patient accrual. However, compared with postoperative observation only, a statistically significant doubling in median survival and a modest improvement in 5-year survival were noted in the patients who received the split-course chemoradiation regimen. The median survival was 21 months in the treated group (n = 21) compared with 11 months in the observation group (n = 22). The 2- and 5-year survival rates were 43% versus 18% and 19% versus 5%, respectively. This trial was subject to considerable criticism because of its small sample size, slow accrual, and premature closure. Furthermore, it was unclear if the derived clinical benefit was because of the combination of chemoradiation and maintenance chemotherapy, or to only one of these therapies.

Similar findings were observed in a follow-up nonrandomized study (no control group) of 30 patients who received the same adjuvant chemoradiotherapy program as in the earlier trial (12). The median survival was 18 months, and the 2-year survival was 46%. Unfortunately, this follow-up study was also subject to criticism, in this case because the treatment group had a better performance status compared with the patients treated in the earlier study. Nevertheless, based on these trials, adjuvant chemoradiation has become standard practice in the United States.

Table 36.1

Published Randomized Trials of Adjuvant Therapy for Pancreatic Cancer

Trial (Ref.)	Treatment	No. of Patients	Results	p Value
GITSG (7)	Observation	22	MS 11 mo	0.035
	Chemoradiation	21	MS 20 mo	
Bakkevold et al. (8)[a]	Observation	30	MS 11 mo	0.02
	Chemotherapy	31	MS 23 mo	
EORTC (9)	Observation	54	MS 12.6 mo	0.099
	Chemoradiation	60	MS 17.1 mo	
Takada et al. (10)	Observation	81	DFS 18.00%	0.02
	Chemotherapy	77	DFS 11.50%	
ESPAC-1 (11)	No chemoradiation	144	MS 17.9 mo	0.05
	Chemoradiation	145	MS 15.9 mo	
	No chemotherapy	142	MS 15.5 mo	0.009
	Chemotherapy	147	MS 20.1 mo	

GITSG, Gastrointestinal Tumor Study Group; MS, median survival; EORTC, European Organisation for Research and
Treatment of Cancer; DFS, 5-year disease-free survival; ESPAC, European Study Group for Pancreatic Cancer
[a]Includes 14 patients with ampullary carcinoma.

In Europe and Asia, however, the value of radiation as an adjunct to chemotherapy continues to be questioned. The European Organisation for Research and Treatment of Cancer (EORTC) initiated a randomized adjuvant trial in 1,987 of patients with pancreatic and periampullary adenocarcinoma (9). A total of 218 patients from 29 centers in Europe who had undergone pancreaticoduodenectomy were randomized to receive either chemoradiation (n = 110) consisting of split-course radiation (40 Gy) and 5-FU continuous infusion (25 mg/kg/day) during the radiation without further adjuvant chemotherapy versus observation alone (n = 108). Two hundred seven patients were eligible for analysis (11 were not eligible because of incomplete resection), of whom 114 (55%) had pancreatic cancer. Twenty-one patients (20%) in the treatment arm did not receive their assigned therapy for various reasons. The median survival for the treatment group was 24.5 months versus 19 months for the observation group ($p = 0.2$). A trend for benefit was seen in the subgroup of patients with pancreatic cancer, with a 2-year survival rate of 34% versus 26% ($p = 0.099$). This was an underpowered study that showed some potential benefit for chemoradiation in the adjuvant setting. The study authors' conclusion, however, was that chemoradiation was not warranted as adjuvant therapy.

Since the publication of the GITSG study, a series of nonrandomized trials of adjuvant chemoradiation have been conducted in single centers in the United States, mostly evaluating postoperative radiation with 5-FU used as radiosensitizer. Whittington and associates (13) conducted a small retrospective study comparing surgery alone (n = 33, historical controls) with varying adjuvant radiation or chemoradiation regimens (n = 39). Compared to surgery alone, chemoradiation seemed to have a beneficial effect in overall survival.

In a larger prospective series by Yeo and associates (14), patients who underwent radical resection (n = 174 with one postoperative death) were offered the options of (a) "standard" chemoradiotherapy (40 to 45 Gy given with two 3-day 5-FU courses and followed by weekly 5-FU for 4 months), (b) "intensive" chemoradiotherapy (50.4 to 57.6 Gy with prophylactic hepatic irradiation 23.4 to 27 Gy given with and followed by infusional 5-FU for 5 of 7 days for 4 months), or (c) observation. Although not randomized, the three groups possessed similar baseline characteristics such as tumor size, lymph node involvement, blood loss, age, and gender. Patients who received adjuvant chemoradiation (n = 120) had an improved median survival of 19.5 versus 13.5 months compared to observation alone. There was no difference in clinical benefit between the standard and intensive adjuvant treatment groups.

In a phase 2 trial, Mehta et al. (15) studied the efficacy and toxicity of adjuvant continuous 5-FU infusion with radiation (45 Gy plus boost to 54 Gy if positive surgical margins). Fifty-two patients underwent radical surgery and were treated with this chemoradiation protocol. No grade 4 or 5 toxicities were observed. Ninety-five percent of the patients were able to complete the prescribed treatment course. The median survival in this cohort was 32 months.

In 2000, investigators at Johns Hopkins University published their single-institutional experience in the management of localized pancreatic cancer. Between 1984 and 1999, 616 patients underwent radical surgery. Treatment with adjuvant chemoradiation was identified as a positive prognostic factor in multivariate analysis (hazard ratio [HR], 0.50; $p < 0.0001$) (3).

Collectively, these aforementioned studies (as well as other smaller studies not included in this review) seem to suggest a beneficial role for adjuvant chemoradiation as a reasonable approach to localized pancreatic cancer. However, in 2004, the much-awaited long-term results of the European Study Group for Pancreatic Cancer (ESPAC-1) adjuvant trial were published (11). This study, which stimulated further controversy, was the largest adjuvant pancreatic trial to date, with accrual of 289 patients from 11 countries. Actually, many more patients were enrolled in the trial, but only data on those who underwent strict randomization were published. The design was a 2 × 2 factorial design randomly assigning 73 patients to chemoradiotherapy alone (20 Gy over a 2-week period plus 5-FU), 75 patients to chemotherapy alone (5-FU), 72 patients to both chemoradiotherapy and chemotherapy, and 69 patients to observation. Because of its design, comparisons could be made between chemoradiation (chemoradiation plus chemoradiation/chemotherapy) versus no chemoradiation (observation plus chemotherapy), and chemotherapy (chemotherapy plus chemoradiation/chemotherapy) versus no chemotherapy (observation plus chemoradiation).

After a median follow-up of 47 months, the results favored adjuvant chemotherapy and not chemoradiation. The median survival was 20.1 months for the chemotherapy-alone group (n = 147) versus 15.5 months for the no-chemotherapy group (n = 142; p = 0.009), with 2- and 5-year estimated survival rates being 40% versus 21%, and 30% versus 8%, respectively, for each treatment group. Surprisingly, chemoradiation (n = 145) was shown to be inferior to no chemoradiation (n = 144) with a median survival of 15.9 versus 17.9 months (p = 0.05). The corresponding estimated 2- and 5-year survival rates were 10% versus 29% and 20% versus 41%, respectively, favoring the no-chemoradiotherapy group. The authors' conclusion was that chemotherapy after radical resection, rather than chemoradio-therapy, should be the new standard of care in the management of localized carcinoma of the pancreas. That is to say, effective treatment doses of chemotherapy should be introduced earlier rather than being delayed by chemoradiation.

The ESPAC-1 trial has provoked considerable controversy, especially in the United States, where adjuvant chemoradiotherapy is considered the standard of care and its administration much more prevalent compared with chemotherapy alone. As a result, this trial has been the subject of several critical reviews. Criticisms of the trial include the fact that a significant proportion of patients did not complete the chemotherapy treatment protocol and that there was a delay in the commencement of chemoradiation after surgery compared with chemotherapy (61 vs. 48 days). Moreover, there was a lack of quality control (i.e., no central review) for radiotherapy planning and delivery, with a significant minority of patients receiving either inadequate or no radiation. Although the study lacked enough power to perform four-arm comparisons, the chemoradiotherapy-alone arm fared worse when compared with the observation arm. This finding raises the question as to whether the outcome was attributable to the ineffectiveness of radiotherapy as a treatment modality in this setting or only to the older generation radiotherapy protocol employed in this trial (16,17).

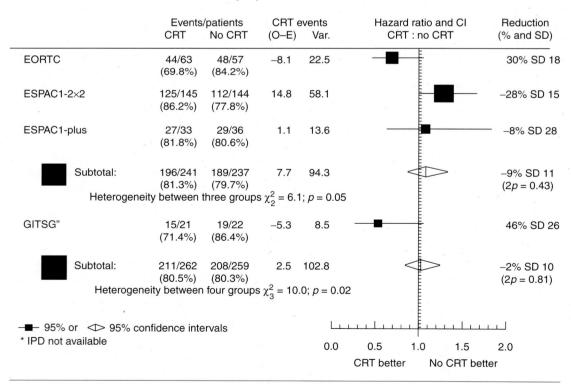

Figure 36.1 Hazard ratio plot of the effect of chemoradiation in the European Organisation for Research and Treatment of Cancer (EORTC) (9), European Study Group for Pancreatic Cancer (ESPAC1) (11), and Gastrointestinal Study Group (GITSG) (7) randomized trials. CRT, adjuvant chemoradiation; O−E, observed minus expected; ◼, individual estimate of the hazard ratio; ◇, pooled stratified estimate of the hazard ratio; IPD, individual patient data. (Reprinted with permission from Macmillan Publishers Ltd.; Stocken DD, Buchler MW, Dervenis C, et al. Meta-analysis of randomised adjuvant therapy trials for pancreatic cancer. *Br J Cancer.* 2005;92:1372–1381.)

In contrast to the conclusions of the ESPAC-1 trial, previous randomized studies examining the role of adjuvant chemotherapy alone versus observation following surgical resection have yielded negative results. A prospective randomized trial conducted by the Norwegian Pancreatic Trials Group (n = 47) employing an adjuvant regimen of 5-FU in combination with mitomycin C and doxorubicin, initially showed a median survival benefit (23 vs. 11 months; $p = 0.02$) for the chemotherapy arm. However, overall survival was the same for the two arms ($p = 0.10$) (8).

Recently, a meta-analysis of randomized adjuvant therapy trials was undertaken by Stocken et al. (18). Five randomized controlled adjuvant trials were identified with a total of 939 patients who had undergone potentially curative resection of pancreatic adenocarcinoma. This meta-analysis also included previously unpublished and newly updated results of the ESPAC1-plus (i.e., an additional 261 patients outside the 2 × 2 factorial trial with 69 patients in the chemoradiation vs. observation comparison and 192 in the chemotherapy vs. observation comparison). The pooled estimate of the HR showed a 25% risk reduction in mortality with adjuvant chemotherapy (HR, 0.75%; 95% confidence interval: 0.64-0.90; $p = 0.001$). The estimated median survival was 19 months in patients treated with chemotherapy versus 13.5 months without. Adjuvant chemoradiation provided no significant clinical benefit compared with no chemoradiation with a HR = 1.09 for risk of death (7−11) (Figures 36.1 and

36.2). However, subgroup analysis seemed to indicate that patients with positive surgical margins may derive benefit from adjuvant chemoradiation but not chemotherapy alone.

These divergent results and points of view (chemotherapy vs. chemoradiotherapy) have led to the design of new clinical trials with emphases differing in Europe and in the United States. In the United States the Gastrointestinal Cancer Committee of the Radiation Therapy Oncology Group (RTOG) designed an adjuvant trial in which patients were randomized to receive continuous infusion 5-FU for 3 weeks or gemcitabine weekly for 3 weeks prior to chemoradiotherapy (with continuous 5-FU). Further 5-FU or gemcitabine per assigned treatment arm was continued as systemic chemotherapy after chemoradiation for an additional 3 months. Gemcitabine, a deoxycytidine analogue, was studied because it had been shown to have clinical activity superior to 5-FU in the treatment of advanced pancreatic cancer (19). The results of this study (RTOG 9704) were presented before the 2006 annual meeting of the American Society of Clinical Oncology (ASCO). From 1998 to 2002, 538 patients were enrolled and 442 patients were eligible and evaluable. The treatment arms were well balanced except for a higher proportion of larger tumors in patients in the gemcitabine arm. Patients with pancreatic head tumors (n = 380) experienced a greater benefit with gemcitabine therapy following surgery and chemoradiotherapy, with a median and 3-year survival of 18.8 months and 31%, respectively, for the gemcitabine arm versus

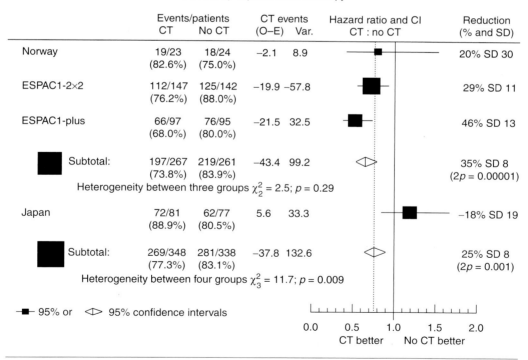

Figure 36.2 Hazard ratio plot of the effect of chemotherapy in the Norwegian (8), European Study Group for Pancreatic Cancer (ESPAC1) (11), and Japanese (10) randomized trials. CT, adjuvant chemotherapy; O−E, observed minus expected; ■, individual estimate of the hazard ratio; ◇, pooled stratified estimate of the hazard ratio. (Reprinted with permission from Macmillan Publishers Ltd.; Stocken DD, Buchler MW, Dervenis C, et al. Meta-analysis of randomised adjuvant therapy trials for pancreatic cancer. *Br J Cancer.* 2005;92:1372–1381.)

16.7 months and 21% for the 5-FU arm ($p = 0.047$). When the analysis included patients with pancreatic body and tail tumors, which in general carry poorer prognoses, no significant difference between the two arms was observed. Nonhematologic toxicity was similar between the two arms, and there was also no difference in febrile neutropenia or infection, although patients in the gemcitabine arm did experience higher hematologic toxicity (20).

The ESPAC, on the other hand, is currently conducting a phase 3 adjuvant clinical trial (ESPAC-3) in which chemoradiotherapy is entirely omitted, based on the conclusions of ESPAC-1. Patients with localized pancreatic cancer will be randomized after surgery to adjuvant 5-FU versus gemcitabine chemotherapy for 6 months. The results of this trial are pending.

In addition, preliminary results of another European chemotherapy-only adjuvant trial were presented at the 2005 ASCO meeting. In this trial, conducted by the Charité Onkologie Clinical Studies in Gastrointestinal Cancers (CONKO-001), 368 patients were enrolled (12 patients were deemed ineligible and excluded). Adjuvant gemcitabine for 6 months was given to 179 patients and 177 patients were in the observation arm. In this well-powered trial, adjuvant gemcitabine was associated with a significant increase in disease-free survival (regardless of surgical margins and/or lymph node status) of 14.2 versus 7.5 months ($p < 0.05$). Updated results on overall survival are pending (21).

Adjuvant Therapy: Current Status

At the present time, it is difficult to propose a standard adjuvant therapy protocol for localized, resected pancreatic cancer given the controversies surrounding the addition of chemoradiotherapy to chemotherapy alone. There seems to be very little doubt that adjuvant chemotherapy with an active regimen (e.g., gemcitabine and other future agents and/or combinations thereof) provides clinical benefit and should be instituted. There also seems to be some consensus that chemoradiotherapy in patients with positive surgical margins will probably be helpful, although definitive data are lacking. The additional role of adjuvant chemoradiotherapy to chemotherapy, especially employing the modern radiation protocols now available, is still vigorously debated, particularly among American and European investigators.

NEOADJUVANT THERAPY

In many of the trials of adjuvant therapy, a significant proportion of patients initially enrolled failed to complete their adjuvant protocol or experienced treatment commencement delays. Prolonged postoperative course and/or patient refusal after surgery are some of the reasons for this phenomenon. In fact, in the United States it has been estimated that only about 40% of patients undergoing radical surgery undergo adjuvant therapy (12% radiation or chemotherapy and 28% chemoradiation) (22).

Consequently, there has been a growing interest in the administration of chemotherapy, radiotherapy, or both, in the preoperative setting, when optimal doses and compliance can be achieved at higher levels. Furthermore, one can also argue that patients whose disease progresses during neoadjuvant therapy represent a subgroup of patients with aggressive, advanced disease for whom attempts at curative resection, with potentially long-term postoperative morbidity and risk of mortality, may be contraindicated.

Early experience with preoperative radiation demonstrated that this therapy can be given safely and may have a salutary impact on local recurrence. A retrospective review by Ishikawa et al. (23) detailed their experience with preoperative radiotherapy (50 Gy) in 18 patients with pancreatic head cancer. All 18 tumors showed some decrease in size and 16 (89%) patients underwent curative resection. In 13 cases, residual tumors showed severely degenerative cancer cells comprising more than one third of the tumor mass, which was seen as a favorable indication of operative curability.

A follow-up retrospective analysis evaluated the effect of preoperative radiation in 54 consecutive patients with resectable pancreatic head cancer. Twenty-three patients received preoperative radiation (50 Gy) and 31 patients did not. No significant differences in baseline characteristics between the two groups were identified. Patients receiving preoperative radiation had a higher 1-year survival (75% vs. 43%; $p < 0.05$), but the 3- and 5-year survival data were not different (28% vs 32% and 22% vs 26%, respectively). Patients treated with preoperative radiation had a lower rate of regional recurrence at 1.5 years postsurgery, but died with higher rates of hepatic metastasis, thus highlighting limitations of neoadjuvant radiation as single modality (24).

Subsequent studies, built on this experience, tested preoperative protocols combining radiation and chemotherapy, mainly 5-FU-based. Much of the early experience with neoadjuvant chemoradiation comes from investigators at the Fox Chase Cancer Center. In one pilot study, 34 patients were treated with preoperative 5-FU, mitomycin, and radiation (50.4 Gy). Surgery was undertaken in 25 patients (9 did not undergo operation: one died of cholangitis, one refused, and 7 had progression of disease), but only 11 patients were able to have potentially curative surgery, and there were 2 perioperative deaths. The median survival of those who survived curative surgery was 45 months and disease-free survival was 27 months. This study suggested that patients with truly localized pancreatic cancer may, in fact, benefit from preoperative chemoradiotherapy (25).

Such encouraging results led to the first multi-institutional phase 2 study of neoadjuvant chemoradiation for localized pancreatic cancer by the Eastern Cooperative Oncology Group (ECOG). The neoadjuvant protocol, as previously described by the Fox Chase Cancer Center investigators, was given to 64 patients with localized pancreatic cancer (stages I to III) deemed resectable by the surgeon. The resection rate of 45% was much lower than previously reported in single-institution retrospective trials (72% to 85%). Moreover, the survival outcome was inferior to that reported in the aforementioned pilot study. The poor results were attributed to entry of patients with more advanced tumors. Although over 80% of patients completed chemoradiation, there were significant toxicities, especially biliary tract complications, due to the tumor or biliary stents (26).

The neoadjuvant use of rapid-fractionation radiation (30 Gy in 3 Gy/fraction) combined with continuous infusion 5-FU was investigated at the M.D. Anderson Cancer Center. The regimen was well tolerated, and 27 of 35 patients enrolled underwent surgery. The resection rate was 57% (20/35) and the median survival was 25 months. In addition, investigators at the M.D. Anderson Cancer Center reported their experience with 132 patients with resectable pancreatic cancer who received preoperative chemoradiation employing either standard or rapid-fractionation radiation. The data indicated that the less toxic, rapid-fractionation radiotherapy lasting 2 weeks instead of the standard $5\frac{1}{2}$ weeks was just as effective as standard radiotherapy (27).

Multiagent chemotherapy with concomitant radiation given preoperatively also has been studied. A protocol using infusion of 5-FU (650 mg/m^2 on days 1 to 5 and 21 to 25) with a bolus of cisplatin (80 mg/m^2 on days 2 and 22) with concurrent radiation has been tested in 19 patients by French investigators. This small study showed that such combination chemotherapy and concurrent radiation was feasible and well tolerated, with 15 patients able to go through radical surgery (28). A multi-institutional phase 2 French trial tested the efficacy of concurrent chemoradiotherapy (50 Gy, with 5-FU 300 mg/m^2/day, 5 days/week for 5 weeks) and cisplatin (20 mg/m^2/day on days 1 to 5 and 29 to 33). A total of 41 patients were enrolled. Ninety-three percent of patients (n = 38) received ≥47 Gy radiation and 73% (n = 30) received ≥75% of the prescribed doses of chemotherapy. Only 26 (63%) patients were able to undergo curative surgery because of local or metastatic progression. Their 2-year survival rate was 31% (29). Although the preoperative protocol was well tolerated, this and other trials continue to underscore the need for more effective agents that will allow a greater proportion of patients to have a chance for curative surgery after neoadjuvant therapy.

As previously stated, gemcitabine has shown superiority over 5-FU in treatment for advanced pancreatic cancer. Moreover, there is ample evidence for the potent radiosensitizing properties of gemcitabine (30). Therefore, this agent is also being evaluated in the neoadjuvant setting. Most recently, results of a multi-institutional phase 2 trial of preoperative chemoradiation using full-dose gemcitabine have been published. Twenty patients with resectable cancer of the pancreas underwent three cycles of full-dose gemcitabine (1,000 mg/m^2) preoperatively. Daily radiation (total of 36 Gy) was started on the second cycle. Ninety-five percent (19/20) of patients were able to tolerate preoperative chemoradiation without interruption. An impressive 85% (17/20) of operated patients underwent curative resection. The surgical complication rate was 24%, with no postoperative deaths. Ninety-four percent (16/17) and 65% (11/17) of patients had clear margins and no lymph node involvement, respectively. One specimen did not contain any evidence of tumor, and three specimens revealed microscopic foci only. With a median follow-up of 18 months, 41% (7/17) of patients are recurrence-free and 41% (7/17) have died. The other patients were alive with metastatic disease at the time of publication (31).

There are no randomized controlled trials in the literature that compare the efficacy of preoperative with postoperative chemotherapy or chemoradiation, although the efficacy seems to be comparable. However, until randomized trials show a clear benefit to neoadjuvant therapy, it cannot be recommended as standard clinical practice in localized resectable cancer of the pancreas, outside of clinical trials.

LOCALLY ADVANCED UNRESECTABLE DISEASE

Unresectable, locally advanced pancreatic cancer, and even suboptimally resected pancreatic cancer with residual tumor left behind is a predictor of poor survival, with a median survival of 6 to 12 months. The principal goals of chemotherapy or chemoradiotherapy in this situation are disease control and/or tumor "downstaging" for a potential curative resection.

Induction therapy has been shown in various relatively small single-institution trials to downstage some initially unresectable tumors. In one of the earliest trials, Pilepich and Miller (32) published the results of preoperative radiation in 17 patients with unresectable or "borderline" resectable disease. Among the 10 patients who underwent surgical exploration following radiation, 6 patients were able to undergo potentially curative radical surgery. Subsequent studies using preoperative chemoradiation or chemotherapy have been published (32–50) (Table 36.2). Resection rates vary between 0% and 64%, with responses to induction therapy ranging between 0% and 59%. Variability across studies, such as definition of resectability, surgical procedures, pathologic evaluation, and induction agents, make comparisons difficult to perform in a meaningful manner. For instance, if the criteria for resectability are very stringent, then it is more likely that induction therapy will show a benefit. In general, however, with our current armamentarium, only a very small minority of truly unresectable patients actually becomes resectable after induction therapy (51).

Although current protocols in the United States for locally advanced disease call for chemoradiation that is 5-FU-based (continuous infusion or capecitabine), the role of gemcitabine has also been explored for reasons previously stated. The optimal dosing of gemcitabine in combination with radiation has yet to be defined. Initial experience with gemcitabine used as a radiosensitizer led to significant toxicity. A phase 1 trial suggested that 600 mg/m^2 was an optimal dose (52), and a confirmatory phase 2 trial using weekly gemcitabine at 600 mg/m^2 with radiation (50.4 Gy) was shown to be well tolerated and effective with a median survival of 7.9 months and a 1-year survival rate of 31.1% (53). Others have shown that even full-dose gemcitabine at 1,000 mg/m^2 weekly with radiation is relatively well tolerated and effective (31).

Most recently, Wilkowski and associates (54) conducted a trial combining gemcitabine and 5-FU and radiation. Thirty-two patients with locally advanced pancreatic cancer were treated with gemcitabine, 300 mg/m^2 on days 1, 15, and 29, and 5-FU as continuous infusion, 350 mg/m^2/day with concurrent radiation (45 to 50 Gy). After chemoradiotherapy, the treatment was continued with an additional two cycles of gemcitabine (1,000 mg/m^2) and cisplatin (50 mg/m^2) applied on days 1 and 15 of a 4-week cycle. Major toxicities were grade 3-4 leukopenia (56.3%) and thrombocytopenia (25%). The treatment seemed to be quite effective, with an overall response rate of 62.5% (20/32). Seven patients underwent definitive curative resection,

Table 36.2

Neoadjuvant Therapy Trials for Locally Advanced Pancreatic Cancer

First Author (Ref.)	No. of Patients	Chemotherapy	Radiation	Response (No.)	Resection (No.)	Median Survival (months) Overall	Resected	Not Resected
Pilepich (32)	17	No	Yes	5	6	8		
Jeekel (33)	20	Yes	Yes	4	2	10		
Jessup (34)	16	Yes	Yes	2	2	8		
Safran (35)	34	Yes	Yes	4	1			
Kamthan (36)	35	Yes	Yes	15	5	15	31	11
Todd (37)	38	Yes	No	15	4	15.5	28	13
Bousquet (38)	7	Yes	Yes	2	2			
Bajetta (39)	32	Yes	Yes	7	5	9		
Wanebo (40)	14	Yes	Yes	9	9		19	9
Snady (41)	68	Yes	Yes	30	20	23.6	32.3	21.2
Kastl (42)	27	Yes	Yes	16	10	11		
White (43)	58	Yes	Yes	19	11	20		
Mehta (44)	15	Yes	Yes	5	9		30	8
Crane (45)	114	Yes	Yes	6	6			
Kim (46)	87	Yes	No	3	1	11	18	
Ammori (47)	67	Yes	Yes	17	9		17.6	11.9
Aristu (50)	47	Yes	Yes	20	9	11	23	10
Joensuu (48)	28	Yes	Yes		20	25	25	14
Moutardier (49)	31	Yes	Yes			8		

Adapted with permission from Mornex F, Girard N, Delpero JR, et al. Radiochemotherapy in the management of pancreatic cancer—part I: neoadjuvant treatment. *Semin Radiat Oncol.* 2005;15:226–234.

with four patients achieving clear margins. The medial survival was 13.6 months for the entire cohort.

Several attempts at elucidating the role of induction chemoradiation versus chemotherapy alone for locally advanced pancreatic cancer have been made. In the United States., a phase 3 trial (ECOG 4021) comparing concurrent gemcitabine and radiation versus gemcitabine alone closed early because of poor accrual. Most recently, however, a trial from Europe comparing induction chemoradiation (5-FU/cisplatin) followed by maintenance gemcitabine versus induction gemcitabine followed by maintenance gemcitabine was stopped early (n = 119) because of decreased survival in the chemoradiation arm. These data, presented at the 2006 ASCO meeting, are preliminary but one could argue that giving the most effective agent early (i.e., gemcitabine) may be accounting for the difference (55).

Rana and associates (56) at the M.D. Anderson Cancer Center explored the possible benefit of consolidative chemoradiation after neoadjuvant chemotherapy. In this retrospective review, 318 patients with locally advanced disease received concurrent chemoradiation therapy. Two hundred forty-five of the patients received induction chemoradiation as initial treatment and 73 patients received a median of 2.5 months of induction chemotherapy prior to chemoradiation. Radiosensitizers included 5-FU, gemcitabine, or capecitabine. Induction chemotherapy was gemcitabine-based. Patients receiving induc-

tion chemotherapy followed by chemoradiation had significant superior overall survival (11.9 vs. 8.5 months), time to local progression (8.4 vs. 6.0 months), and time to distant progression (9.5 vs. 5.8 months).

INTRAOPERATIVE RADIATION

The rationale for intraoperative radiation is that high doses of radiation can be delivered while bowel and other normal tissues can be retracted or shielded. Experience with intraoperative radiation is mostly from single centers with a relatively small number of patients. The value of adjuvant intraoperative radiation seems to rest on the fact that it may reduce local recurrence; however, it does not prevent distant or hepatic disease (57).

THE FUTURE

Various new agents with therapeutic potential are being evaluated in the adjuvant and/or neoadjuvant setting, mostly in phase 1 or 2 stages. Capecitabine is an oral pro-drug of 5-FU that undergoes a multienzymatic transformation with preferential conversion to 5-FU at the tumor site by thymidine phosphorylase (TP). It has been shown to have single-agent activity in advanced pancreatic cancer (58) and has also been used in combination with gemcitabine (59,60). Like 5-FU, capecitabine has radiosensitizing properties with the added advantage of not requiring central venous access and an infusion pump, facilitating the delivery of concurrent chemoradiotherapy. Moreover, intratumoral TP may be induced by radiation within and even outside the radiation field (abscopal effects) (61-63). Higher levels of TP have been associated with greater intratumoral levels of 5-FU and better response in preclinical models testing capecitabine (64).

Saif and associates (65) reported the results of a phase 1 study of capecitabine with concurrent radiation in locally advanced unresectable pancreatic cancer. The dose-limiting toxicity was diarrhea. The use of capecitabine in conjunction with radiation was safe and effective, with a recommended dose for phase 2 trials of 800 mg/m^2 twice daily, Monday through Friday. Three of 15 patients (20%) achieved a partial response. Tumor tissue was obtained by fine-needle aspiration before and after chemoradiation and analyzed for TP, dihydropyrimidine, and tumor necrosis factor-alpha mRNA levels. No significant trends in levels of these factors before and after therapy were observed, nor were there any correlations with response or toxicity noted in the data derived from this small number of patients.

Paclitaxel is another potential radiosensitizer. This agent prevents microtubule depolymerization and leads to the accumulation of tumor cells in the most radiosensitive phase of the cell cycle, the G2/M phase (66,67). Several small phase 1 to 2 trials have been published using different doses of paclitaxel as a radiosensitizer. Overall, it appears that using paclitaxel is at least as effective as 5-FU as radiosensitizer, but paclitaxel may have a bit more toxicity (68-70). One phase 2 trial in particular (RTOG-98-12; n = 109), showed that weekly paclitaxel at 50 mg/m^2 and radiation in locally advanced pancreatic cancer was well tolerated, with an impressive median survival of 11.5 months (70). Larger trials are ongoing to better determine the role of this agent in adjuvant and/or neoadjuvant management.

Bevacizumab is a humanized monoclonal antibody against vascular endothelial growth factor that has been shown to have a significant synergistic effect with chemotherapy in colon, breast, and lung cancers. There is also evidence that blocking the vascular endothelial growth factor pathway may overcome radioresistance (71,72). Crane and associates (73) conducted a phase 1 study using the combination of capecitabine, bevacizumab, and concurrent radiation in 48 patients with locally advanced unresectable disease. Of 46 evaluable patients, 9 (20%) had a response. Tumor-associated duodenal ulcer bleeding (n = 3) and a duodenal perforation were seen in the earlier part of the study. No such events were noted in the later phase of the study when patients with duodenal involvement with tumor were excluded. This regimen was found to be effective and safe, with significant toxicities being uncommon. The recommended capecitabine dose was 825 mg/m^2 twice daily, Monday through Friday, with no final recommendations on the bevacizumab dose until larger trials are done.

Inhibitors of epidermal growth factor receptor (EGFR), cetuximab and erlotinib, have been tested in clinical trials for pancreatic cancer in combination with chemotherapy, most often gemcitabine (74,75). Cetuximab is a monoclonal chimeric antibody against the ligand-binding domain of EGFR. Erlotinib is a tyrosine kinase inhibitor that blocks the signal transduction pathway of EGFR. Erlotinib in combination with gemcitabine has been shown to modestly improve median survival (76). In addition, EGFR inhibitors appear to be effective radiosensitizers (75).

A recent phase 1 study (n = 17) tested the efficacy and toxicity of erlotinib combined with chemoradiation (paclitaxel and gemcitabine). Thirteen patients had locally advanced disease and showed a partial response rate of 46% (6/13). Their median survival was 14 months. The maximum tolerated dose of erlotinib was 50 mg/m^2 with concurrent chemoradiation. The dose-limiting toxicities were diarrhea, dehydration, rash, myelosuppression, and small bowel stricture. Maintenance erlotinib was given at full dose (77).

CONCLUSIONS

The achievement of effective adjuvant and/or neoadjuvant therapy in localized or locally advanced pancreatic cancer is of utmost importance in order to achieve a significant improvement in the otherwise dismal prognosis of this disease. The administration of chemotherapy (either 5-FU or gemcitabine) in the adjuvant setting has been shown to improve survival and is thus warranted. The role of chemoradiation in addition to chemotherapy is an intensely debated topic. In the United States, a majority of practitioners believe in the benefit of chemoradiotherapy in addition to adjuvant chemotherapy, especially when modern radiation protocols are used. Recent trials, however, including the ESPAC-1, have caused some to doubt in the value of additional chemoradiation even in American centers. In Europe, on the other hand, chemoradiation is not considered standard of care. Currently, there are no phase 3 trials nationally or internationally that will satisfactorily answer this question.

Neoadjuvant therapy is an attractive option, especially given the relatively low proportion of patients who actually undergo required adjuvant therapy in a timely fashion. Phase 2 and retrospective evidence suggest that neoadjuvant therapy is at least as effective as adjuvant therapy. However, until randomized phase 3 trials show a clear advantage to neoadjuvant therapy, it cannot be recommended for use except in clinical trials. Moreover, uniform criteria for resectability need to be defined in order to standardize preoperative evaluation and management, as well as to facilitate sound interpretation of future clinical trials.

Lastly, newer agents with potentially higher efficacy are being developed and tested in adjuvant and neoadjuvant protocols. The addition of biologics to standard chemotherapy has added new options to the therapeutic armamentarium. Although progress is being made in small steps, more effective therapies and protocols may be at hand in the near future.

REFERENCES

1. Evans DB, Abbruzzese JL, Willett CG. Cancer of the pancreas. In: DeVita VT Jr, Hellman S, Rosenberg SA (eds). *Cancer: Principles and Practice of Oncology.* 6th ed. Philadelphia: Lippincott Williams & Wilkins; 2001:1126–1161.
2. Whipple A, Parsons W, Mullins C. Treatment of carcinoma of the ampulla of Vater. *Ann Surg.* 1935;102:763–776.
3. Sohn TA, Yeo CJ, Cameron JL, et al. Resected adenocarcinoma of the pancreas-616 patients: results, outcomes, and prognostic indicators. *J Gastrointest Surg.* 2000;4:567–579.

4. Ahmad NA, Lewis JD, Ginsberg GG, et al. Long term survival after pancreatic resection for pancreatic adenocarcinoma. *Am J Gastroenterol.* 2001;96:2609–2615.

5. Sperti C, Pasquali C, Piccoli A, et al. Recurrence after resection for ductal adenocarcinoma of the pancreas. *World J Surg.* 1997;21:195–200.

6. Westerdahl J, Andren-Sandberg A, Ihse I. Recurrence of exocrine pancreatic cancer–local or hepatic? *Hepatogastroenterology.* 1993;40:384–387.

7. Kalser MH, Ellenberg SS. Pancreatic cancer. Adjuvant combined radiation and chemotherapy following curative resection. *Arch Surg.* 1985;120:899–903.

8. Bakkevold KE, Arnesjo B, Dahl O, et al. Adjuvant combination chemotherapy (AMF) following radical resection of carcinoma of the pancreas and papilla of Vater–results of a controlled, prospective, randomised multicentre study. *Eur J Cancer.* 1993;29A:698–703.

9. Klinkenbijl JH, Jeekel J, Sahmoud T, et al. Adjuvant radiotherapy and 5-fluorouracil after curative resection of cancer of the pancreas and periampullary region: phase III trial of the EORTC gastrointestinal tract cancer cooperative group. *Ann Surg.* 1999;230:776–784.

10. Takada T, Amano H, Yasuda H, et al. Is postoperative adjuvant chemotherapy useful for gallbladder carcinoma? A phase III multicenter prospective randomized controlled trial in patients with resected pancreaticobiliary carcinoma. *Cancer.* 2002;95:1685–1695.

11. Neoptolemos JP, Stocken DD, Friess H, et al. A randomized trial of chemoradiotherapy and chemotherapy after resection of pancreatic cancer. *N Engl J Med.* 2004;350:1200–1210.

12. The Gastrointestinal Tumor Study Group. Further evidence of effective adjuvant combined radiation and chemotherapy following curative resection of pancreatic cancer. *Cancer.* 1987;59:2006–2010.

13. Whittington R, Bryer MP, Haller DG, et al. Adjuvant therapy of resected adenocarcinoma of the pancreas. *Int J Radiat Oncol Biol Phys.* 1991;21:1137–1143.

14. Yeo CJ, Abrams RA, Grochow LB, et al. Pancreaticoduodenectomy for pancreatic adenocarcinoma: postoperative adjuvant chemoradiation improves survival. A prospective, single-institution experience. *Ann Surg.* 1997;225:621–636.

15. Mehta VK, Fisher GA, Ford JM, et al. Adjuvant radiotherapy and concomitant 5-fluorouracil by protracted venous infusion for resected pancreatic cancer. *Int J Radiat Oncol Biol Phys.* 2000;48:1483–1487.

16. Choti MA. Adjuvant therapy for pancreatic cancer–the debate continues. *N Engl J Med.* 2004;350:1249–1251.

17. Koshy MC, Landry JC, Cavanaugh SX, et al. A challenge to the therapeutic nihilism of ESPAC-1. *Int J Radiat Oncol Biol Phys.* 2005;61:965–966.

18. Stocken DD, Buchler MW, Dervenis C, et al. Meta-analysis of randomised adjuvant therapy trials for pancreatic cancer. *Br J Cancer.* 2005;92:1372–1381.

19. Burris HA 3rd, Moore MJ, Andersen J, et al. Improvements in survival and clinical benefit with gemcitabine as first-line therapy for patients with advanced pancreas cancer: a randomized trial. *J Clin Oncol.* 1997;15:2403–2413.

20. Regine W, Winter K, Abrams R, et al. RTOG 9704 a phase III study of adjuvant pre and post chemoradiation (CRT) 5-FU vs. gemcitabine (G) for resected pancreatic adenocarcinoma. In: Proceedings from the American Society of Clinical Oncology. June 2-6, 2006; Atlanta, GA. Abstract 4007.

21. Neuhaus P, Oettle S, Post K, et al. A randomised, prospective, multicenter, phase III trial of adjuvant chemotherapy with gemcitabine vs. observation in patients with resected pancreatic cancer. In: Proceedings from the American Society of Clinical Oncology. May 13–17, 2005; Orlando, FL. Abstract 4013.

22. Sener SF, Fremgen A, Menck HR, et al. Pancreatic cancer: a report of treatment and survival trends for 100,313 patients diagnosed from 1985-1995, using the National Cancer Database. *J Am Coll Surg.* 1999;189:1–7.

23. Ishikawa O, Ohhigashi H, Teshima T, et al. Clinical and histopathological appraisal of preoperative irradiation for adenocarcinoma of the pancreatoduodenal region. *J Surg Oncol.* 1989;40:143–151.

24. Ishikawa O, Ohigashi H, Imaoka S, et al. Is the long-term survival rate improved by preoperative irradiation prior to Whipple's procedure for adenocarcinoma of the pancreatic head? *Arch Surg.* 1994;129:1075–1080.

25. Hoffman JP, Weese JL, Solin LJ, et al. A pilot study of preoperative chemoradiation for patients with localized adenocarcinoma of the pancreas. *Am J Surg.* 1995;169:71–78.

26. Hoffman JP, Lipsitz S, Pisansky T, et al. Phase II trial of preoperative radiation therapy and chemotherapy for patients with localized, resectable adenocarcinoma of the pancreas: an Eastern Cooperative Oncology Group Study. *J Clin Oncol.* 1998;16317–16323.

27. Breslin TM, Hess KR, Harbison DB, et al. Neoadjuvant chemodiotherapy for adenocarcinoma of the pancreas: treatment variables and survival duration. *Ann Surg Oncol.* 2001;8:123–132.

28. Moutardier V, Giovannini M, Lelong B, et al. A phase II single institutional experience with preoperative radiochemotherapy in pancreatic adenocarcinoma. *Eur J Surg Oncol.* 2002;28:531–539.

29. Mornex F, Girard N, Scoazec JY, et al. Feasibility of pre-operative combined radiation therapy and chemotherapy with 5-fluorouracil and cisplatin in potentially resectable pancreatic adenocarcinoma: the French SFRO-FFCD 97-04 Phase II trial [published online ahead of print June 21, 2006]. *Int J Radiat Oncol Biol Phys.* 2006;65:1471–1478.

30. Lawrence TS, Chang EY, Hahn TM, et al. Radiosensitization of pancreatic cancer cells by 2′,2′-difluoro-2′-deoxycytidine. *Int J Radiat Oncol Biol Phys.* 1996;34:867–872.

31. Talamonti MS, Small W, Jr., Mulcahy MF, et al. A multi-institutional phase II trial of preoperative full-dose gemcitabine and concurrent radiation for patients with potentially resectable pancreatic carcinoma. *Ann Surg Oncol.* 2006;13:150–158.

32. Pilepich MV, Miller HH. Preoperative irradiation in carcinoma of the pancreas. *Cancer.* 1980;46:1945–1949.

33. Jeekel J, Treurniet-Donker AD. Treatment perspectives in locally advanced unresectable pancreatic cancer. *Br J Surg.* 1991;78:1332–1334.

34. Jessup JM, Steele G Jr, Mayer RJ, et al. Neoadjuvant therapy for unresectable pancreatic adenocarcinoma. *Arch Surg.* 1993;128:559–564.

35. Safran H, King TP, Choy H, et al. Paclitaxel and concurrent radiation for locally advanced pancreatic and gastric cancer: a phase I study. *J Clin Oncol.* 1997;15:901–907.

36. Kamthan AG, Morris JC, Dalton J, et al. Combined modality therapy for stage II and stage III pancreatic carcinoma. *J Clin Oncol.* 1997;15:2920–2927.

37. Todd KE, Gloor B, Lane JS, et al. Resection of locally advanced pancreatic cancer after downstaging with continuous-infusion 5-fluorouracil, mitomycin-C, leucovorin, and dipyridamole. *J Gastrointest Surg.* 1998;2:159–166.

38. Bousquet J, Slim K, Pezet D, et al. Does neoadjuvant radiochemotherapy augment the resectability of pancreatic cancers? [in French]. *Chirurgie.* 1998;123:456–460.

39. Bajetta E, Di Bartolomeo M, Stani SC, et al. Chemoradiotherapy as preoperative treatment in locally advanced unresectable pancreatic cancer patients: results of a feasibility study. *Int J Radiat Oncol Biol Phys.* 1999;45:285–289.

40. Wanebo HJ, Glicksman AS, Vezeridis MP, et al. Preoperative chemotherapy, radiotherapy, and surgical resection of locally advanced pancreatic cancer. *Arch Surg.* 2000;135:81–88.

41. Snady H, Bruckner H, Cooperman A, et al. Survival advantage of combined chemoradiotherapy compared with resection as the initial treatment of patients with regional pancreatic carcinoma. An outcomes trial. *Cancer.* 2000;89:314–327.

42. Kastl S, Brunner T, Herrmann O, et al. Neoadjuvant radiochemotherapy in advanced primarilynon-resectable carcinomas of the pancreas. *Eur J Surg Oncol.* 2000;26:578–582.

43. White RR, Hurwitz HI, Morse MA, et al. Neoadjuvant chemoradiation for localized adenocarcinoma of the pancreas. *Ann Surg Oncol.* 2001;8:758–765.

44. Mehta VK, Fisher G, Ford JA, et al. Preoperative chemoradiation for marginally resectable adenocarcinoma of the pancreas. *J Gastrointest Surg.* 2001;5:27–35.

45. Crane CH, Abbruzzese JL, Evans DB, et al. Is the therapeutic index better with gemcitabine-based chemoradiation than with 5-fluorouracil-based chemoradiation in locally advanced pancreatic cancer? *Int J Radiat Oncol Biol Phys.* 2002;52:1293–1302.

46. Kim HJ, Czischke K, Brennan MF, et al. Does neoadjuvant chemoradiation downstage locally advanced pancreatic cancer? *J Gastrointest Surg.* 2002;6:763–769.

47. Ammori JB, Colletti LM, Zalupski MM, et al. Surgical resection following radiation therapy with concurrent gemcitabine in patients with previously unresectable adenocarcinoma of the pancreas. *J Gastrointest Surg.* 2003;7:766–772.

48. Joensuu TK, Kiviluoto T, Karkkainen P, et al. Phase I-II trial of twice-weekly gemcitabine and concomitant irradiation in patients undergoing pancreaticoduodenectomy with extended lymphadenectomy for locally advanced pancreatic cancer. *Int J Radiat Oncol Biol Phys.* 2004;60:444–452.

49. Moutardier V, Turrini O, Huiart L, et al. A reappraisal of preoperative chemoradiation for localized pancreatic head ductal adenocarcinoma in a 5-year single-institution experience. *J Gastrointest Surg.* 2004;8:502–510.

50. Aristu J, Canon R, Pardo F, et al. Surgical resection after preoperative chemoradiotherapy benefits selected patients with unresectable pancreatic cancer. *Am J Clin Oncol.* 2003;26:30–36.

51. Mornex F, Girard N, Delpero JR, et al. Radiochemotherapy in the management of pancreatic cancer–part I: neoadjuvant treatment. *Semin Radiat Oncol.* 2005;15:226–234.

52. Hoffman JP, McGinn CJ, Szarka C, et al. A Phase 1 study of preoperative gemcitabine (GEM) with radiation therapy (RT) followed by postoperative GEM for patients with localized resectable pancreatic adenocarcinoma (PaC). *Proc Am Soc Clin Oncol.* 1998;17:283a.

53. Moore AM, Cardenes H, Johnson CS, et al. A phase II study of gemcitabine in combination with radiation therapy in patients with localized, unresectable, pancreatic cancer: A Hoosier Oncology Group Trial. In: Proceedings from the American Society of Clinical Oncology; June 5-8, 2004; New Orleans, LA. Abstract 4105.

54. Wilkowski R, Thoma M, Bruns C, et al. Chemoradiotherapy with gemcitabine and continuous 5-FU in patients with primary inoperable pancreatic cancer. JOP 2006;7:349–360.

55. Chauffert B, Mornex F, Bonnetain F, et al. Phase III trial comparing initial chemoradiotherapy (intermittent cisplatin and infusional 5-FU) followed by gemcitabine vs. gemcitabine alone in patients with locally advanced non metastatic pancreatic cancer: A FFCD-SFRO study. In: Proceedings from the American Society of Clinical Oncology; June 2-6, 2006; Atlanta, GA. Abstract 4008.

56. Rana V, Krishnan S, Abbruzzese J, et al. Neoadjuvant chemotherapy improves outcomes of chemoradiation therapy for locally advanced pancreatic cancer. In: Proceedings from the American Society of Clinical Oncology; June 2-6, 2006; Atlanta, GA. Abstract 4036.

57. Bergenfeldt M, Albertsson M. Current state of adjuvant therapy in resected pancreatic adenocarcinoma. *Acta Oncol.* 2006;45:124–135.

58. Cartwright TH, Cohn A, Varkey JA, et al. Phase II study of oral capecitabine in patients with advanced or metastatic pancreatic cancer. *J Clin Oncol.* 2002;20:160–164.

59. Stathopoulos GP, Syrigos K, Polyzos A, et al. Front-line treatment of inoperable or metastatic pancreatic cancer with gemcitabine and capecitabine: an intergroup, multicenter, phase II study. *Ann Oncol.* 2004;15:224–229.

60. Hess V, Salzberg M, Borner M, et al. Combining capecitabine and gemcitabine in patients with advanced pancreatic carcinoma: a phase I/II trial. *J Clin Oncol.* 2003;21:66–68.

61. Sawada N, Ishikawa T, Sekiguchi F, et al. X-ray irradiation induces thymidine phosphorylase and enhances the efficacy of capecitabine (Xeloda) in human cancer xenografts. *Clin Cancer Res.* 1999;5:2948–2953.

62. Blanquicett C, Saif MW, Buchsbaum DJ, et al. Antitumor efficacy of capecitabine and celecoxib in irradiated and lead-shielded, contralateral human BxPC-3 pancreatic cancer xenografts: clinical implications of abscopal effects. *Clin Cancer Res.* 2005;11(24 Pt 1):8773–8781.

63. Blanquicett C, Johnson MR, Heslin M, et al. Housekeeping gene variability in normal and carcinomatous colorectal and liver tissues: applications in pharmacogenomic gene expression studies. *Anal Biochem.* 2002;303:209–214.

64. Schuller J, Cassidy J, Dumont E, et al. Preferential activation of capecitabine in tumor following oral administration to colorectal cancer patients. *Cancer Chemother Pharmacol.* 2000;45:291–297.

65. Saif MW, Eloubeidi MA, Russo S, et al. Phase I study of capecitabine with concomitant radiotherapy for patients with locally advanced pancreatic cancer: expression analysis of genes related to outcome. *J Clin Oncol.* 2005;23:8679–8687.

66. Tishler RB, Schiff PB, Geard CR, et al. Taxol: a novel radiation sensitizer. *Int J Radiat Oncol Biol Phys.* 1992;22:613–617.

67. Liebmann J, Cook JA, Fisher J, et al. In vitro studies of Taxol as a radiation sensitizer in human tumor cells. *J Natl Cancer Inst.* 1994;86:441–446.

68. Pisters PW, Wolff RA, Janjan NA, et al. Preoperative paclitaxel and concurrent rapid-fractionation radiation for resectable pancreatic adenocarcinoma: toxicities, histologic response rates, and event-free outcome. *J Clin Oncol.* 2002;20:2537–2544.

69. Ashamalla H, Zaki B, Mokhtar B, et al. Hyperfractionated radiotherapy and paclitaxel for locally advanced/unresectable pancreatic cancer. *Int J Radiat Oncol Biol Phys.* 2003;55:679–687.

70. Rich T, Harris J, Abrams R, et al. Phase II study of external irradiation and weekly paclitaxel for nonmetastatic, unresectable pancreatic cancer: RTOG-98-12. *Am J Clin Oncol.* 2004;27:51–56.

71. Gorski DH, Beckett MA, Jaskowiak NT, et al. Blockage of the vascular endothelial growth factor stress response increases the antitumor effects of ionizing radiation. *Cancer Res.* 1999;59:3374–3378.

72. Geng L, Donnelly E, McMahon G, et al. Inhibition of vascular endothelial growth factor receptor signaling leads to reversal of tumor resistance to radiotherapy. *Cancer Res.* 2001;61:2413–2419.

73. Crane CH, Ellis LM, Abbruzzese JL, et al. Phase I trial evaluating the safety of bevacizumab with concurrent radiotherapy and capecitabine in locally advanced pancreatic cancer. *J Clin Oncol.* 2006;24:1145–1151.

74. Xiong HQ, Rosenberg A, LoBuglio A, et al. Cetuximab, a monoclonal antibody targeting the epidermal growth factor receptor, in combination with gemcitabine for advanced pancreatic cancer: a multicenter phase II Trial. *J Clin Oncol.* 2004;22:2610–2616.

75. Marshall J. Clinical implications of the mechanism of epidermal growth factor receptor inhibitors. *Cancer.* 2006;107:1207–1218.

76. Moore MJ, Goldstein D, Hamm J, et al. Erlotinib plus gemcitabine compared to gemcitabine alone in patients with advanced pancreatic cancer. A phase III trial of the National Cancer Institute of Canada Clinical Trials Group. *J Clin Oncol.* 2007;25:1960–1966.

77. Iannitti D, Dipetrillo T, Akerman P, et al. Erlotinib and chemoradiation followed by maintenance erlotinib for locally advanced pancreatic cancer: a phase I study. *Am J Clin Oncol.* 2005;28:570–575.

COMMENTARY
Peter J. Rosen

The chapter by Drs. Park and Lenz accurately summarizes the state of the art regarding the adjuvant and neoadjuvant therapy for ductal adenocarcinoma of the pancreas. Whereas the development of moderately effective adjuvant therapies for breast and colorectal cancer has been extensively documented and has become the standard of care, much uncertainty remains regarding pancreas cancer, which, in fact, is most in need of an effective adjuvant (or neoadjuvant) approach.

Pancreatic cancer is now the fourth leading cause of death from cancer in the United States, with nearly 40,000 deaths per year. This is a disease in which the annual incidence and mortality nearly coincide, attesting to the almost certain lethality of the illness. To begin with, only about 10% to 20% of newly diagnosed patients are truly operable with curative intent and even those patients have, at best, a 20% to 30% 5-year life expectancy. Most patients present with metastatic or locally advanced, technically inoperable, tumors. For patients with metastatic disease, median survival is about 6 months with best available therapy, and the situation is only slightly better for patients with locally advanced presentations.

The attempts at developing effective adjuvant therapies for pancreatic cancer have been thwarted by a number of factors. First, the surgical procedure itself, for years, carried an unacceptably high morbidity and mortality rate leaving only a small fraction of patients available for postoperative therapy. Preoperative evaluation was limited by inadequate radiographic and other staging procedures leading to many unnecessary and futile operations with the tumor either left intact or with gross and/or microscopic residual disease. Additionally, the surgical results were often inadequately documented by both the surgeon and pathologist, particularly with respect to the posterior margin of resection, which was often incompletely examined. Finally, the modalities of postoperative therapy were severely limited by the availability of only one, largely ineffective drug, 5-fluorouracil (5-FU), and radiation therapy, which was applied in an inconsistent manner with varying fields, doses, and schedules.

In the past 10 years, there have been some advances that make the testing of adjuvant and neoadjuvant therapies more likely to bear fruit. The surgical procedure has been refined with mortality <2% in experienced hands, and hospital stays of 7 to 10 days. Nevertheless, the recuperative process remains variable, hindering the timely application of postoperative therapies for many patients. Radiographic technology has significantly advanced with the advent of technologies such as spiral computerized tomography and advanced magnetic resonance imaging scanners. Patients who are clearly inoperable are being identified more often and a group of patients with borderline resectability are being identified who might benefit from preoperative or neoadjuvant therapy. Surgeons and pathologists are doing a much better job of carefully documenting the quality of tumor resections. Finally, there has been the development of at least one moderately effective chemotherapeutic agent, gemcitabine, and technical advances such as conformal or intensity-modulated radiation therapy. Thus, the stage is set for more definitive randomized clinical trials in potentially curable pancreatic cancer. Currently these randomized trials remain in short supply.

Prior to reviewing some of the data in more depth, what can we say about the present state of the art? First, it appears clear that adjuvant chemotherapy does extend progression-free survival. Second, the benefit of radiation therapy is not clearly supported by randomized clinical trials. Finally, the role of neoadjuvant therapy is the subject of continued investigation but is not yet clearly proven to benefit patients in the aggregate.

Before one can implement a program of adjuvant therapy it is necessary to have some evidence that drugs or treatment modalities are available that have some impact in the metastatic or advanced disease setting. The advent of gemcitabine for metastatic disease provided the first evidence in over 30 years that a useful drug existed (1). The initial publication showed that, when compared with bolus intravenous 5-FU, gemcitabine was clearly superior, although only modestly effective; median survival was improved to 5.7 months from 4.4 months and 1-year survival occurred in 18% versus only 2% of patients. In addition, clinical benefit was seen in 24% of gemcitabine-treated patients as opposed to 5% for the 5-FU group. Attempts to improve on these figures have been challenging. Despite a variety of combination regimens based on gemcitabine, there has been no convincing advance. The addition of the epidermal growth factor receptor tyrosine kinase inhibitor, erlotinib, did improve survival but by <1 month (2). This meager result led to Food and Drug Administration approval for erlotinib in this setting. More recently, a series of biologic agents have been combined with gemcitabine with negative results. Perhaps the most disappointing was the failure of bevacizumab, an angiogenesis inhibitor found useful in lung, colorectal, and breast cancer in a large phase 3 trial in combination with gemcitabine (3).

The modern history of adjuvant therapy for pancreatic cancer can be traced back to the 1970s and 1980s. The best-known study was a small one conducted by the Gastrointestinal Tumor Study Group (GITSG). This randomized trial could only accrue 43 patients over many years partly because of the dearth of available successfully resected candidates (4). In any event, patients were randomized between bolus 5-FU plus split-course radiation and observation. The median survival was 20 months for the treated arm versus 11 months for the controls. The 2-year survival was 42% and 15%, respectively. 5-FU was continued for 2 years. Importantly, there was no arm that tested chemotherapy alone without radiation. This very small study became the standard of care for decades and remains so for some. Other small, nonrandomized studies did little to clarify the state of the art.

The ESPAC-1 trial (European Study Group for Pancreatic Cancer) was the largest randomized trial published studying adjuvant therapy in pancreas cancer. Unfortunately, the study used a complex 2×2 factorial design supplemented by an additional randomized population and did not employ radiation quality control (5,6). The trial initially randomized patients between chemotherapy, chemoradiation, both treatments, or neither treatment. Subsequently, a group of patients were randomized between chemoradiation versus no chemoradiation and chemotherapy versus no chemotherapy. A total of 550 patients from 76 European hospitals entered the trial. The chemotherapy was 5-FU plus folinic acid and the radiation was 4,000 cGy administered in 20 fractions. The results indicated a superiority of chemotherapy over chemoradiation. The median survival for the chemotherapy-treated patients was 19.7 months (note the similarity to GITSG data) as opposed to 14 months for the no chemotherapy group. Chemoradiation survival was 15.5 months, whereas it was 16.1 months for those not receiving it. Despite the problems with this study, and there are many, it did not establish a role for radiation. It should be added that the bulk of the advantage for chemotherapy was in the R0-resected group.

The cleanest, most straightforward adjuvant study is the recent Charité Onkologie Clinical Studies in Gastrointestinal Cancers (CONKO) trial (7). This is a test of the role of adjuvant gemcitabine versus no therapy for R0- and R1-resected patients. This was a German-Austrian multicenter randomized, placebo-controlled study that enrolled 368 patients. The treated group received a standard 30-minute infusion of gemcitabine at 1,000 mg/m^2 for 3 of 4 weeks for a total of 6 months. An R0 resection was confirmed in 80% of patients. At a median follow-up of 54 months, recurrent disease was documented in 74% of the gemcitabine-treated patients as opposed to 92% of the control patients. Median disease-free survival was 13.4 versus 6.9 for the two arms, respectively. Overall survival at this point was not statistically impacted, although the p value of 0.06 showed a clear trend favoring therapy.

More recent randomized attempts to combine chemotherapy with radiation include the phase 3 Intergroup Trial (RTOG 97-04) that tested before and after chemoradiation 5-FU versus gemcitabine. In this trial 5-FU was given by continuous infusion. Both drugs were administered for 3 weeks prior to and 12 weeks after chemoradiation (8). Radiation was 5,040 cGy with concomitant infusional 5-FU. Five hundred thirty-eight patients enrolled, of which 442 were eligible. Patients with pancreatic head tumors experienced a significantly enhanced survival in the gemcitabine arm (median survival, 20.6 months vs. 16.9 months). Again, there was no control using chemotherapy alone. It should be added at this point that a previous European Organisation for Research and Treatment of Cancer randomized trial did not reveal a statistically significant advantage of combined chemoradiation with 5-FU over observation, although this trial was underpowered to show a small advantage (9).

The observation that it is unclear whether radiation is beneficial is not too surprising in light of the fact that most patients have systemic spread at the time of, or shortly after, diagnosis. Clearly, systemic therapy must be the mainstay of any significant gains in the future.

Neoadjuvant therapy has been espoused by many because of the rapid progression of disease, the prolonged convalescence after surgery, and the potential for improving resectability. Many institutions such as the M.D. Anderson Cancer Center are focusing on this problem, and randomized trials are in the developmental stages.

Finally, what is the future? The potential to exploit a target in the context of tumor vulnerability remains appealing, though elusive, to date. The *RAS* gene is mutated in 90% of cases. Previous trials with farnesyl transferase inhibitors were developed to target *RAS* but that does not seem to have been the true mechanism of action of these drugs. New strategies involving specific *RAS* inhibitors or vaccines directed against *RAS* are being tested. Other similar strategies are in desperate need.

REFERENCES

1. Burris HA, Moore MJ, Andersen J, et al. Improvements in survival and clinical benefit with gemcitabine as first-line therapy for patients with advanced pancreas cancer: a randomized trial. *J Clin Oncol.* 1997;15:2403–2413.

2. Moore MJ, Goldstein D, Hamm J, et al. Erlotinib plus gemcitabine compared with gemcitabine alone in patients with advanced pancreatic cancer: A phase III trial of the National Cancer Institute of Canada Clinical Trials Group. *J Clin Oncol.* 2007;25:1960–1966.

3. Kindler HL, Niedzwiecki, Hollis D, et al. A double-blind, placebo-controlled, randomized phase III trial of gemcitabine plus bevacizumab versus gemcitabine plus placebo in patients with advanced pancreatic cancer: a preliminary analysis of Cancer and Leukemia Group B 80303. In: Proceedings of the 2007 Gastrointestinal Cancers Symposium. January 19-21, 2007; Orlando, FL. Abstract 108. Published online at http://www.asco.org/portal/site/ASCO/menuitem. 34d60f5624ba07fd506fe310ee37a01d/?vgnextoid=76f8201eb61a 7010VgnVCM100000ed730ad1RCRD&vmview=abst_detail_view &confID=45&abstractID=10557.

4. Kalser MH, Ellenberg SS. Pancreatic cancer: adjuvant combined radiation and chemotherapy following curative resection. *Arch Surg.* 1985;120:899–903.

5. Neoptolemos JP, Dunn JA, Stocken DD, et al. Adjuvant chemoradiotherapy and chemotherapy in resectable pancreatic cancer: A randomized controlled trial. *Lancet.* 2001;358:1576–1585.

6. Neoptolemos JP, Stocken DD, Friess H, et al. A randomized trial of chemoradiotherapy and chemotherapy after resection of pancreatic cancer. *N Engl J Med.* 2004;350:1200–1210.

7. Oettle H, Post S, Neuhaus P, et al. Adjuvant chemotherapy with gemcitabine vs. observation in patients undergoing curative-intent resection of pancreatic cancer. *JAMA.* 2007;297;267–277.

8. Regine WF, Winter KA, Abrams R, et al. A phase III Intergroup Trial (RTOG 97-04) of adjuvant pre and post chemoradiation 5-FU vs. gemcitabine for resected pancreatic adenocarcinoma. *Int J Radiat Oncol Biol Phys.* 2006;66(Suppl 1):S23–24.

9. Klinkenbijl JH, Jeekel J, Sahmoud T, et al. Adjuvant radiotherapy and 5-fluorouracil after curative resection of cancer of the pancreas and periampullary region: a phase III trial of the EORTC gastrointestinal tract cancer cooperative group. *Ann Surg.* 1999;230:776–782.

37

Nonhematolymphoid Tumors and Tumorlike Conditions of the Spleen

Leon Morgenstern and Randa Alsabeh

Nonhematolymphoid tumors are uncommon in the spleen as compared with other parenchymatous organs. With advances in imaging, their presence has often become evident as an incidental finding rather than through the occurrence of symptoms. When symptoms do occur, they are primarily due to size, rather than physiologic or functional alteration. The most common complaint is left upper quadrant discomfort or pain. Less common but more dramatic are symptoms due to hemorrhage, rupture, or infection.

Tumorlike conditions of the spleen share the characteristic of relative rarity. They include hamartomas, peliosis, nonparasitic cysts, and pseudotumors. Like tumors, they may be found on imaging studies or on pathologic examination as incidental findings. They also usually become symptomatic only when size causes discomfort or when there is some supervening complicating event such as rupture, hemorrhage, or infection.

Both benign tumors and tumorlike lesions are usually solitary, but less frequently are multiple, or diffuse, involving the entire spleen. Diffuse lesions of the spleen, such as hemangiomatosis, lymphangiomatosis, and hamartomatosis, may present not only with splenic enlargement and accompanying discomfort but can also manifest signs and symptoms of hypersplenism.

Malignant tumors of the spleen are an ominous group of neoplasms with a bleak prognosis. By the time a diagnosis is made, tumors are generally advanced and beyond cure. The best that splenectomy can offer is palliation, with little influence on long-term survival.

Although imaging studies may be helpful in establishing a diagnosis of these conditions, only a pathologic study can do so with absolute certainty. An exception perhaps is the nonparasitic splenic cyst, which has imaging characteristics that are specific enough for a correct diagnosis.

The surgical approach to tumors and tumorlike conditions of the spleen is based on the size of the lesion, the certainty of the diagnosis, and, if the latter is known, the natural history of the condition.

Current surgical approaches include total splenectomy, partial splenectomy, biopsy, and partial or total removal of the lesion. Each of these approaches will be considered for every lesion discussed.

Conditions that produce nonhematolymphoid tumors and tumorlike conditions of the spleen are listed in Table 37.1.

CYSTS

Epithelial (Nonparasitic) Splenic Cysts

Although uncommon, nonparasitic splenic cysts occur with sufficient frequency to warrant description and discussion (1,2). Their etiology and pathogenesis, once thought to be related primarily to trauma, is now considered to be more likely of congenital origin (3). Cysts arising from trauma were labeled "pseudocysts" because an epithelial lining was absent. However, a careful search for such a lining more often than not reveals a remnant of epithelium that identifies them as true cysts. Their congenital origin is further substantiated by their occurrence in accessory spleens, in newborn infants, and in ectopic locations such as the tail of the pancreas. The lining epithelium varies from single to multiple layers of mesothelial, transitional, or most commonly, stratified squamous epithelium that can show keratinization. Cysts may be solitary (most common) or multiple; multiple cysts, when they occur, are usually found in juxtaposition to the major cyst. The size is variable. Smaller cysts may measure ≤1 cm and are detected as incidental findings on imaging studies. They may however grow to "giant" proportions of ≥20 cm. Symptoms related to the cyst are generally not present unless the cyst is large enough to encroach on neighboring organs such as the diaphragm, stomach, kidney, or colon. It is rare that a cyst <5 cm in diameter is symptomatic. The commonest symptom is left upper quadrant discomfort or, more rarely, pain.

Imaging studies show hypoechoic, cystic lesions devoid of intracystic inclusions or lining irregularities. True cysts have a typical appearance of round, uniformly fluid-filled, very well-circumscribed lesions that cannot be mistaken for a neoplasm. The walls may show varying degrees of calcification, but absence of calcification is more common, especially in smaller cysts.

The cyst content varies from clear, straw-colored fluid to turbid or greenish liquid content. A peculiar characteristic is a high level of CA19-9 (4), the genesis of which is unclear.

On gross examination, the inner lining of the cyst is pathognomonic. It is coarsely trabeculated with a glistening, whitish mesh of trabeculae of varying thickness. There is a true capsule of fibrous tissue 1 mm to several millimeters thick. Occasionally the wall of the cyst can show focal or extensive calcifications. The epithelial lining may be difficult to detect, especially in the larger cysts of long duration. A diligent search is usually rewarded with a tell-tale epithelial fragment, but even if this is absent, the gross

Table 37.1

Nonhematolymphoid Tumors and Tumorlike Conditions of the Spleen

Cysts
    Epithelial cysts
    Pseudocysts

Tumorlike conditions
    Hamartoma
    Inflammatory pseudotumor
    Peliosis
    Sclerosing angiomatoid nodular transformation

Diseases simulating splenic tumors
    Sarcoidosis
    Amyloidosis

Nonhematolymphoid tumors
    Dendritic cell tumors
    Muscle tumors
    Lipoma
    Angiomyolipoma
    Fibroma
    Carcinosarcoma
    Fibrosarcoma
    Malignant fibrosis and fibrohistiocytic tumors

Vascular tumors
    Hemangioma
    Littoral cell Angioma
    Lymphangioma
    Hemangiopericytoma
    Hemangioendothelioma
    Angiosarcoma
    Lymphangiosarcoma
    Kaposi sarcoma

Metastatic tumors

characteristics of the cyst are sufficiently specific to warrant the designation of true cysts.

There have been several approaches to the treatment of nonparasitic splenic cysts of the spleen. Nonsurgical treatments such as aspiration with or without injection of sclerosing solutions are ineffective. Marsupialization is needlessly complex and not indicated. A common question when an asymptomatic cyst is discovered is whether or not its removal is indicated. The natural history of splenic cysts, when followed sequentially by periodic imaging studies, is that they enlarge and eventually become symptomatic. Cysts that are ≥5 cm in size should be treated surgically. The traditional and more commonly used approach has been total splenectomy. The recognition that splenectomy has immunologic consequences, particularly in younger individuals, has led to procedures based on splenic conservation rather than extirpation. It is entirely feasible to perform partial splenectomy encompassing the major cyst and adjacent smaller cysts (5). This may be done laparoscopically or by conventional laparotomy. A lesser procedure known as splenic decapsulation

(6,7) removes the dome of the cyst to the level of the bordering normal splenic parenchyma. The interior of the remaining cyst wall is then treated with electrocoagulation or the argon beam coagulator to destroy any residual epithelial elements of the lining. A disadvantage of decapsulation is the possibility of leaving adjacent smaller cysts that may later grow to a clinically significant size. To date no such problems have been reported with splenic decapsulation, which is a technically less demanding procedure.

In addition to the symptoms of pain and impingement on adjacent organs, splenic cysts have been known to rupture, bleed, and become infected. These complications are rare but are still another indication for removal of enlarging cysts.

Pseudocysts

Pseudocysts are a consequence of splenic trauma and are characterized by an absence of epithelial lining. Previously thought to be the most frequent variety of nonparasitic cysts of the spleen, the opposite is now true. The absence of an epithelial lining may be spurious as epithelial linings may be shed or destroyed, especially in cysts of long standing.

The true pseudocyst is a result of subcapsular or intrasplenic hematoma induced by trauma. The larger the hematoma, the more likely the pseudocyst is apt to occur. Pseudocysts of traumatic origin have a shaggy, nontrabeculated interior, with solid elements in various degrees of organization. There is no epithelial lining.

Other characteristics that differentiate the pseudocyst from the true (epithelial lined) cyst are (a) a clear-cut temporal relationship to splenic trauma with imaging evidence to support that causation and (b) the irregular character of the cyst interior as contrasted with the uniform hypoechoic imaging characteristic of the epithelial cyst.

Small traumatic cystic collections can resorb and disappear. Large cystic lesions due to trauma that persist and are symptomatic may require removal. This is usually accomplished by total splenectomy.

Parasitic (Echinococcal) Cysts

The echinococcal or hydatid cyst of the spleen is principally found in those countries where infection caused by the tapeworm *Echinococcus* is common and the definitive hosts, dogs and sheep, are present. Visceral involvement is much more common in the liver (50% to 80%) than in the spleen. In the spleen, the cysts are usually unilocular, but can be multilocular, and may cause pain or discomfort when large enough. The diagnosis is suggested by history and confirmation of the parasitic nature of the cyst by immunologic or serologic tests.

Hydatid disease of the spleen is usually treated by total splenectomy. It is the safer method because it removes any cysts that may not have been detected on imaging as well as the major cyst or cysts being treated. It also avoids the risk of contamination of the peritoneal cavity by removing the cysts intact. Alternatively, especially in children and younger individuals, preservation of the spleen by cystectomy alone has been reported as a feasible method (8,9). The cyst is drained in an isolated operated field, the cyst cavity irrigated with 0.9 NaCl and povidone iodine.

The major portion of the cyst is then resected and omentum is sutured to the cyst edges.

Whether total splenectomy or cystectomy is elected as the procedure of choice, meticulous care must be taken against inadvertent contamination of the peritoneal cavity.

TUMORLIKE LESIONS OF THE SPLEEN

Hamartoma

The term *hamartoma* is derived from the Greek noun *hamartia*, meaning error or defect. It is a developmental aberration resulting in focal or multifocal proliferation of a tissue element normal to the organ in which it develops (10). In the spleen, it presents as a solid, well-demarcated lesion varying in color from dark red to grayish white and varying in size from several millimeters to many centimeters. Microscopically, normal splenic red pulp elements appear in disarray, compacted into a discrete mass (11).

If confirmation of a solitary hamartoma can be made on imaging studies or biopsy (12,13), the lesion may be treated by local resection or partial splenectomy, if indicated by symptoms or size. Removal of solitary hamartomas is indicated because they have been known to rupture (14) and to grow in size.

Occasionally the hamartomas may be distributed diffusely throughout the spleen (hamartomatosis). The enlarged spleen with hamartomatosis may be symptomatic because of its size or may result in hypersplenism (15). In either case, total splenectomy is indicated.

Peliosis

Peliosis is a rare and unusual lesion of the spleen characterized by the presence of multiple blood-filled cavities ranging in size from millimeters to several centimeters (16). The cystlike cavities, lined by fibrous, nonepithelial tissue, may occur in part of or throughout the spleen. The early lesions can be detected only microscopically and represent dilatation of the red pulp sinuses. Large lesions are seen grossly as multiple nodules and are lined histologically by plump endothelial cells.

The etiology is unknown but the association of the condition with the administration of immunosuppressive, steroid, and cytostatic drugs for a variety of conditions points to an autoimmune reactive phenomenon (17). It has been seen following liver transplantation (18), malignancy, sarcoidoses, AIDS, and other diseases. It may also involve the liver, where it can also occur as an incidental finding.

The most serious consequence of peliosis is rupture (19-21), with hemorrhage and hematoperitoneum. Most reported cases are descriptions of this complication. Occasionally peliosis may cause massive splenomegaly. The occurrence of peliosis large enough to be detected in the setting of the conditions mentioned is an indication for total splenectomy.

Inflammatory Pseudotumors

As the name implies, inflammatory pseudotumor in the spleen is a mass that looks like a tumor but is not, with cellular components indicative of acute and chronic inflammation as well as spindle cell elements of varying nature (22). The pseudotumors are usually diagnosed as asymptomatic splenic masses encountered at laparotomy or discovered incidentally during imaging examinations. They are usually solitary, with great variability in size, ranging from millimeters to many centimeters. The etiology is conjectural. Most cases show an association with Epstein-Barr virus (EBV) (23) but they may occur in the absence of EBV. In the spleen, the EBV infected cells are the spindle cells and not the lymphoid cells.

Grossly, the lesion appears as a well-demarcated mass of variegated appearance with nodules of necrosis, hemorrhage, cellularity, and fibrosis. Microscopically there is a profusion of inflammatory cells (granulocytes, lymphocytes, and plasma cells) and spindle cells. Immunohistochemical stains show reactivity with smooth muscle actin in most cases, indicating a fibroblastic origin. Follicular dendritic cell immunoreactivity (CD21) has been also reported in few cases of inflammatory pseudotumor.

A certain diagnosis can be established only on histologic examination. This has been reported on needle biopsy in rare instances (24) but because the imaging and gross characteristics are indistinguishable from neoplastic lesions, total splenectomy is the procedure of choice.

Sclerosing Angiomatoid Nodular Transformation

Another recently described vascular lesion of the spleen is sclerosing angiomatoid nodular transformation (25). This occurs as a solitary mass, commonly discovered as an incidental finding, but less commonly found as a cause of abdominal discomfort, pain, or significant splenomegaly. The masses consist of coalescing nodules of brownish-red tissue within a dense fibrous tissue stroma. Microscopically the nodules appear angiomatoid with slitlike spaces lined with variegated endothelial or spindle cell elements. The fibrous stroma contains inflammatory cells and a variety of hemic elements including plasma cells, lymphocytes, and siderophages. A central calcification may be present.

This lesion is not considered a true neoplasm but malformative red pulp tissue entrapped in an accompanying nonneoplastic stromal proliferative process. Because of the uncertainty of the diagnosis, total splenectomy is indicated. In the cases reported thus far, there have been no instances of recurrent disease after splenectomy.

OTHER DISEASES SIMULATING SPLENIC TUMORS

There are other conditions that on occasion may simulate splenic tumors. Sarcoidosis involving the spleen may present as multiple nodular lesions of low attenuation on imaging, suggesting primary or metastatic neoplasm (26). Amyloidosis may also appear as multifocal areas of low attenuation on computed tomographic studies or of heterogeneous echogenicity on ultrasonography. Spontaneous rupture of the spleen has been reported with primary amyloidosis. Both sarcoidosis and amyloidosis are manifestations of systemic disease and are not in themselves an indication for splenectomy unless complicated by symptomatic splenomegaly (27) or splenic rupture (28).

RARE NONHEMATOLYMPHOID TUMORS

Tumors arising from some nonhematolymphoid elements in the spleen are so rare that reports are almost anecdotal. This is true of dendritic cell tumors, smooth muscle tumors, lipoma (29), angiomyolipoma (30), fibroma (31), carcinosarcoma (32), and fibrosarcoma (33). Only malignant fibrous histiocytoma of the spleen occurs with sufficient frequency to merit discussion here.

Malignant fibrous histiocytoma is a pleomorphic sarcoma, first reported by Govoni et al. (34) in 1982. In most reports (35-37) the patients have been in older age groups, but a huge tumor of this nature has been reported in a child 11 years old (38). Imaging and scanning studies can only provide evidence of a pleomorphic tumor mass. The diagnosis of malignant fibrous histiocytoma can be made only on the basis of histologic and histochemical studies. The tumor is usually composed of pleomorphic spindle cells with a storiform pattern exhibiting increased mitotic activity. The treatment is total splenectomy. The prognosis is guarded; however, some long-term survivors having been reported.

VASCULAR TUMORS

Hemangioma

The commonest benign tumor of the spleen is the hemangioma. It exhibits a broad spectrum of variants in structure and clinical significance, ranging from small incidental findings of no clinical significance to large symptomatic solitary lesions or diffuse involvement of the spleen that are of great clinical significance (39,40). Grossly, they present as well-circumscribed, blue-red spongy nodules that may grow to a size of 10 cm or more. They can be deep within the splenic parenchyma or bulge outward beneath splenic capsule if more superficially located. They are slow-growing, giving rise to symptoms of discomfort or pain when they are significantly large. As they grow larger, they may show areas of fibrosis, infarction, and cystic degeneration.

Histologically, hemangiomas are either of the cavernous or capillary type, rarely an admixture of the two. The cavernous type is much more common; it is composed of thin-walled, blood-filled vascular spaces of varying size lined with plump endothelial cells with intervening thin fibrous septae or splenic red pulp tissue. Capillary hemangiomas exhibit more tightly packed vascular channels without the blood-filled spaces. Hemangiomas are usually CD34 (endothelial marker)-positive and negative for CD8 and CD68.

Rupture with massive bleeding is the most dangerous complication of the larger solitary hemangiomas. They can also be the cause of cytopenia due to hypersplenism or microangiopathic hemolytic anemia consequent to sequestration of clotting factors. The diagnosis of a hemangioma over the size of 5 cm is an indication for splenectomy. It is not a lesion that lends itself to more conservative approaches.

Multiple diffuse hemangiomata in the spleen constitute hemangiomatosis, a rare but serious clinical variant of the benign hemangioma (41). The diffuse lesions may be cavernous or capillary. Conditions that have been reported in association with hemangiomatosis are hypersplenism, Kasabach-Merritt-like syndrome (both with anemia, thrombocytopenia, and coagulation disorder), and portal hypertension (42). Hemangiomatosis of the spleen may be associated with the occurrence of hemangiomata in other parenchymatous organs as well. The diagnosis of diffuse hemangiomatosis is an indication for total splenectomy.

Littoral Cell Angioma

Littoral cell angioma is a rare, recently described, benign vascular neoplasm of the spleen (43). Its distinguishing feature is the cell of origin, namely the littoral cells that occur in the lining of the splenic sinusoids. Although the tumor resembles the hemangioma in gross anatomic and imaging characteristics (44), its distinctive histologic features and histocytic markers set it apart as a unique lesion. It may be solitary but it is more frequently multifocal. Grossly, the spleen shows multiple dark, spongy cystic nodules indistinguishable from hemangiomas. Microscopically, the lesion is relatively well circumscribed and involves the red pulp. The vascular spaces range in appearance from slitlike to cystic and are lined by single layers of flat to tall endothelial cells. Occasionally, the endothelial proliferations are papillary and fill the lumen. Littoral cell angioma cells are negative for the endothelial marker CD34 and CD8 (splenic sinus lining marker) and express the histiocytic marker CD68.

Solitary or multifocal lesions may be discovered as incidental findings or can cause clinically significant splenomegaly with a wide spectrum of syndromes. Among clinical conditions reported with littoral cell angiomas are myelodysplasia (45), aplastic anemia, fever of unknown origin (46), hypersplenism, and an association with visceral neoplasms.

Whether diagnosed as an incidental finding on imaging studies or as splenomegaly with accompanying diverse symptoms, the indication is for total splenectomy. Diagnosis is made with certainty only on histologic study and with histochemical markers.

Lymphangioma

Lymphangiomas are less frequent than hemangiomas in the spleen, but exhibit the same spectrum of variants in structure and clinical import (47). They occur more frequently in children and younger individuals, and more rarely in older age groups. Like hemangiomas, they may occur as solitary lesions, ranging from small subcapsular lesions found incidentally to large symptomatic lesions causing splenomegaly or diffuse lymphangiomatosis (40).

Differentiation from hemangiomas or hemangiomatosis is based primarily on imaging findings (48), including ultrasonography, computed tomography, and magnetic resonance imaging. The content of the cystic components is of course lymph rather than blood, projecting different imaging characteristics. Histologically, lymphangiomas are composed of vascular spaces of varying size, usually lined by flat endothelium. The lining cells express endothelial marker CD31 and are negative for CD34 and CD8.

In children, multiple locations may be involved as part of a generalized developmental defect involving many regions and viscera (49). The solitary lymphangioma can reach a size sufficiently large to cause symptoms of pain or discomfort and become detectable as splenomegaly. More often, the lesions are multiple and subcapsular in location. As with the hemangioma, lymphangiomas may be diffusely distributed within the spleen. Lymphangiomas or lymphangiomatosis do not pose the same dire hematologic sequelae as do hemangiomas. However, they are similarly subject to rupture, an exceedingly rare occurrence.

If the diagnosis of lymphangioma can be made with certainty on small asymptomatic lesions seen on imaging studies, surgical intervention is not indicated. If, however, the lesions are large enough to exhibit splenomegaly or cause symptoms, the indication is for splenectomy.

Angiosarcoma

Angiosarcoma, the malignant counterpart of the hemangioma, occurs much more rarely than its benign relative (50). It is an intensely aggressive neoplasm with an abysmal prognosis. There are few known long-term survivors, metastases are frequent, and rapid deterioration ending in death is the most common outcome after diagnosis.

Angiosarcoma is primarily found in adults, although there are cases reported in children as young as age 2 (51). The most common presenting symptom is abdominal pain caused by the rapidly enlarging spleen, intra-abdominal metastases, or rupture of the neoplasm. By the time the diagnosis is made, the spleen in most cases is very enlarged; a median figure in one large case series being cited as 1,000 g. The gross characteristics of the tumor are variegated with spongy, nodular reddish masses interspersed with areas of hemorrhage, infarction, fibrosis, and occasional focal calcification. Histologically, the degree of differentiation can be quite variable, ranging from well-formed, anastomosing vascular spaces lined by plump atypical endothelial cells to undifferentiated spindle cells with a high degree of pleomorphism and high mitotic activity. The tumor cells express the endothelial markers CD31 and CD34. Metastases to liver, lungs, bone, lymph nodes, and other sites at the time of diagnosis are common.

When the diagnosis is suspected by imaging studies (52), physical signs or at laparotomy, the indication is for splenectomy. Even in the presence of metastases, a spleen that is prone to rupture should be removed. Survival after splenectomy is usually measured in months, with a median survival of about 6 months. Standard chemotherapeutic regimens have been of little benefit, although an occasional response has been reported.

Angiosarcomas of the spleen are among the most aggressive and rapidly lethal neoplasms found in any organ system (53).

Hemangioendothelioma

The hemangioendothelioma differs from angiosarcoma in degree of malignancy, histologic characteristics, and clinical behavior (54). It is best characterized as a malignant neoplasm intermediate between the benign hemangioma and the highly aggressive angiosarcoma. Thus, in its gross and microscopic features, it may resemble both the benign and aggressively malignant lesions. Histologically, the tumor is composed of well-formed vascular channels. It differs from angiosarcoma by absence of necrosis, mild cellular atypia, and low mitotic rate. Some believe that hemangioendotheliomas are examples of well-differentiated splenic angiosarcoma.

As with angiosarcoma, the presenting complaint may be pain secondary to the splenomegaly, anemia, or hematoperitoneum due to splenic rupture. Massively enlarged spleens are common. Also described as part of the presenting symptom complex have been consumptive coagulopathy and hyposplenism.

Although the majority of case reports have been in adults, a number of recent reports have described cases in infancy and childhood (55,56). Metastases to liver, bone, lung, and other organs occur, but they are less frequent than with angiosarcoma, and several long-term survivors have been reported. Splenectomy is indicated when the lesion is suspected or discovered. The prognosis is guarded.

Hemangiopericytoma

Hemangiopericytoma of the spleen is an exceptionally rare tumor in the spleen thought originally to be originating from Zimmerman pericytes, and more commonly found in muscles of the lower extremity. It was first described in the spleen by Guadalajara Jurado (57) et al. in 1989. Controversies exist about its real origin, and the relationship to normal pericytes has not been confirmed.

The neoplasm typically presents with asymptomatic splenomegaly. The characteristic histologic features are proliferating spindle cells in association with dilated vascular channels, appearing grossly as well-defined grayish nodules diffusely scattered throughout the spleen. The biologic behavior may be either benign or malignant, with predominance toward malignancy. Malignant lesions can recur locally or metastasize to the usual preferential sites for vascular malignancies, namely liver and bone.

The diagnosis is made by splenectomy for splenomegaly detected on physical examination or on imaging studies and confirmed by pathologic study. The prognosis is guarded as recurrence or metastasis may appear long after removal of the primary lesion.

METASTATIC TUMORS

Considering the extreme vascularity of the spleen and the volume of blood that traverses it daily, it is surprising that the incidence of metastases to spleen is so low. It is extremely small as compared with the frequency of metastasis to the liver. The reason for this is obscure, although many theories have been propounded.

Melanoma is a neoplasm that seems to have a predilection for metastasis to the spleen when it disseminates. Involvement from other primary malignancies is so unusual that it has occasioned a multitude of case studies reporting such occurrence (58). Metastases to the spleen have been reported from primary lesions of the brain, thyroid, lung, liver, stomach, pancreas, colon, kidney, ovary, and uterus. The metastases may be solitary or multiple involving the splenic parenchyma or the splenic capsule (59). Grossly, metastases appear as well-defined, firm masses of varying size. Splenectomy may be indicated for palliation of symptoms, even if the possibility of cure is improbable. Rupture of splenic metastases causing splenic carcinomatosis has been reported (60,61).

Thus, the spleen has an enhanced resistance to neoplasia, in tumors originating in it or as a site of metastasis to it. No factor explaining this phenomenon has been identified.

SUMMARY

Benign and malignant nonhematolymphoid tumors of the spleen are rare. Vascular tumors are overwhelmingly dominant, as might be expected from the vascular nature of the organ. The commonest benign neoplasm of the spleen is the hemangioma. The most aggressive malignant neoplasm of the spleen is the angiosarcoma. Of the tumorlike conditions of the spleen, the hamartoma is the most frequent, followed by the nonparasitic splenic cyst.

Benign lesions lend themselves to partial splenectomy rather than total removal of the organ. Partial resection is a viable option only when the diagnosis is reasonably certain. Splenic cysts have a distinctive appearance on imaging studies. Needle biopsies performed percutaneously have confirmed other benign diagnoses. When the diagnosis is in doubt, total splenectomy is the procedure of choice. Primary benign tumors and tumorlike conditions offer an excellent prognosis after splenectomy. Malignant tumors of the spleen have a dismal prognosis, with survival after splenectomy measured in months or less. Chemotherapy has proved ineffective, although some anecdotal success have been reported. Solitary metastases to spleen should be treated by splenectomy; diffuse metastatic disease contraindicates it.

Splenectomy, either total or partial, can be performed by open or laparoscopic surgical techniques. The expertise of the operator and the safety of the patient are the primary determinants in choosing one method over the other.

REFERENCES

1. Morgenstern L. Nonparasitic splenic cysts: pathogenesis, classification, and treatment. *J Am Coll Surg.* 2002;194:306–314.
2. Hansen MB, Moller AC. Splenic cysts. *Surg Laparosc Endosc Percutan Tech.* 2004;14:316–322.
3. Burrig KF. Epithelial (true) splenic cysts. Pathogenesis of the mesothelial and so-called epidermoid cyst of the spleen. *Am J Surg Pathol.* 1988;12:275–281.
4. Hulzebos CV, Leemans R, Halma C, et al. Splenic epithelial cysts and splenomegaly: diagnosis and management. *Netherlands J Med.* 1998;53:80–84.
5. Morgenstern L, Shapiro SJ. Partial splenectomy for nonparasitic splenic cysts. *Am J Surg.* 1980;139:278–281.
6. Till H, Schaarschmidt K. Partial laparoscopic decapsulation of congenital splenic cysts: a medium-term evaluation proves the efficiency in children. *Surg Endosc.* 2004;18:626–628.
7. Mackenzie RK, Youngson GG, Mahomed AA. Laparoscopic decapsulation of congenital splenic cysts: a step forward in splenic preservation. *J Pediatr Surg.* 2004;39:88–90.
8. Manouras AJ, Nikolaou CC, Katergiannakis VA, et al. Spleen-sparing surgical treatment for echinococcosis of the spleen. *Br J Surg.* 1997;84:1162.
9. Atmatzidis K, Papaziogas B, Mirelis C, et al. Splenectomy versus spleen-preserving surgery for splenic echinococcosis. *Dig Surg.* 2003;20:527–531.
10. Morgenstern L, McCafferty L, Rosenberg J, et al. Hamartomas of the spleen. *Arch Surg.* 1984;119:1291–1293.
11. Krishnan J, Frizzera G. Two splenic lesions in need of clarification: hamartoma and inflammatory pseudotumor. *Semin Diagn Pathol.* 2003;20:94–104.
12. Elsayes KM, Narra VR, Mukundan G, et al. MR imaging of the spleen: spectrum of abnormalities. *Radiographics.* 2005;25:967–982.
13. Yu RS, Zhang SZ, Hua JM. Imaging findings of splenic hamartoma. *World J Gastroenterol.* 2004;10:2613–2615.
14. Ferguson ER, Sardi A, Beckman EN. Spontaneous rupture of splenic hamartoma. *J La State Med Soc.* 1993;145:48–52.
15. Beham A, Hermann W, Vennigerholz F, et al. Hamartoma of the spleen with haematological symptoms. *Virchows Arch A Pathol Anat Histopathol.* 1989;414:535–539.
16. Tsokos M, Erbersdobler A. Pathology of peliosis. *Forensic Sci Int.* 2005;149:25–33.
17. Gugger M, Gebbers JO. Peliosis of the spleen: an immune-complex disease? *Histopathology.* 1998;33:387–389.
18. Raghavan R, Alley S, Tawfik O, et al. Splenic peliosis: a rare complication following liver transplantation. *Dig Dis Sci.* 1999;44:1128–1131.
19. Rege JD, Kavishwar VS, Mopkar PS. Peliosis of spleen presenting as splenic rupture with haemoperitoneum—a case report. *Indian J Path Microbiol.* 1998;41:465–467.
20. Celebrezze, JP Jr, Cottrell DJ, Williams GB. Spontaneous splenic rupture due to isolated splenic peliosis. *South Med J.* 1998;91:763–764.
21. Ortega-Deballon P, Fernandez-Lobato R, Ortega-Munoz P, et al. Splenic peliosis: a cause of spontaneous splenic rupture. *Surgery.* 1999;126:585–586.
22. Kutok JL, Pinkus GS, Dorfman DM, et al. Inflammatory pseudotumor of lymph node and spleen: an entity biologically distinct from inflammatory myofibroblastic tumor. *Hum Pathol.* 2001;32:1382–1387.
23. Oz Puyan F, Bilgi S, Unlu E, et al. Inflammatory pseudotumor of the spleen with EBV positivity: report of a case. *Eur J Haematol.* 2004;72:285–291.
24. Keogan MT, Freed KS, Paulson EK, et al. Imaging-guided percutaneous biopsy of focal splenic lesions: update on safety and effectiveness. *Am J Roentgenol.* 1999;172:933–937.
25. Martel M, Cheuk W, Lombardi L, et al. Sclerosing angiomatoid nodular transformation (SANT): report of 25 cases of a distinctive benign splenic lesion. *Am J Surg Pathol.* 2004;28:1268–1279.
26. Koyama T, Ueda H, Togashi K, et al. Radiologic manifestations of sarcoidosis in various organs. *Radiographics.* 2004;24:87–104.
27. Zia H, Zemon H, Brody F. Laparoscopic splenectomy for isolated sarcoidosis of the spleen. *J Laparoendosc Adv Surg Techn A.* 2005;15:160–162.
28. Oran B, Wright DG, Seldin DC, et al. Spontaneous rupture of the spleen in AL amyloidosis. *Am J Hematol.* 2003;74:131–135.
29. Easler RE, Dowlin WM. Primary lipoma of the spleen. Report of a case. *Arch Pathol Lab Med.* 1969;88:557–559.
30. Tang P, Alhindawi R, Farmer P. Case report: primary isolated angiomyolipoma of the spleen. *Ann Clin Lab Sci.* 2001;31:405–410.
31. Giardina F, Battocchia A. On a case of fibroma of the spleen. Italian. *Haematologica.* 1968;53:285–292.
32. Westra WH, Anderson BO, Klimstra DS. Carcinosarcoma of the spleen. An extragenital malignant mixed mullerian tumor? *Am J Surg Pathol.* 1994;18:309–315.
33. Gliozzi F, Pola P, Visca T. Primary fibrosarcoma of the spleen (case report) [in Italian]. *Policlinico [Prat].*, 1968;75:118–123.
34. Govoni E, Bazzocchi F, Pileri S, et al. Primary malignant fibrous histiocytoma of the spleen: an ultrastructural study. *Histopathology.* 1982;6:351–361.

35. Mallipudi BV, Chawdhery MZ, Jeffery PJ. Primary malignant fibrous histiocytoma of spleen. *Eur J Surg Oncol.* 1998;24:448–449.

36. Colovic N, Cemerikic-Martinovic V, Colovic R, et al. Primary malignant fibrous histiocytoma of the spleen and liver. *Med Oncol.* 2001;18:293–297.

37. Wick MR, Scheithauer BW, Smith SL, et al. Primary nonlymphoreticular malignant neoplasms of the spleen. *Am J Surg Pathol.* 1982;6:229–242.

38. Yu JW, Law KL, Chi CS, et al. Malignant fibrous histiocytoma of spleen. A case report and literature review [in Chinese]. Zhonghua Yi Xue Za Zhi (Taipei). 1989;44:271–273.

39. Willcox TM, Speer RW, Schlinkert RT, et al. Hemangioma of the spleen: presentation, diagnosis, and management. *J Gastrointest Surg.* 2000;4:611–613.

40. Abbott RM, Levy AD, Aguilera NS, et al. Primary vascular neoplasms of the spleen: radiologic-pathologic correlation. *Radio-Graphics.* 2004;24:1137–1163.

41. Steininger H, Pfofe D, Marquardt L, et al. Isolated diffuse hemangiomatosis of the spleen: case report and review of literature. *Pathol Res Pract.* 2004;200:479–485.

42. Dufau JP, le Tourneau A, Audouin J, et al. Isolated diffuse hemangiomatosis of the spleen with Kasabach-Merritt-like syndrome. *Histopathology.* 1999;35:337–344.

43. Bisceglia M, Sickel JZ, Giangaspero F, et al. Littoral cell angioma of the spleen: an additional report of four cases with emphasis on the association with visceral organ cancers. *Tumori.* 1998;84:595–599.

44. Levy AD, Abbott RM, Abbondanzo SL. Littoral cell angioma of the spleen: CT features with clinicopathologic comparison. *Radiology.* 2004;230:485–490.

45. Ercin C, Gurbuz Y, Hacihanefioglu A, et al. Multiple littoral cell angioma of the spleen in a case of myelodysplastic syndrome. *Hematology.* 2005;10:141–144.

46. Tan YM, Chuah KL, Wong WK. Littoral cell angioma of the spleen. *Ann Acad Med Singapore.* 2004;33:524–526.

47. Morgenstern L, Bello JM, Fisher BL, et al. The clinical spectrum of lymphangiomas and lymphangiomatosis of the spleen. *Am Surg.* 1992;58:599–604.

48. Komatsuda T, Ishida H, Konno K, et al. Splenic lymphangioma: US and CT diagnosis and clinical manifestations. *Abdom Imaging.* 1999;24:414–417.

49. de Perrot M, Rostan O, Morel P, et al. Abdominal lymphangioma in adults and children. *Br J Surg.* 1998;85:395–397.

50. Neuhauser TS, Derringer GA, Thompson LD, et al. Splenic angiosarcoma: a clinicopathologic and immunophenotypic study of 28 cases. *Mod Pathol.* 2000;13:978–987.

51. den Hoed ID, Granzen B, Granzen B, et al. Metastasized angiosarcoma of the spleen in a 2-year-old girl. *Pediatr Hematol Oncol.* 2005;22:387–390.

52. Thompson WM, Levy AD, Aguilera NS, et al. Angiosarcoma of the spleen: imaging characteristics in 12 patients. *Radiology.* 2005;235:106–115.

53. Falk S, Krishnan J, Meis JM. Primary angiosarcoma of the spleen. A clinicopathologic study of 40 cases. *Am J Surg Pathol.* 1993;17:959–970.

54. Kaw YT, Duwaji MS, Knisley RE, et al. Hemangioendothelioma of the spleen. *Arch Pathol Lab Med.* 1992;116:1079–1082.

55. Goyal A, Babu SN, Kim V, et al. Hemangioendothelioma of liver and spleen: trauma-induced consumptive coagulopathy. *J Pediatr Surg.* 2002;37:E29.

56. Suster S. Epithelioid and spindle-cell hemangioendothelioma of the spleen. Report of a distinctive splenic vascular neoplasm of childhood. *Am J Surg Pathol.* 1992;16:785–792.

57. Guadalajara Jurado J, Turegano FF, Garcia MC, et al. Hemangiopericytoma of the spleen. *Surgery.* 1989;106:575–577.

58. Lam KY, Tang V. Metastatic tumors to the spleen: a 25-year clinico-pathologic study. *Arch Pathol Lab Med.* 2000;124:526–530.

59. Klein B, Stein M, Kuten A, et al. Splenomegaly and solitary spleen metastasis in solid tumors. *Cancer.* 1987;60:100–102.

60. Lachachi F, Abita T, Durand Fontanier S, et al. Spontaneous splenic rupture due to splenic metastasis of lung cancer. *Ann Chirurgie.* 2004;129:521–522.

61. Krapohl BD, Komurcu F, Deutinger M. Spleen rupture due to metastasis of thin melanoma (Breslow thickness of 0.75 mm). *Melanoma Res.* 2005;15:135.

COMMENTARY
Angela D. Levy

The opinions and assertions contained herein are the private views of the authors and are not to be construed as official or as reflecting the views of the Departments of the Army or Defense.

Drs. Morgenstern and Alsabeh provide a superlative review of nonhematolymphoid tumors and tumorlike lesions of the spleen. These relatively uncommon lesions are being detected more frequently because the technological advances in sonography, computed tomography (CT), magnetic resonance (MR), and positron emission tomography (PET) imaging with ^{18}F-fluordeoxyglucose (^{18}F-FDG) over the past 2 decades have led to remarkable improvements in our ability to noninvasively image the abdomen. Tissue harmonic and spatial compound imaging have dramatically improved contrast and spatial resolution in abdominal sonography. Multidetector CT technology has revolutionized CT imaging such that high-resolution scanning of the abdomen is now rapidly performed during multiple vascular phases of intravenous contrast enhancement. Rapid MR sequences and phased-array body coils have enabled MR to become a primary abdominal imaging modality because high-resolution MR images can be obtained without significant motion artifact. As a result of the burgeoning imaging technology, sonography, multidetector CT, and MR have become an integral part of the clinical evaluation of patients with abdominal complaints. Consequently, incidental findings in the spleen are more commonly encountered.

IMAGING EVALUATION OF INCIDENTAL SPLENIC MASSES

Patients with incidentally discovered splenic masses rarely have symptoms or laboratory findings that aid in diagnosis. The differential diagnosis of an incidentally discovered splenic mass is often based exclusively on imaging findings, and the subsequent management of the lesion is frequently directed by the suggestions of the radiologist. The most straightforward approach to establishing an imaging differential diagnosis for an incidentally discovered splenic mass is to determine if the mass is solitary or multiple, cystic or solid, and then to examine the mass for imaging features such as intravenous contrast-enhancement pattern, calcification, margin contours, and other findings specific to primary splenic tumors and tumorlike lesions. Finally, the entire scan should be evaluated for evidence of disease in other organs to determine whether or not the splenic mass is part of a multiorgan process.

A solitary cystic mass in the spleen may represent a benign lesion such as an epithelial cyst, pseudocyst, parasitic cyst, or a benign cystic neoplasm such as lymphangioma, and rarely, a cystic hemangioma. Malignant lesions such as metastases or primary splenic sarcomas such as angiosarcomas are much less common and may appear cystic if there is significant intratumoral degeneration or hemorrhage within the lesion or if the metastatic lesion contains a significant mucinous component. Epithelial, or true, splenic cysts are sharply marginated, have a thin wall, and are fluid-filled on imaging studies. They are usually unilocular, do not enhance with intravenous contrast, and only occasionally have mural calcifications. They may have a more complex appearance on sonographic images compared with CT because they may contain low-level internal echoes from fluid that is turbid or viscous, contain thin septations, or have a trabecular wall that is not demonstrable by CT imaging. Pseudocysts have a similar appearance on imaging studies compared with epithelial cysts, but reportedly more commonly have mural calcifications (1). Notably, to suggest the diagnosis of pseudocyst, there should be imaging evidence or a clinical history of prior splenic trauma or infarction to explain the development of a pseudocyst. Pseudocysts may also arise in the spleen as a complication of pancreatitis. However, intrasplenic pancreatic pseudocysts are not generally an incidental finding because the patient will have a clinical history of pancreatitis. Hydatid disease is the most commonly encountered parasitic cyst in the abdomen, but is distinctly uncommon in the spleen. Nevertheless, hydatid cysts should be considered in the differential diagnosis when the splenic cyst is complex with multiple septations, daughter cysts, or membranes. Mural calcification is quite common in hydatid cysts. Lack of intravenous contrast enhancement of the cyst wall is an important feature that helps to distinguish hydatid cysts from cystic neoplasms such as lymphangioma or cystic hemangioma. The finding of daughter cysts or floating membranes within the cyst is highly suggestive of a hydatid cyst. Daughter cysts may be more difficult to visualize when they are closely or tightly packed together. In such cases, they will simulate a multiseptated cyst such as a lymphangioma or cystic hemangioma.

MR imaging can be very useful to help narrow the differential diagnosis when the CT or sonographic findings are nonspecific or when immunologic or serologic tests do not help confirm hydatid disease. The walls of the daughter cysts and internal membranes are low-signal intensity on all MR sequences (2). In less complex echinococcal cysts, a peripheral low-signal intensity rim, which is more evident on T2-weighted images, may be present to help differentiate it from nonparasitic cysts. In contrast, cystic neoplasms such as lymphangiomas and, rarely, hemangiomas, are vascularized. Therefore, the septa and walls surrounding the cystic spaces enhance with intravenous contrast material (3). Lymphangiomas have a subcapsular origin within the spleen because they arise from subcapsular lymphatic tissue. The subcapsular location may be difficult to discern in large le-

sions, but is a very helpful finding to suggest lymphangioma when the lesion is small and incidental (4).

Metastases are frequently included in the differential diagnosis of cystic splenic masses. As a general rule, splenic metastases are very uncommon and when present are usually multiple and occur in the setting of widespread metastatic disease (5). Nevertheless, solitary cystic metastases have been reported (6–8). Splenic metastases may appear cystic when they have extensive necrosis, hemorrhage, or when they are from a mucinous primary. The margins of splenic metastasis are rarely as sharp and as well defined compared with benign cystic lesions. When considering cystic metastasis in the differential diagnosis, other findings suggestive of a malignant process should be carefully sought such as invasion or extension of the mass into the surrounding splenic parenchyma, or extension of the lesion beyond the spleen into the supporting ligaments and connective tissue.

Incidental solitary, solid splenic masses are most commonly benign hemangiomas, particularly when there is no evidence of splenomegaly or findings to suggest lymphoma or metastases. The differential diagnosis includes rarer benign tumors and tumorlike lesions such as hamartoma, inflammatory pseudotumor, and sclerosing angiomatoid nodular transformation as well as rare malignancies such as angiosarcoma, hemangioendothelioma, and hemangiopericytoma.

Hemangiomas are the most frequently occurring benign neoplasms of the spleen and the most common incidentally encountered masses on sonography (4). The imaging features of hemangiomas are variable because they may be solitary or multifocal and solid or cystic. When small and incidentally discovered, their clinical importance primarily lies in differentiating them from more ominous lesions such as lymphoma and metastatic disease. Splenic hemangiomas may have homogenous, marked contrast enhancement, heterogeneous mottled enhancement, or peripheral enhancement with centripetal progression on intravenous contrast material-enhanced CT (9,10). Although it is unusual to identify calcifications within a hemangioma, they are a suggestive finding when present. Calcifications may be small and punctate or curvilinear (11). When CT features are not diagnostic of hemangioma, MR imaging can help distinguish hemangiomas from other solid tumors because hemangiomas are distinctively brighter than the spleen on T2-weighted images because of long T2 relaxation times (12). However, the signal pattern may be more heterogeneous than expected because they may contain areas of fibrosis, infarction, and cystic change. Splenic hamartomas are rare lesions that are usually solitary, homogeneous masses. They have been reported to contain calcifications and to be heterogeneous when cystic degeneration is present secondary to ischemia or hemorrhage (13,14). The most characteristic imaging feature of hamartomas is hypervascularity that is seen on color Doppler sonography. They are featureless on CT because they are typically isoattenuating to normal spleen on unenhanced and intravenous contrast-enhanced CT scans where a contour abnormality may be the only finding (4,15). On MR, they are only minimally hyperintense relative to the normal spleen on T2-weighted and intravenous gadolinium-enhanced T1-weighted images.

Malignant neoplasms should be considered in the differential diagnosis for solid masses that do not meet the imaging criteria of hemangiomas or hamartomas. However, malignant neoplasms occurring within the spleen are rarely incidental findings. Patients typically have symptoms of left upper quadrant pain, fullness, or a palpable left upper quadrant mass. Patients with lymphoma may also have systemic symptoms of weight loss, malaise, and fever. Lymphomas are the most common primary splenic malignancy and are characteristically homogeneous and hypoattenuating following intravenous contrast material administration on CT or MR. Aggressive histologic subtypes of lymphoma may be heterogeneous or have focal areas of cystic change or degeneration on imaging studies. Uncommon primary splenic malignancies such as angiosarcoma, hemangioendothelioma, and hemangiopericytoma have nonspecific imaging features. Although these neoplasms can only be confidently diagnosed after biopsy or splenectomy, recent medical literature has shown that ^{18}F-FDG-PET/CT has a high negative-predictive value for malignancy in assessing solid splenic masses (16). As such, histologic sampling may be warranted for only those splenic masses that are FDG-avid.

Incidental discovery of multiple splenic masses is not a common situation. The most frequent causes of multiple splenic masses are infectious and inflammatory diseases. The majority of patients with multiple splenic masses are symptomatic or clinically suspected of having splenic disease. Bacterial and fungal splenic abscesses are most commonly encountered in patients who are immunosuppressed but may also be seen following trauma or as a result of emboli. The differential diagnosis for multiple splenic masses also includes lymphoma, primary vascular neoplasms, such as littoral cell angioma, and metastases. In general, on cross-sectional imaging, splenic abscesses are round or irregular in shape, have central low attenuation necrosis on CT that is high signal intensity on T2-weighted MR images, and hypoechoic on sonography. Rimlike peripheral enhancement may be seen following intravenous contrast material administration. The margins of splenic abscess may be well defined or ill defined. Larger or more complex abscesses may contain gas, septations, and debris. Similar to bacterial and fungal infections, multifocal vascular neoplasms (with the exception of multiple hemangiomas), lymphoma, and metastases are usually accompanied by clinical symptoms or splenomegaly. On the other hand, granulomatous diseases such as tuberculosis or sarcoid may be an incidental discovery when patients are being imaged for the evaluation of the thoracic manifestations of the disease or for other reasons. Clinical history, thoracic findings, and the presence of associated abdominal lymphadenopathy usually accompany the presence of splenic granulomas in patients with tuberculosis or sarcoid.

In conclusion, evaluation and management of an incidentally discovered splenic mass or masses should begin with the formulation of a differential diagnosis based on the number and composition of the masses (i.e., cystic or solid). If initially discovered on sonography, CT or MR imaging should be performed with and without intravenous contrast material to narrow the diagnostic possibilities or provide a more definitive diagnosis. Simple, solitary cystic lesions are most commonly epithelial cysts. Pseudocysts should be considered when there is supportive clinical history. Hemangiomas are the most common incidentally discovered solid splenic mass. CT and MR findings can usually suggest the diagnosis of hemangioma, whereas the diagnosis of hamartoma can be suggested by sonographic color Doppler findings. If a solid mass is not confirmed to be a hemangioma or hamartoma, ^{18}F-FDG-PET/CT can help select those patients who need to proceed to biopsy or splenectomy for a definitive diagnosis.

REFERENCES

1. Dachman AH, Ros PR, Murari PJ, et al. Nonparasitic splenic cysts: a report of 52 cases with radiologic-pathologic correlation. *AJR Am J Roentgenol.* 1986;147:537–542.
2. von Sinner W, te Strake L, Clark D, Sharif H. MR imaging in hydatid disease. *AJR Am J Roentgenol.* 1991;157:741–745.
3. Wadsworth DT, Newman B, Abramson SJ, et al. Splenic lymphangiomatosis in children. *Radiology.* 1997;202:173–176.
4. Abbott RM, Levy AD, Aguilera NS, et al. From the archives of the AFIP: Primary vascular neoplasms of the spleen: radiologic-pathologic correlation. *Radiographics.* 2004;24:1137–1163.
5. Lee SS, Morgenstern L, Phillips EH, et al. Splenectomy for splenic metastases: a changing clinical spectrum. *Am Surg.* 2000;66:837–840.
6. Cavallaro A, Modugno P, Specchia M, et al. Isolated splenic metastasis from colon cancer. *J Exp Clin Cancer Res.* 2004;23:143–146.
7. Farias-Eisner R, Braly P, Berek JS. Solitary recurrent metastasis of epithelial ovarian cancer in the spleen. *Gynecol Oncol.* 1993;48:338–341.
8. Place RJ. Isolated colon cancer metastasis to the spleen. *Am Surg.* 2001;67:454–457.
9. Ferrozzi F, Bova D, Draghi F, et al. CT findings in primary vascular tumors of the spleen. *AJR Am J Roentgenol.* 1996;166:1097–1101.
10. Ramani M, Reinhold C, Semelka RC, et al. Splenic hemangiomas and hamartomas: MR imaging characteristics of 28 lesions. *Radiology.* 1997;202:166–172.
11. Ros PR, Moser RP Jr, Dachman AH, et al. Hemangioma of the spleen: radiologic-pathologic correlation in ten cases. *Radiology.* 1987;162(1 Pt 1):73–77.
12. Hahn PF, Weissleder R, Stark DD, et al. MR imaging of focal splenic tumors. *AJR Am J Roentgenol.* 1988;150:823–827.
13. Brinkley AA, Lee JK. Cystic hamartoma of the spleen: CT and sonographic findings. *J Clin Ultrasound.* 1981;9:136–138.
14. Zissin R, Lishner M, Rathaus V. Case report: unusual presentation of splenic hamartoma; computed tomography and ultrasonic findings. *Clin Radiol.* 1992;45:410–411.
15. Tang S, Shimizu T, Kikuchi Y, et al. Color Doppler sonographic findings in splenic hamartoma. *J Clin Ultrasound.* 2000;28:249–253.
16. Metser U, Even-Sapir E. The role of ^{18}F-FDG PET/CT in the evaluation of solid splenic masses. *Semin Ultrasound CT MR.* 2006;27:420–425.

38

Colorectal Cancer: Laparoscopic versus Open Surgery

Alan T. Lefor

Over the past 2 decades, laparoscopy has emerged as a valuable tool in the diagnosis and management of many diseases throughout the world. For some conditions, laparoscopy has rapidly become the gold standard in treatment, placing open surgical procedures as a secondary option. One such procedure is laparoscopic cholecystectomy, which has allowed for a dramatic decrease in hospital stay, increased patient comfort, and rapid return to occupation. Indications for laparoscopic colon resection have long included diverticulitis, polyps, and inflammatory bowel disease. Despite the widespread acceptance of laparoscopy for benign conditions, its role in oncology remains more limited and under investigation. Malignancy was formerly considered a contraindication for laparoscopic resection. Issues such as margins of resection, adequacy of lymphadenectomy, and port site recurrences were cited as reasons to avoid laparoscopic resection.

Laparoscopic colon resection was first reported in 1991 (1). Although the use of the laparoscopic technique for benign colon conditions was widely accepted, its use in colon malignancies was much more restrained. In part, this was because of early reports of port site recurrences (2). There were many questions about the value of performing the procedure laparoscopically in terms of patient benefits, oncologic "equivalence" with open resection of colon malignancies, as well as the steep learning curve that applied to the technique for both malignant and benign conditions. However, recent well-designed trials have answered some of these important clinical questions. The list of procedures performed laparoscopically grows exponentially, but the body of evidence supporting its use is growing more slowly. Surgical procedures should maximally benefit the patient, and not be performed just because "we can." Conversely, we must critically evaluate the literature and use the latest techniques when appropriate.

LAPAROSCOPIC PHYSIOLOGY

Cellular/Immune Effects

One of the beneficial effects of laparoscopy is the reduction in postoperative pain, decreased healing time, and decreased adhesion formation. This may easily be attributed to the use of smaller incisions and the lack of retractors holding these incisions open for hours. However, patients who undergo laparoscopic splenectomy and then require an incision for removal of the intact specimen also note decreased pain in their incisions. Implicated in the beneficial effects of laparoscopy is the commonly used CO_2 gas that is used to insufflate the abdominal wall. West and colleagues (3) investigated the effect of different insufflation gases on murine peritoneal macrophage intracellular pH and correlated these alterations with alterations in lipopolysaccharide-stimulated inflammatory cytokine release. Peritoneal macrophages were incubated for 2 hours in air, helium, or CO_2, and the effect on tumor necrosis factor, interleukin (IL)-1 and cytosolic pH were determined. Macrophages incubated in CO_2 produced significantly less tumor necrosis factor and IL-1 compared to incubation in air or helium. In addition, exposure to CO_2, but not air or helium, produced a marked cytosolic acidification. These authors conclude that cellular acidification induced by peritoneal CO_2 insufflation contributes to the diminished local inflammatory response seen in laparoscopic surgery.

Despite reduction in local peritoneal inflammatory response, systemic immunocompetence appears better preserved after laparoscopy than after open procedures. Studies have shown significant decreases in the CD4 and CD8 cell counts in patients undergoing open cholecystectomy while others show a derangement in ratios. Vallina and Velasco (4) studied peripheral lymphocyte populations in 11 patients undergoing laparoscopic cholecystectomy and found a transient decrease in the CD4 to CD8 ratio, with no difference in absolute CD4 and CD8 cell counts, with a return to preoperative ratio within 1 week of surgery.

Effects on Malignant Cells

A common physiologic change during laparoscopy is the exposure of the abdominal contents to high intra-abdominal pressures. Gutt et al. (5) exposed two human tumor cell line (CX-2 colon adenocarcinoma, DAN-G pancreas adenocarcinoma) cultures to 0, 6, and 12 mm Hg CO_2 pressures. The proliferation of colon carcinoma increased significantly with the amount of pressure while the pancreas carcinoma increased with CO_2 exposure independently of ambient pressure. In a rat model, Wittich et al. (6) anesthetized 36 rats, performed laparoscopy under 0, 4, and 16 mm Hg pressure. One milliliter suspension of moderately differentiated colon adenocarcinoma line was injected intraperitoneally and pneumoperitoneum held for 60 minutes. On day 11, the rats were killed and the volume of tumor measured by independent blinded observers. Peritoneal tumor growth increased with higher pressures. In similar studies, other investigators have shown increased rates of metastases.

In a cellular study, an increase in ambient pressure increased tumor *adherence* to matrix proteins, which was mitigated by administration of antibodies to the β_1-integrin subunit (7). In a matrix gel experiment, laparoscopic conditions using both CO_2 and helium caused an increase in tumor *invasiveness* that was abolished with matrix metalloproteinase blockade (8). Other than altering tumor biology to adhere and invade tissues, greater pressure also adversely effects normal host mesothelial cells, decreasing the natural barriers to tumor growth. One hour after performing laparoscopy in mice, electron microscopy of the normal peritoneum surfaces revealed retraction and condensation of mesothelial cells (9). Over the next 12 hours, the intercellular clefts increased in size, exposing the basal membrane. In animals inoculated with tumor, the peritoneal surfaces rapidly became coated with malignant cells, creating wide spread intraabdominal metastases, mimicking human reports of carcinomatosis following laparoscopy. In the pressureless control group, tumor cells remained on top of intact mesothelial cells for a prolonged period prior to invasion in sporadic fashion. The growth of tumor remained localized to the port sites and lower abdomen, similar to that seen in open laparotomy recurrences. The effects of pressure remains multifold, inducing tumor cells to grow bigger, adhere to cells better, and penetrate quicker. Along with peritoneal damage, this has been hypothesized to explain early carcinomatosis following laparoscopy.

Another component of typical laparoscopy is the insufflation gas, CO_2. In cultures, CO_2 in comparison to helium and air, increased ovarian carcinoma cell growth by 52%; however, in animal studies, CO_2 had no impact on tumor growth and metastases (10). In an elegant rat model, the cecal wall was inoculated via a 1-cm abdominal incision with two million viable tumor cells using a 30-gauge needle under microscopic vision (10). Two weeks later, the rats where randomly assigned to laparoscopy or laparotomy. In the laparoscopy group, a standard 5-mm port was inserted and secured using stitches and the abdominal cavity was insufflated for 30 minutes with CO_2. The laparotomy group underwent a midline 4-cm incision, which was remained open for 30 minutes. Four weeks after the second procedure, the rats were analyzed. There was no difference in liver metastases, lung metastases, nodal metastases, wound/port metastases, or cecal tumor weight.

During laparoscopy, abdominal contents, including malignant cells, are exposed to changes in homeostasis, the effects of which have been studied mainly in animal models, wherein controversy exists in the interpretation of the results and the applicability to patients. One common criticism is the lack of significant power with a small number of subjects. Also, many models used tumor inoculums far in excess of what would be represented in humans in nonnaturally occurring locations under extreme environmental conditions. Even the tumor cell lines used varied from study to study, ranging from melanoma to mesothelioma to uncommon lines of colonic adenocarcinoma. Despite a multitude of research, basic questions regarding tumor cell biology remain unanswered, and previous results should be handled with great caution.

PORT SITE METASTASES

A discussion of port site metastases is particularly germane to a discussion of laparoscopic resection of colon cancer, because this was a major issue in restraining the advances in the application of laparoscopy to patients with carcinoma of the colon. As the popularity of laparoscopic treatment of malignancies increased, case reports of port site metastases have increased since an early report in 1978 (11). Port site metastases, broadly defined, is recurrence of tumor at the small wounds created from the transabdominal placement of ports used to pass instruments or retrieve specimens. Prior to any large studies on the true incidence of port site metastases, numerous anecdotal reports suggested that the occurrences of wound metastases far exceeded the experience of laparotomy. Small series suggested that port site metastases occurred in up to 21% (12). From these early concerns, enthusiasm for minimally invasive surgery for malignancy became tempered. As a result, monitoring bodies examined the true incidence of metastasis and laboratory studies attempted to explain the phenomena.

Prior to incriminating laparoscopy, the incidence of wound recurrences during laparotomy needed to be established. Hughes et al. (13) reviewed 1,603 patients with colon carcinoma and found a total of 0.8% rate of recurrence, consisting of 11 instances in the laparotomy scar and 5 in the stoma/drain site. Reilly et al. (14) reviewed 1,711 cases and found a 0.6% recurrence. From these large retrospective studies, the estimated wound recurrence in open cases is <1%.

Early reports of port site recurrences for colorectal carcinoma were discouraging, with a publication of >20% in a series of 14 resections. The American Society of Colon and Rectal Surgeons Laparoscopic registry, in a series of 480 patients, had a port site recurrence rate of 1.1% (15). Zmora and Weiss (16), in 2001, performed an analysis of laparoscopic colorectal resections for carcinoma, including in their review only works that contained more than 50 patients. This was done to prevent biased reports from surgeons on the learning curve. Of 1,737 patients, they identified 17 (0.6%) patients with port site metastases. Unfortunately, many of the early studies were nonprospective, nonrandomized, and with a short follow-up period. Despite the limitations of the earlier studies, the results compare favorably with those of prospective randomized studies. In a U.S. study, Milsom et al. (17) found no port site metastases in 55 patients randomized to laparoscopy.

Upper gastrointestinal malignancies in large series also share low port site metastasis rates. In a prospective study of 1,965 laparoscopic procedures involving 4,299 ports, 0.79% developed port site recurrences, ranging from 15 days postoperatively to 17 months (18). Wound recurrence for open procedures was 0.86%. Of those patients with port site metastases and wound recurrences, a preponderance were in patients with advanced-stage disease at initial presentation, allowing the authors to conclude that port site/wound recurrences is a marker of advanced disease. One particular upper gastrointestinal malignancy, gallbladder carcinoma, continues to have an adverse effect on port sites. In an international survey of 117,840 cholecystectomies for presumed benign disease, 409 nonapparent gallbladder cancers were identified, with a recurrence rate in 70 (17.1%) of the cases (19). Currently, long-term data on the effects of laparoscopy in gynecologic and urologic malignancies are pending.

Given the lack of knowledge of what is the true incidence of port site metastases, it is even more difficult to analyze their significance. In the larger series, port site metastases occurred in association with advanced disease at initial presentation; however, numerous cases have been reported with early disease in a relatively short period. The occurrences with early disease, such as early-stage colon cancer, have been associated with carcinomatosis and adverse outcomes (20). This group of patients otherwise would have done well; only through protocols and diligent studies will the importance be known.

Soon after reports of port site metastases, a number of laboratory studies were made to attempt to explain the phenomenon. One theory is that the constant flow of gas used in creating a pneumoperitoneum seeds the port site by the constant exposure to aerosolized tumor cells. Hewett et al. (21) studied an in vivo pig model using radiolabeled tumor cells inserted into the peritoneum. Under a gamma camera, tumor cells traveled throughout the abdominal cavity faster with pneumoperitoneum. In a later complex study, that group administered radiolabeled human colon cancer cells into the peritoneal cavity of pigs. Ports were inserted and pneumoperitoneum established. After 2 hours, the ports were removed, and the port sites excised and examined (22). The study incorporated two variables. In the first variable, the intra-abdominal tumor inocula increased from 1.5×10^5 to 120×10^5 cells. In the second variable, insufflation pressure increased from 0, 4, 8, and 12 mm Hg. With increased amount of tumor burden ($>2.5 \times 10^6$), tumor cells became detectable at the port sites. In the second portion of their study, as insufflation pressures increased, fewer tumor cells were identified on the port sites. Caution is advised on the interpretation of the second portion of their study given that only eight animals were studied. To test the significance of aerosolized tumor cells, Mathew et al. (23) inserted adenocarcinoma cells into the peritoneum of primary rats; a plastic tubing was then used to vent the gas into the abdominal cavity of a recipient secondary rat. One group of primary rats underwent standard insufflation while the second group underwent gasless laparoscopy. Five of six secondary recipient rats in the insufflation group developed metastases while none of the gasless had this result.

In humans, radiolabeled red blood cells injected into the bed of the gallbladder during standard laparoscopic cholecystectomy migrated to port sites, even though the specimens were removed using a protective bag (24). In the gasless laparoscopic group, no radioactivity was detected at the port sites. During laparoscopy for benign and malignant diseases, Ikramuddin et al. (25) attached a saline suction trap to filter the pneumoperitoneum effluent; normal mesothelial cells were identified in the benign group, and 2 patients of 15 with malignancies had large numbers of malignant cells in the trap. Those two patients had carcinomatosis during the initial laparoscopic procedure, and one of them later developed port site metastasis. Despite some disagreements, it appears that pneumoperitoneum and degree of tumor burden are two independent factors for the development of port site metastases.

Port composition has also been implicated in the enhancement of metastases. Brundell et al. (22) studied different port compositions and the effect of removing and replacing ports, mimicking typical laparoscopy. Significantly more tumor cells adhered to metal ports than to plastic ports. The removal and replacement of a port resulted in significantly more tumor deposition in the wound than if the ports were left in situ the entire duration of the procedure. Brundell et al. concluded that to

Table 38.1

Possible Causes of Tumor Cell Dissemination in Laparoscopic Surgery for Cancer

Possible Cause	Intervention to Potentially Minimize this Cause
Adverse effects of carbon dioxide gas	Use helium, nitrogen, or ambient room air
Dispersion of cells by insufflation gas	Avoid sudden loss of pneumoperitoneum
Tumor spillage from manipulation and instrumentation	Avoid excessive manipulation of the tumor
Tumor spillage at extraction site	Protected tumor extraction (plastic bag)
Immunosuppressive effect of pneumoperitoneum	Irrigation of abdomen with tumoricidal solutions

minimize risks, plastic ports that are secured to prevent dislodgement is mandatory.

Following the recognition of the problem, several investigators attempted to mitigate factors leading to port site metastases. A simple procedural change would be to use plastic bags to remove specimens; however, it has already been shown that aerosolized cells adhere to ports and port sites. To eliminate the effect of pneumoperitoneum, gasless laparoscopy has been recommended, but even then, port site metastases have been reported (26). The literature on changing the insufflation gas to helium or some other agent often generated conflicting results. Wu et al. (27) excised the wound during surgery but this did not completely eliminate metastases; but excising port sites enlarges the wound, and one of the purported advantages of laparoscopy—small wound—would be eliminated. Some authors have irrigated the wound with a variety of agents from lactated Ringer solution, povidone-iodine, to chemotherapeutic agents showing decreased metastasis in animal models (28). Additional studies are recommended prior to using anything other than standard crystalloid irrigation.

Table 38.1 briefly outlines some of the possible causes of port site metastases and some interventions that may help to prevent them. The adoption of some or all of these changes in practice has been part of the evolution of the application of laparoscopy to patients with a variety of malignancies.

LAPAROSCOPY IN THE TREATMENT OF COLORECTAL CANCER

General Considerations

Descriptions of laparoscopic resections have now been reported for practically every major intra-abdominal organ system spanning different surgical subspecialties. Although some of the procedures were palliative in nature, most of the reports are for curative intent. The three major concerns of an operation performed laparoscopically for the treatment of cancer are: (a) laparoscopic maintenance of oncologic resection integrity (e.g., margins of resection, lymph node harvest, evaluation of other intra-abdominal organs), (b) demonstration of feasibility with improved parameters of a resection without undue risk (e.g., decreased hospital stay, decreased cost, more rapid return to work), and (c) absence of a reduction in overall survival (induction of carcinomatosis/metastasis by laparoscopy, port site recurrences). There have been numerous case series of laparoscopic resections of colon cancers as well as three recent well-designed randomized prospective trials. Just because we *can*, does not mean we *should* without valid evidence. However, these recent studies have uniformly demonstrated the safety and efficacy of laparoscopic colon resections for cancer, and this procedure is rapidly becoming the standard in many countries.

Colorectal carcinoma is one of the leading causes of death in the United States; it is also generally a much more curative disease than pancreatic cancer. With a common cancer and growing experience from laparoscopic appendectomy and colon resection for benign disease, laparoscopic colon resection for malignancy was thought be a natural extension of these procedures. Many studies have shown that the resection margins and lymph node retrieval are no different for laparoscopy than laparotomy when attention to detail is maintained. The proposed advantages are decreased pain, ileus, hospital stay, adhesions, and convalescence with an earlier return to work allowing for a lower economic impact.

Prior to the introduction of laparoscopic cholecystectomy, patients were routinely hospitalized for 1 week, followed by prolonged recovery with a large, often painful incision. Suddenly, patients could be sent home safely the next day after laparoscopic cholecystectomy, or even the same day at many centers. Realizing the tremendous potential advantages to both patient and health care organizations, many pioneering surgeons and patients attempted to reap these same benefits from the laparoscopic conduct of other procedures. A case series of laparoscopic colon resections for cancer was published in 1991 (1). However, the early enthusiasm for laparoscopic colon resection for cancer was tempered by the appearance in the literature of case reports of port site recurrences, with incidence rates as high as 21% (29). Since that time, there were hundreds of articles describing the technique, feasibility, and results of laparoscopic resection of the colon for both benign and malignant conditions, but almost no high-level evidence showing either the oncologic equivalence of the laparoscopic procedure to the open procedure or advantages to the laparoscopic procedure.

Meta-Analysis Review

A review of all previous series of laparoscopic colon resections for cancer is beyond the scope of this work, but an excellent review of the existing literature has been published (29) and will be summarized here. Many of the studies reviewed by these authors are nonrandomized, noncontrolled studies, making comparisons between the studies somewhat problematic. However, the authors carefully grouped studies together based on the level of evidence presented.

These authors analyzed a number of factors, including the time until return of bowel function, quality of life (QOL), and length of hospitalization as short-term variables. Several nonrandomized trials showed return of bowel function at 2.6 days compared with 3.5 days for open surgery. Similarly, their review

of randomized trials showed a significantly more rapid return of bowel function in patients who underwent laparoscopic colon resection compared with patients undergoing open resection. QOL studies focused on postoperative pain and the resulting requirements for intravenous analgesia. These authors reviewed many studies and concluded that laparoscopy is superior in reducing pain during the same length of the postoperative period when compared with open surgery. They also point out that further studies are needed for other aspects of QOL to show any potential advantages. Regarding hospital stay, the authors conclude that there is adequate level I evidence to show that laparoscopy for malignancy is associated with more rapid discharge from the hospital compared with open surgery for colon cancer.

Reviewing long-term outcome, the authors evaluated recurrence rates and survival, although they acknowledge the difficulties in comparing the results from many disparate studies. The mean/median follow-up in the various studies reviewed ranges from 16 to 71 months. The authors state that port site recurrence rates do not exceed 1% in most recent studies. Local recurrence rates varied from 1.5% to 4.1%, and distant recurrence rates ranged from 6.1% to 10.3%. Overall, the authors concluded that the studies reviewed support the concept that recurrence rates are equivalent when comparing open surgery with laparoscopic resection of colon cancer. They point out that, in one study, the probability of remaining recurrence-free was statistically significantly higher in the group undergoing laparoscopic resection. A review of survival reported in the studies reviewed demonstrated that case-controlled and cohort studies have not demonstrated any differences in 5-year survival between patients undergoing open resection of colon cancer and those undergoing laparoscopic resection. In one study reviewed, no difference was observed in survival rates between patients undergoing laparoscopy (82%) and open resection (74%). Interestingly, the cancer-related survival was significantly higher in the laparoscopy group (91%) compared with the open resection group (79%; $p = 0.02$). Further analysis showed that the advantage was primarily derived from patients with stage III tumors. Overall, the authors conclude that there are no significant differences in survival for patients undergoing laparoscopic resection of colon cancer compared with those undergoing open resection, with high-level evidence.

This article serves to review the evidence from many of the prior studies of laparoscopic resection of colon cancer (29). The authors conclude that laparoscopic resection of colon cancer affords patients short-term benefits including pain, length of time of ileus, length of hospital stay, morbidity, and disability. They also conclude that laparoscopic resection and open resection of colon cancer have similar long-term outcomes, including recurrence and survival.

LAPAROSCOPIC VERSUS OPEN SURGERY: PROSPECTIVE RANDOMIZED MULTICENTER CONTROLLED TRIALS

Although laparoscopic resection of colon malignancies was adopted by some surgeons very early, there was a paucity of

Table 38.2

Results of Prospective Studies Comparing Laparoscopic Colon Resection with Open Colectomy

Trial (Ref.)	Total No. of Patients	Conversion Rate (%)	Open Resection			Laparoscopic Resection		
			No. of Patients	OR Time (Min)	Time to Discharge (days)	No. of Patients	OR Time (min)	Time to Discharge (days)
COST (30)	865	21	432	95	5	433	150[a]	6[a]
COLOR (33)	1,248	17	621	115	9.3	627	145[a*]	8.2[a]
CLASICC (32)	794	29	268	135	11	526	180[a]	9[a]

OR, operating room; COST, Clinical Outcomes of Surgical Therapy; COLOR, COlon cancer Laparoscopic or Open Resection; CLASICC, Conventional versus Laparoscopic-Assisted Surgery in Colorectal Cancer.
[a] Indicates statistically significant difference between open surgery group and laparoscopic group ($p < 0.05$).

data from large-scale randomized trials to support this change in clinical practice. However, at this time, a number of large, well-designed prospective studies have been completed to compare laparoscopic (or laparoscopically assisted) colon resection with open colectomy. The data from three of these trials will be evaluated and discussed. A summary of salient findings from these three major prospective randomized trials is shown in Table 38.2.

COST Trial

The U.S. National Cancer Institute funded the large randomized controlled Clinical Outcomes of Surgical Therapy (COST) study to evaluate (a) disease-free survival, (b) overall survival, and (c) QOL (30). The study began in 1994 and was specifically designed to evaluate extent of exploration, extent of lymph node resection, and patterns of tumor cell dissemination. Prior observations about port site recurrences served to stimulate interest in this trial. Inclusion criteria included histologically confirmed adenocarcinoma of the colon, age >18 years, and the absence of extensive intra-abdominal adhesions. Patients with advanced local or metastatic disease, rectal or transverse colon cancer, acute bowel obstruction, perforation of a cancer, and severe medical illnesses were excluded from the trial. Postoperative care, including the use of adjuvant chemotherapy, was according to the practice of each individual surgeon. Patients were randomized centrally, and the treatment assignment was balanced with regard to three stratification variables: tumor site, American Society of Anesthesiologists (ASA) class and surgeon.

Quality of Life Data

The QOL component of the COST trial closed in 1999 after the randomization of 449 patients and was subsequently reported in 2002 while data on disease-free survival and overall survival continues to accrue (31). The QOL component measures included Symptoms Distress Scale, Quality of Life Index, and single-item global rating scale at 2 days, 2 weeks, and 2 months postoperatively, in addition to analgesic use and length of stay. The laparoscopic group had statistically less analgesic use ($p < 0.03$) by a small amount and a decrease in hospital stay of 0.8 days ($p < 0.001$). At each point in the study, the only significant difference was the global rating score at 2 weeks. There were *no*

significant differences in QOL at 2 days and 2 months. This is the first of a series of well-designed large trials that reported QOL measures.

Oncologic Outcomes

Patients were assessed for complications at the time of hospital discharge and at 2 and 18 months. Evaluation for tumor recurrence included physical examination and carcinoembryonic antigen testing (every 3 months for the first year, then every 6 months for 5 years), chest radiograph (every 6 months for 2 years, then annually), and colon evaluation (every 3 years). Recurrences were confirmed by imaging or pathologic evaluation. The primary end point was time to tumor recurrence; secondary end points included disease-free survival, complications, variables related to recovery, and QOL.

The final results of this study were published in 2004 and included the "oncologic outcomes" (30). In this trial, 872 patients were randomized to undergo open or laparoscopically assisted colectomy at 48 institutions. The 66 surgeons who participated in the trial were credentialed prior to enrolling any patients. Each surgeon had performed at least 20 laparoscopically assisted colorectal operations. An unedited videotape was submitted for review, and the study organizers looked at oncologic technique, level of mesenteric ligation, avoidance of direct tumor handling, identification of adjacent structures, and the extent of abdominal exploration. The study had rigorous quality control that included a random audit of videotapes with review by an external monitoring committee.

Randomization resulted in 428 patients undergoing open colectomy and 435 patients undergoing laparoscopically assisted resections (there were a small number of patients excluded and a small number of crossover patients). The conversion rate for laparoscopic to open resections was 21%. There were no characteristics of the surgeons identified as significant with regard to the incidence of conversions. Operating time was significantly ($p < 0.001$) longer in the laparoscopic group (mean, 150 minutes) than in the open surgery group (mean, 95 minutes). The extent of resection was similar in both groups. Patients in the laparoscopic group had a significantly ($p < 0.001$) shorter hospital stay (mean, 5 days) than the patients in the open surgery group (mean, 6 days). There were no significant differences in the 30-day mortality, readmission rate, or overall rate of complications.

There were 84 recurrences in the open surgery group and 76 in the laparoscopy group, with a median follow-up of 4.4 years. The cumulative incidence of recurrence in patients who underwent laparoscopic resection was not significantly different from those who underwent open resection ($p = 0.32$). Overall survival was also very similar in the two groups. The authors concluded that there were no significant differences between the two treatment groups in regard to time to recurrence, disease-free survival, or overall survival for any stage. The lack of significant differences was maintained in multivariate analyses adjusted for the various stratification factors. A wound recurrence occurred in one patient in the open surgery group, and there were two port site recurrences in patients in the laparoscopic surgery group.

Overall, this is a well-designed, multicenter, prospective randomized trial that supports the safety of laparoscopic colon resection for patients with colon cancer, in regard to rate of complications, time to recurrence, disease-free survival, and overall survival. Factors relating to the technical conduct of the procedure, such as number of lymph nodes resected, length of bowel and mesentery resected, and bowel margins, also showed no differences in the two treatment groups. The authors acknowledged the rather strict enrollment criteria with respect to surgeon experience and training, and suggest that adherence to these standards in surgical practices should yield similar results. Furthermore, the authors point out that the study was not designed to show whether laparoscopic resection is superior to open resection, only that it is not inferior to open resection. Although the study did not show any particular advantages of laparoscopic colon resection, the authors conclude that laparoscopic colon resection is an acceptable alternative to open colon resection for patients with carcinoma of the colon.

CLASICC Trial

The Conventional versus Laparoscopic-Assisted Surgery in Colorectal Cancer (CLASICC) trial was conducted at 27 centers in the United Kingdom (32). A total of 794 patients with colorectal cancer were randomized to undergo laparoscopic assisted (n = 526) or conventional open colon resection (n = 268). Randomization to laparoscopic surgery was at a 2:1 ratio compared with open surgery to allow for anticipated conversions to open surgery. Patients with lesions of the transverse colon, contraindications to pneumoperitoneum, acute intestinal obstruction, previous malignancy, synchronous lesions, or pregnancy were excluded from the study. Surgeons participating in the trial must have already completed 20 laparoscopic-assisted colon resections to qualify for the study. A total of 32 surgeons participated in the study.

This study defined the short-term end points as positive resection margins, rate of T3-4N1M0 (Dukes C2) tumors, and in-hospital mortality. Other short-term end points included complication rates at 30 days and at 3 months, QOL measurements at 3 months, and transfusion requirements. Long-term end points including survival, recurrence, and QOL will be reported at 3 years and at 5 years.

A total of 253 patients underwent open colon resection and 484 patients underwent laparoscopic-assisted resection, with a conversion rate of 29%. Overall, this report shows significantly shorter operative time in patients undergoing open resection (135 minute open, 180 minutes laparoscopic). The rate of T3-4N1M0 tumors was similar in the two groups (7% open, 6% laparoscopic) as was the in-hospital mortality (5% open, 6% laparoscopic). Rates of positive resection margins were also similar in the two groups.

The time to first bowel movement and time to starting a regular diet was similar in the two groups, but median length of stay was 2 days longer in the patients who underwent open resection compared with those who underwent a laparoscopic resection. Total complication rates were similar in the two groups, including in-hospital complication rates, 30-day complication rates, and 3-month complication rates. There was no difference in the two groups regarding transfusion requirements. Results of QOL surveys were also similar in the two groups, which was evaluated preoperatively and at 2 weeks and at 3 months postoperatively.

This study was somewhat different from others in that patients with carcinoma of the rectum were included. The authors found higher rates of positive margins in patients undergoing laparoscopic anterior resection for carcinoma of the rectum, although the difference was not statistically significant. In addition, total mesorectal excision was undertaken more frequently in the laparoscopic resection group. However, conversion to open resection occurred more frequently in patients undergoing resection of rectal carcinoma compared with those undergoing resection of carcinoma of the colon. Patients who were converted to open surgery from laparoscopic resection also had more complications than those whose resection was completed laparoscopically. For these reasons, the authors suggest caution in the use of laparoscopic anterior resection for patients with carcinoma of the rectum.

Overall, in terms of tumor status, nodal status, QOL, and the defined short-term end points, these authors found no significant differences between laparoscopic resection and open surgery for patients with carcinoma of the colon and rectum. Surgical resection margins were similar in both groups except for patients who had laparoscopic anterior resection for carcinoma of the rectum. The study had no bias in terms of early-stage disease, which may explain the relatively high rate of conversion. They also concluded that the requirement for 20 previous resections to qualify as a surgeon in this study may be somewhat low, in that conversion rates fell through each year of accrual to the study. Lymph node yield was comparable in the two groups. Intraoperative complication rates were similar in the two groups, although as shown previously, patients who undergo conversion to open surgery do have a higher rate of complications. Furthermore, there were no significant differences in the 30-day and 3-month complication rates. Their QOL data are similar to that shown by the COST trial (31) with very small advantages seen in the laparoscopic resection group.

This study concludes that for patients with carcinoma of the colon, laparoscopic-assisted resection is safe, with oncologic results similar to that of open resection, and suggests that local recurrence rates and cancer-related survival will be comparable to patients undergoing conventional open resection. For patients with carcinoma of the rectum, those undergoing laparoscopic resection had a higher rate of total mesorectal excision, but also a slightly increased risk of a positive margin in patients undergoing anterior resection. Although the authors conclude that laparoscopic-assisted resection of colon cancer is reasonable, and should have no long-term differences in outcome compared with open surgery, they state that because of impaired short-term outcomes and pathologic features after laparoscopic anterior resection, these results do not justify routine use of laparoscopic-assisted resection in patients with carcinoma of the rectum.

COLOR Trial

The COlon cancer Laparoscopic or Open Resection (COLOR) trial was conducted in Europe as a multicenter, prospective, randomized trial to assess the safety and benefit of laparoscopic resection compared with open resection for patients with carcinoma of the right or left colon (33). The data regarding short-term outcomes are available now, and 3-year cancer-free survival data will be reported later. All patients with carcinoma of the right or left (above the peritoneal reflection) colon were screened for inclusion in the trial at 29 participating centers. Patients with a body mass index (BMI) >30 kg/m^2, metastatic disease, acute intestinal obstruction, multiple primary tumors, invasion of adjacent structures on preoperative imaging studies, previous malignancies, or contraindications to pneumoperitoneum were excluded from the study.

A total of 627 patients were randomly assigned to laparoscopic resection and 621 patients were randomized to undergo open resection. The two groups were comparable in terms of age, gender, ASA class, BMI, and history of previous abdominal surgery. The extent of resection was similar in both groups. All surgeons had previously completed at least 20 colon resections laparoscopically, and unedited video tapes were reviewed prior to enrollment. Primary outcome is 3-year cancer-free survival, which will be reported later. Secondary outcomes include short-term morbidity and mortality, positive resection margins, local recurrence, port site recurrence, metastases, blood loss, and overall survival.

A review of the operative data showed no significant differences in the two groups with regard to the procedure performed. Operative time was significantly longer (202 minutes) in patients undergoing laparoscopic resection compared with those undergoing open resection (170 minutes). Interestingly, a regression analysis of this data showed a significant decrease in time for the laparoscopic resection with increased numbers of patients at each center. This effect was not seen in patients undergoing open resection. Mean blood loss was significantly less in those undergoing laparoscopic resection (100 mL) compared with those undergoing open resection (175 mL). The conversion rate from laparoscopic to open resection in this series was 19%.

Postoperative pathologic examination of resected specimens showed no differences in the two groups for stage distribution, tumor size, and histologic type. The number of positive resection margins was also similar in both groups. The number of lymph nodes resected was also comparable in both groups.

Patients who underwent laparoscopic resection tolerated oral fluid about 1 day earlier (2.9 days) compared with those who had open surgery (3.8 days). Time to the first bowel movement was also shorter in those who had laparoscopic resection (3.6 days) compared with those who had an open resection

(4.6 days). The hospital stay was a mean of 8.2 days in those who had a laparoscopic resection and 9.3 days in those who had an open resection. All of these differences were statistically significant. There were no differences in the two groups in regard to the occurrence of pulmonary or cardiac events, anastomotic failure, wound or urinary tract infections, or postoperative bleeding. Postoperative death rate was also similar in the two groups.

These short-term outcomes show that although the duration of surgery is longer for laparoscopic resection, patients undergoing laparoscopic resection have less blood loss, tolerate fluid intake earlier, and spend less time in the hospital. Oncologic outcomes such as positive margins, tumor size, and number of lymph nodes resected are equivalent in the two groups. Although we still await the long-term follow-up, these results suggest that laparoscopic resection of the colon is a reasonable procedure and the equivalent oncologic short-term outcomes suggest that the two procedures will result in similar long-term results.

Summary

These three trials all show excellent short-term outcomes for the laparoscopic resection of colon cancer. The three trials generally showed that laparoscopic resection has results comparable to those of open resection in terms of oncologic variables such as margins of resection and number of lymph nodes resected. Operating times were significantly longer for laparoscopic procedures in all three trials, but hospital stays were shorter. Of these three trails, long-term outcome data are available only from the COST trial (30) at this time, and showed similar recurrence and survival rates. There was no significant increase in wound recurrences in any of the trials, which may finally put to rest the concerns about port site metastases seen in so much literature early in the evolution of this technique. Only the CLASICC trial included patients with rectal cancer (32). These authors concluded that laparoscopic-assisted resection of rectal cancer is not justified based on their data. Further studies will be needed to evaluate the effectiveness of this technique in this group of patients.

SURGEON QUALIFICATIONS AND INSTITUTIONAL SETTING

Each of the three randomized prospective trials reviewed in detail here had stringent criteria for surgeons participating in the trials. This is an important component to assure the quality of laparoscopic resection for patients with colon cancer. Codification of such requirements for experience has already begun in some countries. In Japan, the Japan Society of Endoscopic Surgery has devised an Endoscopic Surgical Skill Qualification System to promote safer laparoscopic surgery (34). This includes review of unedited operative videotapes to evaluate both surgical skill and adherence to oncologic principles. There is now a trial in Japan to determine the optimum quality control of surgical skill in laparoscopic surgery. The results of this trial are awaited to help guide this important aspect of laparoscopic surgery.

There has been some interest and concern regarding the type of hospital in which advanced laparoscopic procedures, such as laparoscopic colon resection, are performed. The relatively steep learning curve for laparoscopic colon resection has spurred debate regarding the appropriate hospital setting to perform this advanced procedure. In a nonrandomized study that included a majority of cases performed for nonmalignant disease, Do and coworkers (35) showed that laparoscopic colon resection can be safely performed in a community hospital. Their series of 154 laparoscopic colon resections had a mean operating time of 120 minutes and a mean hospital stay of 5 days. The conversion rate was 9.6%. In regard to the learning curve, they found that the operative time reached a plateau of approximately 2 hours after 30 cases. They concluded that their results were comparable with historical controls in the literature, and stressed the importance of having a group of motivated surgeons.

In another study, the first 50 consecutive laparoscopic colon resections performed at a regional medical center between 2001 and 2003 were compared with the first 50 laparoscopic colon resections performed at a major university medical center during the same time (36). Data were gathered from patient charts in a retrospective manner. These authors hypothesized that there would be no significant differences in outcomes between the two hospitals. Most patients at both institutions underwent surgery for nonmalignant disease, although there were significantly more patients (22%; $p = 0.049$) at the regional medical center with malignancy than at the university hospital (10%). Patients at the regional medical center were significantly older, more commonly female, and had a higher incidence of previous abdominal surgery compared with the university hospital. There were no significant differences in other demographic variables including BMI and ASA class. Overall mean operative times were significantly shorter at the regional medical center (161 minutes) than at the university hospital (237 minutes; $p < 0.0001$). Operative time remained fairly stable at the university hospital over the course of the study, and there was a progressive decline at the regional medical center. The incidence of complications was similar in both groups. Although there were more lymph nodes in the resected specimens at the university hospital compared with the regional medical center, there were no significant differences in margins of resection.

These two studies do not specifically address many issues important when laparoscopic colon resection is performed on patients with malignant disease of the colon, but they do address the very important question of who should perform the procedure and in what setting should it be performed. Success in the adequate performance of this advanced procedure rests in the adequacy of surgeon skill and the support of the institution where it is performed. These studies support the idea that laparoscopic resection of the colon can be safely performed by properly trained surgeons in a variety of health care settings.

TECHNICAL CONSIDERATIONS

Hand-Assisted Laparoscopic Colon Resection

One of the more recent developments in laparoscopic surgery is the use of hand-assisted laparoscopic (HALS) resection, which allows the surgeon to use a gloved hand to facilitate laparoscopic surgery. Using the HALS technique, a hand is inserted into the abdomen through a seal that allows maintenance of the pneumoperitoneum. Thus, the excellent vision afforded by the laparoscope is maintained and the surgeon can also have tactile feedback, which facilitates exposure, retraction, and dissection as well as the rapid control of bleeding. However, this technique necessitates the creation of a relatively large incision, and this may obviate some of the patient-benefits of "minimally invasive" surgery.

A randomized prospective trial was outperformed to evaluate results with HALS compared with routine laparoscopic-assisted colectomy (37). This study sought to evaluate perioperative features such as time and conversion rate, immediate clinical response including time to feeding, postoperative pain and hospital stay, effect on the inflammatory response, oncologic "equivalence," and cost. A total of 54 patients were enrolled in this study, with 27 in the laparoscopic group and 27 in the HALS group. The two groups were well matched for demographic features. The laparoscopic group had a 22% conversion rate, while the HALS group had a 7% conversion rate ($p > 0.05$). Operative time was also similar at 135 minutes for the laparoscopic group and 120 minutes for the HALS group. Intraoperative lavage was performed and malignant cells were not seen in either group. The number of lymph nodes resected was equal in the two groups. The HALS group had a significant increase in inflammatory response as measured by IL-6 level and C-reactive protein levels. There were no differences in the mean operative costs for the two procedures. These authors conclude that the hand-assisted device is helpful in difficult intraoperative situations, and should be considered as an adjunct to conventional laparoscopic procedures when needed.

In another study, Chang et al. (38) reported on 85 patients who underwent conventional laparoscopic sigmoid colon resection and compared the results with 66 patients who underwent hand-assisted laparoscopic sigmoid colon resection. They found shorter operating times in the HALS group compared with the conventional laparoscopy group. There were no significant differences in mortality, hospital stay, or time to feeding. In this series, the conversion rate was 13% for the laparoscopic group.

These studies suggest the need for further studies to evaluate the applicability of HALS in colon resections. It may be particularly useful in more complicated procedures such as rectal resection (39). Studies to date suggest that HALS may have a faster learning curve, and early results suggest that colon resections using HALS are oncologically equivalent to those with conventional laparoscopic resection. At the least, it may be a useful adjunct when difficulties are encountered in conventional laparoscopic resections. The HALS technique can improve retraction and may shorten operative time and improve safety. It may facilitate conversion to an open procedure when needed, and the ability to apply digital pressure in cases of hemorrhage may be very beneficial. Furthermore, the use of tactile sensation may facilitate the identification of additional lesions and significantly change the operative approach (40).

Intracorporeal versus Extracorporeal Anastomoses

The anastomosis following a laparoscopic colon resection can be performed either intracorporeally or extracorporeally. Intracorporeal anastomoses are generally considered to take considerably more technical skill. A study compared 40 patients who had undergone intracorporeal resection with 34 patients who underwent extracorporeal resection in the same institution (41). The two groups were similarly matched for age, weight, gender, and ASA class. The two groups had similar conversion rates, anastomotic distance from the anal verge, estimated blood loss, operating room cost, time to flatus, and total hospital cost. The patients in the intracorporeal resection group had a significantly shorter incision, longer specimen length, higher complication rate, shorter operating room time, time to feeding, and shorter hospital stay. This study suggests that further studies are indicated to evaluate the possible benefits of the intracorporeal technique, although the technical challenges may be a significant barrier to some surgeons.

CONCLUSIONS

Despite early enthusiasm for the laparoscopic resection of cancer of the colon, this procedure's growth was tempered by early concerns about local recurrence. As a result, it was studied intensely in many settings. Although many of the trials were nonrandomized and/or noncontrolled, we now have a large body of evidence to support the notion that the short-term benefits of laparoscopic resection (pain, ileus, length of hospitalization, morbidity, and disability) are in fact superior to the results with open surgery. Furthermore, the long-term results (recurrence and survival) with laparoscopic resection are equivalent to results with open resection. These results can be obtained in a wide range of hospital settings, as long as the surgeons who perform the procedure are appropriately experienced.

This large body of high-level evidence has led to joint endorsement of the technique by the American Society of Colon and Rectal Surgeons and the Society of American Gastrointestinal Endoscopic Surgeons. In part, this endorsement states, "Laparoscopic colectomy for curable cancer results in equivalent cancer related survival compared to open colectomy when performed by experienced surgeons" (29). The slow development of this technique was paralleled by the rapid advances in laparoscopic technology including better video imaging, improved stapling devices, and advancement of techniques that minimize tissue handling. Many patients prefer minimally invasive techniques, and these data support that it is safe to offer this approach to our patients. It should be noted that, at this time, laparoscopic resection of rectal cancer is not justified by some of the available data (32). Further studies are indicated to analyze issues related to cost and quality of life, as well as long-term outcomes from several of the multicenter trials already published (32,33).

REFERENCES

1. Jacobs M, Verdeja JC, Goldstein HS. Minimally invasive colon resection. *Surg Laparosc Endosc.* 1991;1:144–150.
2. Fusco MA, Paluzzi MW. Abdominal recurrence after laparoscopic assisted colectomy for adenocarcinoma of the colon. *Dis Colon Rect.* 1993;36:851–861.
3. West MA, Hackam DJ, Baker J, et al. Mechanism of decreased in vitro murine macrophage cytokine release after exposure to carbon dioxide. *Ann Surg.* 1997;226:179–190.
4. Vallina VL, Velasco JM. The influence of laparoscopy on lymphocyte subpopulations in the surgical patient. *Surg Endosc.* 1996;10:481–484.
5. Gutt NC, Kim ZG, Hollander D, et al. CO2 environment influences the growth of cultured human cancer cells dependent on insufflation pressure. *Surg Endosc.* 2001;15:314–318.
6. Wittich P, Steyerber EW, Simons SH, et al. Intraperitoneal tumor growth is influenced by pressure of carbon dioxide pneumoperitoneum. *Surg Endosc.* 2000;14:817–819.
7. Basson MD, Yu CF, Herden-Kirchoff O, et al. Effects of increased ambient pressure on colon cancer cell adhesion. *J Cell Biochem.* 2000;78:47–61.
8. Ridgway PF, Smith A, Ziprin P, et al. Pneumoperitoneum augmented tumor invasiveness is abolished by matrix metalloproteinase blockade. *Surg Endosc.* 2002;16:533–536.
9. Volz J, Koster S, Spacek Z, et al. The influence of pneumoperitoneum used in laparoscopic surgery on an intraabdominal tumor growth. *Cancer.* 1999;86:770–774.
10. Lecuru F, Agostini A, Camatte S, et al. Impact of pneumoperitoneum on tumor growth. *Surg Endosc.* 2002;16:1170–1174.
11. Dobronte A, Wittmann T, Karacsony G. Rapid development of malignant metastases in the abdominal wall after laparoscopy. *Endoscopy.* 1978;10:127–130.
12. Berends FJ, Kazemier G, Bonjer HJ, et al. Subcutaneous metastases after laparoscopic colectomy. *Lancet.* 1994;344:58.
13. Hughes ES, McDermontt FT, Poligless AL, et al. Tumor recurrence in the abdominal wall scar tissue after large bowel cancer surgery. *Dis Colon Rectum.* 1983;26:571–572.
14. Reilly WT, Nelson H, Schroeder G, et al. Wound recurrence following conventional treatment of colorectal cancer. A rare but perhaps underestimated problem. *Dis Colon Rectum.* 1996;39:200–207.
15. Vukasin P, Ortega AE, Greene FL, et al. Wound recurrence following laparoscopic colon cancer resection: results of the American Society of Colon and Rectal Surgeons laparoscopic registry. *Dis Colon Rectum.* 1996;39:S20–S23.
16. Zmora O, Weiss E. Trocar site recurrence in laparoscopic surgery for colorectal cancer, myth or real concern? *Surg Oncol Clin North Am.* 2001;10:625–638.
17. Milsom JW, Bohm B, Hammerhofer KA, et al. A prospective, randomized trial comparing laparoscopic versus conventional techniques in colorectal cancer surgery: a preliminary report. *J Am Coll Surg.* 1998;187:46–54.
18. Shoup M, Brennan MF, Karpeh MS, et al. Port site metastasis after diagnostic laparoscopy for upper gastrointestinal tract malignancies: an uncommon entity. *Ann Surg Oncol.* 2002;9:632–636.
19. Paolucci V, Schaeff B, Schneider M, et al. Tumor seeding following laparoscopy: International Survey. *World J Surg.* 1999;23:989–997.
20. Neuhaus SJ, Texler M, Hewett PJ, et al. Port site metastases following laparoscopic surgery. *Br J Surg.* 1988;85:735–741.
21. Hewett PJ, Texler ML, Anderson D, et al. In vivo real time analysis of intraperitoneal radiolabeled tumor cell movement during laparoscopy. *Dis Colon Rectum.* 1999;42:868–875.
22. Brundell SM, Tucker K, Brown B, et al. Variables in the spread of tumor cells to trocars and port sites during operative laparoscopy. *Surg Endosc.* 2002;16:1413–1419.
23. Mathew G, Watson DI, Ellis T, et al. The effect of laparoscopy on the movement of tumor cells and metastasis to surgical wounds. *Surg Endosc.* 1997;11:1163–1166.
24. Cavina E, Goletti O, Molea N, et al. Trocar site tumor recurrences: May pneumoperitoneum be responsible? *Surg Endosc.* 1998;12:1294–1296.
25. Ikramuddin S, Lucas J, Ellison C, et al. Detection of aerosolized cells during carbon dioxide laparoscopy. *J Gastrointest Surg.* 1998;2:580–584.

26. Gutt CN, Riemar V, Kim ZG, et al. Impact of laparoscopic colonic resection on tumor growth and spread in an experimental model. *Br J Surg.* 1999;86:1180–1184.

27. Wu JS, Guo LW, Ruiz MB, et al. Excision of trocar sites reduces tumor implantation in an animal model. *Dis Colon Rectum.* 1998;41:1107–1111.

28. Cannis M, Botchorishvili R, Wattiez A, et al. Cancer and laparoscopy, experimental studies: a review. *Eur J Obstet Gynecol.* 2000;91:1–9.

29. Cera S, Wexner SD. Minimally invasive treatment of colon cancer. *Cancer J.* 2005;11:26–35.

30. COST Study Group. A comparison of laparoscopically assisted and open colectomy for colon cancer. *N Engl J Med.* 2004;350:2050–2059.

31. Weeks JC, Nelson H, Gelber S, et al. Short term quality of life outcomes following laparoscopic-assisted colectomy vs open colectomy for colon cancer: a randomized trial. *JAMA.* 2002;287:321–328.

32. Guillou PJ, Quirke P, Thorpe H, et al. Short term endpoints of conventional versus laparoscopic assisted surgery in patients with colorectal cancer (MRC CLASSIC trial): multicentre randomized controlled trial. *Lancet.* 2005;365:1718–1726.

33. COLOR Study Group. Laparoscopic surgery versus open surgery for colon cancer: short-term outcomes of a randomized trial. *Lancet Oncol.* 2005;6:477–484.

34. Okajima M, Ikeda S, Egi H, et al. Laparoscopic surgery for colon cancer: Present status and evaluation. *J Jpn Surg Soc.* 2006;107:81–85.

35. Do LV, LaPlante R, Miller S, et al. Laparoscopic colon surgery performed safely by general surgeons in a community hospital. *Surg Endosc.* 2005;19:1533–1537.

36. Reischenbach DJ, Tackett AD, Harris J, et al. Laparoscopic colon resection early in the learning curve: what is the appropriate setting? *Ann Surg.* 2006;243:730–737.

37. Taragona EM, Gracia E, Garriga J, et al. Prospective randomized trial comparing conventional laparoscopic colectomy with hand assisted laparoscopic colectomy. *Surg Endosc.* 2002;16:234–239.

38. Chang YJ. Hand-assisted laparoscopic sigmoid colectomy: helping hand or hindrance? *Surg Endosc.* 2005;19(5):656–661.

39. Pietrabissa A, Moretto C, Carobbi C, et al. Hand assisted laparoscopic low anterior resection: initial experience with a new procedure. *Surg Endosc.* 2002;16:431–435.

40. Kooby DA. Laparoscopic surgery for cancer: historical, theoretical and technical considerations. *Oncology.* 2006;20:917–928.

41. Bergamaschi R, Tuetch JJ, Pessaux R, et al. Intracorporeal vs laparoscopic assisted resection for uncomplicated diverticulitis of the sigmoid. *Surg Endosc.* 2000;14:520–523.

COMMENTARY
Frederick L. Greene

At the dawn of the laparoscopic revolution in the late 1980s, it was anticipated that this technique would be used for both benign and malignant conditions in the abdomen. It was not until the early 1990s that minimal-access techniques were applied to resection of the colon for benign conditions (1) and this certainly proved to be a beneficial and valuable adjunct to the surgeon per-

forming colonic resection. Early on there was great concern that as a byproduct of the use of carbon dioxide pneumoperitoneum, adverse outcomes would occur because of dispersment of cancer cells and the injudicious techniques used by surgeons for resection of cancer. Over the last several years the application of well-designed clinical trials (2–4) has supported the fact that localized colonic cancer can be safely removed using laparoscopic techniques and that the benefits of minimal-access approaches may indeed have even greater benefit to the cancer patient.

It is important to recognize that the techniques of surgical resection using traditional open methods must be equal to that of minimal-access techniques. Attention to adequate mesenteric dissection and appropriate surgical margins must be the goal of the surgeon who uses laparoscopic maneuvers. The early concerns regarding port site metastases must still be considered, but the anticipated increased number of implantation in trocar sites has not been realized.

One of the great values of having individual surgeons keep data on their cases is to document specific untoward outcomes, and this continues to be a challenge for those who are attempting to perform cancer surgery. The real issue in management of cancer patients is not short-term, 30-day outcomes but 5- and 10-year survivals that depend initially on adequate and appropriate surgical resection. Several of the single-institution and multi-institutional trials have documented appropriate 3-year survival rates and the Clinical Outcomes of Surgical Therapy (COST) trial under the auspices of the National Cancer Institute has recently reported 5-year outcomes (5). The real answer will come from following patients in these trials who have achieved 10- and 15-year outcomes. One of the concerns continues to be the reasonably high percentage of conversion to open procedures that has been reported even in randomized studies in which only qualified surgeons have been invited to participate. The concept of conversion during a cancer operation must be of concern as untoward results during the procedure may have led to conversion. Although data have yet to show an adverse effect in patients who have been converted to open procedures, this factor must be carefully analyzed.

A recent report by Law et al. (6) discusses the impact of laparoscopic resection for colorectal cancer on operative outcomes and survival. This is a prospective database series of 1,134 patients undergoing elective resection for colon and upper rectal cancer from 1996 through 2004. In the time frame of 1996 to 2000, 478 patients had an open surgical resection, while in the later time frame (2000 to 2004) 656 patients underwent either open surgery (n = 401) or laparoscopic resection (n = 255). The results of this study showed that patients treated laparoscopically had more rapid recovery, lower rates of operative mortality, and overall improved 3-year survival. This isolated study showing a favorable 3-year survival rate for the laparoscopic group is not consistent with the randomized clinical trials previously reported. Although it is attractive to anticipate that the protection of immune mechanisms through laparoscopic procedures would lead to an overall better cancer survival rate, the conclusion that minimal-access techniques are better for the cancer patient should not be drawn from an isolated study.

The study by Law et al. (6), however, does confirm that operative mortality and length of stay are favorably affected by laparoscopic approaches. In the previously reported randomized clinical trials, there were no differences in rates of postoperative morbidity or mortality when the laparoscopic and open groups were compared. Once again, selection of techniques should not depend on major differences in morbidity and mortality rates because other factors relating to anesthetic techniques and overall monitoring of patients may have even more influence on short-term outcome.

As surgeons reference monographs as well as reports in journal articles on this topic, reliance on single-institution studies must be considered with some trepidation, especially when these single-institution studies carry a very different message from well-done randomized control trials. The value of a randomized control trial is to provide more accurate estimate of the impact of the practice variable on the measured outcome. The randomized control trial includes a process of randomization as well as adequate numbers of patients to help ensure that selection bias and confounding variables are minimized or eliminated. One of the problems with single-institution studies is the inclusion of patients based on both patient and physician selection. Selection of laparoscopic techniques may well be based on patient acceptance, patient preference, operating room and surgeon availability, and specific tumor characteristics.

There is no doubt that as laparoscopic colectomy is introduced into routine surgical resident training and the training of advanced laparoscopic fellows, the outcomes will continue to be favorable in the short term. There is certainly a benefit from reduced length of stay, decreased time to alimentation, and reduced need for perioperative narcotics. These trends have certainly been beneficial in the 20-year period since laparoscopic cholecystectomy was introduced. The issue, however, is to maintain adequate training and experience in traditional open techniques, especially when laparoscopic approaches are deemed unfavorable. This is a true challenge today for training directors and faculty working with residents and fellows. In addition to training issues, the surgical community, especially those dealing with oncologic issues, should continue to educate insurers and third-party payers that laparoscopic techniques will not be the pre-eminent standard of care when colectomy for cancer is planned. These third-party administrators must understand that there continues to be a role for open operations and that approval for one technique over the other must be avoided in decisions relating insurance coverage.

For surgeons who perform colectomy, whether it is laparoscopic or open, adequate mesenteric resection must be a primary consideration. Data continue to support the fact that the number of lymph nodes resected is a benchmark for adequate surgical care and that even the number of negative nodes resected and examined pathologically is in direct proportion to long-term survival (7). These data are realized from well-done patient databases such as characterized by the National Cancer Data Base supported by the Commission on Cancer of the American College of Surgeons and the American Cancer Society. Although sentinel node concepts have been recommended for staging in colon cancer, the examination of the isolated sentinel node has not become the similar standard as seen in breast cancer management and has been criticized because of the increased number of false-negative findings reported when the isolated sentinel node has been studied (8). Although sentinel nodes have been introduced into breast cancer management in

order to reduce the need for full axillary dissection and resultant complication such as lymphedema, this is not the issue in management of colectomy for colon cancer because adequacy of nodal dissection continues to be the benchmark.

The results of laparoscopic resection for colon cancer cannot be translated to the management of adenocarcinoma of the rectum. Rectal cancer is an entirely different disease and the challenge for the surgeon is to assure that the preoperative localization studies are adequate to assign the tumor to either the colon or rectum. The junction between sigmoid colon and rectum continues to be debated, and upper rectal tumors should be managed differently from tumors in the sigmoid region. The utilization of preoperative radiation is gaining considerable momentum and should be discussed in the venue of a preoperative multidisciplinary conference when patients are diagnosed. Although reports of laparoscopic resection of rectal cancer continue to permeate the peer-reviewed literature, there is yet no adequate randomized control study supporting this technique. Clinical trial groups, especially the American College of Surgeons Oncology Group, are the perfect mechanisms for attaining this information in the long term.

One of the issues that continue to be debated especially in terms of quality is the volume-outcome relationships especially in management of cancer. There is no question that pancreatic and esophageal resection should be performed by surgeons well versed in these procedures and should probably be regionalized to institutions capable of providing adequate care for patients with these diseases. Although there is literature to support that a colectomy should be performed only by surgeons with certain board certification or institutional affiliations, the fact is that adequate colectomy, whether it is performed by open or laparoscopic technique, can have favorable outcomes when surgeons use appropriate and safe techniques. The issue is not necessarily the volume of procedures performed. The overriding issue is to keep an adequate database of one's own outcomes to assure that mortality, morbidity, and 5-year survival benchmarks are met.

Adequate training, whether it is in laparoscopic or open technique, is the prime goal for any surgeon planning to use these procedures in patient management. Individual surgeons will have to decide whether they should take care of patients by using one or the other or both of these technical approaches. As long as randomized control clinical trials show that outcomes are similar for the cancer patient, the application of laparoscopic versus open technique is a critical discussion point between the surgeon and his or her patient.

REFERENCES

1. Jacobs M, Verdeja JC, Goldstein HS. Minimally invasive colon resection. *Surg Laparosc Endosc.* 1991;1:144–150.
2. Nelson H, Sargent DJ, Cost Study Group. A comparison of laparoscopically assisted and open colectomy for colon cancer. *N Engl J Med.* 2004:350; 2050–2059.
3. Guillou PJ, Quirke P, Thorpe H, et al. Short-term endpoints of conventional versus laparoscopic-assisted surgery in patients with colorectal cancer (MRC CLASICC trial): multicentre randomized controlled trial. *Lancet.* 2005;365: 1718–1726.
4. Veldkamp R, Kuhry E, Hop WC, et al. Laparoscopic surgery versus open surgery for colon cancer: short-term outcomes of a randomized trial. *Lancet Oncol.* 2005;6:477–484.

5. Fleshman J, Sargent DJ, Green E, et al. Laparoscopic colectomy for cancer is not inferior to open surgery based on 5-year data from the cost study group trial. *Ann Surg.* 2007;246:655–662.

6. Law WL, Lee YM, Choi HK, et al. Impact of laparoscopic resection for colorectal cancer on operative outcomes and survival. *Ann Surg.* 2007;245:1–7.

7. Le Voyer TE, Sigurdson ER, Hanlon AL, et al. Colon cancer survival is associated with increasing number of lymph nodes analyzed: a secondary survey of Intergroup Trial INT-0089. *J Clin Oncol.* 2003;21:2912–2919.

8. Bembenek A, Rosenberg R, Wagler E, et al. Sentinel lymph node biopsy in colon cancer: a prospective multicenter trial. *Ann Surg.* 2007;245:858–863.

39

Sphincter-Preserving Surgery in the Management of Rectal Cancer

Glenn T. Ault and Robert W. Beart, Jr.

Over 42,000 patients each year are diagnosed with rectal cancer in the United States. There have been recent advances in the oncologic treatment of colon and rectal cancer; however, cure depends on surgical resection. The combined abdominoperineal resection of the rectum (APR) first described by Mayo and popularized by Miles remained the gold standard for cancers of the distal rectum for most of the last century (1). The operation involves removing the rectum, anus, sphincter complex, and a portion of the levator ani and is concluded with the construction of a permanent colostomy. The more recently appreciated efficacy of a much narrower distal margin of resection compared with the heretofore required 5-cm distal margin, the newer technique of total mesorectal excision (TME), and the development and ongoing improvement in stapler technology are the major factors that have resulted in the applicability of sphincter-saving procedures for the majority of patients with distal rectal cancers, usually employing rectosigmoid resection with low rectal anastomosis (low anterior resection) or ultralow coloanal anastomosis (2,3).

In this chapter, we discuss the various factors that must be considered in the preoperative evaluation and staging that would indicate the appropriateness of a sphincter-preserving operation. We outline our technique in the conduct of such operations keeping in mind that performing such an operation simply because it is technically feasible to do so is not always in the patient's best interest. It our goal to shed some light on the techniques and difficult decision-making issues involved when managing low rectal cancers.

GOALS IN THE SURGICAL MANAGEMENT OF RECTAL CANCER

Distal and Proximal Margins

The extent of resection margins in rectal cancer remains controversial. Even though the first line of rectal cancer spread is upward along the course of the lymphatics, tumors below the peritoneal reflection can spread distally in a retrograde manner by intramural or extramural lymphatic and vascular routes. If distal intramural spread occurs, it is usually within 2.0 cm of the tumor, unless the lesion is poorly differentiated or widely metastatic (4-6). A study by Pollett and Nicholls (7) observed no difference in local recurrence rates whether a <2, 2 to 5, or >5 cm margin was achieved.

Two earlier studies also looked at the concept of extramural lymphatic spread. Goligher et al. (8) demonstrated that only 6.5% of patients had metastatic lesions below the primary tumor, whereas 93.5% had no retrograde spread. Of those with retrograde spread, two thirds of patients had metastasis limited to within 6 mm of the distal tumor edge and only 2% had metastasis beyond 2 cm. Dukes (9) published similar results in a study of over 1,500 patients who had undergone APR.

In addition, data from a randomized, prospective trial completed by the National Surgical Adjuvant Breast and Bowel Project demonstrate no significant differences in survival or local recurrence when comparing distal rectal margins of <2, 2 to 2.9, and >3 cm (10).

Based on review of best available current evidence, guidelines for the surgical management of rectal cancer were published by a panel of experts sponsored by the National Cancer Institute (11). A proximal margin of at least 5 cm is recommended. A distal margin length of ≥2 cm is regarded as ideal; however, for tumors of the distal rectum (<5 cm from the anal verge), the minimally acceptable length of the distal margin is 1 cm if necessary to achieve sphincter preservation. Nevertheless, this narrow a margin is not advised in cases of large, bulky tumors or in cases with adverse histologic features, such as poorly differentiated tumors or tumors with lymphovascular or neural invasion. If the distal margin is within 1 to 2 cm, intraoperative confirmation of a disease-free margin by frozen tissue section is imperative. The rationale for these guidelines is based on studies reviewed by the expert panel that have confirmed that distal intramural spread is rare and is found beyond 1 cm in only 4% to 10% of rectal cancers. Moreover, distal spread that does occur beyond 1 cm is associated with tumors of advanced stage or histologically aggressive disease and the associated poor prognosis is not improved by a longer distal margin.

Circumferential (Radial) Margins

It is now widely accepted that the circumferential margin of resection is the most important determinant of local recurrence of distal rectal cancers (12). A significant advance in surgery for rectal cancer has been the widespread acknowledgement of the importance of total TME in achieving clear circumferential margins. Following the mesorectal plane allows for the recovery of the draining nodal tissue and improves circumferential radial margin status by leaving the tumor contained within the envelope of the fascia propria of the rectum.

Although wide anatomic resection of the mesorectal tissue has always been the goal in performing rectal cancer procedures, concerns about actually achieving this goal to obtain clear circumferential margins have now been addressed by the concept and technique of TME (11–13). The traditional surgical technique employs blunt dissection, which often violates the mesorectal circumference, leaving residual mesorectum in the pelvis. Local failures are most often the result of inadequate surgical clearance of the radial margin. With traditional surgery, the incidence of local failure ranges from 14% to 30%, with or without postoperative radiation therapy or chemoradiotherapy (14).

TME in conjunction with low anterior resection or APR involves precise dissection and removal of the entire rectal mesentery, including that distal to the tumor, as an intact unit. Unlike traditional blunt dissection, the rectal mesentery is removed sharply under direct visualization, emphasizing autonomic nerve preservation, complete hemostasis, and avoidance of violation of the mesorectal envelope. Because it is theorized that the field of rectal cancer spread is limited to the mesorectal envelope, its total removal should encompass virtually every tumor satellite, thus improving the likelihood of local control.

Using this technique of TME, several groups have reported local failure rates between 4% and 7% (15–21). The excellent results seen in most (but not all [22]) series with TME may be attributed to improved lateral clearance with removal of potential tumor deposits in the mesentery and decreased risk of tumor spillage from a disrupted mesentery (23).

The completeness of TME appears to influence local control, even if the surgical margins are uninvolved. In one report, for example, both local (11.4% vs. 5.5%) and distant recurrence rates (19.2% vs. 12.2%) were higher in patients with an incomplete excision compared with a complete or nearly complete mesorectal excision (24).

More importantly, improved local control appears to result in better survival. In one of the earliest reports on TME, Heald and associates (25) noted a local recurrence rate of 3.6%, and 86% survival after 9 years of follow-up. Although long-term follow-up data are not yet available from larger series, survival rates ranging from 68% to 74% for Dukes C and 85% to 88% for Dukes B tumors are being reported in series employing TME (19,20).

The notion of the importance of the circumferential radial margin status is not new and was previously reported in a landmark report by Quirke et al. (26) in 1986. In this report, the authors demonstrated an 86% local failure rate after positive circumferential radial margin resections. Other authors have confirmed these findings, with recurrence rates ranging from 22% to 50% following positive circumferential radial margin resections. Evaluation of the Dutch TME data as well as the Mayo/North Central Cancer Treatment Group data has shown that circumferential margins >2 mm are necessary to reduce the risk for local failure after resection of rectal cancer (27–29).

Nodal Clearance

The American Joint Committee on Cancer and a National Cancer Institute-sponsored panel recommended that at least 12 lymph nodes be examined in patients with colon and rectal cancer to confirm the absence of nodal involvement by tumor (11,30,31). This recommendation takes into consideration that the number of lymph nodes examined is a reflection of both the aggressiveness of the lymphovascular mesenteric dissection at the time of surgical resection and the pathologic identification of nodes in the specimen. Retrospective studies have demonstrated that the number of lymph nodes examined in colon and rectal surgery may be associated with patient outcome (32–35). In our experience with patients who have received neoadjuvant therapy and subsequently undergo a rectal dissection, retrieving 12 lymph nodes for examination can be challenging.

Preservation of Sexual and Bladder Function

Traditional rectal surgery has been associated with a significant incidence of sexual and urinary dysfunction. This has been most likely related to damage to the pelvic autonomic sympathetic and parasympathetic nerves by the dissection forces (36). Postoperative impotence and retrograde ejaculation or both have been observed in 25% to 75% of cases, particularly if lateral wall lymphadenectomy and splanchnic nerve resection are performed. After the introduction of TME, with its careful nerve-sparing dissection, impotence has been reported in only 10% to 29% of cases. Masui et al. (37) confirms that autonomic nerve preservation yields good results in terms of morbidity and functional outcome.

There are several points during the rectal dissection at which nerve injury can occur. The clinical consequence of isolated sympathetic nerve injury is retrograde ejaculation. Isolated sympathetic injury can occur at the nerve plexus surrounding the aorta, as well as the pelvic brim where the nerves bifurcate to each side of the pelvis. With meticulous technique, these nerves can be identified as a "wishbone" near the sacral promontory. As dissection descends below the peritoneal reflection, both the sympathetic and parasympathetic nerve fibers are subject to injury. This occurs most commonly at the pelvic sidewall, resulting in impotence and bladder dysfunction. The hypogastric plexus and nervi erigentes can be injured in the anterolateral pelvis. Injuries to these nerves also lead to mixed deficits.

PREOPERATIVE ASSESSMENT OF PATIENTS WITH RECTAL CANCER

Level of the Lesion

The rectum is typically defined as the last 12 to 15 cm of the large intestine. However, the exact site to begin measurement is unclear. Many measure from the anal verge. This measurement can be confounded by the fact that the anal canal can range from 1 to 7 cm in length. Consequently, the level of the tumor can be miscalculated to be located from 1 to 8 cm above the anal canal. We have found the best way to describe the level of the tumor is by using its anatomic relationship to the puborectalis muscle. The distance of the tumor from the puborectalis should be measured using the index finger. If the tumor is not palpable, then the distance can most accurately be assessed using a rigid endoscope. Neither the flexible sigmoidoscope nor colonoscope is accurate in determining the level of the tumor as these instruments may flex as they navigate the valves of Houston. The critical judgment is that if the tumor is not palpable, then intestinal continuity can nearly always be restored with relative ease.

The long-held, unwritten rule that an APR is necessary if a tumor is ≤5 cm from the anal verge is no longer applicable in light of advances in surgical techniques that now allow removal of virtually any tumor in this area without removing the anal canal. Resection of a rectal cancer is generally performed through the abdomen with the removal of the mesorectal lymph nodes. The hypogastric lymph nodes are removed if they are grossly involved. An APR does not improve the outcome as the only additional tissues removed with an APR are the anus, the anal canal, a portion of the levator muscles and ischiorectal fat, areas that are rare sites for retrograde involvement or local recurrence if the sphincter-saving procedure provides a tumor-free margin of resection of a least 1 cm, as previously discussed.

In general, if the lower edge of the tumor does not involve the puborectalis muscle and is at least 2 cm above the anorectal ring, we feel comfortable in counseling the patient preoperatively that a sphincter-preserving procedure can be completed with a very low likelihood of requiring a permanent colostomy.

Recent studies have suggested that in those uncommon patients with very low rectal cancers with limited infiltration of the puborectalis or anal canal, these areas of tumor extension can be resected en bloc with the primary tumor with reconstruction of the anal canal to preserve intestinal continuity (38). We have performed operations such as these in selected patients and have not found them to be technically difficult. Nevertheless, we regard these procedures as experimental, and patients are so advised.

Tumor Fixation

Fixation of the tumor in the pelvis, suggesting invasion of either the pelvic sidewall or the musculature of the pelvic floor, implies a poor prognosis. Appropriate staging studies may help delineate the anatomic relationships. Fixation often hinders the ability to obtain an adequate oncologic resection, with a greater likelihood of local recurrence or anastomotic recurrence. The presence of a fixed tumor may be an indication for preoperative radiotherapy (RT).

TNM Staging Schema

Treatment decisions should be made with reference to the TNM classification, rather than the older Dukes or modified Astler-Coller (MAC) classification schema. The TNM staging system of the American Joint Committee on Cancer is presented in Table 39.1 (30).

Preoperative Staging by Imaging Techniques

Since its inception, computed tomography (CT) has been extensively used to evaluate the extent of the primary tumor. Accuracy rates have been reported as approximately 60% to 80% for staging of the primary tumor and 55% to 85% for determination of nodal status (39). CT scanning remains an important tool for the evaluation of local extension of disease and to evaluate for sites of metastasis elsewhere in the abdomen.

Rectal magnetic resonance imaging (MRI) has also been used for preoperative assessment, but it has not been of particular advantage when compared with CT (40,44). It can delineate bowel wall layers with accuracy similar to endorectal ultrasound. Contrast-enhanced MRI and MRI endoscopy may improve

tumor staging, but the accuracy of lymph node evaluation remains uncertain. Generally, figures for accuracy of tumor staging range from 55% to 95%, with nodal staging accuracy from 72% to 95%. An attempt was made to improve the staging accuracy of MRI with the use of surface MRI coils to allow a higher definition of image with a smaller field of view. Initial reports were promising, but later observations have suggested that the use of the coil does not improve the staging accuracy of MRI, especially when other less expensive, more accurate, modalities are available (45–47). MRI may have benefits for evaluating recurrences secondary to its ability to delineate the fascial planes.

In our practice, we routinely use endorectal ultrasonography (ERUS) for evaluation of the extent of primary rectal tumors. ERUS is also valuable in the assessment of recurrent disease as it allows for full-thickness evaluation of an anastomotic area and is useful in obtaining image-guided biopsies. Each of the layers of the rectum can be sonographically visualized, with the tumor appearing as a hypoechoic variation in the normal anatomic layers. Most studies indicate a sensitivity and specificity for bowel wall involvement >90%. In an analysis from the University of Minnesota in which the ERUS-determined T category of a series of primary rectal tumors was compared with the pathologic T category determined following surgical resection, Garcia-Aguilar et al. (48) found that the overall accuracy of ERUS in assessing the depth of tumor penetration was 69%, with 18% of the tumors overstaged and 13% understaged. The accuracy of ERUS in the diagnosis of lymph node metastases was 64%. None of the patients studied had undergone any neoadjuvant therapy.

The limitations of preoperative nodal staging by MRI or ERUS have been further emphasized by Guillem et al. (49). These investigators reported that among 188 patients with rectal tumors clinically staged T3N0 by ERUS or MRI, 22% had undetected mesorectal lymph node involvement at the time of resection despite preoperative chemoradiotherapy. The actual rate of understaging is likely to have been even higher because preoperative therapy can produce significant downstaging (50).

Histology

A biopsy to confirm the diagnosis of cancer is usually done at the time of discovery of the lesion and is easily accomplished with the use of the rigid proctosigmoidoscope. By and large, tumors with poor differentiation or anaplastic lesions are more aggressive and may require more aggressive combined modality treatment. Saclarides et al. (51) attempted to determine which features were predictors of nodal metastases. They used nine histologic and morphologic features of rectal cancer to determine which were associated with nodal disease. Statistically significant variables were worsening differentiation, increasing depth of penetration, microtubular configuration >20%, the presence of venous invasion or perineural invasion and lymphatic invasion. In analysis of all the variables or combination of factors, the degree of differentiation was the strongest predictor of nodal disease.

MANAGEMENT OF RECTAL CANCER

Perioperative Adjunctive Therapy

The success of combined-modality treatment in the postoperative setting has led to its evaluation in the preoperative treatment of rectal cancer. Clinical trials have essentially focused on

Table 39.1

American Joint Committee on Cancer (AJCC) Staging System for Cancer of the Colon and Rectum

Primary Tumor (T)	Regional Lymph Nodes (N)	Distant Metastasis (M)
TX: Primary tumor cannot be assessed	**NX**: Regional lymph nodes cannot be assessed	**MX**: Distant metastasis cannot be assessed
T0: No evidence of primary tumor	**N0**: No regional lymph node metastasis	**M0**: No distant metastasis
Tis: Carcinoma in situ	**N1**: Metastasis in 1 to 3 regional lymph nodes	**M1**: Distant metastasis
T1: Tumor invades submucosa	**N2**: Metastasis in 4 or more regional lymph nodes	
T2: Tumor invades muscularis propria		
T3: Tumor invades through the muscularis propria into the subserosa, or into nonperitonealized pericolic or perirectal tissue		
T4: Invades other organs or structures, and/or perforates visceral peritoneum		

AJCC Stage Groupings

Stage	Description
0	Tis, N0, M0
I	T1, N0, M0
	T2, N0, M0
IIA	T3, N0, M0
IIB	T4, N0, M0
IIIA	T1, N1, M0
	T2, N1, M0
IIIB	T3, N1, M0
	T4, N1, M0
IIIC	Any T, N2, M0
IV	Any T, any N, M1

Adapted from Greene FL, Page DL, Fleming ID, et al. Colon and rectum. In: *American Joint Committee on Cancer AJCC Cancer Staging Manual.* 6th ed. New York: Springer; 2002:113–124.

two main questions: whether neoadjuvant chemoradiotherapy is better than RT alone and the comparative benefit of preoperative (neoadjuvant) versus postoperative (adjuvant) chemoradiotherapy.

Neoadjuvant Chemoradiotherapy versus Radiotherapy Alone

In phase 2 studies comparing neoadjuvant chemoradiotherapy versus RT, rates of complete pathologic response are higher following preoperative 5-fluorouracil (5-FU)-based chemoradiotherapy than they are in series using moderate- to high-dose (45 to 50 Gy) RT alone (15% to 37% vs. 6% to 12%, respectively) (52-64). Reports are now accumulating that link higher pathologic response rates to improved long-term outcome (65,66).

Several phase 3 randomized trials have directly addressed the question of whether the concurrent administration of chemotherapy with conventional fractionation RT is critical to the success of the neoadjuvant approach (67–70). In 2006, Gerard et al. (67) reported the results of a European trial in which 742 patients with locally advanced (T3-4) rectal cancer accessible to digital rectal examination were randomly assigned to receive preoperative RT alone (45 Gy over 5 weeks) or with concurrent bolus 5-FU (350 mg/m^2 per day) and leucovorin (20 mg/m^2 per day) daily for 5 days during weeks 1 and 5. Patients in both arms were scheduled to receive adjuvant chemotherapy with the same fluorouracil/leucovorin regimen, but only about half of the patients in each group actually received the postoperative chemotherapy. TME was recommended but neither standardized nor controlled in the analysis. At a median of 81 months of follow-up, the combined-modality group had a higher pathologic complete response rate (11.4% vs. 3.6%; $p < 0.05$) and a significantly lower local failure rate (8.1% vs. 16.5%; $p < 0.05$) at 5 years, but the rate of sphincter-preserving surgery

(52% vs. 54%) and 5-year overall survival rates (67% vs. 68%) were similar.

Bosset et al. (68,69) reported the results of the European Organisation for Research and Treatment of Cancer Radiotherapy Group Trial 22921 in which 1011 patients with clinical stage T3 or T4 resectable cancers were randomized to one of four treatment groups: (a) preoperative RT, (b) preoperative chemoradiotherapy, (c) preoperative RT and postoperative chemotherapy, or (d) preoperative chemoradiotherapy and postoperative chemotherapy. Adding fluorouracil-based chemotherapy preoperatively or postoperatively had no significant effected on survival. However, adding chemotherapy to preoperative RT conferred a significant improvement in local control regardless of whether it was administered before or after surgery. Preoperative chemotherapy seemed preferable, however, as adherence to postoperative chemotherapy was poor in that <50% of the patients assigned to this treatment received it according to protocol. Compared with RT alone (RT), patients undergoing preoperative RT plus chemotherapy had a significantly higher rate of pathologic complete response (13.7% vs. 5.3%), significantly less advanced T and N stage, and fewer cases with venous, perineural, or lymphatic invasion (68).

In a third randomized trial, conducted by Bujko et al. (70) in Poland, preoperative short-term RT (5 × 5 Gy fractions) was compared with conventionally fractionated chemoradiotherapy (50.4 Gy plus concomitant bolus 5-FU and leucovorin administered during weeks 1 and 5). In an early report, chemoradiotherapy was associated with significantly higher pathologic complete response rates (16% vs. 1%) and fewer positive radial margins (4% vs. 13%), but a similar sphincter preservation rate. The data were immature as to the impact on local control or survival.

Taken together, the results from these three phase 3 trials support the conclusion that adding chemotherapy to neoadjuvant RT increases the likelihood of a complete pathologic response and improves local control, but the impact on sphincter preservation and survival remains uncertain.

Neoadjuvant versus Adjuvant Chemoradiotherapy

Debate continues regarding the relative merits of adjuvant compared with neoadjuvant combined-modality therapy in the treatment of patients with nonmetastatic rectal carcinoma. Three randomized trails have directly compared the two approaches (65,71–73). The only completed trial that used standard fractionation preoperative RT and modern 5-FU-based chemotherapy was conducted in Germany. The German Rectal Cancer Group randomly assigned 823 patients with clinically staged T3-4 or node-positive rectal cancer to the same chemoradiotherapy regimen administered either preoperatively or postoperatively: 50.4 Gy in 28 daily fractions to the tumor and pelvic lymph nodes concurrent with infusional 5-FU (100 mg/m^2 daily for 5 days during the first and fifth weeks of RT) (71). All patients underwent TME, and four additional cycles of adjuvant single-agent 5-FU (500 mg/m^2 daily for 5 days every 4 weeks). With a 46-month median follow-up, preoperative chemoradiotherapy was associated with a significantly lower pelvic relapse rate compared with postoperative therapy (6% vs. 13%). However, the 5-year disease-free (68% vs. 65%) and overall survival rates (76% vs. 74%) were similar for preoperative and postoperative

therapy, respectively. Stage distribution at surgery was suggestive of significant downstaging effects. Among 194 patients with low-lying tumors who were thought preoperatively to require APR, those undergoing preoperative chemoradiotherapy were twice as likely to undergo a sphincter-sparing operation than an APR (39% vs. 19%).

In the National Surgical Adjuvant Breast and Bowel Project trial (NSABP R-03) patients with operable rectal cancer were assigned to one of two groups (65,72). The first group received preoperative therapy consisting of one cycle of 5-FU and leucovorin, two courses of concomitant 5-FU and leucovorin plus pelvic irradiation, then surgery followed by four cycles of postoperative 5-FU and leucovorin. Patients in the second arm received postoperative therapy, which consisted of surgery, one cycle of 5-FU plus leucovorin, two cycles of 5-FU and leucovorin concomitant with pelvic RT, then four cycles of 5-FU and leucovorin. Accrual did not reach planned levels and the protocol was closed early. In a preliminary analysis that included 267 patients, 23% of those treated preoperatively had a complete clinical response to therapy, and 44% of these were pathologically confirmed (10% of the total). In a later report, preoperative therapy was associated with a higher rate of 3-year disease-free survival (70% vs. 65%) and overall survival (85% vs. 78%), but neither difference was statistically significant.

It has been suggested that patients achieving a complete clinical response to neoadjuvant chemoradiation may be spared operation (74,75). Habr-Gama et al. (75) managed 361 patients with distal rectal cancer with neoadjuvant chemoradiation, including 5-FU, leucovorin, and 5,040 cGy. Patients with a complete clinical response were not immediately operated on and were closely followed. One hundred twenty-two patients were considered to have had a complete clinical response at 8 weeks following the neoadjuvant therapy. Of these, 99 patients sustained a complete clinical response for at least 12 months and were considered stage c0 (27.4%) and were managed nonoperatively. Mean follow-up was 59.9 months. There were 13 (13.1%) recurrences: 5 (5%) endorectal, 7 (7.1%) systemic, and 1 (1%) combined recurrence. All five isolated endorectal recurrences were salvaged. Mean recurrence interval was 52 months for local failure and 29.5 months for systemic failure. There were five cancer-related deaths after systemic recurrences. Overall and disease-free 5-year survival rates were 93% and 85%, respectively. The authors concluded that, although surgery remains the standard treatment for rectal cancer, nonoperative treatment after complete clinical response following neoadjuvant chemoradiation may be safe and associated with good survival rates in a highly selected group of patients.

Preoperative RT does not appear to increase the complication rate from surgical resection (65,71,76). In the German Rectal Cancer Study previously described, the incidence of grade 3 or 4 gastrointestinal toxicity was similar in the preoperative and postoperative chemoradiotherapy groups (28.8% vs. 31.7%, respectively), and the postoperative morbidity rates were not higher with neoadjuvant therapy (71). In contrast, significantly fewer patients undergoing neoadjuvant therapy had chronic anastomotic strictures (2.7% vs. 8.5%).

At the University of Southern California, it is our practice to proceed with neoadjuvant chemoradiation prior to surgery for T2 and more advanced tumors.

Considerations in the Choice of Operation for Rectal Cancer

Sphincter-sparing surgery is now considered the standard of care for patients with rectal cancer. Sphincter preservation can be successfully achieved occasionally by local excision but more commonly by rectosigmoid resection with restoration of intestinal continuity when it is technically feasible, functionally appropriate, and oncologically reasonable. The advent of the circular stapler, in conjunction with improvements in anesthesia, surgical technique, and an increasing understanding of the minimal requirements for margins of resection, has enabled restoration of intestinal continuity after low anterior resection or ultralow resection with coloanal anastomosis for most patients who heretofore would have required APR (77). Invasion of the sphincter complex precludes sphincter preservation, and the relevant issues with respect to the level of the rectal lesion have already been discussed. Other factors that may increase the difficulty of segmental resection with sphincter preservation or may make this approach inadvisable include low-lying bulky tumors, male sex, obesity, and pre-existing fecal incontinence.

Although a sphincter-preserving operation with a low anastomosis may be technically feasible, such a procedure may be associated with functional disturbances that usually resolve but occasionally result in an unacceptable impairment in quality of life. These include bowel urgency, tenesmus, soiling, frequency of bowel movements due to loss of reservoir function, and fecal incontinence (77,78). Persistence of these symptoms may even make a permanent colostomy preferable in selected patients. There is some evidence suggesting that treatment with sphincter-saving procedures is more common and with better outcomes when care is provided in high-volume centers by high-volume surgeons (79,80).

Data from the National Cancer Data Base suggest a decline in frequency of APR for surgical treatment of rectal cancer, with a corresponding increase in the use of sphincter-saving procedures (81). Oncologic outcomes following a low anterior resection are not significantly different from those following APR; however, APR is associated with higher procedure-related morbidity and mortality (82,83) and an inferior quality of life, mainly related to depression and changes in body image (84).

Approaches to Sphincter Preservation

Sphincter preservation may be achieved by one of several operative approaches including local excision under direct vision, transanal excision employing endoscopic microsurgery, and, most commonly, transabdominal resection with an anastomosis above the dentate line (low anterior resection) or combined transabdominal and perineal resection with an ultralow coloanal anastomosis.

Local Excision Under Direct Vision

Patients with early distal rectal cancers with favorable features that are classified as T1 or T2 by depth of invasion have been offered treatment by local excision through the anus (transanal excision), by division of the anal sphincter (transsphincteric or York-Mason procedure), or through a posterior parasacral approach (Kraske resection) (85). The last two procedures are mentioned here primarily for historical reasons, as these approaches are somewhat more extensive than a simple transanal excision and have a greater degree of associated morbidity, mainly because they disrupt the normal musculofascial planes (86).

In performing transanal local excision the goal is complete full-thickness resection of the rectal cancer down to the perirectal fat using electrocautery to achieve a minimum lateral margin of 1 cm and a clear deep margin. Primary closure of the resulting defect is performed. If the margins are found to be positive for tumor, then additional local resection, if feasible, or conventional radical resection should be undertaken.

The customary criteria used to determine suitability for potentially curative local excision include the following:

- Tumor size <4 cm
- Location ≤8 cm from the anal verge
- Well or moderately well-differentiated histology
- Mobile, nonulcerated tumor
- No suspicion of perirectal or presacral nodes (as determined by preoperative staging)
- Tumor involving less than one-third the circumference of the rectal wall
- Tumor stage ≤T2

Enthusiasm for this conservative surgical approach as an alternative to APR or low anterior resection has been curbed by recent reports of high local recurrence rates. In a prospective multi-institutional trial reported by Steele et al. (87), a 20% local recurrence rate was observed for T2 rectal cancers following local excision, despite postoperative radiation therapy. In a series of 125 patients treated by local excision at Memorial Sloan-Kettering Cancer Center (88), the 10-year local recurrence and survival rates were 17% and 74% for T1 rectal cancers and 26% and 72% for T2 cancers. In patients receiving RT, local recurrence was delayed, but overall rates of local and overall recurrence and survival rates were similar to those of patients not receiving RT. Among the 17 patients with isolated local recurrence, 14 underwent salvage resection. Actuarial survival among these surgically salvaged patients was only 30% at 6 years after salvage. Thus, neither adjuvant RT nor salvage surgery was reliable in preventing or controlling local recurrence.

In a report from Mayo Clinic using the National Cancer Data Base, You and associates (89) compared the course of 765 patients who underwent local excision with that of 1,359 patients treated by standard resection. The 5-year local recurrence after local excision and standard resection was 12.5% and 6.9%, respectively, for T1 tumors ($p = 0.003$), and 22.1% and 15.1% for T2 tumors ($p = 0.01$). The 5-year overall survival (T1, 77.4% vs. 81.7%; $p = 0.09$; T2, 67.6% vs. 76.5%; $p = 0.01$) was influenced by age and comorbidities but not the type of surgery.

Local excision may be a reasonable alternative for patients who refuse to have an APR with permanent colostomy, who have significant comorbidities that preclude a major abdominal operation, or who have evidence of distant metastases with a short life expectancy.

In order to improve the efficacy of local excision of early rectal cancers, the American College of Surgeons Oncology Group is enrolling patients in a phase 2 trial (ACOSOG protocol Z6041) in which patients with ultrasound-confirmed T2N0M0 distal rectal cancers receive preoperative chemoradiation with capecitabine and oxaliplatin with 54 Gy pelvic radiation followed by transanal local excision 4 to 6 weeks after completion of the neoadjuvant therapy (90).

Local Excision by Transanal Endoscopic Microsurgery

The traditional transanal approach to local excision is limited to low and midrectal lesions within 8 cm of the anal verge. Minimally invasive endoscopic techniques such as transanal endoscopic microsurgery (TEM) have expanded the possibility of transanal excision to otherwise inaccessible lesions that are within reach of the endoscope (up to 25 cm from the anal verge) (91–103). The apparatus for this procedure consists of a multifunctional endoscopic unit that creates a closed system that simultaneously regulates suction, irrigation, carbon dioxide insufflation, and monitoring of intrarectal pressure. The rectoscope is covered with a sealed locking face piece that has airtight, sealed working ports through which are inserted the instruments necessary for the dissection (100).

Oncologic results appear similar to those obtained with transanal excision of more distal tumors or anterior resection, but patient selection is critical. TEM is most suitable for patients with low-risk T1 tumors; resection of T2 tumors has been associated with high local recurrence rates in most reports (100–102). Although treatment-related morbidity compares favorably with anterior resection, TEM is often associated with transient reduction in anorectal function with full clinical recovery within 1 year (102). Inadvertent entry in to the peritoneal cavity during the procedure is uncommon. Although endoscopic repair of the injury has been reported, conversion to an open procedure may be required (100,103). Given this risk, the utility of full-thickness tumor excision using TEM may be most applicable to lesions below the peritoneal reflection. However, very low lesions, those located in the distal 5 cm of the rectum, may be better addressed with conventional instruments as CO_2 may escape with collapse of the operative field and bleeding may be encountered because of the proximity of the hemorrhoidal veins (100). The technical difficulty of the procedure and the expense of the equipment are factors that currently limit the widespread application of this alternative (100).

Low Anterior Resection

The definition of low anterior resection is variable in the literature. For the purpose of this chapter, low anterior resection is defined as the transabdominal removal of a rectal tumor located at a level such that intestinal continuity can be restored with an anastomosis that is done above the dentate line and below the sigmoid or 15 cm from the anal verge. On digital rectal examination, if the anal sphincter muscles are free of involvement and the tumor is palpated at least one to two cm above the level of the puborectalis muscle, the patient can be confidently counseled that the tumor with the requisite surrounding rectal tissue and associated lymph nodes can be removed with an abdominal dissection with restoration of intestinal continuity and preservation of continence.

We perform this procedure with the patient in the lithotomy position with the buttocks extending beyond the edge of the operating table to allow easy access to the anus. The legs, in

stirrups, are slightly abducted and elevated. The elevation may improve venous drainage and reduce postoperative thromboembolic events. The sigmoid colon is mobilized through a lower midline abdominal incision by incising the lateral peritoneal reflection. In the course of the procedure the ureters are identified and protected. In preparation for restoring bowel continuity employing the double-staple technique, the sigmoid colon is divided with a stapler at least 5 cm above the tumor in its proximal to midportion at level where the diameter of the bowel is sufficient to easily accept a 33-mm end-to-end anastomosis circular stapling device. If the sigmoid at this level is muscular and of too small a diameter, then more proximal colon needs to be mobilized to reach larger diameter bowel or, alternatively, construction of a neoreservoir needs to be considered. The sigmoid mesentery is serially divided, in the course of which the superior hemorrhoidal vessels are exposed and ligated at a point above the bifurcation of the aorta. The mobilization of the rectosigmoid proceeds distalward into the pelvis. Posteriorly, the presacral space is entered and further dissection employs the technique of total mesorectal excision, as previously described. In the course of the dissection the pelvic autonomic nerves are identified and preserved, as previously discussed, in order to reduce the incidence of impotence in men (37,104). Mobilization continues anteriorly by separating the bowel from the vagina in women and the prostate in men. Sharp circumferential dissection continues in order to mobilize the rectum sufficiently beyond the tumor to provide a satisfactory margin of resection. The level of dissection can be periodically assessed during the operation by digital rectal examination as the rectum is easily accessed in the lithotomy position.

When the appropriate level is reached, the rectum is transected after the application of a noncrushing bowel clamp, in preparation for a hand-sewn anastomosis, or preferably with a stapler, in preparation for the double-staple technique of anastomosis. We believe the double-staple technique is the procedure of choice as it is both simple and safe and is a method of performing a low colorectal anastomosis that might otherwise not be technically possible. In this approach, the detached anvil of the circular stapling device is inserted into the lumen of the proximal bowel and secured with a pursestring suture. The shaft of the stapler is then inserted through the anus into the rectal stump. The central trocar is extended and advanced through the rectal staple line or adjacent to it. The anvil is reattached to the shaft of the instrument and the stapler closed by retracting the trocar by rotating the knob on the shaft until the two ends of the bowel are approximated. Thereafter, the stapler is fired to create the circular anastomosis. The adequacy of the anastomosis can be assessed by observing the intactness of the two tissue rings ("doughnuts") removed from the respective ends of the bowel by the stapler and by the absence of bubbles with air insufflation through the anus with the anastomosis submerged in saline. The results of the double-staple technique of anastomosis compare favorably with those of the traditional hand-sewn anastomosis, both with respect to morbidity and local recurrence (105,106).

A tension-free anastomosis requires sufficient length of proximal bowel to reach the residual rectum. If necessary, additional length can be achieved by mobilizing the descending colon and, occasionally, the splenic flexure. The blood supply to the colon must be assessed if achieving adequate length requires division of blood vessels, such as the left colic and sigmoid vessels and the inferior mesenteric vein.

We consider that a tension-free anastomosis has been achieved if the bowel lies along the hollow of the sacrum. If there is any "bowstringing" across the sacrum, then additional mobilization of the colon is necessary. Debate continues as to the indications and benefits of routine pelvic drainage and fecal diversion (107–110). We prefer to lay two suction drains in the pelvis behind the anastomosis. Some have argued that these drains may increase the risk of leak. Our leak rate of 3% seems acceptably low when these drains are used. Others have demonstrated that these drains will control about 50% of leaks should they occur, saving the patient additional procedures. Because the leak rate is low, we do not believe that routine fecal diversion is necessary but, instead, perform a diverting ileostomy selectively if there are any adverse findings, such as complications during construction of the anastomosis and poor initial condition of the patient (110). In addition, if the patient has been radiated preoperatively and the tissues are indurated or in some way abnormal, then we would favor a diverting ileostomy, which should be closed no sooner than 6 weeks after the operation. However, if during the postoperative period there is any evidence of leakage, then additional drainage, usually with CT guidance, or diversion is undertaken promptly to allow healing.

Ultralow Resection with Coloanal Anastomosis

The technique of coloanal anastomosis allows sphincter preservation in patients with tumors with sufficient distal margin but too low to restore bowel continuity by the double-staple technique. Here the rectum is transected just above the anorectal ring. The mucosa above the dentate line is removed transanally, and the proximal colon is drawn down into the anorectal remnant and sutured at the level of dentate line (111).

The abdominal procedure is similar to that described for a low anterior resection. Here the anterior dissection is carried well below the prostate in men and the cervix in women, and the posterior dissection beyond the tip of the coccyx. The more distal the dissection is carried out from above, the easier it is to complete the dissection from below. A laparotomy pad is placed firmly in the presacral space below the level of the coccyx to mark the level of the posterior dissection. Following completion of the abdominal dissection, we turn our attention to the anus. We place a self-retaining anal retractor, such as the Lone Star retractor (Coopersurgical, Trumball, CT), to efface the anus and to achieve optimal exposure. The mucosa is dissected from the anal canal beginning at the dentate line up to the level of the palpable laparotomy pad. We then transect the rectal muscle posteriorly at this level, which should be above the puborectalis muscle. A finger is placed through the defect so created, the laparotomy pad removed, and transection of the rectal muscle laterally on both sides, facilitated by the inserted finger, is carried out. Now a finger is placed through the defect between the anterior pelvic structures and the rectum. These structures are brought down into wound and the anterior portion of the dissection is completed. The specimen is removed and the proximal bowel, previously transected with the stapler, is brought down into the anal canal. Beginning 1 to 2 cm above the staple line, the bowel is anchored to the internal sphincter with interrupted absorbable sutures. Thereafter, the bowel is opened by resecting the staple line, and the full thickness of the bowel wall is sutured to the anoderm with interrupted absorbable sutures. Drainage of these patients is the same as recommended for the low anterior resection. Although we have a lower threshold to divert these patients, particularly if they have had neoadjuvant therapy, if there is sufficient bowel length to avoid any tension, if there is good blood supply, and if the anastomosis has been carried out with ease, diversion is not mandatory.

Restoration of Continuity with a Neoreservoir

Straight colorectal and coloanal anastomoses may result in impaired bowel function, including frequency, urgency, and soiling. The lower the level of the anastomosis, the more adverse the functional outcome (111). Neoreservoirs created either by a colonic J-pouch or by coloplasty appear to provide comparable improvement in bowel function and quality of life scores (111–115). We frequently construct a reservoir when the anastomosis will be within 4 cm of the puborectalis muscle. We currently favor coloplasty as it is less bulky and seems to fit more easily into the pelvis. The anastomosis performed following this procedure must be absolutely tension-free to avoid complications.

Laparoscopic Surgery for Rectal Cancer

Currently, we do not favor laparoscopic resection of the rectum for cancer. A great deal has been written about the influence of laparoscopy on the incidence and patterns of recurrent colorectal cancer. Over a decade was spent resolving this issue for colon cancer. A number of authors have demonstrated that rectal cancer can be removed laparoscopically (116), but until appropriate scientific studies are conducted demonstrating the safety and efficacy of this technique-dependent operation, we favor conducting all rectal cancer operations for T3 and T4 disease with an open technique (117).

Complications of Sphincter-Saving Procedures

Intraoperative Complications

Bleeding

Bleeding from the presacral area is unusual when dissection is carried out in the plane previously described. However, occasionally very large veins in this area are disturbed and bleed vigorously. After applying direct pressure initially, we proceed through a sequence of maneuvers to achieve hemostasis: cautery, direct suture ligation, suture ligation with pledgets, and insertion of thumb tacks. If these efforts are unsuccessful, then a pack can be placed into the presacral space to control the bleeding. Bleeding from the lateral pelvic sidewall is more easily controlled, applying a large Allis clamp and then figure-of-eight 2-0 absorbable sutures on a large needle. The only concern here is that if the sutures are taken very deeply, the sciatic nerve is in some jeopardy. In addition, the ureters must be carefully identified to minimize inclusion or injury. Anteriorly, bleeding from the back of the prostate can occur, but if the dissection is carried out sharply as previously noted, this is unusual. It is a very difficult area to see and, again, packing may be necessary to achieve control. Occasionally the area of an anastomotic staple line continues to bleed. This is somewhat worrisome in that the stapler may not have fired completely, and careful examination is necessary to be sure that there is no leak.

Incomplete Anastomosis

If the staple line is incomplete, the anastomosis can be reinforced with interrupted sutures with confidence that the anastomosis can be made secure. If necessary, a one-layer hand-sewn anastomosis can be performed that is secure, and diversion is not mandatory.

Late Complications

Anastomotic Stricture

Occasionally a stricture will develop at the anastomosis. Therefore, all anastomoses should be checked with a digital examination at approximately 2 weeks after operation. If a diversionary stoma had been created, a contrast study prior to stomal closure should been done to confirm that the anastomosis is well healed. If there is a stricture, it usually can be gently dilated. If it cannot be easily dilated on digital rectal examination, examination under anesthesia is appropriate to see if there is a channel that can be dilated under direct vision.

Anastomotic Leakage with a Sinus Tract

If the anastomosis is not complete at the time of proposed stoma closure, then we would delay closure of the diverting stoma for 6 to 9 months. If the associated sinus tract persists at that point, we proceed with stoma closure and have been gratified to note minimal symptoms from these tracts, which apparently become lined with rectal mucosa. It is important, however, to demonstrate on preoperative contrast enema that the sinus tract drains well back into the rectum. If the sinus tract is strictured at its opening, the stricture should be dilated prior to stoma closure.

Anastomotic Leakage with a Cutaneous Fistula

Occasionally, a fistula through the abdominal wall develops, and it generally occurs along a previous drain tract. In the presence of a stoma, if the fistula persists, closure of the stoma is delayed. We have had some success in closing these low-output fistulas with glue. On rare occasions, we have had to return to the operating room and redo the anastomosis. A rectocutaneous fistula not associated with sepsis that occurs in a nondiverted patient may respond to bowel rest and parenteral nutrition. Otherwise, diversion and possibly drainage may be required.

Stool Frequency and Urgency

Stool frequency and urgency are common for the first 3 months following operation without diversion and for a similar period following closure of a stoma. However, these symptoms generally do not extend beyond this period. If they do, the patient should be evaluated for anal dysfunction as well for inadequate reservoir function. Medications that have been helpful have included fiber, diphenoxylate plus atropine tablets (Lomotil), as well as hyoscyamine and amitriptyline. These latter two drugs also have been useful in irritable bowel syndrome so that response to these agents may reflect some underlying irritable bowel condition.

Tumor Recurrence

The most worrisome postoperative complication is recurrence of the tumor. Local recurrence should occur in <10% of patients, but the rate increases the more distal the tumor and the more advanced the T category. Identification of local recurrence prior to distant spread is important as such localized disease may respond to combined-modality therapy that may consist of radiation, chemotherapy, and salvage surgery, including pelvic exenteration.

Rosen et al. (118) published a meta-analysis of reports assessing the value of intensive follow-up compared with no follow-up for patients after resection of colorectal cancer. "Intensive follow-up" was defined as at least a history and physical examination and carcinoembryonic antigen assay performed a minimum of 3 times a year for at least 2 years. The analysis indicated that the cumulative 5-year survival was 1.16 times higher in the intensively followed group ($p = 0.003$). Two and one-half times more curative re-resections were performed for recurrent cancer in those patients undergoing intensive follow-up ($p = 0.0001$). Those patients in the intensive follow-up group with a recurrence had a 3.62 times higher survival rate than those in the control ($p = 0.0004$). The authors concluded that intensive follow-up detects more recurrent cancers at a stage amenable to curative resection, resulting in an improvement in survival from recurrences and an increased overall 5-year cumulative rate of survival.

In our practice, patients undergo postoperative follow-up evaluations every 3 to 4 months for at least 2 years. These periodic evaluations include a history and physical examination, digital rectal examination, proctoscopic examination, and a carcinoembryonic antigen measurement. Endorectal ultrasound is performed when abnormalities are appreciated on digital rectal examination. However, routine ultrasound may be advisable inasmuch as de Anda et al. (119) reported that among a series of patients with asymptomatic local recurrences, the recurrence was identified only by ultrasound in a third of the patients; the diagnosis had been missed on digital rectal examination and proctoscopy.

REFERENCES

1. Chessin DB, Guillem JG. Abdominoperineal resection for rectal cancer: historic perspective and current issues. *Surg Oncol Clin North Am*. 2005;14:569–586.
2. Jeong SY, Chessin DB, Guillem JG. Surgical treatment of rectal cancer: Radical resection. Surgical Oncology. *Clinics of North America*. 2006;15:95–107.
3. Baik SH, Kim NK, Lee KY, et al. Hand-sewn coloanal anastomosis for distal rectal cancer: Long-term clinical outcomes. *Journal of Gastrointestinal Surgery: Official Journal of the Society for Surgery of the Alimentary Tract*. 2005;9:775–780.
4. Grinell RS. Distal intramural spread of carcinoma of the rectum and rectosigmoid. *Surg Gynecol Obstet*. 1954;99:421–430.
5. Black WA, Waugh JM. The intramural extension of carcinoma of the descending colon, sigmoid, and rectosigmoid: a pathologic study. *Surg Gynecol Obstet*. 1948;87:457–464.
6. Quer EA, Dahlin DC, Mayo CW. Retrograde intramural spread of carcinoma of the rectum and rectosigmoid: a microscopic study. *Surg Gynecol Obstet*. 1953;96:24–30.

7. Pollett WG, Nicholls RJ. The relationship between the extent of distal clearance and survival and local recurrence rates after curative anterior resection for carcinoma of the rectum. *Ann Surg.* 1983;198:159–163.

8. Goligher JC, Dukes CE, Bussey HJ. Local recurrences after sphincter saving excisions for carcinoma of the rectum and rectosigmoid. *Br J Surg.* 1951;39:199–211.

9. Dukes CE. The surgical pathology of rectal cancer. *Proc R Soc Med.* 1943;37:131.

10. Wolmark N, Fisher B, Wieand HS. The prognostic value of the modifications of the Dukes' C class of colorectal cancer. An analysis of the NSABP clinical trials. *Ann Surg.* 1986;203:115–122.

11. Nelson H, Petrelli N, Carlin A, et al. Guidelines 2000 for colon and rectal cancer surgery. *J Natl Cancer Inst.* 2001;93:583–596.

12. Lee SH, Hernandez de Anda E, Finne CO, et al. The effect of circumferential tumor location in clinical outcomes of rectal cancer patients treated with total mesorectal excision. *Diseases of the Colon and Rectum.* 2005;48:2249–2257.

13. Cecil TD, Sexton R, Moran BJ, et al. Total mesorectal excision results in low local recurrence rates in lymph node positive rectal cancer. *Dis Colon Rectum.* 2004;47:1145–1149.

14. Krook, JE, Moertel CG, Gunderson, LL. Et al. Effective surgical adjuvant therapy for high-risk rectal carcinoma. *N Engl J Med.* 1991;324:709–715.

15. Adam IJ, Mohamdee MO, Martin Ig, et al. Role of circumferential margin involvement in the local recurrence of rectal cancer. *Lancet.* 1994;344:707–711.

16. Cawthorn SJ, Parums DV, Gibbs NM, et al. Extent of mesorectal spread and involvement of lateral resection margin as prognostic factors after surgery for rectal cancer. *Lancet.* 1990;335:1055–1058.

17. Arbman G, Milsson E, Hallbook O, et al. Local recurrence following total mesorectal excision for rectal cancer. *Br J Surg.* 1996;83:375–379.

18. Havenga K, DeRuiter MC, Enker WE, et al. Anatomical basis of autonomic nerve preserving total mesorectal excision for rectal cancer. *Br J Surg.* 1996;83:384–388.

19. Enker WE, Thaler HT, Cranor ML, et al. Total mesorectal excision in the operative treatment of carcinoma of the rectum. *J Am Coll Surg.* 1995;191:335–346.

20. MacFarlane JK, Ryall RDH, Heald RJ. Mesorectal excision for rectal cancer. *Lancet.* 1993;341:457–460.

21. Bolognese A, Cardi M, Muttillo IA, et al. Total mesorectal excision for surgical treatment of rectal cancer. *J Surg Oncol.* 2000:21–23.

22. Nagtegaal ID, van de Velde CJ, Jarijnen CA, et al. Low rectal cancer: a call for a change of approach in abdominoperineal resection. *J Clin Oncol.* 2005;23:9257–9264.

23. Guillem JG. Ultra-low anterior resection and coloanal pouch reconstruction for carcinoma of the distal rectum. *World J Surg.* 1997;21:721–227.

24. Nagtegaal ID, van de Velde CJ, van der Worp E, et al. Macroscopic evaluation of rectal cancer resection specimen: clinical significance of the pathologist in quality control. *J Clin Oncol.* 2002;20:1729–1734.

25. Heald RJ, Husband EM, Ryall RD. The mesorectum in rectal cancer surgery—the clue to pelvic recurrence? *Br J Surg.* 1982;69:613.

26. Quirke P, Durdey P, Dixon MF, et al. Local recurrence of rectal adenocarcinoma due to inadequate surgical resection. histopathological study of lateral tumour spread and surgical excision. *Lancet.* 1986;2:996–999.

27. Marijnen CA, Nagtegaal ID, Kapiteijn E, et al. Cooperative investigators of the Dutch Colerectal Cancer Group. Radiotherapy does not compensate for positive resection margins in rectal cancer patients: Report of a multicenter randomized trial. *International Journal of Radiation Oncology, Biology, Physics.* 2003;55:1311–1320.

28. Moore HG, Riedel E, Minsky BD, et al. Adequacy of 1- centimeter distal margin after restorative rectal cancer resection with sharp mesorectal excision and preoperative combined-modality therapy. *Ann Surg Oncol.* 2003;10:80–85.

29. Nagtegaal ID, Marijnen CAA, Kranenbarg EK, et al. Circumferential margin involvement is still an important predictor of local recurrence in rectal carcinoma - not one millimeter but two millimeters is the limit. *American Journal of Surgical Pathology.* 2002;26:350–357.

30. Greene FL, Page DL, Fleming ID, et al. Colon and rectum. In: *American Joint Committee on Cancer AJCC Cancer Staging Manual.* 6th ed. New YouK: Springer; 2002:113–124.

31. Compton CC, Greene FL. The staging of colorectal cancer: 2004 and beyond. *CA Cancer J Clin.* 2004;54:295–308.

32. Swanson RS, Compton CC, Stewart AK, et al. The prognosis of T3N0 colon cancer is dependent on the number of lymph nodes examined. *Ann Surg Oncol.* 2003;10:65–71.

33. Le Voyer TE, Sigurdson ER, Hanlon AL, et al. Colon cancer survival is associated with increasing number of lymph nodes analyzed: a secondary survey of intergroup trial INT-0089. *J Clin Oncol.* 2003;21:2912–2919.

34. Prandi M, Lionetto R, Bini A, et al. Prognostic evaluation of stage B colon cancer patients is improved by an adequate lymphadenectomy: results of a secondary analysis of a large scale adjuvant trial. *Ann Surg.* 2002;235:458–463.

35. Tepper JE, O'Connell MJ, Niedzwiecki D, et al. Impact of number of nodes retrieved on outcome in patients with rectal cancer. *J Clin Oncol.* 2001;19:157–163.

36. Heald RJ. Rectal cancer: anterior resection and local recurrence—a personal view. *Perspect Colon Rectal Surg.* 1988;1:1–26.

37. Masui H, Ike H, Yamaguchi S, et al. Male sexual function after autonomic nerve-preserving operation for rectal cancer. *Dis Colon Rectum.* 1996;39:1140–1145.

38. Fucini C, Elbetti C, Petrolo A, et al. Excision of the levator muscles with external sphincter preservation in the treatment of selected low T4 rectal cancers. *Dis Colon Rectum.* 2002;45:1697–1705.

39. Wiggers T. Staging of rectal cancer. *Br J Surg.* 2003;90:895–896.

40. Cance WG, Cohen AM, Enker WE, et al. Predictive value of a negative computed tomorgraphic scan in 100 patients with rectal carcinoma. *Dis Colon Rectum.* 1991;34:748–751.

41. Clark J, Bankoff M, Carter B, et al. The use of computerized tomography scan in the staging and follow-up study of carcinoma of the rectum. *Surg Gynecol Obstet.* 1984;159:335–342.

42. Koehler PR, Feldber MAM, van Waes PFGM. Preoperative staging of rectal cancer with computerized tomography. *Cancer.* 1984;54:512–516.

43. Shank B, Dershaw DD, Caravelli J, et al. A prospective study of the accuracy of preoperative computed tomographic staging of patients with biopsy-proven rectal carcinoma. *Dis Colon Rectum.* 1990;33:285–290.

44. van Waes PFGM, Koehler PR, Geldber MAM. Management of rectal carcinoma: impact of computed tomography. *AJR Am J Roentgenol.* 1983;140:1137–1142.

45. Beets-Tan RGH, Beets GL, Vliegen RFA, et al. Accuracy of magnetic resonance imaging in prediction of tumour-free resection margin in rectal cancer surgery. *Lancet.* 2001;357:497–504.

46. Heriot AG, Grundy A, Kumar D. Preoperative staging of rectal carcinoma. *British Journal of Surgery.* 1999;86:17–28.

47. Akasu T, Iinuma G, Fujita T, et al. Thin-section MRI with a phased-array coil for preoperative evaluation of pelvic anatomy and tumor extent in patients with rectal cancer. *AJR. American Journal of Roentgenology.* 2005;184:531–538.

48. Garcia-Aguilar J, Pollack J, Lee SH, et al. Accuracy of endorectal ultrasonography in preoperative staging of rectal tumors. *Diseases of the Colon and Rectum*. 2002;45:10–15.

49. Guillem JG, Diaz-Gonzalez JA, Minsky BD, et al. cT3N0 rectal cancer: potential overtreatment with preoperative chemoradiotherapy is warranted. *J Clin Oncol*. 2008;25:368–373.

50. Kachnic LA, Hong TS, Ryan DP. Rectal cancer at the crossroads: the dilemma of clinically staged T3, N0, M0 disease. *J Clin Oncol*. 2008;26:350–351.

51. Saclarides TJ, Bhattacharyya AK, Britton-Kuzel C, et al. Predicting lymph node metastases in rectal cancer. *Diseases of the Colon and Rectum*. 1994;37:52–57.

52. Mendenhall WM, Blan KI, Copeland EM, ed., et al. Does preoperative radiation therapy enhance the probability of local control and survival in high-risk distal rectal cancer? *Ann Surg*. 1992;215:696–706.

53. Myerson RJ, Michalski JM, King ML et al. Adjuvant radiation therapy for rectal carcinoma: predictors of outcome. *Int J Radiat Oncol Biol Phys*. 1995;32:41–50.

54. Chari RS, Tyler DS, Anscher MS, et al. Preoperative radiation and chemotherapy in the treatment of adenocarcinoma of the rectum. *Ann Surg*. 1995;221:778–784.

55. Minsky BD, Cohen AM, Kemeny N, et al. Enhancement of radiation-induced downstaging of rectal cancer by fluorouracil and high-dose leucovorin chemotherapy. *J Clin Oncol*. 1992;10:79–84.

56. Ngan SY, Burmeister BH, Fisher R, et al. Early toxicity from preoperative radiotherapy with continuous infusion 5-fluorouracil for resectable adenocarcinoma of the rectum: a phase II trial for the Trans-Tasman Radiation Oncology Group. *Int J Radiat Oncol Biol Phys*. 2001;50:883–887.

57. Janjan NA, Crane, C, Feig BW, et al. Improved overall survival among responders to preoperative chemoradiation for locally advanced rectal cancer. *Am J Clin Oncol*. 2001;24:107–112.

58. Bosset JF, Manin V, Maingon P, et al. Properative radiochemotherapy in rectal cancer: long-term results of a phase II trial. *Int J Radiat Oncol Biol Phys*. 2000;46:323–327.

59. Rich TA, Skibber JM, Ajani JA, et al. Preoperative infusional chemoradiation therapy for stafe T3 rectal cancer. *Int J Radiat Oncol Biol Phys*. 1995;32:1025–1029.

60. Kim J, Kim J, Cho M, et al. Preoperative chemoradiation using oral capecitabine in locally advanced rectal cancer. *Int J Radiat Oncol Biol Phys*. 2002;54:403–408.

61. Mehta VK, Cho C, Ford JM, et al. Phase II trail of preoperative 3D conformal radiotherapy, protacted venous infusion 5-fluorouracil, and weekly CPT-11, followed by surgery for ultrasound-staged T3 rectal cancer. *Int J Radiat Oncol Biol Phys*. 2003;55:132–137.

62. Gerard JP, Chapet O, Nemoz C, et al. Preoperative concurrent chemoradiotherapy in locally advanced rectal cancer with high-dose radiation and oxaliplatin-containing regimen: The Lyon R0-04 Phase II Trial. *J Clin Oncol*. 2003;21:1119–1124.

63. Valentini V, Coco C, Picciocchi A, et al. Does downstaging predict improved outcome after preoperative chemoradiation for extraperitoneal locally advanced rectal cancer? A long-term analysis of 165 patients. *Int J Radiat Oncol Biol Phys*. 2002;53:664–674.

64. Mohiuddin M, Hayhne M, Regine WF, et al. Prognostic significance of post-chemoradiation stage following preoperative chemotherapy and radiation for advanced/recurrent rectal cancers. *Int J Radiat Oncol Biol Phys*. 2000;48:1075–1080.

65. Roh MS, Colangelo L, Wieand S, et al. Response to preoperative multimodality therapy predicts survival in patients with carcinoma of the rectum (abstract). *Proc Am Soc Clin Oncol*. 2004;23:247a.

66. Ruo L, Tickoo S, Klimstra DS, et al. Long-term prognostic significance of extent of rectal cancer response to preoperative radiation and chemotherapy. *Ann Surg*. 2002;236:75–81.

67. Gerard JP, Conroy T, Bonnetain F, et al. Preoperative radiotherapy with or without concurrent fluoruacil and leucovorin in T3-4 rectal cancers: results of FFCD 9203. *J Clin Oncol*. 2006;24:4260.

68. Bosset JF, Calais G, Mineur L, et al. Enhanced tumorocidal effect of chemotherapy with preoperative radiotherapy for rectal cancer. Preliminary results—EORTC 22921. *J Clin Oncol*. 2005;23:5620–5627.

69. Bosset JF, Collette L, Calais G, et al. Chemotherapy with preoperative radiotherapy in rectal cancer. *N Engl J Med*. 2006;355:1114–1123.

70. Bujko K, Mowacki MP, Nasierowska-Guttmejer A, et al. Sphincter preservation following preoperative radiotherapy for rectal cancer: report of a randomized trial comparing short-term radiotherapy vs. conventionally fractionated radiochemotherapy. *Radiother Oncol*. 2004;72:15–24.

71. Sauer R, Becker H, Hohenberger W, et al. Preoperative versus postoperative chemoradiotherapy for rectal cancer. *N Engl J Med*. 2004;351:1731–1740.

72. Roh MS, Petrilli N, Wieand S, et al. Phase III randomized trial of preoperative versus postoperative multimodality therapy in patients with carcinoma of the rectum: (NSABP-R03) (abstract). *Proc Am Soc Clinic Oncol*. 2001;20:123a.

73. Frykholm GJ, Glimelius B, Pahlman L. Preoperative or postoperative irradiation in adenocarcinoma of the rectum: final treatment results of a randomized trial and an evaluation of late secondary effects. *Dis Colon Rectum*. 1993;36:564–572.

74. Habr-Gama A, Perez RO, Nadalin W, et al. Long-term results of preoperative chemoradiation for distal rectal cancer correlation between final stage and survival. *J Gastrointest Surg*. 2005;9:90–99.

75. Habr-Gama A, Perez RO, Proscurshim I, et al. Patterns of failure and survival for nonoperative treatment of stage c0 distal rectal cancer following neoadjuvant chemoradiation therapy. *J Gastrointest Surg*. 2006;10:1319–1328.

76. Enker WE, Merchant N, Cohen AM, et al. Safety and efficacy of low anterior resection for rectal cancer: 681 consecutive cases from a specialty service. *Ann Surg*. 1999;230:544–552.

77. Baxter NN, Garcia-Aguilar J. Organ preservation for rectal cancer. *J Clin Oncol*. 2007;25:1014–1020.

78. Shibata D, Guillem JG, Lanouette N, et al. Functional and quality of life outcomes in patients with rectal cancer after combined modality therapy, intraoperative radiation therapy, and sphincter preservation. *Dis Colon Rectum*. 2000;43:752–758.

79. Davies RJ. Hospital volume and operative mortality in cancer surgery—A national study—invited critique. *Arch Surg*. 2003;138:726.

80. Dimick JB, Cowan JA, Jr., Upchurch GR, Jr., et al. Hospital volume and surgical outcomes for elderly patients with colorectal cancer in the United States. *Journal of Surgical Research*. 2003;09;114:50–56.

81. Jessup JM, Stewart AK, Menck HR. The National Cancer Data Base report on patterns of care for adenocarcinoma of the rectum, 1985–1995. *Cancer*. 1998;83:2408–2418.

82. Williams NS, Johnston D. Survival and recurrence after sphincter saving resection and abdominoperineal resection for carcinoma of the middle third of the rectum. *Br J Surg*. 1984;71:278–282.

83. Williams NS, Drudey P, Johnston D. The outcome following sphincter-saving resection and abdominoperineal resection for low rectal cancer. *Br J Surg*. 1985;72:595–598.

84. Williams NS, Johnston D. The quality of life after rectal excision for low rectal cancer. *Br J Surg*. 1983;70:460–462.

85. Onaitis M, Ludwig K, Peres-Tamayo A, et al. The Kraske procedure: a critical analysis of a surgical approach for mid-rectal lesions. *J Surg Oncol.* 2006;94:194–202.

86. Gimbel MI, Paty PB. A current perspective on local excision of rectal cancer. *Clin Colorectal Cancer.* 2004;4:26–35.

87. Steele GD, Herndon JE, Bleday R, et al. Sphincter-sparing treatment for distal rectal adenocarcinoma. *Ann Surg Oncol.* 1999;6:443–451.

88. Paty PB, Nash GM, Baron P, et al. Long-term results of local excision for rectal cancer. *Ann Surg.* 2002;236:522–529.

89. You YN, Baxter NN, Stewart A, et al. Is the increasing rate of local excision for stage I rectal cancer in the United States justified? a nationwise cohort study from the National Cancer Database. *Ann Surg.* 2007;245:726–733.

90. Ota D, Nelson H. Local excision of rectal cancer revisited: ACOSOG Protocol Z6041. *Ann Surg Oncol.* 2006;14:271.

91. Neary P, Makin GB, White TJ, et al. Transanal endoscopic microsurgery: a viable operative alternative in selected patients with rectal lesions. *Ann Surg Oncol.* 2003;10:1106–1111.

92. Wang HS, Lin JK, Yang SH, et al. Prospective study of the functional results of transanal endoscopic microsurgery. *Hetpatogastroenterology.* 2003;50:1376–1380.

93. Lee W, Lee D, Choi S, et al. Transanal endoscopic microsurgery and radical surgery for T1 and T2 rectal cancer. *Surg Endos.* 2003;17:1283–1287.

94. Langer C, Liersch T, Suss M, et al. Surgical cure for early rectal carcinoma and large adenoma: transanal endocsopic microsurgery compared to conventional local and radical resection. *Int J Colorectal Dis.* 2003;18:222–229.

95. Araki Y, Isomoto H, Shirouzu K. Video-assisted gasless transanal endoscopic microsurgery: a review of 217 cases of rectal tumors over the past 10 years. *Dig Surg.* 2003;20:48–52.

96. Demartines N, von Flue MO, Harder FH. Transanal endoscopic microsurgical excision of rectal tumors: indications and results. *World J Surg.* 2001;25:870–875.

97. Winde G, Nottberg H, Keller R, et al. Surgical cure for early rectal carcinomas (T1). Transanal endoscopic microsurgery vs. anterior resection. *Dis Colon Rectum.* 1996;39:969–976.

96. Guerrieri M, Feliciotti F, Baldarelli M, et al. Sphincter-saving surgery in patients with rectal cancer treated by radiotherapy and transanl endoscopic microsurgery: 10 years' experience. *Dig Liv Dis.* 2003;35:876–880.

98. Stipa F, Lucandri G, Ferri M, et al. Local excision of rectal cancer with transanal endoscopic microsurgery (TEM). *Anticancer Res.* 2004;24:1167–1172.

99. Smith LE, Ko ST, Saclarides T, et al. Transanal endoscopic microsurgery: initial registry results. *Dis Colon Rectum.* 1996;39:579–584.

100. Saclarides TJ. TEM/local excision: indications, techniques, outcomes, and the future. *J Surg Oncol.* 2007;96:644–650.

101. Whiteford MH. Transanal endoscopic microsurgery (TEM) resection of rectal tumors. *J Gastrointest Surg.* 2007;11:155–157.

102. Suppiah A, Maslekar S, Alabi A, et al. Transanal endoscopic microsurgery in early rectal cancer: time for a trial? *Colorectal Dis.* 2008 (Epub ahead of print).

103. Gavagan JA, Whiteford MH, Swnastrom LL. Full-thickness intraperitoneal excision by transanal endoscopic microsurgery does not increase short term complications. *Am J Surg.* 2004;187:630–634.

104. Chorost MI. Sexual dysfunction, informed consent and multimodality therapy for rectal cancer. *American Journal of Surgery.* 2000;179:271–274.

105. Baran JJ, Goldstein SD, Resnik AM. The double-staple technique in colorectal anastomoses: a critical review. *Am Surg.* 1992;58:270–272.

106. Leff EI, Shaver JO, Hoexter B, et al. Anastomotic recurrences after low anterior resection. Stapled vs. hand-sewn. *Dis Colon Rectum.* 1985;28:164–167.

107. Merad F, Hay JM, Fingerhut A, et al. Is prophylactic pelvic drainage useful after elective rectal or anal anastomsis? A multicenter controlled randomized trial. *French Association for Surgical Research. Surgery.* 1999;125:529–535.

108. Fazio VW. Sump suction and irrigation of the presacral space. *Dis Colon Rectum.* 1978;21:401–405.

109. Karanjia ND, Corder AP, Bearn P, et al. Leakage from stapled low anastomosis after total mesorectal excision for carcinoma of the rectum. *Br J Surg.* 1994;1224–1226.

110. Gastinger I, Marusch F, Steinert R, et al. Working Group "Colon/Rectum Carcinoma". Protective defunctioning stoma in low anterior resection for rectal carcinoma. *The British Journal of Surgery.* 2005;92:1137–1142.

111. Gordon PH. Malignant neoplasms of the rectum. In: Gordon PH, Nivatvongs S, eds. *Neoplasms of the Colon, Rectum, and Anus.* 2nd ed. New York: Informa Healthcare USA, Inc.;2007:20–304.

112. Lazorthes F, Chiotasso P, Gamagami RA, et al. Late clinical outcome in a randomized prospective comparison of colonic J pouch and straight coloanal anastomosis. *Br J Surg.* 1997;84:1449–1451.

113. Z'graggen K, Mauer CA, Birrer S, et al. A new surgical concept for rectal replacement after low anterior resection: the transverse coloplasty pouch. *Ann Surg.* 2001;234:780–785.

114. Fazio VW, Zutshi M, Remzi FH, et al. A randomized multicenter trial to compare long-term functional outcome, quality of life, and complications of surgical procedures for low rectal cancers. *Ann Surg.* 2007;246:481–488.

115. Furst A, Suttner S, Agha A, et al. Colonic J-pouch vs. coloplasty following resection of distal rectal cancer: early results of a prospective, randomized, pilot study. *Dis Colon Rectum.* 2003;46:1161–1166.

116. Pugliese R, Di Lernia S, Sansonna F, et al. Results of laparoscopic anterior resection for rectal adenocarcinoma: retrospective analysis of 157 cases. *Am J Surg.* 2008;195:233–238.

117. Rosen LS, Bilchik AJ, Beart RW, Jr., et al. New approaches to assessing and treating early-stage colon and rectal cancer: summary statement from 2007 Santa Monica conference. *Clin Cancer Res.* 2007;13:6853s–6856s.

118. Rosen M, Chan L, Beart RW, Jr., et al. Follow-up of colorectal cancer: A meta-analysis. *Diseases of the Colon and Rectum.* 1998;41:1116–1126.

119. de Anda EH, Lee SH, Finne CO, et al. Endorectal ultrasound in the follow-up of rectal cancer patients treated by local excision or radical surgery. *Dis Colon Rectum.* 2004;47:818–824.

COMMENTARY
Phillip R. Fleshner

I would like to congratulate the authors on this very well written and insightful Chapter 39 on sphincter preservation in rectal cancer. However, I would like to both expand on a few points and discuss some important issues that have not been addressed.

Current TNM guidelines state that at least 12 nodes should be examined before a patient can be classified as having N0 disease (1). In practice, retrieval of even 12 nodes can be difficult to achieve in many cases, as shown by recent results of the Dutch total mesorectal excision (TME) trial, in which 82% of node-negative patients had <12 nodes examined, regardless of neoadjuvant radiotherapy (2). However, a high motivation to find as many nodes as possible must be maintained, as several studies support the concept that the more nodes that are examined, the more accurate the staging. Caplin and coworkers (3) showed that node-negative patients with less than seven nodes examined had a prognosis similar to that of node-positive patients. In addition, Tepper et al. (4) reported that among node-negative patients, those in whom ≥14 nodes were examined had a better recurrence-free survival compared with those with <8 nodes examined. In addition, it is conceivable that lowering the limit to 12 for the number of nodes that must be found may lead to understaging as specimen prosectors look for the minimum number of nodes and potentially exclude harder-to-find nodes that are closer to the rectal wall.

Routine visual inspection, palpation, and dissection are still the standard of practice for lymph node retrieval, and the extent of examination as well as the enthusiasm of the examiner are some of the most important factors in determining the number of nodes retrieved. In order to address the challenge of lymph node yield, a number of adjunctive methods have been developed, including fat stretching, alcohol treatment, xylene clearance, wintergreen oil/cedar oil clearance, and ether-based methods (5–9). In fact, the most recent protocol for the examination of colorectal cancer specimens from the Cancer Committee of the College of American Pathologists recommends that if fewer than 12 nodes are found with traditional methods, then the use of "visual enhancement techniques" should be considered (10). Although most of the previously mentioned methods require special equipment, the use of noxious volatile compounds, or prolonged treatment of pericolic fat (up to 3 weeks), Newell et al. (11) successfully used GEWF solution (glacial acetic acid, ethanol, distilled water, and formaldehyde), which is an easily prepared, nonnoxious solution with a quick turn-around performance (24 hours), to obtain a significant increase in lymph node yield.

Drs. Ault and Beart state that "current surgical techniques allow us to remove virtually any tumor in this area without removing the anal canal." Although safe anastomoses at the distal rectum or the anal canal have been made possible by advances of mechanical stapling devices and development of the double-stapling technique, the notion that current surgical techniques allow surgeons to remove virtually any tumor without removing the anal canal is not quite a reality. For example, there are limited options besides combined abdominoperineal resection for bulky tumors lying at or below the puborectalis below the anorectal line. Intersphincteric resection (ISR) with coloanal anastomosis, however, has been performed for these tumors in a number of specialized institutions (12–14). Defecatory function is an especially important clinical outcome measure after sphincter-saving resection for low rectal cancer. However, with the ISR technique, the internal anal sphincter is either partially or completely excised, and a variable portion of anoderm is also removed. This raises the question of how anal canal resting pressure and anal sensation are maintained. The maximum resting anal canal pressure is maintained by the internal anal sphincter (15) and, as expected, had fallen by 3 months after ISR in all patients (16). Moreover, it has been reported that patients who have had ISR experience a diminished quality of life because of fecal inconti-

nence compared with those with a conventional coloanal anastomosis (17,18). The use of ISR should be strongly discouraged. Moreover, all patients must know going into any of these operations that there is a chance they will require a permanent colostomy.

The emerging role of positron emission tomography (PET) in the preoperative and postoperative evaluation of these patients requires comment. PET has the distinct advantage of being able to image cellular metabolic changes of cancer before the detection of structural, anatomic changes by conventional imaging modalities, such as ultrasound, computed tomography, and magnetic resonance imaging. This may result in detection of tumor at a stage earlier than that possible by conventional anatomic imaging. For primary disease, it is potentially useful in the assessment of locoregional and metastatic disease, and in the assessment of tumor response to preoperative chemoradiation. A prospective series of 46 patients with primary rectal cancer was studied in order to assess the potential impact of ^{18}F-fluorodeoxyglucose PET on treatment plan. Patients were evaluated with conventional imaging (including endoscopy and computed tomography) followed by PET, and the treatment plan was prospectively recorded before and after the PET scan. PET results altered the preoperative stage in 18 (39%) patients and altered management in 8 (17%) In six patients (13%), operations were cancelled because unresectable metastatic disease was detected, and in two patients (4%), the radiotherapy field was adjusted (19). For suspected recurrent rectal cancer, it may be used as the initial imaging study of the metastatic workup or after equivocal anatomic imaging (20,21).

For patients with stage II or III rectal cancer, data support the use of preoperative concurrent radiation and fluorouracil, and resection performed by total mesorectal excision. Although randomized data are not available to support the use of bevacizumab, capecitabine, cetuximab, irinotecan, or oxaliplatin in the adjuvant treatment of rectal cancer, it is also unclear what role if any these newer cytotoxic and targeted agents will play in the preoperative treatment of these patients. Initial results of the EXPERT trial (a phase 2 study of oxaliplatin [Eloxtin], capecitabine [Xeloda], and preoperative radiotherapy for patients with locally advanced and inoperable rectal cancer) have been recently reported (22). Eligible patients had magnetic resonance imaging–defined poor-risk features including tumor extension within 1 mm or beyond of the mesorectal fascia, T3 tumors at or below the levators, tumor extending ≥5 mm into perirectal fat, and T4 or T1–4 N2 tumors. Sixty-seven patients proceeded to appropriate surgery after an interval of 6 weeks with total mesorectal excision. A pathologic complete response occurred in 24% of patients, and another 48% were noted to have residual microscopic disease only. Further progress in this field depends on the completion of this and other well-designed clinical trials.

Modern rectal surgery is not without morbidity, and many patients wish to avoid the permanent stoma associated with abdominoperineal excision. However, preoperative treatments have developed to such a degree that pathologic complete responses can reach 25% at the time of surgery (23,24). The impressive incidence of pathologic complete responses in recent trials raises the possibility of selecting patients who have a clinical complete response to preoperative treatment and avoiding surgery. Long-term results have been reported by Habr-Gama and colleagues (25) on omission of surgery for selected patients with radiologic and clinical evidence of complete response after neoadjuvant chemoradiotherapy (CRT). Distal resectable rectal tumors in 265 patients were treated with preoperative CRT from 1991 to 2002. Radiotherapy was delivered at a dose of 50.4 Gy in 1.8-Gy fractions for 6 consecutive weeks. Concomitant chemotherapy consisted of fluorouracil and folinic acid on the first 3 days and last 3 days of radiotherapy. Patients were assessed at 8 weeks after completion of CRT. Seventy-one patients (27%) were deemed to have achieved complete response on clinical and radiologic grounds. These patients with complete clinical response did not have surgery, forming an observation group. All other patients proceeded to surgery. At a median follow-up of almost 5 years, overall and disease-free survival was 88% and 83% in the resection group and 100% and 92% in the observation group, respectively. This series was updated in 2005 and again in 2006 (26,27), now extending to 360 patients treated up to 2005, with an additional 28 (now 99 in total) patients classified as having achieved complete clinical response, and, therefore, avoiding surgery. Local recurrence has occurred in three additional patients (five in total) in the CRT group, all amenable to salvage surgery, and none of whom have developed further recurrence. Although the study by Habr-Gama and colleagues (25) is extremely promising, prospective randomized trials are sorely needed.

The importance of complete removal of the lymphovascular tissue surrounding the rectum and a free circumferential margin has been recognized in the management of rectal cancer (28). By sharp meticulous perimesorectal dissection and TME, many centers have reported low local recurrence rates in patients with rectal cancer (29,30). However, routine TME in rectal cancer at all levels has been challenged in view of the increased morbidity associated with TME. The anastomotic leakage rates are high in series of patients with TME (31). Moreover, bowel function will also be adversely affected with a low colorectal or coloanal anastomosis (32). A recent report revealed that partial mesorectal excision for cancer at the upper rectum or rectosigmoid yields similar results when compared with TME for mid and distal rectal cancer in terms of local recurrence and survival. However, TME was associated with a longer operating time, more blood loss, longer hospital stay, a higher leakage rate, and a higher stoma rate (33). Thus, a selective approach using TME for mid and distal rectal cancer is more appropriate and reasonable. For tumors at upper rectum or rectosigmoid, transection of the rectum and mesorectum 4 to 5 cm below the lower border of the tumor following sharp perimesorectal dissection appears to be acceptable. These clinical results corroborate a pathologic study that found that the median extent of distal mesorectal spread (3.6 cm) was greater than the extent of intramural spread (1.2 cm). This article concluded that a 4-cm distal mesorectal margin is necessary to achieve adequate surgical clearance (34).

Laparoscopic resection must prove equivalent to open surgery with solid data before becoming an accepted surgical modality for rectal cancer. Unfortunately, there is a paucity of high-quality evidence to support the practice of laparoscopic resection. Only a single, large, prospective controlled study of laparoscopic surgery has reported on both colon cancer and rectal cancer (35). This study specifically raised concerns regarding laparoscopic resection. In the rectal surgery subgroup, circum-

ferential radial margin positivity was greater in the laparoscopic group when compared with open surgery. This difference was not appreciated in the abdominal perineal laparoscopic procedure group, but was specific to the laparoscopic low anterior resection procedure. The results of additional prospective, randomized trials will ultimately define the appropriate place of laparoscopic resection.

REFERENCES

1. Sobin L, Greene F. TNM classification. *Cancer.* 2001;92:452.
2. Marijnen CA, Nagtegaal ID, Klein Kranenberg E, et al. No downstaging after short-term preoperative radiotherapy in rectal cancer patients. *J Clin Oncol.* 2001;19:1976–1984.
3. Caplin S, Cerottini J, Bosman F, et al. For patients with Dukes' B (TNM stage II) colorectal carcinoma, examination of six or fewer lymph nodes is related to poor prognosis. *Cancer.* 1998;83:666–672.
4. Tepper J, O'Connell M, Niedzwiecki D, et al. Impact of number of nodes retrieved on outcome in patients with rectal cancer. *J Clin Oncol.* 2001;19:157–163.
5. Crucitti F, Doglietto GB, Bellantone R, et al. Accurate specimen preparation is mandatory to detect lymph nodes and avoid understaging in colorectal cancer. *J Surg Oncol.* 1992;51:153–158.
6. Cawthorn SJ, Gibbs NM, Marks CG. Clearance technique for the detection of lymph nodes in colorectal cancer. *Br J Surg.* 1986;73:58–60.
7. Haboubi NY, Clark P, Kaftan SM, et al. The importance of xylene clearance and immunohistochemistry in the accurate staging of colorectal carcinoma. *J R Soc Med.* 1992;85:386–388.
8. Hyder JW, Talbott TM, Maycroft TC. A critical review of chemical lymph node clearance and staging of colon and rectal cancer at Ferguson Hospital, 1977 to 1982. *Dis Colon Rectum.* 1990;33:923–925.
9. Koren R, Siegal A, Klein B, et al. Lymph node-revealing solution: simple new method for detecting minute lymph nodes in colon carcinoma. *Dis Colon Rectum.* 1997;40:407–410.
10. Compton CC. Updated protocol for the examination of specimens from patients with carcinomas of the colon and rectum, excluding carcinoid tumors, lymphomas, sarcomas, and tumors of the vermiform appendix: a basis for checklists. Cancer Committee. *Arch Pathol Lab Med.* 2000;124:1016–1025.
11. Newell KJ, Sawka BW, Rudrick BF, et al. GEWF solution. *Arch Pathol Lab Med.* 2001;125:642–645.
12. Rullier E, Zerbib F, Laurent C, et al. Intersphincteric resection with excision of internal anal sphincter for conservative treatment of very low rectal cancer. *Dis Colon Rectum.* 1999;42:1168–1175.
13. Shirouzu K, Ogata Y, Araki Y, et al. A new ultimate anus-preserving operation for extremely low rectal cancer and for anal canal cancer. *Tech Coloproctol.* 2003;7:203–206.
14. Saito N, Ono M, Sugito M, et al. Early results of intersphincteric resection for patients with very low rectal cancer: an active approach to avoid a permanent colostomy. *Dis Colon Rectum.* 2004;47:459–466.
15. Frenckner B, Euler CV. Influence of pudendal block on the function of the anal sphincters. *Gut.* 1975;16:482–489.
16. Yamada K, Ogata S, Saiki Y, et al. Functional results of intersphincteric resection for low rectal cancer. *Br J Surg* 2007;94:1272–1277.
17. Renner K, Rosen HR, Novi G, et al. Quality of life after surgery for rectal cancer: do we still need a permanent colostomy? *Dis Colon Rectum.* 1999;42:1160–1167.
18. Bretagnol F, Rullier E, Laurent C, et al. Comparison of functional results and quality of life between intersphincteric resection and

conventional coloanal anastomosis for low rectal cancer. *Dis Colon Rectum.* 2004;47:832–838.

19. Heriot AG, Hicks RJ, Drummond EG, et al. Does positron emission tomography change management in primary rectal cancer? A prospective assessment. *Dis Colon Rectum.* 2004;47:451–458.

20. Moore HG, AkhurstT, Larson SM, et al. A case-controlled study of 18-fluorodeoxyglucose positron emission tomography in the detection of pelvic recurrence in previously irradiated rectal cancer patients. *J Am Coll Surg.* 2003;197:22–28.

21. Even-Sapir E, Parag Y, Lerman H, et al. Detection of recurrence in patients with rectal cancer: PET/CT after abdominoperineal or anterior resection. *Radiology.* 2004;232:815–822.

22. Chau I, Brown G, Cunningham D, et al. Neoadjuvant capecitabine and oxaliplatin followed by synchronous chemoradiation and total mesorectal excision in magnetic resonance imaging-defined poor risk rectal cancer. J Clin Oncol. 2006;24:668–674.

23. Mohiuddin M, Winter K, Mitchell E, et al. Randomized phase II study of neoadjuvant combined-modality chemoradiation for distal rectal cancer: Radiation Therapy Oncology Group Trial 0012. *J Clin Oncol.* 2006;24:650–655.

24. Ryan DP, Niedzwiecki D, Hollis D, et al. Phase I/II study of preoperative oxaliplatin, fluorouracil, and external-beam radiation therapy in patients with locally advanced rectal cancer: Cancer and Leukemia Group B 89901. *J Clin Oncol.* 2006;24:2557–2562.

25. Habr-Gama A, Perez RO, Nadalin W, et al. Operative versus nonoperative treatment for stage 0 distal rectal cancer following chemoradiation therapy: long-term results. *Ann Surg.* 2004;240:711–717.

26. Habr-Gama A, Perez RO, Nadalin W, et al. Long-term results of preoperative chemoradiation for distal rectal cancer. Correlation

between final stage and survival. *J Gastrointest Surg.* 2005; 9:90–99.

27. Habr-Gama A. Assessment and management of the complete clinical response of rectal cancer to chemoradiotherapy. *Colorectal Dis.* 2006;8(Suppl 3):21–24.

28. Heald RJ, Husband EM, Ryall RD. The mesorectum in rectal cancer surgery: the clue to pelvic recurrence? *Br J Surg.* 1982;69:613–616.

29. Heald RJ, Moran BJ, Ryall RD, et al. Rectal cancer: the Basingstoke experience of total mesorectal excision, 1978-1997. *Arch Surg.* 1998;133:894–899.

30. Enker WE, Thaler HT, Cranor ML, et al. Total mesorectal excision in the operative treatment of carcinoma of the rectum. *J Am Coll Surg.* 1995;181:335–346.

31. Karanjia ND, Corder AP, Bearn P, et al. Leakage from stapled low anastomosis after total mesorectal excision for carcinoma of the rectum. *Br J Surg.* 1994;81:1224–1226.

32. Karanjia ND, Schache DJ, Heald RJ. Function of the distal rectum after low anterior resection for carcinoma. *Br J Surg.* 1992;79:114–116.

33. Law WL, Chu KW. Anterior resection for rectal cancer with mesorectal excision. A prospective evaluation of 622 patients. *Ann Surg.* 2004;240:260–268.

34. Zhao GP, Zhou ZG, Lei WZ, et al. Pathological study of distal mesorectal cancer spread to determine a proper distal resection margin. *World J Gastroenterol.* 2005;11:319–322.

35. Guillou PJ, Quirke P, Thorpe H, et al. Short term endpoints of conventional versus laparoscopic assisted surgery in patients with colorectal cancer (MRC CLASICC trial): multicentre, randomized controlled trial. *Lancet.* 2005;365:1718–1726.

40

Colorectal Cancer: Adjuvant and Neoadjuvant Therapy

Gregory P. Sarna

Although surgery is clearly the treatment modality with curative potential for locoregional colorectal carcinoma, there is a substantial failure rate in this setting. The Surveillance Epidemiology and End Results (SEER) data (1) on 10-year survival in colon and rectal cancer are available for 1973-1987, an era in which adjuvant therapy was often not given, staging imaging studies were limited, diagnosis was often late, and survival after metastatic disease was poor. In this era, 10-year survival for stage I disease approximated 85%, stage II disease 70%, and stage III disease 40%.

Data on 5-year survival are available from more recent large series, which more accurately define current expectations. Table 40.1 presents survival data for colon cancer and rectal cancer (2-5). These data, with better-staged patients receiving adjuvant/neoadjuvant therapy and better treatment for metastatic disease, are generally superior to earlier data. It is apparent, however, that results in rectal cancer are inferior to those in colon cancer. Colorectal cancer is still a substantial cause of mortality. Estimated deaths from colorectal cancer in the United States in 2006 are 49,960 (6), 9% of all cancer deaths and 34% of estimated colorectal cancer incidence (including patients presenting with metastatic disease). It should be noted that over the past 15 to 20 years, the colorectal cancer incidence rate has been falling (6), likely reflecting the improved prevention of colorectal cancer (largely because of screening colonoscopy). The mortality rate has also improved over time, reflecting this phenomenon as well as therapeutic advances.

Stage, as reflected in Table 1, is an important predictor of survival. It is useful to note that subdividing stage II into stages IIA (T3N0) and IIB (T4N0) and stage III into stages IIIA (T1-2, N1), IIIB (T3-4, N1), and IIIC (T1-4, N2) importantly refines prognosis, and patients with stage IIIA disease may actually fare better than those with stage IIB disease. Clinical trials of adjuvant and neoadjuvant therapy have largely been based on stage. Other factors, however, also are of prognostic importance. Such factors might be of value in determining who is or is not a candidate for adjuvant/neoadjuvant therapy, but trials studying this issue are largely lacking. Possible adverse prognostic factors would include, but are not limited to, aneuploidy and increased "S" phase activity or increased proliferative index (7,8); abnormal gene expression including p53 (9,10), p27 (11) and loss of Bcl-2 (12); pathologic features including lymphatic invasion (13), vascular invasion (13), and high histologic grade (14); increasing numbers of involved lymph nodes (15); thymidylate synthase (TS) overexpression (16,17); increased expression of CD44v6

(18); allelic loss of chromosome 18q (DCC gene) (19,20); high carcinoembryonic antigen (CEA) level preoperatively (21); high lactate dehydrogenase 5 expression (22); high death receptor 4 expression (23); and bowel obstruction (24). Furthermore, it seems likely that gene expression analysis will become important in refining prognosis within a stage and in predicting who will benefit from adjuvant therapy. Such a strategy has been useful in breast cancer (25,26), lymphoma (27), and perhaps lung cancer (28). Promising data are emerging in colorectal cancer (29-32). Surgical factors also may play a prognostic role; for example, the presence of residual disease postoperatively is a clear poor prognostic factor. The type of surgical resection for rectal cancer appears to be important, as total mesorectal excision has been reported to show improved results (33). The number of lymph nodes removed in a patient with negative lymph nodes may correlate with prognosis (34), presumably by improving the validity of N0 status, or by removing lymph nodes whose metastases are occult to the pathologic evaluation.

In addition to *prognostic* variables being potentially useful in refining prognosis and defining who should be a candidate for adjuvant therapy, *predictive* variables may be useful in predicting whether or not cancer cells will be sensitive to a particular chemotherapy and/or whether or not toxicity will be excessive. High TS protein or gene expression may predict resistance to 5-flourouracil (5-FU)-based therapy in metastatic disease, as may high dihydropyrimidine dehydrogenase levels and possibly low thymidine phosphorylase expression (35). Perhaps surprisingly, however, studies of adjuvant therapy with 5-FU-based treatment have shown more benefit in high TS tumors than in low TS tumors (16,17). A variety of factors, including UGT1A1 activity, may predict toxicity of irinotecan; and ERCCI expression may relate to oxaliplatin resistance (36). Those and other issues have been discussed by Iqbal and Lenz (37). Gene expression profiles may also be of use in predicting response to therapy (38).

ADJUVANT THERAPY: GENERAL CONSIDERATIONS

The term *adjuvant therapy*, as applied to colorectal cancer, indicates the use of an additional nonsurgical modality (or modalities) after surgical resection of all known disease. Such surgery would generally be resection of the primary tumor and of regional spread (if present). The term might be applied as well, however, to therapy given after resection of all known metastases

Table 40.1

Survival in Colorectal Cancer as a Function of Stage[a] and Site

5-Year Survival Colon Cancer SEER Data (2) (1991–2000)		5-Year Survival Rectal Cancer				5-Year Relative Survival Rectal Cancer SEER Data (5)[b] (1991–1999)	
		NCDB Data (3) (Relative Survival) (1989–1990)		NCDB Data (4) (Observed Survival) (1987–1993)			
Stage	%	Stage	%	Stage	%	Stage	%
I	93	I	72	IIIA	60	I	92
IIA	85	II	52	IIIB	60	II	70
IIB	72	III	37	IIIC	27	III	53
IIIA	83						
IIIB	64						
IIIC	44						

SEER, Surveillance Epidemiology and End Results; NCDB, National Cancer Data Base.
[a] American Joint Committee on Cancer staging system for cancer of the colon and rectum; see Table 39.1.
[b] Estimated from pooled data.

(e.g., hepatic). Adjuvant therapy would commonly be chemotherapy, but other modalities may also play roles. Radiation therapy would frequently be indicated in rectal cancer (but rarely in colon cancer). Adjuvant therapy may, at least investigationally, be other therapy (e.g., immunotherapy, growth factor/receptor inhibitors, angiogenesis inhibitors). The logic of adjuvant therapy would be as follows:

1. The patient, based on clinical and pathologic findings, is determined to be at substantial risk of relapse, locoregional and/or distant.
2. There exists nonsurgical therapy that is active against metastatic, recurrent, or persistent cancer (usually acting directly, possibly acting indirectly in the case of angiogenesis inhibitors or immunotherapy).
3. Such therapy may be more effective (and potentially curative) in a patient clinically disease-free (but with undetected microscopic disease) than it would be in the setting of gross recurrence.
4. The adjuvant therapy is warranted on the basis of sufficient efficacy and acceptable toxicity. The benefits of treating those patients with occult disease outweigh the risks, cost, and other implications of treating those patients without occult disease.

There are abundant preclinical data and animal models supporting these concepts. There are a variety of biologic explanations for possible superior efficacy of a treatment modality in the setting of occult disease as compared with the setting of gross recurrence. These explanations include (but are not limited to) the following:

1. Less "log kill" would be necessary to eradicate a small tumor burden or lower it to a threshold that can be controlled by host factors.
2. Early disease has had less time to acquire de novo drug (or radiation) resistance.
3. Early disease may have a higher growth fraction and be cytokinetically more sensitive to chemotherapy or radiation therapy.

4. Early disease may be better vascularized and better oxygenated, and may be more sensitive to chemotherapy or radiation therapy on those bases.

As a practical matter, in human tumors, there is a clear role for adjuvant therapy in multiple malignancies, including colorectal cancer.

NEOADJUVANT THERAPY: GENERAL CONSIDERATIONS

The term *neoadjuvant therapy*, as applied to colorectal cancer, would indicate the use of treatment (usually chemotherapy and/or radiation therapy) prior to definitive surgery. As with adjuvant therapy (which may be part of a patient's regimen in addition to neoadjuvant therapy), this may have the goals of improving curability, disease-free survival, or survival in a patient at high risk. It may also have the goal of shrinking tumors preoperatively and, in doing so, facilitating surgery (e.g., by improving operative exposure, by potentially improving margins, or perhaps by allowing a more conservative operation [such as avoiding a colostomy in a patient with rectal cancer]). The neoadjuvant approach is frequently employed in the treatment of head and neck and esophageal cancers, and sometimes in the treatment of locally advanced lung and breast cancer. Neoadjuvant therapy generally would be therapy prior to resection of a primary tumor. The term could be used, however, for treatment of metastatic disease that may be subsequently resected.

STUDIES OF ADJUVANT THERAPY IN COLON CANCER

Early Adjuvant Systemic Therapy Studies

Historically, attempts to treat resected colon carcinomas in the adjuvant setting have progressed from single-agent therapy (predominantly 5-FU, also floxuridine [FUDR] and thiotepa) to combination therapy (usually based on 5-FU). In early randomized controlled trials, single-agent studies of 5-FU generally showed a slight, perhaps clinically insignificant, benefit to therapy. Individual studies showed trends toward "small" improvements in survival (e.g., 5% at 5 years) (39-44) that were generally not statistically significant taken singly. Early single-agent studies were also performed with thiotepa (42,45) and FUDR (46,47), showing no benefit. Early combination chemotherapy studies of both colon and rectal carcinoma using "MOF" (5-FU plus vincristine plus methyl CCNU [semustine]) showed a slight advantage to treatment, although that advantage was temporary (48). That regimen, however was associated with a small risk of iatrogenic myelodysplasia or acute leukemia attributable to the methyl CCNU (49,50), and a subsequent study of radiation therapy and 5-FU plus or minus methyl CCNU in rectal cancer showed no benefit to the methyl CCNU group (51). Early studies of immunotherapy, including BCG and levamisole (alone) (52,53) showed no clear benefit, although a suggestion of slightly improved survival unrelated to cancer control has been seen with BCG (48). In 1988, Buyse et al (54) performed a meta-analysis of controlled trials of adjuvant treatment of colorectal cancer (published up to 1987). In that pooled analysis, they found that adjuvant chemotherapy with 5-FU alone or in combination decreased the odds of death by 10% and increased 5-year survival by 2.3% to 5.7%. When only long-term (>1 year) programs were considered, the odds of death were decreased by 17%, but 5-year survival was increased only by 3.4%.

Overall, 5-FU, alone or in combination as used up to the mid-1980s, can be viewed as being of small benefit. The first studies to show a more significant benefit to adjuvant chemotherapy were the studies of 5-FU plus levamisole. Levamisole was postulated to be immunoaugmentative, and initial studies of combined 5-FU/levamisole in stage III colon cancer showed clear benefit over no therapy, with initial reports of a 25% to 40% decrease in recurrence rate and a 20% to 30% decrease in death rate (55,56). These results were likely due to improved delivery of 5-FU rather than to levamisole, however. Levamisole is ineffective as a single-agent adjuvant therapy (53,55), and subsequent randomized studies (57-61) have shown no benefit to

levamisole. Levamisole has been largely abandoned. It should be noted, however, that one large adjuvant study (3,794 patients, Intergroup 0089) showed no clear differences in efficacy among four arms, with levamisole alone achieving similar results as three regimens based on 5-FU/leucovorin (62).

5-Fluorouracil Plus Leucovorin

Leucovorin (folinic acid, citrovorum factor) has been shown to biomodulate 5-FU and to improve response rates of single-agent 5-FU in metastatic disease (63). In the adjuvant setting, leucovorin-modulated 5-FU, like 5-FU plus levamisole, appears to be of value. Table 40.2 presents results of four pertinent studies. (64–68). All studies show improvement in both survival and disease-free survival in stage C (stage III) disease; benefit is suggested but not clearly demonstrated in stage B (stage II) disease. Three of the four studies use a no-treatment control group; the National Surgical Adjuvant Breast and Bowel Project (NSABP) study uses as the control the MOF regimen previously discussed.

In addition to those studies, a large (>2,000 patients) study of the Nordic Gastrointestinal Tumor Adjuvant therapy group, pooling data with 5-FU/leucovorin and 5-FU/levamisole, found a 5-year survival advantage with adjuvant chemotherapy for stage III colon cancer (55% vs. 48%) but no benefit with stage II disease (69). Overall, 5-FU plus levamisole and 5-FU plus leucovorin have been of comparable benefit (56-58). A pooled analysis (70) of adjuvant 5-FU with leucovorin or levamisole in >3,000 patients has been reported, indicating that for all patients 5-year survival improved from 64% to 71% and 5-year disease free survival improved from 55% to 67%.

Newer Combination Regimens

For *metastatic* colorectal carcinoma, response rates and survival have been improved from results achieved with 5-FU/leucovorin alone by the addition of other agents to the armamentarium. Such other agents would currently include irinotecan (e.g., in the "IFL" or "Folfiri" regimens), oxaliplatin (e.g., in the "Folfox-4" regimen), bevacizumab (Avastin), and cetuximab (Erbitux). Regimens incorporating these new agents have been studied as

Table 40.2

Adjuvant Studies of 5-Fluorouracil (5-FU)/Leucovorin in Colon Cancer

Study Group (Ref.)	No. of Patients	Control Group Treatment	Follow-up (Years)	Disease-free Survival 5-FU/CF vs. Control (%)	Survival 5-FU/CF vs. Control (%)
NSABP (64)	1,081 (292 B, 739 C)	MeCCNU, VCR, 5-FU	3	B: 87 vs. 82 C: 67 vs. 58	B: 95 vs. 93 C: 79 vs. 71
Intergroup (65)	309 (57 B, 252 C)	No therapy	5	74 vs. 58	74 vs. 63
Francini et al. (66)	239 (121 B2, 118 C)	No therapy	4.5	B2: 83 vs. 77 C: 66 vs. 41	B2: 89 vs. 86 C: 62 vs. 42
IMPACT (67,68)	1,668 (1016 B2, 652 C)	No therapy	5 / 3	B2:[a] 76 vs. 73 C:[a] 76 vs. 64	B2: 82 vs. 80 C: 62 vs. 42

CF, ; NSABP, National Surgical Adjuvant Breast and Bowel Project; IMPACT, VCR, vincristine.
[a] Event-free survival.

treatment for metastatic disease and are being studied in the adjuvant setting, with early results available. The "Mosaic" adjuvant study compared Folfox 4 with a like regimen of 5-FU/leucovorin without the oxaliplatin in patients with stage II or III colon cancer. This study, of >2,000 patients, showed in all patients improved 3-year disease-free survival (78% vs. 73%) with the oxaliplatin-based regimen (71). Four-year disease-free survival in stage III disease was improved from 61% to 70%, and in stage II disease free from 81.3% to 85.1% (72). No survival difference is apparent, however, although longer follow-up will be needed. An NSABP study (73) of 2,407 patients found that a 5-FU/leucovorin plus oxaliplatin regimen resulted in 76.5% 3-year disease-free survival as compared with 71.6% with 5-FU/leucovorin alone, again with no clear difference in survival to date. Irinotecan-based regimens, however, have so far failed to show a clear benefit (74,75), albeit with a trend for benefit in one study (76). Longer follow-up of these studies, with attention to survival, and further studies of more complex regimens (e.g., incorporating Avastin and/or Erbitux) will be of interest. Use of Avastin pre- or postoperatively may pose wound-healing or other problems, however.

Who Benefits From Adjuvant Chemotherapy?

Studies have consistently shown benefit to adjuvant chemotherapy in patients with stage III colon cancer, although it is not clear whether all substages (IIIA, IIIB, IIIC) benefit equally. Data in stage II patients are more problematic, as there have been many studies showing small or no benefit to adjuvant therapy in that group. Figueredo et al. (77), in 2004, reviewed 37 studies and 11 meta-analyses and concluded that adjuvant therapy for stage II disease results in a small improvement in disease-free survival, but not necessarily in overall survival. This does not resolve the issue as to benefit in those stage II patients who can be identified as high risk, either from substage (IIB) or other factors (e.g., genetic, histologic). In the pooled analysis by Gill et al. (70) cited earlier (7 studies, 3,302 patients treated with 5-FU—based therapy or no adjuvant therapy), there were 1,440 node-negative patients. Overall survival at 5 years was not improved with adjuvant therapy in the entire lymph node-negative group (81% with treatment vs. 80% without). In the T3N0 and T4N0 subgroup, a modest improvement in 5-year disease-free survival was seen in low-grade, but not high-grade tumors. The large QUASAR study (78) assessed >3,000 patients, 91% of whom were stage II, and found a 1% to 5% survival benefit in the stage II group. Those data reflect 5-FU-based therapy. It is possible that different results could occur with a more complex and modern regimen. The MOSAIC study (71,72) discussed previously showed a slight improvement in disease-free survival in stage II disease with Folfox as compared with 5-FU/leucovorin.

Fluoropyrimidines by Alternative Routes

The approaches cited here generally use adjuvant therapy based on intravenous bolus 5-FU. Alternative routes of adjuvant therapy—intravenous constant infusion, oral, intrahepatic arterial, intraportal vein, and intraperitoneal—have also been studied.

A variety of schedules of constant-infusion 5-FU have been compared in the adjuvant setting to a bolus regimen. These have included infusion over 2 days (79), 8 weeks (80), and 12 weeks (81). In these studies, there was no clear survival benefit to the infusion schedule, although toxicity may have been less. Oral fluoropyrimidine therapy has also been studied. This has largely been capecitabine (Xeloda) (82,83) in the Western world, with comparable efficacy and arguably less toxicity than 5-FU/leucovorin. In Japan, other oral agents have shown utility as compared with no therapy (84), but how they compare with modern therapy is unclear.

Intrahepatic arterial therapy with 5-FU has received limited study as adjuvant treatment of stage II and stage III disease, with 5-year survival reported to be improved from 76% to 89% as compared with a no-therapy control (85). Studies confirming benefit and comparing survival benefit to modern systemic adjuvant therapy, however, are lacking.

Portal vein adjuvant chemotherapy has also been used, based on the premise that newly established hepatic micrometastases may be preferentially vascularized by the portal system rather than the hepatic arterial system. A meta-analysis of approximately 3,800 patients in nine randomized trials, comparing portal vein therapy (generally perioperative 5-FU) with no therapy, has been performed (86). This analysis found a 13% decrease in overall 5-year death rate with treatment (24% vs. 30% in Dukes C disease). Disease-free survival and time to relapse also were shown to be improved. Not all studies, however, show benefit (87-91), and it is not clear that hepatic metastases are decreased in frequency (92). Although there may be efficacy to adjuvant portal vein therapy as compared with no treatment, it is not clear that the portal vein route offers an advantage over systemic adjuvant therapy. A large Italian study (1,084 patients) (93) compared intraportal vein 5-FU to systemic 5-FU/leucovorin and to both intraportal and systemic therapy. It found no clear difference among the treatments.

Intraperitoneal (IP) therapy (e.g., with 5-FU) also has been studied as an adjuvant treatment, with the hope that this would decrease the risk of peritoneal, mesenteric, and omental tumor seeding. This approach appears feasible (94). Results of a randomized study of 241 patients comparing intravenous (IV) 5-FU plus levamisole with IV and IP 5-FU + levamisole indicated a lower relapse rate with the IV/IP approach in stage III, but not stage II disease (95). This should be interpreted, however, with caution, as other studies did not show survival benefit (96,97)

Immunotherapy

Immunotherapy in the adjuvant setting for colorectal cancer has been studied. Studies of adjuvant levamisole have not shown benefit (52,53,56). BCG, too, has failed to show clear benefit as adjuvant nonspecific immunotherapy (98,99). Tumor vaccines have also been studied as adjuvant therapy for colorectal cancer. Although data showing some benefit for this approach in colon, but not rectal, cancer have been reported (100–102), other trials have been negative (103,104). Monoclonal antibody therapy, using a "17-1A antibody" (Panorex) was initially reported to show benefit in Dukes C colon cancer (105), but a subsequent large randomized study showed no benefit (106). Interferon-alpha, when combined with 5-FU, has received study in the adjuvant setting. No clear advantage is seen to that approach (107,108).

Adjuvant Therapy Following and Neoadjuvant Therapy Preceding Metastasectomy

Long-term survival may occur in selected patients with colorectal cancer metastatic to liver or lung who are candidates for and undergo metastasectomy. Adjuvant intrahepatic arterial therapy and intraportal vein therapy have been used following the resection of liver metastases, with (109–111) and without (112,113) additional systemic adjuvant therapy. The results of randomized studies are mixed. A German study of 226 patients found no benefit from adjuvant intrahepatic arterial 5-FU plus leucovorin after resection of liver metastases (114). An Intergroup study of 109 patients found an improved recurrence–free rate (58% vs. 34%) with adjuvant intrahepatic FUDR and systemic infusion of 5-FU as compared with surgery alone (115). Survival, however, was not significantly improved, although a trend existed. A Memorial Sloan-Kettering Cancer Center study compared adjuvant hepatic arterial FUDR plus infusional 5-FU/leucovorin to infusional 5-FU/leucovorin alone (116). The combined intra-arterial and IV approach improved 2-year survival (85% vs. 69%) and hepatic disease-free survival (86% vs. 57%). A more recent study from that institution reported comparable 2-year survival (89%) (117) with hepatic arterial FUDR plus systemic irinotecan, and a pooled analysis (118) of two trials comparing systemic 5-FU/leucovorin with surgery alone after resection of lung or liver metastases favored adjuvant therapy (see Portier et al. [119] for update on one of those studies). Overall, these data argue for a role for adjuvant therapy in this setting, but do not mandate intrahepatic arterial or venous therapy and do not define a best approach.

The issue of neoadjuvant therapy prior to metastasectomy is an emerging but currently unsettled issue. It is not clear whether patients with metastatic disease who are thought to be too extensive to resect can be made resectable by a response to neoadjuvant therapy. Although a radiologic complete response to therapy may occur, it is unlikely to be a pathologic complete response (120), arguing surgery should still encompass all original sites of disease. In patients with resectable disease, one needs to consider the possibility of disease progression on chemotherapy rendering the patient unresectable, or of therapeutic toxicity of chemotherapy increasing the risk of surgery (121). The role of neoadjuvant therapy prior to metastasectomy is currently undefined (122).

Adjuvant Radiation Therapy

Radiation therapy as an adjuvant therapy has received less study in colon cancer than in rectal cancer (see later discussion), presumably because of the decreased importance of local recurrence (vs. systemic recurrence) in colon cancer and the increased toxicity of wide field abdominal radiation. Nevertheless, selected patients with locally advanced colon cancer have a high risk of local recurrence, and radiation might be reasonable in this setting. In a historically controlled study (123), 173 patients with colon (not rectal) cancer were treated with adjuvant radiation therapy. Of these patients, 63 had chemotherapy as well, usually 5-FU daily × 3 in the first and last weeks of radiation. These groups were compared with a historical control of 395 patients. In the control groups, high local failure rates were seen in those with stage B3 and C3 disease (transmural with adherence to or inva-

sion of adjacent structures, essentially T4). In the stage B3/C3 radiation group, local recurrence rate decreased and relapse-free survival improved. Local recurrences were fewer with surgery alone in patients with stage B2 cancer (10%) than those with stage C2 cancer (36%), and there was no clear benefit to radiation in those groups (9% and 30% local recurrences, respectively). Pilot studies of adjuvant whole-abdominal radiation plus infusional 5-FU have been performed by the Southwest Oncology Group (124). Radiation therapy plus IP therapy also has been tested, with no apparent survival benefit (125). Other historically controlled data have suggested increased local control without improved survival (126), and one study suggested poorer local control (127). A more recent randomized study of 222 patients (Intergroup 0130) (128) compared 5-FU/levamisole with 5-FU/levamisole plus radiation for patients with stage B3 and C3 colon carcinomas. This study found no improvement in survival or disease-free survival in the radiation therapy arm. Toxicity was higher with radiation. Overall, it appears local radiation does not improve survival and may or may not improve local control, at the cost of some toxicity.

Conclusions: Colon Cancer

1. Adjuvant chemotherapy is of value for stage III colon cancer, with limited studies and short-term follow-up suggesting that regimens based on 5-FU plus oxaliplatin are most effective as reflected by disease-free survival. With patients for whom a less toxic/complicated regimen is desired, 5-FU/leucovorin or variants thereof (including oral capecitabine) are acceptable, particularly in the absence of clear survival benefit from the oxaliplatin-based regimens.

2. Adjuvant chemotherapy is probably not of substantial value in most patients with stage II colon cancer. It is still unclear whether or not patients with IIB disease or with other genetic or biological high risk factors will benefit.

3. It remains to be seen if adding genetic/biological information to stage can improve the prediction of the need for and expected benefit of adjuvant chemotherapy, and whether genetic/biological factors can determine which particular regimens will be most effective and least toxic.

4. Irradiation plays little role in colon cancer, even in stage B3 and C3 disease (T4 tumors).

5. Adjuvant therapy after metastasectomy is reasonable, but unproven.

6. Although adjuvant therapy by nontraditional routes may have some efficacy, it is not clearly better than more traditional systemic adjuvant therapy. It is less proven and more unwieldy.

STUDIES OF ADJUVANT AND NEOADJUVANT THERAPY IN RECTAL CANCER

Rectal carcinoma differs clinically from colon carcinoma in several ways. Survival and disease-free survival are poorer for rectal carcinoma both overall and stage for stage (129) (Table 1). Rectal carcinoma is more likely than colon cancer to recur locally, and the first site of distant metastasis for rectal cancer is less likely to be liver.

These data would suggest, perhaps, that adjuvant chemotherapy might have a greater potential role in stage II rectal cancer than in stage II colon cancer, that radiation might play a greater role as adjuvant or neoadjuvant therapy in rectal cancer than colon cancer, and that there would be less rationale with rectal cancer for intrahepatic arterial or for intraportal vein adjuvant therapy.

Adjuvant and Neoadjuvant Radiation Therapy

Adjuvant radiation therapy by itself, either preoperative (neoadjuvant) (130–132), postoperative (133,134), or both ("sandwich technique") is of value in decreasing local recurrence rate by roughly 20% to 50%. Many studies have shown little impact on survival (135–140), but there are positive studies, particularly those using preoperative radiation (141–143). A meta-analysis by Camma et al. (144) found a survival benefit with preoperative radiation, while a different meta-analysis (145) failed to find a benefit. It should be noted, however, that regardless of the putative impact on mortality, the improvement of morbidity due to a lower local recurrence rate warrants the adjunctive use of radiation in patients at significant risk of local recurrence. Risk of local recurrence is a function of stage (particularly "T" status) and surgical technique. If a patient has been treated with local excision alone for a T1 rectal cancer, there is a higher risk of local recurrence and death than if the patient had been treated with a radical resection. T1 lesions of the lower rectum have a 22% to 34% incidence of lymph node metastasis, and there is a recurrence rate of 4% to 29% with local excision alone (146). Radiation therapy in this setting is logical, but the benefits are undefined at this time (146). With total mesorectal excision (TME), however, low-stage disease is unlikely to recur locally. The Dutch TME trial (140), comparing preoperative radiation followed by TME with TME alone, found in 244 patients with stage I disease treated by TME alone only a 0.7% local recurrence rate at 2 years. Although that follow-up period is short, local recurrence rate at that point (in the absence of radiation therapy) was 5.7% for stage II disease and 15% for stage III disease. With radiation, 2-year local recurrence rates fell to 1% and 4.3%, respectively. It should be noted that, in patients treated in the Dutch trial with TME who had a positive margin (≤1 mm), neither preoperative nor postoperative radiation therapy improved local control (147). Preoperative radiation therapy did improve local control in patients with a narrow margin (1.1 to 2 mm) or wide margin (>2 mm). Postoperative radiation therapy in patients with positive margins was also found to be inferior to preoperative therapy in the MRC CR07 trial (148). Data on patients treated with TME alone are also available from Memorial Sloan Kettering Cancer Center (149). MSK reported on patients with T2N0 and early (mobile) T3N0 disease. In 97 patients, (pooled, as patients with stage T2 and T3 cancer had similar results), pelvic recurrence rate at 5 years was 7% (with a distant recurrence rate of 24.5%). Patients with an elevated preoperative CEA had a 13% 5-year pelvic recurrence rate (vs. 0% in patients with a normal CEA), and patients with lymphovascular invasion had a 32% 5-year pelvic recurrence rate (vs. 6% in patients without that pathologic finding).

A third study worth noting is that of the North Hampshire Hospital, reported with other studies in an article by Havenga et al. (150). That series encompassed 204 patients (45% with stage III disease, 55% with stage II disease), 97% of whom did not receive radiation and 92% of whom did not receive adjuvant chemotherapy. The actuarial 5-year local recurrence rate in that group is only 3.6% (median follow-up, 45 months). Data on local recurrence rate in early T stage disease from the pre-TME era are available from the NSABP ROI study (134,151). In that study, 5-year local relapse rate was 12% in T1-2/N1 disease without adjuvant therapy, 7% with adjuvant radiation therapy, and 5% with adjuvant chemotherapy. Arguably, in patients with T1-2 N1 disease who are given chemotherapy, radiation is not necessary. Overall, radiation appears appropriate in stage T3 or T4 disease, but not clearly mandatory in patients with stage T1 or T2 disease treated with a TME, particularly when there are good margins, normal preoperative CEA, and no lymphovascular invasion.

The issue of preoperative versus postoperative radiation therapy (with chemotherapy) has been studied in a randomized controlled trial by the German Rectal Cancer Study Group (152). This group compared preoperative chemoradiation plus postoperative chemotherapy with postoperative chemotherapy plus postoperative radiation in over 800 patients with stage T3, T4, or lymph node-positive disease. They found the preoperative approach to be less toxic and more effective as to local control, but without an impact on survival. Similar results have been reported by Frykholm et al. (153).

Adjuvant Chemotherapy

Because of the accepted value of adjuvant radiation therapy in the treatment of rectal carcinoma, most modern adjuvant trials have focused on chemoradiotherapy rather than chemotherapy alone. There are, however, some older studies of adjuvant treatment for rectal cancer that compare chemotherapy alone with no therapy. Examples would be an NSABP study of methyl CCNU, vincristine, and 5-FU (151) and a Gastrointestinal Tumor Study Group study of 5-FU and methyl CCNU (153). They tended to show modest improvement in disease-free and overall survival with chemotherapy as compared with no therapy. A more modern study from the Netherlands of 5-FU/levasimole, however, failed to show survival benefit in rectal cancer (154).

Adjuvant Chemotherapy Plus Radiation Therapy

Combined-modality adjuvant therapy for resected rectal cancer has been the dominant approach in recent years. Early randomized studies (155,156) compared 5-FU/methyl CCNU/radiation with 5-FU/methyl CCNU alone, radiation alone, and no adjuvant therapy. Survival was best in the combined modality arm (59% vs. 44% no therapy, 52% radiation therapy alone, 50% chemotherapy alone) as was local recurrence rate (11% vs. 24% no therapy, 20% radiation alone, 27% chemotherapy alone). Subsequent studies, (51,157) as previously discussed, have shown that methyl CCNU adds little to the regimen and should be avoided. Other large randomized studies have compared the combined-modality approach with either radiation alone or chemotherapy alone in rectal cancer. The North Central Cancer Treatment Group (158) studied 204 patients with rectal cancer and compared radiation therapy alone with a regimen of 5-FU/methyl CCNU followed by further combined radiation/

5-FU followed by 5-FU/methyl CCNU. The combined approach, when compared with radiation therapy alone, decreased 5-year recurrence rates from 63% to 42% and improved 5-year survival from approximately 37% to approximately 55%. The regimens mentioned previously have been superseded by more modern regimens. Intergroup trial 0114 kept radiation constant and compared four variants of adjuvant chemotherapy: bolus 5-FU alone, 5-FU plus leucovorin, 5-FU plus levamisole, and 5-FU plus leucovorin plus levamisole. In a study of approximately 1,700 patients (159), all four regimens were found to be equal in efficacy. A subsequent study, Intergroup 0144 (160), randomized almost 2,000 patients to radiation therapy plus one of three different chemotherapy regimens, with constant-infusion 5-FU and 5-FU/leucovorin approaches being tested. Again, no differences in efficacy were found.

Neoadjuvant Therapy

Preoperative therapy, with radiation plus or minus chemotherapy, has conceptual appeal in the treatment of rectal carcinoma. Radiation prior to surgery should be less toxic to the small bowel, as loops of small bowel would not be expected to be fixed in the pelvic radiation field. Preoperative therapy arguably may increase resectability of locally advanced disease and may allow a sphincter-saving procedure in an otherwise marginal patient. With these benefits in mind, neoadjuvant radiation therapy and combined chemotherapy/radiation therapy have been studied. As previously discussed in the section on radiation therapy, the neoadjuvant approach at this time appears preferable, at least in patients clinically thought to be stage T3, T4, or lymph-node positive. This issue is less clear in patients with disease early enough that radiation may be avoided.

A variety of regimens have been used. The German Neoadjuvant Research Study (152) used 5-FU by constant infusion in 5-day courses in the first and fifth weeks of radiotherapy. Patients, in addition, subsequently received adjuvant therapy of bolus 5-FU, daily × 5 every 4 weeks for four cycles. This study reported a 5-year survival rate of 76% and a 5-year local relapse rate of 6% in a heterogeneous group of patients (largely stage T3, 54% node-positive). Significant downstaging occurred after neoadjuvant therapy (8% complete response, 25% node-positive, 18% stage I). An Italian study (161) used mitomycin C plus a 4-day constant infusion of 5-FU in 83 patients (61 with stage III disease, 22 with stage II disease) and reported 76% 5-year survival, and 60% 10-year survival (66% cancer-related survival) with 8% of patients downstaged to T0-1 pathologic stage. Other regimens based on 5-FU/leucovorin have shown improved local control, but not survival, compared with radiation alone, as reviewed by Ortholan et al. (162). A recent large (1,011 patients) randomized study of patients with clinical stage T3 or T4 resectable rectal cancer has been reported from the European Organisation for Research and Treatment of Cancer (163). All patients received neoadjuvant radiation. One quarter of the group received neoadjuvant radiation alone. Other quarters received neoadjuvant radiation plus neoadjuvant chemotherapy with 5-FU/leucovorin (but no adjuvant therapy), neoadjuvant radiotherapy alone follow by adjuvant chemotherapy, or neoadjuvant radiotherapy with both neoadjuvant and adjuvant chemotherapy. Overall there was no survival advan-

tage seen with neoadjuvant chemotherapy, and a small, not statistically significant, trend for improved survival was seen with adjuvant chemotherapy. Local recurrence rate fell significantly with all chemotherapy regimens. One may quibble with the details of the chemotherapy administered but, as given, this study argues that chemotherapy given either before or after surgery improves local control, but not necessarily survival. More modern chemotherapy regimens are being studied.

The Radiation Therapy Oncology Group trial 0012 (164) evaluated 106 patients with distal T3, T4 tumors treated with constant-infusion 5-FU throughout radiation plus irinotecan weekly × 4, with additional adjuvant therapy for patients not in complete remission. This treatment resulted in a 26% pathologic complete response rate. Survival data are currently lacking. Oxaliplatin-containing regimens have also been tested. "Xelox-RT" (165), using capecitabine and oxaliplatin, has been piloted in 32 patients with 19% complete response, 55% downstaging, and sphincter-sparing surgery in 36% of patients with tumor ≤2 cm from the dentate line. A similar neoadjuvant regimen reported from England (followed by adjuvant capecitabine for 12 weeks) was reported in 77 patients, with a 24% pathologic complete response rate and about 67% 3-year failure free survival (166).

Conclusions: Rectal Cancer

1. If early-stage disease has been treated only with local excision, adjuvant radiation is reasonable, although the benefits are undefined.
2. For pathologic T1 and T2 disease, resected conventionally, and having good prognostic factors (TME resection, CEA normal, no lymphovascular invasion), radiation is likely unnecessary. For the lymph node-positive (stage III) subset, chemotherapy would be appropriate, using colon cancer data as to a choice of regimen. If good prognostic features are absent, radiation therapy maybe relevant.
3. For patients with clinical (e.g., after endoscopic ultrasound) T3, T4, or lymph node-positive disease, neoadjuvant chemoradiation therapy (or neoadjuvant radiation therapy followed by adjuvant chemotherapy) would be appropriate. Data comparing regimens are inadequate, but a capecitabine/oxaliplatin-based regimen has appeal based on convenience/toxicity and the putative advantage of oxaliplatin-based regimens in colon cancer. In patients receiving neoadjuvant therapy, how much (if any) and which adjuvant therapy should be given follow definite surgery is unclear, as is whether the choice of adjuvant therapy should be a function of response to neoadjuvant treatment. If neoadjuvant therapy is not given, adjuvant chemoradiotherapy would be appropriate.
4. Likely, in the future, genetic profiling or other biologic studies of the tumor will refine the need for and choice of adjuvant therapy, (as previously discussed regarding colon cancer).

REFERENCES

1. Gloekler LA, ed. *SEER cancer statistic review 1973–1991.* Bethesda, MD: US Department of Health and Human Services, National Institutes of Health, 1994. NIH publication No. 94–2789.
2. O'Connell JB, Maggard MA, Ko CY. Colon cancer survival rates with the new American Joint Committee on Cancer sixth edition staging. *J Natl Cancer Inst.* 2004;96:1420–1425.

3. Jessup JM, Stewart AK, Menck HR. The National Cancer Data Base Report on Patterns of Care for Adenocarcinoma of the Rectum, 1985–1995. *Cancer.* 1998:2408–2418.

4. Greene FL, Stewart AK, Norton HJ. A New TNM Staging Strategy for Node-Positive (Stage III) Colon Cancer. *Annals of Surgery.* 2002;236:416–421.

5. O'Connell JB, Maggard MA, Liu JH, et al. Are Survival Rates Different for Young and Older Patients with Rectal cancer? *Diseases of the Colon & Rectum.* 2004;47:2064–2069.

6. Jemal A, Siegel R, Ward E, et al. Cancer Statistics, 2008. *CA Cancer J Clin.* 2008;58:71–96.

7. Cascinu S, Ligi M, Graziano F, et al. S-Phase Fraction Can Predict Event Free Survival in Patients with pT2-T3NOMO Colorectal Carcinoma. *Cancer.* 1998;83:1081–1085.

8. Albe X, Vassilakos P, Helfer-Guarnori K, et al. Independent Prognostic Value of ploidy in colorectal cancer. *Cancer.* 1990;66:1168–1175.

9. Zeng ZS, Sarkis AS, Zhang ZF, et al. P53 nuclear overexpression: an independent prediction of survival in lymph node-positive colorectal cancer patients. *J Clin Oncol.* 1994;12:2043–2050.

10. Bosari S, Viale G, Bossi P, et al. Cytoplasmic accumulation of P53 protein: an independent prognostic indicator in colorectal adeocarcinomas. *J Natl Cancer inst.* 1994;86:681–687.

11. Hershko DD, Shapira M. Prognostic Role of P27^{Kip1} Deregulation in Colorectal Cancer. *Cancer.* 2006;107:668–675.

12. Ilyas M, Hao XP, Wilkinson K, et al. Loss of Bcl-2 expression correlates with tumor recurrence in colorectal cancer. *Gut.* 1998;43:383–387.

13. Minsky BD, Mies C, Rich TA, et al. Lymphatic vessel invasion is an independent prognostic factor for survival in colorectal cancer. *Int J Radiat Oncol Biol Phys.* 1989;17:311–318.

14. Chapuis PH, Dent OF, Fisher R, et al. A multivariate analysis of clinical and pathological variables in prognosis after resection of large bowel cancer. *Br J Surg.* 1985;72:698–702.

15. Willett CG, Tepper JE, Chen AM, et al. Failure patterns following curative resection of colonic carcinoma. *Ann Surg.* 1984;200:685–690.

16. Johnston PG, Fisher CR, Rockett HE, et al. The role of thymidylate synthase expression in prognosis and outcome of adjuvant chemotherapy in patients with rectal cancer. *J Clin Oncol.* 1994;12:2640–2647.

17. Edler D, Glimelius B, Hallstrom M, et al. Thymidylate Synthase Expression in Colorectal Cancer: A Prognostic and Predictive Marker of Benefit From Adjuvant Fluorouracil-Based Chemotherapy. 2002;20:1721–1728.

18. Mulder JW, Kruyt PM, Sewnath M, et al. Colorectal cancer prognosis and expression of exon-V6-containing CD44 proteins. *Lancet.* 1994;44:1470–1472.

19. Jen J, Hoguen K, Piantadosi S, et al. Allelic loss of chromosome 18q and prognosis in colon cancer. *N Engl J Med.* 1994;331:213–221.

20. Shibata D, Reale MA, Lavin P, et al. The DCC protein and prognosis in colorectal cancer. *N Engl J Med.* 1996;335:1727–1732.

21. Wolmark N, Fisher B, Wieland S, et al. The prognostic significance of preoperative caricnoembryonic antigen levels in colorectal cancer. *Ann Surg.* 1984;199:375–381.

22. Koukourakis MI, Giatromanolaki A, Sivirdis E, et al. Lactate Dehydrogenase 5 Expression in Operable Colorectal Cancer: Strong Association With Survival and Activated Vascular Endothelial Growth Factor Pathway-A Report of the Tumor Angiogenesis Research Group. *J Clin Oncol.* 2006;24:4301–4308.

23. Van Geelen C, Westra JL, De Vries EG, et al. Prognostic Significance of Tumor Necrosis Factor-Related Apoptosis-Inducing Ligand and Its Receptors in Adjuvantly Treated Stage III Colon Cancer Patients. *J Clin Oncol.* 2006;24:4998–5004.

24. Crucitti F, Sofo L, Doglietto GB, et al. Prognostic factors in colorectal cancer: current status and new trends. *J Surg Oncol Suppl.* 1991;2:76–82.

25. Paik S, Tang G, Shak S, et al. Gene Expression and Benefit of Chemotherapy in Women With Node-Negative, Estrogen Receptor-Positive Breast Cancer. *J Clin Oncol.* 2006;24:3726–3734.

26. Fan C, Oh DS, Wessels L, et al. Concordance among Gene-Expression-Based Predictors for Breast Cancer. *N Engl J Med.* 2006;355:560–569.

27. Lossos IS, Morgensztern D. Prognostic Biomarkers in Diffuse Large B-Cell Lymphoma. *J Clin Oncol.* 2006;24:995–1007.

28. Potti A, Mukherjee S, Petersen R, et al. A Genomic Strategy to Refine Prognosis in Early-Stage Non-Small-Cell Lung Cancer. *N Engl J Med.* 2006;355:570–580.

29. Wang Y, Jatkoe T, Zhang Y, et al. Gene Expression Profiles and Molecular Markers To Predict Recurrence of Dukes' B Colon Cancer. *J Clin Oncol.* 2004;22:1564–1571.

30. O'Connell MJ, Paik S, Yothers G, et al. Relationship between tumor gene expression and recurrence in stage II/III colon cancer: Quantitative RT-PCR assay of 757 genes in fixed paraffin-embedded (FPE) tissue. *JCO.* 2006;24:150s.

31. Johnston PG, Mulligan K, Kay E, et al. A genetic signature of relapse in stage II colorectal cancer derived from formalin fixed paraffin embedded tissue (FFPE) tissue using a unique disease specific colorectal array. *JCO.* 2006;24:150s.

32. Barrier A, Lemoine A, Boelle PY, et al. Colon Cancer Prognosis prediction by gene expression profiling. *Oncogene.* 2005;24:6155–6164.

33. Nagtegaal ID, van de Velde CJH, Marijnen CAM, et al. Low Rectal Cancer: A Call for a Change of Approach in Abdominoperineal Resection. *J Clin Oncol.* 2005;23:9257–9264.

34. Johnson PM, Porter GA, Ricciardi R, et al. Increasing Negative Lymph Node Count Is Independently Associated With Improved Long-Term Survival in Stage IIIB and IIIC Colon Cancer. *J Clin Oncol.* 2006;24:3570–3575.

35. Meropol NJ, Gold PJ, Diasio RB, et al. Thymidine Phosphorylase Expression Is Associated With Response to Capecitabine Plus Irinotecan in Patients With Metastatic Colorectal Cancer. *J Clin Oncol.* 2006;24:4069–4077.

36. E Reed. ERCCI Measurements in Clinical Oncology. *N Engl Med.* 2006;355:1054–1055.

37. Iqbal S, Lenz HJ. Individualized chemotherapy based on genetic and genomic profiling. *Curr Colorectal Cancer Rep.* 2005;I:91–102.

38. Ghadimi BM, Grade M, Difilippantonio MJ, et al. Effectiveness of Gene Expression Profiling for Response Prediction of Rectal Adenocarcinomas to Preoperative Chemoradiotherapy. *J Clin Oncol.* 2005;23:1826–1838.

39. Higgins GA, Dwight RW, Smith JV, et al. Fluorouracil as an adjuvant to surgery in carcinoma of the colon. *Arch Surg.* 1971;102:339–343.

40. Higgins GA Jr, Humphrey E, Juler GL, et al Adjuvant chemotherapy in the surgical treatment of large bowel cancer. *Cancer.* 1976;38:1461–1467.

41. Higgins GA, Dwight RW, Walsh WS, et al. Preoperative radiation therapy as an adjuvant to surgery for carcinoma of the colon and rectum. *Am J Surg.* 1968;115:241–246.

42. Higgins GA, Donaldson RC, Humphrey EW, et al. Adjuvant therapy for large bowel cancer. Update of Veterans Administration Surgical Oncology Group Trial. *Surg Clin North Am.* 1981;61:1311–1320.

43. Grage TB, Hill GJ, Cornell GN, et al. Adjuvant chemotherapy in large bowel cancer-updated analysis of single agent chemotherapy. In: Jones SE, Salmon SE, eds. *Adjuvant Therapy of Cancer II.* New York: Grune & Stratton; 1979:587–594.

44. Grage TB, Moss SE. Adjuvant chemotherapy in cancer of the colon and rectum: demonstration of effectiveness of prolonged 5-FU chemotherapy in a prospectively controlled randomized trial. *Surg Clin North Am.* 1981;61:1321–1329.

45. Dixon WJ, Longmire WP Jr, Holden WD. Use of triethylenethio-phosphoramide as an adjuvant to the surgical treatment of gastric and colorectal carcinoma: ten-year follow-up. *Ann Surg.* 1971;173:26–39.

46. Veterans Administration Adjuvant Cancer Chemotherapy Cooperative Group. The use of 5-fluorodeoxyuridine (FUDR) as a surgical adjuvant in carcinoma of the stomach and colorectum. *Arch Surg.* 1963;86:926–931.

47. Dwight RW, Humphrey EW, Higgins GA, et al. FUDR as an adjuvant to surgery in cancer of the large bowel. *J Surg Oncol.* 1973;5:243–249.

48. Smith RE, Colangelo L, Wieand HS, et al. Randomized Trial of Adjuvant Therapy in Colon Carcinoma: 10-Year Results of NSABP Protocol C-01. *J Natl Cancer Inst.* 2004;96:1128–1132.

49. Fisher B, Wolmark N, Rockette H, et al. Postoperative adjuvant chemotherapy or radiation therapy for rectal cancer. Results from NSABP protocol R-01. *J Natl Cancer Inst.* 1988;80:20–29.

50. Wolmark N, Fisher B, Rockette H, et al. Postoperative adjuvant chemotherapy or BCG for colon cancer: results from NSABP protocol C-01. *J Natl Cancer Inst.* 1988;80:30–36.

51. Gastrointestinal Tumor Study Group. Radiation therapy and flu-orouracil with semustine for the treatment of patients with surgical adjuvant adenocarcinoma of the rectum. *J Clin Oncol.* 1992;10:549–557.

52. Arnaud JP, Buyse M, Nordlinger B, et al. Adjuvant chemotherapy of poor prognosis colon cancer with levamisole: results of an EORTC double-blind randomized clinical trial. *Br J Surg.* 1989;76:284–289.

53. Chlebowski RT, Lillington L, Nystrom JS, et al. Late mortality and levamisole adjuvant therapy in colorectal cancer. *Br J Cancer.* 1994;69:1094–1097.

54. Buyse M, Zeleniuch-Jacquotte A, Chalmers T. Adjuvant therapy of colorectal cancer. *JAMA.* 1988;259:3571–3578.

55. Moertel CG, Fleming TR, MacDonald HS, et al. Fluorouracil plus levamisole as effective adjuvant therapy after resection of stage III colon carcinoma: a final report. *Ann Int Med.* 1995;122:321–326.

56. Laurie JA, Moertel CG, Fleming TR, et al. Surgical adjuvant therapy of large-bowel carcinoima: an evaluation of levamisole and the combination of levamisole and fluorouracil. *J Clin Oncol.* 1989;7:1447–1456.

57. Wolmark N, Rockette H, Mamounas EP, et al. the relative efficacy of 5-FU + leucovorin (FU-LV), 5-FU + levamisole (5-FU-LEV), and 5-FU leucovorin + levamisole (5-FU-LU-LEV) in patients with Dukes's B and C carcinoma of the colon: first report of NSABP C-04. *Proc Am Soc Clin Oncol.* 1996;15:205 (abstract 460).

58. O'Connell MJ, Laurie JA, Kahn M, et al. Prospective randomized trial of postoperative adjunct chemotherapy in patients with high-risk colon cancer. *J Clin Oncol.* 1998;16:295–300.

59. Haller DG, Catalano PJ, MacDonald JS, et al. Fluorouracil (FU) leucovorin (LV) and levamisole adjuvant therapy for colon cancer: preliminary result INT-0089. *Proc Am Soc Clin Oncol.* 1996;15–211. (Abstract 486).

60. QUASAR Collaborative Group. Comparison of fluorouracil with additional levamisole, higher-dose folinic acid, or both, as adjuvant chemotherapy for colorectal cancer: a randomized trial. *Lancet.* 2000;35:1588–1596.

61. Cascinu S, Catalano V, Piga A, et al. The role of levamisole in the adjuvant treatment of stage III colon cancer patients: a randomized trial of 5-fluorouracil and levamisole versus 5-fluorouracil alone. *Cancer Invest.* 2003;21:701–707.

62. Haller DG, Catalano PJ, Macdonald JS, et al. Phase III Study of Fluorouracil, Leucovorin, and Levamisole in High-Risk Stage II and III Colon Cancer: Final Report of Intergroup 0089. *J Clin Oncol.* 2005;23:8671–8678.

63. Advanced Colorectal Cancer Meta-Analysis Project. Modulation of fluorouracil by leucovorin in patients with advanced colorectal cancer; evidence in terms of response rate. *J Clin Oncol.* 1992;10:896–903.

64. Wolmark N, Rockett H, Fisher B, et al. The benefits of leucovorin-modulated fluorouracil as postoperative adjuvant therapy for primary colon cancer: results from National Surgical Adjuvant Breast and Bowel Protocol C-03. *J Clin Oncol.* 1993;11:1879–1887.

65. O'Connell M, Mailliard J, Kahn MJ, et al. Controlled trial of fluorouracil and low-dose leucovorin given for 6 months as postoperative adjuvant therapy for colon cancer. *J Clin Oncol.* 1997;15:246–250.

66. Francini G, Petrioli R, Lorenzini L, et al. Folinic acid and 5 fluorouracil as adjuvant chemotherapy in colon cancer. *Gastroenterology.* 1994;106:899–906.

67. Impact Investigators. Efficacy of adjuvant fluorouracil and folinic acid in colon cancer. *Lancet.* 1995;345:939–944.

68. Impact B2 Investigators. Efficacy of adjuvant fluorouracil and folinic acid in B2 colon cancer. *J Clin Oncol.* 1999;17:1356–1363.

69. Glimelius B, Dahl O, Cedermark B, et al. Adjuvant chemotherapy in colorectal cancer: A joint analysis of randomized trials by the Nordic Gastrointestinal Tumor Adjuvant Therapy Group. *Acta Oncologica.* 2005;44:904–912.

70. Gill S, Loprinzi CL, Sargent DJ, et al. Pooled Analysis of Fluorouracil-Based Adjuvant Therapy for Stage II and III Colon Cancer: Who Benefits and by How Much? *J Clin Oncol.* 2004;22:1797–1806.

71. Andre T, Boni C, Mounedji-Boudiaf L, et al. Oxaliplatin, fluorouracil, and leucovorin as adjuvant treatment for colon cancer. *N Engl J Med.* 2004;350:2343–2351.

72. de Gramont A, Boni C, Navarro M, et al. Oxaliplatin/5FU/LV in the adjuvant treatment of stage II and stage III colon cancer: Efficacy results with a median follow-up of 4 years. *J Clin Oncol.* 2005;23:246s.

73. Wolmark N, Wieand HS, Kuebler JP, et al. A phase III trial comparing FULV to FULV + oxaliplatin in stage II or III carcinoma of the colon: Results of NSABP Protocol C-07. *J Clin Oncol.* 2005;23:1092s.

74. Saltz LB, Niedzwiecki D, Hollis D, et al. Irinotecan plus fluorouracil/leucovorin (IFL) versus fluorouracil/leucovorin alone (FL) in stage III colon cancer (intergroup trial CALGB C89803). *J Clin Oncol.* 2004;22:245s.

75. Ychou M, Raoul JL, Douillard JY, et al. A phase III randomized trial of LV5FU2 +. CPT-11 vs. LV5FU2 alone in adjuvant high risk colon cancer (FNCLCC Accord02/FFCD9802). *J Clin Oncol.* 2005;23:246s.

76. Van Cutsem E, Labianca R, Hossfeld D, et al. Randomized phase III trial comparing infused irinotecan/5-fluorouracil (5-FU)/folinic acid (IF) versus 5-FU/FA (F) in stage III colon cancer patients (pts). (PETACC3). *J Clin Oncol.* 2005;23:1090s

77. Figueredo A, Charette ML, Maroun J, et al. Adjuvant Therapy for Stage II Colon Cancer: A Systematic Review From the Cancer Care Ontario Program in Evidence-Based Care's Gastrointestinal Cancer Disease Site Group. *J Clin Oncol.* 2004;22:3395–3407.

78. Gray RG, Barnwell H, Hills R, et al. QUASAR: A randomized study of adjuvant chemotherapy (CT) vs. observation including 3238 colorectal cancer patients. *J Clin Oncol.* 2004:245s.

79. Andre T, Colin P, Louvet C, et al. Semimonthly Versus Monthly Regimen of Fluorouracil and Leucovorin Administered for 24 or

36 Weeks as Adjuvant Therapy in Stage II and III Colon Cancer: Results of a Randomized Trial. *J Clin Oncol.* 2003;21:2896–2903.

80. Poplin EA, Benedetti JK, Estes NC, et al. Phase III Southwest Oncology Group 9415/Integroup 0153 Randomized Trial of Fluorouracil, Leucovorin, and Levamisole Versus Fluorouracil Continuous Infusion and Levamisole for Adjuvant Treatment of Stage III and High-Risk Stage II Colon Cancer. *J Clin Oncol.* 2005;23:1819–1825.

81. Chau I, Norman AR, Cunningham D, et al. A randomized comparison between 6 months of bolus fluorouracil/leucovorin and 12 weeks of protracted venous infusion fluorouracil as adjuvant treatment in colorectal cancer. *Ann Oncol.* 2005;16:549–557.

82. Twelves C, Wong A, Nowacki MP, et al. Capecitabine as Adjuvant Treatment for Stage III Colon Cancer. *N Engl J Med.* 2005;352:2696–2704.

83. Scheithauer W, McKendrick J, Begbie S, et al. Oral capecitabine as an alternative to i.v. 5-fluorouracil-based adjuvant therapy for colon cancer: safety results of a randomized, phase III trial. *Annals of Oncology.* 2003;14:1735–1743.

84. Meta-Analysis Group of the Japanese Society for Cancer of the Colon and Rectum and the Meta-Analysis Group in Cancer. Efficacy of Oral Adjuvant Therapy After Resection of Colorectal Cancer: 5-Year Results From Three Randomized Trials. *J Clin Oncol.* 2004;22:484–492.

85. Sadahiro S, Suzuki T, Ishikawa K, et al. Prophylactic Hepatic Arterial Infusion Chemotherapy for the Prevention of Liver Metastasis in Patients with Colon Carcinoma. A Randomized Controlled Trial. *Cancer.* 2004:590–597.

86. Piedbois P, Buyse M, Gray R, et al. Portal vein infusion is an effective adjuvant treatment for patients with colorectal cancer. *Proc Am Soc Clin Oncol.* 1996;14:192 (Abstract 444).

87. Beart RW, Moertel CG, Wieand HS, et al. Adjuvant therapy for resectable colorectal carcinoma with fluorouracil administered by portal vein infusion. *Arch Surg.* 1190;125:897–901.

88. Fielding L, Hittinger R, Grace R, et al. Randomized controlled trial of adjuvant chemotherapy by portal vein perfusion after curative resection for colorectal adenocarcinoma. *Lancet.* 1992;340:502–506.

89. Nitti D, Wils J, Sahmoud T, et al. Final results of a phase III clinical trial on adjuvant intraportal infusion with heparin and –fluorouracil (5-FU) in resectable colon cancer (EORTC GITCCG 1983–1987). *Eur J Cancer.* 1997;33:1209–1215.

90. Rougier O, Sahmoud T, Nitti D, et al. Adjuvant portal-vein infusion of fluorouracil and heparin in colorectal cancer: a randomized trial. *Lancet.* 1998;351:1677–1681.

91. AXIS Collaborators Randomized clinical trial of adjuvant radiotherapy and 5-fluorouracil infusion in colorectal cancer (AXIS). *Br J Surg.* 2003;90:1200–1212.

92. Wolmark N, Rockette H, Petrelli N, et al. Long-term results of the efficacy of perioperative portal vein infusion of 5-FU for treatment of colon cancer: NSABP C-02. *Proc Am Soc Clin Oncol.* 1994;13:194 (Abstract 561).

93. Labianca R, Fossati R, Zaniboni A, et al. Randomised Trial of Intraportal and/or systemic Adjuvant Chemotherapy in Patients With Colon Carcinoma. *J Natl Cancer Inst.* 2004;96:750–758.

94. Graf W, Westlin JE, Pahiman L, et al. Adjuvant intraperitoneal 5-fluorouracil and intravenous leucovorin after colorectal cancer surgery: a randomized phase II placebo-controlled study. *Int J Colorectal Dis.* 1994;9:35–39.

95. Scheithauer W, Kornek GV, Marczell A, et al. Combined intravenous and intraperitoneal chemotherapy with flurouracil + leucovorin vs. fluorouracil + levamisole for adjuvant therapy of resected colon carcinoma. *Br J Cancer.* 1998;77:1349–1354.

96. Nordlinger B, Rougier P, Arnaoud JP, et al. Adjuvant regional chemotherapy and systemic chemotherapy versus systemic chemotherapy alone in patients with stage II-III colorectal cancer: a multicentre randomised controlled phase III trial. *Lancet Oncol.* 2005;6:459–468.

97. Vaillant JC, Nordlinger B, Deuffic S, et al. Adjuvant Intraperitoneal 5-Fluorouracil in High-Risk Colon Cancer. A Multicenter Phase III Trial. *Annals of Surgery.* 2000;231:449–456.

98. Gastrointestinal Tumor Study Group. Prolongation of the disease-free interval in surgically treated rectal carcinoma. *N Engl J Med.* 1985;312:1465–1472.

99. Wolmark N, Fisher B, Rockette H, et al. Postoperative adjuvant chemotherapy or BCG for colon cancer: results from NSABP Protocol C-01. *J Natl Cancer Inst.* 1988;80:30–36.

100. Hoover HC, Brandhorst HS, Peters LC, et al. Adjuvant active specific immunotherapy for human colorectal cancer: 6.5 year median follow-up of a phase III prospectively randomized trial. *J Clin Oncol.* 1993;11:390–339.

101. Uyl-de Groot CA, Vermorken JB, Hanna MG Jr., et al. Immunotherapy with autologous tumor cell-BCG vaccine in patients with colon cancer: a prospective study of medical and economic benefits. *Vaccine.* 2005;23:2379–2387.

102. Hanna MG Jr, Hoover HC Jr, Vermorken JB, et al. Adjuvant active specific immunotherapy of stage II and stage III colon cancer with an autologous tumor cell vaccine: first randomized phase III trials show promise. *Vaccine.* 2001;19:2576–2582.

103. Schirrmacher V, Ockert D, Beck N, et al. Newcastle disease virus infected intact autologous tumor cell vaccine for adjuvant active specific immunotherapy of resected colorectal carcinoma. *Proc Am Assoc Cancer Res.* 1995;36:A1336.

104. Harris JE, Ryan L, Hoover HC, et al. Adjuvant Active Specific Immunotherapy for Stage II and III Colon Cancer With an Autologous Tumor Cell Vaccine: Eastern Cooperative Oncology Group Study E5283. *J Clin Oncol.* 2000;18:148–157.

105. Harris J, Ryan L, Adams G, et al. Survival and relapse in adjuvant autologous tumor vaccine therapy for Dukes' B and C colon cancer-EST 5283. *Proc Am Soc Clin Oncol.* 1994;13:294 (Abstract 995).

106. Punt CJ, Nagy A, Douillard JY, et al. Edrecolomab alone or in combination with fluorouracil and folinic acid in the adjuvant treatment of stage III colon cancer: a randomised study. *Lancet.* 2002;360:671–677.

107. Fountzilas G, Zisiadis A, Dafni U, et al. Fluorouracil (FU) and leucovorin (LV) with or without interferon α-2a (IFN) as adjuvant treatment in high risk colon cancer. *Proc ASCO.* 1999;18:239a

108. Gennatas C, Vlahonikolis J, Dardoufas C, et al. Surgical adjuvant therapy of rectal carcinoma: a controlled evaluation of fluorouracil, leucovorin and radiation therapy with or without interferon Alfa-2b. *Proc ASCO.* 1999;18:240a (Abstract 921).

109. Kemeny N, Conti JA, Sigurdson E, et al. A pilot study of hepatic artery floxuridine combined with systemic 5-fluorouracil and leucovorin. *Cancer.* 1993;71:1964–1971.

110. Safi F, Hepp G, Link KH, et al. Simultaneous adjuvant regional and systemic chemotherapy after resection of liver metastases of colorectal cancer. *Proc Am Soc clin Oncol.* 1995;14:217 (Abstract 544).

111. Alberts SR, Mahoney MR, Donohue J, et al. Systemic capecitabine and oxaliplatin administered with hepatic arterial infusion (HAI) of floxuridine (FUDR) following complete resection of colorectal metastases (M-CRC) confined to the liver: A North Central Cancer Treatment Group (NCCTG) phase II intergroup trial. *J Clin Oncol.* 2006;24:152s.

112. Curley SA, Roh MS, Chase JL, et al. Adjuvant hepatic arterial infusion chemotherapy after curative resection of colorectal liver metastases. *Am J Surg.* 1993;166:743–746.

113. Lorenz M, Encke A. Adjuvant regional treatment after resection of colorectal liver metastases. *Rev Oncol.* 1993;3:24.

114. Lorenz, M, Muller HH, Schramm H, et al. Randomized trial of surgery versus surgery followed by adjuvant hepatic arterial infusion with 5-fluorouracil and folinic acid for liver metastases (Arbeitsgruppe Lebermetastasen). *Ann Surg.* 1998;228:756–762.

115. Kemeny MM, Adak S, Lipsitz S, et al. Results of the Intergroup [Eastern Cooperative Oncology Group (ECOG) and Southwest Oncology Group (SWOG)] prospective randomized study of surgery alone versus continuous hepatic artery infusion of FUDR and continuous systemic infusion of 5-FU after hepatic resection for colorectal liver metastases. *Proc Am Soc Clin Oncol.* 1999;18:264a (Abstract 1012).

116. Kemeny N, Cohen A, Huang Y, et al. Randomized study of hepatic arterial infusion (HAI) and systemic chemotherapy (SYS) versus SYS alone as adjuvant therapy after resection of hepatic metastases from colorectal cancer. *Proc Am Soc Clin Oncol.* 1999;18:263a (Abstract 1011).

117. Kemeny N, Jarnagin W, Gonen M, et al. Phase I/II Study of Hepatic Arterial Therapy With Floxuridine and Dexamethasone in Combination With Intravenous Irinotecan As Adjuvant Treatment After Resection of Hepatic Metastases From Colorectal Cancer. *J Clin Oncol.* 2003;21:3303–3309.

118. Mitry E, Fields A, Bleiberg H, et al. Adjuvant chemotherapy after potentially curative resection of metastases from colorectal cancer. A meta-analysis of two randomized trials. *J Clin Oncol.* 2006;24:152s.

119. Portier G, Elias D, Bouche O, et al. Multicenter Randomized Trial of Adjuvant Fluorouracil and Folinic Acid Compared With Surgery Alone After Resection of Colorectal Liver Metastases: FFCD ACHBTH AURC 9002 Trial. *J Clin Oncol.* 2006;24:4976–4982.

120. Benoist S, Brouquet A, Penna C, et al. Complete response of colorectal liver metastases after chemotherapy: does it mean cure? *J Clin Oncol.* 2006;24:3939–3945.

121. Bilchik AJ, Poston G, Curley SA, et al. Neoadjuvant Chemotherapy for Metastatic Colon Cancer: A Cautionary Note. *J Clin Oncol.* 2005;23:9073–9078.

122. Leichman L. Neoadjuvant Chemotherapy for Disseminated Colorectal Cancer: Changing the Paradigm. *J Clin Oncol.* 2006;24:3817–3818.

123. Willett CG, Fung CY, Kaufman DS, et al. Postoperative radiation therapy for high-risk colon carcinoma. *J Clin Oncol.* 1993;11:1112–1117.

124. Fabian C, Giri S, Estes N, et al. Adjuvant Continuous infusion 5-FU, whole abdominal radiation, and tumor-bed boost in high-risk stage III colon carcinoma: a Southwest Oncology Group Study. *Int J Radiat Oncl Biol Phys.* 1995;32:457–464.

125. Palermo JA, Richards F, Lohman KK, et al. Phase II trial of adjuvant radiation and intraperitoneal 5-fluorouracil for locally advanced colon cancer: results with 10-year follow-up. Int J Radiat Oncol Biol Phys 2000;47:725–733.

126. Willett CG, Goldberg S, Shellito PC, et al. Does postoperative irradiation play a role in the adjuvant therapy of stage T4 colon cancer? *Cancer J Sci Am.* 1999;5:242–247.

127. Niloofar A, Mosalaei A, Shapour O, et al. Role of external irradiation in high-risk resected colon cancer. *Indian J Cancer.* 2005;42:133–137.

128. Martenson JA Jr., Willett CG, Sargent DJ, et al. Phase III study of adjuvant chemotherapy and radiation therapy compared with chemotherapy alone in the surgical adjuvant treatment of colon cancer: results of intergroup protocol 0130. *J Clin Oncol.* 2004;22:3277–3283.

129. Tominaga T, Sakabe T, Koyama Y, et al. Prognostic factors for patients with colon or rectal carcinoma treated with resection only. *Cancer.* 1996;78:403–408.

130. Gerard A, Buyse M, Nordlinger B, et al. Preoperative radiotherapy as adjuvant treatment in rectal cancer: final results of a randomized study of the European Organization for Research and Treatment of Cancer (EORTC). *Ann Surg.* 1988;208:606–614.

131. Cedermark B, Johansson H, Rutqvist LE, et al. The Stockholm I Trial of Preoperative Short Term Radiotherapy in Operable Rectal Cancer: a prospective randomized trial. *Cancer.* 1995;75:2269–2275.

132. Cedermark B, Theve NO, Rieger A, et al. Preoperative short-term radiotherapy in rectal carcinoma: a preliminary report of a prospective study. *Cancer.* 1985;55:1182–1185.

133. Gastrointestinal Tumor Study Group. Survival after postoperative combination treatment of rectal cancer. *N Engl J Med.* 1986;315:1294–1295.

134. Fisher B, Wolmark N, Rockette H, et al. Postoperative adjuvant chemotherapy for rectal cancer; results from NSABP protocol R-01. *J Natl Cancer Inst.* 1988;80:21–29.

135. Sause W, Martz K, Noyes D, et al. RTOG 81-15 ECOG 83-23 evaluation of preoperative radiation therapy in operable rectal carcinoma. *Int J Radiat Oncol Biol Phys.* 1990;19:179 (Abstract).

136. Mohiuddin M, Derdel J, Marks G, et al. Results of adjuvant radiation therapy in cancer of the rectum. Thomas Jefferson University Hospital experience. *Cancer.* 1985;55:350–353.

137. Gunderson LL, Dosorety D, Blitzer DH, et al. Low dose preoperative irradiation for resectable rectal and rectosigmoid carcinoma. *Cancer.* 1983;52:446–451.

138. Shank B, Enker W, Santant J, et al. Local control with preoperative radiotherapy alone versus 'sandwich' radiotherapy for rectal carcinoma. *Int J Radiat Oncol Biol Phys.* 1987;13:111–115.

139. Wolmark N, Wieand HS, Hyams DM, et al. Randomized Trial of Postoperative Adjuvant Chemotherapy With or Without Radiotherapy for Carcinoma of the Rectum: National Surgical Adjuvant Breast and Bowel Project Protocol R-02. *J Natl Cancer Inst.* 2000;92:388–396.

140. Kapiteijn E, Marijnen CAM, Nagtegaal ID, et al. Preoperative Radiotherapy Combined With Total Mesorectal Excision For Resectable Cancer. *N Engl J Med.* 2001;345:638–646.

141. Folkesson J, Birgisson H, Pahlman L, et al. Swedish Rectal Cancer Trial: Long Lasting Benefits From Radiotherapy on Survival and Local Recurrence Rate. *J Clin Oncol.* 2005;23:5644–5650.

142. Delaney CP, Lavery IC, Brenner A, et al. Preoperative Radiotherapy Improves Survival for Patients Undergoing Total Mesorectal Excision for Stage T3 Low Rectal Cancers. *Ann Surgery.* 2002;236:203–207.

143. Martling A, Holm T, Hemming J, et al. The Stockholm II Trial on Preoperative Radiotherapy in Rectal Carcinoma. Long-term follow-up of a population-based study. *Cancer.* 2001;92:896–902.

144. Camma C, Giunta M, Fiorica F, et al. Preoperative Radiotherapy for Resectable Rectal Cancer: A Meta-analysis. *JAMA.* 2000;284:1008–1015.

145. Colorectal Cancer Collaborative Group. Adjuvant radiotherapy for rectal cancer: a systematic overview of 8,507 patients from 22 randomized trials. *Lancet.* 2001;358:1291–1304.

146. Sasson AR, Mulcahy MF, Paty PB. Update in the Management of Rectal Cancer. *ASCO Education Book.* 2006;192–198.

147. Marijnen CAM, Nagtegaal ID, Kapiteijn E, et al. Radiotherapy does not compensate for positive resection margins in rectal cancer patients: reports of a multicenter randomized trial. *Int J Rad Oncol Biol Phys.* 2003;55:1311–1320.

148. Sebag-Montefiore D, Steele R, Quirke P, et al. Routine short course pre-op radiotherapy or selective post-op chemoradiotherapy for

resectable rectal cancer? Preliminary results of the MRC CR07 randomized trial. *JCO.* 2006;24:148s.

149. Nissan A, Stojadinovic A, Shia J, et al. Predictors of Recurrence in Patients With T2 and Early T3, N0 Adenocarcinoma of the Rectum Treated by Surgery Alone. *J Clin Oncol.* 2006;24:4078–4084.

150. Havenga K, Enker WE, Norstein J, et al. Improved survival and local control after total mesorectal excision or D3 lymphadenectomy in the treatment of primary rectal cancer: an international analysis of 1411 patients. *Eur J Surg Oncology.* 1999;25:368–374.

151. Gunderson LL, Sargent DJ, Tepper JE, et al. Impact of T and N Stage and Treatment on Survival and Relapse in Adjuvant Rectal Cancer: A Pooled Analysis. *J Clin Oncol.* 2004;22:1785–1796.

152. Sauer R, Becker H, Hohenberger W, et al. Preoperative versus Postoperative Chemoradiotherapy for Rectal Cancer. *N Engl J Med.* 2004:1731–1740.

153. Frykholm GJ, Glimelius B, Pahlman L. Preoperative or postoperative irradiation in adenocarcinoma of the rectum: final treatment results of a randomized trial and an evaluation of late secondary effects. *Dis Colon Rectum* 1993;36:564–572.

154. Zoetmulder FAN, Taal BG, Van Tinteren H. Adjuvant 5FU plus levamisole improves survival in stage II and III colonic cancer, but not in rectal cancer. Interim analysis of the Netherlands Adjuvant Colorectal Cancer Project (NACCP). *Proc ASCO.* 1999;18:266a.

155. Douglass HO, Stablein DM, Mayer RJ. Ten years follow-up of first generation of surgical adjuvant rectal cancer studies of the gastrointestinal tumor study group. In Hamilton J, Elliot J, eds. *NIH Consensus Development Conference: adjuvant therapy for patients with colon and rectum cancer.* Bethesda, MD: National Institutes of Health; 1990:35–40.

156. Douglas HO Jr. Results of surgical adjuvant trials of the Gastrointestinal Tumor Study Group. In: Wanebo HJ, ed. *Colorectal Cancer,* St Louis, MO: Mosby-Year Book, 1993;363–374.

157. O'Connell M, Martenson J, Wieand H, et al. Improving adjuvant therapy for rectal cancer by combining protracted-infusion fluorouracil with radiation therapy after curative surgery. *N Engl J Med.* 1994;331:502–507.

158. Krook JE, Moertel CG, Gunderson LL, et al. Effective surgical adjuvant therapy for high risk rectal carcinoma. *N Engl J Med.* 1991;324:709–715.

159. Tepper JE, O'Connell M, Niedzwiecki D, et al. Adjuvant Therapy in Rectal Cancer: Analysis of Stage, Sex, and Local Control-Final Report of Intergroup 0114. *J Clin Oncol.* 2002;20:1744–1750.

160. Smalley SR, Benedetti JK, Williamson SK, et al. Phase III Trial of Fluorouracil-Based Chemotherapy Regimens Plus Radiotherapy in Postoperative Adjuvant Rectal Cancer: GI INT 0144. *J Clin Oncol.* 2006;24:3542–3547.

161. Coco C, Valentini V, Manno A, et al. Long-Term Results After Neoadjuvant Radiochemotherapy for Locally Advanced Resectable Extraperitoneal Rectal Cancer. *Dis Colon Rectum.* 2006;49:311–318.

162. Ortholan C, Francois E, Thomas O, et al. Role of Radiotherapy With Surgery for T3 and Resectable T4 Rectal Cancer: Evidence From Randomized Trials. *Dis Colon Rectum* 2006;49:302–310.

163. Bosset J, Collette L, Calais G, et al. Chemotherapy with Preoperative Radiotherapy in Rectal Cancer. *N Engl J Med.* 2006;355:1114–1123.

164. Mohiuddin M, Winter K, Mitchell E, et al. Randomized phase ii study of neoadjuvant combined-modality chemoradiation for distal rectal cancer: Radiation Therapy Oncology Group Trial 0012. *J Clin Oncol.* 2006;24:650–655.

165. Rodel C, Grabenbauer GG, Papadopoulos T, et al. Phase I/II Trial of Capecitabine, Oxaliplatin, and Radiation for Rectal Cancer. *J Clin Oncol.* 2003;21:3098–3104.

166. Chau I, Brown G, Cunningham D, et al. Neoadjuvant Capecitabine and Oxaliplatin Followed by Synchronous Chemoradiation and Total Mesorectal Excision in Magnetic Resonance Imaging–Defined Poor-Risk Rectal Cancer. *J Clin Oncol.* 2006;24:668–674.

COMMENTARY
Robert W. Decker

In the first decade of the 21st century, colorectal cancer continues to be a major health problem, with new diagnoses in 2007 estimated to be 153,760 and deaths exceeding 52,000, per data from the National Center for Health Statistics (1). My colleague, Dr. Sarna, has done an excellent job of enumerating many of the salient issues we are dealing with in optimizing management of this disease. Specifically he has focused on the merits of treating patients with stage III colon cancer with postoperative adjuvant therapy, as well as reiterating the dubious benefit of treating patients with stage II disease. In rectal cancer he concluded that patients with stage T1 or T2 disease who have undergone state-of-the-art resection may be spared adjuvant radiation therapy, while patients with T3 or T4 disease, or N+ disease, would be appropriate candidates for neoadjuvant chemoradiotherapy. He has thoroughly reviewed the development of the adjuvant programs currently being used clinically, with the methodical demonstration of increasing benefits for these regimens, from 5-fluorouracil and levamisole, to 5-fluorouracil and leucovorin, and currently to the addition of oxaliplatin to this combination, with 48-hour infusions competing with protracted oral therapy (with capecitabine), but all demonstrating the benefits of adjuvant therapy. This topic is also well reviewed recently by Meyerhardt and Mayer (2). I will attempt to delve further into discussions of novel therapies, as well as extend the discussion on therapy (or not) for patients with stage II and stage IV disease.

The 21st century has seen the advent of several novel agents for the treatment of colorectal cancer, with a resultant doubling or trebling in survival for patients with metastatic disease, such that current data suggest a median survival in the range of 21 months for such patients (3,6). When the first edition of this textbook was written, we did not have oxaliplatin in our therapeutic armamentarium, nor did we have monoclonal antibodies targeting the epidermal growth factor (EGF) receptor (cetuximab, panitumumab) or vascular endothelial growth factor (VEGF; bevacizumab). These "targeted therapies" now have established roles in the treatment of metastatic disease; hence, it is anticipated they may ultimately be used earlier in the course of therapy, that is, in the adjuvant and/or neoadjuvant setting. Presently the response rates for "front-line" treatment of metastatic disease, using a combination of 5-fluorouracil (by 46-hour infusion), with bolus leucovorin, and oxaliplatin ("FOLFOX") exceed 50% even before being combined with bevacizumab (2,3). The relevance of these impressive results relates not just to improved survival, but also that response rates at this level may then lead to the downstaging of patients with earlier stage IV disease and stimulate efforts to pursue curative therapy, with secondary surgical interventions, in patients who previously would be thought to be incurable.

The "flip side" of pursuing the cure of stage IV patients is the identification of patients with early disease, that is, patients with stage II disease, who would ultimately benefit from receiving treatment, given the bodies of evidence that adjuvant treatment of patients with stage II disease as a standard has not been demonstrated to provide enough benefit to employ such an approach routinely (4,5). The answer here lies in development of better prognostic factors and the evolution of molecular analysis of tumors, to help anticipate the behavior (i.e., prognosis) of earlier lesions. Likewise, the corollary of such molecular insights will be the identification of some patients with stage III disease who may have better intrinsic prognoses and thus may not benefit from additional/adjuvant therapy.

WHICH PATIENTS WITH STAGE II COLON CANCER SHOULD RECEIVE ADJUVANT THERAPY?

Dr. Sarna has underscored the modest and nonstatistically significant benefits for adjuvant treatment in patients with stage II disease, as seen in several trials and analyses (4,5). Long-term survival of approximately 80% is typically observed, and the addition of adjuvant therapy may add another 2% to 3% to disease-free survival in these patients, a level that is not statistically significant. Although they adequately represent the data to this point, these trials antedate the use of novel targeted therapies. Patients with stage II disease, however, represent a heterogeneous group sharing the sole distinction of node negativity. Although some tumors only penetrate the muscularis propria, others perforate transmurally or invade adjacent organs. Common factors thought to represent adverse risks include obstruction, perforation, circumferential spread, and invasion of adjacent viscera (i.e., T4 lesions), and the number of negative nodes has also been identified as a factor, as reviewed by Gill et al. (7) and Benson et al. (8). Although some would interpret data on numbers of nodes identified at dissection as conferring a better prognosis, this can also be interpreted that by increasing the "denominator" (number of negative nodes), one is simply confirming that the case in question is truly a stage II, rather than being upstaged when occult node positivity is identified. The benefits of more extensive lymph node dissection has been addressed by Swanson et al. (9) and Chen and Bilchik (10) and present standards suggest that adequate sampling should include at least 12 or 13 lymph nodes. The capability to define nodal negativity with less sampling may be beneficial to the patient by decreasing postoperative morbidity. Thus, sentinel node sampling has become commonplace in treatment of breast cancer as well as melanoma, and has been explored in colon cancer. Whether there is a clinical benefit to diminishing node dissection, as there is with the other diagnoses mentioned (i.e., less lymphedema and discomfort with less axillary dissection in breast cancer), is probably a moot point in colorectal cancer, given the en bloc surgical approach used and the lack of predictive value of sentinel node sampling encountered in this diagnosis.

Although toxicity of treatment in the elderly does not differ substantially from that observed in younger patients, one must also integrate the age and health status, that is, comorbidities, of the patient when weighing the benefits of adjuvant therapy. For example, in a stage II, T3N0 presentation in a healthy 78-year-old patient with a life expectancy of 7 to 10 years, adjuvant therapy offers less benefit in terms of potential years of life gained than treating the same stage tumor in a 40-year-old patient with a life expectancy approaching 50 years. Likewise, the patient with stage III disease who is elderly and/or has serious comorbidities, and thus a diminished life expectancy, may represent a situation in which it may be more appropriate to forego the indicated adjuvant treatment. This may be obvious to some, but it is supported by the strict interpretation of clinical trials, which routinely exclude elderly patients and require "adequate organ function." Thus the results are not necessarily applicable to patients not meeting those qualifications.

TWENTY-FIRST CENTURY THERAPY: "TARGETED" TO SUCCEED

Traditional "chemotherapy" uses cytotoxic agents, that is, medications that kill tumor cells. These agents may have narrow therapeutic indices as they primarily attack growing cells, so toxicity to normal cells may be seen on the basis of their intrinsic growth kinetics; hence, granulocytes, hair, and mucous membranes are frequently affected. Likewise, attacking the DNA of the cells may damage the cells of normal tissues and lead to late secondary consequences such as leukemias and myelodysplasias, as seen with alkylating agents and topoisomerase inhibitors, among others. Clearly an approach that targets the *malignant* cell more specifically is desirable.

Targeted therapies fall primarily into two distinct classes: small molecules that specifically block a protein or proteins crucial to the growth, or malignant phenotype, of the cell, and monoclonal antibodies, that use their extreme specificity to interfere with the function or effect of the target, typically a cell surface receptor or its ligand. The *bcr/abl* gene product, derived from the reciprocal translocation between chromosome 9 and chromosome 12 (the "Philadelphia chromosome"), results in the production of a novel enzyme with tyrosine kinase activity. This was a logical choice to be the first target, as this single chromosomal rearrangement appeared to be the sine qua non leading to the clinical development of chronic myelogenous leukemia. Rather than being a marker for the disease, it provokes the molecular pathophysiologic changes that lead to the malignant phenotype of this disorder.

With the demonstration of clinical activity since human clinical trials were initiated in the late1990s, imatinib has become a model of the potential benefits of translational research and has been a miraculous treatment for patients who previously faced a terminal course after a median of 4 or 5 years; present data reveals that approximately 90% of patients remain in complete remissions after 5 years of therapy, and median survival has not been approached (11). The clinical success of imatinib has been followed by the development, testing, and marketing of numerous other small molecule inhibitors, for example, erlotinib (for lung cancer), sunitinib and sorafenib (renal cell carcinoma), and lapatinib (*HER2*-positive breast cancer), with many others in development. Although these represent significant advances in treating these diseases, tumor cells have multiple, complex cytogenetic or chromosomal abnormalities, and thus the benefits of inhibition of a particular oncogene or its product may be of much less clinical significance. The response rates to treatment with these agents are more modest, although clearly patient selection is crucial and further insights into the molecular characteristics of particular neoplasms should hopefully result in optimizing selection of appropriate therapies and result in improved response rates.

Therapeutic monoclonal antibodies use the extreme specificity of the F(ab) portion of the immunoglobulin molecule to attack a specific target; the identification of unique targets on tumor cells and the absence of these antigens on other sites, including unbound molecules, have been obstacles in their clinical utility. These agents also provide extended exposure to the therapeutic agent given their long plasma half-lives. The development and release of trastuzumab for *HER2*-positive breast cancer, and rituximab for B-cell lymphomas, has led to dramatic improvements in treatment of both diagnoses, and trastuzumab is now indicated for adjuvant treatment of *HER2*-positive breast cancer, while rituximab is routinely incorporated into chemotherapy for B-cell lymphomas, with numerous trials confirming the improved response rates and survival with these agents (12,13).

The first monoclonal antibody targeting the EGF receptor (EGF-R) was cetuximab, and studies in patients with refractory colorectal cancer confirmed efficacy both as a single agent (14) as well as in combination with irinotecan, the latter even in the face of resistance to irinotecan by itself (15). More recently, the fully humanized antibody to EGF-R, panitumumab, also has been approved for treatment of metastatic colorectal cancer. Both of these antibody agents have similar toxicities of skin rash, diarrhea, and asthenia, among others (16). The other cellular protein(s) targeted for treating colorectal cancer are the family of angiogenic factors known as "VEGF," the vascular endothelial growth factor, and its receptor, VEGF-R. When this surface receptor is bound by ligand, it results in dimerization and activation of phosphorylation of multiple gene products stimulating angiogenesis. The anti-VEGF antibody bevacizumab has been shown to increase the efficacy of chemotherapy in treating metastatic colorectal cancer (17) and the use of this agent has now become a first-line therapy for metastatic disease and is being studied in clinical trials as adjuvant therapy in conjunction with chemotherapy. More novel strategies include attacking other members of the VEGF-R family as well as interfering with the ligand itself. Thus clinical trials are underway using some of the small molecule inhibitors referred to previously, as well as using soluble VEGF-R fragments ("VEGF trap") to inhibit tumor angiogenesis.

MOLECULAR DIAGNOSTICS: MORE SPECIFIC IDENTIFICATION OF PATIENTS AT RISK

Improved response rates will be obtained through the combination of more active chemotherapeutic agents and more effective targeted therapies. However, if surgery cures almost half of patients with stage III disease, and half of those receiving adjuvant therapy still relapse, then efforts to identify more precisely those patients who (a) do not need adjuvant therapy (i.e., they are surgically cured), and (b) identifying those patients who may not benefit from conventional or standard adjuvant therapy, and offering them a more individualized or novel therapy, represent important directions for the clinical oncologist to pursue. The advent of molecular diagnostics, identifying patients whose tumors genotypes convey higher or lower risks, has helped discriminate prognoses in patients with early breast cancer, and thus guide the clinician to a more tailored therapeutic approach. In addition, identification of genotypes conveying drug resistance, or sensitivity, should prove useful in formulating a specific therapeutic approach or treatment regimen for such patients, and this has been addressed in detail by Dr. Sarna.

RAMIFICATIONS OF BETTER SYSTEMIC THERAPIES ON SURGICAL TREATMENT APPROACHES: HEPATIC RESECTION FOR STAGE IV DISEASE

The prospect of providing curative therapy for patients with metastatic disease has always been an exciting, although rare, consideration. Typically this occurred when a late, solitary recurrence of the primary tumor has occurred, less often when minimal metastatic disease is recognized at the time of diagnosis. However, with the improvement in response rates to therapy, the broadening of our approach to patients with "early" stage IV disease may be of more clinical benefit. More than 20% of patients with colorectal cancer present with disseminated disease (thus emphasizing the need for better compliance with guidelines for screening colonoscopy, and so forth), most of these with hepatic metastases only. Patients with one or few identifiable lesions at the time of diagnosis form the group that may benefit the most from considering an aggressive initial approach, and potentially a secondary surgical approach to eradicate residual disease following initial treatment. When response rates to primary therapy reach the levels cited, one may anticipate dramatic improvements, or normalization, of previously abnormal scans and tumor markers, that is, "complete responses." However, the surgical resection of metastatic disease is a heroic intervention that must be reserved for the appropriate patients, despite the recent improvements in therapy noted. Various studies have attempted to identify which patients are reasonable candidates to consider such an approach. The primary factors that should be considered include the size and extent, or number, of hepatic metastases, carcinoembryonic antigen level, treatment of synchronous versus metachronous lesions, and the distribution of the lesions in the liver (18,19). Pathologic review showing viable cells in 80% of resected specimens that appeared to be complete responses on imaging, as well as subsequent relapse at sites believed previously to have responded completely, underscore the need to treat each identified lesion fully (20).

If resection is not feasible, then local measures, such as radiofrequency ablation, embolization, or other physical techniques, should be applied, and attempts to identify metastases fully include the use of intraoperative ultrasound and other imaging modalities (18,19). When such approaches are employed, the data suggest that up to 50% of selected patients may enjoy long-term remissions or even cure.

Additional questions being addressed by the medical oncologist concern the role of "adjuvant" therapy after hepatic resection versus "neoadjuvant" therapy prior to such procedures. Although the literature is nebulous on the benefits of such treatments, most of the studies did not use the newest agents, which have the highest response rates and thus should lead to the best long-term results. Given the tolerable toxicity of these treatments and the finding of residual disease at surgery, it is believed that additional systemic therapy is warranted in these situations.

CONCLUSION

I have discussed the myriad novel developments in the medical treatment of colorectal cancer, from the newer and more specific agents available to treat this disease, to the more precise identification of patients who would be the most appropriate candidates for our interventions. The pace of progress in the past decade is unprecedented and should hopefully continue in the coming years. With better and more extensive application of screening, and with improvements in therapeutics, we can be optimistic about the future for our patients with colorectal cancer.

REFERENCES

1. Jemal A, Siegel R, Ward E, et al. Cancer statistics, 2007. *CA Cancer J Clin.* 2007;57:43–66.
2. Meyerhardt J, Mayer RJ. Systemic therapy for colorectal cancer. *N Engl J Med.* 2005;352:476–487.
3. Tournigand C, Andre T, Achille E, et al. FOLFIRI followed by FOLFOX6 or the reverse sequence in advanced colorectal cancer: a randomized GERCOR study. *J Clin Oncol.* 2004;22:229–237.
4. de Gramont A, Boni C, Navarro M, et al. Oxaliplatin/5FU/LV in the adjuvant treatment of stage II and stage III colon cancer: efficacy results with a median follow-up of 4 years. *J Clin Oncol.* 2005;23(Suppl) 3501.
5. Gray RG, Barnwell J, Hills R, et al. QUASAR: a randomized study of adjuvant chemotherapy (CT) vs observation including 3238 colorectal cancer patients. *J Clin Oncol.* 2004;22(Suppl) 3501.
6. Kelly H, Goldberg RM. Systemic therapy for metastatic colorectal cancer: current options, current evidence. *J Clin Oncol.* 2005;23:4553–4560.
7. Gill S, Loprinzi C, Dargent D, et al. Pooled analysis of fluorouracil-based adjuvant therapy for stage ii and iii colon cancer: who benefits and by how much? *J Clin Oncol.* 2004;22:1797–1806.
8. Benson A, Schrag D, Somerfield M, et al. American Society of Clinical Oncology Recommendations on Adjuvant Chemotherapy for Stage II Colon Cancer. *J Clin Oncol.* 2004;22:3408–3419.
9. Swanson R, Compton C, Stewart A, et al. The prognosis of T3N0 colon cancer is dependent on the number of lymph nodes examined. *Ann Surg Oncol.* 2003;10:65–71.
10. Chen S, Bilchik AJ. More extensive nodal dissection improves survival for stages i to iii of colon cancer: a population-based study. *Ann Surg.* 2006;244:602–610.
11. Druker B, Guilhot F, O'Brien S, et al. Five-year follow-up of patients receiving imatinib for chronic myeloid leukemia. *N Engl J Med.* 2006;355:2408–2417.
12. NCCN Clinical Practice Guidelines, non-Hodgkin's lymphoma. *J Natl Compr Canc Netw.* 2004;2:286–336.
13. Romond E, Perez E, Bryant J, et al. Trastuzumab plus adjuvant chemotherapy for operable HER2-positive breast cancer. *N Engl J Med.* 2005;353:1673–84.
14. Saltz L, Meropol N, Loehrer P, et al. Phase II trial of cetuximab in patients with refractory colorectal cancer that expresses the epidermal growth factor receptor. *J Clin Oncol.* 2004;22:1201–1208.
15. Cunningham D, Humblet Y, Siena S, et al. Cetuximab monotherapy and cetuximab plus irinotecan in irinotecan-refractory metastatic colorectal cancer. *N Engl J Med.* 2004;351:337–345.
16. Malik I, Hecht JR, Patnaik A, et al. Safety and efficacy of panitumumab monotherapy in patients with metastatic colorectal cancer (mCRC). *J Clin Oncol.* 2005;23(16 Suppl):251s.
17. Hurwitz H, Fehrenbacher L, Novotny W, et al. Bavacizumab plus irinotecan, fluorouracil, and leucovorin for metastatic colorectal cancer. *N Engl J Med.* 2004;350:2335–2342.
18. Kuvshinoff B, Fong Y. Surgical therapy of liver metastases. *Semin Oncol.* 2007;34:177–185.
19. Adam R, Delvart V, Pascal G, et al. Rescue surgery for unresectable colorectal liver metastases downstaged by chemotherapy: a model to predict long-term survival. *Ann Surg.* 2004;240:644–658.
20. Benoist S, Brouquet A, Penna C, et al. Complete response of colorectal liver metastases after chemotherapy: does it mean cure? *J Clin Oncol.* 2006;24:3939–3945.

41

Pelvic Exenteration: Indications, Techniques, and Results

Robert D. Moore, Alan W. Hackford, and Marvin J. Lopez

*T*otal pelvic exenteration is defined as the complete resection of the pelvic viscera and its draining lymphatic system with the objective of removing all malignant disease within the pelvis. Any discussion about pelvic exenteration would be incomplete without a tribute to the pioneers who developed and subsequently modified the procedure. Before total pelvic exenteration was conceived many "lesser" pelvic operations were developed. Radical hysterectomy was first performed by Wertheim in 1898 (1). The first radical cystectomy was performed by Verhoogen, and the first abdominoperineal resection for rectal cancer, described by Miles, was performed in 1908 (2). Each of these milestones in surgery was developed for primary malignancies of their respective organs. Each of these procedures carries with it a significant amount of morbidity.

Brunschwig (3), credited with the first article on exenterative pelvic surgery, and other pioneers observed that certain pelvic malignancies tended to remain localized, whether primary or as a recurrence. Brunschwig (3) described the procedure mostly in patients with cervical cancer. Appleby (4) and Brintnall and Flocks (5) followed with descriptions of the procedure for rectal carcinoma.

With advancements in anesthesia, sterile technique, and antibiotic therapy that occurred during World War II and in the mid-20th century, even more radical surgical options became feasible. Dr. Eugene Bricker (6), a mentor of the current senior author, gives a fascinating first-hand account of the evolution of radical pelvic surgery in the *Surgical Oncology Clinics of North America* in 1994. In his writings Dr. Bricker describes the different centers that began to develop the techniques after observing that some pelvic carcinomas, particularly cervical and rectal, tended to remain locally advanced longer than other pelvic malignancies.

One of the main challenges of the procedure was developing an adequate substitute for the bladder. Credit for the first successful urinary diversion is usually given to Pawlik who, in 1889, reimplanted the ureters into the vagina of a woman who subsequently lived 16 years (7). Brunschwig (3), in his landmark series, used the wet colostomy by transplanting the ureters to the colon proximal to the colostomy. Appleby (4), as well as Brintnall and Flocks (5), also transplanted the ureters to the colon. Bricker (8) originally used isolated cecum as a bladder substitute. However, he did not obtain good results and soon thereafter pioneered the ileal conduit (9), which is predominantly used today. Of note Gilchrist et al. (10) were able to develop a continent cecal substitute for the bladder, as have others.

After more than 50 years, the technical aspects of the procedure remain largely the same. Some modifications in technique, such as ilioinguinal lymphadenectomy, sacrococcygectomy, and others have been developed since the early procedures. The similarity of the procedure today with that of over 50 years ago is a testament to the innovations of the pioneers of such extensive of pelvic surgery.

PATIENT SELECTION, INDICATIONS, AND CONTRAINDICATIONS

Pelvic exenteration is an option that may be applicable as a component in the current multidisciplinary approach to extensive pelvic malignancy. Selecting the appropriate patients for this procedure and its timing includes the participation not only of the surgical oncologist but frequently the medical oncologist and the radiation therapist. The primary care physician and often a psychiatrist or psychologist also are important participants in the selection process inasmuch as physical deformity, sexual dysfunction, the possibility of failure, and prolonged recovery are all factors that may be associated with this major procedure. Such potential morbidity must be brought to the attention of the patient for whom appropriate counseling and psychological support should be provided before proceeding with surgery. It is also imperative to involve the patient's personal support structure including his or her spouse, family, and friends. Hawighorst (11) found that the most significant contributor to anxiety in patients undergoing pelvic surgery for cancer was not the magnitude of the procedure but the lack of information and dissatisfaction with the patient-physician relationship.

Pelvic exenteration may be indicated for primary tumors, locally recurrent malignancies as salvage surgery, or, in rare cases, as a palliative procedure. During the 1940s and 1950s, pelvic exenteration was performed for a variety of malignant tumors. Although most commonly undertaken for cervical or rectal malignancies, pelvic exenteration was also performed for urologic malignancies, for cancers of the ovary, endometrium, small bowel, and anus, and occasionally even for radiation necrosis (12,13). However, with the advancement in the multidisciplinary approach to cancer, concomitant improvements in nonoperative therapy, and a better understanding of the diseases for which the procedure was previously performed, the indications for pelvic exenteration have become more focused.

Compared to other primary pelvic malignancies, cancer of the uterine cervix and some rectal carcinomas have a propensity to present with locally aggressive disease confined to the central pelvis without systemic metastases and, therefore, are the two most common tumors amenable to resection by pelvic exenteration.

T4 rectal cancer invading the lumen of the bladder or vagina constitutes an indication for exenteration as the primary procedure. When it is known by experience that the extent of the operation is unlikely to be altered by neoadjuvant therapy, including radiation, then it is reasonable to perform the surgery first to avoid the effects of radiation on the dissection. Nevertheless, there is an increasing trend to provide preoperative treatment in an effort to downstage the tumor.

Currently, cervical carcinoma is the indication for more pelvic exenterations than rectosigmoid lesions and accounts for more than half of the gynecologic malignancies treated with pelvic exenteration (13,14). Although advances in chemoradiation have decreased the number of patients requiring radical surgery for cervical carcinoma, stage IVa disease (tumor extending to the mucosa of the bladder or rectum) remains an indication for pelvic exenteration as primary treatment (15).

Carcinoma of the urinary bladder generally is adequately managed by radical cystectomy, and prostate cancer is usually treatable with radiation and hormonal therapy or prostatectomy. However, there are instances that justify the more extensive dissection provided by exenterative surgery (16,17).

Other pelvic malignancies for which exenteration may be feasible include tumors of the vagina, vulva; endometrium, ovary, and pelvic adenocarcinomas arising from an unknown primary site. Pelvic sarcomas are occasionally amenable to radical resection (18,19). In a series, published by Reid et al. (19), 9 of 46 patients with sarcoma of the female genital tract were treated with pelvic exenteration. In this series, the authors demonstrated a role for pelvic exenteration in selected patients despite the propensity for early hematogenous spread. Thus, the surgeon must make every effort to rule out distant spread before performing a pelvic exenteration on these patients.

The same principles applicable in the treatment of primary malignancies also apply to the management of recurrent disease (20). Thus, pelvic exenteration is indicated when recurrent tumor is confined to the pelvis, appears resectable with adequate marginal clearance, and can be performed leaving the patient with satisfactory functional status. As with primary resections, cervical and rectosigmoid cancers are the two most common recurrences amenable to radical salvage surgery.

Pelvic exenteration as a palliative procedure is controversial (21,22). Patients who are incurable by pelvic exenteration should not, as a rule, be subjected to such a morbid procedure. Some important exceptions in which palliative exenteration may be justified include (a) young and good-risk operative candidates who have limited unresectable distant disease associated with a symptomatic pelvic recurrence that is amenable to complete resection, (b) patients with advanced pelvic disease that is infected and unresponsive to percutaneous drainage or antibiotics, (c) patients with fistulas and obstruction that can be relieved by exenterative pelvic surgery, (d) patients with resectable pelvic malignant disease who have transfusion-dependent tumor bleeding, and (e) patients with uncontrolled pain of central or visceral origin but not pelvic parietal pain (22).

Preoperative Evaluation

Patients whose local disease appears to be amenable to pelvic exenteration require thorough evaluation prior to undertaking the procedure. Major comorbid conditions preclude a procedure of this magnitude, and a short disease-free interval is a relative contraindication for patients with recurrent disease. Patients of advanced age, especially those over 65 to 70 years old, must be assessed with respect to their performance status and in the context of even moderate comorbid conditions. Severe malnutrition, progressive leg edema, extensive lymphadenopathy, and fixation of the tumor on pelvic examination under anesthesia are findings on physical examination that suggest advanced and unresectable disease.

An essential part of the preoperative evaluation is extensive radiographic evaluation, to include computed tomography (CT) of the chest, abdomen, and pelvis; magnetic resonance (MRI) of the pelvis; and positron emission tomography (PET). These studies not only determine the presence of metastatic disease but also assist in planning the operation. In primary malignancies, CT scans of the abdomen are useful in assessing the extent of invasion and identifying metastatic disease; however, low sensitivity in detecting lymph node metastases has been reported (23). In assessing patients for possible tumor recurrence, it is often difficult to distinguish recurrent disease from normal postoperative changes on CT imaging. In these cases, it is often more useful to follow a series of scans to determine any changes over time that may suggest a malignancy. For example, a diminishing mass in the presacral region is suggestive of fibrosis, while a mass that enlarges or becomes less well defined are signs worrisome for recurrent malignancy (24). When a question remains, CT-guided biopsies of the region in question have been shown to be helpful in detecting early recurrence (25).

MRI for primary and recurrent pelvic cancer has been studied extensively (26). Although it does not replace CT imaging, MRI improves the visualization of the relationship between the advancing edge of the tumor and the pelvic fascial planes and muscles. MRI has been shown to be useful in evaluating invasion of the pelvic sidewall in patients who have not previously undergone pelvic irradiation (27). Such imaging is important inasmuch as pelvic recurrences confined to the axial location, or axial and anterior locations, are more likely to be completely resectable (R0) than those involving the pelvic sidewall (26).

In addition, MRI is an essential component of preoperative assessment when composite resections are anticipated by virtue of pelvic wall involvement. MRI is also useful in differentiating fibrosis from tumor invasion and adds further anatomic detail to CT in up to 40% of patients. MRI has shown a sensitivity of 97% and a specificity of 98%, compared with 70% and 85% for CT (22,26).

Endorectal coil MRI is useful in staging rectal cancer both by determining local invasion as well as perirectal lymph node involvement (28). Endorectal ultrasound is of limited usefulness in patients with advanced local disease.

Positron emission tomography with $2[^{18}F]$-flouro-2-deoxy-D-glocuse (FDG-PET) is of increasing interest in recent years

Table 41.1

Contraindications to Pelvic Extenteration

Absolute	Relative
Unresectable distant metastasis	Age over 70
Peritoneal carcinomatosis	Periosteal tumor fixation
Proximal pelvic ureteral obstruction	Low pelvic ureteral obstruction
Circumferential pelvic involvement	Severe malnutrition
Tumor invasion of cancellous bone	Nonaxial recurrence
Progressive leg edema	Short disease-free interval
Major comorbid conditions	Moderate comorbid conditions
Sciatic nerve pain	Multiple lymph node metastases
Extensive tumor fixation	

Modified after Lopez M, Barrios L. Evolution of pelvic exenteration. *Surg Oncol Clin North Am.* 2005;14:587–606.

both in the context of assessing local recurrence and in the evaluation of distant metastatic disease. In colorectal cancer, some studies have shown that PET scanning is more sensitive than CT (29). Although there is a paucity of literature regarding PET scanning specifically with regard to pelvic exenteration, there are studies that show its usefulness in the preoperative evaluation of patients with primary or recurrent disease who are candidates for curative resection (30,31). The emergence of fused PET-CT images enhances the value of PET imaging in that the localization of isotopic uptake is facilitated.

Findings on preoperative evaluation that are absolute or relative contraindications to proceeding with pelvic exenteration are summarized in Table 41.1 (22).

NEOADJUVANT THERAPY

The value of neoadjuvant (preoperative) chemoradiotherapy has been well documented in rectal cancer. Its use in downstaging cancers to allow sphincter-sparing procedures has changed the surgical approach to rectal cancers. The same biological and surgical principles may be applied to patients requiring pelvic exenteration for locally advanced rectal cancer. However, the effect that neoadjuvant therapy has on the extent of surgery or the technical aspects of the procedures is debatable. Many surgeons have encountered more difficult dissections associated with preoperative radiation therapy, while others have reported an increased incidence of complications (32). In contrast, Law et al. (33) argue that neither previous irradiation nor surgery has been proven to be an independent risk factor in increasing perioperative morbidity and mortality. Proponents of neoadjuvant therapy for advanced and recurrent rectal cancer cite decreased operative time and an increased percentage of resections with histologically tumor-free margins (R0 resection) (34).

With the advent of new chemotherapy regimens for cervical cancer, many patients whose cancer has been deemed unresectable may be eligible for exenteration after neoadjuvant therapy (35,36). In an encouraging pilot study, Lopez-Graniel et al. (35) treated 17 patients with persistent or locally advanced cervical cancer with neoadjuvant platinum-based chemotherapy. Nine patients responded based on bimanual pelvic examination and underwent pelvic exenteration. Four of the nine patients had achieved pathologic complete responses. At a median follow-up of 11 months, the median survival for the whole group was 11 months, 3 months in the nonoperated group, and 32 months in those subjected to exenteration.

Based on the available evidence demonstrating the downstaging effect of neoadjuvant therapy, patients with locally advanced pelvic malignancy should be considered for preoperative treatment (22).

MAJOR PRINCIPLES IN THE CONDUCT OF THE OPERATION

Confirming Resectability

Despite the extensive preoperative evaluation previously described, contraindications to proceeding with exenteration are often detected at the time of the planned operation. To avoid the morbidity of an unnecessary celiotomy, staging laparoscopy is advocated before exenteration for patients in whom it is technically feasible (22,37). The most compelling reason to use laparoscopy is because the finding of miliary peritoneal implants or a cytologic smear showing malignant cells in peritoneal fluid or lavage, neither of which is recognizable in imaging studies, constitutes a categorical contraindication to pelvic exenteration for cure. In the absence of adverse findings on laparoscopy, a small midline incision is made to allow examination of the viscera including manual palpation and possibly intraoperative ultrasound of the liver. After evaluation of the entire peritoneum and omentum, the whole length of the small bowel is inspected. After ruling out metastatic disease, the incision may need to be extended to facilitate determining the extent of local progression of the tumor.

Urinary tract obstruction is a relative contraindication for pelvic exenteration. The ureteric obstruction occurring at the ureterovesical junction is often resectable because of its central location. However, upper pelvic ureteric obstruction, where the ureter travels in close proximity to the common iliac vessels and the pelvic sidewall, is more likely to be associated with unresectable disease. Tumor surrounding the common iliac vessels is an absolute contraindication for proceeding with exenteration.

Tumor fixation within the pelvis cannot be ascertained without opening the pelvic peritoneum from the promontory of the sacrum along the brim of the pelvis to the bladder on the side where the tumor is closest to the pelvic side wall. Also, sharp mobilization of the posterior part of the rectum down to the sacrorectal ligament and the bladder anterolaterally permits the surgeon to assess mobility and the lateral extent of the tumor. These maneuvers often determine whether complete tumor excision is possible well before transection of the ureters, colon, and visceral blood supply. If the tumor is deemed to be fixed, it is most likely unresectable. However, in some cases of fixation to limited portions of the bony pelvis, an en bloc composite resection may be possible in which portions of the affected bone may be removed (22). In a series of such composite resections, Lopez and Luna-Perez (38) described exenterations that were extended to include portions of the sacrum-coccyx, the ischium, the pubic symphysis, the ischial pubic rami, and hemipelvectomy.

In some cases, vascular invasion is considered only a relative contraindication to proceeding. Major vessel invasion is generally regarded as a sign of unresectability in cases of squamous carcinoma and adenocarcinoma; however, some sarcomas associated with vascular invasion may be resected as long as suitable repair of the vessels is possible (39).

The presence of distant nodal invasion must also be determined. Both manual palpation and frozen section examination of suspicious nodes are useful to determine the presence of nodal disease. Although some advocate opening the para-aortic fascia to inspect the lymph nodes (40), others biopsy only those nodes that are suspicious.

Once the surgeon is completely satisfied with the resectability of the tumor, the operation progresses to the resection stage, with patient in the dorsal-lithotomy or similar position to expose the perineum.

Mobilization and Transection of the Colon

The sigmoid colon is divided with a stapling device, with appropriate attention to achieve a clear proximal margin and adequate lymphadenectomy in cases of rectal cancer. The rectum is mobilized on both sides, and posteriorly the mesorectum is dissected to the tip of the coccyx.

Lateral Pelvic Dissection

The lateral pelvic dissection is carried out in an identical manner on both sides of the pelvis (41). The parietal layer of the endopelvic fascia is first divided medial to the genitofemoral nerve, thereby preserving the nerve. There are no lymph nodes lateral to this nerve, which lies over the psoas muscle. The parietal fascia is then reflected medially. The fascia is contiguous with the vascular sheath of the common and external iliac vessels. This sheath is dissected off these vessels. The testicular or ovarian vessels and round ligament in women are identified, clamped, transected, and ligated. Division of the ureter is usually delayed until the surgeon is certain that a complete exenteration will be performed. Maintaining the ureter intact allows continuous measurement of urinary output and avoids leakage of urine into the operative field. This is particularly important when the urine is infected. The ureters are always ligated distally when they are divided.

After the pelvic fascia has been reflected from the psoas and major vessels, the fascia is dissected from the obturator internus muscle. At this point, the obturator nerve can be seen through an opening adjacent to this fascia. To preserve the nerve, the pelvic fascia is incised over it, and the nerve is reflected laterally. It is then protected laterally with a vein retractor until all pelvic fascia and associated lymph nodes have been reflected away from the obturator internus to the origin of the levator ani. The levator ani originates from the fascia of the obturator internus. The visceral branches of the internal iliac vessels are then systematically ligated and divided. It is not necessary to ligate the hypogastric vessels unless they are involved by tumor. If this is done, care must be taken to avoid the superior gluteal artery that originates on the deep or lateral surface of the internal iliac artery near its origin. This is especially important if the operation is associated with a hemipelvectomy because the blood supply to the posteriorly based flap may be compromised.

The suspensory bladder attachments are transected at this point. The peritoneal incision that was made lateral to the external iliac vessels and medial to the genitofemoral nerve is extended toward the internal abdominal ring onto the lower edge of the midline abdominal incision. The areolar tissue in the prevesical space is dissected away from the pelvic side of the pubis adjacent to the pubic periosteum. Entry into the retropubic vascular perivesical space should be avoided because troublesome bleeding may occur and it is difficult to control. This portion of the operation is generally best performed from the perineal approach. The lymphatic cord passing from the thigh into the pelvis can then be identified; this is composed of fatty, areolar tissue containing the major lymphatics connecting the iliac and femoral lymphatics. It is ligated adjacent to the inguinopectineal triangle to prevent lymph fistulas and lymphoceles from the large volume of fluid that generally flows from the lower extremities into the pelvic space.

The rest of the lateral pelvic dissection depends on the condition of the perivenous tissues and identification of the lumbosacral plexus. This nerve plexus, composed of the fourth and fifth lumbar nerve roots, is situated dorsally and laterally from the obturator nerve, lying adjacent to the caudal fibers of the obturator internus muscle. After identification, the other sacral roots should be avoided by continuing the dissection medially and downward.

After the remaining vascular structures have been transected, the extent of the dissection along the pelvic surface of the levator ani muscle is determined by assessment of the lateral extent of the neoplasm. The levator ani muscle originates from the fascia of the obturator internus muscle. When the levator ani muscle has been circumferentially demonstrated, the rectum mobilized to the coccyx, and the bladder mobilized to the periurethral region, the perineal dissection can begin.

Perineal Dissection

The perineal incision in men extends from the base of the scrotum to the coccygeal region. In women, the amount of skin sacrificed is determined by the type and the proximity of the neoplasm. In some instances, it is necessary to resect the entire vulva, whereas in most cases of carcinoma arising away from the labia, the incision can be made along the labia minor, thereby preserving the major labia for reconstruction. In men, the proximal end of the penile urethra is exposed and the urethra is ligated and divided. In operations for vesical carcinoma, the entire urethra may be dissected from the penis through a ventral incision as prophylaxis against later urethral cancers. In women, the urethra is removed en bloc with the specimen (41).

The remainder of the perineal dissection is carried out in fashion similar to that in a standard abdominoperineal resection. The ischiorectal space is entered, and the dissection is carried to the right and left inferolateral aspects of the levator ani muscle.

The levator muscle is then transected and the abdominal cavity is entered. The levator muscle is then divided circumferentially, the retropubic periosteal attachments are divided, and the specimen is removed through the perineum.

Creation of Colostomy and Urinary Diversion

A sigmoid colostomy is created in the left lower quadrant in the usual manner. Several methods of urinary tract reconstruction are available. In the ileal conduit described by Bricker (9), a segment of distal ileum is isolated to which the ureters are anastomosed. The segment of ileum is then brought through the abdominal wall as a cutaneous ileostomy. More modern methods of urinary diversion include continent conduits and neobladder reconstructions (42).

Intraoperative Radiation Therapy

Data from Memorial Sloan-Kettering Cancer Center suggest that intraoperative high-dose pelvic irradiation may improve local control among patients undergoing pelvic exenteration for recurrent cancer, especially for nonaxial recurrences (22,43,44). In the procedure described by Alektiar et al. (43), brachytherapy applicators are introduced into the tumor bed. The tumor volume is calculated on the basis of CT and MRI scans, ultrasonography, and clinical examination during surgery. Margins from the clips placed at the edges of resection by the surgeon are increased by 1 to 2 cm to obtain a safety margin. Thus, the tumor volume and the margins are defined as the treatment volume with a 100% treatment dose. A total of 20 Gy in a single dose is delivered to the treatment volume. In the authors' experience with 74 patients, the duration of the treatment sessions ranged from 20 to 87 minutes (median, 56 minutes). After completion of the radiotherapy, the applicators are removed, the operating field is irrigated, and wound closure proceeds.

Perineal and Pelvic Reconstruction

The posterior pelvic cavity is drained with closed suction catheters, and the perineal wound is closed primarily. The empty pelvis is frequently the source of considerable morbidity, especially in patients who have had or will have radiation therapy. There are several procedures designed to fill most of the pelvic cavity. The most simple, but not often available, is a large omental pedicle flap based on the gastroepiploic vessels that is transposed through the lateral gutter on the right side after the cecum and ascending colon are mobilized. Often the thickness and length of the omental tissue will fill most of the inner pelvis. Other methods that can be used include placement of absorbable or permanent mesh at the pelvic inlet, pedicle myocutaneous flaps, or free flaps using microvascular reconstruction (41,45–50). These techniques may maintain the small bowel out of the field of subsequent pelvic radiation. Vascularized flaps are also used for vaginal reconstruction (45,46,48,49).

Modifications of Total of Pelvic Exenteration

Modifications of total pelvic exenteration include anterior exenteration, posterior exenteration, and supralevator muscle exenteration (22). The first two types are used almost exclusively in women with recurrent cervical or rectal cancer, owing to the presence of the internal genitalia as a barrier to tumor extension. For women with cervical cancer involving the anterior vaginal wall and vesicovaginal septum, an anterior exenteration often suffices, whereas a posterior exenteration for recurrent low rectal cancer usually includes an extended abdominoperineal resection with en bloc resection of uterus, adnexa, and posterior vaginal wall, thus preserving the bladder. In men, an axial or central pelvic recurrence of rectal cancer generally involves the periprostatic or vesical area, and a partial pelvic exenteration often is not feasible. In the few cases in which a rectal carcinoma invades only the prostate, a combined prostatectomy, approached retropubically, and proctosigmoidectomy may preserve bladder function in the appropriately selected male patients (51). In a supralevator muscle exenteration the pelvic organs are transected at the level of the levator muscles, preserving the urogenital diaphragm as well as the low rectum and anus. This procedure may be performed in selected patients without compromising oncologic principles (52). It may also allow for orthotopic reconstruction of the lower urinary tract (53).

RESULTS OF EXENTERATIVE SURGERY

Postoperative Mortality and Morbidity

In contemporary series, mortality rates range from 0% to 15% (33,34,38,52,54–64) (Table 41.2). These low rates, compared with those of earlier series, are attributable in large part to the availability of parenteral and enteral nutritional support, modern techniques of radiotherapy, and the ability of interventional radiologists to treat various complications without reoperation. Despite these improvements in supportive care, morbidity rates remain high, 37% to 78% in contemporary published series (Table 41.2). The incidence of various complications observed in patients undergoing exenteration for rectal cancer is presented in Table 41.3.

Rectal Cancer

Various factors can be identified as having an adverse impact on the outcome of pelvic exenteration for rectal cancer. These factors include male gender, previous abdominoperineal resection, carcinoembryonic antigen-positive tumors, high *p53* proto-oncogene expression, lymphovascular tumor invasion, advanced patient age at the time of diagnosis, advanced stage of the primary tumor, hydronephrosis, tumor proximity to the pelvic sidewall, and failure to achieve microscopically clear margins of resection (22).

Experience at the University of Texas M.D. Anderson Cancer Center with pelvic exenteration for locally advanced rectal carcinoma was recently reported (63). Forty-five patients were treated for a primary lesion and 27 patients were operated on for recurrent disease. Preoperative chemoradiation was administered to 61 (85%) of the 72 patients. The overall rate of complications was 43%. The 5-year overall survival rate was 48% for all patients. The 5-year overall survival was 65% among those with primary cancers compared with 22% among those with recurrent disease ($p = 0.0007$). The 5-year disease-free survival rate for all patients was 38%; it was 52% among those treated for primary cancers compared with 13% among those treated

Table 41.2

Selected Contemporary Series of Pelvic Exenterations for Rectal Cancer[a]

Study (Ref.)	Year	N	Morbidity (%)	Mortality (%)	5-Year Survival (Recurrent) (%)	5-Year Survival (Primary) (%)	Overall Survival (%)
Law et al. (33)	2000	24	54	0	0	64	44
Kecmanovic et al. (54)	2003	28	43	10	17	32	N/A
Chen and Sheen-Chen (59)	2001	50	37	2	—	49	49
Kakuda et al. (55)	2003	22	68	6	Median survival/ 20 months	—	—
Jimenez et al. (61)	2003	55	78	5	28	77	40
Oliveira et al. (52)	2004	44	62	15	N/A	N/A	41
Gonzalez et al. (62)	2003[b]	45	56	4	32	31	31
Ike et al. (56)	2003[c]	71	66	4	—	54	54
Ike et al. (57)	2003[d]	45	77	13	14	—	14
Wiig et al. (34)	2002	47	38	4	18	36	28
Yamada et al. (60)	2002	64	50	2	23	60	32
Vitelli et al. (58)	2003	26	46	11	N/A	N/A	58
Lopez and Luna-Pérez (38)	2004[e]	19	67	0	44	—	44
Gannon et al. (63)	2007	72	43	0	22 / 13 DFS	65 / 52 DFS	48 / 38 DFS

[a] N/A, not applicable; DFS, disease-free survival.
[b] Transsacral exenteration.
[c] Total pelvic exenteration for primary rectal cancer.
[d] Total pelvic exenteration for recurrent rectal cancer.
[e] Composite exenteration.
Modified after Lopez M, Barrios L. Evolution of pelvic exenteration. *Surg Oncol Clin North Am.* 2005;14:587–606.

Table 41.3

Complications of Pelvic Exenteration for Rectal Cancer

Complication	Rate Range (%)
Wound infection	4–49
Abscess (abdominal, pelvic)	9–38
Fistula (enteral, vaginal, perineal)	3–18
Intestinal obstruction	2–33
Urinary complication	2–20
Anastomotic leaks	2–23
Cardiopulmonary	2–18
Perineal wound dehiscence	4–40
Postoperative bleeding	2–11
Deep vein thrombosis	3–8
Pulmonary embolism	4–5
Stomal hernia	3–5
Sepsis	2–10

Modified after Lopez M, Barrios L. Evolution of pelvic exenteration. *Surg Oncol Clin North Am.* 2005;14:587–606.

for recurrent cancers ($p < 0.01$). The only factor found to be predictive of poor outcome was recurrent presentation.

The most common pattern of recurrence in patients treated for primary disease was distant metastases alone (50% of recurrences). In patients treated for recurrent disease, the most common recurrence pattern was concurrent local recurrence and distant metastases (72% of recurrences). An R0 resection (microscopically clear margins) was achieved in 65 of the 72 of the patients (90%). Of the seven patients who had R1 resections (microscopically involved margins), six were dead of disease at the time of the authors' data collection. Four of the six patients experienced early recurrence of disease and died of it in <12 months. The other two patients died at 37 and 48 months after their resection. All six of these patients had a component of local recurrence, but they died of sequelae of distant disease. The only surviving patient from the R1 resection group had no recurrence at 40 months of follow-up.

Ike et al. (56) correlated the outcome of total pelvic exenteration for primary rectal cancer with tumor stage and lymph node involvement. The 5- and 10-year survival rates according to tumor stage were 65.7% and 58.8% for T3 lesions, and 39% and 39% for T4 lesions, respectively. The difference in survival rates for patients with T3 and T4 lesions was significant ($p = 0.0185$). A multivariate analysis revealed that lymph node metastasis was an independent prognostic factor for survival.

Results of contemporary series of exenterations for rectal cancer are tabulated in Table 41.2.

Gynecologic Malignancies

Sharma et al. (65) recently reported a 20-year experience with pelvic exenteration for gynecologic malignancies at Roswell Park Cancer Institute. Forty-eight patients underwent the operation during this period, all but one for recurrent disease. Thirty-eight patients had cervical cancer; one patient had two primary lesions, endocervical and endometrial; and the remaining patients had vulvar (three patients), endometrial (two patients), ovarian (two patients), or vaginal (two patients) cancers. Forty-five patients had received prior radiation therapy. Mortality from the operation was 4.2%. Early and late postoperative complication rates were 27% and 75%, respectively. Twenty-three patients (48%) required reoperation; the most common indications were for revision of the urinary conduit (43%), drainage of a pelvic abscess (30%), bowel bypass for obstruction (30%), and diversion for a fistula (17%). The median time to reoperation was 13.7 months. Following exenterative surgery, 29 patients (60%) developed recurrent disease. The median time to recurrence was 8 months, with the longest latent interval being 36 months. The site of recurrence was most often in the pelvis, followed by distant recurrences in the liver and lung, and other abdominal sites. The median survival in this series of patients was 35 months; disease-free survival was 32 months; and 5-year survival was 33%.

Marnitz et al. (64) retrospectively analyzed the course of 55 patients who underwent exenterative surgery for cervical cancer between 1998 and 2004. Primary surgery was performed in 20 patients with laparoscopically confirmed stage IVA cervical cancer, while 35 patients with recurrent cervical cancer underwent secondary exenteration. Fifty-one had total exenteration, three had posterior, and one had anterior exenteration. The overall cumulative survival of all patients after exenteration was 36.8% at 5 years with 52.5% in the primary group and 26.7% in the recurrent one ($p = 0.0472$). Complications were noted in 56.9% of patients, most commonly fistulas or gastrointestinal complications. Operative mortality was 5.5%. Survival correlated significantly with the time interval between primary treatment and recurrence (within 1 to 2 years, 16.8% 5-year survival; 2 to 5 years, 28%; >5 years, 83.2%; $p = 0.0105$) as well as with curative or palliative intention (2-year survival rate of 60% in patients with curative intent, 10.5% in those with palliative intent; $p = 0.0001$) and with tumor-free resection margins (2-year survival of 10.2% for positive margins, 5-year survival of 55.2% for negatives ones; $p = 0.0057$). The age, the type of exenteration, the histologic type, and the metastatic spread to pelvic lymph nodes had no significant influence on long-term survival.

CONCLUSIONS

Pelvic exenteration remains a daunting undertaking for both surgeon and patient alike. The surgeon as well as well as the patient must have realistic expectations regarding the feasibility of the procedure, the likelihood of both early and late complications, and the probability of long-term cure or palliation. A compassionate, interactive doctor-patient relationship is particularly important in creating the appropriate supportive environment

that is necessary with a therapeutic strategy of such magnitude (11,66). A multidisciplinary team approach to treatment of patients with advanced lesions deemed amenable to pelvic exenteration is paramount to success. Participants in evaluation and management in addition to the surgical oncologist may include urologists, plastic and reconstructive surgeons, gynecologic oncologists, medical oncologists, radiation oncologists, and, often, psychiatrists. The operation has evolved along with imaging, perioperative care, radiotherapy, and adjuvant and neoadjuvant therapy. This operation must be performed in large centers with dedicated expertise, although there are reports of successes in smaller institutions where trained personnel are available. Because in appropriately selected patients there is a significant chance of cure, prolonged survival, or improvement in the quality of life, pelvic exenteration has retained its place in the armamentarium of the surgical oncologist despite the significant morbidity associated with the procedure.

REFERENCES

1. Hughes SH, Steller MA. Radical gynecologic surgery for cancer. *Surg Oncol Clin North Am.* 2005;14:607–631.
2. Miles WE. A method for performing abdominoperineal excision for carcinoma of the rectum and of the terminal portion of the pelvic colon. *Lancet.* 1908;2:1812–1813.
3. Brunschwig A. Complete excision of pelvic viscera for advanced carcinoma: a one-stage abdominoperineal operation with end colostomy and bilateral ureteral implantation into the colon above the colostomy. *Cancer.* 1948;1:177–183.
4. Appleby LH. Proctocystectomy: the management of colostomy with ureteral transplants. *Am J Surg.* 1950;79:57–60.
5. Brintnall ES, Flocks RH. En masse "pelvic viscerectomy" with ureterointestinal anastomosis. *Arch Surg.* 1961;61:851.
6. Bricker EM. Evolution of radical pelvic surgery. *Surg Oncol Clin North Am.* 1994;3:197–203.
7. Bast RC Jr, Kufe DW, Pollack RE. *Cancer Medicine*, 5th ed. BC Decker: Ontario, Canada, 2000.
8. Bricker EM, Eisman B. Bladder Reconstruction from cecum and ascending colon following resection of pelvic viscera. *Ann Surg.* 1950;132:77–84.
9. Bricker EM. Bladder substitution after pelvic evisceration. *Surg Clin North Am.* 1950;30:1511–1521.
10. Gilchrist RK, Merrick JW, Hamlin HH, et al. Construction of a substitute bladder and urethra. *Surg Gynecol Obstet.* 1950;90:752–760.
11. Hawighorst S. The physician patient relationship before cancer treatment: a prospective longitudinal study. *Gynecol Oncol.* 2004;94:93–97.
12. Kiselow M, Butcher HR Jr, Bricker EM. Results of radical surgical treatment of advanced pelvic cancer: a fifteen year study. *Ann Surg.* 1967;166:428–436.
13. Lawhead RA Jr, Clark DG Smith DH, et al. Pelvic exenteration for recurrent or persistent gynecologic malignancies: a ten year review of the Memorial Sloan-Kettering Cancer Center experience (1972–1981). *Gynecol Oncol.* 1989;22:279–282.
14. Merrick HW. Patient selection and preoperative evaluation for radical pelvic surgery. *Surg Oncol Clin North Am.* 1994;3:205–216.
15. Basil JB, Horowitz IR. Cervical carcinoma: contemporary management. *Obstet Gynecol Clin North Am.* 2001;28:727–742.
16. Roos EJ, van Eijkeren MA, Boon TA, et al. Pelvic exenteration as treatment of recurrent or advanced gynecologic and urologic cancer. *Int J Gynecol Cancer.* 2005;15:624–629.

17. Zincke H. Radical Prostatectomy and exenterative procedures for local failure after radiotherapy with curative intent: comparison of outcomes. *J Urol.* 1992;147:894–895.

18. Lopes A, Pelvic exenteration and sphincter preservation in the treatment of soft tissue sarcomas. *Eur J Surg Oncol.* 2004;30:972–975.

19. Reid GC, Morley GW, Schmidt RW, et al. The role of pelvic exenteration for sarcomatous malignancies. *Obstet Gynecol.* 1989;74:80–84.

20. Moffat FL Jr, Yeung RS, Falk RE, et al. Exenterative surgery for recurrent pelvic neoplasia. *Surg Oncol Clin North Am.* 1994;3:277–290.

21. Yeung RS, Palliative pelvic exenteration. *Surg Oncol Clin North Am.* 1994;3:337–346.

22. Lopez M, Barrios L. Evolution of pelvic exenteration. *Surg Oncol Clin North Am.* 2005;14:587–606.

23. Thompson WN, Halvorsen R, Foster WL Jr, et al. Preoperative and postoperative CT staging of rectosigmoid carcinoma. *Am J Roentgenol.* 1986;146:703–710.

24. Kelvin FM, Korobkin M, Heaston DK, et al. The pelvis after surgery for rectal carcinoma: Serial CT observations with emphasis on non-neoplastic features. *Am J Roentgenol.* 1983;141:959–960.

25. Butch RJ, Wittenberg J, Mueller PR, et al. Presacral masses after abdominoperineal resection for colorectal carcinoma: the need for needle biopsy. *Am J Roentgenol.* 1985;144:309–312.

26. Moore HG, Shoup M, Riedel E, et al. Colorectal cancer pelvic recurrences: determinants of resectability. *Dis Colon Rectum.* 2004;47:1599–1606.

27. Bertram C, Brown G. Endorectal ultrasound and magnetic resonance imaging in rectal cancer staging. *Gastroenterol Clin North Am.* 2002;31:827–839.

28. Toricelli P. Endorectal coil MRI in local staging of rectal cancer. *Radiol Med (Torino).* 2002;(1-2):74–83.

29. Whiteford MH, Whiteford HN, Yee LF, et al. Usefulness of FDG-PET scan in the assessment of suspected metastatic or recurrent adenocarcinoma of the rectum. *Dis Colon Rectum.* 2000;43:759–767.

30. Desai DC, Zervos EE, Arnold MW, et al. Positron emission tomography affects surgical management in recurrent colorectal patients. *Ann Surg Oncol.* 2003:10:59–64.

31. Staib L, Schirrmeister H, Reske SN, et al. Is ^{18}F-flourodeoxy-glucose positron emission tomography in recurrent colon cancer a contribution to surgical decision making? *Am J Surg.* 2000;180:1–5.

32. Mirhashemi R, Averette HE, Estape R, et al. Low colorectal anastamosis after colorectal surgery: a risk factor analysis. *Am J Obs Gynecol.* 2000;182:1375–1379.

33. Law WL, Chu KW, Choi HK. Total pelvic exenteration for locally advanced rectal cancer. *J Am Coll Surg.* 2000;190:78–83.

34. Wiig JN, Poulsen JN, Larsen S, et al. Total pelvic exenteration with preoperative irradiation for advanced and recurrent rectal cancer. *Eur J Surg.* 2002;168:42–48.

35. Lopez-Graniel C, Dolores R, Cetina L, Gonzalez A, et al. Pre-exenterative chemotherapy, a novel therapeutic approach for patients with persistent or recurrent cervical cancer. *BMC Cancer.* 2005;5:118.

36. Sardi JE, Neoadjuvant chemotherapy in gynecologic oncology. *Surg Clin North Am,* 2001;81:965–985.

37. Köhler C, Tozzi R, Possover M, et al. Explorative laparoscopy prior to exenterative surgery. *Gynecol Oncol.* 2002;86:311–315.

38. Lopez M.J, Luna-Pérez P. Composite pelvic exenteration: is it worthwhile? *Ann Surg Oncol.* 2003;11:27–33.

39. Karakousis CP, Surgical treatment of pelvic sarcomas. *Surg Oncol Clin North Am.* 1994;3381–395.

40. Vezeridis MP, Wanebo HJ. Extended radical pelvic surgery including sacral resection. *Surg Oncol Clin North Am.* 1994;3:291–305.

41. Lopez MJ, Spratt JS. Exenterative pelvic surgery. *J Surg Oncol.* 1999;72:102–114.

42. Seigne JD, McDougal WS. Urinary diversion. *Surg Oncol Clin North Am.* 1994;3;307–322.

43. Alektiar KM, Zelefsky MJ, Paty PB, et al. High-dose rate intraoperative brachytherapy for recurrent colorectal cancer. *Int J Radiat Oncol Biol Phys.* 2000;48:219–226.

44. Shoup M, Guillem JG, Alektiar KM, et al. Predictors of survival in recurrent rectal cancer after resection and intraoperative radiotherapy. *Dis Colon Rectum.* 2002;45:585–592.

45. Tobin G. Pelvic, vaginal and perineal reconstruction in radical pelvic surgery. *Surg Oncol Clin North Am.* 1994;3;397–413.

46. McCraw JB, Massey FM, Shanklin KF, et al. Vaginal reconstruction with gracilis myocutaneous flaps. *Plast Reconstr Surg.* 1976;58:176–183.

47. Reddy VR, Stevenson TR, Whetzel TP. 10 year experience with gracilis myofasciocutaneous flap. *Plast Reconstr Surg.* 2005;117 635–639.

48. Tobin GR, Day TG. Vaginal and pelvic reconstruction with distally based rectus abdominus myocutaneous flaps. *Plast Reconstr Surg.* 1988;81:62.

49. Green AE, Escobar PF, Neubaurer, et al. The martius flap neovagina revisited. *Int J Gynecol Cancer.* 2005;15:964–966.

50. Chessin DB, Hartley J, Cohen AM, et al. Rectus flap reconstruction decreases perineal wound complications after pelvic chemoradiation and surgery: a cohort study. *Ann Surg Oncol.* 2005;12:104–110.

51. Campbell SC, Church JM, Fazio VW, et al. Combined radical retropubic prostatectomy and proctosigmoidectomy for en bloc removal of locally invasive carcinoma of the rectum. *Surg Gynecol Obstet.* 1993;176:605–608.

52. Oliveira Poletto AH, Lopes A, Carvalho AL, et al. Pelvic exenteration and sphincter preservation: an analysis of 96 cases. *J Surg Oncol.* 2004;86:122–127.

53. Ungar L, Palvalfi L. Pelvic exenteration without external urinary or fecal diversion in gynecological cancer patients. *Int J Gynecol Cancer.* 2006;16:364–368.

54. Kecmanovic DM, Pavlov MJ, Kovacevic PA, et al. Management of advanced pelvic cancer by exenterations. *Eur J Surg Oncol.* 2003;29:743–746.

55. Kakuda JT, Lamont JP, Chu DZJ, et al. The role of pelvic exenterations in the management of recurrent rectal cancer. *Am J Surg.* 2003;186:660–664.

56. Ike H, Shimada H, Yamaguchi S, et al. Outcome of total pelvic exenteration for primary rectal cancer. *Dis Colon Rectum.* 2003;46:474–480.

57. Ike H, Shimada H, Ohki S, et al. Outcome of total pelvic exenterations for locally recurrent rectal cancer. *Hepatogastroenterology.* 2003;50:700–703.

58. Vitelli CE, Crenca F, Fortunato L, et al. Pelvic exenterative procedures for locally advanced or recurrent colorectal carcinoma in a community hospital. *Tech Coloproctol.* 2003;7:159–163.

59. Chen H, Sheen-Chen S. Total pelvic exenteration for primary local advanced colorectal carcinoma. *World J Surg.* 2001;25:1546–1532.

60. Yamada K, Ishizawa T, Niwa K, et al. Pelvic exenteration and sacral resecion for locally advanced primary and recurrent rectal cancer. *Dis Colon Rectum.* 2002;45:1078–1084.

61. Jiminez RE, Shoup M, Cohen AM, et al. Contemporary outcomes of total pelvic exenteration in the treatment of colorectal cancer. *Dis Colon Rectum.* 2002;45:1078–1084.

62. Gonzalez RJ, McCarter MD, McDermott T, et al. Transsacral exenteration of fixed primary and recurrent anorectal cancer. *Am J Surg.* 2003;186:670–674.

63. Gannon CJ, Zager JS, Chang GJ, et al. Pelvic exenteration affords

safe and durable treatment for locally advanced rectal carcinoma. *Ann Surg Oncol.* 2007; 14: 1870–1877.

64. Marnitz S, Kohler C, Muller M, et al. Indications for primary and secondary exenterations in patients with cervical cancer. *Gynecol Oncol.* 2006;103:1023–1030.

65. Sharma S, Odunsi K, Driscoll D, et al. Pelvic exenterations for gynecological malignancies: twenty-year experience at Roswell Park Cancer Institute. *Int J Gynecol Cancer.* 2005;15:475–482.

66. Wright FC, Crooks D, Fitch M, et al. Qualitative assessment of patient experiences related to extended pelvic resection for rectal cancer. *J Surg Oncol.* 2006;93:92–99.

COMMENTARY
Kimberly A. Varker and Harold J. Wanebo

In their chapter Drs. Moore, Hackford, and Lopez have presented a summary of the technique, indications, and results of pelvic exenteration. The indication for this extensive procedure is most commonly advanced or recurrent cervical carcinoma, other recurrent gynecologic malignancies, or locally advanced primary rectal carcinoma (1). Pelvic exenteration is much less commonly performed for recurrent rectal carcinoma. Landoni et al. (2) reported that 25% of patients with stage IB or IIA cervical cancer will develop disease recurrence after therapy, with the majority being local recurrences. Radiation therapy is not as effective in this circumstance; thus, pelvic exenteration is the only potentially curative therapy for these patients. Similarly, as many as 35% of patients with rectal cancer resected for cure will experience isolated pelvic recurrence. Factors implicated in a higher risk of rectal cancer recurrence include residual disease after resection, mucinous histologic subtype, poorly differentiated tumor, elevated serum carcinoembryonic antigen, extramural venous invasion, and bowel obstruction secondary to tumor (3). Rarely, pelvic exenteration may be performed for localized soft-tissue sarcoma of the pelvis. As pointed out, the use of pelvic exenteration for palliation of drainage, pelvic pain, or rectal bleeding remains somewhat controversial.

As summarized by the authors, absolute contraindications to pelvic exenteration include unresectable distant metastasis, peritoneal carcinomatosis, circumferential involvement, involvement of cancellous bone, and progressive leg edema. Advanced chronological age in itself is not a contraindication to pelvic exenteration, although judgment must be exercised regarding medical comorbidities and fitness of the patient to withstand the operation. As discussed by the authors, there are multiple factors that should be weighed as relative contraindications when deciding whether to embark on the operation. These include factors related to tumor aggressiveness, such as high pelvic ureteral obstruction, periosteal tumor fixation, nonaxial recurrence, and short disease-free interval, as well as host factors such as severe malnutrition. Essential information regarding the decision to operate will be gained from complete history and physical examination with laboratory studies and imaging workup as necessary. Importantly, constitutional symptoms, weight loss,

and significant lower extremity edema all suggest the presence of unresectable disease. Physical examination must also include thorough examination of the draining lymph node basins.

Minimally, the imaging workup should include computed tomography (CT) of the abdomen and pelvis as well as magnetic resonance imaging of the pelvis to rule out involvement of the sacral bone. In the case of recurrent rectal cancer, magnetic resonance imaging may also aid in the differentiation of recurrent disease from postoperative fibrotic change, due to their different signal intensities on T2-weighted images (4). We maintain that tissue biopsy is essential in this circumstance. This may be obtained per vagina in the female, transanally after low anterior resection (AR), or by image-guided biopsy after abdominoperineal resection (3). Involvement of the sacral bone indicates the need for en bloc resection of the tumor with the involved sacrum via abdominosacral resection (ASR) (5,6). Although the authors comment that chest radiograph may be used to search for pulmonary metastases, we routinely employ CT of the chest for this purpose. As discussed, the role of endorectal ultrasound is limited in these cases since by definition the patients all present with advanced disease. Recent studies suggest that 18-fluorodeoxyglucose positron emission tomography (PET) is more sensitive and specific than CT of the abdomen and pelvis for detection of both locoregional recurrences and hepatic metastases from colorectal carcinoma (7–9).

In a study of 114 patients with advanced colorectal cancer (CRC) evaluated independently by CT and PET, patient management was altered by PET in 40% of patients (10). Selzner et al. (11) found that in 76 patients evaluated for resection of hepatic metastases from CRC, sensitivity of contrast-enhanced CT for local recurrence at the primary colorectal resection site was 53%, as compared with 93% for fused PET/CT, and sensitivity of contrast-enhanced CT for other extrahepatic lesions was 64%, as compared with 89% for fused PET/CT. These findings led to altered management in 21% of patients. Similarly, in 58 patients evaluated for recurrent or advanced primary CRC, the sensitivity and specificity of PET for detecting local pelvic recurrence were 91% and 100%, respectively (12). Among 39 patients with normal serum carcinoembryonic antigen and suspected recurrence of CRC that was subsequently pathologically verified, Sariyaka et al. (13) determined that PET had accuracy of 76.9%, negative predictive value of 61.5%, and positive predictive value of 84.6%. In addition, one study of 60 patients who underwent PET scanning an average of 26 months after completion of full-dose (5,000 cGy) external-beam radiation therapy (EBRT) revealed sensitivity of 84%, specificity of 88%, positive predictive value of 76%, and negative predictive value of 92% for detection of recurrent disease, suggesting that PET retains reasonable diagnostic acuity even after radiation therapy (14). PET appears to play an essential role in defining the extent of recurrent CRC, and should be employed in all patients being considered for resection of recurrent disease.

Essentials of the operative approach to pelvic exenteration include first, to carefully exclude the presence of distant metastasis by intraoperative ultrasound of the liver and inspection of the entire small bowel, and to assess resectability by opening the peritoneum along the pelvic inlet and mobilizing the bladder off its retropubic attachments. We also advocate opening the para-aortic fascia in order to sample the paraaortic lymph nodes. The major steps in pelvic exenteration, as well summarized by the authors, include the exposure, mobilization, and transection of the sigmoid colon; the lateral pelvic dissection; the anterior dissection with division of the ureters; the circumferential dissection down to the levator ani muscles; and the perineal dissection with removal of the specimen. After placement of drains, the pelvic defect should be filled by mesh or mobilized omentum. The ostomies are then created and the urinary diversion completed. Care must be taken to ensure that the stomas are well vascularized and tension-free. It is preferable to have an enterostomal therapist measure the patient both supine and sitting, and mark the ideal stoma placement on the abdomen preoperatively. Finally, the wounds are closed.

Serious consideration should be given to the employment of a rectus- or gracilis-based myocutaneous flap for a tension-free wound closure (15,16). Chessin et al. (15) studied a group of 19 patients with anorectal cancer treated by EBRT followed by abdominoperineal resection (APR) and rectus abdominus myocutaneous flap closure, as compared with a control group of 59 patients from the same period treated in an identical manner except for the rectus abdominus flap closure. A significantly lower rate of perineal wound complications occurred in the group of patients undergoing flap closure (15.8% vs. 44.1%; $p = 0.03$), whereas the incidence of other complications was not different between the two groups. We consider a flap closure to be absolutely essential in those cases that require ASR. Our previous experience has demonstrated that closure of the posterior wound after ASR with gluteus myofasciocutaneous flaps is associated with decreased morbidity as compared with primary wound closure (17).

As pointed out, various modifications of the procedure may be required in specific situations. For example, AR alone (preserving rectum) may be performed for posteriorly extending bladder cancer or vulvar cancer invading anteriorly, and posterior resection alone (preserving bladder and urethra) may be performed for low rectal cancer invading the vagina and uterus. Finally, for prostate cancer or a high rectal cancer, a supralevator resection with preservation of the low rectum and anus and creation of a rectosigmoid anastomosis may be performed.

In Table 41.2, the authors summarize results of pelvic exenteration from 14 articles published between 2000 and 2007, including some patients who underwent transsacral exenteration. Within this published experience, the overall morbidity of pelvic exenteration varied between 37% and 78% and mortality between 0% and 15%. The most commonly reported complications specific to pelvic exenteration include complications related to the urinary conduit (leak, obstruction, stenosis, and fistula), wound breakdown, and pelvic abscess or fistula (1). The incidence of postoperative complications may correlate with prior exposure to EBRT. The patient populations as well as the specific procedures reported are often heterogenous; thus, conclusions are difficult to draw regarding overall results. As expected, the reported 5-year survival from pelvic exenteration in this series of reports was higher among procedures performed for primary advanced disease (31% to 77%) as compared with those performed for recurrent disease (0% to 44%).

Special considerations apply in the case of the patient presenting with recurrent rectal cancer. Nonsurgical management options, including EBRT and systemic chemotherapy, do not of-

fer the hope of long-term survival, and additionally often provide only temporary or inadequate palliation of pain (18). Surgical resection is the only modality offering hope of cure, but it is at the expense of considerable morbidity. In a report of a single-institution experience of 90 patients undergoing resection with curative intent for isolated pelvic recurrence after curative colorectal surgery, Henry et al. (19) demonstrated median overall survival of 38 months; however, operative mortality was 4.4% and morbidity was 53%. Similarly, in a recent report of 134 patients with locally recurrent rectal cancer undergoing attempt at curative resection, resection was achieved in 85 patients, with 5-year overall survival of 36% (20). Bowne et al. (21) reported on 100 patients undergoing exploration with curative intent for locoregional recurrence, 25% of whom also had resectable distant disease. Among this challenging group of patients, 56 had an R0 resection including distant sites, with a median survival of 66 months. Finally, as discussed in a recent review article by Heriot et al. (22), the consistent finding among the majority of reports of surgical resection for locally recurrent rectal cancer is that the ability to perform R0 resection is the most important determinant of survival. In turn, this is affected by younger age at recurrence, female gender, and primary surgery having been transanal excision or sphincter-preserving procedure. R0 resection is less likely to be accomplished if the primary surgery resulted in end colostomy, pain was a symptom of recurrence, or there were multiple sites of fixation of the recurrent disease (22). Although the expected 5-year survival is lower than for patients with locally advanced primary disease, the dissection is likely to be more difficult because of disruption of tissue planes by previous surgery and/or radiotherapy, and the incidence of major complications is likely to be higher, treatment options are limited in these patients, and thus we firmly believe that there is a role for aggressive resection of recurrent disease among carefully selected patients.

Recurrent rectal cancer has unique features in comparison to recurrence of endometrial or cervical cancer, and is certainly different from ovarian cancer. We have devised a simple staging system for recurrent rectal cancer based on a slight modification of the American Joint Committee for Cancer staging, which incorporates an "R" to signify recurrence while retaining the local invasive and regional components of the TNM system (3,17). The class of recurrence ranges from a simple anastomotic recurrence (T1-2R; relatively uncommon), to a local recurrence involving the rectal wall (T3R) or peri rectal (or peri anastomotic) soft tissues (T4R). These recurrences may be amenable to resection with reconstruction in the first example (T1-2R) and abdominoperineal resection with wide field pelvic dissection to ensure adequate tumor clearance (R0 resection) in patients with T3R or T4R cancer. Anterior tumor extensions involving the prostate and/or the bladder trigone would necessitate exenterations according to the principles previously discussed. In women, initial anterior extension into vagina and/or the uterus may forestall extension into bladder/trigone and urethra and lessen the need for anterior exenteration permitting wide-field resection of perirectal soft tissue by a lesser technique (APR). Recurrence (T5R) into the posterior pelvis with involvement of musculoskeletal structures (primarily sacrum for central recurrence with or without extension to side walls of pelvis or pelvic outlet) would require resection by an abdominal-sacral resection to obtain an R0 resection.

In our series of 181 recurrent rectal cancer patients examined at a limited time point (2002), there were 86 (48%) patients with local recurrence who were treated with curative intent: 63 (73%) required ASR (abdominal-sacral resection), and 23 patients (27%) had an abdominoperineal resection or an AR with or without exenteration. An additional 23 (13%) had a palliative resection, and 17 (9%) had no surgical therapy. Forty patients (22%) had isolated pelvic perfusion (30 palliative and 10 preoperative, neoadjuvant). Fifteen patients had liver metastases (with local disease controlled by radiation/surgery) and had resection or radiofrequency ablation of dominant lesions. The 5-year survival was 24% with curative re-resection by AR/APR with or without exenteration, 31% with ASR (half of these patients had ASR combined with exenteration), and 24% with resection of liver metastases in the setting of local recurrence controlled by radiotherapy/surgery. There were occasional 5-year survivors in the palliative group, 0% to 5% ,which attests to the unique biology of rectal cancer (Wanebo HJ, Begossi G, unpublished data 2009).

In the large series reported by Moriya et al. (23) the patterns of local recurrence were classified as follows:

1. *Anastomotic* or *perianastomotic recurrence,* for which they recommended an APR.
2. *Perineal recurrence,* which occurs after APR for tumor involving pelvic floor or perineum. Here there is early invasion of coccyx, gluteus maximus, and pelvic wall, which is rarely amenable to re-resection by local excision and may require resection of pelvic wall or intrapelvic organs.
3. *Pelvic recurrence,* which can be subdivided into anterior, lateral, or dorsal recurrence. *Anterior recurrence* refers to locally recurrent rectal cancer, which invades anterior, urogenital organs and requires total pelvic exenteration for bladder invasion. The bladder may be more commonly preserved in women who have some protection from bladder invasion by the intervening uterus and vagina. *Lateral pelvic recurrence* may be secondary to laterally placed nodal metastases present in the mesorectum (or due to an inadequate lymph node dissection) with early pelvic wall invasion. *Dorsal pelvic recurrence* occurs following presacral invasion after APR or low AR with invasion of lateral side wall or sacrum.

In the review by Moriya et al. (23) of 196 consecutive patients having surgery to remove locally recurrent rectal cancer, limited surgery (APR) was done in 62 patients; total pelvic exenteration in 41; total pelvic exenteration with sacrectomy in 69; and 24 patients had unresectable recurrent disease. Of note in this series, less than 6% had RT during treatment of their primary rectal cancer, and 46% had radiation for recurrence. This contrasts with the almost universal application of radiation either of the primary rectal cancer or of the recurrence in most Western series.

As pointed out by Moriya et al. (23), the majority of recurrences after rectal cancer surgery with or without radiation are fixed to pelvic structures and require an extended resection of the musculoskeletal pelvis in conjunction with exenteration (as indicated) to achieve an R0 resection. As also emphasized by the Japanese group, such patients are optimally treated in centers that are experienced in multidisciplinary clinical management

and have surgical teams adept at managing the challenges of the extended pelvic resection needed to extirpate recurrent rectal cancer.

The success with neoadjuvant chemoradiation in treatment of rectal cancers has led to its evaluation for patients with recurrent disease. For example, in a recent study of 103 patients with clinical T3/T4 distal rectal cancers treated with two slightly differing regimens of continuous venous infusion fluorouracil and pelvic hyperfractionated radiation, tumor downstaging was observed in 78% of patients, the overall resectability rate was 93%, and the rate of pathologic complete response was 28% (24). In a randomized study of patients with clinical stage T3 or T4 or node-positive disease, 421 were randomized to preoperative chemoradiation and 402 to postoperative chemoradiation (25). The 5-year cumulative incidence of local relapse for patients receiving preoperative chemoradiation was significantly less than for patients receiving postoperative chemoradiation (6% vs. 13%, respectively). In addition, the incidence of acute toxicity was significantly less in the preoperative treatment group (27% vs. 40% for the postoperative treatment group). Mohiuddin et al. (26) studied 39 patients with recurrent rectal adenocarcinoma following previous adjuvant therapy who underwent reirradiation of the pelvis with concurrent intravenous infusion of 5-fluorouracil. Thirty-one patients had gross total resection of tumor, with 5-year actuarial survival of 24%. Importantly, there was no surgical mortality. Two patients developed delayed wound healing, and six developed late complications. In a multicenter phase 2 study of preoperative hyperfractionated chemoradiation for locally recurrent rectal cancer in previously irradiated patients, Valentini et al. (27) reported complete response in 8.5% of patients, partial response in 35.6%, no change in 52.6%, and progressive disease in 3.4%. The possibility of radical resection was significantly higher among patients who achieved complete or partial response; in turn, 5-year actuarial survival was 66.8% in patients achieving R0 resection as compared with 22.3% in unresected patients or patients undergoing subtotal tumor resection. Finally, Vermaas et al. (28) studied 92 patients with recurrent rectal cancer suitable for resection with curative intent, of whom 59 received preoperative radiotherapy and 33 did not receive preoperative radiotherapy. Complete resection was achieved in 64% of the patients who received preoperative radiotherapy, as compared with 45% of the nonirradiated patients. Local control after preoperative radiotherapy was also significantly higher at both 3 and 5 years. There was no difference in morbidity or reintervention rate between the two groups. These studies demonstrate that preoperative chemoradiation for patients with recurrent rectal cancer is associated with increased likelihood of complete resection, decreased local recurrence rates, and the potential for improved survival. Thus, we advocate preoperative chemoradiation as standard treatment for patients with recurrent rectal cancer.

In summary, pelvic exenteration is a major operative procedure indicated in specific situations including locally advanced cervical cancer, recurrent gynecologic malignancies, and locally advanced or recurrent colorectal carcinoma. Thorough history and physical examination as well as complete imaging workup are necessary in order to determine the complete disease extent and to make determinations concerning the feasibility of resection. Complete R0 resection is the goal among all patients and has been repeatedly shown to be the most important prognostic factor for survival. Major complications involving the gastrointestinal and genitourinary tracts are common; thus, the procedure should be performed in centers with significant experience.

REFERENCES

1. Pawlik TM, Skibber JM, Rodriguez-Bigas MA. Pelvic exenteration for advanced pelvic malignancies. *Ann Surg Oncol.* 2006;13:612–623.

2. Landoni F, Maneo A, Colombo A, et al. Randomised study of radical surgery versus radiotherapy for stage Ib-IIa cervical cancer. *Lancet.* 1997;350:5353–5340.

3. Wanebo HJ, Begossi G, Varker KA. Surgical management of pelvic malignancy: role of extended abdominoperineal resection/exenteration/abdominal sacral resection. *Surg Oncol Clin North Am.* 2005;14:197–224.

4. Huguier M, Houry S. Treatment of local recurrence of rectal cancer. *Am J Surg.* 1998;175:288–292.

5. Wanebo HJ, Marcove RC. Abdominal sacral resection of locally recurrent rectal cancer. *Ann Surg.* 1981;194:458–471.

6. Vezeridis MP, Wanebo HJ. Sacral resection of posterior pelvic malignancy. *Cancer Invest.* 1995;13:375–380.

7. Moore HG, Akhurst T, Larson SM, et al. A case-controlled study of 18-fluorodeoxyglucose positron emission tomography in the detection of pelvic recurrence in previously irradiated rectal cancer patients. *J Am Coll Surg.* 2003;197:22–28.

8. Whiteford MH, Whiteford HM, Yee LF, et al. Usefulness of FDG-PET scan in the assessment of suspected metastatic or recurrent adenocarcinoma of the colon and rectum. *Dis Colon Rectum.* 2000;43:459–467.

9. Arulampalam T, Costa D, Bisvbikis D, et al. The impact of FDG-PET on the management algorithm for recurrent colorectal cancer. *Eur J Nucl Med.* 2001;28:1758–65.

10. Desai DC, Zervos EE, Arnold MW, et al. Positron emission tomography affects surgical management in recurrent colorectal cancer patients. *Ann Surg Oncol.* 2003;10:59–64.

11. Selzner M, Hany TF, Wildbrett P, et al. Does the novel PET/CT imaging modality impact on the treatment of patients with metastatic colorectal cancer of the liver? *Ann Surg.* 2004;240:1027–1034.

12. Ogunbiyi OA, Flanagan FL, Dehdashti F, et al. Detection of recurrent and metastatic colorectal cancer: comparison of positron emission tomography and computed tomography. *Ann Surg Oncol.* 1997;4:613–620.

13. Sariyaka I, Bloomston M, Povoski SP, et al. FDG-PET scan in patients with clinically and/or radiologically suspicious colorectal cancer recurrence but normal CEA. *World J Surg Oncol.* 2007;5:64.

14. Moore HG, Akhurst T, Larson SM, et al. A case-controlled study of 18-fluorodeoxyglucose positron emission tomography in the detection of pelvic recurrence in previously irradiated rectal cancer patients. *J Am Coll Surg.* 2003;197:22–28.

15. Chessin DB, Hartley J, Cohen AM, et al. Rectus flap reconstruction decreases perineal wound complications after pelvic chemoradiation and surgery: a cohort study. *Ann Surg Oncol.* 2005;12:104–110.

16. Reddy VR, Stevenson TR, Whetzel TP. 10-year experience with the gracilis myofasciocutaneous flap. *Plast Reconstr Surg.* 1997;99:635–639.

17. Wanebo HJ, Antoniuk P, Koness RJ, et al. Pelvic resection of recurrent rectal cancer: technical considerations and outcomes. *Dis Colon Rectum.* 1999;42:1438–1448.

18. Wong CS, Cummings BJ, Brierly JD, et al. Treatment of locally recurrent rectal carcinoma—results and prognostic factors. *Int Radiat Oncol Biol Phys.* 1998;40:427–435.

19. Henry LR, Sigurdson E, Ross EA, et al. Resection of isolated pelvic recurrences after colorectal surgery: long-term results and predictors of improved clinical outcome. *Ann Surg Oncol.* 2007;14:1081–1091.

20. Bedrosian I, Giacco G, Pederson L, et al. Outcome after curative resection for locally recurrent rectal cancer. *Dis Colon Rectum.* 2006;49:175–182.

21. Bowne WB, Lee B, Wong WD, et al. Operative salvage for locoregional recurrent colon cancer after curative resection: an analysis of 100 cases. *Dis Colon Rectum.* 2005;48:897–909.

22. Heriot AG, Tekkis PP, Darzi A, et al. Surgery for local recurrence of rectal cancer. *Colorectal Dis.* 2006;8:733–747.

23. Moriya Y, Akasu T, Fujita S, et al. Total pelvic exenteration with distal sacrectomy for fixed recurrent rectal cancer. *Surg Clin North Am.* 2005;14:225–238.

24. Mohiuddin M, Winter K, Mitchell E, et al. Randomized phase II study of neoadjuvant combined-modality chemoradiation for distal rectal cancer: Radiation Therapy Oncology Group Trial 0012. *J Clin Oncol.* 2006;24:650–655.

25. Sauer R, Becker H, Hohenberger W, et al. Preoperative versus postoperative chemoradiotherapy for rectal cancer. *N Engl J Med.* 2004;351:1731–1740.

26. Mohiuddin M, Marks GM, Lingareddy V, et al Curative surgical resection following reirradiation for recurrent rectal cancer. *Int J Radiat Oncol Biol Phys.* 1997;39:643–649.

27. Valentini V, Morganti A, Gambacorta MA, et al. Preoperative hyperfractionated chemoradiation for locally recurrent rectal cancer in patients previously irradiated to the pelvis: a multicentric phase II study. *Int J Radiat Oncol Biol Phys.* 2006;64:1129–1139.

28. Vermaas M, Ferenschild FTJ, Nuyttens JJME, et al. Preoperative radiotherapy improves outcome in recurrent rectal cancer. *Dis Colon Rectum.* 2005;48:918–928.

42

Neuroendocrine Tumors of the Gastroenteropancreatic Axis

Eugene A. Woltering, Jason Cundiff, and John Lyons

GENERAL CONSIDERATIONS FOR NEUROENDOCRINE TUMORS

When considering a multimodality approach to a neuroendocrine tumor (NET) of the gastroenteropancreatic axis, one must first understand the basic biology of these lesions. Words like "islet cell tumor," "carcinoid," and "APUDoma" are commonly used and misused by both pathologists and clinicians. Tumors that are classified as islet cell and carcinoid are derived from a diffuse neuroendocrine system of cells. A.G.E. Pearse (1) was one of the first people to try to understand how these tumors were grouped together. His concept proposed that these tumors would take up amine precursors that were then transformed into amines by intracellular decarboxylation. Although amine precursor uptake (APUD) and decarboxylation refer predominantly to tumors like carcinoids, many people extended this concept to include all amine precursor uptake cells and thus all NETs. However, it is now evident that the cells from diffuse endocrine system cells are indeed different entities according to cytopathologic criteria and display different biologic behaviors. Indeed, if one looks at the diversity of biologic behavior of NETs, the diversity is often greater than the similarities.

Recently, the World Health Organization has adopted a new nomenclature of these NETs (2). Currently, NETs are classified by both their anatomic site of origin and by their embryologic derivation. Key concepts in understanding the biological behavior of a NET include not only the anatomic site of origin, but also the degree of tumor differentiation and the rapidity of tumor cellular proliferation. The classification of NETs is based on the general identification of five major tumor categories. These include well-differentiated and poorly differentiated neoplasms. Solciae et al. (2) classified NETs as well-differentiated endocrine tumors, well-differentiated endocrine carcinomas, poorly differentiated endocrine (small cell) carcinomas, mixed endocrine-exocrine tumors, and tumorlike lesions. These tumor classifications give some indication of tumor prognosis but they do not account for the synthesis or secretion of peptides or amines and thus do not give an insight into the signs and symptoms that are often seen in the clinical presentation of these lesions. For this reason we continue to classify tumors according to the World Health Organization guidelines but speak of these tumors as carcinoid or islet cell tumors.

The term *functional* implies that the tumor hypersecretes an amine or peptide product that results in a clinical manifestation or syndrome. Tumors that have a positive tissue stain for a specific peptide or amine may or may not secrete this substance into the circulation and thus may be functional or nonfunctional. Dr. Robert Zollinger once said that observing the effects of peptide or amine hypersecretion in functional NETs can teach us the physiology of naturally occurring peptides and amines. Thus, NETs became "experiments of nature," teaching us the physiologic effects of peptides and amines (Personal communication). Because there are few "peptide-openic" or "amine-openic" states (clearly, type I diabetes represents a peptide-openic state), it was the elucidation of the physiologic effects of peptide or amine hypersecretion that allowed us to understand the basic physiology of "normal peptide secretion." In addition to "functional tumors" there are subclassifications of NETs known as "nonfunctional." Although nonfunctional tumors can be nonsecreting tumors, they can also be secreting tumors whose peptides do not cause recognizable symptoms or syndromes. An example of this would be the hypersecretion of pancreatic polypeptide by islet cell neoplasms. The hypersecretion of this peptide is not currently associated with a specific clinical symptom complex or syndrome; thus, patients whose tumors hypersecrete pancreatic polypeptide are often misclassified as nonfunctional.

Patients with "carcinoid tumors" have, in general, well-differentiated endocrine tumors composed of serotonin/histamine/amine-containing tumor cells. The diagnosis of carcinoid does not by itself imply the presence of carcinoid syndrome or functionality. Indeed, in most series carcinoid tumors, the syndrome is present in only 10% of patients (3). Well-differentiated endocrine tumors are further subclassified by the most commonly represented tumor cell (e.g., serotonin-producing enterochromaffin tumor cells). Endocrine carcinomas (whose malignant behavior is basically defined by the presence of metastasis) can be well-differentiated or high-grade malignant, poorly differentiated tumors. These latter poorly differentiated endocrine carcinomas have a visual appearance consistent with small cell carcinomas and, in general, lend themselves to treatment with chemotherapy rather than aggressive surgery. The early part of this chapter will use carcinoid tumors as the general example for the diagnosis and subsequent management of NETs. Later sections in this chapter will describe specific islet cell tumors and their syndromes (Table 42.1).

Table 42.1

Signs and Symptoms Associated with Functional Neuroendocrine Tumors of the Gastroenteropancreatic Axis

Clinical Syndromes	Signs and Symptoms	Commonly Associated Serum/Plasma Markers
Zollinger-Ellison	Ulcers, diarrhea	Gastrin
Hypoglycemic	Sweating, loss of conciousness, hypoglycemia	Insulin, proinsulin, C-peptide
Verner-Morrison	Diarrhea, hypokalemia, hypercalcernia	VIP
Glucagonoma	Rash, hypoaminoacidenia, vascular thrombosis, mild diabetes	Glucagon
Somatostatinoma	Gallstones, diabetes, steatorrhea	Somatostatin
Foregut carcinoid	Dry flushing	5-HIAA, histamine, tachykinins, chromogranin A
Midgut carcinoid	Dry flushing, diarrhea righ-sided heart failure, wheezing	5-HIAA, tachykinins, chromogranin A, pancreastatin, neurokinin A
Hindgut carcinoid	Rare	Chromogranin A, BHCG

VIP, vasoactive intestinal polypeptide; 5-HIAA, 5-hydroxy indolacetic acid; BHCG, β-human chorionic gonadotropin.

EVALUATION OF NEUROENDOCRINE TUMORS

An adequate tumor biopsy, proper physical and radiologic evaluation, proper assimilation of this data with clinical syndrome and serum, and plasma or urine markers are probably more important in NETs than in any other form of malignancy. The key concepts that must be discerned from the histologic evaluation of tumor tissue include the degree of tumor differentiation and the rate of proliferation. In some cases, evaluation of tumor tissue should include drug-resistance testing and staining for the presence of certain receptors or signal transduction pathways. Although NETs of the "islet cell" variety are often associated with specific syndromes arising from hypersecretion of a peptide (e.g., gastrin from Zollinger-Ellison/gastrinoma tumors or insulin-proinsulin and C-peptide from hypoglycemic syndromes/insulinomas), in our experience the presence of a positive tumor stain for a specific peptide or amine does not correlate well with the presence of that peptide of amine in the patient's serum or plasma, or necessarily with the presence of a specific tumor-related complex of signs or symptoms (Figure 42.1).

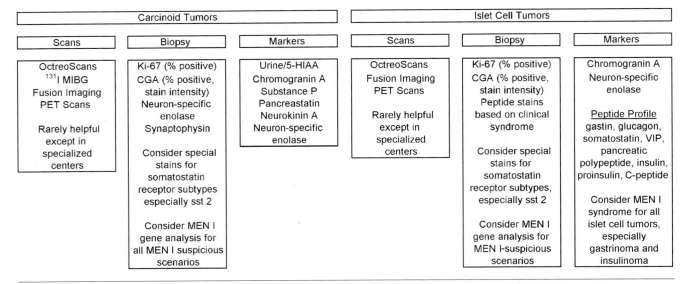

Figure 42.1 Workup of neuroendocrine tumors. Specific tests used in the diagnosis of neuroendocrine tumors. PET, positron emission tomography; CGA, chromogranin A; MEN-1, multiple endocrine neoplasia type 1; 5-HIAA, 5-hydroxyindolacetic acid; VIP, vasoactive intestinal polypeptide.

Laboratory Evaluation of Neuroendocrine Tumors

In addition to peptide or amine secretion from NET cells, chromogranins are often coreleased with peptide hormones and amines, implying the possibility that plasma or serum chromogranin A (CGA) concentrations may be a marker of NET bulk or tumor secretory activity. CGA is a major component of the secretory granules found in NET cells and is involved in angiogenesis. CGA acts as a prohormone and is degraded into a variety of active peptides. The serum concentration of CGA has been shown to reflect the mass of NETs. Because serum levels of CGA closely correlate with tumor burden in patients with NETs, especially in those with carcinoid tumors, CGA measurements are often used to confirm the diagnosis and serial CGA determinations used subsequently to monitor the clinical course and outcome of treatment in patients with NETs (4). CGA is a matrix protein found in dense core vesicles of neuroendocrine cells. It acts as a prohormone and is involved in processing, regulation, secretion, and stabilizing vesicles. Several peptides fragments are contained within the CGA molecule including B-granin, chromostatin, vasostatin, and pancreastatin. Nehar et al (5) showed that measurements of CGA and pancreatic polypeptide levels, in combination, enhance the sensitivity to detect a response to treatment in both functioning and nonfunctioning tumors to >95%. Sondenaa et al (6) found a correlation between tumor weight and plasma CGA levels in nude mice with carcinoid tumors. The octreotide-treated mice had significantly reduced plasma CGA levels when compared with untreated animals. Another study showed CGA levels returned to normal in patients after radical resection of NETs. A normal CGA level in these patients corresponded to a negative postoperative octreotide scan. Pancreastatin, a fragment of the chromogranin molecule, has been cited by some authors (7,8) to be a more sensitive indicator of the presence or growth activity of a tumor than CGA.

However, CGA remains the pivotal tumor marker for the diagnosis and follow-up of functioning and nonfunctioning NETs. The concentration of plasma CGA levels in patients with NETs reflects the degree of neuroendocrine differentiation, the total tumor burden, and when CGA measurements are used in a serial fashion can help assess the effect of medical or surgical interventions. It is critically important that the laboratory measuring serum or plasma marker levels be exquisitely well versed in the performance of these assays. Interlaboratory variations in peptide measurements (different assays, different antibodies, different normal ranges) can lead to misdiagnosis or missteps in the clinical management of the NET patient. It is also critical to determine if the patient is taking prescription or over-the-counter medications that will alter marker levels. A good example of an over-the-counter or prescription medication that will alter CGA and gastrin levels are the proton pump inhibitors (PPIs). By inducing achlorhydria they stimulate the secretion of gastrin. In time, the constant trophic effect of hypergastrinemia induces enterochromaffin like (ECL) cell hyperplasia (4–7,9–12). Those entero chromaffinlike cells, like their carcinoid phylogeny, secrete CGA and its pancreastatin subunit. Following discontinuation of PPIs, the effect on gastrin secretion and CGA elevation can last for months.

We encourage our patients to consistently use the same laboratory and encourage the NET patient community to direct their marker assay analysis to one of several reference laboratories that consistently produce high-quality results that are consistent with the clinical picture. Use of a high-quality, nationally recognized marker measurement source allows patients who seek second or third opinions nationwide to have marker values that are easily comparable across the country.

Not only do markers need to be drawn as an initial diagnostic tool, but subsequent serial measurements of markers can reflect changes in tumor growth patterns, often far earlier than seen on conventional or nuclear medicine scans. Somatostatin analogs are commonly used to treat NETs, especially those that hypersecrete peptides or amines. The acute drop in a marker following treatment with somatostatin analogs does not reflect an abrupt change in the tumor size; however, once patients are on a stable dose of somatostatin analog (3 months or longer of stable therapy on the same dose of a sustained-release product) serial progression of marker values are an accurate reflection of increasing tumor growth (13).

5-Hydroxyindolacetic acid (5-HIAA) is one of the metabolites of serotonin and it is commonly used as a urinary marker for carcinoids, especially those that exhibit carcinoid syndrome. However, a strict diet is required for several days prior to the collection of the 24-hour urine specimen, and ingestion of foods such as bananas, nuts, kiwi, pineapple, aged cheeses, and red wine may produce spuriously high results. In carcinoids, L-tryptophan is connected into 5-hydroxytryptophan (5-HTP) by tryptophan hydroxylase. 5-HTP is then converted to serotonin (5-HT [5-hydrotryptomine]) by dopa-decarboxylase. 5-HT is subsequently converted to the commonly measured 5-HIAA. In rare patients with clear-cut symptoms of carcinoid syndrome and a normal 5-HIAA level, measuring urinary levels of 5-HTP and 5-HT may be necessary. Serum serotonin is occasionally used as a marker for neuroendocrine (carcinoid) tumors that secrete this and other amines. However, when measuring serotonin, the drawing and handling of this specimen is critical for accurate serotonin determination. Serotonin is contained in platelets and hemolysis (due to improper blood-drawing techniques, high-speed centrifugation of the collection tube, and/or prolonged exposure of the serum/plasma to whole blood) may result in spuriously elevated serotonin levels. Plasma measurements of serotonin fluctuate widely and its measurement can be encouraged only in clinical situations in which there is close control and supervision of blood drawing and subsequent specimen handling. Tumors that differentiate along a peptide secreting pathway (islet cell tumors) are also commonly treated with somatostatin analogs and this therapy results in an acute decrease in circulating serum/plasma markers, but again, once stable blood levels have been achieved, serial measurement of these markers becomes a valuable tool in following the clinical progression of these diseases (14).

Thus, when a patient with a possible NET presents to the clinician, one must first have a clinical suspicion that the patient has a NET or a NET syndrome. This clinical suspicion can be heightened by a plethora of nonspecific symptoms, a well-described symptom complex arising from multiple endocrine neoplasia (MEN) syndromes, or highly specific symptoms consistent with hypersecretion of a single peptide (e.g., hypoglycemia with pro-insulin/insulin/C-peptide hypersecretion) (Figure 42.2).

Clinical Presentation	Syndrome	Tumor Type	Sites	Hormones
Flushing	Carcinoid	Carcinoid	Gastric, mid and foregut, pancreas/foregut, adrenal medulla	Serotonin, substance P, NKA, TCT, PP, CGRP, VIP
Diarrhea	Carcinoid	Carcinoid	As above	As above
	WDHHA	VIPoma	Pancreas, mast cells	VIP
	ZE	Gastrinoma	Pancreas, duodenum	Gastrin
	MCT	Medullary carcinoma	Thyroid, pancreas	Clacitonin
	PP	PPoma	Pancreas	PP
Diarrhea/steatorrhea	Somatostatin	Somatostatinoma, neurofibromatosis	Pancreas, duodenum, bleeding GI tract	Somatostatin
Wheezing	Carcinoid	Carcinoid	Gut/pancreas, lung	Serotonin, substance P, chromogranin A
Dyspepsia, ulcer disease, low pH on endoscopy	ZE	Gastrinoma	Pancreas (85%), duodenum (15%)	Gastrin
Hypoglycemia	Whipple triad	Insulinoma	Pancreas	Insulin
		Sarcomas	Retroperitoneal	IGF/binding protein
		Hepatoma	Liver	IGF
Dermatitis	Sweet syndrome	Glucagonoma	Pancreas	Glucagon
	Pellagra	Carcinoid	Midgut	Serotonin
Dementia	Sweet syndrome	Glucagonoma	Pancreas	Glucagon
Diabetes	Glucagonoma	Glucagonoma	Pancreas	Glucagon
	Somatostatin	Somatostatinoma	Pancreas	Somatostatin
Deep venous thrombosis	Somastostatin	Somatostatinoma	Pancreas	Somatostatin
Steatorrhea	Somatostatin	Somatostatinoma	Pancreas	Somatostatin
Cholelithiasis/neurofibromatosis	Somatostatin	Somatostatinoma	Pancreas	Somatostatin
Silent/liver metastases	PPoma	PPoma	Pancreas	PP
Acromegaly/gigantism	Acromegaly	Neuroendocrine tumors	Pancreas	GHRH
Cushing	Cushings	Neuroendocrine tumors	Pancreas	ACTH/CRF
Anorexia, nausea, vomiting	Hypercalcemia	Neuroendocrine tumors	Pancreas	PRHRP
Constipation, abdominal pain		VIPoma	Pancreas	VIP
Pigmentation		Neuroendocrine tumors	Pancreas	VIP
Postgastrectomy	Dumping, syncope, tachycardia, hypotension, borborygmus, explosive diarrhea, diaphoresis, mental confusion	None	Stomach/duodenum	Osmolarity, insulin, GLP

Figure 42.2 The clinical presentation, syndromes, tumor types, sites, and hormones of neuroendocrine tumors. NKA-neurokinin A; TCT-thyrocalcitonin; CGRP-calcitonin gene-related peptide; VIP-vasoactive intestinal polypeptide; WDHHA-watery diarrhea, hypokalemia, hypochlorhydria, and acidosis; VIPoma-VIP-secreting tumor; ZE-Zollinger-Ellison; MCT-medullary carcinoma of the thyroid; GI-gastrointestinal; IGF-insulinlike growth factor; PPoma-pancreatic polypeptide secreting tumor; PP-pancreatic polypeptide; GHRH-growth hormone-releasing hormone; ACTH-corticotropin; CRF-corticotrophin-releasing factor; PRHRP-parathyroid hormone-related peptide; GLP-glucagon-like peptide.

Histologic Evaluation of Neuroendocrine Tumors

The patient's initial workup should consist of an adequate tumor biopsy whenever possible. In patients with carcinoids these biopsies should be stained for Ki-67 (the percent of cells that are actively dividing at the time of tumor excision), the percent of cells that are CGA-positive (as a marker of differentiation of the lesion), and the intensity of the CGA staining in cells that contain CGA. In addition, all NETs should be stained for neuron-specific enolase and synaptophysin. In tumors associated with clinical syndromes that hypersecrete peptides, one should also obtain specific peptide stains that are specific to the syndrome (e.g., gastrin stains in patients with hyperacidity, diarrhea, and non-beta islet cell tumors of the pancreas; vasoactive intestinal polypeptide (VIP) in patients with massive unrelenting diarrhea; glucagon in patients with migratory necrotizing skin rashes, diabetes, and hypoaminoacidemia). Commonly, islet cell tumors will have a discordance between positive tissue and a negative (normal) serum/plasma level of these markers. The designation of a tumor as a gastrinoma or VIP-secreting tumors (VIPoma), or so forth is reserved for those tumors that hypersecrete these peptides into the circulation and the presence of a positive tissue stain should not be used to designate the presence of a specific functional NET. Patients with amine-secreting tumors (carcinoidlike tumors) should undergo 24-hour urinary 5-HIAA collections. These patients should also have CGA, substance P, pancreastatin, neurokinin A, and neuron-specific enolase levels drawn as baseline tumor markers. In patients with NETs of the islet cell variety, one should measure/analyze a battery of peptides, often called a *peptide profile*. These peptide profiles include the measurement gastrin, insulin, C-peptide, VIP, somatostatin, glucagon, ghrelin, and pancreatic polypeptide. When drawing these levels one must remember that an absolute overnight fast must be performed and the patient instructed not to eat, drink, chew gum, brush the teeth, or take oral medications before the blood draw. Timing of marker measurement has to be consistent to ensure that markers are drawn during the same phase of octreotide therapy in patients receiving octreotide long acting, repeatable (LAR). We obtain marker specimens immediately before the next LAR dose (14).

Initial Radiologic and Nuclear Medicine Scanning Protocols for NETs

All patients should undergo an extensive workup for the purpose of trying to discover the site of the primary tumor and the site(s) of metastases. Basic scanning protocols include computed tomography (CT) or magnetic resonance imaging (MRI) scans of the chest, abdomen, and pelvis to obtain anatomic information and nuclear imaging using [111]Indium pentetreotide and, in carcinoid patients, ^{123}I or ^{131}I-MIBG scans to survey the entire body for the location of the primary and metastatic tumor sites. Fusion scans which electronically combine the data from nuclear medicine and CT or MRI images are extremely useful when planning palliative or curative resections or targeted therapy of these lesions. For NETs, OctreoScans (Mallinkrodt Medical, St. Louis, MO are positive in about 80% of cases. Similarly, in patients with NETs of the carcinoid variety, radiolabeled MIBG scans are also positive in about 80% of cases studied. However, in these carcinoidlike lesions, using both OctreoScan and MIBG scanning will lead to the discovery of lesions in approximately 95% of patients (15). Bone scans remain the gold standard for diagnosing bone metastases in patients with NETs; however, OctreoScans can occasionally detect bone metastases missed by conventional bone scans.

THERAPY FOR NEUROENDOCRINE TUMORS

Surgical Considerations for NETs

Surgery remains a mainstay in the treatment of NETs (Figure 42.3). Surgery for these tumors fall into four major categories:

1. Resection of the primary tumor and its regional (nodal) draining basin with curative or palliative intent;
2. Surgical resection of regional or distant metastatic diseases with a cytoreductive intent;
3. Resection of disease for palliation of symptoms without cytoreductive intent;
4. Surgical extirpation of lesions associated with MEN syndromes.

In patients with well-differentiated NETs, resection of the primary and regional nodes is appropriate even in the presence of metastatic disease. Thus, resection of the primary can have either a curative or palliative intent. In a recent series by the Louisiana State University Health Sciences Center group (16), patients with advanced-stage carcinoid (stage II) underwent aggressive surgical approaches to their primary (often previously undiscovered) regional node metastases and hepatic metastases. In this series, the authors reviewed 82 consecutive patients with advanced-stage carcinoid who underwent surgical treatment with the intent to palliate their disease. Of these, 14 (17%) had an undiscovered primary and were explored solely for the purpose of discovery and resection of their primary tumor. Seventy-nine percent of those had their primary discovered. Eight additional patients (10%) presented with signs or symptoms, having undergone prior surgical procedures, but a primary was not discovered during this initial operation. Six of these 8 patients (75%) had their primary tumor diagnosed on repeat exploration.

Most of the patients in this series (55, 67%) had been explored elsewhere and were referred to this multimodality team after their cases were interrupted because their tumor was deemed unresectable. Extensive small bowel involvement was seen in 39 of 82 cases (47.6%). Mesenteric peritoneal/retroperitoneal extension of the tumor or tumor associated desmoplastic reaction was seen in 39 of 82 cases (47.6%). Mesenteric vascular encasement was observed in 12 of 82 cases. Liver metastases were present in 65 of patients (79%) and multilobar involvement was seen in 59 of the 65 cases (91%) with liver metastases. Removal of mesenteric tumor encasing the mesenteric vessels was possible in 10 of 12 cases. Interestingly, 26 of 82 patients were found to have partial or complete intestinal obstruction due to tumor, the tumor-associated desmoplastic reaction, or simple adhesions. Fourteen of these obstructions were not diagnosed preoperatively.

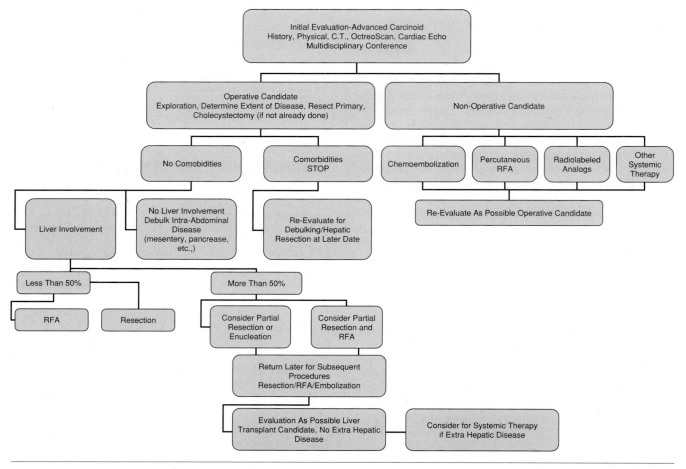

Figure 42.3 Diagnosis and management algorithm for neuroendocrine tumors. CT, computed tomography; RFA, radiofrequency ablation. (Adapted from Boudreaux JP, Putty B, Frey DJ, et al. Surgical treatment of advanced stage carcinoid tumors: lessons learned. *Ann Surg.* 2005;241; 839–846.)

All patients underwent a surgical exploration with the intent to determine the extent of disease, identify the primary tumor if not previously known or removed, perform cholecystectomy if not already done, debulk hepatic or visceral metastases by resection, radiofrequency ablation, or a combination of these procedures. Patients with pancreatic primaries underwent Whipple procedures or distal pancreatectomies when appropriate and occasionally required resection and replacement of the portal vein (n = 4). Other organs occasionally required resection. Hysterectomy or partial gastrectomy was performed when contiguous tumor involvement was present. Oophorectomy was performed when ovarian involvement was suspected by palpation or ultrasound.

The mean follow-up for all patients in this series was 22.8 months with a maximum follow-up range of 72 months. Seventy-five of 82 (91.5%) showed substantial improvement in their symptoms. Fifty-nine of the patients in this series had carcinoid syndrome and 53 of 59 (89.8%) had significant improvement in their clinical syndrome. Thirty-four patients had preoperative 5-HIAA or CGA levels measured and these decreased by an average of 53% postoperatively. Mean pre-/postoperative Karnofsky physical performance scores were 65 and 85, respectively (p <0.0001). Twenty-four of 26 patients

who had an intestinal obstruction were significantly relieved of their obstruction. Twenty-seven patients had significant preoperative pain that required oral, transdermal, or parenteral narcotics. Twenty-seven patients (100%) had significant pain relief and 20 patients (74%) were successfully weaned off narcotics. Even in these very late-stage patients, aggressive surgical extirpation of the primary and regional nodes for curative or palliative intent was done safely. The 30 day postoperative mortality was 0%. Two patients died in the 90 days following surgery: one from a fatal tumor reoccurrence and the other from a late developing pelvic abscess.

For patients with metastases to the mesentery, peritoneum, and retroperitoneum, actuarial 2- and 4-year survival rates were 64% and 44%, respectively. In comparison, 2- and 4-year actuarial survival rates were 77% and 61% for patients without peritoneal, retroperitoneal, or mesenteric metastases ($p = 0.15$). The overall median actuarial survival of this group of advanced stage patients was 51.2 months measured from the time of surgical intervention. Disease-specific actuarial survival of 2 and 4 years was 70% and 55%, respectively. Patients who underwent exploration and were found to have no or unilateral liver metastasis (n = 23) had actuarial survivals at 2 and 4 years of 89%. For those who were found to have bilateral liver metastases (n = 59), the 2- and 4-year survival rates were 68% and 52%. Patients whose primary tumor of origin was in the foregut had 2-year survival rates of 58%, while midgut and hindgut tumors both had 2-year survival rates of 79%. Four-year survival rates for foregut, midgut, and hindgut tumors were 36%, 60%, and 67%, respectively.

Cytoreductive surgery includes primary tumor resection and surgical procedures such as resection of metastases and radiofrequency ablation or cryotherapy. These therapies are designed to either remove or destroy tumor in an effort to control clinical symptoms and potentially to enhance patient survival. Cytoreductive surgery remains the first-line modality in a multimodality approach to patients with NETs. Whenever possible, gross tumors should be removed from the primary site and regional lymphatics.

For islet cell tumors such as benign insulinomas, this may require little more than surgical enucleation without a regional lymph node resection. Although for clearly malignant endocrine cell tumors, a more aggressive surgical approach, including pancreatoduodenectomy (Whipple procedure) may be warranted, even in the face of metastasis.

Many of the neuroendocrine patients who present as candidates for a cytoreductive procedure have been previously treated with somatostatin analogs or will be treated with these agents in the future. One of the most common side effects of chronic somatostatin analog therapy is the development of cholelithiasis or biliary sludge. We believe that when a surgical procedure is planned in the abdomen, a cholecystectomy should be performed (if the exposure allows) in the anticipation of somatostatin analog therapy or subsequent use of embolic procedures (bland or chemoembolization of hepatic metastases). We also believe that surgical options should precede chemoembolization or bland embolization when possible. In our experience, embolization results in an inflammatory response in the liver and results in adhesion of the liver to surrounding structures, especially the diaphragm.

Proper sequencing of systemic local or regional therapy is critically important. This requires a multimodality approach to the treatment of these diseases. Que et al. (17) performed a meta-analysis summarizing 26 years (1973-1999) of the medical literature on cytoreductive procedures on NET metastasis in the liver. In their meta-analysis, the mean 5-year survival rate in 164 carcinoid patients undergoing liver cytoreduction was 71%. One hundred nine patients had carcinoid syndrome and 33 had right-sided heart valve involvement. In this review 52% of these patients had midgut primaries and only 4% had foregut lesions. The remainder of the patients were either unreported or unlocalized. Median survival could not be estimated because of the limited duration of follow-up in many reports. Of the 164 resected carcinoid tumor patients, 43 had no evidence of disease recurrence, with follow-ups ranging from 4 to 36 months. Four additional patients had repeat resections of recurrent disease and were without evidence of disease recurrence at the time of report.

In contrast, the mean survival rates of patients undergoing partial hepatectomy for metastatic islet cell tumors (N = 63) was 82% at 5 years. Twenty-four (38%) of these patients had definable endocrinopathies (14 gastrinoma, 3 VIPoma, 10 glucagonoma, 23 nonfunctional, 7 insulinomas). Median sur-

vival again could not be estimated because of the limited follow-up data from most reported series. Two patients had repeat hepatic resections. Orthotopic liver transplantation for patients with metastatic neuroendocrine disease is considered radical by some clinicians. However, Que et al. (17) showed that patients (N = 93; 43% carcinoid, 44% islet cell, 14% unclassified) undergoing orthotopic liver transplantation for liver-predominant metastatic NET had a 51% 5-year survival and a median survival of 5.1 years. Survival for orthotopic liver transplantation for carcinoid was 44% (median survival, 3.4 years) and for patients with islet cell tumors survival was 43%.

In this meta-analysis, 86% of patients undergoing cytoreductive hepatic procedures had clinical improvement in their carcinoid syndrome and the duration of this response ranged from 4 to 120 months. Three patients had a limited response to surgery and only one patient who underwent cytoreductive surgery failed to exhibit a symptomatic response. Symptomatic response following cytoreductive hepatic surgery for islet cell tumors was again impressive. Of 63 patients, 3 had complete clinical symptomatic responses, 2 patients' responses were not reported, and only 1 of the 63 patients failed to have any clinical symptomatic response. Aggressive cytoreductive procedures often had an unexpected curative outcome with 17 of 63 patients having no evidence of recurrence as judged by hormonal markers and or imaging studies at the time of the publication of this series (17).

Hepatic Arterial Occlusion With Systemic Chemotherapy for NETs

Mayo Clinic investigators (18) studied patients with carcinoid or islet cell neoplasms who had symptoms of specific endocrine syndromes. Patients had their hepatic artery occluded either surgically or percutaneously by embolization. One hundred eleven patients were occluded; 71 of these patients received subsequent chemotherapy with alternating two-drug regimens of doxorubicin plus dacarbazine or streptozocin plus fluorouracil. Objective regressions were seen in 60% of patients treated with hepatic artery occlusion alone and 80% responded when chemotherapy regimens were added. Tumor regressions were associated with marked relief of symptoms; however, the duration of response was very short. The median duration of tumor regression was 4.0 months with occlusion alone, and when systemic chemotherapy was added, the duration of response was 18.0 months. This was not a randomized trial, and thus these groups are not directly comparable. In addition to "bland hepatic artery embolization," some authors have attempted to combine the dearterialization procedure with chemotherapy. These procedures, called *chemoembolization*, mix chemotherapeutic agents in either an oily delivery vehicle or a vehicle such as gel foam powder, designed to permanently occlude hepatic artery while delivering high-dose chemotherapy in a local area. Chemoembolization provides symptomatic responses in most patients, and approximately half the patients have objective tumor responses. However, this is not a nontoxic therapy, and the majority of the patients have abdominal pain, fever, nausea, and vomiting. Major side effects, while rare, can occur when chemoembolic/chemotherapeutic agents are infused into the gastric arterial branches or cystic artery leading to the gallbladder.

Seven series have been reported using chemoembolization for NETs. Objective response rates range from 33% to 80% and the percent of patients who had associated relief of symptoms range from 63% to 100% (19).

The Role of Somatostatin Analogs in Management of Patients with NETs

Somatostatin is a 14-amino acid cyclic peptide discovered originally by Brusseau and Gillemand (20). Although somatostatin exists in a 28-amino acid form, the most biologically active form appears to be somatostatin 14 (21).

Native somatostatin was discovered during the search for a growth hormone (somatomedin) release-inhibiting factor (SRIF). Subsequent studies have shown that somatostatin and its peptidomimetics (analogs) inhibit the secretion of a variety of naturally occurring peptides and amines. It appears that somatostatin and its analogs work by inhibiting not only peptide/amine release from granules within the cells (exocytosis), but they actually also decrease the synthesis of the secretory (peptide/amine) granules. Although somatostatin inhibits the secretion and hypersecretion of peptides and amines, the clinical use of native somatostatin is extremely limited because of the need for continuous intravenous administration, a short duration of action (half-life in the circulation of <3 minutes) and the presence of postinfusion rebound hypersecretion (22). Octreotide acetate is an octapeptide somatostatin analog first reported by Bauer et al. (23). This octapeptide analog of somatostatin had a variety of advantages over native somatostatin that made it clinically useful. First, it was able to be administered subcutaneously because of its longer half-life. Elimination half-lives of approximately 90 to 120 minutes followed subcutaneous administration. Most importantly, rebound hypersecretion of peptides or amines did not occur with this analog. Somatostatin and its analogs exert their suppressive effects through a series of somatostatin receptors. To date, five somatostatin receptors have been discovered and cloned (sst 1-sst 5). Octreotide (SMS 201-995), lanreotide (BIM 23014C) and vapreotide (RC-160) exert their suppressive effects on the release of peptides and amines predominantly via somatostatin receptor subtype 2. Other somatostatin receptors, primarily somatostatin receptor subtype 5, bind to these somatostatin analogs with significantly less affinity. All five somatostatin receptors are part of a superfamily of seven transmembrane domain receptors. These receptors, when occupied, activate the inhibitory subunit of the G protein (G_i) and in turn activate a number of signal transduction pathways, including pathways such as calcium/IP3, tyrosine kinase/phosphatase, and cyclic adenosine monophosphate signal transduction mechanisms (4). Although native somatostatin 14 and 28 bind to essentially all five somatostatin subtypes with high affinity, it is not until recently that a synthetic "universal ligand" was available that bound to multiple somatostatin receptor subtypes with high affinity. Recently, the development of SOM 230 (Novartis Pharmaceuticals, Inc., Basel, Switzerland) has entered clinical trials. This somatostatin analog binds to somatostatin receptor subtypes 1, 2, 3, and 5 with high affinity. It remains unknown if binding to multiple somatostatin receptors offers a significant benefit as compared to the sst 2 preferring analogs.

The Preoperative, Intraoperative and Postoperative Use of Octreotide to Prevent Carcinoid Crisis

Since the discovery of synthetic somatostatin analogs, the list of their uses has increased nearly exponentially over time. One of the most important concepts for the use of octreotide is its preoperative, intraoperative, and postoperative use to prevent carcinoid crisis. Although carcinoid crisis is usually associated with major surgical procedures, the release of serotonin, and the accompanying shocklike picture can be seen in periods of great stress, or when invasive procedures such as bronchoscopy, upper or lower endoscopy are undertaken. A number of regimens have been used to prevent carcinoid crisis, but we currently use a 500-mcg intravenous bolus of octreotide 2 hours prior to the surgical procedure. Immediately after administering this bolus, we institute a 500-mcg/h intravenous infusion of octreotide. This infusion is continued during the operation and for a period postoperatively. Based on the magnitude of the surgical procedure, we taper the octreotide infusion over 4 hours for a minor procedure and taper the infusion over 24 hours for most invasive surgical procedures (16). Intraoperative acute events can be treated with additional 500-to 1,000-mcg bolus injections. The use of pressors such as epinephrine may worsen rather than correct hypotension because epinephrine can cause further degranulation of amines contained within the tumor cells. We have had two cases of malignant hyperthermia that developed during a carcinoid crisis. Control of the hyperthermia was achieved using dantrolene.

Because no corresponding "crisis" has been reported with islet cell tumors, the use of preoperative, intraoperative, and postoperative octreotide infusions are far less commonly used. NETs overexpress somatostatin receptor subtype 2 on their tumor cell surface. This had led to the clinical use of somatostatin analogs to suppress hypersecretion of peptides and amines and, in their radiolabeled form, the use of somatostatin analogs as scanning and therapeutic agents. The use of somatostatin analogs in surgical patients can be considered in three categories: (a) the chronic use for suppression of the signs and symptoms of peptide/amine hypersecretion; (b) preoperative, intraoperative, and postoperative use to prevent carcinoid crisis; and (c) as diagnostic or therapeutic modalities in their radiolabeled form. All patients with symptoms due to the hypersecretion of amines (carcinoid syndrome) or the hypersecretion of peptides (gastrinoma, VIPoma, glucagonoma, growth hormone-producing tumors, and to a significantly lesser extent, insulinomas) may benefit from somatostatin analog therapy. Octreotide acetate is currently available in two forms in the United States: aqueous octreotide is commonly used as a test product to determine the tolerability of somatostatin analog therapy in its chronic, LAR form. Patients who are considered candidates for long-term somatostatin LAR therapy (Novartis Pharmaceuticals, Inc., East Hanover, NJ) should be given the aqueous (subcutaneous) form of octreotide. Although some clinicians use a single injection of octreotide in the morning, and, if well tolerated, followed by an injection of octreotide LAR in the afternoon, more commonly patients are given 200-mcg (1,000 mcg/mL, 0.2 mL) subcutaneous injections 3 times a day for 2 weeks prior to initiation of octreotide LAR therapy. It is important to challenge patients who are considered candidates for LAR therapy, because a small but finite number of patients will either experience an allergic reaction (wheezing, hives/weals) or more commonly, intolerable abdominal pain, borborygmi, flatulence, and/or steatorrhea. Somatostatin analog use is associated with a significant decrease in peptide/amine secretion, and thus pre- and postoperative somatostatin analog therapy marker levels should be obtained. When used acutely, octreotide often suppresses markers by 50% or greater, and some authors have advocated measuring peptides such as gastrin or VIP immediately before and 2 hours after a single subcutaneous injection of 100 mcg. A drop in 50% or more of these markers predicts a long-term response to these agents (13). More commonly, markers are drawn immediately before institution of long-term somatostatin analog therapy, and then after an appropriate period on therapy (to allow octreotide levels to reach steady state, usually 3 months on LAR therapy). Measurement of tumor markers after institution of somatostatin analog therapy is critical to establish a new baseline for subsequent serial measurements of markers to look for tumor progression.

Measurement of Plasma Octreotide Levels as a Guide to Octreotide Therapy for NETS

Traditionally, octreotide has been used in two forms: an aqueous form and an LAR form. Currently, LAR is available in three doses in the United States: 10, 20, and 30 mg. The current recommendations are for patients to begin aqueous Sandostatin therapy for a period of time prior to the administration of their first sustained-release injection to rule out the possibility of an allergic reaction to the medication or that the patient will not tolerate its use. Many patients over time demonstrate an increase of their symptoms or evidence of tumor growth. Recently, Woltering et al. published the results of a study in which they assayed octreotide values in serum and plasma from patients taking LAR at doses of 10, 20, 30, and 60 mg per month. In this publication, the authors point out that the K_d of the somatostatin receptor subtype 2 is approximately 1 nM (1,000 pg/mL) (24). The K_d represents the concentration of octreotide that will saturate half of the sst 2 receptors. In general, it is thought that a concentration of drug 10 times higher than the K_d will completely saturate the receptor. Thus one would expect that plasma octreotide levels of 10 nM (10,000 pg/mL) would completely saturate the sst 2 receptors. Although plasma levels of octreotide in most patients receiving LAR at a dose of 30 mg per month are higher than the K_d, they do not approach the plasma concentrations required for saturation of sst 2 receptors. In the majority of patients receiving 60 mg of LAR per month, the target of 10,000 pg/mL is achieved. There are still a significant number of patients who do not achieve this sst 2 saturating blood level, even on LAR doses of 60 mg per month. Recently, a commercial Sandostatin (octreotide acetate) assay has become available in the United States (Inter Science Institute, Inglewood, CA). Currently, in patients who are experiencing significant symptoms, or in patients who are experiencing tumor growth, we measure plasma octreotide levels in the period immediately before their next LAR dose (trough levels). In these highly symptomatic patients, we

adjust the LAR dose upward (30 mg every 2 weeks or higher) and repeat the octreotide level after three doses of LAR at the new higher dose. This allows steady-state octreotide levels to be achieved. LAR doses are adjusted upward in a sequential fashion until the blood level of 10,000 to 15,000 pg/mL. If this octreotide dose fails to control symptoms or stabilize tumor growth, higher doses of octreotide are not recommended (24).

Chemotherapy of Carcinoid Tumors

In general, most carcinoid tumors present as typical or well-differentiated tumors and, as such, are considered poorly responsive to chemotherapy. Although a number of chemotherapies have been tried in typical carcinoids, the response rates are low and many regimens are highly toxic.

Monotherapy with DTIC, 5-fluorouracil (5-FU), paclitaxel, interferon, and streptozotocin have been commonly used, but all agents have response rates approximating 20% and duration of response intervals of <1 year (18). Recent combination chemotherapy trials in patients with typical carcinoid have yielded disappointing results. Doxorubicin and 5-FU, streptozocin and 5-FU, or streptozocin with dacarbazine all yielded response rates <20% and are associated with significant toxicity. In contrast to the disappointing results of chemotherapy in poorly differentiated carcinoids (atypical, small cell-like) is associated with high response rates but rather short duration of responses (18).

Use of Radiolabeled Somatostatin Analogs as Therapy for NETs

Primary NETs and their metastases overexpress somatostatin receptor subtype 2 (sst 2) and thus these tumors can be visualized after injection of a radiolabeled somatostatin analog. Somatostatin analogs were originally radiolabeled with radioactive iodine; however, the route of excretion of these radioiodinated analogs was predominantly hepatic. The high level of hepatic uptake precluded the identification of liver metastases (25). To obviate the difficulty with hepatic metabolism and excretion, chelated somatostatin analogs were developed. These analogs were radiolabeled with heavy metals such as [111]Indium, ^{177}Lu, and [90]Y. These heavy metals were affixed to the somatostatin analogs with chelating moieties such as DTPA or DOTA. [111]Indium pentetreotide (OctreoScan,) is now considered to be a critical agent for the detection of primary and metastatic NETs (26). For some tumors, such as gastrinomas, the use of an OctreoScan as the first-line scanning agent has been proposed (27). With the development of radiolabeled somatostatin analogs for scanning, the concept arose that these analogs could be used as therapeutic agents. Krenning et al. (28) in the Netherlands was the first to treat a patient with high dose Indium pentetreotide. Woltering et al. (29) were the first to treat a patient in the United States with high-dose radioiodinated somatostatin analogs. Contemporaneously, Anthony et al (30). began using high-dose ^{111}In pentetreotide therapy in the United States. Subsequently other analogs and heavy metals have been tested in clinical trials. Currently, ^{177}Lu-labeled somatostatin analogs seem to be the most effective yet least toxic of the many combinations tested.

CARCINOID AND THE CARCINOID SYNDROME

History

Siegfried Oberndorfer was the first to describe these unusual tumors and referred to them as *benign carcinomas*. During his lifetime, Oberndorfer noted that these tumors were distinct entities and named them *karzinoide* (carcinomalike). The enterochromaffin cells that are the precursors of carcinoid tumors were identified by Kulchinsky in 1897 and the functional nature of Kulchinsky cells was not established until 1922 when Lembeck described the synthesis and secretion of serotonin by these cells (31–38).

Incidence

Modlin et al (39). provided a 5-decade analysis of 13,750 carcinoid tumors. This evaluation included 10,878 carcinoid tumors that were identified by the Surveillance Epidemiology and End Results (SEER) Program of the National Cancer Institute from 1973 to 1999. In addition, these authors reviewed 2,837 carcinoid tumors that were registered previously by two earlier National Cancer Institute programs. From these data, the authors demonstrated that the greatest incidence of carcinoids were in the gastrointestinal tract (67.5%), while 25.3% originated in the bronchopulmonary system. Within the gastrointestinal tract, 41.8% occurred in the small intestine, 27.4% in the rectum, and 8.7% in the stomach. For all sites, age adjusted incidence rates were highest in black males (4.48 per hundred thousand population per year). Five-year survival rates were the best for patients with rectal carcinoids (88.3%) followed by bronchopulmonary (73.5%) and appendicial (71.0%). These tumors were found to be metastatic in 3.9%, 27.5%, and 38.8%, respectively (39). In this study, 12.9% of all patients with carcinoid had distant metastases at the time of diagnosis and the overall 5-year survival rate of all carcinoid tumors regardless of site was 67.2%. The incidence of rectal and gastric carcinoid is increasing; however, this is associated with a concomitant decrease in the incidence of small bowel carcinoids (39).

Since 1950, the percentage of gastric carcinoids among all gastric malignancies has increased from 0.3% to 1.77%. Since 1969, the proportion of gastric carcinoids among all enteric carcinoid lesions has increased from 2.4% to 8.7%. Age-adjusted incidence rates among male, female, and black and white population subsets have all increased during this period, with the greatest increase (800%) noted in white females. The male-to-female ratio has fallen from 0.90 to 0.54. Increased endoscopic surveillance and associated sophisticated pathologic evaluation of gastric biopsies undoubtedly are responsible for some of the observed increase in the incidence of gastric carcinoids. These data allow no specific role to be assigned to the effects of acid-suppressive medications. Many authors have speculated that the widespread use of acid-suppressive medications such as protein pump inhibitors is responsible for this increase in gastric carcinoids. This cannot be concluded from the SEER data, but the role of such agents cannot be discounted as these time frames are somewhat comparable to these agents as is the known biological effect of gastrin on enterochromaffinlike cell proliferation (3). Carcinoids may, however, occur in the bronchus, pancreas, rectum, ovary, lung, and elsewhere. Rarely, carcinoids of the thymus may be associated with MEN syndromes. The tumors grow slowly and often are clinically silent for many years before metastasizing. They frequently metastasize to the regional lymph nodes, liver, and, less commonly, to the bone. The likelihood of metastases relates to tumor size. The incidence of metastases is <15% with a carcinoid tumor <1 cm but rises to 95% with tumors >2 cm (14). In individual cases, size alone may not be the only determinant of lymphatic or distant spread. Lynphatic or vascular invasion, or spread into the fat surrounding the primary tumor, may be an indicator of a more aggressive tumor (14).

The carcinoid syndrome occurs in <10% of patients with carcinoid tumors. It is especially common in tumors of the ileum and jejunum (i.e., midgut tumors) but also occurs with bronchial, ovarian, and other carcinoids. Tumors in the rectum (i.e., hindgut tumors) rarely produce the carcinoid syndrome, even those that have widely metastasized. Tumors may be symptomatic only episodically, and their existence may go unrecognizable for many years. The average time from onset of symptoms attributable to the tumor and the diagnosis is just over 9 years, and diagnosis usually is made only after the carcinoid syndrome occurs. The distribution of carcinoids is Gaussian in nature. The peak incidence occurs in the sixth and seventh decades of life, but carcinoid tumors have also been reported in patients as young as 10 years of age and in those in their ninth decade of life (14).

The major symptoms of carcinoid syndrome consist of flushing, diarrhea, and wheezing. Symptoms less often experienced include right-sided heart failure due to valvular fibrosis, fatigue, joint pain, and skin rash (pellagra) (14). In our opinion, the best treatment option for symptomatic patients is the use of somatostatin analogs in appropriate doses. Following initial treatment with these analogs, most patients will report significant reduction in the intensity and frequency of carcinoid syndrome. In the long term, most patients require upward adjustment of their drug dose to control symptoms.

ISLET CELL TUMORS AND ASSOCIATED SYNDROMES

Gastrinoma and Zollinger-Ellison Syndromes

Zollinger-Ellison syndrome (ZES) refers to a clinical triad of signs and symptoms that includes gastric acid hypersecretion, peptic ulceration, and the presence of a non-beta islet cell tumor of the pancreas. First described in 1955 (40), it is now understood that the syndrome's peptic ulceration is secondary to gastric acid hypersecretion that, in turn, is due to excessive gastrin release from the islet cell tumor. Although Zollinger and Ellison are widely credited for the discovery of gastrinomas, Edkins (41,42) in 1905 provided the first evidence for a gastric acid secretagogue, which he named gastrin. However, the association of this endocrine tumor with hyperacidity was not completed until the 1960s when Gregory and Tracy isolated a "gastrin-like protein" from ZES tumor fragments. Thus, the name "gastrinoma" became associated with the syndrome as it refers to the NET that causes hypergastrinemia, and today the term is used synonymously with ZES Syndrome (43,44).

The incidence of gastrinoma is estimated to be between 0.1 and 3 individuals per 1 million in the United States, and it is present in 0.1% of all patients with peptic ulcer disease (45–46). Approximately 75% of gastrinomas are sporadic, while the remaining 25% are hereditary, associated with MEN-1 (47,48).

MEN-1 is a rare inherited syndrome characterized by tumors of multiple endocrine organs including pituitary, pancreas, and parathyroid (49). The syndrome is inherited as an autosomal dominant trait with high penetrance and variable expression. The gene causing MEN 1, named *menin*, is located at chromosome 11q12–13 and acts as a tumor suppressor (50). Although other functional pancreatic endocrine tumors may occur in the setting of MEN-1, gastrinomas occur the most frequently, 20% to 61% of the time (51). The hypergastrinemia of ZES associated with MEN-1 has also been associated with gastric carcinoids (type II). Those with MEN-1 and ZES have a 20% to 30% risk of developing type II gastric carcinoid, in contrast with patients with sporadic ZES (non-MEN-1-associated) who develop gastric carcinoid in 0% to 1% of cases (52–54).

Sixty-five to 90% of all gastrinomas found at surgery occur in the area of the pancreatic head and the duodenum (55,56). This area, commonly referred to as the "gastrinoma triangle," is represented anatomically by the confluence of the cystic and common bile ducts superiorly, the C-sweep of the duodenum laterally, and the superior mesenteric artery medially. Although it was originally thought that duodenal gastrinomas were less common than pancreatic tumors (57–60), most now think that the duodenal primaries are 3 to 10 times more frequent than their pancreatic counterparts (57,61–63). Recent studies report the frequency of duodenal gastrinomas to be in range of 40% to 50% (56), while the pancreatic primaries comprise closer to 30% to 40% of overall cases (64,65). Less frequent is the occurrence of gastrinoma originating from an abdominal lymph node (9% to 11%) (62,66,67), and extremely uncommon is the presence of an extra-abdominal source (<5%) (68,69). Although gastrin release has been associated with other nongastric malignancies, with the very rare exception of ovarian gastrinomas, these typically do not cause hypergastrinemia, and therefore are not considered to be true gastrinomas by most authorities (70,71).

Pathophysiology

At present, the cell of origin of gastrinomas remains uncertain (72). Duodenal gastrinomas contain many well-differentiated gastrin-containing (G) cells, and their origin may be the gastrin cells in the duodenal crypts and Brunner glands. Pancreatic gastrinomas are more pleomorphic with more heterogeneous cell arrangements. Although G cells are not normally present in the adult pancreas, it has been proposed that multipotential, endocrine-programmed stem cells undergoing differentiation toward G cell are responsible for pancreatic gastrinomas (73,74).

Although gastrinomas tend to be slow-growing, it is estimated that 60% to 90% of them are malignant (75,76). Like other pancreatic NETs, a diagnosis of malignancy cannot be made by histology alone. To be considered malignant, the tumor must evidence invasion, be it local or regional, or show distant organ metastases (76).

Metastases characteristically develop in adjacent lymph nodes, in the liver, subsequently to the bone later in the course of the disease (57,62,77–80). Liver metastasis is currently considered to be the most important predictor for long-term survival as these patients tend to have a worse prognosis (44). There are molecular features that are characteristic of aggressive gastrinomas including increased *HER2/neu* expression (81,82), chromosome 1 or X loss of heterozygosity (83–85), or increased epidermal growth factor receptor expression (81,86). Unfortunately, none of these features is sensitive or specific enough to predict the course of the disease (44). In addition, tumor suppressor genes $p16^{INK4a}$ and *MEN I*, although frequent in gastrinomas, do not predict tumor course (87–89).

There are clinical features that tend to predict a malignant lesion. For instance, malignancy is more likely in females those with very elevated serum gastrin levels, and those with a short disease history (64,90–94). Current studies have shown that both pancreas and duodenal primaries have an equal likelihood of that both locations have an equal rate of malignant disease with being malignant with metastasis about 40% to 70% of the time (48,62,77). Regardless of metastatic potential, duodenal tumors generally tend to be smaller, less likely to metastasize to the liver, and often have a better prognosis than do pancreatic tumors (48,64,66,77,93,95–97).

Presentation

The mean age of presentation for a sporadic gastrinoma is about 50 years of age, while the presentation for an MEN-1-associated gastrinoma is approximately 15 years earlier (98). The most common presenting symptom is epigastric pain caused by ZES-associated peptic ulcer disease, and most patients will have peptic ulceration at the time of diagnosis. Although these ulcers are most commonly solitary proximal duodenal ulcers, patients may have ulcers that are multiple, found in unusual locations (like the distal duodenum or jejunum), and are recurrent despite treatment. Approximately 10% of ZES patients will never elicit any signs or symptoms of peptic ulcer disease.

Secretory diarrhea is the presenting symptom in approximately 20% of ZES patients. ZES-associated gastric acid hypersecretion increases intestinal transit time, causes malabsorption, and is responsible for the diarrhea. Accordingly, the diarrhea usually resolves as the acid secretion is treated.

Symptoms of heartburn and dysphagia may also be present, resulting from esophageal inflammation, stricture, or ulceration. Aggressive and precise acid control is strongly encouraged for ZES patients with these symptoms (98).

Diagnosis

Typically, the physical examination is normal in these patients; therefore, the diagnosis is more frequently made biochemically (98). To that end, the diagnosis may be made when an elevated fasting serum gastrin (>100 pg/mL) exists in the absence of achlorhydria. Patients with gastrinoma will usually have fasting gastrin levels >500 pg/mL, and a level >900 pg/mg is almost pathognomic. In current practice, the most common cause of hypergastrinemia and, thus, the most common cause of false-positive serum gastrin elevations, is the chronic use of PPIs. However, false-positive findings may also occur in the setting of renal failure (99), extensive small bowel resections, G-cell hyperplasia, pernicious anemia, or retained antrum syndrome.

Ideally, patients should be taken off their acid-reducing medications at least 1 week prior to testing. However, the elevated serum gastrin and chromogranin levels induced by achlorhydria as a result of enterochromaffin cell hyperplasia may take months to completely normalize (98). An equivocal gastrin level is observed in nearly 50% of patients with gastrinoma (100). In these cases, a repeat fasting serum gastrin level is recommended, and in this situation discontinuation of acid-suppressing medications is mandatory. A determination of gastric pH when the patient is off acid-suppressive medications is mandatory.

Although other tests including the basal acid output (BAO) and gastric pH levels may be measured, many think that the most useful next test to confirm the diagnosis is the secretin provocative test (99,100). Following an overnight fast, patients are given an intravenous bolus of 2 U/kg of Kabi secretin, and serum gastrin levels are assayed at 0, 2, 5, 10, and 15 minutes following the administration. Typically patients with ZES will experience an increase in their serum gastrin >200 pg/mL from their basal level within 5 minutes of the secretin bolus. Alternatively, a calcium infusion test can be performed in which patients are given a 15-mg/kg infusion of elemental calcium (calcium gluconate or calcium chloride) over 4 hours following a baseline gastrin measurement. Additional gastrin levels are measured at 30 minutes, 1, 2, 3, 4, and 5 hours following the initiation of the infusion. Unfortunately, this test is associated with a significant risk of cardiac arrhythmias and for the most part has been abandoned.

Medical Management

There are two main aims of treatment: control of symptoms secondary to gastric acid hypersecretion and control of the malignant tumor. Once a diagnosis of ZES has been made, the control of gastric acid secretion is the next most important step in its management (100). This is to prevent the potentially dangerous complications of severe ZES-associated peptic ulcer disease (101). In addition, adequate medical control of the gastric acid hypersecretion usually abolishes all clinical symptoms (68,102).

Proton pump inhibitors (PPIs) are currently the drugs of choice in the management of gastric acid hypersecretion in patients with ZES (83,103–104). The most reliable way to ensure the efficacy of this pharmacotherapy is through the measurement of basal acid output (101). Thus, following an initial PPI dose determination and the achievement of a steady-state on this dose, serial BAO levels should be measured every 3 to 4 weeks. Drugs should then be titrated to ensure a BAO goal level of between 1 and 10 mmol/h. More specific recommendations suggest medication adjustment until a basal acid output below 10 mEq/h in uncomplicated ZES and to below 5 mEq/h in complicated ZES (cases status postgastrectomy or associated with gastroesophageal reflux or MEN-1) is achieved (105).

The importance of precise BAO reduction has been supported through studies demonstrating that almost all patients with such careful medical management will both heal their peptic ulcers and prevent ulcer recurrence as long as they continue treatment (103). Although aggressive gastric acid suppression is required, total acid suppression is not considered a goal of therapy. Therefore, the unintended achievement of achlorhydria requires an aggressive decrease (by 50%) of the previously administered PPI dose (101).

Previous studies have demonstrated that the median dosage of omeprazole to control gastric acid hypersecretion in patients with ZES is between 60 and 100mg/day, with one third of patients requiring a more effective divided dose (72,104,106). However, the range of doses of various PPIs that has been effective in clinical trials has been broad and variable, emphasizing the need to individualize the dose through serial monitoring (106,107). In addition, ZES patients should also be evaluated by endoscopic gastric analysis at 3- to 6-month intervals for the first year and at 6 to 12 month intervals in succeeding years (101).

Role of Somatostatin Analogs

Although not considered to be the drugs of first choice to control acid hypersecretion (101), somatostatin analogs have been shown to be effective in the management of gastrinomas. It has been widely reported that the somatostatin analog, octreotide, will decrease serum gastrin levels and lower gastric acid levels in patients with ZES (94,108,109). One author described a mean 87% decrease in serum gastrin with an effective control of gastric acid hypersecretion over a 9- to 12-month period in ZES patients treated with subcutaneous octreotide (110). In addition, tumor stabilization has been reported in 47% of patients and tumor reduction in 6% of patients with malignant gastrinoma being treated with octreoticle (111). Moreover, Mozell et al. found that the mean gastrin suppression secondary to octreotide is persistent for as long as 48 months (112).

Chemotherapy in Gastrinoma

Treatment of gastroenteropancreatic endocrine tumors with classic antitumor chemotherapeutics has yielded equivocal results (101). Newer regimens containing streptozocin resulted in better responses but also higher toxicity (113,114). In addition, a study that looked at 10 patients with metastatic gastrinoma who were treated with streptozocin, fluorouracil, and doxorubicin reported no difference in survival between the four responders and the six nonresponders (115). Taking the current data into account, it is plausible to conclude that chemotherapy is not the first treatment of choice for gastrinomas (101). However, should a practitioner wish to use this modality, some authors have recommended that octreotide be employed prior to the use of chemotherapy (111). Current recommendations for the use of chemotherapy in these patients are for those whose tumors increase in size by >25% as documented by serial imaging and/or for those whose tumor symptoms that are not treatable by other methods (116,117).

The Role of Interferon Alpha

In some studies interferon alpha has been reported to cause tumor stabilization in patients with metastatic gastrinoma; however, use of this reagent has not been shown to prolong survival (118,119). Considering this along with its well-known arsenal of severe adverse effects (101), the use of this reagent should be considered judiciously.

Surgical Management

Historically, surgery for the ZES syndrome was designed to control the severe peptic ulcer disease (101). Because the gastrinoma tumor was rarely localized in these initial operations and because lesser procedures resulted in recurrent symptoms, total gastrectomy was usually advocated (120). Since the advent of medication that reliably manage the gastric acid hypersecretion in these patients, total gastrectomy is no longer indicated. Surgery now focuses on removal of the gastrinoma tumor itself.

Thus, once gastric acid hypersecretion is safely under medical control, the next objective is to localize and treat the gastrinoma tumor (99). The first aim is to attempt to cure the disease through surgical resection and, if this is not possible, to reduce the metastatic potential of the disease (99). Cure is considered a normal fasting serum level of gastrin, interval negative secretin stimulation tests, and no evidence of tumor by imaging studies or OctreoScan (121,122). However, specific surgical management depends on whether or not the patient's gastrinoma is sporadic or hereditary and its association with MEN-1 (99).

Surgery in Sporadic Gastrinoma

Although there has been disagreement in the past regarding the role of surgical resection of gastrinoma (120), Norton et al. (62) published a prospective study following a total of 151 gastrinoma patients who had surgical resection of their tumor. They reported a rate of disease-free survival among patients with sporadic gastrinomas that was 40% at 5 years and 34% at 10 years. The relatively low morbidity (<15%) (56) associated with surgery supports the employment of routine surgical exploration and excision of sporadic gastrinoma when possible. Considering the expanded role of octreotide in the long term management of ZES, cholecystectomy should be considered during all surgical explorations for ZES.

Surgery in Patients with Gastrinoma and MEN-1

Routine surgical exploration in patients with gastrinoma and MEN-1 is controversial for several reasons. First, surgical extirpation of gastrinom a in patients with MEN-1 yields long-term cure rates near zero. In contrast to patients with sporadic gastrinomas, in operative MEN-1/ZES patients Norton et al. (62) found the rate of disease-free survival was 4% at 5 years and 0% at 10 years. Secondly, despite several reports that surgery may reduce the rate of tumor metastasis and increase patient survival (121–123) this has yet to be convincingly demonstrated (120). In addition, no controlled studies have been done to determine the exact timing and role of surgery. Finally, ZES patients with MEN-1 have excellent long-term survival without surgery with survival approximating 52% at 15 years even with metastatic disease (124).

Despite these data, metastatic progression of the primary tumor remains the most important determinant of long-term survival (78,125). Although there are no reliable clinical, laboratory, or tumoral markers that predict the aggressiveness of these tumors, primary tumor size is highly predictive of liver metastasis (77,93,95). Therefore, some authors think that surgery is appropriate in those MEN-1/ZES patients who have a potentially malignant lesion of at least 2 cm based on imaging (120).

Some authors have advocated that in patients with MEN-1, specifically these with parathyroid hyperplasia and ZES, that parathyroidectomy should be the first surgical procedure employed to control gastric acid hypersecretion (126). This has been supported on the basis that parathyroidectomy and the normalization of the serum calcium reduces gastrin secretion and increases the sensitivity of acid secretion to antisecretory reagents (51). Norton et al. (132) found that parathyroidectomy in these patients reduced the basal acid output by 60% and eradicated the clinical evidence of ZES in 20% of these patients postoperatively.

The three forms of MEN have traditionally been considered completely separate entities, each being inherited through entirely distinct genetic traits. Thus, mucosal neuromas are restricted to MEN-2b, pheochromocytoma and medullary thyroid carcinoma are limited to MEN-2, while pituitary tumors and islet cell tumors occur only in MEN-1. Despite this conventional viewpoint, case reports describing ZES in patients with MEN-2 suggest that there may exist a "crossover" between MEN-1and MEN-2 (127,128). In these rare cases, we think that resection of the pheochromocytoma should precede the surgical treatment of the gastrinoma. Furthermore, in contrast to the low cure rate of MEN-1 gastrinomas, the suggestion has been made that the possibility for a curative resection may exist in patients with ZES and MEN-2 (129).

The Role of Pancreaticoduodenectomy

Most experts do not recommend a Whipple procedure (pancreaticoduodenectomy) for the surgical management of gastrinoma (77,12,124,130–133). Whipple procedure is associated with a higher complication and death rate than simple excision or enucleation of pancreatic and duodenal tumors, and it may have long-term sequelae like weight loss, diabetes, and malabsorption. In addition, Whipple resection may make reoperation technically more difficult. This is a potential problem in MEN-1 patients who develop subsequent pancreatic NETs. The increased risk of ascending cholangitis following a Whipple procedure may also render potential chemoembolization of liver metastases more difficult (90). Additionally, Whipple resection does not appear to improve upon the excellent quality and duration of life (122).

There are, however small case series that report a dramatic increase in cure rate in patients undergoing Whipple resection, crediting its improvement on the ability to totally remove the gastrinoma triangle (90,134–136). Thus, currently pancreaticoduodenectomy should be reserved for those patients with a large pancreatic head or duodenal tumor or those with multiple localized lymph nodes. Additional indications may include patients who are not cured after initial removal of a duodenal or pancreatic head gastrinoma by tumor enucleation as assessed by intraoperative secretin test (90,132,135–139). Despite evidence that removal of the gastrinoma triangle yields a greater cure rate, there is currently no proof that the use of a Whipple resection increases the excellent long-term survival of these patients compared with lesser operations (122).

VIPoma and the WDHA Syndrome

The association of pancreatic islet cell tumors and diarrhea was first reported by Priest and Alexander (140). At that time it was thought to be a variant of the ZES syndrome. One year later, Verner and Morrison (141) described two patients with profuse watery diarrhea, hypokalemia, and achlorhydria (WDHA syndrome) associated with a pancreatic islet cell tumor. However, it was not until 1973 that elevated VIP levels were observed and associated with this syndrome (142).

VIP is present in the peripheral and the central nervous systems, where it functions as a nonadrenergic, noncholinergic neurotransmitter or neuromodulator (143). Peripherally, VIP is located in peptidergic neurons of the splanchnic nervous system adjacent to blood vessels in the small intestine, the colon, and the exocrine ducts of the pancreas (144). VIP acts as a neurotransmitter by diffusing across a neurosynaptic cleft and exerting its effects on a target through interactions with a specific adenylate cyclase-coupled receptor.

VIPomas are rare entities accounting for 2% to 7% of all gastroenteropancreatic neuroendocrine tumors (145,146). Despite the widespread presence of VIPs in the gut, roughly 90% of these tumors are located in the pancreas (147). The remaining 10% are extrapancreatic and occur along the along the autonomic nervous system and in the adrenal medulla (148–150). However, extrapancreatic VIPomas have also been observed arising from the retroperitoneum, lungs, esophagus, jejunum, and liver (151–153). The precise cellular origin of this tumor remains controversial, but the neurotransmitter biology of VIPs suggests a neural crest origin (153). This hypothesis is further supported by cases of VIP production from tumors such as neuroblastoma, ganglioneuroblastoma, bronchogenic carcinoma, medullary thyroid carcinoma, and pheochromocytoma (151). Accordingly, VIPomas in children are most commonly either ganglioneuromas or ganglioneuroblastomas, arising from the neural crest tissue of the sympathetic ganglia or the adrenal medulla (150,154–157).

Clinical Features

VIPomas have a reported annual incidence of 1 per 10 million population (145). The mean age for adults at the time of diagnosis is 42 to 51 years (range, 32 to 81 years) (150,158–160). There is a female predominance in some studies (147,150,159), but not others (158,160). Children frequently present between 2 and 4 years of age (150).

It is estimated that 60% of VIPomas are malignant (153). In various series, 37% to 68% of the VIPomas were metastatic to the liver, regional lymph nodes, kidneys, lungs, stomach, or mediastinum at the time of diagnosis or surgery (150,153,161).

Although VIPomas can potentially synthesize a host of other peptides including pancreatic polypeptide, somatostatin, insulin, and glucagon, VIP is the chief secretagogue of these tumors and the major mediator (145,162) of the WDHA syndrome. Thus, the cardinal features of VIPoma are severe, secretory diarrhea, hypokalemia, and dehydration (163).

The secretory diarrhea may be episodic (150,159,164,165), isotonic, and persistent during both fasting (145) and nasogastric suction. It may initially be intermittent, but it typically becomes more severe as the as the tumor enlarges. The volume of diarrhea is >1 L/day in all patients and >3 L/day in most, with daily stool outputs <700 mL excluding the diagnosis. The diarrheal fluid is described as having the appearance of weak tea (165).

The clinical laboratory studies demonstrate hypokalemia in 67% to 100% of VIPoma patients (163). The hypokalemia is often severe, with losses of potassium as great as 400 mEq/day (166) and potassium levels <2.5 mmol/L (154). Other elec-

trolyte abnormalities that are not uncommon include hypercalcemia, hypomagnesemia, and hypophosphatemia. In addition, glucose intolerance and/or frank hyperglycemia has been observed in these patients (142). An erythematous flushing of the head or trunk area is also observed in 14% to 28% of VIPoma patients (164).

Pathophysiology

Physiologically, VIP relaxes the intestinal smooth muscle, generates vasodilation, and stimulates intestinal and exocrine pancreatic secretion (167). Pathologically, VIP inhibits active electrolyte and water absorption in the ileum, and it reverses net colonic absorption to secretion ratios. In addition, VIP-induced anal sphincter relaxation may provoke incontinence, further exacerbating diarrhea with a stool that is isotonic with plasma.

Large fluid volumes that overwhelm the absorptive capacity of the colon result in voluminous diarrhea, profound hypovolemia, and severe electrolyte losses (171). The passive movement of potassium into the stool water as it passes through the small intestine ensures that as much as 50% of potassium presented to the colon may be lost (169). Secondary hyperaldosteronism from VIP-stimulated renin release may further intensify the hypokalemia (172).

Over 72% of patients with VIPomas have associated hypochlorhydria (150). As the parietal cells in gastric mucosal biopsy specimens in these patients are usually normal, this reduction in gastric acid is thought to be secondary to a direct inhibitory effect of VIP on the partial cell mass (147).

VIPomas can directly cause both persistent and intermittent hypercalcemia by stimulating bone resorption via a cyclic adenosine monophosphate-dependent mechanism (173,174). However, hypercalcemia in this setting could also indicate the presence of hyperparathyroidism, MEN-1 and, consequently, the need for genetic testing (175). Alternatively, hypercalcemia has been reported in cases of pancreatic NETs that co-produce calcitonin (176). In addition, some NETs also secrete parathyroid-hormone related protein (PTHrP), another potential cause of hypercalcemia (177–179). Thus, it is important to consider these causes of hyperkalemia and consider testing for intact PTH, PTHrp, and calcitonin (180).

Several theories exist to explain the glucose intolerance seen in patients with VIPoma. These include (a) structural similarities between VIP and glucagon (147), (b) the glycogenolytic effect of VIPs on the liver (181), or (c) an inhibitory effect that hypokalemia has on pancreatic beta cells (182).

VIP is a vasodilator of splanchnic and peripheral vascular beds (147). This effect potentiates the hypotension seen in these patients and may also induce flushing (162).

Diagnosis

A diagnosis of VIPoma syndrome is suspected when a patient presents with classic signs and symptoms of watery diarrhea in the presence of hypokalemia and metabolic acidosis (147). Once the diagnosis of secretory diarrhea is established, it is important to rule out other possible causes including a gastrinoma or other peptide-secreting tumors and/or chronic laxative abuse (183). Accordingly, differentiation from ZES syndrome can be made through a plasma chemistry demonstrating metabolic acidosis, a normal fasting serum gastrin, and a nasogastric aspiration demonstrating hypochlorhydria rather than gastric acid hypersecretion (184). Also, it is important to consider additional possibilities in which diarrhea is associated with other VIP-elevating conditions such as prolonged fasting, inflammatory bowel disease, small bowel resection, radiation enteritis, chronic renal failure, or nonpancreatic VIP-secreting tumors (147,185).

The diagnosis is confirmed when plasma VIP levels are found to be >200 pg/mL (186). Some recommend that fasting VIP levels only be drawn during the active diarrheal state as some VIPoma-WDS patients have normal VIP levels when they are not having diarrhea (162).

Intestinal perfusion studies may occasionally be helpful in the differential diagnosis (159). Net secretion of electrolytes and water occurs in VIPomas instead of a net absorption in perfused small intestinal segments (163,191). This method is reported to be particularly helpful in differentiating VIPomas from surreptitious laxative ingestion because the latter group of patients show normal perfusion results (159,187)

Supportive Therapy and Pharmacotherapy

Death in these patients is usually a result of cardiac arrest secondary to the clinical syndrome's profound metabolic disturbance. Thus, rapid correction of fluid and electrolyte deficits is critical in patients with signs and symptoms of VIPoma. The magnitude and route of administration of fluid therapy should be individualized based on the severity of the symptoms (162).

Currently, octreotide and other somatostatin congeners are the therapy of choice in suppressing the release of hormones from VIPomas (188). These reagents not only suppress hormone release from the tumor but they also have a direct action at the target cell itself, preventing water and electrolyte secretion (189). These two actions together improve the characteristic clinical symptoms in nearly all patients with functional endocrine gastroenteropancreatic tumors (147). Park et al. found that octreotide completely controlled the characteristic watery diarrhoea in 56% of VIPoma patients and significantly improved it in another 28% (146). Moreover, plasma VIP levels fell by about 60% of pretreatment levels.

A marked discrepancy exists in the literature regarding the antitumor effect of somatostatin analogs in the VIPomas. Although some authors have indicated that somatostatin analogs may cause tumor regression in patients with metastatic VIPoma (190,191), other have failed to observe any predictable antitumor activity (192). Although Eriksson and Oberg demonstrated a biochemical response to octreotide in five of nine VIPoma patients, they were unable to show an effect on tumor size (193). Thus individual patients experience considerable variation in their clinical response to octreotide, making it necessary to titrate the dose in order to achieve optimal control of symptoms (24). Recently, octreotide plasma levels have become commercially available and may be useful in optimizing therapy in patients on the LAR formulation of octreotide (24).

In VIPoma patients, the consensus recommendations suggest that an initial dose and subsequent titration regimen depend on the condition of the patient. Patients with life-threatening symptoms should be given a 100-mcg bolus intravenously followed by 50 mcg/hour intravenously until stable

(194). In our experience, this dose can be rapidly titrated upward until control of diarrhea is achieved. For patients with milder symptoms, an initial dose of 100 to 150 mcg subcutaneously every 8 hours is recommended (194). Patients' stool output and electrolyte status should be monitored on a daily or weekly basis, depending on symptom severity. Insufficient doses may be titrated up focusing on the reduction of diarrhea as the treatment end point of rather than normalization of hormone activity (194). Use of the long-acting forms of octreotide is recommended for chronic therapy.

Before the development of octreotide, glucocorticoids constituted the mainstay of medical management of VIP-induced diarrhea (147). They have been reported to produce a 40% to 50% reduction in VIP levels both in vitro and in vivo (195). In our opinion, glucocorticoids may augment the effect of octreotide therapy; however, its use should be limited to patients whose plasma octreotide levels are between 10,000 and 15,000 pg/mL. Octreotide will saturate the sst 2 receptors found on these tumors and will elicit its maximum effect at these plasma levels.

In addition to glucocorticoids, other pharmacologic agents have been employed in the management of VIPoma-induced diarrhea. These have included indomethacin, a prostaglandin inhibitor (196,197), and lithium carbonate (198). Other agents that have been employed include clonidine (199), angiotensin II (200), norepinephrine (201), carbonate phenothiazines (202,203), phosphate buffer (204), metaclopromide (205), and loperamide (206). However, none of these agents has been studied as extensively or in sufficiently large number of patients to warrant their use as an initial form of therapy. At this time, these agents should be considered only in the patient who has failed to respond to other more established drug therapies like somatostatin analogs (147).

Many therapeutic trials have shown variable and often short-lasting response rates of NETs to chemotherapy. Monochemotherapy for carcinoid tumors with either 5-FU or doxorubicin produced an objective clinical response at 3 months in 26% and 21% of patients, respectively (207,208). A similar result is observed in pancreatic NET (209). Combination chemotherapy associating 5-FU, doxorubicin, and streptozotocin gave a response rate of 8% to 40% in carcinoid tumors and of 36% to 54% in pancreatic NET (210–212). With the combination of cisplatin and etoposide, Moertel et al. (213) observed a partial regression in 50% of anaplastic tumors and in 14% of islet cell tumors, but no response in carcinoid tumors. Thus, these tumors are not overly sensitive to chemotherapy, and there is no accepted standard chemotherapy for these tumors to date.

Surgery

Surgical exploration is indicated in nearly all of these patients (214,215). This is because VIPomas like most other islet cell tumors cannot be reliably classified as benign or malignant based on histology alone; thus, surgery is required for accurate staging (144). In addition, complete surgical resection of the tumor offers the only potentially curative therapy available to these patients (144). Therefore, the goals of operative exploration should be (a) meticulous and accurate staging, (b) complete resection if possible, (c) cytoreduction for symptom control, and (d) preparation for nonoperative management if surgery is not feasible (144). Finally, a cholecystectomy should be performed during the abdominal exploration to prevent the subsequent development of gallstones during octreotide therapy.

Studies have shown that metastasectomies can clearly lead to long-term survival in patients with extensive tumor burden (215,216). Also, even if the entire tumor cannot be removed, surgical debulking can provide significant symptom relief (184). In these cases though, it is incumbent on the operating surgeon to carefully individualize the operative approach accounting for the morbidity of the disease and the likely long-term course.

Some nonresective, ablative options for the management of unresectable metastatic disease are available and are garnering interest. Although the experience with these approaches is growing, there is not yet consensus on the optimal incorporation of these modalities into the overall treatment strategy (217–224). The ablative procedures can be done in a variety of ways (cryoablation or radiofrequency ablation, done at open operation, laparoscopically, or with radiologic guidance). In general, there is agreement that these approaches should only be pursued if all, or nearly all, of the known disease can be addressed in some way (144). This is an area of ongoing investigation.

SOMATOSTATINOMAS AND THE SOMATOSTATIN SYNDROME

Somatostatin (originally somatomedin release-inhibiting factor; SRIF) consists of two cyclic peptides of 14 and 28 amino acids (SRIF-14, SRIF 28), respectively. This hormone was originally described in the hypothalamus and was isolated, purified, and sequenced for its ability to inhibit the release of growth hormone (144). It is now understood that somatostatin inhibits numerous endocrine and exocrine functions through somatostatin-producing cells that are widely distributed in normal human tissues (225). Somatostatin inhibits the release of almost all gastrointestinal tract hormones, including insulin, glucagon, gastrin, secretin, cholecystokinin, and motilin. In addition, somatostatin has direct effects on a number of target organs, including inhibition of gastric acid secretion, decreased intestinal motility, and reduced intestinal absorption of fat.

Somatostatinomas are tumors that produce excessive amounts of somatostatin. The first description of a somatostatinoma was in 1977 (226), and since then there have been <100 of these extremely rare cases reported in the literature (227). It is currently estimated that somatostatin-producing tumors account for <1% of all gastroenteropancreatic endocrine neoplasms (146,186) with a prevalence of one in 40 million (186). It should again be stressed that the presence of SRIF in a tumor (immunohistochemical stain) does not necessarily imply the release of this peptide into the circulation.

Although somatostatinomas have been reported in the jejunum, cystic duct, colon, and rectum (228,229), they are typically divided into two basic types based on location: pancreatic somatostatinomas and duodenal somatostatinomas (230). Although two thirds of somatostatinomas originate in the pancreas, the next common site is the duodenum (231). Pancreatic

somatostatinomas are usually larger with an average diameter of 5.1 cm (228). Duodenal somatostatinomas, on the other hand, tend to be smaller, and they are associated with von Recklinghausen disease and with psammoma bodies (228). Although one review found 30% of duodenal and 70% of pancreatic somatostatinomas to be characterized by metastases (229), this difference may be more a result of tumor size than a variation in essential tumor biology (232).

Presentation and Pathophysiology

Overexcretion of somatostatin by tumor tissues results in multisecretory insufficiency and gastrointestinal symptoms collectively termed the *somatostatinoma syndrome* (233). The clinical features associated with the somatostatinoma syndrome are hyperglycemia, cholelithiasis, diarrhea, steatorrhea, and hypochlorhydria (228). In addition, some have referred to the classic triad of this syndrome as hyperglycemia, cholelithiasis, and maldigestion of food (steatorrhea) (234). Patients may also present with abdominal pain, weight loss, and anemia as signs of malignant disease (228).

The somatostatinoma syndrome can be explained by the known actions of somatostatin (234). Somatostatin's suppression of both insulin and glucagon gives rise to mild diabetes; however, hypoglycemia is present in 10% of patients, and this is because of somatostatin's inhibition of growth hormone and impaired carbohydrate absorption (235,236). Cholelithiasis results from the suppression of cholecystokinin-pancreozymin release and the direct inhibition of gallbladder movement (234). Steatorrhea results from somatostatin's suppression of the exocrine function of the pancreas, which prevents intestinal absorption of lipids (164,237).

The symptoms produced by somatostatinomas tend to be less pronounced and less specific than those seen with other endocrine tumors (238). When the classic syndrome symptoms do exist, they are more predictive of a pancreatic somatostatinoma. Although diabetes and cholelithiasis have occasionally been described in duodenal somatostatinomas, these tumors are usually not associated with a secretory syndrome (229,239–241). Instead, most duodenal tumors are located near the ampulla of Vater and may be associated with obstruction of the bile duct, pancreatitis, and gastrointestinal bleeding (229). Thus, their presenting features are more related to local effects of the mass rather than the systemic effects of somatostatin.

Duodenal tumors are also unique for their frequent association with type 1 neurofibromatosis (von Recklinghausen disease) with one half of all reported cases occurring in patients with neurofibromatosis (239–243). Patients with neurofibromatosis also have a 1% incidence of pheochromocytoma. Interestingly, a triad of neurofibromatosis, pheochromocytoma, and duodenal somatostatinoma has been described by. Griffiths et al. (251), who further suggested that this triad may represent a unique form of MEN. Because of lack of evidence of familial transmission, this postulate has not been widely accepted (253). However, it is recommended that patients with neurofibromatosis and evidence of either a pheochromocytoma or a duodenal somatostatinoma undergo an evaluation for the other tumor with either an esophagogastroduodenoscopy or a urinary screen for catecholamines (241).

Somatostatinomas demonstrate evidence of metastasis at diagnosis or operation in 70% to 92% of patients (248,249). There was no difference in the rate of metastases and malignancy between pancreatic and extrapancreatic tumors (238). When Metastasis is present, it usually occurs in the liver, regional lymph nodes and in the bone less frequently (248,249). As with most pancreatic endocrine tumors, the size of the tumor appears to be the critical risk factor for metastasis (233).

Diagnosis

Somatostatinomas are most often found during endoscopy, laparotomy, or abdominal imaging studies for either local obstructive symptoms or nonspecific symptoms that, in retrospect, represent some manifestation of the syndrome (164). CT and MRI are highly effective in detecting pancreatic somatostatinomas but are less sensitive in finding duodenal tumors (250). Endoscopy best demonstrates these.

In patients with a relevant history and the presence of a pancreatic mass, the diagnosis of somatostatinoma can be established by demonstrating elevated plasma somatostatin levels (238). Nearly two thirds of pancreatic somatostatinomas are associated with elevated plasma somatostatin levels (232), often being elevated 50 times normal (186,248). However, duodenal somatostatinomas are frequently nonsecretory, and they are often not demonstrative of elevated somatostatin levels (251).

The presence of normal plasma somatostatin levels in duodenal somatostatinomas may explain why these tumors lack the symptoms of classic clinical syndrome (232). Thus, it may be that the levels of serum somatostatin in duodenal somatostatinoma cases are not sufficiently high enough for the manifestation of symptoms. Another theory recognizes that duodenal somatostatinomas may not only have a lower intrinsic secretory activity but they may also release a less biologically active peptide (252).

Medical and Surgical Treatment

The obstructive clinical manifestations of duodenal somatostatinomas frequently present earlier than the symptoms of pancreatic somatostatinomas. This enables these lesions to be detected and surgically removed at an earlier stage than their pancreatic counterparts (232).

The optimal treatment of somatostatinoma is not certain because of their rarity and the lack of long-term follow-up information (252). Small tumors <2 cm may be locally excised. Intra-arterial methylene blue injection has been reported as an aide to localize very small tumors during operation (240). Pancreaticoduodenectomy, however, is required for larger tumors because of the predilection of these tumors for the head of the pancreas or duodenum (240).

The indolent course of many NETs has allowed extensive resections and even debulking of primary and metastatic disease in unresectable tumors (252). Information on chemotherapeutic drugs is limited, but streptozocin, 5-FU, and doxorubicin have all produced partial responses (231,248,251). Octreotide has reduced symptoms of the syndrome in inoperable patients (253). Survival data are limited, but patients with localized disease and a successful resection can expect long-term survival (36). Soga et al. collected data from international literature and performed statistical analysis on 173 patients with somatotstati-

noma/inhibitory syndrome. They found the average postoperative 5-year survival rate to be 75%. Patients with metastasis experienced a 60% 5-year survival while 100% patients without metastatic disease were alive at 5 year (251). Serial 6-month evaluations of hormone levels and CT of the abdomen are recommended.

INSULINOMA AND HYPOGLYCEMIC SYNDROMES

In 1869, Paul Langerhans first described pancreatic islets as a part of a detailed description of the microscopic structure of the pancreas (254,255). He described nine different types of cells including small, irregularly shaped, polygonal cells without granules, which formed numerous "zellhaufen"—literally cell heaps—measuring 0.1 to 0.24 mm in diameter, throughout the gland. Langerhans refrained from making a hypothesis as to the nature and importance of these cells (256). In 1893, the French histologist Languesse named these spots "ilots de Langerhans" or islets of Langerhans. The insulin-secreting function of these cells was established later (255,257). In 1922, insulin was first discovered by Banting and Best (255,258) in Toronto. Five years later, Wilder et al. (259) were the first to establish an association between hyperinsulinemia and an islet cell tumor. Their discovery was based on a case involving an orthopaedic surgeon with hypoglycemic symptoms. A subsequent exploratory laparotomy performed by William Mayo revealed a pancreatic tumor with multiple liver, lymph node, and mesenteric metastases. An extract prepared from the tumor demonstrated insulinlike activity following injection into a rabbit (258,259).

Insulinomas are the most common islet cell tumors (258,260). Insulinoma tumors secrete insulin, or less commonly proinsulin, which results in the systemic symptoms of hypoglycemia. The majority of insulinomas are intrapancreatic in location. The median age at presentation is 47 years with a female preponderance of 1.4:1 (261). Ninety percent of insulinomas are solitary (258,261). Most insulinomas are benign; only 10% have any evidence of malignancy (258,261). In addition to their highly benign nature, insulinoma tumors are relatively small with 90% being <2 cm in diameter at time of presentation (258,261). Following successful surgical resection, the long-term survival is 88% at 10 years with the exception of MEN-1 patients, who have a higher risk of recurrence (258).

Diagnosis

A high level of clinical suspicion of insulinoma should be triggered when a nondiabetic patient presents with hypoglycemia. However, a profoundly hypoglycemic patient can exhibit a variety of nonspecific neuroglycopenic symptoms including changes in mental status, visual changes, seizures, bizarre behavior, and unconsciousness 258,262–265). A normal plasma glucose concentration obtained during symptoms virtually rules out an insulinoma. The presence of Whipple triad of symptomatic hypoglycemia triggered by fasting (confirmed by a blood glucose <50 mg/dL obtained during symptoms) and relief of symptoms by administration of glucose is highly suggestive for endogenous hyperinsulinemia (258). The diagnostic gold standard for the diagnosis of insulinoma is a supervised 72-hour fast with serial 6-hour interval plasma levels of glucose, insulin, C-peptide, and proinsulin (266). The fast is continued until hypoglycemia is documented or symptoms develop prior to the conclusion of the 72-hour period (266). Patients without hypoglycemia at 70 hours can be urged to exercise to facilitate precipitation of symptoms. Although absolute insulin levels can help in establishing the diagnosis, the ratio of plasma insulin to plasma glucose (I/G ratio) is the most important determination to confirm insulinoma. A patient with an insulinoma will not necessarily maintain high baseline plasma insulin levels; however, the level will be high relative to plasma glucose levels. An I/G ratio >0.3 is generally considered diagnostic of insulinoma (267). Commercially prepared insulin solutions contain no C-peptide, thus low or undetectable plasma C-peptide levels in a hypoglycemic patient with elevated insulin levels indicates an exogenous source of insulin. Sulphonylureas can cause glucose, insulin, and C-peptide patterns indistinguishable from those produced by patients with an insulinoma; therefore, the measurement of plasma sulphonylurea levels are essential to exclude factitious hypoglycemia (258).

Localization

Once the diagnosis of an insulinoma has been clinically confirmed, the critical task is to localize the tumor. The task of localizing an insulinoma is separated into two categories, preoperative and intraoperative investigations. Recent consensus guidelines for the management of gastroenteropancreatic NETs recommend a multimodal approach to detect primary tumors (268). Preoperative evaluation includes transabdominal ultrasonography, CT, MRI, endoscopic ultrasound (EUS), transhepatic portal venous sampling or selective arterial calcium stimulation with hepatic venous sampling, radiolabeled octreotide scanning, and positive emission tomography (PET). Intraoperative evaluation includes extensive mobilization of the head, body, and tail of the pancreas with bimanual palpation and intraoperative ultrasonography (258,269–271).

The sensitivity of transabdominal ultrasonography in the localization of pancreatic insulinomas ranges from 9% to 64% and should not be used as the sole means of detection (258,271–273). EUS has improved accuracy of insulinoma localization in recent years with sensitivities as high as 94% reported (264,279). The availability of linear and curvilinear array EUS has broadened the applicability of endoscopic procedures, allowing for fine-needle aspiration cytology, contrast-enhanced EUS (an abbreviation; multiple manufacturers available) using Levovist and preoperative marking of lesions to facilitate surgical excision (258,274–276). In addition, color-enhanced Doppler transabdominal ultrasonography allows imaging of adjacent vessels. The main limitation of EUS is the limited examination available to evaluate the distal pancreatic body and pancreatic tail. Detection rates of 83% to 100% of head and body lesions are reported with 37% to 60% for pancreatic tail lesions (273).

Historically, arteriography was the most common mode of detection for insulinoma, but improvement in less invasive imaging techniques and the relatively mediocre sensitivities (29% to 64%) have decreased the frequency of its use (277).

Transhepatic portal venous sampling and selective arterial calcium stimulation with hepatic vein sampling has been shown to be highly effective as a localizing technique in several studies (258,278,279). Although this is not a technique that gives precise anatomic localization of an insulinoma, localization of the lesion to a given region of the pancreas is invaluable. In the patient without a discernible lesion identified by available imaging techniques, the presence of a portal venous sampling insulin gradient allows the surgeon to focus the exploration and intraoperative ultrasound examination on specific regions within the pancreas, thereby improving intraoperative accuracy of tumor resection and possibly decreasing operative time (258). The portal venous sampling technique involves percutaneous, transhepatic placement of a portal venous catheter with sequential measurement of insulin levels in the portal vein and its tributaries. Selective arterial calcium stimulation with hepatic venous sampling is a more sensitive and specific provocative test as calcium is a potent stimulator of insulin release from abnormal beta cells and has reported sensitivities over 90% (258,279). This technique involves the placement of a femoral arterial catheter and selective cannulation of the splenic, superior mesenteric, and gastroduodenal arteries. A separate femoral venous catheter is directed into the right hepatic vein. Two milligrams of calcium gluconate are injected locally and insulin measurements taken from the hepatic vein at time of injection, and at 30, 60, and 120 seconds postinjection. A twofold increase in insulin is diagnostic. The sensitivity is further increased when the data from the preoperative studies are combined with intraoperative ultrasonography (258,278). Unfortunately, the invasive, expensive, and technically demanding nature of selective arterial calcium stimulation has prevented its routine use in all patients with a suspected insulinoma.

Technologic developments in CT have greatly increased sensitivities for detection of insulinomas. Diagnostic sensitivity for biphasic thin-section helical CT has been as high as 94% in some studies and combination with EUS has resulted in an overall diagnostic sensitivity up to 100% (258,280). Early arterial phase imaging can be performed to enhance detection. MRI can be very effective in detecting small pancreatic insulinomas. Optimal detection is achieved with fast spin-echo, fat saturation, and dynamic contrast-enhanced techniques with mangafodipir (281–283). Other potentially effective new imaging techniques include [^{11}C]5-hydroxyoytryptophan and ^{18}F-labeled dihydroxyphenylalanine PET scanning (284,285).

Although somatostatin-receptor scintigraphy plays an important role in the localization of most primary gastroenteropancreatic NETs, the relative low density of somatostatin receptors (sst) expressed on insulinoma tumors limits its effectiveness in patients with a suspected insulinoma (25,286). Peptide receptor scintigraphy (OctreoScan) combined with CT or PET scanning (fusion scanning) is being more widely used; however, the lack of sst 2 on insulinomas limits its overall sensitivity (287).

Perhaps the most valuable tool for localization of occult insulinoma is intraoperative ultrasonography (IUS). Several studies have documented the heightened ability of IUS to detect small insulinomas undetectable by palpation alone (264). IUS is performed with a high-resolution probe (7.5 to 10 MHz) and can be combined with color-flow Doppler assessment of adjacent major vessels. Sensitivities of up to 95% have been reported in the detection of pancreatic insulinomas (287,288). With the development of portal venous sampling and selective arterial calcium stimulation with hepatic vein sampling to localize insulinoma tumors to regions of the pancreas, IUS has become indispensable. By locating occult lesions in the head and midbody of the pancreas, morbid radical resections, such as a Whipple pancreaticoduodenectomy, can be avoided in most cases (288,289). The overall advantages of IUS include precise operative localization, enucleation of nonpalpable, nonvisible tumors, and avoidance of ductal and vascular injuries.

Treatment

The definitive treatment and only curative option is surgical resection. Overall cure rates range from 92% to 100% following surgical resection, with prognosis dependent on the stage at presentation and whether complete resection was achieved (258,268–271). Improved outcomes and higher cure rates have been more consistently reported at dedicated, tertiary hepatopancreaticobiliary centers (268). Medical therapy is typically reserved for surgically incurable lesions or with patients who are poor surgical candidates.

Operative Management

Surgical exploration proceeds only after coordination of all preoperative localization data. The pancreas is completely mobilized by an extended Kocher maneuver and division of the peritoneum performed along the inferior border of the pancreas through the lesser sac. Complete exploration with mobilization of the spleen and elevation of the distal pancreatic portion out of the retroperitoneum may be necessary. The entire pancreas is systematically inspected and bimanually palpated. Special attention is provided to areas previously localized by preoperative examinations. Inspection for locoregional spread in the retroperitoneum is also performed. Macroscopically, lesions appear yellow-brown or reddish-brown in color in contrast to the surrounding yellowish pancreatic parenchyma, and most benign insulinomas possess a pseudocapsule with a clear plane of dissection between the tumor and its surrounding soft pancreatic parenchyma (258,268). Following a complete physical inspection, IUS is performed with a high-resolution probe (7.5 to 10 MHz) combined with color-flow Doppler for assessment of major vascular and duct structures. The pancreas is scanned in both transverse and longitudinal planes, anteriorly and posteriorly. Attention should be focused on regions of the pancreas previously localized preoperatively. Insulinoma tumors typically appear as hypoechoic structures on real-time IUS (258,290,291). Techniques for benign resection of insulinomas include enucleation of the tumor and occasionally partial or complete pancreatic resection. Regional node dissection of abnormal nodes or formal node dissection is reserved for clearly malignant lesions. Hepatic metastasectomy may provide significant long-term symptom control. Enucleation is preferred for small benign tumors at least 2 to 3 mm from the main pancreatic duct. Intraoperative and intraductal ultrasonography can be used to gauge the distance between the tumor and duct (290–292). Resection is indicated when tumor is adjacent to pancreatic duct or major vessels. Thus, for insulinomas clearly localized before surgery, at or near the surface of the pancreas, and easily defined at time of surgery, enucleation may be sufficient, provided histopathology demonstrates complete excision and benign features (292–294).

More recently, laparoscopic enucleation of pancreatic tumors has been described. The outcomes have been favorable, with similar operative times, blood loss, and pancreatic fistula rates as with open surgery (291–294). Suspicion of malignancy, as evidenced by macroscopic tissue changes, distal dilatation of the pancreatic duct, or lymph node involvement, mandates aggressive resection (270,292). Usually if enucleation is not feasible, a distal or segmental pancreatectomy is indicated, with distal pancreatectomy (including both with splenectomy and with splenic preservation), pylorus-preserving Whipple procedure, or midbody pancreatectomy all being possible options. Studies have shown patients undergoing distal pancreatectomy with splenic preservation have less perioperative morbidity and decreased infectious complications, compared with conventional pancreatectomy with splenectomy, and should be the operation of choice, when feasible, for distal pancreatic disease other than adenocarcinoma (291,294). Experienced pancreatic surgeons should consider central pancreatectomy in appropriately selected patients with tumors located in the neck of the pancreas and with duct involvement, as it preserves both the spleen and the majority of pancreatic parenchyma (290,291). With advances in laparoscopic techniques, laparoscopic resection of pancreatic insulinomas has been performed successfully. A large retrospective multicenter study demonstrated the feasibility and safety of laparoscopic pancreatic resection in selected patients. The overall laparoscopic conversion rate was 14% and the use of laparoscopic ultrasonography facilitated laparoscopic resection (258,291).

Although blind distal pancreatectomy in cases of undetectable insulinoma was formerly considered to be standard of care, with current preoperative and surgical advances, blind distal pancreatectomy is not a logical approach. Insulinomas not detected during operation are probably not located at the tail of the pancreas but instead reside in the thicker, more complicated anatomic region of the pancreatic head (294,295).

Intraoperative frozen section has limited effectiveness and often cannot assess features of malignancy accurately; thus completeness of resection is best assessed by gross pathologic appearance and should be confirmed by formal histologic examination. If possible, peripheral blood insulin levels can be measured preoperatively, intraoperatively, and 5 minutes following resection with an 8-minute immunochemiluminescent insulin assay (296).

A high proportion of patients with MEN-1 with endogenous hyperinsulinemia (80%) are found to have multiple pancreatic insulinoma tumors. Although the postresection risk of recurrence of hyperinsulinemia in MEN-1 patients is significantly higher than those patients without MEN-1, resection remains the treatment of choice. In these patients, an 80% to 85% subtotal pancreatectomy to the level of the portal vein with enucleation of tumors in the head of the pancreas is recommended to reduce the risk of exocrine and endocrine insufficiency (297).

Malignant Insulinoma

Malignant insulinomas invade locally into surrounding soft tissue or structures, spreading by lymph nodes or liver metastases. The prognosis is determined by the stage of the disease. Malignant pancreatic insulinomas are usually single and are typically larger, most commonly presenting in the 4 to 7 cm diameter size range (298). The absence of hepatic metastases is a major predictor of survival at 3 years (299). For localized disease, formal pancreatic resection and lymphadenectomy are recommended (299). An aggressive approach is recommended in the presence of metastatic disease, with concurrent resection of the primary tumor and synchronous hepatic metastases (258,299,300). Palliative resection is indicated when preoperative evaluation shows that >90% of the tumor burden can be removed, combined with adjunctive ablative techniques. Resection is also indicated for symptom relief after medical management strategies have been exhausted (300). Patients with liver metastases, those with limited metastases outside the liver, those whose primary tumor can be controlled, and those who have a reasonable performance status are candidates for surgical resection (300). Danforth et al. (298) reported a median disease-free survival after curative resection of 5 years, with a recurrence rate of 63%. Palliative resection was associated with a median survival of 4 years, compared with 11 months after biopsy of the tumor only (258).

Adjunctive techniques include hepatic arterial embolization, chemoembolization, local tumor destruction by radiofrequency ablation or cryotherapy systemic chemotherapy, and more recently, radiolabeled somatostatin analog therapy.

Chemotherapy may be used for palliation when ablative techniques have failed or when significant extrahepatic disease is present. Streptozocin-based combinations with 5-FU or doxorubicin remain the first-line standard, but major objective responses are less common than had been previously thought (301). Other choices include intensified doses of 5-FU, dacarbazine, and epirubicin (302). Total response rates of 20% to 35% are reported with symptomatic improvement in 50% of patients (301,302). Second-line agents include interferon-alpha and octreotide. Cisplatin and etoposide are reserved for rapidly dividing tumors. Because of the overall modest success of current chemotherapeutic regimens, patients with advanced disease in need of treatment should be encouraged to enroll in clinical trials testing newer antineoplastic agents or newer treatment strategies (258,301,302).

Selective hepatic artery embolization can help when systemic treatment falters, with response rates of 50% to 90% and a median duration of response of 10 to 15 months. Transcatheter arterial chemoembolization, using doxorubicin and cisplatin-based chemotherapy, is reported to be an effective symptomatic and antiproliferative treatment in patients with progressive tumors (303,304). Combination regimens of transcatheter arterial chemoembolization and systemic chemotherapy have resulted in higher response rates in some studies with improved survival (303,304).

In patients with somatostatin receptor-positive tumors, the use of radiolabeled somatostatin analogs has been attempted in limited series. Local ablation techniques for liver metastases include radiofrequency ablation, cryotherapy, and alcohol injection (258).

Medical Management

Medical management of insulinoma is generally restricted to patients with unresectable metastatic disease, high-risk candidates for surgery, those not suitable for resection, or in those who

have undergone unsuccessful operation with persistent symptoms (258,262,268,305). Dietary management is an important component of any medical management regimen and patients with insulinoma are advised to avoid prolonged fasting and to eat smaller, more frequent meals that include complex carbohydrates. Diazoxide is an antihypertensive drug with hyperglycemic effects. It acts directly on beta cells to suppress insulin secretion and may also have a peripheral hyperglycemic effect. The recommended daily dose is 300 to 800 mg orally. Approximately 50% of patients relate significant symptom control; however, significant side effects of water retention, weight gain, hirsutism, and nausea are reported (306). A diuretic can be given in conjunction with diazoxide to counteract the resulting peripheral edema. Verapamil, propranolol, and phenytoin have all been used with variable success (301,307). Octreotide should be used with caution in patients with insulinomas. The hypoglycemic symptoms can be worsened by the relative lack of type 2 (sst 2) and type 5 (sst 5) receptors recognized by octreotide on beta cells, but a high density of these receptors on the alpha (glucagon) and growth hormone secretory cells that act as natural counter regulators of hypoglycemia. The result is a failure to suppress insulin production compounded by the suppressive effect of octreotide on secretion of glucagons and growth hormone. Therefore, prior to treatment with octreotide, insulinoma patients should have a radiolabeled octreotide scan (OctreoScan) performed to evaluate for presence of octreotide receptors on the tumor (301).

GLUCAGONOMAS AND THE GLUCAGONOMA SYNDROME

In 1942, Becker et al. (308) described the combination of an erosive erythema and cancer of the islet cells of the pancreas for the first time. In 1966, McGavran et al. (309) observed increasing levels of plasma glucagon in a patient with a glucagon-producing alpha cell carcinoma of the pancreas. Wilkinson and associates in 1973 described the rash associated with endocrine tumor as necrolytic migratory erythema. In 1974, Mallinson and colleagues established the association of a cutaneous rash with glucagon-producing tumors of the pancreas when they reported nine patients with the full clinical syndrome and a glucagon-releasing tumor of the pancreas (316,310).

Presentation and Incidence

Glucagon-producing islet cell tumors can present with various clinical manifestations ranging from asymptomatic to full-blown glucagonoma syndrome. Glucagonomas are rare islet cell tumors arising from the alpha-2 cells of the pancreas with distinct clinical manifestations, such as necrolytic migratory erythema, weight loss, diabetes mellitus, thromboembolism, cheilosis, angular stomatitis, diarrhea, and depression. The syndrome also goes by the acronym "4D," which stands for dermatitis, diarrhea, deep vein thromboses, and depression (310,311).

The age range at presentation is generally 20 to 70 years; however, most patients present at between 50 to 70 years of age. There is a female preponderance of 60%, with a reported incidence of 0.2 cases per million per year. Autopsy series have demonstrated an occurrence of 0.8% of microglucagonomas in adult-onset diabetics, suggesting that glucagonomas are more common than clinical diagnosis suggests (312). Most of these tumors occur sporadically, whereas 5% to 17% are associated with MEN-1. Patients suffering from sporadic glucagonomas usually present with symptoms in their fifth decade of life, whereas patients with MEN-1 present symptoms at a younger age (313). Typically the tumors are relatively large at presentation, with an average size between 5 and 10 cm. Glucagonomas usually occur as a single tumor, although multiple tumors or diffuse involvement by a single mass have been found in 10% of patients. The majority of tumors are situated in the pancreatic tail, with the head being the next most common site. Pancreatic body tumors are less common and typically account for <20% of glucagonoma tumors. Approximately 25% of glucagonomas are benign and confined to the pancreas; the remainder are malignant and have metastasized at time of diagnosis (314).

Glucagonoma syndrome is a paraneoplastic process that is pathognomonic for the presence of a glucagonoma tumor. It is characterized by necrolytic migratory erythema (82%), weight loss (70% to 80%), diabetes mellitus (75%), painful cheilosis or angular stomatitis (30% to 40%), diarrhea (15% to 30%), thromboembolism, and depression. Scotomas and changes in visual acuity have been reported in some cases (310–323). The pathophysiology of the syndrome is related to the known actions of glucagon. Glucagon is processed from a large precursor, proglucagon, in a tissue-specific manner in pancreatic alpha cells. In addition to amino acid nutrient stimuli, glucagon is also secreted in response to stressful stimuli, such as hypoglycemia and hypovolemia. In the intestine, proglucagon peptide cleavage results in glicentin, oxyntomodulin, and the glucagonlike peptides I and II. Hyperglycemia, insulin, and somatostatin exert an inhibitory influence. Glucagonomas secrete a disproportionate amount of proglucagonlike material. Glucagon has various important effects on glucose, fat, and protein metabolism (317–318). It stimulates hepatic gluconeogenesis and inhibits glucose breakdown (glycolysis); glycogen synthesis is inhibited. In adequately fed people, glucagon also promotes glycogen breakdown (glycogenolysis) in the liver. In adipose tissue it activates hormone-sensitive lipase, the rate-limiting step in triglyceride degradation.

Glucagon primarily acts on the liver to initiate glycogenolysis and gluconeogenesis, resulting in a rapid increase in endogenous production of glucose. The well-documented catabolic influence of glucagon accounts for the almost uniform weight loss and decrease in muscle mass observed in patients with glucagonomas. The inhibitory effect of glucagon on insulin secretion and action has been well established as the mediator of diabetes in these patients. Glucose intolerance in the glucagonoma syndrome may relate to tumor size. Fasting plasma glucagon levels tend to be higher in patients with large hepatic metastases than in those without hepatic metastases, and in one study all patients with large hepatic metastases had glucose intolerance. Massive hepatic metastases may decrease the ability of the liver to metabolize splanchnic glucagon, thus increasing peripheral plasma glucagon levels. Glucagon may not directly induce hyperglycemia, however, unless metabolism of glucose by the liver is directly compromised. Another factor may be variation in the molecular species of glucagon that is secreted in each case and the biologic potency of that species (317–318).

Necrolytic migratory erythema is a cutaneous condition characterized by temporal waves of irregular erythema, which subsequently erode and become crusted. The condition carries with it the characteristics of a deficiency dermatosis. Necrolytic migratory erythema is the presenting problem in roughly 70% of the patients with a glucagonoma (311–328). The lesions consist of an intense erythema with superficial epidermal necrosis. This leads to shedding of the skin with flaccid bullae and crusted erosions. Central healing occurs, which gives the lesions an annular appearance. Healing can be associated with hyperpigmentation. The lesions primarily affect the perineum and other intertriginous sites. The trunk, legs, perioral skin, and sites of minor trauma can also be involved. Onychoschizia has been reported in some patients. A painful glossitis manifested by an erythematous, mildly atrophic tongue has been associated with these cutaneous lesions. The most specific feature on histologic examination of the skin is necrolysis of the upper epidermis with vacuolated keratinocytes, leading to focal or confluent necrosis. The condition is typically unresponsive to topical steroids, oral antibiotics, and antihistamines. In fact, the histology of the skin is very similar to the biopsy findings in other deficiency states like pellagra, zinc deficiency, and necrolytic acral erythema. The cause of necrolytic migratory erythema has been suggested to be related to the hypoaminoacidemia typically present in patients with glucagonomas; however, the exact cause of the skin rash remains unknown. Biopsy examination of a fresh skin lesion may be the most valuable aid in suggesting the diagnosis of glucagonoma syndrome, but repeated biopsy samples may be necessary to raise this possibility. The differential diagnosis includes several metabolic disorders associated with cutaneous lesions closely resembling necrolytic migratory erythema. These include acrodermatitis enteropathica, zinc deficiency induced by hyperalimentation, essential fatty acid deficiency, the dermatosis of protein calorie malnutrition of kwashiorkor, and pellagra resulting from niacin deficiency. Herpes, eczema, chemical burns, and contact dermatitis may also be considered. Normalization of glucagon concentrations by surgery or somatostatin analogs almost invariably results in rapid disappearance of the skin disorder. Improvement in the rash associated with the glucagonoma syndrome has been reported with amino acid repletion as well as administration of carbohydrate. The skin rash also has been shown to improve with the administration of zinc. Almost invariably, the dermatosis resolves after successful removal of a glucagon-producing tumor, even if the rash has been present for several years. In addition, in those patients who do not undergo curative resection but are treated with chemotherapeutic agents, dermatitis improves as the glucagon levels decrease. However, it is likely from the physiological function of glucagon, as well as from the histopathologic findings on tissue biopsy, that necrolytic migratory erythema is a true deficiency dermatosis (311–330).

Patients with glucagonoma are especially susceptible to thromboembolic events and as high as 50% of the overall mortality related to this condition is secondary to pulmonary embolism. Routine deep venous thrombosis prophylaxis is mandatory, and perioperative heparin administration should be considered because as many as 30% of patients with glucagonoma have evidence of deep venous thrombosis or pulmonary emboli. Unexplained thromboembolic disease in any patient should alert one to the possibility of glucagonoma (331). In our series Coumadin is not effective for prevention of thrombosis, while heparin is routinely effective.

Diagnosis

In previously reported cases of glucagonoma in which plasma glucagon concentrations were measured by radioimmunoassay, fasting plasma glucagon concentrations were 2,100 ± 334 pg/mL. These levels are markedly higher than those reported in normal, fasting subjects (i.e., 150 pg/mL) or in those with other disorders causing hyperglucagonemia, including diabetes mellitus, diabetic ketoacidosis, prolonged starvation, acute pancreatitis, burn injury, acute trauma, bacteremia, cirrhosis, chronic renal insufficiency, or Cushing syndrome, in which fasting plasma glucagon concentrations often are elevated but <500 pg/mL. Generally, serum glucagon levels >1,000 pg/mL are diagnostic for glucagonoma. Patients typically present with hypoaminoacidemia and pronounced cachexia, necessitating hyperalimentation with total parental nutrition and supplemental zinc, trace metals, and insulin. Hyperglycemia, normochromic normocytic anemia, and increased erythrocyte sedimentation rate are other laboratory indicators that are seen (329–330).

As with other islet cell neoplasms, glucagonomas may overproduce multiple hormones. Insulin is the second most common hormone secreted by these tumors. Others include corticotropin, pancreatic polypeptide, parathyroid hormone, or substances with parathyroid hormonelike activity, gastrin, serotonin, VIP, and melanocyte-stimulating hormone, in that order of frequency (318,321).

Radiologic Evaluation

Unlike other pancreatic NETs, the large size of most glucagonomas at time of presentation makes localization with a contrast-enhanced CT scan possible in nearly all instances. Occasionally, MRI, MR angiography, or, rarely, selective portal venous sampling may be required for localization of tumors that are smaller and more difficult to identify. Somatostatin receptor scintigraphy has been used to image glucagonomas that express somatostatin receptors in >80% of cases (333).

Management

Surgical Management

If the diagnosis is made while the tumor is still localized, surgical resection may offer the only likelihood of cure for this disease. Most patients have large, solitary tumors located in the tail of the pancreas and require a distal pancreatectomy. When lymph node or liver metastasis is present, it should be resected (if possible) together with the primary tumor. Although metastases often are present at exploration, a complete surgical resection is possible in 30% of cases. Even if complete removal of tumor is not achievable, palliative debulking may be indicated as a means to control refractory symptoms (333,334). Radiofrequency ablation and hepatic chemoembolization have been used in conjunction with surgery or as an alternative technique to treat symptoms related to hormone excess. Preoperative preparation may require an interval of total parenteral nutrition secondary to preexisting malnutrition induced by the syndrome and aggressive prophylactic measures to prevent venous thrombosis, including low-dose subcutaneous heparin, and intermittent pneumatic compression stockings are mandatory in all patients. Octreotide can be useful in helping to improve the perioperative condition of these patients prior to surgery (332).

Medical Management

Management of metastatic disease is generally conservative. Initial treatment of these tumors includes expectant observation and medical management of symptoms with clinical monitoring and serial CT scans to assess tumor growth. Patients with rapidly progressive disease, with local symptoms caused by tumor bulk, or with uncontrolled symptoms related to hormone secretion require more aggressive medical or surgical intervention. Octreotide may help control hormone secretion and stabilize tumor growth. Patients refractory to octreotide with tumor predominantly in the liver are potential candidates for mechanical ablative techniques, such as hepatic arterial embolization. Radiofrequency ablation and cryosurgical techniques may also be useful, although specific data are limited. Surgical resection of metastatic disease may offer palliative relief of symptoms related to hormone secretion in carefully selected patients. Chemotherapy may be used for palliation when ablative techniques have failed or when significant extrahepatic disease is present (332).

Chemotherapy

Several authors have reported that dacarbazine is a highly effective agent for the treatment of pancreatic islet cell tumors, especially glucagon-secreting tumors. Using either 1,250 mg/m^2 in divided doses over 5 days or a single dose of 650 mg/m^2, Kessinger and colleagues (339) reported two complete responses and two partial responses of elevated serum glucagon in four patients with glucagonomas. Three of four additional patients with malignant islet cell carcinoma associated with glucagonoma syndrome were cited in this report as having responded to dacarbazine alone. In a recently reported prospective study of 48 evaluable patients with advanced islet cell carcinoma, Hahn and colleagues reported 13 patients (27%) with objective responses (including three complete responses) following dacarbazine, 850 mg/m^2 given every 4 weeks. The median survival in all patients was 19 months, and the authors concluded that dacarbazine clearly had beneficial activity in patients with advanced islet cell carcinoma (335–343).

Streptozotocin is a drug that is selectively cytotoxic for pancreatic islet cells. This selective cytotoxicity has provided a rationale for using streptozotocin in neoplastic disorders of pancreatic endocrine cells. In several studies using intravenous and, less commonly, intra-arterial administration, streptozotocin was shown to be active against several pancreatic endocrine cancers, with nearly 40% tumor responses and over 50% hormonal responses reported (344–348). In the case of symptomatic hepatic metastases from glucagonoma, Friesen et al. (344) claim that use of intra-arterial administration of streptozotocin is effective, with reduced incidence of nephrotoxicity, but this has not been confirmed. The relative rarity of gastroenteropancreatic neoplasms has necessitated the combination of several islet cell tumor subtypes in the same study. The experience from these studies suggests that whereas similar responses may be expected from chemotherapy for several tumor subtypes, there may be differences in the response of others. In general, streptozotocin alone has shown little activity against glucagonomas, whereas dacarbazine has demonstrated the most pronounced effectiveness. Various studies have shown limited effectiveness of interferon on hormonal control and tumor reduction, but little specificity toward glucagons-secreting islet cell tumors has been demonstrated.

REFERENCES

1. Pearse AGE. The cytochemistry and ultrastructure of polypeptide hormone-producing cells of the APUD series and the embryologic, physiologic and pathologic implications of the concept. *J Histochem Cytochem.* 1969;17:303–313.

2. Solciae, Kloppings, Lhsobin. *Histologic Typing of Neuroendocrine Tumors.* World Health Organization, New York: Springer-Verlag; 2000.

3. Modlin IM, Lye K, Kidd M. A 50-year analysis of 562 gastric carcinoids: small tumor or larger problem? *Am Jour Gastroenterol.* 2004;99:23–32.

4. Oberg K, Kvols L, Caplin M, et al. Consensus statement on the use of somatostatin analogs for the management of neuroendocrine tumors of the gastroenteropancreatic system. *Ann Onco.* 2004;15:966–973.

5. Nehar D, Lombard-Bohas C, Olivieri S, et al., Interest of Chromogranin A for diagonosis and follow-up of endocrine tumors. 2004;60:644-652.

6. Sondenaa K, Sen J, Heinle F, et al. Chromogranin A, a marker of the therapeutic success of resection of neuroendocrine liver metastases: Preliminary report. *World J Surg* 2004;28:890-895.

7. Calhoun K, Toth-Fejel S, Cheek J, et al. Serum peptide profiles in patients with carcinoid tumors. *Am Jour Surg.* 2003;186:28–31.

8. Desai DC, O'Dorisio TM, Schirmer WJ, et al. Serum pancreastatin levels predict response to hepatic artery chemoembolization and somatostatin analog therapy in metastatic neuroendocrine tumors. *Regulatory Peptides.* 2001;96:113–117.

9. Modlin IM, Lawton JP, Tabg LH, et al. The mastomys gastric carcinoid: aspects of enterochromaffin-like cell function. *Digestion.* 1994;55:31–37.

10. Tang LH, Modlin IM. Somatostatin receptor regulation of gastric carcinoid tumours. *Digestion.* 1996;57: 11–14.

11. Borin JF, Tang LH, Kidd M, et al. Somatostatin receptor regulation of gastric enterochromaffin-like cell transformation to gastric carcinoid. *Surgery.* 1996;120:1026–1032.

12. Kolby L, Wangberg B, Ahlman H, et al. Histamine metabolism of gastric carcinoids in Mastomys natalensis. *Yale Jour Bio & Med.* 1998;71:207–215.

13. Woltering EA, Mozell EJ, O'Dorisio TM, et al. Supression of primary and secondary peptides with somatostatin analog in the therapy of functional endocrine tumors. *Surg Gynecol Obstet.* 1988;167:453–462.

14. Vinik AI, Woltering EA, O'Dorisio TM, et al. Neuroendocrine Tumors: A Comprehensive Guide to Diagnosis and Management. *Inter Science Institute.* 2006.

15. Taal BG, Hoefnagel CA, Valdes Olmos RA, et al. Combined diagnostic imaging with ^{131}I-metaidobenzylguanidine and [111]Inpentetreotide in carcinoid tumours. [*Clinical Trial Journal Article*] *European Journal of Cancer.* 1996;32A:1924–1932.

16. Boudreaux JP, Putty B, Frey DJ, et al. Surgical treatment of advanced stage carcinoid tumors: lessons learned. *Ann Surg.* 2005;241:839–846.

17. Que FG, Sarmiento JM, Nagorney DM. Hepatic surgery for metastatic gastrointestinal neuroendocrine tumors. *Cancer Control.* 2002;9:67–79.

18. Moertel CG, Johnson CM, McKusick MA, et al. The management of patients with advanced carcinoid tumors and islet cell carcinoid tumors. *Annals of Internal Medicine.* 1994;120:102–209.

19. Atwell TD, Charboneau JW, Que FG, et al. Treatment of neuroendocrine cancer metastatic to the liver: the role of ablative techniques. *Cardiovasc Intervent Radiol.* 2005;28:409–421.

20. Brazeau P, Vale W, Burgus R, et al. Hypothalamic polypeptide that inhibits the secretion of immunoreactive pituitary growth hormone. 1973; 179:77–79.

21. Krulichl, Dhariwalap, McCann. Stimulatory and inhibitory effects of purified hypothalamic extracts on growth hormone release from rat pituitary in vitro. *Endocrinology.* 1968;83:83, 73, 90.

22. Lamberts SW. A guide to the clinical use of the somatostatin analogue SMS 201–995 (Sandostatin). [Review] [75 refs] [Journal article. Review Acta endocrinologica. *Supplementum.* 1987;286:54–66.

23. Bauer W, Briner U, Doepfner W, et al. SMS 201–995: A very potent and selective octapeptide analogue of somatostatin with prolonged action. *Life Sciences.* 1982;31:1133–1140.

24. Woltering EA, Mamikunian PM, Zietz S, et al. Effect of octreotide LAR dose and weight on octreotide blood levels in patients with neuroendocrine tumors. *Pancreas.* 2005;31:392–400.

25. Krenning EP, Bakker WH, Breeman WA, et al. Localisation of endorcrine-related tumours with radioiodinated analogue of somatostatin. Lancet 1989; 8632:242–244.

26. Kvols L. Malignant carcinoid and the carcinoid syndrome ACTA Oncologica 1993.

27. de Jong, Bakker WH, Krenning EP, et al. Yttrium-90 and indium-111 labeling, receptor binding and biodistribution of [DOTA0, d-Phe1, Tyr3] octreotide, a promising somatostatin analogue for radionucleide therapy. *Euro Jour Nuc Med.* 1997;24:368–371.

28. Krenning EP, Kooij PP, Bakker WH, et al. Radiotherapy with a radiolabeled somatostatin analog, [^{111}In-DTPA-D-phe1]-octreotide. A Case history. Ann. N.Y. Acad. Sci; 733:496–506.

29. Woltering EA, O'Dorisio MS, Murphy WA, et al. Synthesis and characterization of multiply-tyrosinated, multiply-iodinated somatostatin analogs. *J Peptide Res.* 1999;53:201–213.

30. McCarthy KE, Woltering EA, Anthony LB. In situ radiotherapy with ^{111}In-pentetreotide. State of the art and perspectives. *Quarterly Journal of Nuclear Medicine.* 2000;44:88–95.

31. Oberndorfer S. Beitraege zur pathologischen anatomie der chronischen appendicitis habilitationsschrift. *Mitt au d Grenzgebiet der Mediz und Chirug.* 1906. Bd. 1.

32. Langhans T. Ueber einen drusenpolyp im ileum. *Virchows Arch Pathol Anat.* 1867;38:550–560.

33. Lubarsch O. Ueber dem primaren Krebs des ileum nebst bemerkungen uber das gleichzeitige vorkommen von Krebs und tuberculose. *Virchows Arch Pathol Anat.* 1888;111:280–317.

34. Ransom WB. A case of primary carcinoma of the ileum. *Lancet.* 1890;2:1020–1023.

35. Notthaft A. Ueber die entstechung der carcinoma. *Deutsches Arch Klin Med.* 1895;54:555–587.

36. Obendorfer S. Karzinoide tumoren des dunndarms. *Frankf Z Pathol.* 1907;1:426–432.

37. Michelson K. Zur multiplicitat des primaren carcinoms, I-D, Berlin, Germany 1889.

38. Oberndorfer S. Karzinoide handbuch der speziellen, in Henke F, Lubarsch O (eds): *Handbuch der Speciellen Pathologischen Anatomic und Histologie.* Berlin, Germany: Verlag van Julius Springer; 1928:814–817.

39. Modlin IA. A five decade analysis of 13,715 carcinoid tumors. *Cancer.* 2004;97:934–95

40. Zollinger RM, Ellison EH. Primary peptic ulcerations of the jejunum associated with islet cell tumors of the pancreas. *Ann Surg.* 1955;142:709–723.

41. Edkins JS. On the chemical mechanism of gastric secretion. *Proc R Soc Lond B Biol Sci.* 1905;76:37.

42. Edkins JS. The chemical mechanism of gastric secretion. *J Physiol (Lond).* 1906;34:133–144.

43. Meko JB, Norton JA. Management of patients with Zollinger Ellison syndrome. *Ann Rev Med.* 1995;46:395–411.

44. Gibril F, Jensen RT. Advances in Evaluation and Management of Gastrinoma in Patients with Zollinger-Ellison Syndrome. *Current Gastroenterology Reports.* 2005;7:114–121.

45. Lal G, O'Dorisio T, McDougall R, et al. Cancer of the Endocrine System: Pancreatic Islet Cell Tumors. In Abeloff MD, Armitage JO, Niederhuber JE, Kastan MB, McKenna WG ed. Abeloff's Clinical Oncology, 4th ed, Philadelphia: Churchill Livingstone; 2008.

46. Modlin IM, Jaffe BM, Sank A, et al. The early diagnosis of gastrinoma. *Ann Surg.* 1982;196:512–517.

47. Eriksson B, Skogseid B, Lundqvist G, et al. Medical treatment and long-term survival in a prospective study of 84 patients with endocrine pancreatic tumors. *Cancer.* 1990;65:1883–1890.

48. Jordan PH. A personal experience with pancreatic and duodenal neuroendocrine tumors. *J Am Coll Surg.* 1999;189:470–482.

49. Brandi ML, Gagel RF, Angeli A, et al. Guidelines for diagnosis and therapy of MEN type 1 and type 2. *J Clin Endocrinol Metab.* 2001;86:5658–5671.

50. Chandrasekharappa SC, Guru SC, Manickam P, et al. Positional cloning of the gene for multiple endocrine neoplasia type 1. *Science.* 1997;276:404–407.

51. Jensen RT. Management of the Zollinger-Ellison syndrome in patients with multiple endocrine neoplasia type 1. *J Intern Med.* 1998;243:477–488.

52. Gibril F, Schumann M, Pace A, et al. Multiple endocrine neoplasia type 1 and Zollinger–Ellison syndrome. A prospective study of 107 cases and comparison with 1009 cases from the literature. *Medicine.* 2004;83:43–83.

53. Delle Fave G, Capurso G, Annibale B, et al. Gastric neuroendocrine tumors. *Neuroendocrinology.* 2004;80:16–19.

54. Rindi G, Bordi C, Rappel S, et al. Gastric carcinoids and neuorendocrine carcinomas: pathogenesis, pathology and behavior. *World J Surg.* 1996;20:168–172.

55. Norton JA, Doppman JL, Collen MJ, et al. Prospective study of gastrinoma localization and resection in patients with Zollinger-Ellison syndrome. *Ann Surg.* 1986;204:468–479.

56. Norton JA, Doppman JL, Jensen RT, et al. Curative resection in Zollinger-Ellison syndrome. Results of a 10-year prospective study. *Ann Surg.* 1992;215:8–18.

57. Jensen RT, Gardner JD. Gastrinoma. In: Go VLW, DiMagno ER, Gardner JD, Lebenthal FP, Reber HA, Scheele GA, eds. *The Pancreas: Biology, Pathobiology, and Disease.* 2nd ed. New York: Raven Press, 1993:931–978.

58. Oberhelman HA, Nelsen TS, Johnson AN, et al. Ulcerogenic tumors of the duodenum. *Ann Surg.* 1961;153:214–227.

59. Ellison EH, Wilson SD. The Zollinger–Ellison syndrome: reappraisal and evaluation of 260 registered cases. *Ann Surg.* 1964;160:512–530.

60. Hofmann JW, Fox PS, Wilson SD. Duodenal wall tumors and the Zollinger–Ellison syndrome. Surgical management. *Arch Surg.* 1973;107:334–339.

61. Norton JA, Jensen RT. Resolved and unresolved controversies in the surgical management of patients with Zollinger–Ellison syndrome. *Ann Surg.* 2004;240:757–773.

62. Norton JA, Fraker DL, Alexander HR, et al. Surgery to cure the Zollinger–Ellison syndrome. *N Engl J Med.* 1999;341:635–644.

63. Cadiot G, Lebtahi R, Sarda L, et al. Preoperative detection of duodenal gastrinomas and peripancreatic lymph nodes by somatostatin receptor scintigraphy. *Gastroenterology.* 1996;111:845–854.

64. Thom AK, Norton JA, Axiotis CA, et al. Location, incidence, and malignant potential of duodenal gastrinomas. *Surgery.* 1991; 110:1086–1093.

65. Jensen RT. Zollinger-Ellison syndrome. In: Doherty GM, Skogseid B, eds. *Surgical endocrinology: clinical syndromes.* Philadelphia, PA: Lippincott Williams & Wilkins; 2001:291–344.

66. Norton JA, Alexander HR, Fraker DL, et al. Possible primary lymph node gastrinoma: occurrence, natural history, and predictive factors: a prospective study. *Annals of Surgery.* 2003;237:650–659.

67. Arnold WS, Fraker DL, Alexander HR, et al. Apparent lymph node primary gastrinoma. *Surgery.* 1994;116:1123–1129, discussion 1129.

68. Jensen RT, Gardner JD, Raufman JP, et al. Zollinger-Ellison syndrome: current concepts and management. *Ann Intern Med.* 1983;98:59–75.

69. Primrose JN, Maloney M, Wells M, et al. Gastrin-producing ovarian mucinous cystadenomas: a cause of the Zollinger-Ellison syndrome. *Surgery.* 1998;104:830–833.

70. Jensen RT. Gastrin-producing tumors. *Cancer Treat Res.* 1997;89: 293–334.

71. Rehfeld JF, van Solinge WW. The tumor biology of gastrin and cholecystokinin. *Adv Cancer Res.* 1994;63:295–347.

72. McTavish D, BuckleyMM,Heel RC, et al. Omeprazole. An updated review of its pharmacology and therapeutic use in acid-related disorders. *Drugs.* 1991;42:138–170.

73. Solcia E, Capella C, Buffa R, et al. Endocrine cells of the gastrointestinal tract and related tumors. *Pathobiol Annu.* 1979;9:163–204.

74. Solcia E, Capella C, Buffa R, et al. Pathology of the Zollinger-Ellison syndrome. In: Fenoglio CM, Wolff M, eds. *Progress in surgical pathology.* New York: Masson. 1980:119–123.

75. Li M, Norton J. Gastrinoma. *Curr Treat Opt Oncol.* 2001;2:337–346.

76. Azimuddin K, Chamberlain RS. The surgical mamangement of pancreatic neuroendocrine tumors. *Surgical Clinics of North America.* 2001;81:511–525.

77. Weber HC, Venzon DJ, Lin JT, et al. Determinants of metastatic rate and survival in patients with Zollinger-Ellison syndrome: a prospective long-term study. *Gastroenterology.* 1995;108:1637–1649.

78. Jensen RT. Natural history of digestive endocrine tumors. In Mignon M, Colombel JF, ed. *Recent Advances in the Pathophysiology and Management of Inflammatory Bowel Disease and Digestive Endocrine Tumors.* Paris: John Libbey Eurotext Publishing; 1999:192–219.

79. Gibril F, Doppman JL, Reynolds JC, et al. Bone metastases in patients with gastrinomas: a prospective study of bone scanning, somatostatin receptor scanning, and magnetic resonance image in their detection, frequency, location, and effect of their detection on management. *J Clin Oncol.* 1998;16:1040–1053.

80. Lebtahi R, Cadiot G, Delahaye N, et al. Detection of bone metastases in patients with endocrine gastroenteropancreatic tumors: bone scintigraphy compared with somatostatin receptor scintigraphy. *J Nucl Med.* 1999;40:1602–1608.

81. Corleto VD, Delle Fave G, Jensen RT. Molecular insights into gastrointestinal neuroendocrine tumours: importance and recent advances. *Dig Liver Dis.* 2002;34:668–680.

82. Goebel SU, Iwamoto M, Raffeld M, et al. HER-2/neu Expression and gene amplification in gastrinomas correlations with

tumor biology, growth, and aggressiveness. *Cancer Res.* 2002:62: 3702–3710.

83. Chen YJ, Vortmeyer A, Zhuang Z, et al. X-chromosome loss of heterozygosity frequently occurs in gastrinomas and is correlated with aggressive tumor growth. *Cancer.* 2004;100:1379–1387.

84. Chen YJ, Vortmeyer A, Zhuang Z, et al. Loss of Heterozygosity of Chromosome 1q in Gastrinomas Occurrence and Prognostic Significance. *Cancer Research.* 2003;63:817–823.

85. Guo SS, Wu AY, Sawicki MP. Deletion of Chromosome 1, But Not Mutation of MEN-1, Predicts Prognosis in Sporadic Pancreatic Endocrine Tumors. *World Journal of Surgery.* 2002;26:843–847.

86. Peghini PL, Iwamoto M, Raffeld M, et al. Overexpression of epidermal growth factor and hepatocyte growth factor receptors in a proportion of gastrinomas correlates with aggressive growth and lower curability. *Clin Cancer Res.* 2002;8:2273–2285.

87. Serrano J, Goebel SU, Peghini PL, et al. Alterations in the p16INK4a/CDKN2A tumor suppressor gene in gastrinomas. *J Clin Endocrinol Metab.* 2000;85:4146–4156.

88. Goebel SU, Heppner C, Burns AL, et al. Genotype/Phenotype Correlation of Multiple Endocrine Neoplasia Type 1 Gene Mutations in Sporadic Gastrinomas. *The Journal of Clinical Endocrinology & Metabolism.* 2000;85:116–123.

89. Muscarella P, Melvin WS, Fisher WE, et al. Genetic alterations in gastrinomas and nonfunctioning pancreatic neuroendocrine tumors: an analysis of p16/MTS1 tumor suppressor gene inactivation. *Cancer Res.* 1998;58:237–240.

90. Delcore R, Friesen SR. Role of pancreatoduodenectomy in the management of primary duodenal wall gastrinomas in patients with Zollinger-Ellison syndrome. *Surgery.* 1992;112:1016–1023.

91. Fraker DL, Norton JA, Alexander HR, et al. Surgery in Zollinger-Ellison syndrome alters the natural history of gastrinoma. *Ann Surg.* 1994;220:320–328; discussion 328–330.

92. Pipeleers-Marichal M, Donow C, Heitz PU, et al. Pathologic aspects of gastrinomas in patients with Zollinger-Ellison syndrome with and without multiple endocrine neoplasia type I. *World Journal of Surgery.* 1993;17:481–488.

93. Stabile BE, Passaro E Jr. Benign and malignant gastrinoma. *Am J Surg.* 1985;149:144–150.

94. Berger AC, Gibril F, Venzon DJ, et al. Prognostic value of initial fasting serum gastrin levels in patients with Zollinger-Ellison syndrome. *J Clin Oncol.* 2001;19:3051.

95. Yu F, Venzon DJ, Serrano J, et al. Prospective study of the clinical course, prognostic factors, causes of death, and survival in patients with long-standing Zollinger-Ellison syndrome. *J Clin Oncol.* 1999;17:615–630.

96. Ruszniewski P, Podevin P, Cadiot G, et al. Clinical, anatomical, and evolutive features of patients with the Zollinger-Ellison syndrome combined with type I multiple endocrine neoplasia. *Pancreas.* 1993;8:295–304.

97. Donow C, Pipeleers-Marichal M, Schroder S, et al. Surgical pathology of gastrinoma. Site, size, multicentricity, association with multiple endocrine neoplasia type 1, and malignancy. *Cancer.* 1991; 68:1329–1334.

98. Norton JA. Gastrinoma: advances in localization and treatment. *Surg Oncol Clin N Am.* 1998;7:845–861.

99. Pisegna JR, Sawicki MP. Neuroendocrine pancreas. In: Haskell CM, ed. *Cancer Treatment.* 5th ed. Philadelphia, PA: WB Saunders; 2001:1065–1081.

100. Wolfe MM, Jensen RT. Zollinger-Ellison syndrome. Current concepts in diagnosis and management. *N Engl J Med.* 1987;317: 1200–1209.

101. Tomassetti P, Salomone T, Migliori M, et al. Optimal treatment of Zollinger-Ellison syndrome and related conditions in elderly patients. *Drugs Aging.* 2003;20:1019–1034.

102. Zollinger RM, Ellison EC, Fabri PJ, et al. Primary peptic ulcerations of the jejunum associated with islet cell tumors. Twenty-five-year appraisal. *Ann Surg.* 1980;192:422–430.

103. Maton PN, Vinayek R, Frucht H, et al. Long-term efficacy and safety of omeprazole in patients with Zollinger-Ellison syndrome: a prospective study. *Gastroenterology.* 1989;97:827–836.

104. Maton PN, Frucht H, Vinayek R, et al. Medical management of patients with Zollinger-Ellison syndrome who have had previous gastric surgery: a prospective study. *Gastroenterology.* 1988;94:294–299.

105. Vinayek R, Howard JM, Maton PN, et al. Famotidine in the therapy of gastric hypersecretory states. *Am J Med.* 1986;81:49–59.

106. Raufman JP, Collins SM, Pandol SJ, et al. Reliability of symptoms in assessing control of gastric acid secretion in patients with Zollinger-Ellison syndrome. *Gastroenterology.* 1983;84: 108–113.

107. Metz DC, Strader DB, Orbuch M, et al. Use of omeprazole in Zollinger-Ellison syndrome: a prospective nine-year study of efficacy and safety. *Aliment Pharmacol Ther.* 1983;7:597–610.

108. Lloyd-Davies KA, Rutgersson K, Solvell L. Omeprazole in the treatment of Zollinger-Ellison syndrome: a 4-year international study. *Aliment Pharmacol Ther.* 1988;2:13–32.

109. Hirschowitz BI, Simmons J, Mohnen J. Long-term lansoprazole control of gastric acid and pepsin secretion in ZE and non-ZE hypersecretors: a prospective 10-year study. *Aliment Pharmacol Ther.* 2001;15:1795–1806.

110. Ellison EC, O'Dorisio TM, Sparks J, et al. Observations on the effect of a somatostatin analog in the Zollinger-Ellison syndrome: implications for the treatment of apudomas. *Surgery.* 1986;100:437–444.

111. Ruszniewski P, Laucournet H, Elouaer-Blanc L, et al. Long-acting somatostatin (SMS 201–995) in the management of Zollinger-Ellison syndrome: evidence for sustained efficacy. *Pancreas.* 1988;3:145–152.

112. Ruszniewski P, Ramdani A, Cadiot G, et al. Long-term treatment with octreotide in patients with the Zollinger-Ellison syndrome. *Eur J Clin Invest.* 1993;23:296–301.

113. Shojamanesh H, Gibril F, Louie A, et al. Prospective study of the antitumor efficacy of long-term octreotide treatment in patients with progressive metastatic gastrinoma. *Cancer.* 2002;94:331–343.

114. Mozell EJ, Cramer AJ, O'Dorisio TM, et al. Long-term efficacy of octreotide in the treatment of Zollinger-Ellison syndrome. *Arch Surg.* 1992;127:1019–1024; discussion 1024–1026.

115. Murray-Lyon IM, Eddleston AL, Williams R, et al. Treatment of multiple-hormone-producing malignant islet-cell tumour with streptozotocin. *Lancet.* 1968;2:895–898.

116. Broder LE, Carter SK. Pancreatic islet cell carcinoma. II. Results of therapy with streptozotocin in 52 patients. *Ann Intern Med.* 1973;79:108–118.

117. von Schrenck T, Howard JM, Doppman JL, et al. Prospective study of chemotherapy in patients with metastatic gastrinoma. *Gastroenterology.* 1998;94:1326–1334.

118. Sutliff VE, Doppman JL, Gibril F, et al. Growth of newly diagnosed, untreated metastatic gastrinomas and predictors of growth patterns. *J Clin Oncol.* 1997;15:2420–2431.

119. Rougier P, Mitry E. Chemotherapy in the treatment of neuroendocrine malignant tumors. *Digestion.* 2000;62:73–78.

120. Pisegna JR, Slimak GG, Doppman JL, et al. An evaluation of human recombinant alpha interferon in patients with metastatic gastrinoma. *Gastroenterology.* 1993;105:1179–1183.

121. Oberg K. Advances in chemotherapy and biotherapy of endocrine tumors. *Curr Opin Oncol.* 1998;10:58–65.

122. Norton JA. Surgical treatment and prognosis of gastrinoma. *Best Pract Res Clin Gastroenterol.* 2005;19:799–805.

123. Thompson NW. Current concepts in the surgical management of multiple endocrine neoplasia type 1 pancreatic-duodenal disease. Results in the treatment of 40 patients with Zollinger–Ellison syndrome, hypoglycaemia or both. *J Intern Med.* 1998;243:495–500.

124. Norton JA, Alexander HR, Fraker DL, et al. Does the use of routine duodenotomy affect rate of cure, development of liver metastases or survival in patients with Zollinger–Ellison syndrome (ZES)? *Ann Surg.* 2004;239:617–625.

125. Norton JA, Alexander HR, Fraker DL, et al. Comparison of surgical results in patients with advanced and limited disease with multiple endocrine neoplasia type 1 and Zollinger–Ellison syndrome. *Ann Surg.* 2001;234:495–506.

126. Doherty GM, Olson JA, Frisella MM, et al. Lethality of multiple endocrine neoplasia Type 1. *World J Surg.* 1998;22:581–587.

127. Wilkinson S, The BT, Davey KR, et al. Cause of death in multiple endocrine neoplasia type 1. *Arch Surg.* 1993;128:683–690.

128. Norton JA, Cornelius MJ, Doppman JL, et al. Effect of parathyroidectomy in patients with hyperparathyroidism, Zollinger- Ellison syndrome, and multiple endocrine neoplasia type I: a prospective study. *Surgery.* 1997;102:958–966.

129. Maton PN, Norton JA, Nieman LK, et al. Multiple endocrine neoplasia type II with Zollinger-Ellison syndrome caused by a solitary pancreatic gastrinoma. *JAMA.* 1998;262:535–537.

130. Cameron D, Spiro HM, Landsberg L. Zollinger-Ellison syndrome with multiple endocrine adenomatosis type II. *N Engl J Med.* 1978;299:152–153.

131. Sheppard BC, Norton JA, Doppman JL, et al. Management of islet cell tumors in patients with multiple endocrine neoplasia: a prospective study. *Surgery.* 1989;106:1108–1117.

132. Howard TJ, Zinner MJ, Stabile BE, et al., Gastrinoma excision for cure. A prospective analysis. *Ann Surg.* 1990;211:9–14.

133. Norton JA. Neuroendocrine tumors of the pancreas and duodenum. *Curr Probl Surg.* 1994;31:1–156.

134. Akerstom G, Hessman O, Skogseid B. Timing and extent of surgery in symptomatic and asymptomatic neuroendocrine tumors of the pancreas in MEN1. *Lagenbecks Arch Surg.* 2002;386:558–569.

135. Thompson NW. Management of pancreatic endocrine tumors in patients with multiple endocrine neoplasia type 1. *Surg Oncol Clin North Am.* 1998;7:881–891.

136. Bartsch DK, Langer P, Wild A, et al. Pancreaticoduodenal endocrine tumors in multiple endocrine neoplasia type 1: Surgery or surveillance? *Surgery.* 2000;128:958–966.

137. Stadil F. Treatment of gastrinomas with pancreaticoduodenectomy. In Mignon M, Jensen RT, eds. *Endocrine tumors of the pancreas: recent advances in research and management, Series: frontiers in gastrointestinal research.* Basel, Switzerland: S. Karger. 1995:333–341.

138. Imamura M, Kanda M, Takahashi K, et al. Clinicopathological characteristics of duodenal microgastrinomas. *World J Surg.* 1992;16:703–709.

139. Kato M, Imamura M, Hosotani R, et al. Curative resection of microgastrinomas based on the intraoperative secretin test. *World J Surg.* 2000;24:1425–1430.

140. Preist WM, Alexander MK. Isletcell tumour of the pancreas with peptic ulceration, diarrhoea, and hypokalaemia. *Lancet.* 1957;273:1145–1147.

141. Vermer JV, Morrison AB. Islet cell tumor and a syndrome of refractory watery diarrhea and hypokalemia. *Am J Med.* 1958;25:374–380.

142. Bloom SR, Polak JM, Pearse AG. Vasoactive intestinal peptide and watery-diarrhea syndrome. *Lancet.* 1973;2:14–16.

143. Gozes I, Furman S. Clinical endocrinology and metabolism. Potential clinical appl ications ofvasoactive intestinal peptide: a selected update. *Best Pract Res Clin Endocrinol Metab.* 2004;18:623–640.

144. Doherty GM. *Best Practice & Research Clinical Gastroenterology.* 2005;19:807–817.

145. Krejs GJ. VIPoma syndrome. *Am J Med.* 1987;82:37–48.

146. Debas HT, Mulvihill SJ. Neuroendocrine gut neoplasms. Important lessons from uncommon tumors. *Arch Surg.* 1994;129:965–971.

147. Park SK, O'Dorisio MS, O'Dorisio TM. Vasoactive intestinal polypeptide-secreting tumours: biology and therapy. *Baillieres Clin Gastroenterol.* 1996;10:673–696.

148. Mitchell CH, Sinatra FR, Crast FW, et al. Intractable watery diarrhea, ganglioneuroblastoma, and vasoactive intestinal peptide. *Journal of Pediatrics.* 1976;80:593–595.

149. Jansen-Goemans A, Engelhardt J. Intractable diarrhea in a boy with vasoactive intestinal peptide-producing ganglioneuroblastoma. *Pediatrics.* 1977;59:710–716.

150. Long RG, Bryant MG, Mitchell SJ, et al. Clinicopathological study of pancreatic and ganglioneuroblastoma tumours secreting vasoactive intestinal polypeptide (vipomas). *British Medical Journal.* 1981;282:1767–1771.

151. Said SI, Faloona GR. Elevated plasma and tissue levels of vasoactive intestinal polypeptide in the watery-diarrhea syndrome due to pancreatic, bronchogenic and other tumors. *New England Journal of Medicine.* 1975;293:155–160.

152. Watson KJR, Shulkes A, Smallwood RA, et al. Watery diarrheahypokalemia-achlorhydria syndrome and carcinoma of the esophagus. *Gastroenterology.* 1985;88:798–803.

153. Capella C, Polak JM, Buffa R, et al. Morphologic patterns and diagnostic criteria of VIPproducing endocrine tumors. *Cancer.* 1983;52:1860–1874.

154. Bloom SR, Long RJ, Bryant MG, et al. Clinical, biochemical and pathological studies on 62 vipomas. *Gastroenterology.* 1980;78:1143.

155. Iida Y, Nose O, Kai H, et al. Watery diarrhoea with a vaso-active intestinal peptide-producing ganglioneuroblastoma. *Arch Dis Child.* 1980;55:929–936.

156. Long RG. Vasoactive intestinal polypeptide-secreting tumours (vipomas) in childhood. *J Pediatr Gastroenterol Nutr.* 1983;2:122–126.

157. Kaplan SJ, Holbrook CT, McDaniel HG, et al. Vasoactive intestinal peptide secreting tumors of childhood. *Am J Dis Child.* 1980;134:21–24.

158. Soga J, Yakuwa Y. Vipoma/diarrheogenic syndrome: A statistical evaluation of 241 reported cases. *J Exp Clin Cancer Res.* 1998;17:389.

159. Matsumoto KK, Peter JB, Schultze RG. Watery diarrhea and hypokalemia associated with pancreatic islet cell adenoma. *Gastroenterology.* 1966;50:231.

160. Smith SL, Branton SA, Avino AJ, et al. Vasoactive intestinal polypeptide secreting islet cell tumors: A 15-year experience and review of the literature. *Surgery.* 1998;124:1050.

161. Verner JV, Morrison AB. Endocrine pancreatic islet disease with diarrhea. *Annals of Internal Medicine.* 1974;133:492–500.

162. O'Dorisio TM, Mekhjian HS, Gaginella TS. Medical therapy of VIPomas. Endocrinology and Metabolism *Clinics of North America.* 1989;18:545–556.

163. Jensen RT, Norton JA. Pancreatic Endocrine Tumors. In Feldman M, Friedman LS, Sleisenger MH, ed. *Sleisenger & Fordtran's Gastrointestinal and Liver Disease.* 7th ed. St. Louis, MO:WBSaunders. 2002:988–1016.

164. Jensen RT, Norton JA. Endocrine tumors of the pancreas. In Feldman M, Scharschmidt BF, Sleisenger MH, ed. *Gastrointestinal and Liver Disease.* 6th ed. Philadelphia, PA: WB Saunders: 1998:871.

165. Matuchansky C, Rambaud JC. VIPomas and endocrine cholera: Clinical presentation, diagnosis, and advances in management.

In Mignon M, Jensen RT, ed. *Endocrine Tumors of the Pancreas: Recent Advances in Research and Management*. Series: Frontiers in Gastrointestinal Research, Vol 23. Basel (Switzerland): S Karger. 1995:166–182

166. Grier JF. WDHA (watery diarrhea, hypokalemia, ahclorhydria) syndrome: clinical features, diagnosis, and treatment. *South Med J*. 1995;88:22–24.

167. Walsh JH, Mayer EA. Gastrointestinal hormones. In Sleisenger MH, Fordtran JS, ed. *Gastrointestinal Disease: Pathophysiology, diagnosis, management*. 5th ed. Philadelphia, PA: WB Saunders: 1993:18–44.

168. Wu ZC, O'Dorisio TM, Cataland S, et a1. Effects of pancreatic polypeptide and vasoactive intestinal polypeptide on rat ileal and colonic water and electrolyte transport in vivo. *Digestion Disease Science*. 1979;24:625–630.

169. Krejs GJ, Fordtran JS, Fahrenkrug J, et al. Effect of VIP infusion on water and ion transport in the human jejunum. *Gastroenterology*. 1980;78:722–727.

170. Rood RP, DeLellis RA, Dayal Y, et al. Pancreatic cholera syndrome due to a vasoactive intestinal polypeptide-producing tumor: further insights into the pathophysiology. *Gastroenterology*. 1988;94:813–818.

171. Krejs GJ, Barkley RM, ReadNW, et al. Intestinal secretion induced by vasoactive intestinal polypeptide. *Journal of Clinical Investigation*. 1978;61:1337–1345.

172. Levitan R, Ingelfinger FJ. Effect of d-aldosterone on salt and water absorption from the intact human colon. *J Clin Invest*. 1965;44:801–808

173. Hohmann EL, Levine L, Tashjian AH. Vasoactive intestinal peptide stimulates bone resorption via a cyclic adenosine 3-,5-monophosphate-dependent mechanism. *Endocrinology*. 1983; 112:1233–1239.

174. Holdaway IM, Evans MC, et al. Watery diarrhea syndrome with episodic hypercalcemia. *Aust N Z J Med*. 1977;7:63–65.

175. Cesani F, Ernst R, Walser E, et al. Tc-99m sestamibi imaging of a pancreatic VIPoma and parathyroid adenoma in a patient with multiple type I endocrine neoplasia. *Clin Nucl Med*. 1994;19:532–534.

176. Ichimura T, Kondo S, Okushiba S, et al. A calcitonin and vasoactive intestinal peptide-producing pancreatic endocrine tumor associated with the WDHA syndrome. *Int J Gastrointest Cancer*. 2003;33:99–102.

177. Rizzoli R, Sappino AP, Bonjour JP. Parathyroid hormone-related protein and hypercalcemia in pancreatic neuro-endocrine tumors. *Int J Cancer*. 1990;46:394–398.

178. Wu TJ, Lin CL, Taylor RL, et al. Increased parathyroid hormonerelated peptide in patients with hypercalcemia associated with islet cell carcinoma. *Mayo Clin Proc*. 1997;72:1111–1115.

179. Burgess JR, Wilkinson S, Lowenthal RM. Parathyroid hormone related protein (PTHrP) mediated hypercalcemia complicating enteropancreatic malignancy in multiple endocrine neoplasia type 1 (MEN 1). *Aust N Z J Med*. 2000;30:280–281.

180. Mishra BM. VIPoma. *N Engl J Med*. 2004;351:2558.

181. Go VLW, Korinek JK. Effect of vasoactive intestinal polypeptide on hepatic glucose release. In Said SI, ed. *Vasoactive Intestinal Peptide*. New York: Raven Press. 1982:231.

182. Delvalle T, Yamada T. Secretory tumors of the pancreas. In Sleisenger MH & Fortran JS, ed. *Gastrointestinal Disease: Pathophysiology, Diagnosis, Management*. 4th ed. Philadelphia, PA: WB Saunders: 1989:1884–1900.

183. Morris AI, Tumberg LA. Surreptitious laxative abuse. *Gastroenterology*. 1979;77:780–786.

184. O'Dorisio TM, Vinik AI. Pancreatic polypeptide and mixed peptide-producing tumors of the gastrointestinal tract. In: Colen S, Soloway RD, eds. *Contemporary Issues in Gastroenterology*. Edinburgh: Churchill Livingstone; 1985:117–128.

185. Schiller LR, Rivera LM, Santangelo WC, et al. Diagnostic value of fasting plasma peptide concentrations in patients with chronic diarrhea. *Dig Dis Sci*. 1994;39:2216.

186. Delcore R, Friesen SR. Gastrointestinal neuroendocrine tumors. *Journal of the American College of Surgeons*. 1994;178:187–211.

187. Krejs GJ, Walsh JH, Morawski SG, et al. Intractable diarrhea: Intestinal perfusion studies and plasma VIP concentrations in patients with pancreatic cholera syndrome and surreptitious ingestion of laxatives and diuretics. *Am J Dig Dis*. 1977;22:280–292.

188. Debas HT, Gittes G. Somatostatin analogue therapy in functioning neuroendocrine gut tumors. *Digestion*. 1993;54:68–71.

189. Ruskone A, Rene E, Chayvialle JA, et al. Effect of somatostatin on diarrhea and on small intestinal water and electrolyte transport in a patient with pancreatic cholera. *Digestion Disease Science*. 1982;27:459–466.

190. Clements D, Elias E. Regression of metastatic vipoma with somatostatin analogue SMS 201–995. *Lancet*. 1985;1:874–875.

191. Kraenzlin ME, Ch'ng JLC, Wood SM, et al. Long-term treatment of a VIPoma with somatostatin analogue resulting in remission of symptoms and possible shrinkage of metastases. *Gastroenterology*. 1985;88:185–187.

192. Dunne MJ, Elton R, Fletcher T, et al. Sandostatin and gastroenteropancreatic endocrine tumors-therapeutic characteristics. In O'Dorisio TM, ed. *Sandostatin in the Treatment of Gastroenteropancreatic Endocrine Tumors*. New York: Springer. 1989:93–114.

193. Eriksson B, Oberg K. An update of the medical treatment of malignant endocrine pancreatic tumors. *Acta Oncol*. 1993;32: 203–208.

194. Harris AG, O'Dorisio TM, Woltering EA, et al. Consensus statement: octreotide dose titration in secretory diarrhea. *Digestion Disease Science*. 1995;40:1464–1473.

195. Mekhjian HS, O'Dorisio TM. VIPoma syndrome. *Seminars in Oncology*. 1987;14:282–291.

196. Jaffe BM, Kopen DF, DeSchryver-Kecskemeti K, et al. Indomethacin-responsive pancreatic cholera. *New England Journal of Medicine*. 1977;297:817–821.

197. Albuquerque RH, Owens CW, Bloom SR. A study of vasoactive intestinal polypeptide (VIP) stimulated intestinal fluid secretion in rat and its inhibition by indomethacin. *Experientia*. 1979;35:1496–1497.

198. Pandol SJ, Korman LY, McCarthy DM, et al. Beneficial effect of oral lithium carbonate in the treatment of pancreatic cholera syndrome. *New England Journal of Medicine*. 1980;302:1403–1404.

199. McArthur KE, Anderson DS, Durbin TE, et al. Clonidine and lidamidine to inhibit watery diarrhea in a patient with lung cancer. *Ann Intern Med*. 1982;96:323–325.

200. Rao MB, O'Dorisio TM, George JM, et al. Angiotensin II and norepinephrine antagonize the secretory effect of VIP in rat ileum and colon. *Peptides*. 1984;5:291–294.

201. Field M, McCall I. Ion transport in rabbit ileal mucosa. 3. Effects of catecholamines. *Am J Physiol*. 1973;225:852–857.

202. Donowitz M, Elta G, Bloom SR, et al. Trifluoperazine reversal of secretory diarrhea in pancreatic cholera. *Annals of Internal Medicine*. 1980;93:284–285.

203. Smith PL, Field M. In vitro antisecretory effects of trifluoperazine and other neuroleptics in rabbit and human small intestine. *Gastroenterology*. 1980;78:1545–1553.

204. Van Dyk D, Inbal A, Kraus L, et al. The watery diarrhea syndrome with hypercalcemia-symptomatic response to phosphate buffer. *Hepatogastroenterology*. 1981;28:58–59.

205. Long RG, Bryant MG, Yuille PM, et al. Mixed pancreatic apudoma with symptoms of excess vasoactive intestinal polypcptide

and insulin: improvement of diarrhoea with metoclopramide. *Gut.* 1981;22:505–511.

206. Yamashiro Y, Yamamoto K, Sato M. Loperamide therapy in a child with vipoma-associated diarrhea. *Lancet.* 1982;1:1413.

207. Eriksson B, Oberg K, Alm G, et al. Treatment of malignant endocrine pancreatic tumors with human leucocyte interferon. *Lancet.* 1986;2:1307–1309.

208. Engstrom PF, Lavin PT, Moertel CG, et al. Streptozotocin plus fluorouracil vs doxorubicin therapy for metastatic carcinoid tumor. *J Clin Oncol.* 1984;2:1255–1259.

209. Moertel CG, Lavin P, Hahn G. Phase II trial doxorubicin therapy for advanced islet cell carcinoma. *Cancer Treat Rep.* 1982;66:1567–1569.

210. Moertel CG, Hanley JA, Johnson LA. Streptozotocin alone compared with streptozotocin plus fluorouracil in the treatment of advanced islet cell carcinoma. *N Engl J Med.* 1980;303:1189–1194.

211. Moertel CG, Lefkopoulo M. Lipstiz S, et al. Streptozotocin-doxorubicin, streptozotocin-fluorouracil, or chlorozotocin in the treatment of advanced islet-cell carcinoma. *N Engl J Med.* 1992;326:519–523.

212. Oberg K, Eriksson B. Medical treatment of neuroendocrine gut and pancreatic tumors. *Acta Oncol.* 1989;28:425.

213. Moertel CG, Kvols LK, O'Connell MJ, et al. Treatment of neuroendocrine carcinomas with combined etoposide and cisplatin. *Cancer.* 1991;68:227–223.

214. Wiedenmann B, Jensen RT, Mignon M, et al. Preoperative diagnosis and surgical management of neuroendocrine gastroenteropancreatic tumors: general recommendations by a consensus workshop. *World J Surg.* 1998;22:309–318.

215. Akerstrom G, Hellman P, Hessman O, et al. Surgical treatment of endocrine pancreatic tumours. *Neuroendocrinology.* 2004;80:62–66.

216. Madeira I, Terris B, Voss M, et al. Prognostic factors in patients with endocrine tumours of the duodenopancreatic area. *Gut.* 1998;43:422–427.

217. Ruszniewski P, O'Toole D. Ablative therapies for liver metastases of gastroenteropancreatic endocrine tumors. *Neuroendocrinology.* 2004;80:74–78.

218. Tepel J, Hinz S, Klomp HJ, et al. Intraoperative radiofrequency ablation (RFA) for irresectable liver malignancies. *Eur J Surg Oncol.* 2004;30:551–555.

219. Berber E, Herceg NL, Casto KJ, et al. Laparoscopic radiofrequency ablation of hepatic tumors: prospective clinical evaluation of ablation size comparing two treatment algorithms. *Surg Endosc.* 2004;18:390–396.

220. Sutcliffe R, Maguire D, Ramage J, et al. Management of neuroendocrine liver metastases. *Am J Surg.* 2004;187:39–46.

221. Henn AR, Levine EA, McNulty W, et al. Percutaneous radiofrequency ablation of hepatic metastases for symptomatic relief of neuroendocrine syndromes. *Am J Roentgenol.* 2003;181:1005–1010.

222. Gulec SA, Mountcastle TS, Frey D, et al. Cytoreductive surgery in patients with advanced-stage carcinoid tumors. *Am Surg.* 2002;68:667–671.

223. Berber E, Flesher N, Siperstein AE. Laparoscopic radiofrequency ablation of neuroendocrine liver metastases. *World J Surg.* 2002;26:985–990.

224. Chung MH, Pisegna J, Spirt M, et al. Hepatic cytoreduction followed by a novel long-acting somatostatin analog: a paradigm for intractable neuroendocrine tumors metastatic to the liver. *Surgery.* 2001;130:954–962.

225. Polak JM, Bloom SR. Somatostatin localization in tissues. *Scand J Gastroenterol.* 1986;119:11–21.

226. Larsson LI, Hirsch MA, Holst JJ, et al. Pancreatic somatostatinoma. Clinical features and physiological implications. *Lancet.* 1977;1:666–668.

227. Dayal Y, Ganda O. Somatostatin-producing tumors. In: Dayal Y, ed. *Endocrine Pathology of the Gut and Pancreas.* Boca Raton: CRC Press. 1991:241–277.

228. Soga J, Yakuwa Y. Somatostatinoma/inhibitory syndrome: a statistical evaluation of 173 reported cases as compared to other pancreatic endocrinomas. *J Exp Clin Cancer Res.* 1999;18: 13–22.

229. Mao C, Shah A, Hanson DJ, et al. Von Recklinghausen's disease associated with duodenal somatostatinoma: contrast of duodenal versus pancreatic somatostatinomas. *J Surg Oncol.* 1995;59:67–73.

230. Kelly TR. Somatostatinoma. *Probl Gen Surg.* 1994;11:99–119.

231. Harris GJ, Tio F, Cruz A. Somatostatinoma: a case report and review of the literature. *J Surg Oncol.* 1987;36:8-16.

232. Tanaka S, Yamasaki S, Matsushita H, et al. Duodenal somatostatinoma: A case report and review of 31 cases with special reference to the relationship between tumor size and metastasis. *Pathology International.* 2000;50:146.

233. Scully RE, Mark EJ, McNeely WF, et al. Case records of the Massachusetts General Hospital. *N Engl J Med.* 1989;320:996–1004.

234. Krejs GJ, Orci L, Conlon JM, et al. Somatostatinoma syndrome. Biochemical, morphologic and clinical features. *N Engl J Med.* 1979;301:285–292.

235. Mozell E, Stenzel P, Woltering E, et al. Functional endocrine tumors of the pancreas: clinical presentation, diagnosis and treatment. *Curr Probl Surg.* 1990;27:303–386.

236. Anene C, Thompson JS, Saigh J, et al. Somatostatinoma: atypical presentation of a rare pancreatic tumor. *Am J Gastroenterol.* 1995;90:819–821.

237. Lamberts SW, Vanderlely AJ, Herder WW, et al. Octreotide. *N Eng J Med.* 1996;334:246–254.

238. Öberg K, Eriksson B. Endocrine tumors of the pancreas. *Best Practice & Research Clinical Gastroenterology.* 2005;19:753–781.

239. Dayal Y, Tallberg KA, Nunnemacher G, et al. Duodenal carcinoids in patients with and without neurofibromatosis. *Am J Surg Pathol.* 1986;10:348–357.

240. O-Brien TD, Chejfec G, Prinz RA. Clinical features of duodenal somatostatinomas. *Surgery.* 1993;114:1144–1147.

241. Taccagni GL, Carlucci M, Sironi M, et al. Duodenal somatostatinoma with psammona bodies: an immunohistochemical and ultrastructural study. *Am J Gastroenterol.* 1986;81:33–37.

242. Farr CM, Prince HM, Bezmalinovic Z. Duodenal somatostatinoma with congenital pseudoarthrosis. *J Clin Gastroenterol.* 1991;13:195–197.

243. Hough DR, Chan A, Davidson H. Von Recklinghausen's disease associated with gastrointestinal carcinoid tumors. *Cancer.* 1983;51:2206–2208.

244. Lee HY, Garber PE. Von Reckinghausen's disease associated with pheochromocytoma and carcinoid tumor. *Ohio State Med J.* 1970;66:583–586.

245. Griffiths DFR, Williams GT, Williams ED. Duodenal carcinoid tumors, phaeochromocytoma and neurofibromatosis: islet cell tumor, phaeochromocytoma and the von Hippel-Lindau complex: two distinctive neuroenocrine syndromes. *Q J Med.* 1987;64:769–82.

246. Wheeler M, Curley IR, Williams ED. The association of neurofibromatosis, pheochromocytoma and somatostatin-rich duodenal carcinoid tumor. *Surgery.* 1986;100:1163–1168.

247. Fuller CE, Williams GT. Gastrointestinal manifestations of type I neurofibromatosis (von Recklinghausen's disease). *Histopathology.* 1991;19:1–11.

248. Vinik AI, Stodel WE, Echauser FE, et al. Somatostatinomas, PPomas, neurotensinomas. *Semin Oncol.* 1987;14:263–281.

249. Boden G, Shimoyama R. Somatostatinoma. In: Cohen S, Soloway RD, ed. *Hormone producing tumors of the gastrointestinal tract*. New York: Churchill Livingstone. 1985:194.

250. Tjon A, Tham RT, Jansen JB, et al. Imaging features of somatostatinoma: MR, CT, US and angiography. *J Comput Assist Tomogr*. 1994;18:427–431

251. Soga J, Yakuwa Y. Somatostatinoma/inhibitory syndrome: a statistical evaluation of 173 reported cases as compared to other pancreatic endocrinomas. *J Exp Clin Cancer Res*. 1999;18: 13–22.

252. Green BT, Rockey DC. Duodenal somatostatinoma presenting with complete somatostatinoma syndrome. *J Clin Gastroenterol*. 2001;33:415–417

253. Angeletti S, Corleto VO, Schillaci O, et al. Use of the somatostatin analogue octreotide to localise and manage somatostatinproducing tumors. *Gut*. 1998;42:792–794.

254. Morrison H. Contributions to the microscopic anatomy of the pancreas by Paul Langerhans (Berlin, 1869). *Bull Hist Med*. 1937;5:259–297.

255. Banting FG, Best CH. The internal secretion of the pancreas. *J Lab Clin Med*. 1922;7:251–266.

256. "BookRags Biography on Paul Langerhans." 1 August 2006. http://www.bookrags.com/biography/paul-langerhanswob/index.html.

257. Edis AJ, McIlrath DC, van Heerden JA, et al. Insulinoma–current diagnosis and surgical management. *Curr Probl Surg*. 1976;13:1–45.

258. Tucker ON, Crotty PL, Conlon KC. The management of insulinoma. *Br J Surg*. 2006;93:264–275.

259. Wilder RM, Allan FM, Power MH, et al. Carcinoma of the islands of the pancreas: hyperinsulinism and hypoglycemia. *JAMA*. 1927;89:348–355.

260. Geoghegan JG, Jackson JE, Lewis MP, et al. Localization and surgical management of insulinoma. *Br J Surg*. 1994;81:1025–1028.

261. Service FJ, McMahon MM, O'Brien PC, et al. Functioning insulinoma-incidence, recurrence, and long-term survival of patients: a 60-year study. *Mayo Clin Proc*. 1991;66:711–719.

262. Marx SJ, Agarwal SK, Kester MB, et al. Multiple endocrine neoplasia type 1: clinical and genetic features of the hereditary endocrine neoplasias. *Recent Prog Horm Res*. 1999;54:397–438.

263. Jaroszewski DE, Schlinkert RT, Thompson GB, et al. Laparoscopic localization and resection of insulinomas. *Arch Surg*. 2004;139:270–274.

264. Graves TD, Gandhi S, Smith SJ, et al. Misdiagnosis of seizure: insulinoma presenting as adult-onset seizure disorder. *J Neurol Neurosurg Psychiatry*. 2004;75:1091–1092.

265. Marks V, Teale JD. Hypoglycemic disorders. *Clin Lab Med*. 2001;21:79–97.

266. Service FJ, Natt N. The prolonged fast. *J Clin Endocrinol Metab*. 2000;85:3973–3974.

267. Thompson NW. The surgical treatment of islet cell tumors of the pancreas. T L Dent, editor. In *Pancreatic Disease*, New York: Grune & Stratton. 1981:461.

268. Ramage JK, Davies AH, Ardill J, et al. Guidelines for the management of gastroenteropancreatic neuroendocrine (including carcinoid) tumours. *Gut*. 2005;54:1–16.

269. Hashimoto LA, Walsh RM. Preoperative localization of insulinomas is not necessary. *J Am Coll Surg*. 1999;189:4.

270. Norton JA, Shawker TH, Doppman JL, et al. Localization and surgical treatment of occult insulinomas. *Ann Surg*. 1990;212:615–620.

271. Machado MC, da Cunha JE, Jukemura J, et al. Insulinoma: diagnostic strategies and surgical treatment. A 22-year experience. *Hepatogastroenterology*. 2001;48:854–858.

272. Galiber AK, Reading CC, Charboneau JW, et al. Localization of pancreatic insulinoma: comparison of pre- and intraoperative US with CT and angiography. *Radiology*. 1988;166:405–408.

273. Gorman B, Charboneau JW, James EM, et al. Benign pancreatic insulinoma: preoperative and intraoperative sonographic localization. *AJR Am J Roentgenol*. 1986;147:929–934.

274. McLean AM, Fairclough PD. Endoscopic ultrasound in the localisation of pancreatic islet cell tumours. *Best Pract Res Clin Endocrinol Metab*. 2005;19:177–193.

275. Fritscher-Ravens A, Izbicki JR, Sriram PV, et al. Endosonographyguided, fine-needle aspiration cytology extending the indication for organ-preserving pancreatic surgery. *Am J Gastroenterol*. 2000;95:2255–2260.

276. Kasono K, Hyodo T, Suminaga Y, et al. Contrast-enhanced endoscopic ultrasonography improves the preoperative localization of insulinomas. *Endocr J*. 2002;49:517–522.

277. Gress FG, Barawi M, Kim D, et al. Preoperative localization of a neuroendocrine tumor of the pancreas with EUS-guided fine needle tattooing. *Gastrointest Endosc*. 2002;55:594–597.

278. Doppman JL, Chang R, Fraker DL, et al. Localization of insulinomas to regions of the pancreas by intra-arterial stimulation with calcium. *Ann Intern Med*. 1995;123:269–273.

279. Roche A, Raisonnier A, Gillon-Savouret MC. Pancreatic venous sampling and arteriography in localizing insulinomas and gastrinomas: procedure and results in 55 cases. *Radiology*. 1982;145:621–627.

280. Gouya H, Vignaux O, Augui J, et al. CT, endoscopic sonography, and a combined protocol for preoperative evaluation of pancreatic insulinomas. *AJR Am J Roentgenol*. 2003;181:987–992.

281. Lo CY, Chan FL, Tam SC, et al. Value of intra-arterial calcium stimulated venous sampling for regionalization of pancreatic insulinomas. *Surgery*. 2000;128:903–909.

282. Owen NJ, Sohaib SA, Peppercorn PD, et al. MRI of pancreatic neuroendocrine tumours. *Br J Radiol*. 2001;74:968–973.

283. Hamoud AK, Khan MF, Aboalmaali N, et al. Mangan-enhanced MR imaging for the detection and localisation of small pancreatic insulinoma. *Eur Radiol*. 2004;14:923–925.

284. Orlefors H, Sundin A, Garske U, et al. Whole-body 11C-5- hydroxytryptophan positron emission tomography as a universal imaging technique for neuroendocrine tumors: comparison with somatostatin receptor scintigraphy and computed tomography. *J Clin Endocrinol Metab*. 2005;90:3392–3400.

285. Warner RR, O'dorisio TM. Radiolabeled peptides in diagnosis and tumor imaging: clinical overview. *Semin Nucl Med*. 2002;32:79–83.

286. van der Lely AJ, de Herder WW, Krenning EP, et al. Octreoscan radioreceptor imaging. *Endocrine*. 2003;20:307–311.

287. Virgolini I, Traub-Weidinger T, Decristoforo C. Nuclear medicine in the detection and management of pancreatic islet-cell tumours. *Best Pract Res Clin Endocrinol Metab*. 2005;19:213–227.

288. Hiramoto JS, Feldstein VA, LaBerge JM, et al. Intraoperative ultrasound and preoperative localization detects all occult insulinomas. *Arch Surg*. 2001;136:1020–1026.

289. Yamao K, Okubo K, Sawaka A, et al. Endoluminal ultrasonography in the diagnosis of pancreatic diseases. *Abdom Imaging*. 2003;28:545–555.

290. Bozbora A, Barbaros U, Erbil Y, et al. Is laparoscopic enucleation the gold standard in selected cases with insulinoma? *J Laparoendosc Adv Surg Tech A*. 2004;14:230–233.

291. Mabrut JY, Fernandez-Cruz L, Azagra JS, et al. Laparoscopic pancreatic resection: results of a multicenter European study of 127 patients. *Surgery*. 2005;137:597–605.

292. Kano N, Kusanagi H, Yamada S, et al. Laparoscopic pancreatic surgery: its indications and techniques: from the viewpoint of

limiting the indications. *J Hepatobiliary Pancreat Surg.* 2002;9: 555–558.

293. Doherty GM, Doppman JL, Shawker TH, et al. Results of a prospective strategy to diagnose, localize, and resect insulinomas. *Surgery.* 1991;110:989–996.

294. Huai JC, ZhangW, Niu H, et al. Localization and surgical treatment of pancreatic insulinomas guided by intraoperative ultrasound. *Am J Surg.* 1998;175:18–21.

295. Hirshberg B, Libutti SK, Alexander HR, et al. Blind distal pancreatectomy for occult insulinoma, an inadvisable procedure. *J Am Coll Surg.* 2002;194:761–764.

296. Carneiro DM, Levi JU, Irvin GL III. Rapid insulin assay for intraoperative confirmation of complete resection of insulinomas. *Surgery.* 2002;132:937–942.

297. O'Riordain DS, O'Brien T, van Heerden JA, et al. Surgical management of insulinoma associated with multiple endocrine neoplasia type I. *World J Surg.* 1994;18:488–493.

298. Danforth DN Jr, Gorden P, Brennan MF. Metastatic insulinsecreting carcinoma of the pancreas: clinical course and the role of surgery. *Surgery.* 1984;96:1027–1037.

299. Thompson GB, van Heerden JA, Grant CS, et al. Islet cell carcinomas of the pancreas: a twenty-year experience. *Surgery.* 1988;104:1011–1017.

300. Sarmiento JM, Que FG. Hepatic surgery for metastases from neuroendocrine tumors. *Surg Oncol Clin N Am.* 2003;12:231–242.

301. Brentjens R, Saltz L. Islet cell tumors of the pancreas: the medical oncologist's perspective. *Surg Clin North Am.* 2001;81:527–542.

302. Bajetta E, Ferrari L, Procopio G, et al. Efficacy of a chemotherapy combination for the treatment of metastatic neuroendocrine tumours. *Ann Oncol.* 2002;13:614–621.

303. Kress O,Wagner HJ,Wied M, et al. Transarterial chemoembolization of advanced liver metastases of neuroendocrine tumors - a retrospective single-center analysis. *Digestion.* 2003;68:94–101.

304. Mavligit GM, Pollock RE, Evans HL, et al. Durable hepatic tumor regression after arterial chemoembolization-infusion in patients with islet cell carcinoma of the pancreas metastatic to the liver. *Cancer.* 1993;72:375–380.

305. Perry RR, Vinik AI. Clinical review 72: diagnosis and management of functioning islet cell tumors. *J Clin Endocrinol Metab.* 1995;80:2273–2278.

306. Gill GV, Rauf O, MacFarlane IA. Diazoxide treatment for insulinoma: a national UK survey. *Postgrad Med J.* 1997;73:640–641.

307. Ulbrecht JS, Schmeltz R, Aarons JH, et al. Insulinoma in a 94-year-old woman: long-term therapy with verapamil. *Diabetes Care.* 1986;9:186–188.

308. Becker SW, Kahn D, Rothman S, et al. Cutaneous manifestations of internal malignant tumors. *Arch Dermatol.* 1942;45:1069–1080.

309. McGavran MH, Unger RH, Recant L, et al. A glucagon-secreting alpha-cell carcinoma of the pancreas. *N Engl J Med.* 1966;274: 1408–1413.

310. Mallinson CN, Bloom SR, Warin AP, et al. A glucagonoma syndrome. *Lancet.* 1974;2:1–5.

311. Wilkinson DS. Necrolytic migratory erythema with carcinoma of the pancreas. Transactions of the St John's Hospital Dermatological Society 1973;59:244–250.

312. Binnick AN, Spencer SK, Dennison WL, Jr., et al. Glucagonoma syndrome. Report of two cases and literature review. *Arch Dermatol.* 1977;113:749–754.

313. Chastain MA. The glucagonoma syndrome: a review of its features and discussion of new perspectives. *American Journal of the Medical Sciences.* 2001;321:306–320.

314. Grimelius L, Wilander E. Silver stains in the study of endocrine cells of the gut and pancreas. *Invest Cell Pathol.* 1980;3:3–12.

315. Norton JA. Neuroendocrine tumors of the pancreas and duodenum. *Curr Probl Surg.* 1994;31:77.

316. Simon P. Endocrine tumors of the pancreas. *Endocrinol Metab Clin North Am.* 2006;35:431–447.

317. Boden G. Glucagonomas and insulinomas. *Gastroenterol Clin North Am.* 1989;18:831.

318. Leichter SB. Clinical and metabolic aspects of glucagonoma. *Medicine.* 1980;59:100.

319. Stacpoole PW. The glucagonoma syndrome: Clinical features, diagnosis, and treatment. *Endocr Rev.* 1981;2:347.

320. Unger RH, Orci L. Glucagon and the A Cell. Physiology and pathophysiology. *N Engl J Med.* 1981;304:1575.

321. Conlon JM. The glucagon-like polypeptides - order out of chaos? *Diabetologia.* 1980;18:85–88.

322. Wermers RA, Fatourechi V, Wynne AG, et al. The glucagonoma syndrome. Clinical and pathologic features in 21 patients. *Medicine.* 1996;75:53–63.

323. Nightingale KJ, Davies MG, Kingsnorth AN, et al. Glucagonoma syndrome: survival 24 years following diagnosis. *Digestive Surgery.* 1999;16:68–71.

324. Norton J, Kahan C, Schiebinger R, et al. Acid deficiency and the skin rash associated with glucconoma. *Ann Intern Med.* 1979;91:213.

325. Higgins GA, Recant L, Fischman AB. The glucagonoma syndrome: surgically curable diabetes. *Am J Surg.* 1979;137:142–148.

326. Haneke E. Acquired zinc deficiency mimicking glucagonoma dermatitis. Histology and electron microscopy. *Zeitschrift fur Hautkrankheiten.* 1984;59:902–908.

327. Hoitsma HF, Cuesta MA, Starink TM, et al. Zinc deficiency syndrome versus glucagonoma syndrome. *Archivum Chirurgicum Neerlandicum.* 1979;31:131–140.

328. Hendricks WM. Pellagra and pellagra like dermatoses: etiology, differential diagnosis, dermatopathology, and treatment. *Semin Dermatol.* 1991;10:282–292.

329. Stacpoole PW. The glucagonoma syndrome: clinical features, diagnosis, and treatment. Endocrine Reviews. 1981;2:347–361.

330. Holst JJ. Glucagon-producing tumors. In: Cohen S. Soloway D, eds. *Hormone producing tumors of the gastrointestinal tract.* New York: Churchill Livingstone, 1985:57.

331. Guilarte Lopez-Manas J, Bellot GV, Fernandez PR, et al. Pancreatic glucagonoma and deep vein thrombosis. *Gastroenterol Hepat.* 1998;21:483–485.

332. Vinik A. Glucagonoma syndrome. Endotext.com. 2002.

333. El Rassi Z, Partensky C, Valette PJ, et al. Necrolytic migratory erythema, first symptom of a malignant glucagonoma: treatment by long-acting somatostatin and surgical resection. Report of three cases. *Eur J Surg Oncol.* 1998;24:562–567.

334. Montenegro F, Lawrence GD, Macon W, et al. Metastatic glucagonoma. improvement after surgical debulking. *Am J Surg.* 1980;139:424–427.

335. Thompson NW, Eckhauser FE. Malignant islet-cell tumors of the pancreas. *World J Surg.* 1984;8:940–951.

336. Ajani JA, Kavanaugh J, Patt Y. Roferon and doxorubicin combination active against advanced islet cell or carcinoid tumors. *Proc Am Assoc Cancer Res.* 1989;30:293.

337. Khandekar JD, Oyer D, Miller HJ, et al. Neurologic involvement in glucagonoma syndrome: response to combination chemotherapy with 5-fluorouracil and streptozotocin. *Cancer.* 1979;44:2014–2016.

338. Marlink RG, Lokich JJ, Robins JR, et al. Hepatic arterial embolization for metastatic hormone-secreting tumors. Technique, effectiveness, and complications. *Cancer.* 1990;65:2227–2232.

339. Kessinger A, Foley JF, Lemon HM. Therapy of malignant APUD cell tumors. Effectiveness of DTIC. *Cancer.* 1983;51:790–794.

340. Broder LE, Carter SK. Pancreatic islet cell carcinoma. II. Results of therapy with streptozotocin in 52 patients. *Ann Intern Med.* 1973;79:108–118.

341. Moertel C, Hanley J, Johnson L. Streptozotocin alone compared with streptoxocin plus fluoracil in the treatment of advanced islet-cell carcinoma. *N Engl J Med.* 1980;303:1189.

342. Murray-Lyon I, Eddleston A, Williams R. Treatment of multiple hormone producing malignant islet cell tumour with streptozotocin. *Lancet.* 1968;2:895.

343. Schein P, Kahn R, Gorden P, et al. Streptozotocin for malignant insulinomas and carcinoid tumors. *Arch Intern Med.* 1973;132:555.

344. Friesen SR. Update on the diagnosis and treatment of rare neuroendocrine tumors. *S Surg Clin North Am.* 1987;67:379–393.

COMMENTARY
Edward M. Wolin

Neuroendocrine tumors of the gastrointestinal tract are difficult and confusing tumors to diagnose, particularly in early stages. They are often discovered as incidental findings at operations for other reasons. Thus, carcinoid tumors of the appendix typically are found incidentally at the time of surgery for a clinical diagnosis of acute appendicitis. Otherwise, a high percentage of carcinoid tumors are diagnosed quite late in the course of the disease, particularly when the lesion arises in the pancreas or small bowel. Small bowel carcinoid tumors are particularly hard to diagnose at an early stage because of difficulty in visualizing the small bowel radiographically and endoscopically, and the vagueness of early symptoms. Intermittent abdominal pain associated with partial small bowel obstruction on the basis of direct tumor growth or on the basis of kinking of the small bowel secondary to fibrosis of the mesentery is often mistaken for "irritable bowel syndrome" or other nonspecific conditions. Consequently, the tumor may be present for many years before the proper diagnosis is established. In more advanced cases, the intestinal blood supply can be interrupted by the tumor, leading to ischemia or bowel infarction; or patients may present with intussusception, requiring emergency surgery before a preoperative diagnosis can be established.

Although distal small-bowel carcinoid tumors can sometimes be seen on colonoscopy or small-bowel contrast radiologic studies, the newer techniques of wireless capsule enteroscopy, double-balloon push enteroscopy, or computed tomographic virtual enterography are far more sensitive in making a diagnosis and, therefore, these techniques offer the best chance of diagnosing small bowel carcinoid tumors pre-operatively.

As a result of delayed diagnosis, midgut carcinoid tumors often present with metastatic disease, particularly in the liver, and thus may be associated with the carcinoid syndrome. Eventually approximately 90% of patients with the syndrome will develop flushing and over 80% will develop diarrhea. Over 80% of patients presenting with carcinoid syndrome will prove to have a primary tumor of midgut origin, most commonly arising in distal ileum, with liver metastasis already present at diagnosis.

The carcinoid syndrome usually can be diagnosed on the basis of appropriate diagnostic tests on blood and urine. However, the diagnostic tests used to identify the carcinoid syndrome must be selected and interpreted with great care, as misdiagnosis based on misinterpretation of laboratory tests is common. By the time the diagnosis is made, many patients will have already developed severe manifestations of the carcinoid syndrome associated with extensive liver metastases, including dehydration from severe watery diarrhea, intense flushing, severe malaise, and sometimes impaired cardiac valvular function.

Chromogranin A in the blood will be elevated in approximately 90% of individuals with carcinoid syndrome. When this test is combined with measurements of urinary 5-hydroxyindoleacetic acid (5-HIAA) and blood serotonin, virtually all patients with the syndrome will be detected. However, there are many causes for misinterpretation of the chromogranin A test. Elevated values may be associated with a variety of nonmalignant conditions, such as achlorhydria causing hypergastrinemia (in association with atrophic gastritis, pernicious anemia, proton pump inhibitor therapy, and retained gastric antrum), decreased renal or hepatic function, inflammatory bowel disease, physical stress, and trauma.

However, an elevated level of chromogranin A in conjunction with another specific neuroendocrine marker strongly supports the diagnosis of a neuroendocrine tumor. In a carcinoid tumor, an elevation of chromogranin A would be observed in conjunction with increased levels of blood serotonin or urinary-HIAA. In a gastrinoma, chromogranin A would be increased in conjunction with an elevated gastrin level. In an insulinoma, elevated chromogranin A occurs in association with an increased level of serum insulin. Nonfunctioning neuroendocrine tumors can be diagnosed most accurately if chromogranin A elevation is associated with another neuroendocrine marker of a nonspecific type. Examples of such nonspecific neuroendocrine markers are pancreatic polypeptide, neuron-specific enolase, or alpha/beta subunits of human chorionic gonadotropin.

It should be noted that if a carcinoid tumor is suspected, and the chromogranin A is normal, measurement of pancreastatin is a valuable marker. Pancreastatin is a peptide that is split off the chromogranin molecule, and can be elevated in cases in which the chromogranin A is not elevated.

5-HIAA is a major metabolite of serotonin and is normally increased in the urine of patients with carcinoid syndrome. However, misinterpretation of the urinary 5-HIAA test is a frequent occurrence. Elevated levels of urinary 5-HIAA may result from consumption of high serotonin-containing foods, such as bananas, pineapple products, tomato products, plums, eggplant, avocado, kiwi, and some other types of fruits and nuts. Similarly, elevations of urinary 5-HIAA may be associated with a variety of medications, including cough medications, antihistamines, phenothiazines, antihypertensive medications, benzodiazepines, acetaminophen, muscle relaxants, and monoamine oxidase inhibitors. Therefore, when a urinary 5-HIAA test is ordered, it is important that patients refrain from offending foods and medications for several days prior to obtaining this test.

Octreotide scanning is particularly valuable in diagnosing neuroendocrine tumors; it is positive in over 80% of individuals with carcinoid disease. However, this test also is frequently misinterpreted. The liver is the single most common site of metastasis for midgut neuroendocrine tumors; however, it is exceedingly difficult to distinguish between normal liver and metastatic disease in the liver on scans obtained within the first 2 days after radionuclide injection. Unfortunately, in most institutions scans are rarely appropriately obtained more than 2 days after injection, thereby leading to false-negative results. Thus, liver metastases, which would be easily seen on 7-day delayed scans, or 3-day single photon emission computed tomography (SPECT) scans, are missed on the scans obtained at 2 days.

It should be noted that false-positive octreotide scans also are common. False-positivity can be seen in association with a normal gallbladder, breast, or accessory spleen, and also in connection with recent surgery; recent radiation therapy; recent cerebrovascular accident; autoimmune disease, such as rheumatoid arthritis or lupus; granulomatous disease, such as sarcoid, tuberculosis, or Crohn disease; and occasionally with other types of tumors. Therefore, positive octreotide scans are not entirely specific for neuroendocrine tumors. It should be noted that when a suspected neuroendocrine tumor is not seen on octreotide scanning, there may be a role for positron emission tomography (PET) scanning with radioactively labeled amine precursors. PET scanning used for tumor detection in general oncology is done with ^{18}F-fluoro-deoxy-glucose (FDG). However, this test is usually negative in neuroendocrine or carcinoid tumors, which have a low proliferative rate and low rate of glucose metabolism. However, PET scanning with 11C-5-HTP (hydroxytryptophan) or ^{18}F-DOPA is becoming more generally available, and can detect carcinoid tumors as small as a few millimeters in size.

Intense flushing of the face, neck, and upper body is a hallmark of the carcinoid syndrome. This is most commonly seen with serotonin-producing tumors of the small bowel that are metastatic to liver. However, other types of neuroendocrine tumors can cause flushing syndromes, which can be confused with the carcinoid syndrome. In medullary carcinoma of the thyroid, increased levels of calcitonin can produce intense flushing as can increased levels of catecholamines associated with pheochromocytoma, increased levels of vasoactive intestinal polypeptide associated with VIPoma, and increased levels of neurotensin associated with neurotensinoma of the pancreas. In addition, there are many nonmalignant causes of flushing that can be confused with the flushing of metastatic carcinoid tumor. Flushing can occur as a result of alcohol ingestion, particularly in Asian individuals, and when chlorpropamide is used to treat diabetes mellitus. Other medications that commonly result in flushing include vasodilators such as nitroglycerin, calcium channel blockers, narcotics, amyl and butyl nitrite, cholinergic drugs, and nicotinic acid, among other types of medications. Flushing can result from spicy or sour foods, thermally hot foods, or foods containing nitrites or sulfites. Flushing also can be seen in systemic mastocytosis, menopausal hot flashes, autonomic neuropathy, epilepsy, and anxiety states.

A hallmark of the carcinoid syndrome is profuse watery diarrhea. However, the diarrhea of carcinoid syndrome is often confused with other causes of diarrhea, particularly in patients who have short-gut syndrome as a result of prior bowel resection for primary carcinoid tumor. The diarrhea of the carcinoid syndrome is of the secretory type. In this case, the stool volume is typically >1 L/day. In addition, the diarrhea persists with fasting and when the patient is on intravenous fluids. There is no osmotic gap when stool osmolality is measured.

SUGGESTED READING

Alexander HR Jr, Jensen RT. Pancreatic neuroendocrine tumors. In: DeVita VT Jr, Hellman S, Rosenberg SA, eds. *Cancer: Principles and Practice of Oncology.* Vol 2. 7th ed. Philadelphia: Lippincott, Williams & Wilkins; 2005:1540–1558.

Delcore R, Friesen SR. Gastrointestinal neuroendocrine tumors. *J Am Coll Surg.* 1994;178:187–211.

Vinik A, Perry R. Diffuse hormonal systems and endocrine tumor syndromes. In: Vinik A, ed. Ch 1-13. Endotext.com, medtext.com inc.2004. http://www.endotext.org/guthormones/index/htm. Accessed

Warner RR. Enteroendocrine tumors other than carcinoid: a review of clinically significant advances. *Gastroenterology.* 2005;128:1668–1684.

Warner, RR, O'Dorisio TM. Radiolabeled peptides in diagnosis and tumor imaging: overview. *Semin Nucl Med.* 2002;32:79–83.

43

Gastrointestinal Stromal Tumors

Anthony B. Elkhouiery and David I. Quinn

In the space of the less than decade, a diagnosis of gastrointestinal stromal tumor (GIST) has undergone metaphorical transformation from a nihilistic slow, writhing, clinical death sentence punctuated by gastrointestinal hemorrhage to a disease in which targeted cancer control provides improved quality of life and extended survival for a large proportion of patients and cure for some. Management of this disease is now predicated on a detailed understanding of its unique molecular pathobiology that has led to a pathognomonic immunohistochemical diagnostic test and systemic therapy with a small molecule inhibitor of the kinase product of the c-Kit mutation, imatinib. Early studies of imatinib used targeted therapy with functional imaging in the form of fluorodeoxyglucose (FDG) positron emission tomography (PET) and a novel large-scale randomized phase 2 design that delivered a drug from laboratory concept to patients in record time. Subsequently, therapeutic challenges relate to the integration of surgery into the management of GIST patients and therapy for patients refractory to imatinib. A further group of agents that target a series of other molecules important in the pathogenesis and progression of GIST has activity for patients refractory to imatinib. This group of drugs that target tyrosine kinases of the vascular endothelial receptor, platelet-derived growth factor receptor, and other receptors includes as their first members sunitinib and sorafenib. This chapter will describe the remarkable recent transformation in our understanding of the pathobiology of GIST, which delivered two targeted classes of therapeutics to patients previously orphaned by their diagnosis.

GIST is a relatively new diagnostic entity that is now recognized as the most common mesenchymal tumor of the gastrointestinal tract. Recent historical landmarks in the science and therapy of GIST are summarized in Table 43.1. The age-adjusted annual incidence of GIST was probably between 5 and 15 cases per million in the United States in 2002, although given changing recognition patterns for the condition this may be an underestimate (1). Similar incidence figures are available from Iceland, West Sweden, and the Netherlands (2–4). Surveillance, Epidemiology, and End Results (SEER) and State of Florida data confirm a median age at diagnosis of 63 years and an approximate twofold increase in incidence for African Americans over white Americans (1). These same cohort data suggest that survival has improved with the introduction of imatinib (1). Extrapolation from these data allows an estimate of 5,000 new GIST cases in the United States per year.

The expression of CD117 and other c-Kit alterations has permitted the classification of GIST as a distinct entity (5–7). GIST derives from the enteromotility or "interstitial cells" of Cajal. These cells differentiate and migrate from the notochord to the perialimentary stroma and are responsible for the regulation of gut peristalsis (8,9). Preservation of several genetic elements from the interstitial cells of Cajal into GIST, including CD34, KIT, and smooth muscle myosin heavy chain, provide further evidence for the origin of GIST in these cells (10). Hereditary disposition to GIST has been described as an autosomal dominant pattern in association with germ line gain of function missense or point mutations in the KIT gene and a clinical pattern that may include multiple GISTs, interstitial cell of Cajal hyperplasia, lentigines, melanoma, and angioleiomyoma (11,12). Other reports link familial GIST to Carney's triad and neurofibromatosis type 1 (13–15).

NATURAL HISTORY OF GASTROINTESTINAL STROMAL TUMORS

GISTs have been classically described as smooth muscle sarcomas derived from the pericolonic stromal tissue. GISTs are distributed throughout the gastrointestinal tract, but in most large historical series approximately 60% occur in the stomach, 30% in the small intestine, and 10% elsewhere (5). These tumors may be composed of predominantly spindle (70%) or epithelioid cells (30%) (5). Differentiation within the GIST may occur focally to have myoid, neural, ganglial, or other tissue components. They characteristically grow slowly and have a propensity to produce intermittent bowel obstruction and to periodically outgrow their tenuous and fragile blood supply with resultant infarction and secondary, often significant, hemorrhage. The bleeding is resistant to traditional medical measures but may respond to arterial embolization. A pre-imatinib Swedish population-based study found that 69% of patients presented with clinical symptoms, 21% of the cases were found incidentally at surgery, and 10% were found at autopsy (4).

Response to traditional therapeutic modalities such as radiation therapy and cytotoxic regimens used in soft-tissue sarcomas is rare and transient. Responses to standard soft-tissue sarcoma regimens are reported in <5% of patients with GIST (16,17). Surgical resection remains the principal treatment of primary GIST and currently is the only therapy offering a potential hope for cure. Surgery may also provide significant palliation for a proportion of patients (18). In a series of 200 patients seen at Memorial Sloan Kettering Cancer Center in New York over 16 years in the pre-imatinib era, 46% were localized at diagnosis, 47% had evidence of metastases, and 7% presented with isolated

Table 43.1

Summarized Recent History of Gastrointestinal Stromal Cell Tumors (GISTs)

Year	Event	Ref. No.
1998	"Gain of function" mutations in KIT identified in GIST	63
2000	Phase 1 study of imatinib suggests activity in GIST	64
2001	Phase 2 trial shows major activity for imatinib in GIST but not other soft-tissue sarcomas	36
2001	US FDA approves imatinib for treatment of GIST	65
2002	Randomized phase 2 trial of 400 vs. 600 mg of imatinib daily reports response in >50% of 147 patients accrued	32
2003	Exon-specific mutation of KIT defines response rate	33
2003	Early FDG-PET response is predictive of later RECIST response and 1-year progression-free survival	52
2006	US FDA approves sunitinib for imatinib-refractory GIST	66
2006	Exon-specific mutation of KIT may predict differential response to imatinib or sunitinib with potential for molecular-based therapy selection	44,67
2009	Nilotinib demonstrates activity in GISTs resistant to imatinib and sunitinib	68
2009	Adjuvant imatinib for 1 year after resection for localized GISTs improves RFS (p <0.0001)	69

FDA, Food and Drug Administration; FDG-PET, fluorodeoxyglucose positron emission tomography; RECIST, response evaluation criteria in solid tumors.

local recurrence after prior excision (19). The actuarial 5-year survival for the 80 patients able to undergo complete resection of gross disease was 54%. Survival was predicted by tumor size but not by the presence of positive pathologic margins or the primary site of origin within the gastrointestinal tract (19,20). However, patients with tumors originating in the small bowel appear more likely to present with metastases, especially to the liver, as are patients whose tumors have more mitoses per high-powered microscopic field (21).

Several groups have examined clinicopathologic features such tumor size, mitotic rate, proliferation index, presence of necrosis, and invasion of mucosa or adjacent structures as predictors of outcome in small cohorts and concluded these to be predictive or prognostic (22). Several population-based studies support the use of some of these factors, particularly size and mitotic rate, in defining GIST as high or low risk based on tumor related death (4).

KIT AND CD117

GISTs are characterized by mutations in the protooncogene KIT that lead to constitutive activation of its tyrosine kinase activity (23,24), and CD117 protein expression is reported in 85% of GISTs (25). Interestingly, specific mutations of the KIT gene have not always been associated with the expression of its protein product, CD117 (23). KIT belongs to the type III receptor tyrosine kinase (RTK) subfamily, whose members include platelet-derived growth factor receptors α and β (PDGFRα and PDGFRβ). All type III RTKs contain five immunoglobulin-like domains in their extracellular ligand-binding region followed by a single transmembrane domain and a cytoplasmic tyrosine kinase domain interrupted by a large kinase insert. The ligand of KIT is known as stem cell factor. As for other RTKs, stem cell factor induces dimerization of KIT followed by transautophospho-

rylation of the cytoplasmic tyrosine kinase domain, leading to activation of multiple signaling pathways, such as the PI3K/AKT and mitogen-activated protein kinase pathways but seemingly not c-Jun N-terminal kinase, or STAT pathways (26).

Collaborative research centered at the Dana Farber Cancer Center, Oregon Health and Sciences Campus, and in Finland has defined the role of specific molecule abnormalities in GIST and similar other tumors. The development of CD117 immunohistochemical staining in tumor tissue allowed the entity of GIST to be distinguished from other tumors, particularly retroperitoneal leiomyosarcoma (27). Several other immunohistochemical markers are often expressed in GIST such CD34 and alpha smooth muscle actin. The frequency of expression of these markers varies depending in the site of origin of the GIST within the gastrointestinal tract (27). Desmin is rarely expressed in GIST. These characteristics further help distinguish GIST from leiomyomata, which are typically negative for CD117 and CD34 but positive for SMA and desmin. Gastrointestinal schwannomas are typically negative for CD117 but positive for S100, which is only rarely expressed in GIST of small bowel origin.

Several other tumors can express CD117, such as melanoma and extraskeletal Ewing sarcoma, but these tend to be morphologically distinct from GIST. In addition, very focal CD117 staining can be seen in retroperitoneal leiomyosarcomas and liposarcomas (27). Several studies demonstrate a very consistent molecular signature for GIST compared with other spindle cell tumors (24). Recently, a cell surface molecule of unknown function called DOG1 has been identified in 97.8% of GIST and very few other tumors of similar morphology (28), while protein kinase C theta is reported to be present in almost all GIST (29). Whether DOG1 or protein kinase C theta will have further diagnostic, therapeutic, or clinical utility remains to be seen. In terms of distinguishing clinical features, GISTs tend to metastasize to liver or peritoneum, whereas leiomyosarcomata tend to metastasize to lung. In addition, GIST expresses higher median levels of P-glycoprotein and multidrug resistance protein 1 than leiomyosarcomata (20).

Targeted Therapeutics

Imatinib

Imatinib (formerly STI571; Gleevec in the United States and Glivec in Europe; Novartis Pharma, Basel, Switzerland) inhibits phosphorylation of the c-Kit product in GIST and analogous molecules in other conditions, the bcr/abl kinase product of the t9;22 transformation in chronic myeloid leukemia and of PDGFRβ mutation in dermatofibrosarcoma protuberans (30,31). This effect on signal transduction at the cell membrane translates to a series of intracellular regulators of cell proliferation, apoptosis such as Akt and mitogen-activated protein kinase. In a study of 127 patients with GIST treated with imatinib on a phase 2 trial, 88.2% had activating mutation of KIT and 4.7% had activating mutations of PDGFRα (32,33). Response was predicted based on the presence of exon-specific mutations in the KIT gene. Patients with tumors harboring exon 11 KIT mutations had a response rate of 83.5% compared with response rates of 47.8% in those with exon 9 mutations ($p = 0.0006$).

Patients with no detectable KIT or PDGFRα mutation demonstrated no response to imatinib ($p < 0.0001$ compared with any KIT mutation). Patients with exon 11 KIT mutations also had longer progression-free survival times than other patients (33). Further follow-up and larger assembled cohort will allow these factors to be better dissected in the future (13). Subsequent work has shed light on the mechanism of acquired resistance to imatinib, in which the development of secondary mutations in exon 17 of KIT characterized 46% of tumors in such patients in one series (34), and may predict outcome in response to sunitinib (Table 43.2). Response to imatinib is associated with a variety of pathologic changes including necrosis, cystic and myxoid change, extensive or patchy hypocellularity, and foci of residual viable tumor (35).

In GIST patients, accrued to the first phase 2 trial of imatinib undertaken by the European Organisation for Research and Treatment of Cancer (EORTC), the response rates in 27 patients were 4% complete remission, 67% partial remission, 18% stable disease, and 11% progression, while 73% of GIST patients are free from progression at 1 year (36). No responses were seen in patients with soft-tissue sarcoma treated with imatinib who had a median time to progression of 58 days. In a subsequent larger

Table 43.2

Molecular Markers of Predictive or Prognostic Importance in Gastrointestinal Stromal Cell Tumors (GISTs)

Molecule	Effect	Ref. No.
KIT exon 9 mutant	Increased risk of progression and death on imatinib compared with exon 11 mutants. Decreased in risk of progression with higher imatinib dosing	33,67,70
	Better PFS ($p = 0.0007$) and OS ($p = 0.005$) to sunitinib therapy after failing imatinib compared with exon 11 mutants	44
KIT exon 11 mutant	Worse outcome in pre-imatinib series of GIST	70,74
	Better response to first-line imatinib compared to exon 9 mutants and nonmutants	33,67
	Poorer outcome with sunitinib therapy after imatinib failure than patients with exon 9 or no mutations	44
Absence of KIT or PDGFRα mutation	Increased risk of progression and death on imatinib compared with exon 11 mutants	33,67,70
"Secondary" KIT mutations developing on imatinib therapy	Partial response or stable disease in 65% of patients with exon 13 or 14 mutations vs. 9% with 17 or 18 exon mutations treated with second-line sunitinib ($p = 0.006$)	44, see also 34
Platelet-derived growth factor alpha	D842V at codon 842 in exon 18 is associated with imatinib resistance	60
p16^{INK4A}	p16^{INK4A} loss in 50% of GIST. Loss of p16^{INK4A} predicts poorer survival ($p = 0.012$) and is independently prognostic	75, see also 76 and 77
PTEN	Decreased PTEN expressed may be associated with poorer survival	78
Bcl-2	Increased expression of Bcl-2 associated with a better outcome in patients treated with imatinib	79
Telomerase	Increased telomerase is associated with increased size, proliferative rate, and risk of death	80
Microsatellite DNA alterations: LOH	Poorer OS with increasing LOH ($p = 0.013$). LOH on chromosome 17 particularly detrimental ($p < 0.001$)	81

PFS, progression-free survival; OS, overall survival; LOH, loss of heterozygosity.

United States/Finish experience with 147 patients where patients were randomized to either 400 or 600 milligrams of imatinib per day, 53.7% had a partial response while 27.9% were stable and 4.8% could not be assessed (32). 13.6% of these patients demonstrated early drug resistance with progressive disease. There was no difference in outcome based on dose received although the study was not powered to detect a difference between the two doses prescribed.

A subsequent report on an EORTC, Italian Sarcoma Group, and Australasian Gastrointestinal Trials Group (AGTG)-led phase 3 trial in which 946 patients were randomized to imatinib 400 or 800 mg/day showed no difference in response between the two doses (37). However, there was an increase in progression-free survival in the higher dose group, with progression in 56% of patients on the lower dose compared with 50% on 400 mg twice daily ($p = 0.026$) (37). The American randomized phase II study of imatinib 400 mg vs. 600 mg per day revealed very similar response rates. PFS and overall survival for the two dose levels (38). Similarly, the results of the North American phase III trial support a starting dose for imatinib of 400 mg per day with dose escalation at disease progression depending on patient tolerance (39).

A further issue of clinical importance is whether increasing the dose of imatinib above 400 mg/day may be beneficial based on clinical scenarios such as development of resistance or based on molecular profile. To test the hypothesis that increase in dose from 400 to 800 mg/day might counteract resistance, patients in the EORTC/AGTG phase 3 trial previously described, who were treated with the lower dose and then progressed were offered dose escalation (37,40). One hundred thirty-three patients progressed and were crossed over to the higher dose. Incremental side effects included anemia and fatigue, but 51% were maintained on the increased dose without need for dose reduction (40). The median time to further progression was relatively short at 81 days, with 2% of patients experiencing a partial response and 27% stable disease. However, 18.1% were progression-free at 1 year after cross-over, suggesting that a proportion of patients who progress on the standard lower dose may benefit from dose escalation (40).

Adverse effects associated with imatinib administration are listed in Table 43.3.

Sunitinib

Approximately 12% of GIST patients will be primarily refractory to imatinib and at least 50% of patients will have progressed on this therapy by 2 years. Because the multitargeted tyrosine kinase inhibitor, sunitinib, had demonstrated activity against GIST in phase 1 evaluations (41,42), a phase 3 trial was designed in which 312 patients with advanced GIST, who were either resistant or intolerant to imatinib, were randomized in a ratio of 2:1 to receive sunitinib or placebo with a defined primary end point of progression-free survival (43). Progression-free survival was 24.1 weeks for patients taking sunitinib compared with 6.0 weeks for placebo (hazard ratio, 0.33; $p <0.001$). When results became available, the trial was unblinded and patients taking the placebo were offered sunitinib.

In a study examining the relationship between tumor kinase genotypes and sunitinib clinical activity in patients with

Table 43.3

Adverse Effects Described in Patients with Gastrointestinal Stromal Cell Tumors Who Were Treated in Clinical Trials with Imatinib or Sunitinib[a]

Adverse Effects	Percentage Reported	
	Imatinib	Sunitinib
Edema, periorbital	74.1–84	0
Nausea	52.4–57	31
Vomiting	NR	24
Diarrhea	44.9	40
Myalgia	39.5	NR
Fatigue	34.7–76	42
Rash/skin discoloration	30.6–69	30
Headache	25.9	13
Anemia	92	26
Neutropenia	47	53
Thrombocytopenia		38
Abdominal pain	25.9	33
Gastrointestinal or intra-abdominal hemorrhage	5	3
Decreased left ventricular ejection fraction	NR	10

NR, not reported.
[a]Data derived from references 32, 36, and 71. Other important reported effects from imatinib include exacerbation or induction of hypothyroidism and hypophosphatemia with diminished bone remodeling (72,73).

metastatic imatinib-resistant GIST, 97 such patients were treated with this agent. The partial response rate for GISTs with primary *KIT* exon 9 mutations was 37%, versus 5% for *KIT* exon 11 mutations ($p = 0.003$). Progression-free survival and overall survival were significantly longer for patients with either a primary *KIT* exon 9 mutation or wild type *KIT/PDGFRA* compared with patients with a *KIT* exon 11 mutation (exon 9 vs. 11: progression-free survival, $p = 0.0007$, and overall survival, $p = 0.005$; wild type vs. exon 11: progression-free survival, $p = 0.03$, and overall survival, $p = 0.01$) (44). Hence, the response parameters at a molecular level for sunitinib are inverse to those that predict response to imatinib. Whether the presence of either exon 9 or exon 11 *KIT* mutations in individual tumors should be used to direct first-line therapy to either imatinib for exon 11 mutants and sunitinib for exon 9 mutants is the subject of current study.

The side effects of sunitinib are listed in Table 43.3.

New Kinase Inhibitors

A range of drugs is currently being evaluated for imatinib-resistant disease in GIST. These include sorafenib, nilotinib, and dasatinib (45,46). Sorafenib, a multikinase inhibitor of cell proliferation and angiogenesis, is being studied in a phase 2 trial (NCT000265798) in patients with imatinib- and sunitinib-resistant GISTs.

Nilotinib has 20 times the potency of imatinib as an ABL kinase inhibitor. Dasatinib is a small-molecule, adenosine triphosphate-competitive inhibitor of SRC and ABL tyrosine kinases with the potential to inhibit KIT kinase activity independent of mutation type (47). Src kinase acts downstream from several RTKs, meaning that its inhibition may be therapeutically useful in a number of cancers. On this basis, dasatinib may have extended clinical activity in the presence of imatinib resistance (47). Clinical trials of these drugs in refractory GIST populations are underway.

Radiologic Evaluation

Radiologically, most GISTs are diagnosed by computerized tomography (CT) scanning where tumors are typically well defined, with a heterogeneous rim of soft tissue that enhances less than concurrently imaged normal liver (48). The mean diameter was 13 cm in one study (48). Central attenuation is present in two thirds of lesions prior to therapy. Coexistent ascites is rare even in the presence of peritoneal metastases (48). With imatinib treatment, GIST may display classic progression, stable disease, and partial or complete response by dimensional measurement (49). However, changes in attenuation of lesions is common with two several patterns of response: central necrosis or decreased density, focal cystic changes, calcification, and/or the development of a low attenuation rim below the peripheral surface of the tumor (49,50). Such changes occur commonly in the presence of stable disease on therapy. The development of resistance may be signaled by growth of the lesion, which is often heterogeneous and asymmetric with the development of small knobs of growing tumor with the areas of low attenuation, or by the appearance of a new nodule within a pre-existent mass (51).

Functional imaging with FDG-PET has a potential role in the staging and response evaluation for patients with GIST. In a study of 17 patients with GIST, PET scans using FDG were undertaken prior to therapy and after 8 days of imatinib therapy (52). PET response was seen in 13 patients, with 10 of these patients subsequently meeting the response evaluation criteria in solid tumors on CT scan at 8 weeks. None of the four patients without early PET response went on to have response evaluation criteria in solid tumors. Furthermore, PET response was also associated with a significantly longer progression-free survival at 1 year (92% vs. 12%; $p = 0.00107$) (52). Evidence from other groups also suggests that PET response predates CT response by many months in most cases (49,53).

Role of Surgery in the Tyrosine Kinase Inhibitor Era

There is no doubt that imatinib has resulted in a major change in the natural history of GISTs, whether given with curative or palliative intent (54). The role of imatinib in the neoadjuvant or adjuvant setting for patients judged surgically resectable is the subject of several ongoing clinical trials (55). Imatinib decreases the size of some unresectable tumors and permits resection in a significant proportion of cases (54). The Department of Surgery at Brigham and Women's Hospital and the Dana Farber Cancer Center reported on 69 patients who underwent surgery after imatinib therapy (56). Surgical resection appeared to have little impact in patients with generalized progression; however, patients with stable disease or limited progression did well, with overall 1-year survival in excess of 85%. Individuals with stable disease, limited progression, and generalized progression had no pathologic evidence of disease in 78%, 25%, and 7% of cases, respectively. Patients with limited progression were more likely to have disease progression in the subsequent year (67%) than those with stable disease preoperatively (20%) (56). This suggests that patients with stable disease may be rendered disease-free with surgery, although the current follow-up does not permit conclusions regarding durability.

Experience from Germany suggests that there may be a consolidative role for aggressive surgery in patients presenting with metastatic GIST who have had a major response to imatinib. Investigators from the University of Essen reported a series of 90 patients with metastatic GIST, in whom treatment with imatinib enabled 12 patients with mostly recurrent and extensive disease to be considered for resection of residual disease. Complete resection was achieved in 11 of these patients. However, despite significant radiologic responses, residual tumor was present in all but one of the patients, providing evidence that pathologic complete response to imatinib may be uncommon even in this setting (57). It is likely that the optimal management of patients with GIST, particularly those of gastric origin, will involve both surgery and tyrosine kinase inhibition therapy, with questions relating to the timing, duration, and sequencing of the potential multimodal treatment still to be delineated (58,59).

Molecular Factors Important in Gastrointestinal Stromal Tumors

The role of *KIT* mutations in GIST response and outcome has been discussed previously and summarized in Table 43.2. A very important issue for ongoing research and optimal selection of therapy relates to the two major patterns of *KIT* mutation seen in GIST. Although the hypothesis requires prospective testing, it appears that exon 11 mutants may respond best to imatinib at the standard dose with a relatively poor response to sunitinib as second-line therapy. In contrast, exon 9 mutants respond less well to standard-dose imatinib, but may benefit from either a high initial dose or dose escalation at progression and do well with sunitinib as second-line therapy. The role of earlier use of sunitinib and other tyrosine kinase inhibitors needs to be evaluated.

Expression of another receptor tyrosine kinase, PRGFRα, has been described in GIST with suggested implications for response to therapy. Overall, about 6% of GIST have mutations in *PRGFRα* (60). Of these, approximately two-thirds have an imatinib-resistant substitution D842V at codon 842 in exon 18 of the gene. Most of the remaining one third of patients have mutations across exons 12, 14, and 18 that do not portend a lack of response to this therapy (60). Between 4% and 10% of patients with GIST lack *KIT* expression despite being morphologically and clinically consistent with the tumor entity (21,61). These patients are more likely to have epithelioid cell histology, contain *PDGFRα* oncogenic mutations, and arise in the omentum or peritoneal surfaces (61). A proportion of patients have *KIT* or *PDGFRα* mutations suggesting sensitivity to imatinib, with the important therapeutic implication that the drug should not be withheld in *KIT* (CD117)-negative patients who otherwise fulfill diagnostic criteria (62). Other molecular factors of potential importance in GIST are summarized in Table 43.2.

CONCLUSION

GISTs are archetypal in terms of their molecular pathogenesis, pathology, and response to targeted kinase therapy. The remarkable advances made in our understanding of this entity in the last decade coupled with the translation of this knowledge into patient care represent a paradigm for other cancers and complex diseases. Despite this, the optimal therapy of GIST requires integrated assessment and management by team members that include surgeons, oncologists, and radiologists.

REFERENCES

1. Perez EA, Livingstone AS, Franceschi D, et al. Current incidence and outcomes of gastrointestinal mesenchymal tumors including gastrointestinal stromal tumors. *J Am Coll Surg.* 2006;202:623–629.
2. Tryggvason G, Gislason HG, Magnusson MK, et al. Gastrointestinal stromal tumors in Iceland, 1990-2003: the icelandic GIST study, a population-based incidence and pathologic risk stratification study. *Int J Cancer.* 2005;117:289–293.
3. Goettsch WG, Bos SD, Breekveldt-Postma N, et al. Incidence of gastrointestinal stromal tumours is underestimated: results of a nationwide study. *Eur J Cancer.* 2005;41:2868–2872.
4. Nilsson B, Bumming P, Meis-Kindblom JM, et al. Gastrointestinal stromal tumors: the incidence, prevalence, clinical course, and prognostication in the preimatinib mesylate era–a population-based study in western Sweden. *Cancer.* 2005;103:821–829.
5. Miettinen M, Sarlomo-Rikala M, Lasota J. Gastrointestinal stromal tumors: recent advances in understanding of their biology. *Hum Pathol.* 1999;30:1213–1220.
6. Rubin BP, Singer S, Tsao C, et al. KIT activation is a ubiquitous feature of gastrointestinal stromal tumors. *Cancer Res.* 2001;61:8118–8121.
7. Dorfman DM, Bui MM, Tubbs RR, et al. The CD117 immunohistochemistry tissue microarray survey for quality assurance and interlaboratory comparison: a College of American Pathologists Cell Markers Committee Study. *Arch Pathol Lab Med.* 2006;130:779–782.
8. Huizinga JD, Thuneberg L, Kluppel M, et al. W/kit gene required for interstitial cells of Cajal and for intestinal pacemaker activity. *Nature.* 1995;373:347–349.
9. Sircar K, Hewlett BR, Huizinga JD, et al. Interstitial cells of Cajal as precursors of gastrointestinal stromal tumors. *Am J Surg Pathol.* 1999;23:377–389.
10. Sakurai S, Fukasawa T, Chong JM, et al. Embryonic form of smooth muscle myosin heavy chain (SMemb/MHC-B) in gastrointestinal stromal tumor and interstitial cells of Cajal. *Am J Pathol.* 1999;154:23–28.
11. O'Riain C, Corless CL, Heinrich MC, et al. Gastrointestinal stromal tumors: insights from a new familial GIST kindred with unusual genetic and pathologic features. *Am J Surg Pathol.* 2005;29:1680–1683.
12. Li FP, Fletcher JA, Heinrich MC, et al. Familial gastrointestinal stromal tumor syndrome: phenotypic and molecular features in a kindred. *J Clin Oncol.* 2005;23:2735–2743.
13. Corless CL, Fletcher JA, Heinrich MC. Biology of gastrointestinal stromal tumors. *J Clin Oncol.* 2004;22:3813–3825.
14. Sinha R, Verma R, Kong A. Mesenteric gastrointestinal stromal tumor in a patient with neurofibromatosis. *AJR Am J Roentgenol.* 2004; 183:1844–1846.
15. Levy AD, Patel N, Abbott RM, et al. Gastrointestinal stromal tumors in patients with neurofibromatosis: imaging features with clinicopathologic correlation. *AJR Am J Roentgenol.* 2004;183:1629–1636.
16. Edmonson JH, Marks RS, Buckner JC, et al. Contrast of response to dacarbazine, mitomycin, doxorubicin, and cisplatin (DMAP) plus GM-CSF between patients with advanced malignant gastrointestinal stromal tumors and patients with other advanced leiomyosarcomas. *Cancer Invest.* 2002;20:605–612.
17. Le Cesne A, Judson I, Crowther D, et al. Randomized phase III study comparing conventional-dose doxorubicin plus ifosfamide versus high-dose doxorubicin plus ifosfamide plus recombinant human granulocyte-macrophage colony-stimulating factor in advanced soft tissue sarcomas: a trial of the European Organization for Research and Treatment of Cancer/Soft Tissue and Bone Sarcoma Group. *J Clin Oncol.* 2000;18:2676–2684.
18. Connolly EM, Gaffney E, Reynolds JV. Gastrointestinal stromal tumours. *Br J Surg.* 2003;90:1178–1186.
19. DeMatteo RP, Lewis JJ, Leung D, et al. Two hundred gastrointestinal stromal tumors: recurrence patterns and prognostic factors for survival. *Ann Surg.* 2000;231:51–58.
20. Plaat BE, Hollema H, Molenaar WM, et al. Soft tissue leiomyosarcomas and malignant gastrointestinal stromal tumors: differences in clinical outcome and expression of multidrug resistance proteins. *J Clin Oncol.* 2000;18:3211–3220.
21. Fletcher CD, Berman JJ, Corless C, et al. Diagnosis of gastrointestinal stromal tumors: a consensus approach. *Hum Pathol.* 2002;33:459–465.
22. Bucher P, Taylor S, Villiger P, et al. Are there any prognostic factors for small intestinal stromal tumors? *Am J Surg.* 2004;187:761–766.
23. Lasota J, Jasinski M, Sarlomo-Rikala M, et al. Mutations in exon 11 of c-Kit occur preferentially in malignant versus benign gastrointestinal stromal tumors and do not occur in leiomyomas or leiomyosarcomas. *Am J Pathol.* 1999;154:53–60.
24. Allander SV, Nupponen NN, Ringner M, et al. Gastrointestinal stromal tumors with KIT mutations exhibit a remarkably homogeneous gene expression profile. *Cancer Res.* 2001;61:8624–8628.
25. Sarlomo-Rikala M, Kovatich AJ, Barusevicius A, et al. CD117: a sensitive marker for gastrointestinal stromal tumors that is more specific than CD34. *Mod Pathol.* 1998;11:728–734.
26. Duensing A, Medeiros F, McConarty B, et al. Mechanisms of oncogenic KIT signal transduction in primary gastrointestinal stromal tumors (GISTs). *Oncogene.* 2004;23:3999–4006.
27. Miettinen M, Sobin LH, Sarlomo-Rikala M. Immunohistochemical spectrum of GISTs at different sites and their differential diagnosis with a reference to CD117 (KIT). *Mod Pathol.* 2000;13:1134–1142.
28. West RB, Corless CL, Chen X, et al. The novel marker, DOG1, is expressed ubiquitously in gastrointestinal stromal tumors irrespective of KIT or PDGFRA mutation status. *Am J Pathol.* 2004;165:107–113.
29. Duensing A, Joseph NE, Medeiros F, et al. Protein Kinase C theta (PKCtheta) expression and constitutive activation in gastrointestinal stromal tumors (GISTs). *Cancer Res.* 2004;64:5127–5131.
30. Frolov A, Chahwan S, Ochs M, et al. Response markers and the molecular mechanisms of action of Gleevec in gastrointestinal stromal tumors. *Mol Cancer Ther.* 2003;2:699–709.
31. McArthur GA, Demetri GD, van Oosterom A, et al. Molecular and clinical analysis of locally advanced dermatofibrosarcoma protuberans treated with imatinib: Imatinib Target Exploration Consortium Study B2225. *J Clin Oncol.* 2005;23:866–873.
32. Demetri GD, von Mehren M, Blanke CD, et al. Efficacy and safety of imatinib mesylate in advanced gastrointestinal stromal tumors. *N Engl J Med.* 2002;347:472–480.

33. Heinrich MC, Corless CL, Demetri GD, et al. Kinase mutations and imatinib response in patients with metastatic gastrointestinal stromal tumor. *J Clin Oncol.* 2003;21:4342–4349.

34. Antonescu CR, Besmer P, Guo T, et al. Acquired resistance to imatinib in gastrointestinal stromal tumor occurs through secondary gene mutation. *Clin Cancer Res.* 2005;11:4182–4190.

35. Loughrey MB, Mitchell C, Mann GB, et al. Gastrointestinal stromal tumour treated with neoadjuvant imatinib. *J Clin Pathol.* 2005;58:779–781.

36. Verweij J, van Oosterom A, Blay JY, et al. Imatinib mesylate (STI-571 Glivec, Gleevec) is an active agent for gastrointestinal stromal tumours, but does not yield responses in other soft-tissue sarcomas that are unselected for a molecular target. Results from an EORTC Soft Tissue and Bone Sarcoma Group phase II study. *Eur J Cancer.* 2003;39:2006–2011.

37. Verweij J, Casali PG, Zalcberg J, et al. Progression-free survival in gastrointestinal stromal tumours with high-dose imatinib: randomised trial. *Lancet.* 2004;364:1127–1134.

38. Blanke CD, Demetri GD, von Mehren M, et al. Long-term results from a randomized phase II trial of standard- versus higher-dose imatinib mesylate for patients with unresectable or metastatic gastrointestinal stromal tumors expressing KIT. *J Clin Oncol.* 2008;26:620–625.

39. Blanke CD, Rankin C, Demetri GD, et al. Phase III randomized, intergroup trial assessing imatinib mesylate at two dose levels in patients with unresectable or metastatic gastrointestinal stromal tumors expressing the kit receptor tyrosine kinase: S0033. *J Clin Oncol.* 2008;26:626–632.

40. Zalcberg JR, Verweij J, Casali PG, et al. Outcome of patients with advanced gastro-intestinal stromal tumours crossing over to a daily imatinib dose of 800 mg after progression on 400 mg. *Eur J Cancer.* 2005;41:1751–1757.

41. Faivre S, Delbaldo C, Vera K, et al. Safety, pharmacokinetic, and antitumor activity of SU11248, a novel oral multitarget tyrosine kinase inhibitor, in patients with cancer. *J Clin Oncol.* 2006;24:25–35.

42. Motzer RJ, Hoosen S, Bello CL, Christensen JG. Sunitinib malate for the treatment of solid tumours: a review of current clinical data. *Expert Opin Investig Drugs.* 2006;15:553–561.

43. Demetri GD, van Oosteron AT, Garrett CR, et al. Efficacy and safety of sunitinib in patients with advanced gastrointestinal stromal tumour after failure of imatinib: a randomized controlled trial. *Lancet.* 2006;368:1329–1338.

44. Heinrich MC, Maki RG, Corless CL, et al. Primary and secondary kinase genotypes correlate with the biological and clinical activity of sunitinib in imatinib-resistant gastrointestinal stromal tumor. *J Clin Oncol.* 2008;26:5352–5359.

45. Kantarjian H, Giles F, Wunderle L, et al. Nilotinib in imatinib-resistant CML and Philadelphia chromosome-positive ALL. *N Engl J Med.* 2006;354:2542–2551.

46. Talpaz M, Shah NP, Kantarjian H, et al. Dasatinib in imatinib-resistant Philadelphia chromosome-positive leukemias. *N Engl J Med.* 2006;354:2531–2541.

47. Schittenhelm MM, Shiraga S, Schroeder A, et al. Dasatinib (BMS-354825), a dual SRC/ABL kinase inhibitor, inhibits the kinase activity of wild-type, juxtamembrane, and activation loop mutant KIT isoforms associated with human malignancies. *Cancer Res.* 2006; 66:473–481.

48. Burkill GJ, Badran M, Al-Muderis O, et al. Malignant gastrointestinal stromal tumor: distribution, imaging features, and pattern of metastatic spread. *Radiology.* 2003;226:527–532.

49. Choi H, Charnsangavej C, de Castro Faria S, et al. CT evaluation of the response of gastrointestinal stromal tumors after imatinib mesylate treatment: a quantitative analysis correlated with FDG PET findings. *AJR Am J Roentgenol.* 2004;183:1619–1628.

50. Warakaulle DR, Gleeson F. MDCT appearance of gastrointestinal stromal tumors after therapy with imatinib mesylate. *AJR Am J Roentgenol.* 2006;186:510–515.

51. Shankar S, vanSonnenberg E, Desai J, et al. Gastrointestinal stromal tumor: new nodule-within-a-mass pattern of recurrence after partial response to imatinib mesylate. *Radiology.* 2005;235:892–898.

52. Stroobants S, Goeminne J, Seegers M, et al. 18FDG-Positron emission tomography for the early prediction of response in advanced soft tissue sarcoma treated with imatinib mesylate (Glivec). *Eur J Cancer.* 2003;39:2012–2020.

53. Goldstein D, Tan BS, Rossleigh M, et al. Gastrointestinal stromal tumours: correlation of F-FDG gamma camera-based coincidence positron emission tomography with CT for the assessment of treatment response: an AGITG study. *Oncology.* 2005;69:326–332.

54. Bumming P, Andersson J, Meis-Kindblom JM, et al. Neoadjuvant, adjuvant and palliative treatment of gastrointestinal stromal tumours (GIST) with imatinib: a centre-based study of 17 patients. *Br J Cancer.* 2003;89:460–464.

55. Blanke CD, Corless CL. State-of-the art therapy for gastrointestinal stromal tumors. *Cancer Invest.* 2005;23:274–280.

56. Raut CP, Posner M, Desai J, et al. Surgical management of advanced gastrointestinal stromal tumors after treatment with targeted systemic therapy using kinase inhibitors. *J Clin Oncol.* 2006;24:2325–2331.

57. Bauer S, Hartmann JT, de Wit M, et al. Resection of residual disease in patients with metastatic gastrointestinal stromal tumors responding to treatment with imatinib. *Int J Cancer.* 2005;117:316–325.

58. Wu PC, Langerman A, Ryan CW, et al. Surgical treatment of gastrointestinal stromal tumors in the imatinib (STI-571) era. *Surgery.* 2003;134:656–666.

59. Heinrich MC, Corless CL. Gastric GI stromal tumors (GISTs): the role of surgery in the era of targeted therapy. *J Surg Oncol.* 2005;90:195–207.

60. Corless CL, Schroeder A, Griffith D, et al. PDGFRA mutations in gastrointestinal stromal tumors: frequency, spectrum and in vitro sensitivity to imatinib. *J Clin Oncol.* 2005;23:5357–5364.

61. Medeiros F, Corless CL, Duensing A, et al. KIT-negative gastrointestinal stromal tumors: proof of concept and therapeutic implications. *Am J Surg Pathol.* 2004;28:889–894.

62. Bauer S, Corless CL, Heinrich MC, et al. Response to imatinib mesylate of a gastrointestinal stromal tumor with very low expression of KIT. *Cancer Chemother Pharmacol.* 2003;51:261–265.

63. Hirota S, Isozaki K, Moriyama Y, et al. Gain-of-function mutations of c-kit in human gastrointestinal stromal tumors. *Science.* 1998;279: 577–580.

64. van Oosterom AT, Judson I, Verweij J, et al. Safety and efficacy of imatinib (STI571) in metastatic gastrointestinal stromal tumours: a phase I study. *Lancet.* 2001;358:1421–1423.

65. Dagher R, Cohen M, Williams G, et al. Approval summary: imatinib mesylate in the treatment of metastatic and/or unresectable malignant gastrointestinal stromal tumors. *Clin Cancer Res.* 2002;8:3034–3038.

66. Goodman VL, Rock EP, Dagher R, et al. Approval summary: sunitinib for the treatment of imatinib refractory or intolerant gastrointestinal stromal tumors and advanced renal cell carcinoma. *Clin Cancer Res.* 2007;13:1367–1373.

67. Debiec-Rychter M, Sciot R, Le Cesne A, et al. KIT mutations and dose selection for imatinib in patients with advanced gastrointestinal stromal tumours. *Eur J Cancer.* 2006;42:1093–1103.

68. Montemurro M, Schoffski P, Reichardt P, et al. Nilotinib in the treatment of advanced gastrointestinal stromal tumours resistant to both imatinib and sunitinib. *Eur J Cancer.* 2009 May 19 [Epub ahead of print]. DOI: 10.1016/j.ejca.2009.04.030.

69. Dematteo RP, Ballman KV, Antonescu CR, et al. Adjuvant imatinib mesylate after resection of localised, primary gastrointestinal stromal tumour: a randomised, double-blind, placebo-controlled trial. *Lancet.* 2009;373:1097–1104.

70. Heinrich MC, Owzar K, Corless CL, et al. Correlation of kinase genotype and clinical outcome in the North American Intergroup Phase III Trial of imatinib mesylate for treatment of advanced gastrointestinal stromal tumor: CALGB 150105 Study by Cancer and Leukemia Group B and Southwest Oncology Group. *J Clin Oncol.* 2008;26:5360–5367.

71. Casali PG, Garrett CR, Blackstein ME, et al. Updated results from a phase III trial of sunitinib in GIST patients (pts) for whom imatinib (IM) therapy has failed due to resistance or intolerance. In: Proceedings from the American Society of Clinical Oncology; June 2-6, 2006; Atlanta, GA. Abstract 9513.

72. de Groot JW, Zonnenberg BA, Plukker JT, et al. Imatinib induces hypothyroidism in patients receiving levothyroxine. *Clin Pharmacol Ther.* 2005;78:433–438.

73. Berman E, Nicolaides M, Maki RG, et al. Altered bone and mineral metabolism in patients receiving imatinib mesylate. *N Engl J Med.* 2006;354:2006–2013.

74. Andersson J, Bumming P, Meis-Kindblom JM, et al. Gastrointestinal stromal tumors with KIT exon 11 deletions are associated with poor prognosis. *Gastroenterology.* 2006;130:1573–1581.

75. Schneider-Stock R, Boltze C, Lasota J, et al. Loss of p16 protein defines high-risk patients with gastrointestinal stromal tumors: a tissue microarray study. *Clin Cancer Res.* 2005;11(2 Pt 1):638–645.

76. Ricci R, Arena V, Castri F, et al. Role of p16/INK4a in gastrointestinal stromal tumor progression. *Am J Clin Pathol.* 2004;122:35–43.

77. Perrone F, Tamborini E, Dagrada GP, et al. 9p21 locus analysis in high-risk gastrointestinal stromal tumors characterized for c-kit and platelet-derived growth factor receptor alpha gene alterations. *Cancer.* 2005;104:159–169.

78. Ricci R, Maggiano N, Castri F, et al. Role of PTEN in gastrointestinal stromal tumor progression. *Arch Pathol Lab Med.* 2004;128:421–425.

79. Steinert DM, Oyarzo M, Wang X, et al. Expression of Bcl-2 in gastrointestinal stromal tumors: correlation with progression-free survival in 81 patients treated with imatinib mesylate. *Cancer.* 2006;106:1617–1623.

80. Sakurai S, Fukayama M, Kaizaki Y, et al. Telomerase activity in gastrointestinal stromal tumors. *Cancer.* 1998;83:2060–2066.

81. Schurr P, Wolter S, Kaifi J, et al. Microsatellite DNA alterations of gastrointestinal stromal tumors are predictive for outcome. *Clin Cancer Res.* 2006;12:5151–5157.

COMMENTARY
Chandrajit P. Raut

In the last 10 years, gastrointestinal stromal tumors (GISTs) have been the focus of considerable clinical and laboratory research. The identification of activating oncogenic mutations in genes encoding the KIT or PDGFRA receptor tyrosine kinases coupled with the development of targeted inhibitors that suppress tumor growth, imatinib mesylate (Gleevec) and sunitinib malate (Sutent), has revolutionized the management of these tumors. The advent of effective targeted therapy for GIST has altered, but not diminished, the role of surgery for this disease.

As evidence of the progress in this field, each successive review of the management of this tumor, just months after a prior summary, must update the data on trial results. In the preceding chapter, Drs. Elkhouiery and Quinn have succinctly summarized the major recent milestones in the treatment of GIST in the current era. A key message is the increasing individualization of treatment as therapies continue to advance. This commentary will focus on some of the salient features in determining the most appropriate therapy for localized and advanced disease.

PROGNOSTIC FACTORS

The current risk stratification of primary GIST is based on retrospective studies from the era prior to the regular use of tyrosine kinase inhibitors (TKIs). Three factors predictive of behavior are tumor size, mitotic count, and site of tumor origin (1,2). In general, GISTs originating in the small bowel demonstrate more aggressive behavior than those of comparable size and mitotic rate originating in the stomach. A better understanding of these prognostic factors will allow the treating clinicians to tailor the therapy for each individual patient.

THERAPY FOR LOCALIZED, RESECTABLE, PRIMARY DISEASE

Despite advances in targeted TKIs, surgery remains the principal and only potentially curative treatment for localized, resectable, primary GIST. The goal of surgery is complete macroscopic resection with an intact pseudocapsule and a negative microscopic margin (R0 resection). In general, wedge or segmental resections of the involved stomach or bowel are sufficient for primary tumors. However, anatomic considerations may require a more extensive resection to completely remove the tumor. For instance, large proximal gastric tumors may require a total gastrectomy. Nevertheless, extensive resections are only rarely required for localized, primary GIST. In a series of 140 patients with gastric GISTs, 68% underwent wedge resections, 28% underwent partial gastrectomies, and only 4% needed total gastrectomies (3). Lymphadenectomy is not indicated as lymph nodes are rarely involved.

All GISTs ≥ 2 cm in size should be resected, barring prohibitive comorbidities. Given the propensity of GISTs to recur, none of these should be considered benign (2). Management of GISTs <2 cm in size is more controversial, and the natural history of such tumors is unknown. In two recent series, microscopic GISTs (1 to 10 mm in size) were grossly detected in the proximal stomach in 22.5% of consecutive autopsies in adults older than 50 years in Germany and in 35% of 100 whole stomachs resected for gastric cancer in Japan (4,5). Yet only few of these tumors ever become clinically relevant. In the absence of sufficient data to guide therapy, management of such tumors remains undefined.

At present, microscopic gastric GISTs identified incidentally (usually on imaging or endoscopy) may be followed with serial endoscopy or imaging. Any that are symptomatic (such as those associated with hemorrhage from erosion through the mucosa) should be resected. If a tumor increases in size on serial endoscopy or imaging, it should be resected. Endoscopic resection of small gastric GISTs, although reported, cannot be recommended at this time (6). These tumors frequently involve the muscularis propria; thus, endoscopic resection risks leaving a positive peripheral margin.

Tumors between 1 and 2 cm in size pose an even more difficult management dilemma. Many centers of expertise favor resection. One could argue that with the very low risk of recurrence in patients with tumors <2 cm and a low mitotic rate, all tumors in this category may be observed. However, the mitotic rate cannot be reliably estimated on biopsy results or fine-needle aspiration cytology, and thus observation cannot be recommended based on size alone. Ultimately, the surgeon should carefully discuss the pros and cons of surgery versus observation with the individual patient. Given the higher risk of aggressive behavior in tumors originating at sites other than the stomach, none should be considered "benign" and all should be evaluated for resection.

Laparoscopic or laparoscopy-assisted resection of primary gastric GISTs may be feasible under appropriate circumstances by experienced surgeons for tumors less than 5 cm in size. The limited available supporting data confirm that when performed properly, negative margins are possible and recurrences are rare (7,8). There are no series reporting long-term outcomes with laparoscopy for resection of GISTs at other sites.

NEOADJUVANT AND ADJUVANT THERAPY FOR PRIMARY DISEASE

Although patients with resectable disease should undergo surgery, single-institution retrospective series have demonstrated that recurrence rates are still high. In patients undergoing R0 or R1 resections, 5-year overall survival (OS) rates ranged from 42% to 54% in the pre-TKI era (9-11). Consequently, investigators are evaluating TKIs for neoadjuvant or adjuvant use.

The Radiation Therapy Oncology Group (RTOG) 0312 trial is the only study to examine the use of imatinib as a neoadjuvant agent. In this study, patients with potentially resectable primary GIST measuring ≥5 cm or recurrent tumors at least 2 cm in size received 600 mg of imatinib daily for 8 to 10 weeks, underwent resection, and then received imatinib at the same dose for 2 years. This study has completed accrual, but preliminary data are not yet available.

Four trials evaluating imatinib in the adjuvant setting have completed or nearly completed accrual. The American College of Surgeons Oncology Group (ACOSOG) multicenter Z9000 trial treated patients with 400 mg of imatinib daily for 1 year after surgery for (a) tumors at least 10 cm in size, (b) tumor rupture or hemorrhage, or (c) multiple (more than five) tumors. This study has completed accrual. The primary end point is recurrence-free survival (RFS). The data are currently under analysis.

The SSG XVIII trial from the Scandinavian Sarcoma Group and the Sarcoma Group of the AIO, Germany, is an open-label study randomizing patients to 400 mg of imatinib daily for 1 year versus 3 years after resection. The eligibility criteria are (a) tumor at least 10 cm in size, (b) tumor rupture, (c) mitotic count >10 per 50 high-power fields (HPF), (d) tumor >5 cm and mitotic count >5 per 50 HPF, or (e) primary tumor presenting with synchronous liver or peritoneal metastases. This trial has nearly completed accrual. The primary end point is RFS.

The European Organisation for Research and Treatment of Cancer (EORTC) 62024 study is an open-label study randomizing patients to 400 mg of imatinib daily for 2 years or no adjuvant imatinib after surgery. The eligibility criteria are (a) tumor >5 cm in size, (b) mitotic count >10 per 50 HPF, or (c) tumor <5 cm and mitotic count of 6 to 10 per 50 HPF. This study has also nearly completed accrual. The primary end point is OS.

The results of the ACOSOG Z9001 study were recently reported (12). In this trial, patients with *KIT*-positive primary GISTs at least 3 cm in size were randomized to either 400 mg of imatinib daily or placebo for 1 year after R0/R1 resection. The trial was closed early after planned interim analysis identified significant improvement in RFS in the experimental arm. There was no difference in OS. Future trials should address the optimal duration of adjuvant therapy with imatinib.

The success of TKI therapy should not change the approach to surgery. Despite the early results of the Z9001 trial, the availability of imatinib and sunitinib does not release surgeons from their responsibility in performing an appropriate, oncologically sound operation for resectable, localized primary GIST. However, as the factors predictive of recurrence become increasingly more apparent, sarcoma specialists will be able to determine which patients are likely to benefit from adjuvant therapy after an R0/R1 resection in an effort to reduce the high recurrence rates.

MANAGEMENT OF ADVANCED (UNRESECTABLE OR METASTATIC) DISEASE

Medical Management

Prior to the advent of TKI therapy, the treatment options for patients with metastatic GIST were limited. The tumors are resistant to radiation therapy and fewer than 5% respond to chemotherapy. Surgery is palliative at best.

Presently, a patient with unresectable or metastatic disease should receive imatinib dosed at 400 mg daily as the first line of therapy (13). When unequivocal progression is observed, the dose may be escalated up to 800 mg daily, although the side effects may become more pronounced. Alternatively, the patient may be switched to sunitinib at 37.5 mg daily (13).

In their chapter, Drs. Elkhouiery and Quinn noted that response to imatinib was predicted based on the presence of specific *KIT* exon mutations. In the near future, selection of TKI and dose will likely depend on the specific mutation noted. For instance, patients with *KIT* exon 9 mutations may either start with either imatinib 800 mg daily or sunitinib rather than lower-dose imatinib (14,15). However, such customized therapy based on genotyping needs further validation before it can be widely recommended.

Patients experiencing disease progression when receiving sunitinib should be referred to centers specializing in the management of sarcomas, where protocol therapy may be available. Newer TKIs under investigation in the management of GIST include nilotinib, dasatinib, and AMG 706 (16). Additional targets are also being evaluated. Inhibitors of mTOR and the molecular chaperone HSP90 are under study (16).

Surgery for Advanced Disease after TKI Therapy

In the post-imatinib era, the philosophy on the role of surgery in the management of advanced GIST has begun to change. The majority of patients with advanced GIST experience a partial response or stable disease on TKI therapy. Although >80% of treated patients respond to imatinib, tumors still remain viable and <5% experience pathologic complete responses (17,18). Those who respond to imatinib develop secondary resistance to the drug after a median of 2 years of therapy (19). When drug resistance develops, disease progression may be either limited or generalized (20). Limited disease progression refers to progression at one site of tumor, with other tumor deposits showing continued response to TKI. Generalized disease progression describes progression at more than one site. Experience with sunitinib is more limited, but again drug resistance develops after initial response, leading to disease progression (21).

The effectiveness of TKI therapy provided an opportunity to reconsider options for surgery with cytoreductive rather than palliative intent. Recently, six institutions reported their rates of progression-free survival and OS after surgery in patients with advanced GIST treated with TKI therapy (20,22–26). The definition of resectability is determined by the surgeon, and surgery is commonly extensive. In our institution's experience, liver resections were required in nearly 40% of such cytoreductive operations, and >60% included peritonectomy and/or omentectomy (20). Bowel resections were common, and >60% of patients underwent multivisceral resections (20). Aggressive, complex gastrointestinal operations, including total gastrectomy, pancreaticoduodenectomy, combined abdominoperineal resection of the rectum, and hepatic lobectomy were occasionally necessary to remove all visible disease. The ability to remove all macroscopic disease and the rates of progression-free survival and OS were greatest in patients demonstrating ongoing response to TKI therapy (20). On the other hand, those with generalized progression appeared to derive the least benefit from elective surgery. Thus, it is important to carefully select which patients with advanced disease are offered surgery.

After cytoreductive surgery, patients should resume TKI therapy. Failure to resume imatinib or sunitinib after surgery may lead to rapid recurrence of disease. In a report from Poland, the first five patients undergoing surgery did not restart imatinib, and four of those patients developed recurrent disease (26). The next 19 patients resumed imatinib, and only 1 developed recurrence. An unresolved issue is the length of time to continue TKI therapy postoperatively.

It is crucial to understand that although surgery is feasible, there is still no evidence that outcomes are superior or even equal to those who continue on TKI therapy without surgery. This can only be answered in a randomized clinic trial; such trials are under development in both the United States and Europe.

CONCLUSION

Surgery remains the primary and only potentially curative therapy for GIST. The development of the effective TKIs imatinib and sunitinib has altered the prognosis of metastatic disease. Use of imatinib as a neoadjuvant and adjuvant agent remains an area of active investigation. Surgery may be considered in select patients with advanced GIST on TKI therapy. However, there is no evidence establishing the superiority of surgery plus TKI therapy over TKI therapy alone for advanced disease. As our knowledge of this rare sarcoma improves, we will be able to provide very specific treatment details and indications for neoadjuvant and/or adjuvant therapy in those with localized, resectable primary disease, selection and dosing of targeted agent in those with advanced disease, and surgical therapy for those with advanced disease. As Drs. Elkhouiery and Quinn concluded, the increasing complexity in the management of GISTs requires multidisciplinary management, and affected individuals should be referred to experienced centers.

REFERENCES

1. Fletcher CD, Berman JJ, Corless C, et al. Diagnosis of gastrointestinal stromal tumors: A consensus approach. *Hum Pathol.* 2002;33:459–65.
2. Miettinen M, Lasota J. Gastrointestinal stromal tumors: pathology and prognosis at different sites. *Semin Diagn Pathol.* 2006;23:70–83.
3. Fujimoto Y, Nakanishi Y, Yoshimura K, et al. Clinicopathologic study of primary malignant gastrointestinal stromal tumor of the stomach, with special reference to prognostic factors: analysis of results in 140 surgically resected patients. *Gastric Cancer.* 2003;6:39–48.
4. Agaimy A, Wunsch PH, Hofstaedter F, et al. Minute gastric sclerosing stromal tumors (GIST tumorlets) are common in adults and frequently show c-KIT mutations. *Am J Surg Pathol.* 2007;31:113–120.
5. Kawanowa K, Sakuma Y, Sakurai S, et al. High incidence of microscopic gastrointestinal stromal tumors in the stomach. *Hum Pathol.* 2006;37:1527–1535.
6. Davila RE, Faigel DO. GI stromal tumors. *Gastrointest Endosc.* 2003;58:80–88.
7. Novitsky YW, Kercher KW, Sing RF, et al. Long-term outcomes of laparoscopic resection of gastric gastrointestinal stromal tumors. *Ann Surg.* 2006;243:738–747.
8. Otani Y, Furukawa T, Yoshida M, et al. Operative indications for relatively small (2-5 cm) gastrointestinal stromal tumor of the stomach based on analysis of 60 operated cases. *Surgery.* 2006;139:484–492.
9. Crosby JA, Catton CN, Davis A, et al. Malignant gastrointestinal stromal tumors of the small intestine: a review of 50 cases from a prospective database. *Ann Surg Oncol.* 2001;8:50–59.
10. DeMatteo RP, Lewis JJ, Leung D, et al. Two hundred gastrointestinal stromal tumors: recurrence patterns and prognostic factors for survival. *Ann Surg.* 2000;231:51–58.
11. Pierie JP, Choudry U, Muzikansky A, et al. The effect of surgery and grade on outcome of gastrointestinal stromal tumors. *Arch Surg.* 2001;136:383–389.
12. DeMatteo R, Owzar K, Maki R, et al. Adjuvant imatinib mesylate increases recurrence free survival (RFS) in patients with completely localized primary gastrointestinal stromal tumor (GIST): North American Intergroup Phase III trial ACOSOG Z9001. In: Proceedings from the American Society of Clinical Oncology; Chicago, IL; June 2–5, 2007; Abstract 10079.
13. Demetri GD, Benjamin RS, Blanke CD, et al. NCCN Task Force report: management of patients with gastrointestinal stromal tumor (GIST): update of the NCCN clinical practice guidelines. *J Natl Compr Canc Netw.* 2007;5(Suppl 2):S1–29.
14. Debiec-Rychter M, Sciot R, Le Cesne A, et al. KIT mutations and dose selection for imatinib in patients with advanced gastrointestinal stromal tumours. *Eur J Cancer.* 2006;42:1093–1103.

15. Demetri GD, van Oosterom AT, Garrett CR, et al. Efficacy and safety of sunitinib in patients with advanced gastrointestinal stromal tumour after failure of imatinib: a randomised controlled trial. *Lancet.* 2006;368:1329–1338.

16. Wagner A. Treatment of advanced soft tissue sarcoma: conventional agents and promising new drugs. *J Natl Compr Canc Netw.* 2007;5:401–410.

17. Bauer S, Hartmann JT, de Wit M, et al. Resection of residual disease in patients with metastatic gastrointestinal stromal tumors responding to treatment with imatinib. *Int J Cancer.* 2005;117:316–325.

18. Scaife CL, Hunt KK, Patel SR, et al. Is there a role for surgery in patients with "unresectable" cKIT+ gastrointestinal stromal tumors treated with imatinib mesylate? *Am J Surg.* 2003;186:665–669.

19. Verweij J, Casali PG, Zalcberg J, et al. Progression-free survival in gastrointestinal stromal tumours with high-dose imatinib: randomised trial. *Lancet.* 2004;364:1127–1134.

20. Raut CP, Posner M, Desai J, et al. Surgical management of advanced gastrointestinal stromal tumors after treatment with targeted systemic therapy using kinase inhibitors. *J Clin Oncol.* 2006;24:2325–2331.

21. Heinrich MC, Corless CL, Liegl B, et al. Mechanisms of sunitinib malate resistance in gastrointestinal stromal tumors. In: Proceedings from the American Society of Clinical Oncology; Chicago, IL; June 2–5, 2007; Abstract 10006.

22. Andtbacka RH, Ng CS, Scaife CL, et al. Surgical resection of gastrointestinal stromal tumors after treatment with imatinib. *Ann Surg Oncol.* 2006.

23. Bonvalot S, Eldweny H, Pechoux CL, et al. Impact of surgery on advanced gastrointestinal stromal tumors (GIST) in the imatinib era. *Ann Surg Oncol.* 2006;13:1596–1603.

24. DeMatteo RP, Maki RG, Singer S, et al. Results of tyrosine kinase inhibitor therapy followed by surgical resection for metastatic gastrointestinal stromal tumor. *Ann Surg.* 2007;245:347–352.

25. Gronchi A, Fiore M, Miselli F, et al. Surgery of residual disease following molecular-targeted therapy with imatinib mesylate in advanced/metastatic GIST. *Ann Surg.* 2007;245:341–346.

26. Rutkowski P, Nowecki Z, Nyckowski P, et al. Surgical treatment of patients with initially inoperable and/or metastatic gastrointestinal stromal tumors (GIST) during therapy with imatinib mesylate. *J Surg Oncol.* 2006;93:304–311.

44

Small Bowel Tumors

John H. Donohue and Thomas Schnelldorfer

The small intestines comprise by far the longest segment of the gastrointestinal tract with an enormous surface area for the absorption of nutrients. The mucosal lining is constantly undergoing cell division and turnover. Despite the huge interface with intraluminal carcinogens and billions of mitoses, malignancies of the small intestine are very uncommon. The American Cancer Society (1) estimates that only 6,230 new cases of cancer of the small intestine will be diagnosed in the United States in 2009. This figure is only 2.3% of the 275,720 predicted new digestive tract cancers and 0.4% of the 1.4 million total new cancers that will occur in the United States in 2009. Approximately 1,100 Americans will die of small intestinal cancer, only 0.8% of the gastrointestinal malignancy deaths and 0.2% of all cancer-related patient deaths projected for 2009 (1).

To properly understand cancers of the small bowel, they need to be considered by their histologic type. Nearly all the malignant tumors that occur in the small intestine are of four types: adenocarcinomas, gastrointestinal stromal tumors (GISTs), lymphomas (both mucosal-associated lymphoid tumors [MALTs] and non-MALT lymphomas), and neuroendocrine cancers (almost all of which are carcinoid tumors). Because even common small bowel cancer types are rare, this chapter will be limited to these four forms of malignancies. In each instance, the etiology, presentation, diagnosis, surgical and nonsurgical treatments, and outcomes will be discussed.

ADENOCARCINOMA

Etiology

More than half of all small bowel cancers are adenocarcinomas. The distribution of adenocarcinomas is heavily skewed toward the duodenum, especially the periampullary region of the second portion of the duodenum. Bile acids are the presumed carcinogens, but the exact mechanism has not been elucidated. Patients have a higher risk of small bowel and proximal colon cancers after cholecystectomy (2), presumably because of increased exposure to bile. The lack of bile salt degradation by bacteria in the small intestines (3), in contrast to the colon, is only one factor used to explain the rarity of small bowel carcinomas compared to cancers of the large bowel. Other potential defense mechanisms for the small intestine include the following: (a) less mechanical irritation by liquid chyme compared to solid fecal matter; (b) dilution of intraluminal carcinogens by a large volume of secretions; (c) a rapid transit of fluids that limits exposure time (3); (d) rapid enterocyte turnover that minimizes carcinogen exposure to individual cells (4); (e) significantly lower numbers of bacterial flora, especially anaerobes (3); (f) mucosal microsomal enzymes, such as benzpyrene hydroxylase, which can detoxify carcinogens (5); and (g) a local immune response including high titers of secretory immunoglobulin A (6).

In most patients with small intestine adenocarcinoma, no genetic or acquired predisposition for the malignancy is apparent. An adenoma-carcinoma sequence, comparable to that seen in large intestinal cancers, has been documented. Supporting evidence for this mode of neoplastic progression includes(a) one third of small bowel adenomas contain cancer; (b) benign and malignant tumors have the same anatomic distribution (highest in the duodenum); and (c) benign tumors occur at a younger mean patient age than adenocarcinomas, while the male to female ratios are the same (7). The prevalence of specific genetic anomalies measured in small intestinal adenocarcinomas has widely varied between investigators. Many of the molecular events, primarily mutations of *Ki-ras*, *p53*, and *APC*, are the same in both sporadic colorectal and small intestine cancers (8). Abnormalities of the mismatch repair system have been detected in approximately 20% of sporadic small bowel carcinomas, a finding similar to that for colorectal cancer (9).

Well-recognized, predisposing causes for small bowel adenocarcinoma include several inherited germ line mutations and chronic inflammatory diseases. Patients with familial adenomatous polyposis (FAP, which results from germ line *APC* gene mutations) are at especially high risk of developing periampullary duodenal adenocarcinomas (10). Family members of hereditary nonpolyposis colorectal carcinoma (HNPCC, which occurs mostly as a result of mutations in the mismatch repair enzymes hMLH1 and hMSH2) develop small bowel adenocarcinomas that are evenly distributed throughout the small bowel, in contrast to those in FAP kindreds. Small bowel cancers are commonly diagnosed before colon carcinoma in HNPCC families, while the diagnosis of duodenal cancers in FAP patients usually occurs after total proctocolectomy. Both FAP and HNPCC patients have more than a 100-fold higher risk of small bowel adenocarcinoma compared to the normal population (11). The Peutz-Jeghers syndrome (affected patients have a mutation of the *LKB1* gene, the STK11 serine threonine kinase) was once thought to have no increased risk of gastrointestinal cancer. Newer data suggest patients with Peutz-Jeghers syndrome are 18 times more likely than the general population to develop a bowel malignancy (12). Most cancers arise from a hamartoma that transforms into an adenoma prior to malignant degeneration (13).

Crohn disease is the inflammatory bowel disease most often associated with small bowel adenocarcinoma. The distribution of cancers arising in patients with Crohn disease reflects the frequency of symptomatic inflammatory changes; the ileum is most often involved (~65%), followed by the jejunum (~30%). In contrast to sporadic adenocarcinomas, duodenal adenocarcinomas are uncommon with Crohn disease (14). The risk of adenocarcinoma in patients with Crohn disease seems to be more than 100 times greater than the general population. Chronic and complicated Crohn disease (fistulae, strictures, and excluded bowel loops) appear to heighten the risk of carcinoma development (15). Celiac disease (celiac sprue), the chronic intestinal inflammation caused by dietary gluten exposure, results in an increased incidence of both gastrointestinal and extraintestinal cancers. The two most common types of malignancy in sprue patients are small intestinal lymphomas and small intestinal adenocarcinomas. The calculated incidence of small bowel carcinoma in celiac disease patients is 83-fold higher than baseline. Most adenocarcinomas in sprue patients have been diagnosed in the jejunum (16,17). Rare cases of an ileal carcinoma have been reported in patients long after proctocolectomy for both chronic ulcerative colitis and FAP. Both types of pouch reconstructions (Koch and ileal pouch-anal anastomosis) (18,19) and Brooke ileostomy (20) carry the risk for this adenocarcinoma, usually with a history of chronic, severe inflammation, especially with a pouch.

Clinical Presentation and Diagnosis

Because adenocarcinomas of the small bowel cause no specific symptoms or signs, their diagnosis is frequently delayed. The most common modes of presentation are nonspecific abdominal pain, bowel obstruction, and gastrointestinal hemorrhage (more often occult than clinically apparent). These findings were present in 66%, 40%, and 24% of patients, respectively, in a recent large, single-institution review (21). Obstructive jaundice occurs frequently with periampullary duodenal adenocarcinomas. Systemic complaints, such as weight loss, malnourishment, and decreased performance status, are worrisome for advanced disease.

Because of the nonspecific presentation and rarity of small bowel cancer, the appropriate imaging of the small intestine is frequently not ordered, especially if the standard esophagogastroduodenoscopy and complete colonoscopic examinations are unrevealing. In patients with occult gastrointestinal hemorrhage or progressive symptoms of partial bowel obstruction, the diagnostic evaluation should never be considered complete until a small intestinal source has been excluded. The lack of direct access to most of the small bowel continues to make the diagnosis of small bowel tumors more problematic, but several recent technical advances have improved the diagnostic capabilities.

Carcinomas of the duodenum and proximal jejunum can be directly visualized with standard or extended upper endoscopy. This technology has the advantage of allowing a biopsy to be performed and a specific diagnosis made; whereas upper gastrointestinal radiographs with small bowel follow-through only identify a stricture or intraluminal filling defect. Some terminal ileal cancers can be detected through a patent ileocecal valve during colonoscopy.

Push or Sonde enteroscopy allows more of the proximal jejunum to be visualized and biopsied (22), but much of the small

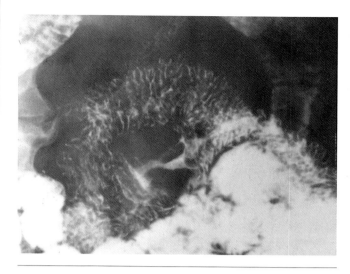

Figure 44.1 Proximal jejunal adenocarcinoma visualized on barium enterography. This demonstrates the classic "apple core" stenosis of the lumen with loss of mucosal folds within the cancer.

intestine is not accessible to currently available endoscopes. Capsule endoscopy has been increasingly used to evaluate the small intestine. Among 562 patients studied for gastrointestinal hemorrhage, capsule endoscopy determined the diagnosis in just 49% of patients, with 50 (9% of the total) having a small bowel tumor (23). At present, this technology's high cost, lack of proven sensitivity, and inability to obtain tissue specimens limits its utility.

A standard barium contrast radiographic study will detect intestinal abnormalities in up to 75% of patients, but <50% of the images will show evidence suggestive of a malignancy (Figure 44.1) (22). Enteroclysis provides a higher detection rate for malignancy (90% vs. 33%) and sensitivity (95% vs. 61%) compared to standard small bowel follow-through (24).

With finer resolution available with multidetector computed tomography (CT), primary small bowel tumors can be more readily detected by CT enterography. Water as the oral contrast plus bolus intravenous iodinated contrast are used with multidetector CT imaging to produce these pictures, which can be reconstructed in three dimensions (25).

Once a small bowel adenocarcinoma is detected by endoscopic or radiographic methods, cross-sectional imaging is performed to better stage the malignancy. CT is still the usual technique of cross-sectional imaging, although oral contrast is of limited use with an obstructing tumor. At least one study (26) has found the sensitivity, specificity, and accuracy of magnetic resonance imaging (MRI; all 95% to 100%) significantly better compared to 71% for all three measures using CT imaging in patients with a bowel obstruction (26).

Surgical Treatment

Because the most common site of metastasis for small bowel carcinomas is regional lymph nodes, appropriate surgical management includes a segmental bowel resection (with 10-cm longitudinal margins) plus excision of the adjacent mesentery. All clinically involved lymph nodes should be removed, although involvement at the base of the mesentery may prevent this. Adherent structures should be removed en bloc when the operation is performed with curative intent. Cancer of the terminal ileum requires a right colectomy.

Jejunal and ileal adenocarcinomas are generally considered separately from duodenal cancers because of different surgical treatments. For 779 jejunal and 602 ileal carcinomas entered in the National Cancer Data Base, the 5-year survival at both sites was 38% with approximately 90% having surgical treatment (curative and palliative) (27). In our institutional operative experience with jejunal and ileal adenocarcinomas, only 65% of the surgical procedures were potentially curative. Five-year survival was 36% following a curative operation and 0% with a palliative procedure (28).

Duodenal adenocarcinomas involving the periampullary region require pancreaticoduodenectomy as a curative procedure. Surgeons 30 years ago advocated a Whipple procedure for all duodenal cancers (29). However, for duodenal cancers of the distal third and fourth portions, this operation does not improve the margins of resection or the harvest of involved nodes along the superior mesenteric vessels. A segmental resection of the distal duodenum has been found to be an equally good operation for distal duodenal cancers (30,31). Resectability rates for duodenal adenocarcinomas range from 50% to 80%, and 5-year survivals of 45% to 60% in single-institution studies (30,32,33) In the National Cancer Data Base review of 1,425 duodenal adenocarcinomas, just over half had a resection and 5-year survival was 28%, a figure significantly lower than that for jejunal and ileal adenocarcinomas (27).

Nonsurgical Therapy

The low prevalence of small bowel adenocarcinomas has limited studies of nonsurgical treatments for this disease. Given similarities between small and large intestinal cancers, some investigators have tried chemotherapy regimens shown to be effective in colorectal carcinoma. Response rates of advanced small intestinal adenocarcinomas to newer drug combinations including 5-fluorouracil, leucovorin, oxaliplatin, and irinotecan should stimulate more investigation in these fields (34). Adjuvant chemoirradiation therapy has been recommended for periampullary duodenal carcinomas (35); however, in retrospective series (30,33), no survival benefit was detected for this treatment. Because no major clinical trials are in progress for this rare disease, nonsurgical treatment of small bowel adenocarcinoma will continue to be variable and empiric.

LYMPHOMA

Etiology

Most lymphomas arise from lymphoid tissues and may involve the small intestine in advanced stages of disease. In contrast, extranodal lymphomas originate in nonlymphoid organs, most commonly in the gastrointestinal tract. Primary small intestinal lymphomas occur most commonly in the ileum, less often in the jejunum, and least frequently in the duodenum. The distribution pattern parallels the amount of mucosal-associated lymphoid tissue in the small bowel (36). Classification of the

Table 44.1
Classification of Primary Gastrointestinal Non-Hodgkin Lymphomas

B-cell lymphoma
  MALT type
    Low-grade
    High-grade ± low-grade component
  IPSID
    Low-grade
    High-grade ± low-grade component
  Mantel-cell (lymphomatous polyposis)
  Burkittlike and Burkitt
  Other lymphomas corresponding to lymph node
    equivalents

T-cell lymphoma
  EATL
  Non-EATL

MALT, mucosa-associated lymphoid tissue; IPSID, immunoproliferative small intestinal disease; EATL, enteropathy-associated T-cell lymphoma.
From Isaacson PG. Gastrointestinal lymphoma. *Hum Pathol.* 1994;25:1020–1029, with permission from Elsevier.

primary gastrointestinal non-Hodgkin lymphomas is listed in Table 44.1.

The most common types of small intestinal lymphoma differ significantly by age and between different parts of the world. In the developed Western countries, higher-grade MALT lymphomas predominate in adult patients. Among children in most of the world, Burkittlike lymphomas of the ileocecal region are the most prevalent (36). In the region around the Mediterranean and to a lesser extent in other parts of Africa, Asia, and South America, immunoproliferation small intestinal disease (IPSID; also known as Mediterranean lymphoma or alpha chain disease) is the most common type of small bowel lymphoma in adults. IPSID occurs most often in young adults of lower socioeconomic classes and generally involves the jejunum first (there is diffuse intestinal infiltration in advanced disease). Patients with early IPSID may respond to broad-spectrum antibiotics; however, late-stage IPSID involves distant sites and has a poor prognosis (37). *Campylobacter jejuni* infection has been documented in the majority (5/7) of IPSID patients tested, implicating *C. jejuni* as a possible immunogenic stimulus for IPSID (38). Although a lymphoproliferative disease of the small intestinal mucosa driven by *C. jejuni* antigens that progresses to high-grade MALT that is not dependent on this stimulus has been proposed, the causative nature of *C. jejuni* in IPSID has not yet been proven (39). The similarities between IPSID and gastric MALT lymphomas caused by *Helicobacter pylori* are plentiful. An infectious cause for IPSID will likely be definitively demonstrated in the near future.

Patients with celiac disease are at significant risk for lymphoma of the small intestine, most commonly a T-cell lymphoma or enteropathy-associated T-cell lymphoma (EATL). Approximately 50% of malignancies arising in celiac patients are lymphomas, with an extraordinary 80% of small bowel origin. In the British Isles, where celiac disease is common, nearly one third of small intestinal lymphomas are EATLs (40). The prevalence of any type of lymphoma in celiac patients is >5%. This risk seems to get substantially higher in older patients who have symptomatic celiac disease (41). Patients with celiac disease have a chronic inflammatory infiltration of the small bowel mucosa. This pathology will often resolve with a gluten-free diet. If these dietary practices are started at an early age, they appear to protect celiac patients from the increased risk of EATL and other malignancies (42). When a patient with celiac sprue no longer responds to a gluten-free diet (refractory sprue) or ulcerative jejunitis develops, a benign monoclonal T-cell population is present. Molecular studies have shown these cells to be clonally identical to those found in the EATLs diagnosed at a later date (43).

Multiple lymphomatous polyposis (MLP) is a rare form of lymphoma with small intestinal involvement in most patients. The ileocecal region is most commonly involved and often a large tumor mass is present. Multiple polyps distributed from the stomach to the rectum give MLP its name. Based on the histologic, immunohistochemical, and molecular phenotypes of MLP, it has been classified as a mantle cell lymphoma of the intestine (44).

Follicular lymphoma of the small bowel is an unusual entity, whereas nodal follicular lymphoma is a common lymphoma diagnosis. This type of small bowel lymphoma usually arises in the distal ileum from a mucosal B-cell population with increased BCL-2 expression due to a translocation between chromosomes 14 and 18 (t 14:18). This is the same molecular abnormality found in nodal follicular lymphoma. Even though the histologic and surface markers of nodal and intestinal follicular lymphomas are the same, the intestinal form rarely spreads to sites distant from the primary tumor (45,46).

Patients with immunosuppression conditions, either inherited (i.e., Wiskott-Aldrich syndrome and ataxia telangiectasia) or acquired (i.e., treatment for solid organ transplantation or human immunodeficiency virus infection) (47) are also at significant risk for non-Hodgkin lymphoma. Primary extranodal lymphomas are more common in these populations than in immunocompetent patients; however, small intestinal lymphomas are rare in these higher risk populations. Primary gastrointestinal Hodgkin disease is rare (late-stage gastrointestinal involvement by nodal Hodgkin disease is not uncommon). An Epstein-Barr virus infection in patients given immunosuppressive drugs for chronic inflammatory bowel disease appears to be the lymphoproliferative stimulus for this very uncommon tumor (48).

Clinical Presentation and Diagnosis

As with other small bowel malignancies, lymphomas frequently have no specific symptoms. Abdominal pain and occult blood loss are common. A palpable mass is more common with a small bowel lymphoma than an adenocarcinoma. An acute perforation from tumor necrosis may occur, but is an infrequent presentation for intestinal lymphomas. If a patient with known celiac disease develops malabsorption despite a gluten-free diet, a lymphoma is likely present. Constitutional or B symptoms—namely weight loss, fatigue, fever, and night sweats—may occur, usually with higher grade and later stage lymphomas.

Most small intestinal lymphomas occur beyond the reach of standard endoscopy, although duodenal or proximal

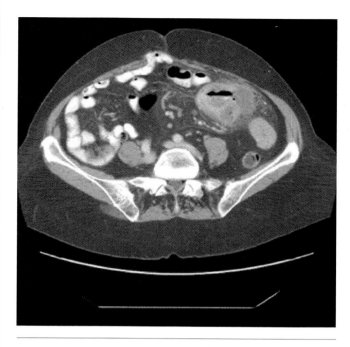

Figure 44.2 Computed tomography scan of a small intestine lymphoma demonstrating the typical findings of circumferentially thickened bowel wall and regional lymphadenopathy.

jejunal biopsies can document evidence of celiac disease or IPSID, narrowing the differential diagnosis when a palpable (or radiographic) abdominal mass is present. Gastrointestinal contrast studies may show a variable (pliable) stricture, luminal compression, or aneurysmal dilatation of the involved bowel. A CT scan or MRI showing a markedly thickened segment or segments of small bowel with marked mesenteric adenopathy is most consistent with lymphoma (Figure 44.2).

Surgical Treatment

For small intestinal lymphomas of limited extent, complete surgical resection is still generally recommended (49). Although the risk of tumor hemorrhage or perforation during chemotherapy for an intact gastrointestinal lymphoma has been given as a reason for resection in the past, these problems have been exceedingly rare during nonsurgical gastric lymphoma treatment (50). Neither controlled data nor large experiences with the nonoperative management of small intestinal lymphoma currently exist. Because surgical intervention is commonly needed to make a diagnosis, resection of the primary lymphoma will continue to be a common practice, as it should for any patient with an obstructing, bleeding, or perforated small bowel lymphoma.

Recent clinical trials involving small intestinal lymphomas have used surgical resection of all tumor, when feasible, plus combination chemotherapy (51,52). Complete clinical responses occur in up to 50% of advanced gastrointestinal lymphomas, irrespective of whether a debulking operation has been performed (53). Patients with limited-extent gastrointestinal lymphomas have the same complete response rate and survival without operative therapy, with partial tumor excision, or with complete lymphoma resection (50).

Table 44.2

Musshoff Gastrointestinal Lymphoma Staging Systems

Stage	Description
IE	GI tumor alone
IIE$_1$	GI tumor and regional nodal involvement (i.e., mesentery, celiac)
IIIE$_2$	GI tumor and extraregional subdiaphragmatic nodal involvement (para-aortic)
IIIE	GI tumor and nodal involvement on both sides of the diaphragm
IVE	GI tumor with other extranodal site(s) of involvement (i.e., bone marrow, liver)

E, extranodal; GI, gastrointestinal.
From Musshoff K. Clinical staging classification of non-Hodgkin's lymphomas [author's translation]. *Strahlentherapie.* 1977;153:218–221, with permission.

Nonsurgical Therapy

All patients with small intestinal lymphoma except those with the most limited low-grade disease should be considered for postoperative adjuvant (or primary) chemotherapy. Intermediate- and high-grade lymphomas (e.g., IPSID, MALT, Burkitt) are generally treated with CHOP (cyclophosphamide, doxorubicin, vincristine, and prednisone) chemotherapy (with or without rituximab, an anti-CD20 antibody), whereas indolent lymphomas (e.g., mantle cell, follicular) respond well to rituximab, an anti-CD20 monoclonal antibody. Intestinal T-cell lymphomas, most of which are EATLs, are not effectively treated by CHOP or its variants (54). Radiation therapy is considered for bulky tumors or advanced disease, but results in significant morbidity (55).

Lymphoma stage at presentation is the most commonly recognized prognostic factor (40,56). The Ann Arbor staging system, as modified by Musshoff (57), is most frequently used (Table 44.2). As mentioned previously, T-cell lymphomas have a worse prognosis, in large part because of their resistance to chemotherapy (40,58). Elderly patients (58,59), constitutional (B) symptoms (58), acute presentation with a perforation (40), and multifocal tumors (40,59) also predict poorer outcomes for patients with small bowel lymphomas. Five-year survival for all patients with small intestinal lymphomas treated with combination therapy ranges from 50% to 70% (60).

GASTROINTESTINAL STROMA TUMORS

Etiology

Once called leiomyomas or leiomyosarcomas, the most common mesenchymal tumor of the gastrointestinal tract is the GIST. These neoplasms are thought to arise from pacemaker cells in the bowel wall (interstitial cells of Cajal) or a pluripotential stem cell. Most GISTs express the KIT tyrosine kinase receptor (CD117) on their surface. Mutations in the *c-Kit* gene, thought to

constitutively activate the tyrosine kinase, are present in most GISTs (most involve exon 11, but also exons 9 and 13 are also mutated). These are believed to be the trigger for tumorigenesis in these neoplasms (61). Several families have been described with germ line *c-Kit* mutations that result in a 91% probability of having a GIST by age 70 and a higher risk of multiple GISTs (62). A small percentage of GIST patients have mutations in platelet-derived growth factor receptor alpha (*PDGFRA*), a Kit-related kinase gene. These mutations in exon 12 or exon 18 result in a constitutively activated PDGFRA molecule (63).

Using Surveillance, Epidemiology and End Results (SEER) data from 1992 to 2000, the yearly incidence of GISTs was 6.8 per million. There is a slight predominance of males affected by GISTs, with a mean age at diagnosis of 63 years. Although the stomach is most commonly involved site (>50%), the small intestine is the next most frequent site with 36% of cases in the database (64). Within the small bowel, the prevalence of GISTs correlates with the length of each segment; the largest number occur in the jejunum, followed by the ileum, and least often occur in the duodenum (65).

Clinical Presentation and Diagnosis

Because of their rapid growth and tumor necrosis, some GISTs are prone to significant hemorrhage. These may present as acute lower gastrointestinal (or rarely upper gastrointestinal) hemorrhage, but more commonly blood loss from GISTs is occult. GISTs commonly reach a larger size and may be easily palpated. Rapid growth, necrosis, or hemorrhage may result in nonspecific abdominal pain. A GIST may compress the bowel lumen, resulting in obstructive symptoms.

Cross-sectional imaging is of more importance in diagnosing GISTs than other small bowel tumors, as they form a distinct round or lobulated mass, usually with a large exenteric component (Figure 44.3). Hepatic and peritoneal metastases can be evaluated equally well with CT or MRI. If the diagnosis of localized GIST has been entertained, percutaneous biopsy should not be performed. This has a significant risk of causing peritoneal seeding.

Surgical Therapy

Complete tumor removal should be attempted whenever feasible. A segmental bowel resection with en bloc removal of any adherent structures is normally sufficient. A limited mesenteric resection is adequate, as GISTs, like most sarcomas, rarely metastasize to lymph nodes. Duodenal GISTs will often require a pancreaticoduodenectomy, but a less extensive operation should be adequate if all tumor is removed with clear margins. Palliative resections may be indicated for bleeding or perforation in some metastatic GIST patients. An ongoing study is assessing the benefit of neoadjuvant imatinib mesylate in reducing GIST size to allow less extensive resections.

Nonsurgical Therapy

If a complete resection of a localized GIST can be performed, the 5-year survival ranges from 50% to 65% (66). Until the introduction of the tyrosine kinase inhibitor imatinib mesylate, there was no effective therapy for metastatic or recurrent GISTs. After a trial of 147 GIST patients showed a 38% partial tumor response,

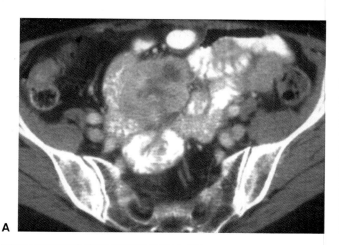
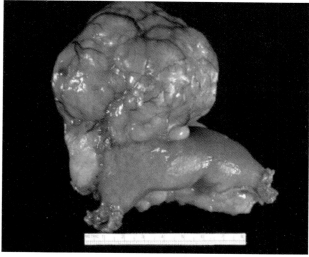

Figure 44.3 (**A**) Computed tomography scan showing a jejunal gastrointestinal stromal tumor (GIST) in the pelvis. This mass has the typical bulky exenteric component with cystic areas due to tumor necrosis. (**B**) Photograph of resected GIST specimen.

the U.S. Food and Drug Administration approved imatinib for advanced GIST treatment (67).

Since that trial, hundreds of additional patients have been treated with imatinib with a 60% to 70% tumor response rate (68). Patients with *Kit* mutations in exon 11 have a much better response rate to imatinib (84%) than those with exon 9 mutations (49%) or no *Kit* mutation (0%) (69). *PDGFRA* mutations also show different sensitivities to imatinib therapy (70). Small intestinal GISTs more commonly have exon 9 *c-Kit* mutations, whereas gastric GISTs most commonly have *c-Kit* mutations in exon 11 (71). This difference in part accounts for the worse prognosis of small bowel GISTs compared to those arising in the stomach.

Currently, imatinib treatment is recommended for metastatic GISTs and should be given as long as tolerated without tumor progression. The use of neoadjuvant and adjuvant imatinib is experimental at present (72). Most GISTs develop

resistance to imatinib by mutations that affect the interaction of the drug with the Kit molecule or bypass this mechanism of tumor inhibition (63). A new tyrosine kinase inhibitor, sunitinib malate, has already been shown effective in some imatinib-resistant GIST patients and has been approved for clinical use. Other tyrosine kinase inhibitors are in development.

The potential for recurrence of GISTs is based on tumor size and the number of mitotic figures (Table 44.3) (73). Certain *Kit* mutations also correlate with patient prognosis (74). Once metastatic disease has developed, tyrosine kinase inhibitors and selective use of tumor debulking may improve the pre-imatinib median survival of 15 months (75). Because complete response of GISTs to imatinib is rare, the long-term outlook for these patients remains bleak.

NEUROENDOCRINE TUMORS

Etiology

Carcinoid neoplasms are the most common neuroendocrine tumor of the gastrointestinal tract. The small intestine represents the most commonly affected site (43% to 45%) followed by the appendix (17% to 28%) and rectum (9% to 20%) (76,77). Carcinoids account for 27% to 44% of all small bowel tumors and are the second most common malignancy of the small intestine after adenocarcinoma (78,79). Large epidemiologic studies show an incidence of one to two cases of small bowel carcinoid tumors per 100,000 population per year, while the prevalence in autopsy series is about 8 per 100,000 population (76,77,80). This discrepancy is best explained by the asymptomatic persistence of many small bowel carcinoids. With improvements in radiographic imaging techniques, the incidence of carcinoid tumors is rising (76). Small bowel carcinoids are predominantly found in the elderly patients beyond the sixth decade without any significant race or gender predominance (76,77,78). The tumor size at clinical presentation is ≤2 cm in >70% of patients (81). Most carcinoid tumors of the small intestine are found in the ileum (75%), followed by duodenum (14%), jejunum (9%),

Table 44.3

Prognostic Index for Localized Gastrointestinal Stromal Tumors

Recurrence Risk	Size (cm)	Metastasis/50 hpf
Very low	<2	<5
Low	2–5	<5
Intermediate	<5	6–10
	5–10	<5
High	>5	>5
	>10	Any
	Any	>10

hpf, high-powered field.
Modified from Fletcher CD, Berman JJ, Corless C, et al. Diagnosis of gastrointestinal stromal tumors: a consensus approach. *Hum Pathol.* 2002;33:459–465, with permission from Elsevier.

and Meckel's diverticulum (2%) (78). Carcinoids are associated with other neoplasms in 29% of patients, with gastrointestinal cancers comprising half of these synchronous tumors plus a variety of other nongastrointestinal malignancies accounting for the other half (78,82,83). These synchronous neoplasms may be explained by the asymptomatic persistence of carcinoid tumors incidentally diagnosed during the treatment of a second symptomatic neoplasm; however, some studies document an increased incidence of metachronous noncarcinoid neoplasms (84).

Carcinoid neoplasms are neuroendocrine tumors arising from amine precursor uptake and decarboxylation (APUD) cells. In the intestine, they originate from the enterochromaffin cells in the base of the crypts of Lieberkühn. Various hormonally active polypeptides and amines are produced by gastrointestinal carcinoid tumor cells. Serotonin, the most common hormonal product, is excreted in the urine after metabolism as 5-hydroxyindole-acetic-acid (5-HIAA). Other commonly secreted hormones include kinins, histamines, and prostaglandins. The pathophysiology of enterochromaffin cell neoplastic transformation has not been identified (85). A family history of a carcinoid tumor in first-degree relatives increases the risk, but most carcinoids occur sporadically. Less than 4% of patients have a family history (86). The association of carcinoid tumors with a mismatch repair protein mutation or a *MEN-1* gene mutation has been described in a few cases (87,88).

Clinical Presentation and Diagnosis

Most small bowel carcinoid neoplasms are diagnosed incidentally at the time of operation for other abdominal disorders. When symptoms occur, they are frequently due to the desmoplastic reaction surrounding the tumor. The mechanism of this peritumoral fibrosis is poorly understood (89). Vague abdominal pain occurs in about 70% of patients. Peritumoral fibrosis can compromise the luminal patency; intestinal obstruction is a presenting symptom in 50% of patients. Less commonly, obstruction results from tumor growth or an intussusception. Rarely, carcinoid patients present with gastrointestinal bleeding or a palpable abdominal mass (90,91).

Carcinoid syndrome occurs in about 20% of patients (92). It is characterized by flushing, predominantly of the face, neck, and upper chest, plus diarrhea. Less common presentations of carcinoid syndrome include pulmonary wheezing and right heart fibrous endocardial thickening resulting in valvular dysfunction. A rare manifestation of small bowel carcinoid tumors is carcinoid-related scleroderma (93). Carcinoid syndrome can be triggered by serotonin-rich foods and stress factors like exercise. Because hepatic monoamine oxidases thoroughly metabolize hormone secretions released into the portal circulation (92), the presence of carcinoid syndrome usually implies the presence of liver metastasis. Exceptions to this rule are very large locoregional tumor burdens with hormonal secretions exceeding the metabolic capacity of the liver or tumor invasion into the retroperitoneum allowing access to the systemic venous circulation.

Because small bowel carcinoid neoplasms can present with various, often obscure symptoms, numerous diagnostic tests are often undertaken prior to establishing the diagnosis. A diagnosis can be accomplished with laboratory testing followed by localization studies to identify the primary neoplasm and metastases. Most centers use plasma chromogranin A or a 24-hour urinary 5-HIAA for laboratory testing. Urinary 5-HIAA is more commonly available, but has a lower sensitivity. 5-HIAA levels may be influenced by the ingestion of serotonin-rich food. Fasting plasma 5-HIAA has replaced the urinary assay in some centers. Chromogranin A is an extremely sensitive diagnostic marker for functional and nonfunctional carcinoid neoplasms and closely correlates to tumor volume. False-positive results may occur in patients with other neuroendocrine tumors, prostate cancer, atrophic gastritis, or in patients given proton pump inhibitors. Localization of the neoplasm with a sensitivity of up to 90% can be accomplished by 111-indium-octreotide scintigraphy. This test is better in detecting small primary or metastatic lesions than conventional imaging because it surveys the whole body with high sensitivity. The sensitivity of octreotide scintigraphy can be enhanced using simultaneous single positron emission CT. If 5-HIAA/chromogranin A testing and octreotide scintigraphy do not reveal evidence of a carcinoid neoplasm, a different diagnosis should be contemplated (94).

Because abnormal symptoms at presentation can be extremely nonspecific, most patients will undergo a CT scan or MRI of the abdomen. The sensitivity of these cross-sectional imaging studies in detecting carcinoid tumors is lower than with octreotide scanning and averages about 80%. Typical findings for a small bowel carcinoid on CT or MRI include a mass with calcifications and peritumoral fibrosis. Traditional contrast examination with barium enterography or enteroclysis has a low yield for diagnosing small bowel carcinoid. Video capsule enteroscopy holds promise, but its ability for precise localization and detection of submucosal tumors is limited. A recent report suggested that capsule enteroscopy is superior in detecting jejunoileal pathology and less invasive than push enteroscopy and Sonde enteroscopy. Capsule enteroscopy also has better sensitivity in identifying small bowel lesions compared to CT scan and barium enterography (95).

Most duodenal carcinoids are found incidentally during upper endoscopy for gastrointestinal symptoms. To better characterize duodenal carcinoids, endoscopic ultrasound with biopsy is mandatory (94). Because of their slow growth and low metabolic rate, conventional positron emission tomography (PET) using ^{18}F-fluorodeoxyglucose (FDG) has very limited indications for carcinoid tumors. Its sensitivity can be augmented with the serotonin precursor ^{11}C-5-HT used as a tracer. Recent limited studies suggest ^{11}C-5-HT PET to be an effective staging tool. Selective mesenteric angiography, formerly used to delineate the relationship of carcinoid neoplasms to the portal vein and mesenteric vessels, has mostly been replaced by CT- or MR-angiography and endoscopic ultrasonography. After a diagnosis of carcinoid is made, adequate staging and operative planning can be achieved with an octreotide scan, cross-sectional imaging with either CT or MRI, and an echocardiogram to rule out carcinoid heart disease (94).

Surgical Treatment

Surgical resection is the only potential curative therapy for isolated small bowel carcinoid neoplasms (96). For operative treatment of jejunoileal carcinoid, segmental excision of the affected bowel should always be en bloc with the mesentery because of a high rate of locoregional spread. Fibrosis around mesenteric lymph node metastases can result in foreshortening and fixation of the mesentery to the retroperitoneum. Although resection of the intestinal tumor might appear straightforward, the associated fibrosis can increase the technical demands for a complete oncologic resection. Injury to major mesenteric vessels due to bulky mesenteric metastases may result in devascularization of a major portion of the small intestine. Up to 25% of carcinoid patients are considered unresectable because of involvement of major mesenteric vessels (97). In selected patients, debulking of the mesentery for cytoreduction should be considered (98). With very small carcinoid tumors, preoperative radionuclide octreotide labeling has a theoretical advantage for intraoperative tumor localization with a gamma probe, but the application of this technique has shown mixed success.

Careful staging of the abdominal cavity is important in order to detect any distant metastases for potential simultaneous operative intervention. More than one primary carcinoid tumor will be present in approximately 30% of patients. Even in the presence of distant metastases, resection of the primary neoplasm is indicated. This prolongs survival by >3 years, decreases symptoms through cytoreduction, and may prevent tumor-induced intestinal obstruction, perforation, or mesenteric ischemia (97). If a complete resection is impossible, tumor debulking may render medical therapy for symptom palliation more effective by decreasing the amount of hormonal secretion. Intestinal bypass should be avoided, if possible, because patients with small bowel carcinoid tumors often survive with advanced disease for several years. A bypass increases the risk for local tumor complications, including obstruction, perforation, or ischemia.

As with other forms of small intestinal malignancies, the operative treatment of duodenal carcinoid neoplasms differs from jejunoileal carcinoid. The close relationship of the duodenum to the pancreas and common bile duct makes simple segmental excision with wide local mesenteric excision impossible. The surgeon, therefore, has to choose between a local excision and pancreaticoduodenectomy. The choice is made according to tumor proximity to the ampulla and the risk of locoregional spread determined by tumor size and depth of invasion measured on endoscopic ultrasonography. A tumor ≤2 cm involving the mucosa or submucosa can be locally excised with a local recurrence rate of about 5% (99). Endoscopic excision is usually reserved for tumors <1 cm, and transduodenal local excision is performed for superficial carcinoids between 1 and 2 cm in diameter. After local excision, close endoscopic follow-up is warranted to ensure complete resection and detect local recurrence early. For larger tumors (>2 cm), tumors extending into the muscularis propria, or tumors in close proximity to the major or minor ampulla not amenable to local excision, a pancreaticoduodenectomy is recommended. Limited data make it unclear whether patients with large tumors or tumors invading into the muscularis receive a therapeutic benefit with pancreaticoduodenectomy. This is especially true because patient survival depends more on the presence of distant metastases at the time of diagnosis than on local tumor recurrence after incomplete resection (99).

Perioperative use of octreotide prevents the occurrence of carcinoid crisis. Carcinoid crisis can be triggered by the induction of general anesthesia or operative intervention. The massive hormone release can lead to life-threatening hypo-or hypertension, arrhythmia, or obstructive pulmonary symptoms. The duration of symptoms is variable and can persist postoperatively. The prophylactic use of octreotide is indicated in patients with preoperative carcinoid syndrome, patients with known hepatic metastatic disease, and any patient with a large tumor burden. The pre-emptive perioperative use of somatostatin analogs for resection of a small primary tumor without metastasis is not standard therapy (100).

The liver is the most common site of distant metastasis from small bowel carcinoid. Most patients have multiple liver metastases. Operative treatment should be considered if at least 90% of the tumor can be excised or ablated. Anatomic hepatic resection is preferred, when possible. For more extensive bilobar hepatic disease, resection in combination with parenchyma-saving techniques, such as wedge resection, enucleation, and radiofrequency ablation, should be entertained. These operations are rarely curative because of residual microscopic or macroscopic tumor, but have significant impact on carcinoid syndrome symptoms. After complete hepatic resection, a 5-year survival rate of 62% can occur, with a 5-year disease-free survival of 18% (101).

For patients in whom safe resection or radiofrequency ablation is not feasible, selective arterial chemoembolization should be entertained. Tumor response rates of 44% have been reported with chemoembolization of carcinoid liver metastases. Five-year survival is approximately 30% (102).

Orthotopic liver transplantation is an option for select patients with unresectable metastatic carcinoid disease isolated to the liver after complete resection of the primary tumor. Experience with liver transplantation for this disease is limited. Five-year survival rates of 47% have been achieved; however, 5-year disease-free survival is only 24% (103). Immunosuppression may promote tumor growth and subsequent recurrence. Low Ki-67 indexes have been proposed as a selection parameter for the transplant recipient (104).

Nonsurgical Therapy

Medical management of metastatic small bowel carcinoid mainly involves symptom palliation from carcinoid syndrome. A variety of single-agent chemotherapeutic agents have shown response rates of only ≤20%. Combination chemotherapy trials have mostly been unsuccessful in improving response rates (105). There is little evidence to advocate chemotherapy for carcinoid tumors except the small subgroup of anaplastic carcinoid tumors. Similarly, external-beam radiation has limited benefit in treating carcinoid tumors. Radiation treatment is used in the palliation of bone, brain, and spinal cord metastases (106). The recent introduction of radiolabeled somatostatin analogs for targeted radiation treatment shows promise in preventing tumor progression and possibly tumor regression (107).

Symptom palliation can best be achieved with long-acting somatostatin analogs. A meta-analysis of approximately 400 patients showed that tumor shrinkage did not occur (median, 0%; range, 0% to 9%), suggesting the absence of any significant inhibitory effect on tumor growth with octreotide therapy (108). Reduction in urinary 5-HIAA levels was observed in 37% of patients (range, 0% to 77%). Symptoms of diarrhea and

Table 44.4

Predictors of Risk for Locoregional and Distant Dissemination of Jejunoileal Carcinoids

Tumor Size (mm)	Incidence of Metastasis (%)	Depth of Invasion	Incidence of Metastasis (%)
≤5	15.8	Intramucosal	33.3
6–10	31.5	Invading submucosa	30.8
11–15	74.6	Invading muscularis propria	37.8
16–20	72.6	Invading subserosa	68.4
>20	73.2	Invading other organs	79.2

From Soga J. Carcinoids of the small intestine: a statistical evaluation of 1102 cases collected from the literature. *J Exp Clin Cancer Res.* 1997;16:353–363, with permission.

flushing were controlled in 71% of patients (range, 40% to 100%). Overall, somatostatin analogs improved symptoms with few side effects. Effective treatment only averages about 12 months because of the development of tachyphylaxis.

Interferon-alpha has been advocated in the therapy of carcinoid tumors. The mechanism of action is indeterminate, but the efficacy of symptom control is similar to octreotide. A meta-analysis of >350 patients treated with interferon-alpha showed a tumor response rate of 10% with reduction in biochemical markers in 42% and symptomatic relief in 75% of patients (108). The combination of octreotide and interferon-alpha has demonstrated improved response rates with reduction of urinary 5-HIAA in 75% of patients, but no reduction in tumor size (108). A recent study reported no significant improvement in survival comparing octreotide alone with the combination of octreotide and interferon-alpha (109). For most patients, interferon-alpha has little benefit, especially with its substantial side effects.

Small bowel carcinoid tumors are slow-growing malignancies. Because of their indolent growth pattern, carcinoid tumors have mistakenly been interpreted in the past as benign. Carcinoid neoplasms of the small bowel have a high incidence of locoregional spread. At the time of diagnosis, 31% to 40% of patients show evidence of regional tumor burden, most commonly involving the mesenteric lymph nodes. Distant disease is found in an additional 22% to 31% (76,78) The most common site of distant metastatic spread is the liver (60%), followed by the peritoneum (29%), and the lung (4%) (81). Despite this biologic aggressiveness, small bowel carcinoids frequently have an indolent course. The overall 5-year cancer-specific survival is 76%. The extent of spread correlates with long-term survival. The 5-year survivals for patients with local, regional, and distant disease are 95%, 85%, and 51%, respectively (76). Factors identified as predictors of risk for locoregional and distant dissemination include tumor size and depth of tumor invasion (Table 44.4) (94). Even jejunoileal tumors of ≤5 mm metastasize in 16% of cases. For jejunoileal tumors of ≤1 cm in diameter, the prevalence of metastatic spread is 30%. For jejunoileal tumors >1 cm, the risk of metastases increases to about 70% (81).

For duodenal carcinoid tumors, a size >2 cm is a risk factor for metastatic spread (110,111) Periampullary duodenal carcinoid neoplasms appear to have a more aggressive course once they metastasize (111,112). The prevalence of metastatic spread for jejunoileal carcinoid tumors involving only the mucosa or submucosa is as high as 33%, whereas if the neoplasms invades the muscularis propria, the prevalence increases to 70% (81). Some studies suggest that the proliferation marker Ki-67 may be useful to determine the potential behavior of intestinal carcinoid tumors (113), but the best indicator of prognosis and malignancy remains the presence of regional or distant metastatic growth.

REFERENCES

1. Jemal A, Siegel R, Ward E, et al. Cancer statistics, 2009. *CA Cancer J Clin.* Published online May 27, 2009. doi:10.3322.
2. Lagergren J, Ye W, Ekbom A. Intestinal cancer after cholecystectomy: is bile involved in carcinogenesis? *Gastroenterology.* 2001;121:542–547.
3. Lowenfels AB. Why are small bowel tumors so rare? *Lancet.* 1973;1:24–26.
4. Bone G, Wright NA. The rarity of small bowel tumors: an alternative hypothesis. *Lancet.* 1973;1:618.
5. Wattenberg LW. Studies of polycyclic hydrocarbon hydroxylases of the intestine possibly related to cancer. Effect of diet on benzpyrene hydroxylase activity. *Cancer.* 1971;28:99–102.
6. Calman KC. Why are small bowel tumours rare? An experimental model. *Gut.* 1974;15:552–554.
7. Sellner F. Investigations on the significance of the adenoma-carcinoma sequence in the small bowel. *Cancer.* 1990;66:701–705.
8. Delaunoit T, Neczyporenko F, Limburg PJ, et al. Pathogenesis and risk factors of small bowel adenocarcinoma: a colorectal cancer sibling? *Am J Gastroenterol.* 2005;100:703–710.
9. Planck M, Ericson K, Piotrowska Z, et al. Microsatellite instability and expression of MLH1 and MSH2 in carcinomas of the small intestine. *Cancer.* 2003;97:1551–1557.
10. Jagelman DG, DeCosse JJ, Bussey HJ. Upper gastrointestinal cancer in familial adenomatous polyposis. *Lancet.* 1988;1:1149-1151.
11. Rodriguez-Bigas MA, Vasen HF, Lynch HT, et al. Characteristics of small bowel carcinoma in hereditary nonpolyposis colorectal carcinoma. International Collaboration Group on HNPCC. *Cancer.* 1998;83:240–244.

12. Giardiello FM, Welsh SB, Hamilton SR, et al. Increased risk of cancer in the Peutz-Jeghers syndrome. *N Engl J Med*. 1987;316:1511–1514.

13. Perzin KH, Bridge MF. Adenomatous and carcinomatous changes in hamartomatous polyps of the small intestine (Peutz-Jeghers syndrome): report of a case and review of the literature. *Cancer*. 1982;49:971–983.

14. Hawker PC, Gyde SN, Thompson H, et al. Adenocarcinoma of the small intestine complicating Crohn's disease. *Gut*. 1982;23:188–193.

15. Senay E, Sachar DB, Keohane M, et al. Small bowel carcinoma in Crohn's disease. Distinguishing features and risk factors. *Cancer*. 1989;63:360–363.

16. Green PH, Jabri B. Celiac disease and other precursors to small-bowel malignancy. *Gastroenterol Clin North Am*. 2002;31:625–639.

17. Swinson CM, Slavin G, Coles EC, et al. Coeliac disease and malignancy. *Lancet*. 1983;1:111–115.

18. Cox CL, Butts DR, Roberts MP, et al. Development of invasive adenocarcinoma in a long-standing Kock continent ileostomy: report of a case. *Dis Colon Rectum*. 1997;40:500–503.

19. Heuschen UA, Heuschen G, Autschbach F, et al. Adenocarcinoma in the ileal pouch: late risk of cancer after restorative proctocolectomy. *Int J Colorectal Dis*. 2001;16:126–130.

20. Godacz TR, McFadden DW, Gabrielson EW, et al. Adenocarcinoma of the ileostomy: the latent risk of cancer after colectomy for ulcerative colitis and familial polyposis. *Surgery*. 1990;107:698–703.

21. Dabaja BS, Suki D, Pro B, et al. Adenocarcinoma of the small bowel: presentation, prognostic factors, and outcome of 217 patients. *Cancer*. 2004;101:518–526.

22. Lewis BS. Radiology versus endoscopy of the small bowel. *Gastroenterol Endosc Clin North Am*. 1999;9:13–27.

23. Cobrin GM, Pittman RH, Lewis BS. Increased diagnostic yield of small bowel tumors with capsule endoscopy. *Cancer*. 2006;107:22–27.

24. Korman MU. Radiologic evaluation and staging of small intestine neoplasms. *Eur J Radiol*. 2002;42:193–205.

25. Horton KM, Fishman EK. Multidetector-row computed tomography and 3-dimensional computed tomography imaging of small bowel neoplasms: current concept in diagnosis. *J Comput Assist Tomogr*. 2004;28:106–116.

26. Beall DP, Fortman BJ, Lawler BC, et al. Imaging bowel obstruction: a comparison between fast magnetic resonance imaging and helical computed tomography. *Clin Radiol*. 2002;57:719–724.

27. Howe JR, Kamell LH, Menck HR, et al. The American College of Surgeons Commission on Cancer and the American Cancer Society. Adenocarcinoma of the small bowel: review of the National Cancer Data Base, 1985–1995. *Cancer*. 1999;86:2693–2706.

28. Ugurlu MM, Asoglu O, Potter DD, et al. Adenocarcinomas of the jejunum and ileum: a 25-year experience. *J Gastrointest Surg*. 2005;9:1182–1188.

29. Spira IA, Ghazi A, Wolff WI. Primary adenocarcinoma of the duodenum. *Cancer*. 1977;39:1721–1726.

30. Bakaeen FG, Murr MM, Sarr MG, et al. What prognostic factors are important in duodenal adenocarcinoma? *Arch Surg*. 2000;135:635–641.

31. Tocchi A, Mazzoni G, Puma F, et al. Adenocarcinoma of the third and fourth portions of the duodenum: results of surgical treatment. *Arch Surg*. 2003;138:80–85.

32. Rose DM, Hochwald SN, Klimstra DS, et al. Primary duodenal adenocarcinoma: a ten-year experience with 79 patients. *J Am Coll Surg*. 1996;183;89–96.

33. Sohn TA, Lillemoe KD, Cameron JL, et al. Adenocarcinoma of the duodenum: factors influencing long-term survival. *J Gastrointest Surg*. 1998;2:79–87.

34. Locher C, Malka D, Boige V, et al. Combination chemotherapy in advanced small bowel adenocarcinoma. *Oncology*. 2005;69:290–294.

35. Chakravarthy A, Abrams RA, Yeo CJ, et al. Intensified adjuvant combined modality therapy for resected periampullary adenocarcinoma: acceptable toxicity and suggestions of improved one-year disease-free survival. *Int J Radiat Oncol Biol Phys*. 2000;48:1089–1096.

36. Isaacson PG. Gastrointestinal lymphoma. *Hum Pathol*. 1994;25:1020–1029.

37. Fine KD, Stone MJ. Alpha-heavy chain disease, Mediterranean lymphoma, and immunoproliferative small intestinal disease: a review of clinicopathological features, pathogenesis, and differential diagnosis. *Am J Gastroenterol*. 1999;94:1139–1152.

38. Lecuit M, Abachin E, Martin A, et al. Immunoproliferative small intestinal disease associated with *Campylobacter jejuni*. *N Engl J Med*. 2004;350:239–248.

39. Paisonnet J, Isaacson PG. Bacterial infection and MALT lymphoma. *N Engl J Med*. 2004;350:213–215.

40. Domizio P, Owen RA, Shepherd NA, et al. Primary lymphoma of the small intestine. A clinicopathological study of 119 cases. *Am J Surg Pathol*. 1993;17:429–442.

41. Freeman HJ. Lymphoproliferative and intestinal malignancies in 214 patients with biopsy-defined celiac disease. *J Clin Gastroenterol*. 2004;38:429–434.

42. Catassi C, Bearzi I, Holmes GK. Association of celiac disease and intestinal lymphomas and other cancers. *Gastroenterology*. 2005;128:S79–S86.

43. Bajdi E, Diss TC, Munson P, et al. Mucosal intra-epithelial lymphocytes in enteropathy-associated T-cell lymphoma, ulcerative jejunitis, and refractory celiac disease constitute a neoplastic population. *Blood*. 1999;94:260–264.

44. Ruskone-Fourmestraux A, Elmer A, Lavergne A, et al. Multiple lymphomatous polyposis of the gastrointestinal tract: prospective clinicopathologic study of 31 cases. Groupe D'etude des Lymphomes Digestifs. *Gastroenterology*. 1997;112:7–16.

45. Le Brun DP, Kamel OW, Cleary ML, et al. Follicular lymphomas of the gastrointestinal tract. Pathologic features in 31 cases and bcl-2 oncogenic protein expression. *Am J Pathol*. 1992;140:1327–1335.

46. Bende RJ, Smit LA, Bossenbroek JG, et al. Primary follicular lymphoma of the small intestine: alpha4 beta7 expression and immunoglobulin configuration suggest an origin from local antigen-experienced B cells. *Am J Pathol*. 2003;162:105–113.

47. Karp JE, Broder S. Acquired immunodeficiency syndrome and non-Hodgkin's lymphomas. *Cancer Res*. 1991;51:4743–4756.

48. Kumar S, Fend F, Quintanilla-Martinez L, et al. Epstein-Barr virus-positive primary gastrointestinal Hodgkin's disease: association with inflammatory bowel disease and immunosuppression. *Am J Surg Pathol*. 2000;24:66–73.

49. Koniaris LG, Drugas G, Katzman PJ, et al. Management of gastrointestinal lymphoma. *J Am Coll Surg*. 2003;197:127–141.

50. Gobbi PG, Dionigi P, Barbieri F, et al. The role of surgery in the multimodal treatment of primary gastric non-Hodgkin's lymphomas. A report of 76 cases and review of the literature. *Cancer*. 1990;65:2528–2536.

51. Ruskone-Fourmestraux A, Aegerter P, Delmer A, et al. Primary digestive tract lymphoma: a prospective multicentric study of 91 patients. Groupe d'Etude des Lymphomes Digestifs. *Gastroenterology*. 1993;105:1662–1671.

52. Daum S, Ullrich R, Heise W, et al. Intestinal non-Hodgkin's lymphoma: a multicenter prospsective clinical study from the German Study Group on Intestinal non-Hodgkin's Lymphoma. *J Clin Oncol*. 2003;21:2740–2746.

53. Salles G, Herbrecht R, Tilly H, et al. Aggressive primary gastrointestinal lymphomas: review of 91 patients treated with the LNH-84 regimen. A study of the Group d'Etude des Lymphomes Agressifs. *Am J Med.* 1991;90:77–84.

54. Wohrer S, Chott A, Drach J, et al. Chemotherapy with cyclophosphamide, doxorubicin, etoposide, vincristine and prednisone (CHOEP) is not effective in patients with enteropathy-type intestinal T-cell lymphoma. *Ann Oncol.* 2004;15:1680–1683.

55. Dragosics B, Bauer P, Radaszkiewicz T. Primary gastrointestinal non-Hodgkin's lymphomas. A retrospective clinicopathologic study of 150 cases. *Cancer.* 1985;55:1060–1073.

56. Amer MH, el-Akkad S. Gastrointestinal lymphoma in adults: clinical features and management of 300 cases. *Gastroenterology.* 1994;106:846–858.

57. Musshoff K. Clinical staging classification of non-Hodgkin's lymphomas (author's transl). *Strahlentherapie.* 1977;153:218–221.

58. Krugmann J, Dimhofer S, Gschwendtner A, et al. Primary gastrointestinal B-cell lymphoma. A clinicopathological and immunohistochemical study of 61 cases with an evaluation of prognostic parameters. *Pathol Res Pract.* 2001;197:385–393.

59. Rosenfelt F, Rosenberg SA. Diffuse histiocytic lymphoma presenting with gastrointestinal tract lesions. The Stanford experience. *Cancer.* 1980;45:2188–2193.

60. Radaszkiewicz T, Dragosics B, Bauer P. Gastrointestinal malignant lymphomas of the mucosa-associated lymphoid tissue: factors relevant to prognosis. *Gastroenterology.* 1992;102:1628–1638.

61. Miettinen M, Lasota J. Gastrointestinal stromal tumors—definition, clinical, histological, immunohistochemical, and molecular genetic features and differential diagnosis. *Virch Arch.* 2001;438:1–12.

62. Robson ME, Glogowski E, Sommer G, et al. Pleomorphic characteristics of a germ-line KIT mutation in a large kindred with gastrointestinal stromal tumors, hyperpigmentation, and dysphagia. *Clin Cancer Res.* 2004;10:1250–1254.

63. Corless CL, Fletcher JA, Heinrich MC. Biology of gastrointestinal stromal tumors. *J Clin Oncol.* 2004;22:3813–3825.

64. Tran T, Davila JA, El-Serag HB. The epidemiology of malignant gastrointestinal stromal tumors: an analysis of 1,458 cases from 1992 to 2000. *Am J Gastroenterol.* 2005;100:162–168.

65. Blanchard DK, Budde JM, Hatch GF 3rd, et al. Tumors of the small intestine. *World J Surg.* 2000;24:421–429.

66. Connolly EM, Gaffney E, Reynolds JV. Gastrointestinal stromal tumours. *Br J Surg.* 2003;90:1178–1186.

67. Dagher R, Cohen M, Williams G, et al. Approval summary: imatinib mesylate in the treatment of metastatic and/or unresectable malignant gastrointestinal stromal tumors. *Clin Cancer Rers.* 2002;8:3034–3038.

68. de Mestier P, des Guetz G. Treatment of gastrointestinal stromal tumors with imatinib mesylate: a major breakthrough in the understanding of tumor-specific molecular characteristics. *World J Surg.* 2005;29:357–361.

69. Heinrich MC, Corless CL, Demetri GD, et al. Kinase mutations and imatinib response in patients with metastatic gastrointestinal stromal tumor. *J Clin Oncol.* 2003;21:4342–4349.

70. Corless CL, Schroeder A, Griffith D, et al. PDGFRA mutations in gastrointestinal stromal tumors: frequency, spectrum and in vitro sensitivity to imatinib. *J Clin Oncol.* 2005;23:5357–5364.

71. Subramanian S, West RB, Corless CL, et al. Gastrointestinal stromal tumors (GISTs) with KIT and PDGFRA mutations have distinct gene expression profiles. *Oncogene.* 2004;23:7780–7790.

72. Blay JY, Bonvalot S, Casali P, et al. Consensus meeting for the management of gastrointestinal stromal tumors. Report of the GIST Consensus Conference of 20–21 March 2004, under the auspices of ESMO. *Ann Oncol.* 2005;16:566–578.

73. Fletcher CD, Berman JJ, Corless C, et al. Diagnosis of gastrointestinal stromal tumors: a consensus approach. *Hum Pathol.* 2002;33:459–465.

74. Taniguchi M, Nishida T, Hirota S, et al. Effect of c-kit mutation on prognosis of gastrointestinal stromal tumors. *Cancer Res.* 1999;59:4297–4300.

75. DeMatteo RP, Lewis JJ, Leung D, et al. Two-hundred gastrointestinal stromal tumors: recurrence patterns and prognostic factors for survival. *Ann Surg.* 2000;231:51–58.

76. Maggard MA, O'Connell JB, Ko CY. Updated population-based review of carcinoid tumors. *Ann Surg.* 2004;240:117–122.

77. Hemminki K, Li X. Incidence of trends and risk factors of carcinoid tumors: a nationwide epidemiologic study from Sweden. *Cancer.* 2001;92:2204–2210.

78. Modlin IM, Lye KD, Kidd M. A 5-decade analysis of 13,715 carcinoid tumors. *Cancer.* 2003;97:934–959.

79. Gabos S, Berkel J, Band P, et al. Small bowel cancer in Western Canada. *Int J Epidemiol.* 1993;22:198–206.

80. Berge T, Linell F. Carcinoid tumors. Frequency in a defined population during a 12-year period. *Acta Pathol Microbiol Scand.* 1976;84:322–330.

81. Soga J. Carcinoids of the small intestine: a statistical evaluation of 1102 cases collected from the literature. *J Exp Clin Cancer Res.* 1997;16:353–363.

82. Gerstle JT, Kauffman GL Jr, Koltun WA. The incidence, management, and outcome of patients with gastrointestinal carcinoids and second primary malignancies. *J Am Coll Surg.* 1995;180:427–432.

83. Habal N, Sims C, Bilchik AJ. Gastrointestinal carcinoid tumors and second primary malignancies. *J Surg Oncol.* 2000;75:301–316.

84. Westergaard T, Frisch M, Melbye M. Carcinoid tumors in Denmark 1978–1989 and the risk of subsequent cancers. *Cancer.* 1995;76:106–109.

85. Modlin IM, Kidd M, Pfragner R, et al. The functional characterization of normal and neoplastic human enterochromaffin cells. *J Clin Endocrinol Metab.* 2006;91:2340–2348.

86. Babovic-Vuksanovic D, Constantinou CL, Rubin J, et al. Familial occurrence of carcinoid tumors and association with other malignant neoplasms. *Cancer Epidemiol Biomarkers Prev.* 1999;8:715–719.

87. Kidd M, Eick G, Shapiro MD, et al. Microsatellite instability and gene mutations in transforming growth factor-beta type II receptor are absent in small bowel carcinoid tumors. *Cancer.* 2005;103:229–236.

88. Gortz B, Roth J, Krahenmann A, et al. Mutations and allelic deletions of the MEN1 gene are associated with a subset of sporadic endocrine pancreatic and neuroendocrine tumors and not restricted to foregut neoplasms. *Am J Pathol.* 1999;154:429–436.

89. Modlin IM, Shapiro MD, Kidd M. Carcinoid tumors and fibrosis: an association with no explanation. *Am J Gastroenterol.* 2004;99:2466–2478.

90. Makridis C, Rastad J, Oberg K, et al. Progression of metastases and symptom improvement from laparotomy in midgut carcinoid tumors. *World J Surg.* 1996;20:900–906.

91. Onaitis MW, Kirshbom PM, Hayward TZ, et al. Gastrointestinal carcinoids: characterization by site of origin and hormone production. *Ann Surg.* 2000;232:549–556.

92. Akerstrom G, Hellman P, Hessman O, et al. Management of midgut carcinoids. *J Surg Oncol.* 2005;89:161–169.

93. Durward G, Blackford S, Roberts D, et al. Cutaneous scleroderma in association with carcinoid syndrome. *Postgrad Med J.*
1995;71:299–300.

94. Modlin IM, Latich I, Zikusoka M, et al. Gastrointestinal carcinoids: the evolution of diagnostic strategies. *J Clin Gastroenterol.*
2006;40:572–582.

95. Triester SL, Leighton JA, Leontiadis GI, et al. A meta-analysis of the
yield of capsule endoscopy compared to other diagnostic modalities in patients with obscure gastrointestinal bleeding. *Am J Gastroenterol.* 2005;100:2407–2418.

96. Loftus JP, van Heerden JA. Surgical management of gastrointestinal
carcinoid tumors. *Adv Surg.* 1995;28:317–336.

97. Hellman P, Lundstrom T, Ohrvall U, et al. Effect of surgery on the
outcome of midgut carcinoid disease with lymph node and liver
metastases. *World J Surg.* 2002;26:991–997.

98. Ohrvall U, Eriksson B, Juhlin C, et al. Method of dissection of
mesenteric metastasis in mid-gut carcinoid tumors. *World J Surg.*
2000;24:1402–1408.

99. Zyromski NJ, Kendrick ML, Nagorney DM, et al. Duodenal carcinoid tumors: how aggressive should we be? *J Gastrointest Surg.*
2001;5:588–593.

100. Kinney MA, Warner ME, Nagorney DM, et al. Perianaesthetic risks
and outcomes of abdominal surgery for metastatic carcinoid tumours. *Br J Anaesth.* 2001;87:447–452.

101. Sarmiento JM, Heywood G, Rubin J, et al. Surgical treatment of
neuroendocrine metastases to the liver: a plea for resection to
increase survival. *J Am Coll Surg.* 2003;197:29–37.

102. Gupta S, Johnson MM, Murthy R, et al. Hepatic arterial embolization and chemoembolization for the treatment of patients with
metastatic neuroendocrine tumors: variables affecting response
rates and survival. *Cancer.* 2005;104:1590–1602.

103. Lehnert T. Liver transplantation for metastatic neuroendocrine carcinoma: an analysis of 103 patients. *Transplantation.*
1998;66:1307–1312.

104. Rosenau J, Bahr MJ, von Wasielewski R, et al. Ki67, E-cadherin,
and p53 as prognostic indicators of long-term outcome after liver
transplantation for metastatic neuroendocrine tumors. *Transplantation.* 2002;73:386–394.

105. Rougier P, Mitry E. Chemotherapy in the treatment of neuroendocrine malignant tumors. *Digestion.* 2000;62:73–78.

106. Schupak KD, Wallner KE. The role of radiation therapy in the
treatment of locally unresectable or metastatic carcinoid tumors.
Int J Radiat Oncol Biol Phys. 1991;20:489–495.

107. Kwekkeboom DJ, Teunissen JJ, Bakker WH, et al. Radiolabeled somatostatin analog [177Lu-DOTA0,Tyr3] octreotate in patients with endocrine gastroenteropancreatic tumors. *J Clin Oncol.*
2005;23:2754–2762.

108. Modlin IM, Latich I, Kidd M, et al. Therapeutic options for gastrointestinal carcinoids. *Clin Gastroenterol Hepatol.* 2006;4:526–547.

109. Kolby L, Persson G, Franzen S, et al. Randomized clinical trial of
the effect of interferon alpha on survival in patients with disseminated midgut carcinoid tumours. *Br J Surg.* 2003;90:687–693.

110. Burke AP, Sobin LH, Federspiel BH, et al. Carcinoid tumors of the
duodenum. A clinicopathologic study of 99 cases. *Arch Pathol Lab
Med.* 1990;114:700–704.

111. Makhlouf HR, Burke AP, Sobin LH. Carcinoid tumors of the ampulla of Vater: a comparison with duodenal carcinoid tumors.
Cancer. 1999;85:1241–1249.

112. Hatzitheoklitos E, Buchler MW, Friess H, et al. Carcinoid of the
ampulla of Vater. Clinical characteristics and morphologic features. *Cancer.* 1994;73:1580–1588.

113. Sokmensuer C, Gedikoglu G, Uzunalimoglu B. Importance of proliferation markers in gastrointestinal carcinoid tumors: a clinicopathologic study. *Hepatogastroenterology.* 2001;48:720–723.

COMMENTARY
Gauree Gupta and Simon K. Lo

The chapter on small bowel tumors written by Drs. Donohue and Schnelldorfer offers a succinct and practical perspective on the diagnosis and management of intestinal tumors. We will attempt to provide some additional information based on new knowledge in this rapidly expanding field of gastroenterology.

For many years the only way to study the small intestine was barium small bowel studies or exploratory laparotomy. The former has since been proven to be highly inaccurate when compared to the newer techniques of capsule endoscopy and double-balloon enteroscopy (1–3), and the latter is an inva-sive procedure that is not well suited as a purely diagnostic maneuver.

Small tumors in the intestine are typically asymptomatic and are traditionally impossible to detect in their early stages. Thus, mass lesions in the small bowel are usually detected in late stages when they cause intestinal obstruction, intussusception, distant metastases or significant gastrointestinal bleeding. The better strategy in dealing with intestinal tumors is to identify these lesions when they are small or in a premalignant stage. The authors believe that this is an achievable goal with the use of the newly available endoscopic modalities.

ENDOSCOPY IN THE NEW MILLENNIUM

Capsule endoscopy was first approved by the Food and Drug Administration for use in the United States in 2001. Since then, hundreds of thousands of these procedures have been done throughout the world. Although the capsule endoscopy litera-ture has focused mainly on the investigation of obscure gastroin-testinal bleeding, it has added to our knowledge on many other conditions, including tumors. Early data showed that 9% of all obscure gastrointestinal bleeding was caused by small bowel tumors (4). The actual incidence of asymptomatic tumors or tumors that cause abdominal pain, diarrhea, or vague obstruc-tive symptoms is uncertain. What is certain is that capsule en-doscopy is the first breakthrough technology that opens up our eyes to smaller and hopefully more treatable masses of the small intestine.

In spite of the availability of this seemingly amazing nonin-vasive procedure, capsule endoscopy has several shortcomings. It lacks the capacity to take samples and determine the pre-cise location of a small bowel lesion, which can pose serious diagnostic and management issues to surgeons and oncologists. Many images of potential tumor captured on capsule endoscopy are imprecise, too dark, or partially obscured by floating de-bris. This imprecision creates a dilemma of whether to explore a patient based on suboptimal findings. Although capsule en-doscopy can visualize a wide area of the small intestine, it has been shown to recognize only 64% of surgically implanted beads

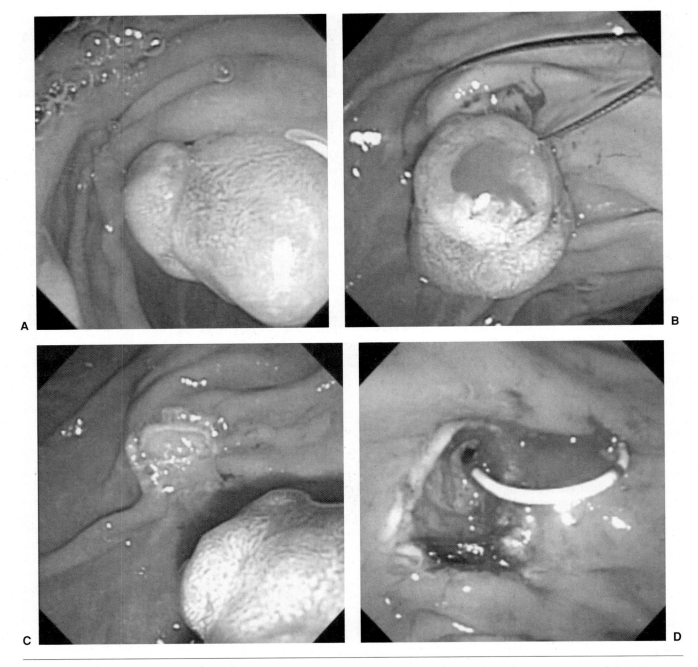

Figure 44C. 1 Endoscopic resection of ampullary adenoma. **(A)** Endoscopic view of the lesion. **(B)** Snare resection of the adenoma. **(C)** The adenoma has been detached from the ampullary tissue. **(D)** A small stent is placed in the pancreatic duct to protect against pancreatitis following the ampullectomy.

on the mucosal surface of the canine small intestine (5). In a multicenter U.S. study involving 130 patients referred for obscure gastrointestinal bleeding, capsule endoscopy missed at least 5 of 17 tumors (29%) and is therefore not the most reliable way to exclude suspected small bowel tumors (6). Nonetheless, the high patient acceptance, lack of radiation risk, and acceptable sensitivity make capsule endoscopy a logical first-line diagnostic test.

Shortly after the introduction of capsule endoscopy, double-balloon enteroscopy (DBE) was invented by Hiro Yamamoto (7).

This form of conventional endoscopy consists of a 200-cm endoscope that is inserted through a 145-cm overtube. DBE relies on traction created by the balloons attached to the tip of the endoscope and its overtube. This traction can either anchor the overtube while pushing the scope forward or secure the endoscope in place while advancing the overtube. When these two balloons are fully inflated, they can hold onto the bowel wall so firmly that a gentle withdrawal of the instrument can pleat and shorten the intestine. After many cycles of pleating and advancement, it is possible to pass the enteroscope through the entire length of a small intestine (8). If an oral or retrograde DBE passage is insufficient to examine the whole small bowel, the bidirectional approach can achieve total enteroscopy in 35% of patients (9). The enteroscope functions like a typical endoscope, with a 2.8-mm instrument channel to perform forceps biopsy, needle injection, polypectomy, and metallic clip placement (10).

Even though DBE can be used like a regular upper endoscope, it is rather labor-intensive to perform the procedure and is impractical to routinely apply on all patients with suspected small bowel disorders. However, it is rapidly becoming the tool of choice for endoscopists in searching for, and marking the location of, small intestinal tumors. In addition to DBE, single-balloon enteroscopy and spiral overtube-assisted enteroscopy are being developed and may further help identify small bowel tumors. Computed tomography (CT) and magnetic resonance enterography are becoming increasingly used for a similar purpose, the combination of capsule endoscopy and DBE is currently the most logical and reliable ways of discovering small bowel tumors (11,12).

INTESTINAL ADENOMAS AND ADENOCARCINOMAS

As Drs. Donohue and Schnelldorfer point out, most small bowel adenomas and adenocarcinomas occur in the duodenum and the ampulla. The risk of having these lesions is significantly higher in patients with familial adenomatous polyposis, Peutz-Jeghers syndrome, (PJS) and hereditary nonpolyposis colon cancer syndrome (13). As is the case in the colon, it is possible to prevent cancer if a duodenal adenoma is successfully removed. The challenge of managing a duodenal adenoma begins with its detection, as an early lesion is usually small and flat. Even as the lesion grows, it tends to spread laterally as a flat lesion rather than develop into a pedunculated polyp. The treatment of a duodenal adenoma is also more difficult than its colonic counterpart. The flat lesion must be removed with one of the mucosectomy techniques rather than a simple polypectomy (14). Perforation and bleeding occur in roughly 1% and 10%, respectively, in endoscopic mucosal resection of flat lesions in the colon and are likely the same in the duodenum (15).

Ampullary adenomas constitute a unique form of adenoma, as they situate in the opening of the pancreatic and bile duct. Assessment of an ampullary adenoma should include an endoscopic ultrasound and endoscopic retrograde cholangiopancreatography (16,17). If the lesion has extended into one of the ductal systems, a surgical resection is mandatory. However, if the lesion is confined to the duodenal portion of the ampulla, then an endoscopic ampullectomy can be safely carried out in most cases (18,19) (Figure 44C.1). Capsule endoscopy seems to have a large blind spot in the duodenum and is not the procedure of choice to survey the duodenum and proximal jejunum. Rather, a push enteroscopy should be performed for this purpose. All adenocarcinomas of the small intestinal must be removed surgically. The assessment of Crohn disease and celiac disease for adenocarcinoma can be very difficult. If there are no obstructive symptoms, capsule endoscopy can be safely performed to look for suspicious lesions. If partial obstruction and capsule

retention are a strong concern, then a DBE and biopsy should be carried out. Once a lesion is detected, India ink tattooing and placement of a metal clip can be done to mark it for future surgical resection.

PEUTZ-JEGHERS SYNDROME

PJS polyps are typically located in the jejunum and are readily reached by a per-oral DBE. Although the risk of small bowel cancer is increased in this condition, most PJS polyps are hamartomas and present clinically by often causing intussusception. Capsule endoscopy is a reasonable tool to screen for PJS polyps (20). Once identified, the polyps can be safely removed during a DBE (21,22). The biggest challenge to performing DBE in PJS patients is getting far into the small intestine because of adhesions caused by a prior surgical resection of the colon or small intestine. Therefore, it is important to perform screening capsule endoscopy early in all PJS patients so that DBE polypectomy can be successfully carried out. If a per-oral DBE attempt fails to reach the polyps, it can be inserted per-rectum to reach the lesions in a retrograde fashion.

INTESTINAL LYMPHOMA

It is difficult to grossly differentiate a lymphoma from adenocarcinoma in the small intestine. Both types of lesion are frequently ulcerated, although adenomatous tissue may be identified around an adenocarcinoma. The less aggressive lymphomas may not be ulcerated and can present as a very subtle cluster of nodules (Figure 44C.2). In the past, many lymphomas were detected only during exploratory surgery. This is no longer the case, as the combined use of capsule endoscopy and DBE can eliminate this uncertainty in most cases (23,24). Whenever a lymphoma is suspected, the endoscopist should obtain fresh, unfixed tissue for special staining in addition to formalin-fixed tissue for routine hematoxylin and eosin staining.

GASTROINTESTINAL STROMAL TUMORS

A large GIST lesion is frequently clinically symptomatic and detected on cross-sectional abdominal imaging; however, <2 cm lesions are commonly missed on these studies. CT enterography, which combines luminal contrast radiography and extraintestinal imaging, is of increasing importance in finding these lesions. However, the best way of finding small GIST lesions is again with the combination of capsule endoscopy and DBE. Small GISTs without superficial ulcerations are also difficult to assess on capsule endoscopy, as the lesions may be mimicked by incidental bulges from adjacent organs or intestinal gas pockets (25,26). DBE has the ability to probe these lesions to determine their firmness and integrity. The recent addition of long-length endoscopic ultrasound probes can be used to differentiate musclelike tumors (including GISTs) from artifacts, lipomas, nonmuscular solid tumors, and cysts or vascular lesion (27,28). Forceps biopsies can obtain tissue from these lesions, but they are typically nondiagnostic because of difficulty in acquiring representative

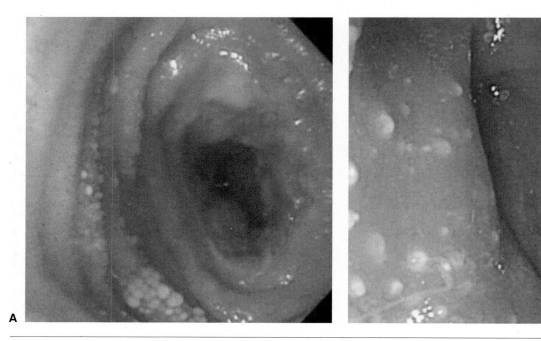

A   **B**

Figure 44C.2 (**A**) Large, circumferential jejunal B-cell lymphoma. (**B**) Some small bowel follicular lymphomas may appear as very innocuous white nodules.

specimens from these tightly formed and mobile lesions (29). Polypectomy of even the smallest GIST lesions is not advisable because of the high risk of perforating the thin wall of the small intestine. Most of these lesions should be inked for planned surgical resection.

CARCINOID TUMORS

Until recently, carcinoids were very difficult lesions to find except for the very large lesions or when they were found at surgery. Situated mostly in the ileum, they are rarely found on small bowel barium studies. As with other small bowel tumors, large carcinoids can be readily identified on CT or magnetic resonance imaging. Small lesions that are <2 cm may be difficult to find. Because most of these lesions are located the distal small bowel, retrograde DBE has been found to be quite sensitive as a diagnostic test (30,31). In our own experience of 20 cases of metastatic neuroendocrine tumors and no obvious findings on CT scans, retrograde DBE was found to be the most sensitive (32). It must be emphasized that most oncologists and gastroenterologists are rather passive in pursuing the primary lesions in the small intestine, stemming from their pessimism on finding these lesions. This type of attitude should be changed in light of the vastly improved sensitivity of radionuclide and endoscopic studies.

In our small bowel endoscopy experience, carcinoid tumors as small as 5 mm have been found on capsule endoscopy and DBE. In spite of the submucosal nature of these lesions, it is easy to obtain tissue for diagnosis with the regular biopsy forceps. Duodenal carcinoids are typically small and nonmalignant. They are usually found incidentally in the duodenal bulb

on routine upper endoscopy. Most lesions are <1 cm and can be removed endoscopically (Figure 44C.3). If an endoscopic ultrasound shows a small, well-circumscribed submucosal carcinoid, an endoscopic attempt may be made to remove the lesion. It must be emphasized that perforation is common because of the very thin duodenum. Endoscopic clip placement may be used to appose the mucosectomy edges to minimize this complication.

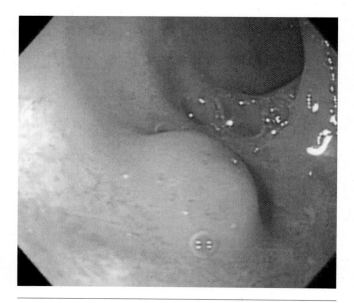

Figure 44C.3 Duodenal carcinoid tumor.

CONCLUSION

Once considered an improbable task, detection of small bowel tumors should no longer be considered a "lucky" find. Large lesions are readily identified on cross-sectional imaging studies and CT enterography. Small lesions should also be routinely detected with the combination of capsule endoscopy and DBE. Both new endoscopic technologies have intrinsic limitations and their accuracies depend on the experience of the endoscopists. Nonetheless, they are important instruments in the diagnosis of all intestinal tumors and allow us to treat these lesions in the smaller and earlier stages.

REFERENCES

1. Guido, C, Saumil, KS, Maria Elena, R, et al. A prospective trial comparing small bowel radiographs and video capsule endoscopy for suspected small bowel disease. *Gastroenterology.* 2002;123:999–1005.
2. Cazzato, I, Cammarota, G, Nista, EC, et al. Diagnostic and therapeutic impact of double-balloon enteroscopy (DBE) in a series of 100 patients with suspected small bowel diseases. *Dig Liver Dis.* 2007;39:483–487.
3. Pasha SF, Leighton JA, Das A, et al. Double-balloon enteroscopy and capsule endoscopy have comparable diagnostic yield in small-bowel disease: a meta-analysis [published online ahead of print March 20, 2008]. *Clin Gastroenterol Hepatol.* 2008;6:671–676.
4. Cobrin G, Pittman R, Lewis B. Increased diagnostic yield of small bowel tumors with capsule endoscopy. *Cancer.* 2006;107:22–27.
5. Appleyard M, Fireman Z, Glukhovsky A, et al. A randomized trial comparing wireless capsule endoscopy with push enteroscopy for the detection of small-bowel lesions. *Gastroenterology.* 2000;119:1431–1438.
6. Mehdizadeh S, Ross A, Gerson L, et al. What is the learning curve associated with double-balloon enteroscopy? Technical details and early experience in 6 U.S. tertiary care centers. *Gastrointest Endosc.* 2006;64:740–750.
7. Yamamoto H, Sekine Y, Sato Y, et al. Total enteroscopy with a nonsurgical steerable double-balloon method. *Gastrointest Endosc.* 2001;53:216–220.
8. Yamamoto H, Kita H, Sunada K, et al. Clinical outcomes of double-balloon endoscopy for the diagnosis and treatment of small-intestinal diseases. *Clin Gastroenterol Hepatol.* 2004;2:1010–1016.
9. May A, Nachbar L, Ell C. Double-balloon enteroscopy (push-and-pull enteroscopy) of the small bowel: feasibility and diagnostic and therapeutic yield in patients with suspected small bowel disease. *Gastrointest Endosc.* 2005;62:62–70.
10. Lo SK, Mehdizadeh S. Therapeutic uses of double-balloon enteroscopy. *Gastrointest Endosc Clin North Am.* 2006;16:363–376.
11. Fletcher JG, Huprich J, Loftus EV Jr, et al. Computerized tomography enterography and its role in small-bowel imaging. *Clin Gastroenterol Hepatol.* 2008;6:283–289.
12. Lohan D, Cronin C, Meehan C, et al. MR small bowel enterography: optimization of imaging timing. *Clin Radiol.* 2007;62:804–807.
13. Hirota WK, Zuckerman MJ, Adler DG, et al. ASGE guideline: the role of endoscopy in the surveillance of premalignant conditions of the upper GI tract. *Gastrointest Endosc.* 2006;63:570–580.
14. Qureshi W, Davila R, Gan SI, et al. The role of endoscopy in ampullary and duodenal adenomas. *Gastrointest Endosc.* 2006;64:849–854.
15. Poppers DM, Haber GB. Endoscopic mucosal resection of colonic lesions: current applications and future prospects. *Med Clin North Am.* 2008;92:687–705.
16. Ito K, Fujita N, Noda Y, et al. Preoperative evaluation of ampullary neoplasm with EUS and transpapillary intraductal US: a prospective and histopathologically controlled study. *Gastrointest Endosc.* 2007;66:740–747.
17. Small AJ, Baron TH. Successful endoscopic resection of ampullary adenoma with intraductal extension and invasive carcinoma (with video). *Gastrointest Endosc.* 2006;64:148–151.
18. Yoon SM, Kim M-H, Kim MJ, et al. Focal early stage cancer in ampullary adenoma: surgery or endoscopic papillectomy? *Gastrointest Endosc.* 2007;66:701–707.
19. Chahal P, Baron TH, Gostout CJ, et al. Predictors of complications following endoscopic ampullectomy. *Gastrointest Endosc.* 2006;63:AB156.
20. Schulmann K, Hollerbach S, Kraus K, et al. Value of capsule endoscopy for the detection of small bowel polyps in patients with hereditary polyposis syndromes (FAP, PJS, FJP). *Gastroenterology.* 2003;124(Suppl 1):A550.
21. Ohmiya N, Taguchi A, Shirai K, et al. Endoscopic resection of Peutz-Jeghers polyps throughout the small intestine at double-balloon enteroscopy without laparotomy. *Gastrointest Endosc.* 2005;61:140–147.
22. Ross AS, Dye C, Prachand VN. Laparoscopic-assisted double-balloon enteroscopy for small-bowel polyp surveillance and treatment in patients with Peutz-Jeghers syndrome. *Gastrointest Endosc.* 2006;64:984–988.
23. Flieger D, Keller R, Fischbach W. Features of intestinal lymphoma in capsule endoscopy. *Gastroenterology.* 2003;124(Suppl 1):A244.
24. Hotta K, Oyama T, Tomori A, et al. Double balloon endoscopy is essential for diagnosis of malignant lymphomas of the small bowel [abstract]. *Gastrointest Endosc.* 2007;65:174.
25. Chong AKH, Chin BWK, Meredith CG. Clinically significant small-bowel pathology identified by double-balloon enteroscopy but missed by capsule endoscopy. *Gastrointest Endosc.* 2006;64:445–449.
26. Schwartz GD, Barkin JS. Small bowel tumors. *Gastrointest Endosc Clin North Am.* 2006;16:267–275.
27. Kunihiro K, Manabe N, Hata J, et al. Gastrointestinal stromal tumor in jejunum: diagnosis using contrast-enhanced ultrasonography and double-balloon enteroscopy. *Dig Dis Sci.* 2006;51:1236–1240.
28. Fukumoto A, Manabe N, Tanaka S, et al. Usefulness of EUS with double-balloon enteroscopy for diagnosis of small-bowel diseases. *Gastrointest Endosc.* 2007;65:412–420.
29. Hoda KM, Rodriguez SA, Faigel DO. EUS-guided sampling of suspected GI stromal tumors. *Gastrointest Endosc.* 2007;65:AB204.
30. Scherubl H, Faiss S, Tschope R, et al. Double-balloon enteroscopy for the detection of midgut carcinoids. *Gastrointest Endosc.* 2005;62:994.
31. Yamaguchi T, Manabe N, Tanaka S, et al. Multiple carcinoid tumors of the ileum preoperatively diagnosed by enteroscopy with the double-balloon technique. *Gastrointest Endosc.* 2005;62:315–318.
32. Cheng D, Han NJ, Mehdizadeh S, et al. What are the most useful tools to search for primary gastrointestinal neuroendocrine tumors (PGI-NET)? *Gastrointest Endosc.* 2007;65:W1358(AB344).

45

Malignant Tumors Arising in Inflammatory Bowel Disease

Thomas A. Ullman

Patients with inflammatory bowel disease (IBD) have an increased risk for colorectal cancer (CRC). Although not always appreciated, this is true not just for patients with ulcerative colitis (UC), but also patients with Crohn disease, particularly those with Crohn colitis. Even though our understanding of the clinical and molecular basis for this association has improved since the first case descriptions and series were reported nearly a century ago, our means of prevention and treatment, primarily colonoscopic surveillance and prophylactic surgery, remain modest at best. CRC still accounts for a large proportion of the premature mortality in both UC and Crohn disease.

This chapter will review the pathogenesis and clinical epidemiology of CRC in IBD, as well as the theoretical and literature-based strategies for CRC prevention. Additionally, the available evidence on the association between Crohn ileitis and small intestinal cancer will be presented.

PATHOGENESIS AND MOLECULAR BASIS OF CANCER IN IBD

Drawing lessons from the molecular changes that account for colon carcinogenesis in familial adenomatosis polyposis and hereditary nonpolyposis CRC, now Lynch syndrome, the genetic and molecular basis of colon carcinogenesis has become better understood in recent years. These lessons have been directly applicable to events involved in the development of sporadic colorectal neoplasia, whose pathways mirror those of the familial cancer syndromes. It is currently believed that most (80% to 85%) sporadic CRCs arise from a pathway that involves *chromosomal instability* resulting in abnormal segregation of chromosomes, aneuploidy, and altered expression of tumor suppressor genes (primarily *APC* and *p53*) and oncogenes (mainly *k-ras*) (Figure 45.1). In this pathway, loss of *APC* function occurs as an initiating or "gatekeeper" event for subsequent molecular alterations that culminate in the development of the adenoma. Loss of *p53* gene function occurs later in the sequence, typically at the transition of the adenoma to carcinoma. The remaining 15% of sporadic CRCs arise through a so-called mutator pathway that involves loss of function of DNA base mismatch repair genes, mainly *hMLH1* and *hMSH2*. In this pathway, loss of mismatch repair gene function results in a phenotype termed *microsatellite instability* (MSI). Sporadic CRCs that demonstrate MSI are often diploid (as opposed to the aneuploid state of chromosomal instability pathway-related tumors), tend to occur in the proximal colon, and frequently display rather unique histologic features such as a medullary or solid growth pattern, signet ring cell histology, a plethora of tumor infiltrating lymphocytes, and an adjacent inflammatory reaction often referred to as a *Crohnlike reaction*. Another distinguishing feature of MSI-positive sporadic CRCs is the better survival of patients with those tumors compared to ones without MSI (1).

IBD-associated CRCs share several features in common with sporadic CRC. First, they both arise from a precursor dysplastic lesion. In the case of sporadic CRC, the dysplastic precursor is a discrete, polypoid growth called an *adenoma*, which typically progresses to cancer by enlarging in size, assuming greater degrees of dysplasia, and often assuming an increasing proportion of villous histology. In chronic colitis, while dysplasia is often polypoid, it may be flat or only slightly raised. Regardless of its growth pattern, colitis-related dysplasia progresses through increasing levels of abnormal development in its path to CRC. Second, stage-based survival of patients with CRC is similar in the two settings. Third, the types of molecular alterations that contribute to the pathogenesis of sporadic CRC are the same ones found in colitis-associated neoplasms (2).

Although the similarities, between colitis-associated neoplasia and sporadic colorectal neoplasia are notable, they differ in several important ways. First, colitis-associated cancers affect individuals at a much younger age. Second, colitis-associated neoplasia, by definition, arises in the setting of long-standing chronic inflammation, whereas sporadic neoplasms occur in the absence of an inflammatory background. Oxidative stress or other insults may lead to earlier or more frequent genetic changes to the colon, but the precise mechanisms by which chronic inflammation leads to neoplasia remain elusive. Third, dysplasias and even cancers in colitis are often multifocal, suggesting more of a precancerous "field change" of the colitic mucosa compared to the colons of patients with sporadic adenomas and colon cancer; the clinical consequence of this difference accounts for the different surgical approach: colitis-associated neoplasms are usually treated with total proctocolectomy, whereas sporadic adenomas and cancers are treated with polypectomy or segmental resection of affected colon. Fourth, although the two settings of colorectal neoplasia might share the several types of molecular changes, the frequency and timing with which these molecular alterations occur is different (Figure 45.1) (3). For example, *APC* mutations are considered to be common and initiating events in sporadic colon carcinogenesis, whereas this molecular alteration is much less frequent and usually occurs late in the

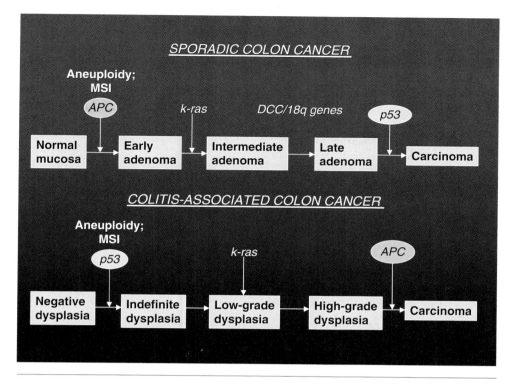

Figure 45.1 Timing in molecular alterations in sporadic colorectal cancer and colitis-associated colorectal cancer. MSI, microsatellite instability. (From Itzkowitz SH, Harpaz N. Diagnosis and management of dysplasia in patients with inflammatory bowel diseases. *Gastroenterology.* 2004;126:1634–1648, with permission.)

colitis-associated dysplasia-carcinoma sequence. Also, in colitis patients, *p53* mutations occur early and have even been detected in mucosa that is nondysplastic or indefinite for dysplasia (4). Likewise, MSI has been detected in nondysplastic mucosa from patients with UC, even those patients with disease of relatively short duration, but not from healthy controls or patients with other types of benign inflammatory colitis (5,6).

COLORECTAL CANCER IN ULCERATIVE COLITIS: EPIDEMIOLOGY AND CLINICAL PRACTICE

Epidemiology

Crohn and Rosenberg (7) first described rectal cancer complicating UC >80 years ago. In their article, they suggested that the malignancy was a complication of the disease. Three years after Crohn and Rosenberg, Bargen (8), at the Mayo Clinic, reported a series of 17 patients with both chronic colitis and CRC. Other cases and series followed, and the crude frequency calculations from these studies served as "evidence" supporting a link between UC and CRC. With the application of modern epidemiologic methods, true incidence calculations, cumulative incidence calculations, and standardized incidence rates confirmed the association between UC and CRC.

Cumulative incidence rates have largely become the standard by which the time-dependent risk of cancer develops in col-

itis. Similarly, standardized incidence rates describe the estimate of the relative risk for developing colon cancer for a segment of a colitis population (such as colitis patients with universal disease) as compared to the general population. Although initial series using this more accurate epidemiologic terminology came from large referral centers in which "incident" cases were referred for evaluation and management because of a suspicion for or even the actual presence of CRC, the use of more appropriate terminology was an advance over the previously used crude rates (9–11). Because of these now-obvious referral biases, however, these first "modern" studies overestimated the true risk of CRC in UC. Subsequent studies from population-based data sources used more realistic calculations for determining the incidence of CRC in UC. Without referral and other selection biases, the cancer incidence calculated in these publications was substantially lower than previously reported (12–16). These studies, however, may have *under*estimated the true risk of cancer in longstanding UC, as they included many patients with UC who had undergone previous colectomy in the denominator of the incidence calculations.

In a meta-analysis of the risk of CRC in UC in which 116 studies were included, Eaden and colleagues (17) found the overall prevalence of CRC to be 3.7% and an overall incidence rate of 3 cases per 1000 person-years duration (95% confidence interval [CI] ranging from 2 to 4 cases per 1000 person-years' duration). The rate increased with each decade of disease, leading to a calculated incidence of 12 per 1000 person-years in the third decade of colitis. These data corresponded to a *cumulative incidence* of CRC of 2% at 10 years, 8% at 20 years, and 18% at 30 years' disease duration (17). It is worth noting, however, that referral centers accounted for 64% of the studies included in the study by Eaden et al. (17); only 13 population-based reports were located by the MedLine search performed as part of the meta-analysis (17). Based on these and older data, typical estimates of CRC incidence usually range between 0.5% and 1% per year after 10 years of colitis.

More recent studies, however, have raised the possibility that prior studies have overestimated the incidence and risk for CRC in this population. In more recent publications from Denmark (18), Hungary (19), Canada (20), and Olmstead County, Minnesota (with its relatively small population) (21), have suggested a CRC in UC incidence of between 1 in 500 to 1 in 1,600 per year, far lower than the 1 in 300 rate calculated in the meta-analysis of Eaden et al. (17). These have corresponded to relative risk calculations ranging from 1.1 to 2.7 times the general population. Although some have argued that these more modern calculations support a declining incidence over calendar time, as seen by Rutter and colleagues (22), no definitive analysis has been performed to support this hypothesis. To what extent such reductions in incidence (if they exist) are a function of colonoscopic surveillance (see later discussion), chemoprevention with mesalamine-based agents or other medicines (also later), or other factors remains unknown.

Risk Factors

A number of clinical variables have been demonstrated to modify the risk for CRC in UC patients. These variables include duration of UC, anatomic extent of disease, age at UC diagnosis, concomitant primary sclerosing cholangitis (PSC), a family history of CRC, and inflammatory activity. The use of certain medications may lessen the risk of developing CRC, but the impact of these potentially chemopreventive agents is modest. Table 45.1 classifies these different risk modifiers.

Duration of Ulcerative Colitis

A number of investigators have demonstrated that the duration of UC correlates with the risk of cancer (9,23–25). Duration of disease, however, can be a rather subjective measurement. Most studies have used the date of UC diagnosis as the point at which the clock starts, but others have argued that the time of symptom onset is a better measure of disease duration. Whichever point is chosen, a number of distortions can be imagined that would impact the findings in any individual study. If *date of diagnosis* is used as a starting point, then patients with long-standing, subclinical disease would appear to have relatively shorter duration of disease, and such subjects would contribute less to any calculation of the effect of disease duration. Conversely, by using *date of first symptoms*, subjects who were without colitis might mistakenly contribute years of disease-free time to calculations of duration. This distinction in the definition of disease duration may be particularly problematic for patients with PSC who frequently have clinically quiescent colitis. Without unanimity in definition, there is variability in the estimate of this factor's effect on subsequent CRC development. In the meta-analysis by Eaden et al. (17), the effect of duration was made clear as the passage of each successive decade resulted in an increase in incidence. In-

Table 45.1

Risk Modifiers of Colorectal Cancer in Ulcerative Colitis

Accepted risk modifiers	
Disease duration	Longer duration increases risk
Extent of disease	Greater extent increases risk
PSC	Presence of PSC increases risk
Age of onset	Early age of onset increases risk
Family history of cancer	Positive family history increases risk
Probable risk modifiers	
Inflammation	Increased inflammation increases risk
Possible risk modifiers	
Sulfasalazine/5-ASA	Use reduces risk
Folic acid	Supplementation reduces risk
Ursodeoxycholic acid	Use reduces risk in UC patients with PSC
Unlikely risk modifier	
Glucocorticoid use	
6-MP/AZA use	

PSC, primary sclerosing cholangitis; 5-ASA, 5-aminosalicylic acid; 6-MP, 6-mercaptopurine; AZA, azathioprine.

cidence was calculated to be 2 per 1,000 patient years (95% CI: 1-4/1,000) at 10 years and 11 per 1,000 (95% CI: 4-28/1,000) at 30 years; the rate at 20 years was intermediate (17).

As the overall curve for cumulative CRC risk starts to meaningfully exceed that of the general population by 8 to 10 years, most clinicians will initiate surveillance colonoscopy once this threshold has been reached. Because many of the studies that were entered into the meta-analysis by Eaden et al. antedated the widespread application of colonoscopic dysplasia surveillance, it remains unclear whether duration of colitis exerts a seeming exponential effect, as the investigators found, or a linear effect, which might result if highest-risk patients are serially removed from the denominator via colectomy from surveillance-identified dysplasia.

Anatomic Extent of Ulcerative Colitis

The length of involved colon also correlates with cancer risk: the greater the surface area of colitis, the greater the cancer risk. Defining the anatomic extent of UC, as with duration of disease, can vary from study to study. In initial reports documenting this independent risk factor, anatomic extent was defined by a barium enema at diagnosis. Flexible endoscopy long ago replaced barium radiography for diagnosing colitis and its extent, but there is no consensus as to whether naked eye findings at colonoscopy or microscopic extent determined histologically should be the gold standard for measuring extent. Additionally, definitions of "pancolitis," "universal colitis," and "extensive colitis" vary within studies, although they are all typically used to describe disease proximal to the splenic flexure. Another feature that invites confusion into the definition of anatomic extent is the timing of the measurement. As extent can change over time

(26), should we take the extent at diagnosis or at some point in follow-up? Like other questions surrounding the issue of extent, this question has been left unresolved, although the majority of studies have used the terms *extent* and *extent at diagnosis* interchangeably. Extent at follow-up has not been well studied as an independent risk factor.

A population-based investigation of a cohort of >3,000 UC patients defined extent of UC by barium enema examination at diagnosis, and demonstrated an impressive gradient of risk as one moves from proctitis (standardized incidence ratio [SIR] of 1.7, 95% CI: 0.8-3.2) to left-sided colitis (SIR, 2.8, 95% CI: 1.6-4.4) to pancolitis (SIR, 14.8, 95% CI: 11.4-18.9) (13). Devroede et al. (9), Greenstein et al. (25), Gyde et al. (24), Katzka et al. (27), Mir-Madjlessi et al. (28), and Gilat et al. (14) all reported similar gradients in their studies. This finding was confirmed, although not directly studied, in the meta-analysis by Eaden et al. (17).

In terms of "how" extent should be defined, it is worth noting that a group from the University of California at San Francisco found CRC in areas proximal to the endoscopically perceived margin of colitis that turned out to have microscopic disease in that region (29). On this basis, clinicians should consider the most proximal extent of disease *microscopically* as the proximal extent of disease, and plan any prevention strategy accordingly.

Age at Onset of Ulcerative Colitis

Age at onset of colitis, as a variable independent of disease duration, has been implicated in some studies to modify the risk of colitic cancer. This hypothesis, however, remains in question. Reporting one of the highest published cumulative rates of CRC in colitis, Devroede and colleagues (9) found that at 35 years of follow-up, 43% of subjects with documented UC prior to age 15 had developed CRC. This study, however, reflected pediatric patients seen at a large referral center; additionally, the number of patients available to analyze after 35 years of follow-up was quite small, with the error surrounding this point estimate correspondingly quite broad. Although some investigators have failed to demonstrate a link between age at onset of colitis and the subsequent development of CRC (14,27), others (13,24) have confirmed the direction if not the magnitude of the findings by Devroede et al. (9). In the previously mentioned study by Ekbom et al. (13), for example, the authors found that the relative risk of cancer in colitis decreased with advancing age—younger patients have a higher risk. This result, however, should come as no surprise because even if the risk of cancer in UC remained constant over a lifetime, by using age-related rates of sporadic cancer in the denominator, relative risks in successive age groups (from youngest to oldest) would necessarily decrease given the known association of age with sporadic CRC. This overall gradient was confirmed by Eaden et al. (17), who found that cumulative rates of CRC were greater than the pooled estimates for CRC among adult colitic patients. Although neither the precise nature nor the precise magnitude of CRC risk for younger patients with UC has been determined, extra caution should be applied to this group of patients given both the suggestion of an increased risk from the medical literature and the obvious increased lifetime risk given a longer life expectancy.

Primary Sclerosing Cholangitis

PSC is a chronic cholestatic liver disease in which there is progressive inflammatory fibrosis of the biliary tree. It is an infrequent complication of IBD, affecting 2% to 8% of patients with UC. However, among patients with PSC, 62% to 72% have underlying IBD. Because the intersection of CRC *and* PSC would be expected to occur in small absolute numbers in patients with UC, it is largely through case-control studies and referral center-based cohort studies that the majority of data have been generated to support an association between PSC and CRC in UC. Although a positive association has not always been noted (30–32), most studies do support such an association, with derived odds ratios from these "positive" studies ranging from 9 to 16 (33–37).

In a population-based study from Sweden, Kornfeld and colleagues (38) found a substantially elevated cumulative incidence of CRC in UC/PSC patients: 33% at 20 years. As previously noted, because colitis activity in PSC is often mild or even subclinical, PSC patients in these studies might well have had a longer duration of disease than was appreciated, making it difficult to tease out the precise, independent contribution of PSC to the development of CRC.

Family History of Colorectal Cancer

Family history of CRC has long been recognized as a risk factor for the development of sporadic CRC. This risk increases according to the number of relatives affected with CRC (39). In UC, only a few clinical studies have been performed to investigate the independent contribution of a positive family history for CRC. An early study by Lashner et al. (40) at the University of Chicago supported family history of CRC as a potential risk factor for CRC in colitis, although the association did not reach statistical significance. A second report from the Cleveland Clinic documented a *lower* rate of positive family history of CRC among UC patients with cancer or dysplasia compared to UC controls without colonic neoplasia, although this finding, too, failed to exclude the null hypothesis (41). Both of these studies, however, were designed to test hypotheses concerning the association between folic acid supplementation and CRC in colitis. Testing for family history as a risk factor was performed as part of a secondary analysis, and these studies did not specify the rigor with which a family history was obtained.

More recently, a handful of studies have suggested an increased risk for CRC in UC when a positive family history of CRC was documented. Nuako and colleagues (42) at the Mayo Clinic were the first to clearly demonstrate this increased risk, calculating an odds ratio of 2.3 (95% CI: 1.1-5.1) in their case-control study. In a population-based study from Scandinavia, Askling and colleagues (43) found a similar elevated risk of 2.5 (95% CIL 1.4-4.4), while Eaden et al. (44) (in the United Kingdom) found an even greater risk (odds ratio, 5.0; 95% CI: 1.1-22.8) in a multivariable model using case-control-derived data. Whatever the absolute magnitude, it appears quite likely that a positive family history confers an increased risk of CRC in UC.

Inflammation

Curiously, although inflammation has been assumed to be a key factor contributing to higher risk of colonic neoplasia in UC, few studies have examined this issue. One well-conducted retrospective case-control study recently reported that histologic inflammation was indeed associated with an increased risk of neoplastic progression based on a retrospective case-control analysis of patients followed at a specialized center (45). A retrospective cohort study from Mount Sinai, New York, has also demonstrated a link between histologic inflammation on dysplasia and cancer risk, with a twofold risk increase for each unit of inflammation derived from a 4-point scale (46).

Pharmacotherapy and Chemoprevention

As with sporadic CRC and interest in cyclooxygenase inhibiting compounds, investigators, clinicians, and patients are actively seeking medications that might *decrease* the risk of developing CRC in UC. Retrospective studies have been performed examining a number of potential chemopreventive agents with mixed results. As is often the case in retrospectively performed studies of medication use, the dose and duration of use that defines exposure can be arbitrarily chosen. Nevertheless, a number of studies have been performed looking at different hypothesized chemopreventive medication with exposure defined in a number of different ways.

Sulfasalazine

Sulfasalazine and the newer 5-aminosalicylic acid (5-ASA) products have been investigated for their chemopreventive effect, mainly by post hoc secondary analyses, yielding conflicting results. In a study designed to investigate the effect of supplemental folic acid on CRC risk, sulfasalazine use was found to have a positive (i.e., predisposing) effect on the development of CRC (slightly but not significantly higher rates of CRC in the exposed group); sulfasalazine-allergic patients, however, were noted to have a substantially lower risk of developing CRC (40). Subsequently, Pinczowski et al. (47) and Eaden et al. (44) were able to demonstrate a protective effect for sulfasalazine or mesalazine, when dose and duration were considered. Tung et al. (48) failed to demonstrate a meaningful protective effect, but this study was limited to high-risk PSC patients.

A number of additional studies with a variety of definitions for exposure have now been performed with conflicting results. Some have shown benefit with exposure to mesalamine-based agents (49,50), while others have been less optimistic (51,52). A meta-analysis has reviewed a number of these studies, but its conclusion that mesalamine is chemopreventive must be taken with some caution owing to the heterogeneity of the included studies as well as the different designs that were used (case-control, retrospective cohort, secondary analyses) (53). Given the lack of unanimity of these studies, it remains in question whether mesalamine-based medications constitute truly chemopreventive agents. Given their utility at preventing flares in patients in remission, however, their use should be advocated in all UC patients.

Folic Acid

Folic acid, which has been demonstrated to have a protective effect in sporadic CRC was twice studied by Lashner et al., once at the University of Chicago (40) and again at the Cleveland Clinic (41). In neither study was a significant protective effect noted, although the point estimates of risk (0.38 and 0.45) sug-

gested the possibility of a chemopreventive effect. Given the low cost and the low risk of adverse events at conventional doses of 400 mcg/day and 1 mg/day, the administration of folic acid as a chemopreventive drug should be strongly considered for all at-risk patients.

Ursodeoxycholic Acid

Ursodeoxycholic acid, an exogenous bile acid used in the treatment of PSC, has also been studied. In UC-PSC patients, an impressive chemopreventive effect has been demonstrated, with a 40% difference in neoplasia noted between the ursodeoxycholic acid-treated group (32%) and the untreated group (72%) (48). This was additionally demonstrated in a randomized clinical trial of ursodeoxycholic acid in which a 74% reduction in dysplasia or CRC was noted (54). Whether this chemopreventive effect can be demonstrated in patients with UC or Crohn colitis who do not have PSC remains unknown, although it is under investigation.

Methods to Reduce Risk/Mortality

Until we discover or develop a meaningful chemopreventive agent and effective strategies to identify a minimal risk subgroup, only two acceptable forms of CRC prophylaxis exist: surgery and dysplasia surveillance. In dysplasia surveillance, high-risk patients are identified by the identification of neoplasia (either dysplasia or cancer) at colonoscopy and are subsequently referred to surgery, while cancer and dysplasia-free patients continue with periodic colonoscopy. The presumption is that only the patients at highest risk will undergo a colectomy, and lower risk patients will be able to maintain a higher quality of life with their colons intact. A third option, watch and wait, with colonoscopy performed only for symptoms, is available, but because of the available evidence that symptomatic cancers are associated with a worse survival than asymptomatic ones (55,56), it is never used in clinical practice.

Surgery

Without question, the most effective method for minimizing CRC risk in UC patients is to perform a total proctocolectomy. This nearly eliminates the risk of colon or rectal cancer, and, while cancers have been reported in case reports and series in patients who have undergone either hand-sewn or stapled anastomoses, the risk of such an event is quite small. In the pre-endoscopic era, this strategy of cancer prevention was often advocated for patients with long-standing colitis, and should still be considered, particularly for patients with medically refractory or difficult disease. As surgery is not without its potential complications and change in quality of life, however, and as the absolute risk of developing a lethal colon cancer may not be sufficiently high to warrant such a radical approach in *all* colitis patients, surgical prophylaxis in asymptomatic patients with long-standing colitis is now viewed with skepticism by both patients and clinicians.

At present, surgical options (for CRC prophylaxis *or* as primary treatment for colitis-related dysplasia or cancer) include total proctocolectomy with creation of an ileal pouch-anal anastomosis (often referred to as a *restorative proctocolectomy*) or total proctocolectomy with end-ileostomy. Subtotal colectomy with ileorectal anastomosis is to be avoided, although there are no studies comparing this procedure with either of the other conventional choices. Pouch surgery is generally reserved for younger patients, as it requires sufficient anal sphincter tone. Following pouch surgery, patients may expect to have five or more bowel movements per day because of pouch size and ileal flow. Possible complications include sexual and bladder dysfunction, incontinence, pouchitis (which usually responds to short courses of antibiotics but may become chronic and refractory), fistula formation, stricture formation, anastomotic leakage, and pouch failure. The overall failure rate (the proportion of patients eventually converted to end-ileostomy) is approximately 5% (57). It should also be noted that the malignant potential of ileal pouch mucosa in colitis patients remains unknown. Initial reports of pouch dysplasia have been reported, and there have been reports of cancer in the cuff of rectal mucosa to which the pouch is anastomosed (58,59). Even though cancer risk following proctocolectomy with Brooke ileostomy is close to nil, the loss of anorectal function and attendant stoma make this option less appealing to most patients who would otherwise be candidates for pouch surgery. Potential complications of total proctocolectomy with end-ileostomy include sexual and bladder dysfunction, stomal fistula, peristomal hernia, and small bowel obstruction (57).

Dysplasia Surveillance

As it results in too many colectomies in patients who would otherwise be unaffected by CRC, prophylactic total proctocolectomy is seldom performed. Even if limited to the high-risk groups of patients with long-standing and extensive UC, with or without PSC or a family history of CRC, a large number of colectomies would be performed in patients who would never develop CRC. What is needed is a tissue marker that better determines those patients at highest risk, those with an imminent risk of CRC. Although imperfect on many levels, mucosal dysplasia serves as such a marker.

In 1967 Morson and Pang (60) first reported the association between mucosal dysplasia and CRC in patients with UC. In their seminal report they noted that rectal dysplasia, then termed *precancer* and identified by blind rectal biopsy of colitis mucosa, heralded the presence of an invasive adenocarcinoma *elsewhere* in the colon. If appropriately discriminating, mucosal dysplasia, it was hypothesized, could be used as a diagnostic test to identify the highest-risk patients to whom surgery would be offered.

Subsequent studies revealed that, although by no means a perfect test, dysplasia was discriminating enough to be tested in clinical practice. Retrospective studies confirmed the findings of Morson and Pang (60), noting the presence of dysplasia either adjacent to or remote from cancer in colitis (61–63). Additionally, cancer foci were discovered in colons resected for the indication of dysplasia (64). These data, along with the advent of flexible fiberoptic instruments with their ability to deliver multiple mucosal samples to the pathologist's microscope, led to the development of protocol-based surveillance programs. Unfortunately, no randomized, controlled trials of surveillance were performed. (This may have been a function of difficulty in defining suitable control patients: would patients allow themselves to be randomized to a "no surgery" or "no endoscopy" arm of a surveillance study? Or to a "prophylactic surgery" arm?) Nevertheless,

based on the clinical characteristics of dysplasia and the results of numerous surveillance programs, as well as the very limited acceptability of other prevention strategies—namely surgery for all long-standing colitis or waiting for cancer symptoms—periodic colonoscopy with biopsy for dysplasia became an accepted form of cancer prevention in UC. In addition to its widespread use in clinical practice, it has been advocated in guidelines statements for colon cancer prevention (65) and UC care (66).

Single-armed surveillance programs have demonstrated the feasibility, although not the efficacy, of conventional surveillance (15,64,67–77). When "control" arms were used in these studies, they included patients in whom surveillance at another institution or referral to the institution for malignancy could be considered as "no surveillance." Nevertheless, the finding that cancers found during surveillance were more often at earlier stages than cancers found in a "watch and wait" strategy contributed to the acceptance of dysplasia surveillance as a form of cancer prevention (55,56). Other key features about surveillance programs worth noting include the presence of advanced-stage cancers despite inclusion in a surveillance program (some resulting from patient dropout and some from progression while under surveillance) (74,77,78); the variable intervals used for surveillance, variable rates of patient dropout, and the substantially varied rates of dysplasia incidence across studies.

For surveillance to be effective, it should reduce CRC mortality in IBD patients. In the absence of prospective controlled studies, a well-designed population-based case-control study sheds light on this issue. Karlen and colleagues (79) compared the exposure to colonoscopy among cases with CRC deaths and alive controls matched for age, gender, disease duration, and disease extent. Their point estimate of cancer mortality reduction from either one or only two previous colonoscopic examinations was a threefold decrease. Although the odds ratio of 0.3 did not reach statistical significance, (95% CI: 0.1-1.3), this is certainly a clinically impressive result. A recent case-control study from the Mayo Clinic confirmed these findings, and even crossed the threshold of statistical significance with an odds ratio of 0.4 for one to two surveillance examination (95% CI: 0.2-0.7) (80). Although these data were not population-based in their orientation, they nevertheless support the notion that surveillance is likely effective. Additional support comes from decision analysis models (81–83) that demonstrate improved outcomes for a population in surveillance compared to no surveillance. As with all such modeled data, there are many assumptions that lack real-world support, such as a lack of dropout while under surveillance and an orderly progression from no dysplasia to low-grade dysplasia to high-grade dysplasia to CRC (81,84,85). Cost-effectiveness analyses have similarly predicted that surveillance was a superior strategy to no surveillance (although prophylactic colectomy, while unacceptable to patients, was the preferred strategy vis-à-vis life-years saved over time).

What, then, might limit the effectiveness of dysplasia surveillance in UC in practice? One factor may be difficulties in histologic interpretation among pathologists. Indeed this was thought to be so substantial a problem after the initial reports of surveillance studies that in 1983, an international group of experts convened to establish true definitions for the evaluation of dysplasia surveillance specimens: no dysplasia, indefinite for dysplasia (with three subtypes), low-grade dysplasia

(LGD), high-grade dysplasia (HGD), and CRC (86). Unfortunately, despite these codified definitions, substantial rates of disagreement, even among expert gastrointestinal pathologists, have been noted (86–89). Rates of disagreement among community pathologists, not surprisingly, have been substantial, too) (87). In these studies, crude rates of agreement have been as low as 40% and as high as 72%, with best agreement when no dysplasia was present; kappa values, which can account for chance agreement were fair to good. Clearly, this system needs less subjectivity and overall improvement.

Lack of perfection from practicing pathologists is not the only reason for surveillance not to reach its potential. Gastroenterologists also fall short of ideal practices. One variable that contributes to lack of uniform clinician practices stems from the uncertainty that surrounds the predictive value of dysplasia. Although there is near-universal agreement that patients found to have HGD should undergo colectomy because of rates of concurrent adenocarcinoma near 50% (62), considerable controversy surrounds the management of LGD. Adding to the controversy is the fact that LGD can be flat or polypoid, unifocal or multifocal, or not repeatedly found on sequential colonoscopic exams. Few studies have directly addressed these variables in patients with LGD.

How to best manage LGD depends in large part on how likely patients with this finding are to either already harbor or progress to more advanced neoplasia (HGD or cancer). More specifically, the essential unanswered question is whether failure to perform a colectomy in patients with LGD results in a poor outcome. In a landmark study from St. Mark's Hospital in which the 1983 definitions of Inflammatory Bowel Disease Morphology Study Group were used (86), the rate of progression to advanced dysplasia from LGD was 54% at 5 years (90). In the same year as the St. Mark's publication, a systematic review of surveillance programs by Bernstein and colleagues noted a 19% rate of cancer at "immediate colectomy" following the discovery of LGD (113). These results were confirmed by studies from the Mayo Clinic (91) and Mount Sinai in New York (78), in which the rates of progression for flat LGD were 33% (95% CI: 9%-56%) and 53% (95% CI), respectively. Furthermore, in the Mount Sinai study, 19% of patients who underwent colectomy within 6 months of their initial flat LGD finding were found to have CRC in their resection specimens. Of those who progressed, cases of node-positive cancer without intervening HGD were found. Neither the number of biopsies positive for LGD nor any other clinical variable were found to be predictive of subsequent progression, with unifocal flat LGD carrying a 5-year rate of progression of 53% (78).

Investigators from the University of Washington where an aggressive biopsy protocol is followed (92) and from The Karolinska Institute, Sweden (93), however, discovered less frequent progression and no cancers. Not all investigators have discovered the same high-risk for LGD as that noted by St. Mark's, Mayo Clinic, and Mount Sinai in New York. A group from Karolinska in Sweden noticed a near-total lack of progression following discovery of LGD, but this group's pathologists did not use the full panoply of IBD Morphology Study Group definitions, as readings of "indefinite" for dysplasia were not allowed. Additionally, a number of patients were included whose discovery of LGD occurred prior to establishment of the Riddell criteria

(94). Additionally, Lim et al. (95) from Leeds, U.K., found little progression from LGD, leading them to conclude that continued surveillance with satisfactory biopsy practices was a safe alternative to surgery. Although the variable rates of progression (perhaps secondary to variable biopsy practices, observer variation in the interpretation of dysplasia, or imperfect follow-up), make it difficult to draw absolute conclusions for the management of patients with flat LGD, early colectomy for LGD that is histologically confirmed by two expert pathologists should be strongly considered at the least. For patients who defer or refuse colectomy for LGD, gastroenterologists must make certain that patients return for follow-up examinations and that surveillance is appropriately performed with an adequate number of biopsies taken to exclude dysplasia.

It should be noted that negative findings on examination following LGD can occur for a number of reasons: (a) the previous examination was a false-positive because of pathologic interpretation error; (b) the present examination is a false-negative because of sampling or interpretation error; or (c) both examinations were accurate. Not finding dysplasia on a repeat colonoscopy following one that detected LGD is no reassurance that dysplasia has regressed or will not "recur" (77). It was estimated that to exclude dysplasia with 95% confidence, 56 biopsies must be performed, and to exclude 90% confidence, 33 biopsies should be taken (96). This number of biopsies is rarely performed even in academic centers (97,98). Eaden et al. (97) noted that 57% of U.K gastroenterologists take fewer than 10 biopsies in a surveillance examination, based on their response to a questionnaire. In a study examining actual gastroenterologists' practices, Ullman and colleagues (78) found that the mean number of evaluable biopsies in patients with LGD was only 17.5. Such undersampling represents another limitation for dysplasia surveillance among gastroenterologists. Whether such practices truly limit the effectiveness of surveillance remains unknown.

The appropriate management of polypoid LGD, like that of flat LGD, is equally challenging. Polypoid dysplastic lesions in UC were labeled DALMs, (dysplasia-associated lesions or masses) by Blackstone and colleagues (68) in 1981. In this study, in which the pond was effectively stocked with patients referred for a suspicion of CRC and may lesions were noted to be >2 cm in diameter, DALMs were noted to harbor a 58% (7 of 12) risk of cancer (68). Despite the impressive cancer risk of DALMs in the report by Blackstone et al., astute clinicians hypothesized that smaller, adenomalike lesions might present a lesser risk. Two simultaneously published studies reported on their experience of treating smaller, sessile lesions with endoscopic resection (without surgery). Rubin and colleagues (99) from Mount Sinai, New York, followed 48 patients with ulcerative or Crohn colitis in whom dysplastic polyps were detected at colonoscopy. In those patients in whom polyps were endoscopically resected and the remaining colon was dysplasia-free, *no* patients progressed to CRC after a mean follow-up of 4.1 years (99). In study from the Brigham and Women's Hospital in Boston by Engelsgjerd et al. (100), none of 24 colitis patients with adenomalike polyps treated with polypectomy developed adenocarcinoma after a mean follow-up of 42.4 months. Odze et al. (101) reported on the continued follow-up of the Brigham group 5 years later, and only one case of CRC developed, this in a patient 7.5 years after her initial polypoid lesion had been resected. Similar results were noted in a recent publication by Rutter and colleagues (22). The need for complete resection of polypoid lesions was underlined in a publication by Vieth et al. (102), in which 10 of 60 patients in whom residual neoplasia was left behind progressed to CRC. These data seem to indicate the relative safety of endoscopic polypectomy in colitis provided the lesions are small, completely resected, and that the rest of the surveillance run is dysplasia-free. When removing a suspicious polyp in a colitic colon, it is important to separately biopsy the mucosa immediately adjacent to the polyp base because if the polyp resides in a bed of dysplasia, colectomy is warranted.

The colitic colon with numerous inflammatory pseudopolyps presents another challenge to the endoscopist. It is wise to remove any polyp that has unusual features. Molecular studies using global gene expression arrays suggest that DALMs can be distinguished from apparently sporadic adenomas (103) holding promise for managing these difficult lesions. Finding a dysplastic lesion in a sea of inflammatory polyps, however, poses a substantial challenge to the endoscopist. It is not surprising that a recent publication found that the presence of inflammatory pseudopolyps carries a substantial (2.5-fold) risk for subsequent CRC (80).

In addition to a lack of certainty among experts as to how to manage flat, LGD and polypoid dysplasia, other impediments to the success of surveillance exist within the gastrointestinal community. Poor understanding of dysplasia and surveillance practices exist among trained gastroenterologists (97,98,104) Indeed, only 19% of respondents correctly identified dysplasia as neoplastic tissue in2-decade-old questionnaire study by Bernstein et al. (104). Whether gastroenterologists' understanding has improved since that time remains uncertain.

Patient factors have also limited the effectiveness colonoscopic surveillance in colitis. Patient dropout or noncompliance with surveillance programs has been demonstrated to be a substantial source of CRC mortality (56,72,74,77).

Despite the limitations of surveillance based on the difficulties of dysplasia interpretation, poor agreement on dysplasia management, suboptimal surveillance performance, and risks of patient dropout, no other acceptable method for cancer prevention in colitis exists. As such, dysplasia surveillance will remain with us until a superior substitute is found. Current recommendations for how surveillance should be performed has been published in a number of different formats (3,105,106). All of these publications agree that four-quadrant biopsies, with each quartet of biopsies in a separate jar, should be taken every 10 cm, with suspicious lesions labeled and placed in a separate jar; examinations should be performed every 1 to 2 years for patients with disease involving one-third or more of their colon after 8 years of disease. Surveillance should begin at diagnosis for all patients with UC and PSC.

Alternatives to Surveillance

Augmentation of white-light surveillance has been proposed using *chromoendoscopy* using the dye stains methylene blue or indigo carmine to better highlight subtle and "flat" lesions. These procedures have demonstrated higher detection rates for dysplasia in head-to-head comparisons (107) with conventional dysplasia surveillance and in back-to-back surveillance in which

each patient serves as his or her own control (108). Whether the introduction and application of chromoendoscopic surveillance will alter outcome for colitis patients remains untested. Other types of advanced endoscopy have been proposed as well, including narrow band imaging and various forms of spectroscopy. To date, none have been subjected to a trial. Molecular markers, whether from serum, RNA or stool, may also hold promise for complementing or replacing dysplasia surveillance, but as yet they have not been incorporated into surveillance protocols.

COLORECTAL CANCER IN CROHN DISEASE

Like UC, colitis in Crohn disease carries a risk for CRC greater than that of the general population. This was not always appreciated, however, as initial reports noted only a small, and sometimes not statistically significant, increase in CRC among patients with Crohn disease (109,110). A number of factors likely contributed to the dilution of the true effect of Crohn disease on colorectal carcinogenesis. First, patients with disease limited to the small bowel were included in some calculations of incidence. Second, patients who had undergone surgery, particularly colectomy, were often included. And finally, a number of investigators performed their analyses without taking into account the duration of disease, or more importantly, the extent of colonic involvement for this often segmental disease. Together, these factors resulted in a long-held belief that Crohn disease carried a *lower* risk for colon cancer than UC. Other studies (111–114) and even reanalysis of original data in which only subjects with long-standing and anatomically substantial Crohn colitis were examined (115) demonstrated that Crohn *colitis* harbored a CRC risk increase similar to that of UC and that both greater duration of colitis and greater length of involved colon increased the risk.

As with UC, earlier disease onset resulted in even greater increases in relative risk of CRC, likely as a function decreased risk in the rate of sporadic CRC used in the denominator of these calculations. Population-based studies from separate continents have demonstrated a clear increase in CRC rates not only when limited to cases of Crohn colitis, but even when all patients with Crohn disease are considered (20,116). A recent meta-analysis by Canavan and colleagues (117) calculated a pooled estimate of CRC relative risk to be 2.5 (95% CI: 1.3-4.7) for all patients with Crohn disease, culled from 12 published articles; for patients with colonic disease (in the 4 reports where it was available), the pooled RR was 4.5 (95% CI: 1.3-14.9). Clearly patients with Crohn disease have a higher risk than the general population.

Similarities Between CRC in Crohn Colitis and UC and Rationale Behind Recommendation for Surveillance

In addition to the greater rate and earlier appearance of CRC in Crohn colitis when compared to the general population, investigators have noted other important similarities between Crohn-related CRC and UC-related CRC (118). These include:

- A higher proportion of mucinous and signet-ring histology
- A greater proportion of synchronous lesions compared with sporadic CRC

- Similar survival rates once detected (also true of sporadic CRC)
- Presence of tumor in areas of macroscopic disease (although this point remains in question for Crohn disease)
- Presence of dysplasia adjacent to and distant from tumor, suggesting a field effect

This latter feature has led a number of experts to recommend a strategy of serial surveillance colonoscopy for patients with long-standing, extensive Crohn colitis as is performed and recommended for UC patients. To date, only one single-practice-based retrospective Crohn surveillance program has been reported in the literature. In this study, Friedman and colleagues (119) demonstrated both the feasibility and practicality of surveillance in patients with Crohn disease with colitis affecting at least one third of their colon for a minimum of 8 years. The authors detected dysplasia or cancer in 16% of their 259 patients over a 16-year period, in which 663 examinations were performed; there were no cancer deaths (119). As this is the only available study describing a surveillance program in Crohn disease, and there is no available control arm (i.e., no surveillance) against which to compare mortality rates, the efficacy of surveillance in Crohn disease is not yet established. Nevertheless, it has been recommended that all patients with extensive Crohn colitis (greater than one third of colon involved) undergo periodic surveillance or be recommended prophylactic surgery after 8 years of disease, as is done with extensive UC. Guidelines have suggested that practices used in surveillance should be similar to those demonstrated to be able to rule out dysplasia in UC (3). The effects of agents thought to be chemopreventive in UC are untested in Crohn disease.

CROHN DISEASE AND ADENOCARCINOMA OF THE SMALL INTESTINE

As with colonic adenocarcinoma in Crohn colitis, an increased risk of small intestine adenocarcinoma has been demonstrated in patients with small bowel Crohn disease. Unlike CRC, the second most common lethal malignancy in the United States, adenocarcinoma of the small intestine is uncommon. Even when evaluated in population-based reports, absolute number are quite small, with the largest such series having only five patients with small bowel adenocarcinoma (20). A summary of these studies is presented in Table 45.2.

Because the absolute rates for these cancers are so small, and the best means of prevention is uncertain if a preclinical, precancerous finding were detected, it would be impractical to perform screening and surveillance in all patients with small bowel Crohn disease. When there is a change in clinical symptoms or a change in barium examinations, however, the possibility of a small bowel malignancy should be entertained, particularly in a patient with long-standing disease.

OTHER MALIGNANCIES

Following case reports and series of extraintestinal malignancies, investigators questioned whether certain neoplasms might be related to either the presence or treatment of IBD. Greenstein and colleagues (120) performed one of the first studies in which relative risks were calculated. Using patients hospitalized for IBD at a tertiary care hospital, the authors determined that there was an increased incidence of leukemias, lymphomas, and squamous cell cancers when compared with published population-based controls (120). Given the source of their sampling, a likelihood of selection and detection biases must be considered. Other referral-based studies examining this issue have demonstrated increased incidence of leukemias (121,122) as well as bile duct (28), and endometrial cancers (28). Despite the large number of Crohn disease and UC patients, low absolute numbers of extraintestinal malignancies with broad confidence intervals have resulted in claims of "significance," when one less case would have resulted in "no significance." Ultimately, population-based analyses of cancer incidence in IBD have replaced the center-specific studies with their inherent biases. One such population-based study came from Ekbom and colleagues (116), who determined that in a cohort from Uppsala, Sweden, there was no increase in the incidence of leukemias, lymphomas, bile duct cancers or uterine cancers. However, an increase was noted in connective tissue cancers and squamous cell cancers of the skin, as well as brain cancers among patients with extensive UC (116). It is worth noting, however, that no adjustments were made for the multiple comparisons in the studies by Ekbom et al. (116).

Other population-based studies have also failed to detect an increased number of extraintestinal malignancies. These include another Swedish study in which patients with Crohn disease from Stockholm County were analyzed (123)—only a slight increase in bladder cancer was found and no increase in leukemias, lymphomas, bile duct cancers, or endometrial cancers was demonstrated—and one from North America (20). In

Table 45.2					
Studies of Small Intestinal Cancer and Crohn Disease					
Year	Study (Ref.)	No. of Patients	Cases	Risk/Odds	95% CI
1992	Ekbom et al. (116)	1,655	1	3.4	0.1–18.6
1993	Munkholm et al. (110)	373	2	50	37.1–65.9
1994	Persson et al. (123)	1,251	4	15.6	4.7–40.1
2001	Bernstein et al. (20)	2,857	5	17.4	4.2–72.9

CI, confidence interval.

this latter population-based study from Manitoba, Canada, that included >6,000 IBD patients, Bernstein and colleagues (20) found an increase in liver and biliary tumors in both Crohn disease and UC (with only five such cases) and a small increase in lymphomas only among men with Crohn disease. As increased rates of lymphoma and other hematologic malignancies have been raised as possible adverse effects of either azathioprine or 6-mercaptopurine use in other conditions (124–126) and rates of these malignancies have been calculated in series from large referral practices and centers (127,128), it is notable that Bernstein and colleagues (20) demonstrated *no* relation to an increased risk of hematologic malignancies and purine analogue use, the first population-based data set to do so. More recently, rare lymphomas (hepatosplenic T-cell lymphomas), particularly in younger patients, have been noted with anti-tumor necrosis factor therapy particularly in combination with purine analog immunomodulators (129).

CONCLUSIONS

CRC remains a major threat to patients with long-standing UC and Crohn colitis. Because of patients' and physicians' desires to avoid unnecessary surgery, prophylactic colectomies are rarely performed in these patients. Instead, caregivers and IBD patients tend to elect a program of dysplasia surveillance in an effort to simultaneously minimize cancer mortality and unnecessary colectomies. Although only circumstantial evidence supports the use of such a strategy as a means of reducing CRC-related mortality, dysplasia surveillance will remain the standard of care until better tests are available. Small intestinal cancer occurs at an increased rate in patients with Crohn enteritis, but the absolute risk remains small. Extraintestinal malignancies are uncommon in IBD but lymphomas, biliary tract cancers, and squamous cell cancers of the skin may occur at an increased rate in IBD patients. The mechanisms for all of these processes remain elusive, but it is hoped that advances in molecular medicine will help to unravel these issues in the future.

REFERENCES

1. Itzkowitz SH, Yio X. Inflammation and cancer IV. Colorectal cancer in inflammatory bowel disease: the role of inflammation. *Am J Physiol Gastrointest Liver Physiol.* 2004;287:G7–17.
2. Itzkowitz SH. Inflammatory bowel disease and cancer. *Gastroenterol Clin North Am.* 1997;26:129–139.
3. Itzkowitz SH, Harpaz N. Diagnosis and management of dysplasia in patients with inflammatory bowel diseases. *Gastroenterology.* 2004;126:1634–1648.
4. Brentnall TA, Crispin DA, Rabinovitch PS, et al. Mutations in the p53 gene: an early marker of neoplastic progression in ulcerative colitis. *Gastroenterology.* 1994;107:369–378.
5. Brentnall TA, Crispin DA, Bronner MP, et al. Microsatellite instability in nonneoplastic mucosa from patients with chronic ulcerative colitis. *Cancer Res.* 1996;56:1237–1240.
6. Suzuki H, Harpaz N, Tarmin L, et al. Microsatellite instability in ulcerative colitis-associated colorectal dysplasias and cancers. *Cancer Res.* 1994;54:4841–4844.
7. Crohn BB, Rosenberg H. The sigmoidoscopic picture of chronic ulcerative colitis. *Am J Med Sci.* 1925;170:220–228.

8. Bargen TA. Chronic ulcerative colitis associated with malignant disease. *Arch Surg.* 1928;17:862–868.
9. Devroede GJ, Taylor WF, Sauer WG, et al. Cancer risk and life expectancy of children with ulcerative colitis. *N Engl J Med.* 1971;285:17–21.
10. Bargen JA, Gage RP. Carcinoma and ulcerative colitis: prognosis. *Gastroenterology.* 1960;39:385–392.
11. Slaney G, Brooke BN. Cancer in ulcerative colitis. *Lancet.* 1959;2:694–698.
12. Rozen P, Baratz M, Fefer F, et al. Low incidence of significant dysplasia in a successful endoscopic surveillance program of patients with ulcerative colitis. *Gastroenterology.* 1995;108:1361–1370.
13. Ekbom A, Helmick C, Zack M, et al. Ulcerative colitis and colorectal cancer. A population-based study. *N Engl J Med.* 1990;323:1228–1233.
14. Gilat T, Fireman Z, Grossman A, et al. Colorectal cancer in patients with ulcerative colitis. A population study in central Israel. *Gastroenterology.* 1988;94:870–877.
15. Leidenius M, Kellokumpu I, Husa A, et al. Dysplasia and carcinoma in longstanding ulcerative colitis: an endoscopic and histological surveillance programme. *Gut.* 1991;32:1521–1525.
16. Langholz E, Munkholm P, Davidsen M, et al. Colorectal cancer risk and mortality in patients with ulcerative colitis. *Gastroenterology.* 1992;103:1444–1451.
17. Eaden JA, Abrams KR, Mayberry JF. The risk of colorectal cancer in ulcerative colitis: a meta-analysis. *Gut.* 2001;48:526–535.
18. Winther KV, Jess T, Langholz E, et al. Long-term risk of cancer in ulcerative colitis: a population-based cohort study from Copenhagen County. *Clin Gastroenterol Hepatol.* 2004;2:1088–1095.
19. Lakatos L, Mester G, Erdelyi Z, et al. Risk factors for ulcerative colitis-associated colorectal cancer in a Hungarian cohort of patients with ulcerative colitis: results of a population-based study. *Inflamm Bowel Dis.* 2006;12:205–211.
20. Bernstein CN, Blanchard JF, Kliewer E, et al. Cancer risk in patients with inflammatory bowel disease: a population-based study. *Cancer.* 2001;91:854–862.
21. Jess T, Loftus EV, Jr., Velayos FS, et al. Risk of intestinal cancer in inflammatory bowel disease: a population-based study from olmsted county, Minnesota. *Gastroenterology.* 2006;130:1039–1046.
22. Rutter MD, Saunders BP, Wilkinson KH, et al. Thirty-year analysis of a colonoscopic surveillance program for neoplasia in ulcerative colitis. *Gastroenterology.* 2006;130:1030–1038.
23. Edwards F, Truelove S. The course and prognosis of ulcerative colitis. III and IV. *Gut.* 1964;5:1.
24. Gyde SN, Prior P, Allan RN, et al. Colorectal cancer in ulcerative colitis: a cohort study of primary referrals from three centres. *Gut.* 1988;29:206–217.
25. Greenstein AJ, Sachar DB, Smith H, et al. Cancer in universal and left-sided ulcerative colitis: factors determining risk. *Gastroenterology.* 1979;77:290–294.
26. Langholz E, Munkholm P, Davidsen M, et al. Changes in extent of ulcerative colitis: a study on the course and prognostic factors. *Scand J Gastroenterol.* 1996;31:260–266.
27. Katzka I, Brody RS, Morris E, et al. Assessment of colorectal cancer risk in patients with ulcerative colitis: experience from a private practice. *Gastroenterology.* 1983;85:22–29.
28. Mir-Madjlessi SH, Farmer RG, Easley KA, et al. Colorectal and extracolonic malignancy in ulcerative colitis. *Cancer.* 1986;58:1569–1574.
29. Mathy C, Schneider K, Chen YY, et al. Gross versus microscopic pancolitis and the occurrence of neoplasia in ulcerative colitis. *Inflamm Bowel Dis.* 2003;9:351–355.

30. Gurbuz AK, Giardiello FM, Bayless TM. Colorectal neoplasia in patients with ulcerative colitis and primary sclerosing cholangitis. *Dis Colon Rectum*. 1995;38:37–41.

31. Loftus EV, Jr., Sandborn WJ, Tremaine WJ, et al. Risk of colorectal neoplasia in patients with primary sclerosing cholangitis. *Gastroenterology*. 1996;110:432–440.

32. Nuako KW, Ahlquist DA, Sandborn WJ, et al. Primary sclerosing cholangitis and colorectal carcinoma in patients with chronic ulcerative colitis: a case-control study. *Cancer*. 1998;82:822–826.

33. Brentnall TA, Haggitt RC, Rabinovitch PS, et al. Risk and natural history of colonic neoplasia in patients with primary sclerosing cholangitis and ulcerative colitis [see comments]. *Gastroenterology*. 1996;110:331–338.

34. Broome U, Lindberg G, Lofberg R. Primary sclerosing cholangitis in ulcerative colitis–a risk factor for the development of dysplasia and DNA aneuploidy? *Gastroenterology*. 1992;102:1877–1880.

35. Broome U, Lofberg R, Veress B, et al. Primary sclerosing cholangitis and ulcerative colitis: evidence for increased neoplastic potential. *Hepatology*. 1995;22:1404–1408.

36. D'Haens GR, Lashner BA, Hanauer SB. Pericholangitis and sclerosing cholangitis are risk factors for dysplasia and cancer in ulcerative colitis. *Am J Gastroenterol*. 1993;88:1174–1178.

37. Marchesa P, Lashner BA, Lavery IC, et al. The risk of cancer and dysplasia among ulcerative colitis patients with primary sclerosing cholangitis. *Am J Gastroenterol*. 1997;92:1285–1288.

38. Kornfeld D, Ekbom A, Ihre T. Is there an excess risk for colorectal cancer in patients with ulcerative colitis and concomitant primary sclerosing cholangitis? A population based study [see comments]. *Gut*. 1997;41:522–525.

39. Burt RW. Familial risk and colorectal cancer. *Gastroenterol Clin North Am*. 1996;25:793–803.

40. Lashner BA, Heidenreich PA, Su GL, et al. Effect of folate supplementation on the incidence of dysplasia and cancer in chronic ulcerative colitis. A case-control study [see comments]. *Gastroenterology*. 1989;97:255–259.

41. Lashner BA, Provencher KS, Seidner DL, et al. The effect of folic acid supplementation on the risk for cancer or dysplasia in ulcerative colitis. *Gastroenterology*. 1997;112:29–32.

42. Nuako KW, Ahlquist DA, Mahoney DW, et al. Familial predisposition for colorectal cancer in chronic ulcerative colitis: a case-control study. *Gastroenterology*. 1998;115:1079–1083.

43. Askling J, Dickman PW, Karlen P, et al. Family history as a risk factor for colorectal cancer in inflammatory bowel disease. *Gastroenterology*. 2001;120:1356–1362.

44. Eaden J, Abrams K, Ekbom A, et al. Colorectal cancer prevention in ulcerative colitis: a case-control study. *Aliment Pharmacol Ther*. 2000;14:145–153.

45. Rutter M, Saunders B, Wilkinson K, et al. Severity of inflammation is a risk factor for colorectal neoplasia in ulcerative colitis. *Gastroenterology*. 2004;126:451–459.

46. Gupta RB, Harpaz N, Itzkowitz S, et al. Histologic inflammation is a risk factor for progression to colorectal neoplasia in ulcerative colitis: a cohort study. *Gastroenterology*. 2007;133:1099–1105.

47. Pinczowski D, Ekbom A, Baron J, et al. Risk factors for colorectal cancer in patients with ulcerative colitis: a case-control study. *Gastroenterology*. 1994;107:117–120.

48. Tung BY, Emond MJ, Haggitt RC, et al. Ursodiol use is associated with lower prevalence of colonic neoplasia in patients with ulcerative colitis and primary sclerosing cholangitis. *Ann Intern Med*. 2001;134:89–95.

49. van Staa TP, Card T, Logan RF, et al. 5-Aminosalicylate use and colorectal cancer risk in inflammatory bowel disease: a large epidemiological study. *Gut*. 2005;54:1573–1578.

50. Rubin DT, LoSavio A, Yadron N, et al. Aminosalicylate therapy in the prevention of dysplasia and colorectal cancer in ulcerative colitis. *Clin Gastroenterol Hepatol*. 2006;4:1346–1350.

51. Bernstein CN, Blanchard JF, Metge C, et al. Does the use of 5-aminosalicylates in inflammatory bowel disease prevent the development of colorectal cancer? *Am J Gastroenterol*. 2003;98:2784–2788.

52. Terdiman JP, Steinbuch M, Blumentals WA, et al. 5-Aminosalicylic acid therapy and the risk of colorectal cancer among patients with inflammatory bowel disease. *Inflamm Bowel Dis*. 2006.

53. Velayos FS, Terdiman JP, Walsh JM. Effect of 5-aminosalicylate use on colorectal cancer and dysplasia risk: a systematic review and metaanalysis of observational studies. *Am J Gastroenterol*. 2005;100:1345–1353.

54. Pardi DS, Loftus EV, Jr., Kremers WK, et al. Ursodeoxycholic acid as a chemopreventive agent in patients with ulcerative colitis and primary sclerosing cholangitis. *Gastroenterology*. 2003;124:889–893.

55. Choi PM, Nugent FW, Schoetz DJ, Jr., et al. Colonoscopic surveillance reduces mortality from colorectal cancer in ulcerative colitis. *Gastroenterology*. 1993;105:418–424.

56. Connell WR, Lennard-Jones JE, Williams CB, et al. Factors affecting the outcome of endoscopic surveillance for cancer in ulcerative colitis [see comments]. *Gastroenterology*. 1994;107:934–944.

57. Becker JM. Surgical therapy for ulcerative colitis and Crohn's disease. *Gastroenterol Clin North Am*. 1999;28:371–390, viii–ix.

58. Stern H, Walfisch S, Mullen B, et al. Cancer in an ileoanal reservoir: a new late complication? *Gut*. 1990;31:473–475.

59. Thompson-Fawcett MW, Marcus V, Redston M, et al. Risk of dysplasia in long-term ileal pouches and pouches with chronic pouchitis. *Gastroenterology*. 2001;121:275–281.

60. Morson BC, Pang LS. Rectal biopsy as an aid to cancer control in ulcerative colitis. *Gut*. 1967;8:423–434.

61. Cook MG, Goligher JC. Carcinoma and epithelial dysplasia complicating ulcerative colitis. *Gastroenterology*. 1975;68:1127–1136.

62. Ransohoff DF, Riddell RH, Levin B. Ulcerative colitis and colonic cancer. Problems in assessing the diagnostic usefulness of mucosal dysplasia. *Dis Colon Rectum*. 1985;28:383–388.

63. Taylor BA, Pemberton JH, Carpenter HA, et al. Dysplasia in chronic ulcerative colitis: implications for colonoscopic surveillance. *Dis Colon Rectum*. 1992;35:950–956.

64. Dickinson RJ, Dixon MF, Axon AT. Colonoscopy and the detection of dysplasia in patients with longstanding ulcerative colitis. *Lancet*. 1980;2:620–622.

65. Levin B, Lennard-Jones J, Riddell RH, et al. Surveillance of patients with chronic ulcerative colitis. WHO Collaborating Centre for the Prevention of Colorectal Cancer. *Bull World Health Organ*. 1991;69:121–126.

66. Kornbluth A, Sachar DB. Ulcerative colitis practice guidelines in adults. American College of Gastroenterology, Practice Parameters Committee. *Am J Gastroenterol*. 1997;92:204–211.

67. Brostrom O, Lofberg R, Ost A, et al. Cancer surveillance of patients with longstanding ulcerative colitis: a clinical, endoscopical, and histological study. *Gut*. 1986;27:1408–1413.

68. Blackstone MO, Riddell RH, Rogers BH, et al. Dysplasia-associated lesion or mass (DALM) detected by colonoscopy in long-standing ulcerative colitis: an indication for colectomy. *Gastroenterology*. 1981;80:366–374.

69. Lashner BA, Silverstein MD, Hanauer SB. Hazard rates for dysplasia and cancer in ulcerative colitis. Results from a surveillance program. *Dig Dis Sci*. 1989;34:1536–1541.

70. Lashner BA, Kane SV, Hanauer SB. Colon cancer surveillance in chronic ulcerative colitis: historical cohort study. *Am J Gastroenterol*. 1990;85:1083–1087.

71. Lennard-Jones JE, Morson BC, Ritchie JK, et al. Cancer in colitis: assessment of the individual risk by clinical and histological criteria. *Gastroenterology*. 1977;73:1280–1289.

72. Lennard-Jones JE, Melville DM, Morson BC, et al. Precancer and cancer in extensive ulcerative colitis: findings among 401 patients over 22 years. *Gut*. 1990;31:800–806.

73. Lofberg R, Brostrom O, Karlen P, et al. Colonoscopic surveillance in long-standing total ulcerative colitis–a 15-year follow-up study. *Gastroenterology*. 1990;99:1021–1031.

74. Lynch DA, Lobo AJ, Sobala GM, et al. Failure of colonoscopic surveillance in ulcerative colitis [see comments]. *Gut*. 1993;34:1075–1080.

75. Nugent FW, Haggitt RC, Gilpin PA. Cancer surveillance in ulcerative colitis [see comments]. *Gastroenterology*. 1991;100:1241–1248.

76. Rutegard J, Ahsgren L, Stenling R, et al. Ulcerative colitis. Cancer surveillance in an unselected population. *Scand J Gastroenterol*. 1988;23:139–145.

77. Woolrich AJ, DaSilva MD, Korelitz BI. Surveillance in the routine management of ulcerative colitis: the predictive value of low-grade dysplasia. *Gastroenterology*. 1992;103:431–438.

78. Ullman T, Croog V, Harpaz N, et al. Progression of flat low-grade dysplasia to advanced neoplasia in patients with ulcerative colitis. *Gastroenterology*. 2003;125:1311–1319.

79. Karlen P, Kornfeld D, Brostrom O, et al. Is colonoscopic surveillance reducing colorectal cancer mortality in ulcerative colitis? A population based case control study. *Gut*. 1998;42:711–714.

80. Velayos FS, Loftus EV, Jr., Jess T, et al. Predictive and protective factors associated with colorectal cancer in ulcerative colitis: A case-control study. *Gastroenterology*. 2006;130:1941–1949.

81. Gage TP. Managing the cancer risk in chronic ulcerative colitis. A decision-analytic approach. *J Clin Gastroenterol*. 1986;8:50–57.

82. Delco F, Sonnenberg A. A decision analysis of surveillance for colorectal cancer in ulcerative colitis. *Gut*. 2000;46:500–506.

83. Inadomi JM. Cost-effectiveness of colorectal cancer surveillance in ulcerative colitis. *Scand J Gastroenterol Suppl*. 2003:17–21.

84. Delco F, Sonnenberg A. A decision analysis of surveillance for colorectal cancer in ulcerative colitis. *Gut*. 2000;46:500–506.

85. Provenzale D, Kowdley KV, Arora S, et al. Prophylactic colectomy or surveillance for chronic ulcerative colitis? A decision analysis [see comments]. *Gastroenterology*. 1995;109:1188–1196.

86. Riddell RH, Goldman H, Ransohoff DF, et al. Dysplasia in inflammatory bowel disease: standardized classification with provisional clinical applications. *Hum Pathol*. 1983;14:931–968.

87. Eaden J, Abrams K, McKay H, et al. Inter-observer variation between general and specialist gastrointestinal pathologists when grading dysplasia in ulcerative colitis. *J Pathol*. 2001;194:152–157.

88. Dixon MF, Brown LJ, Gilmour HM, et al. Observer variation in the assessment of dysplasia in ulcerative colitis. *Histopathology*. 1988;13:385–397.

89. Melville DM, Jass JR, Morson BC, et al. Observer study of the grading of dysplasia in ulcerative colitis: comparison with clinical outcome. *Hum Pathol*. 1989;20:1008–1014.

90. Connell WR, Talbot IC, Harpaz N, et al. Clinicopathological characteristics of colorectal carcinoma complicating ulcerative colitis. *Gut*. 1994;35:1419–1423.

91. Ullman TA, Loftus EV, Jr., Kakar S, et al. The fate of low grade dysplasia in ulcerative colitis. *Am J Gastroenterol*. 2002;97:922–927.

92. Brentnall T, Bronner M, Rubin C, et al. Natural history and management of low-grade dysplasia in ulcerative colitis. *Gastroenterology*. 1999;116:A382.

93. Befrits R, Ljung T, Jaramillo E, et al. Low grade dysplasia in flat colonic mucosa in patients with extensive longstanding inflammatory bowel disease—a follow-up study. *Gastroenterology*. 1999;116:A376.

94. Befrits R, Ljung T, Jaramillo E, et al. Low-grade dysplasia in extensive, long-standing inflammatory bowel disease: a follow-up study. *Dis Colon Rectum*. 2002;45:615–620.

95. Lim CH, Dixon MF, Vail A, et al. Ten year follow up of ulcerative colitis patients with and without low grade dysplasia. *Gut*. 2003;52:1127–1132.

96. Rubin CE, Haggitt RC, Burmer GC, et al. DNA aneuploidy in colonic biopsies predicts future development of dysplasia in ulcerative colitis. *Gastroenterology*. 1992;103:1611–1620.

97. Eaden JA, Ward BA, Mayberry JF. How gastroenterologists screen for colonic cancer in ulcerative colitis: an analysis of performance. *Gastrointest Endosc*. 2000;51:123–128.

98. Ullman T, White J, Harpaz N, et al. Assessment of Biopsy Practices in Colonoscopic Surveillance in Ulcerative Colitis. *Gastroenterology*. 2001;120:A–446.

99. Rubin PH, et al. Colonoscopic polypectomy in chronic colitis: conservative management after endoscopic resection of dysplastic polyps. *Gastroenterology*. 1999;117:1295–1300.

100. Engelsgjerd M, Farraye FA, Odze RD. Polypectomy may be adequate treatment for adenoma-like dysplastic lesions in chronic ulcerative colitis [see comments]. *Gastroenterology*. 1999;117:1288–1294; discussion 1488–1491.

101. Odze RD, Farraye FA, Hecht JL, et al. Long-term follow-up after polypectomy treatment for adenoma-like dysplastic lesions in ulcerative colitis. *Clin Gastroenterol Hepatol*. 2004;2:534–541.

102. Vieth M, Behrens H, Stolte M. Sporadic adenoma in ulcerative colitis: endoscopic resection is an adequate treatment. *Gut*. 2006;55:1151–1155.

103. Selaru FM, Xu Y, Yin J, et al. Artificial neural networks distinguish among subtypes of neoplastic colorectal lesions. *Gastroenterology*. 2002;122:606–613.

104. Bernstein CN, Weinstein WM, Levine DS, et al. Physicians' perceptions of dysplasia and approaches to surveillance colonoscopy in ulcerative colitis [see comments]. *Am J Gastroenterol*. 1995;90:2106–2114.

105. Rubin DT, Turner JR. Surveillance of dysplasia in inflammatory bowel disease: The gastroenterologist-pathologist partnership. *Clin Gastroenterol Hepatol*. 2006;4:1309–1313.

106. Itzkowitz SH, Present DH. Consensus conference: Colorectal cancer screening and surveillance in inflammatory bowel disease. *Inflamm Bowel Dis*. 2005;11:314–321.

107. Kiesslich R, Fritsch J, Holtmann M, et al. Methylene blue-aided chromoendoscopy for the detection of intraepithelial neoplasia and colon cancer in ulcerative colitis. *Gastroenterology*. 2003;124:880–888.

108. Rutter MD, Saunders BP, Schofield G, et al. Pancolonic indigo carmine dye spraying for the detection of dysplasia in ulcerative colitis. *Gut*. 2004;53:256–260.

109. Gollop JH, Phillips SF, Melton LJ, 3rd, et al. Epidemiologic aspects of Crohn's disease: a population based study in Olmsted County, Minnesota, 1943–1982. Gut 1988;29:49–56.

110. Munkholm P, Langholz E, Davidsen M, et al. Intestinal cancer risk and mortality in patients with Crohn's disease. *Gastroenterology*. 1993;105:1716–1723.

111. Weedon DD, Shorter RG, Ilstrup DM, et al. Crohn's disease and cancer. *N Engl J Med*. 1973;289:1099–1103.

112. Greenstein AJ, Sachar DB, Smith H, et al. A comparison of cancer risk in Crohn's disease and ulcerative colitis. *Cancer*. 1981;48:2742–2745.

113. Bernstein CN, Shanahan F, Weinstein WM, et al. Are we telling patients the truth about surveillance colonoscopy in ulcerative colitis? *Lancet*. 1994;343(8889).

114. Gillen CD, Walmsley RS, Prior P, et al. Ulcerative colitis and Crohn's disease: a comparison of the colorectal cancer risk in extensive colitis. *Gut.* 1994;35:1590–1592.

115. Ekbom A, Helmick C, Zack M, et al. Increased risk of large-bowel cancer in Crohn's disease with colonic involvement. *Lancet.* 1990;336:357–359.

116. Sachar DB. Cancer in Crohn's disease: dispelling the myths. *Gut.* 1994;35:1507–1508.

117. Ekbom A, Helmick C, Zack M, et al. Extracolonic malignancies in inflammatory bowel disease. *Cancer.* 1991;67:2015–2019.

118. Canavan C, Abrams KR, Mayberry J. Meta-analysis: colorectal and small bowel cancer risk in patients with Crohn's disease. *Aliment Pharmacol Ther.* 2006;23:1097–1104.

119. Choi PM, Zelig MP. Similarity of colorectal cancer in Crohn's disease and ulcerative colitis: implications for carcinogenesis and prevention. *Gut.* 1994;35:950–954.

120. Friedman S, Rubin PH, Bodian C, et al. Screening and surveillance colonoscopy in chronic Crohn's colitis. *Gastroenterology.* 2001;120:820–826.

121. Greenstein AJ, Gennuso R, Sachar DB, et al. Extraintestinal cancers in inflammatory bowel disease. *Cancer.* 1985;56:2914–2921.

122. Mir Madjlessi SH, Farmer RG, Weick JK. Inflammatory bowel disease and leukemia. A report of seven cases of leukemia in ulcerative colitis and Crohn's disease and review of the literature. *Dig Dis Sci.* 1986;31:1025–1031.

123. Cuttner J. Increased incidence of acute promyelocytic leukemia in patients with ulcerative colitis. *Ann Intern Med.* 1982;97:864–865.

124. Persson PG, Karlen P, Bernell O, et al. Crohn's disease and cancer: a population-based cohort study. *Gastroenterology.* 1994;107:1675–1679.

125. Wilkinson AH, Smith JL, Hunsicker LG, et al. Increased frequency of posttransplant lymphomas in patients treated with cyclosporine, azathioprine, and prednisone. *Transplantation.* 1989;47:293–296.

126. Opelz G, Henderson R. Incidence of non-Hodgkin lymphoma in kidney and heart transplant recipients. *Lancet.* 1993;342:1514–1516.

127. Silman AJ, Petrie J, Hazleman B, et al. Lymphoproliferative cancer and other malignancy in patients with rheumatoid arthritis treated with azathioprine: a 20 year follow up study. *Ann Rheum Dis.* 1988;47:988–992.

128. Loftus EV, Jr., Tremaine WJ, Habermann TM, et al. Risk of lymphoma in inflammatory bowel disease. *Am J Gastroenterol.* 2000;95:2308–2312.

129. Korelitz BI, Mirsky FJ, Fleisher MR, et al. Malignant neoplasms subsequent to treatment of inflammatory bowel disease with 6-mercaptopurine. *Am J Gastroenterol.* 1999;94:3248–3253.

130. Mackey AC, Green L, Liang LC, et al. Hepatosplenic T cell lymphoma associated with infliximab use in young patients treated for inflammatory bowel disease. *J Pediatr Gastroenterol Nutr.* 2007;44:265–267.

COMMENTARY
David A. Etzioni and Ann C. Lowry

For patients with inflammatory bowel disease (IBD), the increased relative risk of developing a gastrointestinal malignancy is certainly the addition of insult to injury. The initial approach to a patient with a suspected or established diagnosis of IBD is always to gain an understanding of the patient's disease manifestation. IBD is broadly categorized into two main types, Crohn's disease and ulcerative colitis, but this distinction may not serve all patients well. A third category of colitis, indeterminate colitis, encompasses a spectrum of clinical findings that does not fit neatly into either category.

The preceding chapter by Dr. Ullman is an excellent synthesis of existing literature regarding the pathogenesis of dysplasia/carcinoma in the gastrointestinal tract of patients with IBD, as well as of surveillance strategies targeted at early detection. In this commentary, the focus will be on the surgical treatment of malignancies arising in the context of IBD, with specific attention to how treatment options vary among ulcerative colitis, Crohn's disease, and indeterminate colitis.

ULCERATIVE COLITIS

Patients with ulcerative colitis are at increased risk for developing colorectal carcinoma. Despite prevention efforts, dysplasia and carcinoma are still identified in patients with ulcerative colitis. The following discussion of surgical treatment presents the management of colonic disease separately from that of the rectum because of differences in their biology and the consequences of treatment.

Indications for Surgical Management

The development of dysplasia or carcinoma in a patient with ulcerative colitis constitutes a landmark event in the disease process. Unlike similar disease arising in a patient without IBD, these findings generally occur in the context of multifocal changes, a "field change." Treatment decisions must address the entire large intestine not only in terms of the dysplasia/carcinoma at hand, but also in terms of the need for future surveillance.

The development of carcinoma of the colon or rectum in a patient with ulcerative colitis is a firm indication for colectomy. Dysplasia (flat vs. raised) and sporadic adenoma are more controversial indications for surgery.

Flat Dysplasia

Professional guidelines uniformly recommend that IBD patients with a surveillance biopsy showing high-grade dysplasia (HGD) should be offered a colectomy (1–3). Considerable differences of opinion exist, however, regarding the management of low-grade dysplasia (LGD).

The Crohn's and Colitis Foundation of America recommendations state that a finding of focal LGD on surveillance biopsy should prompt the discussion of competing options: colectomy versus continued surveillance (1). These recommendations also raise the important distinction between a unifocal finding (LGD in a single biopsy specimen) versus multifocal results (LGD in two or more biopsy specimens); they advise that patients with multifocal disease should be ". . . strongly encouraged to undergo prophylactic total proctocolectomy." Guidelines from the American Society of Gastrointestinal Endoscopy and the American Society of Colon and Rectal Surgeons do not specifically address the management of unifocal LGD detected on surveillance biopsy (2,3).

A recommendation for colectomy on the basis of LGD seems dramatic, but has basis in evidence. In a series of 46 ulcerative colitis patients surveyed at St. Mark's Hospital, approximately 20% of patients with LGD undergoing colectomy had carcinoma in the resected specimen. In the same series, 5 of 11 patients (45%) with HGD were found to have carcinoma in their colectomy specimen (4). Another series of 46 patients with ulcerative colitis and LGD treated at Mt Sinai in New York noted a 53% progression to more advanced neoplasia (HGD or carcinoma) at 5 years (5). Opposing this body of evidence, a Swedish group from the Karolinska Hospital published data on 60 patients with IBD and LGD followed for a mean of 10 years. They noted no progression from LGD to HGD or carcinoma in their cohort (6). Results from similar studies have reported intermediate results, finding neoplastic progression in 10% to 19% of patients with LGD (6,7). At minimum, it can be inferred that LGD implies a distinctly increased risk for developing/harboring HGD or carcinoma.

Dysplasia-Associated Mass and Sporadic Adenoma

The implication of a mass lesion in the large intestine of a patient with ulcerative colitis is another area of significant controversy. An important distinction is whether or not the lesion has associated dysplasia in the surrounding mucosa. Patients with ulcerative colitis can sporadically develop isolated adenomatous polyps that do not imply a field change within the colon. This concept is supported by several studies that monitored the natural history of sporadic adenomas in patients with IBD (8–10).

A dysplasia-associated lesion or mass arising within a field of dysplasia is generally considered an indication for a colectomy (1,3). However, in selected clinical situations in which biopsies from tissue surrounding a dysplastic lesion do not show dysplasia, some have argued that continued surveillance is adequate (2,11). Unfortunately, limited data exist to accurately define the risk of synchronous/metachronous carcinoma in these situations. Most surgeons consider this condition an indication for surgery.

The finding of a dysplasia-associated lesion or mass or a sporadic adenoma, if not treated with colectomy, should trigger an increased intensity of surveillance (12).

Surgical Management of Colonic Dysplasia and Carcinoma

There are several surgical options for patients with ulcerative colitis, each with different anatomic and functional implications. These strategies, often lumped under the basket term *colectomy*, are different than those that would be offered a patient without IBD. The rationale for a more radical surgical treatment is the need to treat (or survey) all of the at-risk colorectal mucosa.

Options include (a) total proctocolectomy with end ileostomy, (b) total proctocolectomy with ileoanal reservoir/anal anastomosis, and (c) total abdominal colectomy with ileorectal anastomosis. Choosing the most appropriate option for a specific patient hinges on several factors, including the amount of at-risk mucosa that remains after the procedure, burden of neoplasia, gastrointestinal function, quality of life, and the need for postoperative surveillance.

Restorative Proctocolectomy

Total proctocolectomy with construction of an ileal pouch-anal anastomosis (restorative proctocolectomy) is considered by most experts to be the procedure of choice for patients with ulcerative colitis requiring surgery. With this option, nearly the entirety of at-risk colorectal mucosa is removed with preservation of the anal sphincter mechanism, thereby providing a mechanism for continence. Restorative proctocolectomy can be performed in one, two, or three stages depending on the specific clinical situation. Because surgery for dysplasia or carcinoma is usually elective, the operative choice is between one and two stages.

With a one-stage or a two-stage procedure, the initial surgery entails total proctocolectomy and creation of an ileoanal reservoir. In a two-stage procedure a diverting ileostomy is placed 10 to 20 cm proximal to the ileoanal reservoir. The major drawback of a one-stage procedure is that pouch complications (most importantly, leak) are more dramatic and difficult to manage nonoperatively. The addition of a temporary diverting ileostomy is widely believed to be a safer option. Opinions vary widely regarding whether or not this increased risk is justified by the avoidance of a second-stage procedure (13,14).

In planning a restorative proctocolectomy, another major technical consideration is whether or not to perform a mucosectomy. During a mucosectomy, all mucosa above the dentate line is removed. There are documented cases of carcinoma occurring in the anal transition zone above the dentate line, which theoretically would have been avoided with a mucosectomy technique (15,16). On the other hand, even a mucosectomy does not guarantee removal of all the at-risk mucosa, as there have been reports of carcinoma arising in residual mucosal elements (17).

The alternative to mucosectomy is a double-stapled anastomosis, leaving behind 1 to 2 cm of rectal mucosa. Proponents of this technique argue that the procedure is technically easier and results in better functional outcomes (18,19). The residual anorectal mucosa poses specific drawbacks, not only for progression to dysplasia/carcinoma, but also ongoing inflammation due to the continued underlying disease process (20). One series from the Cleveland Clinic documented a 3.1% progression to LGD in the anal transition zone (mean follow-up, 2.3 years) with the stapled technique, prompting a recommendation for frequent surveillance (21,22). Inflammation of the residual rectal mucosal "cuff" is a problem for approximately 16% of patients, and may necessitate medical therapy (23).

Patients who successfully undergo restorative proctocolectomy generally enjoy good quality of life and continence. In a prospective study of 391 patients with a mean age of 33.7 years, Michelassi et al. (24) reported an average of five to six bowel movements per day within 1 year of surgery. Two thirds of their patients reported being fully continent.

Total Proctocolectomy and End Ileostomy

Total proctocolectomy with end ileostomy removes all the colorectal mucosa, including the entire anoderm. After this type of procedure the risk of developing a colorectal carcinoma is zero, thereby obviating the need for postoperative surveillance. Gastrointestinal function is necessarily routed into either a continent or an incontinent (Brooke) ileostomy.

Several institutions have accumulated a body of experience with the continent ileostomy. The Cleveland Clinic recently reported their experience with 330 patients using the Koch pouch technique. During a median follow-up period of 11 years, they noted a 10-year pouch survival of 87%, but with an average of 2.9 surgical revisions (25). Other approaches show promise, including the T-pouch technique currently employed at the University of Southern California (25). In general, the experience with continent ileostomy is a tradeoff between improved control over stoma function, and an increased need for subsequent surgical care.

Total Abdominal Colectomy and Ileorectal Anastomosis

With total abdominal colectomy and ileorectal anastomosis (IRA), a patient with ulcerative colitis may be spared the surgical and physiological burden of proctectomy. As a procedure for dysplasia or carcinoma it is certainly incomplete: the entire rectal mucosa is left behind, necessitating frequent future surveillance.

An IRA has significant benefits: the lesser extent of surgery and the ability to maintain anal sphincter function/continence in addition to the avoidance of risk of sexual and urinary dysfunction related to a proctectomy. Its long-term success in patients with ulcerative colitis is questionable, however. At 10 years, proctectomy is necessary in approximately 30% to 50% of patients, with failures due to recurrent inflammation, dysplasia, carcinoma, and technical complications (26,27). Patients with an IRA also must be willing to submit to frequent surveillance with flexible endoscopy.

In the context of a diagnosis of colonic dysplasia/carcinoma, an IRA should be entertained only in patients of prohibitive operative risk and rectal sparing in terms of disease activity and dysplasia (28). Patients who present with colon cancer and obvious nodal involvement or metastatic disease may be well served by an IRA as the recovery is generally faster, and chemotherapy could be started earlier.

Surgical Management of Rectal Dysplasia and Carcinoma

Evidence of dysplasia/carcinoma in the rectum mandates a set of treatment options that is distinctly different from ones appropriate for colonic disease.

With dysplasia in the rectum, total abdominal colectomy and ileorectal anastomosis would not be adequate treatment. Along the same lines of reasoning, a restorative proctocolectomy should be performed with mucosectomy in order to minimize the likelihood of persistent/recurrent dysplasia. Total proctocolectomy and end ileostomy is a viable alternative to restorative proctocolectomy, depending on specific patient characteristics and preferences.

Decision making for patients with rectal carcinoma is much more complicated because of the higher risk of local recurrence and frequent use of adjuvant therapies. The risk of local recurrence is much higher particularly in patients with T3/T4 or N1/N2 disease. Because of this, adjuvant chemotherapy and radiation are central elements of treatment of rectal cancer.

Current practice for all patients with rectal cancer includes preoperative radiation and chemotherapy for those staged as T3/T4 or N1 (stage IIa or higher). Postoperative therapy would be offered if the pathologic stage was higher than the preoperative clinical staging. Unfortunately, radiation treatment (either pre- or postoperative) raises concerns about reconstruction with a restorative proctocolectomy. Radiation therapy increases the risk of incontinence even in patients without IBD undergoing treatment for rectal cancer. Given the sensitivity of the small intestine to radiation, it would be difficult to recommend postoperative radiation following a restorative proctocolectomy. In addition, postoperative follow-up for recurrent pelvic disease would be more difficult.

Ideally, surgical planning would depend on preoperative staging, and patients meeting criteria for preoperative adjuvant treatment would receive therapy according to standard protocols. Patients with early-stage disease (T1/T2 and N0) would be offered either a restorative proctocolectomy or a total proctocolectomy and end ileostomy. This approach is fraught with some hazard, however, from inaccuracies with conventional staging technologies. In a recent meta-analysis, Bipat et al. (29) compared the accuracy of computed tomography, magnetic resonance imaging, and endorectal ultrasound in staging rectal cancer. They found that these imaging techniques discerned perirectal tissue invasion (T3 status) with sensitivity of 79% to 90% and specificity of 75% to 78%. Evaluation of nodal status is also less than perfect: a recent review by Skandarajah and Tjandra (30) reported an estimated accuracy of 73%. Although these techniques are the current standard for staging and treatment recommendations, there is a risk that the pathologic stage will be different.

Regardless of stage, the optimal oncologic procedure is a total proctocolectomy with an end ileostomy with consideration of neoadjuvant therapy for those patients with a preoperative stage of IIa or higher. However, many patients will seek a restorative procedure. If so, patients with early disease must be counseled regarding the risk of very difficult decisions if the pathologic stage is higher. For patients with higher stage disease, an ileoanal reservoir could be entertained if the cancer responds well to the preoperative treatment. This option should be considered only with significant discussion and counseling regarding the risks, both in terms of local recurrence and functional results.

CROHN'S DISEASE

With regard to the detection and treatment of gastrointestinal malignancies, Crohn's disease is distinctly different from ulcerative colitis. Appropriate surgical therapy for ulcerative colitis, whether for dysplasia/carcinoma or for refractory inflammation, must treat the entire large intestine. In rare cases, the rectum is left in situ with an ileorectal anastomosis, but these situations are unusual and necessitate a lifetime of close surveillance.

Decision making for patients with Crohn's disease is more complicated because of the nature of the disease, specifically its propensity to induce focal disease anywhere in the gastrointestinal tract. Surgical treatment of Crohn's disease may be performed for a broad range of indications, including obstruction, perforation, fistula, and carcinoma. The diagnosis of dysplasia/carcinoma is frequently not known at the time of surgery; the management of a postoperative (unsuspected) diagnosis of dysplasia/carcinoma will be addressed separately.

Indications for Surgical Management

As with ulcerative colitis, there is considerable controversy regarding the treatment of dysplasia in Crohn's disease; multifocal LGD and HGD are well-accepted indications for surgery. Unifocal LGD is more controversial. The development of carcinoma in the colon of a patient with Crohn's disease is a clear indication for colectomy.

Surgical Management of Colonic Dysplasia/ Carcinoma Known Preoperatively

Because of the nature of Crohn's disease, the surgical considerations are somewhat different from ulcerative colitis. Disease activity is more often segmental and the entire gastrointestinal tract is at risk for recurrence of symptomatic disease. Therefore, segmental resections are more acceptable with Crohn's disease than in ulcerative colitis. In treating Crohn's disease and colorectal dysplasia/carcinoma, the most difficult determination is the extent of surgery necessary for adequate treatment.

Segmental versus Extended Colectomy

Theoretically, the treatment of dysplasia/carcinoma arising in a patient with Crohn's disease can be either a segmental or an extended colectomy (subtotal colectomy, total abdominal colectomy, or total proctocolectomy). The decision making would ideally be informed by studies documenting rates of recurrence for each approach. Unfortunately, these prospective analyses simply do not exist.

Professional guidelines allow room to consider either a segmental or an extended colectomy for a patient with Crohn's and colonic dysplasia/carcinoma (1,31,32). One small study raises concern about segmental colectomy for this indication. A series of 22 patients with colorectal carcinoma and Crohn's disease found that 19 (86%) had adjacent dysplasia and 9 (41%) had distant dysplasia. Of course, the extent of colitis must also be considered in determining the extent of colectomy.

Proctectomy

Proctectomy is not mandatory for a colonic malignancy in a patient with Crohn's disease, but this issue deserves some discussion. Adding a proctectomy to a total abdominal colectomy poses significant surgical morbidity, including risks of sexual dysfunction (impotence, retrograde ejaculation, dyspareunia), and bladder dysfunction. The rectal remnant can be used in an ileorectal anastomosis or defunctionalized as a blind rectal remnant (Hartmann pouch). Restorative proctocolectomy is contraindicated in Crohn's disease because of the risk of developing symptomatic disease in the ileoanal pouch.

IRA is an attractive option for patients with Crohn's disease for a number of reasons. The rectum is less likely to have active disease and restorative proctocolectomy is not an option. Patients who undergo IRA should have a rectum that is relatively spared from inflammation. Also, it is imperative to consider the status of the patient's perineum. A patient with poor sphincter function or severe perianal Crohn's disease will not be well served by this procedure.

If an IRA is not performed with total abdominal colectomy, a Hartmann pouch is left behind. This option avoids the complications of a proctectomy, but this rectal remnant can pose problems in the form of occasional drainage, diversion colitis, need for periodic endoscopic surveillance, and risks of carcinoma arising in the rectum (despite surveillance) (33,34). Decision making for each patient must include an informed discussion of these issues.

Surgical Management of Colonic Carcinoma Unsuspected at the Time of Surgery

A patient with Crohn's disease may occasionally be found to have dysplasia or carcinoma in the specimen removed for symptomatic disease. In a series of 222 patients with Crohn's disease undergoing colectomy (partial or total) from the University of Minnesota, 3 patients had a preoperative diagnosis of dysplasia and 1 had a preoperative diagnosis of adenocarcinoma. Failure of medical therapy (54%) and complications of Crohn's disease (44%) were the indications for surgery in the other patients. Adenocarcinoma was diagnosed postoperatively in four patients without a preoperative diagnosis of dysplasia/carcinoma (35).

Should such a patient return to the operating room for an extended colectomy? The answer to this question needs to be tailored to the specific risks posed to the patient. Assuming that the initial carcinoma was resected to appropriate margins, the intent of further surgery would be to reduce/eliminate the risk of a metachronous carcinoma in the residual colon and rectum. Factors to consider would include the age/health status of the patient, the stage/prognosis of the carcinoma, and the patient's wishes regarding undergoing additional resection and reconstruction. At a minimum, such a patient should enter into an intensive surveillance program.

Surgical Management of Rectal Dysplasia and Carcinoma

The treatment of rectal dysplasia/carcinoma in a patient with Crohn's disease is similar to treatment for patients with ulcerative colitis. Surgical planning should begin with accurate staging to determine whether or not a patient is well served by neoadjuvant therapy.

Unlike ulcerative colitis, proctectomy alone is a consideration for rectal dysplasia/carcinoma in a patient with Crohn's disease (36). This choice is appropriate only when there is no dysplasia or active disease in the abdominal colon. Preservation of the abdominal colon would be particularly beneficial in a patient with previous significant small intestine resection, to reduce the risk of diarrhea and dehydration.

Surgical Management of Small Bowel Carcinoma

Patients with Crohn's disease are at increased risk for the development of small bowel adenocarcinoma. A recent meta-analysis calculated a 27-fold risk, but an actual incidence rate is difficult to ascertain because of the rarity of this neoplasm in a non-Crohn's population (37). Surgical treatment is relatively straightforward compared with disease in the colon or rectum, and generally entails resection with wide margins and an appropriate nodal harvest (38).

INDETERMINATE COLITIS

Approximately 10% to 15% of patients with IBD cannot be clearly categorized as having Crohn's disease or ulcerative colitis (39). Although many of these patients will develop, over time, a firm diagnosis of Crohn's or ulcerative colitis, some will elude definitive categorization. The concept of indeterminate colitis is useful in determining appropriate surgical therapy for these patients.

The indications for surgical therapy in a patient with indeterminate colitis are similar to those seen with Crohn's or with ulcerative colitis. The diagnosis raises several questions regarding the surgical management of colonic dysplasia/carcinoma. Management of rectal disease is comparable to methods of treatment in Crohn's disease and ulcerative colitis.

Surgical Management of Colonic Dysplasia/Carcinoma

With indeterminate colitis, surgical options need to be considered carefully, given the uncertainty of the diagnosis. Patients with indeterminate colitis are candidates for any of the reconstructive options available to a patient with ulcerative colitis (total proctocolectomy, ileorectal anastomosis, restorative proctocolectomy), with two important qualifications.

First, it is incumbent on the treating physician to eliminate a potential diagnosis of Crohn's disease before constructing an ileoanal reservoir. Therefore, in cases of ongoing uncertainty, a common approach is to perform a total abdominal colectomy with end ileostomy, leaving the rectal remnant in place. Based on histopathologic examination of the colonic specimen, a definitive diagnosis can often be made before an ileoanal reservoir is fashioned.

Second, patients with a diagnosis of indeterminate colitis that persists after total abdominal colectomy are still candidates for restorative proctocolectomy. However, this topic is controversial, even among experts in colorectal surgery (40,41). One large series of patients with ileoanal pouch/anal anastomosis documented 5-year pouch failure rates of 19% for patients with indeterminate colitis, compared with 8% for patients with ulcerative colitis (42).

CONCLUSION

Determining the best therapy to manage dysplasia/carcinoma in patients with IBD involves complex decision making. The choice of which (if any) surgical treatment to offer represents a balance between the risk of recurrence/progression of disease and the physiological consequences of surgery.

The first challenge for physicians is to optimize interpretation of the pathology and communication among the members of a multidisciplinary treatment team. At the current time, each step in the care pathway for these patients is plagued with critical controversies and variations in care.

Adherence to evidence-based guidelines would improve care. As mentioned in the chapter by Dr. Ullman, endoscopists often do not biopsy the number of sites needed to represent the entire colorectum (5,43). Biopsy specimens find inconsistent interpretation; one recent study noted poor interobserver agreement (kappa <0.4) between pathologists evaluating surveillance biopsies for LGD (7). This finding is not unique (7,44–48).

Once a diagnosis of dysplasia is made, there is poor consensus regarding whether or not a colectomy is indicated. Studies within and outside the United States have shown wide variability in terms of physician adherence to guidelines regarding treatment (43,49). Even though there is agreement that the presence of carcinoma requires surgery, the optimal surgical option is not clear. Surgeons also lack universal agreement regarding the technical aspects of surgical care (one-stage vs. two-stage, mucosectomy vs. double-staple, segmental vs. extended colectomy, and so forth).

Historically, patients with IBD-associated colitis were advised to proceed with total proctocolectomy and end ileostomy after 8 to 10 years of active disease. Over time, surveillance has gained wide acceptance as an alternative to empiric proctocolectomy. Despite the best efforts of the multidisciplinary team of physicians who manage IBD patients, definitive evidence that these efforts improve outcomes remains elusive (50). This finding should inspire clinical scientists to develop quality of care benchmarks, hopefully ones that reflect true consensus in the field. Future research should focus on identifying and resolving key areas of controversy in a way that allows for an evidence-based pattern of practice for patients with IBD.

REFERENCE

1. Itzkowitz SH, Present DH. Consensus conference: Colorectal cancer screening and surveillance in inflammatory bowel disease. *Inflamm Bowel Dis.* 2005;11:314–321.
2. Leighton JA, Shen B, Baron TH, et al. ASGE guideline: endoscopy in the diagnosis and treatment of inflammatory bowel disease. *Gastrointest Endosc.* 2006;63:558–565.
3. Cohen JL, Strong SA, Hyman NH, et al. Practice parameters for the surgical treatment of ulcerative colitis. *Dis Colon Rectum.* 2005;48:1997–2009.
4. Rutter MD, Saunders BP, Wilkinson KH, et al. Thirty-year analysis of a colonoscopic surveillance program for neoplasia in ulcerative colitis. *Gastroenterology.* 2006;130:1030–1038.
5. Ullman T, Croog V, Harpaz N, et al. Progression of flat low-grade dysplasia to advanced neoplasia in patients with ulcerative colitis. *Gastroenterology.* 2003;125:1311–1319.
6. Befrits R, Ljung T, Jaramillo E, et al. Low-grade dysplasia in extensive, long-standing inflammatory bowel disease: a follow-up study. *Dis Colon Rectum.* 2002;45:615–620.
7. Lim CH, Dixon MF, Vail A, et al. Ten year follow up of ulcerative colitis patients with and without low grade dysplasia. *Gut.* 2003;52:1127–1132.
8. Engelsgjerd M, Farraye FA, Odze RD. Polypectomy may be adequate treatment for adenoma-like dysplastic lesions in chronic ulcerative colitis. *Gastroenterology.* 1999;117:1288–1294.
9. Rubin PH, Friedman S, Harpaz N, et al. Colonoscopic polypectomy in chronic colitis: conservative management after endoscopic resection of dysplastic polyps. *Gastroenterology.* 1999;117:1295–1300.
10. Odze RD, Farraye FA, Hecht JL, et al. Long-term follow-up after polypectomy treatment for adenoma-like dysplastic lesions in ulcerative colitis. *Clin Gastroenterol Hepatol.* 2004;2:534–541.

11. Itzkowitz SH, Harpaz N. Diagnosis and management of dysplasia in patients with inflammatory bowel diseases. *Gastroenterology*. 2004;126:1634–1648.

12. Odze RD. Adenomas and adenoma-like DALMs in chronic ulcerative colitis: a clinical, pathological, and molecular review. *Am J Gastroenterol*. 1999;94:1746–1750.

13. Williamson ME, Lewis WG, Sagar PM, Holdsworth PJ, Johnston D. One-stage restorative proctocolectomy without temporary ileostomy for ulcerative colitis: a note of caution. *Dis Colon Rectum*. 1997;40:1019–1022.

14. Heuschen UA, Hinz U, Allemeyer EH, et al. One- or two-stage procedure for restorative proctocolectomy: rationale for a surgical strategy in ulcerative colitis. *Ann Surg*. 2001;234:788–794.

15. Sequens R. Cancer in the anal canal (transitional zone) after restorative proctocolectomy with stapled ileal pouch-anal anastomosis. *Int J Colorectal Dis*. 1997;12:254–255.

16. Baratsis S, Hadjidimitriou F, Christodoulou M, et al. Adenocarcinoma in the anal canal after ileal pouch-anal anastomosis for ulcerative colitis using a double stapling technique: report of a case. *Dis Colon Rectum*. 2002;45:687–692.

17. Laureti S, Ugolini F, D'Errico A, et al. Adenocarcinoma below ileoanal anastomosis for ulcerative colitis: report of a case and review of the literature. *Dis Colon Rectum*. 2002;45:418–421.

18. Tekkis PP, Fazio VW, Lavery IC, et al. Evaluation of the learning curve in ileal pouch-anal anastomosis surgery. *Ann Surg*. 2005;241:262–268.

19. Ziv Y, Fazio VW, Church JM, et al. Stapled ileal pouch anal anastomoses are safer than handsewn anastomoses in patients with ulcerative colitis. *Am J Surg*. 1996;171:320–323.

20. Rauh SM, Schoetz DJ Jr, Roberts PL, et al. Pouchitis: is it a wastebasket diagnosis? *Dis Colon Rectum*. 1991;34:685–689.

21. Ziv Y, Fazio VW, Sirimarco MT, et al. Incidence, risk factors, and treatment of dysplasia in the anal transitional zone after ileal pouch-anal anastomosis. *Dis Colon Rectum*. 1994;37:1281–1285.

22. Das P, Johnson MW, Tekkis PP, et al. Risk of dysplasia and adenocarcinoma following restorative proctocolectomy for ulcerative colitis. *Colorectal Dis*. 2007;9:15–927.

23. Shen B, Lashner BA, Bennett AE, et al. Treatment of rectal cuff inflammation (cuffitis) in patients with ulcerative colitis following restorative proctocolectomy and ileal pouch-anal anastomosis. *Am J Gastroenterol*. 2004;99:1527–1531.

24. Michelassi F, Lee J, Rubin M, et al. Long-term functional results after ileal pouch anal restorative proctocolectomy for ulcerative colitis: a prospective observational study. *Ann Surg*. 2003;238:433–445.

25. Nessar G, Fazio VW, Tekkis P, et al. Long-term outcome and quality of life after continent ileostomy. *Dis Colon Rectum*. 2006;49:336–344.

26. Leijonmarck CE, Lofberg R, Ost A, et al. Long-term results of ileorectal anastomosis in ulcerative colitis in Stockholm County. *Dis Colon Rectum*. 1990;33:195–200.

27. Oakley JR, Lavery IC, Fazio VW, et al. The fate of the rectal stump after subtotal colectomy for ulcerative colitis. *Dis Colon Rectum*. 1985;28:394–396.

28. Pastore RL, Wolff BG, Hodge D. Total abdominal colectomy and ileorectal anastomosis for inflammatory bowel disease. *Dis Colon Rectum*. 1997;40:1455–1464.

29. Bipat S, van Leeuwen MS, Comans EF, et al. Colorectal liver metastases: CT, MR imaging, and PET for diagnosis–meta-analysis. *Radiology*. 2005;237:123–131.

30. Skandarajah AR, Tjandra JJ. Preoperative loco-regional imaging in rectal cancer. *ANZ J Surg*. 2006;76:497–504.

31. Stucchi AF, Aarons CB, Becker JM. Surgical approaches to cancer in patients who have inflammatory bowel disease. *Gastroenterol Clin North Am*. 2006;35:641–673.

32. Greenstein AJ. Cancer in inflammatory bowel disease. *Mt Sinai J Med*. 2000;67:227–240.

33. Leteurtre E, Kosydar P, Gambiez L, et al. Excluded rectum during Crohn's diseases: what is the risk of dysplasia? [in French]. *Gastroenterol Clin Biol*. 1999;23:477–482.

34. Lavery IC, Jagelman DG. Cancer in the excluded rectum following surgery for inflammatory bowel disease. *Dis Colon Rectum*. 1982;25:522–524.

35. Maykel JA, Hagerman G, Mellgren AF, et al. Crohn's colitis: the incidence of dysplasia and adenocarcinoma in surgical patients. *Dis Colon Rectum*. 2006;49:950–957.

36. Sjodahl RI, Myrelid P, Soderholm JD. Anal and rectal cancer in Crohn's disease. *Colorectal Dis*. 2003;5:490–495.

37. Jess T, Gamborg M, Matzen P, et al. Increased risk of intestinal cancer in Crohn's disease: a meta-analysis of population-based cohort studies. *Am J Gastroenterol*. 2005;100:2724–2729.

38. Delaney CP, Fazio VW. Crohn's disease of the small bowel. *Surg Clin North Am*. 2001;81:137–158.

39. Guindi M, Riddell RH. Indeterminate colitis. *J Clin Pathol*. 2004;57:1233–1244.

40. Schoetz DJ Jr. Is ileoanal the proper operation for indeterminate colitis: the case against. *Inflamm Bowel Dis*. 2002;8:366–369.

41. Wolff BG. Is ileoanal the proper operation for indeterminate colitis: the case for. *Inflamm Bowel Dis*. 2002;8:362–369.

42. McIntyre PB, Pemberton JH, Wolff BG, et al. Indeterminate colitis. Long-term outcome in patients after ileal pouch-anal anastomosis. *Dis Colon Rectum*. 1995;38:51–54.

43. Eaden JA, Ward BA, Mayberry JF. How gastroenterologists screen for colonic cancer in ulcerative colitis: an analysis of performance. *Gastrointest Endosc*. 2000;51:123–128.

44. Eaden J, Abrams K, McKay H, et al. Inter-observer variation between general and specialist gastrointestinal pathologists when grading dysplasia in ulcerative colitis. *J Pathol*. 2001;194:152–157.

45. Dixon MF, Brown LJ, Gilmour HM, et al. Observer variation in the assessment of dysplasia in ulcerative colitis. *Histopathology*. 1988;13:385–397.

46. Odze RD, Goldblum J, Noffsinger A, et al. Interobserver variability in the diagnosis of ulcerative colitis-associated dysplasia by telepathology. *Mod Pathol*. 2002;15:379–386.

47. Melville DM, Jass JR, Morson BC, et al. Observer study of the grading of dysplasia in ulcerative colitis: comparison with clinical outcome. *Hum Pathol*. 1989;20:1008–1014.

48. Connell WR, Lennard-Jones JE, Williams CB, et al. Factors affecting the outcome of endoscopic surveillance for cancer in ulcerative colitis. *Gastroenterology*. 1994;107:934–944.

49. Bernstein CN, Weinstein WM, Levine DS, et al. Physicians' perceptions of dysplasia and approaches to surveillance colonoscopy in ulcerative colitis. *Am J Gastroenterol*. 1995;90:2106–2114.

50. Collins PD, Mpofu C, Watson AJ, et al. Strategies for detecting colon cancer and/or dysplasia in patients with inflammatory bowel disease. *Cochrane Database Syst Rev*. 2006:CD000279.

46

Surgical Management of Primary Malignant and Benign Tumors of the Liver

Gagandeep Singh, Lea Matsuoka, Rick Selby, and Nicolas Jabbour

Benign tumors of the liver affect nearly 20% of the population in the United States; 250,000 people per year in the United States are diagnosed with primary or secondary liver cancer (1). The number of benign lesions of the liver are correspondingly increasing as the use of diagnostic imaging increases. The major benign lesions include cystic tumors such as simple cysts, cystadenomas, and echinococcal cysts. Major benign solid lesions include hepatic adenomas, focal nodular hyperplasia, and hemangiomas. In this chapter we discuss the clinical presentation, diagnosis, pathology, and treatment of these most common benign lesions.

Hepatocellular carcinoma causes 500,000 deaths yearly worldwide and the incidence in the United States has been rising. Trends from the hepatitis C epidemic predict the incidence of hepatocellular carcinoma will continue to increase for the next 10 years. Attempts to battle this problem include strategies for prevention and treatment. Surveillance of patients with cirrhosis is now common, but how effective are the current screening methods? Additionally, the detection of hepatocellular carcinoma at an earlier stage would be of no benefit without effective treatment options. Multiple treatment modalities including liver transplantation, liver resection, radiofrequency ablation, chemical ablation, and transarterial and systemic chemotherapy have been extensively studied and used. We discuss the benefits and risks of the multiple treatment modalities and offer an algorithm for the management of hepatocellular carcinoma.

BENIGN CYSTIC TUMORS OF THE LIVER

Simple Cysts

Clinical Presentation

Simple hepatic cysts are the most common cystic lesions of the liver. They are congenital, formed from aberrant or excessive bile ducts that become obstructed or fail to fuse with extrahepatic ducts. Simple cysts are more common in women above the age of 50 years. The majority are asymptomatic and discovered incidentally. When symptomatic, the most common complaints are abdominal pain or an abdominal mass.

The majority of simple cysts are solitary. Patients may also have multicystic livers or polycystic liver disease (PCLD). PCLD has been defined as more than six liver cysts or cysts that encompass >50% of the liver parenchyma (2,3). PCLD is usu-

ally asymptomatic, although large cysts may cause symptoms. The disease manifests during adulthood and is associated with intracranial aneurysms and mitral valve abnormalities (4). Renal cysts are rare with PCLD, although patients with polycystic kidney disease commonly have liver cysts.

Diagnosis

Ultrasound has >90% sensitivity and specificity in the diagnosis of simple hepatic cysts (5). These lesions appear as unilocular, anechoic masses with smooth margins and a thin wall. Back wall enhancement is often noted and there are no septations found in the lesion. On computed tomography (CT) scan simple cysts appear as nonenhancing lesions that are the same density as water. Lack of septations within the mass on ultrasound and CT scan is 100% predictive of a simple cyst (3). CT scans are additionally useful to determine the proximity of the cyst to vessels and biliary structures, although invasion into adjacent structures is rare. The cyst on magnetic resonance imaging (MRI) appears hypointense on T1-weighted images and hyperintense on T2-weighted images. Liver function tests are usually normal.

Pathology

Simple hepatic cysts appear bluish and are filled with clear, straw-colored fluid. Microscopically they are lined with simple cuboidal epithelium.

Treatment

Asymptomatic simple cysts may be followed routinely (Figure 46.1). Surgical treatment is recommended for cysts that are symptomatic. Percutaneous aspiration has a 100% recurrence rate and is performed only to secure a diagnosis or as a therapeutic test (5). The current recommended therapy is laparoscopic unroofing of the cyst (6) (Figure 46.2). During surgery the cyst fluid should be sent for Gram stain, culture analysis, and cytology, and biopsies should be performed on the cyst wall.

PCLD is treated conservatively, with surgery only in symptomatic patients. Surgical treatment is unroofing of the cysts, with possible liver resection or transplantation for more severe disease.

Cystadenoma and Cystadenocarcinoma of the Liver

Clinical Presentation

Cystadenomas are most commonly found in the liver parenchyma and less often in the extrahepatic biliary ducts. The

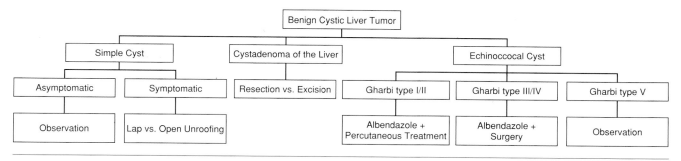

Figure 46.1 Management algorithm for benign cystic lesions of the liver. Lap, laparoscopic.

pathogenesis is unclear, and may be congenital in origin from abnormal bile ducts or from aberrant germ cells. The disease tends to occur in women 30 to 50 years old. These cystic tumors are often large and symptomatic, causing abdominal pain or presentation with an abdominal mass.

Ten percent of cystadenomas are malignant (5) and there is a 25% chance of malignant degeneration (7).

Diagnosis

On ultrasound and CT scan, cystadenomas appear as multiloculated cystic lesions with papillary projections. MRI displays variable signal intensities on T1- and T2-weighted imaging, depending on the protein content of the fluid and soft-tissue components.

It is difficult to distinguish cystadenomas and cystadenocarcinomas radiologically unless there are clear signs of invasion. However, the combination of internal nodularity and septations, wall hemorrhage, and hemorrhagic fluid has been associated with cystadenocarcinomas (8). Cytologic features of malignancy found by examining the cyst wall can definitively diagnose cystadenocarcinoma.

Pathology

Grossly, cystadenomas are often large and have a smooth, thin wall with variable septations and nodularity. Cystadenocarcinomas often have a thicker wall with multiple polypoid protrusions. Cystadenomas are composed of cuboidal to columnar epithelium, with the majority containing a densely cellular spindle cell stroma resembling ovarian stroma. Cystadenocarcinomas are of two types. The first type is seen only in women, arises from a previous cystadenoma, contains spindle-cell stroma, and follows an indolent course. The second type is a more aggressive tumor seen in both male and female patients and lacks the spindle-cell stroma (8, 9).

Treatment

Cystadenomas carry the risk of malignant degeneration, enlargement, and infection and should undergo complete resection (Figure 46.1). Partial resection commonly leads to recurrence of the cystadenoma. Enucleation may also be performed for cystadenomas (10). Cystadenocarcinomas require hepatic resection.

Echinococcal Cyst
Clinical Presentation

Cystic echinococcosis of the liver, also known as *hydatid disease*, is most commonly caused by the tapeworm *Echinococcus granulosus*, which is a parasitic infection endemic in Eastern Europe, Asia, South America, and the Mediterranean. Humans become accidental hosts on ingestion of the ova, which are found in the feces of dogs. The most common site of infection is the liver.

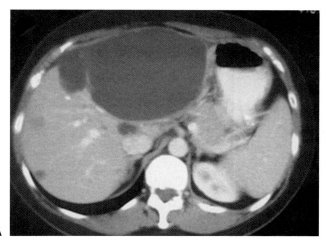

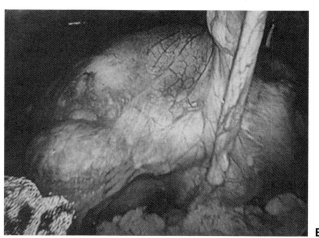

Figure 46.2 (**A**) Large hepatic cyst compressing stomach. (**B**) Laparoscopic view of same hepatic cyst just prior to excision.

The majority of patients with echinococcal cyst (EC) are asymptomatic, although the cysts may cause abdominal pain, fever, or hepatomegaly. Rupture of the EC into the peritoneal cavity can cause anaphylactic shock, and EC may also invade the biliary tract or pleural space. Up to one third of patients have multiple cysts [11].

Diagnosis

Diagnosis is made by the combination of radiologic and serologic studies. The Gharbi ultrasound classification is commonly employed and thought to represent the evolution of the disease. A type I EC is a pure fluid collection, representing an uncomplicated cyst. A type II cyst is composed of a fluid collection with a split wall, seen either inside or immediately outside the cyst. Type III cysts are fluid collections containing multiple septations. Type IV cysts have heterogenous echo patterns, and a type V EC has a reflecting thick wall [12].

The appearance of EC on CT is a well-defined lesion with calcified rim, septations, and daughter cysts. On MRI, the outer fibrous pericyst appears hypointense on T1- and T2-weighted imaging, while the inner matrix is hypointense on T1 and hyperintense on T2. Daughter cells within the EC appear hypointense compared to the matrix on both T1- and T2-weighted imaging.

If biliocystic communication is suspected based on elevated liver function tests or symptoms of cholangitis, endoscopic retrograde cholangiopancreatography should be performed. Endoscopic retrograde cholangiopancreatography can define the communication between the EC and biliary system and sphincterotomy can be performed in the face of an obstructed duct.

Eosinophilia is commonly seen in patients with EC. There are multiple tests for specific detection of the parasitic antigen, including protein electrophoresis for DD5, enzyme-linked immunosorbent assay (ELISA)-immunoglobulin (Ig) G and IgE, latex agglutination, indirect hemagglutination, and Western blot. For screening purposes, ELISA-IgG or Western blot is recommended, while protein electrophoresis for DD5 can be used for confirmation [13].

Pathology

EC are composed of three layers: (a) an outer pericyst, which is compressed hepatic tissue; (b) the ectocyst, a thin interleaved membrane; and (c) an endocyst, which is the inner germinal layer. On gross examination the cyst fluid is clear or pale yellow, and multiple daughter cysts look similar to a bunch of grapes.

Treatment

Surgery has traditionally been the cornerstone of therapy for EC, as albendazole (the antiparasitic agent of choice) given alone is effective in <30% of patients [14]. The goals of treatment are to avoid spillage of cyst contents and to prevent recurrence.

Percutaneous treatment of EC has recently been advocated for univesicular and multivesicular cysts of Gharbi type I and II (Figure 46.1). Percutaneous treatment results in shorter hospital stays and less complications in these patients and is as effective as cystectomy [14]. Percutaneous methods have also been advocated for infected cysts and EC found in pregnant or high surgical risk patients [15].

Gharbi type III and IV EC are treated with traditional surgical therapy. Surgical therapy involves either tissue-sparing methods that remove the parasite and leave some of the pericyst behind, or removal of the entire pericyst by total pericystectomy or liver resection [16]. Intraparenchymal cysts are most often treated by partial cystectomy and omentoplasty [17]. Additionally, the advent of laparoscopy has made possible a laparoscopic approach in infected and complex EC, resulting in shorter hospital stays and no recurrence [18]. Albendazole is given before percutaneous and operative treatment. Gharbi type V EC requires no intervention as these cysts likely represent empty cyst cavities. Ultrasound-guided radiofrequency ablation of the germinal layer has also been described for complex EC [19].

BENIGN SOLID TUMORS OF THE LIVER

Hepatic adenoma

Clinical Presentation

Hepatic adenomas (HAs) occur mostly in 20- to 40-year-old women. These lesions have a 20% to 25% risk of rupture of bleeding [20], and patients commonly present with abdominal pain. The first report of the association of HA and oral contraceptive was by Baum et al. [21] in 1973. Since that time, it has become well known that HAs are associated with estrogen and progesterone. Understandably, HAs have a tendency to grow and rupture during pregnancy, and the risks to the mother and fetus are extremely high [22].

There is a low risk of malignant transformation [23] that has yet to be precisely defined. HA may rarely be seen in men using anabolic steroids and in patients with glycogen storage diseases [24].

Diagnosis

HAs are usually solitary lesions that are hypervascular because of multiple sinusoids and subcapsular feeding arteries. CT scan will show a heterogeneous mass created by areas of hemorrhage, fat, and necrosis. There is early peripheral enhancement with centripetal movement, representing the subcapsular vessels. On MRI, HA shows up bright on T1-weighted images and hyperintense relative to the liver on T2-weighted images. Dynamic contrast-enhanced MRI will similarly show early enhancement of the mass due to the subcapsular feeding vessels. Liver function tests are usually normal.

Pathology

On gross examination, HAs are circumscribed, smooth, and soft. The mass is an orange or yellow color, often with focal areas of hemorrhage, necrosis, or fat. Microscopically, HAs are composed of sheets of hepatocytes separated by sinusoids with an absence of bile ducts. These hepatocytes are normal but contain large amounts of glycogen or lipid, creating the yellowish color of the mass. HAs may contain few Kupffer cells that have little or no function [25]. There is often a pseudocapsule formed by the compression of adjacent tissue.

Treatment

Resection is the rule for HA because of the risks of rupture, bleeding, and malignant transformation (Figure 46.3). Although

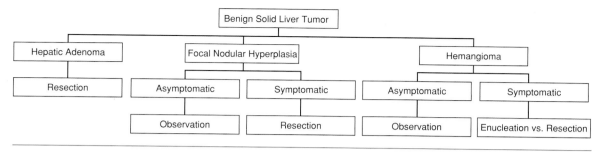

Figure 46.3 Management algorithm for benign solid lesions of the liver.

there have been reports of complete resolution of HA following the cessation of oral contraceptives (26), resection is still the recommended therapy. Some advocate resection only for lesions >5 cm (27). Smaller lesions may then be observed with serial ultrasound examinations, cessation of oral contraceptives, and avoidance of pregnancy. Radioablation may be considered in high-risk patients. In pregnant patients, resection preferably during the second trimester has been recommended for HAs >5 cm (28), as there have been no reports of rupture in HAs smaller than 6.5 cm. Approximately one third of ruptured HAs occur postpartum, so mothers should continue to be closely followed after giving birth (22).

Focal Nodular Hyperplasia

Clinical Presentation

Focal nodular hyperplasia (FNH) tends to be discovered incidentally in women of childbearing age. It is the second most common benign solid tumor of the liver, caused by a hyperplastic response to congenital vascular malformations (7). Unlike HA, FNH has no risk of malignancy. The association between FNH and oral contraceptives is questionable; oral contraceptives are likely not associated with the development of FNH but may cause progression of the lesion. Pregnancy does not increase the risk of bleeding or symptoms in patients with FNH (29).

Diagnosis

CT scan and dynamic contrast-enhanced MRI show homogenous enhancement of the mass with a hypodense central stellate scar. Specific to FNH is the presence of Kupffer cells and thus the uptake of tracer in 99m-technetium-sulfur-colloid scans. These scans can be useful in differentiating HA and FNH in the absence of an obvious stellate scar.

Pathology

On gross examination FNH is made up of a fibrous central scar radiating into surrounding liver tissue and forming multiple nodules. The majority of FNH are solitary and <5 cm (30). Microscopically, the scar is composed of fibrous tissue, inflammatory cells, and tortuous arteries. The surrounding nodules contain proliferating bile ducts but no portal veins or terminal hepatic venules (31). The presence of bile ducts in FNH is in contrast to HAs, which have an absence of bile ducts.

Treatment

The treatment for FNH is observation (Figure 46.3). Resection is indicated in cases in which the etiology is in question, if the patient is symptomatic, or if the lesion is enlarging.

Hemangioma

Clinical Presentation

Hepatic hemangiomas are the most common benign solid lesion of the liver. These lesions are usually incidentally found in middle-aged women, are most commonly located in the subcapsular area of the right lobe, and measure <5 cm (31). If larger, they may cause nonspecific abdominal pain as a result of tumor expansion, hemorrhage, or localized thrombosis. Although there are case reports of spontaneous and traumatic rupture of hemangiomas (32,33), hemorrhage is very uncommon.

Rarely, giant hemangiomas may lead to Kasabach-Merritt syndrome, a consumptive coagulopathy. Patients with this syndrome may have thrombocytopenia, disseminated intravascular coagulopathy, bleeding, and abdominal pain. Symptoms are usually precipitated by surgical or dental procedures.

Diagnosis

Hemangiomas are usually solitary but 5% to 10% of patients have multiple lesions (7). Ultrasound performed on hemangiomas demonstrates a round or lobular mass that is well circumscribed with vascular features. Sensitivity of ultrasound for hemangiomas is 60% to 75% and specificity is 60% to 80% (7). CT scan images of hepatic hemangiomas typically show peripheral nodular enhancement that progresses centripetally with time. Delayed images show uniformly enhanced masses. Sensitivity of CT scan ranges from 75% to 85% while specificity ranges from 75% to 90% (7). MRI, with a sensitivity and specificity of 85% to 95% for hemangiomas, display bright intensity on T2-weighted imaging and a pattern similar to that of CT scan (7). Single photon emission CT with technetium-labeled red blood cells have diagnostic accuracy similar to that of MRI if the hemangiomas are >3 cm and close to the liver surface (31). Liver function tests are within normal limits.

Pathology

On gross examination, hemangiomas are well-circumscribed masses that are dark in color and have a spongy consistency secondary to venous engorgement. Usually a clear plane exists between the lesion and the surrounding normal parenchyma. Microscopically, hemangiomas are composed of multiple vascular

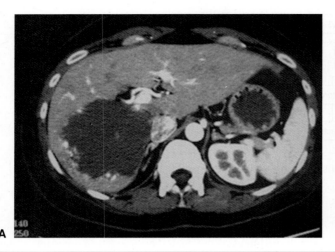
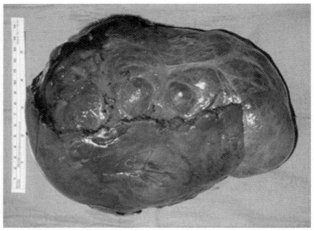

Figure 46.4 **(A)** Large hemangioma in the right lobe of liver. **(B)** Hemangioma removed by enucleation and partial hepatectomy.

channels with a single cell layer of endothelial cells and a collagenous wall. Blood supply is from the hepatic artery.

Treatment

Surgical treatment should be considered only for patients who are symptomatic or to definitively rule out cancer (Figure 46.3). Other possible causes of the patient's symptoms must be thoroughly investigated and excluded. Enucleation or resection of the hemangioma is recommended (Figure 46.4). Enucleation has been associated with less blood loss and fewer complications compared with anatomic resection, and is the recommended treatment for amenable lesions with secure diagnosis (34,35). If surgical removal of the hemangioma is not feasible because of multiple lesions or hilar involvement, then embolization (36) or transplantation (37,38), although an extreme measure, may be considered.

HEPATOCELLULAR CARCINOMA

Epidemiology and Risk Factors

Hepatocellular carcinoma (HCC) is the fifth most common solid tumor in the world (following lung, breast, colon/rectum, and stomach cancer), with worldwide prevalence highest in southeast Asia and Africa (39–41). HCC is responsible for 500,000 deaths every year worldwide and has been a rising trend in the United States. The incidence of HCC in the United States was 1.4/100,000 in 1976-1980 and this number rose to 2.4/100,000 in 1991–1995 and to 3.0/100,000 in 1996–1998 (42,43). The incidence is expected to continue to increase until the year 2015–2019 because of the chronic hepatitis C epidemic (41).

Men are at higher risk for developing HCC compared to women, and in developed countries risk increases after the age of 45 until the age of 70 years (39). The cause of HCC is usually chronic liver disease, caused mainly by alcohol and hepatitis infection. Alcohol use accounts for 32% to 45% of all HCC in the United States (44). Chronic alcohol use of >80 g/day for >10 years increases the risk for developing HCC fivefold and the risk of HCC in an alcoholic cirrhotic liver is 1% per year.

Hepatitis C infection increases the risk of HCC 20-fold, while the annual incidence of HCC in a patient with hepatitis B is 470/100,000 (45,46). The combination of alcohol and hepatitis C infection increases the risk of HCC by more than either factor alone. Hereditary hemochromatosis (20-fold increased risk), primary biliary cirrhosis, alpha-1 antitrypsin deficiency, and diabetes (two- to threefold increased risk) have also been shown to increase the risk of developing HCC (47–50).

Clinical Presentation and Surveillance

The establishment of surveillance programs for the detection of HCC in patients with cirrhosis has led to the diagnosis of tumors before they become symptomatic, as early HCC is clinically silent. Larger tumors typically cause right upper quadrant pain and nonspecific symptoms such as malaise, weight loss, and anorexia (51,52). Many patients with large tumors replacing a significant portion of the liver parenchyma, invading the portal or hepatic vein, or compressing the intrahepatic vasculature will present with hepatic decompensation and liver failure. On physical examination, hepatomegaly is common and a vascular bruit may be evident secondary to the vascularity of the mass. Tumor rupture is rare and causes severe pain, hypotension, and peritonitis. Similarly, only 1% to 12% of patients initially present with symptoms of obstructive jaundice (53). Paraneoplastic syndromes causing hypoglycemia, hypercalcemia, polycythemia, and hypercholesterolemia have been reported (54).

The United States has no official screening criteria for patients at risk for developing HCC. Alpha-fetoprotein (AFP) levels and ultrasound are the modalities most commonly used to screen patients for HCC. The screening interval ranges from every 4 to 12 months, with most centers performing surveillance every 6 months because it is the estimated median doubling time of HCC (55). Ultrasound as a screening tool for HCC has a sensitivity of 48% to 80% and a specificity of >90% (39,56). Prospective cohort studies evaluating the utility of AFP for screening found sensitivities ranging from 39% to 65% and specificities ranging from 76% to 90% (57). Most centers both perform ultrasound and measure AFP levels in patients, and the combination has been reported to have a sensitivity of 50% to 85% and specificity of 70% to 90% (58).

It is as yet unclear whether or not surveillance increases survival in patients with HCC. A few studies published in the early 1990s found that screening cirrhotic patients for HCC did not increase the rate of detection of resectable, potentially curable tumors (59,60). However, other studies have concluded that screening patients with cirrhosis does detect HCC at an earlier stage, which theoretically could lead to improved treatment options and ultimately survival (61–63). The only randomized, controlled trial was performed in Qidong, China (64). The study period was 1989 to 1995, and men with chronic hepatitis B were randomized into screening and no-screening arms. Screening involved measuring AFP levels every 6 months. The study found that surveillance led to earlier diagnosis of HCC, but failed to impact 5-year survival because therapy at the time was ineffective. The problem with many of these studies is that they span several years and do not account for improvements in diagnosis and treatment. These studies also have differences in equipment and technical factors, and often use different cutoff levels in terms of AFP measurements. Sangiovanni et al. (65) compared cirrhotic patients receiving surveillance for HCC in two time periods and found that the outcome of patients under surveillance has improved in recent years. With the improvements in treatment options, it may be that the increases in earlier diagnosis seen with surveillance will lead to increases in survival.

A study by Colli et al. (56) reviewed all studies performed to evaluate surveillance for HCC and reported pooled values for ultrasound, CT, and MRI. The pooled sensitivity and specificity for ultrasound was 48% and 97% while that of CT and MRI were 67% and 92%, and 81% and 85%, respectively. The authors supported the use of ultrasound in patients with cirrhosis and a high likelihood of developing HCC, but considered ultrasound inadequate for screening purposes based on the low sensitivity. MRI, because of its high sensitivity, may prove to be a better modality in the surveillance of cirrhotic patients. Various tumor markers are being evaluated for use in detecting HCC in cirrhotic livers, such as lens culinaris-agglutinin reactive fraction (AFP-L3), which is a variant of AFP and more specific for tumors. In the studies thus far performed, AFP-L3 has sensitivity from 36% to 96% and specificity from 89% to 94% (57). The data are encouraging but further studies validating this tumor marker need to be performed.

Radiologic Findings

Typical ultrasound findings of HCC include a mosaic pattern, peripheral halo, lateral shadow, and posterior echo enhancement (66). The mosaic pattern results from multiple internal regions of hemorrhage, fat, necrosis, and fibrosis found within the tumor, separated by fibrous septations. The lateral shadow is seen because of the pseudocapsule surrounding the lesion. Mosaic patterns tend to be discovered in larger nodules, while small nodules have a uniform internal echo pattern.

On CT scan the mosaic pattern of larger tumors and the surrounding fibrous capsule will also be evident. Calcifications are sometimes seen but are not common. The most characteristic finding of HCC on CT scan is contrast enhancement during the arterial phase (67). HCC will have lower attenuation than liver parenchyma on the unenhanced CT. Extension of the tumor mass into the venous and biliary system may be seen, and diffuse enhancement during the arterial phase will differentiate tumor from benign thrombus. Additionally, clusters of tumor nodules close to the tumor margin are representative of HCC.

Lesions such as hemangiomas, transient focal enhancement during the arterial phase, or regenerative nodules can mimic HCC on imaging. Cirrhotic livers are notoriously difficult to image because of their distorted architecture. A false-positive rate of 8% has been reported in patients with cirrhosis and HCC detected by CT scan (68). Hemangiomas enhance during the arterial phase, but will also enhance during the portal venous phase, while HCC typically shows tumor washout. Transient focal enhancement is often caused by arterial-portal shunting so a peripheral, wedge-shaped mass is noted that does not cause bulging of the capsule. Regenerative nodules and HCC have considerable overlap on imaging studies. Regenerative nodules are supplied mainly by portal veins, but as the transition from regenerative nodule to dysplastic nodule to HCC progresses, the supply from the hepatic artery tends to increase (69). Hence, examining the enhancement of the lesion can sometimes make the distinction between regenerative nodule and HCC. Regenerative nodules should enhance similar to the liver parenchyma, while HCC will have marked enhancement during the arterial phase. Additionally, some HCC will have a visible capsule, while regenerative nodules do not (66). Follow-up CT scans of questionable lesions may help confirm the benign nature of these lesions or show progression typical of HCC.

Lipiodol CT has been reported to have sensitivities from 40% to >90% in the detection of HCC (70). Lipiodol is a lipid-based iodine contrast agent that is infused through the hepatic artery and retained for weeks in neoplastic lesions. Studies comparing helical CT and lipiodol CT show that helical CT is superior in terms of sensitivity and specificity, but indicate lipiodol CT is better at detecting intrahepatic metastatic lesions (70,71).

There is no significant difference between dynamic helical CT and dynamic MRI in detecting hypervascular HCC (66). MRI will also show the typical contrast enhancement during the arterial phase of contrast administration. On MRI the mosaic pattern seen by ultrasound and CT is also evident, seen best by T2-weighted imaging. On T1-weighted imaging the capsule appears hypointense while T2-weighted imaging will show a hypointense inner layer and a hyperintense outer layer (72). The HCC capsule has an inner fibrous layer and outer water-rich layer accounting for the MRI imaging results. Differences in tumor signal intensity are common because of the differences in free water contained in the tumor.

Staging

There are over ten classifications of HCC in use today and no one system is uniformly accepted. Some classification systems use clinical and radiologic characteristics such as the Okuda, Barcelona Clinic Liver Cancer, and Cancer of the Liver Italian Program (CLIP) classifications. Other systems incorporate anatomic and histologic features of the tumor at resection, such as the American Joint Committee on Cancer/Union Internationale Centre le Cancer and Liver Cancer Study Group of Japan.

Table 46.1

Modified TNM Classification and Milan and Proposed University of California at San Francisco (UCSF) Criteria for Liver Transplantation

Modified TNM classification and staging system[a] (Clark et al.)

Class	
TX, NX, MX	Not assessed
T0, N0, M0	Not found
T1	One nodule ≤1.9 cm
T2	One nodule 2.0–5.0 cm; two or three nodules, all <3.0 cm
T3	One nodule >5.0 cm; two or three nodules, at least one >3.0 cm
T4a	Four or more nodules, any size
T4b	T2, T3, or T4a plus gross intrahepatic portal or hepatic vein involvement
N1	Regional (portal hepatis) node involvement
M1	Metastatic disease, including extrahepatic portal or hepatic vein involvement
Stage	
I	T1
II	T2
III	T3
IVA1	T4a
IVA2	T4b
IVB	Any N1, M1
Milan criteria	
1 lesion ≤5 cm or 2–3 lesions each ≤3 cm	
Proposed UCSF criteria	
Single tumor ≤6.5 cm or ≤3 nodules with the largest lesion ≤4.5 cm and total diameter ≤8 cm	

Data derived from Clark HP, Carson WF, Kavanagh PV, et al. Staging and current treatment of hepatocellular carcinoma. *Radiographics.* 2005;25:S3–S23.

Furthermore, the United Network of Organ Sharing recognizes the modified tumor-node-metastasis (TNM) system (Table 46.1).

The CLIP classification system has been validated and found to be a better predictor of survival following surgery than the Child-Pugh score, Okuda, and TNM systems (73,74). It seems most prudent to use a clinical staging system such as the CLIP classification system at diagnosis and another such as the modified TNM following surgery. Furthermore, patients are also staged according to the Milan or proposed University of California at San Francisco (UCSF) criteria in determining whether they may be eligible for liver transplantation (Table 46.1).

Therapeutic Modalities

The choice of therapy depends on many factors, including the stage of the tumor, the underlying condition of the liver, and the patient. In the United States, only 25% to 40% of HCC are treated with curative intent, with the remaining patients receiving palliative or supportive treatment (75). Therapeutic modalities for HCC include liver resection, liver transplantation, radiofrequency thermal ablation (RFA), ethanol ablation, and transcatheter arterial chemoembolization (TACE). These various modalities and appropriate situations in which they should be employed are discussed.

Liver Resection versus Liver Transplantation

The treatment of HCC involves consideration of the tumor as well as the underlying condition of the liver. More than 80% of HCC develop in cirrhotic livers and the remaining 20% arise in livers without evidence of cirrhosis. In the absence of cirrhosis, if the lesion lends itself to resection, aggressive surgical therapy is the norm. For patients with advanced cirrhosis, liver transplantation for HCC makes theoretical sense, as it removes the tumor as well as the underlying cirrhosis. Early results of liver transplantation for HCC were dismal, with survival rates far below those of liver transplantation performed for benign disease. With limited liver allografts, transplantation for HCC could not be supported. However, in 1996 Mazzaferro et al. (76) established the Milan criteria for liver transplantation for HCC. The criteria included single tumors ≤5 cm and up to three tumors with each measuring ≤3 cm (Figure 46.5). Under these criteria, the authors reported 4-year survival rates of 75% and recurrence-free survival of 83% in patients with underlying cirrhosis. Liver transplantation for HCC under the Milan criteria thus yielded survival results comparable to those of transplantation performed for benign disease. The Milan criteria have been verified by other studies (77) and liver transplantation for HCC

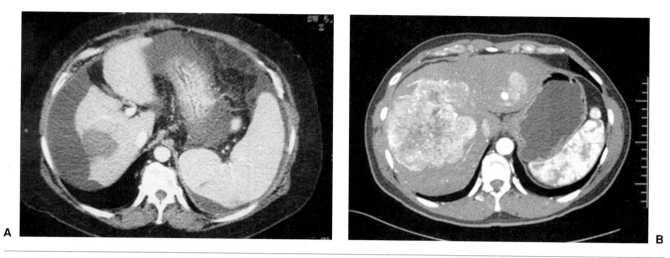

Figure 46.5 **(A)** Hepatocellular carcinoma in a cirrhotic patient within Milan criteria, a candidate for transplant. **(B)** Hepatocellular carcinoma in a cirrhotic patient exceeding Milan criteria limits.

in patients with Child's class B and C cirrhosis meeting these criteria has become the standard of care (Figure 46.6). Yao et al. (78) from UCSF described what is now known as the UCSF criteria: single tumor ≤6.5 cm or ≤hree or more nodules with the largest lesion ≤4.5 cm and total diameter ≤8 cm. Under the UCSF criteria, patients had a 5-year survival rate of 75% following transplantation. The authors suggest that with further validation, the selection criteria for transplantation for HCC may be extended.

The question now is, what is the optimal treatment for patients with HCC and Child's class A cirrhosis? Studies looking at liver resection for HCC falling under transplantation criteria found similar survival rates as liver transplantation (79,80). Specifically, Poon et al. (80) reported a 5-year survival rate of 70% in 135 patients with Child's class A cirrhosis and Milan criteria. However, the problem is HCC has a tendency to be multicentric, and thus 5-year recurrence rates following liver resection for HCC have been reported to be 50% to 70% (75,81). Poon et al. (80) found that 79% of recurrences were eligible for transplantation and suggest the option of salvage transplantation in recurrences following liver resection. Additionally, several studies have attempted to determine ways to measure adequacy

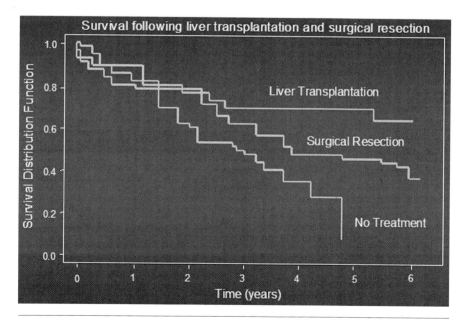

Figure 46.6 Survival curve for liver transplantation (Child's B/C), liver resection (Child's A), and no treatment. (Adapted from Llovet JM, Fuster J, Bruix J. Intention-to-treat analysis of surgical treatment for early hepatocellular carcinoma: resection versus transplantation. *Hepatology.* 1999;30:1434–1440.)

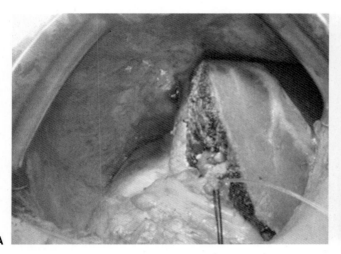
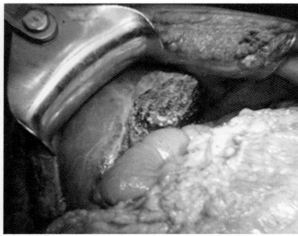

Figure 46.7 (**A**) Completed living donor right hepatectomy. (**B**) Completed living donor liver transplantation.

of functional reserve in patients potentially undergoing liver resection. The Makuuchi criteria determines the extent of safe hepatic resection based upon the presence of ascites, bilirubin levels, and the plasma retention rate of indocyanine green at 15 minutes (82,83). Grazi et al. (84) propose the presence of ascites, portosystemic encephalopathy, and esophageal varices as absolute contraindications for liver resection. They additionally use a lidocaine (MEGX) value of <25 mcg/L as a risk factor for postoperative liver insufficiency. The key message is that results after liver resection for HCC in patients with adequate liver function reserve and absence of portal hypertension are comparable to that following liver transplantation and should be the first treatment consideration in this era of liver allograft shortage.

Major Principles of Liver Resection

When determining the extent of surgical resection of the liver for HCC, several concerns must be addressed. What is the extent of disease? Is the operation curative or palliative? What is the overall status of the patient? There are five major anatomic liver resections performed that are based on Couinaud liver segments and termed according to Goldsmith and Woodburne. An extended right hepatectomy involves segments 4 to 8; an extended left hepatectomy involves segments 2, 3, 4, 5, and 8; a right lobectomy involves segments 5 to 8; and a left lobectomy involves removal of segments 2 to 4. Additionally, unisegmentectomy or bisegmentectomy may be performed in appropriate situations. It is always advisable to encircle the portal vein and hepatic artery for vascular control (Pringle maneuver), which may be administered in intermittent 10- to 20-minute intervals. Parenchymal dissection is performed using the cautery, Kelley clamp-crushing technique, staplers, or ultrasonic dissectors.

Living Donor Liver Transplantation

Living donor liver transplantation (LDLT) in patients meeting Milan criteria yield survival results similar to cadaveric liver transplantation (85,86) (Figure 46.7). However, the Milan criteria were judged against results following liver transplantation for benign disease. Comparable outcomes justified the incorporation of HCC meeting Milan criteria in the organ allocation scheme. LDLT is a different situation and some suggest that the criteria may be extended. Todo and Furukawa (86) retrospectively examined 1,389 patients who underwent LDLT for HCC in Japan. The authors found that 60% of recipients who exceeded Milan criteria lived for at least 3 years. The option of LDLT may also be considered for salvage therapy in patients who go into liver failure following hepatic resection. However, the risk to the living donor is of paramount concern and further studies need to be performed to define the exact role of LDLT in the treatment of HCC.

Local Ablation Therapy

Local ablation therapy can be used in Child's class A or B cirrhotic patients who are not candidates for liver resection or transplantation. Patients may have a single lesion measuring <5 cm or up to three lesions, each measuring <3 cm. Contraindications include ascites, hemostasis disorders, platelets <40,000, PT <40%, or extrahepatic spread (87). Chemical ablation therapy using ethanol has been the more widely used standard treatment, but RFA is proving to be more effective.

Ethanol

Ethanol ablation is usually performed under ultrasound guidance and requires an average of four sessions for complete tumor necrosis. Tumor necrosis is caused by the direct infusion of denaturing material such as ethanol into the tumor. Complete responses have been reported in 90% to 100% of lesions <2 cm, 70% of lesions 3 to 5 cm, and 50% of lesions >5 cm (87). Complication rates occur in 1.7% to 3.2% of patients and mortality has been reported in 0.1% (88,89). Major complications of the procedure include liver abscess, liver failure, hemorrhage, cholangitis, biloma, and tumor seeding along the needle tract. Although complete response rates are positive, local recurrence rates range from 27% to 44% 2 years following treatment (90,91). Five-year survival rates are 32% to 47% (89,92). Fibrous septa within the tumors limit the spread of ethanol and there can be diffusion of ethanol outside the lesion, creating the need for multiple sessions and increasing the unpredictability of necrosis.

Radiofrequency Thermal Ablation

RFA uses direct current to create heat and irreversible cellular damage of the tumor. The goal of RFA is to destroy all visible tumor with a 1-cm margin. It is best for lesions that provide clear targets and are not adjacent to the gallbladder or hilum (risk of thermal injury to the biliary tract). RFA causes complete necrosis of small tumors in 88% to 98% of cases and in 80% to 90% of lesions 3 to 5 cm, following a single treatment session (87). Severe complications are reported in 0% to 12% of cases and mortality ranges from 0.1% to 0.5% (87). Complications include bleeding, liver abscess, intestinal perforation, pneumothorax, biliary stenosis, and needle tract seeding. The zone of necrosis caused by RFA can be altered by the blood flow of adjacent vessels that dissipate the heat.

Multiple randomized, controlled studies have been performed comparing RFA and ethanol ablation. Lin et al. (93) compared RFA with ethanol ablation in patients with Child's class A and B cirrhosis and HCC <4 cm. The study found that fewer sessions were needed to achieve complete necrosis with RFA compared with ethanol ablation, and RFA had significantly lower tumor progression rates and higher survival rates. Three-year overall survival was 74% in the RFA group and 50% in the ethanol ablation group, while 3-year disease-free survival was 37% and 17%, respectively. Lencioni et al. (94) performed a similar randomized, controlled study in cirrhotic patients with a single HCC <5 cm or up to three lesions each <3 cm. They found significantly better local recurrence-free survival in the RFA group compared with the ethanol ablation group after 2 years (96% vs. 62%). RFA is favored over chemical ablation with ethanol because it effectively achieves large areas of necrosis, is predictable, has improved survival rates, and can be performed with fewer treatment sessions. Studies have also shown the utility of RFA as a bridge in patients waiting for liver transplantation (95,96).

Transcatheter Arterial Chemoembolization

TACE is the administration of cytotoxic drugs via the hepatic artery, followed by embolization. The most common individual agent used is doxorubicin and the most common combination regimen is doxorubicin, cisplatin, and mitomycin C (97). These drugs are often combined with lipiodol, which allows the drugs to be selectively retained in the tumor for up to months following administration. Administering intraarterial therapy alone is not more effective than intravenous chemotherapy (97). However, the addition of embolization causes tumor ischemia, which increases tissue permeability and thus the concentration of the drugs in the tumor. The decrease in blood flow additionally increases the exposure time of the drugs in the tumor. Contraindications to therapy with TACE include Child's class C cirrhosis, severe thrombocytopenia or leukopenia, cardiac and renal insufficiency, ascites, portal vein occlusion, or atypical arterial

anatomy (98). These conditions increase the risk of complications following treatment, most notably liver failure. A postembolization syndrome is seen in 80% to 90% of TACE procedures and produces abdominal pain, fever, nausea, and vomiting (97). Other possible complications include cholecystitis, pancreatitis, gastric erosions, liver abscess, bile duct injury, and liver failure.

TACE has been shown to be effective in unresectable HCC. In two recent randomized controlled trials, lipiodol chemoembolization significantly increased survival in patients with unresectable HCC when compared with patients receiving symptomatic treatment (99,100). TACE has also been used to downstage tumors to allow resection with 5-year survival rates of 56% (101). For patients on the waiting list for liver transplantation for HCC, dropout rates of 20% to 25% have been reported (102,103). In an intention-to-treat analysis, Llovet et al. (103) concluded that dropouts from the waiting list significantly decreased the long-term outcome of liver transplantation for HCC. A prospective study that administered TACE to patients on the waiting list reported a 5-year survival after transplantation of 93%, a mean waiting list time of 200 days, and no patients were removed from the waiting list (102). Thus, TACE can be used not only as a palliative treatment in unresectable HCC, but to downstage tumors and as a bridge to liver transplantation.

Systemic Therapy

Systemic therapy in the treatment of advanced HCC has not been shown to be effective and is poorly tolerated in patients with cirrhosis. The two most effective single chemotherapeutic agents are 5-fluorouracil and doxorubicin, with response rates of 15% to 35% (98,104). Randomized, controlled studies have reported tamoxifen, antiandrogens, and interferon-alpha to be ineffective in prolonging survival in advanced HCC (105–108). Small studies have been reported using megestrol, octreotide, and pravastatin, but further studies need to be performed before any conclusions are drawn (87).

Small studies assessing the effect of systemic or intraarterial chemotherapy following curative resection have been performed. These studies show that adjuvant chemotherapy following resection for HCC does not confer an overall or disease-free survival benefit (109). Newer agents targeting tumor signaling pathways in cancer cells are being developed and tested and will hopefully lead to improved treatment for patients with advanced HCC.

Fibrolamellar Carcinoma

Fibrolamellar carcinoma of the liver (FLC) is a variant of HCC with different characteristics and an improved prognosis. FLC accounts for only 1% to 9% of cases of HCC but composes up to 35% of cases in patients younger than 50 years of age (110). FLC tends to be diagnosed in the second or third decades of life and the majority is of white race. Additionally, there is usually no evidence of underlying liver disease.

FLC presents most commonly as a solitary, large mass. The abundant fibrous portions of the tumor often coalesce to form a central scar. On CT scan the parenchyma of the tumor enhances on arterial and portal phases while the scar remains hypointense. This hypointense scar is well visualized using MRI, and can be used to differentiate FLC from FNH, which has a hyperintense

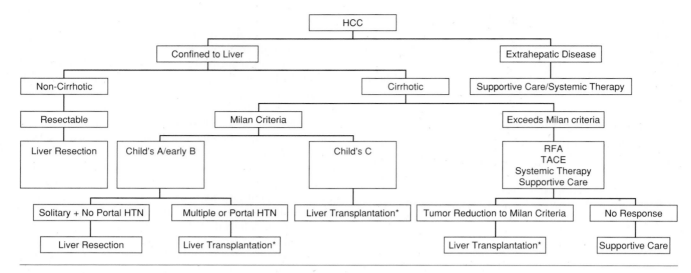

Figure 46.8 Management algorithm for hepatocellular carcinoma (HCC). HTN, hypertension. *Patients listed for liver transplantation may receive transcatheter arterial chemoembolization (TACE) and/or radiofrequency thermal ablation (RFA) while on the waiting list.

scar on imaging studies (110). The AFP levels are usually normal. Microscopically, FLC is composed of well-differentiated malignant cells arranged in sheets or cords and thick, fibrous bands throughout the tumor.

In a large population-based study, a greater proportion of patients with FLC underwent curative therapy compared with patients with HCC, and patients with FLC had significantly better survival rates (111). Aggressive surgical therapy, which entails a curative liver resections whenever feasible, has been the recommended standard of care for patients with FLC (112).

Decision Making: Which Modality to Use and When?

A schematic for the management of HCC is shown in Figure 46.8. In patients with disease confined to the liver, the first assessment made should determine the extent of underlying liver cirrhosis. A noncirrhotic patient with resectable disease should undergo liver resection. In patients with cirrhosis, the next step is to classify their disease as meeting or exceeding Milan criteria (solitary ≤5 cm or ≤three or more lesions, each ≤3 cm). In patients with Child's A or early B cirrhosis who have a solitary lesion and no evidence of portal hypertension, liver resection should be performed. In patients with Child's A or early B cirrhosis who have multiple lesions or portal hypertension, liver resection is likely to lead to hepatic decompensation. Therefore, liver transplantation is the best option. Child's C cirrhotic patients usually have portal hypertension and will not tolerate surgical resection. These patients with Child's C cirrhosis that meet Milan criteria will benefit from liver transplantation.

Patients with cirrhosis and HCC exceeding Milan criteria may be candidates for RFA, TACE, systemic, or supportive therapy, depending on individual circumstances. Following RFA or TACE therapy, patients whose tumors are reduced to within Milan criteria may appeal to become possible candidates for liver transplantation. Additionally, patients on the waiting list for liver transplantation may be candidates for TACE therapy or

RFA to prevent tumor progression. LDLT is a viable option in lieu of cadaveric liver transplantation, but the precise limits for transplantable disease with LDLT remains to be defined. Some centers experienced with LDLT are adopting an aggressive philosophy in transplanting patients with HCC using living donors as opposed to being placed on the wait list for a cadaveric donor.

CONCLUSIONS

The diagnosis of benign liver lesions involves a variety of imaging modalities, such as ultrasound and CT scan. Once the diagnosis is secure the management of these lesions is fairly straightforward. Simple cysts are treated if symptomatic, cystadenomas are always removed because of the risk of malignancy, and ECs are treated according to the Gharbi ultrasound classification (Figure 46.1). With regard to benign solid liver lesions, HAs are always resected because of the risk of spontaneous rupture and the remote possibility of malignant transformation, while FNHs and hemangiomas are resected only when symptomatic (Figure 46.3).

The diagnosis and treatment of HCC is much more confusing and difficult. As discussed, although surveillance for HCC in patients with cirrhosis is widespread, the utility of current screening methods leaves much to be desired. Newer tumor markers such as AFP-L3 are being studied, and the results from screening with MRI show increased sensitivity. In the future, different tumor markers, radiologic studies, or DNA and protein gene arrays may lead to earlier diagnosis and an increase in the survival of this disease.

Improvements in patient selection and operative technique have led to much improved 5-year survival rates. Noncirrhotic patients with resectable lesions undergo liver resection, while the Milan and proposed UCSF criteria have set standards for the optimal selection of patients for liver transplantation for HCC. The role of LDLT needs to be closely examined and clarified, as do the roles of RFA and TACE therapy. The advent of targeted and gene therapy will hopefully add to the armamentarium of options for patients with advanced HCC (113,114). As survival rates after surgery, interventional treatments, or a combination of modalities continue to improve, the current patient criteria should be expanded in an attempt to increase the number of patients treated with curative intent.

REFERENCES

1. Gibbs JF, Litwin AM, Kahlenberg MS. Contemporary management of benign liver tumors. *Surg Clin North Am.* 2004;84:463–480.

2. Arnold HL, Harrison SA. New advances in evaluation and management of patients with polycystic liver disease. *Am J Gastroenterol.* 2005;100:2569–2582.

3. Hansman MF, Ryan JA, Holmes JH, et al. Management and long-term follow-up of hepatic cysts. *American Journal of Surgery.* 2001;181:404–410.

4. Tahvanainen E, Tahvanainen P, Kaariainen H, et al. Polycystic liver and kidney diseases. *Annals of Medicine.* 2005;37:546–555.

5. Cowles RA, Mulholland MW. Solitary hepatic cysts. *J Am Coll Surg.* 2000;191:311–321.

6. Katkhouda N, Mavor E. Laparoscopic management of benign liver disease. *Surgical Clinics of North America.* 2000;80:1203–+.

7. Trotter JF, Everson GT. Benign Focal Lesions of the Liver. *Clinics in Liver Disease* 2001;5:17–42.

8. Buetow PC, Buck JL, Pantongragbrown L, et al. Biliary Cystadenoma and Cystadenocarcinoma—Clinical-Imaging-Pathological Correlation with Emphasis on the Importance of Ovarian Stroma. *Radiology.* 1995;196:805–810.

9. Devaney K, Goodman ZD, Ishak KG. Hepatobiliary Cystadenoma and Cystadenocarcinoma—A Light-Microscopic and Immunohistochemical Study of 70 Patients. *American Journal of Surgical Pathology.* 1994;18:1078–1091.

10. Pinson CW, Munson JL, Rossi RL, et al. Enucleation of Intrahepatic Biliary Cystadenomas. *Surg Gynecol Obstet.* 1989;168:534–537.

11. Yagci G, Ustunsoz B, Kaymakcioglu N, et al. Results of surgical, laparoscopic, and percutaneous treatment for hydatid disease of the liver: 10 Years experience with 355 patients. *World Journal of Surgery.* 2005;29:1670–1679.

12. Gharbi HA, Hassine W, Brauner MW, et al. Ultrasound Examination of the Hydatic Liver. *Radiology.* 1981;139:459–463.

13. Manterola C, Cuadra A, Munoz S, et al. In a diagnostic test study the validity of three serodiagnostic test was compared in patients with liver echinococcosis. *Journal of Clinical Epidemiology.* 2005;58:401–406.

14. Khuroo MS, Wani NA, Javid G, et al. Percutaneous drainage compared with surgery for hepatic hydatid cysts. *New England Journal of Medicine.* 1997;337:881–887.

15. Dervenis C, Delis S, Avgerinos C, et al. Changing concepts in the management of liver hydatid disease. *Journal of Gastrointestinal Surgery.* 2005;9:869–877.

16. Jabbour N, Shirazi SK, Genyk Y, et al. Surgical management of complicated hydatid disease of the liver. *Am Surg.* 2002;68:984–988.

17. Ezer A, Nursal TZ, Moray G, et al. Surgical treatment of liver hydatid cysts. *HPB Surgery.* 2006;8:38–42.

18. Bickel A, Lobcrant N, Singer-Jordan J, et al. The laparoscopic approach to abdominal hydatid cysts—A prospective nonselective study using the isolated hypobaric technique. *Archives of Surgery.* 2001;136:789–795.

19. Brunetti E, Filice C. Radiofrequency thermal ablation of echinococcal liver cysts. *Lancet.* 2001;358:1464.

20. Kim J, Ahmad SA, Lowy AM, et al. An algorithm for the accurate identification of benign liver lesions. *American Journal of Surgery.* 2004;187:274–279.

21. Baum JK, Bookstein JJ, Holtz F, et al. Possible association between benign hepatomas and oral contraceptives. *Lancet.* 1973;2:926–929.

22. Cobey FC, Salem RR. A review of liver masses in pregnancy and a proposed algorithm for their diagnosis and management. *American Journal of Surgery.* 2004;187:181–191.

23. Foster JH, Berman MM. The Malignant Transformation of Liver-Cell Adenomas. *Archives of Surgery.* 1994;129:712–717.

24. Labrune P, Trioche P, Duvaltier I, et al. Hepatocellular adenomas in glycogen storage disease type I and III: A series of 43 patients and review of the literature. *Journal of Pediatric Gastroenterology and Nutrition.* 1997;24:276–279.

25. Grazioli L, Federle MP, Brancatelli G, et al. Hepatic adenomas: Imaging and pathologic findings. *Radiographics.* 2001;21:877–892.

26. Aseni P, Sansalone CV, Sammartino C, et al. Rapid disappearance of hepatic adenoma after contraceptive withdrawal. *Journal of Clinical Gastroenterology.* 2001;33:234–236.

27. Terkivatan T, de Wilt JHW, de Man RA, et al. Indications and long-term outcome of treatment for benign hepatic tumors—A critical appraisal. *Archives of Surgery.* 2001;136:1033–1038.

28. Jabbour N, Brenner M, Gagandeep S, et al. Major hepatobiliary surgery during pregnancy: safety and timing. *Am Surg.* 2005;71:354–358.

29. Mathieu D, Kobeiter H, Maison P, et al. Oral contraceptive use and focal nodular hyperplasia of the liver. *Gastroenterology.* 2000;118:560–564.

30. Brunt EM. Benign tumors of the Liver. *Clinics in Liver Disease.* 2001;5:1–15.

31. Choi BY, Nguyen MH. The diagnosis and management of benign hepatic tumors. *Journal of Clinical Gastroenterology.* 2005;39:401–412.

32. Corigliano N, Mercantini P, Amodio PM, et al. Hemoperitoneum from a spontaneous rupture of a giant hemangioma of the liver: Report of a case. *Surgery Today.* 2003;33:459–463.

33. Hotokezaka M, Kojima M, Nakamura K, et al. Traumatic rupture of hepatic hemangioma. *Journal of Clinical Gastroenterology.* 1996;23:69–71.

34. Gedaly R, Pomposelli JJ, Pomfret EA, et al. Cavernous hemangioma of the liver—Anatomic resection vs enucleation. *Archives of Surgery.* 1999;134:407–411.

35. Yoon SS, Charny CK, Fong Y, et al. Diagnosis, management, and outcomes of 115 patients with hepatic hemangioma. *J Am Coll Surg.* 2003;197:392–402.

36. Deutsch GS, Yeh KA, Bates WB, et al. Embolization for management of hepatic hemangiomas. *Am Surg.* 2001;67:159–164.

37. Ferraz AA, Sette MJ, Maia M, et al. Liver transplant for the treatment of giant hepatic hemangioma. *Liver Transpl.* 2004;10:1436–1437.

38. Kumashiro Y, Kasahara M, Nomoto K, et al. Living donor liver transplantation for giant hepatic hemangioma with Kasabach-Merritt syndrome with a posterior segment graft. *Liver Transpl.* 2002;8:721–724.

39. Sherman M. Hepatocellular carcinoma: Epidemiology risk factors, and screening. *Seminars in Liver Disease.* 2005;25:143–154.

40. Parkin DM, Bray F, Ferlay J, et al. Estimating the world cancer burden: GLOBOCAN 2000. *International Journal of Cancer.* 2001;94:153–156.

41. Wilson JF. Liver cancer on the rise. *Annals of Internal Medicine.* 2005;142:1029–1032.

42. El Serag H, Davila JA, Petersen NJ, et al. The continuing increase in the incidence of hepatocellular carcinoma in the United States: An update. *Annals of Internal Medicine.* 2003;139:817–823.

43. El Serag HB, Mason AC. Rising incidence of hepatocellular carcinoma in the United States. *New England Journal of Medicine.* 1999;340:745–750.

44. Morgan TR, Mandayam S, Jamal MM. Alcohol and hepatocellular carcinoma. *Gastroenterology.* 2004;127(5):S87–S96.

45. Sherman M, Peltekian KM, Lee C. Screening for Hepatocellular-Carcinoma in Chronic Carriers of Hepatitis-B Virus—Incidence and Prevalence of Hepatocellular-Carcinoma in A North-American Urban-Population. *Hepatology.* 1995;22:432–438.

46. Sun CA, Wu DM, Lin CC, et al. Incidence and cofactors of hepatitis C virus-related hepatocellular carcinoma: A prospective study of 12,008 men in Taiwan. *Am J Epidemiol.* 2003;157:674–682.

47. Caballeria L, Pares A, Castells A, et al. Hepatocellular carcinoma in primary biliary cirrhosis: similar incidence to that in hepatitis C virus-related cirrhosis. *Am J Gastroenterol.* 2001;96:1160–1163.

48. Davila JA, Morgan RO, Shaib Y, et al. Diabetes increases the risk of hepatocellular carcinoma in the United States: a population based case control study. *Gut.* 2005;54:533–539.

49. Elmberg M, Hultcrantz R, Ekbom A, et al. Cancer risk in patients with hereditary hemochromatosis and in their first-degree relatives. *Gastroenterology.* 2003;125:1733–1741.

50. Eriksson S, Carlson J, Velez R. Risk of Cirrhosis and Primary Liver-Cancer in Alpha-1-Antitrypsin Deficiency. *New England Journal of Medicine.* 1986;314:736–739.

51. Di Bisceglie AM. Epidemiology and clinical presentation of hepatocellular carcinoma. *Journal of Vascular and Interventional Radiology.* 2002;13:S169–S171.

52. Kaczynski J, Hansson G, Wallerstedt S. Clinical features in hepatocellular carcinoma and the impact of autopsy on diagnosis. A study of 530 cases from a low-endemicity area. *Hepato-Gastroenterology.* 2005;52:1798–1802.

53. Qin LX, Tang ZY. Hepatocellular carcinoma with obstructive jaundice: diagnosis, treatment and prognosis. *World Journal of Gastroenterology.* 2003;9:385–391.

54. Luo JC, Hwang SJ, Wu JC, et al. Clinical characteristics and prognosis of hepatocellular carcinoma patients with paraneoplastic syndromes. *Hepato-Gastroenterology.* 2002;49:1315–1319.

55. Schafer DF, Sorrell MF. Hepatocellular carcinoma. *Lancet.* 1999;353:1253–1257.

56. Colli A, Fraquelli M, Casazza G, et al. Accuracy of ultrasonography, spiral CT, magnetic resonance, and alpha-fetoprotein in diagnosing hepatocellular carcinoma: A systematic review. *Am J Gastroenterol.* 2006;101:513–523.

57. Marrero JA. Screening Tests for Hepatocellular Carcinoma. *Clinics in Liver Disease.* 2005;9:235–251.

58. De Masi S, Tosti ME, Mele A. Screening for hepatocellular carcinoma. *Digestive and Liver Disease* 2005;37:260–268.

59. Colombo M, Defranchis R, Delninno E, et al. Hepatocellular-Carcinoma in Italian Patients with Cirrhosis. *New England Journal of Medicine.* 1991;325:675–680.

60. Pateron D, Ganne N, Trinchet JC, et al. Prospective-Study of Screening for Hepatocellular-Carcinoma in Caucasian Patients with Cirrhosis. *Journal of Hepatology.* 1994;20:65–71.

61. Taura N, Hamasaki K, Nakao K, et al. Clinical benefits of hepatocellular carcinoma surveillance: A single-center, hospital-based study. *Oncology Reports.* 2005;14:999–1003.

62. Yuen MF, Cheng CC, Lauder IJ, et al. Early detection of hepatocellular carcinoma increases the chance of treatment: Hong Kong experience. *Hepatology.* 2000;31:330–335.

63. Zoli M, Magalotti D, Bianchi G, et al. Efficacy of a surveillance program for early detection of hepatocellular carcinoma. *Cancer.* 1996;78:977–985.

64. Chen JG, Parkin DM, Chen QG, et al. Screening for liver cancer: results of a randomised controlled trial in Qidong, China. *J Med Screening.* 2003;10:204–209.

65. Sangiovanni A, Del Ninno E, Fasani P, et al. Increased survival of cirrhotic patients with a hepatocellular carcinoma detected during surveillance. *Gastroenterology.* 2004;126:1005–1014.

66. Murakami T, Mochizuki K, Nakamura H. Imaging evaluation of the cirrhotic liver. *Seminars in Liver Disease.* 2001;21:213–224.

67. Baron RL, Brancatelli G. Computed tomographic imaging of hepatocellular carcinoma. *Gastroenterology.* 2004;127:S133–S143.

68. Brancatelli G, Baron RL, Peterson MS, et al. Helical CT screening for hepatocellular carcinoma in patients with cirrhosis: Frequency and causes of false-positive interpretation. *American Journal of Roentgenology.* 2003;180:1007–1014.

69. Lim JH, Kim EY, Lee WJ, et al. Regenerative nodules in liver cirrhosis: Findings at CT during arterial portography and CT hepatic arteriography with histopathologic with histopathologic correlation. *Radiology.* 1999;210:451–458.

70. Nakayama A, Imamura H, Matsuyama Y, et al. Value of lipiodol computed tomography and digital subtraction angiography in the era of helical biphasic computed tomography as preoperative assessment of hepatocellular carcinoma. *Ann Surg.* 2001;234:56–62.

71. Zheng XH, Guan YS, Zhou XP, et al. Detection of Hypervascular Hepatocellular Carcinoma: Comparison of Multi-Detector CT with Digital Subtraction Angiography and Lipiodol CT. *World Journal of Gastroenterology.* 2005;11:200–203.

72. Kadoya M, Matsui O, Takashima T, et al. Hepatocellular-carcinoma—correlation of MR imaging and histopathologic findings. *Radiology.* 1992;183:819–825.

73. Cancer of the Liver Program (CLIP) Investigators. A New Prognostic System for Hepatocellular Carcinoma: A Retrospective Study of 435 Patients. *Hepatology.* 1998;28:751–755.

74. Farinati F, Rinaldi M, Gianni S, et al. How should patients with hepatocellular carcinoma be staged? Validation of a new prognostic system. *Cancer.* 2000;89:2266–2273.

75. Llovet JM, Schwartz M, Mazzaferro V. Resection and liver transplantation for hepatocellular carcinoma. *Seminars in Liver Disease.* 2005;25:181–200.

76. Mazzaferro V, Regalia E, Doci R, et al. Liver transplantation for the treatment of small hepatocellular carcinomas in patients with cirrhosis. *New England Journal of Medicine.* 1996;334:693–699.

77. Bismuth H, Majno PE, Adam R. Liver transplantation for hepatocellular carcinoma. *Seminars in Liver Disease* 1999;19:311–322.

78. Yao FY, Ferrell L, Bass NM, et al. Liver transplantation for hepatocellular carcinoma: Expansion of the tumor size limits does not adversely impact survival. *Hepatology.* 2001;33:1394–1403.

79. Fong Y, Sun RL, Jarnagin W, et al. An Analysis of 412 Cases of Hepatocellular Carcinoma at a Western Center. *Ann Surg.* 1999;229:790–800.

80. Poon RT, Fan ST, Lo CM, et al. Long-Term Survival and Pattern of Recurrence After Resection of Small Hepatocellular Carcinoma in Patients with Preserved Liver Function. *Ann Surg.* 2002;235:373–382.

81. Ercolani G, Grazi GL, Ravaioli M, et al. Liver resection for hepatocellular carcinoma on cirrhosis. *Ann Surg.* 2003;237:536–543.

82. Miyagawa S, Makuuchi M, Kawasaki S, et al. Criteria for Safe Hepatic Resection. *American Journal of Surgery.* 1995;169:589–594.

83. Makuuchi M, Kosuge T, Takayama T, et al. Surgery for Small Liver Cancers. *Seminars in Surgical Oncology.* 1993;9:298–304.

84. Grazi GL, Ercolani G, Pierangeli F, et al. Improved results of liver resection for hepatocellular carcinoma on cirrhosis give the procedure added value. *Ann Surg.* 2001;234:71–78.

85. Kaihara S, Kiuchi T, Ueda M, et al. Living-donor liver transplantation for hepatocellular carcinoma. *Transplantation.* 2003;75:S37–S40.

86. Todo S, Furukawa H. Living donor liver transplantation for adult patients with hepatocellular carcinoma—Experience in Japan. *Ann Surg.* 2004;240:451–459.

87. Beaugrand M, N'kontchou G, Seror O, et al. Local/regional and systemic treatments of hepatocellular carcinoma. *Seminars in Liver Disease.* 2005;25:201–211.

88. DiStasi M, Buscarini L, Livraghi T, et al. Percutaneous ethanol injection in the treatment of hepatocellular carcinoma—A multicenter survey of evaluation practices and complication rates. *Scandinavian Journal of Gastroenterology.* 1997;32:1168–1173.

89. Livraghi T, Giorgio A, Marin G, et al. Hepatocellular-carcinoma and cirrhosis in 146 patients—long-term results of percutaneous ethanol injection. *Radiology.* 1995;197:101–108.

90. Khan KN, Yatsuhashi H, Yamasaki K, et al. Prospective analysis of risk factors for early intrahepatic recurrence of hepatocellular carcinoma following ethanol injection. *Journal of Hepatology.* 2000;32:269–278.

91. Koda M, Murawaki Y, Mitsuda A, et al. Predictive factors for intrahepatic recurrence after percutaneous ethanol injection therapy for small hepatocellular carcinoma. *Cancer.* 2000;88:529–537.

92. Lencioni R, Bartolozzi C, Carmella D, et al. Treatment of Small Hepatocellular-Carcinoma with Percutaneous Ethanol Injection—Analysis of Prognostic Factors in 105 Western Patients. *Cancer.* 1995;76:1737–1746.

93. Lin S, Lin C, Lin C, et al. Radiofrequency Ablation Improves Prognosis Compared With Ethanol Injection for Hepatocellular Carcinoma </= 4 cm. *Gastroenterology.* 2004;127:1714–1723.

94. Lencioni RA, Allgaier HP, Cioni D, et al. Small hepatocellular carcinoma in cirrhosis: Randomized comparison of radio-frequency thermal ablation versus percutaneous ethanol injection. *Radiology.* 2003;228:235–240.

95. Mazzaferro V, Battiston C, Perrone S, et al. Radiofrequency ablation of small hepatocellular carcinoma in cirrhotic patients awaiting liver transplantation—A prospective study. *Ann Surg.* 2004;240:900–909.

96. Fontana RJ, Hamidullah H, Nghiem H, et al. Percutaneous radiofrequency thermal ablation of hepatocellular carcinoma: A safe and effective bridge to liver transplantation. *Liver Transpl.* 2002;8:1165–1174.

97. Lau WY, Yu SCH, Lai ECH, et al. Transarterial chemoembolization for hepatocellular carcinoma. *J Am Coll Surg.* 2006;202:155–168.

98. Clark HP, Carson WF, Kavanagh PV, et al. Staging and Current Treatment of Hepatocellular Carcinoma. *Radiographics.* 2005;25:S3–S23.

99. Llovet JM, Real MI, Montana X, et al. Arterial embolisation or chemoembolisation versus symptomatic treatment in patients with unresectable hepatocellular carcinoma: a randomised controlled trial. *Lancet.* 2002;359:1734–1739.

100. Lo CM, Ngan H, Tso WK, et al. Randomized controlled trial of transarterial lipiodol chemoembolization for unresectable hepatocellular carcinoma. *Hepatology.* 2002;35:1164–1171.

101. Fan JT, Yu ZY, Wu YQ, et al. Improved Survival with Resection after Transcatheter Arterial Chemoembolization (TACE) for Unresectable Hepatocellular Carcinoma. *Digestive Surgery.* 1998;15:674–678.

102. Graziadei IW, Sandmueller H, Waldenberger P, et al. Chemoembolization followed by liver transplantation for hepatocellular carcinoma impedes tumor progression while on the waiting list and leads to excellent outcome. *Liver Transpl.* 2003;9:557–563.

103. Llovet JM, Fuster J, Bruix J. Intention-to-Treat Analysis of Surgical Treatment for Early Hepatocellular Carcinoma: Resection Versus Transplantation. *Hepatology.* 1999;30:1434–1440.

104. Burroughs A, Hochhauser D, Meyer T. Systemic treatment and liver transplantation for hepatocellular carcinoma: two ends of the therapeutic spectrum. *Lancet Oncol.* 2004;5:409–418.

105. Chow PKH, Tai BC, Tan CK, et al. High-dose tamoxifen in the treatment of inoperable hepatocellular carcinoma: A multicenter randomized controlled trial. *Hepatology.* 2002;36:1221–1226.

106. CLIP Group (Cancer of the Liver Italian Programme). Tamoxifen in Treatment of Hepatocellular Carcinoma: a Randomised Controlled Trial. *Lancet.* 1998;352:17–20.

107. Grimaldi C, Bleiberg H, Gay F, et al. Evaluation of antiandrogen therapy in unresectable hepatocellular carcinoma: Results of a European organization for research and treatment of cancer multicentric double-blind trial. *Journal of Clinical Oncology.* 1998;16:411–417.

108. Llovet JM, Sala M, Castells L, et al. Randomized controlled trial of interferon treatment for advanced hepatocellular carcinoma. *Hepatology.* 2000;31:54–58.

109. Schwartz JD, Schwartz M, Mandeli J, et al. Neoadjuvant and adjuvant therapy for resectable hepatocellular carcinoma: review of the randomised clinical trials. *Lancet Oncology.* 2002;3:593–603.

110. McLarney JK, Rucker PT, Bender GN, et al. Fibrolamellar carcinoma of the liver: Radiologic-pathologic correlation. *Radiographics.* 1999;19:453–471.

111. El Serag HB, Davila JA. Is fibrolamellar carcinoma different from hepatocellular carcinoma? A US population-based study. *Hepatology.* 2004;39:798–803.

112. Pinna AD, Iwatsuki S, Lee RG, et al. Treatment of fibrolamellar hepatoma with subtotal hepatectomy or transplantation. *Hepatology.* 1997;26:877–883.

113. Caruso M, Panis Y, Gagandeep S, et al. Regression of Established Macroscopic Liver Metastasis After In Situ Transduction of a Suicide Gene. *Proceedings of the National Academy of Sciences (USA).* 1993;90:7024–7028.

114. Gagandeep S, Ott M, Nisen PD, et al. Overexpression of Mad transcription factor inhibits proliferation of cultured human hepatocellular carcinoma cells along with tumor formation in immunodeficient animals. *JG Med.* 2000;2:117–127.

COMMENTARY
Linda L. Wong

The incidence of hepatocellular cancer (HCC) continues to rise: the incidence in the 1970s was 1.4 per 100,000, the incidence in the late 1990s was 3.0 per 100,000, and the incidence continues to rise into the 2000s (1). The increase has been clearly identified in those above age 40 years, and the greatest increase is seen in white men ages 45 to 54 years. As mentioned by the authors of the preceding chapter, the increase in incidence of HCC has paralleled the rise in incidence of hepatitis C, and the high rate of HCC is expected to double in the next 10 to 20 years (2). However, the next epidemic of chronic liver disease to cause cirrhosis and HCC will be nonalcoholic steatohepatitis (NASH). An estimated 20% of the population in the United States is obese, and this is a trend not likely to decrease any time soon. Fatty liver disease and nonalcoholic liver disease that accompany the metabolic syndrome of obesity, dyslipidemia, hypertension, and insulin resistance will flourish and the cirrhosis related to these diseases will only further fuel the incidence of HCC. HCC was once a disease primarily of underdeveloped countries related to hepatitis B and aflatoxin, but may soon become an epidemic in developed counties.

Although it has always been a given tenet that the best treatments for HCC have been surgical ones, most patients will not be candidates for any type of surgical intervention. Liver transplantation is the best treatment for limited HCC of small size with underlying cirrhosis; superior long-term survival without recurrence can be achieved with transplantation. Large HCC or HCC in the absence of underlying cirrhosis and good synthetic function is best treated with liver resection. The larger HCCs have a higher likelihood of having vascular invasion and subsequent disease recurrence (3). Larger HCC and extensive multifocal disease are thus not appropriate for liver transplant because of concern about disease recurrence under immunosuppression. Although the exact size and extent of disease that is appropriate for transplant is controversial and not been completely delineated, the current accepted criteria for liver transplant, as the authors of the chapter have mentioned, are the Milan criteria (single tumor <5 cm or three or less tumors all <3 cm). Ablative techniques are used for nontransplant candidates or as a bridge to transplant. Systemic chemotherapy or chemoembolization are clearly not as effective as the surgical and ablative techniques and are reserved for nonsurgical candidates.

One might conclude that the key to optimal treatment would be to find HCC early and transplant as many patients as possible. Unfortunately, in spite of efforts to increase the supply of liver donors, the number of available livers cannot possibly keep up with the burgeoning demand. In 2007, there were over 17,000 patients waiting for liver transplant, and in 2006 only 5,365 deceased donor liver transplants and 249 living donor liver transplants were performed. About 6.8% of all liver transplants in 2005 were done in the face of HCC. This has progressively increased from 1% to 2% of all transplants a decade ago. Five-year survival for liver transplant for HCC has recently been calculated to be 54.3%. Although this is an excellent result for patients with HCC, this is the lowest 5-year survival rate when compared with liver transplantation for nonmalignant diseases. The overall 5-year survival for liver transplantation for all indications is 66.7% (4). So at the moment, are we justified in using a precious resource such as the donor liver for so many patients with HCC when these patients will have an inferior outcome compared with the thousands of patients waiting for livers who have nonmalignant diseases? Living liver donors may help, but careful donor identification/evaluation, potential donor morbidity, and proper credentialing and data collection of centers has prompted transplant centers to proceed vigilantly in this area.

The answer to this epidemic of HCC may not be only in the surgeon's ability to resect or transplant this disease. First, we need to identify HCC as early as possible so that patients may be candidates for resection or transplant. Requirements for a successful screening program for any disease include the following: (a) the disease must be common and have a severe outcome; (b) the screening test should be widely available and noninvasive, inexpensive, and easily applied; (c) the at-risk population should be well defined and should accept the need for screening; (d) the physicians caring for the at-risk population should also accept the need for screening; and (e) there should be effective treatment available (5). Although screening patients with viral hepatitis B and C with alpha fetoprotein levels and ultrasound of the liver will fulfill many of these criteria, there are very few randomized, controlled trials that have been done to evaluate the impact of surveillance. Despite the lack of evidence from controlled studies, most gastroenterologists advocate screening those patients at risk for HCC.

Another area that may have a more profound effect on the incidence of HCC is strategies to prevent the diseases that predispose one to HCC. In 1984, a large-scale program in Taiwan was initiated to vaccinate all newborns for hepatitis B. Initial report from Taiwan's National Cancer Registry showed that the annual incidence of HCC in children ages 6 to 14 years declined from 0.7 to 0.36 per 100,000 between 1986 and 1990 and 1990 and 1994. The mortality from HCC also declined. By 2000, they reported that the annual incidence in children ages 6 to 9 years had a decline in incidence from 0.52 to 0.13 per 100,000 when comparing children born before 1986 versus 1986 and 1988 (6,7).

Treatment of viral hepatitis B and C may also have an impact on prevention of HCC. Liaw et al. (8) randomized 651 patients with hepatitis B to receive the nucleoside analog, lamivudine, or a placebo. The primary end point was time to disease progression defined by hepatic decompensation, HCC, spontaneous bacterial peritonitis, bleeding gastroesophageal varices, or death related to liver disease. HCC developed in 3.4% of patients receiving lamivudine versus 7.4% of those receiving placebo. The study had to be terminated after a mean of 32.4 months because of a significant difference between the treatment groups in the number of end points reached. Other studies are emerging that indicate that persistent elevation of hepatitis B-DNA levels and hepatitis B e-antigen positivity are associated the highest risk for HCC (9,10). Newer antiviral agents for hepatitis B that specifically target viral replication may have a profound effect on development of HCC in the future.

There is also evidence that treatment of hepatitis C with interferon may reduce the incidence of HCC. A large retrospective cohort study of 738 patients indicated that patients who received interferon (n = 594) had a lower incidence of HCC than those who did not (n = 144). Both those who had a sustained response and a transient response to interferon appeared to have this reduced incidence of HCC (11). Several other smaller retrospective studies seem to confirm this, but it was difficult to determine if patients who were selected for interferon treatment were earlier in the course of their disease/fibrosis and were thus inherently less likely to develop HCC (12,13). More recently, several randomized studies demonstrated reduction or delays in the incidence of HCC (14,15). Treatment of viral hepatitis C as well as B may have a great impact on the incidence of HCC in the future. Thus, it is imperative that primary care physicians recognize those patients who are at risk for having viral hepatitis so they may not only treat the viral disease but prevent HCC.

As for the emerging epidemic of fatty liver disease and NASH, the United States continues to do what it can to improve diet and encourage exercise in the population. This may come in the form of better labeling of foods, banning of trans fats, changing school lunches, and public education on proper diet and exercise. Public education on nutrition has occurred for many decades; despite this, the percentage of Americans who are obese or overweight has continued to increase. This is not a problem unique to the United States as many developed countries are facing similar problems. Within the last 5 years, we have also seen an astronomical increase in the use of bariatric surgery to combat this condition. There is some early evidence that gastric bypass does improve the steatosis, necroinflammatory activity, and hepatic fibrosis associated with NASH (16,17). Reduced fibrosis and inflammation would have a theoretic benefit on hepatocarcinogenesis, but whether bariatric surgery has the ability to ultimately change the incidence of HCC in this population is unknown.

Thus, HCC is about to become an epidemic. Although surgeons are proud of their success with liver transplantation for HCC, this approach may not be enough to control the disease. Among 232 patients with HCC referred to the Transplant Center in Honolulu, only 15% were deemed qualified for a liver transplant, and only 8.2% actually underwent liver transplantation (18). The SEER database (Surveillance, Epidemiology and End-Results) of the National Cancer Institute has 7,389 patients with HCC followed from 1977 to 1996. Overall 1-year survival increased from 14% in the period 1977–1981 to 23% in the period 1992–1996. Five-year survival increased from 2% to 5% between these two periods. During the period 1987–1991, only 0.8% of patients underwent radical surgery, and these patients had a 1-year survival of 59% and 5-year survival of 35% (19). A more recent review of the SEER Medicare database in 1992–1999 identified 2,963 patients with HCC with continuous Medicare enrollment. Of these patients, 13% received potentially curative therapy (transplant, 0.9%; resection, 8.2%; local ablation, 4.1%), 4% received transarterial chemoembolization, 57% received other palliative therapy, and 26% received no specific therapy (20). To truly impact this disease, we need to improve our ability to detect HCC at an early stage and allow for potentially curative therapies, or we need to find ways to completely prevent HCC.

REFERENCE

1. El-Serag HB, Davila JA, Petersen NJ, et al. The continuing increase in the incidence of hepatocellular carcinoma in the United States: an update. *Ann Intern Med.* 2003;139:817–823.
2. El-Serag HB. Hepatocellular carcinoma and hepatitis C in the United States. *Hepatology.* 2002;36:S74–83.
3. Pawlik TM, Delman KA, Vauthey JN, et al. Tumor size predicts vascular invasion and histologic grade: Implications for selection of surgical treatment for hepatocellular carcinoma. *Liver Transpl.* 2005;11:1086–1092.
4. www.unos.org
5. Prorok PC. Epidemiologic approach for cancer screening: problems in design and analysis of trials. *Am J Pediatr Hematol Oncol.* 1992;14:117–128.
6. Chang MH, Chen CJ, Lai MS, et al. Universal hepatitis B vaccination in Taiwan and the incidence of hepatocellular carcinoma in children. Taiwan Childhood Hepatoma Study Group. *N Engl J Med.* 1997;336:1855–1859.
7. Hung K, Lin S. Nationwide vaccination: a success story in Taiwan. *Vaccine.* 2000;18:s35–38.
8. Liaw YF, Sung JJ, Chow WC, et al. Lamivudine for patients with chronic hepatitis B and advanced liver disease. *N Engl J Med.* 2004;351:1521–1531.
9. Chen CJ, Yang HI, Su J, et al. Risk of hepatocellular carcinoma across a biological gradient of serum hepatitis B viral DNA level. JAMA 2006;295:65–73.
10. Yang HI, Lu SN, Liaw YF, et al. Hepatitis B e-Antigen and the risk of hepatocellular cancer. *N Engl J Med.* 2002;347:168–174.
11. Tanaka H, Tsukuma H, Kasahara A, et al. Effect of interferon therapy on the incidence of hepatocellular carcinoma and mortality of patients with chronic hepatitis C: a retrospective cohort study of 738 patients. *Int J Cancer.* 2000;87:741–749.
12. Miyajima I, Sata M, Kumashiro R et al. The incidence of hepatocellular carcinoma in patients with chronic hepatitis C after interferon treatment. *Oncol Rep.* 1998;5:201–204.
13. Hayashi K, Kumada T, Nakano S et al. Incidence of hepatocellular carcinoma in chronic hepatitis C after interferon therapy. *Hepatogastroenterology.* 2002;49:508–512.
14. Soga K, Shibasaki K, Aoyagi Y. Effect of interferon on incidence of hepatocellular carcinoma in patients with chronic hepatitis C. Hepatogastroenterology. 2005;52:1154–1158.
15. Hino K, Kitase A, Satoh Y, et al. Interferon retreatment reduces or delays the incidence of hepatocellular carcinoma in patients with chronic hepatitis C. *J Viral Hepat.* 2002;9:370–376.
16. Klein S., Mittendorfer B, Eagon JC, et al. Gastric bypass surgery improves metabolic and hepatic abnormalities associated with nonalcoholic fatty liver disease. *Gastroenterology.* 2006;130:1564–1572.
17. deAlmeida SR, Rocha PR, Sanches MD, et al. Roux-en-Y gastric bypass improves the nonalcoholic steatohepatitis (NASH) of morbid obesity. *Obes Surg.* 2006;16:270–278.
18. Wong LL, Tsai N, Limm W et al. Liver transplant for hepatocellular cancer: a treatment for the select few. *Clin Tranplant.* 2004;18:205–210.
19. El-serag HB, Mason AC, Key C. Trends in survival of patients with hepatocellular carcinoma between 1977 and 1996 in the United States. *Hepatology.* 2001;33:62–65.
20. El-Serag HB, Siegel AB, Davila JA, et al. Treatment and outcomes of treating of hepatocellular carcinoma among Medicare recipients in the United States: a population-based study. *J Hepatol.* 2006;44:158–166.

47

Surgical Management of Metastatic Liver Disease

Jeffrey M. Farma, Hiroomi Tada, and John M. Daly

The liver is a common site of metastatic disease for many different malignancies. This chapter focuses primarily on the evaluation and management of hepatic metastases from colorectal carcinoma and the surgical approaches to their treatment. Surgical treatment modalities include hepatic resection, local ablation techniques, and regional infusion therapies. This chapter will also touch on the application of these and other strategies in the management of metastatic tumors from neuroendocrine tumors, other gastrointestinal cancers, sarcoma, melanoma, and breast cancer.

It is estimated that 146,970 new cases of colorectal cancer will be diagnosed in the United States in 2009 and that 49,920 patients will die of the disease in this year. About 20% of the patients will have metastatic disease at the time of initial diagnosis (1). Although many of these patients develop liver metastases in the course of their disease, the liver is the only site of recurrence in 23% (2). Many of these patients are potential candidates for locoregional therapy including surgical resection. Without resection, the median survival of patients with liver metastases treated with aggressive systemic chemotherapy ranges from 11 to 20 months, depending on tumor burden, and 5-year survival of patients with even solitary liver metastases is rare (3–6). The natural course of the disease, if left untreated, has a median survival of 6 to 12 months (7). However, in selected patients undergoing surgical resection, 5-year survival rates of 25% to 48% have been reported with operative mortalities between 1.3% and 5% (8–11). Therefore, treatment of metastatic colorectal cancer limited to the liver in selected patients may alter the natural history of the disease.

EVALUATION OF THE PATIENT WITH LIVER METASTASES

Preoperative Evaluation

Over the past decade there has been a dramatic change in the quality of imaging modalities, providing increased opportunities to detect recurrent cancer earlier. The initial evaluation of a patient with liver metastases from colorectal cancer should include liver function tests, a carcinoembryonic antigen (CEA) level, a chest radiograph, and computerized tomography (CT) scans of the chest, abdomen, and pelvis to identify any additional sites of metastatic disease. Additional modalities may include dynamic enhanced magnetic resonance imaging (MRI), ultrasound and 2-[^{18}F]-fluro-2-deoxyglucose (^{18}FDG) positron emission tomography (PET). Evidence of local colon recurrence can be assessed by barium enema, colonoscopy, CT, and/or PET scan. In one study of 132 patients who were thought to have isolated liver metastases, 25 patients were found to have other sites of distant spread (primarily lung metastases) on their preoperative evaluation. Even when all preoperative studies were negative, 26% of the remaining 107 patients had extrahepatic disease discovered at the time of laparotomy (12). The most common sites of intra-abdominal, extrahepatic disease were the celiac and porta hepatis lymph nodes (12,13). Other studies have shown similar rates of unsuspected extrahepatic disease ranging from 21% to 54% (14–16).

In addition to identifying extrahepatic disease, preoperative studies are aimed at assessing the extent and resectability of the metastases (Table 47.1). The number, size, and segmental location of liver lesions as well as their proximity to major arterial, venous, portal, and biliary structures can now be more accurately determined prior to surgery. Current high-resolution multidetector dynamic CT has the capability of providing very detailed images of the liver with three-dimensional vascular reconstructions, which have made formal angiography generally unnecessary. Using triple-phase evaluation, the arterial, and portal venous phases may be used to better delineate tumors with varying degrees of vascularity (17). In a recent meta-analysis comparing different noninvasive imaging methods to detect hepatic metastases from gastrointestinal tract cancers, Kinkel et al. (18) found a mean weighted sensitivity for CT of 72% in approximately 1,700 patients imaged. Others have reported sensitivities between 69% and 73% and specificities of 86% to 96% with helical CT (Table 47.2) (19,20). CT portography has a sensitivity ranging from 83% to 94% with a false-positive rate of 15% (21–23). CT portogram can accurately detect small lesions or additional metastases that alter the surgical approach or preclude resection, but has largely been replaced by CT angiography (21).

MRI has improved dramatically with increases in computing power and image acquisition. By employing phase-array surface coils, smaller field of views, thinner slices, and higher resolution can be used for improved tumor detection. In addition to gadolinium, newer contrast agents including mangafodipir trisodium, a hepatocyte-selective contrast agent, and superparamagnetic iron oxide have helped to further delineate liver architecture and pathology (17). The sensitivity of MRI in the detection of liver metastases ranges from 76% to 82%, and has been shown to be increased to 86.8% with the addition of superparamagnetic iron oxide-enhanced MRI (18,20,24,25).

Table 47.1

Factors Determining Resectability of Hepatic Lesions

Factor	Considerations
Number of lesions	Four or fewer lesions
Location of lesions	Proximity to major vascular structures
	Type of resection required
	Ability to obtain clear margins (>1 cm)
Extrahepatic disease	Generally precludes hepatic resection

The use of PET has been studied to evaluate patients considered to be at high risk for harboring extrahepatic metastatic disease. Using a positron emitting ^{18}F-labeled analog of glucose FDG, investigators have been studying the increase in glucose metabolism in tumor cells as compared with normal tissue. Increased uptake can be reported and measured as the standardized uptake value, which is the ratio of activity in a tissue divided by the decay-corrected activity injected into the patient (26). Multiple studies using PET for detection of metastatic disease in the abdomen and liver have found superior sensitivities to both CT and MRI (18). Fong et al. (27) evaluated preoperative PET in a group of 40 patients. PET had a sensitivity of 91% and a specificity of 79% for detecting extrahepatic disease, but PET detection was limited with liver and peritoneal tumors <1 cm in size. In a recent meta-analysis of 229 patients, PET was helpful in the identification of extrahepatic disease in 20% of patients, and influenced management in 27% of patients who were candidates for partial liver resection (28). Selzner et al. (29) compared the combination of PET/CT with standard contrast CT in 76 patients being evaluated for resection of liver metastases from colorectal cancer. They found comparable detection of intrahepatic metastases with sensitivity of PET/CT 95% and CT 91%; however, PET/CT was superior in diagnosing intrahepatic recurrence in

Table 47.2

Radiographic Evaluation of Liver Metastases

Modality	Sensitivity (%)	Specificity (%)
Ultrasound	20–88	60–70
Contrast-enhanced ultrasound	91	
Intraoperative ultrasound	82–98	70–80
CT	69–73	86–96
CT portogram	83–94	80–90
Magnetic resonance imaging	76–87	80–90
Positron emission tomography	91–95	79

CT, computed tomography.

patients with prior hepatectomy, local recurrence, and extrahepatic lesions (sensitivity 100%, 93%, and 89%, respectively).

A recent study compared the use of contrast-enhanced ultrasound with standard CT and MRI in patients with liver metastases and known extrahepatic tumors. The investigators evaluated 125 patients and found 31.4% more lesions when contrast was used as compared with unenhanced sonography. They also reported this modality to be as accurate at detecting metastatic liver disease (91.2%) when compare to triple-phase CT (89.2%) and MRI (30).

Intraoperative Evaluation

The resectability rate of liver metastases from colorectal cancer is only 50% to 70%, despite extensive preoperative studies. Gibbs and colleagues (13) have assessed the intraoperative factors determining unresectability in 62 patients. The most common factor was extrahepatic disease, found in 40% of patients, primarily in the porta hepatis and celiac lymph nodes, and they advocate routine biopsy of these nodes at the time of exploration. Other factors include the prohibitive extent of liver resection required (31%), more than four metastatic lesions (13%) or satellitosis (10%), and extensive hepatic parenchymal disease (6%). One group looked at the use of diagnostic laparoscopy and laparoscopic ultrasonography as an adjunct to preoperative imaging studies prior to resection in 50 patients. On the basis of diagnostic laparoscopy and laparoscopic ultrasonography, 38% of patients were deemed unresectable, and an additional 13% of the patients that went on to open exploration were thought to be unresectable based on intraoperative ultrasonography (28).

The evaluation at laparotomy is critical and should include a thorough exploration of the abdomen and pelvis, with particular attention to the porta hepatis and celiac lymph nodes, as well as assessment of the liver itself. In addition to palpation, numerous studies have demonstrated the benefit of intraoperative ultrasound (IOUS) and advocate its use to confirm the number and location of known hepatic lesions and identify any additional unsuspected metastases (31,32). The sensitivity of IOUS reported in several studies ranges from 82% to 98% and has been shown to be superior to that of preoperative ultrasonography, conventional or dynamic CT scanning, CT portogram, and palpation alone (33). IOUS is able to detect smaller lesions (0.5 to 1.5 cm), approximately 5% to 10% of lesions often missed by CT scan, and deep lesions not identified by palpation (33–35). Further, IOUS can define proximal venous anatomy and evaluate the adequacy of resection margins. In one series, information obtained by IOUS changed the operative management in 49% of cases (32,36). However, with recent advances in preoperative imaging techniques, some authors have questioned the benefit of IOUS. Jarnagin et al. (37) evaluated the use of IOUS in 111 patients. Although additional tumors were found using IOUS (45%), the majority of patients underwent resection with no modification in the planned procedure.

HEPATIC RESECTION FOR COLORECTAL METASTASES

Patients with isolated hepatic metastases may be candidates for liver resection, local ablation, and regional infusion therapies,

Table 47.3

Treatment Options for Patients with Hepatic Metastases

Disease at Presentation	Management Options
Liver disease only	
Few lesions, any size, favorable anatomy	Hepatic resection
Multiple, bilobar lesions, unfavorable anatomy	Ablation combined with resection
	Chemoembolization
Diffuse disease	Systemic chemotherapy ± HAI
	Chemoembolization
	Isolated hepatic perfusion
Liver and extrahepatic disease	Systemic chemotherapy

HAI, hepatic artery infusion pump.

depending on the location and extent of their disease (Table 47.3) and their medical comorbidities.

Patient Selection

Many clinical, operative, and pathologic factors have been evaluated in an attempt to improve the selection of patients for hepatic resection (9,10,38–44). Age and gender are not important factors, although comorbid disease may be prohibitive in the elderly patient (45). As in all major surgery, the patient's general medical condition must be evaluated to avoid serious cardiac or pulmonary complications. Adson and coworkers (46) demonstrated a clear relationship between initial cancer stage and overall survival following resection of liver metastases. In 1999, Fong et al. (47) determined a clinical risk score in 1,001 patients who underwent liver resection for metastatic colorectal cancer. Using multivariate analysis they identified seven significant and independent factors predictive of poor long-term prognosis. These factors included a positive margin of resection, the presence of extrahepatic disease, a node-positive primary tumor, a disease-free interval of <12 months, more than one metastasis, largest tumor metastasis >5 cm, and a preoperative CEA level

>200 ng/mL. Five of these factors determine the clinical risk score (node positive primary, disease-free interval <12 months, more than one metastasis, largest tumor >5 cm, CEA >200), and was found to be highly predictive of prognosis, with no 2-year survivors in patients with a score of 5. Recently, a computer model (OncoSurge) was created by an expert panel who reviewed 252 cases to better identify individual patient resectability and assist in devising future optimal treatment strategies (48).

In the current era of liver surgery, there does not appear to be a consensus limiting the size or number of lesions resected, as long as there is adequate hepatic reserve and negative margins. As such, some centers have reported resections of up to 80% of the liver to obtain an adequate resection, with low perioperative mortality (49). Several studies report significantly better prognosis when three or fewer nodules are resected compared to four or more, but other studies do not confirm this finding (10,38,50,51). Several studies have evaluated resection of four or fewer compared with five or more metastases, with promising results even with more extensive resections (8,52–55). Although the results regarding the absolute number of lesions to be resected are variable, there is general agreement that patients with fewer lesions have a better prognosis, whereas those with more than four lesions may have less favorable long-term outcomes.

Patients with no evidence of extrahepatic disease are candidates for hepatic resection of their metastases, either by wedge or anatomic resection, as long as there is an adequate hepatic reserve and a reasonable expectation of obtaining 1-cm margins (Table 47.3). Patients with extrahepatic disease found preoperatively or during exploration should be considered for systemic chemotherapy. Patients with numerous bilateral lesions and no extrahepatic disease may be candidates for regional infusional therapy. Ablative techniques such as radiofrequency ablation (RFA), either alone or in combination with resection, may be an option for patients with limited lesions in a bilobar distribution. Local ablation may also be considered for lesions excluded from resection because of anatomic considerations (8).

Surgical Planning

The operative approach for resection should be guided by the anatomy of the liver, with the goals of obtaining adequate margins and minimizing the incidence of postoperative liver failure by preserving normal liver parenchyma (Table 47.4). An ongoing

Table 47.4

Operative Approaches to Hepatic Resection Based on Disease

Operative Approach	Pattern of Disease
Wedge resection	Single or multiple superficial nodules Unilobar or bilobar
Anatomic resection (lobectomy, extended lobectomy, trisegmentectomy)	Multiple, unilobar metastases Bilobar lesions (amenable trisegmentectomy) Large, bulky lesion Deep or central metastases
Anatomic plus wedge resection (or anatomic resection with local ablation)	Large or deep lesion with smaller, superficial metastasis in contralateral lobe Multiple unilobar metastases with single lesion in contralateral lobe

trend in liver resection includes segmental liver resections based on the anatomic segments as described by Couinaud (9,10,56–60). In some series, wedge resection is associated with a higher incidence of positive margins as compared with anatomic dissection, while others suggest there is no difference in margin status, survival, or pattern of recurrence (61,62). In addition, there are increasing numbers of reports presenting data on the feasibility of safe and adequate resection using laparoscopic techniques (63–65).

Another operative consideration is the management of synchronous versus metachronous metastases. Synchronous liver metastases are found in 15% to 25% of patients with primary colorectal cancer (6,66). When resectable liver metastases are identified preoperatively in a good candidate, a combined procedure or a staged approach can be employed. Many series recommend a strategy of staging the procedures, with resection of the liver metastases 2 to 3 months after resection of the primary colon cancer (43,45,67). Major anatomic resections performed in combination with colon resection have been associated with a significant risk of septic and gastrointestinal complications, including anastomotic dehiscence, small-bowel obstruction, perforation, and ischemic colitis (43,45,68,69). However, the strategy for a combined approach has been recently re-evaluated (70,71). Martin et al. (72) looked at 134 patients who underwent simul-taneous resection compared with a similar group of 106 patients who underwent a staged approach. They found there to be fewer complications, fewer hospital days, and equivalent perioperative mortality in the group treated with simultaneous resection.

Operative Procedures and Perioperative Management

The liver is exposed through an extended right subcostal incision, and a thorough abdominal and pelvic exploration is performed to confirm the absence of extrahepatic disease, with particular attention to the porta hepatis and celiac axis. Any suspicious extrahepatic lesions should be biopsied, with an intraoperative frozen section performed. Hepatic resection should be aborted if extrahepatic metastatic disease is identified. In the absence of extrahepatic disease, the liver is fully mobilized and examination is performed using IOUS to confirm the number and location of the lesions, and to define the vascular anatomy. A final decision is made regarding resectability and the type of resection to be performed (Table 47.4 and Figure 47.1). If the lesions are deemed unresectable because of technical considerations or lack of adequate hepatic reserve, local ablation or placement of a hepatic arterial infusion pump can be considered (Table 47.3).

Resection is performed using the continuous ultrasonic surgical aspirator or finger-fracture of the hepatic parenchyma after

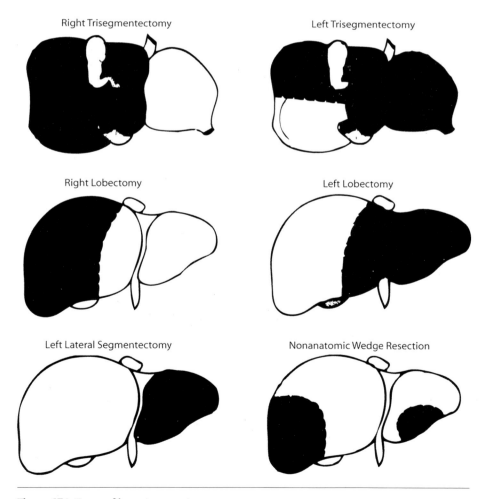

Figure 47.1 Types of hepatic resection.

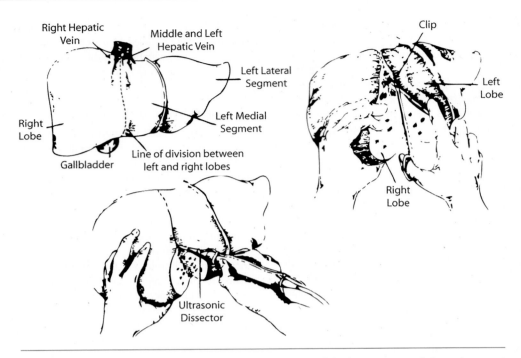

Figure 47.2 Technique of hepatic lobectomy. The branches of the hepatic artery, biliary duct, and portal vein are divided. Glisson's capsule is scored along the line of demarcation and the resection is performed using the continuous ultrasonic surgical aspirator. Vessels and biliary radicals are either clipped or suture-ligated.

scoring Glisson's capsule with cautery. Communication with the anesthesiologist to maintain a low central venous pressure (<5 mm Hg) is important to minimize back bleeding from the hepatic veins. Small vessels and biliary radicals are clipped as they are encountered, and larger branches are suture ligated or stapled as they are encountered (Figure 47.2). In formal resections, the hepatic vein(s) can be oversewn or stapled with a vascular stapler. The argon beam coagulator can be helpful in achieving hemostasis of the raw surface of the liver. Temporary vascular occlusion can be performed using total vascular isolation, Longmire clamping, or the Pringle maneuver. Intermittent inflow occlusion can be performed for up to 45 minutes at a time, but should be minimized to decrease the incidence of postoperative hepatic failure. Usually total hepatic isolation is not necessary and may be associated with increased transfusion requirements and complications (73). At the completion of the procedure, the liver surface is examined and any biliary radicals identified are clipped or oversewn. Closed suction drains may or may not be necessary.

Laparoscopic liver resection was initially described in France, and other institutions have subsequently demonstrated that minimally invasive techniques can be feasible and safe (63,74–77). A multicenter study from Europe evaluated laparoscopic resection for malignant disease in 37 patients, with reasonable 2-year outcomes despite multiple specimens having margins <1 cm (75). Buell et al. (65) reported results in 17 patients who underwent 21 resections laparoscopically for both benign and malignant disease, with varied anatomic resections performed. Their operative approach included a hand-assist device, and two 5- or 12-mm ports, with the addition of a laparoscopic ultrasound probe and ultrasound dissector. Hepatic

transection is performed with an endovascular articulating stapler. Bongiovanni et al. (78) recently reviewed their experience with 89 patients treated with laparoscopic liver resection for both benign and malignant disease, and demonstrated comparable results at 3-year follow-up as compared with laparotomy. Evaluation of larger numbers of patients with longer follow-up is needed to determine the utility of these techniques with respect to operative morbidity, mortality, and oncologic outcome.

Postoperatively, patients are initially observed for signs of coagulopathy and bleeding. The administration of vitamin K and fresh-frozen plasma is begun if the prothrombin time exceeds 18 seconds or if nonsurgical bleeding develops. After major lobectomy, liver regeneration results in hypophosphatemia. Patients are generally given 50 mmol/day of phosphorus to maintain normal serum phosphorus levels. If a nasogastric tube has been placed, it can be removed quickly to improve pulmonary function. Clinical monitoring of liver function is performed and the patient's diet is advanced as tolerated. Generally, the postoperative length of stay after major resection is in the range of 6 to 9 days.

If persistent or increasing hyperbilirubinemia occurs, a nuclear medicine scan can be obtained to evaluate for the presence of biliary leak or obstruction. Additionally, endoscopic retrograde cholangiopancreatography can be performed if this is inconclusive and a stent placed if a bile leak is demonstrated. A rare but potentially devastating complication of liver resection is portal vein thrombosis. This complication should be suspected in patients with a significant deterioration in hepatic function with associated ascites, tachycardia, and cardiopulmonary compromise. Routine use of surveillance duplex ultrasonography is generally not recommended, although duplex ultrasound, CT

Table 47.5			
Survival after Curative Hepatic Resection for Colorectal Metastases			
Study (Ref.)	No. of Patients	Operative Morality (%)	5-/10-year Survival (%)
Mutsaerts et al. (184) 2005	102	—	29
Abdalla et al. (185) 2004	190	—	58
Bramhall et al. (186) 2003	212	2.8	28
Liu et al. (187) 2002	72	4	32
Choti et al. (188) 2002	226	0.9	40/26
Fong et al. (47) 1999	1,001	3	37/22
Bradley et al. (83) 1999	134	4	36/23
Nakamura et al. (82) 1999	79	—	49/33
Jamison et al. (86) 1997	280	4	27
Jenkins et al. (189) 1997	131	4	25
Rees et al. (81) 1997	89	0.9	37
Fong et al. (190) 1997	577	4	35
Nordlinger et al. (43) 1996	1,568	2	28
Pinson et al. (80) 1996	95	4	32
Wanebo et al. (51) 1996	74	7	24
Scheele et al. (10) 1995	434	4.4	33/20
Gayowski et al. (38) 1994	204	0	32

angiography, or MRI/magnetic resonance angiography may help confirm the diagnosis. Supportive care and anticoagulation are generally recommended, although no large series on the management of this complication have been reported. Thrombolysis or reoperation in patients with deteriorating hepatic function despite anticoagulation may be considered.

Surgical Outcomes

The perioperative mortality for hepatic resection with curative intent ranges from 0% to 9% in recent series, with rates of <5% at major centers (Table 47.5) (10,11,38,47,51,79–86). The major operative morbidity ranges from 13% to 35% with an average of 23%. The complications most often contributing to operative mortality are hepatic failure and hemorrhage. Other hepatic complications include biliary leak resulting in fistula (3% to 4%) and abscess (1% to 9%) (9,10,43,45,87–89). Specific attention should be directed at oversewing small biliary radicals and securing the major bile duct at the completion of the resection to prevent a biloma. Most bile collections and abscesses can be drained percutaneously and persistent biliary leaks treated with endoscopic stenting. Significant perioperative bleeding mandates reoperation.

The 5- and 10-year survival for patients undergoing curative hepatic resection for colorectal metastases ranges from 24% to 58% (Table 47.5). The survival data in these tables reflect patients undergoing complete resection of all metastases with pathologically clear margins. The data from several of these series underscore the significance of obtaining adequate surgical margins. Scheele and coworkers (10) report a 33% 5-year tumor-free survival in 350 patients resected for cure with negative surgical margins. The 10-year actuarial survival in this group was 23.6%. In this same series, 65 patients underwent curative resection but had histologically positive margin, with a median survival of 14.4 months. A more recent series by Fong et al. (47) analyzed 1,001 patients treated with hepatic resection for metastatic colon cancer. They reported median survival of 45 months with 5- and 10-year survival rates of 37% and 22%, respectively, in patients with negative margins. However, in the group of patients with positive margins, they found a 20% 5-year survival with a median survival of 23 months. Their overall 30-day hospital mortality was 2.8%. This also underscores what appears to be a long-term survival benefit of hepatic resections performed at high-volume centers (>25 cases/year) as compared to low-volume centers (85). With improved preoperative imaging and center experience with aggressive resections, the trend has been a decrease in mortality with an increase in long-term survival.

A number of clinical and pathologic factors are thought to influence the prognosis following liver resection for colorectal metastases. By far the most significant factors determining prognosis are the absence of extrahepatic disease and clear surgical margins (≥1 cm). There is some debate comparing anatomic versus wedge resection, but clearly margin status is most important. Few studies have included an evaluation of intraoperative blood loss, but several have found a correlation between blood loss or perioperative transfusion and survival (39,41,90). Further, Doci et al. (45) found a significant correlation between blood transfusion and postoperative complications. Kooby et al. (91) retrospectively reviewed 1,351 patients undergoing liver resection and found operative mortalities of 1.2%, 2.5%, and 11.1% in patients receiving no transfusion, one or two units, or more than two units, respectively. Pathologic factors such as satellite lesions or aneuploid tumors are also associated with a poorer prognosis (39). Yamaguchi and coworkers (50) found that aneuploid tumors had a recurrence rate of 56%, compared with diploid tumors with an 18% recurrence rate.

Recently, some authors have advocated proceeding with hepatic resection even in the presence of extrahepatic disease (92,93). Elias et al. (93) reported results in 75 patients who underwent R0 resection of extrahepatic disease in conjunction with hepatic resection. Sites of extrahepatic disease included peritoneal implants, ovarian metastases, hilar lymph nodes, local recurrence, retroperitoneal lymph nodes, lung, and abdominal wall. Their operative mortality was 2.7% with a morbidity of 25%. At a median follow-up of 4.9 years, the overall survival was 45% and 28% at 3 and 5 years, respectively. They found that R0 resection could not be accomplished in 50% of patients explored, and negative prognostic factors included more than five liver lesions and multiple extrahepatic sites of disease.

Recurrence of colorectal carcinoma occurs in 60% to 80% of patients following hepatic resection. The lung is the most common site of extrahepatic metastasis, found in >50% of patients with recurrent disease, followed by other intra-abdominal sites such as porta hepatis or retroperitoneal lymph nodes and the adrenal glands (15,94). Most commonly, hepatic recurrences occur at sites other than the resection bed. Resection bed recurrence is found in only 15% to 30% of patients with liver-only disease, which may relate to the surgical margin obtained at the original resection (94,95). In their series of 109 patients with negative margins of resection, Sugihara and coworkers (15) reported 34 of 64 patients with recurrences in the liver, of which 91% were detected within the first 18 months. Ten of these pa-tients had a recurrence in the initial resection bed in the liver despite a previous negative margin.

REPEAT HEPATIC RESECTION

Overall, approximately one third of patients undergoing resection for hepatic metastases will have long-term survival. Of the patients who have recurrences, about 30% to 40% recur in the liver only, and the remainder develop disseminated disease, including peritoneum, lung, bone, brain, and other abdominal/pelvic sites (9,83). Because resection is the only modality that offers a chance of cure, patients who have recurrent disease limited to the liver should be considered for additional liver-directed therapy, including repeat hepatic resection (Table 47.6). There have been numerous small, single-institution series, reviewed by Wanebo and coworkers (96), that demonstrate the technical feasibility of repeat hepatic resection. Several larger single- and multi-institutional series confirm that the operative mortality is low and the morbidity is similar to that reported for initial resections, with long-term survival in some patients (Table 47.6) (82,97–101). To minimize complications, patients should be carefully selected for repeat liver resection, especially with regard to hepatic reserve. Use of indocyanine green or galactose tolerance tests can be helpful in determining adequate hepatic reserve.

The median survival following second hepatectomy ranges from 30 to 46 months. The overall survival following second liver resection approximates the results seen following initial resection. The 3-year survival is reported as 32% to 68%, with 5-year survival of 31% to 44% (98,100,101). Nordlinger and associates (98) reported recurrences in 66% of 116 patients undergoing second resection for colorectal metastases. Eighty-four percent of these recurrences involved the liver. The prognostic factors for outcome are similar for the first and second resections. In the series of 170 patients from the Registry of Repeat Resection

Table 47.6

Repeat Hepatic Resection for Colorectal Metastases

Study (Ref.)	No. of Patients	Operative Mortality (%)	Morbidity (%)	Median Survival (mo.)	3-/5-year Survival (%)
Shaw et al. (191) 2006	66	0	18	—	68/44
Adam et al. (192) 2003[a]	60	0	25	—	32
Petrowsky et al. (193) 2002	126	1.6	28	37	51/34
Suzuki et al. (194) 2001	26	0	27	31	62/32
Muratore et al. (195) 2001	29	3.4	7	—	35/—
Yamamoto et al. (196) 1999	75	0	11	30	48/31
Adam et al. (197) 1997	64	0	20	46	60/41
Tuttle et al. (99) 1997	23	0	22	39.9	—/32
Fernandez-Trigo et al. (100) 1995	170	—	19	34	45/32
Que et al. (101) 1994	21	5	Low	40	43 (4 yr)
Fong et al. (97) 1994	25	0	28	30	—
Nordlinger et al. (98) 1994	116	0.9	25	30	33/—

[a] Third hepatectomy.

of Hepatic Metastasis, the absence of extrahepatic disease and negative surgical margins were important factors in predicting long-term survival after second hepatic resection for colorectal metastases. The interval between first and second resection, the type of resection, and the number of metastases did not have a significantly impact on outcome (100).

LOCAL TUMOR ABLATION

Local ablative techniques include ethanol injection, cryotherapy, and RFA. These techniques provide an adjunct to hepatic resection for the treatment of liver metastases (102–104). The main indications for local ablation include unresectable lesions due to multiplicity, bilobar distribution, or anatomic limitations. Ablation may also be used as a less invasive procedure in patients with comorbid medical conditions or limited hepatic reserve that prohibits hepatic resection (Table 47.7). Additionally, ablation has been used in conjunction with resection in the treatment of contralateral lobe lesions.

Percutaneous Ethanol Injection

Percutaneous ethanol injection with 98% sterile alcohol has been shown to be effective in treating small hepatocellular carcinomas. Using ultrasound or CT guidance, intratumoral injections can be performed. The alcohol induces coagulative necrosis with subsequent small vessel thrombosis and fibrosis of surrounding parenchyma (105). Injections can be performed during a single session or repeated over the course of several weeks. Effectiveness has been less promising when treating metastases from colorectal cancer.

Cryoablation

Cryotherapy destroys tumors along with a margin of adjacent normal liver tissue using a liquid nitrogen-cooled probe inserted directly into the metastasis with the aid of IOUS. The subzero temperatures result in the formation of intracellular ice crystals, denaturation of cellular proteins, reduction of cell volume, and destruction of tumor vasculature (106,107). In a small phase 1 trial, cryoablated lesions were immediately resected, showing that the IOUS findings correlated well with the histologic findings and confirming adequate margins (103). Cryoablated

Table 47.7

Indications for Local Ablation

Variable	Indication for Ablation
Tumor characteristics	Multiple bilateral lesions
	Central lesion not amenable to anatomic resection
	Contralateral nodules in patient undergoing hepatic lobectomy
Host factors	Comorbid medical disease
	Limited hepatic reserve
	Cirrhosis
	Prior liver resection

lesions persist as abnormal densities on serial CT scans, which can be problematic. Few patients have had subsequent histologic confirmation of disease control; biopsy of the persistent cryoablated site usually shows scar tissue (102,108).

The operative approach is quite similar to that for hepatic resection. Use of the Bair Hugger warming device (Arizant, Inc., Eden Prairie, MN) has been shown to minimize hypothermia (109). IOUS is used to identify additional hepatic metastases to be treated, define the anatomy of the lesions, and monitor the progress of the freezing process. Prior to the first freeze, the patient is given mannitol and sodium bicarbonate to minimize complications from myoglobinuria. Large lesions require the placement of multiple probes and lesions as large as 10 to 12 cm have been treated successfully. Freezing is continued until the freeze front extends 1 to 2 cm beyond the edges of the lesion, usually for a median of 8 minutes. The period of thawing is of approximately the same duration as the freeze cycle and a minimum of two freeze-and-thaw cycles is recommended based on experimental animal data (110).

Polk and coworkers (111) have described a technique of cryo-assisted hepatic resection, maintaining an ice ball with alternating freeze-and-thaw cycles every minute during the hepatic dissection. The plane of dissection is on or near the ice ball and the probe can be used as a handle to facilitate exposure. This approach is thought to improve the likelihood of obtaining clear margins during wedge resection, to facilitate resection in anatomically difficult areas, and to allow minimal resection of normal parenchyma in patients with limited hepatic reserve.

The overall operative mortality is <5%, although there were no operative deaths reported in combined series of 250 patients (103). The major morbidity rate ranges from 6% to 38% and includes the "cryoshock phenomenon" of disseminated intravascular coagulation, multisystem organ failure, severe coagulopathy, and hepatic hemorrhage requiring reoperation (102,108). Myoglobinuria and asymptomatic right pleural effusions are common minor complications that are seen in most patients. Another series of 136 patients with otherwise unresectable disease underwent cryosurgery, with a median survival of 30 months and an operative mortality of 3.6% (108).

Radiofrequency Ablation

The use of RFA, a modified electrocautery technique, has become increasingly more common compared with cryosurgical ablation in treating liver metastases given the cost, availability, and ability to perform laparoscopically, percutaneously, or in an open fashion. The probe functions by passage of an alternating high-frequency current through the tissue. At 50°C to 52°C, cells undergo coagulation necrosis in 4 to 6 minutes. At temperatures >60°C, necrosis is immediate. Using IOUS, a monopolar array needle electrode is placed directly into the tumor nodule. Probes have been developed with an ability to ablate tumors up to 7 cm in diameter in 30 minutes. Numerous studies have looked at the use of RFA in the treatment of multiple histologies as well as in conjunction with resection and hepatic artery infusion (HAI) pumps.

Larger lesions require repeated applications to span the area of the metastasis. Selected patients with small peripheral lesions may be treated percutaneously, although general anesthesia may

Table 47.8

Recurrence and Survival after Radiofrequency Ablation (RFA)

Study (Ref.)	Patients/ Lesions (N)	Mean Follow-up (mo)	Recurrence at RFA site (%)	New Metastases (%)	Overall Survival (%)
Hildebrand et al. (198) 2006	81/426	21.2	17	23.9	40 (3 yr)
Navarra et al. (199) 2005	57/297	20.5	30	40	52.5 (3 yr)
Bleicher et al. (200) 2003	153/447	11	20.9	—	—
Machi (201) 2001	46/204	20.5	8.8	45.7	—
Solbiati et al. (113) 2001	117/179	24	39	66	36
Curley et al. (112) 1999	123/169	15	1.8	27.6	—

still be required to alleviate the pain associated with the procedure. RFA is may be used to treat lesions in proximity to major vascular structures as the heat-sink effect of blood flow prevents endothelial injury (105). Multiple institutions have evaluated RFA in terms of morbidity, mortality, and long-term follow-up (Table 47.8). Curley and associates (112) recently reported a series of 123 patients with unresectable liver tumors (61 with colorectal metastases) treated with RFA, with no deaths and an overall complication rate of 2.4%. After 15 months of follow-up, the tumor had recurred at the site of treatment in 3 of 169 lesions treated (1.8% local failure rate) and new disease has developed in 28%. Other groups have looked at long-term follow-up after RFA treatment. Solbiati et al. (113) reported long-term results in 117 patients treated with RFA for metachronous colorectal metastases to liver. Median survival was 36 months, with estimated 2- and 3-year survival rates of 69% and 46%, respectively. Of all lesions treated, 39% developed local recurrence after treatment and 66% of patients developed new metastases at follow-up.

In 2003, Livraghi et al. (114) reported the morbidity of percutaneous RFA performed in 41 Italian institutions. In this large series, a total of 2,320 patients were treated, the majority with hepatocellular carcinoma, and 501 patients had metastatic colorectal cancer. Mortality was 0.3% and 2.2% of patients had additional major complications including peritoneal hemorrhage, neoplastic seeding, intrahepatic abscesses, and intestinal perforation. The number of RFA sessions significantly correlated with higher rates of major complications. Minor complications were observed in <5% of patients, demonstrating the safety of this technique in a large series.

Pawlik et al. (8) published their results of 154 patients with four or more colorectal metastases treated with resection (29%), RFA alone (7.5%), or resection in combination with RFA (63.5%). The 5-year actuarial survival and overall survival in all patients was 21.5% and 50.9%, respectively. Increasing studies have shown similar improved results using RFA alone or in combination with surgery for the treatment of unresectable metastases.

HEPATIC ARTERY INFUSION

HAI of chemotherapeutic agents using an implantable pump is an option for patients with unresectable liver metastases from colorectal carcinoma. The basis of regional therapy using HAI is the fact that tumor deposits in the liver are selectively perfused by branches of the hepatic artery while the primary blood supply to the normal liver is through the portal vein (115). Thus, chemotherapeutic agents with high hepatic extraction administered through the hepatic artery target tumor metastases preferentially while diminishing systemic toxicity. Sigurdson and coworkers (116) showed that ^{3}H-FUDR (5-fluoro-2-deoxyuridine) is concentrated 15-fold in tumor cells when injected via the hepatic artery when compared with portal vein delivery, whereas the drug was uniformly distributed in the normal parenchyma when infused through either route.

Regional hepatic chemotherapy also maximizes local drug exposure while minimizing systemic toxicities by using agents primarily cleared by the liver. FUDR, the primary drug initially used for HAI of colorectal metastases, is an antimetabolite that is catabolized to 5-fluorouracil (5-FU) when given intra-arterially. FUDR is cleared primarily by the liver on first pass (94% to 99% of FUDR compared with 19% to 55% of 5-FU), and much higher effective doses can be delivered locally, limiting systemic effects. The main toxicities of HAI are related to local effects on the liver and upper gastrointestinal tract (117–126). Liver function tests should be monitored closely in patients treated with HAI. Hepatic toxicity is initially manifested by an elevation in transaminases. Initially, these changes are reversible and liver function tests normalize when the FUDR is withheld. A certain percentage of patients, however, develop irreversible biliary strictures or more diffuse biliary sclerosis with findings similar to those of idiopathic sclerosing cholangitis (127). Focal strictures can be managed with ductal drainage by endoscopic retrograde cholangiopancreatography or a percutaneous transhepatic route. CT scan should exclude external compression of the ducts by bulky, metastatic porta hepatis lymph nodes prior to placement of pump.

Gastritis and ulcer disease are associated with HAI and are thought to be due to chemotherapy perfusion through collateral branches to the stomach and duodenum. Careful dissection and ligation of all branches to the stomach, duodenum, pancreas, and bile ducts distal to the cannulation site are necessary to prevent these complications. Methylene blue or fluorescein can be injected through the pump catheter intraoperatively to assure appropriate placement of the catheter. A postoperative nuclear medicine injection through the pump should be performed prior to chemotherapy infusion to confirm proper position.

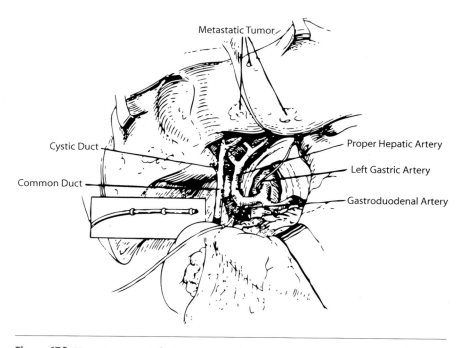

Figure 47.3 Hepatic artery infusion pump placement. Cholecystectomy is performed to avoid the risk of chemical cholecystitis. The catheter is ligated in place in the gastroduodenal artery (GDA) with the tip just at the junction of the GDA and the proper hepatic artery. The right gastric artery and branches of the proximal GDA are divided. (From Niederhuber JE, Ensminger WD, DeVita VT, et al. Treatment of metastatic cancer to the liver. In: DeVita VT, Hellman S, Rosenberg SA (eds) *Cancer Principles and Practice of Oncology*, ed. 4. Philadelphia: JB Lippincott; 1993: 2201–2224, with permission.)

Surgical Considerations

All patients who are candidates for pump placement should have a preoperative study to define the vascular anatomy. The option of hepatic infusion pump placement should be discussed with patients for whom hepatic resection is planned should liver disease prove unresectable. Patients with extrahepatic disease on exploration are not candidates for an infusion pump, but should be considered for systemic chemotherapy.

The hepatic infusion pump may be placed using either a right subcostal or upper midline incision. After exploration, cholecystectomy is performed to prevent chemical cholecystitis. Most commonly, the catheter is placed in the gastroduodenal artery (GDA) to the junction of the common hepatic and proper hepatic arteries, and the GDA is ligated distal to the insertion site (Figure 47.3). Vascular anomalies, however, are common and require adjustment of the surgical approach. In the usual situation, the junction of the common hepatic, proper hepatic, and GDAs is exposed and the GDA is dissected for 2 cm to the first portion of the duodenum. The right gastric artery is ligated, as are all branches distal to the infusion site that feed the stomach, duodenum, pancreas, or bile duct. After creating the subcutaneous pocket for the pump, the catheter is passed through the abdominal wall. The GDA is ligated distally and the catheter is advanced in a retrograde fashion through the GDA and secured at the junction with the common hepatic artery (Figure 47.3). Protrusion of the catheter into the common hepatic artery may result in turbulent flow, with unequal distribution

of the chemotherapeutic agent or thrombosis of the vessel itself. Uniform perfusion of the liver can be confirmed at the completion of the procedure by injecting half-strength fluorescein through the sideport and viewing with the Wood's lamp. Postoperatively, a technetium perfusion scan is obtained to confirm correct catheter placement and liver perfusion prior to dosing chemotherapeutic agents.

Apart from the hepatotoxicity already mentioned, most complications are related to technical considerations. Dissection of side branches of the GDA and proper hepatic arteries must be complete. Care must be taken in the exact placement of the tip of the catheter at the junction of the GDA and the common hepatic artery. Uniform perfusion of the liver should be confirmed at the completion of the procedure. A recent large single-institution series evaluated complications in 544 patients treated with HAI. Incidence of pump failure was 9% and 16% at 1 and 2 years, respectively. Pump complications occurred in 22% of patients with an increased rate in patients with variable vascular anatomy (128).

Results

There have been a number of randomized clinical trials reviewed elsewhere that have studied HAI versus systemic chemotherapy in patients with unresectable metastatic disease isolated to the liver (129–137). Essentially, all have demonstrated a significantly higher response rate in patients treated with HAI (42% to 62%) compared with those treated with systemic chemotherapy

(10% to 38%), although the difference in survival was not statistically significant. These trials, however, were limited by small numbers of patients and frequent crossover design. Two randomized European trials demonstrated a statistically significant overall survival in the HAI arms, (15 vs. 11 months, and 13.5 vs. 7.5 months) (129,138). However, treatments within the control arms in these trials are generally considered inadequate. Some consideration has been given to HAI as an adjunct to hepatic resection, with an infusion pump placed at the time of resection. Several trials are underway to address this issue. Trials reported to date have shown mixed results, with two trials supporting the implantation of hepatic artery pumps at the time of resection (139–144). Kemeny et al (144). randomized 156 patients to receive FUDR and dexamethasone via HAI plus systemic fluorouracil with or without leucovorin, or similar systemic therapy alone after liver resection. At 2 years, actuarial overall survival was 86% with combined therapy and 72% with systemic therapy alone ($p = 0.03$), with rates of hepatic-free recurrence of 90% and 60%, respectively. Most patients, however, recur in extrahepatic sites and would require systemic chemotherapy. Patients with isolated liver recurrence after resection may be candidates for repeat hepatic resection or for HAI at that time (15,94,145).

Recently the Cancer and Leukemia Group B (CALGB) 9481 study results were published. In this multi-institutional study, 135 patients with hepatic metastases from colorectal cancer were randomly assigned to receive HAI with FUDR, leucovorin, and dexamethasone versus systemic fluorouracil and leucovorin. In this study overall survival was significantly longer for HAI versus systemic chemotherapy (median, 24.4 vs. 20 months) with response rates of 47% versus 24%, respectively. Quality of life assessment demonstrated improved physical functioning in the HAI arm at 3 and 6 months. However, although a survival benefit was realized in the HAI arm, the control arm did not use an oxaliplatin- or irinotecan-based systemic chemotherapy, which has been shown to improve overall survival (146). HAI needs to be further evaluated in the clinical setting with newer hepatic selective agents, and to determine its role in combination with other treatments.

NEOADJUVANT CHEMOTHERAPY

Historically, the response rate of colorectal liver metastases to systemic 5-FU and leucovorin has been low, and therefore generally ineffective for use in a neoadjuvant strategy. Modern combination chemotherapy regimens containing oxaliplatin, irinotecan, and bevacizumab have resulted in improved response rates, and several studies have shown that previously unresectable liver metastases were rendered resectable after a course of systemic therapy. Similar results have also been reported with regional chemotherapy via hepatic arterial infusion. As a result, neoadjuvant chemotherapy in the treatment of isolated liver metastases has become increasingly more common. A comprehensive review of neoadjuvant chemotherapy prior to liver resection for unresectable metastases was recently compiled by Leonard et al. (147).

Bismuth et al. (148) reported the results of an aggressive multimodal treatment strategy of systemic chemotherapy using an oxaliplatin-containing regimen and a broad array of surgical resection techniques including two-stage hepatectomy, portal vein embolization, and extrahepatic resections in selected patients. They demonstrated that 53 of 330 patients (16%) with initially unresectable colorectal liver metastases ultimately underwent potentially curative resections. The mean duration of chemotherapy was approximately 8 months before a treatment plateau was achieved and surgery was performed. This impressive series reported no operative deaths and a cumulative 5-year survival rate of 40%. Subsequent studies evaluating systemic oxaliplatin and/or irinotecan in combination with 5-FU and leucovorin have reported similar response rates of up to 40% in "downstaging" unresectable liver metastases (149–151).

HAI, either alone or in combination with systemic chemotherapy, results in similar rates of tumor downstaging, although it remains to be seen whether HAI provides additional benefits to modern systemic chemotherapy alone. Therefore, in patients with initially unresectable liver-only metastases, it is reasonable to monitor their response to chemotherapy and routinely reassess for potentially curative surgical therapy.

Given the results in initially unresectable patients, the question remains whether to extend a neoadjuvant approach to patients with resectable colorectal liver metastases. The rationale for treating patients with chemotherapy prior to liver resection includes the ability to assess tumor response and tumor biology, downstaging tumors to facilitate resection and preserve normal hepatic parenchyma, and exclude patients with rapidly progressive disease from surgery. In a retrospective analysis of patients with four or more metastatic lesions, Adam et al. (152) reported that progression on chemotherapy was associated with significantly worse outcomes following liver resection (8% 5-year survival) compared to those with tumors responsive or stabilized by chemotherapy (37% and 30% 5-year survival, respectively). On multivariate analysis, progression during chemotherapy was an important predictor of decreased survival, leading the authors to suggest that initial control of metastatic disease with modern chemotherapy was preferable to immediate surgical treatment. Such a strategy allows for selection of those patients with favorable biologic responses for subsequent surgical therapy.

A neoadjuvant approach to all patients with liver metastases raises several important questions, particularly in those with isolated resectable lesions. In these patients, is it acceptable to treat systemically if the risk of tumor growth might preclude a potentially curative resection? Does chemotherapy lead to morbidity that makes surgery impossible in some patients? In patients who remain resection candidates following systemic treatment, are there more complications following major hepatic resection in patients treated with systemic chemotherapy? Does chemotherapy make extended resections less feasible because of parenchymal damage and steatosis that decreases regenerative capacity following hepatectomy? A retrospective analysis by Parikh et al. (153) found that steatosis was indeed higher in patients treated with 5-FU/leucovorin/irinotecan compared with 5-FU/leucovorin and no chemotherapy. However, they did not find an increase in morbidity and mortality, including hepatic failure, in patients treated preoperatively with 5-FU/leucovorin/irinotecan, leading the authors to suggest that a neoadjuvant approach may be a therapeutic option for patients with multiple hepatic metastases. However, in the absence of further prospective data regarding role of neoadjuvant chemotherapy and liver resection, an individualized approach with medical decision making involving the medical oncologist and surgeon appears to be the most appropriate strategy.

HEPATIC METASTASES FROM NONCOLORECTAL PRIMARY TUMORS

Metastatic Neuroendocrine Tumors

Extended survival has been reported in several small series in patients after resection of primary neuroendocrine tumors and hepatic metastases. Frequently, systemic symptoms from carcinoid syndrome and other paraneoplastic syndromes can be managed with the administration of somatostatin. Curative resection is frequently impossible secondary to multiple, bilobar metastases; however, when possible, surgical debulking and palliation should be considered. Neuroendocrine tumors, particularly carcinoids, are generally slow-growing, thus tumor debulking may portend to long-term survival. In addition, the symptoms of carcinoid syndrome depend on peptide release from total tumor mass; thus, debulking may palliate symptoms. Treatment with locoregional therapies have also been reported, including RFA and chemoembolization (154).

Norton et al. (155) reported on 18 patients with liver neuroendocrine tumors in which ten patients with carcinoid syndrome had resolution of symptoms with an actuarial 5-year survival of 80% after resection. In 2001, Yao et al. (156) reviewed their experience with 36 patients, 18 patients with islet cell tumors of the pancreas and 18 patients with carcinoid, who were treated with resection and hepatic chemoembolization. Similarly, they reported an actuarial 5-year survival of 70%, and emphasized the importance of surgical resection for hopes of long-term survival. Chamberlain et al. (157) evaluated 85 patients with carcinoid and functional or nonfunctional islet cell tumors, treated with medical therapy, hepatic artery embolization, or surgical resection. The 3- and 5-year survival with surgical resection was 83% and 76%, respectively.

Metastatic Breast Cancer

Isolated metastases to the liver from a primary breast cancer are rare and occur in approximately 5% of patients with metastatic disease. Even with systemic chemotherapy or hormonal therapy, long-term survival is uncommon. There have been a few small retrospective studies that have evaluated the role of liver resection in this subset of patients with metastatic breast cancer. In these studies, median survival ranges from 24 to 44 months, with 5-year survivals ranging from 22% to 38% (158–163). In addition, some authors have looked at the role of local ablation or chemoembolization of these lesions.

Metastatic Sarcoma

There are little data available regarding resection of metastatic sarcoma to the liver, compared with evidence supporting lung metastasectomy for sarcoma. One of the largest reviews was published by the Memorial Sloan-Kettering Cancer Center analyzing their experience over a 19-year period. Of 331 patients identified, 56 underwent complete resection for gastrointestinal stromal tumors or gastrointestinal leiomyosarcomas. At a median of

39 months they reported actuarial 1-, 3-, and 5-year survivals of 88%, 50%, and 30%, respectively. This was compared with patients who did not undergo resection who had a 5-year survival of 4%. They concluded that, when technically feasible, complete resection of lesions is associated with prolonged survival (164).

Metastatic Melanoma

There is a paucity of clinical information regarding the utility of liver resection with metastatic melanoma. Rose et al. (165) prospectively reviewed the experience at the John Wayne Cancer Institute and Sydney Melanoma Unit with patients who had metastatic melanoma to the liver. Of 1,750 patients who had hepatic metastases, 34 (2%) were identified who underwent exploration with planned resection. Of these patients, 71% underwent resection, with a median disease-free and overall survival of 12 and 28 months, respectively. Complete resection with negative margins significantly improved disease-free survival. Other small studies have reported on select patients with long-term survival after resection of liver metastases from melanoma. Similarly, metastatic disease from ocular melanoma has a poor prognosis because of disseminated metastases. However, there have been anecdotal reports in the literature in a select subset of these patients who have isolated metastases and who are amenable to resection, and has been associated with long-term survival (166,167).

FUTURE APPROACHES

New approaches to the management of colorectal metastases to the liver are being developed and studied for efficacy. These approaches fall into three broad categories: local ablative; chemotherapy administration, systemic, and regional; and regional gene therapy.

There is a subset of patients who are deemed unresectable based on poor hepatic reserve. Numerous authors have begun to look at techniques to improve hepatic reserve prior to hepatectomy. One method is preoperative selective portal vein embolization (PVE). This technique is performed with the hope of inducing selective hypertrophy of the nondiseased portion of liver. This method is used to increase potential candidates for resection and decrease postoperative liver failure (168–170). Farges et al. (170) evaluated PVE in 55 patients. They found no beneficial effect on postoperative course in patients with a normal liver function; however, they found a significant decrease in postoperative complications in patients with chronic liver disease after PVE.

Because many patients have recurrence in extrahepatic sites following "curative" resection, it is clear that the potential benefit of adjuvant systemic chemotherapy following liver resection needs to be addressed. Efforts are ongoing to identify the significant prognostic variables and to determine which patients are most at risk for recurrence. In addition to using HAI following resection to minimize local recurrence, the combination of systemic and HAI of chemotherapy postresection is being evaluated in clinical trials.

Approaches to the management of unresectable hepatic disease from colorectal or other cancers are also under investigation. Isolated hepatic perfusion (IHP) is a procedure that allows complete isolation of the liver from the systemic circulation using an extracorporeal circuit consisting of a roller pump, reservoir, heat exchanger, and oxygenator. The technique of IHP was designed based on the experience with isolated limb perfusion for melanoma and sarcoma. Once the liver is placed on the bypass circuit, high doses of therapeutic agents can be delivered via the hepatic artery at levels that would normally be limited by systemic toxicities. In addition, regional hyperthermia can be administered, enhancing vascular permeability and allowing increased selective delivery of the therapeutic agent (171).

There are limited systemic toxicities. Some agents that have been studied in clinical trials include 5-FU, mitomycin C, melphalan, and tumor necrosis factor. Fifty-one patients with metastatic colorectal cancer to the liver were treated on a trial combining IHP with melphalan (1.5 mg/kg) with or without tumor necrosis factor (1 mg), with some patients receiving postoperative continuous HAI of FUDR (0.2 mg/kg/day) and leucovorin (15 mg/m^2/day) (172). Twenty-four of 31 patients who had IHP alone had a partial response (77%); the median duration of response for IHP alone was 8.5 months with a median overall survival of 16 months. In the group treated with IHP followed by HAI therapy, 14 of 19 patients (74%) had a partial response; the median duration of response in this group was 14.5 months with a median overall survival of 27 months. Alexander et al. (173) demonstrated efficacy of IHP with melphalan in 25 patients who had progressive disease after systemic treatment with irinotecan. There was 1 complete response and 14 partial responses in 25 patients (60%), with a median duration of 12 months. The median overall survival was 12 months (range, 1 to 47 months), and the 2-year survival was 28%. In addition IHP has been studied in the setting of metastatic ocular melanoma to the liver (174–176). In 2003, results of 29 patients treated with a 60-minute IHP using 1.5 mg/kg melphalan were published. There were 3 patients (10%) who achieved a complete response, 15 patients (52%) who had a partial response with a mean duration of 10 months, for an overall response rate of (62%). At a median follow-up of 30.7 months, the median actuarial progression-free and overall survivals were 8 and 12.1 months, respectively.

Several groups have developed a percutaneous catheter-based technique of isolated hepatic perfusion using a double-balloon vena cava catheter for hepatic venous isolation (177–179). Pingpank et al. (180) recently published their results from a phase 1 trial using percutaneously placed catheters and hepatic venous hemofiltration using a double-balloon catheter positioned in the retrohepatic inferior vena cava using a 30-minute melphalan infusion. In the 28 patients treated, melphalan delivery was feasible with limited, manageable toxicity. There was an overall radiographic response of 30% in treated patients. In addition, of the ten patients treated with ocular melanoma, a 50% response rate was seen, with complete response in two patients.

Regional gene therapy is being applied to the treatment of primary and metastatic liver tumors (181). Issues of the optimal vector for delivery and expression, route of administration, and specific transgene delivered are under investigation. Retrovirus or adenovirus can be administered by intratumoral injection, intra-arterially using a percutaneous catheter or HAI pump, or intravenously through the portal vein or a peripheral vein. Different types of genes are being studied, including suicide genes such as thymidine kinase (TK) or cytosine deaminase; immunostimulatory molecule or cytokine genes; and tumor suppressor genes such as *p53*. Animal studies have been reported using rat or murine models with subcapsular colon cancer liver nodules injected with HSVI-TK retroviral producer cells or adenovirus with the 112 and/or TK transgenes, with evidence of regression (182). Antisense therapy remains another alternative. Gene therapy is an exciting modality under active investigation that can be applied to the treatment of colorectal liver metastases (183).

REFERENCES

1. Jemal A, Siegel R, Ward E, et al. Cancer statistics, 2009. *CA Cancer J Clin.* Published online. doi: 10.3322/caac.20006.
2. Greenlee RT, Murray T, Bolden S, et al. Cancer statistics, 2000. *CA Cancer J Clin.* 2000;50:7–33.
3. Hurwitz H, Fehrenbacher L, Novotny W, et al. Bevacizumab plus irinotecan, fluorouracil, and leucovorin for metastatic colorectal cancer. *N Engl J Med.* 2004;350:2335–2342.
4. Bilchik AJ, Poston G, Curley SA, et al. Neoadjuvant chemotherapy for metastatic colon cancer: a cautionary note. *J Clin Oncol.* 2005;23:9073–9078.
5. Rothenberg ML, Oza AM, Bigelow RH, et al. Superiority of oxaliplatin and fluorouracil-leucovorin compared with either therapy alone in patients with progressive colorectal cancer after irinotecan and fluorouracil-leucovorin: interim results of a phase III trial. *J Clin Oncol.* 2003;21:2059–2069.
6. Ballantyne GH, Quin J. Surgical treatment of liver metastases in patients with colorectal cancer. *Cancer.* 1993;71:4252–4266.
7. Bengmark S, Hafstrom L, Olsson A. The natural history of primary and secondary liver tumours. V. The prognosis for conventionally treated patients with liver metastases. *Digestion.* 1972;6:321–329.
8. Pawlik TM, Abdalla EK, Ellis LM, et al. Debunking dogma: surgery for four or more colorectal liver metastases is justified. *J Gastrointest Surg.* 2006;10:240–248.
9. Fong Y, Cohen AM, Fortner JG, et al. Liver resection for colorectal metastases. *J Clin Oncol.* 1997;15:938–946.
10. Scheele J, Stang R, Altendorf-Hofmann A, et al. Resection of colorectal liver metastases. *World J Surg.* 1995;19:59–71.
11. Jarnagin WR, Gonen M, Fong Y, et al. Improvement in perioperative outcome after hepatic resection: analysis of 1,803 consecutive cases over the past decade. *Ann Surg.* 2002;236:397–406; discussion 406–397.
12. Lefor AT, Hughes KS, Shiloni E, et al. Intra-abdominal extrahepatic disease in patients with colorectal hepatic metastases. *Dis Colon Rectum.* 1988;31:100–103.
13. Gibbs JF, Weber TK, Rodriguez-Bigas MA, et al. Intraoperative determinants of unresectability for patients with colorectal hepatic metastases. *Cancer.* 1998;82:1244–1249.
14. Jarnagin WR, Fong Y, Ky A, et al. Liver resection for metastatic colorectal cancer: assessing the risk of occult irresectable disease. *J Am Coll Surg.* 1999;188:33–42.
15. Sugihara K, Hojo K, Moriya Y, et al. Pattern of recurrence after hepatic resection for colorectal metastases. *Br J Surg.* 1993;80:1032–1035.
16. Kemeny MM. Hepatic resection: when, what kind, and for which patients. *J Surg Oncol Suppl.* 1991;2:54–58.
17. Choi J. Imaging of hepatic metastases. *Cancer Control.* 2006;13:6–12.
18. Kinkel K, Lu Y, Both M, et al. Detection of hepatic metastases from cancers of the gastrointestinal tract by using noninvasive imaging methods (US, CT, MR imaging, PET): a meta-analysis. *Radiology.* 2002;224:748–756.

19. Kamel IR, Lawler LP, Fishman EK. Comprehensive analysis of hypervascular liver lesions using 16-MDCT and advanced image processing. *AJR Am J Roentgenol.* 2004;183:443–452.

20. Bhattacharjya S, Bhattacharjya T, Baber S, et al. Prospective study of contrast-enhanced computed tomography, computed tomography during arterioportography, and magnetic resonance imaging for staging colorectal liver metastases for liver resection. *Br J Surg.* 2004;91:1361–1369.

21. Soyer P, Levesque M, Elias D, et al. Preoperative assessment of resectability of hepatic metastases from colonic carcinoma: CT portography vs sonography and dynamic CT. *AJR Am J Roentgenol.* 1992;159:741–744.

22. Soyer P, Bluemke DA, Hruban RH, et al. Hepatic metastases from colorectal cancer: detection and false-positive findings with helical CT during arterial portography. *Radiology.* 1994;193:71–74.

23. Vogel SB, Drane WE, Ros PR, et al. Prediction of surgical resectability in patients with hepatic colorectal metastases. *Ann Surg.* 1994;219:508–514; discussion 514–506.

24. Wernecke K, Rummeny E, Bongartz G, et al. Detection of hepatic masses in patients with carcinoma: comparative sensitivities of sonography, CT, and MR imaging. *AJR Am J Roentgenol.* 1991;157:731–739.

25. Heiken JP, Weyman PJ, Lee JK, et al. Detection of focal hepatic masses: prospective evaluation with CT, delayed CT, CT during arterial portography, and MR imaging. *Radiology.* 1989;171:47–51.

26. Graham MM, Peterson LM, Hayward RM. Comparison of simplified quantitative analyses of FDG uptake. *Nucl Med Biol.* 2000;27:647–655.

27. Fong Y, Saldinger PF, Akhurst T, et al. Utility of 18F-FDG positron emission tomography scanning on selection of patients for resection of hepatic colorectal metastases. *Am J Surg.* 1999;178:282–287.

28. Rahusen FD, Cuesta MA, Borgstein PJ, et al. Selection of patients for resection of colorectal metastases to the liver using diagnostic laparoscopy and laparoscopic ultrasonography. *Ann Surg.* 1999;230:31–37.

29. Selzner M, Hany TF, Wildbrett P, et al. Does the novel PET/CT imaging modality impact on the treatment of patients with metastatic colorectal cancer of the liver? *Ann Surg.* 2004;240:1027–1034; discussion 1035.

30. Dietrich CF, Kratzer W, Strobe D, et al. Assessment of metastatic liver disease in patients with primary extrahepatic tumors by contrast-enhanced sonography versus CT and MRI. *World J Gastroenterol.* 2006;12:1699–1705.

31. Bismuth H, Castaing D, Garden OJ. The use of operative ultrasound in surgery of primary liver tumors. *World J Surg.* 1987;11:610–614.

32. Parker GA, Lawrence W, Jr., Horsley JS, 3rd, et al. Intraoperative ultrasound of the liver affects operative decision making. *Ann Surg.* 1989;209:569–576; discussion 576–567.

33. Knol JA, Marn CS, Francis IR, et al. Comparisons of dynamic infusion and delayed computed tomography, intraoperative ultrasound, and palpation in the diagnosis of liver metastases. *Am J Surg.* 1993;165:81–88.

34. Soyer P, Levesque M, Elias D, et al. Detection of liver metastases from colorectal cancer: comparison of intraoperative US and CT during arterial portography. *Radiology.* 1992;183:541–544.

35. Machi J, Isomoto H, Kurohiji T, et al. Accuracy of intraoperative ultrasonography in diagnosing liver metastasis from colorectal cancer: evaluation with postoperative follow-up results. *World J Surg.* 1991;15:551–557.

36. Staren ED, Gambla M, Deziel DJ, et al. Intraoperative ultrasound in the management of liver neoplasms. *Am Surg.* 1997;63:591–597.

37. Jarnagin WR, Bach AM, Winston CB, et al. What is the yield of intraoperative ultrasonography during partial hepatectomy for malignant disease? *J Am Coll Surg.* 2001;192:577–583.

38. Gayowski TJ, Iwatsuki S, Madariaga JR, et al. Experience in hepatic resection for metastatic colorectal cancer: analysis of clinical and pathologic risk factors. *Surgery.* 1994;116:703–711.

39. Rosen CB, Nagorney DM, Taswell HF, et al. Perioperative blood transfusion and determinants of survival after liver resection for metastatic colorectal carcinoma. *Ann Surg.* 1992;216:493–504; discussion 504–495.

40. Savage AP, Malt RA. Survival after hepatic resection for malignant tumours. *Br J Surg.* 1992;79:1095–1101.

41. Cady B, Stone MD, McDermott WV, Jr., et al. Technical and biological factors in disease-free survival after hepatic resection for colorectal cancer metastases. *Arch Surg.* 1992;127:561–569.

42. Scheele J, Stangl R, Altendorf-Hofmann A, et al. Indicators of prognosis after hepatic resection for colorectal secondaries. *Surgery.* 1991;110:13–29.

43. Nordlinger B, Guiguet M, Vaillant JC, et al. Surgical resection of colorectal carcinoma metastases to the liver. A prognostic scoring system to improve case selection, based on 1568 patients. Association Francaise de Chirurgie. *Cancer.* 1996;77:1254–1262.

44. Schindl M, Wigmore SJ, Currie EJ, et al. Prognostic scoring in colorectal cancer liver metastases: development and validation. *Arch Surg.* 2005;140:183–189.

45. Doci R, Gennari L, Bignami P, et al. Morbidity and mortality after hepatic resection of metastases from colorectal cancer. *Br J Surg.* 1995;82:377–381.

46. Adson MA, van Heerden JA, Adson MH, et al. Resection of hepatic metastases from colorectal cancer. *Arch Surg.* 1984;119:647–651.

47. Fong Y, Fortner J, Sun RL, et al. Clinical score for predicting recurrence after hepatic resection for metastatic colorectal cancer: analysis of 1001 consecutive cases. *Ann Surg.* 1999;230:309–321.

48. Poston GJ, Adam R, Alberts S, et al. OncoSurge: a strategy for improving resectability with curative intent in metastatic colorectal cancer. *J Clin Oncol.* 2005;23:7125–7134.

49. Fong Y. Surgical therapy of hepatic colorectal metastasis. *CA Cancer J Clin.* 1999;49:231–255.

50. Yamaguchi A, Kurosaka Y, Kanno M, et al. Analysis of hepatic recurrence of colorectal cancer after resection of hepatic metastases. *Int Surg.* 1993;78:16–19.

51. Wanebo HJ, Chu QD, Vezeridis MP, et al. Patient selection for hepatic resection of colorectal metastases. *Arch Surg.* 1996;131:322–329.

52. Ercolani G, Grazi GL, Ravaioli M, et al. Liver resection for multiple colorectal metastases: influence of parenchymal involvement and total tumor volume, vs number or location, on long-term survival. *Arch Surg.* 2002;137:1187–1192.

53. Bolton JS, Fuhrman GM. Survival after resection of multiple bilobar hepatic metastases from colorectal carcinoma. *Ann Surg.* 2000;231:743–751.

54. Weber SM, Jarnagin WR, DeMatteo RP, et al. Survival after resection of multiple hepatic colorectal metastases. *Ann Surg Oncol.* 2000;7:643–650.

55. Minagawa M, Makuuchi M, Torzilli G, et al. Extension of the frontiers of surgical indications in the treatment of liver metastases from colorectal cancer: long-term results. *Ann Surg.* 2000;231:487–499.

56. Fortner JG, Blumgart LH. A historic perspective of liver surgery for tumors at the end of the millennium. *J Am Coll Surg.* 2001;193:210–222.

57. Bartlett D, Fong Y, Blumgart LH. Complete resection of the caudate lobe of the liver: technique and results. *Br J Surg.* 1996;83:1076–1081.

58. Lui WY, Chau GY, Loong CC, et al. Hepatic segmentectomy for curative resection of primary hepatocellular carcinoma. *Arch Surg.* 1995;130:1090–1097.

59. Hemming AW, Scudamore CH, Davidson A, et al. Evaluation of 50 consecutive segmental hepatic resections. *Am J Surg.* 1993;165:621–624.

60. Bismuth H, Houssin D, Castaing D. Major and minor segmentectomies "reglees" in liver surgery. *World J Surg.* 1982;6:10–24.

61. DeMatteo RP, Palese C, Jarnagin WR, et al. Anatomic segmental hepatic resection is superior to wedge resection as an oncologic operation for colorectal liver metastases. *J Gastrointest Surg.* 2000;4:178–184.

62. Zorzi D, Mullen JT, Abdalla EK, et al. Comparison between hepatic wedge resection and anatomic resection for colorectal liver metastases. *J Gastrointest Surg.* 2006;10:86–94.

63. Are C, Fong Y, Geller DA. Laparoscopic liver resections. *Adv Surg.* 2005;39:57–75.

64. Ballantyne GH. Laparoscopic-assisted colorectal surgery: review of results in 752 patients. *Gastroenterologist.* 1995;3:75–89.

65. Buell JF, Thomas MJ, Doty TC, et al. An initial experience and evolution of laparoscopic hepatic resectional surgery. *Surgery.* 2004;136:804–811.

66. Bengmark S, Hafstrom L. The natural history of primary and secondary malignmant tumors of the liver. *Cancer.* 1969;23:198–202.

67. Kemeny MM. Expressing the surgery first position on treatment of synchronous colorectal metastases in the asymptomatic patient. *Ann Surg Oncol.* 2006;13:140–141.

68. Steele G, Jr., Bleday R, Mayer RJ, et al. A prospective evaluation of hepatic resection for colorectal carcinoma metastases to the liver: Gastrointestinal Tumor Study Group Protocol 6584. *J Clin Oncol.* 1991;9:1105–1112.

69. Nordlinger B, Quilichini MA, Parc R, et al. Hepatic resection for colorectal liver metastases. Influence on survival of preoperative factors and surgery for recurrences in 80 patients. *Ann Surg.* 1987;205:256–263.

70. Fujita S, Akasu T, Moriya Y. Resection of synchronous liver metastases from colorectal cancer. *Jpn J Clin Oncol.* 2000;30:7–11.

71. Lyass S, Zamir G, Matot I, et al. Combined colon and hepatic resection for synchronous colorectal liver metastases. *J Surg Oncol.* 2001;78:17–21.

72. Martin R, Paty P, Fong Y, et al. Simultaneous liver and colorectal resections are safe for synchronous colorectal liver metastasis. *J Am Coll Surg.* 2003;197:233–241; discussion 241–232.

73. Buell JF, Koffron A, Yoshida A, et al. Is any method of vascular control superior in hepatic resection of metastatic cancers? Longmire clamping, pringle maneuver, and total vascular isolation. *Arch Surg.* 2001;136:569–575.

74. Cherqui D, Husson E, Hammoud R, et al. Laparoscopic liver resections: a feasibility study in 30 patients. *Ann Surg.* 2000;232:753–762.

75. Gigot JF, Glineur D, Santiago Azagra J, et al. Laparoscopic liver resection for malignant liver tumors: preliminary results of a multicenter European study. *Ann Surg.* 2002;236:90–97.

76. Fong Y, Jarnagin W, Conlon KC, et al. Hand-assisted laparoscopic liver resection: lessons from an initial experience. *Arch Surg.* 2000;135:854–859.

77. Lesurtel M, Cherqui D, Laurent A, et al. Laparoscopic versus open left lateral hepatic lobectomy: a case-control study. *J Am Coll Surg.* 2003;196:236–242.

78. Bongiovanni M, Cassoni P, De Giuli P, et al. p27(kip1) immunoreactivity correlates with long-term survival in pleural malignant mesothelioma. *Cancer.* 2001;92:1245–1250.

79. Pedersen IK, Burcharth F, Roikjaer O, Baden H. Resection of liver metastases from colorectal cancer. Indications and results. *Dis Colon Rectum.* 1994;37:1078–1082.

80. Pinson CW, Wright JK, Chapman WC, et al. Repeat hepatic surgery for colorectal cancer metastasis to the liver. *Ann Surg.* 1996;223:765–773; discussion 773–766.

81. Rees M, Plant G, Bygrave S. Late results justify resection for multiple hepatic metastases from colorectal cancer. *Br J Surg.* 1997;84:1136–1140.

82. Nakamura S, Suzuki S, Konno H. Resection of hepatic metastases of colorectal carcinoma: 20 years' experience. *J Hepatobiliary Pancreat Surg.* 1999;6:16–22.

83. Bradley AL, Chapman WC, Wright JK, et al. Surgical experience with hepatic colorectal metastasis. *Am Surg.* 1999;65:560–567.

84. Fan ST, Lo CM, Liu CL, et al. Hepatectomy for hepatocellular carcinoma: toward zero hospital deaths. *Ann Surg.* 1999;229:322–330.

85. Fong Y, Gonen M, Rubin D, et al. Long-term survival is superior after resection for cancer in high-volume centers. *Ann Surg.* 2005;242:540–547.

86. Jamison RL, Donohue JH, Nagorney DM, et al. Hepatic resection for metastatic colorectal cancer results in cure for some patients. *Arch Surg.* 1997;132:505–511.

87. Schlag P, Hohenberger P, Herfarth C. Resection of liver metastases in colorectal cancer: competitive analysis of treatment results in synchronous versus metachronous metastases. *Eur J Surg Oncol.* 1990;16:360–365.

88. Fortner JG, Silva JS, Golbey RB. Multivariate analysis of a personal series of 247 consecutive patients with liver metastases from colorectal cancer: I, Treatment by hepatic resection. *Ann Surg.* 1984;196:306–316.

89. Fong Y. Hepatic colorectal metastasis: current surgical therapy, selection criteria for hepatectomy, and role for adjuvant therapy. *Adv Surg.* 2000;34:351–381.

90. Stephenson KR, Steinberg SM, Hughes KS, et al. Perioperative blood transfusions are associated with decreased time to recurrence and decreased survival after resection of colorectal liver metastases. *Ann Surg.* 1988;208:679–687.

91. Kooby DA, Stockman J, Ben Porat L, et al. Influence of transfusions on perioperative and long-term outcome in patients following hepatic resection for colorectal metastases. *Annals of Surgery.* 2003;237:860–869.

92. Elias D, Lasser P, Ducreux M, et al. Liver resection (and associated extrahepatic resections) for metastatic well-differentiated endocrine tumors: a 15-year single center prospective study. *Surgery.* 2003;133:375–382.

93. Elias D, Sideris L, Pocard M, et al. Results of R0 resection for colorectal liver metastases associated with extrahepatic disease. *Ann Surg Oncol.* 2004;11:274–280.

94. Harned RK, 2nd, Chezmar JL, Nelson RC. Recurrent tumor after resection of hepatic metastases from colorectal carcinoma: location and time of discovery as determined by CT. *AJR Am J Roentgenol.* 1994;163:93–97.

95. Doci R, Gennari L, Bignami P, et al. One hundred patients with hepatic metastases from colorectal cancer treated by resection: analysis of prognostic determinants. *Br J Surg.* 1991;78:797–801.

96. Wanebo HJ, Chu QD, Avradopoulos KA, et al. Current perspectives on repeat hepatic resection for colorectal carcinoma: a review. *Surgery.* 1996;119:361–371.

97. Fong Y, Blumgart LH, Cohe A, et al. Repeat hepatic resections for metastatic colorectal cancer. *Ann Surg.* 1994;220:657–662.

98. Nordlinger B, Vaillant JC, Guiguet M. Survival benefit of repeat liver resections for recurrent colorectal metastases: 143 cases. *J Clin Oncol.* 1994;12:1491–1496.

99. Tuttle TM, Curley SA, Roh MS. Repeat hepatic resection as effective treatment of recurrent colorectal liver metastases. *Ann Surg Oncol.* 1997;4:125–130.

100. Fernandez-Trigo V, Shamsa F, Sugarbaker PH. Repeat liver resections from colorectal metastasis. *Surgery.* 1995;117:296–304.

101. Que FG, Nagorney DM. Resection of 'recurrent' colorectal metastases to the liver. *Br J Surg.* 1994;81:255–258.

102. Ravikumar TS, Kane R, Cady B, et al. A 5-year study of cryosurgery in the treatment of liver tumors. *Arch. Surg.* 1991;126:1520–1524.

103. Steele G, Jr. Cryoablation in hepatic surgery. *Semin Liver Dis.* 1994;14:120–125.

104. Onik GM, Atkinson D, Zemel R, et al. Cryosurgery of liver cancer. *Seminars in Surgical Oncology.* 1993;9:309–317.

105. Khatri VP, McGahan J. Non-resection approaches for colorectal liver metastases. *Surg Clin North Am.* 2004;84:587–606.

106. Rubinsky B, Lee CY, Bastacky J, et al. The process of freezing and the mechanism of damage during hepatic cryosurgery. *Cryobiology.* 1990;27:85–97.

107. Farrant J, Walter CA. The cryobiological basis for cryosurgery. *J Dermatol Surg Oncol.* 1977;3:403–407.

108. Weaver ML, Ashton JG, Zemel R. Treatment of colorectal liver metastases by cryotherapy. *Seminars in Surgical Oncology.* 1998;14:163–170.

109. Onik GM, Chambers N, Chernus SA, et al. Hepatic cryosurgery with and without the Bair Hugger. *J Surg Oncol.* 1993;52:185–187.

110. Ravikumar TS, Steele G, Jr., Kane R, et al. Experimental and clinical observations on hepatic cryosurgery for colorectal metastases. *Cancer Res.* 1991;51:6323–6327.

111. Polk W, Fong Y, Karpeh M, et al. A technique for the use of cryosurgery to assist hepatic resection. *J Am Coll Surg.* 1995;180:171–176.

112. Curley SA, Izzo F, Delrio P, et al. Radiofrequency ablation of unresectable primary and metastatic hepatic malignancies: results in 123 patients. *Ann Surg.* 1999;230:1–8.

113. Solbiati L, Livraghi T, Goldberg SN, et al. Percutaneous radiofrequency ablation of hepatic metastases from colorectal cancer: long-term results in 117 patients. *Radiology.* 2001;221:159–166.

114. Livraghi T, Solbiati L, Meloni MF, et al. Treatment of focal liver tumors with percutaneous radio-frequency ablation: complications encountered in a multicenter study. *Radiology.* 2003;226:441–451.

115. Breedis C, Young G. Blood supply of neoplasms of the liver. *American Journal of Pathology.* 1954;30:969–985.

116. Sigurdson ER, Ridge JA, Kemeny N, et al. Tumor and liver drug uptake following hepatic artery and portal vein infusion in man. *J Clin Oncol.* 1987;5:1836–1840.

117. Ensminger WD, Rosowsky A, Raso V, et al. A clinical-pharmacologic evaluation of hepatic arterial infusions of 5-fluoro-2'-deoxyuridine and 5-fluorouracil. *Cancer Res.* 1978;38:3784–3792.

118. Niederhuber JE, Ensminger W, Gyves J, et al. Regional chemotherapy of colorectal cancer metastatic to the liver. *Cancer.* 1984;53:1336–1343.

119. Balch CM, Urist MM. Intraarterial chemotherapy for colorectal liver metastases and hepatomas using a totally implantable drug infusion pump. *Recent Results Cancer Res.* 1986;100:234–247.

120. Kemeny N, Daly J, Oderman P, et al. Hepatic artery pump infusion: toxicity and results in patients with metastatic colorectal carcinoma. *J Clin Oncol.* 1984;2:595–600.

121. Shepard KV, Levin B, Karl RC, et al. Therapy for metastatic colorectal cancer with hepatic artery infusion chemotherapy using a subcutaneous implanted pump. *J Clin Oncol.* 1985;3:161–169.

122. Cohen AM, Kaufman SD, Wood WC, et al. Regional hepatic chemotherapy using an implantable drug infusion pump. *Am J Surg.* 1983;145:529–533.

123. Hohn DC, Stagg RJ, Friedman MA, et al. A randomized trial of continuous intravenous versus hepatic intraarterial floxuridine in patients with colorectal cancer metastatic to the liver: The Northern California oncology group trial. *Journal of Clinical Oncology.* 1989;7:1646–1654.

124. Kemeny MM, Goldberg D, Beatty JD, et al. Results of a prospective randomized trial of continuous regional chemotherapy and hepatic resection as treatment of hepatic metastases from colorectal primaries. *Cancer.* 1986;57:492–498.

125. Schwartz SI, Jones LS, McCune CS. Assessment of treatment of intrahepatic malignancies using chemotherapy via an implantable pump. *Ann Surg.* 1985;201:560–567.

126. Weiss GR, Garnick MB, Osteen RT, et al. Long-term hepatic arterial infusion of 5-fluorodeoxyuridine for liver metastases using an implantable infusion pump. *J Clin Oncol.* 1983;1:337–344.

127. Kemeny MM, Battifora H, Blayney DW, et al. Sclerosing cholangitis after continuous hepatic artery infusion of FUDR. *Annals of Surgery.* 1985;202:176–181.

128. Allen PJ, Nissan A, Picon AI, et al. Technical complications and durability of hepatic artery infusion pumps for unresectable colorectal liver metastases: an institutional experience of 544 consecutive cases. *J Am Coll Surg.* 2005;201:57–65.

129. Allen-Mersh TG, Earlam S, Fordy C, et al. Quality of life and survival with continuous hepatic-artery floxuridine infusion for colorectal liver metastases. *Lancet.* 1994;344:1255–1260.

130. Grage TB, Vassilopoulos PP, Shingleton WW, et al. Results of a prospective randomized study of hepatic artery infusion with 5-fluorouracil versus intravenous 5-fluorouracil in patients with hepatic metastases from colorectal cancer: A Central Oncology Group study. *Surgery.* 1979;86:550–555.

131. Martin JK, O'Connel MJ, Wieand HS, et al. Intra-arterial floxuridine vs systemic fluorouracil for hepatic metastases from colorectal cancer. *Arch Surg.* 1990;125:1022–1027.

132. Wagman LD, Kemeny MM, Leong L, et al. A prospective, randomized evaluation of the treatment of colorectal cancer metastatic to the liver. *J Clin Oncol.* 1990;8:1885–1893.

133. Chang AE, Schneider PD, Sugarbaker PH, et al. A prospective randomized trial of regional versus systemic continuous f-luorodeoxyuridine chemotherapy in the treatment of colorectal liver metastases. *Annals of Surgery.* 1987;206:685–693.

134. Kemeny N, Daly J, Reichman B, et al. Intrahepatic or systemic infusion of fluorodeoxyuridine in patients with liver metastases from colorectal carcinoma. *Ann Intern Med.* 1987;107:459–465.

135. Daly JM, Kemeny NE, DeVita VT, et al. Metastatic cancer to the liver. In: DeVita VT, Hellman S, Rosenberg SA (eds) *Cancer: Principles and Practice of Oncology*, ed. 5. Philadelphia: Lippincott-Raven, 1997:2551–2570.

136. Hohn DC, Stagg RJ, Friedman MA, et al. A randomized trial of continuous intravenous versus hepatic intraarterial floxuridine in patients with colorectal cancer metastatic to the liver: the Northern California Oncology Group trial. *J Clin Oncol.* 1989;7:1646–1654.

137. Cohen AD, Kemeny NE. An update on hepatic arterial infusion chemotherapy for colorectal cancer. *Oncologist.* 2003;8:553–566.

138. Rougier P, LaPlanche A, Huguier M, et al. Hepatic arterial infusion of floxuridine in patients with liver metastases from colorectal carcinoma: Long-term results of a prospective randomized trial. *Journal of Clinical Oncology.* 1992;10:1112–1118.

139. Lorenz M, Måller HH, Schramm H, et al. Randomized trial of surgery versus surgery followed by adjuvant hepatic arterial infusion with 5-fluorouracil and folinic acid for liver metastases of colorectal cancer. *Ann Surg.* 1998;228:756–762.

140. Rudroff C, Altendorf-Hoffmann A, Stangl R, et al. Prospective randomized trial on adjuvant hepatic-artery infusion chemotherapy after RO resection of colorectal liver metastases. *Langenbecks Arch Surg.* 1999;384:243–249.

141. Lorenz M, Staib-Sebler E, Loch B. The value of postoperative hepatic arterial infusion following curative liver resection. *Anticancer Research.* 1997;17:3825–3833.

142. Ambiru S, Miyazaki H, Ito H. Adjuvant regional chemotherapy after hepatic resection for colorectal metastases. *Br J Surg.* 1999;86:1025–1031.

143. Berlin J, Merrick HW, Smith TJ, et al. Phase II evaluation of treatment of complete resection of hepatic metastases from colorectal cancer and djuvant hepatic arterial infusion of floxuridine. *American Journal of Clinical Oncology.* 1999;22:291–293.

144. Kemeny N, Huang Y, Cohen AM, et al. Hepatic arterial infusion of chemotherapy after resection of hepatic metastases from colorectal cancer. *N Engl J Med.* 1999;341:2039–2048.

145. Hughes KS, Simon R, Songhorabodi S. Resection of the liver for colorectal carcinoma metastases: A multi-institutional study of indications for resection. *Surgery.* 1988;103:278–288.

146. Kemeny NE, Niedzwiecki D, Hollis DR, et al. Hepatic arterial infusion versus systemic therapy for hepatic metastases from colorectal cancer: a randomized trial of efficacy, quality of life, and molecular markers (CALGB 9481). *J Clin Oncol.* 2006;24:1395–1403.

147. Leonard GD, Brenner B, Kemeny NE. Neoadjuvant chemotherapy before liver resection for patients with unresectable liver metastases from colorectal carcinoma. *J Clin Oncol.* 2005;23:2038–2048.

148. Bismuth H, Adam R, LÇvi F, et al. Resection of nonresectable liver metastases from colorectal cancer after neoadjuvant chemotherapy. *Ann Surg.* 1996;224:509–522.

149. Giacchetti S, Itzhaki M, Gruia G, et al. Long-term survival of patients with unresectable colorectal cancer liver metastases following infusional chemotherapy with 5-fluorouracil, leucovorin, oxaliplatin and surgery. *Ann Oncol.* 1999;10:663–669.

150. Pozzo C, Basso M, Cassano A, et al. Neoadjuvant treatment of unresectable liver disease with irinotecan and 5-fluorouracil plus folinic acid in colorectal cancer patients. *Ann Oncol.* 2004;15:933–939.

151. Adam R, Avisar E, Ariche A, et al. Five-year survival following hepatic resection after neoadjuvant therapy for nonresectable colorectal. *Ann Surg Oncol.* 2001;8:347–353.

152. Adam R, Pascal G, Castaing D, et al. Tumor progression while on chemotherapy: a contraindication to liver resection for multiple colorectal metastases? *Ann Surg.* 2004;240:1052–1061; discussion 1061–1054.

153. Parikh AA, Gentner B, Wu TT, et al. Perioperative complications in patients undergoing major liver resection with or without neoadjuvant chemotherapy. *J Gastrointest Surg.* 2003;7:1082–1088.

154. Sutton R, Doran HE, Williams EM, et al. Surgery for midgut carcinoid. *Endocr Relat Cancer.* 2003;10:469–481.

155. Norton JA. Endocrine tumours of the gastrointestinal tract. Surgical treatment of neuroendocrine metastases. *Best Pract Res Clin Gastroenterol.* 2005;19:577–583.

156. Yao KA, Talamonti MS, Nemcek A, et al. Indications and results of liver resection and hepatic chemoembolization for metastatic gastrointestinal neuroendocrine tumors. *Surgery.* 2001;130:677–682; discussion 682–675.

157. Chamberlain RS, Canes D, Brown KT, et al. Hepatic neuroendocrine metastases: does intervention alter outcomes? *J Am Coll Surg.* 2000;190:432–445.

158. Singletary SE, Walsh G, Vauthey JN, et al. A role for curative surgery in the treatment of selected patients with metastatic breast cancer. *Oncologist.* 2003;8:241–251.

159. Schneebaum S, Walker MJ, Young D, et al. The regional treatment of liver metastases from breast cancer. *J Surg Oncol.* 1994;55:26–32.

160. Raab R, Nussbaum KT, Behrend M, et al. Liver metastases of breast cancer: results of liver resection. *Anticancer Res.* 1998;18:2231–2233.

161. Santoro E, Vitucci C, Carlini M, et al. [Liver metastasis of breast carcinoma. Results of surgical resection. Analysis of 15 operated cases]. *Chir Ital.* 2000;52:131–137.

162. Pocard M, Pouillart P, Asselain B, et al. [Hepatic resection for breast cancer metastases: results and prognosis (65 cases)]. *Ann Chir.* 2001;126:413–420.

163. Selzner M, Morse MA, Vredenburgh JJ, et al. Liver metastases from breast cancer: long-term survival after curative resection. *Surgery.* 2000;127:383–389.

164. DeMatteo RP, Shah A, Fong Y, et al. Results of hepatic resection for sarcoma metastatic to liver. *Ann Surg.* 2001;234:540–548.

165. Rose DM, Essner R, Hughes TM, et al. Surgical resection for metastatic melanoma to the liver: the John Wayne Cancer Institute and Sydney Melanoma Unit experience. *Arch Surg.* 2001;136:950–955.

166. Feldman ED, Pingpank JF, Alexander HR, Jr. Regional treatment options for patients with ocular melanoma metastatic to the liver. *Ann Surg Oncol.* 2004;11:290–297.

167. Aoyama T, Mastrangelo MJ, Berd D, et al. Protracted survival after resection of metastatic uveal melanoma. *Cancer.* 2000;89:1561–1568.

168. Covey AM, Tuorto S, Brody LA, et al. Safety and efficacy of preoperative portal vein embolization with polyvinyl alcohol in 58 patients with liver metastases. *AJR Am J Roentgenol.* 2005;185:1620–1626.

169. Liu H, Fu Y. Portal vein embolization before major hepatectomy. *World J Gastroenterol.* 2005;11:2051–2054.

170. Farges O, Belghiti J, Kianmanesh R, et al. Portal vein embolization before right hepatectomy: prospective clinical trial. *Ann Surg.* 2003;237:208–217.

171. Di Filippo F, Anza M, Rossi CR, et al. The application of hyperthermia in regional chemotherapy. *Semin Surg Oncol.* 1998;14:215–223.

172. Bartlett DL, Libutti SK, Figg WD, et al. Isolated hepatic perfusion for unresectable hepatic metastases from colorectal cancer. *Surgery.* 2001;129:176–187.

173. Alexander HR, Jr., Libutti SK, Pingpank JF, et al. Isolated hepatic prefusion for the treatment of patients with colorectal cancer (CRC) liver metastases after irinotecan-based therapy. *Ann Surg Oncol.* 2005;12:138–144.

174. Alexander HR, Libutti SK, Bartlett DL, et al. A Phase I-II study of isolated hepatic perfusion using melphalan with or without tumor necrosis factor for patients with ocular melanoma metastatic to liver. *Clin Cancer Res.* 2000;6:3062–3070.

175. Alexander HR, Libutti SK, Pingpank JF, et al. Hyperthermic Isolated Hepatic Perfusion (IHP) Using Melphalan for Patients with Ocular Melanoma Metastatic to Liver. *Clin Cancer Res.* 2003;9:6343–6349.

176. Noter SL, Rothbarth J, Pijl ME, et al. Isolated hepatic perfusion with high-dose melphalan for the treatment of uveal melanoma metastases confined to the liver. *Melanoma Res.* 2004;14:67–72.

177. van Etten B, Brunstein F, van Ijken MG, et al. Isolated Hypoxic Hepatic Perfusion With Orthograde or Retrograde Flow in Patients With Irresectable Liver Metastases Using Percutaneous Balloon Catheter Techniques: A Phase I and II Study. *Ann Surg Oncol.* 2004;11:598–605.

178. Ravikumar TS, Pizzorno G, Bodden W, et al. Percutaneous hepatic vein isolation and high-dose hepatic arterial infusion chemotherapy for unresectable liver tumors. *J Clin Oncol.* 1994;12:2723–2736.

179. Lowy AM, Curley SA. Clinical and preclinical trials of isolated liver perfusion for advanced liver tumors: primary liver tumors. *Surg Oncol Clin North Am.* 1996;5:429–441.

180. Pingpank JF, Libutti SK, Chang R, et al. A Phase I feasibility study of hepatic arterial melphalan infusion with hepatic arterial melphalan infusion with hepatic venous hemofiltration using

percutaneously placed catheters in patients with unresectable hepatic malignancies. *Amer Soc Clin Oncol Proc.* 2003;22:282.

181. Panis Y, Rad ARK, Boyer O, et al. Gene therapy for liver tumors. *Surgical Oncology Clinics of North America.* 1996;5:461–473.

182. Caruso M, Panis Y, Gagandeep S, et al. Regression of established macroscopic liver metastases after in situ transduction of a suicide gene. *Proceedings of the National Academy of Sciences of the United States of America.* 1993;90:7024–7028.

183. Chen SH, Chen SHL, Wang Y, et al. Combination gene therapy for liver metastasis of colon carcinoma in vivo. *Proceedings of the National Academy of Science USA.* 1995;92:2577–2581.

184. Mutsaerts EL, van Ruth S, Zoetmulder FA, et al. Prognostic factors and evaluation of surgical management of hepatic metastases from colorectal origin: a 10-year single-institute experience. *J Gastrointest Surg.* 2005;9:178–186.

185. Abdalla EK, Vauthey JN, Ellis LM, et al. Recurrence and outcomes following hepatic resection, radiofrequency ablation, and combined resection/ablation for colorectal liver metastases. *Ann Surg.* 2004;239:818–825; discussion 825–817.

186. Bramhall SR, Gur U, Coldham C, et al. Liver resection for colorectal metastases. *Ann R Coll Surg Engl.* 2003;85:334–339.

187. Liu CL, Fan ST, Lo CM, et al. Hepatic resection for colorectal liver metastases: prospective study. *Hong Kong Med J.* 2002;8:329–333.

188. Choti MA, Sitzmann JV, Tiburi MF, et al. Trends in long-term survival following liver resection for hepatic colorectal metastases. *Ann Surg.* 2002;235:759–766.

189. Jenkins LT, Millikan KW, Bines SD, et al. Hepatic resection for metastatic colorectal cancer. *The American Surgeon.* 1997;63:605–610.

190. Fong Y, Blumgart LH, Fortner JG, et al. Pancreatic or liver resection for malignancy is safe and effective for the elderly. *Ann Surg.* 1995;222:426–434; discussion 434–427.

191. Shaw IM, Rees M, Welsh FK, et al. Repeat hepatic resection for recurrent colorectal liver metastases is associated with favourable long-term survival. *Br J Surg.* 2006;93:457–464.

192. Adam R, Pascal G, Azoulay D, et al. Liver resection for colorectal metastases: the third hepatectomy. *Ann Surg.* 2003;238:871–883; discussion 883–874.

193. Petrowsky H, Gonen M, Jarnagin W, et al. Second liver resections are safe and effective treatment for recurrent hepatic metastases from colorectal cancer: a bi-institutional analysis. *Ann Surg.* 2002;235:863–871.

194. Suzuki S, Sakaguchi T, Yokoi Y, et al. Impact of repeat hepatectomy on recurrent colorectal liver metastases. *Surgery.* 2001;129:421–428.

195. Muratore A, Polastri R, Bouzari H, et al. Repeat hepatectomy for colorectal liver metastases: A worthwhile operation? *J Surg Oncol.* 2001;76:127–132.

196. Yamamoto J, Kosuge T, Shimada K, et al. Repeat liver resection for recurrent colorectal liver metastases. *Am J Surg.* 1999;178:275–281.

197. Adam R, Bismuth H, Castaing D, et al. Repeat hepatectomy for colorectal liver metastases. *Ann Surg.* 1997;225:51–62.

198. Hildebrand P, Kleemann M, Roblick UJ, et al. Radiofrequency-ablation of unresectable primary and secondary liver tumors: results in 88 patients. *Langenbecks Arch Surg.* 2006;391:118–123.

199. Navarra G, Ayav A, Weber JC, et al. Short- and-long term results of intraoperative radiofrequency ablation of liver metastases. *Int J Colorectal Dis.* 2005;20:521–528.

200. Bleicher RJ, Allegra DP, Nora DT, et al. Radiofrequency ablation in 447 complex unresectable liver tumors: lessons learned. *Ann Surg Oncol.* 2003;10:52–58.

201. Machi J, Uchida S, Sumida K, et al. Ultrasound-guided radiofrequency thermal ablation of liver tumors: percutaneous, laparoscopic, and open surgical Machi approaches. *J Gastrointest Surg.* 2001;5:477–489.

202. Niederhuber JE, Ensminger WD, DeVita VT, et al. Treatment of metastatic cancer to the liver. In: DeVita VT, Hellman S, Rosenberg SA (eds) *Cancer Principles and Practice of Oncology,* ed. 4. Philadelphia: JB Lippincott; 1993:2201–2224.

COMMENTARY
Michael A. Choti

Since first reported more than 40 years ago (1), surgical therapy for patients with metastatic liver disease has gained increasing acceptance as a potentially curative option. For colorectal cancer in particular, surgical therapy of hepatic metastases remains the only therapy with potential for cure. Although recent advances in systemic chemotherapy have led to improved tumor response rates, the median survival of unresected patients still ranges from 12 to 24 months and survival beyond 5 years is uncommon (2–4). In contrast, long-term survival and potential cure following surgical resection for hepatic colorectal metastases have been demonstrated in numerous studies. In this accompanying chapter, Drs. Farma, Tada, and Daly provide a comprehensive overview of the issues relating to the surgical management of patients with hepatic metastatic disease. The authors summarize the importance of preoperative and intraoperative assessment, describe the operative techniques and outcomes of liver resection, and review other locoregional approaches such as tumor ablation and hepatic arterial chemotherapy.

Management paradigms for the surgical approach to hepatic colorectal metastases have changed significantly in recent years (5). Specifically, the definition of what is resectable disease has undergone a paradigm shift. Traditionally, clinicopathologic factors have been used to define whether hepatic colorectal metastases were amenable to surgical resection. Criteria contraindicating resection focused on the lesions to be removed rather than the liver that would remain. These included the presence of four or more metastases, presence of additional extrahepatic disease, large size of the hepatic metastasis, and an anticipated resection margin of <1 cm. Subsequent studies by other investigators, to varying degrees, corroborated some of these findings. With time, these clinicopathologic and morphologic factors were used as the determining criteria to decide which patients with colorectal liver metastases had "resectable" disease. However, based on more recent data, the usefulness of clinicopathologic factors in deciding who is resectable is of limited value. Specifically, seemingly established prognostic factors and clinical scoring systems failed to accurately predict those who derive long-term benefit from liver resection (6,7).

Conventional clinicopathologic factors—although perhaps generally instructive with regard to prognosis—should not be used to define resectability criteria in patients with colorectal liver metastases. Rather, current data have precipitated a shift in the definition of resectability from criteria based on the characteristics of the metastatic disease to new criteria based on whether a macroscopic and microscopic complete or R0 resection of the liver lesion, as well as any extrahepatic disease, can be performed. In addition, decisions on resectability are contingent on whether an adequate liver remnant will be left following surgery. Instead of resectability being defined by what is removed, decisions concerning resectability are largely based on what remains after resection. Resectability is now defined by four main criteria:

1. The disease needs to be amenable to complete resection (R0), including intra- and extrahepatic disease sites.
2. At least two adjacent liver segments need to be spared.
3. Vascular inflow and outflow, as well as biliary drainage to the remaining segments, must be preserved.
4. The volume of the liver remaining after resection must be adequate.

These new criteria of resectability depend less on rigid parameters such as tumor number, size, or location and more on clinical judgment and preoperative imaging. Particularly in cases that are difficult or borderline, resectability should be based on high-quality imaging and assessed by an experienced hepatobiliary surgeon.

In spite of what can be considered a broader definition of resectable disease, many patients are not initially resectable. Several strategies, however, can be employed in order to expand the number of patients eligible for surgical therapy. These can be divided into three general approaches: (a) decrease tumor size, (b) increase the remnant liver volume, or (c) apply combined modality local therapy.

Newer systemic combination chemotherapeutic and biologic regimens not only have demonstrated improved survival in unresectable patients, but also often achieve significant radiographic tumor responses. This improved tumor response to chemotherapy has allowed up to 20% of patients previously deemed unresectable patients to be "converted" to resectable status following tumor downsizing (8). Use of preoperative chemotherapy in this setting should be distinguished from neoadjuvant chemotherapy prescribed for patients with initially resectable disease. Adam et al. (9) reported that liver resection of unresectable colorectal liver metastases downsized by combination chemotherapy resulted in a 5-year survival rate of 33%. Other investigators (10,11) have substantiated these findings, and resection of initially unresectable liver metastases following systemic chemotherapy has become increasingly more common. As such, patients with initially unresectable disease who respond to chemotherapy should be reassessed for surgical therapy. By reconsidering resection of initially unresectable patients, long-term survival may be achieved in patients who otherwise would have poor outcomes.

When treating patients with initially unresectable disease with preoperative chemotherapy, the question often arises as to whether one should treat to maximal response or discontinue chemotherapy as soon as the disease within the liver is found to be resectable. In the setting of unresectable disease, the goal of preoperative chemotherapy is to convert the intrahepatic disease to a resectable status based on the criteria outlined here. As such, in general, preoperative chemotherapy should be stopped once the disease has been downsized to the point where hepatic resection is feasible. This is recommended in part because prolonged courses of preoperative chemotherapy may have a detrimental effect on the hepatic parenchyma. Some studies

have associated the use of oxaliplatin with an increased incidence of hepatic sinusoidal changes (12,13), while others have suggested that irinotecan may be associated with steatosis (13) and steatohepatitis (14). The liver injury, which is exacerbated with prolonged chemotherapy duration, can result in increased perioperative morbidity (14). Another reason to limit preoperative chemotherapy is the risk of lesions achieving a complete radiologic response. Although perhaps counterintuitive, such a response can lead to the inability to find and resect all original sites of disease. In one study, Benoist et al.(15) examined metastatic sites in which complete radiologic response occurred. Of 66 lesions evaluated, the majority could not be identified intraoperatively. Moreover, they found persistent tumor on pathologic examination or follow-up in 83% of cases, confirming that pathologic complete responses are uncommon. Based on these data, resection should be performed on all original sites of disease and inability to identify all sites at surgery may result in poorer outcomes.

In summary, these findings suggest that preoperative chemotherapy potentially can be a powerful tool to convert otherwise unresectable patients, but its use should be individualized and monitored. Thus, chemotherapy that has effectively downsized previously unresectable lesions should not be continued indefinitely. Rather, the patient should be referred back to a hepatic surgeon for reconsideration of resection.

Another means by which resectability can be increased is through a strategy of increasing the hepatic reserve of the remnant liver. In general, 20% to 25% of the total liver volume appears to be the minimum safe volume that can be left following extended resection in patients with normal underlying liver. In patients with liver injury such as steatosis, steatohepatitis, or cirrhosis, including that associated with chemotherapy, the remnant liver should be greater (16,17). Computed tomography or magnetic resonance imaging can now provide an accurate, reproducible method for preoperatively measuring the volume of the future liver remnant. One method that can be employed to increase the hepatic remnant in cases in which insufficient liver reserve is anticipated is with the use of preoperative *portal vein embolization* (PVE). By embolizing the portal vein of the portion of the liver to be resected, atrophy occurs in these segments with compensatory hypertrophy of the contralateral (remnant) liver (17). Typically, at least 5 weeks should be allowed to elapse following PVE in order to allow time for sufficient hypertrophy. Repeat cross-sectional imaging with liver volumetrics can document the achievement of adequate remnant volume. In some cases, additional waiting time can be employed, including with concomitant use of chemotherapy during this period if needed. A second approach that can be applied in patients requiring extensive bilateral resection is the *two-stage hepatectomy*. In such procedures, a limited unilateral resection of some disease can be performed at initial operation, followed by a contralateral major hepatectomy to remove the remaining disease (18). Again, the interval between operations allows for compensatory hypertrophy of the planned remnant liver. The initial procedure can be combined with contralateral portal vein ligation or followed by contralateral PVE in order to promote the remnant hypertrophy, and chemotherapy may be employed between operations. The selective use of PVE or two-stage resection may enable safe and potentially curative hepatic resection in a subset of patients with advanced colorectal metastases who would otherwise have been marginal candidates for resection because of an inadequate future liver remnant or significant underlying liver disease.

As reviewed in the accompanying chapter, methods for local ablation have been developed in recent years with a goal of increasing the number of patients eligible for liver-directed therapy. Combining hepatic resection with ablation can expand the number of patients who may be candidates for liver-directed surgical therapy, particularly as larger lesions that are less effectively treated with ablation can be resected and small lesions can be ablated. However, ablation should not be viewed as a replacement for resection, but more as a supplement or extension of localized therapy in unresectable patients. In general, patients with resectable colorectal liver metastasis should undergo resection and not ablation. The main indication for ablation is in patients who do not meet the criteria for resectability, but are candidates for liver-directed therapy based on the presence of liver-only disease. As with the criteria for resectability, only those patients in whom complete "margin-negative" ablation can be achieved should be considered for this therapy. As with resection, incomplete or cytoreductive therapy should not be advocated outside a clinical trial.

The role of liver resection for hepatic metastases from noncolorectal tumors has not been studied as well as that for metastases from colorectal cancer. Although patients with endocrine metastases (19) or those with imatinib-responsive gastrointestinal stromal tumors (20) appear to derive a survival benefit from surgical therapy of metastatic disease, the role of resection of metastases from other primary tumor types is less clear. Several recent reports do suggest that an aggressive surgical approach may benefit selected patients. In 2006, Adam et al. (21) published a retrospective analysis of hepatic resections performed in more than 1,400 patients with noncolorectal, nonendocrine liver metastases from 41 centers in France. The authors reported an overall 5-year survival of 36%. In addition, they found improved outcomes from some primary sites such as breast, renal, and adrenal malignancies compared with those with primary tumors from upper gastrointestinal cancer or melanoma. Squamous cell histology was associated with poor survival, whereas young age and a prolonged disease-free interval were associated with better survival. Based on these data, liver surgery for noncolorectal, nonendocrine metastases can be considered in highly selected circumstances with a variety of tumor types. Specifically, in cases with favorable biology and in which the metastatic disease is well controlled or responding to systemic therapy, surgical therapy may be able to offer some patients an improvement in long-term survival.

REFERENCES

1. Woodington GF WJ. Results of resection of metastatic tumors of the liver. *Am J Surg.* 1963;105:24-29.
2. Funaioli C, Longobardi C, Martoni AA. The impact of chemotherapy on overall survival and quality of life of patients with metastatic colorectal cancer: a review of phase III trials. *J Chemother.* 2008;20:14–27.
3. Hurwitz H, Fehrenbacher L, Novotny W, et al. Bevacizumab plus irinotecan, fluorouracil, and leucovorin for metastatic colorectal cancer. *N Engl J Med.* 2004;350:2335–2342.
4. Tournigand C, Cervantes A, Figer A, et al. OPTIMOX1: a randomized study of FOLFOX4 or FOLFOX7 with oxaliplatin in a stop-and-Go fashion in advanced colorectal cancer: a GERCOR study. *J Clin Oncol.* 2006;24:394–400.
5. Pawlik TM, Schulick RD, Choti MA. Expanding criteria for resectability of colorectal liver metastases. *Oncologist.* 2008;13:51–64.
6. Pawlik TM, Abdalla EK, Ellis LM, et al. Debunking dogma: surgery for four or more colorectal liver metastases is justified. *J Gastrointest Surg.* 2006;10:240–248.
7. Tomlinson JS, Jarnagin WR, DeMatteo RP, et al. Actual 10-year survival after resection of colorectal liver metastases defines cure. *J Clin Oncol.* 2007;25:4575–4580.
8. Folprecht G, Grothey A, Alberts S, et al. Neoadjuvant treatment of unresectable colorectal liver metastases: correlation between tumour response and resection rates. *Ann Oncol.* 2005;16:1311–1319.
9. Adam R, Avisar E, Ariche A, et al. Five-year survival following hepatic resection after neoadjuvant therapy for nonresectable colorectal. *Ann Surg Oncol.* 2001;8:347–353.
10. Christophi C, Nikfarjam M, Malcontenti-Wilson C, et al. Long-term survival of patients with unresectable colorectal liver metastases treated by percutaneous interstitial laser thermotherapy. *World J Surg.* 2004;28:987–994.
11. Capussotti L, Muratore A, Mulas MM, et al. Neoadjuvant chemotherapy and resection for initially irresectable colorectal liver metastases. *Br J Surg.* 2006;93:1001–1006.
12. Rubbia-Brandt L, Audard V, Sartoretti P, et al. Severe hepatic sinusoidal obstruction associated with oxaliplatin-based chemotherapy in patients with metastatic colorectal cancer. *Ann Oncol.* 2004;15:460–466.
13. Pawlik TM, Olino K, Gleisner AL, et al. Preoperative chemotherapy for colorectal liver metastases: impact on hepatic histology and postoperative outcome. *J Gastrointest Surg.* 2007;11:860–868.
14. Vauthey JN, Pawlik TM, Ribero D, et al. Chemotherapy regimen predicts steatohepatitis and an increase in 90-day mortality after surgery for hepatic colorectal metastases. *J Clin Oncol.* 2006;24:2065–2072.
15. Benoist S, Brouquet A, Penna C, et al. Complete response of colorectal liver metastases after chemotherapy: does it mean cure? *J Clin Oncol.* 2006;24:3939–3945.
16. Ferrero A, Viganò L, Polastri R, et al. Postoperative liver dysfunction and future remnant liver: where is the limit? Results of a prospective study. *World J Surg.* 2007;31:1643–1651.
17. Ribero D, Abdalla EK, Madoff DC, et al. Portal vein embolization before major hepatectomy and its effects on regeneration, resectability and outcome. *Br J Surg.* 2007;94:1386–1394.
18. Adam R, Miller R, Pitombo M, et al. Two-stage hepatectomy approach for initially unresectable colorectal hepatic metastases. *Surg Oncol Clin North Am.* 2007;16:525–536.
19. Chen H, Hardacre JM, Uzar A, et al. Isolated liver metastases from neuroendocrine tumors: does resection prolong survival? *J Am Coll Surg.* 1998;187:88–92.
20. DeMatteo RP, Maki RG, Singer S, et al. Results of tyrosine kinase inhibitor therapy followed by surgical resection for metastatic gastrointestinal stromal tumor. *Ann Surg.* 2007;245:347–352.
21. Adam R, Chiche L, Aloia T, et al; Association Française de Chirurgie. Hepatic resection for noncolorectal nonendocrine liver metastases: analysis of 1,452 patients and development of a prognostic model. *Ann Surg.* 2006;244:524–535.

48

Liver Tumors: Multimodality Treatment of Hepatic Metastases

Liselot B. J. van Iersel, Hans Gelderblom, Johannes W. R. Nortier, and Cornelis J. H. van de Velde

The liver is one of the most common sites for metastatic disease. The liver is involved in approximately 40% of adult patients with primary extrahepatic malignant disease who come to autopsy (1). The most common origin of hepatic metastasis is colorectal cancer. Liver metastases are diagnosed in 10% to 25% of patients at the time of resection of their primary colorectal tumor and eventually up to 70% of patients with colorectal cancer develop liver metastases (2). In approximately 30% of the patients, the liver is the only site of metastatic disease (3,4). Neuroendocrine tumors and uveal melanomas, although rare, are the second most common origin of metastases confined to the liver (5). Gastrointestinal neuroendocrine tumors are predominantly carcinoids (55%), consisting mainly of midgut carcinoids (50% to 70%), which have the greatest potential for metastasizing to the liver. Carcinoid syndrome is characterized by flushing, diarrhea, asthma, and bronchospasms and develops in about 10% of all patients with carcinoid tumors and approximately 50% of patients with hepatic metastases (6,7). Uveal melanoma is the most common primary intraocular tumor in adults, with an incidence of 5 to 7 per 1 million per year in the Western population (8). As many as 50% of patients will ultimately develop metastases, of which more than half are confined to the liver (9,10). Other primary tumors that may initially metastasize to the liver only include gastrointestinal sarcoma and even more rarely, renal cell carcinoma, Wilms tumor, and breast cancer. Although liver metastases from other primary tumors such as cancers of the lung, breast, stomach, and cutaneous melanoma may occur more frequently, dissemination usually occurs simultaneously to other visceral organs.

Treatment directed at both the primary tumor and liver metastasis is thought to improve survival, although randomized studies of local versus systemic therapy in patients with operable liver metastases are lacking. If the metastases are confined to the liver, there are several locoregional treatment options, including partial hepatic resection, local ablative therapy, administration of chemotherapy by hepatic artery infusion (HAI), and isolated hepatic perfusion with high-dose chemotherapy. Curative resection of colorectal and neuroendocrine cancer liver metastases is possible in <10% of patients because of the number, location, or size of the metastases (11,12). After neoadjuvant treatment with modern systemic chemotherapy regimens, another 12% to 14% of colorectal cancer patients with liver metastases are suitable for hepatic resection (13). If patients are ineligible for locoregional treatment, palliative systemic chemotherapy is often the only treatment option for liver metastases. Here we discuss treatment options for liver metastases not amendable to surgical resection.

LOCAL ABLATIVE THERAPY

Several local ablative techniques are available for the treatment of liver metastases. Radiofrequency ablation (RFA) is most often applied. Other therapies include cryotherapy, hepatic artery embolization, percutaneous alcohol injection (PAI), microwave coagulation therapy (MCT), laser-induced thermotherapy (LITT), photodynamic therapy, and radiotherapy. Local ablative therapies provide the possibility of local disease control without systemic toxicity.

Radiofrequency Ablation

The major advantage of RFA is the selective destruction of tumor tissue without significant damage to vascular structures, limiting the loss of large areas of normal liver tissue. In RFA, the needle electrodes deliver a high-frequency alternating current to the tissue, causing hyperthermia of the tissue, resulting in irreversible cellular damage with breakdown of proteins and cell membranes, inducing coagulative necrosis. The RFA electrodes can be either single probes, inducing a cylindrical necrotic lesion, or multitined expandable electrodes that induce spherical lesions. Under optimal conditions current RFA devices can provide spherical lesions of up to 7 cm in diameter (14). During RFA treatment, an adequate necrotic margin surrounding the tumor should be achieved, similar to hepatic resection. To achieve a sufficient margin, especially in tumors over 3 cm in diameter, multiple insertions are often required, emphasizing the critical importance of correct placement of the electrodes. Mulier et al. (15) performed an analysis of several probes, concluding that different probes induced hepatic lesions of varying size and geometry, often with a diameter smaller than suggested. Electrodes are usually placed under ultrasound guidance, either percutaneously, laparoscopically, or in an open procedure. If correct placement of electrodes is hindered (large tumors, compromised electrode accessibility) or when there is an increased risk of complications (tumors close to large vessels, diaphragm, or to adjacent internal organs), an open procedure may be beneficial. The presence of major complications depends on the RFA technique used; abscess formation is reported as the most frequent complication.

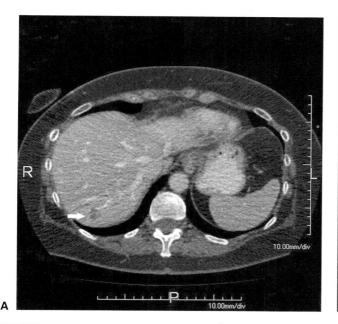
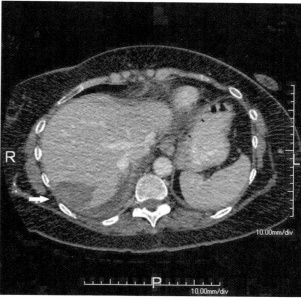

Figure 48.1 Computed tomographic scan of patient before **(A)** and 3 months after **(B)** radiofrequency ablation of a colorectal liver metastasis with a cooled-tip electrode. Note the increase of size of the ablated lesion without evidence of focal enhancement.

Follow-up usually consists of imaging at regular intervals by contrast-enhanced computed tomography (CT) scans or magnetic resonance images, although some centers use positron emission tomography scans. On postoperative CT, liver metastases treated by RFA typically appear larger than the size of the original lesion, which can be falsely interpreted as progression of disease (Figure 48.1). This is the result of inclusion of a rim of normal liver surrounding the lesion (16). Even though the occasional enhancement of the rim may be present, no focal enhancement should be observed along the margin of treatment, as this would indicate incomplete treatment. During follow-up scans the lesion may remain stable or gradually decrease in size.

RFA can be applied in combination with surgical resection if there is bilobar distribution of liver tumors that cannot all be surgically removed, widening the applicability of surgical resection. RFA has also been applied on its own in liver metastases from a diverse origin, but most studies focus around colorectal liver metastases, neuroendocrine tumors, and breast cancer. Results are often difficult to interpret because reports include different tumor types treated with a variety of techniques, and additional treatments such as chemotherapy obscure the primary effect of RFA treatment.

In colorectal cancer liver metastases, RFA has resulted in complete response rates of 52% to 95%. It can offer palliation by prolongation of disease-free and overall survival to, respectively, 50% and 94% at 1 year, with a median survival time of approximately 30 to 34 months after diagnosis of liver metastases. Possibly it can even result in curation, although at present the limited follow-up in most studies does not allow a meaningful determination of survival rates. Local recurrence rates (lesion-based) vary between 2.0% and 39%, depending on which method is applied (17–27). Several studies have shown local recurrence rates

to be less if an open or laparoscopic technique is applied, as compared with the percutaneous method (28,29). Over 90% of the recurrent disease occurs outside the treated area both intra- and extrahepatically, emphasizing the local nature of the treatment. Optimal results in RFA are achieved in an experienced center, using an open technique, on three or less liver metastases, not located near any large vascular structures, and <5 cm in diameter (27,30,31).

Treatment of neuroendocrine liver metastases is directed at the improvement of the disabling hormonal symptoms through reduction of tumor burden. Ideally, tumor load is reduced by hepatic resection, but only <10% of patients are suitable for this procedure (11). Several studies have been reported on the use of RFA for neuroendocrine liver metastases (32–34). In the largest published study, the laparoscopic ablation of 234 hepatic lesions in 34 patients is reported (35). Symptoms were relieved in 95% of the patients, with a significant or complete symptom control in 80% for a mean duration of 10 months. New liver metastases developed in 28% of these patients, new extrahepatic disease in 25%, and local liver recurrence in 13%, at a mean follow-up of 1.6 years. In neuroendocrine cancer patients undergoing RFA, adequate measures should be taken to block hormone secretion, because during RFA the release of hormones can possibly result in systemic complications (36).

Little is known about the results of RFA of liver metastases in breast cancer patients. Metastatic breast cancer is usually considered a disseminated disease that requires systemic, rather than local therapy. Nevertheless in 5% to 12% of breast cancer patients, metastases are confined to the liver and 3-year survival rates after hepatic resection have been reported ranging from 35% to 71% (37–39). Livraghi et al. (40) reported the results of percutaneous RFA in 24 breast cancer patients with no or stable extrahepatic disease. Complete necrosis, as evaluated by spiral

CT, was achieved in 92% of lesions. After a median follow-up of 10 months, 10 of 24 patients were alive and disease-free.

Although hepatic resection still remains the gold standard for local treatment of liver metastases from all primary tumors, RFA can be applied when resection is not possible, because of bilobar distribution or intimate association with major blood vessels, or when the medical condition of the patient or previous hepatic resection inhibits a large open procedure. The possibility of curation and the large percentage of extrahepatic recurrences after RFA have resulted in the common practice of combining systemic treatment with RFA, even though the benefits of combining both treatments have not been thoroughly examined. The true value of RFA remains to be seen; so far there have been no prospective comparisons between RFA and open resection of liver metastases. Currently the only randomized clinical trial comparing RFA plus chemotherapy and chemotherapy alone in colorectal cancer liver metastases is the currently ongoing European Organisation for Research and Treatment of Cancer-Chemotherapy and Local ablation versus Chemotherapy (EORTC-CLOCC) trial (for additional information see www.eortc.org).

Other Ablative Treatment Modalities

In cryoablation, a probe through which liquid nitrogen circulates is inserted in the lesion, repeatedly freezing and thawing the surrounding tumor tissue. The resulting formation of intra- and extracellular ice crystals causes tumor destruction. Cryoablation is most frequently applied in the treatment of hepatocellular carcinoma and to a lesser extent in colorectal cancer liver metastases. In colorectal cancer patients, there is a median survival of around 26 months after cryoablation has been reported. The morbidity rate is considerable, ranging from 10% to 30%, with bleeding of the liver as the most serious complication (41–44). Several studies comparing cryotherapy with RFA have shown high rates of local recurrences and complications after cryoablation (45,46). In addition, RFA probes are of smaller diameters than those used in cryotherapy. Therefore, cryotherapy has been replaced by other ablative treatment modalities in most centers and the use of RFA now greatly exceeds that of cryotherapy.

Hepatic arterial ligation and (chemo)embolization are based on the principle that, in contrast to normal liver parenchyma, established liver metastases derive most of their blood supply from the hepatic artery (47,48). Although ligation and embolization were considered promising treatments at introduction several decades ago, no studies have shown substantial benefit in the treatment of liver metastases (49). Therefore, many centers have abandoned this technique.

PAI is mainly applied in the treatment of hepatocellular carcinoma with tumor response rates up to 80%, but its role in the treatment of liver metastases seems limited (50). During PAI, sterile ethyl alcohol is injected through a needle that is placed in the tumor under ultrasound guidance. The injected alcohol will cause chemical coagulative necrosis, resulting in formation of fibrotic tissue and thrombosis of small intratumoral vessels. A study of 40 patients with liver metastases from various primary tumors including colorectal, breast, and neuroendocrine origin, revealed complete necrosis in 56% on spiral CT of treated tumors and a median overall survival of 21 months (51). As shown by the poor results of PAI in colorectal liver metastases, with no necrosis induced in a series of 22 colorectal tumors, the more solid aspect of colorectal liver metastases can impair the adequate injection of sufficient volumes of alcohol in the tumor (52). Therefore, the use of PAI in the treatment of liver metastases is limited to metastases that can be adequately injected.

MCT and LITT resemble the RFA technique, as they are based on the generation of heat in the tumor and are therefore considered thermal ablation techniques. In MCT heat is generated through a microwave-emitting needle, producing dielectric heat by stimulation of water molecules within cells. The rapid agitation of water molecules produces frictional heating and coagulative necrosis (53). Like RFA and LITT, MCT can be performed percutaneously, laparoscopically, or during an open procedure. The major drawback of MCT is it produces zones of only 10 to 25 mm of coagulative necrosis, requiring multiple needle insertions for adequate treatment. Few studies have been performed using MCT as a treatment modality in liver metastases. In colorectal cancer liver metastases, studies have shown tumor response up to 87% with a mean survival of 27 months, but patient numbers are small (54,55). In LITT heat is not generated by high-frequency current but by a laser applicator that delivers light energy through optical fibers inserted in the target tissue. The resulting coagulative necrosis leads to tumor destruction (53). Mack et al. (56,57) and Vogl et al. (58) reported the largest series of 705 patients, including 57% colorectal cancer patients, 18% breast cancer patients, 5% hepatocellular carcinoma patients, and 20% other patients. The rate of clinically relevant complications such as pleural effusion, intrahepatic abscess and intra-abdominal bleeding was 1.3%. The tumor response rate was 99.3% after 3 months, with a mean survival rate in colorectal cancer and breast cancer patients of 41.8 and 51.6 months, respectively.

Similar to LITT, PDT makes use of optical fibers and laser light, but the antitumor effect is not based on generation of heat but of reactive oxygen species. In PDT, a photosensitizing agent is administered systemically and will, with varying specificity, localize in tumor tissue (59,60). On illumination of the tumor by light of an appropriate wavelength, the photosensitizer is excited by photons to an unstable higher energy level. Once the photosensitizer returns to its ground state energy level, the absorbed energy is transformed to oxygen, leading to the formation of reactive oxygen species, which are cytotoxic and cause direct tumor cell and vascular damage, resulting in both apoptosis and necrosis (61). PDT has been successfully applied in a rat model for liver metastases (62,63). Results of a phase 1 trial in 24 patients show PDT to be safe, feasible, and effective in treatment of colorectal liver metastases (64).

Application of external radiotherapy for the treatment of liver metastases has been limited by low tolerance of the normal liver parenchyma and absence of an obvious survival benefit in studies involving whole-liver irradiation (65). Recently two alternative techniques to deliver radiation more selectively have been developed involving radioactive isotopes, that is, SIR-spheres and three-dimensional planning software (Sirtex Medical, Ltd., North Ryde, Australia). In selective internal radiation therapy, radioactive spheres are delivered selectively to the tumor through injection in the hepatic artery. Gray et al. (66) performed a randomized clinical trial in 74 colorectal cancer patients comparing a single administration of SIR-spheres combined with HAI of fluorodeoxyuridine (FUDR) with HAI of

FUDR alone. Treatment with SIR-spheres was associated with a significantly better response rate (44% vs. 17.6%; $p = 0.01$) and median time to progression (15.9 vs. 9.7 months; $p = 0.001$). Grade 3-4 treatment related toxicity was similar for both groups. In stereotactic radiotherapy, improvements in positioning and three-dimensional planning software have enabled treatment of a specific focus in the liver with a single high dose of radiotherapy with minimal damage to healthy liver tissue (53,67). A phase 1/2 trial in 60 liver tumors show the technique is safe and local tumor control was achieved in 98% of tumors (68).

CHEMOTHERAPY

Systemic Chemotherapy

For most patients with extrahepatic metastases, systemically administered chemotherapy is the only treatment option. The effect of systemic treatment depends on the origin of the primary tumor; ideally, palliation and/or survival benefit is achieved. Other determinants of the effect of systemic treatment include age, performance status, and extent of the disease. Possible benefits need to be weighed against toxicity profiles of the respective agents. A specific challenge in metastatic cancer patients with hepatic metastases is liver dysfunction, especially as most chemotherapeutics have a substantial hepatic metabolism.

Until recently, the standard first-line treatment for metastatic colorectal cancer consisted of 5-fluorouracil (5-FU)-based schedules, resulting in response rates around 15%, median time to progression of 5 months, and overall survival of 12 months (69). In the past decade several new agents have become available, including oxaliplatin, irinotecan, and the monoclonal antibodies bevacizumab and cetuximab. Irinotecan combined with 5-FU/leucovorin has shown an increase in terms of progression-free survival, survival, and quality of life compared with 5-FU/leucovorin alone in both first- and second-line therapy (70–73). The combination of oxaliplatin with 5-FU/leucovorin also showed an improved response rate, increase in progression-free survival, and overall survival in first- and second-line therapy (74–76). Already the first large trials have been reported treating patients with combinations of the regimens described here. Tournigand et al. (77) conducted a phase 3 crossover study of first-line chemotherapy with 5-FU/leucovorin with oxaliplatin in one arm and 5-FU/leucovorin with irinotecan in the other arm, resulting in maximum medium survival of 21.5 months. Even more recently Koopman et al. showed that both combination treatment and sequential treatment with capecitabine, irinotecan, and oxaliplatin yields similar results (78). The introduction of bevacizumab, a monoclonal antibody directed against vascular endothelial growth factor (VEGF), has further improved treatment options in metastatic colorectal cancer. Hurwitz et al. reported that the addition of bevacizumab to bolus irinotecan and 5-FU/leucovorin as a first-line treatment resulted in increased survival, response rate, and duration of response (79). Similarly, panitumumab/cetuximab, monoclonal antibodies against epidermal growth factor receptor (EGRF), have further improved survival in combination with either irinotecan or oxaliplatin, especially in patients without K-ras mutation (80,81). Now oncologists are faced with the challenge of choosing the optimal treatment schedule for advanced colorectal cancer for each individual patient. Currently,

the combination of fluoropyrimidine-based chemotherapy with oxaliplatin and bevacizumab is considered standard first-line treatment in metastatic colorectal cancer. The addition of panitumumab of cetuximab to a schedule with bevacizumab increases toxicity without improving survival and thus should be reserved for second-line treatment (82,83).

The presence of liver metastasis in advanced breast cancer is considered an ominous sign. Most patients with liver metastases have extrahepatic disease as well, leaving systemic treatment as the only available treatment option. Breast cancer liver metastases tend to be negative for hormone receptors, limiting the use of hormonal therapy (80). Initially most patients received either cyclophosphamide, 5-FU, methotrexate, or anthracycline combinations as first-line therapy, with response rates around 35% (81). Today both taxanes and fluoropyrimidines are added as second- or even third-line treatment. In HER2-overexpressing breast cancer patients, trastuzumab, a HER2-targeted monoclonal antibody, can be considered as first-line therapy. Response rates between 50% to 80% have been reported in combination with either paclitaxel, docetaxel or vinorelbine (82–86).

In neuroendocrine cancer metastases, results of systemically administered agents have been disappointing with response rates around 30% to 40% for cytostatic drugs and 11% for interferon-α (87–89). Symptomatic relief can be achieved through somatostatin analogs such as octreotide. Symptomatic improvement occurs in up to 70% of patients, but objective tumor response is <10% and drug resistance can develop in 3 to 12 months (90–93). Recently, attention has shifted to the development of radiolabeled somatostatin analogs. Valkema et al. (94) reported the response after peptide receptor radionuclide therapy with [^{90}Y-DOTA^0, Tyr^3] octreotide in 56 patients with advanced neuroendocrine tumors. Overall, 58% of patients experienced improvement of symptoms, and the median progression-free survival was 29 months with a median overall survival of nearly 37 months.

No standard systemic agent is available for the treatment of metastatic uveal melanoma. Several studies have reported response rates of <1% to 10% to conventional systemic chemotherapy (95,96). Results with immunotherapy, for example, interferon-α and interleukin-2, are equally disappointing with no or only minor responses (97,98). Currently, regional treatment options offer the best disease control in metastatic uveal melanoma.

Regional Chemotherapy

HAI is a therapeutic option for patients with isolated liver metastases who are not suitable for surgical resection or local ablation. Similar to hepatic arterial ligation and embolization, HAI of chemotherapy is based on the principle that, in contrast to normal liver parenchyma, liver metastases derive most of their blood supply from the hepatic artery (47,48). As a result, high drug concentrations can be achieved at the tumor site while the liver parenchyma is relatively spared. HAI has mainly been applied in colorectal cancer liver metastases and hepatocellular carcinoma, although there have been some reports of HAI in breast cancer and melanoma patients (99–102). Early infusion trials administered chemotherapy using percutaneously placed catheters, requiring bed rest and hospitalization during infusion of the chemotherapy. When a totally implantable pump was introduced, HAI chemotherapy changed into a more convenient ambulatory treatment. All techniques require an angiogram to assess vascular anatomy before catheter placement. Most studies show around 20% to 40% of patients cannot receive infusion treatment because of abnormal vasculature inhibiting perfusion of the entire liver (103–105). Catheters and pumps can be placed through laparotomy or laparoscopy. Laparotomy enables assessment of extrahepatic metastases and ligation of arterial collaterals to decrease incidence of extrahepatic perfusion and chemical gastritis or duodenitis (106,107). Complications associated with catheter placement include death, hepatic misperfusion, catheter obstruction, and hepatic artery thrombosis, with complications rates being less for implantable pumps as compared with ports (106,108,109).

FUDR and 5-FU are the drugs most often used for HAI. An ideal drug for HAI has to fulfill several criteria including a steep dose-response curve, high total-body clearance, and minimal liver toxicity. Both FUDR and 5-FU have a steep dose-response curve, but FUDR has a higher hepatic extraction rate when continuously infused (95% for FUDR vs. 19% to 90% for 5-FU) (110). Although higher hepatic extraction rates lead to increased regional drug exposure, it also implies limited systemic exposure. Considering approximately 50% of patients treated with HAI have extrahepatic disease progression, some centers prefer HAI with 5-FU to obtain both local and systemic disease control (111). Treatment-related toxicities include chemical hepatitis, biliary sclerosis, and peptic ulceration. Kemeny et al. (112) reported an increase in response and survival rate and a decrease in hepatotoxicity if dexamethasone is added to FUDR. Several randomized studies involving HAI with FUDR or 5-FU in colorectal cancer patients have reported significantly higher tumor response rates compared with systemic administration (HAI, 41%; systemic, 14%; $p <0.0001$) (103,104,113). In 1996, two meta-analysis combining the results of ten randomized trials appeared, comparing HAI with either systemic treatment or best supportive care (111,114). The Meta-Analysis Group in Cancer studied seven randomized trials and, when combining the results of the five trials comparing HAI with systemic treatment, concluded that although HAI showed superior response rates compared with systemic treatment (41% vs. 14%) there was no significant survival benefit and treatment-related hepatotoxicity was considerable. Harmantas et al. (114) studied six randomized trials and reported a modest survival benefit for HAI over systemic treatment. These studies have two major drawbacks. First, in three of the analyzed randomized trials, patients were allowed to cross over from systemic treatment to HAI, possibly obscuring any survival benefit. Second, the drug doses and schedules varied substantially between HAI and systemic treatment groups. A recent randomized study in which 290 colorectal cancer patients were included also did not show significant differences in tumor response, progression-free survival, and overall survival between patients who had received 5-FU/leucovorin either systemically or by HAI, while the HAI group reported a worse quality of life compared with the systemically treated group (115). On the other hand, Kemeny et al. (116) published the results of a trial in 135 colorectal cancer patients and reported a significant survival benefit (median overall survival 24.4 vs. 20 months; $p = 0.0034$) and increased physical functioning in patients receiving HAI compared with systemic treatment.

Recently, several new drugs (e.g., oxaliplatin and irinotecan) have been safely introduced in HAI (117–122). Results of a phase 1/2 study on biweekly HAI with oxaliplatin combined with systemic 5-FU en leucovorin according to the de Gramont schedule were recently reported by Ducreux et al. (123). A total of 28 previously untreated patients with colorectal cancer with isolated liver metastases were treated with this schedule; the objective response rate was 64% and the median overall survival was 27 months. Grade 3 or 4 neutropenia occurred in ten patients and there were two treatment-related deaths.

Results of HAI in liver metastases from origin other than colorectal are scarce. There have been several, mainly Japanese, case reports of successful HAI in breast cancer patients (124–126). Peters et al. (127) reported the use of HAI with fotemustine, an alkylating agent, in 101 uveal melanoma patients with liver metastases. Fotemustine was infused in the hepatic artery for a 4-week induction period and then as a maintenance treatment every 3 weeks until disease progression. A median of eight infusions per patient were delivered. Catheter-related complications occurred in 23% of patients. The overall response rate was 36%, with a median overall survival of 15 months and a 2-year survival rate of 29%.

Theoretically, HAI of chemotherapy can offer several advantages, but its role in the treatment of liver metastases is still unclear. Compared with local ablative treatments, HAI of chemotherapy can offer the additional benefit of both local and systemic disease control. Although multiple trials have been conducted in colorectal cancer patients, results in liver metastases other than colorectal cancer liver metastases are too limited to draw any conclusions. In colorectal cancer liver metastases, meta-analysis and recent randomized trials show conflicting results, but most trial designs did not allow for correct comparison of both treatment groups. Moreover, recent developments in new systemic drugs like oxaliplatin, irinotecan, and bevacizumab have improved results substantially in the systemic treatment over liver metastases. Whether these agents have a role in HAI remains to be investigated.

Isolated Hepatic Perfusion

Isolated hepatic perfusion (IHP) involves complete vascular isolation of the liver to allow local treatment of the liver. During this procedure the blood circulation of the liver is temporarily isolated from the systemic circulation. Inflow catheters are inserted in the common hepatic artery and the portal vein, and an outflow catheter in the infrahepatic caval vein, while the suprahepatic caval vein is occluded by a surgical clamp (Figure 48.2). Subsequently, the catheters are connected to heart-lung machine and the anticancer drug is administered in this isolated circuit. Leakage to the systemic circulation is monitored in order to prevent inadvertently high systemic exposure. After perfusion of the liver with the drug for a certain period (1 hour in most IHP trials), the liver is flushed with clean perfusate to wash out the anticancer drug, after which the natural blood circulation is restored (128).

The major advantage of IHP is the ability to treat the liver with drug levels that would be toxic when administered systemically; doses of anticancer drugs up to fourfold the maximum systemically tolerated dose have been administered (128). Furthermore, agents that cannot be administered systemically

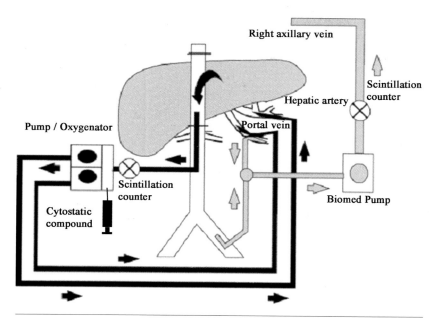

Figure 48.2 Isolated hepatic perfusion circuit with extracorporeal venovenous bypass.

because of their toxicity, such as tumor necrosis factor-alpha (TNF-α), can be used in IHP (129,130). Finally, hyperthermia can be applied by heating the perfusate solution, which is known to enhance antitumor efficacy of several anticancer drugs (131).

IHP is a treatment option in patients with isolated liver metastases not amendable to surgical resection or local ablation. Although most experience has been obtained with colorectal liver metastases, several studies have reported the treatment of uveal melanoma and neuroendocrine cancer liver metastases (129,130,132–136).

Various drugs have been used in IHP studies, including 5-FU, mitomycin C, cisplatin, and melphalan with or without TNF-α (Table 48.1). In most studies, mild hyperthermia up to 40°C is applied during IHP; hyperthermia alone (42°C to 42.5°C) has been applied in only one study. Recent clinical studies have mainly employed IHP with melphalan. Melphalan is an alkylating agent with a steep dose-response curve that is effective against colorectal cancer after relatively short exposure time, and is therefore a very interesting drug for IHP. In most centers granulocyte colony-stimulating factor is administered as a preventive measure because of minimal leakage in nearly all perfusions.

Two large trials have been reported in colorectal cancer patients. Bartlett et al. (136) have reported IHP in 51 patients with different treatment schedules, including IHP with high doses of melphalan alone and moderately high doses of melphalan combined with TNF-α or followed by monthly hepatic intra-arterial infusion of FUDR and leucovorin. Results of these studies show response rates up to 74%, a median time to progression up to 14.5 months, and a median survival of 27 months. Rothbarth et al. (135) performed a phase 1/2 trial in 73 colorectal cancer patients with high-dose melphalan, achieving an overall response rate of 59%, median time to progression of 7.7 months, and a median overall survival of 28.8 months. In uveal melanoma patients, IHP has resulted in response rates of 50% to 62%, with a median overall survival of 9.9 to 12 months (129,132,134). Although overall survival is limited as compared with IHP in

colorectal cancer patients, it is considerable compared with a median survival of 2 to 8 months in uveal melanoma patients without treatment (137,138). Grover et al. (133) reported the experience with IHP in 13 neuroendocrine cancer patients with a overall response rate of 50% and median progression-free survival of 7 months. The nature and incidence of major complications was similar in all trials independent of primary origin of liver metastases. Mortality rate varied between 2% and 5% and major complications consisted of bleeding and hepatoxicity, including veno-occlusive disease.

The current IHP technique is an expensive, demanding, and technically difficult procedure with considerable morbidity and mortality, which is not suitable for repetition. In a select group of patients who had a long disease-free interval after the first treatment episode, repetitive treatment with IHP might be beneficial. There have been several attempts to develop minimally invasive procedures for high-dose drug administration. Clinical and experimental studies have been described involving chemofiltration under complete hepatic venous isolation after HAI of drugs, allowing administration of high doses of intrahepatic chemotherapy with either 5-FU or doxorubicin (139–141). In this technique, the liver is partially cut off from the systemic circulation by occluding the inferior caval vein above and below the hepatic veins using a four-lumen/two-balloon catheter, which collects the blood from the hepatic veins. After the drug is infused in the hepatic artery, the hepatic venous blood is bypassed to a charcoal hemoperfusion filter for extracorporeal drug elimination before it returns to the patient's systemic circulation. Recently, Pingpank et al. (142) reported a phase 1 study using the technique previously described. This study demonstrated that treatment with high-dose melphalan is feasible, but complete extraction of melphalan by charcoal hemoperfusion is not possible, limiting the maximum tolerated dose.

Complete isolation of the liver using minimally invasive techniques is still experimental. Although animal studies show the technique to be technically feasible, recently performed

Table 48.1

Isolated Hepatic Perfusion Studies

Study (Ref.)	Year	No. of Patients	Primary Tumor	Treatment	Drug Dose
Aigner et al. (152)	1984	32	Colorectal carcinoma (29), miscellaneous (3)	5-Fluorouacil	750–1250 mg
Skibba et al. (153)	1986	8	Colorectal carcinoma (5), melanoma (2), miscellaneous (1)	Hyperthermia 42°C–42°C without drug	—
Schwemmle et al. (154)[a]	1987	50	Colorectal carcinoma (45), miscellaneous (4), falsely diagnosed (1)	5-Fluorouacil (47) Mitomycin C (17) Cisplatin (4)	300–1250 mg 5–50 mg 50 mg
Hafström et al. (155)	1994	29	Colorectal carcinoma (4), melanoma (10), miscellaneous (15)	Melphalan (29) Cisplatin (20)	0.5 mg/kg 0.2–0.7 mg/kg
Marinelli et al. (156)	1996	9	Colorectal carcinoma	Mitomycin C	30 mg/m^2
De Vries et al. (157)	1998	9	Colorectal carcinoma	Melphalan (9) TNF-α (9)	1 mg/kg 0.4–0.8 mg
Alexander et al. (130)	1998	34	Colorectal carcinoma (26), ocular melanoma (4), miscellaneous (4)	Melphalan (34) TNF-α (34)	1.5 mg/kg 1.0 mg
Oldhafer et al. (158)	1998	12	Colorectal carcinoma (6), ocular melanoma (2), miscellaneous (4)	Melphalan (6), TNF-α (6) Mitomycin C (6)	60–140 mg 200–300 mcg 20–50 mg
Lindner et al. (159)	1999	11	Colorectal carcinoma (5) Ocular melanoma (2) Miscellaneous (4)	Melphalan (11) TNF-α (11)	0.5 mg/kg 30–200 mcg
Vahrmeijer et al. (128)	2000	24	Colorectal carcinoma	Melphalan	0.5–4.0 mg/kg
Alexander et al. (129)	2000	22	Ocular melanoma	Melphalan (22) TNF-α (11)	1.5–2.5 mg/kg 1.0 mg
Bartlett et al. (136)[b]	2001	51	Colorectal carcinoma	Melphalan (51) TNF-α (32)	1.5 mg/kg 1.0 mg
Rothbarth et al. (135)	2003	73	Colorectal carcinoma	Melphalan	200 mg
Alexander et al. (132)[c]	2003	29	Ocular melanoma	Melphalan	1.5 mg/kg
Noter et al. (134)	2004	8	Ocular melanoma	Melphalan	200 mg
Alexander et al. (160)[d]	2005	25	Colorectal carcinoma	Melphalan	1.5 mg/kg

TNF-α, tumor necrosis factor-alpha

[a] Overlapping patient groups, also reported by Aigner et al. (152).

[b] Sixteen patients previously included in the study of Alexander et al. (130).

[c] Overlapping patient groups, also reported by Alexander et al. (129).

[d] Overlapping patient groups, also reported by Alexander et al. (130) and Bartlett et al. (136).

phase 1 trials have disappointing results (143). Savier et al. (144) reported treatment of four patients with three successive courses of chemotherapy by IHP, in which the first course was given at laparotomy and the next two courses percutaneously. Percutaneous isolation of the liver was achieved by placing an occlusion catheter in the portal vein according to the transhepatic Seldinger technique and a double-balloon catheter in retrohepatic caval vein through the saphenous vein; finally, the hepatic artery was occluded by traction of a silicon-lined nylon thread that was positioned around the common hepatic artery during previous laparotomy. Melphalan (15 to 45 mg) was administered through a catheter in the gastroduodenal artery, which had also been inserted during the previous laparotomy. Although isolated perfusion was achieved by this method, considerable leakage to the systemic circulation occurred during IHP. The resulting systemic toxicity was acceptable and did not result in mortality in this study, but this would probably not be the case in the current clinical IHP programs in which up to 6 times higher melphalan doses are administered. van Etten et al. (145) reported a phase 1/2 study in 18 patients using two techniques. In the first eight patients the portal vein was occluded and outflow was via the hepatic veins into an intracaval double-balloon catheter, resulting in on average 56% leakage. In the next ten patients, retrograde outflow perfusion, with a triple balloon blocking outflow into the caval vein and allowing outflow via the portal vein was performed. Although this resulted in less leakage, retrograde perfusion still had an average 35% leakage.

Melphalan has been the only agent applied in major clinical trials over the past 10 years. Over the past few years, new agents such as irinotecan, oxaliplatin, and bevacizumab have been introduced in the systemic treatment of colorectal metastases, increasing response rates, disease-free survival, and overall survival (77,79,146,147). Ideally, some of the development in the systemic treatment of colorectal cancer metastases can be incorporated in IHP. For successful application in IHP, a drug has to fulfill several conditions. First, as IHP is a regional treatment, the drug should be a direct working agent or can be transformed to its active agent in the liver. Second, increased concentrations of the drug should lead to an increased response. Third, as IHP is a short treatment the drug should cause rapid irreversible tumor cell cytotoxicity. Finally, liver toxicity should be minimal. Irinotecan may not be applicable in IHP as it is not a direct agent and the bioactivation to its active metabolite is slow (148). The monoclonal antibody bevacizumab may not be suitable, considering it is not directly cytotoxic and has been shown to impair wound healing (149). Oxaliplatin is rapidly absorbed and transformed by nonenzymatic pathways to its biologically active species, and substantial dose-dependent DNA adduct formation occurs within 1 hour (150,151). In studies in which oxaliplatin is administered systemically, neurotoxicity, hematologic toxicity, and nephrotoxicity are dose-limiting, while hepatoxicity is rarely mentioned. Possibly, the introduction of one of the agents described here can lead to increased response and survival rates in isolated hepatic perfusion.

Despite encouraging results in recent trials, IHP should still be considered an experimental treatment. No prospective trials have been reported comparing IHP with either systemic treatment or local ablative treatment, and little is known about the role of adjuvant systemic treatment. Whether IHP will eventually become a standard treatment option is highly dependent on the introduction of new drugs in order to further increase effectiveness, as recently shown for systemic treatment, and the development of minimally invasive techniques allowing repetitive treatment.

SUMMARY

The treatment of liver metastases poses a difficult challenge for most physicians. Considering the associated morbidity and mortality, aggressive local treatment is warranted. Although studies comparing systemic treatment with resection are lacking, resection remains the preferred treatment of choice, but if resection is not possible because of size, location, multifocality of lesions, or limited hepatic reserve, regional treatment can be considered. In patients with a limited number of metastases in the liver, RFA should be the only first treatment of choice because of superior experience and results, as compared with other local ablative treatments and regional chemotherapy. In metastatic chemosensitive tumors, for example, colorectal and breast cancer, local treatment should be considered in combination with systemic

treatment because of a high number of extrahepatic recurrences. If local ablation is impossible and patients can tolerate surgery, HAI or isolated hepatic perfusion can be considered. IHP offers the advantage of high local drug exposure, which may offer increased local and systemic disease control if combined with systemic treatment. For patients who have both hepatic and extrahepatic metastases, systemic treatment is indicated.

REFERENCES

1. Johnson PJ. The clinical features and natural history of malignant liver tumours. *Baillieres Clin Gastroenterol*. 1987;1:17–34.
2. Jessup JM, McGinnis LS, Steele GD Jr., et al. The National Cancer Data Base. Report on colon cancer. *Cancer*. 1996;78:918–926.
3. Weiss L, Grundmann E, Torhorst J, et al. Haematogenous metastatic patterns in colonic carcinoma: an analysis of 1541 necropsies. *J Pathol*. 1986;150:195–203.
4. Welch JP, Donaldson GA. The clinical correlation of an autopsy study of recurrent colorectal cancer. *Ann Surg*. 1979;189:496–502.
5. Sutcliffe R, Maguire D, Ramage J, et al. Management of neuroendocrine liver metastases. *Am J Surg*. 2004;187:39–46.
6. Shebani KO, Souba WW, Finkelstein DM, et al. Prognosis and survival in patients with gastrointestinal tract carcinoid tumors. *Ann Surg*. 1999;229:815–821.
7. Moertel CG, Sauer WG, Dockerty MB, et al. Life history of the carcinoid tumor of the small intestine. *Cancer*. 1961;14:901–912.
8. Egan KM, Seddon JM, Glynn RJ, et al. Epidemiologic aspects of uveal melanoma. *Surv Ophthalmol*. 1988;32:239–251.
9. Folberg R. Tumor progression in ocular melanomas. *J Invest Dermatol*. 1993;100:326S–331S.
10. Assessment of metastatic disease status at death in 435 patients with large choroidal melanoma in the Collaborative Ocular Melanoma Study (COMS): COMS report no. 15. *Arch Ophthalmol*. 2001;119:670–676.
11. Ihse I, Persson B, Tibblin S. Neuroendocrine metastases of the liver. *World J Surg*. 1995;19:76–82.
12. Scheele J, Stang R, Altendorf-Hofmann A, et al. Resection of colorectal liver metastases. *World J Surg*. 1995;19:59–71.
13. Bismuth H, Adam R, Levi F, et al. Resection of nonresectable liver metastases from colorectal cancer after neoadjuvant chemotherapy. *Ann Surg*. 1996;224:509–520.
14. Feliberti EC, Wagman LD. Radiofrequency ablation of liver metastases from colorectal carcinoma. *Cancer Control*. 2006;13:48–51.
15. Mulier S, Miao Y, Mulier P, et al. Electrodes and multiple electrode systems for radiofrequency ablation: a proposal for updated terminology. *Eur Radiol*. 2005;15:798–808.
16. Goldberg SN, Gazelle GS, Compton CC, et al. Treatment of intrahepatic malignancy with radiofrequency ablation: radiologic-pathologic correlation. *Cancer*. 2000;88:2452–2463.
17. Bilchik AJ, Rose DM, Allegra DP, et al. Radiofrequency ablation: a minimally invasive technique with multiple applications. *Cancer J Sci Am*. 1999;5:356–361.
18. Jiao LR, Hansen PD, Havlik R, et al. Clinical short-term results of radiofrequency ablation in primary and secondary liver tumors. *Am J Surg*. 1999;177:303–306.
19. Oshowo A, Gillams A, Harrison E, et al. Comparison of resection and radiofrequency ablation for treatment of solitary colorectal liver metastases. *Br J Surg*. 2003;90:1240–1243.
20. Parikh AA, Curley SA, Fornage BD, et al. Radiofrequency ablation of hepatic metastases. *Semin Oncol*. 2002;29:168–182.
21. Scaife CL, Curley SA. Complication, local recurrence, and survival rates after radiofrequency ablation for hepatic malignancies. *Surg Oncol Clin North Am*. 2003;12:243–255.

22. Wood TF, Rose DM, Chung M, et al. Radiofrequency ablation of 231 unresectable hepatic tumors: indications, limitations, and complications. *Ann Surg Oncol.* 2000;7:593–600.

23. Curley SA, Izzo F, Delrio P, et al. Radiofrequency ablation of unresectable primary and metastatic hepatic malignancies: results in 123 patients. *Ann Surg.* 1999;230:1–8.

24. Bilchik AJ, Wood TF, Allegra D, et al. Cryosurgical ablation and radiofrequency ablation for unresectable hepatic malignant neoplasms: a proposed algorithm. *Arch Surg.* 2000;135:657–662.

25. Bleicher RJ, Allegra DP, Nora DT, et al. Radiofrequency ablation in 447 complex unresectable liver tumors: lessons learned. *Ann Surg Oncol.* 2003;10:52–58.

26. de Baere T, Elias D, Dromain C, et al. Radiofrequency ablation of 100 hepatic metastases with a mean follow-up of more than 1 year. *AJR Am J Roentgenol.* 2000;175:1619–1625.

27. Solbiati L, Livraghi T, Goldberg SN, et al. Percutaneous radiofrequency ablation of hepatic metastases from colorectal cancer: long-term results in 117 patients. *Radiology.* 2001;221:159–166.

28. Mulier S, Ni Y, Jamart J, et al. Local recurrence after hepatic radiofrequency coagulation: multivariate meta-analysis and review of contributing factors. *Ann Surg.* 2005;242:158–171.

29. Kuvshinoff BW, Ota DM. Radiofrequency ablation of liver tumors: influence of technique and tumor size. *Surgery.* 2002;132:605–611.

30. Berber E, Pelley R, Siperstein AE. Predictors of survival after radiofrequency thermal ablation of colorectal cancer metastases to the liver: a prospective study. *J Clin Oncol.* 2005;23:1358–1364.

31. Sutherland LM, Williams JA, Padbury RT, et al. Radiofrequency ablation of liver tumors: a systematic review. *Arch Surg.* 2006;141:181–190.

32. Hellman P, Ladjevardi S, Skogseid B, et al. Radiofrequency tissue ablation using cooled tip for liver metastases of endocrine tumors. *World J Surg.* 2002;26:1052–1056.

33. Henn AR, Levine EA, McNulty W, et al. Percutaneous radiofrequency ablation of hepatic metastases for symptomatic relief of neuroendocrine syndromes. *AJR Am J Roentgenol.* 2003;181:1005–1010.

34. Wessels FJ, Schell SR. Radiofrequency ablation treatment of refractory carcinoid hepatic metastases. *J Surg Res.* 2001;95:8–12.

35. Berber E, Flesher N, Siperstein AE. Laparoscopic radiofrequency ablation of neuroendocrine liver metastases. *World J Surg.* 2002;26:985–990.

36. Wettstein M, Vogt C, Cohnen M, et al. Serotonin release during percutaneous radiofrequency ablation in a patient with symptomatic liver metastases of a neuroendocrine tumor. *Hepatogastroenterology.* 2004;51:830–832.

37. Zinser JW, Hortobagyi GN, Buzdar AU, et al. Clinical course of breast cancer patients with liver metastases. *J Clin Oncol.* 1987;5:773–782.

38. Gillams AR. The use of radiofrequency in cancer. *Br J Cancer.* 2005;92:1825–1829.

39. Hoe AL, Royle GT, Taylor I. Breast liver metastases–incidence, diagnosis and outcome. *J R Soc Med.* 1991;84:714–716.

40. Livraghi T, Goldberg SN, Solbiati L, et al. Percutaneous radiofrequency ablation of liver metastases from breast cancer: initial experience in 24 patients. *Radiology.* 2001;220:145–149.

41. Neeleman N, Wobbes T, Jager GJ, et al. Cryosurgery as treatment modality for colorectal liver metastases. *Hepatogastroenterology.* 2001;48:325–329.

42. Ruers TJ, Joosten J, Jager GJ, et al. Long-term results of treating hepatic colorectal metastases with cryosurgery. *Br J Surg.* 2001;88:844–849.

43. Sheen AJ, Poston GJ, Sherlock DJ. Cryotherapeutic ablation of liver tumours. *Br J Surg.* 2002;89:1396–1401.

44. Sotsky TK, Ravikumar TS. Cryotherapy in the treatment of liver metastases from colorectal cancer. *Semin Oncol.* 2002;29:183–191.

45. Adam R, Hagopian EJ, Linhares M, et al. A comparison of percutaneous cryosurgery and percutaneous radiofrequency for unresectable hepatic malignancies. *Arch Surg.* 2002;137:1332–1339.

46. Tait IS, Yong SM, Cuschieri SA. Laparoscopic in situ ablation of liver cancer with cryotherapy and radiofrequency ablation. *Br J Surg.* 2002;89:1613–1619.

47. Sigurdson ER, Ridge JA, Kemeny N, et al. Tumor and liver drug uptake following hepatic artery and portal vein infusion. *J Clin Oncol.* 1987;5:1836–1840.

48. Wang LQ, Persson BG, Stenram U, et al. Influence of portal branch ligation on the outcome of repeat dearterializations of an experimental liver tumor in the rat. *J Surg Oncol.* 1994;55:229–234.

49. Hunt TM, Flowerdew AD, Birch SJ, et al. Prospective randomized controlled trial of hepatic arterial embolization or infusion chemotherapy with 5-fluorouracil and degradable starch microspheres for colorectal liver metastases. *Br J Surg.* 1990;77:779–782.

50. Livraghi T, Giorgio A, Marin G, et al. Hepatocellular carcinoma and cirrhosis in 746 patients: long-term results of percutaneous ethanol injection. *Radiology.* 1995;197:101–108.

51. Giovannini M, Seitz JF. Ultrasound-guided percutaneous alcohol injection of small liver metastases. Results in 40 patients. *Cancer.* 1994;73:294–297.

52. Amin Z, Bown SG, Lees WR. Local treatment of colorectal liver metastases: a comparison of interstitial laser photocoagulation (ILP) and percutaneous alcohol injection (PAI). *Clin Radiol.* 1993;48:166–171.

53. Izzo F. Other thermal ablation techniques: microwave and interstitial laser ablation of liver tumors. *Ann Surg Oncol.* 2003;10:491–497.

54. Shibata T, Niinobu T, Ogata N, et al. Microwave coagulation therapy for multiple hepatic metastases from colorectal carcinoma. *Cancer.* 2000;89:276–284.

55. Seki T, Wakabayashi M, Nakagawa T, et al. Percutaneous microwave coagulation therapy for solitary metastatic liver tumors from colorectal cancer: a pilot clinical study. *Am J Gastroenterol.* 1999;94:322–327.

56. Mack MG, Straub R, Eichler K, et al. Percutaneous MR imaging-guided laser-induced thermotherapy of hepatic metastases. *Abdom Imaging.* 2001;26:369–374.

57. Mack MG, Straub R, Eichler K, et al. Breast cancer metastases in liver: laser-induced interstitial thermotherapy–local tumor control rate and survival data. *Radiology.* 2004;233:400–409.

58. Vogl TJ, Straub R, Eichler K, et al. Colorectal carcinoma metastases in liver: laser-induced interstitial thermotherapy–local tumor control rate and survival data. *Radiology.* 2004;230:450–458.

59. Boyle RW, Dolphin D. Structure and biodistribution relationships of photodynamic sensitizers. *Photochem Photobiol.* 1996;64:469–485.

60. Bugelski PJ, Porter CW, Dougherty TJ. Autoradiographic distribution of hematoporphyrin derivative in normal and tumor tissue of the mouse. *Cancer Res.* 1981;41:4606–4612.

61. Fingar VH. Vascular effects of photodynamic therapy. *J Clin Laser Med Surg.* 1996;14:323–328.

62. Rovers JP, Schuitmaker JJ, Vahrmeijer AL, et al. Interstitial photodynamic therapy with the second-generation photosensitizer bacteriochlorin a in a rat model for liver metastases. *Br J Cancer.* 1998;77:2098–2103.

63. Rovers JP, Saarnak AE, Molina A, et al. Effective treatment of liver metastases with photodynamic therapy, using the second-generation photosensitizer meta-tetra(hydroxyphenyl)chlorin (mTHPC), in a rat model. *Br J Cancer.* 1999;81:600–608.

64. van Duijnhoven FH, Rovers JP, Engelmann K, et al. Photodynamic therapy with 5,10,15,20-tetrakis(m-hydroxyphenyl) bacteriochlorin for colorectal liver metastases is safe and feasible: results from a phase I study. *Ann Surg Oncol.* 2005;12:808–816.

65. Russell AH, Clyde C, Wasserman TH, et al. Accelerated hyperfractionated hepatic irradiation in the management of patients with liver metastases: results of the RTOG dose escalating protocol. *Int J Radiat Oncol Biol Phys.* 1993;27:117–123.

66. Gray B, Van Hazel G, Hope M, et al. Randomised trial of SIR-Spheres plus chemotherapy vs. chemotherapy alone for treating patients with liver metastases from primary large bowel cancer. *Ann Oncol.* 2001;12:1711–1720.

67. Blomgren H, Lax I, Naslund I, et al. Stereotactic high dose fraction radiation therapy of extracranial tumors using an accelerator. Clinical experience of the first thirty-one patients. *Acta Oncol.* 1995;34:861–870.

68. Herfarth KK, Debus J, Lohr F, et al. Stereotactic single-dose radiation therapy of liver tumors: results of a phase I/II trial. *J Clin Oncol.* 2001;19:164–170.

69. Van Cutsem E, Twelves C, Cassidy J, et al. Oral capecitabine compared with intravenous fluorouracil plus leucovorin in patients with metastatic colorectal cancer: results of a large phase III study. *J Clin Oncol.* 2001;19:4097–4106.

70. Saltz LB, Cox JV, Blanke C, et al. Irinotecan plus fluorouracil and leucovorin for metastatic colorectal cancer. Irinotecan Study Group. *N Engl J Med.* 2000;343:905–914.

71. Cunningham D, Pyrhonen S, James RD, et al. Randomised trial of irinotecan plus supportive care versus supportive care alone after fluorouracil failure for patients with metastatic colorectal cancer. *Lancet.* 1998;352:1413–1418.

72. Douillard JY, Cunningham D, Roth AD, et al. Irinotecan combined with fluorouracil compared with fluorouracil alone as first-line treatment for metastatic colorectal cancer: a multicentre randomised trial. *Lancet.* 2000;355:1041–1047.

73. Rougier P, Van Cutsem E, Bajetta E, et al. Randomised trial of irinotecan versus fluorouracil by continuous infusion after fluorouracil failure in patients with metastatic colorectal cancer. *Lancet.* 1998;352:1407–1412.

74. Becouarn Y, Ychou M, Ducreux M, et al. Phase II trial of oxaliplatin as first-line chemotherapy in metastatic colorectal cancer patients. Digestive Group of French Federation of Cancer Centers. *J Clin Oncol.* 1998;16:2739–2744.

75. de Gramont A, Figer A, Seymour M, et al. Leucovorin and fluorouracil with or without oxaliplatin as first-line treatment in advanced colorectal cancer. *J Clin Oncol.* 2000;18:2938–2947.

76. Giacchetti S, Perpoint B, Zidani R, et al. Phase III multicenter randomized trial of oxaliplatin added to chronomodulated fluorouracil-leucovorin as first-line treatment of metastatic colorectal cancer. *J Clin Oncol.* 2000;18:136–147.

77. Tournigand C, Andre T, Achille E, et al. FOLFIRI followed by FOLFOX6 or the reverse sequence in advanced colorectal cancer: A randomized GERCOR study. *Journal of Clinical Oncology.* 2004;22:229–237.

78. Cunningham D, Humblet Y, Siena S, et al. Cetuximab monotherapy and cetuximab plus irinotecan in irinotecan-refractory metastatic colorectal cancer. *N Engl J Med.* 2004;351:337–345.

79. Hurwitz H, Fehrenbacher L, Novotny W, et al. Bevacizumab plus irinotecan, fluorouracil, and leucovorin for metastatic colorectal cancer. *New England Journal of Medicine.* 2004;350:2335–2342.

80. Mano MS, Cassidy J, Canney P. Liver metastases from breast cancer: management of patients with significant liver dysfunction. *Cancer Treat Rev.* 2005;31:35–48.

81. Pentheroudakis G, Fountzilas G, Bafaloukos D, et al. Metastatic breast cancer with liver metastases: a registry analysis of clinicopathologic, management and outcome characteristics of 500 women. *Breast Cancer Res Treat.* 2005;1–8.

82. Fountzilas G, Tsavdaridis D, Kalogera-Fountzila A, et al. Weekly paclitaxel as first-line chemotherapy and trastuzumab in patients with advanced breast cancer. A Hellenic Cooperative Oncology Group phase II study. *Ann Oncol.* 2001;12:1545–1551.

83. Leyland-Jones B, Gelmon K, Ayoub JP, et al. Pharmacokinetics, safety, and efficacy of trastuzumab administered every three weeks in combination with paclitaxel. *J Clin Oncol.* 2003;21:3965–3971.

84. Esteva FJ, Valero V, Booser D, et al. Phase II study of weekly docetaxel and trastuzumab for patients with HER-2-overexpressing metastatic breast cancer. *J Clin Oncol.* 2002;20:1800–1808.

85. Raff JP, Rajdev L, Malik U, et al. Phase II study of weekly docetaxel alone or in combination with trastuzumab in patients with metastatic breast cancer. *Clin Breast Cancer.* 2004;4:420–427.

86. Burstein HJ, Harris LN, Marcom PK, et al. Trastuzumab and vinorelbine as first-line therapy for HER2-overexpressing metastatic breast cancer: multicenter phase II trial with clinical outcomes, analysis of serum tumor markers as predictive factors, and cardiac surveillance algorithm. *J Clin Oncol.* 2003;21:2889–2895.

87. Moertel CG, Kvols LK, O'Connell MJ, et al. Treatment of neuroendocrine carcinomas with combined etoposide and cisplatin. Evidence of major therapeutic activity in the anaplastic variants of these neoplasms. *Cancer.* 1991;68:227–232.

88. Rivera E, Ajani JA. Doxorubicin, streptozocin, and 5-fluorouracil chemotherapy for patients with metastatic islet-cell carcinoma. *Am J Clin Oncol.* 1998;21:36–38.

89. Oberg K. Interferon in the management of neuroendocrine GEP-tumors: a review. *Digestion.* 2000;62:92–97.

90. Kvols LK, Moertel CG, O'Connell MJ, et al. Treatment of the malignant carcinoid syndrome. Evaluation of a long-acting somatostatin analogue. *N Engl J Med.* 1986;315:663–666.

91. Oberg K. Endocrine tumors of the gastrointestinal tract: systemic treatment. *Anticancer Drugs.* 1994;5:503–519.

92. Oberg K, Norheim I, Theodorsson E. Treatment of malignant midgut carcinoid tumours with a long-acting somatostatin analogue octreotide. *Acta Oncol.* 1991;30:503–507.

93. Vinik A, Moattari AR. Use of somatostatin analog in management of carcinoid syndrome. *Dig Dis Sci.* 1989;34:14S–27S.

94. Valkema R, Pauwels S, Kvols LK, et al. Survival and response after peptide receptor radionuclide therapy with [90Y-DOTA0,Tyr3]octreotide in patients with advanced gastroenteropancreatic neuroendocrine tumors. *Semin Nucl Med.* 2006;36: 147–156.

95. Bedikian AY, Legha SS, Mavligit G, et al. Treatment of uveal melanoma metastatic to the liver: a review of the M. D. Anderson Cancer Center experience and prognostic factors. *Cancer.* 1995;76:1665–1670.

96. Flaherty LE, Unger JM, Liu PY, et al. Metastatic melanoma from intraocular primary tumors: the Southwest Oncology Group experience in phase II advanced melanoma clinical trials. *Am J Clin Oncol.* 1998;21:568–572.

97. Agarwala SS, Hellstrand K, Gehlsen K, et al. Immunotherapy with histamine and interleukin 2 in malignant melanoma with liver metastasis. *Cancer Immunol Immunother.* 2004;53:840–841.

98. Bedikian AY. Metastatic uveal melanoma therapy: current options. *Int Ophthalmol Clin.* 2006;46:151–166.

99. Ikeda T, Adachi I, Takashima S, et al. A phase I/II study of continuous intra-arterial chemotherapy using an implantable reservoir for the treatment of liver metastases from breast cancer: a Japan Clinical Oncology Group (JCOG) study 9113. JCOG Breast Cancer Study Group. *Jpn J Clin Oncol.* 1999;29:23–27.

100. Cantore M, Fiorentini G, Aitini E, et al. Intra-arterial hepatic carboplatin-based chemotherapy for ocular melanoma metastatic to the liver. Report of a phase II study. *Tumori*. 1994;80: 37–39.

101. Egerer G, Lehnert T, Max R, et al. Pilot study of hepatic intraarterial fotemustine chemotherapy for liver metastases from uveal melanoma: a single-center experience with seven patients. *Int J Clin Oncol*. 2001;6:25–28.

102. Leyvraz S, Spataro V, Bauer J, et al. Treatment of ocular melanoma metastatic to the liver by hepatic arterial chemotherapy. *J Clin Oncol*. 1997;15:2589–2595.

103. Kemeny N, Daly J, Reichman B, et al. Intrahepatic or systemic infusion of fluorodeoxyuridine in patients with liver metastases from colorectal carcinoma. A randomized trial. *Ann Intern Med*. 1987;107:459–465.

104. Lorenz M, Muller HH. Randomized, multicenter trial of fluorouracil plus leucovorin administered either via hepatic arterial or intravenous infusion versus fluorodeoxyuridine administered via hepatic arterial infusion in patients with nonresectable liver metastases from colorectal carcinoma. *J Clin Oncol*. 2000;18:243–254.

105. O'Connell MJ, Nagorney DM, Bernath AM, et al. Sequential intrahepatic fluorodeoxyuridine and systemic fluorouracil plus leucovorin for the treatment of metastatic colorectal cancer confined to the liver. *J Clin Oncol*. 1998;16:2528–2533.

106. Curley SA, Chase JL, Roh MS, Hohn DC. Technical considerations and complications associated with the placement of 180 implantable hepatic arterial infusion devices. *Surgery*. 1993;114:928–935.

107. Daly JM, Kemeny N, Oderman P, et al. Long-term hepatic arterial infusion chemotherapy. Anatomic considerations, operative technique, and treatment morbidity. *Arch Surg*. 1984;119:936–941.

108. Campbell KA, Burns RC, Sitzmann JV, et al. Regional chemotherapy devices: effect of experience and anatomy on complications. *J Clin Oncol*. 1993;11:822–826.

109. Burke D, Fordy C, Earlam SA, et al. Hepatic arterial cannulation for regional chemotherapy is safe in patients with a liver metastasis volume of less than 1 litre. *Br J Cancer*. 1997;75:1213–1216.

110. Barber FD, Mavligit G, Kurzrock R. Hepatic arterial infusion chemotherapy for metastatic colorectal cancer: a concise overview. *Cancer Treat Rev*. 2004;30:425–436.

111. Reappraisal of hepatic arterial infusion in the treatment of nonresectable liver metastases from colorectal cancer. Meta-Analysis Group in Cancer. *J Natl Cancer Inst*. 1996;88:252–258.

112. Kemeny N, Seiter K, Niedzwiecki D, et al. A randomized trial of intrahepatic infusion of fluorodeoxyuridine with dexamethasone versus fluorodeoxyuridine alone in the treatment of metastatic colorectal cancer. *Cancer*. 1992;69:327–334.

113. Rougier P, Laplanche A, Huguier M, et al. Hepatic arterial infusion of floxuridine in patients with liver metastases from colorectal carcinoma: long-term results of a prospective randomized trial. *J Clin Oncol*. 1992;10:1112–1118.

114. Harmantas A, Rotstein LE, Langer B. Regional versus systemic chemotherapy in the treatment of colorectal carcinoma metastatic to the liver. Is there a survival difference? Meta-analysis of the published literature. *Cancer*. 1996;78:1639–1645.

115. Kerr DJ, McArdle CS, Ledermann J, et al. Intrahepatic arterial versus intravenous fluorouracil and folinic acid for colorectal cancer liver metastases: a multicentre randomised trial. *Lancet*. 2003;361:368–373.

116. Kemeny NE, Niedzwiecki D, Hollis DR, et al. Hepatic arterial infusion versus systemic therapy for hepatic metastases from colorectal cancer: a randomized trial of efficacy, quality of life, and molecular markers (CALGB 9481). *J Clin Oncol*. 2006;24:1395–1403.

117. Fiorentini G, Rossi S, Dentico P, et al. Irinotecan hepatic arterial infusion chemotherapy for hepatic metastases from colorectal cancer: a phase II clinical study. *Tumori*. 2003;89:382–384.

118. Fiorentini G, Lucchi SR, Giovanis P, et al. Irinotecan hepatic arterial infusion chemotherapy for hepatic metastases from colorectal cancer: results of a phase I clinical study. *Tumori*. 2001;87:388–390.

119. Fiorentini G, Rossi S, Dentico P, et al. Oxaliplatin hepatic arterial infusion chemotherapy for hepatic metastases from colorectal cancer: a phase I-II clinical study. *Anticancer Res*. 2004;24:2093–2096.

120. Kern W, Beckert B, Lang N, et al. Phase I and pharmacokinetic study of hepatic arterial infusion with oxaliplatin in combination with folinic acid and 5-fluorouracil in patients with hepatic metastases from colorectal cancer. *Ann Oncol*. 2001;12:599–603.

121. Guthoff I, Lotspeich E, Fester C, et al. Hepatic artery infusion using oxaliplatin in combination with 5-fluorouracil, folinic acid and mitomycin C: oxaliplatin pharmacokinetics and feasibility. *Anticancer Res*. 2003;23:5203–5208.

122. Mancuso A, Giuliani R, Accettura C, et al. Hepatic arterial continuous infusion (HACI) of oxaliplatin in patients with unresectable liver metastases from colorectal cancer. *Anticancer Res*. 2003;23:1917–1922.

123. Ducreux M, Ychou M, Laplanche A, et al. Hepatic arterial oxaliplatin infusion plus intravenous chemotherapy in colorectal cancer with inoperable hepatic metastases: a trial of the gastrointestinal group of the Federation Nationale des Centres de Lutte Contre le Cancer. *J Clin Oncol*. 2005;23:4881–4887.

124. Tekin K, Kocaoglu H, Bayar S. Long-term survival after regional chemotherapy for liver metastases from breast cancer. A case report. *Tumori*. 2002;88:167–169.

125. Hashimoto K, Nio Y, Koike M, et al. [A case of liver metastases of breast cancer successfully treated by combination chemotherapy using hepatic arterial infusion of docetaxel and systemic administration of trastuzumab]. *Gan To Kagaku Ryoho*. 2004;31:1391–1393.

126. Fujito T, Maeura Y, Matsuyama J, et al. [A case of multiple liver metastases from breast cancer in which we confirmed disappearance of cancer cells after hepatic resection following hepatic arterial infusion chemotherapy]. *Gan To Kagaku Ryoho*. 2002;29:2354–2357.

127. Peters S, Voelter V, Zografos L, et al. Intra-arterial hepatic fotemustine for the treatment of liver metastases from uveal melanoma: experience in 101 patients. *Ann Oncol*. 2006;17:578–583.

128. Vahrmeijer AL, van Dierendonck JH, Keizer HJ, et al. Increased local cytostatic drug exposure by isolated hepatic perfusion: a phase I clinical and pharmacologic evaluation of treatment with high dose melphalan in patients with colorectal cancer confined to the liver. *Br J Cancer*. 2000;82:1539–1546.

129. Alexander HR, Libutti SK, Bartlett DL, et al. A phase I-II study of isolated hepatic perfusion using melphalan with or without tumor necrosis factor for patients with ocular melanoma metastatic to liver. *Clin Cancer Res*. 2000;6:3062–3070.

130. Alexander HR Jr, Bartlett DL, Libutti SK, et al. Isolated hepatic perfusion with tumor necrosis factor and melphalan for unresectable cancers confined to the liver. *J Clin Oncol*. 1998;16:1479–1489.

131. van der ZJ, Kroon BB, Nieweg OE, et al. Rationale for different approaches to combined melphalan and hyperthermia in regional isolated perfusion. *Eur J Cancer*. 1997;33:1546–1550.

132. Alexander HR, Jr., Libutti SK, Pingpank JF, et al. Hyperthermic isolated hepatic perfusion using melphalan for patients with ocular melanoma metastatic to liver. *Clin Cancer Res*. 2003;9:6343–6349.

133. Grover AC, Libutti SK, Pingpank JF, et al. Isolated hepatic perfusion for the treatment of patients with advanced liver metastases

from pancreatic and gastrointestinal neuroendocrine neoplasms. *Surgery.* 2004;136:1176–1182.

134. Noter SL, Rothbarth J, Pijl ME, et al. Isolated hepatic perfusion with high-dose melphalan for the treatment of uveal melanoma metastases confined to the liver. *Melanoma Res.* 2004;14: 67–72.

135. Rothbarth J, Pijl ME, Vahrmeijer AL, et al. Isolated hepatic perfusion with high-dose melphalan for the treatment of colorectal metastasis confined to the liver. *Br J Surg.* 2003;90:1391–1397.

136. Bartlett DL, Libutti SK, Figg WD, et al. Isolated hepatic perfusion for unresectable hepatic metastases from colorectal cancer. *Surgery.* 2001;129:176–187.

137. Kath R, Hayungs J, Bornfeld N, et al. Prognosis and treatment of disseminated uveal melanoma. *Cancer.* 1993;72:2219–2223.

138. Eskelin S, Pyrhonen S, Hahka-Kemppinen M, et al. A prognostic model and staging for metastatic uveal melanoma. *Cancer.* 2003;97:465–475.

139. Curley SA, Byrd DR, Newman RA, et al. Reduction of systemic drug exposure after hepatic arterial infusion of doxorubicin with complete hepatic venous isolation and extracorporeal chemofiltration. *Surgery.* 1993;114:579–585.

140. Ravikumar TS, Pizzorno G, Bodden W, et al. Percutaneous hepatic vein isolation and high-dose hepatic arterial infusion chemotherapy for unresectable liver tumors. *J Clin Oncol.* 1994;12:2723–2736.

141. Ku Y, Iwasaki T, Fukumoto T, et al. Percutaneous isolated liver chemoperfusion for treatment of unresectable malignant liver tumors: technique, pharmacokinetics, clinical results. *Recent Results Cancer Res.* 1998;147:67–82.

142. Pingpank JF, Libutti SK, Chang R, et al. Phase I study of hepatic arterial melphalan infusion and hepatic venous hemofiltration using percutaneously placed catheters in patients with unresectable hepatic malignancies. *J Clin Oncol.* 2005;23:3465–3474.

143. van IJken MG, de Bruijn EA, de Boeck G, et al. Isolated hypoxic hepatic perfusion with tumor necrosis factor-alpha, melphalan, and mitomycin C using balloon catheter techniques: a pharmacokinetic study in pigs. *Ann Surg.* 1998;228:763–770.

144. Savier E, Azoulay D, Huguet E, et al. Percutaneous isolated hepatic perfusion for chemotherapy: a phase 1 study. *Arch Surg.* 2003;138:325–332.

145. van Etten B, Brunstein F, van IJken MG, et al. Isolated hypoxic hepatic perfusion with orthograde or retrograde flow in patients with irresectable liver metastases using percutaneous balloon catheter techniques: a phase I and II study. *Ann Surg Oncol.* 2004;11:598–605.

146. Douillard JY. Irinotecan and high-dose fluorouracil/leucovorin for metastatic colorectal cancer. *Oncology (Williston Park).* 2000;14:51–55.

147. de Gramont A, Figer A, Seymour M, et al. Leucovorin and fluorouracil with or without oxaliplatin as first-line treatment in advanced colorectal cancer. *J Clin Oncol.* 2000;18:2938–2947.

148. Chabot GG, Abigerges D, Catimel G, et al. Population Pharmacokinetics and Pharmacodynamics of Irinotecan (Cpt-11) and Active Metabolite Sn-38 During Phase-I Trials. *Annals of Oncology.* 1995;6:141–151.

149. Scappaticci FA, Fehrenbacher L, Cartwright T, et al. Surgical wound healing complications in metastatic colorectal cancer patients treated with bevacizumab. *Journal of Surgical Oncology.* 2005;91:173–180.

150. Extra JM, Marty M, Brienza S, et al. Pharmacokinetics and safety profile of oxaliplatin. *Seminars in Oncology.* 1998;25:13–22.

151. Raymond E, Faivre S, Woynarowski JM, et al. Oxaliplatin: Mechanism of action and antineoplastic activity. *Seminars in Oncology.* 1998;25:4–12.

152. Aigner KR, Walther H, Tonn JC, et al. [Isolated liver perfusion in advanced metastases of colorectal cancers]. *Onkologie.* 1984;7: 13–21.

153. Skibba JL, Quebbeman EJ. Tumoricidal effects and patient survival after hyperthermic liver perfusion. *Arch Surg.* 1986;121:1266–1271.

154. Schwemmle K, Link KH, Rieck B. Rationale and indications for perfusion in liver tumors: current data. *World J Surg.* 1987;11:534–540.

155. Hafstrom LR, Holmberg SB, Naredi PL, et al. Isolated hyperthermic liver perfusion with chemotherapy for liver malignancy. *Surg Oncol.* 1994;3:103–108.

156. Marinelli A, de Brauw LM, Beerman H, et al. Isolated liver perfusion with mitomycin C in the treatment of colorectal cancer metastases confined to the liver. *Jpn J Clin Oncol.* 1996;26:341–350.

157. de Vries MR, Borel R, I, van de Velde CJ, et al. Isolated hepatic perfusion with tumor necrosis factor alpha and melphalan: experimental studies in pigs and phase I data from humans. *Recent Results Cancer Res.* 1998;147:107–119.

158. Oldhafer KJ, Lang H, Frerker M, et al. First experience and technical aspects of isolated liver perfusion for extensive liver metastasis. *Surgery.* 1998;123:622–631.

159. Lindner P, Fjalling M, Hafstrom L, et al. Isolated hepatic perfusion with extracorporeal oxygenation using hyperthermia, tumour necrosis factor alpha and melphalan. *Eur J Surg Oncol.* 1999;25:179–185.

160. Alexander HR, Jr., Libutti SK, Pingpank JF, et al. Isolated hepatic perfusion for the treatment of patients with colorectal cancer liver metastases after irinotecan-based therapy. *Ann Surg Oncol.* 2005;12:138–144.

COMMENTARY
David J. Gallagher and Nancy E. Kemeny

In the preceding chapter the authors provide a menu of the available treatment modalities for hepatic metastases. The topics covered are systemic chemotherapy, partial hepatic resection, local ablative therapy, administration of chemotherapy by hepatic artery infusion (HAI), and isolated hepatic perfusion with high-dose chemotherapy. Surgical resection remains the treatment of choice, when possible; but for unresectable disease, the standard of care is less clear. There are many variables to consider, making it difficult to provide a "one size fits all" consensus approach for patients. In this commentary we discuss a number of treatment options, outline our suggested approach to patients with unresectable hepatic metastases, and emphasize that cure is now a reasonable goal for selected patients.

The majority of evidence for the management of hepatic metastases comes from the treatment of colorectal cancer. It is not surprising that the most common site of distal metastasis from colorectal cancer is the liver, perhaps because venous drainage from the colon flows via the portal vein to the liver (1). What is not known is whether colon cancer cells have unique characteristics that allow them to grow in the liver, in preference to other organs. Approximately 15% of patients will have liver metastases at the time of primary diagnosis and another 60% of patients treated for colorectal cancer will develop liver metastases during or after treatment of their primary disease (2). With 940,000 new colon cancer cases per year worldwide, it is obvious why improved treatment modalities are a priority. A minority of patients with liver metastases (approximately 20%) (3) will have disease that is suitable for complete resection at the time of diagnosis, rendering these patients macroscopically clear of disease. Complete surgical resection is associated with 30% survival at 5 years (4). Optimal results from surgery are achieved with a low clinical risk score: lymph node negative; no more than one metastatic lesion; size of lesion <5 cm; if the preoperative carcinoembryonic antigen is <200 mg/dL; and if the disease free interval is >12 months (5). These factors are not an absolute contraindication to surgery, and each patient needs to be considered on a case-by-case basis. However, most patients present with unresectable disease for which initial surgery is not an option. Strategies such as portal vein embolization, staged resections, and neoadjuvant chemotherapy increase the number of patients who can undergo potentially curable surgery. In addition, local ablative therapy and adjuvant chemotherapy may complement surgery and improve survival.

SYSTEMIC CHEMOTHERAPY

Historically, the median survival for patients with metastatic colorectal cancer to the liver is 6 to 12 months. A number of new agents are now available, including irinotecan (Camptosar), a topoisomerase inhibitor, and oxaliplatin (Eloxatin), a platinum compound with in vivo and in vitro activity against colon cancer cell lines and the ability to synergize with 5-fluorouracil (5-FU) (6,7). Phase 3 studies have demonstrated the superiority of 5-FU with leucovorin (LV) in combination with irinotecan over 5-FU plus LV alone (8). When irinotecan/5-FU/LV irinotecan/bolux 5-FU/LV (IFL) was compared with oxaliplatin plus 5-FU/LV (FOLFOX), the response rate increased from 35% to 45%, and survival increased from 15 to 19.5 months, respectively (9). When irinotecan is combined with infusional 5-FU as opposed to bolus (FOLFIRI instead of irinotecan, 5-FU, and leucovorin [IFL]), results are similar to those obtained with FOLFOX (10). The addition of novel targeted agents such as bevacizumab (an antivascular endothelial growth factor monoclonal antibody) and cetuximab (an antiepidermal growth factor receptor antibody) can enhance the efficacy of cytotoxic chemotherapeutic agents (11,12). Bevacizumab plus IFL has a median survival of 20.3 months versus 15.5 months with IFL alone. It is not clear if addition of bevacizumab to FOLFOX increases survival (13).

Even with the newer systemic therapies, the 2-year survival rate is generally <40%, and drops rapidly with ≤5% surviving at 5 years (14). Getting a patient to resection therefore remains the main goal of systemic treatment and requires close follow-up of patients while on therapy. An alternative approach is the use of HAI chemotherapy.

HEPATIC ARTERIAL INFUSION

The rationale for the use of HAI is based on the fact that tumor residing within the hepatic parenchyma is fed primarily by the hepatic artery, whereas normal liver tissue is supplied by the portal vein (15). Therefore, direct infusion of chemotherapy into the hepatic artery may expose the tumor to higher drug concentrations. This method of administration also allows for minimal systemic toxicity by bypassing the effect of first-pass metabolism. We disagree with the authors' review of complications from pump placement including "death." That review is based on old data, and complications such as catheter obstruction and hepatic artery thrombosis are now rare as confirmed by more recent evidence showing much lower complication rates with long duration of pump function, and no deaths related to pump placement in 544 consecutive cases at a single institution (16).

Ten randomized studies have compared HAI with systemic chemotherapy, and nine showed an increase in response rate in favor of HAI (17). Improvements were seen in overall survival, but these were not significant, possibly because of the crossover option permitted in some studies and to the small sample sizes in others. Contrary to what is reported in this chapter, a meta-analysis as well as a recently published trial by Cancer and Leukemia Group B (CALGB) that incorporated dexamethasone with fluorodeoxyuridine (FUDR) in the HAI group did demonstrate an increase in median survival in favor of HAI (18). The meta-analysis showed an increase in median survival of 16 versus 12 months in favor of HAI (19). In the CALGB trial, the HAI group had a significant improvement in survival over the systemic group (24.4 vs. 20 months, respectively). These results demonstrated that regional therapy alone can improve survival over systemic 5-FU/LV and the survival obtained with HAI alone was similar to that seen with newer systemic agents.

NEOADJUVANT CHEMOTHERAPY

For patients with borderline resectability, chemotherapy can be given preoperatively, but in order to minimize toxicity it should only be used for short periods of time. As soon as response is noted, surgery should be performed. Several systemic chemotherapy studies have retrospectively evaluated resectability after chemotherapy. Adam et al. (20) reviewed the records of 1,104 patients with unresectable disease who received mainly FOLFOX as neoadjuvant chemotherapy; 12.5% became resectable and the 5-year survival rate of these patients was 34%, similar to what could be achieved with patients who were initially resectable, with a 71% recurrence rate in the liver. Rougier at al. (21) treated 23 patients with cetuximab and FOLFIRI and 7 (30%) became resectable.

For patients who are resectable, this approach is not without risk, and toxicity from systemic chemotherapy can complicate surgery. There are reports of increased incidence of steatosis, sinusoidal abnormalities, veno-occlusive disease, and steatohepatitis in this setting. Complications can arise with both irinotecan and oxaliplatin (22,23). Recently, a 20% incidence of steatohepatitis was reported in patients receiving preoperative irinotecan versus 4.4% in those who received no prior chemotherapy, and an 18.9% incidence of sinusoidal dilatation in those receiving preoperative oxaliplatin versus 1.9% in those receiving no prior chemotherapy. Patients with steatohepatitis had an increased 90-day mortality (14.7% vs. 1.6%; $p = 0.001$) (24). A prospective study of six cycles of neoadjuvant FOLFOX showed a significantly increased risk of sinusoidal lesions but not of steatosis or steatohepatitis. Sensory neuropathy appeared to predict sinusoidal lesions, but so far with only 29 patients evaluable, liver damage had no substantial impact on surgical outcome (25).

A recent study examining the use of pre- and/or postoperative bevacizumab concluded that clinical experience thus far does not indicate a statistically significantly increased risk of perioperative complications with the incorporation of bevacizumab into perioperative treatment paradigms. However, this was a very small study and more information is needed to be sure that bevacizumab is safe in the preoperative setting. Given the long half-life of bevacizumab and the potential for antivascular endothelial growth factor therapy to impede wound healing and/or liver regeneration, a window of 6 to 8 weeks between bevacizumab administration and surgery is favored (26). Another retrospective review found that neither the neoadjuvant use of bevacizumab nor the time to surgery affected complication rates (27).

Another issue complicating neoadjuvant chemotherapy in patients who are resectable is that if metastases disappear on computed tomography (CT) scan, these areas may be difficult to find at surgery. Nordlinger et al. (28) reviewed 586 patients, and 38 patients had disappearance of at least one lesion on CT. Pathologic examinations of sites that were considered to have a complete response showed that in 12 of 15 of these lesions (80%) there were still viable tumor cells on pathologic examination. Thirty-one sites that could not be resected were closely followed, and in 23 (74%) a recurrence developed.

ADJUVANT CHEMOTHERAPY

In the review by Adam et al. (20), 71% of patients recurred in the liver after liver resection. It appears that postresection treatment is necessary. One study combining two European trials using postoperative systemic 5-FU/LV versus no postoperative chemotherapy following curative resection found that, although there was a trend toward improved progression-free survival, there was no significant difference in progression-free or overall survival between the groups (29). A small study of 29 patients addressed the efficacy of systemic irinotecan posthepatic resection. The 2-year overall survival rate in this study was 85%; however, the patients were in a better risk category, having fewer metastases and a longer disease-free interval (30).

A number of ongoing trials are addressing the issue of perioperative chemotherapy. In an European Organisation for Research and Treatment of Cancer (EORTC) study looking at pre- and postoperative FOLFOX versus observation, 364 patients have been randomized to six cycles of FOLFOX before and after surgery versus surgery alone. At recent follow-up, in the preoperative chemotherapy group, 7.7% progressed prior to surgery and 11% could not undergo resection. In the control group, 4% were not able to undergo resection (31). For unresectable disease, the North Central Cancer Treatment Group and National Surgical Adjuvant Breast and Bowel Project are conducting a phase 2 trial of FOLFOX and cetuximab. N. D. Anderson Cancer Center, with Genentech, has initiated a study of FOLFIRI and bevacizumab and the National Cancer Institute, among others, is investigating FOLFOX with bevacizumab and erlotinib.

In the adjuvant setting, four large randomized trials have addressed the issue of HAI therapy. At the Memorial Sloane-Kettering Cancer Center, patients were randomized after liver resection to HAI FUDR and dexamethasone plus systemic 5-FU with or without LV versus systemic chemotherapy alone. After a median follow-up of 10 years, 10-year survival was 41% for the HAI plus systemic chemotherapy group and 27% for the systemic therapy alone group, and overall median survivals were 68.4 versus 58.8 months, respectively. Median time to hepatic recurrence has not been reached in the HAI plus systemic arm but was 32.5 months for systemic treatment alone (p <0.01). Median progression-free survival was 31 months and 17 months for HAI plus systemic therapy versus systemic therapy alone, respectively ($p = 0.02$) (32). This benefit for HAI plus systemic therapy versus systemic therapy alone was supported by two other studies (33,34). A fourth randomized trial from Germany found no benefit for adjuvant HAI versus no adjuvant treatment but in this study only 87 patients (77%) were actually treated with HAI therapy for various reasons, including extrahepatic disease and technical complications. When the actually treated patients were compared with those receiving no therapy, median survival was 44.8 versus 39.7 months, median time to hepatic progression was 44.8 versus 23.3 months, and median time to any progression was 20 versus 12.6 months, respectively (35).

Newer agents have also been combined with HAI in the adjuvant setting. In a phase 1 study of systemic irinotecan and HAI FUDR/dexamethasone with a median follow-up of 5.2 years, the 2-year survival rate was 89% and the 5-year survival rate was 58% (36). Another phase 1 trial using systemic FOLFOX plus HAI therapy has a minimum follow-up of 26.9 months, and presently a 2-year survival of 98% (37). New studies at Memorial Sloane-Kettering Cancer Center are looking at the feasibility of adding bevacizumab to HAI and systemic therapy after liver resection.

SECOND-LINE CHEMOTHERAPY

The authors of the preceding chapter discuss first-line chemotherapy only. In patients who progress on first-line chemotherapy, the ability to achieve a response with second-line therapy is low. In the study by Tournigand (10) for patients who progressed on first-line treatment, there was a 15% response with FOLFOX versus 4% with FOLFIRI. Cetuximab was approved based on the results of a European phase 2 trial in patients with advanced colorectal cancer who had failed irinotecan (63% also failed oxaliplatin). Patients were randomized to cetuximab and irinotecan or cetuximab alone. The response rates were 22.9% and 10.8%, median time to progression 4.1 and 1.5 months, and median survival 8.6 and 6.9 months, respectively, for the combined therapy versus cetuximab alone (11). In the BOND-2 trial, bevacizumab was added to each arm (38). Again, all patients had failed irinotecan and the majority (85%) had also failed oxaliplatin treatment. The response rates were 23% and 35% and time to tumor progression was 4.0 and 5.8 months for the two-drug group versus the bevacizumab, cetuximab, and irinotecan group.

In the second-line setting, HAI-based therapy has produced much higher response rates than systemic therapy in small, single-institution studies. A trial using FUDR/LV/dexamethasone in both chemotherapy-naïve and previously treated patients produced response rates of 72% and 52% and median survivals of 23 and 13.5 months, respectively, for the chemotherapy-naïve and previously treated patients (39). HAI FUDR/dexamethasone plus mitomycin administered through the pump sideport produced a 70% response rate in previously treated patients, with a median survival of 19 months after the start of HAI therapy (40). Combined treatment with HAI and systemic therapy has also been investigated in this patient population. A phase 1 study of HAI FUDR combined with systemic irinotecan in previously treated patients (45% had previously received irinotecan but none had received prior oxaliplatin) reported a response rate of 74%, a time to disease progression of 8.1 months, and a median survival of 20 months (41). A phase 1 trial of systemic oxaliplatin plus 5FU/LV or oxaliplatin plus irinotecan with concurrent HAI FUDR/dexamethasone in 36 previously treated patients (74% had received prior irinotecan) produced response rates of 86%, with a median survival of 36 months and a 1-year survival of 80% (42).

In the United States, FOLFOX plus bevacizumab has emerged as the most commonly used first-line therapy based on the effectiveness of FOLFOX over IFL (43). It is not clear how best to treat patients who progress on FOLFOX. A recent study investigating HAI plus systemic irinotecan in patients who had all failed treatment with systemic oxaliplatin, and 28% of whom had previous irinotecan as well, showed a partial response of 43.9%, a median survival of 20 months, from time of initiation of treatment, with 16 patients alive at most recent follow-up. Survival from initiation of treatment for their metastatic disease was 32 months. Finally, 18% of patients to date have proceeded to surgical resection or ablation (44).

LOCAL ABLATIVE THERAPY

Local ablative therapy also aims to further increase the resectability rate. Techniques such as cryotherapy and radiofrequency ablation (RFA) can be used to cope with the technical limitations of surgery but have their own disadvantages. Cryotherapy often fails to kill all tumor cells, and in one study, 75% of patients treated with cryotherapy developed an elevated carcinoembryonic antigen within 6 months (45). RFA is more commonly used, but its widespread use has preceded full analysis of outcome with this modality. The authors recommend this modality as the preferred regional therapy citing a complete response rate of 52% to 94%. However, as studies often report outcome per lesion rather than per patient and reports relate to different tumor types treated with different ablation techniques, one has to be cautious when assessing this treatment. A more recent study not reviewed in this chapter reports a recurrence rate of 84% with RFA alone. Resection alone was significantly superior to RFA alone. Resection plus RFA analyzed in a retrospective manner appeared to offer a significant survival benefit to systemic chemotherapy (46). RFA is commonly used as an adjunct to surgery in unresectable patients but it is not known if this approach is superior to treatment with newer systemic agents or HAI. The EORTC are currently exploring a related question with a randomized phase 2 trial of chemotherapy (one of three

FOLFOX and bevacizumab combinations) with or without RFA in patients with unresectable liver metastases secondary to colorectal adenocarcinoma.

CONCLUSIONS

Improvements in surgical technique and perioperative care have led to a reduction in perioperative mortality (now at 0% to 2% in specialized units) and an increase in 5-year survival (30% to 40%) following hepatic metastasectomy (47). The addition of perioperative chemotherapy and adjunctive surgical techniques has made cure a realistic goal for a select group of initially unresectable patients. However, for the remainder and even for those surgical candidates, in whom the risk of recurrence remains high, further progress is required.

Clinical trials of new systemic agents and new combinations of systemic and intrahepatic chemotherapy are ongoing. Different methods of treatment such as the use of chemotherapy-free intervals (such as with OPTIMOX-1 and -2) aimed at reducing toxicity and improving both quality life and outcome are promising. Novel therapies such as selective internal radiation therapy are entering the clinical armamentarium. The use of positron emission tomography scans as a preoperative assessment of patients with a high clinical risk score improves patient selection for surgery and survival (48).

In reality, the problem is not a shortage of options, rather it is a lack of clarity regarding the correct option for an individual patient. The variable presentation of patients with hepatic metastases makes a consensus treatment protocol difficult to construct, and management of these patients requires the multidisciplinary involvement of medical oncologists, radiologists, and hepatobiliary surgeons. A new multidisciplinary decision tool (Onco-Surge) has been developed for this purpose. Unless ongoing studies show a benefit for preoperative chemotherapy, clearly resectable patients should be resected up front. If chemotherapy is given, it should be for a short period to avoid hepatic toxicity. Because of the high risk of relapse, adjuvant therapy should be administered. Where available, patients should be enrolled on clinical trials investigating new agents, either alone or in combination with HAI therapy. The challenges for the future are to match patients with the most beneficial of the different treatment options available by using molecular and other prognostic indicators, and thereby work toward continually increasing the cure rate in this disease.

REFERENCES

1. Kemeny N, Kemeny MM, Lawrence TS. Liver metastases. In: Abeloff MD, Armitage JO, Niederhuber JE, et al (eds). *Clinical Oncology*, 3rd ed. Philadelphia: Elsevier; 2004:1141–1178.
2. Jewel A, Tiwari RC, Murray T, et al. Cancer statistics 2004. *CA Cancer J Clin.* 2004;54:8–29.
3. Adam R. Chemotherapy and surgery: new perspectives on the treatment of unresectable liver metastases. *Ann Oncol.* 2003;14(suppl 2): ii13–ii16
4. Fong Y, Cohen AM, Fortner JG, et al. Liver resection for colorectal metastases. *J Clin Oncol.* 1997;15:938–946.
5. Jarnigan WJ, Conlon K, Bodniewicz J, et al. A clinical scoring system predicts the yield of diagnostic laparoscopy in patients

with potentially resectable hepatic colorectal metastases. *Cancer.* 2001;91:1121–1128.

6. Tashiro T, Kawada Y, Sakurai Y, et al. Antitumor activity of a new platinum complex, oxalate (trans-I-1,2-diaminocyclohexane) platinum (II): new experimental data. *Biomed Pharmacother.* 1989;43:251–260.

7. Mathe G, Kidani Y, Segiguchi M, et al. Oxalato-platinum or 1-OHP, a third-generation platinum complex: an experimental and clinical appraisal and preliminary comparison with cis-platinum and carboplatinum. *Biomed Pharmacother.* 1989;43:237–250.

8. Saltz LV, Cox JV, Blanke C, et al. Irinotecan plus fluorouracil and leucovorin for metastatic colorectal cancer. Irinotecan Study Group. *N Engl J Med.* 2000;343:905–914.

9. Goldberg RM, Seargent DJ, Morton RF, et al. A randomised controlled trial of flourouracil plus leucovorin, irinotecan and oxaliplatin combinations in previously untreated metastatic colorectal cancer. *J Clin Oncol.* 2004;22:23–30.

10. Tournigand C, Andre T, Achille E, et al. Folfiri followed by Folfox 6 or the reverse sequence in advanced colorectal cancer: a randomized GERCOR study. *J Clin Oncol.* 2004;22:229–237.

11. Hurwitz H, Fehrenbacher L, Novotny W, et al. Bevacizumab plus irinotecan, fluorouracil, and leucovorin for metastatic colorectal cancer. *N Engl J Med.* 2004;350:2335–2342.

12. Cunningham D, Humblet Y, Siena S, et al. Cetuximab monotherapy and cetuximab plus irinotecan in irinotecan-refractory metastatic colon cancer. *N Engl J Med.* 2004;351:337–345.

13. Saltz LB, Clarke S, Diaz-Rubio E, et al. Bevacizumab in addition to XELOX or FOLFOX 4: Efficacy results XELOX1/NO16966, a randomized phase III trial in the first line treatment of metastatic colorectal cancer. In: Proceedings from the American Society of Clinical Oncology Gastrointestinal Cancers Symposium; January 19–21, 2007; Orlando, Florida. Abstract 238.

14. Giacchetti S, Itzhaki M, Gruia G, et al. Longterm survival of patients with resectable colorectal cancer liver metastases following infusional chemotherapy with 5-flourouracil, leucovorin, oxaliplatin and surgery. *Ann Oncol.* 1999;10:663–669.

15. Breedis C, Young G: The blood supply of neoplasms in the liver. *Am J Pathol.* 1954;30:969–977.

16. Allen PJ, Nissan A, Picon AI, et al. Technical complications and durability of hepatic artery infusion pumps for unresectable hepatic metastases: An institutional experience of 544 consecutive cases. *J Am Coll Surg.* 2005;201:1;57–65.

17. Kemeny N. Management of liver metastases from colorectal cancer. *Oncology.* 2006;20:1161–1176.

18. Kemeny NE, Niedzwiecki D, Hollis DR, et al. Hepatic arterial infusion vs systemic therapy for hepatic metastases from colorectal cancer: a randomized trial of efficacy, quality of life, and molecular markers (CALGB 9481). *J Clin Oncol.* 2006;24:1395–1403.

19. Meta-analysis Group in Cancer. Reappraisal of hepatic arterial infusion in the treatment of nonresectable liver metastases from colorectal cancer. *J Natl Cancer Inst.* 1996;88:252–258.

20. Adam R, Delvart V, Pascal G, et al. Rescue surgery for unresectable liver metastases downstaged by chemotherapy: a model to predict long term survival. *Ann Surg.* 2004;240:644–658.

21. Rougier P, Raoul J-L, Van Laethem J-L, et al. Cetuximab + FOLFIRI as first-line treatment for metastatic colorectal cancer. In: Proceedings from the American Society of Clinical Oncology; June 5-8, 2004; New Orleans, LA. Abstract 3513.

22. Rubbia-Brandt L, Audard V, Sartoretti P, et al. Severe hepatic sinusoidal obstruction associated with oxaliplatin-based chemotherapy in patients with metastatic colorectal cancer. Ann Oncol. 2004;15:460–466.

23. Parikh AA, Gentner D, Wu TT, et al. Perioperative complications in patients undergoing major liver resection with or without neoadjuvant chemotherapy. *J Gastrointestin Surg.* 2003;7:1082–1088.

24. Vauthey JN, Pawlik TM, Ribero D, et al. Chemotherapy regimen predicts steatohepatitis and an increase in 90-day mortality after surgery for hepatic colorectal metastases. *J Clin Oncol.* 2006;24:2065–2072.

25. Julie C, Lutz P, Aust D, et al. Pathological analysis of hepatic injury after oxaliplatin-based neoadjuvant chemotherapy of colorectal cancer liver metastases: results of the EORTC intergroup phase III study 40983. In: Proceedings from the American Society of Clinical Oncology Gastrointestinal Cancers Symposium; January 19–21, 2007; Orlando, Florida. Abstract 241.

26. D'Angelica M, Kornprat P, Gonen M, et al. Lack of evidence for increased operative morbidity after hepatectomy with perioperative use of bevacizumab: a matched case control study [published online ahead of print November 11, 2006]. *Ann Surg Oncol.* 2006;14:759-765.

27. Kesmodel SB, Ellis LM, Lin E, et al. Complication rates following hepatic surgery in patients receiving neoadjuvant bevacizumab for colorectal cancer liver metastases. In: Proceedings from the American Society of Clinical Oncology Gastrointestinal Cancers of Symposium; January 19–21, 2007; Orlando, Florida. Abstract 234.

28. Nordlinger B, Brouqet A, Penna C, et al. Complete radiological response of colorectal liver metastases (LM) after chemotherapy: does it mean cure? *J Clin Oncol.* 2006;(24):3939–3945.

29. Mitry E, Fields A, Bleiberg H, et al. Adjuvant chemotherapy after potentially curative resection of metastases from colorectal cancer. A meta-analysis of two randomized trials [abstract 3524]. *J Clin Oncol.* 2006';24):152S.

30. Mackey HJ, Billingsley K, Gallinger S, et al. A multicenter phase II study of "adjuvant" irinotecan following resection of colorectal hepatic metastases. *Am J Clin Oncol.* 2005;28:6;548–554.

31. Gruenberger T, Sorbye H, Debois M, et al. Tumor response to preoperative chemotherapy using FOLFOX-4 for respectable colorectal cancer metastases. Interim results of EORTC group randomized phase III study of 40983 [abstract 3500]. *J Clin Oncol.* 2006;24(18S):146S.

32. Kemeny NE, Huang Y, Cohen AM, et al. Hepatic arterial infusion of chemotherapy after resection of hepatic metastases from colorectal cancer. *N Engl J Med.* 1999;341:2039–2048.

33. Kemeny MM, Addak S, Gray B, et al. Combined-modality treatment for resectable metastatic colorectal cancer to liver: surgical resection of hepatic metastases in combination with continuous infusion of chemotherapy?an intergroup study. J Clin Oncol. 2002;20:1499–1505.

34. Lygidakis NJ, Sgourakis G, Vlachos L, et al. Metastatic disease of colorectal origin: the value of locoregional immunochemotherapy combined with systemic chemotherapy following liver resection. Results of a prospective randomized study. *Hepatogastroenterology.* 2001;48:1685–1691.

35. Lorenz M, Muller HH, Schramm H, et al. Randomized trial of surgery vs surgery followed by adjuvant hepatic artery infusion of 5-flourouracil and folinic acid for hepatic metastases from colorectal cancer. German Cooperative Group on Hepatic Metastatses (Arbsitsgruppe Lebermetastasen). *Ann Surg.* 1998;228:756–762.

36. Kemeny N, Jarnigan W, Gonen M, et al. Phase I/II study of hepatic arterial therapy with floxuridine and dexamethasone in combination with intravenous irinotecan as adjuvant treatment after resection of hepatic metastases from colorectal cancer. *J Clin Oncol.* 2003;21:3303–3309.

37. Kemeny NE, Jarnigan W, Gönen M, et al. Phase I trial of hepatic arterial infusion (HAI) with Floxuridine (FUDR) and dexamethasone in combination with systemic oxaliplatin (OXAL), fluorouracil (FU) + leucovorin (LV) after resection of hepatic

metastases from colorectal cancer [abstract 3579]. *J Clin Oncol.* 2005;23(16S):265S.

38. Saltz LB, Lenz HJ, Hochster H, et al. Randomized phase II study of cetuximab/bevacizumab/irinotecan (CBI) versus cetuximab/bevacizumab (CB) in irinotecan refractory colorectal cancer [abstract]. *J Clin Oncol.* 2005;23:3508.

39. Kemeny N, Conti JA, Cohen A, et al. Phase II study of hepatic arterial floxuridine, leucovorin and dexamethasone for unresectable liver metastases from colorectal cancer. *J Clin Oncol.* 1994;12:2288–2295.

40. Kemeny N, Eid A, Stockman J, et al. Hepatic arterial infusion of floxuridine and dexamethasone plus high-dose mitomycin C for patients with unresectable hepatic metastases from colorectal carcinoma. *J Surg Oncol.* 2005;91:97–101.

41. Kemeny N, Gönen M, Sullivan D, et al. Phase I study of hepatic arterial infusion of floxuridine and dexamethasone with systemic irinotecan for unresectable hepatic metastases from colorectal cancer. *J Clin Oncol.* 2001;19:2687–2695.

42. Kemeny N, Jarnigan W, Paty P, et al. Phase I trial of systemic oxaliplatin combination chemotherapy with hepatic arterial infusion in patients with unresectable liver metastases from colorectal cancer. *J Clin Oncol.* 2005;23:4888–4896.

43. Terstriep S, Grothey A. First- and second-line therapy of metastatic colorectal cancer. *Expert Rev Anticancer Ther.* 2006;6:921–930.

44. Gallagher DJ, Capanu M, Kemeny N, et al. Retrospective Analysis of Hepatic Arterial Infusion (HAI) plus systemic CPT-11 in patients with unresectable hepatic metastases from colorectal cancer, previously treated with systemic FOLFOX or XELOX. In: Proceedings from the American Society of Clinical Oncology Gastrointestinal Cancers Symposium; January 19–21, 2007; Orlando, Florida. Abstract 238.

45. Morris DL, Ross WB. Australian experience with cryoablation of liver tumors: metastases. *Surg Oncol Clin North Am.* 1996;5:391–397.

46. Abdalla EK, Vauthey J-N, Ellis L, et al. Recurrence and outcomes following hepatic resection, radiofrequency ablation and combined resection/ablation for colorectal metastases. *Ann Surg.* 2004;239;818–827.

47. Adam R. Chemotherapy and surgery in the treatment of colorectal liver metastases: The Golden Alliance. In: Proceedings from the American Society of Clinical Oncology Gastrointestinal Cancers Symposium; January 19–21, 2007; Orlando, Florida. Abstract 238.

48. Taylor RA, Tuorto SJ, Akhurst TJ, et al. Evaluation with positron emission tomography before hepatic resection for metastatic colorectal cancer improves survival in patients with a high clinical risk score. In: Proceedings from the American Society of Clinical Oncology Gastrointestinal Cancers Symposium; January 19–21, 2007; Orlando, Florida. Abstract 240.

49

Primary Vascular Tumors

Ajay Jain, Heitham T. Hassoun, and Julie A. Freischlag

Neoplasms of vascular tissues, especially benign growths such as hemangiomas or angiodysplasias, are relatively common and occur in nearly every organ system. However, the focus of this chapter will be on primary vascular tumors, which are rare, with only a few hundred cases of all varieties having been reported in the medical literature. These neoplasms may (a) be benign or malignant; (b) arise from large arteries or veins, small blood vessels, or lymph vessels; and (c) may arise from any part of the vessel wall. Because of their rarity, these malignancies are often not included in the initial differential diagnosis of mass lesions, and therefore diagnosis can often be delayed. In addition, because of their low incidence the pathogenesis, clinical characteristics and optimal management have not been clearly defined.

TUMORS OF LARGE ARTERIES AND VEINS

When considering primary vascular tumors of large arteries and veins, they are usually malignant and much more common in veins than arteries. The most common malignancies are sarcomas, and there are two major types. The first type is the sarcoma that arises from progenitor cells of vascular endothelium, and is referred to generally as *intimal* sarcomas. The second type of tumor arises from mesenchymal elements of the vessel wall, and is referred to as a *mural* sarcoma. Burke and Virmani (1) characterized the clinical, pathologic, and immunohistochemical characteristics of tumors arising from the aorta, vena cava, and pulmonary vessels. They found that in general, most tumors arising from the aorta and pulmonary artery had characteristics typical of intimal sarcomas, while tumors of the vena cava and pulmonary veins tended to be mural sarcomas. However, this is not always the case, and because the histopathologic spectrum of these vascular sarcomas is not completely understood, they are often characterized by the vessel of origin.

Primary Tumors of Large Veins

Two thirds of all primary neoplasms of major blood vessels occur in large veins. More than 90% of these tumors are of smooth muscle cell origin and most (~85%) are malignant (i.e., leiomyosarcoma). Signs and symptoms on clinical presentation depend on the site of luminal obstruction. Peripheral tumors cause pain, swelling, or a palpable mass, while symptoms caused by central tumors are more variable and depend on size and location. More than half of large vein tumors arise in the inferior vena cava (IVC), while the remainder generally occur in the saphenous, ileofemoral, jugular, or pulmonary veins in decreasing order.

Primary IVC tumors are more common in women than in men with an incidence in males versus females from 1:5 to 1:6 (2–4). They typically present in the fifth decade of life, and although not as uncommon as primary tumors of the aorta, they are still quite rare (5). Approximately 400 cases have been reported in the literature to date. Most primary vena cava tumors are sarcomas, and they tend to arise from mesenchymal elements of the vessel wall (mural type tumors). Most often these mesenchymal cells are precursor smooth muscle cells. Growth of these tumors can be intraluminal or extraluminal, and involvement of adjacent organs has been well described (6).

Caval sarcomas almost always arise in the IVC, and sarcomas of the IVC are often characterized by the anatomic segment of origin because data suggest that tumor location affects prognosis. In one of the largest reported case series, 3% of tumors involved level 1 of the IVC (from the right atrium to the origin of the hepatic veins), 33% involved level 2 (below the hepatic veins to include the origin of renal veins), and 8% involved level 3 (below the renal veins) (6) (Figure 49.1).

On gross examination, these IVC tumors are fleshy, lobulated, and have a gray-white color (Figure 49.2). Intraluminal and extraluminal elements are both classically present. When incised, areas of necrosis and hemorrhage can often be identified, and the tissue architecture often has a whorled appearance. Histologically, these tumors are made up of dense bundles of spindle-shaped cells and are typically pleomorphic, with hyperchromic and irregular nuclei. These cells often contain large amounts of eosinophilic cytoplasm on hematoxylin and eosin staining, while immunostaining is typically positive for desmin and actin (7,8). No formal staging system for IVC leiomyosarcomas exists, but the staging system for retroperitoneal sarcomas (based on the number of mitotic figures/high-power field) is often used (6,9).

In a review of 211 cases of leiomyosarcoma of the IVC, Hilliard and colleagues (6) determined that the most common presenting symptom was abdominal pain or a mass. Other common symptoms included Budd-Chiari syndrome from hepatic vein compression (17%) and deep vein thrombosis (4%). Rarely, these tumors have also presented with renal insufficiency in instances when renal vein involvement was present. Intraluminal growth and pulmonary embolization of tumor thrombus has also been described (10). Unfortunately, the clinical presentation of caval tumors is often at an advanced stage.

The diagnosis of primary IVC tumor can be suggested with noninvasive imaging such as computed tomography (CT) scan (Figure 49.3), or magnetic resonance imaging (MRI). Venography can demonstrate the presence of an intraluminal filling

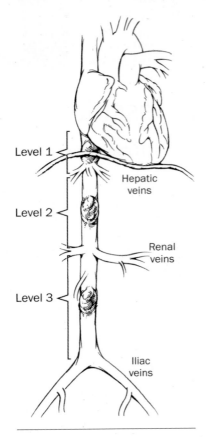

Figure 49.1 Inferior vena cava tumor classification.

defect, but cannot reliably distinguish tumor from benign causes such as deep vein thrombosis. CT and MRI can both accurately demonstrate intraluminal filling defects in the vena cava, and both methods can also demonstrate mass effects and displacement of adjacent organs or structures. Differential enhancement may help to distinguish tumor from clot (especially on T1-weighted images using MRI), and these methods may also identify tumor metastases (11).

It is generally agreed that surgical resection provides the only chance for long-term cure of primary vena caval tumors. Hollenbeck and colleagues (12) reported the results of 25 patients with vena caval leiomyosarcoma, of whom 21 underwent surgical resection. The authors noted that patients who successfully underwent complete resection had significantly better survival than patients who did not (3- and 5-year survival of 76% and 33% for resected patients vs. 0% 3-year survival for unresectable patients).

Although resection of the vena cava is warranted, the operation can be extensive and the anatomic relationships with the hepatic veins and renal veins must be taken into consideration. Tumors in the upper levels of the vena cava (levels 1 and 2) can abut or encompass the hepatic or renal veins. For high level 1 tumors that abut or extend into the right atrium, cardiopulmonary bypass or circulatory arrest may be necessary in order to safely facilitate complete tumor resection (13). For retrohepatic tumors, complete mobilization of the liver from the

diaphragm and IVC may be necessary, in addition to use of a pringle maneuver and venovenous bypass for total venous exclusion of the liver. It is not uncommon for level 2 caval tumors to encompass the proximal renal veins, and to compress adjacent structures such as the adrenal glands, kidneys, or liver. True invasion of adjacent organs is relatively rare, and every attempt should be made to resect the entire tumor. This may necessitate partial hepatectomy, unilateral nephrectomy, or adrenalectomy. If the renal vein origins are involved, they can also be resected and reimplanted into a synthetic tube graft at the time of reconstruction. Level 3 vena caval tumors are generally the least challenging to resect, as they tend to be farther away from major structures such as the renal and hepatic veins. Proximal and distal control of the cava is not as difficult, and venovenous bypass is typically not necessary. Following resection, the vena cava can by repaired primarily if the postresection defect is small enough, or it can be reconstructed with a synthetic (i.e., polytetrafluoroethylene) graft. Additionally, if there is complete occlusion of the vena cava by tumor, and venography demonstrates adequate collateral flow, the cava can also be ligated following resection (14).

The role of adjuvant chemotherapy and radiation therapy is controversial. There is no randomized, prospective data that support the use of adjuvant chemotherapy and radiation therapy in the management of IVC leiomyosarcomas. Although the data regarding the use of adjuvant therapy for these tumors are quite limited, some insight may be gleaned from data regarding the management of retroperitoneal sarcomas. Although there is a clear role for the use of radiation in the treatment of sarcomas of the extremities, the use of radiation in the management of retroperitoneal sarcomas is more controversial. Radiation doses used to treat retroperitoneal sarcomas are typically lower than those used to manage extremity sarcomas because of the increased risk of visceral toxicity. Nevertheless, there is a good body of evidence that adjuvant radiation decreases the 5-year incidence of local recurrence of retroperitoneal sarcomas, although it does not seem to impact survival. There is no convincing data that chemotherapy increases long-term survival after resection of retroperitoneal sarcomas (15,16). Although the data regarding the use of adjuvant chemoradiation in the treatment of vena caval leiomyosarcomas are much more limited than the data with retroperitoneal sarcomas, there are anecdotal reports in the literature that adjuvant therapy may be beneficial (17,18).

When completely resected, IVC tumors have a 5-year survival of 30% to 56% (12,13,19). As with all sarcomas, local recurrence remains a vexing problem. Despite aggressive management, approximately 50% of patients will develop either local recurrence or distant metastases after complete resection (20,21). When metastases occur, they are most frequently in the liver, followed by the lung. Metastases to regional lymph nodes, kidney, and bones have also been documented (6). As with all sarcomas, the major determinant of long-term cure is completeness of resection with negative surgical margins. Palliative resection/debulking offers no survival benefit and resection should not be attempted if attainment of negative margins is deemed impossible or if distant metastases are noted on preoperative workup. There is some evidence to suggest that the location of the primary lesion may determine prognosis. Analysis of the International Registry of Vena Cava Leiomyosarcoma

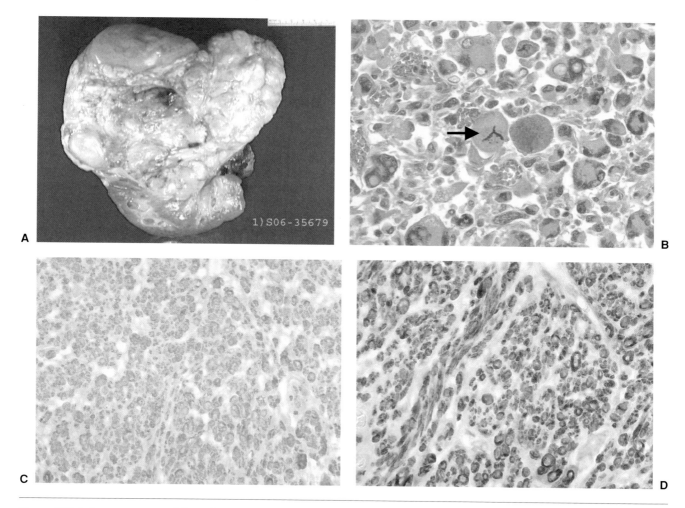

Figure 49.2 Leiomyosarcoma of the inferior vena cava (IVC). (**A**) Gross specimen reveals characteristic fleshy, lobulated, and gray-white appearance. (**B**) Hematoxylin and eosin stain reveals pleomorphic cells with hyperchromic and irregular nuclei. A mitotic figure can be identified (*arrow*). These tumors stain for desmin (**C**) and actin (**D**) on immunohistochemistry analysis. The dense bundles of spindle shaped cells typical of IVC leiomyosarcomas can be seen in image provided by Elizabeth Montgomery (**D**). (See color plates.)

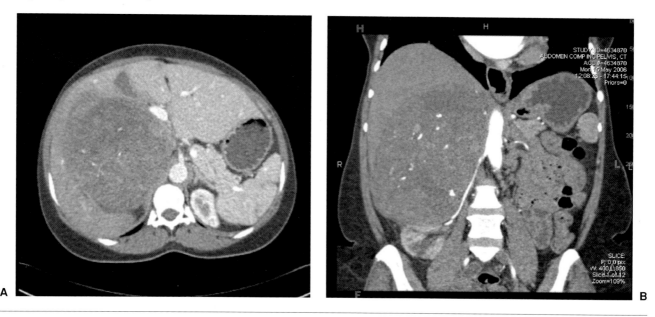

Figure 49.3 Computed tomographic scan of abdomen in patient with a large inferior vena cava tumor on axial (**A**) and sagittal (**B**) images. This tumor displaces the portal vein anteriorly, and the right renal artery inferiorly. Provided by Elizabeth Montgomery.

database has revealed that patients with upper segment tumors that were complicated by lower extremity edema, caval occlusion, or Budd-Chiari syndrome has a worse prognosis. This registry has also noted intraluminal tumor growth to be a negative prognostic sign (20,21). Regardless of the tumor location, there is a clear role for surgery if the possibility of attaining negative margins exists.

Primary Tumors of Large Arteries

Primary tumors of large arteries are also rare, as only 180 cases have been reported in the world literature since the initial description by Brodowski in 1873. More than 90% of these tumors arise from the aorta, and nearly all are malignant. Grossly, these tumors are often intraluminal, and aneurysmal dilatation of the aorta is often seen. Descriptions of the actual lesion vary, but the tumor may often mimic severe atherosclerotic changes of the aortic wall. Tumor elements often have a gray color, and can be rubbery, polypoid, and have hemorrhagic or necrotic elements (22).

Classification of aortic tumors is difficult. In 1972, Salm (23) and colleagues classified these tumors by morphologic characteristics. They described three distinct subtypes: (a) intraluminal: polypoid growths into the vessel lumen with an area of focal attachment to the vessel wall; (b) intimal angiosarcomas: grow along the surface of the vessels and do not project much into the lumen; and (c) adventitial sarcoma: characterized by outward growth from the aorta and invasion of surrounding structures. With further experience and evolution of advanced histologic and immunologic techniques, it has become clear that this gross characterization of aortic tumors is overly simple, and characterization of these lesions is now histologic.

Under microscopy, the tumor can appear very similar to a complex atherosclerotic plaque. Viable tumor cells are seen at the periphery of the tumors with central areas of tumor necrosis and fibrin deposition. Histologically, these tumors are a mixed group, with poorly defined histologic and immunologic characteristics. Most of these aortic tumors originate from precursor cells in the intima of the aorta. Even within intimal sarcomas, there is wide histologic variation. Some authors have suggested that they key to understanding the pathogenesis and prognosis of intimal tumors is to characterize these differences. Sebenik and colleagues (22) have suggested that two variants of intimal sarcoma (undifferentiated and differentiated intimal sarcomas) are actually two distinct disease processes that should be characterized separately. These histologic differences may predict different clinical courses. For instance, undifferentiated intimal sarcomas generally appear a decade later and are associated with 50% shorter survival than differentiated intimal sarcomas. Other sarcoma variants have also been described, including intimal myofibroblastic sarcomas, which contain elements of mesenchymal tissue, and tumors arising from the aortic adventitia have also been described (23).

Aortic malignancies occur most commonly in middle-aged patients with a mean age of 54 years, and tend to be more common in men than women (24). They typically come to medical attention with symptoms caused by peripheral or mesenteric embolization of tumor thrombus. These symptoms can be as vague as generalized fatigue or malaise, but can also include extremity claudication, abdominal pain, or back pain (25–27). Stroke from

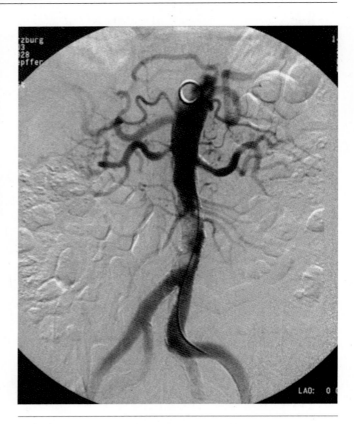

Figure 49.4 Digital subtraction aortography reveals a large infrarenal aortic filling defect from an aortic sarcoma. These lesions often mimic complex atherosclerotic plaques. (Reprinted with permission from ref. 25.)

embolism to cerebral vasculature has also been described (28). These symptoms are identical to symptoms caused by atherosclerotic disease and therefore, the diagnosis of a primary aortic malignancy is often not suspected. Nonspecific symptoms such as back pain could be indicative of metastatic spread to the bones, and carries a graver prognosis.

Because aortic malignancies commonly present with peripheral arterial ischemic symptoms, the workup often proceeds to CT, magnetic resonance angiography, or conventional angiography. On these studies, aortic tumors can mimic more commonly occurring occlusive or aneurysmal disease secondary to atherosclerotic changes (29) (Figure 49.4). As a result, the diagnosis of primary aortic malignancy is usually not made until the pathologic specimen is examined. If the diagnosis is kept in the differential, it may be possible to diagnose these tumors preoperatively.

All patients with evidence of embolic disease should receive an echocardiogram to exclude a mural thrombus or other intracardiac source. If no cardiac source for peripheral embolic disease is found, then CT or magnetic resonance angiography should be obtained to evaluate for potential aortic pathology. On MRI, atheromatous material and tumor have different radiologic enhancement (30). Additionally, infiltration of the wall of the aorta or invasion of other structures and organs can be evaluated with a high level of sensitivity, and MRI can also reveal potential bony metastases (28).

Once the diagnosis of aortic tumor has been established, it is generally agreed that surgical management offers the best chance for cure. Treatment classically consists of en bloc resection of the vessel and contiguous structures, reconstruction with a prosthetic graft, and postoperative chemoradiation therapy (31). Most authors recommend wide resection of the affected vasculature with reconstruction using synthetic graft providing that the patient is able to withstand the operation and does not have evidence of advanced metastatic disease. If tumors are found incidentally in pathologic specimens after endarterectomy, thrombectomy, or revascularization, most authors agree that reoperation and wide resection is indicated.

The role of chemotherapy and radiation therapy has not been clearly established. Because aortic sarcomas are so rare, no prospective, randomized, controlled trials exist to shed light on whether there is clinical benefit to adjuvant therapy. There are data that suggest radiation therapy may increase disease-free survival after resection of angiosarcomas in other locations (e.g., skin). However, it is not clear whether this actually improves overall survival (32). In addition to decreasing local recurrence, radiation has also been used to palliate bony metastases. The role of chemotherapy in the management of aortic sarcomas is even more uncertain. Most currently used adjuvant chemotherapy regimens are doxorubicin-based. In European studies, doxorubicin alone has been used as adjuvant chemotherapy, while in the United States protocols have used doxorubicin in conjunction with isofosfamide, mesna, and dacarbazine. Despite the lack of definitive evidence, there are many advocates of palliative or adjuvant radiation and chemotherapy. In a few small case series, some authors have claimed that aortic sarcomas can be controlled with radiation or chemotherapy if limited metastasis or unresectable local recurrence is present (33,34).

Overall, despite all modalities of treatment, long-term survival for primary aortic malignancies remains dismal. Although surgery and adjuvant therapies may provide some palliation from this aggressive disease, there are no objective data that either actually improves survival. Autopsy studies show that distant metastasis to bone, kidneys, liver, the adrenal glands, and lungs can be found in 80% of patients (35). Mean overall survival is around 16 months while mean survival at 5 years is a dismal 8% (36).

TUMORS OF SMALL BLOOD VESSELS AND LYMPHATICS

In addition to major blood vessels, primary vascular malignancies can occur in smaller vessels throughout the body. Like tumors found in large arteries and veins, these tumors tend to be sarcomas, but the histologic subtypes are varied. Overall, these vascular sarcomas make up <1% of all known sarcomas. The majority of these tumors are angiosarcomas that arise from endothelial cells in blood vessels from almost every major organ, but most commonly in the skin. They are particularly common in the head and neck area (37–43) (Figure 49.5). Angiosarcomas tend to be aggressive tumors that most commonly occur in the seventh decade of life. Metastasis via both vascular and lymphatic routes is common, and 53% of patients die by 11 months (44). Although the etiologic factors that lead to angiosarcomas

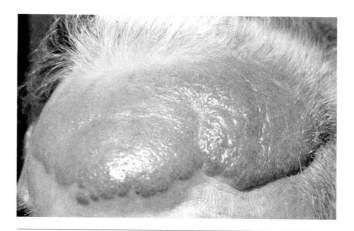

Figure 49.5 Angiosarcoma of the scalp. These tumors most commonly present in the skin of the head and neck regions in elderly patients. (See color plates.)

have not been completely elucidated, radiation and chronic lymphedema have been associated with its occurrence (43).

Other major small vessel tumor subtypes include malignant hemangiopericytomas, epithelioid hemangioendotheliomas, and lymphangiosarcomas. Hemangiopericytomas arise from a blood vessel cell type known as the *Zimmerman pericyte*, which are modified smooth muscle cells located outside the basement membrane. These tumors can occur anywhere in the body, but most frequently occur in the pelvis and retroperitoneum. Epithelial hemangioendotheliomas arise from endothelial cells and often show significant atypia and mitotic activity. These tumors are usually less aggressive than angiosarcomas, and seem to occur more commonly in women. Lymphangiosarcomas are angiosarcomas that arise from lymph vessels in the setting of chronic lymphedema. Most often this occurs in the upper extremity of patients with chronic lymphedema postmastectomy, and is termed *Stewart-Treves syndrome*. These tumors occur on average 10 years after mastectomy and present as blue or purple elevations on chronically edematous skin (45,46).

There are few data regarding the contemporary management and outcomes of malignant vascular tumors of small blood vessels and lymphatics. Leowardi and colleagues (46) recently published a relatively large single-institution observational study regarding the management of 43 malignant vascular tumors (30 primary, 13 recurrent) in a variety of locations. In their series, 90% of patients with these tumors presented with clinical symptoms that were most commonly reported as pain or a palpable mass lesion. Other symptoms cited by the authors included extrusion, hemorrhage, weight loss, and fatigue. Complete resections were performed in 32 patients, and microscopically negative margins were achieved in 23 patients (53.5%). Median survival for all patients was 21.4 months. In their study, tumor location was the best predictor of survival following surgical resection. Patients with tumors located in the extremities and trunk had the best 5-year survival (67.1% and 60.4%, respectively), while patients with intra-abdominal and retroperitoneal tumors had poor survival (22.1% and 14.7%, respectively). The presence of metastatic disease was also a poor prognostic indicator. The histologic subtypes of the resected malignant vascular tumors did not affect 5-year survival, as all seemed to be equally aggressive.

REFERENCES

1. Burke AP, Virmani R. Sarcomas of the great vessels. A clinicopathologic study. *Cancer.* 19931;71:1761–1773.

2. Griffin AS, Sterchi JM. Primary leiomyosarcoma of the inferior vena cava: a case report and review of the literature. *J Surg Oncol.* 1987;34:53–60.

3. Dzsinich C, Gloviczki P, van Heerden JA, et al.Primary venous leiomyosarcoma: a rare but lethal disease. *J Vasc Surg.* 1992;15:595–603.

4. Bailey RV, Stribling J, Weitzner S, et al. Leiomyosarcoma of the inferior vena cava: report of a case and review of the literature. *Ann Surg.* 1976;184:169–173.

5. Monig SP, Gawenda M, Erasmi H, et al. Diagnosis, treatment and prognosis of the leiomyosarcoma of the inferior vena cava. Three cases and summary of published reports. *Eur J Surg.* 1995;161:231–235.

6. Hilliard NJ, Heslin MJ, Castro CY. Leiomyosarcoma of the inferior vena cava: three case reports and review of the literature. *Ann Diagn Pathol.* 2005;9:259–266.

7. Yuzer Y, Zeytunlu M, Makay O, et al. Leiomyosarcoma of the inferior vena cava: report of a case. *Surg Today.* 2004;34:370–373.

8. Parwani AV, Yang B, Erozan YS, et al. Pathologic quiz case: a 54-year-old man with hypertension. Primary high-grade leiomyosarcoma of the IVC. *Arch Pathol Lab Med.* 2003;127:e423–424.

9. Weiss S, Goldblum J, eds. *Enzinger and Weiss's Soft Tissue Tumors.* St. Louis, MO: Mosby; 2001.

10. Gowda RM, Gowda MR, Mehta NJ, et al. Right atrial extension of primary venous leiomyosarcoma: pulmonary embolism and Budd-Chiari syndrome at presentation-a case report. *Angiology.* 2004;55:213–216.

11. Hemant D, Krantikumar R, Amita J, et al. Primary leiomyosarcoma of the inferior vena cava, a rare entity. Imaging features. *Australis Radiol.* 2001;45:448–451.

12. Hollenbeck ST, Grobmyer SR, Kent KC, et al. Surgical treatment and outcomes of patients with primary inferior vena cava leiomyosarcoma. *J Am Coll Surg.* 2003;197:575–579.

13. Laas J, Schmid C, Allhoff E, et al. Tumor-related obstruction of the inferior vena cava extending into the right heart–a plea for surgery in deep hypothermic circulatory arrest. *Eur J Cardiothorac Surg.* 1991;5:653–656.

14. Dew J, Hansen K, Hammon J, et al. Leiomyosarcoma of the inferior vena cava: surgical management and clinical results. *Am Surg.* 2005;71:497–501.

15. Mendenhall WM, Zlotecki RA, Hochwald SN, et al. Retroperitoneal soft tissue sarcoma. *Cancer.* 200515;104:669–675.

16. Lewis JJ, Leung D, Woodruff JM, et al. Retroperitoneal soft-tissue sarcoma: analysis of 500 patients treated and followed at a single institution. *Ann Surg.* 1998;228:355–365.

17. Abisi S, Morris-Stiff GJ, Scott-Coombes D, et al. Leiomyosarcoma of the inferior vena cava: clinical experience with four cases. *World J Surg Oncol.* 2006;;4:1.

18. Alektiar KM, Hu K, Anderson L, et al. High-dose-rate intraoperative radiation therapy (HDR-IORT) for retroperitoneal sarcomas. *Int J Radiat Oncol Biol Phys.* 2000;47:157–163.

19. Kulaylat MN, Karakousis CP, Doerr RJ, et al. Leiomyosarcoma of the inferior vena cava: a clinicopathologic review and report of three cases. *J Surg Oncol.* 1997;65:205–217.

20. Mingoli A, Cavallaro A, Sapienza P, et al. International registry of inferior vena cava leiomyosarcoma: analysis of a world series on 218 patients. Anticancer Res. 1996 Sep-Oct;16(5B):3201–3205.

21. Mingoli A, Feldhaus RJ, Cavallaro A, Stipa S. Leiomyosarcoma of the inferior vena cava: analysis and search of world literature on 141 patients and report of three new cases. *J Vasc Surg.* 1991;14:688–699.

22. Sebenik M, Ricci A Jr, DiPasquale B, et al.Undifferentiated intimal sarcoma of large systemic blood vessels: report of 14 cases with immunohistochemical profile and review of the literature. *Am J Surg Pathol.* 2005;29:1184–1193.

23. Salm R. Primary fibrosarcoma of aorta. *Cancer.* 1972;29:73–83.

24. Shuster TA, Dall'Olmo CA, Spadone D, et al. Abdominal aortic sarcoma: report of a case with long-term survival and review of the literature [published online ahead of print August 19, 2002]. *Ann Vasc Surg.* 2002;16:545–549.

25. Thalheimer A, Fein M, Geissinger E, et al. Intimal angiosarcoma of the aorta: report of a case and review of the literature. *J Vasc Surg.* 2004;40:548–553.

26. Tulsyan N, Valentin MD, Ombrellino M, et al. Recurrent aortic angiosarcoma–a case report and review of the literature. *Angiology.* 2006;57:123–125.

27. Kwon TW, Kim DK, Kim GE, et al. Sarcoma of the abdominal aorta involving marginal arteries of the small intestine: a case report. *Ann Vasc Surg.* 2005;19:719–723.

28. Mohsen NA, Haber M, Urrutia VC, et al. Intimal sarcoma of the aorta. *AJR Am J Roentgenol.* 2000;175:1289–1290.

29. Hagspiel KD, Hunter YR, Ahmed HK, et al. Primary sarcoma of the distal abdominal aorta: CT angiography findings [published online ahead of print May 12, 2004]. *Abdom Imaging.* 2004;29:507–510.

30. Higgins R, Posner MC, Moosa HH, et al. Mesenteric infarction secondary to tumor emboli from primary aortic sarcoma. Guidelines for diagnosis and management. *Cancer.* 1991;68:1622–1627.

31. Abularrage CJ, Weiswasser JM, White PW, et al. Aortic angiosarcoma presenting as distal arterial embolization. *Ann Vasc Surg.* 2005;19:744–748.

32. Brand CU, Yawalkar N, von Briel C, et al. Combined surgical and X-ray treatment for angiosarcoma of the scalp: report of a case with a favourable outcome. *Br J Dermatol.* 1996;134:763–765.

33. Bohner H, Luther B, Braunstein S, et al. Primary malignant tumors of the aorta: clinical presentation, treatment, and course of different entities. *J Vasc Surg.* 2003;38:1430–1433.

34. Majeski J, Crawford ES, Majeski EI, et al. Primary aortic intimal sarcoma of the endothelial cell type with long-term survival. *J Vasc Surg.* 1998;27:555–558.

35. Seelig MH, Klingler PJ, Oldenburg WA, et al. Angiosarcoma of the aorta: report of a case and review of the literature. *J Vasc Surg.* 1998;28:732–737.

36. Chiche L, Mongredien B, Brocheriou I, et al. Primary tumors of the thoracoabdominal aorta: surgical treatment of 5 patients and review of the literature. *Ann Vasc Surg.* 2003;17:354–364.

37. Kurian KC, Weisshaar D, Parekh H, et al. Primary cardiac angiosarcoma: case report and review of the literature. *Cardiovasc Pathol.* 2006;15:110–112.

38. Catena F, Santini D, Di Saverio S, et al. Skin angiosarcoma arising in an irradiated breast: case-report and literature review. *Dermatol Surg.* 2006;32:447–455.

39. Leowardi C, Hormann Y, Hinz U, et al. Ruptured angiosarcoma of the liver treated by emergency catheter-directed embolization. *World J Gastroenterol.* 2006;12:804–808.

40. Fodor J, Orosz Z, Szabo E, et al. Angiosarcoma after conservation treatment for breast carcinoma: our experience and a review of the literature. *J Am Acad Dermatol.* 2006;54:499–504.

41. Brown CJ, Falck VG, MacLean A. Angiosarcoma of the colon and rectum: report of a case and review of the literature. *Dis Colon Rectum.* 2004;47:2202–2207.

42. Allison KH, Yoder BJ, Bronner MP, et al. Angiosarcoma involving the gastrointestinal tract: a series of primary and metastatic cases. *Am J Surg Pathol.* 2004;28:298–307.

43. McIntosh BC, Narayan D. Head and neck angiosarcomas. *J Craniofac Surg.* 2005;16:699–703.

44. Meis-Kindblom JM, Kindblom LG. Angiosarcoma of soft tissue: a study of 80 cases. *Am J Surg Pathol.* 1998;22:683–697.

45. O'Hara CD, Nascimento AG. Endothelial lesions of soft tissues: a review of reactive and neoplastic entities with emphasis on low-grade malignant ("borderline") vascular tumors. *Adv Anat Pathol.* 2003;10:69–87.

46. Leowardi C, Hinz U, Hormann Y, et al. Malignant vascular tumors: clinical presentation, surgical therapy, and long-term prognosis. *Ann Surg Oncol.* 2005;12:1090–1101.

COMMENTARY
Bruce L. Gewertz

This commentary will focus on the most common primary vascular tumors—leiomyosarcomas of the inferior vena cava (IVC). As pointed out in the preceding chapter, even these tumors are rare. Although fewer than 500 cases have been documented in published clinical series, doubtless numerous others have been treated in sporadic personal experiences. The major diagnostic challenge is differentiating such primary vascular tumors from the slightly more common retroperitoneal soft-tissue sarcomas with secondary compression of the IVC. Both types of malignancies can present with an abdominal mass, pain, and lower extremity swelling, and occur in patients in the fifth decade of life. It is well recognized that the prognosis is slightly better in soft-tissue sarcomas even in those patients with vascular involvement (5-year survival >50% in soft-tissue sarcomas vs. 30% to 50% in primary caval tumors) (1,2,3).

Over the last decade, precise diagnosis of caval tumors has been greatly advanced by computerized tomography and magnetic resonance imaging. Still, the less sophisticated tests of ascending and descending cavography frequently provide valuable information about the nature and extent of the tumors. Phlebography can often complete the anatomic classification of the tumors, which depends on the proximal extent of the process; specifically, the involvement of the renal and hepatic veins (level 1, infrarenal; level 2, suprarenal below major hepatic veins; level 3, suprarenal with hepatic vein involvement) (3). In some patients, celiac angiography may also be useful, especially if hepatic involvement is suspected.

In a number of recent and relatively large clinical series (>25 patients), it is increasingly clear that complete resection of these tumors at the initial operation is the only chance for cure (1–2). Although it would be reasonable to think that tumor grade may have some influence on prognosis, no such relationship has been demonstrated either because of the actual biologic behavior or the relatively small number of reports, which may limit statistical power.

To date, the benefits of postoperative radiation and chemotherapy are not well defined. Some centers recommend both modalities because of the generally unfavorable outlook for these lesions. Others treat selectively, using chemotherapy in most patients and reserving radiation for local recurrence.

Given the central role of complete resection in providing the best chance of cure, any discussion of these lesions must properly focus on the operative approach. Adequate preoperative assessment allows selection of the best incision and exposure. Midline abdominal incisions are satisfactory for tumors confined to the infra- or perirenal cava. In lesions involving the hepatic veins, an extended right subcostal incision with extension into a median sternotomy affords ideal exposure (2).

Because primary caval tumors rarely extend into the aorta or other viscera, resection of level 1 lesions involving only the infrarenal cava are generally straightforward. Irrespective of the extent of the tumor, the entire infrarenal cava should be resected. Even though it may seem possible in some lateral tumors to resect only the involved portion of the vessel and use an autologous vein patch for reconstruction, such minimalist resections should be avoided because of the primacy of complete initial removal in producing a cure. Historically, simple resection with caval ligation has been advocated. Unfortunately, significant lower extremity edema may occur after ligation, leading most surgeons to now prefer reconstruction of the cava with prosthetic grafts (1,2).

This author prefers externally reinforced, but thin-walled polytetrafluoroethylene, for caval replacement. An omental flap is often used to separate the graft from the bowel. I also create an autogenous arteriovenous fistula between the femoral artery and vein to increase flow through the graft in the immediate postoperative period. The short loop can be placed in a superficial position in the groin such that ligation can be performed easily. Postoperative use of anticoagulation is not clearly indicated, although I have usually maintained low-dose heparin in the immediate postoperative period followed in 5 days by warfarin to maintain an international normalized ratio of 1.5 to 2.

The resection of juxtarenal lesions (level 2) is more complicated because of the likelihood of renal vein involvement. Nonetheless, the principle of complete resection should be applied and clean margins should never be sacrificed. Because of the short right renal vein, autotransplantation (or even unilateral nephrectomy) may be needed in some patients.

The operative management of level 3 tumors is obviously more complicated and far more challenging. Every ancillary technique to minimize intraoperative venous hypertension should be considered including the venovenous bypasses now widely used in liver transplantation. Hypothermic perfusion of the liver may also be helpful in complex reconstructions; cardiopulmonary bypass and total circulatory arrest have also been used (2,3). The principle difficulty of these resections is achieving tumor-free margins while maintaining enough of a caval cuff that incorporates the orifices of the major hepatic veins. This may require careful "syndactylization" of these veins prior to venous anastomosis. After reconstitution of venous outflow, it is important to critically assess the degree of venous congestion in the liver and consider partial hepatectomy if the poor outflow is not remediable.

In summary, the chance to positively impact the survival of patients with these unusual lesions is fully dependent on the adequacy of the initial surgical resection. Every ancillary technique should be considered to produce the superior exposure and unhurried environment that favors complete resection.

REFERENCES

1. Dew J, Hansen K, Hammon J, et al. Leiomyosarcoma of the inferior vena cava: surgical management and clinical results. *Am Surg.* 2005;71:497–501.

2. Kieffer E, Alaoui M, Piette JC, et al. Leiomyosarcoma of the inferior vena cava: experience in 22 cases. *Ann Surg.* 2006;244:289–295.

3. Schwarzbach MH, Hormann Y, Hinz U, et al. Clinical results of surgery for retroperitoneal sarcoma with major blood vessel involvement. *J Vasc Surg.* 2006;44:46–55.

4. Illuminati G, Calio' FG, D'Urso A, et al. Prosthetic replacement of the infrahepatic inferior vena cava for leiomyosarcoma. *Arch Surg.* 2006;141:919–924.

50

Diagnosis and Management of Thyroid Cancer

James A. Lee and Orlo H. Clark

With over 30,000 new cases diagnosed each year, the incidence of thyroid cancer is increasing faster than any other cancer in the United States at a rate of 4.3% per year (1). Thyroid cancer accounts for 95% of all endocrine cancers and is by far the most common endocrine malignancy. Excluding ovarian cancer, it is also the most lethal endocrine cancer (1,2). Although the majority of patients with thyroid cancer have a good prognosis, 5% to 10% of patients eventually succumb to their disease (3). In general, thyroid cancer is best considered under the rubric of well-differentiated versus poorly differentiated or anaplastic cancers as the prognosis and treatment for each differs radically.

WELL-DIFFERENTIATED THYROID CANCERS

Classification and Epidemiology

Well-differentiated thyroid cancers (WDTCs) comprise up to 98% of all cases of thyroid cancer and include tumors arising from follicular cells (papillary, follicular, and Hürthle cell cancers) and parafollicular cells (medullary thyroid cancer). Incidence rates of the different subtypes of differentiated thyroid cancers vary depending on ethnicity and geography, but generally the incidence is between 0.5 and 10 cases per 100,000 women (3). Fewer than 10% of cases occur in patients younger than 21 years old (4).

Papillary Thyroid Cancer

Papillary thyroid cancer (PTC) accounts for 80% of all thyroid cancer cases. PTC has a peak incidence in the third decade of life and has a 2:1 female to male predilection. The peak age of presentation is between 38 and 45 years old. Risk factors for PTC include exposure to ionizing radiation, family history of thyroid cancer, and high-iodine diets. Up to 85% of PTCs are multifocal on final pathologic examination (5–8). In most series, 30% to 40% of patients will have cervical lymph node metastases at the time of diagnosis. However, up to 80% of patients may have micrometastatic nodal disease when prophylactic node dissection is performed (7–11). Distant metastases are uncommon, with only 2% to 14% of patients presenting with lung, bone, or liver disease (5,6,8). The overall 20-year survival for PTC is >90% and only 20% of patients will have clinically significant recurrent disease (9,12–15). Occult or minimal PTCs are PTCs that are <1 cm. The prevalence of occult PTC greatly depends on the region studied, age of the patient, and number of histologic sections examined and is estimated at 0.45% to 36% (16). Surprisingly, autopsy studies reveal that up to 16% of patients with

occult PTC will have cervical lymph node metastases (10). Because of the uniformly excellent prognosis (0% to 0.4% mortality rate), many physicians advocate conservative treatment with thyroid lobectomy and isthmusectomy followed by thyroid hormone suppression for most occult PTC (17–19). Exceptions to this rule include patients with a radiation history, family history of thyroid cancer, angioinvasive tumors, contralateral nodules or cancer, lymph node metastases, or multifocal PTC on pathologic examination of the removed lobe. Approximately 1% of all PTC will dedifferentiate to anaplastic thyroid cancer (18,19).

The follicular variant of PTC is an emerging subset of PTC. Histologically, these tumors must have at least 80% follicular architecture while having some or all of the classic nuclear features of PTC, which include nuclear grooving, Orphan Annie eye nuclei, intranuclear inclusion bodies, and hyperchromatic nuclei. Fortunately, these tumors have a disease course and prognosis similar to PTC.

Follicular Thyroid Cancer

Follicular thyroid cancer (FTC) comprises 10% to 20% of all thyroid cancer cases. Approximately 20% of patients with a follicular neoplasm on fine-needle aspiration biopsy will have FTC. Often associated with benign thyroid disease and iodine deficiency, the incidence of FTC has been decreasing with the salt iodination program in the United States. FTC is not associated with radiation exposure. FTC also tends to occur in women, although patients are typically older (fourth and fifth decades of life) and present with slightly later stage disease than patients with PTC. Unlike PTC, most FTC is unifocal, with 90% having a single lesion (20). Because FTC spreads hematogenously, <10% of patients will have cervical lymph node metastases. However, up to 33% of patients will have distant metastasis to the lungs, bone, or liver. Although patients with FTC have an overall worse 10-year survival rate than patients with PTC, the prognosis is similar when matched for age (20,23). Patients without recurrence of FTC within 12 years of operation are considered cured and lifelong surveillance is not necessary. Patients with minimally invasive FTC (tumors with limited capsular invasion or angioinvasion) have an excellent prognosis (20,24).

Hürthle Cell Cancer

The exact genealogy of Hürthle cell cancer (HCC) is debatable, with various experts classifying it as a variant of FTC, a variant of PTC, or as a distinct subtype. HCC demonstrates unique histologic features that include oxyphilic, polygonal oncocytes with hyperchromatic nuclei. HCC accounts for 3% of all thyroid cancers and has a strong female predilection with a peak incidence in the fifth to sixth decades of life. Radiation exposure and a family history of HCC are known risk factors for HCC. Patients with HCC have a 25% rate of lymph node metastases, 10% rate of radioactive iodine (RAI) uptake (vs. 70% for PTC and 80% for FTC), and a 30% recurrence rate (25). In contrast to PTC and FTC, HCC is a somewhat more aggressive cancer (correlating with DNA ploidy) with a 30% 20-year mortality rate (16,26).

Medullary Thyroid Cancer

Although medullary thyroid cancer (MTC) accounts for only 7% to 8% of all thyroid cancers, it comprises 15% of thyroid cancer deaths. The parafollicular cells or "C cells" give rise to MTC; therefore, these tumors are almost always found laterally in the upper to middle portion of the thyroid. MTC has a sporadic form (85% unilateral with a single focus) and a hereditary form (90% multifocal and bilateral). Over 50% of patients will have disease in regional lymph nodes (especially in the central neck) at the time of diagnosis, and this rate increases to over 80% in patients with a palpable primary (27,28). The prognosis for MTC is worse than for PTC with a 78% 10-year survival that plummets to a 35% 5-year survival with the presence of distant metastases (27). Patients with occult MTC have a better prognosis but should undergo completion thyroidectomy with neck dissection for patients with an elevated basal or pentagastrin-stimulated calcitonin, microcarcinomas >5mm in diameter, or if they are difficult to follow.

Hereditary MTCs occur in 25% of cases and are associated with point mutations in the *RET* proto-oncogene. Interestingly, up to 10% of spontaneous MTC cases may have de novo mutations in the *RET* proto-oncogene as well. Hereditary MTC is divided into familial MTC (FMTC) and multiple endocrine neoplasia type 2A and 2B (MEN-2A and -2B). MEN-2A accounts for two thirds of hereditary MTC. The diagnosis of FMTC is confirmed when three or more family members have MTC without the manifestations of MEN-2A or -2B (i.e., pheochromocytoma and hyperparathyroidism or Marfanoid habitus and ganglioneuromas respectively). All patients with MTC should undergo genetic testing for *RET* mutations. A missense mutation occurs in codon 634 in 80% of patients with MEN-2A, and more aggressive MTC is seen with mutations in codons 883, 918, and 922 (27,29). Approximately 98% of patients with MEN-2B have a mutation in codons 918 (95%) or 883 (3%). Patients with MEN-2B have the most aggressive MTCs. If the *RET* mutation screen is negative, there is a <1% chance that the patient has hereditary MTC (27). The families of MTC patients with a *RET* mutation should undergo testing for the specific mutation found in the index case. All patients with MTC should be screened for a pheochromocytoma and primary hyperparathyroidism prior to thyroidectomy as up to 20% of patients will have these disorders. For patients with MEN-2A, up to 42% will have a pheochromocytoma and 35% will have hyperparathyroidism. Patients with MEN-2B develop pheochromocytomas in 50% and neurogangliomas in nearly 100% of cases (27,30).

Diagnosis and Risk-assessment
Presentation

A palpable thyroid nodule is the most common presentation for patients with differentiated thyroid cancers. A history of voice change, hemoptysis, compressive symptoms (dysphagia, stridor, dyspnea), rapid growth, significant radiation to the head and neck, and personal or family history of thyroid cancer increase the patient's risk of cancer. Flushing and diarrhea are suggestive of MTC, and patients with these symptoms generally have a worse prognosis (27,30). Radiation exposure has both an age- and dose-related effect on the risk of developing thyroid cancer. Patients who received low doses of ionizing radiation, up to 60 Gray, have a 1% to 13% chance of developing thyroid cancer. In addition, multiple studies have shown that the younger the patient at the time of exposure (especially those younger than 5 years), the greater the risk of WDTC (31–35). In contrast, patients over 20 years at the time of exposure have only a minimally increased risk of thyroid cancer. Radiation-induced malignancies have a peak incidence at 20 to 30 years postexposure, but can occur as soon as 4 years and as late as 50 years postexposure (36–39). A patient with a thyroid nodule and a history of neck irradiation has a 40% chance of having thyroid cancer, with 60% of these cancers found in the dominant nodule (40,41). Radiation-induced PTC tends to be multicentric but is of similar aggressiveness as non-radiation-induced PTC (36).

The most common nonmedullary familial thyroid cancer, familial PTC accounts for 5% of all PTC and is typically diagnosed at an earlier age (35 to 38 years old) than nonfamilial PTC (3). Familial PTC tends to be multifocal with a higher recurrence rate of 33% (42,43). Furthermore, familial PTC may be more aggressive, especially in families with more than three affected members (43).

Concerning physical examination signs include a fixed or invasive nodule, palpable lymph nodes, and hoarse voice. Up to one third of patients with PTC will have palpable cervical lymphadenopathy (44). A normal or elevated thyroid-stimulating hormone (TSH) can rule out a hyperfunctioning nodule, which has only a 1% chance of being malignant. High elevations in serum thyroglobulin (especially in the setting of a sonographically normal-sized thyroid) are often indicative of metastatic disease. Levels >300 may signify the presence of pulmonary or bony metastases, with levels >1,000 typically indicating bony disease (45). Elevated serum calcitonin or carcinoembryonic antigen (CEA) levels are suggestive of MTC and, like thyroglobulin, often reflects tumor volume (27). Calcitonin levels >1,000 typically signify liver metastases, the most common distant metastatic site. These liver metastases are often military and not well seen on computed tomography or magnetic resonance imaging scan. Patients with a calcitonin doubling time <6 months had a 10-year survival of 8% compared with 100% with doubling times >2 years (46). High CEA levels are also associated with a worse prognosis.

Fine-Needle Aspiration Biopsy

Aside from surgical removal of the thyroid, fine-needle aspiration biopsy (FNAB) is the best means of differentiating between the varieties of thyroid pathology and is the diagnostic test of choice. Typically the dominant nodule is biopsied, but other nodules or lymph nodes may be biopsied if there are suspicious features on physical examination or ultrasound. On cytologic review, the FNAB is classified as inadequate, benign, malignant (papillary, medullary, or anaplastic thyroid cancer), or indeterminate (follicular or Hürthle cell neoplasm). An inadequate sampling should be repeated. A reading of benign disease has a 95% to 97% accuracy and false-negative rate of 2-6% (44). PTC is readily distinguished on FNAB based on classic cellular features such as nuclear grooving, Orphan Annie eye nuclei, intranuclear inclusion bodies, and hyperchromatic nuclei. A reading of malignancy has 97% to 99% accuracy. Unfortunately, follicular and Hürthle cell cancers have no pathognomonic cellular features, and therefore examination of the entire capsule for evidence of invasion or angioinvasion is necessary. Therefore, FNAB cannot make the diagnosis of FCC or HCC and can only be classified as a "suspicious" or "indeterminate" neoplasm. An indeterminate reading carries a 20% risk of cancer for a follicular neoplasm and 35% for Hürthle cell neoplasm. An indeterminate reading is an indication for a diagnostic lobectomy and isthmusectomy. If the patient has FTC or HCC on permanent histology, then completion thyroidectomy is usually warranted. Special stains for calcitonin and thyroglobulin may help in the diagnosis of medullary cancer or metastatic thyroid cancer in a lymph node, respectively. Combining FNAB with molecular marker analysis is an area of active research that may deliver increasing diagnostic accuracy.

Cervical Ultrasound

Cervical ultrasound (USG) is a crucial part of the evaluation of patients with thyroid nodules or suspected thyroid cancer. With improvements in resolution and increasing operator experience, USG can often be used to make the diagnosis of thyroid cancer prior to FNAB or excision. The classic sonographic findings of thyroid cancer include solid, hypoechoic nodules with either small or coarse echogenic foci, irregular borders, and/or refractive shadows from the edges of the nodule. Up to 63% to 90% of PTCs are solid and hypoechoic, although 13% will have a cystic component (47,48). Almost all MTCs are hypoechoic. Unfortunately, 55% of benign nodules are also hypoechoic. Internal calcifications, which are intensely echogenic, are more specific signs of malignancy. In particular, microcalcifications, which usually do not cause acoustic shadowing, have a specificity of 93% to 95% for cancer and a positive predictive value of 70% (47,49). Although punctate calcifications are quite specific for the Psammoma bodies seen in PTC, coarse calcifications may be seen in both PTC as well as MTC. In MTC, these coarse calcifications are caused by calcification of amyloid deposits and are seen predominantly in the center of the nodule. In contrast, coarse calcifications in PTC are typically calcified foci of fibrosis or degeneration. Although coarse calcifications may also be seen in multinodular goiters, benign lesions typically have dense, peripheral calcifications that increase with frequency and density the longer the goiter has been present (50). Irregular borders are suggestive of cancer, but not universally present. Indeed, many PTCs will have a sonographically smooth and intact capsule (47). Shadowing at the edges of a nodule is worrisome for cancer, but may also be present in benign cystic lesions (47). Hypervascularity within the nodule is also associated with an increased risk of malignancy (30). Finally, invasion into surrounding structures is a clear indication of malignancy. Of course, these same characteristics suggest regional metastatic disease when seen in cervical lymph nodes and make ultrasound an important adjunct to surveillance for recurrence. In fact, USG may reveal metastatic disease as small as a few millimeters. USG-guided FNAB can confirm the diagnosis of lymph node metastases.

Risk Assessment

Over the years, many scoring systems have been developed to gauge the prognosis of patients with thyroid cancer. The most important favorable prognostic factors appear to be small tumor size (<4 cm), absence of invasion or metastases, young age (between 16 and 45 years), and female sex. Tumor characteristics that convey a worse prognosis include aneuploidy, decreased RAI uptake, decreased cAMP response to TSH, increased epidermal growth factor binding, *p53* mutations, increased *c-myc* expression, and combined *N-ras* and *gsp* mutations (51–58). Although the presence of lymph nodes increases recurrence, it has minimal impact on tumor-specific mortality (52). Most scoring systems use a combination of prognostic factors to segregate patients into high and low risk groups. AGES (age, grade of tumor, extrathyroidal invasion or metastases, and tumor size) was one of the first scoring systems that fell out of favor because there was no uniform scheme for determining grade among pathologists. The MACIS system (metastases, age, completeness of resection, invasion, and tumor size) is perhaps the most widely known system and reliably predicts outcomes in patients with PTC (59). In contrast to the TNM scores for other cancers, the TNM classification for thyroid cancer also takes into account the patient's age (those younger than 45 years have a maximum stage of I or II and those over 45 years can be any stage I to IV). These scoring systems, and many others, all take into account age and tumor size.

Typically, high-risk patients have a 40% to 50% mortality versus a 2% to 5% mortality for low-risk patients (7,9,59). Fortunately, up to 85% of patients fall into this low-risk group (60). Interestingly, a subset of low-risk patients is at higher risk for recurrence, which may be predicted based on age (<16 or >45 years), histologic subtype (tall-cell, columnar variant, diffusesclerosing, HCCs, and poorly differentiated tumors), large tumors (>4 cm), and those with extrathyroidal invasion or distant metastases. Unfortunately, all of these prognostic scores depend on intraoperative findings and therefore cannot be used to plan the extent of surgical resection needed.

Treatment

Total Thyroidectomy Versus Isthmusectomy and Lobectomy

The guiding principle of operative therapy is complete resection of the primary tumor. However, the extent of surgical excision is somewhat controversial. Most physicians agree that total or near-total thyroidectomy is indicated for high-risk patients and patients with a clinically significant radiation exposure or family history of thyroid cancer. For low-risk patients, some groups advocate lobectomy and isthmusectomy instead of total thyroidectomy. Proponents of less extensive resection cite the excellent prognosis of these patients with either procedure, the minimal clinical significance of multicentricity, and the increased number of recurrent laryngeal nerves and parathyroids at risk for injury during total thyroidectomy (16). Certainly for occult PTC or microinvasive FTC (capsular invasion only), multiple studies have failed to show a survival benefit with total thyroidectomy versus lobectomy and isthmusectomy (36). In contrast, advocates for total or near-total thyroidectomy claim that more extensive resection has multiple advantages that include (a) easier detection and treatment of recurrence because it allows for RAI ablation of thyroid remnants, (b) increased sensitivity of thyroglobulin as a marker of persistence or recurrence (after total thyroidectomy, thyroglobulin levels should be <2 ng/mL), (c) eliminated risk of recurrence in the contralateral lobe, (d) lower recurrence rate after total thyroidectomy, (e) improved survival in patients with PTC >1.5 cm and invasive FTC, (f) improved survival rates in high-risk patients, and (g) decreased need for reoperation (16,61). Indeed, most retrospective studies demonstrated a significantly lower recurrence rate after total thyroidectomy with all stages of thyroid cancer (62–64). Although there is only a 7% recurrence rate in the contralateral lobe, approximately 50% of these patients will die from their disease (61). Perhaps the most compelling argument for total thyroidectomy is that all of the scoring systems rely on intraoperative data to assess the risk of the patient. Therefore, it is impossible to determine preoperatively which patients will be adversely affected by a less complete resection. Of note, one of the few uses of external-beam radiation therapy for thyroid cancer is to treat gross residual disease postoperatively (e.g., after shaving tumor off the trachea or esophagus).

Prophylactic Versus Therapeutic Lymph Node Dissection

Most experts recommend therapeutic compartment-based lymph node dissection rather than prophylactic neck dissection (i.e., when there is no evidence of lymph node metastases by ultrasound or physical examination). Although up to 80% of patients with PTC will have microscopic lymph node disease at the time of diagnosis in prophylactic node dissection studies, most of these will not become clinically significant. As mentioned, only 20% to 30% of patients will ultimately have clinically significant lymph node metastases. Furthermore, many studies demonstrate that survival and recurrence rates are equivalent in patients with and without lymph node disease, although matted nodes carry a worse prognosis (9,10,61,64). These studies also demonstrate that patients with PTC have nearly identical survival rates when treated with prophylactic lymph node dissection or observation alone. The presence of palpable cervical lymph nodes is a clear indication for therapeutic lymph node dissection. Intraoperative discovery of lymph node metastases should be confirmed by frozen section and a central and lateral neck dissection should be performed. Abnormal lymph nodes identified by ultrasound examination should also be removed. So-called berry picking has a higher rate of recurrence than compartment-based neck dissection and should be discouraged. Prophylactic neck dissection may increase the frequency of complications, especially hypoparathyroidism. This risk of hypoparathyroidism has prompted some groups to routinely autotransplant parathyroids after prophylactic neck dissection. Despite these risks, prophylactic neck dissection has certain indications. For example, some Japanese surgeons advocate prophylactic neck dissection because RAI is not commonly used in Japan (8). Also, in cases of known HCC, some surgeons perform prophylactic central neck dissections because HCC has a high rate of lymph node metastases but does not tend to concentrate RAI limiting postoperative treatment options (36,61).

Operative Therapy for MTC

For patients with MTC, the best chance of cure is to eliminate all disease at the initial operation. Therefore, most experts agree that total thyroidectomy with prophylactic central compartment lymph node dissection is indicated. If the primary tumor is palpable or >1.5 cm, lateral neck dissection is added as 80% of these patients have positive lateral neck nodes (28). Some surgeons also advocate contralateral lateral neck dissection.

In familial or MEN-related cases, operative intervention should occur before the age of potential malignant transformation. Ideally, total thyroidectomy should be performed before 5 to 6 years old with MEN 2A and shortly after birth in patients with MEN 2B and certain specific codon mutations that predict a very aggressive disease course (65,66). Central neck dissection is not necessary in patients under 6 years with negative ultrasound findings and normal calcitonin level (67). For patients with very high calcitonin levels preoperatively, some surgeons recommend a diagnostic laparoscopy to verify the presence of the typical miliary liver disease that is usually not apparent on computed tomography. Reoperations for recurrent disease are usually palliative as calcitonin levels rarely become undetectable.

Thyroid-Stimulating Hormone Suppression with Thyroid Hormone

TSH is a potent stimulator of thyrocyte growth and function. In a classic feedback inhibition loop, high levels of circulating thyroid hormone stimulate the pituitary to decrease TSH production. As such, suppressing TSH levels with exogenous thyroid hormone has been shown to inhibit the growth of malignant thyroid tissue both in vitro and in patients (52,64,68,69). Retrospective studies have shown decreased rates of tumor progression and recurrence in patients with suppressed TSH levels postoperatively (64,70,71). Although it is clear that patients benefit from TSH suppression, controversy exists as to the optimal level of suppression. By definition, TSH suppression induces a state of mild hyperthyroidism. In the elderly or patients with pre-existing medical conditions (especially cardiac disease), this iatrogenic hyperthyroidism may not be tolerable. A careful risk-benefit analysis must be made for each patient, weighing the benefits of tumor inhibition against side effects such as accelerated bone loss, atrial fibrillation, cardiac hypertrophy, and angina. For example, TSH suppression seems to cause bone loss in postmenopausal women but not premenopausal women or men. Bisphosphonates seem to halt this hypermetabolic bone loss. TSH suppression to <0.1 mU/L for low-risk patients and around 0.05 mU/l for high-risk patients is the general recommendation for the first 5 years after surgery. Thereafter, this suppression may be decreased to a TSH range of 0.1 to 0.5 mU/L if the patient has no evidence of disease.

Follow-up

Patients with WDTC should be monitored closely for recurrent disease. Postoperatively, patients should have a clinical examination and assessment including serum TSH, serum thyroglobulin, cervical ultrasound, and RAI scan at 6 months and 1 year after

Table 50.1

Probable Location of Recurrent Disease Based on Suppressed and Stimulated Thyroglobulin Levels

Location	Suppressed	Stimulated
Cervical	>10	<100
Mediastinal	>10	<200
Pulmonary	100	300
Bone	1,000	>1,000

Adapted from results published by Robbins RJ, Srivastava S, Shaha A, et al. Factors influencing the basal and recombinant human thyrotropin-stimulated serum thyroglobulin in patients with metastatic thyroid carcinoma. *J Clin Endocrinol Metab.* 2004;89:6010–6016.

the operation. If the RAI scan demonstrates any uptake, than RAI ablation with posttreatment scanning is also recommended for all but low-risk patients. If the patient is disease-free for 1 to 2 years, then subsequent follow-up may occur annually. Because recurrences can occur up to 50 years later, follow-up should be life-long.

Thyroglobulin

Thyroglobulin is a protein precursor to thyroid hormone and is made almost exclusively by benign or malignant thyroid cells. Therefore, elevations in thyroglobulin after total thyroidectomy or thyroid ablation are highly specific for persistent or recurrent thyroid cancer. In addition, the overall level of thyroglobulin can be used to predict tumor burden and location (Table 50.1). Thyroglobulin production is up-regulated by TSH stimulation. For this reason, measuring thyroglobulin during periods of elevated TSH levels after thyroid hormone withdrawal or the administration of recombinant TSH is more sensitive for detecting disease than when TSH levels are suppressed (72). In fact, only 60% of disease will be detected while patients are suppressed with thyroid hormone (73). Elevated stimulated thyroglobulin levels are so good at detecting recurrent or persistent disease, that some experts suggest that follow-up with stimulated thyroglobulin levels and ultrasound scanning is sufficient to follow low-risk patients (52,74–77). However, Robbins et al. (76) suggest that RAI scanning initially also adds valuable information in high-risk patients.

Antithyroglobulin antibodies are markers of autoimmune thyroid disease. The presence of these antibodies reduces the utility of thyroglobulin monitoring because they falsely lower, and rarely increase, the thyroglobulin levels. Up to 15% of women and 3% of men in the general population have antithyroglobulin antibodies. These antibodies are present in about 30% of patients with thyroid cancer (73). Some investigators use antithyroglobulin antibodies as a surrogate marker for thyroglobulin and have noted a correlation between decreasing antibody levels and declining tumor burden (73). Because of the confounding nature of antithyroglobulin antibodies, it is important to draw concomitant antibody and thyroglobulin levels for correlation. Calcitonin and CEA levels should be followed in patients with MTC.

Radioactive Iodine Ablation

Radioiodine ablation is recommended for patients with PTCs >1.5 cm, multifocal tumors, lymph node metastases, and those with elevated thyroglobulin levels after total thyroidectomy. Invasive follicular and Hürthle cell cancer also warrant radioiodine therapy. We routinely use 30 to 50 mCi of RAI in low-risk patients and 100 to 200 mCi in high-risk patients. Patients should have a TSH, thyroglobulin, and pregnancy test prior to 131-iodine scanning and ablation therapy, as well as posttreatment imaging

Postoperatively, RAI may be used to ablate the thyroid remnant as well as residual disease. Ablating the thyroid remnant increases the sensitivity of thyroglobulin as a marker for recurrence. Without residual normal thyroid tissue, the serum thyroglobulin level should be undetectable or <2 ng/mL and subsequent elevations suggest persistent or recurrent disease. Furthermore, remnant ablation increases the ability of RAIs to destroy metastases. Thyroid cells collect and organify iodine to produce thyroid hormone. Because of differential expression of the sodium-iodine symporter (NIS), normal thyroid cells trap iodine 100 times more efficiently than thyroid cancer cells. This increased avidity for iodine by normal thyrocytes means that RAI will preferentially collect in normal rather than malignant thyrocytes. Therefore, higher doses of RAI need to be administered to achieve the same desired therapeutic effect in patients with residual normal thyroid.

In order to optimize RAI uptake, clinicians drive up the patient's TSH level to >30 mU/L either by withdrawal of thyroid hormone to induce a state of hypothyroidism or by injections of recombinant TSH (rTSH). With hormone withdrawal, patients must stop taking thyroxine for 4 to 6 weeks prior to RAI. To reduce the period of hypothyroidism, many clinicians maintain patients on tri-iodothyronine up until 2 weeks prior to RAI at which time they are completely deprived of thyroid hormone. Patients should be placed on a low iodine diet 2weeks prior to RAI to deplete endogenous iodine stores. In contrast, treatment with rTSH requires no period of hypothyroidism and is of particular benefit to the elderly and those who cannot tolerate the hypothyroid state. rTSH therapy has few side effects, but has caused rapid enlargement of tumor in rare instances (78). Multiple prospective trials demonstrate that RAI scanning in combination with serum thyroglobulin measurement after rTSH has approximately the same sensitivity and specificity as thyroid hormone withdrawal (79–82).

Controversy exists as to whether or not a small "scanning dose" of RAI should be used to perform a diagnostic scan prior to giving a larger, "ablative dose" of RAI if disease is detected. The arguments against routine diagnostic scans are that small doses often do not uncover disease that later becomes evident on posttherapy scans and that thyrocyte "stunning" may occur. Stunning occurs when low-dose RAI damages but does not destroy thyroid cells. This damage decreases the ability of the cell to trap further RAI given as an ablative dose. The frequency of stunning varies from trial to trial but increases with increased initial 131-iodine dose and increased time between diagnostic and therapeutic doses (52,83,84). To overcome this effect, some groups have proposed scanning with 123-iodine, which does not appear to cause stunning, or to forgo diagnostic scans altogether (52). We concur with the latter recommendation.

After complete thyroid resection and/or ablation, patients with a positive findings on RAI scan or elevated thyroglobulin level should be suspected of having recurrent or occult disease. Reoperation is indicated for patients with gross disease. For patients with residual or metastatic thyroid cancer, RAI ablation is a critical adjunctive therapy to treat disease before it becomes radiologically apparent or clinically significant. RAI ablation is most helpful in treating patients with pulmonary micrometastases and is also indicated in patients with a high risk of recurrence based on local invasion, positive margins, or aggressive histology. MTC only rarely responds to RAI therapy.

Cervical Ultrasound

As discussed previously, the sensitivity of ultrasound has increased to a point where it has become an integral part of patient follow-up. In fact, ultrasound has become so sensitive that it often uncovers subcentimeter cervical disease that previously would have gone undetected. What percentage of these sonographically identified recurrences will become clinically significant has yet to be determined.

Positron Emission Tomography Scan

Positron emission tomography (PET) scans identify metabolically active lesions by highlighting tissue that consumes relatively larger quantities of radiolabeled glucose (18 fluorodeoxyglucose). As such, PET scans are useful for detecting malignant disease. In patients who have elevated thyroglobulin levels but negative findings on an RAI scan, PET scans have become useful to identify the location of disease. Studies have shown that up to 60% to 94% of recurrences in patients with negative RAI scans will be seen on PET (85). These PET-positive, RAI-negative tumors have dedifferentiated and lost the ability to trap or organify iodine, and therefore usually have a worse prognosis (86–88). In contrast, the majority of relatively well-differentiated RAI scan-positive tumors will not be detected by PET (87). Although promising, PET scanning has not yet been widely used to screen for recurrent disease.

ANAPLASTIC THYROID CANCER

Epidemiology

Anaplastic thyroid cancer (ATC) is rare and accounts for only 1% of all thyroid cancers, but up to half of thyroid cancer deaths in the United States. A portion of ATC is believed to arise from WDTC that dedifferentiates into this aggressive and highly lethal form of thyroid cancer. Patients with ATC typically present later in life (mean age, 60 years) with a rapidly enlarging, firm, fixed thyroid mass. ATC may invade into the trachea, larynx, esophagus, carotid artery, and jugular vein. Patients may also have hoarseness because of direct tumor invasion into the recurrent laryngeal nerve. Symptoms of tracheal deviation, dysphagia, dysphonia, and dyspnea are common. Unfortunately, regional lymph node metastases are present in 84% and distant metastases to the lungs, bone, brain, and adrenal gland occur in 75% of patients (27,30). ATC is invariably a progressive disease that is ultimately lethal within months of diagnosis.

Diagnosis

The differential diagnosis for ATC includes aggressive forms of WDTC (especially MTC) and lymphoma. Lymphoma comprises only 1% of thyroid cancers and also presents as a rapidly enlarging thyroid mass that causes local symptoms. A clinical suspicion of ATC can be confirmed by FNAB. Immunophenotyping can help rule out lymphoma. Serum calcitonin and CEA levels can rule out MTC. It is crucial to differentiate lymphoma from ATC because the former is readily treated by chemotherapy or radiation therapy. Practically speaking, patients with ATC present in such extremis or dramatic fashion that waiting for the results of these special stains is often not an option.

Treatment

As mentioned, long-term survival for ATC is nearly nonexistent. However, surgical resection for palliation, especially when near-complete surgical resection seems possible, is one of the mainstays of treatment and may improve the quality of the remaining days of life by relieving compressive symptoms. Although tracheostomy is indicated in cases of a compromised airway, palliative tracheostomy is more controversial (27,89). Although some groups, including our group, advocate combination therapy with surgical resection, chemotherapy, and radiation, most series report median survivals of 2.5 to 9 months (90). The 2-year survival is <20% (27,89).

REFERENCES

1. Estimated new cancer cases and deaths for 2006. http://seercancergov/csr. Accessed May 5, 2006.
2. Robbins J, Merino MJ, Boice JD Jr, et al. Thyroid cancer: a lethal endocrine neoplasm. *Ann Intern Med.* 1991;115:133–147.
3. Busnardo B, De Vido D. The epidemiology and etiology of differentiated thyroid carcinoma. *Biomed Pharmacother.* 2000;54:322–326.
4. Gow KW, Lensing S, Hill DA, et al. Thyroid carcinoma presenting in childhood or after treatment of childhood malignancies: an institutional experience and review of the literature. *J Pediatr Surg.* 2003;38:1574–1580.
5. Carcangiu ML, Zampi G, Pupi A, et al. Papillary carcinoma of the thyroid. A clinicopathologic study of 241 cases treated at the University of Florence, Italy. *Cancer.* 1985;55:805–828.
6. Hay ID. Papillary thyroid carcinoma. *Endocrinol Metab Clin North Am.* 1990;19:545–576.
7. Mazzaferri EL. Papillary thyroid carcinoma: factors influencing prognosis and current therapy. *Semin Oncol.* 1987;14:315–332.
8. Mizukami Y, Noguchi M, Michigishi T, et al. Papillary thyroid carcinoma in Kanazawa, Japan: prognostic significance of histological subtypes. *Histopathology.* 1992;20:243–250.
9. DeGroot LJ, Kaplan EL, McCormick M, et al. Natural history, treatment, and course of papillary thyroid carcinoma. *J Clin Endocrinol Metab.* 1990;71:414–424.
10. Harwood J, Clark OH, Dunphy JE. Significance of lymph node metastasis in differentiated thyroid cancer. *Am J Surg.* 1978;136:107–112.
11. Moreno-Egea A, Rodriguez-Gonzalez JM, Sola-Perez J, et al. Multivariate analysis of histopathological features as prognostic factors in patients with papillary thyroid carcinoma. *Br J Surg.* 1995;82:1092–1094.
12. Asakawa H, Kobayashi T, Komoike Y, et al. Prognostic factors in patients with recurrent differentiated thyroid carcinoma. *J Surg Oncol.* 1997;64:202–206.

13. Coburn M, Teates D, Wanebo HJ. Recurrent thyroid cancer. Role of surgery versus radioactive iodine (I131). *Ann Surg.* 1994;219:587–593.

14. Hamy A, Mirallie E, Bennouna J, et al. Thyroglobulin monitoring after treatment of well-differentiated thyroid cancer. *Eur J Surg Oncol.* 2004;30:681–685.

15. Hay ID, Ryan JJ, Grant CS, et al. Prognostic significance of nondiploid DNA determined by flow cytometry in sporadic and familial medullary thyroid carcinoma. *Surgery.* 1990;108:972–980.

16. Jossart GH, Clark OH. Well-differentiated thyroid cancer. *Curr Probl Surg.* 1994;31:933–1012.

17. DeGroot LJ. Radiation and thyroid cancer. *Proc Inst Med Chic.* 1976;31:95–96.

18. Allo MD, Christianson W, Koivunen D. Not all "occult" papillary carcinomas are "minimal." *Surgery.* 1988;104:971–976.

19. Crile G Jr. Changing end results in patients with papillary carcinoma of the thyroid. *Surg Gynecol Obstet.* 1971;132:460–468.

20. Emerick GT, Duh QY, Siperstein AE, et al. Diagnosis, treatment, and outcome of follicular thyroid carcinoma. *Cancer.* 1993;72:3287–3295.

21. Brennan MD, Bergstralh EJ, van Heerden JA, et al. Follicular thyroid cancer treated at the Mayo Clinic, 1946 through 1970: initial manifestations, pathologic findings, therapy, and outcome. *Mayo Clin Proc.* 1991;66:11–22.

22. Jorda M, Gonzalez-Campora R, Mora J, et al. Prognostic factors in follicular carcinoma of the thyroid. *Arch Pathol Lab Med.* 1993;117:631–635.

23. Mueller-Gaertner HW, Brzac HT, Rehpenning W. Prognostic indices for tumor relapse and tumor mortality in follicular thyroid carcinoma. *Cancer.* 1991;67:1903–1911.

24. Crile G Jr, Pontius KI, Hawk WA. Factors influencing the survival of patients with follicular carcinoma of the thyroid gland. *Surg Gynecol Obstet.* 1985;160:409–413.

25. D'Avanzo A, Treseler P, Ituarte PH, et al. Follicular thyroid carcinoma: histology and prognosis. *Cancer.* 2004;100:1123–1129.

26. Grossman RF, Clark OH. Hürthle cell carcinoma. *Cancer Control.* 1997;4:13–17.

27. Nix PA, Nicolaides A, Coatesworth AP. Thyroid cancer review 3: management of medullary and undifferentiated thyroid cancer. *Int J Clin Pract.* 2006;60:80–84.

28. Moley JF, DeBenedetti MK. Patterns of nodal metastases in palpable medullary thyroid carcinoma: recommendations for extent of node dissection. *Ann Surg.* 1999;229:880–888.

29. Moore FD, Dluhy RG. Prophylactic thyroidectomy in MEN-2A–a stitch in time? *N Engl J Med.* 2005;353:1162–1164.

30. Zarnegar R, Clark OH. Thyroid cancer. In: Cameron, ed. *Current Surgical Therapy.* 9th ed. New York: Elsevier; 2007.

31. Crawford JD. Hyperthyroidism in children. A reevaluation of treatment. *Am J Dis Child.* 1981;135:109–110.

32. DeGroot LJ. Effects of irradiation on the thyroid gland. *Endocrinol Metab Clin North Am.* 1993;22:607–615.

33. MacDougal IR. Which therapy for Graves' hyperthyroidism in children? *Nucl Med Commun.* 1989;10:855–857.

34. Rivkees SA, Sklar C, Freemark M. Clinical review 99: The management of Graves' disease in children, with special emphasis on radioiodine treatment. *J Clin Endocrinol Metab.* 1998;83:3767–3776.

35. Takeichi N, Ezaki H, Dohi K. A review of forty-five years study of Hiroshima and Nagasaki atomic bomb survivors. Thyroid cancer: reports up to date and a review. *J Radiat Res (Tokyo).* 1991;32(suppl):180–188.

36. Caron NR, Clark OH. Well differentiated thyroid cancer. *Scand J Surg.* 2004;93:261–271.

37. Belfiore A, Garofalo MR, Giuffrida D, et al. Increased aggressiveness of thyroid cancer in patients with Graves' disease. *J Clin Endocrinol Metab.* 1990;70:830–835.

38. Ron E, Doody MM, Becker DV, et al. Cancer mortality following treatment for adult hyperthyroidism. Cooperative Thyrotoxicosis Therapy Follow-up Study Group. *JAMA.* 1998;280:347–355.

39. Tezelman S, Grossman RF, Siperstein AE, et al. Radioiodine-associated thyroid cancers. *World J Surg.* 1994;18:522–528.

40. Attie JN, Moskowitz GW, Margouleff D, et al. Feasibility of total thyroidectomy in the treatment of thyroid carcinoma: postoperative radioactive iodine evaluation of 140 cases. *Am J Surg.* 1979;138:555–560.

41. Ready AR, Barnes AD. Complications of thyroidectomy. *Br J Surg.* 1994;81:1555–1556.

42. Grossman RF, Tu SH, Duh QY, et al. Familial nonmedullary thyroid cancer. An emerging entity that warrants aggressive treatment. *Arch Surg.* 1995;130:892–899.

43. Triponez F, Wong M, Sturgeon C, et al. Does familial non-medullary thyroid cancer adversely affect survival? *World J Surg.* 2006;30:787–793.

44. Tallini G. Molecular pathobiology of thyroid neoplasms. *Endocrinol Pathol.* 2002;13:271–288.

45. Robbins RJ, Srivastava S, Shaha A, et al. Factors influencing the basal and recombinant human thyrotropin-stimulated serum thyroglobulin in patients with metastatic thyroid carcinoma. *J Clin Endocrinol Metab.* 2004;89:6010–6016.

46. Jackson CE, Norum RA, Talpos GB, et al. Clinical value of calcitonin and carcinoembryonic antigen doubling times in medullary thyroid carcinoma. *Henry Ford Hosp Med J.* 1987;35:120–121.

47. Jun P, Chow LC, Jeffrey RB. The sonographic features of papillary thyroid carcinomas: pictorial essay. *Ultrasound Q.* 2005;21:39–45.

48. Reading CC, Charboneau JW, Hay ID, et al. Sonography of thyroid nodules: a "classic pattern" diagnostic approach. *Ultrasound Q.* 2005;21:157–165.

49. Papini E, Guglielmi R, Bianchini A, et al. Risk of malignancy in nonpalpable thyroid nodules: predictive value of ultrasound and color-Doppler features. *J Clin Endocrinol Metab.* 2002;87:1941–1946.

50. Komolafe F. Radiological patterns and significance of thyroid calcification. *Clin Radiol.* 1981;32:571–575.

51. Duh QY, Siperstein AE, Miller RA, et al. Epidermal growth factor receptors and adenylate cyclase activity in human thyroid tissues. *World J Surg.* 1990;14:410–418.

52. Ringel MD, Ladenson PW. Controversies in the follow-up and management of well-differentiated thyroid cancer. *Endocrinol Relat Cancer.* 2004;11:97–116.

53. Goretzki PE, Lyons J, Stacy-Phipps S, et al. Mutational activation of RAS and GSP oncogenes in differentiated thyroid cancer and their biological implications. *World J Surg.* 1992;16:576–581.

54. Goretzki PE, Simon D, Roher HD. G-protein mutations in thyroid tumors. *Exp Clin Endocrinol.* 1992;100:14–16.

55. Ito T, Seyama T, Mizuno T, et al. Unique association of p53 mutations with undifferentiated but not with differentiated carcinomas of the thyroid gland. *Cancer Res.* 1992;52:1369–1371.

56. Jhiang SM, Mazzaferri EL. The ret/PTC oncogene in papillary thyroid carcinoma. *J Lab Clin Med.* 1994;123:331–337.

57. Romano MI, Grattone M, Karner MP, et al. Relationship between the level of c-myc mRNA and histologic aggressiveness in thyroid tumors. *Horm Res.* 1993;39:161–165.

58. Siperstein AE, Zeng QH, Gum ET, et al. Adenylate cyclase activity as a predictor of thyroid tumor aggressiveness. *World J Surg.* 1988;12:528–533.

59. Hay ID, Bergstralh EJ, Goellner JR, et al. Predicting outcome in papillary thyroid carcinoma: development of a reliable prognostic scoring system in a cohort of 1779 patients surgically treated at one

institution during 1940 through 1989. *Surgery*. 1993;114:1050–1058.

60. Schlumberger MJ. Papillary and follicular thyroid carcinoma. *N Engl J Med*. 1998;338:297–306.

61. Kebebew E, Clark OH. Differentiated thyroid cancer: "complete" rational approach. *World J Surg*. 2000;24:942–951.

62. Hay ID, Grant CS, Bergstralh EJ, et al. Unilateral total lobectomy: is it sufficient surgical treatment for patients with AMES low-risk papillary thyroid carcinoma? *Surgery*. 1998;124:958–964.

63. Kebebew E, Duh QY, Clark OH. Total thyroidectomy or thyroid lobectomy in patients with low-risk differentiated thyroid cancer: surgical decision analysis of a controversy using a mathematical model. *World J Surg*. 2000;24:1295–1302.

64. Mazzaferri EL, Jhiang SM. Long-term impact of initial surgical and medical therapy on papillary and follicular thyroid cancer. *Am J Med*. 1994;97:418–428.

65. Brandi ML, Gagel RF, Angeli A, et al. Guidelines for diagnosis and therapy of MEN type 1 and type 2. *J Clin Endocrinol Metab*. 2001;86:5658–5671.

66. Machens A, Niccoli-Sire P, Hoegel J, et al. Early malignant progression of hereditary medullary thyroid cancer. *N Engl J Med*. 2003;349:1517–1525.

67. Skinner MA, Moley JA, Dilley WG, et al. Prophylactic thyroidectomy in multiple endocrine neoplasia type 2A. *N Engl J Med*. 2005;353:1105–1113.

68. McGriff NJ, Csako G, Gourgiotis L, et al. Effects of thyroid hormone suppression therapy on adverse clinical outcomes in thyroid cancer. *Ann Med*. 2002;34:554–564.

69. Clark OH, Gerend PL, Cote TC, et al. Thyrotropin binding and adenylate cyclase stimulation in thyroid neoplasms. *Surgery*. 1981;90:252–261.

70. Cooper DS, Specker B, Ho M, et al. Thyrotropin suppression and disease progression in patients with differentiated thyroid cancer: results from the National Thyroid Cancer Treatment Cooperative Registry. *Thyroid*. 1998;8:737–744.

71. Pujol P, Daures JP, Nsakala N, et al. Degree of thyrotropin suppression as a prognostic determinant in differentiated thyroid cancer. *J Clin Endocrinol Metab*. 1996;81:4318–4323.

72. Lo Gerfo P, Colacchio TA, Colacchio DA, et al. Effect of TSH stimulation on serum thyroglobulin in metastatic thyroid cancer. *J Surg Oncol*. 1980;14:195–200.

73. Mazzaferri EL, Robbins RJ, Spencer CA, et al. A consensus report of the role of serum thyroglobulin as a monitoring method for low-risk patients with papillary thyroid carcinoma. *J Clin Endocrinol Metab*. 2003;88:1433–1441.

74. Cailleux AF, Baudin E, Travagli JP, et al. Is diagnostic iodine-131 scanning useful after total thyroid ablation for differentiated thyroid cancer? *J Clin Endocrinol Metab*. 2000;85:175–178.

75. Mazzaferri EL, Kloos RT. Is diagnostic iodine-131 scanning with recombinant human TSH useful in the follow-up of differentiated thyroid cancer after thyroid ablation? *J Clin Endocrinol Metab*. 2002;87:1490–1498.

76. Robbins RJ, Chon JT, Fleisher M, et al. Is the serum thyroglobulin response to recombinant human thyrotropin sufficient, by itself, to monitor for residual thyroid carcinoma? *J Clin Endocrinol Metab*. 2002;87:3242–3247.

77. Wartofsky L. Using baseline and recombinant human TSH-stimulated Tg measurements to manage thyroid cancer without diagnostic ^{131}I scanning. *J Clin Endocrinol Metab*. 2002;87:1486–1489.

78. Robbins RJ, Voelker E, Wang W, et al. Compassionate use of recombinant human thyrotropin to facilitate radioiodine therapy: case report and review of literature. *Endocr Pract*. 2000;6:460–464.

79. Haugen BR, Pacini F, Reiners C, et al. A comparison of recombinant human thyrotropin and thyroid hormone withdrawal for the detection of thyroid remnant or cancer. *J Clin Endocrinol Metab*. 1999;84:3877–3885.

80. Robbins RJ, Pentlow KS. Coming of age: recombinant human thyroid-stimulating hormone as a preparation for ^{131}I therapy in thyroid cancer. *J Nucl Med*. 2003;44:1069–1071.

81. Robbins RJ, Robbins AK. Clinical review 156: Recombinant human thyrotropin and thyroid cancer management. *J Clin Endocrinol Metab*. 2003;88:1933–1938.

82. Schlumberger M, Ricard M, Pacini F. Clinical use of recombinant human TSH in thyroid cancer patients. *Eur J Endocrinol*. 2000;143:557–563.

83. Hurley JR. Management of thyroid cancer: radioiodine ablation, "stunning," and treatment of thyroglobulin-positive, ^{131}I scan-negative patients. *Endocr Pract*. 2000;6:401–406.

84. Kao CH, Yen TC. Stunning effects after a diagnostic dose of iodine-131. *Nuklearmedizin*. 1998;37:30–32.

85. Khan N, Oriuchi N, Higuchi T, et al. PET in the follow-up of differentiated thyroid cancer. *Br J Radiol*. 2003;76:690–695.

86. Larson SM, Robbins R. Positron emission tomography in thyroid cancer management. *Semin Roentgenol*. 2002;37:169–174.

87. Lind P, Kresnik E, Kumnig G, et al. 18F-FDG-PET in the follow-up of thyroid cancer. *Acta Med Austriaca*. 2003;30:17–21.

88. Tiepolt C, Beuthien-Baumann B, Hliscs R, et al. 18F-FDG for the staging of patients with differentiated thyroid cancer: comparison of a dual-head coincidence gamma camera with dedicated PET. *Ann Nucl Med*. 2000;14:339–345.

89. Are C, Shaha AR. Anaplastic thyroid carcinoma: biology, pathogenesis, prognostic factors, and treatment approaches. *Ann Surg Oncol*. 2006;13:453–464.

90. Ekman ET, Lundell G, Tennvall J, et al. Chemotherapy and multimodality treatment in thyroid carcinoma. *Otolaryngol Clin North Am*. 1990;23:523–527.

COMMENTARY 1
Glenn D. Braunstein

Drs. Lee and Clark have provided an excellent overview of the classification, epidemiology, diagnosis, and treatment of thyroid cancer. Therefore, I am going to confine my remarks to selected issues concerning differentiated thyroid carcinoma, the most common form of the disease, and the one whose incidence has had a dramatic increase over the past 3 decades.

WHY IS THE INCIDENCE OF THYROID CANCER INCREASING?

During the 30-year period between 1973 and 2002, the incidence of thyroid cancer increased 2.4-fold, from 3.6 to 8.7 per 100,000 population. The increase is virtually confined to the most common form of well-differentiated thyroid cancer, papillary, which increased 2.9-fold from 2.7 to 7.7 per 100,000. There was no significant change in the incidence of follicular, medullary, or anaplastic thyroid carcinoma over this time period.

Papillary microcarcinomas measuring ≤1 cm made up almost half of the increase, while over 85% of the cancers accounting for the increase were ≤2 cm. Of importance, there was no difference in the mortality from thyroid cancer over this period, which remained at about 0.5 deaths per 100,000 (1). This increase could be due to exposure to an environmental carcinogen such as radiation, or to an ascertainment bias due to the increasing use of ultrasound for screening for carotid atherosclerosis, total-body, or chest computed tomography (CT) scans that include the lower neck in the field, positron emission tomography scanning for staging or monitoring other neoplastic diseases, and diagnostic magnetic resonance imaging of the head, neck, or cervical spine. The finding of a thyroid nodule by any of these modalities often prompts a fine-needle aspiration (FNA) of the lesion, leading to the discovery that the thyroid harbors a carcinoma. The lack of a concomitant increase in mortality from thyroid cancer, coupled with the fact that many of the cancers that are being discovered are small and nonpalpable, strongly argues that the increase is due to the findings of "incidentalomas" (2). An autopsy study carried out >20 years ago demonstrated the presence of "occult" papillary thyroid cancers in 36% of patients who did not have clinical thyroid cancer during their lifetime (3). Thus, the present "outbreak" of thyroid cancer most likely represents the use of sensitive tools to detect the occult disease that has always been present in a high proportion of the population. The key is to identify those patients whose tumors may cause morbidity or mortality ("clinical carcinomas") and those whose tumors will remain "occult."

DOES SIZE MATTER?

The prevalence of thyroid carcinoma in a patient with a palpable nodule is about 5%, and the prevalence is the same for nonpalpable nodules of the same size detected incidentally (4,5). There is a relationship between papillary and follicular tumor size and mortality, with a 30-year mortality of 0.4% for tumors <1.5 cm, 7% for tumors between 1.5 and 4.4 cm, and 18% for tumors >4.5 cm (6). Several studies of papillary microcarcinomas have indicated that about a third are multifocal, up to 20% have local tumor extension into the surrounding tissue, 12% to 50% have cervical lymph node metastasis, distant metastasis are present in 1.6% to 2.5%, and the mortality rate is ≤1% (7,8). In a study of 366 patients with papillary carcinoma and 134 with follicular carcinoma, cervical lymph node involvement and extrathyroidal tissue invasion was found in papillary carcinomas ≥5 mm and in follicular carcinomas that were ≥2 cm or larger, while for both tumor types pulmonary metastasis were unlikely for tumors <2 cm and bone metastasis were not generally found until the primary tumors were 3 to 4 cm (9). A recent study of 243 patients with papillary microcarcinomas showed that 0.8% of patients with tumors <5 mm had cervical lymph node involvement, and distant metastasis and tumor recurrence following surgery and radioactive iodine ablation were seen only in tumors >8 mm (10).

The mortality rate following therapy for papillary thyroid microcarcinomas is very low, but it is unknown what the mortality rate would be if the tumors were left untreated. One study of "watchful waiting" in a subgroup of 162 of 732 patients with papillary microcarcinoma showed that the tumors in a few patients spontaneously disappeared, about 11% increased in size by >1 cm, and 1.2% spread to cervical lymph nodes during the observation period, but over 70% did not change or decreased in size during the follow-up of up to 10 years (11). Clearly, a method is desperately needed to discriminate between occult tumors that are nonaggressive and will remain occult from those microcarcinomas that will result in morbidity and possibly mortality.

WHAT IS THE ROLE OF ULTRASOUND IN THE DIAGNOSIS AND MANAGEMENT OF THYROID CANCER?

The decrease in the cost of high-resolution ultrasound units and the development of ultrasound training courses by national societies including the American Thyroid Association, the Endocrine Society, and the American Association for Clinical Endocrinologists has resulted in thyroid ultrasonography no longer being performed exclusively by radiologists. Increasingly, endocrinologists are using thyroid ultrasound as an extension of the thyroid physical examination. It has become an essential tool for examining the thyroid for nodules, determining the characteristics of the nodules in order to decide which to biopsy, to aid in the performance of the FNA, and in the follow-up of nodule size and morphology. As previously noted, the prevalence of carcinoma in nonpalpable lesions is the same as in palpable lesions of the same size. In addition, the cancer rate for patients with multiple nodules is the same as that in patients with solitary nodules (12). Therefore, ultrasound is a valuable tool for examining nodules in order to decide which nodule(s) to biopsy.

The characteristics of nodules that increase the suspicion of carcinoma include the presence of microcalcifications, irregular margins, absence of a perinodular halo of compressed blood vessels, hypoechogenicity of a solid nodule, a nodule that is more tall than wide, and increased intranodular blood flow (12–14). Nodules with several of these characteristics, regardless of size, should be biopsied. Even in palpable nodules, biopsies should be carried out under ultrasound guidance, which has been shown to reduce the rates of both nondiagnostic and false-negative biopsies (4,15). This is especially important for lesions with cystic degeneration, as the ultrasound can help guide the placement of the needle into the solid portion of the nodule or into a mural nodule in a primarily cystic lesion.

Preoperative ultrasound mapping of the cervical lymph nodes before thyroidectomy has been shown to be useful. In one study, such mapping detected unappreciated abnormal lymph nodes in 20% of the patients prior to the initial thyroidectomy. In those undergoing initial surgery, patients with preoperative mapping had a cervical lymph node recurrence rate of 6% at 3 years. Indeed, preoperative mapping, before thyroidectomy and prior to reoperation, altered the surgical procedure 39% of the time (16).

Finally, ultrasound has been invaluable in detecting persistent or recurrent disease in the neck following thyroidectomy with or without radioactive iodine ablation. It has 94% sensitivity for detecting residual disease in the neck, while a diagnostic ^{131}I whole-body scan has a sensitivity of 45% and a

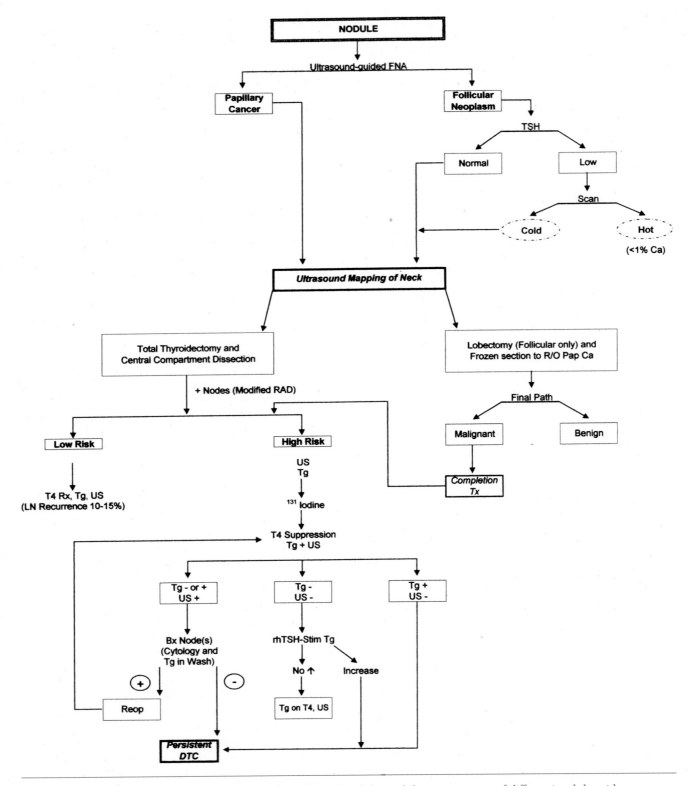

Figure 50 C.1 Algorithm for the evaluation of suspicious thyroid nodules and the management of differentiated thyroid cancer. FNA, fine-needle aspiration; TSH, thyroid-stimulating hormone; Pap Ca, papillary carcinoma; RAD, radical neck dissection; US, ultrasound; Tg, thyroglobulin level; rhTSH, recombinant human DTC, differentiated thyroid cancer.

serum thyroglobulin of ≥2 ng/mL off thyroid hormone has only a 57% sensitivity (17). The ultrasound characteristics of cervical lymph nodes with metastatic thyroid cancer include a round rather than oval shape; hyperechoic echogenicity in comparison to the surrounding strap muscles, absence of a hilus due to tumor infiltration of the sinuses; cystic change; microcalcifications; increased vascularity in the peripheral and central zones; and indentation of the jugular vein (18).

Ultrasound-guided FNA of the abnormal lymph nodes allows confirmatory tissue diagnosis of metastatic disease. Cytology on the lymph node aspirates has 85% sensitivity for detecting the disease. Following an aspirate, the needle should be washed in 1 mL of normal saline, and the thyroglobulin measured. The combination of cytology and elevated levels of thyroglobulin in the lymph node has 96% sensitivity for detecting nodal metastasis (17). I have used this technique to detect metastatic papillary carcinoma in cervical lymph nodes measuring 5 mm. Because 20–30% of patients with well-differentiated thyroid carcinoma will have a recurrence over 40 years of follow-up, and there is an approximate 10% mortality rate over 40 years, the detection of residual disease in the neck has resulted in patients undergoing functional neck compartment dissections in an attempt to eradicate all persistent disease. However, the question that is unanswered is whether this approach is too aggressive for the majority of patients who will not succumb to the cancer.

HOW SHOULD PATIENTS BE MANAGED?

We have generally followed the algorithm presented in Figure 50C.1 for managing patients. In a patient with a thyroid nodule, we biopsy any suspicious nodule, irrespective of size, or the dominant nodule in a multinodular goiter without a suspicious lesion. All biopsies are done under ultrasound guidance. If the FNA reveals a follicular neoplasm, we perform a thyroid-stimulating hormone (TSH) test. A low TSH suggests that the nodule may be overproducing thyroid hormone. Therefore, we perform a radioactive iodine uptake and scan. If the nodule is warm or hot, indicating that it is overactive, we recommend radioactive iodine treatment to destroy it. Such nodules have <1% chance of being a carcinoma. If the nodule is cold or the TSH is normal, we recommend thyroid surgery. The patient is given the option of a total thyroidectomy or a lobectomy, as long as if he or she is willing to undergo a completion thyroidectomy should the final pathologic examination reveal the lesion to be a carcinoma. If a lobectomy is chosen, we perform a frozen section in order to rule out the lesion being a follicular variant of papillary carcinoma, which would warrant an immediate total thyroidectomy. If the FNA is indicative of a papillary carcinoma, we recommend a total thyroidectomy. Prior to the procedure, a high-resolution ultrasound examination of the neck is performed for lymph node mapping, as previously discussed.

Total thyroidectomy for papillary carcinomas is accompanied by a central compartment dissection in order to detect lymph node metastasis, even if no abnormal nodes are seen on preoperative ultrasound, as the central compartment may be difficult to visualize while the thyroid is in the neck. Abnormal lymph nodes detected by preoperative ultrasound are removed through functional neck dissections of the involved compartments.

Radioactive iodine is administered to patients with lesions >1.5 cm, multifocal tumors, invasion of the surrounding soft tissue, or metastasis to cervical lymph nodes or distant metastasis. Low-risk patients without these characteristics are placed on suppressive doses of thyroxine, with the goal to keep the serum TSH level at about 0.1 mU/L. Disease status is monitored with serum thyroglobulin determinations and neck ultrasounds. We anticipate a 10% to 15% detection of disease involving the lymph nodes in this population at some time. For the higher-risk patients, following radioactive iodine, we attempt to reduce the TSH to <0.1 mU/L with thyroxine, as data from the National Thyroid Cooperative Study has shown decreased disease progression when the TSH is kept below 0.1 mU/L as opposed to levels between 0.1 and 5 mU/L (19). Disease is monitored with serum thyroglobulins during thyroxine suppression and neck ultrasounds. If the thyroglobulin is elevated, persistent or recurrent disease is present. If the ultrasound reveals an abnormal lymph node, we perform a biopsy for cytology and thyroglobulin analysis. If either or both are positive, persistent or recurrent disease is diagnosed. If the serum thyroglobulin on thyroxine suppression is undetectable and the neck ultrasound is negative, we perform a stimulation test with recombinant human TSH (rh-TSH). In this test, the thyroglobulin level is measured 72 hours following two doses of rh-TSH. If the thyroglobulin remains undetectable, then there is no evidence of disease. A rise above 2 ng/mL is indicative of residual disease. We do not routinely perform a radioactive iodine whole-body scan as part of this test in low-risk patients as the thyroglobulin measurement is a more sensitive indication of persistent disease (20).

Once residual disease is diagnosed, we attempt to localize it with neck ultrasound, magnetic resonance imaging of the mediastinum with gadolinium, a high-resolution CT of the chest without contrast, and in some instances with a rh-TSH-stimulated positron emission tomography/CT scan. Further treatment depends on the findings but may include repeat neck surgery, surgical removal of isolated metastasis, additional radioactive iodine, external-beam radiotherapy, or a trial of one of the newer targeted therapies for thyroglobulin-positive/radioactive iodine scan-negative patients with progressive disease (21).

REFERENCES

1. Davies L, Welch HG. Increasing incidence of thyroid cancer in the United States, 1973-2002. *JAMA.* 2006;295:2164–2167.
2. Ezzat S, Sarti DA, Cain DR, Braunstein GD. Thyroid incidentalomas. *Arch Intern Med.* 1994;154:1838–1840.
3. Harach HR, Franssila KO, Wasenius VM. Occult papillary carcinoma of the thyroid: a "normal" finding in Finland. *Cancer.* 1985;56:531–538.
4. Carmeci C, Jeffrey RB, McDougall IR, et al. Ultrasound-guided fine-needle aspiration biopsy of thyroid masses. *Thyroid.* 1998;8:283–289.
5. Hagag P, Strauss S, Weiss M. Role of ultrasound-guided fine-needle aspiration biopsy in evaluation of nonpalpable thyroid nodules. *Thyroid.* 1998;8:989–995.
6. Mazzaferri EL, Jhiang SM. Long-term impact of initial surgical and medical therapy on papillary and follicular thyroid cancer. *Am J Med.* 1994';97:418–428.

7. Mazzaferri EL. Managing small thyroid cancers. *JAMA.* 2006;295: 2179–2182.

8. Burman KD. Editorial: micropapillary thyroid cancers: should we aspirate all nodules regardless of size? *J Clin Endocrinol Metab.* 2006;91:2043–2046.

9. Machens A, Holzhausen HJ, Dralle H. The prognostic value of primary tumor size in papillary and follicular thyroid carcinoma. *Cancer.* 2005;103:2269–2273.

10. Roti E, Rossi R, Trasforini G, et al. Clinical and histological characteristics of papillary thyroid microcarcinoma: results of a retrospective study in 243 patients. *J Clin Endocrinol Metab.* 2006;9:2171–2178.

11. Ito Y, Uruno T, Nakano K, et al. An observation trial without surgical treatment in patients with papillary microcarcinoma of the thyroid. *Thyroid.* 2003;13:381–387.

12. Papini E, Guglielmi R, Bianchini A, et al. Risk of malignancy in nonpalpable thyroid nodules: predictive value of ultrasound and color-Doppler features. *J Clin Endocrinol Metab.* 2002;87:1941–1946.

13. Kim EK, Park CS, Chung WY, et al. New sonographic criteria for recommending fine-needle aspiration biopsy of nonpalpable solid nodules of the thyroid. *Am J Roentgenol.* 2002;178:687–691.

14. Shimura H, Haraguchi K, Hiejima Y, et al. Distinct diagnostic criteria for ultrasonographic examination of papillary thyroid carcinoma: a multicenter study. *Thyroid.* 2005;15:251–258.

15. Danese D, Sciacchitano S, Farsetti A, et al. Diagnostic accuracy of conventional versus sonography-guided fine-needle aspiration biopsy of thyroid nodules. *Thyroid.* 1998;8:15–21.

16. Kouvaraki MA, Shapiro SE, Fornage D, et al. Role of preoperative ultrasonography in the surgical management of patients with thyroid cancer. *Surgery.* 2003;134:946–955.

17. Frasoaldati A, Pesenti M, Gallo M, et al. Diagnosis of neck recurrences in patients with differentiated thyroid carcinoma. *Cancer.* 2003;97:90–96.

18. Ahuja A, Ying M. Sonography of neck lymph nodes. Part II: abnormal lymph nodes. *Clin Radiat.* 2003;58:359–366.

19. Cooper DS, Specker B, Ho M, et al. Thyrotropin suppression and disease progression in patients with differentiated thyroid cancer: results from the notational thyroid cancer treatment cooperative registry. *Thyroid.* 1998;8:737–744.

20. Mazzaferri EL, Robbins J, Spencer CA, et al. A consensus report of the role of serum thyroglobulin as a monitoring method for low-risk patients with papillary thyroid carcinoma. *J Clin Endocrinol Metab.* 2003;88:1433–1441.

21. Cooper DS, Doherty GM, Haugen BR, et al. Management guidelines for patients with thyroid nodules and differentiated thyroid cancer. *Thyroid.* 2006;16:1–33.

COMMENTARY 2
Jatin P. Shah

Carcinoma of the thyroid is a unique human neoplasm. Thyroid cancer is not a single entity but is a spectrum of a variety of different histologic entities with unique biological behavior and diverse prognosis. Fortunately, a great majority of patients with thyroid carcinoma have well-differentiated thyroid cancer with excellent prognosis. Microscopic dissemination of primary tumor with multifocal intrathyroidal primary lesions and occult metastasis to cervical lymph nodes is very common; however, these unique features do not create an adverse impact on prognosis in most patients (1–3).

Drs. Lee and Clark present a comprehensive review of the diagnosis and management of patients with cancer of the thyroid gland and suggest a relatively uniform surgical approach in all patients. However, adopting this philosophy will probably result in gross overtreatment for a great majority of patients with low-risk thyroid cancer and outstanding prognoses. Clearly, overtreatment of low-risk thyroid cancer has no impact on prognosis but has increased cost of treatment and may even have a potentially higher rate of complications and sequelae of therapy.

PATHOLOGY

It is important to appreciate that nearly 80% of all patients with thyroid cancer have well-differentiated thyroid carcinoma. These include papillary carcinoma, follicular carcinoma, and Hürthle cell carcinomas. Approximately 5% of patients have medullary carcinoma and 2% to 3% of patients have anaplastic carcinoma of the thyroid gland. This leaves approximately 10% to 12% of patients who have aggressive variants of thyroid cancer such as tall cell variant of thyroid carcinoma, insular carcinoma, and poorly differentiated thyroid carcinomas (4). It is in this group of patients for whom aggressive treatment and aggressive adjuvant therapy have a role to play as it would favorably impact on prognosis. A majority of the patients with well-differentiated thyroid carcinoma carry an outstanding overall prognosis, while prognosis is uniformly dismal in patients with anaplastic thyroid cancer.

A majority of patients with well-differentiated thyroid carcinoma will be cured after initial treatment, and these patients carry on a normal lifestyle and lifespan. The biological behavior of more aggressive variants of thyroid carcinoma follow a tumor progression model whereby well-differentiated carcinoma progresses on to metaplastic changes leading to the less well-differentiated variants of thyroid carcinoma, poorly differentiated thyroid carcinoma, and eventually to anaplastic carcinoma. This biological behavior is supported by the observation that in many patients with poorly differentiated thyroid carcinomas, areas of well-differentiated tumors are demonstrated under histologic scrutiny (5,6). Similarly, patients with well-differentiated thyroid carcinoma who develop multiple recurrences show progressive metaplastic transformation into the less differentiated variants of thyroid cancer, eventually leading to transformation into anaplastic carcinoma (7). Exploiting this biological behavior of thyroid cancer greatly facilitates clinical management and helps the clinician to be selective in implementing aggressive therapeutic strategies.

PROGNOSTIC FACTORS AND RISK GROUP STRATIFICATION

The importance of prognostic factors and risk group stratification in clinical management of thyroid carcinoma cannot be overemphasized. Drs. Lee and Clark indicate that risk group stratification can be undertaken only after surgical treatment. On the other hand, risk group stratification is easily assessed prior to implementation of any surgical intervention based on patient and tumor characteristics. The well-known independent parameters of prognosis are patients' age and gender as well as the size of the tumor, the histologic nature of the tumor, presence or absence of extrathyroidal extension, and distant metastasis. Note that extent of surgery of the primary tumor, cervical lymph node metastasis, and adjuvant therapy with radioactive iodine are not statistically significant independent parameters of prognosis on multivariate analyses (8-10). Thus, based on these patient and tumor factors, one can easily stratify patients into low-, high-, and intermediate-risk categories (11).

SURGICAL TREATMENT

In selection of initial surgical treatment, risk group stratification simplifies the decision regarding extent of surgery and preoperative discussion with the patient. Needless to say, the extent of surgery is clearly dictated by operative findings. Unifocal intraglandular well-differentiated thyroid carcinoma confined to one lobe with negative sonogram for any other nodularity in the contralateral side is appropriately treated by ipsilateral extracapsular thyroid lobectomy. In these low-risk patients, more extensive surgery or adjuvant therapy has no impact on subsequent biological behavior of the cancer and long-term survivorship. Matched-pair analysis of patients undergoing lobectomy and total thyroidectomy show equivalent 30-year survivorship as well as local, regional, and distant failure rates (12). Thus, optimal surgical therapy for low-risk patients with single intrathyroidal unifocal nodule confined to one lobe requires thyroid lobectomy as initial definitive treatment. The presence of contralateral nodules, regardless of whether or not they are malignant, will warrant the need for total thyroidectomy. Similarly, patients who fall into the intermediate- or high-risk category, with more aggressive tumors, will require total thyroidectomy and adjuvant treatment, depending on the histologic nature of the primary tumor, the iodine avidity of the cancer, or the presence or absence of residual disease following surgery in the neck. Extent of surgery has not influenced the subsequent behavior of thyroid cancer in low-risk patients. Twenty-year survivorship in low-risk patients is 99% (13). Similarly, cause-specific mortality at 10 years in low-risk patients in the Mayo Clinic series was zero (2).

Total thyroidectomy is indicated for diffuse bilateral disease, thyroid cancer with gross extrathyroidal extension, patients who present with distant metastases, patients with massive bilateral cervical nodal metastases, and in children with papillary carcinoma in whom radioiodine therapy is indicated by high risk of occult pulmonary metastases. Clearly, total thyroidectomy should be performed if the need for radioactive iodine therapy is thought to be necessary. Patients with invasion of the larynx, trachea, esophagus, and recurrent laryngeal nerves may need more radical operations. If the indication for surgery is cancer, then the appropriate operation is "total extracapsular thyroidectomy." The practice of doing "subtotal" and "near-total" thyroidectomy should be condemned.

RADIOIODINE THERAPY

Routine ablation of thyroid tissue following total thyroidectomy is not warranted in all patients. Clearly, patients in the low-risk

group who have undergone total thyroidectomy have no benefit from radioiodine ablation (2). Ablation of all thyroid tissue will certainly facilitate monitoring the behavior of thyroid cancer with serial thyroglobulin evaluations. However, if surgical thyroidectomy is complete and the postoperative thyroglobulin level is <2, then radioiodine ablation is not necessary. Use of radioactive iodine is not without its sequelae and consequences. Chronic sialadenitis, dryness of mouth, and potential risk of development of multiple primary tumors are a few of the adverse effects of radioiodine therapy (14). Thus, routine use of radioiodine therapy without specific indications is not advisable and can indeed be harmful (15).

Our philosophy is to measure postoperative thyroglobulin in low-risk patients who have undergone total thyroidectomy approximately 6 weeks following surgery. If the basal thyroglobulin level is <2, then we do not advocate radioiodine ablation. These low-risk patients can be simply followed with serial thyroglobulin values as the risk of recurrent disease and death from thyroid cancer in these patients is miniscule.

OVERAGGRESSIVE FOLLOW-UP STRATEGIES

Overaggressive use of serial thyroglobulin assays and ultrasound examination of the central compartment will invariably detect minute and often occult metastatic deposits in lymph nodes less than a few millimeters in diameter. Discovery of such small, inconsequential metastatic deposits will produce extreme apprehension and anxiety in many low-risk patients. Embarking on surgical excision for these inconsequential, minute metastatic deposits can be hazardous and is likely to be accompanied by significant complications as a result of potential risk of injury to the blood supply to the parathyroid glands and to recurrent laryngeal nerves. Thus, extreme discretion needs to be exercised in embarking on overzealous follow-up strategies in low-risk patients. We at Memorial Sloan-Kettering Cancer Center have exercised significant restraint in embarking on fine-needle aspiration cytology of small and stable lymph nodes <1 cm in diameter during postoperative follow-up. Identification of subcentimeter lymph nodes would be followed by serial ultrasounds, and only if progression in the size of such lymph nodes is demonstrated or if a lymph node >1 cm in diameter is detected, would we advocate fine-needle aspiration cytology for confirmation of diagnosis to justify surgical intervention. Under these circumstances, a formal central compartment lymph node dissection of levels VI and VII should be performed.

Exploiting the biological behavior of thyroid cancer in diagnosis and selection of therapy is very valuable and cost-effective. Simple identification of minute amounts of recurrent or metastatic thyroid cancer in regional lymph nodes in low-risk patients has no impact on prognosis but will be a cause for significant anxiety on the part of the patient. Exercise of restraint in overzealous follow-up strategies is essential to deliver cost-effective treatment in a great majority of low-risk patients. Clearly, genetic markers of aggressive behavior in patients with differentiated carcinoma are desperately needed to implement aggressive therapeutic strategies on those few patients in whom a well-differentiated thyroid cancer may cause local recurrence and potential mortality. Such strategy would prevent the blanket use of excessive surgery and aggressive adjuvant therapy in a majority of such patients without any proven benefit.

REFERENCES

1. Shah JP, Loree T, Dharkar D, et al. Prognostic factors in differentiated carcinoma of the thyroid. Am J Surg. 1992;164:658–661.
2. Hay ID, Thompson GB, Grant CS, et al. Papillary thyroid carcinoma managed at the Mayo Clinic during six decades (1940-1999): temporal trends in initial therapy and long-term outcome in 2444 consecutively treated patients. World J Surg. 2002;26:879–885.
3. Hughes CJ, Shaha AR, Shah JP, et al. Impact of lymph node metastasis in differentiated carcinoma of the thyroid. Surgery. 1995;118:1131–1138.
4. Sywak M, Pasieka JL, Ogilvie T. A review of thyroid cancer with intermediate differentiation. J Surg Oncol. 2004;86:44–54.
5. Rosai J. Poorly differentiated thyroid carcinoma: introduction to the issue, its landmarks, and clinical impact. Endocr Pathol. 2004;15: 293–296.
6. Rosai J, Saxen EA, Woolner L. Undifferentiated and poorly differentiated carcinoma. Semin Diagn Pathol. 1985;2:123–136.
7. Hutter RV, Tollefsen HR, De Cosse JJ, et al. Spindle and giant cell metaplasia in papillary carcinoma of the thyroid. Am J Surg. 1965;110:660–668.
8. Cady B. Our AMES is true: how an old concept still hits the mark: or, risk group assignment points the arrow to rational therapy selection in differentiated thyroid cancer. Am J Surg. 1997;174:462–468.
9. McConahey WM, Hay ID, Woolner LB, et al. Papillary thyroid cancer treated at the Mayo Clinic, 1946 through 1970: initial manifestations, pathologic findings, therapy, and outcome. Mayo Clin Proc. 1986;61:978–996.
10. Hay ID, Bergstralh EJ, Goellner JR, et al. Predicting outcome in papillary thyroid carcinoma: development of a reliable prognostic scoring system in a cohort of 1,779 patients surgically treated at one institution during 1940 through 1989. Surgery. 1993;114:1050–1058.
11. Shaha AR, Shah JP, Loree TR. Risk group stratification and prognostic factors in papillary carcinoma of thyroid. Ann Surg Oncol. 1996;3:534–538.
12. Shah JP, Loree TR, Dharker D, et al. Lobectomy vs. total thyroidectomy for differentiated carcinoma of the thyroid. A matched pair analysis. Am J Surg. 1993;166:331–335.
13. Shaha AR, Shah JP, Loree TR. Low risk differentiated thyroid cancer. The need for selective treatment. Ann Surg Oncol. 1997;4:328–333.
14. Rubino C, de Vathaire F, Dottorini ME, et al. Second primary malignancies in thyroid cancer patients. Br J Cancer. 2003;89: 1638–1644.
15. Jonklaas J, Sarlis NJ, Litofsky D, et al. Outcomes of patients with differentiated thyroid carcinoma following initial therapy. Thyroid. 2006;16:1229–1242.

51

Surgical Management of Primary Lung Cancer

Robert J. McKenna Jr.

Although surgery has been the mainstay of treatment for lung cancer for over 60 years, during the last decade there have been substantial changes in the approach. For many years, lung surgery was simply a major resection through a posterolateral thoracotomy incision. Current additional treatment options include minimally invasive surgery, new surgical techniques, and multimodality therapies. These changes require a different understanding and approach to evaluation of the potential candidate for an operation.

DIAGNOSTIC EVALUATION AND PRETREATMENT PLANNING

Diagnosis

The use of needle biopsy to diagnose a lung mass is somewhat controversial (1). Some centers routinely biopsy lung masses. The author does not because there are some false-negative biopsy results and the test usually cannot prove that a mass is benign. Therefore, suspicious masses are resected whether the biopsy result is diagnostic for cancer or if it is nondiagnostic.

The positron emission tomography (PET) scan is often incorporated into the standard workup of a pulmonary mass. If the mass does not enhance on PET scan, there is a minimal chance that it could be cancer. False-negative PET scans occur in masses <10 mm and bronchioalveolar cancers (2).

Radiologic Evaluation

The era of multimodality treatment for lung cancer has increased the importance of staging for the lung cancer patient (Table 51.1). Patients with stage IA disease with a good performance status are candidates for resection and follow-up. Patients with stage IB through stage IIIA disease are candidates for multimodality treatment with postoperative chemotherapy. If patients are shown to have N2 disease prior to resection, they usually receive preoperative chemotherapy and then resection. Therefore, accurate staging is critically important for determining the optimal treatment of the patient.

The evaluation begins with a thorough history and physical examination. Any neurologic or bone symptoms necessitate a magnetic resonance image of the brain or a bone scan. These tests may also be indicated for patients with unexplained weight loss or more advanced tumors on computed tomography (CT) scan.

The workup routinely includes radiologic intrathoracic staging. The surgeon needs to view the CT scan of the chest for many reasons. The size and relationship of the primary tumor

to the pulmonary vessels, the fissures, chest wall, and the bronchi help with operative planning. For example, for a centrally located tumor in the anterior segment of the right upper lobe, the relationship of the tumor to the artery will determine the need for a pneumonectomy or a lobectomy. The physiologic tolerance of a pneumonectomy must be assessed.

Evaluation of the mediastinum is critical to the operative planning for a lung cancer. Generally, the sensitivity and specificity of CT evaluation of mediastinal nodes are both about 60% (3). The PET scan is often incorporated into the standard staging of a lung cancer. The literature reports that the PET scan may identify unsuspected distant metastatic disease in 10% of patients. The PET scan is better than the CT for evaluation of the mediastinum (sensitivity, 85%; specificity, 70%). In our experience with over 1,000 PET scans for lung cancer, the false-positive rate is 30%, so surgeons often will confirm the status of the mediastinal node rather than rely on the PET scan.

There is no substitute for pathologic staging. A cervical mediastinoscopy is a short operation that allows biopsy of paratracheal (level 2 and 4), pretracheal (level 3), subcarinal (level 7), and tracheobronchial angle (level 10) nodes. This is usually an outpatient operation done under general anesthesia. Biopsy of para-aortic (level 5) and aortopulmonary window (level 6) nodes usually require an anterior mediastinotomy. This is often, although not always, an outpatient operation performed with general anesthesia. Because this operation is more painful than a mediastinoscopy, the patient may remain in the hospital overnight.

Physiologic Evaluation

Patients routinely have pulmonary function tests prior to a resection. The postoperative forced expiratory volume in 1 second (FEV_1) should be >40%. For patients with marginal pulmonary status, a quantitative ventilation-perfusion scan is often helpful. The lateral and oblique views are studied to determine how functional is the section to be removed. If a pneumonectomy is contemplated, the perfusion scan will tell the surgeon how much function is on the side to be resected. Exercise pulmonary function tests and VO_2 max may be helpful.

ROLE FOR SURGERY FOR THE TREATMENT OF LUNG CANCER

At the present time, surgery has the highest cure rate for any treatment available for lung cancer, and it has a role for the

Table 51.1

Staging System for Lung Cancer

Definition of TNM

Primary tumor (T)

TX	Primary tumor cannot be assessed or tumor proven by the presence of malignant cells in sputum or bronchial washings but not visualized by imaging or bronchoscopy
	No evidence of primary tumor
	Carcinoma in situ
	Tumor ≤3 cm in greatest dimension, surrounded by lung or visceral pleura, without bronchoscopic evidence of invasion more proximal than the lobar bronchus,[a] (i.e., not in the main bronchus)
T2	Tumor with any of the following features of size or extent:
	More than 3 cm in greatest dimension
	Involves main bronchus, ≥2 cm distal to the carina
	Invades the visceral pleura
	Associated with atelectasis or obstructive pneumonitis that extends to the hilar region but does not involve the entire lung
T3	Tumor of any size that directly invades any of the following: chest wall (including superior sulcus tumors), diaphragm, mediastinal pleura, parietal pericardium; or tumor in the main bronchus <2 cm distal to the carina, but without involvement of the carina; or associated atelectasis or obstructive pneumonitis of the entire lung
T4	Tumor of any size that invades any of the following: mediastinum, heart, great vessels, trachea, esophagus, vertebral body, carina; or separate tumor nodules in the same lobe; or tumor with malignant pleural effusion[b]

Regional lymph nodes (N)

NX	Regional lymph nodes cannot be assessed
N0	No regional lymph node metastasis
N1	Metastasis to ipsilateral peribronchial and/or ipsilateral hilar lymph nodes, and intrapulmonary nodes including involvement by direct extension of the primary tumor
N2	Metastasis to ipsilateral mediastinal and/or subcarinal lymph node(s)
N3	Metastasis to contralateral mediastinal, contralateral hilar, ipsilateral or contralateral scalene, or supraclavicular lymph node(s)

Distant metastasis (M)

MX	Distant metastasis cannot be assessed
M0	No distant metastasis
M1[c]	Distant metastasis present

Stage grouping

Occult carcinoma	TX	N0	M0
Stage 0	Tis	N0	M0
Stage IA	T1	N0	M0
Stage IB	T2	N0	M0
Stage IIA	T1	N1	M0
Stage IIB	T2	N1	M0
	T3	N0	M0
Stage IIIA	T1	N2	M0
	T2	N2	M0
	T3	N1	M0
	T3	N2	M0
Stage IIIB	Any T	N3	M0
	T4	Any N	M0
Stage IV	Any T	Any N	M1

[a] Note: The uncommon superficial tumor of any size with its invasive component limited to the bronchial wall, which may extend proximal to the main bronchus, is also classified T1.

[b] Note: Most pleural effusions associated with lung cancer are due to tumor. However, there are a few patients in whom multiple cytopathologic examinations of pleural fluid are negative for tumor. In these cases, fluid is nonbloody and is not an exudate. Such patients may be further evaluated by videothoracoscopy (VATS) and direct pleural biopsies. When these elements and clinical judgment dictate that the effusion is not related to the tumor, the effusion should be excluded as a staging element and the patient should be staged T1, T2, or T3.

[c] Note: M1 includes separate tumor nodule(s) in a different lobe (ipsilateral or contralateral).

From the *American Joint Committee on Cancer Staging Manual.* 6th ed. New York: Springer, 2002:171, with permission.

Table 51.2

Usual Treatment of Lung Cancer by Stage

Stage	Treatment of Choice
1A	Lobectomy
1B	Lobectomy plus adjuvant treatment
2A and 2B	Lobectomy plus adjuvant treatment
3A	Neoadjuvant treatment and lobectomy
3B	Usually nonsurgical treatment
4	Nonsurgical treatment

treatment of all four stages of lung cancer. Table 51.2 shows the most common treatment by stage. For stages IA through IIIA, surgery is the primary treatment. Recent studies have shown that neoadjuvant and adjuvant treatment may add slightly to the cure rate of an operation. That will be discussed later in the chapter.

Lobectomy

For many years, a lobectomy has been the standard resection for lung cancer. In the 1940s and 1950s, a pneumonectomy was the standard resection until surgical techniques improved and studies showed that a lobectomy offered the same results.

As operative techniques improved further, there was interest in sublobar resection (segmentectomy and wedge resection). The only randomized trial to compare lobar resection with sublobar resection for the treatment of stage IA (T1N0) non-small cell lung cancer (NSCLC) was reported in 1995 by the Lung Cancer Study Group (4). A threefold increase in local recurrence was found in patients who underwent a procedure that was less than a lobectomy. In a nonrandomized study comparing lobectomy and lesser resections, Warren and Faber (5) reported a 22% local recurrence rate for patients with stage I disease after lesser resection versus 4.9% after lobar resection. Therefore, for several decades the preferred treatment for NSCLC has been a lobectomy.

Pneumonectomy

The goal of any cancer operation must be complete resection of the cancer. There has never been proof that an incomplete or partial resection benefited patients. In some cases, therefore, complete resection requires a pneumonectomy. This procedure carries a higher risk than a lobectomy, and a right pneumonectomy has a higher mortality than a left pneumonectomy (10% vs. 3.3%). Darling et al. (6) concluded that the higher risk of a bronchopleural fistula for a right versus left pneumonectomy (9 [13.2%]) vs. left, 6 [5.0%]; $p = 0.0472$) accounts for the higher mortality. In addition, a right pneumonectomy after preoperative chemotherapy and radiation has been reported to increase the mortality rate to 23.9%) (7).

Sleeve Resections

There are cases in which creative procedures can provide clear margins around the cancer without the need for a pneumonectomy. An example is a sleeve resection of the right upper lobe with transection of the main stem bronchus and the intermedi-ate bronchus and reimplantation of the intermediate bronchus into the proximal main stem or the trachea. The vessels and the fissures are handled in the standard fashion for a lobectomy. By preserving seven of the ten segments that would have been resected with a pneumonectomy, a right upper lobe sleeve resection provides better quality of life without compromising the survival rate (8).

Many different sleeve resections are possible. For example, if a left upper lobe cancer is attached to the main left pulmonary artery at the origin of the anterior trunk, a vascular sleeve resection is possible. A carcinoid tumor at the origin of the middle lobe bronchus can be resected with a sleeve resection of the middle lobe and the superior segment of the lower lobe. This removes only three segments, rather than the alternative procedure, a lower and middle lobectomy, that would remove seven segments.

Extended Resections

If a lung cancer extends beyond the limits of the lobe into the mediastinum or the chest wall, a more radical resection than a standard lobectomy may be justified. For a T3N0 tumor that extends to the chest wall, lobectomy with chest wall resection provides a 39.6% 5-year survival, whereas the survival is only 7.1% with N1 or N2 nodes (9). Similar results are possible for resection of tumors invading the diaphragm or pericardium. A localized tumor invading the superior vena cava may be resected for cure (10). There are even reports of 20% 5-year survivals for resection of a lobe and vertebral bodies when the bone is invaded (11). There are very few tumors that are amenable to such a resection, and this type of procedure requires a multimodality team for the pulmonary resection, spinal resection, and the reconstruction. It is only worth considering if the radiologic evaluation suggests that the tumor can be completely resected. Usually the tumor should not extend past the midline.

Segmentectomy/Wedge Resection

Recently, CT screening detection of ever smaller peripheral NSCLC again raised the question of a lesser resection. Published series suggest that lesser resections may offer similar results to a lobectomy for tiny, peripheral stage IA NSCLC (12,13) especially for subpleural bronchioalveolar cancers, which have a much lower incidence of nodal metastases than the other types of NSCLC (14).

ADJUVANT BRACHYTHERAPY AND EXTERNAL-BEAM RADIATION

The higher incidence of local recurrence has been the primary factor leading North American surgeons to abandon resections less than a lobectomy. Adjuvant treatments may reduce the incidence of local recurrence. In the 1980s, Miller and Hatcher (15) treated a series of patients with compromised pulmonary function (FEV$_1$ = 35% to 40% predicted). Coned-down radiation (4,500 rad) to the margin of resection reduced the recurrence rate from 20% to 7.5% for the radiated vs. nonradiated group.

Recently, adjuvant brachytherapy has been evaluated. In a nonrandomized series comparing lobectomy with wedge resection for stage IA (T1N0) disease, the mean and median survivals were 95.8 and 85 months for lobectomy and 82.2 and 55.8 months for lesser resections. These were not significantly different ($p = 0.97$) (16). However, for tumors 2 to 3 cm in size, the median survival was significantly better after lobectomy, (70 vs. 44.7 months; $p = 0.003$) (17). Brachytherapy (125-iodinne seeds in a mesh on the margin of resection for the wedge resections) decreased local recurrence rates from 18.6% to 2%, compared with patients who did not receive adjuvant brachytherapy (16).

RADIATION AS PRIMARY TREATMENT

Primary radiation therapy is an alternative to the surgical treatment of lung cancer, but the results are poor. Of 71 node-negative patients who received at least 60 Gy to their cancers, 3- and 5-year survival rates were 19% and 12% (18). A different series of 141 patients with stage I disease demonstrated 2- and 5-year survival rates of 39% and 13%, respectively (18). In another series of 60 patients with stage I or II cancers treated with radiation therapy, local progression occurred in 53% of patients, with a median progression-free survival of 18.5 months and an overall median survival of 20 months (19). The overall median survival was 18 months.

New Approaches for Radiation

Stereotactic radiation has been used for years for the brain and is now available for lung tumors. This requires a special machine with respiratory gating. A large radiation dose is concentrated on pulmonary tumors in the hope that this delivery system will have better efficacy than traditional radiation therapy. The experience is currently too early to evaluate the results (20). Brachytherapy seeds can be placed percutaneously with CT guidance, but there are no data to show the results (21).

Radiofrequency Ablation

Radiofrequency ablation (RFA) has been used for tumors in other organs and recently has been used for lung tumors (22). Its use has primarily been limited to patients who are not surgical candidates. For example, we use RFA for patients with marginal pulmonary function, poor performance status, or patients with metachronous bronchioalveolar cancers. Local recurrence rates are high for tumors >4 cm, but RFA appears to be effective for small tumors (22). Currently, however, no long-term follow-up data exist. Until long-term outcomes are available, RFA should be reserved for patients who are deemed to be at increased risk with pulmonary resection.

VIDEO-ASSISTED THORACIC SURGERY VERSUS OPEN PULMONARY RESECTIONS

Video-assisted thoracic surgery (VATS) lobectomies have been performed since 1992 (23). Although some surgeons still have concerns, many articles in the literature now prove the safety and ability to perform standard anatomic dissection and node dissection by VATS. Between 1992 and 2005, we performed 1,315

VATS lobectomies in 700 women (54.1%) and 605 men (45.9%), with a mean age of 71.2 years, with a 0.8% mortality rate. The mean length of stay was 4.78 days and the median length of stay was 3 days. On the first postoperative day, 70 patients (5.3%) were discharged, and on the second postoperative day, 260 patients (19.8%) were discharged No complications occurred in 84.7% of the patients. Conversion to a thoracotomy occurred in 28 patients (2.5%). In 2003, 89% of our lobectomies were performed with VATS. These data clearly show that lobectomies can be safely performed by VATS. The survival for VATS lobectomies is the same survival as has been reported for lobectomy via a thoracotomy.

The literature even suggests that VATS may have advantages over thoracotomy for lobectomy, although there are no current large randomized, prospective series to compare thoracotomy and VATS approaches for lobectomy. Demmy and Curtis (24) showed that the VATS approach has less blood loss, a shorter hospitalization (5.3 ± 3.7 vs. 12.2 ± 11.1 days; $p = 0.02$), shorter chest tube duration (4.0 ± 2.8 vs. 8.3 ± 8.9 days; $p = 0.06$), and earlier returns to full preoperative activities (2.2 ± 1.0 vs. 3.6 ± 1.0 months; $p <0.01$). There was less pain 3 weeks after the lobectomy for the VATS group (none or mild, 63% vs. 6%; severe, 6% vs. 63%; $p <0.01$). A randomized trial from Germany showed fewer complications after the VATS approach (14.2% vs. 50%) (25). Cost, as measured by anesthesia charges, laboratory charges, and hospital charges, were less with the VATS approach (26).

So, why are <10% of lobectomies in the United States performed via VATS? A switch from thoracotomies to VATS is a large leap. Few centers perform VATS lobectomies, so the faculty needs to learn the procedure to teach residents. This process will take time.

COMBINED LUNG VOLUME REDUCTION SURGERY AND LUNG CANCER SURGERY

The advent of lung volume-reduction surgery (LVRS) has allowed pulmonary resections in patients who were previously physiologically inoperable. We have operated on patients with an FEV_1 as low as 400 mL. LVRS is typically performed for patients with upper lobe emphysema that is resected to allow the better parenchyma in the lower lobes to allow more effective function. For selected patients, LVRS improves pulmonary function, exercise capacity, quality of life, and survival (27). When patients have severe emphysema and a cancer, they can undergo operations for both diseases. If the emphysema and the cancer is in the same area, then a lobectomy can be performed and LVRS on the opposite side. If the emphysema is in the upper lobes and the cancer is in the lower lobe, then upper lobe LVRS and a wedge resection of the lower lobe can be performed.

ADJUVANT THERAPY

Until 2004, there was no evidence that adjuvant treatment was effective for lung cancer. Two randomized, prospective studies have shown a 5% to 10% improvement in survival for patients with resected stage IB to IIIA NSCLC (28,29).

A randomized, prospective study by the Lung Cancer Study Group showed that radiation reduced the incidence of local recurrence but did not alter survival (30). There is still no proof of benefit for radiation after pulmonary resection.

NEOADJUVANT THERAPY

In two randomized, prospective studies, neoadjuvant treatment has now been shown to improve survival for patients with stage III NSCLC (31,32). These studies used chemotherapy alone. There are phase 2 studies that use chemotherapy and radiation therapy preoperatively, but there is no phase 3 trial that compares preoperative chemotherapy with preoperative chemotherapy and radiation. Both impact the operation after neoadjuvant treatment. After preoperative chemotherapy and radiation, the chance of a pneumonectomy is 30% (33) and the risk of a right pneumonectomy in that setting is 25% (9).

Operations after neoadjuvant treatment are different compared with operations when no preoperative treatment has been given. The operations are certainly technically more challenging. Operating around vessels is difficult because the normal planes around vessels have been obliterated. The lymph node areas are usually matted, making dissections challenging. The morbidity and mortality of an operation after neoadjuvant treatment is comparable to that for a lobectomy without neoadjuvant treatment (34). In our experience, a lobectomy can usually be performed by VATS after preoperative chemotherapy, but not after preoperative chemotherapy and radiation. When the patient has received preoperative radiation therapy, a flap (usually an intercostal muscle flap) is placed on the bronchial stump.

LYMPH NODE DISSECTION OR SAMPLING

Most thoracic surgeons agree that mediastinal lymph nodes need to be evaluated pathologically, but there is disagreement about the extent of the nodal removal. The PET scan and the CT scan are not accurate enough. Sentinel node biopsies are common for breast cancer evaluation, but not for lung cancer evaluation. Nodal removal is important for prognosis (because patients with nodal disease have a worse survival), therapy (because some patients with nodal mets are long-term survivors), and treatment implications (because it is now common to offer postoperative chemotherapy to patients with N1 or N2 disease). Some surgeons perform selective nodal sampling (35), while others perform formal nodal dissections (36). Currently, there is no accepted standard as to the extent of lymphadenectomy.

CONCLUSION

Patients with early-stage NSCLC should be treated with complete surgical resection whenever possible. The current standard pulmonary resection is an anatomic lobectomy. Lesser resections are currently thought to increase the local recurrence rate and compromise the potential for cure. The lobectomy should include removal of mediastinal lymph nodes by either sampling or dissection. The data regarding the use of VATS for a lobectomy suggests that it should be used more often for the treatment of lung cancer. Adjuvant radiotherapy has not improved survival in patients with resected NSCLC, while postoperative chemotherapy has now been shown to slightly improve survival. More clinical trials, earlier diagnosis, and better systemic treatment are needed if the prognosis for lung cancer is to change dramatically.

REFERENCES

1. Mohammed TL, White CS, Yankelevitz DF. Percutaneous needle biopsy in single lung patients. *J Comput Assist Tomogr.* 2006;30:267–269.
2. Bunyaviroch T, Coleman RE. PET evaluation of lung cancer. *J Nucl Med.* 2006;47:451–469.
3. McKenna RJ Jr, Libshitz HI, Mountain CF, et al. Roentgenographic evaluation of mediastinal nodes for preoperative assessment in lung cancer. *Chest.* 1985;88:206–210.
4. Ginsberg RJ, Rubinstein LV. Randomized trial of lobectomy versus limited resection for T1 N0 non-small cell lung cancer. Lung Cancer Study Group. *Ann Thorac Surg.* 1995;60:615–622.
5. Warren WH, Faber LP. Segmentectomy vs. lobectomy in patients with stage I pulmonary carcinoma: 5 year survival and patterns of intrathoracic recurrence. *J Thorac Cardiovasc Surg.* 1994;107:1087–1094.
6. Darling G, Abdurahman A, Yi QL, et al. Risk of a right pneumonectomy: role of bronchopleural fistula. *Ann Thorac Surg.* 2005;79:433–437.
7. Martin J, Ginsberg RJ, Abolhoda A, et al. Morbidity and mortality after neoadjuvant therapy for lung cancer: the risks of right pneumonectomy. *Ann Thorac Surg.* 2001;72:1149–1154.
8. Fadel E, Yildizeli B, Chapelier AR, et al. Sleeve lobectomy for bronchogenic cancers: factors affecting survival. *Ann Thorac Surg.* 2002;74:851–858.
9. Lin YT, Hsu PK, Hsu HS, et al. En bloc resection for lung cancer with chest wall invasion. *J Clin Med Assoc.* 2006;69:157–161.
10. Shargall Y, de Perrot M, Keshavjee S, et al. 15 years single center experience with surgical resection of the superior vena cava for non-small cell lung cancer. *Lung Cancer.* 2004;45:357–363.
11. DeMeester TR, Albertucci M, Dawson PJ, et al. Management of tumor adherent to the vertebral column. *J Thorac Cardiovasc Surg.* 1989;97:373–378.
12. Kodama K, Doi O, Higashiyama M, et al. Intentional limited resection for selected patients with T1 N0 M0 non-small-cell lung cancer: a single-institution study. *J Thorac Cardiovasc Surg.* 1997;114:347–353.
13. Landreneau RJ, Sugerbaker DJ, Mark MJ, et al. Wedge resection versus lobectomy for stage I non-small cell lung cancer. *J Thorac Cardiovasc Surg.* 1997;113:691–700.
14. Okada M, Yoshikawa K, Hatta T, et al. Is segmentectomy with lymph node assessment an alternative to lobectomy for non-small cell lung cancer of 2 cm or smaller? *Ann Thorac Surg.* 2001;71:956–960.
15. Miller JI, Hatcher CR. Limited resection of bronchogenic carcinoma in the patient with marked impairment of pulmonary function. *Ann Thorac Surg.* 1987;44:340–343.
16. Fernando HC, Santos RS, Benfield JR. Lobar and sublobar resection with and without brachytherapy for small stage IA non-small cell lung cancer. *J Thorac Cardiovasc.* 2005;129:261–267.
17. Kupelian PA, Komaki R, Allen P. Prognostic factors in the treatment of node-negative non-small cell lung carcinoma with radiotherapy alone. *Int J Radiat Oncol Biol Phys* 1996;36;:607–613.

18. Sibley GS, Jamieson TA, Marks LB, et al. Radiotherapy alone for medically inoperable stage I non–small cell lung cancer: the Duke experience. *Int J Radiat Oncol Biol Phys* 1998;40:149–154.

19. Zierhut D, Bettscheider C, Schubert K, et al. Radiation therapy of stage I and II non–small cell lung cancer (NSCLC). *Lung Cancer.* 2001;34(Suppl 3):S39–S43.

20. Whyte R, Crownover R, Murphy MJ, et al Stereotactic radiosurgery for lung tumors: preliminary report of a phase I trial *Ann Thorac Surg.* 2003;75:1097–1101.

21. Martinez-Monge R, Garran C, Vivas I, et al. Percutaneous CT-guided 103Pd implantation for the medically inoperable patient with T1N0M0 non-small cell lung cancer: a case report. *Brachytherapy.* 2004;3:179–181.

22. El-Sherif A, Luketich J, Landreneau RJ, et al New therapeutic approaches for early stage non-small cell lung cancer. *Surg Oncol.* 2005;14:27–32.

23. McKenna RJ Jr, Houck W, Fuller CB. Video-assisted thoracic surgery lobectomy: experience with 1,100 cases. *Ann Thorac Surg.* 2006;81:421–426.

24. Demmy TL, Curtis JJ. Minimally invasive lobectomy directed toward frail and high-risk patients: a case-control study. *Ann Thorac Surg.* 1999;68:194–200.

25. Hoksch B, Ablassmaier B, Walter M, et al. Complication rate after thoracoscopic and conventional lobectomy. *Zentralblatt fur Chirurgie.* 2003;128:106–110.

26. Nakajima J, Takamoto S, Kohno T, et al. Costs of videothoracoscopic surgery versus open resection for patients with lung carcinoma. *Cancer.* 2000;89(11 Suppl):2497–2501.

27. McKenna RJ Jr, Fischel RJ, Brenner M, et al. Combined operations for lung volume reduction surgery and lung cancer. *Chest.* 1996;110:885–888.

28. Douillard J, Rosell R, Delena M, et al. ANITA: phase III adjuvant vinorelbine and cisplatin versus observation in completely resected (stage I-III) non-small cell lung cancer patients: final results after 70-month median follow-up. *J Clin Oncol.* 2005;23(Suppl 16):624s

29. Strauss GM, Herndon J, Maddaus MA, et al. Randomized clinical trial of adjuvant chemotherapy with paclitaxel and carboplatin following resection in stage IB non-small cell lung cancer (NSCLC): report of Cancer and Leukemia Group B (CALGB) Protocol 9633. *J Clin Oncol.* 2004;22(Suppl):7019.

30. Weisenburger T, Gail M, for the Lung Cancer Study Group. Effects of postoperative mediastinal radiation on completely resected stage II and III epidermoid carcinoma of the lung. *N Engl J Med.* 1986;315:1377–1381.

31. Rosell R, Gomez-Codina J, Camps C, et al. A randomized trial comparing preoperative chemotherapy plus surgery with surgery alone in patients with non-small cell lung cancer. *N Engl J Med.* 1994;330:153–158.

32. Roth JA, Fossella F, Komaki R, et al. A randomized trial comparing preoperative chemotherapy plus surgery with surgery alone in patients with resectable non-small cell lung cancer. *J Natl Cancer Inst.* 1994;86:673–680.

33. Rusch V, Albain K, Crowley J, et al. Surgical resection of stage IIIA and stage IIIB non-small cell lung cancer after intensive preoperative chemoradiotherapy: a Southwest Oncology Group study. *J Thorac Cardiovasc Surg.* 1993;105:97–104.

34. Takizawa T, Terashima M, Koike T, et al. Mediastinal lymph node metastasis in patients with clinical stage I peripheral non-small-cell lung cancer. J Thorac Cardiovasc Surg. 1997;113:248–252.

35. Naruke T, Tsuchiya R, Kondo H. Lymph node sampling in lung cancer: how should it be done? *Eur J Cardiothorac Surg.* 1999;16(Suppl 1):S17–S24.

36. Keller S, Adak H, Wagner H et al. Mediastinal lymph node dissection improves survival in patients with stages II and IIIa non-small cell lung cancer. Eastern Cooperative Oncology Group. *Ann Thorac Surg.* 2000;70:358–365.

COMMENTARY
Larry R. Kaiser

Although it garners nowhere near the press coverage that breast cancer receives, carcinoma of the lung accounts for more deaths in both women and men than any other malignancy. More deaths result from lung cancer in the United States than from breast cancer, colorectal cancer, and prostate cancer combined. There seemingly remains an undercurrent that holds to the view that because so many lung cancers are smoking-related, patients who develop the disease somehow are "getting what they brought upon themselves." There can be no question that lung cancer, for the most part, is much more prevalent in those who smoke than in those who do not, but approximately 15% of lung cancers occur in nonsmokers.

Lung cancers are categorized into two major groups: small cell and, for lack of a better term, non-small cell. By far the majority of lung cancers are of the non-small cell type, accounting for at least 85%. Small cell lung cancer, in the era before effective chemotherapy, usually resulted in death in a matter of weeks, and is assumed to be a systemic disease at the time of presentation. The rare small cell lung cancer will present as a solitary pulmonary nodule but the majority present with bulky intrathoracic disease with or without evidence of systemic spread. With the presumption of systemic disease, all but the few isolated small cell lung cancers are treated initially with multidrug platinum-based chemotherapy, most commonly cis-platinum or carboplatin in combination with etoposide, followed by radiation therapy for those with so-called limited disease, that is disease confined to the thorax (1). Patients with extensive-disease small cell lung cancer are treated with chemotherapy alone with radiation therapy reserved for the treatment of symptomatic metastases. From the time of diagnosis, the median survival ranges from 14 to 20 months for limited-disease small cell and 8 to 13 months for extensive disease. For non-small cell lung cancers, prognostic variables include tumor stage, presence or absence of lymph node involvement, and a number of clinical factors including overall performance status.

SCREENING

Intuitively it makes sense that early diagnosis at least for non-small cell lung cancer should result in more people being cured, yet the overall mortality for lung cancer has not changed significantly in many years. Despite the belief that earlier diagnosis should be an advantage, the American Cancer Society currently does not recommend yearly chest radiographs as a screening modality to detect early lung cancers, based on data from studies published in the late 1970s. Recently these data have been called into question by the use of low-dose computed tomographic (CT) scanners as a screening tool. In a large collaborative study in which over 30,000 asymptomatic persons considered at risk for lung cancer were screened, a diagnosis of lung cancer was made in 484 participants. Of these, 412 (85%) had clinical stage I disease and the estimated 10-year survival rate for this group was 88% (2). There is no doubt that low-dose CT scanning is capable of detecting early lung cancer, but the question remains as to whether a screened population has a better overall survival than a nonscreened population, recognizing that a number of cancers will appear between screening intervals and a significant percentage of cancers detected will already be at an advanced stage. The current study did not enroll a control group and was not a prospective randomized trial; thus we still have no basis on which to say that screening with early identification of lung cancer will decrease overall lung cancer mortality, although the thought remains an intriguing one. A randomized trial of lung cancer screening currently is underway and being conducted under the auspices of the Mayo Clinic.

DIAGNOSIS AND IMAGING

Unfortunately most patients with lung cancer are found to have disseminated disease at the time of presentation, and even with currently available chemotherapy, including the newer targeted therapies such as the epidermal growth factor receptor inhibitors, as well as radiation therapy delivered following sophisticated treatment planning, few if any of these patients can be cured. From a surgical standpoint we have the advantage of dealing with a selected patient population, those with either local disease or locally advanced disease along with a few exceptions. The prototypical patient is the individual with a solitary pulmonary nodule, the so-called coin lesion that is found on a chest radiograph that is being done for some other purpose, often as a preoperative study prior to an elective procedure. Once a lesion is identified on a chest radiograph the patient should be sent for a chest CT scan to be done with contrast to better delineate mediastinal and hilar lymph nodes. The chest CT scan serves to further delineate the clinical stage of the disease. I look for additional pulmonary nodules, bony abnormalities, enlarged lymph nodes either in the hilum of the lung or the mediastinum, and evidence of metastatic disease, specifically in the liver and adrenal glands, two common sites of metastatic disease.

The recent advent of integrated positron emission tomography (PET)-CT scanners has obviated the need for a stand-alone CT scan in many centers, and patients benefit from both the anatomic delineation provided by the CT scan and the metabolic information provided by the PET component. Integrated PET-CT provides a statistically significant advantage over CT alone in assessing lymph node involvement both at the N1 (hilar) and N2 (mediastinal) nodal locations (3). Interestingly, sensitivity (TP/FN + TP [true positive/false-negative + true positive]) is not improved with PET-CT, but specificity (TN/FP + TN [true negative/false-positive + true negative]) and accuracy are significantly better. How this translates operationally varies

among surgeons, but in our hands a positive finding on PET-CT scan in a node that is not markedly enlarged prompts a mediastinoscopy to confirm metastatic disease based on the significant false-positive incidence. However, a negative PET-CT finding often leads to thoracotomy without a confirming mediastinoscopy because of the low incidence of false-negative results. Considering that integrated PET-CT is now state of the art in most institutions, continued validation of the results will be important.

STAGING AND PREOPERATIVE TREATMENT

Surgical resection remains the treatment of choice for patients with local or locally advanced disease. Once a patient has been clinically determined to have stage I or stage II disease, a decision must be made as to whether further invasive staging is warranted. As mentioned, a PET-positive mediastinal lymph node should prompt mediastinoscopy to document histologically the presence of metastatic disease. If ipsilateral mediastinal lymph node disease is present in the absence of contralateral nodal disease, current treatment involves preoperative chemotherapy with or without radiation therapy. Often this decision is based on whether the lymph node disease is contained within the lymph node(s) or extends beyond the capsule of the lymph node. Bulky mediastinal lymph node disease should mandate consideration of combined radiation therapy and chemotherapy, in some instances given concurrently as a preoperative regimen if operation is being contemplated. Many would argue that in the case of bulky lymph node involvement, definitive chemoradiation without operation should be the treatment of choice.

Taylor and colleagues (4) looked at 107 patients with stage IIIA disease who were treated over a 10-year period at the M.D. Anderson Cancer Center with either induction chemotherapy followed by resection or concurrent chemoradiation. In this nonrandomized study, no statistically significant differences were found in local control, overall disease-free survival, or distant metastasis-free survival between the two treatment groups. Median survival time was 31 months and 27 months, and the 5-year overall survival rate was 33% and 30% in the chemotherapy/surgery and chemoradiation groups, respectively. However patients in the chemotherapy/surgery group who had a significant response to induction chemotherapy had a significantly improved 5-year overall survival (50%) compared with those who had stable or progressive disease (16%; $p = 0.0001$).

There are few randomized clinical trials comparing a nonsurgical approach with induction therapy followed by resection in patients with stage IIIA disease. In a meta-analysis of randomized controlled trials of surgery for non-small cell lung cancer, Wright and colleagues (5) started with 1,681 citations identified as potentially relevant, that after systematic review yielded 11 trials that fit criteria for inclusion. Looking at trials that compared chemotherapy plus radiotherapy with chemotherapy plus surgery in patients with stage IIIA disease shows a 4-year survival advantage for patients undergoing resection. Several additional trials that are ongoing should help to further clarify the value, or lack thereof, for surgical resection in patients with locally advanced disease.

POSTOPERATIVE ADJUVANT THERAPY

Dr. McKenna mentions the change in thinking about postoperative adjuvant therapy based on several recent trials (6–8). For the past 3 or 4 years, medical oncologists have taken an aggressive approach to postoperative adjuvant therapy for essentially all resected patients, with the exception of those with stage Ia disease. Despite the modest improvement in survival demonstrated by these "positive" studies, patients routinely get the "hard sell" from medical oncologists based on the rationalization that even with the small difference, a significant number of patients could benefit based on the large numbers of patients who develop lung cancer. A recent update to one of the studies has shown that at least one group, those with stage Ib (N0) disease, previously thought to benefit from adjuvant therapy, actually do not, based on longer follow-up (9). It remains to be seen whether this update will influence the behavior of medical oncologists in recommending adjuvant therapy to this group.

ISSUES REGARDING SURGICAL RESECTION

There is no argument that operation for early-stage disease (stage I and II) is a well-established therapy and is associated with longer survival than treatment with nonoperative approaches. As Dr. McKenna points out, some controversy continues to exist over the optimal surgical approach. Anatomic lobectomy long has been considered the "gold standard" for surgical resection and this was reinforced by the Lung Cancer Study Group randomized trial comparing lobectomy with lesser resection that showed a threefold increase in local recurrence among those who underwent either a nonanatomic wedge excision or an anatomic segmentectomy (9). This increased incidence of local recurrence also translated into poorer 5-year survival for the group undergoing limited resection. Unless it is thought that the patient's pulmonary function will not allow it, a lobectomy should be performed and lesser resections should be viewed as a compromise. However, what we have learned from our experience with lung volume-reduction surgery is that many patients previously thought to be inoperable on the basis of poor pulmonary function not only can have an operation, and specifically a lobectomy, but their function might actually be improved by a resection, depending on the location of their tumor vis a vis the location of lung tissue most involved by emphysema.

VIDEO-ASSISTED THORACIC SURGERY VERSUS OPEN LOBECTOMY

The technique for performing lobectomy was discussed in detail by Dr. McKenna, and specifically video-assisted thoracic surgery (VATS) lobectomy, for which he has been the major proponent. A standard lobectomy involves a thoracotomy incision with rib spreading that results in significant postoperative pain. Patient-controlled epidural analgesia is commonly used for the management of postoperative pain in the postthoracotomy patients with excellent results. VATS lobectomy, for the most part, avoids rib spreading and has been touted as causing less postoperative pain,

although rigorous trials supporting this contention are lacking. What is clear is that there is no oncologic disadvantage to performing a VATS lobectomy and the procedure may be performed with no increase in morbidity or mortality.

The type of VATS lobectomy most commonly performed is a hybrid operation with standard instruments used through a "utility" incision with the majority of the visualization provided by the thoracoscope. Proponents of this approach maintain that a standard mediastinal lymph node dissection also can be performed as in an open procedure. It is argued that patients have a shorter hospital stay following VATS lobectomy, but hospital stay can be influenced by a variety of variables including patient motivation. It must also be kept in mind that the majority of the costs for a surgical hospitalization are expended during the first and second day of the stay, and decreasing the hospital stay by 0.5 to 1 day results in minimal cost savings but does allow for the bed to be filled by another patient. In our experience, as opposed to many laparoscopic procedures, patients do express a strong desire to have their operation performed with VATS technique, and this may account for why only a minority of lobectomies currently are performed in this fashion, as Dr. McKenna has noted, no doubt to his disappointment.

OUTCOMES AND SURGICAL VOLUME

Finally, it is useful to make a few comments about outcomes in patients with lung cancer. As surgeons, we are fortunate in seeing a select population of patients with lung cancer, that is, those patients with either local or locally advanced disease with few exceptions, and thus our view of survival is somewhat jaded. When one views the entire population of patients with lung cancer, there has been little improvement in overall survival over the past 40 years. What we have done significantly better than our predecessors is more accurately stage patients and thus be able to look at survival more critically based on extent of disease. This applies mainly to clinical staging, which is so dependent on imaging modalities that have improved so markedly over the past few years. The addition of later generations of CT scanners as well as the advent of PET scans and fusion PET/CT has allowed us to precisely stage patients with accuracy that coincides closely with the pathologic staging following surgical resection. The recognition that lymph node sampling, or preferentially lymph node dissection, is necessary for complete staging at the time of operation also has allowed us to get a better handle on survival in patients with local or locally advanced disease. A negative lymph node dissection in a patient with a 2.5-cm lesion allows us to definitively state that this patient has stage Ia disease, and in series of patients in which this has been done, to obtain a true picture of survival for accurately staged patients.

Interestingly, it has been recognized that survival differences may be observed based on where the operation is performed and who does the operation. We know that survival following certain operations depends on either surgeon volume, hospital volume, or both. This has been well shown for pancreatic surgery and esophageal resections, among other procedures. In a landmark article, Bach and colleagues (10) demonstrated that patients who undergo resection for lung cancer at hospitals that perform large numbers of such procedures not only experience less morbidity and early mortality, but are likely to survive longer than patients who are operated on at hospitals with a low volume of lung resections. This improved survival results even after taking into account the higher incidence of postoperative morbidity and early mortality at the low-volume hospitals. These results were based on a study of Medicare patients with local or locally advanced disease who underwent operation at hospitals that participate in the Nationwide Inpatient Sample, which included 2,118 patients at 76 hospitals that were entered into the Surveillance, Epidemiology, and End Results Program (SEER) database. Five years after surgery, 44% of patients who underwent operations at high-volume hospitals were alive, compared with 33% of those who underwent operation at hospitals with the lowest volume ($p < 0.001$). These data are somewhat sobering and beg the question as to whether pulmonary resections should be performed only in hospitals in which a high volume of these procedures are performed. These results should certainly make referring physicians look critically at where they are sending patients for resections, and they should cause patients to question their doctors along these lines.

Lung cancer has been and continues to be the source of more deaths from cancer among both men and women, and thus deserves greater attention on the part of the medical profession, government funding agencies, pharmaceutical companies, politicians and activists, and the general public.

REFERENCES

1. Pujol JL, Carestia L, Daures JP, et al. Is there a case for cisplatin in the treatment of small-cell lung cancer? A meta-analysis of randomized trials of a cisplatin-containing regimen versus a regimen without this alkylating agent. *Br J Cancer.* 2000;83:8–15.

2. The International Early Lung Cancer Action Program Investigators. Survival of patients with stage I lung cancer detected on CT screening. *N Engl J Med.* 2006;355:1763–1771.

3. Shim SS, Lee KS, Dim BT, et al. Non-small cell lung cancer: prospective comparison of integrated FDG PET/CT and CT alone for preoperative staging. *Radiology.* 2005;236:1011–1019.

4. Taylor NA, Liao Z, Cox JD, et al. Equivalent outcome of patients with clinical Stage IIIA non-small call lung cancer treated with concurrent chemoradiation compared with induction chemotherapy followed by surgical resection. *Int J Radiat Oncol Biol Phys.* 2004;58:204–212.

5. Wright G, Manser RL, Byrnes G, et al. Surgery for non-small cell lung cancer: systematic review and meta-analysis of randomised controlled trials. *Thorax.* 2005;61:597–603.

6. Strauss GM, Herndon JE 2nd, Maddaus MA, et al. Adjuvant paclitaxel plus carboplatin compared with observation in stage IB non-small-cell lung cancer: CALGB 9633 with the Cancer and Leukemia Group B, Radiation Therapy Oncology Group, and North Central Cancer Treatment Group Study Groups. *J Clin Oncol.* 2008;26: 5043–5051.

7. Winton TL, Livingston R, Johnson D, et al. Vinorelbine plus cisplatin vs. observation in resected non-small-cell lung cancer. *N Engl J Med.* 2005;352:2589–2597.

8. Douillard JY, Rosell R, De Lena M, et al. Adjuvant vinorelbine plus cisplatin versus observation in patients with completely resected stage IB-IIIA non-small-cell lung cancer (Adjuvant Navelbine International Trialist Association [ANITA]): a randomised controlled trial. *Lancet Oncol.* 2006;7:719–727.

9. Ginsberg RJ, Rubenstein LV, for the Lung Cancer Study Group. Randomised trial of lobectomy versus limited resection in T1N0 lung cancer. *Ann Thorac Surg.* 1995;60:615–623.

10. Bach PB, Cramer LD, Schrag D, Downey RJ, et al. The influence of hospital volume on survival after resection for lung cancer. *N Engl J Med.* 2001;345:181–188.

52

Adjuvant Chemotherapy for Early-Stage Non-Small Cell Lung Cancer

Ronald B. Natale

Lung cancer is the leading cause of cancer-related deaths worldwide. The turn of the 21st century marked the surpassing of 1 million deaths per year, 85% of which were due to the non-small cell lung cancer (NSCLC) subtype (1). Traditionally, complete surgical resection of early-stage NSCLC has been considered the only treatment with a curative potential. However, 5-year survival rates ranged from 70% in patients with stage IA disease to about 20% in patients with completely resected stage IIIA disease (2). In the overwhelming majority of cases, the failure to cure early-stage lung cancer results from the growth and progression of micrometastatic disease that is clinically undetectable at the time of surgery (3,4). Given the success of adjuvant chemotherapy in patients with breast or colorectal cancer, it is possible that chemotherapy administered postoperatively to patients with completely resected early-stage NSCLC could improve survival. This chapter will review the results of clinical trials of adjuvant chemotherapy, the evolving standard of care based on recent successful trials, and the most promising future directions.

EARLY CLINICAL TRIALS

Early efforts to explore the role of adjuvant chemotherapy following surgery in the 1960s and 1970s failed to demonstrate any benefit owing to poor trial design, heterogeneous and generally small patient populations, and drugs with minimal efficacy. However, by the 1980s, investigators began to explore the use of cisplatin-based chemotherapy regimens that had shown moderate effectiveness in patients with advanced or metastatic NSCLC in the early-stage disease setting. Several clinical trials, notably those conducted by the Lung Cancer Study Group (LCSG), began to demonstrate positive, albeit mixed, results. In LCSG-772, 141 patients with completely resected stage II or III adenocarcinoma or large cell undifferentiated carcinoma were randomized postoperatively to either six cycles of combination cyclophosphamide, doxorubicin, and cisplatin (CAP) or putative immunotherapy with intrapleural bacillus Calmette-Guerin (BCG) and levamisole. Although the outcome initially favored the adjuvant CAP arm with a significant delay in median time to recurrence and a 15% survival advantage at 1 year (77% vs. 62%), longer follow-up (8.5 years median) demonstrated only a nonsignificant trend favoring the adjuvant chemotherapy arm (5). The LCSG-791 trial randomized patients with positive surgical margins or metastases to the highest paratracheal lymph node station (level 2) to postoperative radiation therapy alone

or radiation therapy and adjuvant chemotherapy. Although the 1-year survival rate favored the combined modality arm by 14%, the relapse and death rates were similar at 2 years and the median survival time of 17 months was identical in both arms of the study (6). In LCSG-801 (7), 283 patients with completely resected T2N0 or T1N1 NSCLC were randomized to four postoperative cycles of CAP or standard observation. Although CAP failed to improve 5-year survival (55% in each arm), only about one half (53%) of the patients randomized to CAP received all four planned cycles of therapy. Finally, a Finnish trial reported a statistically significant 11% improvement in 5-year survival in patients with completely resected T13N0 NSCLC randomized to adjuvant CAP chemotherapy versus observation. Notably, over 60% of patients suffered grade 3 or 4 gastrointestinal toxicities and failed to complete all of the planned chemotherapy (8).

These mixed results prompted a meta-analysis conducted by The Non-Small Cell Lung Cancer Collaborative Group (9). The analysis included 9,387 completely resected NSCLC patients, 7,151 of whom had died, from 52 randomized clinical trials performed between January 1, 1965, and December 31, 1991. Overall, adjuvant chemotherapy demonstrated a 13% reduction in the risk of death and an absolute 5% improvement in 5-year survival. Confirmation of the benefit from cisplatin-based chemotherapy, however, was the most important result of this analysis. Adjuvant chemotherapy with alkylating agents produced an inferior survival rate compared with observation, with a 15% increased risk of death (hazard ratio [HR], 1.15; $p = 0.005$), whereas adjuvant platinum-based chemotherapy used in eight of the trials (1,394 patients) produced a 13% reduction in risk of death (HR, 0.87; $p = 0.08$) and absolute improvement in survival of 3% at 2 years and 5% at 5 years. These findings renewed interest in the study of adjuvant chemotherapy in early-stage NSCLC and emphasized the need for larger trials, more homogenous and well-staged patients, and more effective and tolerable chemotherapy regimens. The latter became feasible with the emergence of improved second- and third-generation platinum-based regimens and supportive care measures that addressed various toxicities.

SECOND- AND THIRD-GENERATION PLATINUM-BASED REGIMENS

In the 1980s, second-generation platinum-based regimens in which agents such as etoposide, vinblastine, vindesine, and mitomycin/ifosfamide were added to a platinum compound (usually cisplatin but occasionally carboplatin) were proven to produce, for the first time, modest but significant improvements in survival and quality of life in patients with advanced or metastatic NSCLC. The 1990s saw the development of third-generation platinum-based regimens that substituted vinorelbine, paclitaxel, gemcitabine, or docetaxel for the second agent in platinum doublets because of proven further increases in survival. Also, carboplatin began to be substituted for cisplatin, allowing outpatient administration without the prolonged and copious intravenous normal saline hydration routinely used to protect against cisplatin-induced nephrotoxicity and with significant reductions in nausea, vomiting, ototoxicity, and peripheral neurotoxicity. Furthermore, improvements in supportive care that addressed common chemotherapy-associated adverse effects such as nausea and vomiting, anemia, and life-threatening febrile neutropenia led to better patient tolerance and compliance with planned treatment programs. These new regimens and the growing use of selected supportive care drugs were thought to have a greater potential to improve survival outcomes in patients with early-stage resected NSCLC. Consequently, several large European, worldwide, and North American clinical trials were launched (Table 52.1) (10–16).

Despite the renewed enthusiasm, however, the first two reports to emerge from these new efforts were disappointing. The Adjuvant Lung Project Italy (ALPI) trial randomized 1,209 patients with completely resected stage I to IIIA NSCLC to an aggressive postoperative chemotherapy regimen consisting of three cycles of mitomycin, vindesine, and cisplatin every 3 weeks or to observation (10). Stratification included tumor size, lymph node involvement, and intended radiotherapy. Unfortunately, only 65% of patients completed the planned three cycles of postoperative chemotherapy, with grade 3 or 4 neutropenia occurring in 16% and 12% of patients, respectively. Furthermore, there was a significant imbalance in the subset of patients who received planned postoperative radiotherapy between the two

arms of the study (65% in the chemotherapy arm and 85% in the nonchemotherapy arm). With a 64.5 month median follow-up time, there was no observed difference in recurrence rates, time to recurrence, or survival time between the two arms.

In the Big Lung Trial (BLT), patients were randomized to three cycles of chemotherapy (choosing from any of four presumably equivalent regimens consisting of vinorelbine/cisplatin, vindesine/cisplatin, mitomycin/ifosfamide/cisplatin, or mitomycin/vinblastine/ifosfamide) before or after surgery or to postoperative observation (11). Although the complex design of this trial attempted to satisfy differing treatment preferences among the participating European centers, patient accrual was slow and the study was closed with only 381 patients. No improvement in disease-free survival or overall survival was observed. Furthermore, chemotherapy-associated toxicity was severe with less than half of the patients receiving three unmodified courses of planned chemotherapy, 30% of patients suffering grade 3 toxicities or greater, and six patients suffering treatment-related deaths.

The International Adjuvant Lung Trial (IALT) is the largest study of adjuvant chemotherapy that has been conducted to date (12). This international collaborative effort planned to enroll 3,300 patients with completely resected stage I, II or IIIA NSCLC to surgery alone or three or four cycles of postoperative cisplatin-based chemotherapy in order to have the statistical power to confirm a 5% absolute survival benefit for chemotherapy at 5 years (from 50% to 55%). Each center determined its own policy for postoperative chemotherapy (from an agreed group of four chemotherapy regimens including etoposide/cisplatin, vindesine/cisplatin, mitomycin/ifosfamide/cisplatin, or vinorelbine/cisplatin) and radiotherapy before randomization. Although the study was closed with only 1,867 patients because of slow accrual, IALT met its primary statistical end point. With a median follow-up of 56 months, there was a statistically significant improvement in survival with a 14% decreased relative risk in dying in the adjuvant chemotherapy arm and an

Table 52.1

Major Randomized Adjuvant Clinical Trials

Trial (Ref.)	No. of Patients	Stages	Chemotherapy	Absolute Difference % 5-YeAr Survival (Adjuvant -Control)	Hazard Ratio (95% CI)	p Value
ALPI et al. (10)	1,209	I, II, IIIA	MVdP	3	0.96 (0.81–1.13)	0.589
BLT et al. (11)	381	I, II, IIIA	Platin-based	0	1.02 (0.75–1.35)	0.98
IALT et al. (12)	1,867	I, II, IIIA	PE or PVinca	4.5	0.86 (0.76–0.98)	<0.03
NCI-C et al. (13)	482	IB, II[a]	PVin	15	0.70 (0.52–0.92)	0.012
CALGB et al. (15)	344	IB	CarboPac	2	0.80 (0.60–1.07)	0.10
ANITA et al. (16)	840	IB, II, IIIA	PVin	8.6	0.80 (0.66–0.96)	0.017

CI, confidence interval; ALPI, Adjuvant Lung Project Italy; MVdP, mitomycin/vindesine/cisplatin; BLT, Big Lung Trial; platin-based, cisplatin combined with vinorelbine, vindesine, mitomycin/ifosfamide or mitomycin/vinblastine/ ifosfamide; IALT, International Adjuvant Lung Cancer Trial; PE, cisplatin/etoposide; PVinca, cisplatin combined with vinblastine, vindesine or vinorelbine; NCI-C, National Cancer Institute of Canada; PVin, cisplatin/vinorelbine; CALGB, Cancer and Acute Leukemia B; CarboPac, carboplatin/paclitaxel mitomycin/vinblastine/ifosfamide; ANITA, Adjuvant Navelbine International Trialist Association; PVin, cisplatin/vinorelbine.
[a] Excluding T3N0.

absolute 4.1% improvement in 5-year survival (44.5% vs. 40.4%). Part of the limited success of this trial may have resulted from the fact that 74% of patients received at least 240 mg/m^2 of cisplatin (somewhat higher than the ALPI and BLT trials) and that only seven patients (0.8%) randomized to adjuvant chemotherapy suffered fatal toxicities.

Despite the apparent success of the IALT trial, the mixed results of these three mostly European studies, the heterogeneity of the patients populations especially with regard to surgical staging and type of surgery performed, the variable use of postoperative radiotherapy, and the multiple chemotherapy regimens used, some of which were considered suboptimal by the time the trials were completed, limited the acceptance of adjuvant chemotherapy for patients with completely resected NSCLC. These drawbacks were to be answered by two North American and one additional European trial using more homogeneous patient populations and third-generation platinum-based doublets.

The National Institute of Canada Clinical Trials Group (NCIC-CTG) conducted a study (JBR10) in which 482 patients with completely resected stages IB or II NSCLC (excluding T3N0) were randomized to surgery alone or surgery followed by four cycles of vinorelbine (25 mg/m^2 weekly for 16 weeks) and cisplatin (50 mg/m^2 days 1 and 8 every 4 weeks) (13). Patients were stratified according to nodal status (N0 vs. N1) and *ras* mutation status (present vs. absent vs. unknown) prior to randomization. The two arms of the study were well balanced for the important prognostic factors (e.g., stage, gender, performance status, prior weight loss). Again, patient tolerance was a major issue in this study with only 58% of patients receiving at least three of the planned four cycles of chemotherapy. Chemotherapy doses had to be reduced or omitted in 77% of patients and over 50% required delays in treatment. Febrile neutropenia occurred in 7% of patients receiving chemotherapy and two patients died of drug-related toxicity. Despite these problems, however, there was a highly significant improvement in median survival in the adjuvant chemotherapy arm from 73 to 94 months ($p = 0.011$) and a large reduction (over 40%) in the relative risk of dying from recurrent lung cancer (HR, 0.69; $p = 0.04$). There was a 15% absolute improvement in 5-year survival favoring the adjuvant chemotherapy arm (69% vs. 54%; $p = 0.03$).

The Cancer and Leukemia Group B (CALGB) evaluated the role of a relatively well-tolerated platinum-based regimen, carboplatin and paclitaxel, in patients with completely resected stage IB NSCLC (CALGB 9633) (14,15). The trial was planned for 384 patients to be randomized postoperatively to observation versus four cycles of carboplatin (AUC 6) plus paclitaxel (200 mg/m^2) every 3 weeks. However, the study was closed early with 344 patients because an interim analysis demonstrated an absolute 12% survival advantage at four years for the adjuvant chemotherapy arm (71% versus 59%, $p = 0.028$) as well as over a 40% relative improvement in failure free survival (HR = 0.69, $p = 0.02$) favoring adjuvant chemotherapy. In contrast to the previous studies, chemotherapy was well tolerated with 85% of patients completing 4 planned cycles of treatment and 55% receiving all 4 cycles at full doses. There were no treatment-related deaths. Unfortunately, with additional follow-up, the survival curves nearly came together at 5 years. With updated analysis, the initially reported 8% absolute improvement in survival at 3 years and 4 years (79% vs. 71% and 69% vs. 61%, respectively) narrowed to only 2% at 5 years (59% vs. 57%). This trial no longer shows a statistically significant overall survival benefit for adjuvant chemotherapy (HR, 0.80; $p = 0.10$) (15). Interestingly, a subset analysis, which serves for hypothesis generation only, demonstrated an adjuvant chemotherapy-associated improvement in survival for patients with primary tumors ≥4.0 cm in diameter (HR, 0.62; $p = 0.01$).

Confirmation of the beneficial role of adjuvant chemotherapy in early-stage NSCLC came with the results of Adjuvant Navelbine International Trialist Association (ANITA) trial (16). In this study, 840 patients with completely resected stage IB-IIIA NSCLC were randomly assigned to observation or to vinorelbine 30 mg/m^2/weekly for 16 weeks plus cisplatin 100 mg/m^2 every 4 weeks. Moderate to severe (grade 3-4) chemotherapy adverse effects included neutropenia, febrile neutropenia, nausea or vomiting, or asthenia in 85%, 9%, 27%, and 28% of patients, respectively. Treatment-related fatal toxic effects occurred in 7 patients (2%). Only 50% of treated patients completed all four planned cycles of chemotherapy and only 61% completed three cycles. However, despite toxicities, dose attenuations, or discontinuations, adjuvant chemotherapy produced a highly significant improvement in median survival (65.7 months vs. 43.7 months; HR, 0.80; $p = 0.017$) and overall survival. The absolute overall survival benefit for patients assigned to chemotherapy compared with controls was 8.6% at 5 years.

URACIL/TEGAFUR-BASED ADJUVANT TRIALS IN JAPAN

Uracil/Tegafur (UFT) is an oral prodrug of 5-fluorouracil that has been studied in six single-agent randomized adjuvant clinical trials in Japan in daily doses for up to 2 years (17–22). Although the effectiveness of this agent in patients with advanced or metastatic NSCLC is marginal (23), some studies have suggested that this prolonged treatment schedule may provide for a long continuous suppression of micrometastatic disease and that additional benefit derives from an antiangiogenic effect or an inhibitory effect on the development of second primary lung tumors (24,25). A meta-analysis that included 2,003 patients with stage I NSCLC randomized to surgery followed by observation or UFT showed a significant survival benefit, with an overall pooled HR of 0.74 (95% confidence interval: 0.61-0.88; $p = .001$) (26). Interestingly, the difference in survival was greater in the adjuvant arm compared with the observation arm at 7 years of follow-up (77.2% vs. 69.5%, respectively; $p = .001$) than at 5 years of follow-up (81.5% vs. 76.5%, respectively; $p = .011$). To date, however, there are no confirmatory data on the use of UFT in the postoperative setting in patients with NSCLC outside of Japan and, given the agent's marginal activity in patients with advanced disease, questions have been raised regarding possible pharmacogenetic differences that may favor the usefulness of this agent in Japanese compared with non-Japanese patients.

DISCUSSION

Until 2005, surgery alone was the worldwide standard of care for the treatment of patients with early-stage operable NSCLC. However, the results of several meta-analyses and the accumulating data from several large, well-designed, and well-executed

Table 52.2

Subset Analysis by Stage in Recent Adjuvant Clinical Trials

Trial (Ref.)	Overall Hazard Ratio (*p* Value)	Hazard Ratio (CI) by Stage		
		I B	II A-B	III A
IALT et al. (12)	0.86 (<0.03)	0.95 (0.74–1.23)	0.93 (0.72–1.20)	0.79 (0.66–0.95)
NCI-C et al. (13)	0.69 (0.04)	0.94	0.59	Not tested
CALGB et al. (15)	0.80 (0.10)	0.80 (0.6–1.07)	Not tested	Not tested
ANITA et al. (16)	0.79 (0.013)	1.10 (0.76–1.57)	0.71 (0.49–0.94)	0.69 (0.53–0.90)

CI, confidence interval; IALT, International Adjuvant Lung Cancer Trial; IALT, International Adjuvant Lung Cancer Trial; NCI-C, National Cancer Institute of Canada; CALGB, Cancer and Acute Leukemia B; ANITA, Adjuvant Navelbine International Trialist Association.

clinical trials have established a significant survival benefit with the postoperative administration of platinum-based chemotherapy regimens. It is estimated that adoption of this new standard of care could result in saving over 10,000 lives per year worldwide. As should be expected, however, several questions regarding patient and chemotherapy regimen selection remain.

As is the case in patients with breast or colorectal cancers, the benefit of adjuvant chemotherapy in patients with completely resected NSCLC appears to be greater in the subset of patients with more advanced localized disease (stages II and III), and who therefore are at higher risk of disease recurrence following surgery alone, than in patients with stage I disease. As summarized in Table 52.2, subset analysis by stage of disease for the various contemporary randomized clinical trials of adjuvant chemotherapy fails to demonstrate a survival benefit in patients with stage IB disease. The CALGB trial (15) that focused exclusively on patients with stage IB disease came the closest to achieving a statistically significant improvement in survival but ultimately was a negative trial. Therefore, it is reasonable to conclude at this time that there is insufficient evidence to recommend the routine use of adjuvant platinum-based chemotherapy in patients with stage IA or IB NSCLC.

Another issue relates to which platinum species is used, cisplatin or carboplatin, in the adjuvant setting. In patients with advanced or metastatic NSCLC, meta-analyses have demonstrated no statistically significant difference in survival in randomized trials comparing cisplatin-based versus carboplatin-based combinations, although the HR of 1.10 favored cisplatin over carboplatin (27). Because of the more favorable toxicity profile and patient tolerance of carboplatin over cisplatin (less nausea and vomiting and virtual absence of renal toxicity, ototoxicity and peripheral neurotoxicity), and the ease of administration of carboplatin compared with cisplatin (no need for rigorous intravenous hydration schemas with carboplatin), carboplatin has increasingly become the platinum drug of choice for the palliative treatment of patients with advanced or metastatic NSCLC.

However, the slight, albeit statistically insignificant, advantage of cisplatin over carboplatin in the advanced or metastatic disease setting in which the goal is palliation, could result in a more meaningful advantage in the early-stage setting in which cure is the goal. More important than this theoretical advantage is the fact that all of the positive platinum-based adjuvant clinical trials have used cisplatin rather than carboplatin. The CALGB

adjuvant clinical trial in patients with stage IB NSCLC has been the only trial to use a carboplatin-based regimen. It should be noted that the carboplatin plus paclitaxel regimen used in the CALGB trial produced the best HR of any regimen in the stage IB patient population and came the closest to achieving a statistically significant difference. Therefore, the lack of evidence supporting the use of carboplatin in the adjuvant setting does not mean that it is inactive, only that it is unproven.

At the present time cisplatin-based chemotherapy regimens should be considered the adjuvant treatment of choice. Furthermore, the total cumulative dose of cisplatin may also be important. A meta-analysis of five cisplatin-only adjuvant clinical trials (28) demonstrated that improved survival was associated with total cumulative doses of cisplatin $>300 \, mg/m^2$. Carboplatin can be recommended only for those patients in whom comorbidities, age (e.g., the elderly over 75 or 80 years of age), pre-existing renal problems, peripheral neuropathy, or hearing loss, or in whom peripheral neurotoxicity must be avoided (e.g., patients who need unaffected tactile sensation in their hands or feet).

FUTURE DIRECTIONS

The success of adjuvant chemotherapy in patients with completely resected NSCLC has raised tremendous interest among investigators worldwide to further improve the survival benefit with additional strategies. The major efforts fall into two areas of investigation that will certainly come together in the near future, namely, specialized patient selection based on tumor-specific molecular characteristics and biologically targeted agents.

Although the TNM staging system uses clinical and pathologic data to stratify patients into various risk categories, there is no doubt that within each stage and substage there is tremendous variance in survival outcome. Although the benefits of adjuvant chemotherapy are greater in patients with higher stages of locally advanced disease, the benefits vary from marginal to significant and are enjoyed by a minority of patients within each stage. Hence, in trials conducted thus far, the survival outcome of patients receiving postoperative chemotherapy separates from the surgery-alone arm by a small amount and results in absolute survival difference of 5% to 10% at 5 years. Unfortunately, all of the treated patients are exposed to the adverse effects of platinum-based chemotherapy while only a subset enjoys the benefit.

Several strategies have been explored to improve the selection of patients for the adjuvant chemotherapy regimens currently available using tumor-specific molecular characteristics. One has involved quantitative assessment of DNA adduct repair pathway, excision repair cross-complementing 1 (ERCC1). ERCC1 is thought to be responsible for repair of cisplatin-induced interstrand and intrastrand cross-links (DNA adducts) and several studies have shown an association between ERCC1 expression and cisplatin resistance (29,30). Most notably, in one of these studies, patients with tumors expressing low levels of ERCC1 achieved a significantly longer median survival than patients with tumors expressing high levels following treatment with cisplatin-based chemotherapy (14.2 vs. 4.7 months; $p = 0.005$). However, there were only 56 patients with advanced or metastatic disease in this trial. The need for testing the predictive value of ERCC1 tumor expression in a larger clinical trial was recently answered by an analysis of 761 patient tumor specimens from the 1,867 patients in IALT. ERCC1 expression was determined by a semiquantitative immunohistochemical score using an ERCC1 monoclonal antibody. High ERCC1 expression was identified in 44% of tumors and interestingly correlated with older age, nonadenocarcinomas, and pleural invasion. Patients with low ERCC1-expressing tumors had a 14-month improvement in median survival following postoperative treatment with a cisplatin-containing regimen compared with the postoperative observation group (56 vs. 42 months; HR, 0.65; $p = 0.002$). In contrast, postoperative cisplatin-based chemotherapy did not produce an improvement in median survival compared with the observation control group (50 vs. 55 months; HR, 1.14; $p = 0.04$). In addition, the analysis confirmed the prognostic value of high ERCC1 tumor expression; although patients with low ERCC1 tumor expression had a significantly improved survival with postoperative cisplatin-based chemotherapy, untreated patients had a significantly poorer survival compared with untreated patients with high ERCC1 tumor expression (42 vs. 55 months) (31).

Another molecular strategy has been to explore large data sets of gene expression and to search for patterns of gene expression that are prognostic and that might allow selection of patients at highest risk of disease recurrence for adjuvant chemotherapy treatment. At this time, the "Metagene" assay is the most advanced of the various attempts to exploit the power gene chip technology (32) for this purpose. First, differential tumor gene expression using an Affymetrix chip was performed in 89 patients with completely resected early-stage lung cancer in which about 50% had disease recurrence in <2.5 years and the other 50% had disease-free survival >5 years. A highly discriminatory set a genes was identified and then applied to the postoperative observation group from CALGB trial 9633. Remarkably, in this analysis the Metagene demonstrated 90% accuracy in identifying a high-risk group of patients with stage IB NSCLC with a 5% 5-year survival and a low-risk group with a 90% 5-year survival. The CALGB is now initiating a clinical trial in which patients with completely resected stage IA or IB lung cancer with high risk of disease recurrence will be selected for postoperative treatment with a cisplatin-based chemotherapy regimen versus postoperative observation.

Biologically targeted agents bring the greatest hope of improving survival beyond what has been accomplished with cytotoxic chemotherapy agents. When these novel agents are found to produce benefit in patients with advanced or metastatic disease, it is only logical to incorporate them into the postoperative treatment strategy. The current most promising agents undergoing this evolution are the epidermal growth factor receptor-tyrosine kinase inhibitor, erlotinib, and the vascular endothelial growth factor monoclonal antibody, bevacizumab. The former has demonstrated significant single-agent activity in the second- and third-line setting in patients with advanced or metastatic disease (33), but no survival improvement when combined with standard platinum-based chemotherapy in the first-line treatment setting (34,35). Based on these observations, it is being studied in a randomized, placebo-controlled, clinical trial primarily following adjuvant chemotherapy in patients with completely resected early-stage lung cancer. The latter, bevacizumab, is the only targeted agent proven to prolong survival when combined with standard platinum-based chemotherapy in patients with advanced or metastatic non-squamous cell NSCLC (36). It is now being studied in a randomized controlled clinical trial combined with standard cisplatin-based chemotherapy in patients with stage IB (tumors >4.0 cm in diameter), IIA, B, or IIIA NSCLC.

SUMMARY

Recent multi-institutional, multinational clinical trials and meta-analyses have established a new standard of care supporting the use of postoperative cisplatin-based chemotherapy for patients with completely resected stage IIA, IIB, and IIIA NSCLC. Adjuvant chemotherapy produces an absolute 5% to 10% improvement in 5-year survival in these patients, which translates to a 15% to 20% reduced risk of dying from recurrent metastatic disease. Data are suggestive, but not definitive, that cisplatin- or carboplatin-based regimens may also improve survival in patients with stage IB disease. In Japan the use of oral UTF for 1 to 2 years following surgery in patients with this stage of disease has been well established and should be confirmed in a non-Japanese trial. Ongoing investigations will determine whether patients with completely resected early-stage NSCLC can be better selected for postoperative chemotherapy based on molecular determinants of risk of recurrence. This approach will allow patients who are unlikely to have recurrence to be spared exposure to cytotoxic chemotherapy regimens that would otherwise contribute little or no benefit to their survival. Additional molecular studies may allow the selection of specific chemotherapy regimens rather than the current empiric approach of using one regimen for all patients. Finally, biologically targeted agents are also being studied in the adjuvant setting with the expectation that significant additional advances in survival will soon be achieved.

REFERENCES

1. Parkin DM, Bray FI, Devesa SS. Cancer burden in the year 2000: the global picture. *Eur J Cancer*. 2001;37(suppl 8):S4–S66.
2. Mountain CF. Revisions in the international system for staging lung cancer. *Chest*. 1997;111:1710–1717.
3. Feld R, Rubinstein LV, Weisenberger TH. Sites of recurrence in resected stage I non-small cell lung cancer: a guide for future studies. *J Clin Oncol*. 1984; 2:1352–1358.

4. Immerman SAC, Vanecko RM, Fry WA, et al. Site of recurrence in patients with stages I and II carcinoma of the lung resected for cure. *Ann Thorac Surg.* 1981;32:23–27.

5. Holmes E, Gail M. Surgical adjuvant therapy for stage II and stage III adenocarcinoma and large cell undifferentiated carcinoma. *J Clin Oncol.* 1986;4:710–715.

6. Lad T, Rubinstein L, Ahmad S. The benefit of adjuvant treatment for resected locally advanced non-small cell lung cancer: the Lung Cancer Study Group. *J Clin Oncol.* 1988;6:9–17.

7. Feld R, Rubinstein L, Thomas P. Adjuvant chemotherapy with cyclophosphamide, doxorubicin, and cisplatin in patients with completely resected stage I non-small cell lung cancer: the Lung Cancer Study Group. *J Natl Cancer Inst.* 1993;85:299–306.

8. Nilranen A, Niitamo-Korhonen S, Kouri M, et al. Adjuvant chemotherapy after radical surgery for non-small cell lung cancer: a randomized study. *J Clin Oncol.* 1992;10:1927–1932.

9. Non-small Cell Lung Cancer Collaborative Group. Chemotherapy in non-small cell lung cancer: a meta-analysis using updated data on individual patients from 52 randomised clinical trials. *BMJ.* 1995;311:899–909.

10. Scagliotti GV, Fossati R, Torri V, et al. Chemotherapy for completely resected stage I, II, or IIIA non small cell lung cancer. *J Natl Cancer Inst.* 2003;95:1453–1461.

11. Waller D, Peake MD, Stephens RJ, et al. Chemotherapy for patients with non small cell lung cancer: the surgical setting of the Big Lung Trial. *Eur J Cardiothorac Surg.* 2004;26:173–182.

12. Arriagada R, Bergman B, Dunant A, et al; International Adjuvant Lung Cancer Trial Collaborative Group. Cisplatin-based adjuvant chemotherapy in patients with completely resected non small cell lung cancer. *N Engl J Med.* 2004;350:351–360.

13. Winton T, Livingston R, Johnson D, et al; National Cancer Institute of Canada Clinical Trials Group; National Cancer Institute of the United States Intergroup JBR.10 Trial Investigators. Vinorelbine plus cisplatin versus observation in resected non small cell lung cancer. *N Engl J Med.* 2005;352:2589–2587.

14. Strauss GM, Herndon J, Maddaus MA, et al; for the CALGB, Radiation Therapy Oncology Group, and North Central Cancer Treatment Group. Randomized clinical trial of adjuvant chemotherapy with paclitaxel and carboplatin following resection in stage IB non small cell lung cancer (NSCLC); report of the Cancer and Leukemia Group B (CALGB) protocol 9633. In: Proceedings from the American Society of Clinical Oncology; June 5-8, 2004; New Orleans, LA. Abstract 7019.

15. Strauss GM, Herndon J, Maddaus MA, et al; for the CALGB, RTOG and NCCTG. Adjuvant chemotherapy in stage IB non small cell lung cancer (NSCLC): update of CALGB protocol 9633. In: Proceedings from the American Society of Clinical Oncology; May 13–17, 2005; Orlando, FL. Abstract 7181.

16. Douillard JY, Rosell R, De Lena M, et al. Adjuvant vinorelbine plus cisplatin versus observation in patients with completely resected stage IB-IIIA non-small cell lung cancer (Adjuvant Navelbine International Trialist Association [ANITA]): a randomised controlled trial. *Lancet Oncol.* 2006;7:719–727.

17. Wada H, Hitomi S, Teramatsu T, et al. Adjuvant chemotherapy after complete resection in non-small cell lung cancer. *J Clin Oncol.* 1996;14:1048–1054.

18. Nakagawa M, Tanaka F, Tsubota N, et al. A randomized phase III trial of adjuvant chemotherapy with UFT for completely resected pathologic stage I non-small cell lung cancer: the West Japan study group for lung cancer surgery (WJSG), the 4th study. *Ann Oncol.* 2005;16:75–80.

19. Endo C, Saito Y, IwanaminH, et al. A randomized trial of postoperative UFT therapy in p stage I, II non-small cell lung cancer: Northeast Japan study group for lung cancer surgery. *Lung Cancer.* 2003;40:181–186.

20. Tada H, Yasumitsu T, Iuchi K, et al. Randomized study of adjuvant chemotherapy for completely resected non-small cell lung cancer. *Proc Clin Oncol* 2002; 21:313a.

21. Imaizumi M. A randomized trial of postoperative adjuvant chemotherapy for p-stage I non-small cell lung cancer (4th cooperative study). *Lung Cancer.* 2003;5:41–52.

22. Kato H, Ichinose Y, Ohta M, et al. A randomized trial of adjuvant chemotherapy with uracil-tegafur for adenocarcinoma of the lung. *N Engl J Med.* 2004;350:1713–1721.

23. Keicho N, Saijo N Shinkai T, et al. Phase II study of UFT in patients with advanced non-small cell lung cancer. *Jpn J Clin Oncol.* 1986;16:143–146.

24. Tanaka F, Yanagihara K, Otake Y, et al. Angiogenesis and the efficacy of postoperative administration of UFT in pathologic stage I non-small cell lung cancer. *Cancer Sci.* 2004;95:371–376.

25. Wada H, Miyahara R, Tanaka F, et al. Postoperative adjuvant chemotherapy with PVM (cispaltin, vindesine and mitomycin C) and UFT (uracil + tegafur) in resected stage I-II NSCLC (non-small cell lung cancer): a randomized clinical trial. *Eur J Cardiothorac Surg.* 1999;15:438–443.

26. Hamada C, Tanaka F, Ohta M, et al. Meta-analysis of postoperative adjuvant chemotherapy with tegafur-uracil in non-small cell lung cancer. *J Clin Oncol.* 2005;23:4999–5006.

27. Ardizzoni A, Boni L, Tiseo M, et al. Cisplatin-versus carboplatin-based chemotherapy in first-line treatment of advanced non small cell lung cancer: an individual patient data meta-analysis. *J Natl Cancer Insi.* 2007;99:847–857.

28. Pignon JP, Tribodet H, Scagliotti GV, et al. and the Lung Adjuvant Cisplatin Evaluation (LACE) Collaborative Group. Lung Adjuvant Cisplatin Evaluation (LACE): a pooled analysis of 5 randomized trials including 4,584 patients. In: Proceedings from the American Society of Clinical Oncology; June 2–6, 2006; Atlanta, GA. Abstract 7008.

29. Lord RV, Brabender J, Gandara, et al. Low ERCC! Expression correlates with prolonged survival after cisplatin plus gemcitabine chemotherapy in non-small cell lung cancer. *Clin Cancer Res.* 2002';8:2286–2291.

30. Rosell R, Feloip E, Taron M, et al. Gene expression as a predictive marker of outcome in stage IIB-IIIa-IIIB non-small cell lung cancer after induction gemcitabine-based chemotherapy followed by resectional surgery. *Clin Cancer Res.* 2004;10:4215S–4219S.

31. Olaussen KA, Dunant A, Fouret P, et al. IALT Bio Investigators. DNA repair by ERCC1 in non-small cell lung cancer and cisplatin-based adjuvant chemotherapy. *N Engl J Med.* 2006;355:983–991.

32. Potti A, Mukherjee S, Petersen R, et al. A genomic strategy to refine prognosis in early-stage non-small cell lung cancer. *N Engl J Med.* 2006;355:570–580.

33. Shepherd FA, Rodrigues Pereira J, Tan EH, et al. Erlotinib in previously treated non-small cell lung cancer. *N Engl J Med.* 2005; 353:123–132.

34. Gatzemeier U, Pluzanska A, Szczesna A, et al. Results of a phase III trial of erlotinib (OSI-774) combined with cisplatin and gemcitabine (GC) chemotherapy in advanced non-small cell lung cancer (NSCLC). *J Clin Oncol.* 2004;22:619s.

35. Herbst RS, Prager D, Hermann R, et al. TRIBUTE: a phase III trial of erlotinib hydrochloride (OSI-774) combined with carboplatin and paclitaxel chemotherapy in advanced non-small cell lung cancer. *J Clin Oncol.* 2005;23:5892–5899.

36. Sandler A, Gray R, Perry MC, et al. Paclitaxel-carboplatin alone or with bevacizumab for non-small cell lung cancer. *N Engl J Med.* 2006;355:2542–2550.

COMMENTARY
Chandra P. Belani

Even after adequate surgical resection, the majority of the patients with non-small cell lung cancer (NSCLC) develop recurrence of disease, necessitating the need for additional therapy (1). It appears that factors contributing to the failure of previous adjuvant therapy trials include trial design, accuracy of preoperative staging, chemotherapy agents selected, and dosage, as well as a lack of statistical power in the studies.

NSCLC may well be a systemic disease for which there now appears to be a clear role for systemic therapy both in surgically resected disease and also in potentially resectable disease. The presence of disseminated micrometastatic disease at the time of resection is the likely reason for the high rate of recurrence despite complete removal of all macroscopic disease. Such micrometastatic disease has been detected by employing methods such as immunohistochemistry and the polymerase chain reaction in patients with radiologically localized lung cancer (2). Ohgami et al. (2) found that micrometastatic cancer cells were frequently present in the bone marrow of patients with operable NSCLC and that those patients with cytokeratin 18-positive cells in their bone marrow demonstrated a significantly earlier recurrence than those without such cells ($p = 0.0083$). The outcome for such patients can only be improved by eradication of micrometastatic disease in addition to optimal surgical resection. This goal provides the rationale for the use of adjuvant therapy for patients even with early-stage NSCLC following surgical resection.

Thus, the need for systemic therapy in patients with early-stage NSCLC is evident, based on the high incidence of recurrent disease at systemic sites. Recent data (3–6) as described in detail by Dr. Natale demonstrate that adjuvant chemotherapy should now be considered the unequivocal standard of care for the treatment of patients with completely resected early-stage NSCLC, with the exception of patients with stage IA disease and stage IB disease with tumors <4 cm, as either the prognosis is relatively favorable or there is currently no evidence that adjuvant therapy is efficacious in this subset of patients. An ongoing debate involves the role of carboplatin-based regimens in this setting. It is our belief that cisplatin-based regimens are preferred in the adjuvant therapy setting. However, the administration of planned doses of systemic chemotherapy in the postoperative setting remains a challenge. Inadequate dose delivery has been reported in several trials testing postoperative chemotherapy, with an average of only 50% to 70% of patients receiving the planned course of treatment.

Available data indicate that >90% of patients who receive neoadjuvant (preoperative) chemotherapy undergo the planned surgical resection. Although recent trials of adjuvant therapy have demonstrated promising results, no study to date has compared the utility of adjuvant chemotherapy versus neoadjuvant chemotherapy. Neoadjuvant therapy provides the opportunity to improve the delivery of chemotherapy over the adjuvant setting. It also has the advantage of downstaging the disease before surgery and decreasing tumor-seeding during surgery. In addition, patients with rapidly progressive disease can be identified while receiving neoadjuvant therapy, thus avoiding the need for surgery. Neoadjuvant therapy with molecularly targeted agents may also provide information on in vivo effects such as alteration in molecular factors and downstream signaling events in tumor tissue at resection, paving the road for individualized approaches.

PATIENT SELECTION TO OPTIMIZE ADJUVANT THERAPY

The explosion of knowledge regarding the molecular etiology of lung cancer has yielded much that is promising, but so far significant patient benefit has not materialized. For example, the expression of *k-ras*, *p53*, and Ki-67 was prospectively evaluated in subgroups of patients included in the ALPI trial and, unfortunately, no relevant prognostic implication was found (7). Genetic alterations affecting the *p53* gene are among the commonest changes during malignant progression of several types of tumors, including NSCLC. However, studies that explore the prognostic role of *p53* mutations in NSCLC reported highly conflicting results and no definitive information can be obtained from those studies (8). CALGB 9633 (4,6) evaluated the prevalence of ten molecular biological markers (growth factors *HER-2/neu* and *K-ras* codon 12 mutations, cell cycle factors Ki-67 and Rb, apoptosis factors *p53* and *bcl-2*, angiogenesis factor VIII, and adhesion protein CD-44 plus motility factor gelsolin) to determine the influence of adjuvant chemotherapy on cancer-free survival relative to marker expression in these patients, and results are awaited. It should be noted that the largest biomarker study retrospectively performed in 515 cases of resected stage I NSCLC failed to show any significant association between survival and the expression of an extensive panel of biomarkers, including epidermal growth factor receptor, angiogenesis *HER2/neu*, *bcl-2*, and *p53* (9).

The excision repair cross complementing gene (*ERCC*) 1 is a DNA repair enzyme that is often overexpressed in patients with NSCLC. In such patients, cisplatin-based regimens are associated with lesser efficacy, potentially because of the more effective repair of cisplatin-DNA adducts. Tumor samples from 761 patients who participated in IALT study were analyzed for *ERCC1* expression by immunohistochemistry (10). For the 56% of the patients without *ERCC1* expression, there was a significant survival benefit with adjuvant chemotherapy, whereas those with overexpression did not derive any survival advantage with cisplatin-based adjuvant chemotherapy. Based on these observations, prospective studies are being planned to select patients for adjuvant chemotherapy based on *ERCC1* expression. Other potential predictive markers including ribonucleotide reductase M1 (RRM1) are also being evaluated to select the optimal adjuvant chemotherapy. The lung Metagene model published by the Duke Group may predict the risk of recurrence better than the traditional clinicopathologic factors (11) and the recent information on identification of a three-gene classifier STX1A, HIF1A, and CCR7 for early-stage NSCLC may have a potential value in selecting appropriate adjuvant therapy for resected NSCLC patients independent of stage (12).

These data are of great interest and raise many issues with respect to future management of patients with early-stage NSCLC. Should all patients with surgically resected NSCLC be considered for adjuvant chemotherapy? We are also looking for the "advance" that will allow us to separate potential patients who do not require any additional therapy after curative surgical resection from those in whom individualized treatment approaches will improve their outcome.

REFERENCES

1. Jemal A, Thomas A, Murray T, Thun M. Cancer statistics, 2002. *CA Cancer J Clin*. 2002;52:23–47.
2. Ohgami A, Mitsudomi T, Sugio K, et al. Micrometastatic tumor cells in the bone marrow of patients with non-small cell lung cancer. *Ann Thorac Surg*. 1997;64:363–367.
3. Arriagada R, Bergman B, Dunant A, et al. Cisplatin-based adjuvant chemotherapy in patients with completely resected non-small-cell lung cancer. *N Engl J Med*. 2004; 350:351–360.
4. Strauss GM, Herndon J, Maddaus MA, et al. Randomized clinical trial of adjuvant chemotherapy with paclitaxel and carboplatin following resection in stage IB non-small cell lung cancer (NSCLC): report of Cancer and Leukemia Group B (CALGB) Protocol 9633. In: Proceedings from the American Society of Clinical Oncology; June 5-8, 2004; New Orleans, LA. Abstract 7019.
5. Douillard JY, Rosell R, Delena M, et al. ANITA: phase III adjuvant vinorelbine (N) and cisplatin (P) versus observation (OBS) in completely resected (stage I-III) non-small-cell lung cancer (NSCLC) patients (pts): final results after 70-month median follow-up. On behalf of the Adjuvant Navelbine International Trialist Association. J Clin Oncol 2004;23:624s (Abstract 7013).
6. Strauss GM, Herndon JE, Maddaus MA, et al. Adjuvant chemotherapy in stage IB non-small cell lung cancer (NSCLC): Update on Cancer and Leukemia Group B (CALGB) protocol 9633. J Clin Oncol 2004; 24:365s (Abstract 7007).
7. Scagliotti GV, Fossati R, Torri V, et al. Chemotherapy for completely resected stage I, II, or IIIA non small cell lung cancer. *J Natl Cancer Inst*. 2003;95:1453–1461.
8. Saintigny P, Le Pimpec-Barthes F, Bernaudin JF. Micro-metastases and non-small cell lung cancer [in French] *Rev Mal Respir*. 2004; 21:105–116.
9. Pastorino U, Andreola S, Tagliabue E, et al. Immunocytochemical markers in stage I lung cancer: relevance to prognosis. *J Clin Oncol*. 1997;15:2858–2865.
10. Olaussen KA, Dunant A, Fouret P, et al. DNA repair by ERCC1 in non-small-cell lung cancer and cisplatin-based adjuvant chemotherapy. *N Engl J Med*. 2006;355:983–991.
11. Potti A, Mukherjee S, Petersen R, et al. A genomic strategy to refine prognosis in early-stage non-small cell lung cancer. *N Engl J Med*. 2006;355:570–580.
12. Lau SK, Boutros PC, Pintilie M, et al. Three-gene prognostic classifier for early-stage non small-cell lung cancer. *J Clin Oncol*. 2007;25:5562–5569.

53

Surgical Management of Metastatic Lung Disease

John C. Kucharczuk and Larry R. Kaiser

On initial consideration, the idea of pulmonary resection to treat metastatic disease appears unlikely to benefit the patient, especially if multiple lesions are present. For that matter the mere idea that resection of metastatic disease, specifically hematogenous metastatic disease, can be associated with long-term survival itself seems counterintuitive. Nevertheless, over the past 100 years pulmonary metastasectomy has developed into an acceptable treatment modality for a select group of patients with specific malignancies who have lung metastases. This practice, however, is not grounded in rigorous evidence-based evaluation, but rather has developed gradually on a foundation of case reports, case series, and case registries. The intent of this chapter is to outline the current status of pulmonary metastatectomy and highlight the situations and patient characteristics most likely to be associated with a beneficial outcome.

HISTORICAL REVIEW

From a historical perspective the first reported attempt at resection of distant metastases was performed in Germany in 1882 (1). Weinlechner reported removal of two distant metastatic nodules in the upper lobe of the lung during the removal of a chest wall sarcoma. It is interesting that the first attempt at pulmonary metastasectomy was performed in a patient with a sarcoma, as this group has repeatedly been identified as a population who benefit most significantly from aggressive resection of isolated pulmonary metastasis. Unfortunately, Weinlechner's patient died 24 hours following operation and thus received no long-term benefit from the pulmonary resection. It was not until 1927 that Divis (2) in the Scandinavian literature reported resection of a pulmonary metastasis as a separate procedure. Not long after this report, Franz Torek (3) performed and reported resection of two pulmonary metastases in the right lower lobe of a woman 2 years following a hysterectomy for adenocarcinoma. Barney and Churchill (4) reported one of the first long-term survivors following pulmonary resection for metastatic disease in a patient with a renal cell carcinoma. The patient survived for 23 years following the procedure and died from unrelated causes. Following these initial case reports came a relatively large and landmark case series from Alexander and Haight (5), who in 1947 reported on 24 cases of surgically treated solitary lung metastases. This series included 16 carcinomas and 8 sarcomas. Of the 24 patients, 11 developed recurrent disease, 1 died, and 12 were disease-free 1 to 12 years following resection. This report ultimately came to be recognized as a seminal

article because the authors put forth the basic tenets for resection of pulmonary metastases that still hold true today. The primary tumor must be controlled prior to embarking on resection of metastatic disease and there should be no evidence of additional metastatic disease outside the chest. In addition, the patient must be medically fit enough to tolerate a pulmonary resection.

Almost 20 years later, surgeons at the Mayo Clinic reported their experience with over 220 operations for metastatic tumors in the lung following these basic tenets (6). The series included a mix of carcinomas (80%) and sarcomas (20%) with an overall survival at 5 years of 30%. The Mayo group also added a fourth tenet of pulmonary metastasectomy: the concept of parenchymal sparing but complete resection, acknowledging that patients may have recurrence and thus be candidates for additional pulmonary resection at a later time. Complete resection implies that all metastatic disease be removed. Few attempts were made at multiple resections for pulmonary metastases until Beattie (7) and coworkers in 1991 noted the value of multiple sequential resections in the treatment of osteogenic sarcoma and the potential for long-term survival with repeated resections. Recently, some have even advocated repeated surgical removal of pulmonary metastases by third and even fourth time repeat operations (8). In the past 20 years, centers with the most experienced clinicians have taken a very aggressive approach toward resection of both solitary and multiple pulmonary metastases arising from an array of primary neoplasms with good long-term survival in up to 40% of patients treated.

PATHOLOGY

Malignant tumors may metastasize in three ways: hematogenous, lymphogenic, and direct invasion. Underlying tumor biology and host resistance determine mechanisms of spread, location(s) of metastases, and extent of growth. Blood-borne metastases most frequently are found in the lung and liver. Tumor cells are filtered out in the lungs or may preferentially adhere to the underlying capillary endothelium. Tumor cells may travel by lymphatics and occupy a discrete position within the lung or may involve diffusely the entire lung, as is seen with lymphangitic spread. Rarely, metastases may metastasize to other organs; however, metastases can develop in draining pulmonary lobar, hilar, or mediastinal lymph nodes depending on the underlying histology. Direct invasion of metastases into other structures may occur as the metastasis grows.

DIAGNOSIS

Metastatic disease to the lung is usually asymptomatic, although some patients may present with cough and occasionally with hemoptysis, especially if there is an endobronchial component. Most commonly, the diagnosis of pulmonary metastasis is made following a surveillance chest radiograph or computed tomography (CT) scan. Surveillance imaging depends to a great extent on the primary tumor; sarcomas, well recognized to metastasize to lung, are followed with CT scans done on a routine basis. Where previously chest radiographs were the most frequently employed imaging modality to follow patients with a known propensity to develop pulmonary metastatic disease, it is now recognized that helical CT scanning is a far more sensitive modality and is the imaging study of choice. If a nodule or a question of a nodule is seen on chest radiograph, a CT scan with or without contrast is the definitive study as it will not only confirm the presence of a suspected lesion, but will also show any other lesions that may be present.

In the past, full lung tomography was used to assess the possibility of metastatic disease; however, this modality is mentioned only as a historical footnote since the advent of CT scans has rendered this modality obsolete. We have not had occasion to see full lung linear tomograms in almost 20 years. CT scanning can demonstrate nodules as small as 1 to 2 mm, but this level of sensitivity creates more problems than it solves because many of these tiny nodules ultimately prove to be nonmalignant. Once a nodule is identified, it becomes necessary to continue to follow it with repeat CT scans usually done at 3-month intervals. Growth of the nodule or the appearance of additional nodules is highly suggestive of metastatic disease. The first recognition of a nodule suggestive of metastatic disease should prompt a follow-up CT scan in 2 to 3 months and resection should be considered once stability of metastatic disease is demonstrated in the absence of extrathoracic metastatic disease. One must keep in mind that a new solitary nodule does not necessarily represent metastatic disease, but may be a primary lung cancer and thus should be treated as such. Most commonly, the only way to distinguish a primary lung cancer from a metastatic nodule is by excision, and even then the pathologist may not be able to establish a diagnosis with certainty, especially when the patient has had another adenocarcinoma.

SCREENING FOR LUNG METASTASIS

Generally, pulmonary metastases do not cause symptoms; most are found on radiographic screening studies. Thus, the rate at which lung metastases are identified depends on the biology of the tumor itself, which determines the rate of occurrence of lung metastasis for a given primary tumor, and the rate and interval at which screening studies are obtained. Considerations taken into account when ordering a screening study for lung metastasis should include (a) the histology of the primary, (b) the accuracy of the imaging modality in detecting lung metastases, (c) the radiation dose, and (d) the cost effectiveness of the study. To guide clinical screening decisions, the American College of Radiology (9) (ACR) published a guideline entitled "Screening for Pulmonary Metastases." Because data from multivariate analysis were lacking, the American College of Radiology convened

Table 53.1

Primary Malignancy: Bone and Soft-Tissue Sarcoma (9)

Radiologic Procedure	Appropriateness Rating[a]	Comments
Roentgenogram, chest, PA and lateral	9	If performed as a baseline
CT, chest	9	Initial evaluation or surveillance
FDG-PET, whole body	5	—
MRI, chest	2	—

PA, posteroanterior; CT, computed tomography; FDG-PET, fluorodeoxyglucose-positron emission tomography; MRI, magnetic resonance imaging.

[a]Appropriateness criteria scale: 1 through 9, with 1 = least appropriate and 9 = most appropriate.

From Mohammed TL, Chowdhry AA, Khan A, et al., Expert Panel on Thoracic Imaging. Screening for pulmonary metastases. [online publication]. Reston, VA: American College of Radiology; 2006.

an Appropriateness Criteria Panel and used a modified Delphi technique to arrive at a consensus. The recommendations are given by tumor type in Tables 53.1 through Table 53.5. They should be used as a guide in screening for lung metastases.

TREATMENT OF PULMONARY METASTASES

The majority of patients who are found to have pulmonary metastatic disease present with disease at other sites. In these

Table 53.2

Primary Malignancy: Renal Cell Carcinoma

Radiologic Procedure	Appropriateness Rating[a]	Comments
Roentgenogram, chest, PA and lateral	8	—
CT, chest	7	Depends on the stage of the disease
MRI, chest	2	—
FDG-PET, whole body	1	—

PA, posteroanterior; CT, computed tomography; FDG-PET, fluorodeoxyglucose-positron emission tomography; MRI, magnetic resonance imaging.

[a]Appropriateness criteria scale: 1 through 9, with 1 = least appropriate and 9 = most appropriate.

From Mohammed TL, Chowdhry AA, Khan A, et al., Expert Panel on Thoracic Imaging. Screening for pulmonary metastases. [online publication]. Reston, VA: American College of Radiology; 2006.

Table 53.3
Primary Malignancy: Testicular Cancer

Radiologic Procedure	Appropriateness Rating[a]	Comments
Roentgenogram, chest, PA and lateral	8	—
CT, chest	7	Recommended if abdominal disease is present
FDG-PET, whole body	3	—
MRI, chest	3	—

PA, posteroanterior; CT, computed tomography; FDG-PET, fluorodeoxyglucose-positron emission tomography; MRI, magnetic resonance imaging.
[a]Appropriateness criteria scale: 1 through 9, with 1 = least appropriate and 9 = most appropriate.
From Mohammed TL, Chowdhry AA, Khan A, et al., Expert Panel on Thoracic Imaging. Screening for pulmonary metastases. [online publication]. Reston, VA: American College of Radiology; 2006.

patients treatment is either palliative or "curative," recognizing that few solid tumors actually are cured with systemic chemotherapy once metastatic disease is present. However, recent efforts with antiangiogenic agents and targeted therapies may change that outlook. Numerous trials are ongoing but a discussion of these newer agents and the current trials is beyond the scope of this chapter (10,11).

Chemotherapy

The value of chemotherapy for the treatment of pulmonary metastases is controversial. For the most part, the addition

Table 53.4
Primary Malignancy: Malignant Melanoma

Radiologic Procedure	Appropriateness Rating[a]	Comments
Roentgenogram, chest, PA and lateral	9	If performed as a baseline
CT, chest	8	Initial evaluation or surveillance
FDG-PET, whole body	5	—
MRI, chest	2	—

PA, posteroanterior; CT, computed tomography; FDG-PET, fluorodeoxyglucose-positron emission tomography; MRI, magnetic resonance imaging.
[a]Appropriateness criteria scale: 1 through 9, with 1 = least appropriate and 9 = most appropriate.
From Mohammed TL, Chowdhry AA, Khan A, et al., Expert Panel on Thoracic Imaging. Screening for pulmonary metastases. [online publication]. Reston, VA: American College of Radiology; 2006.

Table 53.5
Primary Malignancy: Head and Neck Carcinoma

Radiologic Procedure	Appropriateness Rating[a]	Comments
Roentgenogram, chest, PA and lateral	9	If performed as a baseline
CT, chest	9	Initial evaluation or surveillance
FDG-PET, whole body	5	—
MRI, chest	2	—

PA, posteroanterior; CT, computed tomography; FDG-PET, fluorodeoxyglucose-positron emission tomography; MRI, magnetic resonance imaging.
[a]Appropriateness criteria scale: 1 through 9, with 1 = least appropriate and 9 = most appropriate.
From Mohammed TL, Chowdhry AA, Khan A, et al., Expert Panel on Thoracic Imaging. Screening for pulmonary metastases. [online publication]. Reston, VA: American College of Radiology; 2006.

of chemotherapy in the patient with resectable pulmonary metastatic disease has not altered survival significantly. Most of the experience with pulmonary resection of metastatic disease has been in patients with sarcoma. For other malignancies, the data are difficult to interpret, as there is a significant selection bias because the number of patients who present with isolated pulmonary metastatic disease is already a selected population. This is especially true with colorectal cancer metastatic to the lung.

The incidence of pulmonary metastases in patients with primary osteogenic sarcoma treated with surgical resection and adjuvant chemotherapy has declined significantly compared with those patients treated with resection alone (12,13). Bacci and Lari (14) noted that in patients who receive adjuvant chemotherapy for primary osteogenic sarcoma, surgical resection of pulmonary metastases may be accomplished in a larger proportion of patients than it can be in those who did not receive adjuvant chemotherapy (51% vs. 29%). The situation with soft-tissue sarcoma differs somewhat. In what is likely the largest series reported to date, Canter and colleagues (15) from Memorial Sloan-Kettering Cancer Center reviewed 1,897 patients with extremity soft-tissue sarcomas culled from their prospective sarcoma database accumulated over a 15-year period. They noted that 508 patients (27%) developed lung metastases and 138 (7%) underwent pulmonary resection of metastatic disease. Fifty-three patients who underwent resection also received perioperative chemotherapy, and the median postmetastasis disease-specific survival in this group was 24 months compared with 33 months in those treated with resection alone. It must be noted that the age at diagnosis and the disease-free interval were significantly different between patients who received perioperative chemotherapy and those who did not, but all other prognostic factors were equivalent. The authors concluded that systemic chemotherapy has minimal, if any, long-term impact on the outcome of patients undergoing pulmonary resection for metastatic soft-tissue sarcoma of the extremity.

Attempts have been made to mount an international study randomizing patients with pulmonary metastatic disease from soft-tissue sarcoma to preoperative chemotherapy followed by resection versus resection alone to definitively answer the question. Unfortunately such a study has never been able to be completed because of low accrual and the time projected that it would take to complete such a study. It is safe to say that conventional chemotherapy for metastatic sarcoma provides for only a narrow therapeutic window with the exception of a few responsive pathologic subtypes. In assessing opportunities for improving the therapeutic ratio for patients with sarcoma, Wunder and colleagues (16) note that targeting underlying molecular events in specific sarcomas may be a worthwhile strategy, particularly based on the dramatic benefits seen in patients with gastrointestinal stromal tumors treated with imatinib. These types of targeted therapies represent an area of active research not just in sarcoma but in other tumors as well.

Despite some of the promising results with sarcoma, the same cannot be said for melanoma. To date, no adjuvant therapy has resulted in improved overall survival, although the occasional patient with metastatic disease can be salvaged with aggressive treatment of metastatic disease, especially regional recurrent disease.

Radiation Therapy

Currently, radiation therapy is used for the palliation of symptoms of advanced metastatic disease and is rarely used for the treatment of pulmonary metastases. Prophylactic lung radiation has been performed for osteogenic sarcoma because of the high propensity for these patients to develop metastatic disease in the lung. Burgers et al. (17) showed that patients receiving prophylactic lung irradiation for primary osteogenic sarcoma developed pulmonary metastases at a rate similar to that of patients having adjuvant chemotherapy.

Radiofrequency Ablation

Following its successful use for hepatic tumors, radiofrequency ablation (RFA) has been adapted for use in treating lung lesions, both primary and metastatic. During the past few years there have been a number of reports describing the use of RFA for lung nodules. Most of these reports have been feasibility trials, but we are now seeing some intermediate-term results (18). Simon and colleagues (19) included 18 patients with colorectal metastases in their series and noted that 57% were alive at a median follow-up of 27 months. The Radiofrequency Ablation of Pulmonary Tumors Response Evaluation (RAPTURE) trial included 53 patients with metastatic lesions with an overall 2-year survival of 62% and a cancer-specific survival of 82% (20).

RFA has been demonstrated to be a safe modality for the local control of tumors in the lung. Where it will fit into the armamentarium of treatment modalities available for metastatic disease in the lung of varying histologies remains to be determined. A head-to-head comparison of RFA and operative resection has yet to be undertaken, and currently RFA should be reserved for the compromised patient in whom resection is contraindicated. The efficacy is better for smaller lesions, those <3 cm in size.

PREOPERATIVE EVALUATION

Depending on the primary tumor, patients are followed longitudinally with various imaging studies often determined by the bias of the medical oncologist or the other physicians caring for the patient. Most commonly, patients are referred for consideration of surgical resection of pulmonary metastatic disease at the first sign of a pulmonary nodule or nodules as seen on a CT scan. Depending on the interval between scans, the new finding of a pulmonary nodule should begin a process that ultimately may lead to resection, assuming other criteria ultimately are met. The initial recognition of an abnormality on the chest CT scan should not immediately prompt a decision for pulmonary resection. An interval scan in 2 to 3 months often provides additional information that may greatly benefit the patient. It is desirable to document a period of relatively stability of metastatic disease prior to embarking on resection in order to derive the maximal benefit. Given this short interval, what was presumed to be a solitary lesion may now be seen to be accompanied by additional lesions or not. The appearance of numerous tiny lesions precludes definitive resection and it is far better to find this out prior to subjecting the patient to a thoracotomy.

An interval in which the metastatic disease can be documented to be relatively stable in terms of number of lesions makes it more likely that complete resection of all disease will be accomplished. We prefer to avoid subjecting a patient to pulmonary resection only to find that several months later new lesions appear. This issue of timing has been looked at in more detail. Tanaka et al. (21) reviewed 68 patients who underwent complete resection of pulmonary metastatic disease and found that both the interval from metastasectomy until subsequent recurrence and the interval from detection of pulmonary metastases until resection were independent prognostic factors. Significantly shorter survival was seen in patients who underwent pulmonary resection within 3 months of detection than in those who underwent surgery beyond 3 months. They noted many cases of early relapse following resection when the interval from detection of pulmonary metastatic disease was short, likely representing disease that was present at the time of resection but not clinically apparent.

Prior to making a determination as to whether a given patient is a candidate for resection of pulmonary metastatic disease, a thorough evaluation must be performed that includes a determination that the primary tumor is under control and that there is no evidence of other metastatic disease outside the lungs. In addition, it must be determined that the patient can physiologically tolerate a pulmonary resection. Depending on the site and type of the primary tumor, physical examination and imaging studies, in addition to endoscopy in certain situations, are all used to establish that the primary tumor has been controlled and that there is no evidence of residual or locoregional recurrent disease. A complete body survey, often in the form of a positron emission tomography (PET) scan or more recently a PET/CT fusion scan, should be used to rule out extrathoracic sites of disease. If the brain is a suspected site of metastatic disease, magnetic resonance imaging is the imaging modality of choice. Patients should also undergo standard spirometry with a determination of flows and lung volumes in order to characterize their pulmonary function and ensure they have the physiologic reserve to tolerate the proposed pulmonary resection that may even include bilateral staged thoracotomies. Patients with severe underlying pulmonary dysfunction who are marginal candidates from a physiologic perspective probably should be excluded from resection of asymptomatic pulmonary metastases as their life expectancy may be as equally limited by their lung dysfunction as it is by their metastatic disease.

Several criteria have been proposed in an attempt to predict which patients will derive the most benefit from resection of pulmonary metastatic disease and thus guide patient selection. These criteria include the disease-free interval, the time from resection of the primary tumor until the diagnosis of pulmonary metastases, and the number of lung metastases present. Unfortunately, analysis of these and other factors have been inconclusive, with some studies demonstrating predictive prognostic value and others showing no benefit. In an attempt to more precisely delineate some of these criteria for soft-tissue sarcomas, Smith and colleagues (22) from Roswell Park Cancer Institute reviewed their series of 94 soft-tissue sarcoma patients with pulmonary metastases, all of whom had been followed for at least 5 years. Most of the primary tumors were intermediate to high grade and half of them were extremity sarcomas. Thirty-four of the patients had extrapulmonary disease at the time of the pulmonary resection, and all extrapulmonary disease was completely resected. The mean disease-free interval from the time of the original diagnosis until the development of metastatic disease was 25 months (median, 15 months). The actual 5-year disease-free survival and overall survival for all patients were 5% and 15%, respectively. For the 74 patients who were able to have a resection of all pulmonary disease (R0 resection), disease-free survival and overall survival were 7% and 18%, respectively. Patient characteristics, tumor features, local recurrence, and adjuvant therapy did not affect overall survival; however, an R0 resection and a prolonged disease-free interval were associated with improved overall survival.

This has been seen in other studies, but currently no specific criteria exist to definitively predict which patients will derive the maximum benefit from pulmonary resection. The presence of extraparenchymal disease, that is, pleural masses or mediastinal involvement, clearly is associated with a poor prognosis, even following resection of all presumed metastatic disease. Although a longer disease-free interval and fewer pulmonary metastases likely are associated with a better outcome, no useful cutoff can be identified to exclude patients from surgical consideration. That being said, van Geel et al. (23) looked at data from ten related studies that looked at prognostic factors in patients with pulmonary metastases from soft-tissue sarcoma. Although the data did not permit a rigorous meta-analysis using standard techniques, they were able to conclude that a disease-free interval from time of diagnosis to the development of pulmonary metastatic disease of 7 months or less was associated with a poor prognosis despite resection of the metastatic disease. Based on this combined data, the number of metastases did not emerge as an important prognostic indicator.

The most important selection criterion remains the ability to completely resect all metastatic disease. In most instances the decision to offer resection of pulmonary metastatic disease to a given patient is based on the surgeon's judgment and, to some extent, institutional bias. The timing of resection may also be particularly important.

Selection of Surgical Approach

The choice of operative approach for the resection of metastatic disease depends on a number of factors, including the presence or absence of bilateral disease, the size of the lesions, and the surgeon's preference, with no single approach being the "right" approach. Additionally, questions arise as to the role, if any, for mediastinoscopy to assess mediastinal lymph node involvement, the need for intraoperative palpation of the lung to identify metastases that may not be imaged by CT scan, and the role of minimally invasive approaches, such as thoracoscopy.

Mediastinal lymph node involvement in patients undergoing lung metastasectomy portends a very poor prognosis. In one recent study, the estimated overall 5-year survival was 60% in patients with no nodal involvement, 17% for those with N1 (intrapulmonary or hilar) nodal involvement, and 0% for those with N2 (ipsilateral mediastinal) disease (24). Unlike patients with lung cancer, there is no consensus on the role of mediastinoscopy and no agreement on whether lymph node dissection or sampling should be performed at the time of pulmonary metastasectomy. Nevertheless, mediastinoscopy likely has a role in more accurate staging and may influence the decision to proceed with metastasectomy (25). Our current practice is to perform mediastinoscopy on a selective basis on patients who are candidates for pulmonary metastasectomy. Our selection criteria include mediastinal adenopathy >1.5 cm in short axis by CT scan and/or increased activity by fluorodeoxyglucose (FDG)-PET scanning. Patients who have suspicious mediastinal lymph nodes that are subsequently confirmed as positive at mediastinoscopy are excluded from pulmonary metastasectomy. Those with suspicious intrapulmonary or hilar (N1) lymph nodes undergo lymph node dissection at the time of pulmonary resection of metastatic disease.

Once the decision has been made that resection of metastatic disease is feasible, a decision needs to be made regarding what incision should be used to access the chest. Available options include unilateral thoracotomy, sternotomy, bilateral anterior thoracotomy, thoracosternotomy, and video-assisted thoracoscopy. The best approach is always one tailored to the patient, and the site and extent of the disease. Currently, the main controversy in choice of approach centers on the ability to perform bimanual palpation of the lung to locate radiographically occult sites of metastasis. This issue was brought to the forefront with the advent of video-assisted thoracic surgery, improved CT scanning, and questioning of the need to palpate the entire lung rather than directed minimally invasive resection based on preoperative localization by CT scan.

Over 10 years ago a well-designed prospective clinical trial was carried out at the Memorial Sloan-Kettering Cancer Center in which patients underwent preoperative CT scanning in an attempt to identify all metastatic lesions and then underwent resection presumably of all metastatic lesions. Immediately following the thoracoscopic resection, the chest was opened and bimanual palpation of the lung carried out to see if any palpable metastatic disease remained (26). The trial was stopped when 14 of the first 18 patients were found to have additional lesions at thoracotomy that had been missed during the video-thoracoscopic procedure. This trial led many surgeons to espouse that resection of metastatic disease should be performed only via thoracotomy because of the high likelihood that disease could be missed without the benefit of palpation of the lung. One has to keep in mind, however, that this study was performed long before the advent of the helical CT scanners, which have the ability to detect even tiny metastatic lesions.

More recently, however, several published case series have shown good outcomes and long-term survival following thoracoscopic resection of metastatic disease (27,28). Many have thought that with improved CT scan technology, especially the addition of helical CT scanning, the need for manual lung palpation, that is the hallmark of the open thoracotomy approach, has lessened. Unfortunately, there have also been recent publications suggesting that even with high-resolution and helical CT scans (29), there are still significant limitations in identification and characterization of all nodules, particularly when they are ≤6 mm in size (30).

We have taken what we believe to be a common sense approach to this issue. We offer a thoracoscopic approach to patients with a solitary, peripherally located pulmonary nodule, especially after an interval of follow-up in which the lesion has remained as a solitary one over several months. During the thoracoscopic procedure, we incise the inferior pulmonary ligament to provide lung mobility and perform digital palpation of the rest of the lung in an attempt to rule out occult metastases. The index finger inserted through one of the thoracoscopic ports provides a reasonably thorough palpation of the lung as the lung can be moved to the palpating finger. In patients with more than one pulmonary nodule, we offer an open approach with manual palpation of the entire lung to rule out other sites of metastatic disease. This practice is supported in the literature by other thoracic surgery units (31).

For bilateral lesions, median sternotomy often is the approach of choice as long as all of the radiographically apparent nodules are considered resectable by an experienced surgeon. For larger lesions, especially if the left lower lobe is involved, bilateral staged thoracotomies may be the preferred approach. The left lower lobe is difficult to manipulate with the median sternotomy approach because retraction of the heart in an effort to expose the left lower lobe often results in hypotension that is not well tolerated. Certainly, most peripheral nodules can be localized and wedge excised via sternotomy, and most anatomic resections (i.e., lobectomy for centrally located lesions), with the exception being left lower lobectomy, can be readily performed via median sternotomy. In a patient with bilateral lesions for whom a left lower lobe segmentectomy or lobectomy may be required, we generally perform bilateral staged thoracotomies with the procedures spaced at a 4- to 6-week interval.

A modification of the median sternotomy, the thoracosternotomy, may occasionally be used for the resection of metastatic disease (32). The standard thoracosternotomy or "clamshell" incision enjoyed resurgence in popularity when it was routinely employed for bilateral lung transplants in the early 1990s. The incision is composed of bilateral anterior thoracotomies with a transverse sternotomy providing access to both pleural spaces. This incision can be further modified as a unilateral thoracoster-

notomy or "hemi-clamshell" approach, which provides better access from an anterior approach than a median sternotomy alone.

DISEASE-SPECIFIC RECOMMENDATIONS AND RESULTS

Sarcoma

Osteosarcoma mostly affects children and young adults with a high predilection to metastasize to the lung preferentially. At time of initial diagnosis, 20% of patients will have radiographically detectable synchronous lung metastases (33) and 50% will develop lung metastasis some time during the course of their disease (34). Unfortunately, the presence or the development of lung metastases decreases the overall survival rates by 50%. The initial management of osteosarcoma is systemic chemotherapy and control of the primary tumor by surgical resection. Control of the primary tumor is mandatory even if the patient presents with evidence of pulmonary metastatic disease. Although most surgeons base a decision regarding resection of lung metastases on a number of criteria, including primary tumor size, number of metastases and location, these factors play little role in long-term survival and outcome after pulmonary resection.

Kempf-Bielack et al. (35) reviewed a series of 576 patients with recurrent osteosarcoma following complete surgical remission as a result of combined modality therapy. These authors found that improved prognosis was associated with complete resection of the metastatic disease, prolonged disease-free interval, a solitary secondary lesion, unilateral compared to bilateral pulmonary disease, the absence of pleural disruption, and the administration of polychemotherapy. Hartling and associates (36) studied 137 patients under the age of 21 with pulmonary metastases from osteosarcoma. In this report, the only characteristics that were associated with an increased likelihood of 5-year overall survival after pulmonary resection were primary tumor necrosis greater than 98% after neoadjuvant chemotherapy ($P < .05$) and a disease-free interval before developing lung metastases of more than one year ($P < .001$). No statistically significant difference in overall survival or disease-free survival was found based on the number of pulmonary metastases resected. Primary tumor size, site, or extension; chemotherapy; early versus late metastases; unilateral versus bilateral metastases; and resection margins were additional features that also did not significantly affect survival.

The current optimal approach to these patients is a multimodality strategy that includes aggressive surgical resection of all gross pulmonary disease following systemic chemotherapy and complete resection of the primary tumor. Patients receive additional adjuvant chemotherapy following pulmonary resection in an attempt to control any microscopic residual disease.

In patients with soft-tissue sarcomas, local recurrence is common and metastases seem to preferentially target the lungs (37,38). Several studies have suggested that patients with isolated lung metastases may be cured by pulmonary metastasectomy (39). Our current practice is to offer these patients aggressive pulmonary resection according to the basic tenets articulated earlier that include absence of locally recurrent disease, resectable pulmonary metastatic disease, and the ability to tolerate the necessary pulmonary resection. With complete resection of pulmonary metastatic disease, 5-year survival rates would be expected to be in the 30% to 50% range. Further supporting the concept of resecting pulmonary metastatic sarcoma is a recent combined analysis from M.D. Anderson and Memorial Sloan-Kettering Cancer Centers that suggests pulmonary resection is also the most cost-effective treatment when compared with ongoing chemotherapy and hospitalizations, as well as quality of life and longevity (40).

Colorectal Cancer

Because of the high incidence of colon and rectal cancers as well as their propensity to metastasize to the lung, the number of patients presenting with pulmonary metastatic disease is large. However, only about 10% of patients with metastatic colorectal cancer who have isolated metastatic disease to the lung prove to be candidates for pulmonary resection. Many of these patients will also have liver metastases, but a small percentage of patients will have isolated pulmonary lesions without hepatic metastases. According to the National Comprehensive Cancer Network (NCCN) Clinical Practice Guidelines in Oncology, surgery remains the mainstay of treatment in patients with isolated pulmonary metastases (41). There is substantial evidence from retrospective case series demonstrating that resection of colorectal pulmonary metastases can be performed safely with minimal mortality and acceptable morbidity. A recent large review of 20 published series that included 1,684 patients demonstrated improved survival following resection of colorectal metastatic lung lesions with a 5-year median survival of 52.5% with a range of 38.3% to 63.7% (42). Interestingly, the authors also found that the importance of several clinical factors, including the distribution of pulmonary metastases, previous pulmonary resection, the technical aspects of the surgical approach, and the role of minimal invasive surgery, could not be clearly determined. Disease-free interval was reported as an independent prognostic indicator in only two studies. No significant difference in outcome was seen between patients with and without a history of previously resected liver metastases at the time of pulmonary resection, with 5-year survival rates reported between 30% and 42%. The number of metastases resected was not predictive of long-term outcome nor was chemotherapy of prognostic significance in the population of patients undergoing resection of pulmonary metastatic disease. Furthermore, although the elevated preoperative serum carcinoembryonic antigen level was found to be associated with a poorer overall prognosis, patients with elevated levels still fared better following pulmonary resection as compared with those who had not undergone lung resection. Because improvements in chemotherapy for colorectal cancer have markedly improved prognosis, it is difficult to distinguish the contribution that resection of metastatic disease plays.

As mentioned previously, the more common situation encountered is the patient with concomitant synchronous or metachronous hepatic and pulmonary colorectal metastases. Although the basic tenets that have been laid out for pulmonary metastasectomy dictate that all extrathoracic disease is controlled, it does not necessarily exclude patients with disease at more than one extrathoracic site that potentially can be controlled. This seems to be the situation in a cohort of patients with both liver and lung metastases in whom both sites are amenable to complete resection. With aggressive resection of both hepatic and pulmonary colorectal metastases, the Memorial Sloan-Kettering Cancer Center group was able to achieve disease-specific survival rates of 91%, 55%, 31%, and 19% at 1, 3, 5, and 10-years (43). Based on this information, our current approach is to offer aggressive resection of both hepatic and pulmonary metastases, especially in patients with solitary or a small volume of easily resected hepatic disease. Patients undergo hepatic resection first, followed by restaging prior to undergoing pulmonary resection of metastatic nodules.

Melanoma

Overall, the outcome for patients with pulmonary metastatic disease from malignant melanoma is poor. Most commonly, pulmonary metastases occur in addition to metastases at other visceral sites and overall long-term survival is poor. Pulmonary resection plays three distinct roles in melanoma. The first is to render a patient "radiographically disease-free" in order to allow them to qualify for a clinical trial. The second is to obtain tumor as part of a clinical trial to create an autologous tumor vaccine. The third is to render the patient "disease-free surgically" in an attempt to influence their overall long-term survival.

Peterson and colleagues (44) identified 1,720 patients with lung metastases in a prospective database of 14,057 patients with melanoma. They noted a median survival of 7.3 months after the development of pulmonary metastases and a survival advantage of 12 months for patients undergoing resection of metastatic disease in those with a disease-free interval longer than 5 years (Figure 53.1). Significant predictors of survival in patients with lung metastases included nodular histologic type, disease-free interval, number of pulmonary metastases, presence of extrathoracic metastatic disease, and resection of pulmonary metastatic disease. Current 5-year survival ranges from 4.5% to 25%. Patients with multiple pulmonary metastases have poor long-term survival (45). To date, no adjuvant therapy has resulted in improved overall survival for patients with malignant melanoma.

Renal Cell Carcinoma

There are approximately 54,000 cases of renal cell carcinoma each year in the United States and about 13,000 deaths each year from this disease (46). About 30% of patients with renal cell carcinoma have metastases on initial presentation, and in most of these, survival is limited (47). Traditionally, an attempt at compete surgical metastasectomy was the only option for patients with stage IV renal cell carcinoma. Recently, however, new approaches including cytokine therapy (48), antiangiogenic therapy (49,50), and small molecule inhibitor therapy have gained momentum. Traditional cytotoxic chemotherapy plays little role because of the very low response rates.

Despite the introduction of new treatment modalities, pulmonary metastasectomy continues to play a significant role in the management of patients with stage IV renal cell carcinoma due to lung metastases. Pfannschmidt et al. (51) reported a series of 191 patients who underwent pulmonary resection for metastatic renal cell carcinoma with a complete resection achieved in 149 patients. The overall 5-year survival for the entire group was

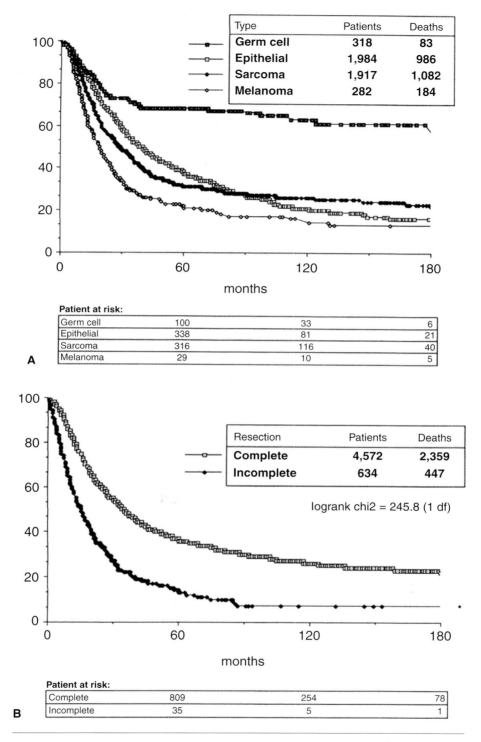

Figure 53.1 (**A**) Overall survival according to tumor type. (**B**) Overall survival: complete versus incomplete resection. (From Pastorino U, Buyse M, Friedel G, et al. Long-term results of lung metastasectomy: prognostic analyses based on 5260 cases. J Thorac Cardiovasc Surg. 1997;113:37–49.)

36.9%, but patients with fewer than seven metastases resected had overall survival of 46.8% versus only 14.5% for those with more than seven metastases. For patients undergoing a complete resection who had a disease-free interval <23 months, the 5-year survival was 24.7% versus 47% for those in whom the disease-free interval was >23 months. By multivariate analysis, the authors were able to show that the number of metastases, the presence or absence of lymph node metastases, and the disease-free interval all were significant prognostic indicators.

A recent review of the Cleveland Clinic experience found that the most important predictor of survival was complete surgical resection of all lung metastases, with a 5-year survival of 45% for patients undergoing complete resection and 8% for those patients with incomplete resection (52). The authors concluded that pulmonary resection of metastatic disease of renal cell origin was safe and that preoperative determination of resectablity was crucial. Our current practice is to work closely with a medical oncologist who has a particular interest and knowledge of the available treatments for renal cell carcinoma. We evaluate the patient's ability to tolerate complete resection from a pulmonary perspective. We also do the appropriate imaging studies to rule out other sites of distant disease. This information is used to develop a multidisciplinary consensus as to the next step in treatment that can include resection, novel systemic treatment, or a combination of both.

Germ Cell Tumors

Germ cell tumors constitute a diverse group of relatively uncommon tumors. They are related by the fact that they originate from precursor cells of the sperm or the egg. They can arise anywhere in the body and can be either benign or malignant. This group includes testicular germ cell tumors, ovarian germ cell tumors, and extragonadal germ cell tumors. Metastases from malignant germ cell tumors can occur to the lung from any of the primary tumor sites. Treatment is generally specific for the type of germ cell tumor involved. After control of the primary site, and either three or four cycles of systemic platinum-based chemotherapy, patients with residual disease are referred for surgical consideration. Usually the level of the serum tumor markers, if previously elevated, has normalized. There are a few exceptions when patients with serum markers that have not normalized are referred for surgical resection.

Multiple studies have demonstrated the importance of resecting residual masses following first-line or salvage chemotherapy for nonseminomatous germ cell tumors (53). The intent is to resect all residual disease as completeness of resection and the histology of the resected specimens are the two factors most predictive of long-term outcome. Overall multimodality treatment results are excellent. In men with testicular tumors and lung metastases who undergo multimodality treatment including pulmonary metastasectomy and resection of other residual disease, over 85% will achieve long-term survival (54).

Breast Cancer

The mainstay of treatment in patients with stage IV breast cancer is chemotherapy and resection of the primary tumor. That being said, a small number of patients with breast cancer and a solitary lung nodule will come to surgical resection.

Isolated lung metastases are reported to occur in 10% to 20% of all women with breast carcinoma. Planchard and associates (55) looked at 125 consecutive patients who underwent pulmonary resection for lung metastases from breast cancer. Ninety-six of these patients had a complete resection and the median number of resected lesions was 1 (range, 1 to 16). The median disease-free interval from the time of the treatment of the primary tumor to the development of metastatic disease was 3 years. Three-, 5-, and 10-year actuarial survival was 58%, 45%, and 30%, respectively. The median survival from time of pulmonary resection was 4.2 years. The size of the largest metastasis (≤20 mm versus >20 mm) and the disease-free interval (≤3 years versus >3 years) were highly significant prognostic indicators of survival. Whether patient selection or the actual resection of metastatic disease had the most influence on survival could not be determined, but the 5-year survival certainly is respectable. In most of these cases, the intent is to secure a diagnosis and rule out a concomitant primary lung cancer (56). Review of the International Registry of Lung Metastases (see later discussion) identified 467 metastasectomies for breast cancer from a total of 5,206 pulmonary resections for lung metastases (57). Examination of the registry data suggested that pulmonary resection could be carried out with a low morbidity and mortality. Complete resection was also associated with better long-term results of chemotherapy and immunotherapy in select groups.

In some cases in which there is a solitary pulmonary nodule, a distinction between a metastatic breast cancer and a primary lung carcinoma cannot be made, even with sophisticated pathologic testing. In these cases, we proceed to complete resection (i.e., lobectomy) in good-risk candidates whose pulmonary function tests suggest they can tolerate a lobar pulmonary resection.

Head and Neck Cancers

Patients with head and neck primary cancers are at high risk for other primary aerodigestive malignancies, especially esophageal cancer, as the risk factors for both are similar. Unfortunately, it is often impossible to distinguish a primary lung cancer from a metastatic head and neck cancer even with very sophisticated pathologic testing. Liu et al. (58) reported on 83 patients with head and neck cancers who underwent 94 pulmonary resections for presumed metastatic disease. There were 68 patients who had complete resection, and the median disease-free interval was 27 months. Actuarial overall survival at 5 years was 50%, but it was 64% for glandular tumors and only 34% for squamous cell carcinomas. Patients with adenoid cystic carcinomas had >80% 5-year survival, although none of the patients remained disease-free.

Although the role of metastasectomy in head and neck cancer is questionable, the role of surgery in primary lung cancer is well documented. Therefore, in the case of a solitary malignant lung nodule, even if it is the same histologic type as the primary head and neck cancer, usually squamous carcinoma, we generally evaluate and treat as a primary lung cancer. In those patients with multiple nodules throughout different lobes, treatment must be individualized based on the number of lesions, location, and the overall health of the patient.

Recent knowledge dealing with the resection of metastatic disease in the lung has been greatly enhanced based on data accumulated in a large, multicenter registry, the International Registry of Lung Metastases. The registry, started in 1991, included patients accrued from 18 major thoracic surgery centers in 9 different countries. By 1996, the registry had accumulated 5,206 cases. Outcome data presented according to site of the primary were published in 1997 (59). Primary tumor types in the registry included 2,260 epithelial neoplasms, 2,173 sarcomas, 363 germ cell tumors, and 328 melanomas. Figure 53.1 shows overall survival according to tumor type. The goal of the registry was to determine common characteristics important in selecting patients for lung metastasectomy across a variety of primary tumor types. Multivariate analysis suggested that a

disease-free interval of >3 years from the primary tumor to the diagnosis of lung metastasis and the finding of a solitary lung metastasis were important individual predictors of long-term survival. They also concluded that pulmonary metastasectomy was a safe and potentially curative procedure for certain tumor types. Interestingly, there has not been a follow-up to the initial report.

CONCLUSIONS

Isolated and resectable metastases to the lungs represent a unique biology among the host, the primary neoplasm, and the

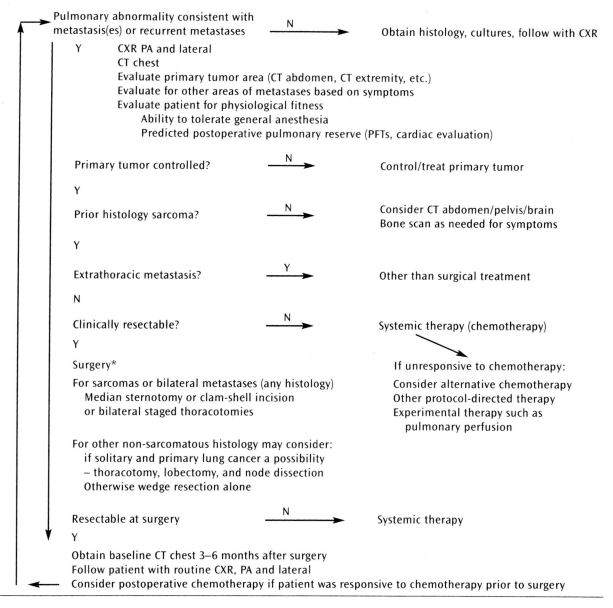

*The response to salvage chemotherapy after development of sarcomatous pulmonary metastases has not been shown to be associated with improved survival after resection compared to resection alone.

Figure 53.2 Algorithm for the management of suspected pulmonary metastases. CXR, chest x-ray; PA, posteroanterior; CT, computed tomography.

metastases. The combination forms a self-selected group that may benefit from surgical resection. Many of these patients can achieve long-term survival associated with complete resection of their pulmonary metastatic disease. Whether the long-term survival is more closely related with the self-selection and the biology of the tumor, or the resection of the metastatic disease itself, cannot be determined with certainty. Complete resection is the most significant predictor of long-term survival, regardless of the primary tumor histology. Patients with resectable lung metastases should undergo resection to render them disease-free as long as the preoperative assessment indicates that a complete resection can be accomplished. In order to determine this, a period of observation confirming a finding of disease stability, that is, the lack of an explosion of additional metastatic disease whether in the lung or elsewhere, usually is recommended. The issue of timing of surgical resection of pulmonary metastasis may be more important than previously realized, as pointed out by Tanaka et al. (21). An algorithm for the management of pulmonary metastases is presented in Figure 53.2.

The future surgical treatment of pulmonary metastases likely will be defined by improved diagnosis and better systemic treatments. Hopefully, a tumor's molecular signature and comparison to the primary will enable us to distinguish between metastatic lesions and primary lung malignancies. It is also likely that these molecular signatures will identify new targets for therapeutic intervention. At present, however, we remain guided by the basic tenets set forth by Alexander and Haight (5) over 60 years ago. The tenets then as now are (a) initial control of the primary tumor, (b) absence of other metastatic disease outside the lungs, and (c) physiologic suitability to undergo a pulmonary resection.

Despite a lack of randomized clinical trials demonstrating efficacy of resection of metastatic disease, numerous case series have established metastasectomy as part of the treatment regimen for a number of tumors. Data from the International Registry further supports the use of this modality in selected patients with pulmonary metastatic disease. This view, however, is not uncontested and we would be remiss in not mentioning a dissenting viewpoint. Treasure (60) and Treasure et al. (61) have questioned the entire practice of pulmonary metastasectomy and they believe that the concept is based on weak evidence. They opine that as the surgical procedures are becoming more extensive and more frequent, there is an increasing amount of harm done as a consequence. According to them, the lack of any prospective randomized clinical trials along with poor data provided even in the observational trials, begs the question as to whether there is any significant efficacy in resecting pulmonary metastatic disease. The authors of a recent review looking at resection of colorectal metastases state that randomized trials comparing metastasectomy with nonsurgical treatment are not possible at this point (40). Treasure (60,61) concludes that even a "generous" review of the literature indicates a lack of clarity as to the objectives, the rationale for metastasectomy is "insecure," and the evidence available does not address the question of whether the benefit exceeds the potential harm. It must be said that at the present time, Treasure stands as the "lone voice in the wilderness" as current practice in most centers includes the resection of metastatic disease.

Despite the existence of the registry data that included large numbers of patients, perhaps it is not too late to either conduct either rigorous observational trials that include the total number of patients, both operated and nonoperated, or even randomized clinical trials to once and for all establish whether metastasectomy truly is of value in prolonging life. The literature is littered with surgical procedures once in vogue that are now only mentioned to be condemned. Those of us in surgery need to get beyond what Horton (62) implied over 10 years ago in an editorial entitled, "Surgical research or comic opera: questions, but few answers."

ACKNOWLEDGMENTS

The authors acknowledge the contributions of Joe B. Putnam Jr. and Jack A. Roth, who contributed the chapter on pulmonary metastases in the first edition of this book. The present authors have used portions of that chapter in the current work.

REFERENCES

1. Weinlechner JW. Zur Kasuistik der Tumoren and der Brustwant und deren Behandlung. *Wien Med Wochenschr.* 1882;32:589–591, 624–628, 1882.
2. Divis G. Deitrag Zur Operativen Behandlung der Lungeschwulste. *Acta Chirur Scand.* 1927;62:329–341.
3. Torek F. Removal of metastatic carcinoma of the lung and mediastinum. *Arch Surg.* 1930;21:1416–1424.
4. Barney JD, Churchill EJ. Adenocarcinoma of the kidney with metastasis to the lung cured by nephrectomy and lobectomy. *J Urol.* 1939;42:269–276.
5. Alexander J, Haight C. Pulmonary resection for solitary metastatic sarcomas and carcinomas. *Surg Gynecol Obstet.* 1947;85:129–146.
6. Thomford NR, Woolner LB, Clagett OT. The surgical treatment of metastatic tumors in the lungs. *J Thorac Cardiovasc Surg.* 1965;49:357–363.
7. Beattie EJ, Harvey JC, Marcove R, et al. Results of multiple pulmonary resections for metastatic osteogenic sarcoma after two decades. *J Surg Oncol.* 1991;46:154–155.
8. Kandioler D, Kromer E, Tuchler H, et al. Long-term results after repeated surgical removal of pulmonary metastases. *Ann Thorac Surg.* 1998;65:909–912.
9. Mohammed TL, Chowdhry AA, Khan A, et al., Expert Panel on Thoracic Imaging. Screening for pulmonary metastases. [online publication]. Reston, VA: American College of Radiology; 2006.
10. Demmy TL, Dunn KB. Surgical and nonsurgical therapy for lung metastasis: indications and outcomes. *Surg Oncol Clin North Am.* 2007;16:579–605.
11. Strumberg D, Clark JW, Awada A, et al. Safety, pharmacokinetics and preliminary antitumor activity of sarafenib: a review of four phase I trials in patients with advanced refractory solid tumors. *Oncologist.* 2007;12:426–437.
12. Ferguson WS, Goorin AM. Current treatment of osteosarcoma. *Cancer Invest.* 2001;19:292–315.
13. Pastorino U. Lung metastasectomy: why, when, how. *Crit Rev Oncol Hematol.* 1997;26:137–145.
14. Bacci G, Lari S. Adjuvant and neoadjuvant chemotherapy in osteosarcoma. *Chir Organi Mov.* 2001;86:253–268.
15. Canter RJ, Qin LX, Downey RJ, et al. Perioperative chemotherapy in patients undergoing pulmonary resection for metastatic

soft-tissue sarcoma of the extremity: a retrospective analysis. *Cancer.* 2007;110:2050–2060.

16. Wunder JS, Nielson RG, O'Sullivan B, et al. Opportunities for improving the therapeutic ratio for patients with sarcoma. *Lancet Oncol.* 2007;8:513–24.

17. Burgers JM, van Glabbeke M, Busson A, et al. Osteosarcoma of the limbs. Report of the EORTC-SIOP 03 trial 20781 investigating the value of adjuvant treatment with chemotherapy and/or prophylactic lung irradiation. *Cancer.* 1988;61:1024–1031.

18. Fernando HC. Radiofrequency ablation to treat non-small cell lung cancer and pulmonary metastases. *Ann Thorac Surg.* 2008;85:S780–S784.

19. Simon CJ, Dupuy DE, DiPetrillo TA, et al. Pulmonary radiofrequency ablation; long-term safety and efficacy in 153 patients. *Radiology.* 2007;243:268–275.

20. Lencioni R, Crocetti L, Cioni R, et al. Response to radiofrequency ablation of pulmonary tumors: a prospective, intention-to-treat, multicentre clinical trial the (RAPTURE study) [published online ahead of print June 17, 2008]. *Lancet Oncol.* 2008;9:621–628.

21. Tanaka Y, Maniwa Y, Nishio W, et al. The optimal timing to resect pulmonary metastasis. *Eur J Cardiothorac Surg.* 2008;33:1135–1138.

22. Smith R, Pak Y, Kraybill W, Kane JM. Factors associated with actual and long-term survival following soft tissue sarcoma pulmonary metastasectomy [published online ahead of print February 21, 2008]. *Eur J Surg Oncol.* 2009;35:356-361.

23. Van Geel AN, van Der Sijp JRM, Schmitz PI. Which soft tissue sarcoma patients with lung metastases should not undergo pulmonary resection? *Sarcoma.* 2002;6:57–60.

24. Veronesi G, Petrella F, Leo F, et al. Prognostic role of lymph node involvement in lung metastasectomy. *J Thorac Cardiovasc Surg.* 2007;133:976–972.

25. Meno A, Milton R, Thore J, et al. The value of video-assisted mediastinoscopy in pulmonary metastasectomy. *Eur J Cardiothorac Surg.* 2007;32:351–355.

26. McCormack P, Bains M, Begg C, et al. Role of videoassisted thoracic surgery in the treatment of pulmonary metastases: results of a prospective trial. *Ann Thorac Surg.* 1996;62:213–217.

27. Mutsaerts E, Zoetmulder F, Meijer S, et al. Long term survival of thoracoscopic metastasectomy vs metastasectomy by thoracotomy in patients with a solitary pulmonary lesion. *Eur J Surg Oncol.* 2002;28:864–868.

28. Mutsaerts E, Zoetmulder F, Meijer S, et al. Outcome of thoracoscopic pulmonary metastasectomy evaluated by confirmatory thoracotomy. *Ann Thorac Surg.* 2001;72:230–233.

29. Parsons A, Ennis E, Yankaskas B, et al. Helical computed tomography inaccuracy in the detection of pulmonary metastases: can it be improved? *Ann Thorac Surg.* 2007;84:1830–1837.

30. Margaritora S, Porziella V, D'Andrilli A, et al. Pulmonary metastases: can accurate radiological evaluation avoid thoracotomic approach? *Eur J Cardiothorac Surg.* 2002;21:1111–1114.

31. Ludwig C, Cerinza J, Passlick B, et al. Comparison of the number of pre-, intra- and postoperative lung metastases. *Eur J Cardiothorac Surg.* 2008;33:470–472.

32. Bains MS, Ginsberg RJ, Jones II WG, et al. The clamshell incision: an improved approach to bilateral pulmonary and mediastinal tumors. *Ann Thorac Surg.* 1994;58:30–33.

33. Chi S, Conklin L, Qin J et al. The patterns of relapse in osteosarcoma. *Pediatr Blood Cancer.* 2004;42:46–51.

34. Torre W, Rodriquez-Spiteri N, Sierrasesumaga L. Current role for resection of thoracic metastases in children and young adults-do we need different strategies for this population? *Thor Cardiovasc Surg.* 2004;52:90–95.

35. Kempf-Bielack B, Dielack S, Jurgens H, et al. Osteosarcoma relapse after combined modality therapy an analysis of unselected patients I the Cooperative Osteosarcoma Study Group. *J Clin Oncol.* 2005;23:559–568.

36. Harting M, Blakely M, Jaffe N, et al. Long-term survival after aggressive resection of pulmonary metastases among children and adolescents with osteosarcoma. *J Pediatr Surg.* 2006;41:194–195.

37. Potter D, Glenn J, Kinsella E, et al. Patterns of recurrence in patients with high-grade soft-tissue sarcomas. *J Clin Oncol.* 1985;3:353–366.

38. Billingsley K, Burt M, Jara E, et al. Pulmonary metastases from soft-tissue sarcoma: analysis of patterns of disease and postmetastasis survival. *Ann Surg.* 1993;229:602–612.

39. Temple L, Brennan M. The role of pulmonary metastasectomy in soft tissue sarcoma. *Semin Thorac Cardiovasc Surg.* 2002;114:35–44.

40. Porter G, Cantor S, Walsh G, et al. Cost-effectiveness of pulmonary resection and systemic chemotherapy in the management of metastatic soft tissue sarcoma: a combined analysis from the University of Texas M.D. Anderson and Memorial Sloan-Kettering Cancer Center. *J Thorac Cardiovasc Surg.* 2004;127:1366–1372.

41. National Comprehensive Cancer Network. Clinical Practice Guidelines in Oncology. v.2. 2009 Colon Cancer. http://www.nccn.org/professionals/physcians_gls/PDF/colon.pdf. Accessed May 23, 2009.

42. Pfannschmidt J, Dienemann H, Hoffmann H. Surgical resection of pulmonary metastases from colorectal cancer: a systematic review of published series. *Ann Thorac Surg.* 2007;84:324–338.

43. Miller G, Biernacki P, Kemeny N, et al. Outcomes after resection of synchronous or metachronous hepatic and pulmonary colorectal metastases. *J Am Coll Surg.* 2007;205:231–238.

44. Peterson R, Hanish S, Haney J, et al. Improved survival with pulmonary metastasectomy: an analysis of 1720 patients with pulmonary metastatic melanoma. *J Thorac Cardiovasc Surg.* 2007;133:104–110.

45. Pogrebniak HW, Stovroff M, Roth JM, et al. Resection of pulmonary metastases for malignant melanoma: results of a 16-year experience. *Ann Thorac Surg.* 1988;46:20–23.

46. American Cancer Society.*Cancer Facts and Figures 2008.* Atlanta, GA: American Cancer Society, 2008.

47. Golimbu M, Joshi P, Sperber A, et al. Renal cell carcinoma: survival and prognostic factors. *J Urol.* 1986;27:291–301.

48. Flanigan RC, Salmon SE, Blumenstein BA, et al. Nephrectomy followed by interferon alfa-2b compared with interferon alfa-2b alone for metastatic renal-cell cancer. *N Engl J Med.* 2001;345:1655–1659.

49. Motzer RJ, Hutson TE, Tomczak P, et al. Sunitinib versus interferon alfa in metastatic renal-cell carcinoma. *N Engl J Med.* 2007;356(2):115–24.

50. Motzer RJ, Michaelson MD, Redman BG, et al. Activity of SU11248, a multitargeted inhibitor of vascular endothelial growth factor receptor and platelet-derived growth factor receptor, in patients with metastatic renal cell carcinoma. *J Clin Oncol.* 2006;24:16–24.

51. Pfannschmidt J, Hoffmann H, Muley T, et al. Prognostic factors for survival after pulmonary resection of metastatic renal cell carcinoma. *Ann Thorac Surg.* 2002;74:1653–1657.

52. Murthy S, Kim K, Rice T, et al. Can we predict long-term survival after pulmonary metastasectomy for renal cell carcinoma? *Ann Thorac Surg.* 2005;79:996–1003.

53. Feldman DR, Bosl GJ, Sheinfeld J, et al. Medical treatment of advanced testicular cancer. *JAMA.* 2008;299:672–684.

54. Liu D, Abolhoda A, Burt M, et al. Pulmonary metastasectomy for testicular germ cell tumors: a 28-year experience. *Ann Thorac Surg.* 1998;66:1709–1714.

55. Planchard D, Soria JC, Michiels S, et al. Uncertain benefit from surgery in patients with lung metastases from breast carcinoma. *Cancer.* 2004;100:28–35.

56. Tanaka F, Li M, Hanaoka N, et al. Surgery for pulmonary nodules in breast cancer patients. *Ann Thorac Surg.* 2005;79:1711–1715.

57. Fruedek G, Pastorino U, Ginsberg R, et al. Results of lung metastasectomy from breast cancer: prognostic criteria on the basis of 467 cases of the international registry of lung metastases. *Eur J Cardiothorac Surg.* 2002;22:335–344.

58. Liu D, Labow DM, Dang N, et al. Pulmonary metastasectomy for head and neck cancers. *Ann Surg Oncol.* 1999;6:572–578.

59. Pastorino U, Buyse M, Friedel G, et al. Long-term results of lung metastasectomy: prognostic analyses based on 5260 cases. *J Thorac Cardiovasc Surg.* 1997;113:37–49.

60. Treasure T. Pulmonary metastasectomy: a common practice based on weak evidence. *Ann R Coll Surg Engl.* 2007;89:744–748.

61. Treasure T, Internullo E, Utley M. Resection of pulmonary metastases: a growth industry. *Cancer Imaging.* 2008;8:121–124.

62. Horton R. Surgical research or comic opera: questions, but few answers. *Lancet.* 1996;347:984–985.

COMMENTARY
Howard Silberman

Drs. Kucharczuk and Kaiser have presented a comprehensive review of the contemporary management of pulmonary metastases. In this Commentary, various aspects of diagnosis, prognosis, and treatment are emphasized or further discussed.

A new pulmonary lesion, especially a solitary one, detected on chest imaging in a patient with a history of cancer *may* be a metastasis from the original primary tumor, but, alternatively, such a lesion may actually be a new, primary lung lesion, benign or malignant. The histology of the primary tumor determines the likelihood that a newly detected pulmonary lesion represents metastatic disease (1). A patient with a primary lung cancer must not be denied the opportunity for aggressive treatment because of assumptions about the nature of the new pulmonary finding. In a review of patients previously treated for an extrathoracic malignancy who were found to have a new lung lesion, Adkins et al. (2) reported that the nodule represented metastatic disease in 46% of patients, a new lung primary in 32%, and benign disease in 18%.

DIAGNOSIS AND STAGING

Positron emission tomography (PET) scanning has emerged as an important procedure in the diagnosis and staging of patients with pulmonary metastases (1,3). Pastorino et al. (3) evaluated the role of PET scanning in the preoperative assessment of ap-

parently operable lung metastases. Eighty-six patients with a previously treated malignancy and proven or suspected lung metastases, who were deemed resectable on the basis of computed tomography (CT), were investigated with 89 preoperative PET procedures. Primary tumor sites were gastrointestinal in 32 cases, sarcoma in 13, urologic in 14, breast in 8, head and neck in 7, gynecologic in 5, thymus in 5, and other sites in 5. Seventy lung lesions were resected in 68 patients. Only 54 of the 70 lesions proved to be lung metastases; 7 were primary lung tumors and 9 were benign lesions. Of importance is the fact that in 19 cases (21%) eligibility for pulmonary resection was excluded on the basis of PET scan results because of extrapulmonary metastases (11 cases), primary site recurrence (2 cases), mediastinal adenopathy (2 cases), or benign disease (4 cases). All mediastinal node metastases (7 cases) were detected by PET with a sensitivity, accuracy, and negative predictive value for mediastinal staging of 100%, 96%, and 100%, respectively, versus 71%, 92%, and 95% of the CT scan. In the group of patients who underwent lung resection, PET sensitivity for detection of lung metastasis was 87%. Thus, in this series PET scanning proved to be a valuable staging procedure and had a significant impact on clinical judgment in that therapeutic management was altered in a high proportion of cases on the basis of this examination.

It is usually desirable to pathologically confirm the nature of pulmonary lesions deemed to be metastatic. Diagnostic material for cytologic, histologic, or immunohistochemical analysis (4), for detection of molecular markers (4), or for in vitro chemosensitivity testing can be obtained by fine-needle aspiration or core-needle biopsy under CT or ultrasound guidance (5—10) or by video-assisted thoracoscopic excision (8,11,12) Such an initial evaluation may well facilitate subsequent therapeutic decisions. A solitary nodule proven to represent a primary lung lesion will be more widely resected than the wedge resection often undertaken for a metastatic lesion. Patients with several metastatic nodules, especially those with a short disease-free interval following resection of the primary tumor, may benefit from a period of chemotherapy during which the stability of disease within the lung can be assessed and the development of extrathoracic dissemination can be identified. Progression of disease in the interim would preclude any benefit from local resection of the lung nodules.

PROGNOSIS

Factors that in most series appear to contribute to an adverse outcome following pulmonary metastasectomy include incomplete resection, short disease-free interval (DFI), multiple pulmonary lesions, and mediastinal nodal involvement. In addition, outcome varies considerably with the nature of the primary malignancy.

Chen et al. (13) reported that among 41 patients who underwent complete resection of pulmonary metastases from breast cancer, overall survival was 51% at 5 and 10 years. On multivariate analysis, fewer than four lung lesions and a DFI of >3 years were statistically significant favorable prognostic factors for overall survival ($p = 0.023$ and 0.024, respectively). Friedel et al. (14) analyzed data collected by the International Registry of Lung Metastases from 467 patients with pulmonary metastasis from breast cancer and confirmed the salutary impact of a DFI ≥3 years, but patients with single and multiple metastatic lesions had similar outcomes.

In the management of pulmonary lesions metastatic from squamous cell cancers of the head and neck, Liu and associates (15) reported incomplete resection, age >50 years, and a DFI of ≤2 years were significant adverse prognostic factors. Chen et al. (16) found that among 20 patients with pulmonary metastases from head and neck cancers who had undergone complete pulmonary resection, women fared significantly better as did those with a DFI of ≥12 months and a nonsquamous cell primary tumor.

Kane et al. (17) found that, in contrast to patients with metachronous metastases from soft-tissue sarcomas, pulmonary resection provided no survival benefit to 17 patients undergoing resection of synchronous metastases. These findings further emphasize the relationship of prognosis and DFI.

Casali and associates (18) reviewed the course of 142 patients with primary epithelial tumors treated with lung metastasectomy. Twelve percent of the patients had mediastinal node metastases. Mediastinal nodal status negatively affected survival at univariate analysis (5 years, 32% for node-positive and 40% for node-negative patients; $p = 0.013$). Disease-free survival also was significantly different according to nodal status: 5-year disease-free survival 17% and 28% for node-positive and node-negative patients, respectively ($p = 0.053$). Systemic recurrences were more frequent in patients with nodal involvement ($p = 0.058$). The authors concluded that inasmuch as patients with pulmonary metastases and nodal involvement had a poor prognosis and relapsed early after pulmonary metastasectomy, nodal status should be considered in the selection of patients for lung metastasectomy.

The International Registry of Lung Metastases was established to assess the long-term results of pulmonary metastasectomy (19). Analysis of data from 5,206 cases is summarized in Table 53C.1, in which the relative risks of death, that is, the hazard rates for each level of the variable relative to the rest of the population, as well as 95% confidence limits estimated by the Cox proportional hazard model, are tabulated. The relative risks of death for each variable were adjusted for all the other variables of interest: sex, age, DFI, number of metastases, and tumor type. There was a trend to poorer prognosis (relative risk of death >1) associated with shorter DFI and greater number of metastases. The best outcomes observed among patients were DFIs ≥36 months, single metastases, and germ cell or Wilms tumors. Melanoma was the tumor associated with the worst prognosis.

NONSURGICAL TREATMENT MODALITIES

Nonsurgical ablative modalities being evaluated for the treatment of pulmonary metastases with curative intent include radiofrequency ablation (discussed by Drs. Kucharczuk and Kaiser), stereotactic radiosurgery (SRS), and cryotherapy.

Stereotactic Radiosurgery

Conventional radiotherapy in the treatment of primary lung cancer is associated with poor response rates (20). Dose escalation to improve outcome provided by conventional fractionated radiotherapy is limited by two factors: prolonged treatment time allowing accelerated tumor cell repopulation and increased exposure of functional lung tissue to radiation resulting in impaired pulmonary function (21). SRS is the application of very high doses of ionizing radiation in larger-than-traditional fractionation to much smaller-than-traditional radiotherapy fields, often with the integration of advanced modalities for tumor imaging and devices for tumor immobilization (22). Thus, SRS potentially addresses the need for dose escalation within a short treatment time with sparing of functional lung tissue (21). Several investigators have reported their experience with the application of SRS in the management of metastatic pulmonary lesions (21,23–25).

Wulf et al. (21) reported their results using stereotactic radiotherapy in the management of 41 patients with 51 metastatic pulmonary lesions. The median follow-up was 9 months (range, 2 to 37 months). Five local failures were observed, leading to a crude local control rate for all targets of 90%. All local failures occurred within the first year after treatment, at 5, 7, 8, 8, and 11 months. The actuarial local control rate for the 51 metastases was 80% at ≥12 months. The overall survival rate was 85% after 12 months and 33% after 24 months. Most patients had systemic disease progression. The freedom from systemic progression rate was 35% after 12 months and 23% after 24 months.

Pennathur et al. (25) reported their preliminary experience in the management of 32 medically inoperable patients, 27 with non-small cell lung cancer and 5 with pulmonary metastases. Treatment was delivered using the CyberKnife Radiosurgery System (Accuray, Inc., Sunnyvale, CA). The CyberKnife is a frameless system that provides image-guided robotic SRS that is capable of directing ablative doses to limited treatment volumes. The system delivers the prescribed dose using radiation beams from many different angles converging on the tumors, with real-time target tracking through combined orthogonal radiograph imaging with respiratory and skeletal structure tracking (23). The authors observed an initial complete response rate in 7 (22%) of the 32 patients. The estimated 1-year overall survival rate for the patients with metastatic disease was 80%.

Brown et al. (23), at the University of Miami, treated 35 patients, 33 to 91 years of age and with 69 histologically proven pulmonary metastases, with the CyberKnife system. Fourteen patients had multiple metastases and were treated for two to eight pulmonary lesions. Each patient was determined to have technically resectable lesions but was deemed ineligible for surgery because he or she lacked adequate respiratory reserve, had severe cardiac dysfunction or chronic heart disease, pulmonary hypertension, advanced diabetes mellitus with severe end-organ damage, vascular disease, general frailty, or severe cerebral disease. Tumors >5 cm in diameter were excluded for treatment with curative intent. A complete response was defined as a disappearance of the lesion determined by chest PET/CT scan with fluorodeoxyglucose (FDG)-negative status, and a partial response as the presence of a residual abnormality on PET/CT scan and a reduction of FDG. Stable disease was represented by no significant change in the size of the tumor or FDG level. Progressive disease was defined as an enlarging lesion on PET/CT scan or increasing FDG activity not attributable to radiation pneumonitis or fibrosis. All of the patients tolerated the radiosurgery well,

Table 53C.1

Adjusted Relative Risks of Death (RRD) after Pulmonary Metastasectomy[a]

Variable	No.	RRD	95% Confidence Interval
Disease-free interval (mo)			
Synchronous	474[b]	0.952	(0.820–1.104)
1–11	909[b]	1.401	(1.263–1.555)
12–23	1040[b]	1.217	(1.104–1.343)
24–35	622[b]	1.007	(0.892–1.136)
36+	1416[b]	0.637	(0.575–0.705)
No. of lesions			
0	47	1.034	(0.678–1.575)
1	2169	0.764	(0.681–0.818)
2	738	1.070	(0.953–1.200)
3	487	1.021	(0.885–1.178)
4	235	1.316	(1.091–1.587)
5	214	1.183	(0.971–1.442)
6	125	1.328	(1.029–1.715)
7	88	1.251	(0.947–1.652)
8–9	118	1.206	(0.932–1.561)
10	73	1.677	(1.262–2.229)
11–19	179	1.083	(0.880–1.334)
20+	90	1.270	(0.935–1.725)
Tumor type			
Teratoma	203	0.373	(0.272–0.510)
Wilms	25	0.503	(0.232–1.088)
Embryonal	92	0.571	(0.373–0.829)
Uterus	83	0.796	(0.555–1.142)
Bowel	645	0.831	(0.721–0.959)
Other bone sarcoma	223	0.965	(0.789–1.180)
Breast	396	1.117	(0.945–1.320)
Head and neck	247	0.898	(0.735–1.096)
Kidney	372	0.928	(0.790–1.091)
Osteosarcoma	734	0.990	(0.863–1.136)
Synovial sarcoma	174	1.026	(0.833–1.264)
Leiomyosarcoma	156	1.098	(0.878–1.374)
Other epithelial	184	1.120	(0.900–1.393)
Other soft sarcoma	421	1.238	(1.078–1.422)
Histiocytoma	186	1.150	(0.937–1.412)
Lung	53	1.374	(0.913–2.067)
Melanoma	282	2.034	(1.728–2.394)

[a]Adjusted by sex, age, disease-free interval, number of metastases, and tumor type.
[b]Numbers indicate number of patients undergoing complete metastasectomy.
From Long-term results of lung metastasectomy: prognostic analyses based on 5206 cases. The International Registry of Lung Metastases. *J Thorac Cardiovasc Surg.* 1997;113:37–49, with permission.

with fatigue as the main side effect. Of the 35 treated patients, 27 (77%) were still alive at a median 18-month (range, 2 to 41 months) follow-up. Local control was 71% with 25 tumors showing a complete response, 16 showing a partial response, and 7 stable with disease. Eight had progressive disease.

Thus, early experience with limited follow-up data suggests that SRS in the management of pulmonary metastases is feasible, safe, and achieves good rates of local disease control with limited toxicity to surrounding tissues. Currently, SRS has been offered only to patients deemed at high risk for operative resection.

Cryotherapy

Several preliminary reports indicate the feasibility of image-guided percutaneous cryoablation of pulmonary lesions (26,27). Kawamura et al. (26) treated 35 pulmonary tumors in 20 patients in 22 sessions of cryoblation. In all cases, cryoablation was performed percutaneously under CT guidance with local anesthesia. No major complications were encountered. Seven (20%) of the 35 tumors locally recurred in 7 (35%) of the 20 patients during a 9- to 28-month follow-up period. One year Kaplan-Meier survival was 89.4%.

The comparative efficacy of surgical resection and these nonsurgical ablative modalities has not been studied. It may be that a combination of surgical resection, nonsurgical ablative techniques, with or without adjunctive chemotherapy, may prove most effective, especially in patients with multiple pulmonary nodules wherein the peripheral nodules can be resected with minimal sacrifice of pulmonary tissue and the deeper-seated lesions managed with a nonsurgical ablative technique.

REFERENCES

1. Quiros RM, Scott WJ. Surgical treatment of metastatic disease to the lung. *Semin Oncol.* 2008;35:1341–1346.
2. Adkins PC, Wesselhoeft CW Jr, Newman W, et al. Thoracotomy on the patient with previous malignancy: metastasis or new primary? *J Thorac Cardiovasc Surg.* 1968;56:351–361.
3. Pastorino U, Veronesi G, Landoni C, et al. Fluorodeoxyglucose positron emission tomography improves preoperative staging of resectable lung metastasis. *J Thorac Cardiovasc Surg.* 2003;126:1906–1910.
4. Okasaka T, Usami N, Mitsudomi T, et al. Stepwise examination for differential diagnosis of primary lung cancer and breast cancer relapse presenting as a solitary pulmonary nodule in patients after mastectomy. *J Surg Oncol.* 2008;98:510–514.
5. Anderson JM, Murchison J, Patel D. CT-guided lung biopsy: factors influencing diagnostic yield and complication rate. *Clin Radiol.* 2003;58:791–797.
6. Hsu WH, Chiang CD, Hsu JY, et al. Ultrasound-guided fine-needle aspiration biopsy of lung cancers. *J Clin Ultrasound.* 1996;24:225–233.
7. Laurent F, Latrabe V, Vergier B, et al. Percutaneous CT-guided biopsy of the lung: comparison between aspiration and automated cutting needles using a coaxial technique. *Cardiovasc Intervent Radiol.* 2000;23:266–272.
8. Miller JC, Shepard JA, Lanuti M, et al. Evaluating pulmonary nodules. *J Am Coll Radiol.* 2007;4:422–426.
9. Shaham D. Semi-invasive and invasive procedures for the diagnosis and staging of lung cancer. I. Percutaneous transthoracic needle biopsy. *Radiol Clin North Am.* 2000;38:525–534.
10. Yang PC. Ultrasound-guided transthoracic biopsy of the chest. *Radiol Clin North Am.* 2000;38:323–343.
11. Decamp MM Jr. The solitary pulmonary nodule: aggressive excisional strategy. *Semin Thorac Cardiovasc Surg.* 2002;14:292–296.
12. Rena O, Papalia E, Ruffini E, et al. The role of surgery in the management of solitary pulmonary nodule in breast cancer patients. *Eur J Surg Oncol.* 2007;33:546–550.
13. Chen F, Fujinaga T, Sato K, et al. Clinical features of surgical resection for pulmonary metastasis from breast cancer [published online ahead of print June 18, 2008]. *Eur J Surg Oncol.* 2009;35:393–397.
14. Friedel G, Pastorino U, Ginsberg RJ, et al. Results of lung metastasectomy from breast cancer: prognostic criteria on the basis of 467 cases of the International Registry of Lung Metastases. *Eur J Cardiothorac Surg.* 2002;22:335–344.
15. Liu D, Labow DM, Dang N, et al. Pulmonary metastasectomy for head and neck cancers. *Ann Surg Oncol.* 1999;6:572–578.
16. Chen F, Sonobe M, Sato K, et al. Pulmonary resection for metastatic head and neck cancer. *World J Surg.* 2008;32:1657–1662.
17. Kane JM, Finley JW, Driscoll D, et al. The treatment and outcome of patients with soft tissue sarcomas and synchronous metastases. *Sarcoma.* 2002;6:69–73.
18. Casali C, Stefani A, Storelli E, et al. Prognostic factors and survival after resection of lung metastases from epithelial tumours. *Interact Cardiovasc Thorac Surg.* 2006;5:317–321.
19. Long-term results of lung metastasectomy: prognostic analyses based on 5206 cases. The International Registry of Lung Metastases. *J Thorac Cardiovasc Surg.* 1997;113:37–49.
20. Sibley GS, Jamieson TA, Marks LB, et al. Radiotherapy alone for medically inoperable stage I non-small-cell lung cancer: the Duke experience. *Int J Radiat Oncol Biol Phys.* 1998;40:149–154.
21. Wulf J, Haedinger U, Oppitz U, et al. Stereotactic radiotherapy for primary lung cancer and pulmonary metastases: a noninvasive treatment approach in medically inoperable patients. *Int J Radiat Oncol Biol Phys.* 2004;60:186–196.
22. Cesaretti JA, Pennathur A, Rosenstein BS, et al. Stereotactic radiosurgery for thoracic malignancies. *Ann Thorac Surg.* 2008;85:S785–S791.
23. Brown WT, Wu X, Fowler JF, et al. Lung metastases treated by CyberKnife image-guided robotic stereotactic radiosurgery at 41 months. *South Med J.* 2008;101:376–382.
24. Muacevic A, Drexler C, Wowra B, et al. Technical description, phantom accuracy, and clinical feasibility for single-session lung radiosurgery using robotic image-guided real-time respiratory tumor tracking. *Technol Cancer Res Treat.* 2007;6:321–328.
25. Pennathur A, Luketich JD, Burton S, et al. Stereotactic radiosurgery for the treatment of lung neoplasm: initial experience. *Ann Thorac Surg.* 2007;83:1820–1824.
26. Kawamura M, Izumi Y, Tsukada N, et al. Percutaneous cryoablation of small pulmonary malignant tumors under computed tomographic guidance with local anesthesia for nonsurgical candidates. *J Thorac Cardiovasc Surg.* 2006;131:1007–1013.
27. Wang H, Littrup PJ, Duan Y, et al. Thoracic masses treated with percutaneous cryotherapy: initial experience with more than 200 procedures. *Radiology.* 2005;235:289–298.

54

Urologic Cancers: Surgical Management of Kidney, Bladder, Prostate, and Testis Cancers

Polina Reyblat, Donald G Skinner, and John P Stein

KIDNEY TUMORS

Angiomyolipoma

Renal angiomyolipoma (AML; hamartoma) is a benign solid tumor of the kidney that can be sporadic or associated with tuberous sclerosis. In the general population, AML is a solitary tumor, predominantly unilateral, and most commonly seen in female patients. In patients with tuberous sclerosis it occurs in up to 80% of the affected population.

Classically, AMLs present with a triad of flank pain, palpable mass, and gross or microhematuria. Other presenting symptoms include nausea, vomiting, fever, hypertension, anemia, renal failure, and hypotension secondary to hemorrhage. Flank pain is the most common complaint (41%), followed by hematuria (11%) in symptomatic AML. Retroperitoneal hemorrhage due to spontaneous rupture of the AML can be a life-threatening presentation of the disease. Up to 15% of patients with symptomatic AML present with hemorrhage. AML is the second most common cause of renal retroperitoneal bleeding after renal cell carcinoma (RCC). AML also commonly presents as an incidental finding on radiologic studies. Overall, 15% to 25% of AMLs under 4 cm are symptomatic at presentation, in contrast to 50% to 80% of AMLs over 4 cm that are symptomatic at the time of diagnosis (1).

AMLs have unique radiographic characteristics that aid in the diagnosis. Computerized tomography (CT) is the ideal radiographic method to diagnose AML. The CT diagnosis of AML depends on identifying fat within the renal lesion. Fat imaged by CT, with negative density of −20 to −80 Hounsfield units, is pathognomonic for AML in the renal lesion. In contrast, it is exceedingly unusual—almost uncommon enough to be described as a case report—to have fat content with negative Hounsfield units in a RCC. Lesions that contain only minimal amount of fat represent a diagnostic difficulty, and frequently patients with these lesions choose to undergo surgery because of diagnostic uncertainty. On magnetic resonance imaging (MRI), the fat component of AML has high signal intensity on unenhanced T1-weighted images and lower intensity on T2-weighted images, while it is generally isointense in comparison to retroperitoneal fat.

Management of AML depends on degree of symptoms, size, multiplicity, renal function, and ability of imaging modalities to establish a diagnosis with certainty. Indications for intervention include suspicion for malignancy, spontaneous hemorrhage causing significant symptoms and hemodynamic instability, pain, and risk of rupture. Preservation of renal function

remains of significant concern, especially in multicentric and bilateral lesions. In 1986, Oesterling et al. (2) proposed a threshold of 4 cm as cutoff for intervention. This threshold has been evaluated in subsequent studies and a review of literature suggested that although there is an increased risk of hemorrhage because of large tumor size, significant number of larger lesions remain asymptomatic. Therefore, in addition to size, other parameters such as comorbidity, renal reserve, pregnancy plans, activity level, and occupation should be considered at the time of treatment decision making.

Expectant management of asymptomatic AML should include annual or semiannual CT or ultrasound scanning to evaluate disease stability versus progression. Patients manifesting acute hemorrhage and hemodynamic instability are best managed by angiographic embolization. Patients with poor renal reserve and poor surgical candidates should be managed by angiographic embolization as well. Nephron-sparing approaches are the primary goal in management of patients with multiple lesions. Prophylactic intervention may be advocated for larger tumors, in women of childbearing age, and in patients with inadequate follow-up or access to medical care.

Oncocytoma

Renal oncocytomas constitute approximately 5% of all renal tumors, but may represent up to 20% of all solid renal masses under 4 cm in contemporary nephrectomy series (3). Oncocytomas are usually solitary and unilateral, although several cases of bilateral and multiple oncocytomas have been described. Oncocytomas affect men twice as often as women, and 50% of tumors are currently discovered incidentally (3).

The diagnosis of oncocytomas is predominately pathologic. There are no reliable clinical or imaging characteristics. No precise features appear on ultrasound, intravenous pyelogram, CT, or MRI to distinguish oncocytomas from a malignant lesion. Features such as stellate central scar on CT, "spoke wheel" appearance of feeding arteries on angiography, and "lucent rim sign" of the capsule suggest the diagnosis, but are not pathognomonic and cannot be reliably used in clinical decision making.

Renal biopsy and aspiration have limited diagnostic value. Limitations relate to difficulty distinguishing oncocytomas from the granular form of RCC (4), the well-known inaccuracy of renal needle biopsy with false-negative rate up to 25% to 30% (5), and the documented coexistence of RCC in the same lesion or other locations in the same kidney from 10% (3) to 32% (6).

Given these diagnostic uncertainties, most urologists advocate surgical treatment of these lesions. Nephron-sparing approach (if anatomically feasible) and laparoscopic techniques have been widely employed more recently.

Renal Cell Carcinoma

In the United States, an estimated 57,760 new cases of adenocarcinoma of the kidney are expected to be diagnosed, with 12,980 deaths occurring from this disease, in 2009 (7). RCC accounts for approximately 2.5% of adult cancers and constitutes 85% of primary malignant renal tumors. RCC is the second most prevalent and the most malignant urologic cancer, ultimately killing 35% of affected individuals. RCC is most commonly seen in patients in their 40s to 60s, and is twice as common in men as it is in women.

Etiology

The etiology of RCC is not well understood. To date, only tobacco use remains a significant risk factor for RCC, with most investigations demonstrating twofold increase in risk for development RCC (8). Other etiologic factors such as obesity and hypertension appear to increase risk for RCC in men (9). RCC also occurs in approximately 10% of patients with acquired cystic disease of the kidneys, a condition that develops in uremic patients on dialysis.

RCC can be sporadic and inherited. Two inherited patterns have been established. Von Hippel-Lindau disease a rare autosomal-dominant disorder with a mutation in the tumor suppressor gene located on chromosome 3, 3p25-26. Alteration of both copies of the *VHL* gene triggers up-regulation of the expression of vascular endothelial growth factor, the proangiogenic growth factor in RCC, contributing to the pronounced neovascularity of RCC.

Patients with the second hereditary form of RCC, hereditary papillary RCC (HPRCC) suffer from bilateral multifocal tumors of papillary histologic appearance. HPRCC has been mapped to chromosome 7 and it has been shown that up-regulation of proto-oncogene *MET* is a triggering event in HPRCC.

Among sporadic forms of RCC, clear cell RCC is most common and is associated with structural changes of chromosome 3.

Presentation

Renal tumors may remain asymptomatic until quite late in the disease because of the renal topography and expansile capacities of the retroperitoneum. Because of the advances and widespread use of CT and ultrasonographic imaging, approximately 50% to 60% of renal masses are diagnosed incidentally, with the majority of these still in the early stages of the disease. The classic triad of renal mass—palpable mass, flank pain, and gross hematuria—is exceedingly rare, and is often associated with an advanced disease.

Approximately 60% of symptomatic patients will present with gross or microhematuria. A variety of paraneoplastic syndromes related to the renal tumors subsequently earned the disease the name of *internist tumor*. The most common paraneoplastic syndromes are hypercalcemia (20% of patients), secondary to parathyroid hormone-related protein production or, less commonly, osteolytic metastatic involvement; hypertension (40% of patients), most likely secondary to renin hypersecretion; and erythrocytosis (3% of patients) due to overproduction of erythropoietin. Stauffer syndrome, a hepatic dysfunction that presents with elevated alkaline phosphatase and bilirubin, prolonged prothrombin time, and hypoalbuminemia in the absence of liver metastasis, is a fascinating paraneoplastic presentation of RCC. The presence of paraneoplastic syndromes at diagnosis does not appear to have a negative prognostic value, although failure of resolution of these abnormalities carries a negative prognostic significance (10).

Staging/Prognosis

Complete staging process should include a thorough history and physical examination, complete blood count, comprehensive metabolic panel, prothrombin time, and complete metastatic evaluation. The extent of the metastatic workup is dictated by the clinical picture and laboratory abnormalities. Basic metastatic workup of all cases should include chest radiograph, detailed review of the CT scan, and liver function test. CT scanning is important for further staging of the disease, evaluation of tumor location in relationship to renal hilum, renal vein and inferior vena cava involvement, extension into Gerota's fat, as well as evaluation of retroperitoneum, liver, and chest. Bone scan is reserved for patients with elevated alkaline phosphatase as well as patients with bone pain. Head CT is warranted for patients with clinical suggestion of brain involvement. MRI remains the best radiographic study to evaluate possible tumor thrombus extension into renal vein and vena cava seen in 10% to 15% of patients.

Renal biopsy, although not routinely recommended, is sometimes necessary. Biopsy of renal masses quite often returns as nondiagnostic. In cases with a history of other primary tumor (especially lung, breast, gastrointestinal tumor, or lymphoma) needle biopsy may be warranted.

The standard TNM staging system revised in 2002 is used for RCC evaluation. Criteria for staging are outlined in Table 54.1. The pathologic stage is the most important prognostic factor. Patients with organ-confined disease (stage I and II) demonstrate 5-year survival rates of 70% to 90% and a reduction of 15% to 20% in survival is associated with invasion of the perinephric fat. Involvement of vena cava, renal vein, adrenal vein, or regional lymph nodes (stage III) reduces overall survival into the range of 30% to 45%, but depends on the extent of the tumor thrombus. Stage IV disease (T4, N2, or metastatic disease) shows dismal prognosis with 5-year survival under 15%. Significant effort has been made to create various mathematical models to incorporate other factors such as grade, microscopic invasion, aneuploid DNA content, and performance status into prognostic algorithm to provide an individual patient with a more precise prognostic picture (11).

Treatment

Localized Disease

Radical nephrectomy, first described by Robson in 1963, remains the standard treatment for localized disease. The goal is to remove the tumor with a wide margin of unaffected tissue. Radical nephrectomy by definition includes en bloc removal of the

Table 54.1

Tumor, Nodes, and Metastases Clinical Classification (2002)

pT—Primary Tumor

pTx	Primary tumor cannot be assessed
pT0	No evidence of primary tumor
pT1a	<4.0 cm; limited to kidney
pT1b	4–7 cm; limited to kidney
pT2	>7.0 cm; limited to the kidney
pT3	Tumor extends into major veins or invades adrenal gland or perinephric tissues but not beyond Gerota fascia
pT3a	Tumor invades adrenal gland or perinephric tissues but not beyond Gerota fascia
pT3b	Tumor grossly extends into renal vein(s) or vena cava below diaphragm
pT3c	Tumor grossly extends into vena cava above diaphragm
pT4	Tumor invades beyond Gerota fascia

N—Regional Lymph Nodes

NX	Regional lymph nodes cannot be assessed
N0	No regional lymph node metastasis
N1	Metastasis in a single regional lymph node
N2	Metastasis in more than one regional lymph node

M—Distant Metastasis

Mx	Distant metastasis cannot be assessed
M0	No distant metastasis
M1	Distant metastasis

(From *Comprehensive Textbook of Genitourinary Oncology* Vogelzang et al., 3rd ed LWW 2006, with permission.)

kidney, Gerota's fascia, including the ipsilateral adrenal, proximal ureter, and retroperitoneal regional lymph nodes. However, resection of the ipsilateral adrenal gland as well as an extensive lymphadenectomy has been actively debated in the recent literature.

Various approaches to nephrectomy provide access to the kidney and renal vasculature. Radical nephrectomy can be performed via anterior subcostal, flank, and thoracoabdominal incision. The authors have advocated a thoracoabdominal incision for large and upper pole renal tumors because of its excellent exposure to the upper pole, adrenal gland, and the great vessels. This incision also allows wide exploration of the abdomen and resection of pulmonary or hepatic lesions in the same procedure. Exposure to the great vessels is also facilitated with this approach for an appropriate retroperitoneal lymphadenectomy.

After decades of evaluation, the role of lymphadenectomy in the management of RCC remains controversial. Initial observations demonstrated that between 18% and 33% of patients undergoing radical nephrectomy have metastatic involvement at the time of surgery (12). Contemporary series suggest that the true incidence of isolated lymph node metastases in clinically localized disease is less, and the location of such metas-

tases is unpredictable. Although several institutional series have suggested a therapeutic benefit for extended lymphadenectomy, there remains a lack of randomized data to support its routine use. Despite this, there remains a role for lymphadenectomy in individuals with high risk of lymph node metastasis or known lymphadenopathy for whom few other options exist for aggressive, potentially curative therapy (13).

RCC has a predisposition for the development of venous thrombi extending into the renal vein, inferior vena cava, hepatic vein, and occasionally the right atrium. Surgical approach to the thrombi depends on the extent and level of the tumor involvement. In general, tumor thrombus does not invade the wall of the vessel and can be removed without vascular resection. Cardiopulmonary bypass is typically required for the removal of a thrombus at the level of the atrium.

Adrenalectomy was a mandatory part of the treatment for the RCC as was described by Robson in 1963. However, in the past decade with an increase in the diagnosis of the early-stage small renal tumors, and advancement in imaging technology in which adrenal involvement can be better evaluated, the necessity of ipsilateral adrenalectomy has been repeatedly questioned. The incidence of ipsilateral adrenal involvement has been quoted as 1.2% to 10% and numbers significantly dropping to as low as 0.6% to 1% as the size of kidney tumor decreases. A recent retrospective review of 511 patients who underwent radical nephrectomy (with ipsilateral adrenalectomy) suggests that adrenalectomy can be omitted in treatment of small T1 tumors with no radiologic evidence of adrenal involvement and in lower pole tumors (14).

Laparoscopic nephrectomy, first performed by Clayman et al. (15) in 1990, has gained widespread acceptance as a form of treatment for T1 and some T2 (7 to 13 cm) tumors. A number of studies have demonstrated oncologic effectiveness of laparoscopic nephrectomy, which appears to be equivalent to the open radical nephrectomy (16).

In the early 1980s a nephron-sparing approach was initially advocated and limited to cases with a unilateral kidney, bilateral tumors, and patients with declining renal function. Long-term survival data have shown comparable results to radical nephrectomy. Subsequently, the use of nephron-sparing nephrectomy extended to cases with a normal opposite kidney. Extended survival among patients with lesions under 4 cm remained in the range >90% (17). Local recurrence of tumor in the same kidney ranges from 0% to 10% and is as low as 0% to 3% in tumors under 4 cm (18,19). With advancement of laparoscopic and robotic technology technique and equipment, laparoscopic and robot-assisted robot nephron-sparing approaches have gradually become an accepted treatment modality for small and peripherally located tumors. Oncologic outcomes of laparoscopic nephron-sparing nephrectomy mirror those of open series in the short follow-up studies published to date (2,20).

Additional therapeutic approaches are being explored for the treatment of small lesions in older individuals with multiple comorbidities. Cryoablation with liquid nitrogen or argon gas can be performed percutaneously, laparoscopically, or via an open approach. Radiofrequency ablation has also been used in a small group of patients with RCC. Both approaches are safe and have minimal morbidity (21). As follow-up is approaching 5 years, the oncologic effectiveness of these methods is being analyzed and evaluated. Observation can also be used in smaller lesions in individuals with severe comorbidities.

Surveillance for recurrent malignancy is tailored to the initial stage of the disease. For T1 lesions, annual history, physical examination, and selective blood tests are indicated with no need for additional imaging. For patients with T2 node-negative disease, an annual chest radiograph and a biannual CT scan of the abdomen and pelvis is indicated. Radiologic surveillance intensifies in patients who have undergone partial nephrectomy because of potential risk of a local recurrence.

Disseminated Disease

Approximately one third of the patients with RCC will present with advanced or metastatic disease. Initially, nephrectomy was used only as a palliative procedure. Utility of the surgical treatment for advanced disease has subsequently been evaluated in two randomized clinical trials performed by the Southwest Oncology Group and in a European study. Collectively, these studies demonstrate a significant increase in survival in patients undergoing nephrectomy followed by adjuvant therapy (22). These results have created a shift in the treatment approach to metastatic RCC in patients with good performance status. Patients presenting with solitary metastatic site that is amendable to surgical resection can be candidates for combined nephrectomy and metastatic lesion resection.

BLADDER CANCER

Bladder cancer represents the second most common genitourinary tumor, and is the fourth most prevalent noncutaneous malignancy in the United States. There are over 70,980 new cases diagnosed each year and over 14,330 bladder cancer related deaths (7). Bladder cancer affects men 3 times as often as women, and is more common in whites than in African Americans.

Epidemiologic data linking cigarette smoking to bladder cancer dates back to the 1950s (23). Cigarette smoking increases the risk of bladder cancer by two- to threefold. Occupational exposure to benzidine, beta-naphthylamine, and 4-aminobiphenyl places workers in chemical, dye, leather, petroleum, and rubber industries at increased risk for bladder cancer. Prior treatment with cyclophosphamide, as well as exposure to pelvic radiation for pelvic malignancies, also increases the risk of bladder cancer. On the contrary, increased total fluid intake appears to decrease the risk of bladder cancer by diluting the carcinogens in urine and by decreasing duration of contact with urothelium (24).

Approximately 90% of patients in the United States with bladder cancer have transitional cell carcinoma (TCC). Squamous carcinoma accounts for <10% of bladder cancers and is associated with chronic irritation and infection, bladder calculi, and chronic indwelling catheters. In Egypt and parts of Africa, where squamous cell carcinoma of the bladder is the predominant cell type, infection with *Schistosoma haematobium* is the principal causative agent. Adenocarcinoma of the bladder accounts for <2% of the bladder cancer cases.

Bladder cancer development is a complex multistep process involving steps in activation of oncogenes and loss of tumor suppression genes. It has been suggested that loss of heterozygosity of chromosome 9 may be an early step in initiation and progression; deletions or alterations of the *p53* gene on chromosome 17 are present in 30% to 40% of muscle-invasive bladder cancers and are thought to be related to a more invasive phenotype. Other genes and proteins controlling cell cycle, regulating angiogenesis, and growth factors all play important role in bladder cancer tumorigenesis (25,26).

Presentation and Diagnosis

The diagnosis of superficial bladder cancer can be elusive because the symptoms mimic those of other common urologic conditions. Approximately three fourths of patients with bladder cancer present with painless, intermittent hematuria. It is estimated that approximately 20% of patients evaluated for gross hematuria will be diagnosed with bladder cancer. Similarly, of patients presenting with microscopic hematuria, up to 10% will be diagnosed with bladder cancer. The most recent Best Policy Panel of the American Urological Association has accounted for this in their recommended workup of asymptomatic microscopic hematuria (27). Furthermore, the panel recommended that for all patients without risk factors for primary renal disease, a urologic evaluation including radiographic imaging of the upper urinary tract followed by cystoscopy should be performed. Although urine cytology is best used for the follow-up of patients with known bladder cancer, it is our belief that bladder washings should be evaluated at the time of cystoscopy. Irritative voiding symptoms are also a common mode of presentation, particularly in patients with diffuse carcinoma in situ (CIS) or invasive bladder tumors. Bone pain from metastatic disease, flank pain from ureteral obstruction, or retroperitoneal metastasis can be presenting symptoms in patients with advanced disease.

The upper urinary tracts are evaluated with intravenous pyelogram, CT, MRI, or ultrasound. The presence of a bladder mass may be suggested by imaging, but cystoscopy remains the "gold standard" in diagnosis and evaluation of bladder lesions. To complete the evaluation of a bladder mass, transurethral resection of the bladder tumor (TURBT) is performed. The goals of TURBT are to provide tissue samples for pathologic staging and to perform a complete resection that may be therapeutic with superficial lesions. The treatment approach to bladder tumors that invade the muscularis propria or beyond differs dramatically from the treatment of bladder tumors that remain superficial or superficially invasive into the lamina propria. Therefore, it is important for the resection specimen to include muscularis propria.

Staging and Grading

As early as 1947, Jewett observed an increase in local and distant metastasis as the depth of the primary bladder tumor increased. Later, Jewett (28) noted the correlation of the depth of invasion to the 5-year survival. These observations served as the basis for the initial Jewett staging system. Currently, bladder tumors are staged based on the American Joint Committee on Cancer TNM staging system (Table 54.2). Pure noninvasive superficial papillary lesions (Ta) have no involvement of the lamina propria and demonstrate a neovascular core with 8 to 20 layers. T1 lesions invade the lamina propria. Tumors invading the muscularis propria are designated as T2. T3 tumors extend beyond bladder muscle and into perivesical fat. T4 tumors invade adjacent organs or the stroma of the prostate. CIS is a flat, high-grade, epithelial lesion

Table 54.2		
TNM Staging Systems for Bladder Carcinoma		
Primary tumor (T)	Tx	Primary cannot be assessed
	T0	No evidence of primary tumor
	Ta	Noninvasive papillary tumor
	Tis	Carcinoma *in situ*
	T1	Tumor invades subepithelial connective tissue
	T2	Tumor invades muscle
	PT2a	Tumor invades superficial muscle (inner half)
	PT2b	Tumor invades deep muscle (outer half)
	T3	Tumor invades perivesical tissue
	PT3a	Tumor invades perivesical tissue microscopically
	PT3b	Tumor invades perivesical tissue macroscopically (extravesical mass)
	T4	Tumor invades any of the following: prostate, uterus, vagina, pelvic wall, abdominal wall
	T4a	Tumor invades prostate, uterus, vagina
	T4b	Tumor invades pelvic wall, abdominal wall
Regional lymph node (N)	NX	Regional lymph nodes cannot be assessed
	N0	No regional lymph node metastases
	N1	Metastasis in a single lymph node, 2 cm or less in greatest dimension
	N2	Metastasis in a single lymph node, more than 2 cm but not more than 5 cm in greatest dimension; or multiple lymph nodes, none more than 5 cm in greatest dimension
	N3	Metastasis in a lymph node, more than 5 cm in greatest dimension
Distant metastasis (M)	MX	Distant metastasis cannot be assessed
	M0	No distant metastases
	M1	Distant metastasis

(From *Comprehensive Textbook of Genitourinary Oncology* Vogelzang et al. 3rd ed LWW 2006, with permission.)

with anaplastic features and lack of cellular polarity. Although CIS is by definition noninvasive, it generally exhibits a more aggressive behavior. Bladder carcinomas are also stratified on the basis of grade. Tumor grade is an important prognostic factor for tumor recurrence and progression. Traditionally, urothelial tumors have been classified as grades 1, 2, and 3. A new classification system using only low- and high-grade classification has been recently proposed. Currently, both systems are employed and no consistent conversion scale exists. Nonetheless, higher-grade urothelial neoplasm correlates with higher rates of recurrence and progression.

Superficial Transitional Cell Carcinoma (Ta, Tis, T1)

Approximately 80% of bladder cancers are so-called superficial at diagnosis. The natural history of superficial bladder cancer is difficult to predict because of its heterogeneity. Two features that characterize superficial bladder cancer are recurrence and progression. The risks for recurrence and progression are related to histologic grade, depth of invasion, multiplicity, tumor size, tumor morphology, presence of vascular or lymphatic invasion, and presence of CIS. Nearly 60% to 90% of patients with superficial disease will have a tumor recurrence if treated by transurethral resection (TUR) alone (29).

The primary goals of treating patients with superficial disease include eradicating existing disease, preventing tumor recurrence, and progression or metastases. TUR is the preferred initial treatment of superficial disease. This allows for histopathologic assessment of the lesion. Furthermore, there may also be a therapeutic benefit of an appropriate TURBT. Treatment with TUR of superficial bladder cancer can be followed by intravesical chemotherapy or immunotherapy in those with high-risk tumors for recurrence and progression. Patients with low-grade, noninvasive small tumors (<3 cm) and solitary tumors are at low risk of progression and may be treated by TUR alone.

Most T1 bladder cancers are high-grade lesions with a propensity for recurrence, progression, and possibly death. Caution should be employed in the treatment of these lesions, as they are frequently understaged or misclassified (30). In cases that lack muscle in the initial resected TUR specimen, up to half of these lesions are subsequently associated with either residual tumor burden or muscle-invasive disease at the time of repeat resection (31,32). One third of T1 patients show eventual progression to muscle-invasive disease. The presence of concomitant CIS confers a worse prognosis, with up to 80% progressing to muscle-invasive disease (33). It is our belief that high-grade T1 disease, particularly those tumors associated with CIS and/or showing lymphovascular invasion, represents a potentially lethal disease that warrants consideration for early radical cystectomy.

Intravesical Therapy

High rates of recurrence of superficial urothelial cancer have led to the application of intravesical chemotherapeutic or immunotherapeutic agents. Intravesical therapy can be used as a prophylactic modality to prevent or delay recurrence and progression or as a therapeutic modality to cure residual disease in the cases of incomplete TUR. In the United States the attenuated strain of the *Mycobacterium bovis*, known as Bacillus Calmette-Guérin (BCG), is most commonly used for intravesical immunotherapy. Chemotherapeutic agents such as thiotepa, mitomycin C, and doxorubicin are also used for intravesical therapy, but appear less effective in preventing recurrence than BCG and do not impact progression. The exact mechanism of BCG is unknown, but appears to be immunologically mediated. BCG has been shown to be effective both therapeutically and prophylactically. It is efficacious against CIS, with complete response rates in the 36% to 70% range. Recurrence rates are reduced by approximately half after BCG treatment compared with TUR alone. The most commonly used BCG regimen is 6 weekly administrations of BCG followed by 6 weeks of no treatment. At 12 weeks, if cancer is not identified on follow-up cystoscopy, BCG may be also administered in maintenance fashion weekly for 3 weeks at 3 months, 6 months, and every 6 months for up to 3 years (34). The only studies to suggest a benefit with BCG and tumor progression are those that have used maintenance therapy.

Unfortunately, side effects such as urgency, frequency, and hematuria are often significant and <20% of patients will tolerate full-course maintenance therapy. Reduced concentrations of BCG with the addition of alpha-interferon have been reported to reduce side effects with similar efficacy with intermediate follow-up.

Follow-up

Because a large proportion of patients with superficial TCC of the bladder have recurrence, close and careful follow-up is important in order to diagnose and treat recurrences early, and to prevent and/or treat the sequela of tumor progression. Historically, follow-up is performed in 3-month intervals using cystoscopy and urinary cytology. Upper tracts are evaluated on an annual basis initially, and at less frequent intervals if patient remains recurrence-free for >2 years. Presence of recurrence at the first 3-month cystoscopy examination is ominous and requires a careful re-evaluation regarding grade and degree of invasion, as well as consideration for more aggressive therapy.

The clinician must carefully weigh the risks of tumor recurrence and progression against the toxicity of treating the patient with local and conservative therapies. Moreover, the clinician must astutely know when to abandon these therapies and proceed to a more aggressive line of treatment that may improve survival. Indications for radical cystectomy include progression to muscle-invasive disease, failed intravesical therapy for high-grade disease, poor tolerance of intravesical therapy, persistent high-grade tumor, endoscopically uncontrollable tumor, and involvement of prostatic ducts or stromal invasion.

Because of the excellent clinical outcomes and avoidance of potential understaging, progression, and metastatic spread of the disease, radical cystectomy should be considered for high–risk patients. Surgery achieves a high cure rate for superficial TCC with 5-year recurrence-free survival rates of >75% for patients with clinical stage T1 tumors undergoing cystectomy (35). In addition, improvements in urinary diversion and nerve-sparing technique have significantly decreased the social implications of

cystectomy and have provided an excellent treatment option for high-risk patients.

Invasive Transitional Cell Carcinoma

Muscle-invasive TCC of the bladder refers to the tumors involving the muscularis propria. Twenty percent to 25% of patients with newly diagnosed bladder cancer present with muscle invasion. Fewer than 15% of these patients survive 2 years if left untreated. Prior to the definitive treatment of high-grade invasive TCC of the bladder, a comprehensive evaluation is performed to identify those with metastatic disease. The most frequent site of metastasis is to the pelvic or regional lymph nodes. Complete metastatic workup involves CT of the abdomen and pelvis, chest radiograph and bone scan for the patients with bony pain, or elevated alkaline phosphatase. Although CT scan is accurate in evaluation of distant metastasis, it is quite unreliable in detecting pelvic lymphadenopathy, seen in 25% of patients at cystectomy (35). Radical cystectomy and lymph node dissection remains the optimal way to pathologically stage and define the primary bladder tumor and regional lymph nodes, which provide risk assessment in those with invasive bladder cancer.

Radical Cystectomy

Radical cystectomy is the gold standard for invasive bladder cancer as it provides the best survival results and the lowest local recurrence rates (35). Radical cystectomy should include a bilateral pelvic iliac lymph node dissection. Radical cystectomy in male patients includes the removal of the prostate and seminal vesicles. Reasons for removal of the prostate are high incidence of direct extension of TCC into the prostatic urethra or stroma and presence of concomitant prostatic adenocarcinoma. Radical cystectomy in women includes removal of the cervix, uterus, fallopian tubes, and ovaries, with preservation of the anterior vaginal wall in the majority of women.

Radical cystectomy provides accurate pathologic staging of the primary bladder tumor and the regional lymph nodes that may then influence decision for the adjuvant chemotherapy based on pathologic criteria. Approximately 20% to 35% of patients with negative findings on preoperative workup will have involvement of regional lymph nodes, an incidence that reflects our inability to accurately stage bladder cancer using imaging modality. Pathologic staging allows for better assessment of patients' prognosis and planning of adjuvant therapy. To date, chemotherapy alone or coupled with bladder-sparing surgery has yet to demonstrate equivalent recurrence and long-term survival rates compared with radical cystectomy.

Improvements in medical, surgical, and anesthetic technique have dramatically reduced morbidity and mortality associated with radical cystectomy. Prior to the 1970s, mortality rate of radical cystectomy was nearly 20%, which has diminished to 2% in contemporary cystectomy series (36). Although early postoperative complications are fairly common (25% to 30%), the majority are easily identified and treated.

Lymphadenectomy is an integral part of the surgical treatment of bladder cancer. Data demonstrate that the completeness of lymph node dissection relates to long-term disease-free survival. Recent studies have indicated that the actual number of nodes removed in node-positive and node-negative patients plays a predictive role in patient survival. In the review of 244 patients with node-positive disease, patients with ≤15 lymph nodes removed had 25% 10-year recurrence-free survival compared with 36% survival rate in patients in whom ≥15 lymph nodes were removed. The total number of positive lymph nodes (lymph node burden) has a prognostic value as well. In the same study, recurrence-free survival was significantly higher in patients with fewer than eight positive lymph nodes (40% vs. 10%). The concept of lymph node density (number of positive lymph nodes/number of lymph nodes removed) introduced by our institution also has prognostic value. Patients with lymph node density of <20% had a significantly higher survival than those with lymph node density >20% (43% vs. 17%) (37).

Urinary diversion following cystectomy involves reconnecting ureters to an intestinal segment. There are essentially three methods for urinary diversion: ileal conduit, continent cutaneous, and orthotopic bladder reconstruction. The type of diversion selected depends on multiple factors, including patient's renal function, dexterity, tumor presence at the urethral margin, and history of prior radiation to the pelvic floor. The development of orthotopic urinary tract reconstruction has helped decrease the social implications of cystectomy and improve the quality of life of the patients after removal of the bladder. Orthotopic diversion allows patients a more normal voiding, good continence, and eliminates the need for urostomy appliance or intermittent catheterization (38).

Conclusion

Urothelial cancer of the bladder represents a wide spectrum of disease defined by various recurrence and progression rates. Diagnosis and treatment modalities of bladder cancer continue to evolve. Early diagnosis, close follow-up, and timely treatment will improve overall survival.

Radical cystectomy with an appropriate lymphadenectomy provides the best survival rates with lowest local recurrence for invasive bladder cancer. It also allows precise staging and prognostic information. It allows identifying patients who should be considered for adjuvant systemic chemotherapy. Technical advances in orthotopic reconstruction now provide patients reasonable alternative to native bladder.

PROSTATE CANCER

Prostate cancer is the most commonly diagnosed noncutaneous cancer and the second leading cause of cancer deaths in American men. An estimated 192,280 new cases of prostate cancer were diagnosed in 2009. Prostate cancer accounts for 27,350 deaths annually (7). The lifetime risk for a male to be diagnosed with prostate cancer is 1 in 6.

Several risk factors for the development of prostate cancer have been identified. Increasing age, African American race (with incidence of 1.6-fold and mortality rate of 2.6 times that of whites), and positive family history (with twofold increase in risk with a first-degree relative).

Various dietary and nutritional factors have been evaluated regarding their impact on development of prostate cancer. There are data suggesting a protective effect of low-fat/high-fiber diet, lycopene, selenium, vitamin E, and soy-derived products (39).

Clinical data available to date are insufficient to warrant formal recommendations to patients.

The potential preventive effects of finasteride (5-alpha-reductase inhibitor) on the development of prostate cancer have been evaluated by the Prostate Cancer Prevention trial that enrolled >18,000 men. It suggested a 24% reduction in the prevalence of prostate cancer in the finasteride group over a 7-year period. It must be noted, however, that tumors of higher Gleason score were observed in the finasteride group (40).

Pathology

Over 95% of prostate cancers are adenocarcinomas. The remaining 5% are affected predominantly by TCC and, rarely, neuroendocrine carcinomas or sarcomas. Sixty to seventy percent of prostate cancers originate from the peripheral zone, while 10% to 20% arise from the transitional and only 10% from the central zone. Prostate cancer is multifocal within the gland.

In the United States, prostatic adenocarcinoma is evaluated using the grading system proposed by Gleason in the 1970s. Five distinct grades are recognized, ranging from 1 to 5 (from well differentiated to poorly differentiated). Because prostate cancer is usually heterogeneous and more than one grade may be present in one specimen, a pathologist assigns a primary grade to the most prevalent grade in the specimen and a secondary grade to the second most prevalent grade in the specimen. As Gleason grades range from 1 to 5, the total sum ranges from 2 (1 + 1) to 10 (5 + 5). Behavior of Gleason 3 + 4 tumors differs from 4 + 3 tumors, suggesting that grade of the predominant tumor has important prognostic significance (41). The presence of tertiary Gleason 5 in the biopsy or prostatectomy specimen, even in focal amounts, is a powerful predictor of biochemical relapse (42).

The clinical staging of prostate cancer is based on the recently revised TNM staging system that uses clinical assessment of prostate-specific antigen (PSA) and digital rectal examination (DRE) to assign clinical stages T1 through 4 (Table 54.3).

The pattern of disease progression is well characterized. Local extension through the prostate capsule is generally followed by invasion of the seminal vesicles. Locoregional lymph node metastasis commonly affects the obturator lymph nodes chain, and local pelvic lymph nodes. The axial skeleton is the most common site of distant metastasis, with the lumbar spine most frequently affected. Metastatic bone lesions are usually osteoblastic. Lung, liver, and adrenal are typical sites of widely metastatic prostate cancer.

Screening

Prostate screening is controversial and an actively debated topic in medicine (3). Serum PSA has been used for screening of prostate cancer along with a DRE. A cutoff of 4 ng/mL has been traditional; however, approximately 25% of men diagnosed with prostate cancer have a PSA level of <4 ng/mL, and 27% of men with PSA values of 3.1 to 4.0 ng/mL are found to have prostate cancer (4).

Diagnosis and Evaluation

The initial diagnosis of prostate cancer is made by prostate biopsy, typically prompted by an abnormal DRE and/or elevated

Table 54.3

The 2002 American Joint Committee on Cancer/International Union Against Cancer Prostate Cancer TNM Staging Classification

Stage	Definition
Clinical (T)	
TX	Primary tumor cannot be assessed
T0	No evidence of primary tumor
T1	Clinically inapparent tumor not palpable or visible by imaging
T1a	Tumor incidental histologic finding in ≤5% of tissue resected
T1b	Tumor incidental pathologic finding in >5% of tissue resected
T1c	Tumor identified by needle biopsy (elevated PSA level)
T2	Tumor confined within the prostate[a]
T2a	Tumor involves half of one lobe or less
T2b	Tumor involves more than half of one lobe but not both
T2c	Tumor involves both lobes
T3	Tumor extends through prostate capsule[b]
T3a	Extracapsular invasion (unilateral or bilateral)
T3b	Tumor invades seminal vesicle(s)
T4	Tumor is fixed or invades adjacent structures other than the seminal vesicle(s): bladder neck, external sphincter, rectum, levator muscles, pelvic wall, or all the above
Pathologic (pT)	
pT2[c]	Organ confined
pT2a	Unilateral, involving half of one lobe or less
pT2b	Unilateral, involving more than half of one lobe but not both lobes
PT2c	Bilateral
pT3	Extraprostatic extension
pT3a	Extraprostatic extension
pT3b	Seminal vesicle invasion
pT4	Invasion of bladder, rectum
Regional lymph node (N)	
NX	Regional lymph nodes cannot be assessed
N0	No regional node metastasis
N1	Metastasis in regional lymph node or nodes
Distant metastasis[d] (M)	
MX	Distant metastasis cannot be assessed
M0	No distant metastasis
M1	Distant metastasis
M1a	Nonregional lymph nodes
M1b	Bone(s)
M1c	Other site(s)

PSA, prostate-specific antigen.

[a] Tumor found in one or both lobes by needle biopsy, but not palpable or reliably visible by imaging, is classified T1c.

[b] Invasion into the prostatic apex or into (but not beyond) the prostatic capsule is classified as T2, not T3.

[c] There is no pathologic T1 classification.

[d] When more than one site of metastasis is present, the most advanced category is used; pM1c is most advanced.

Used with the permission of the American Joint Committee on Cancer (AJCC), Chicago, Illinois. The original source for this material is the *AJCC Cancer Staging Manual*, 6th ed. New York: Springer-Verlag; 2002; www.springeronline.com

PSA level. Prostate biopsy is well-tolerated routine office procedure performed with use of local anesthetic. Typically, an 8- to 12-biopsy scheme is used to systematically evaluate the prostate gland. In addition to a diagnostic tool, the prostate biopsy is a predictor of clinical outcome. D'Amico et al. (43) in their study of a cohort of 960 patients showed that biochemical control rate was significantly higher (87% vs. 11%) in patients with 1 or 2 positive cores versus 4 to 6 positive cores, respectively. Correlation between the number of positive prostate biopsy cores to extracapsular invasion and margin positivity has also been demonstrated (44).

Bone scan is a widely used modality to evaluate the presence and extent of metastatic bony spread of prostate cancer. It should be implemented in patients with PSA >10 ng/mL or Gleason ≥8. CT of the pelvis has a limited diagnostic value and is generally not recommended in patients with low-grade, clinically localized prostate cancer, with a PSA <20 ng/mL. MRI has not been used widely in the past. Data supporting the superior quality of an endorectal coil MRI for evaluation of extracapsular disease in patients with clinically localized prostate cancer has been suggested but remains controversial (45).

Pretreatment Risk Stratification

Prior to treatment, the assessment of the potential for cure with a given type of treatment, estimated disease-free survival, and possibility of locally advanced disease at the time of initiation of therapy, need to be evaluated and discussed with the patient. The risk of recurrence after radical prostatectomy increases with the stage of disease. A 5-year disease-free survival exceeds 85% in T1c disease, which decreases to 70% to 80% in patients with palpable cT2 disease (46). Serum PSA level generally correlates with tumor volume and also with postoperative and posttreatment outcomes.

As the number of patients with T1c prostate cancer increases, the need for counseling and decision-making tools to assists clinicians and patients predicting posttreatment outcomes became necessary. In the early 1990s, Partin et al. (47,48) used regression analysis, and combined PSA, DRE, and Gleason score as predictors of final pathologic stage. Using the Partin tables, one can use pretreatment PSA, Gleason score, and DRE to predict postprostatectomy outcomes such as probability of having organ-confined disease on the pathologic specimen, as well as possibility of positive lymph nodes, seminal vesicles involvement, or presence of extraprostatic disease.

A continuous nomogram model of prediction was created by Kattan and colleagues (49). The initial Kattan nomogram was designed to predict probability of remaining free of biochemical recurrence at 5 years after radical prostatectomy based on PSA, clinical stage, and biopsy Gleason sum. Recently, this predictive value of nomogram was extended to 10 years (50). These models can be used by clinicians and patients, and are available as a Web-based calculation (www.nomograms.org).

Another stratification system was developed to simplify pretreatment risk stratification. This three-group system categorizes patients into low-risk (T1c or T2a and Gleason sum 2 to 6, and PSA <10 ng/mL), intermediate risk (T2b or Gleason sum 7 or PSA >10 and <20 ng/mL), and high-risk (T2c or Gleason >8, or PSA >20 ng/mL) groups (51).

Surgical Treatment and Outcomes of Localized Prostate Cancer

Patients diagnosed with low-risk, localized prostate cancer face several treatment options including watchful waiting or active surveillance, radical prostatectomy, and various forms of radiation therapy. Prior to selecting treatment, the patient must be informed and has to decide whether active treatment designed to eradicate cancer is desirable or one of the observation protocols are preferred.

Observation or "watchful waiting," also called *active surveillance*, is a pathway by which treatment is deferred until PSA rises substantially or symptoms occur. Choosing observation may reduce overtreatment of clinically insignificant disease, and avoid or postpone treatment-related side effects. On the other hand, while under observation, tumor may progress beyond a curable stage, and may require more aggressive or additional treatment with potentially greater side effects. Observation is generally contraindicated in high-grade tumors and in those patients with an expected survival of >10 years.

External beam radiation therapy (EBRT) techniques have been refined over the last decade. Development of three-dimensional conformal radiation reportedly allows treatment to be delivered more precisely to the tumor and reduces the bladder, rectal, and erectile side effects. For patients with low-risk prostate cancer receiving treatment with EBRT, 5-year PSA-progression-free outcome is reported to be 70% to 85% (52). Radiation therapy may be preferred in patients with significant comorbidities. Disadvantages of EBRT include significant risk of delayed impotence, lack of knowledge of true pathologic stage, and irritable bowel and bladder symptoms. EBRT is contraindicated in patients with previous pelvic irradiation, active inflammatory disease of the rectum, low bladder capacity, and chronic diarrhea.

Brachytherapy approaches for prostate cancer uses radioisotope-loaded seeds placed in the prostate. Cancer control rates for low risk are comparable to those from EBRT and achieve 87% at 10 years (53). Advantages of brachytherapy include plausibility for patients with significant comorbidities. Disadvantages are similar to those of EBRT. Brachytherapy is contraindicated in patients with previous pelvic irradiation, history of TUR of prostate, large-volume gland, significant voiding symptoms, chronic diarrhea, and inflammatory bowel disease.

Radical prostatectomy is an excellent treatment option for localized prostate cancer that provides effective long-term cancer control, and allows precise staging of the disease, including lymph node status. It also has been demonstrated to be superior to watchful waiting in a randomized control study from the Scandinavian Prostate Cancer Study Group in which radical prostatectomy reduced disease-specific mortality, overall mortality, and the risks of metastasis and local progression. The absolute reduction in the risk of death after 10 years was small, but the reductions in the risks of metastasis and local tumor progression were substantial (54).

Excellent cancer control of localized disease after radical prostatectomy has been demonstrated in many series. The 10-year cancer-specific survival has shown to be between 90% and 97% in large institutional series, and progression-free rates of 70% to 80% at 5 years and 60% to 70% at 10 years are achieved

(55–57). It is clear that an active treatment aimed at cure of localized prostate cancer provides better outcome than observation alone for patients with life expectancy >10 years. Superiority of one type of treatment over another has not been evaluated in a randomized fashion to date.

Surgical Management of Locally Advanced Prostate Cancer

Prostate cancer is considered locally advanced once the cancer is identified beyond the prostatic capsule (T3a), invades the seminal vesicles (T3b), or invades adjacent organs such as bladder or rectum (T4). The management of T3 disease has been debated and has remained controversial through the years. Historically, surgical management of T3 prostate cancer has not been considered a treatment of choice by some. Nonetheless, a growing retrospective body of evidence was supporting improved disease-free survival in patients with T3 disease that received a multimodality form of therapy that includes surgical resection. At our institution, we advocate surgical treatment of T3 prostate cancer followed by radiation therapy to the prostatic bed to improve disease-specific survival and reduce local recurrence (58,59). Recently, the first randomized trial comparing radical prostatectomy with radical prostatectomy with postoperative radiation supported previous findings from multiple retrospective observational studies and demonstrated biochemical progression-free survival of 74% in postoperative radiation therapy group versus 52% in radical prostatectomy-alone group at 5 years (60).

We believe, based on data available, that the surgical treatment allows improved staging and excellent control of local disease. A multimodal therapy including adjuvant radiation and perioperative hormonal or chemotherapy improves overall survival and impedes biochemical progression of locally advanced prostate cancer.

Radical Prostatectomy

The retropubic approach to radical prostatectomy was pioneered by Millin in 1947. Over time, this technique was modified but did not gain widespread use because of the significant complications of bleeding, incontinence, and impotence. Subsequently, a series of anatomic discoveries has improved the surgeon's ability to remove the prostate and substantially reduce perioperative morbidity (46). Delineation of the anatomy of the dorsal vein complex improved hemostasis and allowed precise anatomic dissection in a relatively bloodless field. With an understanding of the anatomy of the pelvic plexus and its branches to the corpora cavernosa, modifications in the surgical technique also made it possible to preserve sexual function. Improvements in the understanding of periprostatic anatomy have permitted wider margins of excision for improved cancer control (46). The three goals of the urologic surgeon, in order of importance, are cancer control, preservation of urinary control, and preservation of sexual function. Although 3- and 5-year oncologic outcomes appear to be similar. Longer follow-up and perhaps randomized control studies will be necessary to truly justify superiority of one approach over another (61).

Early Complications

Through improved understanding of periprostatic anatomy, increased surgeons skills, and improved intraoperative and perioperative care, mortality from radical prostatectomy is exceedingly rare (<0.3%). Other complications of major pelvic surgery not specific to radical prostatectomy include myocardial infarction (0.1% to 0.4%), pulmonary embolism (0.75%), and deep venous thrombosis (1.1%). Intraoperative hemorrhage requiring blood transfusion is seen in <5%. Rectal injury is exceedingly rare (<0.5%) although somewhat more common in laparoscopic approach, and is generally repaired primarily. A diverting colostomy is required in irradiated bowel only. Injury to obturator nerve (<0.5%) and ureteral injury (<0.5%) should be identified and repaired intraoperatively. The majority of patients experience an uneventful postoperative course, resume ambulation and bowel function during the first day after surgery, and are routinely discharged within 48 hours after surgery with urinary catheter in place for 1 or 2 weeks.

Late complications such as anastomotic stricture, incisional hernia, lymphocele, pelvic abscess, and ileus are seen in <1%.

Urinary Function

Immediately after radical prostatectomy and following catheter removal (7–14 days postoperatively), approximately 80% of patients will have some degree of incontinence. At 24 months after surgery, 93% to 97% of patients achieve complete urinary continence (62,63). Higher rates of incontinence correlated with advanced age in the majority of reports. Treatment options for postprostatectomy incontinence include bulking agent injections at the urinary sphincter for minimal incontinence, male urinary sling procedure for mild-to-moderate symptoms, and artificial urinary sphincter for severe incontinence.

Erectile Function

Until the development of nerve-sparing prostatectomy, men undergoing radical prostatectomy were expected to become impotent. With the nerve-sparing technique modification, erectile function can be preserved in ≥70% of appropriately selected patients (64). There are emerging data suggesting the improvement of erectile function after radical prostatectomy with the early use of erectogenic medications (65).

Conclusion

In conclusion, prostate cancer is a remarkably prevalent tumor that affects nearly a quarter of a million patients and their families every year. In some patients it remains stable and responds well to curative treatment; in others, it behaves aggressively and is resistant to many forms of treatment. Major advances have been made to identify and stratify patients according to their disease characteristics and tailor their therapy appropriately. Men with localized prostate cancer and life expectancy of ≥10 years should be considered for definitive treatment. Long-term experience with radical prostatectomy has shown this to be an excellent choice for cure of localized disease. Men with locoregional disease or disease with high-risk features require aggressive, multimodal therapy to obtain local as well as systemic control of the disease progression. Radical prostatectomy as a mainstay of treatment for localized and locoregional disease has been demonstrated to be a surgery with low morbidity and mortality. Recovery of continence and potency are very dependent on surgical technique.

TESTIS CANCER

Testicular cancer, although relatively rare, is the most common neoplasm in men 15 to 35 years of age. In 2009, an estimated 8,400 men were diagnosed with testis cancer. Germ cell testicular tumors account for 95%. Testicular tumors of germ cell origin are classified into seminoma and nonseminomatous germ cell tumors. Seminoma generally affects older men and rarely presents with elevation of human chorionic gonadotropin (HCG). Nonseminomatous germ cell tumors include embryonal and yolk sac tumors (20%), teratoma (5%), and choriocarcinoma (1%). Embryonal and yolk sac tumors produce alpha-fetoprotein (AFP); choriocarcinoma produces HCG. Mixed germ cell tumors contain various combinations of the mentioned cell types. Although the cause of testicular cancer is unknown, cryptorchidism and maternal exposure to estrogen compounds during pregnancy have been associated with an increased risk of testicular tumors.

Presentation

A painless testicular mass is the most common presentation of testicular tumors. Nonetheless, 32% of patients with a testicular tumor have testicular pain on presentation (66). History of trauma, infection, and hydrocele must not distract a physician from a complete testicular evaluation, including testicular ultrasound. Seventy percent of testicular tumors are discovered by patient self-examination (66). Occasionally patients present with symptoms of metastatic disease: malaise, weight loss, fatigue, abdominal or back pain, obstructive renal colic, lower extremity edema, seizures, and palpable lymphadenopathy. In addition, patients with pulmonary metastasis can present with cough, hemoptysis, or shortness of breath.

The gold standard for imaging of the testis is scrotal ultrasound. Infection, inflammation, and trauma can cause changes in testicular parenchyma that may appear indistinguishable from the neoplasm. In these cases a 2-week course of anti-inflammatory or antimicrobial therapy may be instituted and followed by a repeat testicular study.

Patterns of Spread

Testicular tumors (with the exception of choriocarcinoma) tend to spread in a stepwise fashion following the lymphatic drainage to the retroperitoneum. The right testis lymphatics drain to the intra-aortocaval area at the level of renal hilum and then in the following order: precaval, preaortic, paracaval, right common iliac, and right external iliac nodes. The left testis lymphatics drain into the para-aortic area just below the renal hilum, followed by the preaortic, left common iliac, and left external iliac lymph nodes. Left-sided disease does not cross over to the right-sided drainage area; however, right-to-left drainage is rather common. Based on this lymphatic mapping, modified templates for retroperitoneal lymph node dissection (RPLND) have been described. Other sites of metastasis in decreasing frequency are lung, supraclavicular lymphadenopathy, liver, brain, bone, kidney, adrenal, gastrointestinal tract, and spleen.

Clinical Staging

Complete workup of the patient with suspected testicular tumor should include CT of the abdomen and pelvis, plain chest radiograph, tumor markers (AFP, bHCG, and lactate dehydrogenase). If chest radiograph is abnormal or CT of the abdomen reveals metastasis, a CT of chest is generally indicated to evaluate the possibility and extent of chest involvement. Testis cancer staging system employs determination of the primary pathology, radiographic imaging, and serum tumor marker status (Table 54.4).

After the clinical diagnosis of a testicular cancer has been established and tumor markers are obtained, a radical orchiectomy is performed via an inguinal approach to avoid cross-contamination of inguinal lymphatics with testicular lymphatics. Pathologic evaluation should document percentage of each cell type and the T stage of the lesion.

Serum markers are useful in making the diagnosis, suggesting tumor pathology as well as following response to treatment, disease progression, and/or relapse. Lactate dehydrogenase is a nonspecific marker and is used to estimate tumor bulk. AFP and HCG levels are repeated after orchiectomy. The half-life of AFP is 5 days and that of HCG is about 48 hours. Typically, five biological half-lives should elapse for a tumor marker to adequately clear from the body.

SEMINOMA

Stage I/IIa

Approximately 70% of patients with seminoma have stage I disease at presentation. Seminomas are known to be highly radiosensitive; currently, the standard of treatment for stage I seminoma is adjuvant retroperitoneal radiation therapy. Disease-free survival in this clinical scenario exceeds 95%. Surveillance has been shown to have similar survival rates (>95%) with 18% relapse at 5 years (67). Several factors have been shown to correlate with relapse of stage I seminoma on surveillance: size of primary tumor >4 cm, lymphovascular invasion, and invasion of rete testis. The authors prefer the use of adjuvant radiation for stage I seminoma.

Stage IIb/IIc/III

Cisplatinum-based chemotherapy is used in these patients with excellent outcomes. Approximately 90% of the patients with advanced seminoma will demonstrate response to chemotherapy. The main predictor of survival is metastasis limited to pulmonary and retroperitoneal location.

Residual retroperitoneal disease presents in two radiographic forms. One is as a dense desmoplastic sheath reaction tightly adhering to the retroperitoneum and great vessels. Retroperitoneal dissection in this case is difficult and often accompanied by perioperative morbidity. Histology of this dissection is predominantly fibrotic and protracted period of regression is not uncommon. The second form of bulky disease presents as well delineated, circumscribed, and amendable to resection masses. Resection is supported in masses >3 cm (68).

Table 54.4

Testicular Cancer Staging System of the American Joint Committee on Cancer and the International Union Against Cancer: Definition of Tumor, Node, Metastasis (TNM) System

Primary tumor (T)	Description
pTX	Primary tumor cannot be assessed (if no radical orchiectomy has been performed, TX is used)
pT0	No evidence of primary tumor (e.g., histologic scar in testis)
pTis	Intratubular germ cell neoplasia (carcinoma *in situ*)
pT1	Tumor limited to the testis and epididymis and no vascular/lymphatic invasion. Tumor may invade the tunica albuginea but not the tunica vaginalis
pT2	Tumor limited to the testis and epididymis with vascular/lymphatic invasion or tumor extending through the tunica albuginea with involvement of tunica vaginalis
pT3	Tumor invades the spermatic cord with or without vascular/lymphatic invasion
pT4	Tumor invades the scrotum with or without vascular/lymphatic invasion

Regional lymph nodes (N)

Clinical

NX	Regional lymph nodes cannot be assessed
N0	No regional lymph node metastasis
N1	Lymph node mass 2 cm or less in greatest dimension; or multiple lymph node masses, none more than 2 cm in greatest dimension
N2	Lymph node mass, more than 2 cm but not more than 5 cm in greatest dimension; or multiple lymph node masses, any one mass greater than 2 cm but not more than 5 cm in greatest dimension
N3	Lymph node mass more than 5 cm in greatest dimension

Pathologic

pN0	No evidence of tumor in lymph nodes
pN1	Lymph node mass, 2 cm or less in greatest dimension and ≤5 nodes positive, none >2 cm in greatest dimension
pN2	Lymph node mass, more than 2 cm but not more than 5 cm in greatest dimension; more than 5 nodes positive, none >5 cm; evidence of extranodal extension of tumor
pN3	Lymph node mass more than 5 cm in greatest dimension; more than 5 nodes positive, none >5 cm; evidence of extranodal extension of tumor

Distant metastases (M)

M0	No evidence of distant metastases
M1	Nonregional nodal or pulmonary metastases
M2	Nonpulmonary visceral metastases

Serum Tumor Markers (S)

	LDH	hCG (mIU/mL)	AFP (ng/mL)
S0	≤N	≤ N	≤N
S1	<1.5 N	<5,000	<1,000
S2	1.5–10 N	5,000–50,000	1,000–10,000
S3	>10 N	>50,000	>10,000

Testis Cancer

Stage Grouping	T	N	M	S
Stage 0	pTis	N0	M0	S0
Stage I	T1–T4	N0	M0	SX
IA	T1	N0	M0	S0
IB	T2	N0	M0	S0
	T3	N0	M0	S0
	T4	N0	M0	S0
IS	Any T	N0	M0	S1–3
Stage II	Any T	Any N	M0	SX
IIA	Any T	N1	M0	S0
	Any T	N1	M0	S1
IIB	Any T	N2	M0	S1
IIC	Any T	N3	M0	S0
	Any T	N3	M0	S1
Stage III	Any T	Any N	M1	SX
IIIA	Any T	Any N	M 1	S0
	Any T	Any N	M1	S1
IIIB	Any T	Any N	M0	S2
	Any T	Any N	M1	S2
IIC	Any T	Any N	M0	S3
	Any T	Any N	M1a	S3
	Any T	Any N	M1b	Any S

AFP, alpha-fetoprotein; hCG, human chorionic gonadotropin; LDH, lactate dehydrogenase; N, upper limit of normal for the LDH assay.

(From *Comprehensive Textbook of Genitourinary Oncology* Vogelzang et al. 3rd ed LWW 2006, with permission.)

NONSEMINOMATOUS GERM CELL TUMOR

Stage 1A

Patients with stage 1A (low-stage) disease have three treatment options: surveillance, RPLND, or primary short-course chemotherapy. Overall survival for stage 1 disease approaches 100%. Typical surveillance protocols are rigorous. Surveillance includes periodic chest radiographs, tumor markers, and CT scans. Patients are evaluated monthly during year 1, every 2 months in year 2, every 3 months in year 3, every 4 months in year 4, and every 6 months thereafter. CT scans are obtained every 3 months for the first 2 years and every 6 months in the third to fifth years. Relapses, in general, occur more frequently in the retroperitoneum alone, and most of these patients re-present with stage IIB tumors (nodes of 2 to 5 cm). These patients thus require three or four cycles of chemotherapy often followed by RPLND, with survival rates that are widely variable in the literature.

Not all patients with low-stage disease are good candidates for the observation regimen. We believe only patients with low recurrence risk are appropriate candidates for observation. High risk factors for recurrence are presence of lymphovascular invasion, persistent elevation of serum markers after orchiectomy, presence of >40% of embryonal carcinoma in the orchiectomy specimen, and presence of choriocarcinoma in the orchiectomy specimen. The majority of relapses occur in the first 2 years of observation. It is important to note that although observation appears to be the least invasive option for selected group of patients, the intensity of observation protocol makes compliance quite difficult. It is a treating physician's responsibility to limit surveillance to compliant patients with low-risk disease.

RPLND, first performed in 1906, has undergone significant revision and improvements to limit side effects without altering efficacy. Initially, the en bloc dissection spanned the area from the diaphragm to the level of bifurcation of the common iliac arteries and laterally from ureter to ureter. This dissection, although relatively safe, rendered patients without the ability to ejaculate. Also, on the histologic review, 30% of stage I patients were upstaged to stage II, but the remaining 70% had no evidence of tumor on the final pathology. Modified templates were introduced in the early 1980s (69,70) (Figures 54.1 and 54.2), followed by development of nerve-sparing techniques (71); that, in combination, allowed preservation of emission without compromising cancer control. A short course of chemotherapy can also be used in stage 1A disease, but the potential short- and long-term side effects must be discussed and patients must be aware that chemotherapy is ineffective for teratoma. Patients with stage 1B disease can be offered template RPLND or chemotherapy. The authors have strongly advocated nerve-sparing RPLND as this provides a diagnostic and therapeutic approach to low-stage disease with minimal side effects.

Laparoscopic Retroperitoneal Lymph Node Dissection

In the past decade, laparoscopic approaches in urologic diseases have become increasingly more accepted among surgeons and patients. Early acceptance of laparoscopic RPLND centered on

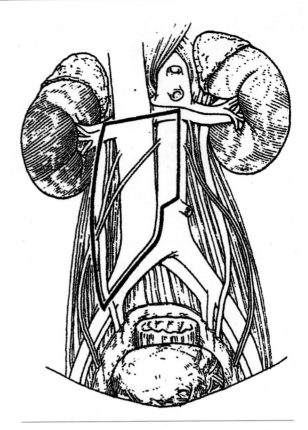

Figure 54.1 Template of dissection for right-modified nerve-sparing retroperitoneal lymph node dissection. (From Vogelzang NJ, Scardino PT, Shipley WU, eds. *Comprehensive Textbook of Genitourinary Oncology*, 3rd ed. Philadelphia: Lippincott Williams & Wilkins; 2005, with permission.)

its use as a staging tool for clinical stage I tumors. Patients with nonseminomatous tumors, normalized tumor markers, no contraindications for laparoscopy, and who would otherwise be considered for surveillance (patients with low risk for recurrence) have been the typical candidates for the laparoscopic approach.

Overall, laparoscopic RPLND is being gradually accepted by the urologic community as an appropriate staging tool for stage I disease when performed by experienced laparoscopic surgeon. As the technique of laparoscopic RPLND is being developed to duplicate the open counterpart (72) and long-term follow-up from laparoscopic centers of excellence accumulates for extended laparoscopic RPLND as a therapeutic modality for low-stage disease (73), laparoscopic RPLND may gain acceptance as an appropriate treatment option for stage I disease. However, it is emphasized that most of the experience of laparoscopic RPLND exists primarily as a staging modality for low-volume disease as most patients with disease are treated with systemic chemotherapy following laparoscopic RPLND. The therapeutic benefit of laparoscopic RPLND remains to be defined.

Stage IIA/IIB

Individuals with stage IIA/IIB disease account for approximately 40% of patients with nonseminomatous germ cell tumors.

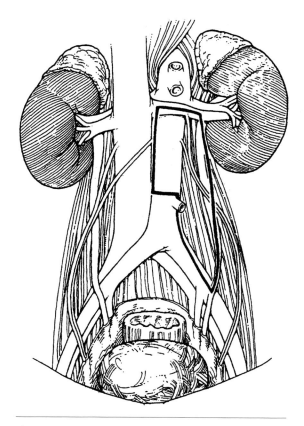

Figure 54.2 Template of dissection for left-modified nerve-sparing retroperitoneal lymph node dissection. (From Vogelzang NJ, Scardino PT, Shipley WU, eds. *Comprehensive Textbook of Genitourinary Oncology,* 3rd ed. Philadelphia: Lippincott Williams & Wilkins; 2005, with permission.)

Initially, two treatment options were offered: primary chemotherapy or primary RPLND. Observed recurrence for N1 disease was in the range of 15%, 30% to 50% for N2, and as high as 50% to 90% in N3 disease. Such high recurrence in post-RPLND cohort with clinical N2 and higher disease shifted the treatment algorithm to avoid primary RPLND in patients with stage IIB disease and to treat these patients initially with systemic chemotherapy.

Primary RPLND in stage IIA disease is commonly performed using modified templates with nerve-sparing approach. Postoperative mortality is low (<0.5%) and operative complications are in the range of 10%. If histologic outcome is negative, the observation protocol is implemented. Patients who demonstrate positive lymph nodes with viable cancer (nonteratoma) in the RPLND sample can either follow observation protocol and receive chemotherapy at the time of recurrence (three to four cycles), or can undergo immediate adjuvant chemotherapy (two cycles). Limitation of primary RPLND to patients with stable markers and clinical stage I and IIA resulted in significantly reduced risk of relapse after RPLND (74).

Stage IIc/III

Prior to the introduction of platinum-based multidrug chemotherapy regimen, survival of disseminated germ cell tumor was poor. After the introduction of platinum-based therapy, overall survival of patients with extensive disease improved dramatically. Surgical resection of any residual tumor after completion of chemotherapy is essential. Surgical resection normally takes place once the serum tumor markers have normalized. Full bilateral RPLND template is generally performed in this setting. Preoperatively, postchemotherapy RPLND patients need to be informed that an intraoperative decision regarding resection of adjacent organs such as kidney or bowel may be required. Only complete resection of tumor gives patients survival benefit; therefore, resection of all palpable and visible disease is mandated. Incision depends on location of the tumor in the individual patient. The authors prefer the thoracoabdominal approach for most patients. Initially, prospective dissection of vessels away from tumor and lymphatics is performed, followed by dissection of tumor and lymphatics away from the posterior body wall. Complications of postchemotherapy RPLND are more frequent and significant than in a primary RPLND setting. Pulmonary complications are of concern as the majority of the patients receive bleomycin as part of the chemotherapeutic regimen. No supplemental oxygen should be administered and fluid status of the patient needs to be closely monitored to avoid the pulmonary congestion or irreversible adult respiratory distress syndrome.

In general postchemotherapy residual masses are found to pathologically contain teratoma in 40%, scar and/or necrosis in 40%, and residual primitive viable tumor in 20%. If mature teratoma or necrosis is found, only observation is required. The presence of active primitive disease in the residual mass will require additional/salvage chemotherapy because nearly 50% of these patients will recur following surgical resection. Salvage chemotherapy following surgery can cure nearly 75% of these patients.

Testis cancer is not only chemosensitive but also a "surgery-sensitive" disease. Advances in surgical technique and postoperative care allow the approach of retroperitoneal lymph node dissection with significantly reduced morbidity, even in a high-risk setting. Today the application of multiple forms of therapy provides excellent outcomes and cure. Management choices need to be explained to patients including risks, benefits, and long-term morbidities. Future advances in treatment of testicular cancer will concentrate on further reduction in treatment-related morbidities while maintaining excellent oncologic outcomes.

REFERENCES

1. Nelson CP, Sanda MG. Contemporary diagnosis and management of renal angiomyolipoma. *J Urol.* 2002;168:1315–1325.
2. Oesterling JE, Fishman EK, Goldman SM, et al. The management of renal angiomyolipoma. *J Urol.* 1986;135:1121–1124.
3. Dechet CB, Bostwick DG, Blute ML, et al. Renal oncocytoma: multifocality, bilateralism, metachronous tumor development and coexistent renal cell carcinoma. *J Urol.* 1999;162:40–42.
4. Weiss LM, Gelb AB, Medeiros LJ. Adult renal epithelial neoplasms. *Am J Clin Pathol.* 1995;103:624–635.
5. Dechet CB, Zincke H, Sebo TJ, et al. Prospective analysis of computerized tomography and needle biopsy with permanent sectioning to determine the nature of solid renal masses in adults. *J Urol.* 2003; 169:71–74.

6. Licht MR, Novick AC, Tubbs RR, et al. Renal oncocytoma: clinical and biological correlates. *J Urol.* 1993;150:1380–1383.

7. Jemal A, Siegel R, Ward E, et al. Cancer statistics, 2006. *CA Cancer J Clin* 2006;56:106–130.

8. McLaughlin JK, Lindblad P, Mellemgaard A, et al. International renal-cell cancer study. I. Tobacco use. *Int J Cancer.* 1995;60:194–198.

9. Chow WH, Gridley G, Fraumeni JF Jr, et al. Obesity, hypertension, and the risk of kidney cancer in men. *N Engl J Med.* 2000;343:1305–1311.

10. Robson CJ. The natural history of renal cell carcinoma. *Prog Clin Biol Res.* 1982;100:447–452.

11. Zisman A, Pantuck AJ, Dorey F, et al. Mathematical model to predict individual survival for patients with renal cell carcinoma. *J Clin Oncol.* 2002;20:1368–1374.

12. Skinner DG, Lieskovsky G, Pritcher TR. Technique of radical nephrectomy. Saunders, 1988.

13. Phillips CK, Taneja SS. The role of lymphadenectomy in the surgical management of renal cell carcinoma. *Urol Oncol.* 2004;22:214–224.

14. Tsui KH, Shvarts O, Barbaric Z, et al. Is adrenalectomy a necessary component of radical nephrectomy? UCLA experience with 511 radical nephrectomies. *J Urol.* 2000;163:437–441.

15. Clayman RV, Kavoussi LR, Soper NJ, et al. Laparoscopic nephrectomy: initial case report. *J Urol.* 1991;146:278–282.

16. Portis AJ, Yan Y, Landman J, et al. Long-term followup after laparoscopic radical nephrectomy. *J Urol.* 2002;167:1257–1262.

17. Lau WK, Blute ML, Weaver AL, et al. Matched comparison of radical nephrectomy vs nephron-sparing surgery in patients with unilateral renal cell carcinoma and a normal contralateral kidney. *Mayo Clin Proc.* 2000;75:1236–1242.

18. Uzzo RG, Novick AC. Nephron sparing surgery for renal tumors: indications, techniques and outcomes. *J Urol.* 2001;166:6–18.

19. Hafez KS, Novick AC, Campbell SC. Patterns of tumor recurrence and guidelines for followup after nephron sparing surgery for sporadic renal cell carcinoma. *J Urol.* 1997;157:2067–2070.

20. Moinzadeh A, Gill IS, Finelli A, et al. Laparoscopic partial nephrectomy: 3–year followup. *J Urol.* 2006;175:459–462.

21. Gill IS, Remer EM, Hasan WA, et al. Renal cryoablation: outcome at 3 years. *J Urol.* 2005;173:1903–1907.

22. Flanigan RC, Salmon SE, Blumenstein BA, et al. Nephrectomy followed by interferon alfa-2b compared with interferon alfa-2b alone for metastatic renal-cell cancer. *N Engl J Med.* 2001;345:1655–1659.

23. Levin ML, Lilienfeld AM, Moore GE. The association of smoking with cancer of the urinary bladder in humans. *AMA Arch Intern Med.* 1956;98:129–135.

24. Michaud DS, Spiegelman D, Clinton SK, et al. Fluid intake and the risk of bladder cancer in men. *N Engl J Med.* 1999;340:1390–1397.

25. Esrig D, Elmajian D, Groshen S, et al. Accumulation of nuclear p53 and tumor progression in bladder cancer. *N Engl J Med.* 1994;331:1259–64.

26. Chatterjee SJ, Datar R, Youssefzadeh D, et al. Combined effects of p53, p21, and pRb expression in the progression of bladder transitional cell carcinoma. *J Clin Oncol.* 2004;22:1007–1013.

27. Grossfeld GD, Wolf JS Jr, Litwan MS, et al. Asymptomatic microscopic hematuria in adults: summary of the AUA best practice policy recommendations. *Am Fam Physician.* 2001;63:1145–1154.

28. Jewett HJ. Infiltrating carcinoma of the bladder; relation of early diagnosis to five-year survival rate after complete extirpation. *JAMA.* 1952;148:187–189.

29. Lutzeyer W, Rubben H, Dahm H. Prognostic parameters in superficial bladder cancer: an analysis of 315 cases. *J Urol.* 1982;127:250–252.

30. Van Der Meijden A, Sylvester R, Collette L, et al. The role and impact of pathology review on stage and grade assessment of stages Ta and T1 bladder tumors: a combined analysis of 5 European Organization for Research and Treatment of Cancer Trials. *J Urol.* 2000;164:1533–1537.

31. Freeman JA, Esrig D, Stein JP, et al. Radical cystectomy for high risk patients with superficial bladder cancer in the era of orthotopic urinary reconstruction. *Cancer.* 1995;76:833–839.

32. Schips L, Augustin H, Zigeuner RE, et al. Is repeated transurethral resection justified in patients with newly diagnosed superficial bladder cancer? *Urology.* 2002;59:220–223.

33. Sylvester RJ, van der Meijden AP, Oosterlinck W, et al. Predicting recurrence and progression in individual patients with stage Ta T1 bladder cancer using EORTC risk tables: a combined analysis of 2596 patients from seven EORTC trials. *Eur Urol.* 2006;49:466–475.

34. Lamm DL, Blumenstein BA, Crissman JD, et al. Maintenance bacillus Calmette-Guerin immunotherapy for recurrent TA, T1 and carcinoma in situ transitional cell carcinoma of the bladder: a randomized Southwest Oncology Group Study. *J Urol.* 2000;163:1124–1129.

35. Stein JP, Lieskovsky G, Cote R, et al. Radical cystectomy in the treatment of invasive bladder cancer: longterm results in 1,054 patients. *J Clin Oncol.* 2001;19:666–675.

36. Quek ML, Stein JP, Daneshmand S, et al. A critical analysis of perioperative mortality from radical cystectomy. *J Urol.* 2006;175:886–890.

37. Stein JP, Cai J, Groshen S, et al. Risk factors for patients with pelvic lymph node metastases following radical cystectomy with en bloc pelvic lymphadenectomy: concept of lymph node density. *J Urol.* 2003;170:35–41.

38. Stein JP, Skinner DG. Orthotopic urinary diversion. In: Walsh PC, Retik AB, Vaughan ED, et al., eds. *Campbell's Urology.* 8th ed. Philadelphia: WB Saunders; 2003;3835–3867.

39. Sonn GA, Aronson W, Litwin MS. Impact of diet on prostate cancer: a review. *Prostate Cancer Prostatic Dis.* 2005;8:304–310.

40. Thompson IM, Goodman PJ, Tangen CM, et al. The influence of finasteride on the development of prostate cancer. *N Engl J Med.* 2003;349:215–224.

41. Chan TY, Partin AW, Walsh PC, et al. Prognostic significance of Gleason score 3 + 4 versus Gleason score 4 + 3 tumor at radical prostatectomy. *Urology.* 2000;56:823–827.

42. Hattab EM, Koch MO, Eble JN, et al. Tertiary Gleason pattern 5 is a powerful predictor of biochemical relapse in patients with Gleason score 7 prostatic adenocarcinoma. *J Urol.* 2006;175:1695–1699.

43. D'Amico AV, Whittington R, Malkowicz SB, et al. Clinical utility of percent-positive prostate biopsies in predicting biochemical outcome after radical prostatectomy or external-beam radiation therapy for patients with clinically localized prostate cancer. *Mol Urol.* 2000;4:171–175.

44. Huland H, Hammerer P, Henke RP, et al. Preoperative prediction of tumor heterogeneity and recurrence after radical prostatectomy for localized prostatic carcinoma with digital rectal, examination prostate specific antigen and the results of 6 systematic biopsies. *J Urol.* 1996;155:1344–1347.

45. D'Amico AV, Schnall M, Whittington R, et al. Endorectal coil magnetic resonance imaging identifies locally advanced prostate cancer in select patients with clinically localized disease. *Urology.* 1998;51:449–454.

46. Walsh P. Anatomic radical retropubic prostatectomy. In: Walsh PC, Retic AB, Vaughan ED, et al., eds. *Campbell's Urology.* 8th ed. Philadelphia: WB Sounders; 2003;3107–3129.

47. Partin AW, Yoo J, Carter HB, et al. The use of prostate specific antigen, clinical stage and Gleason score to predict pathological

stage in men with localized prostate cancer. *J Urol.* 1993;150:
110–114.

48. Partin AW, Mangold LA, Lamm DM, et al. Contemporary update of prostate cancer staging nomograms (Partin Tables) for the new millennium. *Urology.* 2001;58:843–848.

49. Kattan MW, Eastham JA, Stapleton AM, et al. A preoperative nomogram for disease recurrence following radical prostatectomy for prostate cancer. *J Natl Cancer Inst.* 1998;90:766–771.

50. Stephenson AJ, Scardino PT, Eastham JA, et al. Preoperative nomogram predicting the 10-year probability of prostate cancer recurrence after radical prostatectomy. *J Natl Cancer Inst.* 2006;98:715–717.

51. D'Amico AV, Moul J, Carroll PR, et al. Cancer-specific mortality after surgery or radiation for patients with clinically localized prostate cancer managed during the prostate-specific antigen era. *J Clin Oncol.* 2003;21:2163–2172.

52. Shipley WU, Thames HD, Sandler HM, et al. Radiation therapy for clinically localized prostate cancer: a multi-institutional pooled analysis. *JAMA.* 1999;281:1598–1604.

53. Grimm PD, Blasko JC, Sylvester JE, et al. 10-year biochemical (prostate-specific antigen) control of prostate cancer with (125)I brachytherapy. *Int J Radiat Oncol Biol Phys.* 2001;51:31–40.

54. Bill-Axelson A, Holmberg L, Ruutu M, et al. Radical prostatectomy versus watchful waiting in early prostate cancer. *N Engl J Med.* 2005;352:1977–1984.

55. Hull GW, Rabbani F, Abbas F, et al. Cancer control with radical prostatectomy alone in 1,000 consecutive patients. *J Urol.* 2002;167:528–534.

56. Han M, Partin AW, Zahurak M, et al. Biochemical (prostate specific antigen) recurrence probability following radical prostatectomy for clinically localized prostate cancer. *J Urol.* 2003;169:517–523.

57. Roehl KA, Han M, Ramos CG, et al. Cancer progression and survival rates following anatomical radical retropubic prostatectomy in 3,478 consecutive patients: long-term results. *J Urol.* 2004;172:910–914.

58. Freeman JA, Lieskovsky G, Cook DW, et al. Radical retropubic prostatectomy and postoperative adjuvant radiation for pathological stage C (PcN0) prostate cancer from 1976 to 1989: intermediate findings. *J Urol.* 1993;149:1029–1034.

59. Petrovich Z, Lieskovsky G, Stein JP, et al. Comparison of surgery alone with surgery and adjuvant radiotherapy for pT3N0 prostate cancer. *BJU Int.* 2002;89:604–611.

60. Bolla M, van Poppel H, Collette L, et al. Postoperative radiotherapy after radical prostatectomy: a randomised controlled trial (EORTC trial 22911). *Lancet.* 2005;366:572–578.

61. Tooher R, Swindle P, Woo H, et al. Laparoscopic radical prostatectomy for localized prostate cancer: a systematic review of comparative studies. *J Urol.* 2006;175:2011–2017.

62. Kundu SD, Roehl KA, Eggener SE, et al. Potency, continence and complications in 3,477 consecutive radical retropubic prostatectomies. *J Urol.* 2004;172:2227–2231.

63. Lepor H, Kaci L, Xue X. Continence following radical retropubic prostatectomy using self-reporting instruments. *J Urol.* 2004;171:1212–1215.

64. Burnett AL. Erectile dysfunction following radical prostatectomy. *JAMA.* 2005;293:2648–2653.

65. Mulhall J, Land S, Parker M, et al. The use of an erectogenic pharmacotherapy regimen following radical prostatectomy improves recovery of spontaneous erectile function. *J Sex Med.* 2005;2:532–542.

66. Kennedy BJ, Schmidt JD, Winchester DP, et al. National survey of patterns of care for testis cancer. *Cancer.* 1987;60:1921–1930.

67. Tyldesley S, Voduc D, McKenzie M, et al. Surveillance of stage I testicular seminoma: British Columbia Cancer Agency experience 1992 to 2002. *Urology.* 2006;67:594–598.

68. Quek ML, Simma-Chiang V, Stein JP, et al. Postchemotherapy residual masses in advanced seminoma: current management and outcomes. *Expert Rev Anticancer Ther.* 2005;5:869–874.

69. Pizzocaro G, Salvioni R, Zanoni F. Unilateral lymphadenectomy in intraoperative stage I nonseminomatous germinal testis cancer. *J Urol.* 1985;134:485–489.

70. Richie JP. Modified retroperitoneal lymphadenectomy for patients with clinical stage I testicular cancer. *Semin Urol.* 1988;6:216–222.

71. Donohue JP, Thornhill JA, Foster RS, et al. Retroperitoneal lymphadenectomy for clinical stage A testis cancer (1965 to 1989): modifications of technique and impact on ejaculation. *J Urol.* 1993;149:237–243.

72. Allaf ME, Bhayani SB, Link RE, et al. Laparoscopic retroperitoneal lymph node dissection: duplication of open technique. *Urology.* 2005;65:575–577.

73. Bhayani SB, Ong A, Oh WK, et al. Laparoscopic retroperitoneal lymph node dissection for clinical stage I nonseminomatous germ cell testicular cancer: a long-term update. *Urology.* 2003;62:324–327.

74. Stephenson AJ, Bosl GJ, Motzer RJ, et al. Retroperitoneal lymph node dissection for nonseminomatous germ cell testicular cancer: impact of patient selection factors on outcome. *J Clin Oncol.* 2005;23:2781–2788.

COMMENTARY
R. Houston Thompson and Michael L. Blute

Drs. Reyblat, Skinner, and Stein from the University of Southern California (USC) present a well-written overview of the most common urologic malignancies observed in the United States. It is appropriately organized by organ system, and our commentary will generally follow that of the previous chapter. It should be noted that the authors from USC have considerable experience with the surgical management of urologic cancers and their opinions in the previous chapter should be considered knowledgeable and up to date. For example, the USC experience with bladder cancer introduced the urologic community to lymph node density and emphasized the importance of a complete and thorough lymph node dissection at the time of radical cystectomy. However, in the spectrum of urologic malignancies, surgical management and nuances thereof often differ, if only slightly, from one institution to another. Perhaps this is related to the dogma that surgery and technical considerations inherent with operations are mostly learned from mentors as opposed to textbooks or journal articles. As such, we will highlight important similarities practiced at USC and the Mayo Clinic and point out differences that may or may not be associated with improvements in patient quality of life or long-term outcome.

KIDNEY TUMORS

Angiomyolipoma

Angiomyolipomas (AMLs) are the only enhancing tumors of the kidney that are diagnosed radiographically, and are inherently benign. Thus, any renal lesion that contains fat on computed tomography (CT) is an AML unless other suspicious features are present to suggest concomitant renal cell carcinoma (RCC). It is not infrequent for a patient to be referred for surgical removal of a small "renal mass" and on careful inspection of the CT, fat is present within the renal mass, and thus observation is recommended. On the contrary, any enhancing tumor arising from the kidney that does not contain fat should be considered RCC until proven otherwise. The USC authors addressed the unusual situation of a lipid-poor AML, and even with optimal imaging techniques, these lesions are often removed surgically because of the diagnostic uncertainty.

In general, we advocate angiographic embolization for any AML that presents with spontaneous hemorrhage, regardless of whether or not significant symptoms or hemodynamic instability are present. Unlike RCCs, AMLs do not necessarily form a prominent capsule or pseudocapsule, which makes surgical resection via a partial nephrectomy slightly more difficult. However, embolization of the mass usually results in a prominent tumor capsule and is associated with a technically easier partial nephrectomy, should surgical intervention become warranted. That being said, we agree with the USC group in that preservation of renal function is paramount. It is only in extreme situations that an entire kidney should be removed for an AML.

In the case of an incidental AML that is <4 cm and without features suspicious for RCC, we tend to follow these with ultrasound evaluation every 6 months for 1 year and then annually. AMLs are characteristically hyperechoic on ultrasound, which are distinguished from a renal calculus by the lack of acoustic shadowing. During follow-up, partial nephrectomy is indicated if the tumor grows to <4 cm or if rapid growth is demonstrated, especially in a women planning pregnancy (AMLs can rapidly grow and rupture with estrogen surges).

Oncocytoma

Oncocytomas are the most common benign tumor of the kidney. Unfortunately, all imaging techniques, and even renal biopsy, cannot reliably distinguish a renal mass as benign without concomitant RCC (1,2). Thus, most oncocytomas are diagnosed pathologically, preferably through a nephron-sparing approach. Occasionally, oncocytomas are difficult to distinguish pathologically from the chromophobe subtype of RCC. Therefore, during a partial nephrectomy, if a frozen-section pathologic analysis is consistent with oncocytoma, care must be taken to achieve a negative margin because permanent section pathology may be changed to a malignant chromophobe RCC.

At the Mayo Clinic, we have examined the relationship between tumor size and histology for 2,770 consecutive patients undergoing partial and radical nephrectomy for a solitary and localized renal cortical tumor (i.e., the most common type of presentation) (3). A unique feature of our Kidney Cancer Registry is that all patients have had their pathologic specimen reviewed by a single urologic pathologist (John C. Cheville, MD). In this consecutive group of 2,770 patients, 13% of tumors removed surgically were benign, of which 73% were oncocytomas, followed by AML, papillary adenoma, metanephric adenoma, and benign tumor–not otherwise specified (3). However, among patients with a tumor <1 cm, 46% were benign, and among patients with a tumor 1 to 3 cm, 22% were benign (3). In contrast,

94% of patients with a tumor >7 cm had RCC. Furthermore, for the subset of patients with clear cell RCC, the most common histologic subtype, only 8% of patients with tumors <3 cm were of high nuclear grade compared with 62% of patients with tumors >7 cm (3). Thus, we conclude that patients with smaller tumors, especially <3 cm, are more likely to have benign tumors or low-grade RCC and the tables presented in the article can be useful for preoperative patient counseling (3).

Renal Cell Carcinoma

The etiology of RCC was well addressed by Dr. Reyblat and colleagues. One additional recently recognized syndrome associated with RCC is the Birt-Hogg-Dubé syndrome. This autosomal-dominant disorder is associated with fibrofolliculomas, cutaneous mucinous papules on the face and neck, spontaneous pneumothorax, along with multiple and bilateral benign and malignant renal tumors (4). Because both Birt-Hogg-Dubé syndrome and hereditary leiomyoma RCC syndrome have characteristic cutaneous lesions often on the face and scalp, these areas should be examined in patients with a renal mass, especially those presenting with multiple or bilateral tumors.

Historically, RCC patients presented with symptoms related to the underlying tumor and was therefore labeled the "internist tumor" (5). With the widespread use of cross-sectional imaging, approximately two thirds of contemporary renal mass patients present with an incidental tumor, and RCC may be more appropriately labeled the "radiologist's tumor." The workup of an incidental renal mass is addressed in the previous chapter and focuses on the pattern of metastatic spread in descending order: lung, bone, liver, lymph nodes, followed by brain. Of note, positron emission tomography scan is not very useful with RCC, especially in low-grade tumors, in part due to obscurity from 18-fluoro-2-deoxyglucose concentration in the collecting system (6). However, CT angiography can be particularly helpful for preoperative planning in cases of complex partial nephrectomy.

We agree with the USC group that renal biopsy is not routinely indicated for renal tumors because of its high false-negative rate (1). In cases of suspected sarcoma or urothelial carcinoma of the kidney, biopsy may help identify patients for neoadjuvant chemotherapy; however, this situation is rare.

The TNM staging system for RCC has sparked growing interest in the literature, more so than any other urologic malignancy (7). The T1 tumor classification was recently subdivided into T1a (<4 cm) and T1b (4 to 7 cm) categories (8) and recommendations have been made to subdivide the T2 tumor classification based on a 10 cm size cutoff (9). Direct adrenal gland invasion, currently within the pT3a tumor classification, is more appropriately grouped with pT4 patients (10). The impact of renal sinus fat invasion is a recently recognized adverse pathologic feature that is both underreported and may be responsible for outcome differences noted with tumor size (11–14). Additionally, we have developed a scoring algorithm that is based on pathologic features (tumor stage, size, grade and necrosis; the SSIGN score) predictive of cancer-specific survival in a multivariate analysis (15), which has been externally validated with an international cohort (16). This prognostic model can be used in the immediate postoperative setting for risk assessment or in the dynamic setting incorporating the length of disease-free follow-up during surveillance (17).

The USC group advocates a thoracoabdominal incision for RCC, especially for large tumors arising from the upper pole. At the Mayo Clinic, if a laparoscopic approach is not taken, we have trended away from this incision in favor of the flank incision or subcostal approach if a retroperitoneal lymph node dissection is warranted. This obviates the need for a chest tube and may decrease postoperative pain and speed recovery. Furthermore, complicated tumor thrombectomy can be performed successfully through a subcostal or midline incision without entering the pleural cavity (18). Nevertheless, the thoracoabdominal approach allows for excellent exposure with access to the renal hilum and great vessels along with the ability to treat concomitant chest lesions.

Surgical resection remains the only curative treatment for renal tumors, although the operative approach continues to evolve. Radical nephrectomy including ipsilateral adrenalectomy became the standard of therapy in the late 1960s. However, this was challenged in the 1980s by several reports demonstrating favorable results with open partial nephrectomy (19,20). During the last decade, partial nephrectomy has been accepted as a safe and effective alternative to radical nephrectomy and many urologists now believe that partial nephrectomy is standard of care for small renal tumors even in the setting of a normal contralateral kidney (21–24). However, the application of partial nephrectomy has yet to become widespread as contemporary data demonstrate that partial nephrectomy remains underused in the United States and abroad (25,26).

As treatment of renal tumors continues to evolve, less invasive approaches have found new applications in our field. Laparoscopy has become an increasingly important part of our surgical armamentarium. Several groups have now reported their results with laparoscopic partial nephrectomy accompanied with diminished postoperative pain, shorter hospitalization, and satisfactory oncologic outcomes. However, as more complex laparoscopic procedures are being performed, the reported warm ischemia times appear to be longer compared with partial nephrectomy done via an open approach (21). Even in the most skilled laparoscopic hands, collecting system repair and parenchymal defect closure result in longer ischemia times compared with the open approach (21). Furthermore, in a recent multi-institutional review of 1,800 partial nephrectomies at the Mayo Clinic, Cleveland Clinic, and Johns Hopkins, laparoscopic partial nephrectomy was associated with significantly increased risk of postoperative complications, longer ischemia times, and the need for additional procedures (27). The kidney is exquisitely sensitive to warm ischemia as metabolic activities are predominantly aerobic. Consistent with this, most studies in humans have supported a maximal renal tolerance of approximately 30 minutes (21,28,29). In fact, we recently reported a multi-institutional investigation of 537 patients with a solitary kidney, demonstrating that warm ischemia >20 minutes was associated with an increased risk of acute renal failure, chronic renal insufficiency, and permanent dialysis (29). Thus, as we strive to reduce the frequency of overtreatment of small renal tumors via radical nephrectomy, it is paramount not to lose sight of the goal of renal preservation, which includes limiting warm ischemia.

BLADDER CANCER

As well described in the previous chapter, bladder cancer is more common in men and often presents with hematuria. However, we have noticed that women often present to the urologist in a delayed fashion. It is not uncommon for women to be referred for hematuria that has been treated with antibiotics for months, and sometimes years, before a cystoscopy is performed. Urinary tract infections with associated hematuria are much more common in women, and we agree that an initial trial of empiric antibiotics along with urine culture is prudent. However, follow-up of women with hematuria, especially those with a negative urine culture, is mandatory to avoid delay in diagnosis of bladder cancer.

The American Urologic Association guidelines for asymptomatic microscopic hematuria define microhematuria as three or more red blood cells per high-power field from two of three properly collected specimens (30). For patients without evidence of renal parenchymal dysfunction (i.e., significant proteinuria, red blood cell casts), recommendations were made for upper tract imaging (intravenous pyelogram or CT urogram), cystoscopy, and urine cytology in all patients except those patients considered "low risk." However, low risk only includes patients <40 years old, without a smoking history, no chemical exposure, no irritative voiding symptoms, no previous gross hematuria, *and* no history of a urologic disorder or disease (30). It is rare that we find a patient who qualifies as low risk and thus, cystoscopy, cytology, and upper tract imaging should be obtained on all patients with asymptomatic microscopic hematuria. However, it is important to remember that while cytology is highly specific for transitional cell carcinoma (TCC), especially carcinoma in situ, it not very sensitive. Therefore, a negative cytology does not rule out TCC. There are numerous other urine tests used for detection and monitoring of patients with TCC. In general, all of the tests are more sensitive and less specific than cytology and none of the tests should be routinely obtained prior to a diagnosis of TCC. We have found urinary fluorescence in situ hybridization (Abbot Laboratories, Abbot Park, IL) to be useful in monitoring response to Bacillus Calmette-Guerin (BCG) vaccine therapy; however urinary fluorescence in situ hybridization is not clinically useful prior to the diagnosis of TCC (31).

TCC, also known as *urothelial carcinoma*, is the predominant histology in the United States. TCC with mixed features such as squamous differentiation, glandular differentiation, or micropapillary TCC are much more aggressive and treated with upfront cystectomy without delay. The one exception is TCC with small cell differentiation (and perhaps plasma cell differentiation), which represent an aggressive variant and should treated with upfront chemotherapy followed by consolidative cystectomy. Pure adenocarcinoma is rare and requires workup of potential metastatic disease to the bladder or further investigation of the urachus.

Optimal treatment of superficial TCC is well delineated by the USC group. At the Mayo Clinic, patients undergoing transurethral resection of a bladder tumor receive an immediate postoperative intravesical instillation of thiotepa (60 mg diluted in 30 mL for 30 minutes duration) (32). Other groups have used mitomycin C; however, a single dose of immediate postoperative intravesical chemotherapy is effective at reducing the risk of recurrence by about 40% (33). BCG should not be used immediately postoperatively because of the high risk of systemic absorption and BCG sepsis. Most patients with pT1 TCC at our institution undergo repeat transurethral resection approximately 4 weeks later because of the significant number of understaged patients. Additionally, we strongly agree with the USC group that high-risk patients with pT1 TCC should be considered for early cystectomy because of the elevated risk of recurrence and progression. Additionally, patients with superficial TCC who recur after BCG therapy should undergo surgical extirpation. We have seen patients referred for cystectomy with years of recurrent TCC refractory to multiple courses of BCG and find development of lymphadenopathy or extravesical disease.

We agree with the USC group that radical cystectomy remains the gold standard for invasive bladder TCC. Others support sensitizing chemotherapy with radiation; however, we agree with the authors that upfront cystectomy allows for immediate treatment and identification of high-risk patients for adjuvant chemotherapy. This remains a matter of debate as neoadjuvant platinum-based chemotherapy for muscle-invasive TCC is associated with an approximately 5% improvement in survival at 5 years (33–35). Although the data for adjuvant chemotherapy are not as robust, we agree with the USC authors in that neoadjuvant chemotherapy may overtreat a significant proportion of patients and delay definitive therapy for the few who do not respond. However, for patients with unambiguous invasive bladder cancer that is clinical stage T3 or greater or involving regional lymph nodes, we prefer upfront chemotherapy followed by consolidative surgical resection.

PROSTATE CANCER

Optimal prostate-specific antigen (PSA) cutoff values are frequently debated. It is now clear that the traditional cutoff of 4 ng/mL for all patients is no longer applicable. Lower PSA thresholds will identify more patients with cancer; however, the increase in patients requiring prostate biopsy and potential increase in detection of insignificant cancers remains confounding. At the Mayo Clinic, we use age-adjusted PSA values for prostate cancer screening. More importantly, we have been using PSA kinetics for both screening and evaluation of biochemical recurrence following definitive therapy (36).

Following definitive treatment for prostate cancer, a number of tools exist for patient risk stratification. We previously created a postoperative prognostic algorithm, termed *GPSM*, incorporating features predictive of biochemical recurrence in a multivariate model, namely Gleason score, PSA value, seminal vesicle involvement, and margin status. The GPSM score is calculated as follows:

GPSM = [sum Gleason score] + [+1 for PSA 4–10 ng/mL,

+2 for PSA 10.1–20 or + 3 for PSA > 20] + 2 for

seminal vesicle involvement + 2 for a positive margin

This algorithm represents the easiest of all tools to calculate and does not require a computer, calculator, palm pilot, or neural network to compute. We recently updated the prognostic ability of the GPSM algorithm using a more contemporary cohort of patients, demonstrating that the model remains predictive

of biochemical recurrence and is the first algorithm to predict cancer-specific survival immediately following radical prostatectomy (37). Thus, we found that patients with a GPSM score of ≥10 were significantly more likely to die of prostate cancer compared with patients with a GPSM score of <10 (at 15 years 13% vs. 2%, hazard ratio, 6.5; *p* <0.001). We currently employ this algorithm for identification of high-risk patients for adjuvant trials. This information is additionally useful when counseling patients after surgery. For example, it is reassuring to inform a patient with a positive margin who has a GPSM score <10 that, based on the Mayo Clinic data, his chance of dying from prostate cancer in the next 15 years is only 2%, although further therapy may be necessary during follow-up.

Over the years, we have strongly advocated radical prostatectomy as part of a multimodal approach for high-risk prostate cancer (38–42). Recent analysis of our experience with high-risk clinical stage T3 prostate cancer patients treated by initial radical retropubic prostatectomy demonstrated that 27% of patients actually harbored organ-confined (pT2) disease and cancer-specific survival at 10 and 15 years was 90% and 79%, respectively (40). Furthermore, among 500+ patients with lymph node metastases treated with initial radical retropubic prostatectomy, 10-year cancer-specific survival was 86% and local control was achieved in 89% of patients, supporting the efficacy of initial surgery in preventing long-term pelvic complications and removal the potential source of late dissemination (43). We believe that the greatest threat to a patient's long-term quality of life is failure to control the primary tumor. It is important to note that salvage prostatectomy, or surgery after radiation, is associated with a higher incidence of postoperative complications (44). Thus, in patients with surgically resectable high risk or locally advanced prostate cancer, we prefer to perform extirpation prior to radiation.

TESTIS CANCER

Tumor markers are critical in the evaluation of testis cancer patients and have a few absolutes. First, pure seminoma never produces alpha fetal protein (AFP) and any "pure seminoma" with a truly elevated AFP should be treated as a mixed germ cell tumor. Second, choriocarcinoma always produces beta human chorionic gonadotropin (bHCG), which can also be present in about 10% of pure seminoma, although it is usually quite elevated with choriocarcinoma. Third, patients with persistent marker elevation after radical orchiectomy and before retroperitoneal lymph node dissection (RPLND) should always receive primary chemotherapy (45). It is also important to be cognizant of potential "false" elevations in testis tumor markers. Elevation in bHCG can also occur with marijuana use or in situations of elevated levels of luteinizing hormone (from bilateral orchiectomy or unilateral orchiectomy with contralateral atrophy) secondary to cross-reactivity in some assays for bHCG. Elevations in AFP can occur with liver dysfunction, such as postchemotherapy hepatitis, and is normally elevated in infants younger than 6 to 12 months old.

We agree with the USC group that radiation is indicated for most patients with stage I seminoma and that nerve-sparing RPLND should be recommended for most patients with high-risk stage I nonseminomatous germ cell tumor, along with patients harboring stage IIa nonseminomatous germ cell tumor, assuming tumor markers normalize following orchiectomy. A nerve-sparing primary RPLND preserves emission and antegrade ejaculation in >97% of patients, allows for pathologic diagnosis of the primary landing spots, cures 50% to 75% of patients with pathologic stage II disease, and is associated with acceptable short- and long-term morbidity (46). Additionally, primary RPLND for pathologically confirmed N1 disease can obviate the need for chemotherapy, providing cure for about 80% of patients (45). It is important to recognize that chemotherapy can be associated with both short-term side effects and long-term toxicities, some now just being discovered in survivorship studies. Nephrotoxicity, neurotoxicity, diminished fertility, and vascular complications including coronary artery disease are recognized potential complications from cisplatin (46). Etoposide is associated with therapy-induced leukemia in about 3 of every 1,000 patients (46). Bleomycin can lead to pulmonary fibrosis and long-term risk of secondary cancers from the combination presented here are just beginning to be discovered (46).

Postchemotherapy RPLND is well addressed by the USC group, and we echo the notion that all palpable and viable tumor must be resected. These cases are inherently challenging, especially for seminoma, and should generally be performed at tertiary care facilities where ancillary surgical services are readily available and anesthesiologists are experienced with managing the postchemotherapy patient. In general, we perform postchemotherapy RPLND through a midline incision as opposed to the thoracoabdominal approach done at USC. Additionally, we agree with the USC group that testis cancer is both a chemosensitive and "surgery-sensitive" disease. However, there is one setting in which testis cancer is quite resistant to chemotherapy: Patients who relapse >2 years following an initial cure harbor disease that is highly resistant to chemotherapy and should undergo aggressive surgical resection, one of the only times when surgery is indicated in the presence of an elevated marker (47,48).

REFERENCES

1. Dechet CB, Sebo T, Farrow G, et al. Prospective analysis of intraoperative frozen needle biopsy of solid renal masses in adults. *J Urol.* 1999;162:1282–1289.
2. Dechet CB, Bostwick DG, Blute ML, et al. Renal oncocytoma: multifocality, bilateralism, metachronous tumor development and coexistent renal cell carcinoma. *J Urol.* 1999;162:40–42.
3. Frank I, Blute ML, Cheville JC, et al. Solid renal tumors: an analysis of pathological features related to tumor size. *J Urol.* 2003;170: 2217–2220.
4. Lindor NM, Hand J, Burch PA, et al. Birt-Hogg-Dubé syndrome: an autosomal dominant disorder with predisposition to cancers of the kidney, fibrofolliculomas, and focal cutaneous mucinosis. *Int J Dermatol.* 2001;40:653–656.
5. Motzer RJ, Bander NH, Nanus DM. Renal-cell carcinoma. *N Engl J Med.* 1996;335:865–875.
6. Thompson RH, Hartman RP, Lowe VJ, et al. Applications of positron emission tomography imaging, intraoperative ultrasonography, magnetic resonance imaging, and angiography in the evaluation of renal masses. *Curr Urol Rep.* 2004;5:30–34.
7. Thompson RH, Cheville JC, Lohse CM, et al. Reclassification of patients with pT3 and pT4 renal cell carcinoma improves prognostic accuracy. *Cancer.* 2005;104:53–60.
8. Greene FL, Page DL, Fleming ID, et al. *AJCC Cancer Staging Manual,* 6th ed. New York: Springer Verlag, 2002.
9. Frank I, Blute ML, Leibovich BC, et al. pT2 classification for renal cell carcinoma. Can its accuracy be improved? *J Urol.* 2005;173: 380–384.
10. Thompson RH, Leibovich BC, Cheville JC, et al. Should direct ipsilateral adrenal invasion from renal cell carcinoma be classified as pT3a? *J Urol.* 2005;173:918–921.
11. Thompson RH, Leibovich BC, Cheville JC, et al. Is renal sinus fat invasion the same as perinephric fat invasion for pT3a renal cell carcinoma? *J Urol.* 2005;174:1218–1221.
12. Bonsib SM. The renal sinus is the principal invasive pathway: a prospective study of 100 renal cell carcinomas. *Am J Surg Pathol.* 2004;28:1594–1600.
13. Thompson RH, Blute ML, Krambeck AE, et al. Patients with pT1 renal cell carcinoma who die from disease after nephrectomy may have unrecognized renal sinus fat invasion. *Am J Surg Pathol.* 2007; 31:1089–1093.
14. Bonsib SM. T2 clear cell renal cell carcinoma is a rare entity: a study of 120 clear cell renal cell carcinomas. *J Urol.* 2005;174: 1199–1202.
15. Frank I, Blute ML, Cheville JC, et al. An outcome prediction model for patients with clear cell renal cell carcinoma treated with radical nephrectomy based on tumor stage, size, grade and necrosis: the SSIGN score. *J Urol.* 2002;168:2395–2400.
16. Ficarra V, Martignoni G, Lohse C, et al. External validation of the Mayo Clinic Stage, Size, Grade and Necrosis (SSIGN) score to predict cancer specific survival using a European series of conventional renal cell carcinoma. *J Urol.* 2006;175:1235–1239.
17. Thompson RH, Leibovich BC, Lohse CM, et al. Dynamic outcome prediction in patients with clear cell renal cell carcinoma treated with radical nephrectomy: the D-SSIGN score. *J Urol.* 2007;177: 477–480.
18. Blute ML, Leibovich BC, Lohse CM, et al. The Mayo Clinic experience with surgical management, complications and outcome for patients with renal cell carcinoma and venous tumour thrombus. *BJU Int.* 2004;94:33–41.
19. Novick AC, Streem S, Montie JE, et al. Conservative surgery for renal cell carcinoma: a single-center experience with 100 patients. *J Urol.* 1989;141:835–839.
20. Zincke H, Engen DE, Henning KM, et al. Treatment of renal cell carcinoma by in situ partial nephrectomy and extracorporeal operation with autotransplantation. *Mayo Clin Proc.* 1985;60: 651–652.
21. Thompson RH, Leibovich BC, Lohse CM, et al. Complications of contemporary open nephron sparing surgery: a single institution experience. *J Urol.* 2005;174:855–858.
22. Leibovich BC, Blute ML, Cheville JC, et al. Nephron sparing surgery for appropriately selected renal cell carcinoma between 4 and 7 cm results in outcome similar to radical nephrectomy. *J Urol.* 2004;171: 1066–1070.
23. Huang WC, Levey AS, Serio AM, et al. Chronic kidney disease after nephrectomy in patients with renal cortical tumours: a retrospective cohort study. *Lancet Oncol.* 2006;7:735–740.
24. Lau WK, Blute ML, Weaver AL, et al. Matched comparison of radical nephrectomy vs nephron-sparing surgery in patients with unilateral renal cell carcinoma and a normal contralateral kidney. *Mayo Clin Proc.* 2000;75:1236–1242.
25. Miller DC, Hollingsworth JM, Hafez KS, et al. Partial nephrectomy for small renal masses: an emerging quality of care concern? *J Urol.* 2006;175:853–857.

26. Nuttall M, Cathcart P, van der Meulen J, et al. A description of radical nephrectomy practice and outcomes in England: 1995–2002. *BJU Int.* 2005;96:58–61.

27. Gill IS, Kavoussi LR, Lane BR, et al. Comparison of 1,800 laparoscopic and open partial nephrectomies for single renal tumors. *J Urol.* 2007;178:41–46.

28. Novick AC. Renal hypothermia: in vivo and ex vivo. *Urol Clin North Am.* 1983;10:637–644.

29. Thompson RH, Frank I, Lohse CM, et al. The impact of ischemia time during open nephron sparing surgery on solitary kidneys: a multi-institutional study. *J Urol.* 2007;177:471–476.

30. Grossfeld GD, Litwin MS, Wolf JS Jr, et al. Evaluation of asymptomatic microscopic hematuria in adults: the American Urological Association best practice policy–part II: patient evaluation, cytology, voided markers, imaging, cystoscopy, nephrology evaluation, and follow-up. *Urology.* 2001;57:604–610.

31. Kipp BR, Karnes RJ, Brankley SM, et al. Monitoring intravesical therapy for superficial bladder cancer using fluorescence in situ hybridization. *J Urol.* 2005;173:401–404.

32. Zincke H, Utz DC, Taylor WF, et al. Influence of thiotepa and doxorubicin instillation at time of transurethral surgical treatment of bladder cancer on tumor recurrence: a prospective, randomized, double-blind, controlled trial. *J Urol.* 1983;129:505–509.

33. Parekh DJ, Bochner BH, Dalbagni G. Superficial and muscle-invasive bladder cancer: principles of management for outcomes assessments. *J Clin Oncol.* 2006;24:5519–5527.

34. Advanced Bladder Cancer (ABC) Meta-Analysis Collaboration. Neoadjuvant chemotherapy in invasive bladder cancer: update of a systematic review and meta-analysis of individual patient data advanced bladder cancer (ABC) meta-analysis collaboration. *Eur Urol.* 2005;48:202–206.

35. Advanced Bladder Cancer (ABC) Meta-Analysis Collaboration. Neoadjuvant chemotherapy in invasive bladder cancer: a systematic review and meta-analysis. *Lancet.* 2003;361:1927–1934.

36. Sengupta S, Myers RP, Slezak JM, et al. Preoperative prostate specific antigen doubling time and velocity are strong and independent predictors of outcomes following radical prostatectomy. *J Urol.* 2005;174:2191–2196.

37. Thompson RH, Blute ML, Slezak JM, et al. Is the GPSM scoring algorithm for patients with prostate cancer valid in the contemporary era? *J Urol.* 2007;178:459–463.

38. Lau WK, Bergstralh EJ, Blute ML, et al. Radical prostatectomy for pathological Gleason 8 or greater prostate cancer: influence of concomitant pathological variables. *J Urol.* 2002;167:117–122.

39. Inman BA, DiMarco DS, Slezak JM, et al. Outcomes of Gleason score 10 prostate carcinoma treated by radical prostatectomy. *Urology.* 2006;68:604–608.

40. Ward JF, Slezak JM, Blute ML, et al. Radical prostatectomy for clinically advanced (cT3) prostate cancer since the advent of prostate-specific antigen testing: 15-year outcome. *BJU Int.* 2005;95:751–756.

41. Cheng L, Zincke H, Blute ML, et al. Risk of prostate carcinoma death in patients with lymph node metastasis. *Cancer.* 2001;91:66–73.

42. Seay TM, Blute ML, Zincke H. Long-term outcome in patients with pTxN+ adenocarcinoma of prostate treated with radical prostatectomy and early androgen ablation. *J Urol.* 1998;159:357–364.

43. Boorjian SA, Thompson RH, Saddiqui S, et al. Long-term outcome after radical prostatectomy for patients with lymph node positive prostate cancer in the PSA era. *J Urol.* 2007;178:864–870.

44. Ward JF, Sebo TJ, Blute ML, et al. Salvage surgery for radiorecurrent prostate cancer: contemporary outcomes. *J Urol.* 2005;173:1156–1160.

45. Rabbani F, Sheinfeld J, Farivar-Mohseni H, et al. Low-volume nodal metastases detected at retroperitoneal lymphadenectomy for testicular cancer: pattern and prognostic factors for relapse. *J Clin Oncol.* 2001;19:2020–2025.

46. Foster RS, Donohue JP. Retroperitoneal lymph node dissection for the management of clinical stage I nonseminoma. *J Urol.* 2000;163:1788–1792.

47. George DW, Foster RS, Hromas RA, et al. Update on late relapse of germ cell tumor: a clinical and molecular analysis. *J Clin Oncol.* 2003;21:113–122.

48. Baniel J, Foster RS, Einhorn LH, et al. Late relapse of clinical stage I testicular cancer. *J Urol.* 1995;154:1370–1372.

55

Adjuvant and Neoadjuvant Treatment for Genitourinary Cancers

Toni K. Choueiri, Snehal G. Thakkar, and Derek Raghavan

In the past 30 years, there has been an increased use of chemotherapy early in the course of management of genitourinary malignancy in an attempt to improve cure rates by reducing the viability and size of the primary tumor and by addressing occult micrometastases. Our increasing knowledge of the natural and treated history of genitourinary cancers, and an improved precision in prognostication, has allowed us to tailor the use of systemic treatment more accurately to those localized tumors with a greater chance of systemic spread and relapse.

In this chapter, we review the evolution of prognostic markers and the development and use of systemic chemotherapy as aids to the management of clinically localized tumors with potentially increased risk of distant spread or relapse.

TESTICULAR CANCER

Dramatic progress in the management of testicular cancer has been made in the past 30 years and the expectations of cure have changed completely. Prior to 1970s, the 5-year survival rate from advanced or metastatic testicular cancer did not exceed 50% to 70% (1). Currently the 5-year survival rate exceeds 95% in both seminomatous and nonseminomatous germ cell tumors (NSGCTs) (2). The factors that led to this major achievement include a better understanding of the biology of the disease, the identification of specific tumor markers, the more precise radiographic staging, the improvements in surgical techniques, and the introduction of platinum-based combination chemotherapy. This section will focus on chemotherapy as an adjuvant therapy in patients with NSGCT and in seminoma. We have not focused on adjuvant radiotherapy for NSGCT as studies >20 years ago, from the Royal Marsden Hospital (3) and the Danish Testicular Cancer Study Group (DATECA) (4), conclusively demonstrated that adjuvant radiotherapy reduces local relapse rate in the retroperitoneum without influencing overall survival. For seminoma, adjuvant radiotherapy still has a place, and this is discussed in detail later.

ADJUVANT CHEMOTHERAPY FOR CLINICAL STAGE I AND PATHOLOGIC STAGE II NONSEMINOMATOUS GERM CELL TUMORS

Definition and Rationale

For men with testicular germ cell tumors, adjuvant chemotherapy refers to systemic treatment that is delivered following radical inguinal orchiectomy alone for clinical stage I (CS I) disease, or after a retroperitoneal lymph node dissection (RPLND) for pathologic stage II (PS II) disease. The term *CS I disease* refers to tumor that appears to be confined to the testis after negative radiographic staging with normal serum tumor markers.

The reported relapse rate after radical orchiectomy alone for CS I NSGCT is 26% to 35%, depending on the protocol of staging, the length of follow-up, and the experience of the investigators (5–10). The high success rate reported for cisplatin-based chemotherapy in the setting of metastatic disease has led to the investigation of a shorter course of chemotherapy to prevent relapse in patients with CS I disease. The theoretical goal of this adjuvant chemotherapy is to minimize the risk of relapse and to allow the avoidance of a RPLND and/or the longer course of chemotherapy usually administered for patients who relapse on surveillance. However, given that the majority of patients with CS I NSGCT are cured of their disease following radical orchiectomy, considerable attention has been devoted in the last 2 decades to identifying clinical and pathologic parameters associated with the presence of occult metastasis in the retroperitoneum or distant sites. This would allow better selection of "high-risk" patients for additional therapy after orchiectomy. That said, it is our belief that this is not the optimal route of treatment, and we prefer to observe those patients who do not undergo radical RPLND and to treat them at the time of relapse. This avoids the unnecessary use of chemotherapy for any patients who are not destined ultimately to relapse, thus avoiding unnecessary late effects (11).

High-Risk Early-Stage NSGCT

The most commonly reported risk factors for occult metastasis in the retroperitoneum or at distant sites are the presence of lymphovascular invasion and a predominant component of embryonal carcinoma. The definition of embryonal carcinoma predominance in the literature varies from 45% to 90% (12,13). The reported rate of relapse for patients with lymphovascular invasion and embryonal carcinoma predominance varies from 50% to 90% and 30% to 80%, respectively (6,8,10,12–18). In the absence of these two risk factors, the reported rate of occult metastasis is 0% to 19%. Other identified risk factors from these series include advanced pT stage (19), absence of mature teratoma (16), absence of yolk sac tumor (8), and percentage of MIB-1 staining (15).

Adjuvant Chemotherapy for High-Risk CS I Disease

Adjuvant chemotherapy in patients with high-risk CS I disease has been investigated in at least nine case series and phase 2 trials, almost all of which have used two cycles of bleomycin, etoposide, and cisplatin (BEP) chemotherapy (20–28). Several of these trials have used the lower European etoposide dose of 360 mg/m^2 per cycle (120 mg/m^2/day for days 1 to 3) while others have used the current standard dose of 500 mg/m^2 per cycle (100 mg/m^2/day for days 1 to 5). The published results suggest that primary cisplatin-based chemotherapy, predominantly using two cycles of BEP, results in very low early relapse rates in men with early-stage, high-risk NSGCT. However, only limited long-term follow-up data are available, with little definitive information about late relapses and late toxicity (23,25). In such patients, it is possible to reduce the recurrence rate from 30% to 50% to about 2.5%. This approach has been adopted by many European institutions as being preferable to RPLND (29). The largest three trials are summarized here.

The Medical Research Council (MRC) prospectively evaluated 114 patients with CS I NSGCT who were estimated to have ≥50% risk of relapse based on having three or more MRC adverse prognostic factors. The MRC prognostic factors had been prospectively validated earlier and included involvement of vascular or lymphatic structures, absence of yolk sac elements, presence of undifferentiated elements, or malignant teratoma (6,8). With a median of only 4 years of follow-up, two men (1.7%) were reported to have relapsed at 7 and 18 months, one of whom was found later not to have a germ cell tumor after a reference histopathologic review (22).

The Anglian Germ Cell Tumor Group studied, in a nonrandomized fashion, 382 men with high-risk NSGCT who underwent either surveillance between 1978 and 2000 (234 men) or two cycles of BOP (bleomycin, vincristine, and cisplatin) or BEP (148 men) between 1986 and 2000. From 1986, adjuvant chemotherapy was offered to patients at a high risk of relapse. High-risk men where defined as having at least two MRC risk factors (i.e., constituting a potentially different risk group from the preceding series). After a median follow-up of only 33 months, six patients (4%) assigned to the chemotherapy group had relapsed (26). In contrast, 30% of patients assigned to observation subsequently relapsed (28% early and 2% late relapses) after a median of follow-up of 83 months. The introduction of adjuvant

treatment only for high-risk patients made it possible to reduce the overall relapse rate of the total cohort of patients with CS I disease from 36% to 15.7% (p <0.001) (26).

Subsequently, the MRC completed a second trial evaluating two cycles of BOP in 115 men with a high risk of relapse based on the presence of vascular invasion. After a median follow-up of 70 months, three relapses occurred (2.6%), although one of these was an isolated brain lesion with normal serum tumor markers. The lesion did not change with adjuvant chemotherapy and a subsequent biopsy revealed no evidence of neoplasm (28).

We have reviewed these three trials (22,26,28) and six other published studies (20,21,23–25,27) and have found a 0% to 4% relapse rate with adjuvant chemotherapy after orchiectomy (Table 55.1). These data suggest that primary chemotherapy is associated with a very low early relapse rate, compared to observation (26% to 35% relapse rate) or RPLND (12% to 15% relapse rate (17,18). However, none of the previous studies provide a direct comparison of the three strategies, making it difficult to draw any definitive conclusions, and this is compounded by the lack of long-term follow-up data.

The early published results are provocative, but adjuvant chemotherapy is not considered standard of care for CS I NSGCT in the United States, although it is used routinely in parts of Europe. Although some American authorities argue that RPLND is the best option for high-risk men, their European counterparts assert that the high post-RPLND relapse rates seen in these men makes RPLND an inferior choice. Although it is true that RPLND and primary chemotherapy result in nearly 100% disease-specific survival (with relatively short follow-up in the latter instance), we believe that time has validated RPLND, with a paucity of late effects. As yet, the true incidence of late effects of two to three cycles of adjuvant chemotherapy has not been clearly defined, but it is clear that three cycles of standard BEP chemotherapy may be associated with significant late complications, some of which may be life-threatening (11,30). Thus we routinely advise our patients to avoid adjuvant chemotherapy for CS I NSGCT unless there are unusual circumstances, although we do inform them that adjuvant chemotherapy is used in some centers, defining the known risk-benefit ratio for them (31).

Adjuvant Chemotherapy After RPLND for PS II NSGCT

A disadvantage of administering adjuvant chemotherapy to all men with PS II (node-metastatic) disease is the risk of overtreatment. Eighty to 90 percent of men with PS IIA disease who have normal serum tumor markers prior to RPLND are cured with surgery alone; in comparison, relapse-free survival rates are up to 65% for PS IIB disease and <50% with nodal masses over 5 cm in diameter (32–34).

In the largest published study, Williams et al. (34) randomly assigned 195 patients, the majority of whom had high-volume nodal metastases, to be treated with adjuvant chemotherapy after RPLND (two cycles of a platinum-containing regimen) or to surveillance with chemotherapy (three or four cycles) given at relapse. Of the patients assigned to surveillance, 48 of 98 (49%) relapsed. However, all but three of these patients were successfully salvaged with chemotherapy. In contrast, 6 of 97 patients assigned to initial chemotherapy relapsed. With a median

Table 55.1

Published Reports of Primary Chemotherapy in Clinical Stage I Nonseminomatous Germ Cell Tumors

Study (Ref.)	No. of Patients	Risk Factors	Chemotherapy Regimen	Median Follow-up (months)	No. of Relapses	Relapse Interval (months)
Abratt et al. 1994 (20)	20	≥2 MRC risk factors	2 cycles BEP (E 360)	31	0	—
Cullen et al. 1996 (22)	114	≥3 MRC risk factors	2 cycles BEP (E 360)	48	2	7, 18
Pont et al. 1996 (21)	74	LVI	2 cycles BEP (E 500)	70	2	8, 27
Ondrus et al. 1998 (24)	18	LVI	2 cycles BEP (E 360)	36	0	—
Bohlen et al. 1999 (23)	58	LVI, EC, pT3-4	2 cycles BEP (E 360) 2 PVB (20 patients)	93	2	22, 90
Amato et al. 2004 (27)	68	VI, AFP >80, >80% EC	2 cycles CEB (E 360)	38	1	21
Chevreau et al. 2004 (25)	40	LVI EC	2 cycles BEP (E 360) 2 PVB (2 patients)	113	0	—
Oliver et al. 2004 (26)	148	≥2 MRC risk factors	1 cycle BEP (n = 28) 2 cycles BEP (46 patients) or 2 cycles BOP (n = 74). (E 360)	33	6	Not reported
Dearnaley et al. 2005 (28)	115	LVI	2 cycles BOP	70	3	3, 6, 26

MRC, Medical Research Council; BEP, bleomycin, etoposide, and cisplatin; E 360, an etoposide dose of 360 mg/m^2 per cycle; LVI, lymphovascular invasion; EC, embryonal carcinoma; PVB, cisplatin, vinblastine, and bleomycin; CEB, carboplatin, etoposide, and bleomysin; AFP, alpha-fetoprotein; E 500, an etoposide dose of 500 mg/m^2 per cycle; BOP, bleomycin, vincristine, and cisplatin.

follow-up of 4 years, survival rates were not significantly different between the two groups. Of note, one third of patients undergoing RPLND had persistently elevated serum tumor markers, and these patients accounted for half of the relapses. By today's standard, these patients should have had immediate chemotherapy and would not have been observed (32,35).

Two contemporary series from the Memorial Sloan Kettering Cancer Center showed that patients with high-volume nodal (PS IIB and IIC) disease who underwent two cycles of etoposide and cisplatin after RPLND had a 99% relapse-free survival after 8 years of follow-up (36). On the other hand, patients with low-volume disease (PS IIA) had only a 10% relapse rate with RPLND only (37).

These data have led to the general recommendation of closely monitoring patients with PS IIA disease following RPLND, while those with higher stage disease are given two to three cycles of adjuvant cisplatin and etoposide with or without bleomycin. Patients with stage IIA disease who are thought to be unlikely to comply with a surveillance schedule following RPLND are often treated with two cycles of adjuvant chemotherapy as treatment appears to reduce the risk of relapse from 10% to 20% to <2% (38–40). Once again, the paucity of data relating

to late relapse and delayed toxicity (including significant cardiovascular complications and second malignancies [41]) should make the clinician cautious when considering the use of adjuvant chemotherapy, and clearly defined, evidence-based indications should be implemented when this strategy is being considered.

ADJUVANT CHEMOTHERAPY IN CS I SEMINOMA

Approximately 15% to 20% of men with stage I seminoma who undergo surveillance after orchiectomy will develop recurrent stage II or III disease within 3 to 4 years (42). Tumor size and invasion of the rete testis have been found to be significant risk factors for relapse (43).

Because of the extreme radiosensitivity of seminoma and its utility in relapsed patients, radiation was explored as an adjuvant therapy in this disease long before the use of chemotherapy. Results were excellent, with <5% relapse at 5 years (44,45). The somewhat inconvenient schedule of radiation therapy (RT), as well as the potential for causing secondary malignancies and other side effects, prompted an interest in adjuvant chemotherapy. Cisplatin-based combination chemotherapy had already been used in advanced germ cell tumors, but was initially considered to be more toxic than radiation if used in CS I seminoma.

Several uncontrolled series have evaluated two courses of adjuvant single-agent carboplatin (46,47) and reported very few relapses at a relatively short follow-up of 5 to 6 years. A pooled analysis of published series with one or two courses of carboplatin showed <3% relapse rate in 521 patients with 100% disease-specific survival (48). The only randomized phase 3 trial that compared RT with a single dose of carboplatin (dosed at an area under the concentration × time curve of 7) was recently reported. With a median of 4 years of follow-up, this combined European Organisation for Research and Treatment of Cancer (EORTC) and MRC study showed that relapse-free survival was 95.9% in the RT arm and 94.8% in the carboplatin arm in 1,447 treated patients (no statistically significant difference). No disease-related or treatment-related deaths were reported in the carboplatin group, while only one was reported with RT. Ten patients receiving RT developed second germ cell cancers compared with only two allocated to carboplatin (49). Although this trial results suggest the potential equivalence of adjuvant carboplatin and RT for stage I seminoma, the duration of follow-up is short, and mature results are needed before a final conclusion can be drawn about these data. In addition, there was a worrisome trend of relapse in the para-aortic region with nodes ≥3 cm in the carboplatin arm (9 of 29 relapses as compared to 1 of 36 postradiation relapses). It appears also that one course of chemotherapy is associated with a more disease recurrence than two courses. In the pooled analysis previously mentioned (48), there was 4.4% relapse rare with one course compared with 2.9% in men treated with two courses of carboplatin.

Although most European institutions have adapted adjuvant chemotherapy as a gold standard following orchiectomy, most North American centers recommend RT or surveillance rather than chemotherapy for CS I seminoma, based primarily on the short follow-up with the carboplatin data and the uncertainty of long-term side effects (50). In our institution, we do not routinely employ adjuvant chemotherapy for CS I seminoma, preferring to use programs of adjuvant radiotherapy or active surveillance.

TRANSITIONAL CELL CARCINOMA OF THE BLADDER

Transitional cell carcinoma (TCC) is the most common histologic subtype of bladder cancer. Radical cystectomy with or without lymph node dissection has long been the gold standard for muscle invasive bladder cancer (51). Despite potentially curative surgery and the advances in surgical techniques, 50% of patients continue to relapse and most of these die of their disease, probably because of the presence of occult micrometastatic disease at initial presentation (52). Recent advances in understanding the underlying molecular mechanisms of bladder cancer have revealed significant heterogeneity between superficial and invasive disease. Although noninvasive disease is characterized by a

loss of heterozygosity of chromosome 9 (53), mutations in the p53 tumor suppressor gene (54) play an essential role in invasion and metastasis. Clinically, bladder cancer is also far from being a homogeneous entity as there is no unique pattern of spread that is characteristic of this disease. Bladder cancer may extend locally to the surrounding tissue and organs but also can metastasize via the lymphatic or blood vessels to distant sites (55).

Both advanced pathologic stage and lymph node involvement are associated with higher risk of recurrence (56). Other adverse prognostic factors for recurrence include the presence of carcinoma in situ (57), DNA aneuploidy (58), expression of epidermal growth factor receptor (59), perhaps the presence of high glutathione levels in the tumor (60), absence of retinoblastoma protein expression (61), and absence of p21 expression (62).

The identification of active chemotherapy agents in metastatic disease led many investigators to explore both neoadjuvant chemotherapy and classic adjuvant systemic therapy in patients with high-risk disease in order to decrease systemic progression and improve overall survival.

NEOADJUVANT CHEMOTHERAPY

The administration of neoadjuvant chemotherapy has many advantages. In theory, systemic chemotherapy may reduce the extent of local tumor, while treating occult metastases (63). It can also provide effective therapy when the burden of disease is less extensive and the patient performance status is optimal. In addition, a major advantage of this approach is the ability to assess the response of the primary lesion, which is of potential prognostic significance after cystectomy. In one study, patients with a major pathologic response (p stage <2) after neoadjuvant chemotherapy had a 5-year survival of 75% in contrast to 20% for the remaining nonresponding patients (p stage ≥2). The survival of patients with a major pathologic response was independent of the type of chemotherapy received (MVAC [methotrexate, vinblastine, doxorubicin, and cisplatin] in comparison with cisplatin plus methotrexate) or number of chemotherapy courses (64). A disadvantage of this approach is the potential delay of effective therapy if the tumor is innately chemoresistant or if the regimen is too toxic so that the patient discontinues therapy. Another disadvantage is the relative discordance between clinical and pathologic staging; in this setting, chemotherapy may not be needed if clinical understaging has occurred after cystectomy. In one report, 57% of patients treated with neoadjuvant cisplatin based chemotherapy had a clinical complete remission (CR), defined as T0 on cystoscopy. However, only 30% of patients were found to be in pathologic CR (pCR) at subsequent cystectomy, confirming the inadequacy of clinical staging in the assessment of chemotherapy response (65).

Early phase 2 trials with chemotherapy showed the feasibility of the approach and promising activity, based on tumor downstaging and some early survival data (66,67). However, most of the subsequent randomized trials (68,69) and an early meta-analysis failed to support a significant survival benefit from this strategy (70). However, most of these early reports, including the meta-analysis, used single-agent cytotoxic therapy regimens or chemotherapy regimens that are not currently considered as standard therapy in advanced bladder cancer.

Studies in the late 1980s showed higher response rates from the use of multiagent, cisplatin-based combination chemotherapy in the metastatic setting. The MVAC regimen was shown to confer a survival benefit over single-agent cisplatin in metastatic bladder cancer (71). The success of cisplatin-based, multiagent chemotherapy in advanced disease led clinicians to evaluate this concept in the neoadjuvant setting. Initial retrospective studies with MVAC demonstrated that tumor downstaging after neoadjuvant chemotherapy was associated with improved survival in patients with muscle-invasive bladder cancers, but only for those with extravesical disease (T3B or higher) (67). A series of more recent, randomized controlled trials showed somewhat mixed results with regard to survival benefit from neoadjuvant chemotherapy in bladder cancer, but nevertheless established this approach as one of the new standards of clinical care for advanced bladder cancer.

The Nordic Cooperative Bladder Cancer Study Group conducted two randomized studies. The first (Nordic I) randomized 311 patients with locally advanced bladder cancer (T1 grade 3, T2–T4a, NX, M0) to neoadjuvant chemotherapy (two cycles of cisplatin and doxorubicin) or no chemotherapy. Local therapy consisted in radical cystectomy after brief radiation (4 Gy daily for 5 consecutive days). A small improvement in overall survival ($p = 0.1$) with neoadjuvant chemotherapy was noted. In a subset analysis, patients with T3 and T4a tumors had a 15% absolute overall survival benefit ($p = 0.03$) (72). Of importance, the probability value is likely to have been influenced substantially by the relatively small case numbers.

The Nordic Cystectomy II trial studied 317 patients with stages T2–T4a, NX, M0 bladder cancer. Patients were randomly assigned to receive either three cycles of cisplatin and methotrexate, or no treatment prior to cystectomy. Despite a statistically significant improvement in tumor downstaging (26% with chemotherapy vs. 11% in the controls; $p = 0.001$) at 5.3 years of follow-up, there was no evident survival advantage ($p = 0.2$), a finding that may be explained by an inferior chemotherapy regimen or perhaps because of relatively small case numbers for this type of randomized clinical trial (73).

The Italian Bladder Tumor Study Group (GISTV) has completed two trials of neoadjuvant chemotherapy for bladder cancer (to date, to our knowledge, neither has been published in peer-reviewed form). In the first trial, 153 patients were randomized to MVEC (methotrexate, vinblastine, epirubicin, and cisplatin) before cystectomy or to cystectomy alone. At 33 months, there was no survival benefit. The accuracy of clinical compared with pathologic staging was only 42%, with over one third of patients being understaged (74). In the second trial, Bassi et al. (75) randomly assigned 206 patients to receive either four cycles of neoadjuvant MVAC or cystectomy alone. Again, at 5 years there was no survival benefit in patients who received neoadjuvant treatment. Both Italian trials lacked statistical power to show a survival advantage.

A study from Egypt, published only in an abstract format, randomly assigned 196 patients to receive neoadjuvant chemotherapy with two cycles of treatment with CMV (cisplatin, methotrexate, and vinblastine) followed by cystectomy, or cys-

tectomy alone. A preliminary report of a disease-free survival (DFS) after 5 years favored the chemotherapy arm (62% survived with chemotherapy vs. 42% without; $p = 0.013$) (76).

Of more importance, an international consortium study conducted by the MRC and the EORTC and other national groups compared radiotherapy or cystectomy (as definitive therapy) with or without initial CMV chemotherapy (77). This trial, the largest to date, enrolled 976 bladder cancer patients from 106 institutions in 20 countries with T2 G3, T3, T4a, N0–NX, M0 disease, and was designed to detect a difference in survival of at least 10% at 3 years. A total of 484 patients underwent cystectomy, 414 received external-beam radiotherapy, and 77 patients were treated with combined modality. Toxicities were generally acceptable, but with mortality from chemotherapy and surgery being 1% and 3.7%, respectively. Neoadjuvant chemotherapy was associated with a higher rate of pCR (pT0) in primary tumors (32.5% with chemotherapy vs. 12.3% no chemotherapy). The hazard ratio (HR) analysis demonstrated a 15% reduction in the risk of death with the chemotherapy regimen, equating to an absolute 3-year survival difference of 5.5% (95% confidence interval [CI]: –0.5 to 11.0; $p = 0.075$; 3-year survival was 55.5% for chemotherapy and 50.0% for local therapy alone). The authors concluded that this trial was "negative" because the result did not achieve the predefined level of clinical difference of 10%. Several factors may explain why the survival improvement was less than anticipated. The chemotherapeutic regimen used in this study is not considered a standard of care, although CMV has never been compared to MVAC regimen in a randomized trial. Moreover, >40% of patients in each group received RT alone, a practice that is considered inferior to cystectomy in North America (77). A subsequent update of this trial in 2002 reported that the favorable impact of neoadjuvant chemotherapy on survival was maintained over a median follow-up of 8 years (78).

The North American US Intergroup (INT-0080) carried out a randomized study to evaluate the role of neoadjuvant MVAC plus cystectomy compared with cystectomy alone (79). Over an 11-year period only 317 patients with T2-T4a N0M0 were enrolled in this multi-institutional trial. Although at least one third of patients had severe hematologic and gastrointestinal toxicity, no deaths were attributed to chemotherapy and there appeared to be no increase rates of postoperative complications. With a median follow-up of 8.4 years, an intention-to-treat analysis demonstrated a median survival of 46 months in the surgery-alone group compared with 77 months in the chemotherapy group. (HR, 0.74; CI: 0.55-0.95). Overall survival between the groups was significantly different when a one-sided log rank test was used, but this difference was reduced with a two-sided test ($p = 0.06$). Of note, 38% of patients treated with combined modality were in pT0 stage compared with only 15% of patients who had cystectomy alone ($p < 0.001$). At 5 years, 85% of patients with pT0 were alive, suggesting that the survival benefit is strongly related to downstaging of the tumor. Although this study showed a survival benefit from neoadjuvant chemotherapy, several caveats should be considered such as the modest difference in absolute death rate and the possibility of stage migration with the slow accrual (79).

Despite the fact that all the previously mentioned trials are plagued with many problems such as poor design, execution,

Table 55.2

Selected Randomized Trials of Neoadjuvant Chemotherapy in Bladder Cancer

Study (Ref.)	Sample Size	No. of Patients	Definitive Treatment	Chemotherapy Regimen	Survival	Comments
Nordic I Malmstrom et al. 1996 (72)	325	T1 G3, T2-T4a, Nx, M0	Low-dose XRT (20 Gy) + Cystectomy	Cisplatin + doxorubicin × 2	At 5 years: OS: 59% vs. 51% ($p = 0.1$)	OS benefit in T3/T4 ($p = 0.03$)
Nordic II Sherif et al. 2002 (73)	317	T2 G3, T2-T4, Nx, M0	Cystectomy	Cisplatin + methotrexate × 2	At 5 years: OS: 53% vs. 46% ($p = 0.2$)	Tumor downstaging pT0: 26% vs. 11% ($p = 0.001$)
Italian Study Group I Cortesi et al. 1995 (74)	171	T2-T4, N0, M0	Cystectomy	MVEC	At 33 months: no difference in OS or DFS	Accuracy of clinical vs. pathologic staging is 42% only
Italian Study Group II Bassi et al. 1999 (75)	206	T2-T4, Nx, M0	Cystectomy	MVAC × 4	At 5 years: OS: 55% vs. 54%	One third of patients received suboptimal chemotherapy because of toxicity
Abol Enein et al. 1997 (76)	196	T2-T4, Nx, M0	Cystectomy	Carboplatin + methotrexate vinblastine × 2	At 5 years: DFS: 62% vs. 42% ($p = 0.013$)	14% pT0 in chemotherapy patients
Hall et al. 1999 (77,78)	976	T2 G3, T2-T4a, Nx, M0	XRT (60 Gy) or cystectomy	CMV × 3	At 3 years: 55.5% vs. 50% ($p = 0.075$)	32.5% pT0 in chemotherapy patients
SWOG 8710 Grossman et al. 2003 (79)	317	T2 G3, T2-T4a, N0, M0	Cystectomy	MVAC × 3	At 5 years: 57% vs. 43% ($p = 0.06$)	Tumor downstaging pT0: 38% vs. 15% ($p < 0.001$)

XRT, external-beam radiation therapy; OS, overall survival; MVEC, methotrexate, vinblastine, epirubicin, and cisplatin; DFS, disease-free survival; MVAC, methotrexate, vinblastine, doxorubicin, and cisplatin; MRC, Medical Research Council; EORTC, European Organisation for Research and Treatment of Cancer; CMV, cisplatin, methotrexate, and vinblastine; SWOG, Southwest Oncology Group.

and accrual, the use of one-sided probability values, different chemotherapy regimens, small survival advantage, the conclusion remains that neoadjuvant chemotherapy, mostly specifically the MVAC regimen, reduces the death rate for deeply invasive bladder cancer at a statistically significant level. A summary of selected randomized neoadjuvant studies is presented in Table 55.2.

A recent meta-analysis in a 2005 Cochrane database review included 3,005 individuals enrolled in 11 randomized trials comparing neoadjuvant chemotherapy with local therapy alone. Chemotherapy with cisplatin-based combinations showed a significant benefit in overall survival with a 14% reduction in risk of death, and a 5% (from 45% to 50%) absolute benefit at 5 years (HR, 0.86; 95% CI: 0.77-0.95; $p = 0.003$). This survival benefit was achieved irrespective of the type of surgical or radiotherapy treatment administered (80). There was also a significant DFS benefit associated with platinum-based combination chemotherapy (HR, 0.78; 95% CI: 0.71-0.86; $p < 0.0001$), equivalent to a 9% absolute improvement at 5 years. Another meta-analysis from Canada included 2,605 patients and showed that platinum-based combination chemotherapy produced an

absolute improvement in overall survival of 6.5% from 50% to 56.5% ($p = 0.006$) (81).

Neoadjuvant Chemotherapy for Bladder Preservation

Neoadjuvant chemotherapy with or without bladder radiation or chemoradiation has been administered to patients with muscle-invasive bladder cancer as a bladder-preserving strategy. Many phase 2 studies showed the feasibility of this approach in carefully selected individuals (lower T stage, absence of hydronephrosis or nodal metastases) who achieve a pCR with neoadjuvant chemotherapy. Overall, 60% of patients achieved long-term survival, two thirds of whom had preserved normal bladder function (82–85). However, it should be noted that there is heavy case selection in these series, and there is often the continued addition of new patients in serial updates, making the long-term survival data less robust.

The Radiation Therapy Oncology Group (RTOG) studied, in a randomized trial, the impact of two cycles of neoadjuvant CMV chemotherapy on a chemoradiation regimen that used concurrent 39.6-Gy pelvic irradiation with concurrent cisplatin 100 mg/m^2 for two courses 3 weeks apart (86). Neoadjuvant chemotherapy, most specifically the MVAC regimen, was not shown to increase the rate of CR or 5-year overall survival over that achieved with standard induction therapy. This study did not complete the planned accrual of 174 patients to detect a 20% difference in bladder-intact survival, and therefore lacked statistical power. On subgroup analysis, patients without hydronephrosis displayed a trend toward improved overall survival (54 vs. 33%; $p = 0.02$) and bladder-intact survival (43 vs. 26%; $p = 0.06$). However, one should be cautious when interpreting subgroup analysis results.

We believe that, in 2009, the state of the art of treatment for deeply invasive transitional cell cancer of the bladder should be neoadjuvant MVAC chemotherapy, followed by cystectomy. At the present time, it is not possible to comment on the respective merits of neoadjuvant chemotherapy/cystectomy versus radical cystectomy followed by adjuvant chemotherapy. Investigators at the M.D. Anderson Cancer Center attempted to resolve this issue in a comparison of neoadjuvant chemotherapy followed by cystectomy versus cystectomy plus adjuvant chemotherapy (87,88). This trial accrued 140 patients who were randomized to receive MVAC chemotherapy before or after radical cystectomy. Despite the fact that 28% of patients achieved pCR with neoadjuvant chemotherapy, there was no survival difference identified between the two arms ($p = 0.54$). However, as patients receiving neoadjuvant chemotherapy were also treated with two cycles of adjuvant MVAC, this trial really did not address the neoadjuvant versus adjuvant question, but simply showed that the timing of surgery, within a sequence of several cycles of chemotherapy, is probably not important.

ADJUVANT CHEMOTHERAPY

The use of adjuvant therapy in bladder cancer holds the theoretical benefit of preventing relapse after definitive therapy by treating micrometastatic disease. Adjuvant therapy offers the advantage of an accurate pathologic staging (56), therefore limiting chemotherapy-induced toxicity to only those patients who truly require it. Additionally, a strategy of adjuvant chemotherapy also limits the unnecessary delay for potentially curative surgery.

A retrospective analysis from the M.D. Anderson Cancer Center (89) analyzed 71 high-risk bladder cancer patients (pelvic visceral invasion, lymphovascular invasion, lymph node metastases, extravesical tumor extension) who received adjuvant chemotherapy with cyclophosphamide, doxorubicin and cisplatin (CISCA regimen) after radical cystectomy. A significant DFS benefit was observed in the adjuvant group when compared with 62 control patients with similar high-risk features (70% vs. 37%, respectively; $p = 0.00012$), but overall survival was not addressed. Despite the fact that no clear conclusions can be drawn from a retrospective review, the potential of adjuvant chemotherapy in the context of high-risk patients was intriguing. Subsequent prospective trials were initiated to confirm the potential advantage of this approach.

Skinner et al. (90) randomized 91 patients to adjuvant chemotherapy versus observation following cystectomy. The chemotherapy regimen was heterogeneous and included CISCA regimen, single-agent cisplatin, and other chemotherapy regimens selected by clonogenic survival assays. Median survival was 4.3 years in the chemotherapy arm versus 2.4 years in the control arm ($p = 0.0062$ by Wilcoxon test). However, the 3-year survival with adjuvant chemotherapy (66%) was not statistically superior ($p = 0.09$) to surgery alone (50%). This trial has been heavily criticized for the lack of statistical power, the extremely low accrual rate (91 patients over 8 years) with the potential selection bias, the lack of adherence to predefined chemotherapy regimens, and the use of Wilcoxon statistics that emphasizes early, nonsustained, survival differences (55).

A subsequent trial conducted in Germany by Stockle et al. (91) randomized 49 patients with locally advanced bladder carcinoma (pT3b, pT4a and/or pN1 or pN2) to observation (with no standard option of receiving any chemotherapy upon relapse) or three cycles of MVAC or MVEC. This trial was prematurely closed secondary to an interim analysis that demonstrated a significant progression-free survival (PFS) advantage for those patients receiving chemotherapy (63% vs. 13%; $p = 0.0015$), which was especially pronounced in those patients with node-positive disease. Unfortunately, this trial has also been criticized because of many methodologic flaws. It took 3.5 years to accrue 49 patients, and of the 26 patients in the chemotherapy group, 8 did not receive treatment. A subsequent update added nonrandomized patients to the first report and analyzed 166 patients, 80 of whom underwent adjuvant chemotherapy (92). A significant PFS ($p = 0.004$) continued to be observed. However, the second report is seriously flawed owing to the obvious case selection bias in a nonrandomized comparison. Finally, the fact that the patients on the observation arm were not permitted to receive chemotherapy at any time after surgery made it a study of "any" chemotherapy rather than adjuvant chemotherapy.

A trial by the Swiss Group for Cancer Research (93) randomized 77 patients with muscle-invasive bladder cancer to observation or cisplatin monotherapy (three courses of 90 mg/m^2 of cisplatin given for 3 consecutive days at monthly intervals). The 5-year overall survivals in both groups were similar (54% for the cisplatin group vs. 57% for the controls; $p = 0.65$). The small numbers of patients as well as the fact that 19% of patients allocated to chemotherapy did not receive it, make the results of this study difficult to interpret.

A study reported by Freiha et al. (94) from Stanford University randomly allocated patients with extravesical disease after cystectomy (pT3b, T4 with or without lymph node involvement) to observation or to treatment with adjuvant CMV chemotherapy. This study was closed early (after 55 patients were accrued) because of a large DFS benefit favoring the chemotherapy arm (37 vs. 12 months; $p = 0.01$). Unfortunately, however, this did not translate into a statistically significant difference in median survival between the two groups (63 vs. 36 months; $p = 0.32$). This is another example of an underpowered study with early closure before achieving the predetermined target of 80 patients.

Finally, it is worth mentioning that investigators in Taiwan have also reported their experience with cystectomy for invasive bladder cancer, followed by six cycles of CMV chemotherapy. Long-term survival reached only 50%, suggesting the absence of any substantial impact on survival from adjuvant chemotherapy, at least in this selected population of patients (95).

There is no current consensus on the true role of adjuvant chemotherapy for invasive bladder cancer. Clinical trials have been flawed but generally have suggested a PFS benefit (17% to 50%) without a statistically significant overall survival benefit (96). Final recommendations will require the completion of clinical studies that are currently in progress. One trial conducted by the EORTC, comparing adjuvant chemotherapy with MVAC and gemcitabine after cystectomy versus delayed chemotherapy at relapse, was inconclusive due to early closure because of poor accrual. Consequent upon preliminary data from the University of Southern California, selection of candidates for adjuvant chemotherapy based on molecular factors is an interesting concept that has been tested in a Southwest Oncology Group (SWOG) trial. Patients with T1-2 disease and overexpression/mutation of *p53*, a tumor suppressor gene correlated with tumor progression, are treated with three cycles of MVAC. In addition, the Cancer and Leukemia group B (CALGB) and the Eastern Cooperative Oncology Group (ECOG) have decided that gemcitabine/cisplatin (GC) chemotherapy should be the standard arm in a randomized trial. This intergroup study plans to enroll 800 high-risk patients at cystectomy to be randomized to either GC or dose-dense doxorubicin/gemcitabine followed by paclitaxel/cisplatin. The rationale behind this trial is based on the Norton-Simon hypothesis, wherein dose-dense therapy leads to greater tumor kill than conventionally dosed regimens. The potential problem in this trial is that no true standard of adjuvant chemotherapy has been defined, and it is not clear that GC should really be viewed as a control arm in the adjuvant setting.

For patients presenting after radical cystectomy with node-positive disease, the potential benefits and risks need to be discussed and documentation regarding such discussion should be carefully entered into the chart. We do not have a "standard" approach in this setting, although we tend to use adjuvant chemotherapy more liberally in younger, healthier patients, and in those with more extensive lymph node involvement. In this setting, we make clear that a standard of care has not been defined in the adjuvant context. However, it should not be forgotten that Stein and Skinner (96) have demonstrated that patients with lymph node metastases can be cured by surgery alone, and this observation should be considered when contemplating the role of adjuvant chemotherapy.

PROSTATE CANCER

Neoadjuvant and Adjuvant Therapy

Patients with prostate cancer are at risk of developing local and systemic disease recurrence, presumably owing to the presence of occult micrometastatic disease at initial presentation (97). The identification of novel biological, targeted, and chemotherapeutic agents with activity in advanced prostate cancer has led many clinical investigators to evaluate the concept of both adjuvant and neoadjuvant therapy in patients with locally advanced disease in an attempt to decrease systemic progression.

The administration of systemic therapy in the neoadjuvant setting has a number of advantages, including the potential to achieve a pathologically determined complete remission at the time of surgery, and the delivery of systemic therapy while the burden of micrometastatic disease is minimal. Potential disadvantages of this approach include unnecessarily treating individuals whose disease is overstaged and the time delay to radical

prostatectomy (RP) if systemic therapy is either ineffective or results in significant therapy-related toxicity. Furthermore, several predictive models can be used to better identify patients at significant risk who may benefit from multimodality approaches. These nomograms have been extensively tested, validated, and are used daily by many clinicians around the world. Adjuvant treatment also theoretically diminishes relapse rates from eradication of micrometastatic sites and has the advantage of definitive staging and no time delay to curative treatment.

New approaches, using more targeted, and thereby, less toxic drugs in the neoadjuvant and adjuvant setting are in progress. Several of the targeted agents include growth factor inhibitors, angiogenesis inhibitors, antioxidants, and inducers of apoptosis. The use of systemic therapy (hormonal and chemotherapy) has been well studied. This section will focus on the use of neoadjuvant and adjuvant therapy in patients with prostate cancer.

Neoadjuvant Therapy in Prostate Cancer
Neoadjuvant Hormonal Therapy Prior to Radical Prostatectomy

Since the early report by Huggins et al. (98) in 1941, androgen deprivation therapy (ADT) has gained widespread use in patients with metastatic prostate cancer. Whether an impact of hormones could be demonstrated in earlier disease had yet to be studied. Preclinical studies, including one by Gleave et al. (99), demonstrated a 50% reduction in local recurrence rates when mice had been castrated prior to definitive resection. A further, more recent analysis with similar animal models again demonstrated a significant delay ($p < 0.001$) in tumor recurrence with early castration (100).

A complete pathologic assessment is the ideal standard to compare disease stage and to predict outcomes. However, this is limited in the neoadjuvant setting because of the low accuracy of clinical staging (101,102). Other prognostic factors including tumor stage, tumor grade, and preoperative prostate-specific antigen (PSA) have been shown to correlate with pathologic stage (103). Using these factors, patients with low-risk tumors (Gleason score ≤6, PSA ≤10, stage <T2b) would benefit least from neoadjuvant therapy (103–106).

In intermediate and higher risk patients, several randomized trials have attempted to quantify potential benefits (Table 55.3). The majority of these studies used a 3-month neoadjuvant treatment period prior to definitive therapy. Labrie et al. (107) enrolled 161 patients with intermediate and high-risk prostate cancer patients to receive combined androgen blockade (CAB) with flutamide and luteinizing hormone-releasing hormone agonist or observation. This study demonstrated a significant impact on the postoperative positive surgical margins for patients treated in a neoadjuvant fashion with CAB as compared with controls (3% vs. 8%; $p < 0.001$), but with no overall survival benefit. A similar patient population enrolled in the European Study Group trial, treated with CAB, suggested no survival benefit in the whole cohort despite a benefit in decreasing positive surgical margins in patients with T2 tumors as compared with T3 tumors (108).

Additionally, Soloway et al. (109) reported on 5-year follow up data outlining the results of their experience after neoadjuvant

Table 55.3

Neoadjuvant Hormonal Therapy Prior to Surgery in Prostate Cancer[a]

Study (Ref.)	Sample Size	Clinical Stage	GS (Mean Therapy vs. Control)	Pre-PSA (ng/mL) (Mean Therapy Group vs. Mean Control)	Neoadjuvant Therapy	Post-PSA (ng/mL) (Mean Therapy Group vs. Mean Control)	Positive Margins (Therapy vs. Control)	Seminal Vesicle Involvement	Lymph Node Involvement (Therapy vs. Control)
Labrie et al. 1997 (107)	161	T2-3	NR	NR	CAB	NR	7.8% vs. 33.8% (p <0.001)	NR	NR
Witjes et al. 1997 (108)	354	T2-3	NR	20 vs. NR	CAB	0.08 vs. NR	27% vs. 46% (p <0.01)	NR	13% vs. 23% (p = 0.01)
Soloway et al. 2002 (109)	303	T2b	6.1 vs. 5.8	14.3 vs. 12.5	CAB	NS (used 0.4 as cutoff)	18% vs. 48% (p <0.001)	15% vs. 22% (p = NS)	6% vs. 9% (p = NS)
Klotz et al. 2000 (113)	213	T1b-2c	15% vs. 12%[a]	45% vs. 41%[b]	Antiandrogen	Not specifically reported	28% vs. 65% (p = 0.001)	10% vs.12% (p = NR)	7% vs. 3% (p = NS)

GS, Gleason score; PSA, prostate-specific antigen; NR, not reported; CAB, combined androgen blockade (flutamide plus luteinizing hormone-releasing hormone agonist); NS, not significant.

[a]Reported as ≥8.

[b]Reported as ≥10.

[c]Results combined for positive margins and/or seminal vesicle involvement.

CAB. Consistent with the previous reports there was a significant improvement in the positive margin status between patients treated with CAB and controls (18% vs. 48%; p <0.001). Unfortunately, the study also did not demonstrate an improved survival outcome. In fact, patients treated with CAB who had negative surgical margins had an increased rate of biochemical failure compared with controls with negative surgical margins after surgery. A possible explanation may be due to the inability of the pathologist to accurately characterize the margins of the androgen-ablated prostate tissue after resection (110). It is also possible that the failure to achieve true overall survival benefit from this approach to neoadjuvant treatment was because of the limited duration of treatment, as surgeons often prefer to reduce toxic side effects associated with their surgery (e.g., impotency from hormones that might confound the apparent limited effects of nerve-sparing prostatectomy).

At least two studies have reported on the long-term use of neoadjuvant therapy (>3 months) (111,112). In the PROSIT study, patients were randomized to neoadjuvant treatment of with CAB (luteinizing hormone-releasing hormone plus bicalutamide) for 3 or 6 months followed by RP, or RP alone. The rates of positive surgical margins were significantly less in the neoadjuvant group (control vs. 3 months, 47% vs. 26%, $p = 0.003$; control vs. 6 months, 47% vs. 19%, p <0.001), although not significantly different between the two neoadjuvant groups (3 months vs. 6 months; 26% vs. 19%; $p = 0.295$).

A study by the Canadian Uro-Oncologic Group (CUOG) randomized patients to either 3 or 8 months of neoadjuvant therapy with cyproterone acetate followed by RP (113). After only 1 year of follow-up, positive margins were significantly lower in the 8-month group as compared to the 3-month group (12% vs. 23%; $p = 0.0106$), as was the incidence of positive lymph nodes (0.4% vs. 3.1%; $p = 0.038$). Unfortunately, in the absence of a control group, no direct comparison could be made between neoadjuvant therapy and immediate RP. Although more mature results are pending, an extended duration of neoadjuvant ADT therapy seems reasonable.

A meta-analysis published in 2000 analyzed the routine use of neoadjuvant hormonal therapy prior to RP (114). Although six of the seven studies reviewed noted a decrease in the positive surgical margins rate, no significant improvement in outcome to support the routine administration of neoadjuvant hormonal therapy before prostatectomy was observed.

Despite the abundance of data, no definitive conclusion can be made as to the role of neoadjuvant hormonal therapy prior to RP. Although neoadjuvant ADT impacts the rate of positive surgical margins, benefits in survival have not been demonstrated. As such, the routine use of neoadjuvant hormonal therapy prior to definitive RP is not recommended outside a clinical trial context.

Neoadjuvant Chemotherapy Prior to Radical Prostatectomy

In 1996, a palliative benefit with chemotherapy was demonstrated with a combination of mitoxantrone and prednisone in hormone-refractory prostate cancer patients, although no survival benefit was noted in view of the cross-over design of the study (115). In 2004, two subsequent randomized phase 3 trials were reported (SWOG 9916 and TAX 327) comparing docetaxel

(plus estramustine in SWOG 9916) to standard mitoxantrone in hormone-refractory prostate cancer patients (116,117). A modest 2 to 2.5 months of improvement in median survival in the docetaxel arm (given every 3 weeks) was reported in both studies (SWOG 9916: 17.5 vs. 15.6 months, $p = 0.02$; TAX 327: 18.9 vs. 16.5 months, $p = 0.009$). The HR for death in both studies demonstrated an approximate 20% reduction in death with the docetaxel regimen (SWOG 9916 HR = 0.80, TAX 327 HR = 0.76). The global experience with the modern generation of cytotoxic agents suggests that there is anticancer efficacy against prostate cancer, and that modest clinical, palliative, and survival gains can be achieved from the use of such treatment. Of interest, the level of activity of these agents against prostate cancer is quite similar to that shown against breast cancer in the 1970s, which culminated in the routine implementation of cytotoxic regimens as adjuvant treatment for node-positive breast cancer.

Numerous phase 1/2 trials were initiated in early prostate cancer treatment including the neoadjuvant setting after the initial clinical benefit for chemotherapy was established in 1996. Two trials in particular reported on the single-agent use of a taxane (docetaxel) in the neoadjuvant setting. Dreicer et al. (118) and Febbo et al. (119) reported trials from the Cleveland Clinic and the Dana Farber Cancer Institute, respectively. Although similar in design, the study by Dreicer et al. used high-dose docetaxel for a short course (60 mg/m^2 weekly $\times$ 6 weeks), as compared to Febbo et al., who used a standard dose of docetaxel for a prolonged period (36 mg/m^2 weekly $\times$ 6 months). No pCR was demonstrated for any patient in either study on histologic examination of the prostate. This was consistent with the results of other neoadjuvant trials. To date, no phase 3 randomized controlled trials have been completed to address outcomes when using neoadjuvant chemotherapy. A conglomerate of phase 1/2 clinical trials has only confirmed that neoadjuvant chemotherapy trials are feasible and safe to perform.

Currently, the CALGB 90203 study is planning to enroll 700 high-risk patients (as defined from the Kattan nomogram to have a 60% biochemical failure at 5 years [106]) to receive docetaxel with prednisone for six cycles in an attempt to answer the question regarding the potential benefit of neoadjuvant chemotherapy in high-risk prostate cancer. In addition, the Dana Farber Cancer Institute has neared accrual for a phase 2 neoadjuvant study with docetaxel and vascular endothelial growth factor (VEGF) inhibitor bevacizumab. Other than in the context of a clinical trial, we do not recommend the routine use of neoadjuvant chemotherapy in the treatment of prostate cancer.

Adjuvant Therapy in Prostate Cancer

Adjuvant Hormonal Therapy After Radical Prostatectomy

Several studies have attempted to address the issue of early hormonal therapy in patients who have undergone definitive therapy with RP. Approximately 40% of men with localized prostate cancer are treated initially with RP (120). The early use of hormonal therapy in these patients was initially reported in the 1960s. The evaluation from the Veterans Administration Cooperative Group reported that early hormonal ablation after RP did not impact overall survival (121). However, newer hormonal agents renewed interest in hormonal manipulation in the adjuvant setting for prostate cancer (122,123). Subsequent trials again addressing this issue were undertaken.

Myers et al. (124) reported on 62 patients with a median follow-up of >10 years on the use of adjuvant hormonal manipulation after a retropubic RP. In their report, 62 patients with lymph node-positive adenocarcinoma of the prostate were divided with respect to DNA ploidy status and the use of early hormonal manipulation. The results were significant in that those patients with diploid (normal DNA) cancers who received early hormones had a statistically significant improved DFS (p <0.001) and tumor-specific mortality ($p = 0.03$). In patients with nondiploid tumors (tetraploid or aneuploid), DFS and tumor-specific mortality were not significantly improved ($p = 0.06$ and $p = 0.46$, respectively). Although this was a small study, the benefit of early hormonal manipulation on a subset of patients was intriguing. Further evaluation as to the impact of DNA ploidy in prostate cancer has yet to be determined (125,126).

A subsequent retrospective analysis was carried out by the Mayo Clinic and reported in 1998 (127). In this analysis, 790 men who were treated with RP and found to have node-positive disease were reviewed. Of the 790 patients, 96 were followed with observation alone (9 of the 96 had received additional RT). Patients with diploid tumors had a statistically significant improvement in disease-specific mortality when treated with hormonal therapy beyond 10 years (p <0.002).

A prospective trial by Messing et al. (128) randomized 98 patients with node-positive disease between 1988 and 1993 to either ADT (either surgical castration or biochemical with monthly goserelin injections) or observation following RP. After a follow-up of 7 years, an overall survival and cancer-specific survival was noted, with 65% of the patients alive in the observation arm versus 85% in the treatment arm ($p = 0.02$). Seventy-seven percent in the ADT group and 18% in the observation group had no evidence of recurrent disease at the time of last follow-up (p <0.001). Several limitations of this study must be acknowledged, including that the accrual goal of 220 patients was not attained. In addition, pathology review was not centralized, contributing potentially to an imbalance between the two arms and a selection bias. One must be cautious when interpreting these results pending longer-term survival data, although it appears that these investigators have defined a new standard of care as they form the basis of several ongoing randomized trials incorporating adjuvant hormonal care as the standard arm.

Further investigation of the role of adjuvant ADT has been undertaken in the Early Prostate Cancer study. Patients with T1-4NxM0 prostate cancer were enrolled in a multicenter, international, randomized clinical trial. The evaluation of high-dose bicalutamide (150 mg daily) as an adjuvant to RP or radiation as well as a comparison to watchful waiting was undertaken. The long-term results of the North American arm of the trial (0023) were recently reported after a median 7.7-year follow-up (129). Eligible patients enrolled in North America (3,292 patients: ≈80% RP, ≈20% radiotherapy) demonstrated no significant difference in mortality between treatment and control groups (12.9% vs. 12.3%) as well as no difference in objective progression (15.4% vs. 15.3%). There was, however, a significant benefit in the treatment group for time to PSA progression

(HR, 0.80; p <0.001). These findings were not consistent with the results of the of the experience in other sites (Europe, Scandinavia, and others) that demonstrated significant improved objective PFS with the use of adjuvant bicalutamide (129). However, the North American trial did not enroll patients who were followed with watchful waiting, making the comparison between different sites and arms difficult.

Adjuvant Chemotherapy After Radical Prostatectomy

The role of chemotherapy as an adjuvant treatment for high-risk prostate cancer has been the focus of several trials. Early adjuvant chemotherapy studies have reported inconclusive results. One study published by the National Prostate Cancer Project (NPCP) randomized patients to either estramustine, cyclophosphamide, or observation for 2 years following definitive RT (Protocol 900) or RP (Protocol 1000) (130,131). Adjuvant cyclophosphamide had no significant impact in either protocol. In the estramustine arms, however, adjuvant treatment after radiation in node-positive patients had improved recurrence rates, compared with observation (60% vs. 81%; p <0.05). Unfortunately, this trial was underpowered to make definitive conclusions (132).

A second small, nonrandomized, under-powered study by Wang et al. (133) compared hormonal therapy with or without chemotherapy with mitoxantrone and prednisone in 96 patients with pT3-T4 disease. The results significantly favored overall survival in the chemotherapy arm (median overall survival, 84 vs. 41 months; $p = 0.028$).

Two large randomized trials are currently underway to definitively address this issue, including the SWOG 9921 (adjuvant androgen deprivation vs. androgen deprivation plus mitoxantrone/prednisone) and the TAX 3501 (arm 1, androgen deprivation; arm 2, androgen deprivation plus docetaxel; arm 3, no adjuvant therapy).

Although there is no clear consensus, most uro-oncologists in centers of excellence in North America recommend the use of adjuvant hormonal therapy in patients with lymph node-positive disease who have undergone RP with lymphadenectomy. The exact duration of therapy is not known, although most patients in the study by Messing et al. (128) underwent lifelong androgen deprivation. The results of the current randomized trials assessing duration of hormonal therapy for advanced disease will probably shape clinical practice in the adjuvant setting.

In patients without lymph node-positive disease, there is no conclusive evidence to support the use of adjuvant hormonal therapy after definitive therapy with RP. The role for adjuvant chemotherapy in this context is still under investigation.

Adjuvant ADT After Radiation Therapy

One of the earlier trials assessing the role of hormonal therapy after definitive radiation was the RTOG 8531 study. This study randomized 945 patients with locally advanced prostate cancer (lymph node-positive disease or cT3) to receive ADT indefinitely as an adjunct to definitive radiation. The updated results from this study after a median follow-up of 7.6 years demonstrated a statistically significant improvement in overall survival (49% vs. 39%; $p = 0.002$) and disease-specific mortality (24% vs. 39%; p <0.001) favoring the adjuvant treatment group (134,135).

This study had some limitations because 139 patients received a prior RP and, in addition, this trial was conducted in the pre-PSA era, making translation to current practice more difficult (134).

A subsequent landmark trial by the EORTC did have more conclusive results. The EORTC 22863 enrolled 415 node-negative patients with T3/4 tumors or high-grade (grade 3) T1/2 tumors and was reported by Bolla et al. (137). This study randomized patients to either adjuvant hormonal therapy with goserelin for a total of 3 years or observation after definitive radiation (136). The most updated results from this study did confirm an overall survival benefit for adjuvant hormonal therapy (78% vs. 62%; $p = 0.0002$) as well as a DFS benefit (74% vs. 40%; $p = 0.0001$).

D'Amico et al. (98) randomized 206 patients with clinically localized prostate cancer to receive hormonal therapy or observation after definitive radiation. Eligible patients included those with a PSA of at least 10 ng/mL, a Gleason score of at least 7, or radiographic evidence of extraprostatic disease. Hormonal therapy with leuprolide or goserelin combined with a nonsteroidal anti-androgen flutamide was begun 2 months prior to irradiation initiation and continued for a total of 6 months. After a median follow-up of about 4.5 years there was statistically significant advantage favoring the combination treatment group in terms of freedom from salvage therapy (82% vs. 57%; $p = 0.002$), cancer-specific mortality (0% vs. 5%; $p = 0.02$), and overall survival (88% vs. 78%; $p = 0.04$). Because of the small number of patients, the outcomes hinge on the behavior of a few patients, hence introducing a potential bias. In fact, a large single-institution retrospective review refutes these data and suggests that adjuvant hormonal therapy, despite any type of definitive radiation, does not impact low- or intermediate-risk patients (138). Nevertheless, this is still a model for future trials in the treatment of intermediate-risk disease (and possibly high-risk patients as defined in the RTOG 8531, RTOG 9413, and EORTC studies) wherein patients can potentially be treated with shorter hormonal therapy courses (98,139).

The consensus among many genitourinary oncology clinicians at this time is to use adjuvant hormonal therapy as per D'Amico et al. (98) for 6 months in the intermediate disease setting after definitive RT. In the high-risk patients, the data are not so clearly defined. The general understanding is that there is a definitive benefit for adjuvant hormonal therapy after definitive radiation in this group. The duration of therapy is still up for debate. Pending future studies, at least 6 months of adjuvant ADT after definitive RT should be considered as standard in high-risk patients.

RENAL CELL CARCINOMA

Renal cell carcinoma (RCC) accounts for >30,000 new cases of cancer and >12,000 deaths in the United States annually (140). One third of RCC patients have metastatic disease at the time of diagnosis (141). The 5-year overall survival of all RCC patients is 40% to 45% and has not appreciably improved in over 30 years (142). The prognosis for patients with RCC is primarily dependent on disease stage. Organ-confined disease (pathologic stage pT1-2) confers the best prognosis, with 5-year cancer-specific survival rates after nephrectomy ranging from

71% to 97% (143). For patients with locally advanced tumors, 5-year cancer-specific survival rates after nephrectomy decrease to 20% to 53% (143), and once RCC has metastasized, the 5-year survival rate is <10% (144,145).

Moreover, metastatic disease has been shown to be resistant to chemotherapy (146), radiotherapy (147), and hormonal therapy (148). Biologic therapies such as interferon-alpha (IFN-α) and interleukin-2 (IL-2) demonstrated objective responses in 15% to 25% of patients with disseminated metastases with only 5% of patients experiencing durable complete remissions (149). In addition to tumor stage, clearly defined prognostic factors, both prior to surgery and after surgery have been identified, including tumor grade, performance status, histology, and more recently genetic and molecular markers like carbonic anhydrase IX, PTEN, pAKT, and others (150). Integrated staging systems and nomograms based on the TNM staging and other clinical factors have also been developed to better stratify patients into prognostic categories (151,152). Based on these prognostic determinants, high-risk tumors can be identified around the time of surgery, giving rise to consideration of the role of adjuvant treatment.

Adjuvant Therapy
Biologic Therapies

In view of the reported activity of biologic agents in metastatic RCC and the high risk of recurrence for patients with locally advanced disease, investigators evaluated the role of adjuvant IFN-α or IL-2 or after complete resection of the primary tumor. Unfortunately, at least five randomized trials failed to demonstrate a survival benefit from this approach (153–157).

The largest trial, conducted by the ECOG, randomly assigned 283 patients with stage T3b, T3c, T4, and/or N1 to N3 disease to IFN-α therapy or observation. At a median follow-up of 10.4 years, adjuvant IFN-α was not associated with a significant improvement in either disease-free or overall survival with even a trend toward a worse survival in the treatment arm (median survival was 7.4 years in the observation arm and 5.1 years in the treatment arm; log-rank $p = .09$) (153). The reasons patients treated with IFN-α tended toward worse initial survival were not readily apparent from toxicity data because there were no lethal toxicities from treatment (153).

Similarly, an Italian trial randomized 247 patients to receive IFN-α or to observation following nephrectomy for Robson stages II or III RCC. The 5-year overall and event-free survival probabilities were 66.5% and 67%, respectively, for controls and 66% and 56.7%, respectively, for the treated group; the differences were not statistically significant ($p = .861$ for overall and $p = .107$ for event-free survival with the log-rank test) (154).

IFN-α was tested in a third randomized trial from Germany that assigned 203 patients with resected stage III disease or a completely resected local recurrence or solitary metastasis to IFN-α plus 5-fluorouracil, 8 weeks of low-dose subcutaneous IL-2, or no treatment (155). After a median 4.3 years of follow-up, the 8-year survival was inferior in the adjuvant treatment arm compared with observation arm (58 vs. 66%, respectively; log rank $p = 0.0278$).

IL-2, the only cytokine approved by the Food and Drug Administration in the metastatic setting, was used in a Cytokine

Working Group trial phase 3 trial in which 69 patients were randomized to receive one cycle of high-dose IL-2 or were observed. Early closure occurred when an interim analysis determined that the 30% improvement in 2-year DFS could not be achieved despite full accrual. Median DFS was 19.5 months in the treated arm versus 30 months in the observation arm ($p = 0.4$). Overall survival was also not different between the two arms (156).

Autologous Tumor Vaccines

Autologous tumor cell vaccines have been used as an adjuvant in high-risk patients. At least two different vaccines have been assessed in randomized phase 3 clinical trials:

A German trial randomly assigned 558 patients with resected pT2-3bpN0-3M0 RCC to 6-monthly intradermal injections of autologous tumor cell vaccine or no adjuvant therapy (158). At 4.5 years of follow-up, vaccine therapy was associated with significantly better 5-year PFS (77% vs. 68%; $p = 0.02$, log rank test). In subgroup analysis, benefit was seen in patients with T3 tumors (5-year PFS, 68% vs. 50%; $p = 0.02$), but not T2 tumors (5 -year PFS, 81% vs. 75%; $p = 0.2$). Despite this observation, some methodologic issues impede the interpretation of use of tumor vaccine as a new standard for adjuvant therapy. Three of these issues include the number of patients lost after the randomization step (174/553, 32%), the imbalance of this loss (99 from the vaccine group, 75 from controls), and absence of tabulation of overall survival.

An alternative approach has used peptides from individual tumors in conjunction with heat shock proteins to generate a vaccine. This has been used as an adjuvant in a randomized phase 3 trial involving 728 patients. A preliminary analysis did not demonstrate an improvement in overall survival, and additional analyses are being conducted with more follow-up (159).

Novel Targeted Therapies

Over the last few years, RCC has become a cancer model for targeted therapeutics based on the growing understanding of the underlying molecular pathways in this disease. Clear cell RCC, which comprises 75% to 80% of all histologic RCC subtypes, is characterized by the inactivation of the von Hippel-Lindau tumor suppressor gene, which results in the dysregulation of hypoxia response genes, including an overproduction of VEGF and other growth factors that promote tumor angiogenesis, growth, and metastasis. In advanced RCC, substantial clinical activity has been reported with VEGF blockade employing a variety of approaches, including antibodies and small-molecule VEGF receptor inhibitors (160).

Two agents, both VEGF receptor inhibitors, sunitinib and sorafenib, were recently approved by the Food and Drug Administration for use in advanced RCC, based on a PFS benefit in cytokine-refractory disease (161,162). Given the perception that these antiangiogenic agents may also work in a minimal disease setting, exploration of these agents in the adjuvant setting in RCC seems logical, and indeed several trials are currently ongoing. An ECOG-led Intergroup trial will randomize RCC patients who are at high risk for recurrence after nephrectomy to 1 year of treatment with placebo, sorafenib, or sunitinib with a primary end point of DFS. Additionally, the SORCE trial, led by the MRC, will randomize over 1,800 high-risk RCC patients after nephrectomy to placebo therapy for 3 years, sorafenib for 3 years, or sorafenib for 1 year followed by placebo for 2 years. This trial will test both the utility of sorafenib in this setting and the optimal duration of use. It should be noted, however, that treatment of patients outside a clinical trial is inappropriate given the lack of clinical data and potentially serious toxicities.

CONCLUSION

Adjuvant and neoadjuvant chemotherapy have been studied in genitourinary malignancies in an attempt to improve survival, especially in patients at higher risk for recurrence. Although chemotherapy achieves nearly 100% disease-specific survival in early-stage NSGCT, long-term toxicities are a major concern and overall survival is not different from a RPLND or an "active surveillance" approach. In bladder cancer, neoadjuvant cisplatin-based chemotherapy is the standard of care based on convincing data from well-designed randomized controlled trials. Unfortunately, perioperative chemotherapy in prostate cancer is still investigational and trials are underway, although a clear benefit from adjuvant hormonal therapy has been identified.

Finally, there is no defined role for adjuvant or neoadjuvant chemotherapy in kidney cancer. Novel antiangiogenic trials are ongoing in this disease and may provide, if positive, the first evidence of benefit for systemic treatment in the perioperative setting with this malignancy. Of importance, our improved understanding of the biology of metastasis and of its markers may help us to rationalize this potentially important approach to the care of high-risk, clinically localized genitourinary malignancy.

REFERENCES

1. Loehrer PJ Sr, Williams SD, Einhorn LH. Status of chemotherapy for testis cancer. *Urol Clin North Am.* 1987;14:713–720.
2. Ries LAG, Eisner MP, Kosary CL, et al. (eds.). *SEER Cancer Statistics Review, 1975–2002*, National Cancer Institute. Bethesday, MD, http://seer.cancer.gov/csr/1975_2002/, based on November 2004 SEER data submission, posted to SEER web site 2005.
3. Peckham MJ, Barrett A, Horwich A, et al. Orchiectomy alone for stage I testicular non-seminoma: a progress report on the Royal Marsden Hospital study. *Br J Urol.* 1983;55:754–759.
4. Rorth M, Jacobsen GK, von der Maase H, et al. Surveillance alone versus radiotherapy after orchiectomy for clinical stage I nonseminomatous testicular cancer. Danish Testicular Cancer Study Group. *J Clin Oncol.* 1991;9:1543–1548.
5. Raghavan D, Colls B, Levi J, et al. Surveillance for stage I nonseminomatous germ cell tumours of the testis: the optimal protocol has not yet been defined. *Br J Urol* 1988;61(6):522–526.
6. Freedman LS, Parkinson MC, Jones WG, et al. Histopathology in the prediction of relapse of patients with stage I testicular teratoma treated by orchidectomy alone. Lancet 1987;2(8554):294–298.
7. Sturgeon JF, Jewett MA, Alison RE, et al. Surveillance after orchidectomy for patients with clinical stage I nonseminomatous testis tumors. *J Clin Oncol* 1992;10(4):564–568.
8. Read G, Stenning SP, Cullen MH, et al. Medical Research Council prospective study of surveillance for stage I testicular teratoma. Medical Research Council Testicular Tumors Working Party. *J Clin Oncol* 1992;10(11):1762–1768.
9. Daugaard G, Petersen PM, Rorth M. Surveillance in stage I testicular cancer. *APMIS.* 2003;111:76–85.

10. Sogani PC, Perrotti M, Herr HW, et al. Clinical stage I testis cancer: long-term outcome of patients on surveillance. J Urol 1998; 159(3):855–858.

11. Raghavan D. "Active surveillance" for stage I testis cancer: attaining maturity at 21 years. Eur J Cancer 2000;36(15):1891–1894.

12. Heidenreich A, Sesterhenn IA, Mostofi FK, et al. Prognostic risk factors that identify patients with clinical stage I nonseminomatous germ cell tumors at low risk and high risk for metastasis. Cancer 1998;83(5):1002–1011.

13. Nicolai N, Miceli R, Artusi R, et al. A simple model for predicting nodal metastasis in patients with clinical stage I nonseminomatous germ cell testicular tumors undergoing retroperitoneal lymph node dissection only. J Urol 2004;171(1):172–176.

14. Albers p, Siener R, Kliesch S, et al. Risk factors for relapse in clinical stage I nonseminomatous testicular germ cell tumors: results of the German Testicular Cancer Study Group Trial. J Clin Oncol 2003;21(8):1505–1512.

15. Vergouwe Y, Steyerberg EW, Eijkemans MJ, et al. Predictors of occult metastasis in clinical stage I nonseminoma: a systematic review. J Clin Oncol 2003;21(22):4092–4099.

16. Alexandre J, Fizazi K, Mahe C, et al. Stage I non-seminomatous germ-cell tumours of the testis: identification of a subgroup of patients with a very low risk of relapse. Eur J Cancer 2001;37(5): 576–582.

17. Hermans BP, Sweeney CJ, Foster RS, et al. Risk of systemic metastases in clinical stage I nonseminoma germ cell testis tumor managed by retroperitoneal lymph node dissection. J Urol. 2000;163:1721–1724.

18. Stephenson AJ, Bosl GJ, Bajorin DF, et al. Retroperitoneal lymph node dissection in patients with low stage testicular cancer with embryonal carcinoma predominance and/or lymphovascular invasion. J Urol 2005;174(2):557–560; discussion 60.

19. Raghavan D, Vogelzang NJ, Bosl GJ, et al. Tumor classification and size in germ-cell testicular cancer: influence on the occurrence of metastases. Cancer 1982;50(8):1591–1595.

20. Abratt RP, Pontin AR, Barnes RD, et al. Adjuvant chemotherapy for stage I non-seminomatous testicular cancer. S Afr Med J 1994;84(9):605–607.

21. Pont J, Albrecht W, Postner G, et al. Adjuvant chemotherapy for high-risk clinical stage I nonseminomatous testicular germ cell cancer: long-term results of a prospective trial. J Clin Oncol 1996;14(2):441–448.

22. Cullen MH, Stenning SP, Parkinson MC, et al. Short-course adjuvant chemotherapy in high-risk stage I nonseminomatous germ cell tumors of the testis: a Medical Research Council report. J Clin Oncol 1996;14(4):1106–1113.

23. Bohlen D, Borner M, Sonntag RW, et al. Long-term results following adjuvant chemotherapy in patients with clinical stage I testicular nonseminomatous malignant germ cell tumors with high risk factors. J Urol 1999;161(4):1148–1152.

24. Ondrus D, Matoska J, Belan V, et al. Prognostic factors in clinical stage I nonseminomatous germ cell testicular tumors: rationale for different risk-adapted treatment. Eur Urol 1998;33(6): 562–566.

25. Chevreau C, Mazerolles C, Soulie M, et al. Long-term efficacy of two cycles of BEP regimen in high-risk stage I nonseminomatous testicular germ cell tumors with embryonal carcinoma and/or vascular invasion. Eur Urol. 2004;46:209–215.

26. Oliver RT, Ong J, Shamash J, et al. Long-term follow-up of Anglian Germ Cell Cancer Group surveillance versus patients with Stage 1 nonseminoma treated with adjuvant chemotherapy. Urology 2004;63(3):556–561.

27. Amato RJ, Ro JY, Ayala AG, et al. Risk-adapted treatment for patients with clinical stage I nonseminomatous germ cell tumor of the testis. Urology 2004;63(1):144–148; discussion 8–9.

28. Dearnaley DP, Fossa SD, Kaye SB, et al. Adjuvant bleomycin, vincristine and cisplatin (BOP) for high-risk stage I nonseminomatous germ cell tumours: a prospective trial (MRC TE17). Br J Cancer 2005;92(12):2107–2113.

29. Schmoll HJ, Souchon R, Krege S, et al. European consensus on diagnosis and treatment of germ cell cancer: a report of the European Germ Cell Cancer Consensus Group (EGCCCG). Ann Oncol 2004;15(9):1377–1399.

30. Boyer M, Raghavan D. Toxicity of treatment of germ cell tumors. Semin Oncol 1992;19(2):128–142.

31. Raghavan D, Boyer M. Active surveillance for stage I nonseminomatous germ cell testis tumors: practice and pitfalls. Prog Clin Biol Res 1990;350:309–318.

32. Rabbani F, Sheinfeld J, Farivar-Mohseni H, et al. Low-volume nodal metastases detected at retroperitoneal lymphadenectomy for testicular cancer: pattern and prognostic factors for relapse. J Clin Oncol 2001;19(7):2020–2025.

33. Donohue JP, Einhorn LH, Perez JM. Improved management of nonseminomatous testis tumors. Cancer. 1978;42:2903–2908.

34. Williams SD, Stablein DM, Einhorn LH, et al. Immediate adjuvant chemotherapy versus observation with treatment at relapse in pathological stage II testicular cancer. N Engl J Med 1987;317(23):1433–1438.

35. Davis BE, Herr HW, Fair WR, et al. The management of patients with nonseminomatous germ cell tumors of the testis with serologic disease only after orchiectomy. J Urol 1994;152(1):111–113; discussion 4.

36. Kondagunta GV, Sheinfeld J, Mazumdar M, et al. Relapse-free and overall survival in patients with pathologic stage II nonseminomatous germ cell cancer treated with etoposide and cisplatin adjuvant chemotherapy. J Clin Oncol 2004;22(3):464–467.

37. Stephenson AJ, Bosl GJ, Motzer RJ, et al. Retroperitoneal lymph node dissection for nonseminomatous germ cell testicular cancer: impact of patient selection factors on outcome. J Clin Oncol 2005;23(12):2781–2788.

38. Beck SD, Foster RS, Bihrle R, et al. Impact of the number of positive lymph nodes on disease-free survival in patients with pathological stage B1 nonseminomatous germ cell tumor. J Urol 2005;174(1):143–145.

39. Behnia M, Foster R, Einhorn LH, et al. Adjuvant bleomycin, etoposide and cisplatin in pathological stage II non-seminomatous testicular cancer. the Indiana University experience. Eur J Cancer 2000;36(4):472–475.

40. NCCN practice guidelines for testicular cancer. National Comprehensive Cancer Network. Oncology (Williston Park) 1998;12(11A):417–462.

41. Raghavan D. Hidden by HIPAA: the costs of cure. J Clin Oncol 2005;23(16):3663–3665.

42. Sharda NN, Kinsella TJ, Ritter MA. Adjuvant radiation versus observation: a cost analysis of alternate management schemes in early-stage testicular seminoma. J Clin Oncol. 1996;14:2933–2939.

43. Warde P, Specht L, Horwich A, et al. Prognostic factors for relapse in stage I seminoma managed by surveillance: a pooled analysis. J Clin Oncol 2002;20(22):4448–4452.

44. Giacchetti S, Raoul Y, Wibault P, Droz JP, Court B, Eschwege F. Treatment of stage I testis seminoma by radiotherapy: long-term results–a 30-year experience. Int J Radiat Oncol Biol Phys 1993;27(1):3–9.

45. Bauman GS, Venkatesan VM, Ago CT, et al. Postoperative radiotherapy for Stage I/II seminoma: results for 212 patients. Int J Radiat Oncol Biol Phys 1998;42(2):313–317.

46. Reiter WJ, Brodowicz T, Alavi S, et al. Twelve-year experience with two courses of adjuvant single-agent carboplatin therapy for clinical stage I seminoma. *J Clin Oncol* 2001;19(1):101–104.

47. Steiner H, Holtl L, Wirtenberger W, et al. Long-term experience with carboplatin monotherapy for clinical stage I seminoma: a retrospective single-center study. *Urology* 2002;60(2):324–328.

48. Oliver T DK, Steiner H. Pooled analysis of phase 2 reports of 2 vs 1 course of carboplatin as adjuvant for stage I seminoma. *J Clin Oncol* 2005;23:395s.

49. Oliver RT, Mason MD, Mead GM, et al. Radiotherapy versus single-dose carboplatin in adjuvant treatment of stage I seminoma: a randomised trial. *Lancet* 2005;366(9482):293–300.

50. Loehrer PJ, Sr., Bosl GJ. Carboplatin for stage I seminoma and the sword of Damocles. *J Clin Oncol* 2005;23(34):8566–8569.

51. Richie JP. Surgery for invasive bladder cancer. *Hematol Oncol Clin North Am.* 1992;6:129–145.

52. Raghavan D, Shipley WU, Garnick MB, et al. Biology and management of bladder cancer. *N Engl J Med* 1990;322(16):1129–1138.

53. Spruck CH, 3rd, Ohneseit PF, Gonzalez-Zulueta M, et al. Two molecular pathways to transitional cell carcinoma of the bladder. *Cancer Res* 1994;54(3):784–788.

54. Esrig D, Elmajian D, Groshen S, et al. Accumulation of nuclear p53 and tumor progression in bladder cancer. *N Engl J Med* 1994;331(19):1259–1264.

55. Raghavan D, Quinn D, Skinner DG, et al. Surgery and adjunctive chemotherapy for invasive bladder cancer. *Surg Oncol* 2002;11(1–2):55–63.

56. Stein JP, Lieskovsky G, Cote R, et al. Radical cystectomy in the treatment of invasive bladder cancer: long-term results in 1,054 patients. *J Clin Oncol* 2001;19(3):666–675.

57. van Gils-Gielen RJ, Witjes WP, Caris CT, et al. Risk factors in carcinoma in situ of the urinary bladder. Dutch South East Cooperative Urological Group. *Urology* 1995;45(4):581–586.

58. Tribukait B, Gustafson H, Esposti PL. The significance of ploidy and proliferation in the clinical and biological evaluation of bladder tumours: a study of 100 untreated cases. *Br J Urol* 1982;54(2):130–135.

59. Sauter G, Haley J, Chew K, et al. Epidermal-growth-factor-receptor expression is associated with rapid tumor proliferation in bladder cancer. *Int J Cancer* 1994;57(4):508–514.

60. Pendyala L, Velagapudi S, Toth K, et al. Translational studies of glutathione in bladder cancer cell lines and human specimens. *Clin Cancer Res* 1997;3(5):793–798.

61. Cordon-Cardo C, Wartinger D, Petrylak D, et al. Altered expression of the retinoblastoma gene product: prognostic indicator in bladder cancer. *J Natl Cancer Inst.* 1992;84:1251–1256.

62. Stein JP, Ginsberg DA, Grossfeld GD, et al. Effect of p21WAF1/CIP1 expression on tumor progression in bladder cancer. *J Natl Cancer Inst* 1998;90(14):1072–1079.

63. Raghavan D. Chemotherapy and cystectomy for invasive transitional cell carcinoma of bladder. *Urol Oncol* 2003;21(6):468–474.

64. Splinter TA, Scher HI, Denis L, et al. The prognostic value of the pathological response to combination chemotherapy before cystectomy in patients with invasive bladder cancer. European Organization for Research on Treatment of Cancer–Genitourinary Group. *J Urol* 1992;147(3):606–608.

65. Scher HI, Yagoda A, Herr HW, et al. Neoadjuvant M-VAC (methotrexate, vinblastine, doxorubicin and cisplatin) effect on the primary bladder lesion. *J Urol* 1988;139(3):470–474.

66. Dreicer R, Kollmorgen TA, Smith RF, Williams RD. Neoadjuvant cisplatin, methotrexate and vinblastine for muscle-invasive bladder cancer: long-term followup. *J Urol* 1993;150(3):849–852.

67. Schultz PK, Herr HW, Zhang ZF, et al. Neoadjuvant chemotherapy for invasive bladder cancer: prognostic factors for survival of patients treated with M-VAC with 5-year follow-up. *J Clin Oncol* 1994;12(7):1394–1401.

68. Wallace DM, Raghavan D, Kelly KA, et al. Neo-adjuvant (pre-emptive) cisplatin therapy in invasive transitional cell carcinoma of the bladder. *Br J Urol* 1991;67(6):608–615.

69. Martinez-Pineiro JA, Gonzalez Martin M, Arocena F, et al. Neoadjuvant cisplatin chemotherapy before radical cystectomy in invasive transitional cell carcinoma of the bladder: a prospective randomized phase III study. *J Urol.* 1995;153:964–973.

70. Ghersi D, Stewart LA, Parmar M. Does neoadjuvant cisplatin-based chemotherapy improve the survival of patients with locally advanced bladder cancer: a meta-analysis of individual patient data from randomized clinical trials. Advanced Bladder Cancer Overview Collaboration. *Br J Urol* 1995;75(2):206–213.

71. Loehrer PJ, Sr., Einhorn LH, Elson PJ, et al. A randomized comparison of cisplatin alone or in combination with methotrexate, vinblastine, and doxorubicin in patients with metastatic urothelial carcinoma: a cooperative group study. *J Clin Oncol* 1992;10(7):1066–1073.

72. Malmstrom PU, Rintala E, Wahlqvist R, et al. Five-year followup of a prospective trial of radical cystectomy and neoadjuvant chemotherapy: Nordic Cystectomy Trial I. The Nordic Cooperative Bladder Cancer Study Group. *J Urol* 1996;155(6):1903–1906.

73. Sherif A, Rintala E, Mestad O, et al. Neoadjuvant cisplatin-methotrexate chemotherapy for invasive bladder cancer–Nordic cystectomy trial 2. *Scand J Urol Nephrol* 2002;36(6):419–425.

74. Cortesi E. Neoadjuvant treatment for locally advanced bladder cancer: A randomized prospective clinical trial. In: Proceedings from the American Society of Clinical Oncology; 1995. Abstract 623.

75. Bassi P, Pappagallo GL, Sperandio P, et al. Neoadjuvant M-VAC chemotherapy of invasive bladder cancer: results of a multicenter phase III trial. *J Urol* 1999;161:264 (abstract 1021).

76. Abol-Enein H, El-Mekresh M, El-Baz M, et al. Neo-adjuvant chemotherapy in the treatment of invasive transitional bladder cancer: a controlled, prospective randomized study. *Br J Urol.* 1997;79(suppl 4):43.

77. Neoadjuvant cisplatin, methotrexate, and vinblastine chemotherapy for muscle-invasive bladder cancer: a randomised controlled trial. International collaboration of trialists. Lancet 1999;354(9178):533–540.

78. Hall RR. Updated results of a randomised controlled trial of neoadjuvant cisplatin, methotrexate and vinblastine chemotherapy for muscle invasive bladder cancer. *Proc Am Soc Clin Oncol* 2002;21:178a (abstract 710).

79. Grossman HB, Natale RB, Tangen CM, et al. Neoadjuvant chemotherapy plus cystectomy compared with cystectomy alone for locally advanced bladder cancer. *N Engl J Med* 2003;349(9):859–866.

80. Neoadjuvant chemotherapy for invasive bladder cancer. Cochrane Database Syst Rev 2005(2):CD005246.

81. Winquist E, Kirchner TS, Segal R, et al. Neoadjuvant chemotherapy for transitional cell carcinoma of the bladder: a systematic review and meta-analysis. *J Urol* 2004;171(2 Pt 1):561–569.

82. Herr HW, Bajorin DF, Scher HI. Neoadjuvant chemotherapy and bladder-sparing surgery for invasive bladder cancer: ten-year outcome. *J Clin Oncol* 1998;16(4):1298–1301.

83. Sternberg CN, Pansadoro V, Calabro F, et al. Can patient selection for bladder preservation be based on response to chemotherapy? Cancer 2003;97(7):1644–1652.

84. Kachnic LA, Kaufman DS, Heney NM, et al. Bladder preservation by combined modality therapy for invasive bladder cancer. *J Clin Oncol* 1997;15(3):1022–1029.

85. Rodel C, Grabenbauer GG, Kuhn R, et al. Combined-modality treatment and selective organ preservation in invasive bladder cancer: long-term results. *J Clin Oncol.* 2002;20:3061–3071.

86. Shipley WU, Winter KA, Kaufman DS, et al. Phase III trial of neoadjuvant chemotherapy in patients with invasive bladder cancer treated with selective bladder preservation by combined radiation therapy and chemotherapy: initial results of Radiation Therapy Oncology Group 89-03. *J Clin Oncol* 1998;16(11): 3576–3583.

87. Logothetis C, Swanson D, Amato R, et al. Optimal delivery of perioperative chemotherapy: preliminary results of a randomized, prospective, comparative trial of preoperative and postoperative chemotherapy for invasive bladder carcinoma. *J Urol* 1996;155(4):1241–1245.

88. Millikan R, Dinney C, Swanson D, et al. Integrated therapy for locally advanced bladder cancer: final report of a randomized trial of cystectomy plus adjuvant M-VAC versus cystectomy with both preoperative and postoperative M-VAC. *J Clin Oncol* 2001;19(20):4005–4013.

89. Logothetis CJ, Johnson DE, Chong C, et al. Adjuvant cyclophosphamide, doxorubicin, and cisplatin chemotherapy for bladder cancer: an update. *J Clin Oncol* 1988;6(10):1590–1596.

90. Skinner DG, Daniels JR, Russell CA, et al. The role of adjuvant chemotherapy following cystectomy for invasive bladder cancer: a prospective comparative trial. *J Urol* 1991;145(3):459–464; discussion 64–67.

91. Stockle M, Meyenburg W, Wellek S, et al. Advanced bladder cancer (stages pT3b, pT4a, pN1 and pN2): improved survival after radical cystectomy and 3 adjuvant cycles of chemotherapy. Results of a controlled prospective study. *J Urol* 1992;148(2 Pt 1):302–306; discussion 6–7.

92. Stockle M, Meyenburg W, Wellek S, et al. Adjuvant polychemotherapy of nonorgan-confined bladder cancer after radical cystectomy revisited: long-term results of a controlled prospective study and further clinical experience. *J Urol.* 1995;153:47–52.

93. Studer UE, Bacchi M, Biedermann C, et al. Adjuvant cisplatin chemotherapy following cystectomy for bladder cancer: results of a prospective randomized trial. *J Urol* 1994;152(1):81–84.

94. Freiha F, Reese J, Torti FM. A randomized trial of radical cystectomy versus radical cystectomy plus cisplatin, vinblastine and methotrexate chemotherapy for muscle invasive bladder cancer. *J Urol* 1996;155(2):495–499; discussion 9–500.

95. Wei CH, Hsieh RK, Chiou TJ, et al. Adjuvant methotrexate, vinblastine and cisplatin chemotherapy for invasive transitional cell carcinoma: Taiwan experience. *J Urol* 1996;155(1):118–121.

96. Stein JP, Skinner DG. Radical cystectomy for invasive bladder cancer: long-term results of a standard procedure. *World J Urol* 2006.

97. D'Amico AV, Manola J, Loffredo M, et al. 6-month androgen suppression plus radiation therapy vs radiation therapy alone for patients with clinically localized prostate cancer: a randomized controlled trial. *JAMA* 2004;292(7):821–827.

98. Huggins C, Stevens RE Jr, Hodges CV. Studies on prostatic cancer. II. The effects of castration on advanced carcinoma of the prostate gland. *Arch Surg* 1941;43:209–223.

99. Gleave ME, Sato N, Goldenberg SL, et al. Neoadjuvant androgen withdrawal therapy decreases local recurrence rates following tumor excision in the Shionogi tumor model. *J Urol.* 1997;157:1727–1730.

100. So AI, Bowden M, Gleave M. Effect of time of castration and tumour volume on time to androgen-independent recurrence in Shionogi tumours. *BJU Int* 2004;93(6):845–850.

101. Frazier HA, Robertson JE, Humphrey PA, et al. Is prostate specific antigen of clinical importance in evaluating outcome after radical prostatectomy. *J Urol* 1993;149(3):516–518.

102. Khan MA, Partin AW, Mangold LA, et al. Probability of biochemical recurrence by analysis of pathologic stage, Gleason score, and margin status for localized prostate cancer. *Urology* 2003;62(5): 866–871.

103. Partin AW, Yoo J, Carter HB, et al. The use of prostate specific antigen, clinical stage and Gleason score to predict pathological stage in men with localized prostate cancer. *J Urol* 1993;150(1): 110–104.

104. D'Amico AV, Whittington R, Malkowicz SB, et al. Biochemical outcome after radical prostatectomy, external beam radiation therapy, or interstitial radiation therapy for clinically localized prostate cancer. *Jama* 1998;280(11):969–974.

105. Nelson CP, Dunn RL, Wei JT, et al. Contemporary preoperative parameters predict cancer-free survival after radical prostatectomy: a tool to facilitate treatment decisions. *Urol Oncol* 2003;21(3): 213–218.

106. Kattan MW, Eastham JA, Stapleton AM, et al. A preoperative nomogram for disease recurrence following radical prostatectomy for prostate cancer. *J Natl Cancer Inst* 1998;90(10):766–771.

107. Labrie F, Cusan L, Gomez JL, et al. Neoadjuvant hormonal therapy: the Canadian experience. *Urology.* 1997;49(3A suppl):56–64.

108. Witjes WP, Schulman CC, Debruyne FM. Preliminary results of a prospective randomized study comparing radical prostatectomy versus radical prostatectomy associated with neoadjuvant hormonal combination therapy in T2-3 N0 M0 prostatic carcinoma. The European Study Group on Neoadjuvant Treatment of Prostate Cancer. *Urology* 1997;49(3A Suppl):65–69.

109. Soloway MS, Pareek K, Sharifi R, et al. Neoadjuvant androgen ablation before radical prostatectomy in cT2bNxMo prostate cancer: 5-year results. *J Urol* 2002;167(1):112–116.

110. Reuter VE. Pathological changes in benign and malignant prostatic tissue following androgen deprivation therapy. Urology 1997;49(3A Suppl):16–22.

111. Gleave ME, Goldenberg SL, Chin JL, et al. Randomized comparative study of 3 versus 8-month neoadjuvant hormonal therapy before radical prostatectomy: biochemical and pathological effects. *J Urol* 2001;166(2):500–506; discussion 6–7.

112. Selli C, Montironi R, Bono A, et al. Effects of complete androgen blockade for 12 and 24 weeks on the pathological stage and resection margin status of prostate cancer. *J Clin Pathol* 2002;55(7):508–513.

113. Klotz L, Gleave M, Goldenberg SL. Neoadjuvant hormone therapy: the Canadian trials. *Mol Urol* 2000;4(3):233–237; discussion 9.

114. Scolieri MJ, Altman A, Resnick MI. Neoadjuvant hormonal ablative therapy before radical prostatectomy: a review. Is it indicated? *J Urol* 2000;164(5):1465–1472.

115. Tannock IF, Osoba D, Stockler MR, et al. Chemotherapy with mitoxantrone plus prednisone or prednisone alone for symptomatic hormone-resistant prostate cancer: a Canadian randomized trial with palliative end points. *J Clin Oncol* 1996;14(6):1756–1764.

116. Petrylak DP, Tangen CM, Hussain MH, et al. Docetaxel and estramustine compared with mitoxantrone and prednisone for advanced refractory prostate cancer. *N Engl J Med.* 2004;351:1513–1520.

117. Tannock IF, de Wit R, Berry WR, et al. Docetaxel plus prednisone or mitoxantrone plus prednisone for advanced prostate cancer. *N Engl J Med* 2004;351(15):1502–1512.

118. Dreicer R, Magi-Galluzzi C, Zhou M, et al. Phase II trial of neoadjuvant docetaxel before radical prostatectomy for locally advanced prostate cancer. *Urology* 2004;63(6):1138–1142.

119. Febbo PG, Richie JP, George DJ, et al. Neoadjuvant docetaxel before radical prostatectomy in patients with high-risk localized prostate cancer. *Clin Cancer Res* 2005;11(14):5233–5240.

120. Mettlin CJ, Murphy GP, McDonald CJ, et al. The National Cancer Data base Report on increased use of brachytherapy for the treatment of patients with prostate carcinoma in the U.S. Cancer 1999;86(9):1877–1882.

121. Treatment and survival of patients with cancer of the prostate. The Veterans Administration Co-operative Urological Research Group. *Surg Gynecol Obstet* 1967;124(5):1011–1017.

122. Leuprolide versus diethylstilbestrol for metastatic prostate cancer. The Leuprolide Study Group. *N Engl J Med* 1984;311(20):1281–1286.

123. Crawford ED, Eisenberger MA, McLeod DG, et al. A controlled trial of leuprolide with and without flutamide in prostatic carcinoma. *N Engl J Med* 1989;321(7):419–424.

124. Myers RP, Larson-Keller JJ, Bergstralh EJ, et al. Hormonal treatment at time of radical retropubic prostatectomy for stage D1 prostate cancer: results of long-term followup. *J Urol* 1992;147(3 Pt 2):910–915.

125. Haggarth L, Auer G, Busch C, et al. The significance of tumor heterogeneity for prediction of DNA ploidy of prostate cancer. *Scand J Urol Nephrol*. 2005;39:387–392.

126. Sieh W, Edwards KL, Fitzpatrick AL, et al. Genetic Susceptibility to Prostate Cancer: Prostate-specific Antigen and its Interaction with the Androgen Receptor (United States). *Cancer Causes Control* 2006;17(2):187–197.

127. Seay TM, Blute ML, Zincke H. Long-term outcome in patients with pTxN+ adenocarcinoma of prostate treated with radical prostatectomy and early androgen ablation. *J Urol* 1998;159(2):357–364.

128. Messing EM, Manola J, Sarosdy M, et al. Immediate hormonal therapy compared with observation after radical prostatectomy and pelvic lymphadenectomy in men with node-positive prostate cancer. *N Engl J Med* 1999;341(24):1781–1788.

129. McLeod DG, See WA, Klimberg I, et al. The bicalutamide 150 mg early prostate cancer program: findings of the North American trial at 7.7-year median followup. *J Urol* 2006;176(1):75–80.

130. Schmidt JD, Gibbons RP, Murphy GP, et al. Adjuvant therapy for clinical localized prostate cancer treated with surgery or irradiation. *Eur Urol* 1996;29(4):425–433.

131. Schmidt JD, Gibbons RP, Murphy GP, et al. Evaluation of adjuvant estramustine phosphate, cyclophosphamide, and observation only for node-positive patients following radical prostatectomy and definitive irradiation. Investigators of the National Prostate Cancer Project. *Prostate* 1996;28(1):51–57.

132. Nakabayashi M, Oh WK. Chemotherapy for high-risk localized prostate cancer. *BJU Int.* 2006;97:679–683.

133. Wang J, Halford S, Rigg A, et al. Adjuvant mitozantrone chemotherapy in advanced prostate cancer. *BJU Int* 2000;86(6):675–680.

134. Pilepich MV, Caplan R, Byhardt RW, et al. Phase III trial of androgen suppression using goserelin in unfavorable-prognosis carcinoma of the prostate treated with definitive radiotherapy: report of Radiation Therapy Oncology Group Protocol 85–31. *J Clin Oncol* 1997;15(3):1013–1021.

135. Pilepich MV, Winter K, Lawton CA, et al. Androgen suppression adjuvant to definitive radiotherapy in prostate carcinoma–long-term results of phase III RTOG 85–31. *Int J Radiat Oncol Biol Phys* 2005;61(5):1285–1290.

136. Bolla M, Gonzalez D, Warde P, et al. Improved survival in patients with locally advanced prostate cancer treated with radiotherapy and goserelin. *N Engl J Med* 1997;337(5):295–300.

137. Bolla M, Collette L, Blank L, et al. Long-term results with immediate androgen suppression and external irradiation in patients with locally advanced prostate cancer (an EORTC study): a phase III randomised trial. Lancet 2002;360(9327):103–106.

138. Ciezki JP, Klein EA, Angermeier K, et al. A retrospective comparison of androgen deprivation (AD) vs. no AD among low-risk and intermediate-risk prostate cancer patients treated with brachytherapy, external beam radiotherapy, or radical prostatectomy. Int *J Radiat Oncol Biol Phys* 2004;60(5):1347–1350.

139. D'Amico AV, Schultz D, Loffredo M, et al. Biochemical outcome following external beam radiation therapy with or without androgen suppression therapy for clinically localized prostate cancer. *Jama* 2000;284(10):1280–1283.

140. Jemal A, Siegel R, Ward E, et al. Cancer statistics, 2006. *CA Cancer J Clin.* 2006;56:106–130.

141. Motzer RJ, Bander NH, Nanus DM. Renal-cell carcinoma. *N Engl J Med* 1996;335(12):865–875.

142. Robson CJ, Churchill BM, Anderson W. The results of radical nephrectomy for renal cell carcinoma. *J Urol* 1969;101(3):297–301.

143. Frank I, Blute ML, Leibovich BC, et al. Independent validation of the 2002 American Joint Committee on cancer primary tumor classification for renal cell carcinoma using a large, single institution cohort. *J Urol* 2005;173(6):1889–1892.

144. Motzer RJ, Mazumdar M, Bacik J, et al. Survival and prognostic stratification of 670 patients with advanced renal cell carcinoma. *J Clin Oncol* 1999;17(8):2530–2540.

145. Mekhail TM, Abou-Jawde RM, Boumerhi G, et al. Validation and extension of the Memorial Sloan-Kettering prognostic factors model for survival in patients with previously untreated metastatic renal cell carcinoma. *J Clin Oncol* 2005;23(4):832–841.

146. Yagoda A, Petrylak D, Thompson S. Cytotoxic chemotherapy for advanced renal cell carcinoma. *Urol Clin North Am* 1993;20(2):303–321.

147. Onufrey V, Mohiuddin M. Radiation therapy in the treatment of metastatic renal cell carcinoma. Int *J Radiat Oncol Biol Phys* 1985;11(11):2007–2009.

148. Kjaer M. The role of medroxyprogesterone acetate (MPA) in the treatment of renal adenocarcinoma. Cancer Treat Rev 1988;15(3):195–209.

149. Bukowski RM. Cytokine therapy for metastatic renal cell carcinoma. *Semin Urol Oncol.* 2001;19:148–154.

150. Lam JS, Leppert JT, Figlin RA, et al. Role of molecular markers in the diagnosis and therapy of renal cell carcinoma. Urology 2005;66(5 Suppl):1–9.

151. Zisman A, Pantuck AJ, Dorey F, et al. Improved prognostication of renal cell carcinoma using an integrated staging system. *J Clin Oncol* 2001;19(6):1649–1657.

152. Kattan MW, Reuter V, Motzer RJ, et al. A postoperative prognostic nomogram for renal cell carcinoma. *J Urol* 2001;166(1):63–67.

153. Messing EM, Manola J, Wilding G, et al. Phase III study of interferon alfa-NL as adjuvant treatment for resectable renal cell carcinoma: an Eastern Cooperative Oncology Group/Intergroup trial. *J Clin Oncol* 2003;21(7):1214–1222.

154. Pizzocaro G, Piva L, Colavita M, et al. Interferon adjuvant to radical nephrectomy in Robson stages II and III renal cell carcinoma: a multicentric randomized study. *J Clin Oncol* 2001;19(2):425–431.

155. Atzpodien J, Schmitt E, Gertenbach U, et al. Adjuvant treatment with interleukin-2- and interferon-alpha2a-based chemoimmunotherapy in renal cell carcinoma post tumour nephrectomy: results of a prospectively randomised trial of the German Cooperative Renal Carcinoma Chemoimmunotherapy Group (DGCIN). *Br J Cancer* 2005;92(5):843–846.

156. Clark PE, Peereboom DM, Dreicer R, et al. Phase II trial of neoadjuvant estramustine and etoposide plus radical prostatectomy for locally advanced prostate cancer. Urology 2001;57(2):281–285.

157. Porzsolt F, et al. Adjuvant therapy of renal cell cancer with interferon alpha-2a. *Proc Am Soc Clin Oncol* 1992;11:202a.

158. Jocham D, Richter A, Hoffmann L, et al. Adjuvant autologous renal tumour cell vaccine and risk of tumour progression in patients

with renal-cell carcinoma after radical nephrectomy: phase III, randomised controlled trial. *Lancet.* 2004;363:594–599.

159. Antigenics press release. http://www.antigenics.com/news/2006/0607.phtml aoJ, 2006.
160. Choueiri TK, Bukowski RM, Rini BI. The Current Role of Angiogenesis Inhibitors in the Treatment of Renal Cell Carcinoma. Semin Oncol 2006;33(5):596–606.
161. Motzer RJ, Rini BI, Bukowski RM, et al. Sunitinib in patients with metastatic renal cell carcinoma. *Jama* 2006;295(21):2516–2524.
162. Escudier B, Szczylik C, Eisen Tea. Randomized phase III trial of the Raf kinase and VEGFR inhibitor sorafenib (BAY 43–9006) in patients with advanced renal cell carcinoma (RCC). In: Proceedings from the American Society of Clinical Oncology; May 13–17, 2005; Orlando, FL. Abstract 4510.

COMMENTARY
Przemyslaw Twardowski and Robert A. Figlin

Drs. Choueiri, Thakkar, and Raghavan should be commended for their detailed, meticulous review of the role of neoadjuvant and adjuvant chemotherapy in the treatment of genitourinary malignancies. It is probably the most comprehensive, well-referenced, and up-to-date work summarizing the current "state of the art" on that subject. In addition, it provides an interesting historical perspective on the accomplishments and shortcomings of several decades of clinical trials that determined the existing guidelines for adjuvant systemic therapy of genitourinary cancers.

TESTICULAR CANCER

This chapter illustrates the remarkable progress that has been achieved in the treatment of testicular cancer in the last 30 years. Testicular cancer became the prototypical success story of the application of modern chemotherapy. In fact, in the face of very modest progress in the treatment of other solid tumors, some cynics have suggested that testicular cancer is the only reason justifying the existence of clinical medical oncologists. Although this judgment may be excessively harsh toward our field, until recently it was not without some merit.

With cure rates exceeding 95%, the focus of recent clinical research has shifted from maximizing therapeutic efficacy to minimizing the side effects of effective therapy. One of the emerging trends in the treatment of early stage (I) testicular cancer is the gradual increase in the application of brief adjuvant systemic chemotherapy at the expense of more traditional treatment approaches like radiation therapy in seminoma or retroperitoneal lymph node dissection (RPLND) in nonseminomatous germ cell tumors. This strategy has been adopted more readily in Europe, with American counterparts being more cautious in interpreting the results of recent clinical trials.

In the context of this chapter, which deals primarily with the issue of perioperative chemotherapy, the authors focused their attention on post-RPLND chemotherapy in patients with stage II nonseminomatous germ cell tumors. It is worth mentioning that the roles of RPLND and chemotherapy in that setting are evolving and chemotherapy (without RPLND) is increasingly recognized as a viable treatment option, with RPLND reserved for patients with residual radiographic abnormalities. This is reflected in the recent treatment guidelines for testicular carcinoma published by the National Comprehensive Cancer Network, Inc. (NCCN) (1). It appears to the authors of the NCCN guidelines that the trend of increasing reliance on adjuvant chemotherapy in testicular cancer will continue as the clinical data matures and the advantages of high efficacy and lower morbidity of modern chemotherapy become apparent after long-term follow-up. One of the most interesting and important areas of translational research in the next decade will focus on the discovery and validation of molecular predictive factors and imaging techniques that will augment currently used clinical and pathologic features allowing for much more precise selection of patients that are at risk of cancer relapse and need adjuvant therapy, while reducing the problem of overtreatment of patients who are cured with primary therapy (2).

BLADDER CANCER

Paraphrasing Winston Churchill's famous statement praising aviators of Battle of Britain, "Never in the field of human conflict was so much owed by so many to so few" (3), it has to be admitted that research of adjuvant chemotherapy in bladder cancer represents an area in which an effort by so many investigators over such a long period of time provided so little useful information. This is not intended to be a criticism of the investigators, but reflects widespread frustration with difficulties in conducting robust clinical trials that would establish the evidence-based recommendations for the use of adjuvant therapy in urothelial malignancies. Transitional carcinoma of the bladder is a chemotherapy-sensitive tumor. The response rates for metastatic disease with platinum-containing combination chemotherapy regimens (50% partial response and 20% complete response) (4) at least match or exceed what is reported in the setting of breast, colon, ovarian, and lung cancers, malignancies in which the benefit of adjuvant chemotherapy has been proven. It is certainly possible to hypothesize the existence of unique biological factors that would make adjuvant chemotherapy for urothelial cancers less effective, but the more likely scenario is that we have not been able to execute clinical trials of sufficient quality and power to show the benefit.

Here are some basic statistical considerations for the design of adjuvant clinical trials for bladder cancer: Approximately 50% of patients with invasive transitional cell carcinoma of the bladder will be cured with surgery; therefore, the potential benefit is limited to the remaining 50% of patients. Assuming that the "complete response" using cisplatin-based regimens in the adjuvant setting is about the same as in metastatic disease (20%), only about 10% of patients (20% of 50%) will benefit. A trial to detect a 10% absolute difference in survival between adjuvant therapy and no-adjuvant therapy after cystectomy would require randomizing approximately 650 patients in order to achieve sufficient statistical power. Most of the adjuvant trials reported and discussed in this chapter accrued fewer than 100 patients, making the trials significantly underpowered to detect an expected difference in survival.

The issue of neoadjuvant therapy was addressed by several trials described in this chapter and at least two of these trials were of high quality and power to provide more solid evidence of the benefit of chemotherapy in high-risk patients. Based on that, neoadjuvant therapy is considered by many experts in the field to be the current standard of care for patients with muscle invasive or locally advanced bladder cancer (5). For a variety of reasons, only a fraction of patients are being currently treated in that fashion. Because of continuous perceptions of high toxicity of chemotherapy in that setting (not supported by data), questions about the real benefits of chemotherapy (perpetuated by ongoing controversies of adjuvant data) and concerns about delaying surgery, the majority of patients with muscle-invasive bladder cancer undergo upfront cystectomy and are referred for evaluation by medical oncologists later. The oncology practice patterns and conversations with colleagues suggest that the majority of oncologists "half-heartedly" offer adjuvant chemotherapy to younger patients with stage T3 and T4 and lymph node-positive tumors; however, lack of solid evidence of benefit makes those decisions and discussions with patients very difficult.

There are two ongoing large randomized clinical trials mentioned in the review that will hopefully provide more answers regarding the indications for adjuvant chemotherapy in bladder cancer: The European Organisation for Research and Treatment of Cancer (EORTC) trial is randomizing high-risk patients to observation versus a chemotherapy regimen of choice (MVAC [methotrexate, vinblastine, doxorubicin, and cisplatin] or "high-dose MVAC" or cisplatin with gemcitabine). This trial expects to accrue 660 patients. The other trial comparing cisplatin/gemcitabine with Adriamycin/gemcitabine followed by cisplatin and taxol is being conducted by Cancer and Leukemia Group B and is planning to accrue 800 patients. Based on the experience from the past, it remains to be seen whether those high accrual targets can be met.

To make the issue even more complex, it is becoming increasingly recognized that surgical factors can have a major impact on the outcome of patients with bladder cancer (6). The retrospective analysis of the neoadjuvant intergroup trial 0080 showed that the number of lymph nodes removed at the time of radical cystectomy (less than ten vs. more than ten) was an independent predictor of survival after cystectomy adjusting for pathologic stage, age, chemotherapy, and node status. Because there is significant variability in the number of lymph nodes removed during cystectomy by different surgical centers and individual surgeons, it is important to take this into account in the analysis and design of clinical trials of adjuvant therapy for bladder carcinoma. Standardized surgical approach using more extensive lymphadenectomy is being advocated by urologic oncologists. The previously mentioned EORTC adjuvant trial is prospectively stratifying patients based on the number of lymph nodes removed, hopefully addressing that variability.

PROSTATE CANCER

The area of clinical research in prostate cancer presents a distinctive set of challenges because of the rather indolent nature of the disease and a very long time needed to complete clinical trials and document important clinical end points. By the time clinical trial results are published, new drugs and technologies are being routinely implemented, making previously tested hypotheses less relevant. An example is the Rapid Plan progress radiation techniques allowing for administration of significantly higher-dose intensity of radiation to the prostate area, resulting in better treatment outcomes compared to doses given just a few years ago (7). That immediately raises the question of whether the benefit of adjuvant hormone therapy seen in the past is just compensating for "inadequate radiation therapy." Another example is a completed Southwest Oncology Group protocol using postoperative adjuvant mitoxantrone, a chemotherapeutic drug that was a standard at the time of a trial design but has since shown to be inferior to docetaxel, at least in the metastatic setting.

Neoadjuvant and adjuvant androgen-deprivation therapy for prostate cancer has been established as a standard of care in patients undergoing definitive radiation therapy for localized, intermediate, and high-risk disease (8,9). There is a continuing debate about the timing and duration of that therapy and clinical trials have not elucidated whether the beneficial effect of androgen deprivation is independent of radiation or there is a specific interaction between radiation and hormone therapy that accounts for that benefit.

The role of perioperative androgen deprivation therapy in patients treated with prostatectomy is much less defined. As noted in this chapter, several neoadjuvant trials using short-term androgen deprivation reported a decrease in the rate of a positive surgical margin, but demonstrated no effect on other important clinical outcomes like disease progression and survival. The one positive adjuvant postsurgical trial frequently cited and also mentioned in this chapter was published by Messing et al. (10). It is an important trial showing survival benefit of indefinite androgen ablation in patients treated with prostatectomy who were found to have lymph node involvement. One major criticism of this study is its relatively small size (98 patients) and absence of confirmatory data, making it difficult for some experts in the field to accept it as a definitive "standard of care."

Nevertheless, a relatively simple general pattern appears to be emerging from the analysis of adjuvant and neoadjuvant androgen deprivation trials: Long duration of therapy provides benefits, while with short duration of therapy, little or no benefits are seen. This may be an oversimplification but it is consistent with preclinical studies in which prolonged androgen deprivation leads to ongoing apoptosis of cancer cells partially mediated by an antiangiogenic effect (11).

It is also worth noting that the benefits of adjuvant hormonal therapy in breast cancer continue to increase with treatment lasting ≥ 5 years (12). Unfortunately, prolonged androgen deprivation therapy is associated with significant side effects and increased risk of osteoporosis, cardiovascular problems, and diabetes (13). The full impact of protracted hormone therapy on quality of life and other medical problems continues to be investigated, and it would be of major interest to establish "minimum effective duration" of adjuvant therapy and to develop better treatment strategies to minimize side effects. Examples include the use of antiosteoporosis measures like bisphosphonates, exercise and dietary programs to prevent weight gain, and possibly the development of new, more potent antiandrogens that would more effectively block the prostate cancer androgen receptor without a need for inducing castrated levels of testosterone. As with other disease sites, discovery of molecular markers that will allow for accurate selection of patients that are at high risk of cancer relapse and truly need adjuvant therapy represents one of the important goals of prostate cancer research. Chemotherapy in the adjuvant setting is being evaluated in conjunction with radiation and surgery, but we will have to wait for the results of these studies for several more years. Until then, adjuvant chemotherapy for prostate cancer should be reserved for patients participating in clinical trials.

RENAL CARCINOMA

Therapy of advanced renal cell carcinoma is undergoing rapid transformation with the recent Food and Drug Administration approval of sorafenib (Nexavar) and sunitinib (Sutent), both targeted agents that work via inhibiting specific receptor tyrosine kinase activities and are associated with relatively mild toxicity. Kidney cancer now represents one of the first common solid tumors for which rationally designed targeted therapies constitute the main therapeutic option. This is the direct result of very comprehensive understanding of molecular abnormalities responsible for the pathophysiology of this disease. The inactivation of the von Hippel-Lindau tumor-suppressor gene leading to overexpression of hypoxia-regulated genes including vascular endothelial growth factor and platelet-derived growth factor is of particular importance in renal cell carcinoma and especially in the clear cell histologic variant. The role of other kidney cancer pathways and signal transduction molecules like mTOR is not only better understood, but multiple agents inhibiting those pathways are already available and showing efficacy in metastatic disease (14).

Of equal importance is the development and refinement of predictive models identifying patients at high risk of relapse after local therapy. Those models incorporate not only the usual clinical and pathologic variables (performance status, TNM stage, tumor grade, and necrosis), but molecular markers based on microarray tissue analysis. Several markers including Ki-67, Ep-CAM, p53, and carbonic anhydrase IX have been found to be significantly associated with tumor recurrence, and many others are being studied using large tissue and clinical databases collected over the last 2 decades (15). These recent discoveries provide us with extremely useful tools to design adjuvant clinical trials in patients with renal cell carcinoma. We have now significantly more effective and less toxic agents than were available when previous negative adjuvant trials were conducted, and can more accurately select patients for high risk of recurrence, allowing for robust statistical power of the studies with smaller number of patients, and we can expect the results of clinical trials to be available in relatively shorter periods of time.

It can be argued that the foundations for progress in therapy of renal cell carcinoma are stronger than in the majority of other solid tumors because of a better understanding of the molecular biology of this disease. We are probably not too far away from selecting therapy for individual kidney cancer patients based on the identification of the main "driving" pathway responsible for tumor growth and progression. The hint of that is already seen in therapy of metastatic disease where mTOR inhibitors may soon become front-line therapy in aggressive tumors while tyrosine kinase inhibitors may be initially used for patients with more indolent cancers, reflecting the different importance of specific pathways in distinctive clinical settings. One can imagine that these observations will become very applicable to the design of future adjuvant clinical trials. At this point, the interest in immunotherapy for kidney cancer has decreased being supplanted by rapid progress in targeted treatments. However, it is unlikely that the durable complete responses seen in selected patients treated with interleukin-2, indicating the potentially powerful impact of immune modulation on this disease, will be forgotten.

There is an ongoing effort to improve tumor vaccine efficacy focusing on eliminating the inhibitory pathways like the CTLA4 molecule that interferes with costimulatory signals provided by the interaction of B7 on dendritic cells. Several investigators are evaluating carbonic anhydrase IX as a candidate tumor-associated antigen for renal cell carcinoma with promising preclinical data (16). Future testing of immunotherapies in the adjuvant setting for renal cell carcinoma will require more progress at the basic science level and ultimately may necessitate a combinational approach. There is an emerging evidence of interactions between angiogenic factors and immune system. One example includes the vascular endothelial growth factor-mediated inhibition of activity of dendritic cells (17); therefore, combinations of antiangiogenic agents and immune therapies may provide an attractive possibility of enhancing anti-tumor immune response.

In summary, the chapter by Drs Choueiri, Thakkar, and Raghavan is an extremely useful resource for physicians interested in expanding their understanding of adjuvant therapy of genitourinary malignancies. It also provides invaluable background for the development of new concepts and ideas that will move this area of medical oncology forward.

REFERENCES

1. National Comprehensive Cancer Network, Inc., Testicular Cancer Practice Guidelines in Oncology, Version http://www.nccn.org/professionals/physician_gls/PDF/testicular.pdf, Version 2, 2009. Accessed 5/22/2009.
2. Hussain A. Germ cell tumors. *Curr Opin Oncol.* 2005;17:268–274.
3. Winston Churchill speech in House of Commons. August 20, 1940.
4. Siefker-Radtke A. Systemic chemotherapy options for metastatic bladder cancer. *Expert Rev Anticancer Ther.* 2006;6:877–885.
5. Bajorin DF. Plenary debate of randomized phase iii trial of neoadjuvant MVAC plus cystectomy versus cystectomy alone in patients with locally advanced bladder cancer. *J Clin Oncol.* 2001;19(suppl):17s–20s.
6. Herr HW, Faulkner JR, Grossman HB, et al. Surgical factors influence bladder cancer outcomes: a Cooperative Group rReport. *J Clin Oncol.* 2004;22,:2781–2789.
7. Peeters ST, Heemsbergen, WD, Koper PC, et al. Dose-response in radiotherapy for localized prostate cancer: results of the Dutch multicenter randomized phase III trial comparing 68 Gy of radiotherapy with 78 Gy. *J Clin Oncol.* 2006;24:1975–1977.
8. D'Amico AV, Manola J, Loffredo M, et al. Six-month androgen suppression plus radiation therapy vs radiation therapy alone for patients with clinically localized prostate cancer: a randomized controlled trial. *JAMA.* 2004;292:821–827.

9. Bolla M, Collette L, Blank L, et al. Long-term results with immediate androgen suppression and external irradiation in patients with locally advanced prostate cancer (an EORTC study): a phase III randomized trial. *Lancet.* 2002;360:103–106.

10. Messing EM, Manola J, Yao J, et al. Eastern Cooperative Oncology Group study EST 3886. Immediate versus deferred androgen deprivation treatment in patients with node-positive prostate cancer after radical prostatectomy and pelvic lymphadenectomy. *Lancet Oncol* 2006;7:472–479.

11. Buttyan R, Ghafar MA, Shabsigh A. The effects of androgen deprivation on the prostate gland: cell death mediated by vascular regression. *Curr Opin Urol.* 2000;10:415–420.

12. Sacco M, Valentini M, Belfiglio M, et al. Randomized trial of 2 versus 5 years of adjuvant tamoxifen for women aged 50 years or older with early breast cancer: Italian Interdisciplinary Group for Cancer Evaluation Study of Adjuvant Treatment in Breast Cancer, 01. *J Clin Oncol.* 2003;21:2276–2281.

13. Keating NL, O'Malley AJ, Smith MR. Diabetes and cardiovascular disease during androgen deprivation therapy for prostate cancer. *J Clin Oncol.* 2006;24:4448–4456.

14. Twardowski P, Figlin R. Emerging targeted therapies in renal cell carcinoma. *Monographs in Renal Cell Carcinoma.* 2006;1:10–13.

15. Lam JS, Belldegrun AS, Figlin RA. Adjuvant treatment for renal cell carcinoma. *Expert Opin Pharmacother.* 2006;7:705–720.

16. Vissers JL, De Vries IJ, Engelen LP, et al. Renal cell carcinoma-associated antigen G250 encodes naturally processed epitope presented by human leukocyte antigen-DR molecules to CD4(+) T lymphocytes. *Int J. Cancer.* 2002;100:441–444.

17. Laxmanan S, Robertson SW, Wang E, et al. Vascular endothelial growth factor impairs the functional ability of dendritic cells through Id pathways. *Biophys Biochem Res Commun.* 2005;334:193–198.

56

Surgical Management of Ovarian Cancer

Ilana Cass

EPIDEMIOLOGY

Epithelial ovarian cancer is the most lethal of all gynecologic malignancies. In 2008, the American Cancer Society estimated that 21,650 women would be diagnosed with ovarian cancer in the United States and that 15,520 would succumb to their disease (1). The lifetime risk of ovarian cancer is 1 in 55. Ovarian cancer is the fifth leading cause of cancer-related deaths in American women, following behind lung, breast, colon, and pancreas cancer.

ETIOLOGY AND RISK FACTORS

Several theories have been proposed to explain the etiology of ovarian cancer. The most common theory is "incessant ovulation," which suggests that ovulatory trauma to the ovarian epithelium predisposes to malignant transformation (2). Epidemiologic studies suggest that women who have more ovulatory events have higher rates of ovarian cancer, such as women who are nulliparous, those with polycystic ovarian syndrome, or those with early menarche or late menopause (3,4). Pregnancy, breast-feeding, and oral contraceptives have all been shown to decrease the risk of ovarian cancer. The use of oral contraceptive pills for >5 years decreases the risk of ovarian cancer by 50% and the benefit appears to persist for years after discontinuation (5).

Transuterine or transtubal passage of chemical carcinogens introduced through the vagina is another theory of ovarian carcinogenesis. Animal and some epidemiologic data have shown that asbestos exposure has been associated with higher rates of ovarian pathology. In 1979, Longo and Young (6) proposed that talc placed on sanitary napkins could be introduced into the upper genital tract. Although some studies have found higher rates of ovarian cancer among women who use talc, this association is controversial (7). Bilateral tubal ligation has been shown to decrease the risk of ovarian cancer, which may relate to obstruction of the transtubal passage of potential carcinogens or may relate to more subtle disruptions of blood supply to the adnexa from the broad ligament (8,9)

Prolonged use of ovulation induction agents has been associated with an increased risk of ovarian cancer, although subsequent analysis reveals that women who conceive and carry full-term pregnancies with these agents have a risk of ovarian cancer comparable to that of the general population. Those women with primary ovarian infertility who never conceive despite the use of ovulation-inducing agents appear to have an increased risk of ovarian cancer (10–12).

HEREDITARY OVARIAN CANCER SYNDROMES

The single largest risk factor for the development of ovarian cancer is a family history of breast and ovarian cancer. In addition to personal history of cancer and ethnicity, obtaining a complete family history from both maternal and paternal sides of the family is an important tool to assess the likelihood of carrying a breast cancer gene (BRCA) mutation.

Although the lifetime risk of developing ovarian cancer in the general population is 1% to 2%, a first-degree relative who has had ovarian cancer increases a woman's risk of ovarian cancer to 4% to 5%. Two affected relatives increases the lifetime risk to 7% (13).

Approximately 10% of all ovarian cancers are attributed to familial syndromes, which appear to be transmitted in an autosomal-dominant fashion. Two major syndromes responsible for familial ovarian cancer that have been described include hereditary breast-ovarian cancer syndrome and hereditary nonpolyposis colorectal cancer (HNPCC).

Hereditary Breast-Ovarian Cancer Syndrome

Hereditary breast-ovarian cancer syndrome is characterized by early onset of disease, and breast cancer may involve both breasts. Germline mutations in BRCA genes are responsible for the majority of hereditary breast-ovarian cancer syndrome. The prevalence of BRCA mutations in the general population is approximately 0.4%. Certain ethnic groups or geographic areas have higher frequencies of BRCA mutations including Ashkenazi Jews, French Canadians, and Russian populations from the Baltic area (14). Germline BRCA mutations occur in 2.5% of healthy, unaffected Ashkenazi Jewish women (15).

The presence of a germline mutation in BRCA confers a significantly elevated risk of developing breast or ovarian cancer. BRCA1 or BRCA2 mutations are associated with a 80% risk of developing breast cancer by the age of 70. BRCA1 mutations confer a higher risk of ovarian cancer than BRCA2 mutations, which is also characterized by an earlier age of onset. The risk of developing ovarian cancer for BRCA1 mutation carriers by age 70 is 39% to 54% in contrast to 22% to 27% among BRCA2 mutation carriers (16,17).

Current strategies to reduce the risk of developing ovarian, primary peritoneal, or fallopian tube cancer in high-risk women with hereditary BRCA1 or BRCA2 mutations include surveillance, chemoprevention, and surgery. The recommended screening procedures include semiannual pelvic examination, transvaginal ultrasound, and serum CA 125 levels beginning at ages 35 years or 5 to 10 years earlier than the earliest age of first diagnosis of ovarian cancer in the family (18,19) To date, these screening procedures have a limited ability to detect ovarian cancer at an early, more curable stage of disease and there is no evidence that screening has reduced the mortality or significantly improved the survival associated with ovarian cancer in high-risk populations. The low prevalence of ovarian cancer and the high likelihood of a positive screening test necessitating further invasive surgical evaluation are obstacles in ovarian cancer screening (20–22). Future cancer screening programs will likely need to incorporate multiple screening markers and algorithms that can better discriminate between pathologic conditions and the normal fluctuations of CA 125 and ovarian cyst formation over time (23).

Oral contraceptives have been the mainstay of chemoprevention for the hereditary BRCA mutation carrier, although the benefit and magnitude of reduced risk have not been reported as consistently as for the general low-risk population. A reduced risk of ovarian cancer has been observed for ever-use and for longer duration use (>5 years) in some studies (24–27). Some studies have suggested, however, that oral contraceptive use may be associated with an increased risk of breast cancer in women with BRCA mutations. Although it is reasonable for women with mutations in BRCA1 or BRCA2 to use oral contraceptives, the risks and benefits for both chemoprevention and reproductive control should be carefully weighed by the patient and her physician.

Other potential chemopreventative agents that have been studied include fenretinide, a synthetic vitamin A analogue with antitumor effects, and high-potency progestins. Fenretinide, 200 mg per day, did appear to reduce the incidence of ovarian cancer during the 5 years of treatment, but no protective effect was seen after discontinuation of the drug (28,29). Parity, a prior history of any gynecologic surgery, especially with removal of some portion of the ovary, tubal ligation, and hysterectomy have also been associated with a reduction in the risk of ovarian cancer among BRCA mutation carriers (9,27,30–32).

Given the limitations of current ovarian cancer screening approaches, prophylactic risk-reducing surgery, including removal of the ovaries and as much of the fallopian tube as possible, should be strongly considered after the conclusion of childbearing. This procedure has been shown to reduce the risk of ovarian, fallopian tube, and peritoneal carcinoma by approximately 85% to 90% in women with known BRCA mutations and decreased mortality (33–37). Prophylactic bilateral salpingo-oophorectomy also reduces the risk of breast cancer by 50% to 70% (33,34,36,38). This protection appears to be maximized if patients are premenopausal at the time of prophylactic surgery (33). The effect of long-term hormone-replacement therapy on breast cancer risk reduction in the patient following a prophylactic bilateral salpingo-oophorectomy is not known. Data suggest that short-term use of hormone-replacement therapy does not significantly diminish the protective effect of prophylactic surgery (39).

As women with BRCA1 mutations have a 10% to 21% chance of developing ovarian cancer by age 50, it is prudent for women with BRCA1 mutations to consider *risk-reducing salpingo-oophorectomy* around the fourth decade. For BRCA2 mutation carriers, the risk of ovarian cancer by age 50 is approximately 2% to 3% (16). However, women with BRCA2 mutations have a 26% to 34% chance of developing breast cancer by age 50, and the maximum benefit of removing the ovaries on breast cancer risk reduction is achieved the earlier the ovaries are removed. Women with mutations in the BRCA gene need to individualize the timing of salpingo-oophorectomy based on their life factors, desire for fertility, or natural hormones, as well as their age-dependent breast and ovarian cancer risks.

Laparoscopy and laparotomy are both options for risk-reducing salpingo-oophorectomy. Laparoscopy allows for minimally invasive surgery while a thorough inspection of peritoneal surfaces may still be performed. Peritoneal washings should be taken. The ovarian vessels should be isolated and ligated proximal to the end of identifiable ovarian tissue to ensure that all ovarian tissue is complete removed. Removal of specimens using an endoscopic-contained bag optimizes specimen preservation. Intraoperative pathology review includes a close examination for possible occult disease. If cancer is identified at the time of surgery, surgical staging with lymphadenectomy and omentectomy may be performed at the time of risk-reducing surgery, providing appropriate preoperative consent has been obtained.

Occult disease may be identified through careful gynecologic pathology review. Rather than taking only one or two sections from each ovary, the complete ovaries and tubes should be serially sectioned and evaluated, as this procedure has been demonstrated to improve the detection of occult disease (40). Approximately 5% of women with BRCA mutations will have occult carcinoma at the time of prophylactic surgery (33–35,37,41). Primary tubal carcinomas occur commonly among these occult cases with a frequency that is approximately a log fold higher than that seen in the general population. This underscores the need to remove as much of the fallopian tube as possible at the time of prophylactic surgery (40,42). Despite the microscopic tumors identified, they are often high grade, and information from the peritoneal lavage may reflect the aggressiveness of the disease (43).

Hysterectomy may be considered with risk-reducing salpingo-oophorectomy especially when there are other medical conditions for the removal of the uterus and cervix. (44). Although there is a small risk of endometrial cancer and a theoretical increased risk of cancer in the cornual fallopian tube, salpingo-oophorectomy alone confers a significant cancer risk reduction with less surgical risk and postoperative recovery (45,46). Endometrial carcinoma does not appear to be part of the BRCA-associated spectrum of disease based on small series (47,48). Those women taking tamoxifen may have their endometrial cancer risk lowered by performing concurrent hysterectomy, and unaffected women may have their future hormone therapy regimens simplified. There is limited information on hormonal replacement in BRCA1/2 mutation carriers, and needs to be individualized with respect to menopausal effects and breast cancer risks.

Hereditary Nonpolyposis Colorectal Carcinoma

HNPCC, or Lynch II syndrome, is a much less common cause of familial ovarian cancer, accounting for 2% of cases (49,50).

HNPCC is characterized by mutations in DNA mismatch repair genes including *MLH1*, *MSH2*, and *MSH6* that predispose individuals to colorectal carcinoma and cancers of the endometrium, ovary, and other gastrointestinal or genitourinary cancers. Women with HNPCC mutations are more likely to present with endometrial or ovarian cancer than colorectal cancer. The lifetime risk of ovarian cancer for a woman who carries a HNPCC mutation is 12% and the risk of endometrial cancer approaches 60% (51–53). Surgical prophylaxis with removal of the uterus, tubes, and ovaries has been shown to reduce mortality in women with HNPCC syndrome, although the optimum timing of the procedure remains unclear (54). Given the early onset of ovarian and endometrial cancer in these women, consideration of surgical prophylaxis is warranted after childbearing is complete.

HISTOLOGICL CLASSIFICATION OF OVARIAN CANCER

The World Health Organization has classified the different types of ovarian carcinoma based on the histogenesis of the ovary into epithelial, germ cell, sex-cord stromal, metastases to the ovary, and rare neoplasms of other origin (55,56) (Table 56.1).

Epithelial Carcinomas

Epithelial ovarian carcinoma is the most common type of ovarian cancer and comprises 90% of all ovarian malignancies in women (57). The single-cell ovarian epithelium is derived from the mesothelial lining that lines the pelvic cavity. During embryogenesis this same mesothelial lining gave rise to the müllerian ducts that formed the uterus, fallopian tubes, endocervix, and upper vagina. Serous carcinomas occur most commonly and are characterized by cystic and solid bilateral ovarian masses. Microscopically, the serous carcinomas resemble fallopian tube epithelium with glands and papilla formation. Psammoma bodies are seen in 30% of cases (58). The majority of serous carcinomas are poorly differentiated, high-grade carcinomas with sheets of malignant cells and marked nuclear atypia and mitoses. Clinical prognosis has been shown to correlate with tumor grade and the degree of differentiation. The tumor marker CA 125 is elevated in 75% to 80% of advanced-stage serous carcinomas (59).

Mucinous carcinomas make up about 15% of ovarian carcinomas. On gross inspection, mucinous carcinomas are frequently large, unilateral, multiloculated tumors. Microscopically, mucinous tumors are lined by cells that resemble the lining of the endocervix or colon. In the latter, a metastases from a gastrointestinal primary must be excluded as these patients have a uniformly worse prognosis (60). CA 19-9 is frequently elevated in mucinous carcinomas while CA 125 is modestly elevated. Pseudomyxoma peritonei is a variant of ovarian mucinous carcinoma with abundant extracellular mucin and admixed with mucinous epithelial cells that results in copious mucinous ascites. Pseudomyxoma is most frequently associated with well-differentiated or low-malignant potential ovarian mucinous carcinomas (see later discussion). The majority of cases of pseudomyxoma peritonei arise from the appendix with concurrent or secondary involvement of the ovary (61–63). The mainstay of treatment is cytoreductive surgery, and multiple treatment modalities with systemic and intraperitoneal chemotherapy have

Table 56.1

World Health Organization Histologic Classification of Ovarian Neoplasms

I. Surface epithelial tumors
   A. Serous tumors
   B. Mucinous tumors
      1. Endocervical-like
      2. Intestinal type
   C. Endometrioid tumors
   D. Clear cell tumors
   E. Transitional cell tumors
   F. Squamous cell tumors
   G. Mixed epithelial tumors
   H. Undifferentiated and unclassified carcinoma
II. Sex cord-stromal tumors
   A. Granulosa-stromal cell tumors
      1. Granulosa cell tumors (adult and juvenile)
      2. Tumors in the thecoma—fibroma group
         a. Thecoma
         b. Fibroma
         c. Cellular fibroma
         d. Fibrosarcoma
         e. Sclerosing stromal tumor
   B. Sertoli/stromal-cell tumors
      1. Sertoli cell tumors
      2. Sertoli-Leydig cell tumors
   C. Sex cord tumors with annular tubules
   D. Gynandroblastoma
   E. Unclassified
   F. Steroid (lipid) cell tumors
      1. Stromal luteoma
      2. Leydig cell tumor
      3. Steroid cell tumor, not otherwise specified
III. Germ cell tumors
   A. Dysgerminoma
   B. Yolk sac tumor (endodermal sinus tumor)
   C. Embryonal carcinoma
   D. Polyembryoma
   E. Choriocarcinoma
   F. Teratoma
      1. Immature
      2. Mature
      3. Struma ovarii
      4. Carcinoid tumors
   G. Mixed germ cell tumors
IV. Gonadoblastoma
V. Miscellaneous
   A. Small cell carcinoma
   B. Malignant lymphomas, leukemias, plasmacytomas
   C. Unclassified
   D. Metastatic tumors

From Scully RE. *Histologic Typing of Ovarian Tumors.* 2nd ed. New York: Springer-Verlag; 1999.

been described to improve patient survival (64). Patients have a high recurrence rate, with variable times to recurrence. Most series agree that when patients have recurrent disease, repeat laparotomy is required to relieve symptoms. The overall 5-year survival rate is 50%, and most patients die from bowel obstruction.

Endometrioid carcinomas resemble the lining of the uterus with frequent extracellular mucin production and squamous differentiation. There appears to be an association between ovarian endometrioid adenocarcinoma and endometriosis in approximately 5% to 10% of cases in which the carcinoma seems to arise from foci of endometriosis that has undergone malignant transformation (65). There are similar patterns of molecular alterations observed between endometriosis and endometrioid ovarian adenocarcinomas, suggesting that in select cases they may represent a continuum of carcinogenesis. Ovarian endometrioid adenocarcinoma presents with endometrial adenocarcinomas in 10% to 25% of cases. Distinguishing synchronous carcinomas from metastatic lesions from one site to the other can be a challenge and frequently relies on a combination of histopathologic features and the distribution of disease within the uterus and ovary (7,66).

Clear cell carcinomas are uniformly high-grade lesions with a poor prognosis. Microscopically, tumors have clear cells that result from abundant intracellular glycogen and hobnail cells. There is also an association between ovarian clear cell carcinoma and endometriosis in which it appears extraovarian endometriosis has undergone malignant transformation.

Tumors of Low Malignant Potential (Atypical Proliferating Tumors)

Ovarian tumors of low malignant potential (LMP), also known as *atypical proliferating tumors*, comprise a group of tumors showing greater epithelial proliferation than that seen in benign serous cystadenoma, although they are by definition noninvasive. Recognized by the International Federation of Gynecology and Obstetrics in 1971, LMP ovarian tumors account for approximately 15% of all epithelial ovarian cancers; mean age of occurrence is 40 years. A meta-analysis performed by the Collaborative Ovarian Cancer Group found that, as with malignant epithelial ovarian cancer, parity, multiple births, history of breast-feeding, and oral contraceptive use are protective against LMP tumors. A history of infertility and use of infertility drugs increase the risk of developing an LMP tumor, although the data are weak and controversial (67).

LMP ovarian tumors have been described for all epithelial ovarian subtypes; the most common types are serous and mucinous tumors. The absence of stromal invasion is an absolute criterion for making the diagnosis. Careful examination of the tissue blocks is necessary to minimize the potential for omitting an area of invasive carcinoma in LMP tumors. Approximately 20% to 30% of ovarian tumors diagnosed as LMP at frozen section prove to be invasive carcinomas on review of the permanent section (68).

Stage for stage, the 5-year survival rate for patients with LMP epithelial ovarian tumors is far better than that for patients with malignant epithelial ovarian cancer. A review of the literature by several investigators revealed a survival rate of >95% in patients with stage I LMP ovarian tumors. Furthermore, Trimble and Trimble (69) found that a majority of patients with LMP tumors actually died with the disease, not from it, as invasive carcinoma developed in only 8 of 953 patients (0.8%) with a mean follow-up of 7 years.

The primary surgical treatment for patients with LMP tumors who have completed childbearing is identical to the recommendation for invasive ovarian disease, including a total abdominal hysterectomy, bilateral salpingo-oophorectomy, tumor debulking, and full staging. An appendectomy should be performed in patients with a mucinous LMP tumor because of the association with a synchronous primary appendiceal neoplasm. In younger patients with early-stage disease and a desire for future childbearing, conservative surgery with preservation of the uterus, the contralateral ovary, and in some cases the ipsilateral ovary (i.e., cystectomy) may be the appropriate treatment. Consultation with a gynecologic oncologist and pathologist can identify those patients who are candidates for conservative management. Several studies, both cohort and observational, have reported excellent outcome with conservative management of such patients (70). One of the largest studies reports a 12% recurrence rate for patients treated conservatively with either unilateral salpingo-oophorectomy (n = 110) or ovarian cystectomy (n = 74) versus 2.5% for patients treated with definitive hysterectomy and bilateral salpingo-oophorectomy. Recurrences or progression to carcinoma (1.5%) were more common among patients with invasive implants or advanced stage disease. The feasibility of performing a cystectomy for an LMP ovarian tumor and conserving the rest of the ovarian tissue in early-stage disease has been described, but requires further study (71).

Presently, there is no evidence to suggest that adjuvant chemotherapy in early-stage disease or in patients with optimal cytoreduction of advanced disease improves survival in patients with LMP tumors. In fact, patients may be more likely to die from the side effects of adjuvant therapy than from the disease itself. Platinum-based therapy may be appropriate for a select group of patients with micropapillary serous tumors and invasive serous implants, based on the high rates of recurrence in these patients. However, patients must be counseled that available literature does not demonstrate improved survival with chemotherapy (72,73).

Germ Cell Tumors

Germ cell tumors account for 20% of all ovarian tumors and typically occur in young women. Germ cell tumors are the most common ovarian neoplasm for women under the age of 30. The typical presentation is from abdominal/pelvic pain. Less often, these tumors present with ovarian torsion, ovarian capsular rupture, and, rarely, hemoperitoneum. Most germ cell tumors are benign and only 2% to 3% are composed of malignant germ cell elements. The most common benign germ cell tumor is a mature cystic teratoma. The most common malignant germ cell tumors are the dysgerminoma, endodermal sinus tumor, and the immature teratoma. These ovarian cancers generally present with unilateral ovarian involvement and are highly curable with appropriate conservative surgery and chemotherapy. Elevations in serum tumor markers are frequently associated with germ cell cancers and are useful in assessing response to therapy and possible disease recurrence. These markers include alpha-fetoprotein, lactate dehydrogenase, human chorionic gonadotropin, and CA 125 (7).

Sex Cord-Stromal Tumors

Stromal cell tumors accounts for 8% of ovarian tumors. This category of tumors includes a wide array of tumors derived from sex cords (granulosa and Sertoli cells) and from gonadal stroma (theca and Leydig cells). The most common sex cord-stromal tumors are granulosa cell tumors and fibrothecomas. These tumors have a potential for sex steroid hormone secretion, most commonly the hormone estrogen. With the exception of juvenile granulosa cell tumors, most sex cord-stromal tumors present in women in their fifth decade. Early-stage tumors are treated with surgery while chemotherapy is generally reserved for women with advanced stage or recurrent cancers.

Patterns of Spread and Staging Epithelial Ovarian Cancer

Ovarian cancer spreads via four principle routes: direct extension, peritoneal dissemination, retroperitoneal lymphatics, and hematogenous dissemination. Exfoliation of cancer cells from the ovarian surface disseminate into the peritoneal cavity. Malignant cells can circulate in the normal flow of peritoneal fluid along the right paracolic gutter to the undersurface of the right hemidiaphragm that results in tumor nodules. Multifocal nodules are generally superficially invasive and may involve adjacent pelvic structures and the abdominal cavity. Such peritoneal spread can occur even in the absence of gross ovarian capsule involvement. Ascites occurs in approximately two thirds of patients. Ascites results from decreased plasma oncotic pressure and the third-spacing of fluid into the peritoneal cavity, increased fluid production from peritoneal surfaces damaged by tumor infiltration, and decreased absorption of fluid by tumor-obstructed lymphatics (74,75). Ovarian lymphatics drain primarily to the para-aortic, iliac, and obturator lymph nodes (76,77).

The objectives of primary surgery for patients with ovarian cancer are to establish a diagnosis, stage disease, cytoreduce, and palliation of symptoms. Historically the diagnosis of ovarian cancer is rarely made prior to surgery because concerns that biopsy of suspicious pelvic masses may seed the abdominal wall and that resulting tumor spill may cause further spread of disease. Staging is performed surgically to assess the spread and extent of disease (Tables 56.2 and 56.3) (78). An adequate vertical incision is generally required to provide adequate exposure and examination of the abdominal and pelvic cavities. Any ascites is collected on entry into the abdominal cavity. In the absence of widespread disease, pelvic washings are obtained and sent for cytologic evaluation. Random biopsies are taken from peritoneal surfaces including the gutters, right diaphragm, cul de sac, and other sites commonly involved with disease. Any suspicious areas or adhesions are biopsied. An infracolic omentectomy is generally performed to rule out occult disease. In the absence of gross upper abdominal disease >2 cm in diameter (stage IIIC), lymph node sampling is performed to rule out lymph node metastases, which would also upstage the patient to stage IIIC disease.

Table 56.2

Elements of Ovarian Cancer Staging

Adequate vertical incision
Abdominal and pelvic washings
Inspection and palpation of all abdominal and pelvic surfaces
Random peritoneal biopsies
Biopsy/resection of peritoneal adhesions
Removal of affected ovary
Removal of remaining ovary, uterus, and fallopian tubes[a]
Total abdominal hysterectomy and bilateral salpingo-oophorectomy
Omentectomy
Appendectomy
Pelvic and para-aortic lymph node sampling

[a] May forgo in selected patients.
From Chu CS, Rubin SC. Epidemiology, staging and clinical characteristics. Reproduced from Bristow RE, Karlan BY, eds. *Surgery for Ovarian Cancer: Principles and Practice.* London: Taylor and Francis; 2006:1–38.

In the context of disease that is clinically confined to the pelvis, great care is taken to avoid rupture of the ovarian mass and intraoperative spread of disease. Hysterectomy and removal of the contralateral ovary are performed except in the case of certain histologies, patient age, and clinical extent of disease. Young women with unilateral germ cell, stromal, or low malignant potential tumors who desire future fertility may have staging that preserves the uterus and contralateral ovary. Conservative therapy of low malignant-potential tumors with ovarian cystectomy has been recommended in the young patient, although the risk of recurrence appears to be higher than that observed with complete removal of the affected ovary (71). Complete surgical staging is paramount given that disease that appears clinically confined to the pelvis will be upstaged by virtue of occult nodal, peritoneal, or omental disease in 30% of patients who undergo comprehensive staging (79) (Table 56.4).

OPTIMAL SURGICAL CYTOREDUCTION

The majority of women will present with regional spread of disease and only 20% of patients will have disease confined to the pelvis at diagnosis (80). In this context, survival is multifactorial but there are two factors that are clinician-driven that strongly predict clinical outcome: surgical cytoreduction and platinum-taxane-based combination chemotherapy. Despite widely metastatic disease, the majority of patients with advanced ovarian cancer can achieve clinical remission through cytoreductive surgery and adjuvant chemotherapy because of the relatively chemosensitive nature of ovarian cancer.

The surgical management of ovarian cancer evolved from isolated oophorectomy in the 18th and 19th centuries to the concept of cytoreductive surgery in the 20th century. The value of omentectomy to remove a common site of metastatic disease

Table 56.3

International Federation of Gynecology and Obstetrics Staging of Ovarian Cancer

Stage	Definition
I	Growth limited to the ovaries
IA	Growth limited to one ovary; no ascites present containing malignant cells; no tumor on the external surfaces; capsule intact
IB	Growth limited to both ovaries; no ascites present containing malignant cells; no tumor on the external surfaces; capsules intact
IC	Tumor stage IA or TB, but with tumor on the surface of one or both ovaries; or with capsule ruptured; or with ascites present containing malignant cells, or with positive peritoneal washings
II	Growth involving one or both ovaries with pelvic extension
IIA	Extension and/or metastases to the uterus and/or tubes
IIB	Extension to other pelvic tissues
IIC	Tumor stage IIA or IIB but with tumor on the surface of one or both ovaries; or with capsule(s) ruptured; or with ascites present containing malignant cells, or with positive peritoneal washings
III	Tumor involving one or both ovaries with peritoneal implants outside the pelvis and/or positive retroperitoneal or inguinal nodes; superficial liver metastasis equals stage III; tumor is limited to the true pelvis but with histologically verified malignant extension to small bowel or omentum
IIIA	Tumor grossly limited to the true pelvis with negative nodes with histologically confirmed microscopic seeding or abdominal peritoneal surfaces
IIIB	Tumor of one or both ovaries; histologically confirmed implants of abdominal peritoneal surfaces, none exceeding 2 cm in diameter; nodes negative
IIIC	Tumor of one or both ovaries; histologically confirmed implants of abdominal peritoneal surfaces, none exceeding 2 cm in diameter; nodes negative
IV	Growth involving one or both ovaries with distant metastasis; if pleural effusion is present, there must be positive cytologic test results to allot a case to stage IV; parenchymal liver metastasis equals stage IV

Modified from Heintz AP, Odicino F, Maisonneuve P, et al. Carcinoma of the ovary. FIGO 6th Annual Report on the Results of Treatment in Gynecological Cancer. *Int J Gynaecol Obstet.* 2006;95(suppl 1):S161–S192.

Table 56.4

Frequency (%) of Malignant Ovarian Carcinoma (Including Low Malignant Potential Tumors) SEER 1992–1999*

Classification	%	Age Median	Stage Disease at Diagnosis* (%)		
			Localized	Regional	Distant
All epithelial	95.3	61	25.7	10.4	60.6
Serous	41.4	60			
Mucinous	13.7	52			
Endometrioid	12.8	58			
Clear	3.8	55			
Other epithelial	23.5	70			
Germ cell	2.6	26	54.2	15	28.7
Stromal cell	1.2	50	57.3	15	22.2
Other ovary	0.8	70	14.6	5.5	30.7

Localized–cancer confined entirely to ovary; Regional–cancer has extended into surrounding organs or tissues; Distant–cancer has spread to parts of the body remote from the ovary.
*Modified after Quirk and Natarajan[57]

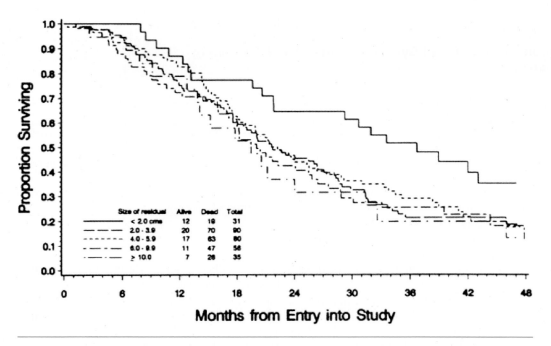

Size of residual	Alive	Dead	Total
< 2.0 cms	12	19	31
2.0 - 3.9	20	70	90
4.0 - 5.9	17	63	80
6.0 - 9.9	11	47	58
≥ 10.0	7	28	35

Figure 56.1 Survival by maximum diameter of residual disease. (From Hoskins et al. (86)).

was described and led to the concept of removing the primary tumor and metastases in order to improve patient outcome and symptoms (81,82). Munnell (83) introduced the concept that "maximal surgical effort" led to improved survival for patients whose tumors were largely resected compared with those patients who had only partial removal or biopsy. Griffiths (84) published a pivotal study in 1975 that quantified residual tumor volume following cytoreductive surgery and showed an inverse correlation between patient outcome and residual tumor diameter in 102 patients with stage II and II invasive epithelial cancer of the ovary. Patients with no residual tumor had a mean survival of 39 months while patients with residual tumor of 0.5 to 1.5 cm had a mean survival of 18 months. Patients who were left with >1.5 cm of tumor had a mean survival of 11 months and no patient survived beyond 25 months regardless of extensive surgical debulking. These findings suggest that surgical resection is of limited utility unless minimal/no residual tumor remains (84,85).

The definition of optimal surgical cytoreduction has evolved as more data have emerged to support the ability of aggressive surgical intervention to achieve minimal residual disease and improve patient outcome. Historically there have been opposing viewpoints regarding the relative importance of surgical effort versus the inherent biologic predisposition of the tumor on patient outcome. It has been suggested that improved patient outcome occurs more as a function of the inherent aggressiveness of the tumor, which determines its resectability and chemosensitivity rather the surgeon's operative effort. The positive impact of combination platinum-based chemotherapy on patient survival with advanced-stage disease has been shown in many prospective, randomized studies, while the relative effect of maximal surgical effort has been more difficult to quantify.

Large retrospective reviews have demonstrated the importance of optimal surgical cytoreduction and minimal residual

disease after primary surgery. Hoskins et al. (86) reported findings from Gynecologic Oncology Group studies that suboptimal debulking surgery (>2 cm residual disease) offered patients no improvement in survival regardless of the diameter of residual disease (Figure 56.1). In contrast, patients with stage III disease with ≤2 cm residual tumor had significantly improved survival compared to patients with >2 cm residual disease. Another Gynecologic Oncology Group study of 349 patients with optimally cytoreduced stage III disease (≤1 cm of residual disease) subsequently treated with platinum-based combination chemotherapy found that the volume of initial extrapelvic disease was a more significant predictor of survival than the amount of residual disease following cytoreductive surgery. Hoskins et al. (87) concluded that cytoreduction of large-volume disease to small-volume disease (≤1 cm) did not confer the same prognosis as that for patients with small initial tumor volume. However, further analysis suggested that the site and number of tumor implants of extrapelvic disease may influence survival.

A multivariate analysis performed in another retrospective review of 282 patients with advanced-stage ovarian carcinoma treated at the Memorial Sloan Kettering Cancer Center identified patient age, ascites, and residual disease ≤1 cm as significant prognostic factors that correlated with survival. Patients with ≤1 cm of residual disease had a median survival of 55 months compared with 28 months for those patients with >1 cm of disease. There was no significant difference between patients with 1 to 2 cm and >2 cm of disease. These data lend support to the current Gynecologic Oncology Group definition of optimal cytoreduction in which the largest residual tumor nodule measures ≤1 cm (88).

The probability of achieving optimal surgical cytoreduction (≤1 cm) was examined in 163 consecutive patients with advanced-stage ovarian cancer by Eisenkop et al. (89). Predictors of optimal cytoreduction in a multivariate analysis included performance status, stage, and the number of tumor implants on the intestinal serosa. Although poor performance status, stage IV disease, and a large number (>75) of metastatic implants decreased the likelihood of optimal cytoreduction, >60% of these patients still had complete surgical cytoreduction. The same authors analyzed the relationship between use of extended surgical procedures to achieve complete surgical cytoreduction on survival in an expanded cohort of 213 advanced-stage ovarian cancer patients. Extrapelvic bowel resection, modified posterior exenteration, diaphragm stripping or resection, lymph node debulking, and/or extensive peritoneal implant ablation were required in 209 patients (98%). Median operative time was 180 minutes with a mean estimated blood loss of 980 mL and a median hospital stay of 12 days. Median survival was 75.8 months with 1.9% perioperative death rate. Patient survival was not influenced by the use of any specific operative procedure or any specific intra-abdominal tumor location in this cohort of completely cytoreduced patients (90,91).

As expected, the aggressive surgical procedures necessary to achieve optimal cytoreduction often result in significant patient morbidity with prolonged operative time, additional blood loss, and longer hospitalization. Chi et al. (92) described the morbidity of incorporating more comprehensive debulking of upper abdominal disease on 140 patients with advanced stage (III/IV) ovarian/peritoneal and fallopian tube cancer using diaphragm stripping/resection, splenectomy, partial liver resection, and distal pancreatectomy. Patients who underwent more extensive procedures had significantly higher rates of optimal cytoreduction compared with patients treated with standard hysterectomy/bilateral salpingo-oophorectomy/omentectomy (76% vs. 50%) with higher estimated mean blood loss, 880 versus 460 mL (p <0.001) and loner mean operative time 264 versus 174 minutes (p <0.001). There were no significant differences in the frequency of complications, with a reported 6% rate of major complications including one death in the standard surgery arm, although the authors provided no information on the performance status or presence of comorbidities.

The majority of patients with stage IV disease appear to benefit from the same aggressive surgical efforts in an attempt to achieve optimal surgical cytoreduction. A cumulative total of 231 women with stage IV ovarian cancer were evaluable for response in three contemporaneous retrospective series (93–95). Approximately half of patients presented with cytologically confirmed pleural effusions, 16% to 20% with parenchymal liver disease and the remainder had a variety of metastatic sites including the abdominal/chest wall, extraperitoneal genital tract, and supraclavicular nodes. Optimal surgical cytoreduction (≤2 cm residual disease) was successful in 30% to 42% and was not influenced by the site of metastases. Median survival time was significantly longer for patients who were optimally cytoreduced compared with women with bulky residual disease, 25 to 40 months versus 15 to 18 months. Survival estimates of women with optimally cytoreduced disease were similar between patients with pleural effusion only and other stage IV patients. Further analysis of survival in one study found that neither the site nor the number of extraperitoneal metastases influenced survival. The size of extrapelvic disease did not impact survival in a subgroup of 23 of the 31 optimally cytoreduced patients in the same series (95).

Although the studies were retrospective with incomplete information regarding chemotherapy, the consistent finding of improved survival among optimally surgically cytoreduced stage IV patients supports a role for an aggressive surgical approach whenever possible (96). The presence of intrahepatic or extraperitoneal metastatic disease should not be a contraindication to surgical exploration in the appropriate patient. Bristow et al. (97) reported a median survival of 50 months for 6 of 37 (16%) stage IV patients who had optimal surgical cytoreduction (<1 cm of residual disease) of both intrahepatic and extrahepatic sites compared with 7.6 months for the 20 patients left with bulky residual disease at both sites. Even among patients with unresectable liver metastases, optimal cytoreduction of extrahepatic sites resulted in improved survival of median 27 months. Significant postoperative complications occurred in approximately 20% of patients including five patients (6%) who expired within 30 days of surgery. It is noteworthy that four of these patients had poor performance status of three with significant comorbidities (97).

A meta-analysis by Bristow et al. (98) demonstrated the importance of optimal surgical cytoreduction in ovarian cancer patients (Figure 56.2). Fifty-three studies comprising 6,885 patients with advanced-stage ovarian carcinoma treated with combination platinum-based chemotherapy following primary surgery were analyzed for variables that influence survival. The majority of studies used a definition of ≤2 cm residual disease to define maximal surgical cytoreduction. Maximal cytoreduction was the strongest predictor of patient survival in multiple linear regression analysis. Comparing estimated actuarial survival, patient cohorts with >75% maximal cytoreduction had a 50% increase in the median survival compared with cohorts with <25% maximal cytoreduction, 33.9 months versus 22.7 months. The

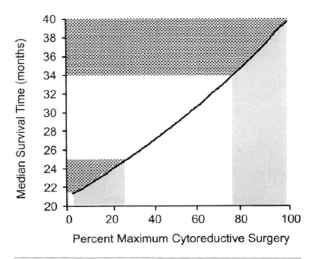

Figure 56.2 Simple linear regression analysis: de-logged median survival time plotted against percent maximal cytoreductive surgery. Gray area, maximal cytoreductive surgery ≤25% and >75%. Cross-hatched area, corresponding range of median survival times. (From Bristow RE, Tomacruz RS, Armstrong DK, et al. Survival effect of maximal cytoreductive surgery for advanced ovarian carcinoma during the platinum era: a meta-analysis. *J Clin Oncol* 2002;20(5):1248–1259.

authors concluded that referral of patients with presumed ovarian cancer to expert referral centers for primary surgery with experience in surgical cytoreduction was warranted to optimize patient survival (98).

Surgical outcome data in women with ovarian cancer suggest that specialized care is associated with superior outcome. Women cared for by specialists have higher rates of optimal surgical cytoreduction, higher compliance with published guidelines regarding appropriate surgical staging and use of adjuvant chemotherapy, and a reduction in the risk of death (99,100). Disease-directed therapy based on complete surgical staging in women with clinically early-stage disease found to have more advanced-stage disease largely explains the survival benefit of women cared for by gynecologic oncologists compared with other surgeons (101). Carney et al. (102) analyzed patterns of care for 848 women with ovarian cancer from a statewide tumor registry in Utah and found that the percentage of cases managed by a gynecologic oncologist varied by patient age. Thirty-six percent of women under the age of 40 years were seen by a gynecologic oncologist in comparison to 55% of women ages 40 to 59 and 43% of women ages 60 to 69. Among cases of advanced-stage disease, women cared for by a gynecologic oncologist had significantly improved survival compared with those who were not; median survival 26 versus 15 months, respectively.

Two companion studies evaluated the impact of surgeon specialty and hospital and surgeon procedure volume on the care of over 2,000 American elderly ovarian cancer patients (>65 years) in population-based cohorts using Surveillance, Epidemiology, and End Results (SEER) data registries linked to Medicare claims. SEER registries ascertain incident cancer cases in five states and six metropolitan areas that collectively represent 14% of the U.S. population (103,104). The authors found that the minority (33%) of patients were cared for by gynecologic oncologists while the majority was treated by general gynecologists (45%) or general surgeons (22%). The authors concluded that while patient age and stage were the most significant factors affecting patient outcome, high-volume surgeons in high-volume hospitals achieved marginally better surgical outcomes, which support the recommendations of professional societies to maximize access for women with known or suspected ovarian cancer to expert care centers (105,106).

INTERVAL CYTOREDUCTION

Survival for patients undergoing suboptimal surgical cytoreduction resulting in residual disease >2 cm remains poor, with a 21% 5-year survival rate according to the 2003 statistics of the International Federation of Gynecology and Obstetrics (107). Interval surgical cytoreduction following a short course of chemotherapy, typically two to three cycles, for women left with residual disease after primary surgical exploration has been proposed to improve the chemosensitivity of residual disease and improve patient outcome. Patients with disease progression (5% to 15%) receiving chemotherapy were not eligible for interval cytoreduction as further surgical effort has shown minimal survival benefit (108). Optimal cytoreduction following the interval cytoreduction has been reported in 63% to 80% of patients (85). Two large prospective, randomized trials on interval cytoreduc-

tion, Gynecologic Cancer Cooperative Group of the European Organisation for Research and Treatment (EORTC-GCG) 55865 (109) and Gynecologic Oncology Group 152 (110), found conflicting results on the impact of further surgery on patient survival. Both studies involved patients with advanced-stage disease of similar ages.

The EORTC study enrolled 425 patients with suboptimal resection of tumor at primary surgery. One hundred forty patients were randomized to surgery followed by an additional three cycles of cisplatin and cyclophosphamide chemotherapy in comparison to 138 patients who received chemotherapy alone. Overall and progression-free survival was significantly improved in patients randomized to interval cytoreduction, with a calculated reduction in risk of death of 33% compared to patients who had no surgery. Further analysis revealed that this survival advantage was seen only in patients who achieved optimal residual disease (<1 cm) following induction chemotherapy and interval surgery. Patients whose residual tumors were >1 cm after chemotherapy and interval surgery had identical median survival to those patients who had chemotherapy alone, 19.4 months versus 20 months (109).

The Gynecologic Oncology Group (GOG) study randomized 550 women with advanced-stage residual disease >1 cm following primary attempted surgical cytoreduction to three cycles of cisplatin and paclitaxel followed by interval cytoreduction or three additional cycles of chemotherapy. Interval cytoreductive surgery did not improve overall or progression-free survival (110).

The dissimilar results of these two trials may reflect different degrees of initial surgical effort. The GOG trial required maximal surgical effort at laparotomy with removal of as much tumor as possible. In this study 95% of the primary operations were performed by gynecologic oncologists, whereas the type of surgeon and extent of surgery was not described in the EORTC trial. This presumed maximal surgical effort made at primary surgery in the GOG trial resulted in a study population of women with unresectable residual tumor, in contrast to the EORTC study in which less primary surgical effort resulted in a study population of patients with remaining disease that was potentially resectable. Additionally, the more effective cisplatin and paclitaxel chemotherapy used in the GOG study may have minimized the benefit of secondary surgery compared with the earlier regimen of chemotherapy in the EORTC trial (85). Both studies confirmed the poor prognosis for women whose tumors could not be resected after maximal primary and interval surgical effort with intervening platinum-based chemotherapy (109,110).

NEOADJUVANT CHEMOTHERAPY

Although it is difficult to determine the relative contribution of tumor biology versus surgical effort to optimal surgical cytoreduction, it is clear that suboptimal cytoreduction offers the patient with ovarian cancer little benefit. Neoadjuvant chemotherapy in lieu of primary surgery has been proposed as an alternative to avoid the morbidity of an unsuccessful surgical procedure for patients considered at the highest risk of having primarily unresectable tumor. Pathologic confirmation of the diagnosis by biopsy is mandatory before offering patients neoadjuvant chemotherapy. Cytology diagnosis from ascites or a pleural effusion may be used as a surrogate for biopsy in suspected cases of advanced ovarian cancer when combined with appropriately elevated tumor markers and clinical disease distribution.

Efforts to identify a group of patients with preoperative factors or risks that render the likelihood of optimal cytoreduction have had variable success. The predictive ability of radiologic criteria, preoperative CA 125, volume of ascites, and distribution of abdominal/peritoneal tumor have all been proposed to distinguish between optimal and suboptimal surgical candidates with disappointing results (85,97). The limited reproducibility of results from small retrospective populations and poor predictive value of such radiologic criteria diminish the accurate preoperative identification of patients destined to have a suboptimal cytoreduction (111–113). A recent multi-institutional cross-validation study of CT predictors of suboptimal primary cytoreduction found that 64% to 86% of patients predicted to undergo suboptimal cytoreduction actually underwent optimal cytoreduction (114). A reliable, predictive model of surgical outcome for advanced-stage patients must incorporate multiple factors, including an individual surgeon's philosophy and experience with maximal surgical effort, reproducible radiologic assessment of disease distribution, as well as appropriate postoperative care.

The identification of patient factors that predict suboptimal surgical cytoreduction is also difficult. Data suggest that older patients are less likely to undergo maximal cytoreductive surgery, but chronological age itself should not be a contraindication to cytoreductive surgery. Performance status correlates more accurately with surgical outcome. Neoadjuvant chemotherapy has shown benefit in women with severe systemic disorders by reducing the extent of disease and improving patient performance status before undertaking surgical cytoreduction. Advocates of neoadjuvant chemotherapy have reported additional benefits, including an increased rate of optimal cytoreduction, less extensive surgery with reduced blood loss, lower morbidity, and reduced hospital stay in patients treated with chemotherapy first followed by surgery without compromising patient prognosis (115–117). Vergote et al. (117) retrospectively compared 112 patients treated with standard primary surgery followed by chemotherapy from 1980 to 1988 with 173 women treated between 1989 and 1997 who were assigned to either neoadjuvant chemotherapy (43%) or primary surgery (57%) based laparoscopic and/or radiologic assessment of tumor burden, stage IV disease, and performance status. The actuarial crude 3-year survival was superior in the second period than the first, 42% versus 26%. However, patients in the second period treated with primary surgery had significantly longer 3-year survival than those treated with primary chemotherapy, 53% versus 25%. Eighty-four percent of women deemed to have unresectable disease by laparoscopic assessment underwent an optimal surgical cytoreduction following primary chemotherapy; however, 18 patients (37%) assigned to primary chemotherapy never underwent an attempted interval surgical procedure. Schwartz et al. (116) compared the outcome of 59 consecutively treated women who received neoadjuvant chemotherapy for medical comorbidities or disease presumed to be unresectable to conventionally treated women during the same period. Although it did not achieve statistical significance, median overall survival of patients treated

with neoadjuvant chemotherapy was approximately half of that observed for women treated with primary surgery, 1.07 versus 2.18 years, respectively.

A recent meta-analysis reviewed available studies to better address the survival outcome of patients treated with neoadjuvant chemotherapy and to try to identify prognostic variables within this patient population. Twenty-one studies comprising 835 patients were included. Studies were largely retrospective, with 16 different platinum-based chemotherapy regimens (85,118). The median overall survival for the cohort ranged from 10 to 42 months, with a weighted median survival of 24.5 months. A significant detrimental impact on survival was noted when patients received more cycles of chemotherapy before attempted cytoreductive surgery. Each incremental increase in preoperative chemotherapy cycles was associated with a decrease in median survival of 4.1 months. Median overall survival was improved in those cohorts treated with platinum-taxane therapy and more recent year of publication (118).

The authors concluded that neoadjuvant chemotherapy in lieu of primary cytoreduction is associated with inferior patient survival. Although reported optimal surgical cytoreduction rates for patients with advanced-stage ovarian cancer range from 30% to 90%, most high-volume centers describe optimal cytoreductive surgery is possible in 75% of patients (119). The median survival for cohorts in which optimal surgical cytoreduction is achieved 75% of the time is 36.8 months (98). Considering this equation it is necessary to search for reliable selection criteria that can identify patients with surgically unresectable disease without depriving good surgical candidates the opportunity for optimal surgical cytoreduction. Given the significant survival benefit of optimal surgical cytoreduction, which is unparalleled by neoadjuvant chemotherapy and interval cytoreduction, it is advised that surgical exploration should be offered to all patients who are medically fit for surgery. This finding must be reinforced in light of the widespread implementation of neoadjuvant chemotherapy and perception by some that neoadjuvant chemotherapy and standard primary cytoreductive surgery followed by chemotherapy have equivalent patient outcomes. A questionnaire distributed among full members of the Society of Gynecologic Oncologists found that, although the majority chose treatment with surgical resection over chemotherapy as primary treatment for patients with advanced-stage disease, 50% agreed that the two approaches were equivalent (120). Multi-institutional prospective trials comparing neoadjuvant to conventional therapy are underway and hope to address whether preoperative models exist that can predict surgical outcome and the impact on patient survival. In the interim, neoadjuvant chemotherapy should be reserved for the patient whose medical comorbidities severely limit the patient's ability to tolerate surgical cytoreduction (96).

SECONDARY CYTOREDUCTION

The natural history of advanced-stage ovarian cancer is that disease will recur in the majority of cases. The rationale behind cytoreductive surgery followed by chemotherapy in these circumstances remains more controversial. Theoretically, repeat or secondary cytoreductive surgery can enhance the response to chemotherapy in the appropriate patients by reducing tumor volume and improving chemotherapy pharmacokinetics as is proposed in the newly diagnosed patient. The limited success of chemotherapy in the setting of recurrent disease has contributed to the controversy regarding the benefit of secondary cytoreductive surgery. Conclusions from available retrospective studies have been hampered by small numbers of heterogeneous patient populations treated with variable chemotherapy regimens over wide intervals of time (121). Nonetheless, aggregate data suggest that there is a benefit for secondary cytoreduction in the appropriately selected patient. Secondary cytoreduction is reported feasible in 37% to 87% of patients who underwent the procedure with acceptable morbidity and median overall survival after secondary cytoreduction of 16.3 to 35.9 months. For those patients who achieved macroscopic resection of all residual disease at secondary cytoreduction, median survival was reported from 29 to 100 months (122–124).

Although consensus is lacking, studies have found that predictors of successful secondary cytoreduction include prolonged disease-free interval, ideally >12 months, good performance status, *primary* optimal cytoreductive surgery, absence of large-volume ascites, and a limited number of sites of recurrence (121,125). The Arbeitsgemeinschaft Gynaekologische Onkologie Ovarian Committee (AGO OC) and AGO-OVAR conducted a retrospective analysis of hospital records from 267 patients who had secondary cytoreductive surgery for recurrent ovarian cancer from 2000 to 2003. The authors found that the only patients who benefited from secondary cytoreduction were those who had complete resection of tumor, which was feasible in 49.8% of patients. Three variables predicted surgical outcome at secondary cytoreduction: performance status, residual disease after primary surgery, and volume of ascites. AGO is currently applying these findings in a prospective trial that evaluates a predictive model for surgical outcome in secondary cytoreductive surgery (125).

POSTOPERATIVE CHEMOTHERAPY

Combination platinum-taxane-based chemotherapy has been the cornerstone of postoperative care for patients with ovarian cancer. Platinum agents, such as cisplatin and carboplatin, are the most active agents in ovarian cancer and have been incorporated into treatment for over 3 decades. Carboplatin has largely replaced cisplatin in the treatment of newly diagnosed disease because of its ease of administration and better side effects profile (126,127). Two large randomized trials in patients with advanced ovarian cancer demonstrated that combination platinum-taxane therapy prolonged both progression-free and overall survival compared with regimens that did not contain taxanes (128,129). The median survival for patients left with >1 cm residual who received with paclitaxel and cisplatin therapy was 37 months compared with 25 months for those patients who received cyclophosphamide and cisplatin (p <0.001) (128). For patients with advanced-stage disease who had optimal surgical cytoreduction, the median overall survival for patients treated with paclitaxel-carboplatin regimen approached 5 years and resulted in complete pathologic remission in more than half of patients (126). It is estimated that the inclusion of taxanes in first-line therapy of patients with advanced-stage ovarian cancer

has reduced the risk of death by 30% (130). Although the majority of patients tolerate paclitaxel/carboplatin without difficulty, peripheral neuropathy has been the principal nonhematologic toxicity associated with paclitaxel that can impair patients' quality of life. Docetaxel combined with carboplatin appears to have less neurotoxicity with equivalent efficacy compared to paclitaxel/carboplatin, although it did result in greater myelosuppression (131). Even in the context of advanced-stage ovarian cancer, 70% to 80% of patients achieve clinical remission with platinum/taxane combination chemotherapy defined as normal physical examination, CA 125, and imaging studies largely due to the chemosensitive nature of ovarian cancer.

INTRAPERITONEAL CHEMOTHERAPY

Intraperitoneal administration of chemotherapy has long been advocated as a treatment for ovarian cancer based on the distribution of disease within the abdominal-pelvic cavity and the high local concentrations of chemotherapy that can be delivered via the intraperitoneal route. The pharmacologic advantage of intraperitoneal route is considerable with concentrations that are 20- to more than 100-fold higher for drugs such as cisplatin and paclitaxel when given via intraperitoneal catheter compared with standard intravenous therapy. Because drugs delivered via the intraperitoneal route penetrate to a depth of only millimeters below the peritoneal surface, the intraperitoneal treatment of patients has been most effective in those patients with minimal residual peritoneal disease (132).

Three large, randomized multicenter trials comparing cisplatin-combination intraperitoneal chemotherapy to standard intravenous therapy for patients with optimally cytoreduced patients with advanced-stage disease found an 8- to 16-month survival advantage for patients treated with intraperitoneal chemotherapy and a 21% reduction in the risk of death (133–136). The most recent study randomized 415 newly diagnosed, optimally cytoreduced, stage III ovarian cancer patients to control intravenous cisplatin/paclitaxel versus experimental intravenous paclitaxel on day 1, intraperitoneal cisplatin on day 2, and intraperitoneal paclitaxel on day 8. At a median follow-up of 50 months, the intravenous/intraperitoneal patients had a median improved overall survival of 15.9 months (135). The intravenous/intraperitoneal regimen was, however, significantly less tolerable than standard intravenous therapy. Significant abdominal pain, hematologic, metabolic, and neurological toxic effects were seen more commonly in the experimental arm, as well as catheter-related problems. Of the 205 eligible women randomized to intravenous/intraperitoneal therapy, only 42% of patients completed all six cycles. Forty of these women (34%) discontinued experimental treatment because of catheter-related complications including occlusion, catheter infection, or leakage or leaking from the vagina (137). The authors suggested that successful intraperitoneal treatment can be optimized by the use of single-lumen venous catheters as well as avoiding the placement of devices at the time of left-sided colon/rectosigmoid resection if the peritoneal cavity is grossly contaminated. Extensive adhesions and significant obesity may also limit successful intraperitoneal access and distribution of drug delivery. Given the significant survival advantage seen among patients treated with intraperitoneal therapy, efforts should be made to optimize intraperitoneal drug selection, dosing, and delivery strategies to improve its tolerability for ovarian cancer patients.

REFERENCES

1. Jemal A, Siegel R, Ward E, et al. Cancer statistics, 2006. *CA Cancer J Clin.* 2008;56:106–130.
2. Fathalla MF. Incessant ovulation: a factor in ovarian neoplasia? *Lancet.* 1971;2:163.
3. Parazzini F, Tavani A, Ricci E, et al. Menstrual and reproductive factors and hip fractures in post menopausal women. *Maturitas* 1996;24(3):191–196.
4. Wu ML, Whittemore AS, Paffenbarger RS, Jr., et al. Personal and environmental characteristics related to epithelial ovarian cancer. I. Reproductive and menstrual events and oral contraceptive use. *Am J Epidemiol* 1988;128(6):1216–1227.
5. Whittemore AS, Harris R, Itnyre J. Characteristics relating to ovarian cancer risk: collaborative analysis of 12 US case-control studies. II. Invasive epithelial ovarian cancers in white women. Collaborative Ovarian Cancer Group. *American Journal of Epidemiology* 1992;136(10):1184–1203.
6. Longo DL, Young RC. Cosmetic talc and ovarian cancer. *Lancet* 1979;2(8150):1011–1012.
7. Chu CS, Rubin SC. Epidemiology, staging and clinical characteristics. In: Bristow RE, Karlan BY, eds. *Surgery for Ovarian Cancer: Principles and Practice.* London: Taylor and Francis; 2006:1–38.
8. Hankinson SE, Hunter DJ, Colditz GA, et al. Tubal ligation, hysterectomy, and risk of ovarian cancer. A prospective study. *JAMA.* 1993;270(23):2813–2818.
9. Kreiger N, Sloan M, Cotterchio M, et al. Surgical procedures associated with risk of ovarian cancer. *Int J Epidemiol* 1997;26(4):710–715.
10. Bristow RE, Karlan BY. The risk of ovarian cancer after treatment for infertility. *Curr Opin Obstet Gynecol* 1996;8(1):32–37.
11. Rossing MA, Daling JR, Weiss NS, et al. Ovarian tumors in a cohort of infertile women. *N Engl J Med.* 1994;331:771–776.
12. Whittemore AS, Wu ML, Paffenbarger RS, Jr., et al. Epithelial ovarian cancer and the ability to conceive. *Cancer Res* 1989;49(14):4047–4052.
13. Kerlikowske K, Brown JS, Grady DG. Should women with familial ovarian cancer undergo prophylactic oophorectomy? *Obstet Gynecol* 1992;80(4):700–707.
14. Szabo CI, King MC. Population Genetics of BRCA1 and BRCA2. *Am J Hum Genet* 1997;60:1013–1020.
15. Struewing JP, Hartge P, Wacholder S, et al. The risk of cancer associated with specific mutations of BRCA1 and BRCA2 among Ashkenazi Jews. *N Engl J Med* 1997;336(20):1401–1408.
16. King MC, Marks JH, Mandell JB. Breast and ovarian cancer risks due to inherited mutations in BRCA1 and BRCA2. *Science* 2003;302(5645):643–646.
17. Chen S, Iversen ES, Friebel T, et al. Characterization of BRCA1 and BRCA2 mutations in a large United States sample. *J Clin Oncol* 2006;24(6):863–871.
18. Burke W, Daly M, Garber J, et al. Recommendations for follow-up care of individuals with an inherited predisposition to cancer. II. BRCA1 and BRCA2. *Cancer Genetics Studies Consortium. JAMA* 1997;277(12):997–1003.
19. Daly MB. Genetic/Familial High-Risk Assessment: Breast and Ovarian Cancer. V.1.2007. National Comprehensive Cancer Network (NCCN) Clinical Practice Guidelines in Oncology. Published online at http://www.nccn.org/professionals/physician_gls/PDF/genetics_screening.pdf
20. Stirling D, Evans DG, Pichert G, et al. Screening for familial ovarian cancer: failure of current protocols to detect ovarian cancer at an early stage according to the International Federation of Gynecology and Obstetrics system. *J Clin Oncol.* 2005;23:5588-5596.
21. Oei AL, Massuger LF, Bulten J, et al. Surveillance of women at high risk for hereditary ovarian cancer is inefficient. *Br J Cancer* 2006;94(6):814–819.
22. Olivier RI, Lubsen-Brandsma MA, Verhoef S, et al. CA125 and transvaginal ultrasound monitoring in high-risk women cannot prevent the diagnosis of advanced ovarian cancer. *Gynecologic Oncology* 2006;100(1):20–26.
23. Skates SJ, Menon U, MacDonald N, et al. Calculation of the Risk of Ovarian Cancer From Serial CA-125 Values for Preclinical Detection in Postmenopausal Women. *J Clin Oncol* 2003;21(10 Suppl):206–210.
24. Whittemore AS, Balise RR, Pharoah PD, et al. Oral contraceptive use and ovarian cancer risk among carriers of BRCA1 or BRCA2 mutations. *Br J Cancer* 2004;91(11):1911–1915.
25. Narod S, Risch H, Moslehi R, et al. Oral contraceptives and the risk of hereditary ovarian cancer. *New England Journal of Medicine* 1998;339:424–428.
26. Modan B. BRCA1 mutations and survival in women with ovarian cancer [letter; comment]. *New England Journal of Medicine* 1997;336(17):1255; discussion 6–7.
27. McGuire V, Felberg A, Mills M, et al. Relation of contraceptive and reproductive history to ovarian cancer risk in carriers and noncarriers of BRCA1 gene mutations. *Am J Epidemiol* 2004;160(7):613–618.
28. De Palo G, Mariani L, Camerini T, et al. Effect of fenretinide on ovarian carcinoma occurrence. *Gynecologic Oncology* 2002;86(1):24–7.
29. De Palo G, Veronesi U, Camerini T, et al. Can fenretinide protect women against ovarian cancer? *J Natl Cancer Inst.* 1995;87:146-147.
30. Modan B, Hartge P, Hirsh-Yechezkel G, et al. Parity, oral contraceptives, and the risk of ovarian cancer among carriers and noncarriers of a BRCA1 or BRCA2 mutation. *N Engl J Med* 2001;345(4):235–240.
31. Narod SA, Sun P, Ghadirian P, et al. Tubal ligation and risk of ovarian cancer in carriers of BRCA1 or BRCA2 mutations: a case-control study. *Lancet* 2001;357(9267):1467–1470.
32. Rutter JL, Wacholder S, Chetrit A, et al. Gynecologic surgeries and risk of ovarian cancer in women with BRCA1 and BRCA2 Ashkenazi founder mutations: an Israeli population-based case-control study. *J Natl Cancer Inst* 2003;95(14):1072–1078.
33. Rebbeck TR, Lynch HT, Neuhausen SL, et al. Prophylactic oophorectomy in carriers of BRCA1 or BRCA2 mutations. *N Engl J Med* 2002;346(21):1616–1622.
34. Kauff ND, Satagopan JM, Robson ME, et al. Risk-reducing salpingo-oophorectomy in women with a BRCA1 or BRCA2 mutation. *N Engl J Med* 2002;346(21):1609–1615.
35. Leeper K, Garcia R, Swisher E, et al. Pathologic findings in prophylactic oophorectomy specimens in high-risk women. *Gynecologic Oncology* 2002;87(1):52–56.
36. Domchek SM, Friebel TM, Neuhausen SL, et al. Mortality after bilateral salpingo-oophorectomy in BRCA1 and BRCA2 mutation carriers: a prospective cohort study. *Lancet Oncol* 2006;7(3):223–229.
37. Finch A, Beiner M, Lubinski J, et al. Salpingo-oophorectomy and the risk of ovarian, fallopian tube, and peritoneal cancers in women with a BRCA1 or BRCA2 Mutation. *JAMA.* 2006;296(2):185–192.
38. Eisen A, Lubinski J, Klijn J, et al. Breast cancer risk following bilateral oophorectomy in BRCA1 and BRCA2 mutation carriers:

an international case-control study. *J Clin Oncol.* 2005;23:7491–7496.

39. Rebbeck TR, Friebel T, Wagner T, et al. Effect of short-term hormone replacement therapy on breast cancer risk reduction after bilateral prophylactic oophorectomy in BRCA1 and BRCA2 mutation carriers: the PROSE Study Group. *J Clin Oncol* 2005;23(31):7804–7810.

40. Powell CB, Kenley E, Chen LM, et al. Risk-reducing salpingo-oophorectomy in BRCA mutation carriers: role of serial sectioning in the detection of occult malignancy. *J Clin Oncol* 2005;23(1):127–132.

41. Lu KH, Garber JE, Cramer DW, et al. Occult ovarian tumors in women with BRCA1 or BRCA2 mutations undergoing prophylactic oophorectomy. *J Clin Oncol* 2000;18(14):2728–2732.

42. Medeiros F, Muto MG, Lee Y, et al. The tubal fimbria is a preferred site for early adenocarcinoma in women with familial ovarian cancer syndrome. *Am J Surg Pathol* 2006;30(2):230–236.

43. Colgan TJ, Murphy J, Cole DE, et al. Occult carcinoma in prophylactic oophorectomy specimens: prevalence and association with BRCA germline mutation status. *Am J Surg Pathol* 2001;25(10):1283–1289.

44. Paley PJ, Swisher EM, Garcia RL, et al. Occult cancer of the fallopian tube in BRCA-1 germline mutation carriers at prophylactic oophorectomy: a case for recommending hysterectomy at surgical prophylaxis. *Gynecologic Oncology* 2001;80(2):176–180.

45. Lavie O, Hornreich G, Ben-Arie A, et al. BRCA germline mutations in Jewish women with uterine serous papillary carcinoma. *Gynecol Oncol.* 2004;92:521–524.

46. Cass I, Holschneider C, Datta N, et al. BRCA-mutation-associated fallopian tube carcinoma: a distinct clinical phenotype? *Obstet Gynecol* 2005;106(6):1327–1334.

47. Levine DA, Lin O, Barakat RR, et al. Risk of endometrial carcinoma associated with BRCA mutation. *Gynecologic Oncology* 2001;80(3):395–398.

48. Goshen R, Chu W, Elit L, et al. Is uterine papillary serous adenocarcinoma a manifestation of the hereditary breast-ovarian cancer syndrome? *Gynecologic Oncology* 2000;79(3):477–481.

49. Aaltonen LA, Peltomaki P, Leach FS, et al. Clues to the pathogenesis of familial colorectal cancer. *Science* 1993;260(5109):812–816.

50. Leach FS, Nicolaides NC, Papadopoulos N, et al. Mutations of a mutS homolog in hereditary nonpolyposis colorectal cancer. *Cell* 1993;75(6):1215–1225.

51. Watson P, Vasen HF, Mecklin JP, et al. The risk of endometrial cancer in hereditary nonpolyposis colorectal cancer. *Am J Med* 1994;96(6):516–520.

52. Lu KH, Dinh M, Kohlmann W, et al. Gynecologic cancer as a "sentinel cancer" for women with hereditary nonpolyposis colorectal cancer syndrome. *Obstet Gynecol* 2005;105(3):569–574.

53. Aarnio M, Sankila R, Pukkala E, et al. Cancer risk in mutation carriers of DNA-mismatch-repair genes. *Int J Cancer* 1999;81(2):214–218.

54. Schmeler KM, Lynch HT, Chen LM, et al. Prophylactic surgery to reduce the risk of gynecologic cancers in the Lynch syndrome. *N Engl J Med* 2006;354(3):261–269.

55. Scully RE. *Histologic Typing of Ovarian Tumors.* 2nd ed. New York: Springer-Verlag; 1999.

56. Robboy SJ, Duggan M, Kurman RJ. The female reproductive system. In: Rubin E FJ, ed. *Pathology.* 2nd ed. Philadelphia: LB Lippincott; 1988, 972–981.

57. Quirk JT, Natarajan N. Ovarian cancer incidence in the United States, 1992–1999. *Gynecologic Oncology* 2005;97(2):519–523.

58. Aure JC, Hoeg K, Kolstad P. Psammoma bodies in serous carcinoma of the ovary. A prognostic study. *Am J Obstet Gynecol* 1971;109(1):113–118.

59. Bast RC, Jr., Klug TL, St John E, et al. A radioimmunoassay using a monoclonal antibody to monitor the course of epithelial ovarian cancer. *N Engl J Med* 1983;309(15):883–887.

60. Seidman JD, Kurman RJ, Ronnett BM. Primary and metastatic mucinous adenocarcinomas in the ovaries: incidence in routine practice with a new approach to improve intraoperative diagnosis. *Am J Surg Pathol* 2003;27(7):985–993.

61. Ronnett BM, Kurman RJ, Zahn CM, et al. Pseudomyxoma peritonei in women: a clinicopathologic analysis of 30 cases with emphasis on site of origin, prognosis, and relationship to ovarian mucinous tumors of low malignant potential. *Hum Pathol* 1995;26(5):509–524.

62. Wertheim I, Fleischhacker D, McLachlin CM, et al. Pseudomyxoma peritonei: a review of 23 cases. *Obstet Gynecol* 1994;84(1):17–21.

63. Young RH, Gilks CB, Scully RE. Mucinous tumors of the appendix associated with mucinous tumors of the ovary and pseudomyxoma peritonei. A clinicopathological analysis of 22 cases supporting an origin in the appendix. *Am J Surg Pathol* 1991;15(5):415–429.

64. Sugarbaker PH, Chang D. Results of treatment of 385 patients with peritoneal surface spread of appendiceal malignancy. *Ann Surg Oncol.* 1999;6:727–731.

65. Ness RB. Endometriosis and ovarian cancer: thoughts on shared pathophysiology. *Am J Obstet Gynecol* 2003;189(1):280–294.

66. Walsh C, Holschneider C, Hoang Y, et al. Coexisting ovarian malignancy in young women with endometrial cancer. *Obstet Gynecol* 2005;106(4):693–699.

67. Harris R, Whittemore AS, Itnyre J. Characteristics relating to ovarian cancer risk: collaborative analysis of 12 US case-control studies. III. Epithelial tumors of low malignant potential in white women. Collaborative Ovarian Cancer Group. *Am J Epidemiol* 1992;136(10):1204–1211.

68. Houck K, Nikrui N, Duska L, et al. Borderline tumors of the ovary: correlation of frozen and permanent histopathologic diagnosis. *Obstet Gynecol* 2000;95(6 Pt 1):839–843.

69. Trimble CL, Trimble EL. Management of epithelial ovarian tumors of low malignant potential. *Gynecologic Oncology* 1994;55(3 Pt 2):S52–S61.

70. Lim-Tan SK, Cajigas HE, Scully RE. Ovarian cystectomy for serous borderline tumors: a follow-up study of 35 cases. *Obstet Gynecol* 1988;72(5):775–781.

71. Zanetta G, Chiari S, Rota S, et al. Conservative surgery for stage I ovarian carcinoma in women of childbearing age. *Br J Obstet Gynaecol* 1997;104(9):1030–1035.

72. Seidman JD, Kurman RJ. Ovarian serous borderline tumors: a critical review of the literature with emphasis on prognostic indicators. *Hum Pathol* 2000;31(5):539–557.

73. Gershenson DM. Contemporary treatment of borderline ovarian tumors. *Cancer Invest* 1999;17(3):206–210.

74. Feldman GB, Knapp RC, Order SE, et al. The role of lymphatic obstruction in the formation of ascites in a murine ovarian carcinoma. *Cancer Res.* 1972;32:1663-1666.

75. Holm-Nielsen P. Pathogenesis of ascites in peritoneal carcinomatosis. *Acta Pathol Microbiol Scand* 1953;33(1):10–21.

76. Buchsbaum HJ, Brady MF, Delgado G, et al. Surgical staging of carcinoma of the ovaries. *Surg Gynecol Obstet* 1989;169(3):226–232.

77. Burghardt E, Girardi F, Lahousen M, et al. Patterns of pelvic and paraaortic lymph node involvement in ovarian cancer. *Gynecologic Oncology* 1991;40(2):103–106.

78. Heintz AP, Odicino F, Maisonneuve P, et al. Carcinoma of the ovary. FIGO 6th Annual Report on the Results of Treatment in Gynecological Cancer. *International Journal of Gynaecology and Obstetrics:*

the Official Organ of the International Federation of Gynaecology and Obstetrics 2006;95 Suppl 1:S161–S192.

79. Young RC, Decker DG, Wharton JT, et al. Staging laparotomy in early ovarian cancer. *JAMA* 1983;250(22):3072–3076.

80. Heintz AP, Odicino F, Maisonneuve P, et al. Carcinoma of the ovary. *J Epidemiol Biostat* 2001;6(1):107–138.

81. Meigs J. *Tumors of the Female Pelvis*. New York: MacMIllan; 1934.

82. Pemberton F. Carcinoma of the Ovary. *Am J Obstet Gynecol* 1940;40:751–763.

83. Munnell EW. The changing prognosis and treatment in cancer of the ovary. A report of 235 patients with primary ovarian carcinoma 1952–1961. *Am J Obstet Gynecol* 1968;100(6):790–805.

84. Griffiths CT. Surgical resection of tumor bulk in the primary treatment of ovarian carcinoma. *Natl Cancer Inst Monogr.* 1975;42:101–104.

85. Holschneider C, Berek JS. Cytoreductive Surgery:principles and rationale. In: Bristow RE, Karlan BY, ed. *Surgery for Ovarian Cancer: Principles and Practice*. London: Taylor and Francis; 2006, 87–125.

86. Hoskins WJ, McGuire WP, Brady MF, et al. The effect of diameter of largest residual disease on survival after primary cytoreductive surgery in patients with suboptimal residual epithelial ovarian carcinoma. *Am J Obstet Gynecol* 1994;170(4):974–979; discussion 9–80.

87. Hoskins WJ, Bundy BN, Thigpen JT, et al. The influence of cytoreductive surgery on recurrence-free interval and survival in small-volume stage III epithelial ovarian cancer: a Gynecologic Oncology Group study. *Gynecologic Oncology* 1992;47(2):159–166.

88. Chi DS, Liao JB, Leon LF, et al. Identification of prognostic factors in advanced epithelial ovarian carcinoma. *Gynecologic Oncology* 2001;82(3):532–537.

89. Eisenkop SM, Friedman RL, Wang HJ. Complete cytoreductive surgery is feasible and maximizes survival in patients with advanced epithelial ovarian cancer: a prospective study. *Gynecologic Oncology* 1998;69(2):103–108.

90. Eisenkop SM, Spirtos NM. Procedures required to accomplish complete cytoreduction of ovarian cancer: is there a correlation with "biological aggressiveness" and survival? *Gynecologic Oncology* 2001;82(3):435–441.

91. Eisenkop SM, Spirtos NM, Friedman RL, et al. Relative influences of tumor volume before surgery and the cytoreductive outcome on survival for patients with advanced ovarian cancer: a prospective study. *Gynecologic Oncology* 2003;90(2):390–396.

92. Chi DS, Franklin CC, Levine DA, et al. Improved optimal cytoreduction rates for stages IIIC and IV epithelial ovarian, fallopian tube, and primary peritoneal cancer: a change in surgical approach. *Gynecol Oncol.* 2004;94:650-654.

93. Liu FS, Ho ESC, Shih RT, et al. Mutational analysis of the BRCA1 tumor suppressor gene in endometrial carcinoma. *Gynecologic Oncology* 1997;66(3):449–453.

94. Curtin JP, Malik R, Venkatraman ES, et al. Stage IV ovarian cancer: impact of surgical debulking. *Gynecologic Oncology* 1997;64(1):9–12.

95. Liu PC, Benjamin I, Morgan MA, et al. Effect of surgical debulking on survival in stage IV ovarian cancer. *Gynecol Oncol* 1997;64:4–8.

96. Schwartz PE. Cytoreductive surgery for the management of stage IV ovarian cancer. *Gynecologic Oncology* 1997;64(1):1–3.

97. Bristow RE, Montz FJ, Lagasse LD, et al. Survival impact of surgical cytoreduction in stage IV epithelial ovarian cancer. *Gynecologic Oncology* 1999;72(3):278–287.

98. Bristow RE, Tomacruz RS, Armstrong DK, et al. Survival effect of maximal cytoreductive surgery for advanced ovarian carcinoma during the platinum era: a meta-analysis. *J Clin Oncol* 2002;20(5):1248–1259.

99. Engelen MJ, Kos HE, Willemse PH, et al. Surgery by consultant gynecologic oncologists improves survival in patients with ovarian carcinoma. *Cancer* 2006;106(3):589–598.

100. Junor EJ, Hole DJ, McNulty L, et al. Specialist gynaecologists and survival outcome in ovarian cancer: a Scottish national study of 1866 patients. *Br J Obstet Gynaecol* 1999;106(11):1130–1136.

101. Bristow RE, Zahurak ML, del Carmen MG, et al. Ovarian cancer surgery in Maryland: volume-based access to care. *Gynecol Oncol.* 2004;93:353-360.

102. Carney ME, Lancaster JM, Ford C, et al. A population-based study of patterns of care for ovarian cancer: who is seen by a gynecologic oncologist and who is not? *Gynecologic Oncology* 2002;84(1):36–42.

103. Earle CC, Schrag D, Neville BA, et al. Effect of surgeon specialty on processes of care and outcomes for ovarian cancer patients. *J Natl Cancer Inst* 2006;98(3):172–180.

104. Schrag D, Earle C, Xu F, et al. Associations between hospital and surgeon procedure volumes and patient outcomes after ovarian cancer resection. *J Natl Cancer Inst* 2006;98(3):163–171.

105. Morgan RJ Jr, Alvarez RD, Armstrong DK, et al: Ovarian cancer. Clinical Practice Guidelines in Oncology. *J Natl Compr Cancer Netw* 2006; 4: 912–939.

106. Guidelines for referral to a gynecologic oncologist: rationale and benefits. The Society of Gynecologic Oncology. *Gynecol Oncol* 2000;78(3Pt2):S1–13.

107. Heintz AP, Odicino F, Maisonneuve P, et al. Carcinoma of the ovary. *International Journal of Gynaecology and Obstetrics: the Official Organ of the International Federation of Gynaecology and Obstetrics* 2003;83 Suppl 1:135–166.

108. Morris M, Gershenson DM, Wharton JT. Secondary cytoreductive surgery in epithelial ovarian cancer: nonresponders to first-line therapy. *Gynecologic Oncology* 1989;33(1):1–5.

109. van der Burg ME, van Lent M, Buyse M, et al. The effect of debulking surgery after induction chemotherapy on the prognosis in advanced epithelial ovarian cancer. Gynecological Cancer Cooperative Group of the European Organization for Research and Treatment of Cancer. *N Engl J Med* 1995;332(10):629–634.

110. Rose PG, Nerenstone S, Brady MF, et al. Secondary surgical cytoreduction for advanced ovarian carcinoma. *N Engl J Med.* 2004;351:2489–2497.

111. Nelson BE, Rosenfield AT, Schwartz PE. Preoperative abdominopelvic computed tomographic prediction of optimal cytoreduction in epithelial ovarian carcinoma. *J Clin Oncol* 1993;11(1):166–172.

112. Qayyum A, Coakley FV, Westphalen AC, et al. Role of CT and MR imaging in predicting optimal cytoreduction of newly diagnosed primary epithelial ovarian cancer. *Gynecologic Oncology* 2005;96(2):301–306.

113. Meyer JI, Kennedy AW, Friedman R, et al. Ovarian carcinoma: value of CT in predicting success of debulking surgery. *AJR Am J Roentgenol* 1995;165(4):875–878.

114. Axtell AE, Lee MH, Bristow RE, et al. Multi-institutional reciprocal validation study of computed tomography predictors of suboptimal primary cytoreduction in patients with advanced ovarian cancer. *J Clin Oncol* 2007;25(4):384–389.

115. Pecorelli S, Odicino F, Favalli G. Interval debulking surgery in advanced epithelial ovarian cancer. *Best Pract Res Clin Obstet Gynaecol* 2002;16(4):573–583.

116. Schwartz PE, Rutherford TJ, Chambers JT, et al. Neoadjuvant chemotherapy for advanced ovarian cancer: long-term survival. *Gynecologic Oncology* 1999;72(1):93–99.

117. Vergote I, De Wever I, Tjalma W, et al. Neoadjuvant chemotherapy or primary debulking surgery in advanced ovarian

carcinoma: a retrospective analysis of 285 patients. *Gynecologic Oncology* 1998;71(3):431–436.

118. Bristow RE, Chi DS. Platinum-based neoadjuvant chemotherapy and interval surgical cytoreduction for advanced ovarian cancer: a meta-analysis. *Gynecol Oncol.* 2006;103:1070–1076.

119. Bristow RE, Eisenhauer EL, Santillan A, et al. Delaying the primary surgical effort for advanced ovarian cancer: A systematic review of neoadjuvant chemotherapy and interval cytoreduction. *Gynecologic Oncology* 2007;104(2):480–490.

120. Chen L, Learman LA, Weinberg V, et al. Discordance between beliefs and recommendations of gynecologic oncologists in ovarian cancer management. *Int J Gynecol Cancer* 2004;14(6):1055–1062.

121. Munkarah AR, Coleman RL. Critical evaluation of secondary cytoreduction in recurrent ovarian cancer. *Gynecologic Oncology* 2004;95(2):273–280.

122. Eisenkop SM, Friedman RL, Spirtos NM. The role of secondary cytoreductive surgery in the treatment of patients with recurrent epithelial ovarian carcinoma. *Cancer* 2000;88(1):144–153.

123. Zang RY, Li ZT, Tang J, et al. Secondary cytoreductive surgery for patients with relapsed epithelial ovarian carcinoma: who benefits? *Cancer* 2004;100(6):1152–1161.

124. Munkarah A, Levenback C, Wolf JK, et al. Secondary cytoreductive surgery for localized intra-abdominal recurrences in epithelial ovarian cancer. *Gynecologic Oncology* 2001;81(2):237–241.

125. Harter P, Bois A, Hahmann M, et al. Surgery in recurrent ovarian cancer: the Arbeitsgemeinschaft Gynaekologische Onkologie (AGO) DESKTOP OVAR trial. *Ann Surg Oncol* 2006;13(12):1702–1710.

126. Ozols RF, Bundy BN, Greer BE, et al. Phase III trial of carboplatin and paclitaxel compared with cisplatin and paclitaxel in patients with optimally resected stage III ovarian cancer: a Gynecologic Oncology Group study. *J Clin Oncol.* 2003;21:3194–3200.

127. du Bois A, Luck HJ, Meier W, et al. A randomized clinical trial of cisplatin/paclitaxel versus carboplatin/paclitaxel as first-line treatment of ovarian cancer. *J Natl Cancer Inst* 2003;95(17):1320–1329.

128. McGuire WP, Hoskins WJ, Brady MF, et al. Cyclophosphamide and cisplatin compared with paclitaxel and cisplatin in patients with stage III and stage IV ovarian cancer. *N Engl J Med* 1996;334(1):1–6.

129. Piccart MJ, Bertelsen K, James K, et al. Randomized intergroup trial of cisplatin-paclitaxel versus cisplatin-cyclophosphamide in women with advanced epithelial ovarian cancer: three-year results. *J Natl Cancer Inst* 2000;92(9):699–708.

130. Cannistra SA. Cancer of the ovary. *N Engl J Med* 2004;351(24):2519–2529.

131. Vasey PA, Jayson GC, Gordon A, et al. Phase III randomized trial of docetaxel-carboplatin versus paclitaxel-carboplatin as first-line chemotherapy for ovarian carcinoma. *J Natl Cancer Inst* 2004;96(22):1682–1691.

132. Cannistra SA. Intraperitoneal chemotherapy comes of age. *N Engl J Med* 2006;354(1):77–79.

133. Alberts DS, Liu PY, Hannigan EV, et al. Intraperitoneal cisplatin plus intravenous cyclophosphamide versus intravenous cisplatin plus intravenous cyclophosphamide for stage III ovarian cancer. *N Engl J Med* 1996;335(26):1950–1955.

134. Markman M, Bundy BN, Alberts DS, et al. Phase III trial of standard-dose intravenous cisplatin plus paclitaxel versus moderately high-dose carboplatin followed by intravenous paclitaxel and intraperitoneal cisplatin in small-volume stage III ovarian carcinoma: an intergroup study of the Gynecologic Oncology Group, Southwestern Oncology Group, and Eastern Cooperative Oncology Group. *J Clin Oncol.* 2001;19:1001–1007.

135. Armstrong DK, Bundy B, Wenzel L, et al. Intraperitoneal cisplatin and paclitaxel in ovarian cancer. *N Engl J Med* 2006;354(1):34–43.

136. National Cancer Institute. Clinical announcement—intraperitoneal chemotherapy for ovarian cancer. Available at URL:http://ctep.cancer.gov.highlights/clin_annc_010506.pdf (2006).

137. Walker JL, Armstrong DK, Huang HQ, et al. Intraperitoneal catheter outcomes in a phase III trial of intravenous versus intraperitoneal chemotherapy in optimal stage III ovarian and primary peritoneal cancer: a Gynecologic Oncology Group Study. *Gynecologic Oncology* 2006;100(1):27–32.

COMMENTARY
Christian Marth

Surgery is the cornerstone of ovarian cancer treatment. Long-term survival is inversely correlated with residual tumor at the end of the surgical procedure. The less tumor remaining, the longer the patient will survive. Therefore, complete removal of all intraperitoneal tumor deposits has been advocated. Bowel resection, splenectomy, and removal of the diaphragmatic peritoneum have been recommended in order to improve cytoreduction. Despite the fact that epithelial ovarian cancer metastasizes primarily and predominantly via the peritoneal and lymphatic routes, less attention has been paid to surgery of the retroperitoneum. Indeed in the chapter written by Dr. Ilana Cass, the role of the lymphatics has not been sufficiently emphasized. In the last 20 years, interest has been focussed on the role of lymph node involvement.

ROLE OF LYMPHADENECTOMY IN THE MANAGEMENT OF OVARIAN CANCER

In 1974, Knapp and Friedman (1) first reported their experience with aortic lymph node metastases in patients with early ovarian cancer treated by lymphadenectomy. Thereafter, other articles have extended our knowledge about the routes and the incidence of lymphatic spread. Aortic and pelvic lymph nodes are considered the nodal groups that are primarily involved. Burghardt et al. (2) reviewed a series of 123 ovarian cancer patients and reported positive lymph nodes in about 62%. Similar results were obtained by other authors. di Re et al. (3) performed a retrospective analysis of 488 patients with untreated advanced ovarian cancer. A systematic pelvic and paraaortic lymphadenectomy was performed in 248 of the patients. Only selective sampling or node biopsy was performed in 33 and 47 patients, respectively. Node metastases were found in 194 (59%) of the 328 patients from whom nodal tissue was available for study. The incidence of metastatic nodes significantly increased with more advanced stages, with serous histology and with a greater amount of residual tumor. Patients with negative nodes survived significantly longer than those who had node metastases.

This well-known, prognostic importance of lymph node involvement has led to the hypothesis that removal of involved nodes might be beneficial. For 2 decades there has been a debate on the value of including systematic aortic and pelvic lymphadenectomy as part of the initial ovarian cancer-debulking procedure in patients with advanced disease. Moreover, some investigators have suggested that the retroperitoneal space may represent a sanctuary for chemoresistance, and therefore lymph nodes might not be adequately treated with chemotherapy (3).

In a large population-based study, the efficacy of lymphadenectomy was evaluated in clinical stage I ovarian cancer by Chan and associates (4). The 5-year disease-specific survival of all women with clinical stage I ovarian cancer who underwent lymphadenectomy was 93% compared with 87% for those who did not have a lymphadenectomy (p <0.001). Lymphadenectomy, however, was not associated with improved survival in patients <50 years of age (93% vs. 94%). In contrast, patients ≥50 years of age who underwent lymphadenectomy experienced an improvement in the survival rate from 82% to 92% (p <0.01). In addition, the extent of node resection (0 nodes, fewer than 10, and 10 or more) correlated with an increased rate of survival among patients with stage Ic disease, from 72.8% to 86.7% to 90.1% (p <0.001), respectively, but only a nonstatistically significant improvement was observed in stage Ia and Ib disease. Because this was not a prospective, randomized trial, the survival differences observed may simply be the result of the comparison of patients with true stage I disease after optimal staging procedure with inaccurately staged patients with true stage III disease. To overcome such inherent flaws of retrospective trials, prospective randomized trials are required.

Panici et al. (5) studied the role of systematic aortic and pelvic lymphadenectomy in patients with optimally debulked advanced ovarian cancer. These investigators conducted the first randomized clinical trial to determine whether systematic aortic and pelvic lymphadenectomy improves progression-free and overall survival compared with resection of bulky nodes only. From January 1991 through May 2003, 427 eligible patients with International Federation of Gynecology and Obstetrics stage IIIB-C and IV epithelial ovarian carcinoma were randomly assigned to undergo systematic pelvic and para-aortic lymphadenectomy (n = 216) or resection of only bulky nodes, including all nodes >1 cm (n = 211). Adequate systematic lymphadenectomy required the removal of at least 25 pelvic and 15 para-aortic nodes. Progression-free survival and overall survival were analyzed after a median follow-up period of 68.4 months. The adjusted risk for first event was statistically significantly lower in the systematic lymphadenectomy arm (hazard ratio, 0.75; 95% confidence interval [CI]: 0.59-0.94; p = 0.01) than in the no-lymphadenectomy arm, corresponding to 5-year progression-free survival rates of 31.2% and 21.6% and to median progression-free survival of 29.4 and 22.4 months in the systematic lymphadenectomy and control arms, respectively. The risk of death, however, was similar in both arms (hazard ratio, 0.97; 95% CI: 0.74-1.29; p = 0.85), corresponding to 5-year overall survival rates of 48.5% and 47% and to median overall survival of 58.7 and 56.3 months in the experimental and control groups, respectively. Median operating time was significantly longer, and the percentage of patients requiring blood transfusions was significantly higher in the systematic lymphadenectomy arm than in the no-lymphadenectomy arm. Significant increases in perioperative and late morbidity,

including lymph cysts and lymphedema, were also observed among patients undergoing systematic lymphadenectomy (28% vs. 18%). This increased morbidity must be weighed in judging the appropriateness of more radical surgery in a given patient.

In a randomized trial of patients with ovarian carcinoma macroscopically confined to the pelvis, those receiving systematic lymphadenectomy were compared with a control group receiving lymph node sampling only. The investigators, Maggioni and associates (6), found a higher proportion of patients had metastatic involvement of pelvic and/or para-aortic nodes in the lymphadenectomy group than in the control group (22% vs. 9%, respectively). However, systematic lymphadenectomy was neither associated with an improvement in progression-free nor overall survival. Again, median operating time in the lymphadenectomy arm was longer and the blood loss higher than in the control arm; 14% more patients received blood transfusions in the experimental group.

These trials do not support the inclusion of systematic lymphadenectomy as part of maximal surgical debulking in the current management of ovarian cancer. Further trials are necessary to be certain about the role of lymphadenectomy in ovarian cancer. It would be worthwhile to perform a trial in optimally debulked, macroscopically negative, patients who would be randomized to receive or not receive systematic lymphadenectomy. Such a study would finally determine whether removal of additional tumor material from the lymph nodes results in improved progression-free and overall survival.

Lymph nodes are not an inert harbor for tumor cells, but they play a major role in cell immunity. Regional lymph nodes are active in the immune defense against cancer cells and are considered the first line of immune defense against metastases by the lymphatic route. An important question is whether removal of lymph nodes, especially those unaffected by metastatic disease, reduces the efficacy of the regional immune system. Activated monocytes, macrophages, and leukocytes important in the innate immune system can be directly cytotoxic to tumor cells either through antibody-mediated mechanisms, such as antibody-dependent cell-mediated cytotoxicity and phagocytosis, or through direct cellular mechanisms. Tumor-associated, antigen-specific immunity has been demonstrated in ovarian cancer. Nonetheless, immune-based therapies for ovarian cancer generally have been clinically ineffective, as they have been for most epithelial tumors. Failure of current strategies to induce significant antitumor immunity relates at least in part to the capacity of the tumor to activate tumor-mediated processes.

However, we should not conclude that lymph node-mediated immunity has no surveillance activity in ovarian cancer patients. In fact, Zhang et al. (7) reported that the presence of intratumoral T cells correlated with improved clinical outcome in advanced ovarian carcinoma. This conclusion was based on immunohistochemical analyses of frozen specimens from patients with advanced-stage disease to assess the distribution of tumor-infiltrating T cells. These tumor-specific T cells can be used to establish functional tumor-associated, antigen-specific T-cell lines that kill autologous tumor cells in vitro and in vivo. However, it is clear that established tumors can induce immune tolerance to escape destruction, although the mechanisms are not well defined. Regulatory T cells mediate homeostatic tolerance by suppressing autoreactive T cells, and the presence of these regulatory T cells has been shown to be associated with poor progression-free and overall survival in ovarian cancer patients (8,9). In another study of cell-mediated immunity in ovarian cancer, Marth et al. (10) reported that activation of macrophages measured by urinary neopterine excretion is associated with poor outcome.

In summary, the role of lymph node immunity in ovarian cancer survival remains uncertain. At present, we cannot exclude the possibility that removal of immunocompetent cells and tissues from cancer patients can be harmful, especially in cases in which the majority of lymph nodes resected are free of metastatic disease. The indications for systematic para-aortic and pelvic lymphadenectomy are not established.

REFERENCES

1. Knapp RC, Friedman EA. Aortic lymph node metastases in early ovarian cancer. *Am J Obstet Gynecol.* 1974; 119 (8):1013–1017.
2. Burghardt E, Pickel H, Lahousen M, et al. Pelvic lymphadenectomy in operative treatment of ovarian cancer. *Am J Obstet Gynecol.* 1986;155:315–319.
3. di Re F, Baiocchi G, Fontanelli R, et al. Systematic pelvic and paraaortic lymphadenectomy for advanced ovarian cancer: prognostic significance of node metastases. *Gynecol Oncol.* 1996; 62:360–365.
4. Chan JK, Munro EG, Cheung MK, et al. Association of lymphadenectomy and survival in stage I ovarian cancer patients. *Obstet Gynecol.* 2007;109:12–19.
5. Panici PB, Maggioni A, Hacker N, et al. Systematic aortic and pelvic lymphadenectomy versus resection of bulky nodes only in optimally debulked ovarian cancer: a randomized clinical trial. *J Natl Cancer Inst.* 2005;97:560–566.
6. Maggioni A, Benedetti Panici P, Dell'Anna T, et al. Randomised study of systematic lymphadenectomy in patients with epithelial ovarian cancer macroscopically confined to the pelvis. *Br J Cancer.* 2006;95:699–704.
7. Zhang L, Conejo-Garcia JR, Katsaros D, et al. Intratumoral T cells, recurrence, and survival in epithelial ovarian cancer. *N Engl J Med.* 2003;348:203–213.
8. Curiel TJ, Coukos G, Zou L, et al. Specific recruitment of regulatory T-cells in ovarian carcinoma fosters immune privilege and predicts reduced survival. *Nat Med.* 2004;10:942–949.
9. Wolf D, Wolf AM, Rumpold H, et al. The expression of the regulatory T cell–specific forkhead box transcription factor FoxP3 is associated with poor prognosis in ovarian cancer. *Clin Cancer Res.* 2005;11:8326–8331.
10. Marth C, Weger A, Müller-Holzner E, et al. The prognostic value of nuclear roundness and neopterin in ovarian cancer. *Eur J Cancer.* 1993;29:1863–1868.

57

Cancers of the Biliary Tract: Surgical Management of Cancer of the Gallbladder and Bile Ducts

Steven C. Stain and Ankesh Nigam

Cancers of the gallbladder and extrahepatic bile ducts are uncommon, with an estimate of 1.2 and 1.7 cancers diagnosed per 100,000 persons in the United States (1,2). As many of these tumors are unresectable at the time of diagnosis, palliative therapy is often indicated. The choice of therapy (attempt at surgical resection or palliative biliary decompression) should be based on accurate staging, with particular attention to bilateral involvement of vascular or biliary structures. The use of adjuvant chemotherapy or radiation therapy has often been employed, although there are not definitive studies that prove efficacy.

TUMORS OF THE GALLBLADDER

Incidence

Carcinoma of the gallbladder is the most common extrahepatic biliary tract malignancy and the fifth most common gastrointestinal cancer (3). There is an increased female-to-male ratio of 2.5:1 to 3:1, and the incidence varies significantly between ethnic groups within the United States and throughout the world. The highest incidence of gallbladder cancer worldwide was shown in women from Delhi, India (21.5 per 100,000), followed by South Karachi, Pakistan (13.8 per 100,000), and Quito, Ecuador (12.9 per 100,000) (4). There are significant variations of gallbladder incidence among ethnic groups in the Unites States, with Hispanic white women in California (8.2 per 100,000) and New Mexico (5.4 per 100,000) having the highest reported incidence among U.S. reporting tumor registries. Hispanic white women had a three- to fivefold higher incidence than non-Hispanic white women in the same areas. By comparison, SEER (Surveillance Epidemiology End Results) data from 1993–1997, reported an incidence of 1.52 per 100,000 among U.S. black males and 0.87 among U.S. white males (4).

Etiology

The association between gallstones and gallbladder carcinoma was observed by Charles Mayo (5) in 1903 (6). Gallbladder cancer is more frequent in patients with gallstones, especially if the gallstones are symptomatic and large (7,8). Risk factors associated with the development of gallbladder carcinoma include female sex, obesity, and carbohydrate intake, all of which are associated with gallstone disease (7). However the risk of gall-

bladder carcinoma is so low that prophylactic cholecystectomy is not recommended (9). Ransohoff and Gracie (10) estimated that the risk of developing gallbladder cancer is 0.02% per year for persons older than 50 years of age. Gallbladder polyps, especially when they are >10 mm, are considered a predisposing factor for cancer, and when identified, warrant cholecystectomy, even in asymptomatic patients (5). The presence of an anomalous pancreaticobiliary junction, often associated with a choledochal cyst, is associated with a marked increase in gallbladder cancer (11).

The sequence of molecular changes leading to neoplastic transformation of the gallbladder epithelium is unknown. Many studies have focused on the *ras*, *TP53*, and *p16*^{INK4}/*CDKN2* gene abnormalities and deletions ("loss of heterozygosity") at several chromosomal regions harboring tumor suppressor genes (12). Bacterial infection of bile, with or without gallstone disease, occurs in up to 80% of patients with gallbladder cancer (13). Epidemiologic studies have suggested a significant positive association between gallbladder cancer and the carrier state of *Salmonella typhi* and *Salmonella paratyphi* (4).

Adenomatous changes, squamous metaplasia, and calcifications (porcelain gallbladder) have all been reported to be associated with gallbladder cancer. The incidence of cancer arising in calcified gallbladders is not clearly delineated and has been estimated from 12% to 61% (14). In a careful review of 25,900 gallbladder specimens from the Massachusetts General Hospital (1962–1999), Stephen and Berger (15) identified only 44 patients (0.2%) with calcified gallbladders. There was a positive association with cancer, but the incidence was much lower than previously reported. No patients with diffused intramural calcification had cancer, and cancer was found in only 2 of 27 patients with selective mucosal wall calcification (7%). Similarly, Towfigh et al. (16) reported porcelain gallbladders in 15 of 10,742 gallbladder specimens from the UCLA Medical Center (1955–1998), and none of the 15 patients had cancer. Based on the more recent data, it would seem the association is not as strong as previously reported.

Pathology

The most common histology of gallbladder cancer is adenocarcinoma. Albores-Saavedra et al. (17) reviewed the SEER database for the years 1973–2001 and identified 8,773 cases of gallbladder cancer. Adenocarcinoma and carcinoma (not otherwise specified) composed 80.1% of the cases. Other histologic types included adenosquamous carcinoma (2.4%), mucinous carcinoma (2.7%), and papillary adenocarcinoma (4.5%).

More differentiated tumors, and those associated with adjacent metaplasia have better prognosis. The gross morphology of papillary, tubular, and nodular forms are also important prognostic factors. In general, papillary tumors are less likely to invade the liver and spread to adjacent lymph nodes. Nodular tumors are more likely to infiltrate into the adjacent liver and exhibit early metastases to lymph nodes (18).

Clinical Features

The most common symptom of patients with gallbladder cancer is abdominal pain, and the clinical presentation may be indistinguishable from patients with biliary colic or acute cholecystitis. Piehler and Chrichlow (19) reviewed data from 6,222 patients with primary gallbladder carcinoma and found that 76% of symptomatic patients had pain, 38% jaundice, 32% nausea and vomiting, and 39% weight loss.

Diagnostic Studies

Symptoms of right upper quadrant abdominal pain should prompt ultrasonography for the presumptive diagnosis of symptomatic cholelithiasis. The first preoperative diagnosis of gallbladder cancer based on ultrasound was by Olken et al. (20) in 1978. As ultrasound is an operator-dependent modality, there are conflicting data regarding the sensitivity and specificity of transabdominal sonography to identify gallbladder carcinoma. Several reports have recommended an aggressive approach to clinical management of ultrasonographically detected gallbladder polyps. Polyp size may be indicative of malignant potential, and cholecystectomy for gallbladder polyps >10 mm has been recommended (21,22). Damore et al. (23) reviewed 41 patients with ultrasound-diagnosed gallbladder polyps (all <10 mm) and no patients had carcinoma. Csendes et al. (24) provided long-term follow-up of 111 patients with gallbladder polyps <10 mm. No patients with a polyp <10 mm had cancer in a cholecystectomy specimen or developed cancer over a 71-month follow-up. Finally, Terzi et al. (25) examined the histopathologic data of 100 patients with gallbladder polyps and found that 23 of the 26 patients (88%) with cancer had polyps >10 mm. Conversely, only 3 of 66 patients (4.5%) with polyps <10 mm had cancer. Using size >10 mm as measured by transabdominal ultrasound as a cutoff, Chattopadhyaya et al. (26) found 100% sensitivity and 86.95% specificity with a positive predictive value of 50% in the diagnosis of polypoid lesions of the gallbladder.

For most patients with a suspicion of gallbladder based on ultrasound, the next recommended test is computed tomography (CT) scan (Figure 57.1). Abdominal CT may give information regarding hepatic invasion, and remote and lymph node metastases, which provide evidence of unresectability (27). Preoperative CT has an overall accuracy of 83% to 86%; however, although advanced disease is accurately and reliably detected on CT, the ability to identify early disease by CT remains disappointing (28). Magnetic resonance imaging (MRI) may provide additional information such as focal gallbladder wall thickening with an eccentric mass, direct liver invasion, lymphadenopathy, and biliary tract invasion. As compared with operative and

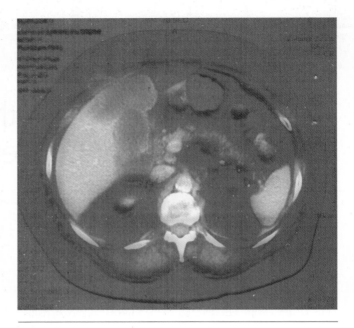

Figure 57.1 Computed tomography scan of gallbladder cancer.

biopsy finding in 34 patients, Schwartz et al. (29) found MRI to be 100% sensitive for direct hepatic invasion and 92% sensitive for lymph node metastases.

Cholangiography is an important diagnostic component of the preoperative evaluation of the jaundiced patient with gallbladder cancer. Jaundice in the presence of gallbladder cancer predicts advanced disease and indicates involvement of the common hepatic or bile duct by direct invasion or lymph node metastases. Both endoscopic retrograde cholangiography and percutaneous cholangiography can provide the typical finding of a long stricture of the hepatic duct in patients with gallbladder cancer. Increasingly, magnetic resonance cholangiopancreatography has been used to noninvasively image the biliary tract, and may be useful in preoperative assessment and planning (29)

There have been recent reports of the application of endoscopic ultrasound-guided fine-needle aspiration (FNA) for the diagnosis of bile duct and gallbladder cancer (30–32). The modality offers the opportunity for a preoperative diagnosis in patients considered for resection but, more importantly, may establish a tissue diagnosis prior to palliative therapy, excluding the need for operation in patients considered unresectable.

Despite increased accuracy of cross-sectional imaging techniques (CT and MRI), the full extent of disease is commonly underestimated. The most common causes of understaging preoperatively are undetected peritoneal seeding, small hepatic metastases, and microscopically involved regional lymph nodes. Donahue (33) has recommended that diagnostic laparoscopy should be routinely performed before exploratory laparotomy for patients with known or suspected gallbladder cancer. Weber et al. (34) performed laparoscopy on 44 patients with potentially resectable tumors based on preoperative imaging, and 21 (48%) were unresectable by laparoscopy because of peritoneal implants in 15 patients or liver metastases in 6 patients. To further identify unresectable disease, fluorodeoxyglucose (FDG)-positive emission tomography (PET) scan has been studied for patients with gallbladder cancer. In small series, several groups have suggested FDG-PET may have utility in patients with gallbladder cancer (35,36).

Staging

Gallbladder cancer spreads by direct hepatic invasion and by locoregional then distant lymph node metastases. The two most common staging systems used for gallbladder cancer are the Nevin system and the American Joint Committee on Cancer and the Internal Union Against Cancer (AJCC/UICC) TNM staging system. Nevin et al. (37) described a staging system composed of five stages of gallbladder cancer, later modified by Donahue et al. (38). This system divided tumors into invasion of the mucosa (stage I); invasion of the muscularis and mucosa (stage II); invasion of the subserosa, muscularis, and mucosa (stage III); transmural invasion with cystic lymph node metastases (stage IV); or extension into the liver bed or distant spread (stage V). The most recent version of the AJCC staging system is shown in Table 57.1. Both systems (Nevin and AJCC) correlate with survival, although Fong et al. (39) argue that because patients with bulky direct invasion of the liver may be cured by surgery, the modified Nevin system may be more useful for selection of patients for adjuvant therapy or stratification of patients for clinical trials (39).

Gallbladder cancer that invades the biliary tree with subsequent jaundice is a poor prognostic sign and defines a subset of patients with aggressive disease. Hawkins et al. (40) reported the 7-year experience from Memorial Sloan-Kettering Cancer Center of 240 patients with gallbladder cancer. Of the 82 patients (34%) with jaundice, only 6 could be resected, and there were no disease-free survivors at 2 years. The authors concluded that routine operative exploration of these patients is not warranted. For such patients, palliative treatment by biliary stenting may provide the most rational treatment.

Operative Treatment

The only effective treatment for carcinoma of the gallbladder is operative resection. At present, most gallbladder cancer patients present for treatment with incurable disease. If a gallbladder cancer appears completely resectable and the patient is fit enough to tolerate the planned procedure, a curative resection should be planned (33). If the entire burden of disease cannot be removed, the patient is incurable and palliative treatment should be pursued. Even in the face of nodal metastases or hepatic invasion that can be resected, long-term survival is exceptionally rare.

Although all preoperatively suspected gallbladder cancers should have open operation, nearly half of early gallbladder cancers are diagnosed after operation (41,42). There are three distinct presentations for patients with gallbladder cancer: preoperative suspected cancer based on imaging studies, an unsuspected diagnosis made by the pathologist after cholecystectomy for symptomatic cholelithiasis, or evaluation for further resection for transmural cancer after cholecystectomy.

Preoperative Suspicion of Gallbladder Cancer

The first consideration in selection of treatment for patients with preoperative suspected gallbladder carcinoma is to determine unresectability. Patients with stage IVB disease based on distant

Table 57.1

The American Joint Committee on Cancer Staging System for Gallbladder Cancer[a]

T category	
Tis	Carcinoma in situ
T1	Tumor invades lamina propria or muscle layer
	T1a: invades lamina propria T1b: invades the muscle layer
T2	Tumor invades perimuscular connective tissue; no extension beyond serosa or into the liver
T3	Tumor perforates the serosa (visceral peritoneum) and/or directly invades the liver and/or adjacent organs
T4	Tumor invades main portal vein or hepatic artery or invades multiple extrahepatic organs
N category	
N0	No regional lymph node metastasis
N1	Regional lymph node metastasis
Distant metastasis (M)	
M0	No distant metastasis
M1	Distant metastasis
Staging system	
0	Tis, N0, M0
IA	T1, N0, M0
IB	T2, N0, M0
IIA	T3, N0, M0
IIB	T1,2,3, N1, M0
III	T4, any N, M0
IV	Any T, any N, M1

[a]Adapted from Greene FL, Page DL, Fleming ID, et al, eds, for the American Joint Committee on Cancer. *AJCC Cancer Staging Manual.* 6th ed. New York, NY: Springer-Verlag; 2002.

metastases (M1) are not candidates for curative resection. Because patients who exhibit gross evidence of nodal metastases beyond the hepatoduodenal ligament (N2) will not be cured, even with radical extirpative operations, these patients are usually not treated surgically (33). All other patients, with stages 0-IVA cancers can be considered operative candidates, recognizing that very few patients with nodal metastases are cured in Western series.

Fong et al. (39) reported the Memorial Sloan-Kettering Cancer Center experience of 410 patients evaluated with gallbladder cancer. By multivariate analysis, only N category of disease and T category of disease remained as independent predictors of adverse long-term outcome. Thirty-six of the 102 patients were treated by resection with curative intent. Only two survived more than 5 years, and both subsequently died of recurrent disease. Taner et al. (43) analyzed the Mayo Clinic experience of 131 patients with gallbladder cancer. Patients who underwent a radical cholecystectomy had a significantly longer median survival

(24 months) than those treated by simple cholecystectomy (6 months) for all stages except stage 1 (AJCC).

The standard operative procedure of radical cholecystectomy at both Memorial Sloan-Kettering Cancer Center and the Mayo Clinic consists of subsegmental resections of segments IVB and V adjacent to the gallbladder, including at least 2 cm of normal liver parenchyma beyond the cancer, and a regional lymphadenectomy encompassing the lymph nodes within the hepatoduodenal ligament, those behind the head of the pancreas, and along the common hepatic artery medial to the celiac axis and, for most patients, common bile duct excision. Hepatic lobectomy has been advocated for bulky tumor involvement of the liver. En bloc resection of the extrahepatic bile duct with bilioenteric reconstruction is indicated to achieve a complete regional node dissection when all known disease can be resected. Shimuzu et al. (44) reported hepatoduodenal ligament involvement in 30 of 50 patients with transmural gallbladder cancer. The utility of a "radical" approach has been supported by data demonstrating that simple cholecystectomy for T2 tumors is associated with a 5-year survival of 20% to 40%, while radical resections were associated with 5-year survival upward of 80% (39,45–50).

Western series have generally reported a dismal outcome among patients with lymphatic metastases (46,49,51). Fong et al. (39) reported a 16% 5-year survival of patients with N1 disease and no 5-year survivors with N2 disease. Extensive regional lymphadenectomy to include para-aortic nodes has been recommended by some authors, but other Japanese surgeons report no long-term survivors if the superior mesenteric, celiac, or para-aortic lymph nodes contain metastases (52,53). Several Japanese groups have demonstrated the ability to perform combined major hepatic and pancreatic resections with an apparent improvement in survival (54–58). These results have not been replicated outside Japan, and few Western surgeons have advocated such an approach.

Postoperative Diagnosis of Incidental Gallbladder Cancer

In the instance of incidentally found cancer, treatment should be based on the degree of tumor invasion of the gallbladder wall (Table 57.1). T1a tumors are localized to the mucosa and T1b tumors are localized to the muscularis layer. The preponderance of recent literature suggests that T1a lesions that are incidentally discovered after laparoscopic cholecystectomy require no further treatment (9,59–61). The treatment of incidentally identified T1b gallbladder cancers after cholecystectomy is controversial, with some authors recommending a second radical hepatic bed resection with or without bile duct excision, and other studies showing no benefit to a second operation (9,59–62). In a survey of members of the Japanese Society of Biliary Surgery, Ouchi et al. (61) identified 498 gallbladder cancer patients treated with laparoscopic cholecystectomy. Thirty of 67 patients with T1b disease had additional excisions, and the 5-year survival was 95% of patients with T1b tumors; there was no difference between those who had simple laparoscopic cholecystectomy and those who underwent additional resection. Despite these data, the clinical practice guidelines from the National Comprehensive Cancer Network recommends hepatic resection and lymphadenectomy with consideration of excision of the bile duct and port sites for T1b or greater gallbladder cancers (63).

Postoperative Diagnosis of Transmural Gallbladder Cancer

The data regarding reresection after prior noncurative surgical therapy are selective, as referral centers evaluate and often treat a subset of patients with potentially resectable disease, albeit after careful repeat radiologic staging. Available data, however, would suggest there is a subset of patients who may benefit from repeat exploration. In the Memorial Sloan-Kettering Cancer Center series, 80 of 248 patients (32%) with a previous exploration had curative resections (39). Thirty-two of these patients had T2 tumors, and their 5-year survival was 61%, compared with 16 potentially curable patients not offered reresection or who refused resection whose 5-year survival was 19%. Although the group treated 31 T3 and 15 T4 patients with reresection, most of these patients had nodal metastases, 58% and 69%, respectively. As previously stated, a few patients with nodal lymph node metastases can be cured (16% 5-year survival with N1 disease). In the final analysis, advanced T category did not preclude long-term survival, with 21% and 28% 5-year survival for T3 and T4 tumors. Radical reresection would seem indicated for early-stage (T2) tumors, but can result in long-term survival for tumors with bulky liver involvement (T3 or T4).

Excision of port sites after laparoscopic cholecystectomy has been advocated because of the possibility of port-site dissemination of disease (64). This occurrence is not unique to the laparoscopic wound and has been well described after laparotomy (65). These port site excisions are more likely to be more of a staging procedure than a therapeutic one (39).

Adjuvant Therapy

During the 1980s and 1990s a number of reports appeared on the effect of drugs on the management of patients who presented with locally advanced bile duct or gallbladder cancer. A large number of agents, including fluorouracil, mitomycin, methotrexate, etoposide, doxorubicin, and cisplatin, have been tested as single or combination therapies without appreciable effects (9). Single-institution studies using 5-fluorouracil with adjuvant external-beam radiation therapy have suggested some improvement in survival compared to historical controls (66,67). Controlled trials are needed to determine if there is a significant benefit. As there is currently no effective therapy adjuvant therapy for gallbladder cancer known, effective systemic therapy is desperately needed to have an impact for most patients with carcinoma of the gallbladder (68).

TUMORS OF THE BILE DUCT

Bile duct tumors are found in three primary sites: (i) proximal to the cystic duct insertion into the common hepatic duct, (ii) midbile duct tumors in the region of the cystic duct, and (iii) at the lower end of the common bile duct tumor. The diagnostic workup and treatment of distal bile duct tumors is essentially the same as that for lesions of the pancreatic head (see Chapter 35). This section will focus primarily on the diagnosis and treatment of hilar and midbile duct tumors, which have similar diagnostic and therapeutic determinations. These lesions are usually malignant, although up to 10% may be benign. The term *malignant masquerade* was first coined by associates of Blumgart in 1985 (Hadjis et al. [69]) and further characterized by Corvera et al. [70]) to describe a benign fibroinflammatory process of the hilum of liver that is clinically indistinguishable from hilar cholangiocarcinoma. Corvera et al. reported the experience of 275 proximal nontraumatic biliary strictures and found that 22 (8%) were benign. Histologic examination identified five different benign processes: lymphoplasmacytic sclerosing pancreatitis and cholangitis, primary sclerosing cholangitis, granulomatous disease, nonspecific fibrosis/inflammation, and stone disease. Most patients, however, with proximal or midbile duct strictures in the absence of previous cholecystectomy have malignant strictures.

Incidence

Worldwide, cholangiocarcinoma accounts for almost 3% of all gastrointestinal cancers (71,72). It is useful to separate the intrahepatic cholangiocarcinoma from extrahepatic cholangiocarcinoma when examining the epidemiology of these tumors. In the United States, there are approximately 5,000 cases of cholangiocarcinoma diagnosed per year, equally divided between intrahepatic cholangiocarcinomas and extrahepatic cholangiocarcinomas. Welzel et al. (73) calculated the age-adjusted incidence rate population per year in the United States from the SEER-9 registry at 0.8 per 100,000 between 1992 and 2000. An earlier analysis of SEER data from 1973 to 1987 suggested the rates of extrahepatic cholangiocarcinoma were slightly lower in blacks and in women (74). Data have suggested that current coding practices of hilar cholangiocarcinomas in tumor registries may result in overreporting of intrahepatic cholangiocarcinomas by 13% and underreporting of extrahepatic cholangiocarcinomas by as much as 15% (73).

Etiology

Most cases of cholangiocarcinoma develop in what is believed to be a normal liver. However, in approximately 10% of cases, the identification of tumor is preceded by an identifiable risk chronic inflammatory disease of the bile ducts (71). Several risk factors have been associated with the development of cholangiocarcinoma. The strongest associations have been reported are conditions associated with chronic biliary inflammation in patients with conditions such as primary sclerosing cholangitis, liver fluke infestation, hepatolithiasis, and conditions of biliary stasis such as choledochal cysts or the presence of anomalous pancreatobiliary junction. Additional established risk factors for development of cholangiocarcinoma include thorotrast exposure, liver cirrhosis, and hepatitis C viral infection. Accumulated data suggest there also may be increased risk of cancer in patients infected with *Clonorchis sinensis*, human immunodeficiency virus, hepatitis B, and environmental exposure to dioxin or vinyl chloride (75).

The prevalence of cholangiocarcinoma in patients with primary sclerosing cholangitis is high, with a reported lifetime risk between 9% and 23% (75). However, the risk of developing cholangiocarcinoma does not seem to be related to the duration of primary sclerosing cholangitis (76–78). Broome et al. reported a series of 305 Swedish patients with primary sclerosing cholan-

gitis, in which 8% developed cholangiocarcinoma. Burak et al. (79) studied 161 patients followed at the Mayo clinic with primary sclerosing cholangitis. During the study period of a median of 11.5 years, only 11 patients (6.8%) developed cholangiocarcinoma, at a rate of 0.6% per year, but no association was found between the duration of primary sclerosing cholangitis and the development of cholangiocarcinoma.

Although the relationship between the *C. sinensis* liver fluke and cholangiocarcinoma remains only probable, the role of *Opisthorchis viverrini* liver fluke as an etiologic factor has been clearly established (80,81). In a population-based study from Northeast Thailand, Honjo et al. (81) identified that elevated levels of antibodies to *O. viverrini* was strongly associated, with a nearly 30-fold increase in the risk of cholangiocarcinoma. An increase in cases of cholangiocarcinoma associated with *C. sinensis* have been reported among Asian immigrants to the United States, and in case-control studies from Pusan, Korea, an area with an extremely high prevalence of *C. sinensis* infestation (80,82–85).

The incidence of biliary tract malignancy in patients with choledochal cysts has been reported at between 10% and 30% (86–89). The pathogenesis of cholangiocarcinoma among patients with choledochal cysts may be caused by the carcinogenic pancreatic reflux due to the anomalous pancreaticobiliary junction, and in some series the anomalous union has a more grave clinical course that the presence of choledochal cyst alone (87,90).

A variety of mutations in the oncogenes, as well as tumor suppressor genes, has been described in specimens of biliary tract tumors. Several studies have demonstrated mutations resulting in overexpression of K-*ras*, *p53*, and COX-2 genes (3,91). K-*ras* has been implicated in aggressive hilar intrahepatic cholangiocarcinoma, with elevated expression in metastatic lymph nodes (92). K-*ras* expression was found to correlate with poor prognosis; however, the mutation was found in only 14.3% of biliary tract cancers (93). It has also been demonstrated that high levels of *p53* expression correlated with higher-grade tumors and decreased patient survival (94). Immunohistochemical studies demonstrate enhanced COX-2 expression in cholangiocarcinoma cells and precancerous bile duct lesions, but not in normal biliary epithelial cells (95). The mechanism of COX-2 activation appears to involve the tyrosine kinase receptor epidermal growth factor and mitogen-activated protein MAPK cascade.

Although detection of mutations and gene products may suggest the prognosis of patients with biliary tract cancer, future studies are needed to further delineate the cellular and molecular pathways of cholangiocarcinoma pathogenesis. As seen with other cancers, mutations and phenotypic changes are also seen under non malignant conditions, precluding their routine use in clinical practice. There are no tumor markers specific for cholangiocarcinoma. The carbohydrate antigen 19–9 (CA19–9) commonly used has low specificity and can be increased with benign conditions such as bacterial cholangitis, primary biliary cirrhosis, or alcoholic liver disease.

Pathology

The usual histology of a hilar or proximal bile duct cancer is a well-differentiated adenocarcinoma, termed *cholangiocarcinoma*.

Extrahepatic cholangiocarcinoma, the frequent cause of proximal malignant bile duct strictures, appear as a sclerosing mass of tumor, up to approximately 4 cm in length with an increase in ductal wall thickness to 1 cm. The mass often extends into surrounding liver tissue or adjacent portal vein or hepatic artery. Tumors involving the middle region of the ductal system, immediately proximal to the pancreas, are generally nodular, sclerosing discrete tumors, but often presenting as an intraluminal, sharply demarcated spherical mass. Tumors in the distal 2 cm of the common bile duct are most frequently papillary adenocarcinomas, and are often friable, pink, or greyish white masses.

Clinical Features

Cholangiocarcinoma, a malignant neoplasm of the biliary epithelium, was initially described by Durand-Fardel in 1840, and a lesion in the hepatic duct was reported in 1878 (91,96). In 1957, Altemeier et al. (97) reported three cases of sclerosing carcinoma of the major intrahepatic ducts; however, it was Klatskin (98) who first drew attention to the definite clinical features of hilar bile duct carcinoma (97–99). His article, entitled "Adenocarcinoma of the Hepatic Duct and Bifurcation within the Porta Hepatis: An Unusual Tumor with Distinctive Clinical and Pathologic Features," described 13 cases, and emphasized the fact that such type tumor was often small, with clear margins, and that even without metastatic spread, patients often died of prolonged biliary obstruction and liver failure rather than tumor growth.

Bile duct cancers usually produce obstruction of the biliary tree. Jaundice may be absent in the early stages, when the obstruction is unilateral, segmental, or incomplete. Proximal dilatation of the biliary tree above an obstructing lesion usually occurs and is accompanied by elevation of the alkaline phosphatase. Minor or intermittent degrees of biliary obstruction may causes significant elevations of alkaline phosphatase and should raise the suspicion of biliary pathology, even in the absence of jaundice, and should prompt investigation of the biliary tree. Long-standing unilateral biliary obstruction or portal venous occlusion can lead atrophy of the ipsilateral lobe with compensatory hyperplasia of the contralateral lobe (100,101).

The typical age of presentation for patients with cholangiocarcinoma is in the seventh decade, with a male-to-female ratio of 1.3:1 (102). The dominant symptom of bile duct cancer is jaundice, although biliary cancers may be silent for months. There may be a prodrome of malaise, pruritus, anorexia, or weight loss. Abdominal pain is usually mild or absent, and cholangitis is infrequent without prior biliary tract manipulation. Physical examination most often shows jaundice, accompanied by dark urine and pale stools.

Assessment of Resectability

Although most clinical series of patients with bile duct tumors focus on the survival benefits of resection, it should be noted that <30% of patients with hilar cholangiocarcinoma are resectable at the time of diagnosis. In general, criteria for unresectability are:

1. Patients deemed unfit for resection
2. Bilateral tumor extension beyond secondary biliary radicles
3. Encasement of portal vein proximal to the bifurcation
4. Lobar atrophy with contralateral biliary or portal venous encasement

5. Unilateral biliary tumor extension with contralateral portal venous encasement
6. Metastases to lung, liver, peritoneum, or nodes beyond porta hepatis

Preoperative radiologic evaluation should define the majority of patients who are clearly unresectable. Although there are operative methods for palliative bilioenteric bypass to segmental ducts, if known to be clearly unresectable, these patients may be best treated by percutaneous transhepatic intubation (103).

Evaluation

Ultrasound is the initial radiologic test for patients with jaundice or unexplained elevation of alkaline phosphatase. CT is complementary to ultrasound, and may be more sensitive in detection of a hilar mass; cross-sectional images may depict the relationship of the tumor to vascular structures in planning hepatic resection. Cholangiography is essential to delineate the longitudinal extent of tumor. Percutaneous cholangiography better demonstrates the proximal extent of tumor involvement of hilar lesions than endoscopic retrograde cholangiopancreatography. The manipulation of the biliary tree with either modality may increase the chance of cholangitis. Hochwald et al. (104) reported an increased incidence of postoperative infectious complications after preoperative biliary stenting; however, the group from Johns Hopkins has reported good results with prolonged preoperative biliary decompression using silastic stents that are used for reconstruction (105). Magnetic resonance cholangiopancreatography is replacing percutaneous and endoscopic cholangiography because it is noninvasive, does not require biliary manipulation, provides excellent images of biliary anatomy, and can also give details of the relationship to the portal venous and hepatic arterial anatomy that may identify unresectability (102,106–108) (Figure 57.2). Duplex sonography may also be useful, as it is noninvasive and, in experienced hands, a skilled operator not only can identify the site of biliary obstruction, but also the

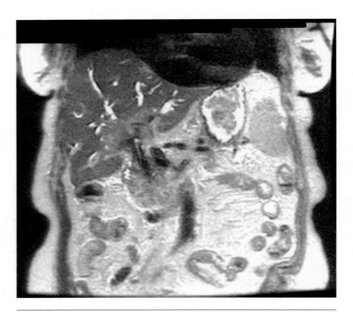

Figure 57.2 Magnetic resonance cholangiogram of hilar cholangiocarcinoma.

presence or absence of portal venous involvement. Hann et al. (109) reported 93% sensitivity and 99% specificity in detecting portal venous involvement in patient with malignant hilar obstructions.

Newer modalities for the diagnostic evaluation of bile duct tumors include staging laparoscopy, 2-deoxy-[^{18}F]fluoro-D-glucose PET, and endoscopic ultrasonography (EUS) with FNA (110). Weber et al. (34) studied the use of laparoscopy for 56 patients with hilar cholangiocarcinoma at Memorial Sloan-Kettering Cancer Center and found that the overall yield of laparoscopy was only 25%, which argues against its routine use. Several authors have reported small series using PET scan for bile duct tumors for distinguishing malignant from benign biliary strictures or extrahepatic disease (36,111,112). Anderson et al. (36) warns that these results should be interpreted with caution in patients with primary sclerosing cholangitis, those with stents in place, as well as patients with known granulomatous disease. EUS-FNA offers several advantages over traditional CT-guided FNA for cytology or endoscopic retrograde cholangiography brushings for establishing the diagnosis of cholangiocarcinoma. Two prospective studies, by Eloubedi et al. (113) and Fritscher-Ravens et al. (114), analyzed the results of EUS-FNA in series of 28 and 48 patients, respectively, with suspected cholangiocarcinomas. Both articles reported high sensitivity (86% and 89%) and specificity (100%). The precise role of EUS-FNA remains to be defined, as most surgical series have recommended operative exploration based on cross-sectional imaging and cholangiography, and reserved cytologic confirmation for patients in whom palliative therapy is indicated.

Staging

In 1975, Bismuth and Corlette described a staging system for hilar cholangiocarcinoma based on tumor involvement of the common hepatic duct (Type I), hepatic duct bifurcation (Type II), unilateral extension into the right hepatic duct (Type IIIa), unilateral extension into the left hepatic duct (Type IIIb), or bilateral extension into sectoral ducts (Type IV) (115). Although there have been several modifications, this remains an important classification of the proximal tumor extension. The sixth edition of the staging manual by American Joint Committee on Cancer (AJCC) and the Internal Union Against Cancer (UICC), was published in 2002 (116). Although the sixth edition adopted similar TNM classification and staging system as the fifth edition, the new classification did focus on the importance of vascular invasion and lymph nodes metastases (Table 57.2) (116,117). Jarnagin has proposed a new clinical T-staging system combining extent of bile duct involvement, presence of portal vein invasion, and lobar atrophy. The authors argue the proposed system can better determine resectability and stratify patients into treatment groups and predict the need for hepatic resection (102).

Techniques of Resection

Resection may be local, including the common bile duct, cystic duct, gallbladder, and common hepatic and proximal ducts to a clear margin above the tumor with the clearance of the hepatoduodenal ligament including the related lymph nodes. For more extensive tumors, hepatic resection may be required, and there has been a growing body of literature that documents not only

Table 57.2

The American Joint Committee on Cancer Staging System for Extrahepatic Bile Duct Cancer

T category	
Tis	Carcinoma in situ
T1	Tumor confined to the bile duct histologically
T2	Tumor invades beyond the wall of the bile duct
T3	Tumor invades the liver, gallbladder, pancreas, and/or unilateral branches of the portal vein or hepatic artery
T4	Tumor invades main portal vein or its branches bilaterally, common hepatic artery or adjacent structures such as colon, stomach, or abdominal wall
Regional lymph nodes (N)	
N0	No regional lymph node metastasis
N1	Regional lymph node metastasis
Distant metastasis (M)	
M0	No distant metastasis
M1	Distant metastasis
Staging system	
0	Tis, N0, M0
IA	T1, N0, M0
IB	T2, N0, M0
IIA	T3, N0. M0
IIB	T1,2,3 N1, M0
III	T4, any N, M0
IV	Any T, any N, M1

^{a}Adapted from Greene FL, Page DL, Fleming ID, et al, eds, for the American Joint Committee on Cancer. *AJCC Cancer Staging Manual*. 6th ed. New York, NY: Springer-Verlag; 2002.

the safety of hepatic resection in experienced hands, but that hepatic resection is frequently necessary to obtain tumor-free margins for hilar cholangiocarcinoma. Liver resection is indicated when the lesion extends unilaterally into either the right or left liver, but leaves the contralateral portion with an intact biliary drainage and blood supply. The initial exploration should be complete, with an evaluation for peritoneal and hepatic deposits or metastases to lymph nodes beyond the porta hepatis, which would indicate unresectability.

Local Resection

Without evidence of distal spread, the bile duct is transected early in the dissection, reflected cephalad with the tumor, associated connective tissue, and periductal lymph nodes. The portal vein and hepatic artery are skeletonized under direct vision, and the dissection is continued superiorly to a site above the tumor. Some groups have used preoperatively placed biliary stents, which may aid in reconstruction. If there is no invasion of the quadrate lobe (segment IV), the hilar plate is lowered by incising the tissue at the base of the quadrate lobe, extending the

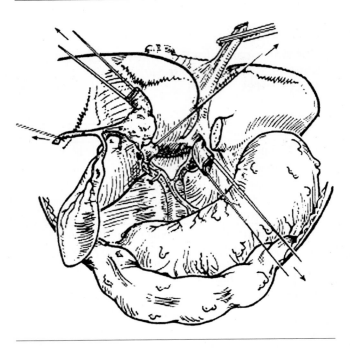

Figure 57.3 Local resection of hilar cholangiocarcinoma. (From Blumgart LH, Fong Y, eds. *Surgery of the Liver and Biliary Tract,* 3rd ed, with permission.)

dissection anterior to the left hepatic duct. Further exposure of the left hepatic duct may be obtained by dividing the bridge of liver tissue at the base of the umbilical fissure. The left hepatic duct can be traced beyond the tumor, transected, and sent for histologic examination (Figure 57.3). There is a relatively shorter segment of right hepatic duct before dividing into anterior and posterior sectoral ducts, and may require the individual ducts to be divided separately for tumor clearance. Biliary continuity is re-established by a Roux-en-Y hepaticojejunostomy in an end-to-side fashion using single-layer absorbable sutures.

Hepatic Resection

The need for a hepatic resection may be evident by preoperative imaging demonstrating unilateral ductal and/or vascular involvement. The initial operative evaluation and hilar dissection are similar to the techniques used in a local resection. If tumor clearance can be achieved along the left hepatic duct and there is tumor extension beyond the right hepatic duct division to sectoral ducts, then an extended right hepatectomy (trisegmentectomy) will be required. Before proceeding with resection, it is important to assess the involvement of the caudate lobe; if necessary, the caudate lobe is resected in continuity. After dissection of the hilum, the proximal extent of the tumor into the bile duct and portal vein can be assessed. If the portal vein bifurcation is clear, the relevant hepatic artery can be ligated and the corresponding right or left portal vein divided. Completion of the hepatic parenchymal resection proceeds using standard techniques, with bilioenteric reconstruction.

Results of Resection

Nakeeb et al. (118) reported the Johns Hopkins experience of treating 196 patients with "perihilar" cholangiocarcinoma. In this series, 109 of the group (56%) underwent resection, and the majority of patients (86%) had local resection of the bile duct without partial hepatectomy. The perioperative mortality and morbidity were 3.6% and 47%, respectively. In this series treated primarily by local resection, only 28 patients (26%) had negative microscopic margins, and the median survival of patients who had resection was 19 months.

Jarnagin et al. (102) reported a series of 225 patients with hilar cholangiocarcinoma from Memorial Sloan-Kettering Cancer Center in which 160 patients underwent exploration with a curative intent. Eighty patients were resected, including 62 who required a hepatic resection. This series highlights the fact that even in a tertiary center with experienced hepatobiliary surgeons, a resection with curative intent was possible in only 50% of those patients who were explored, and only 36% of all patients. An R0 resection (negative margins) could be achieved in 62 patients. Forty-four of the 62 patients with negative margins had a hepatic resection, and 18 were treated by resection of extrahepatic biliary apparatus only (supraduodenal bile duct, cholecystectomy subhilar lymphadenectomy). The large number of patients resected in this series over a relatively short time (80 patients in 9 years) provides the modern benchmark for comparison of all other therapies. The operative mortality was 10%, and 64% of patients had perioperative complications. Infections were the most frequent complication, and the authors reported that positive intraoperative bile cultures doubled the incidence of postoperative infections (79% vs. 33%; $p < 0.04$), and positive bile cultures correlated with the presence of preoperatively placed biliary stents (84% with stents vs. 12% without stents; $p < 0.00001$). Median survival for all patients was 16 months, and was significantly longer in patients who had resection (35 vs. 10 months; $p < 0.00001$). Patients treated by hepatic resection survived longer than those who underwent bile duct excision alone (46 vs. 28 months; $p < 0.04$). The actuarial 5-year survival rate was 37% in patients who underwent hepatic resection and 0% for those treated with bile duct excision alone. It should be noted that the only actual 5-year survivors were patients treated by partial hepatectomy. Multivariate analysis of this series of patients who had a R0 resection identified partial hepatectomy as the only independent predictor of survival after resection with negative margins. The authors cautiously suggest that hepatic resection should be considered for all patients.

Orthotopic Liver Transplantation

Early experience with orthotopic liver transplantation for cholangiocarcinoma resulted in high rates of tumor recurrence and shortened survival. Five-year survival rates from single-institution series were 20% to 30% and, until recently, cholangiocarcinoma was considered a contraindication for liver transplantation (119–122). Separate series from the Mayo Clinic and the University of Nebraska have reported improved results for patients with hilar cholangiocarcinoma by treating patients with neoadjuvant chemoradiation therapy. The Nebraska group reported tumor progression in five patients; however, long-term tumor-free survival was achieved in 45% of the 11 transplanted patients (123). The Mayo Clinic protocol used external-beam radiotherapy (targeted dose of 4,500 cGy in 30 fractions) combined with intravenous fluorouracil, 500 mg/m^2, as a daily bolus for the first 3 days of radiation (124). Transluminal boost of radiation was delivered using transcatheter iridium-192 brachytherapy wire, with a target dose of 2,000 to 3,000 cGy. Patients had a staging laparotomy before transplantation, and only operatively confirmed stage I or II disease underwent liver transplant. Seventy-one patients were enrolled in the protocol; 61 had operative staging and 38 have had transplant at the time of the report. The survival for all 71 patients enrolled in the transplant protocol was 79%, 61%, and 58% at 1, 3, and 5 years after enrollment in the protocol, respectively. Survival for the 38 patients who underwent liver transplantation was 92%, 82%, and 82% at 1, 3, and 5 years after transplantation. Although promising, the inherent supply-demand limitations for liver transplantation will be the greatest obstacle to this therapy (125).

ADJUVANT THERAPY

It is difficult to find convincing evidence for a survival benefit to administration of adjuvant therapy after complete resection of hilar cholangiocarcinoma. An analysis of 46 patients treated in a nonrandomized fashion at the Mayo Clinic did not show a survival advantage to those patients receiving adjuvant chemotherapy (126). Several noncontrolled trials have suggested a benefit to postoperative radiation (127–129). Pitt et al. (130) had reported a series of 50 patients randomized to receive radiotherapy or no adjuvant therapy and found no survival difference. Potentially chemosensitizing agents were not administered in this trial; however, the mean and median survival in several multimodality regimens was less than that observed in their randomized trial. The lack of convincing survival benefit of adjuvant therapy after complete resection suggests the application should be limited to clinical trials.

PALLIATIVE TREATMENT

Jaundice is the predominant symptom of patients with advanced gallbladder cancer or bile duct cancer, and palliation should be directed at relief of jaundice. If unresectability can be determined preoperatively, transtumoral drainage by percutaneous or endoscopic stents can provide relief of jaundice. Percutaneous transhepatic drainage is preferred for high biliary obstructions, and metallic expandable stents have a longer duration of patency (6 to 8 months) than plastic stents. If late occlusion occurs, the stents can be recanalized. If unresectability is identified at the time of exploration, surgical bypass to the left hepatic or segment III duct is an option, and can also provide durable relief of jaundice.

A recently employed modality for palliation of cholangiocarcinoma has been photodynamic therapy plus stenting. The photosensitizing drug sodium porfimer is injected intravenously, followed by photoactivation using an endoscopic retrograde transtumoral intubation and insertion of a 400-mcm thin quartz fiber (131). Witzigman et al. (132) reported a series of patients with hilar cholangiocarcinoma that included 68 unresectable patients treated with photodynamic therapy and stenting compared with 56 patients who had stenting alone. Photodynamic therapy and stenting resulted in longer median survival (12 vs. 6.4 months; $p <0.01$) compared with stenting alone.

CONCLUSION

Cancers of the gallbladder and bile ducts present difficult treatment dilemmas because most are incurable at the time of diagnosis. Advances in preoperative staging may help select proper candidates for operative exploration, and surgical resection offers the only hope for long-term survival. Hepatic resection with negative margins can be performed with acceptable mortality and morbidity at tertiary centers, and should be considered for fit patients without preoperatively documented signs of unresectability. The role of transplantation for cholangiocarcinoma remains to be determined. Although there has yet to be a significant survival advantage with adjuvant chemotherapy or radiotherapy, further improvements in survival will likely require novel approaches, best identified from carefully constructed clinical trials.

REFERENCES

1. Ries LAG, Harkins D, Krapcho M, et al., eds. *SEER Cancer Statistics Review, 1975–2003.* Bethesda, MD: National Cancer Institute. Available at http://seer.cancer.gov/csr/1975_2003/. Accessed August 8, 2006.
2. Urbach DR, Swanstrom LL, Khajanchee YS, et al. Incidence of cancer of the pancreas, extrahepatic bile duct and ampulla of Vater in the United States, before and after the introduction of laparoscopic cholecystectomy. *Am J Surg.* 2001;181:526–528.
3. Abdalla EK, Vauthey JN. Biliary tract cancer. *Curr Opinion Gastroenterology* 2001;17:450–457.
4. Randi G, Franceschi S, La Vecchia C. Gallbladder cancer worldwide: geographical distribution and risk factors. *Int J Cancer* 2005;118:1591–1602.
5. Mayo WJ, A study of 534 operations upon the gallbladder and bile passages: tabulated reports of 547 operated cases. *Boston Med Surg J* 1903:cxlviii:545–547.
6. Pitt HA, Dooley WC, Yeo CJ, et al. Malignancies of the biliary tree 1995.;32:1–90.
7. Zatonski WA, Lowenfels AB, et al. Epidemiologic aspects of gallbladder cancer: a case control study of the SEARCH Program of the International Agency for Research on Cancer. *J Natl Cancer Inst* 1997;89:1132–1138.
8. Lowenfelds AB, Walker AM, Althaus DP, et al. Gallstone growth, size, and risk of gallbladder cancer: an interracial study. *In J Epidemiol* 1989;18:50–54.
9. de Groen PC, Gories GJ, LaRusso NF, et al. Biliary tract cancers. *New Engl J Med.* 1999;341:1368–1378.
10. Ransohoff DF, Gracie WA. Treatment of gallstones. *Ann Intern Med* 1993;119:606–619.
11. Chijiiwa K, Tanaka M. Polypoid lesion of the gallbladder: indications of carcinoma and outcome after surgery for malignant polypoid lesion. *Int Surg* 1994;79:106–109.
12. Lazcano-Ponce EC, Miguel JF, Munoz N, et al. Epidemiology and molecular pathology of gallbladder cancer. *CA Cancer J Clin* 2001;51:349–364.
13. Csendes A, Becerra M, Burdiles P, et al. Bacteriological studies of bile from the gallbladder in patients with carcinoma of the gallbladder, cholelithiasis, common bile duct stones and no gallstones disease. *Eur J Surg* 1994;160:363–367.
14. Corsetti RL, Wanebo HJ. Gallbladder cancer. In: Cameron JS, ed. *Current Surgical Therapy.* St. Louis, MO: Mosby; 1998;462–468.
15. Stephen AE, Berger DL. Carcinoma in the porcelain gallbladder: a relationship revisited. *Surgery* 2001;129:699–703.

16. Towfigh S, McFadden Cortina GR, et al. Porcelain gallbladder is not associated with gallbladder carcinoma. *Am Surgeon* 2001;67:7–10.

17. Albores-Saavedra J, Tuck M, McLaren BK, et al. Papillary carcinomas of the gallbladder: analysis of noninvasive and invasive types. *Arch Pathol Lab Med* 2005;129905–129909.

18. Sumiyoshi K, Nagai E, Chijiiwa K, et al. Pathology of carcinoma of the gallbladder. *World J Surg* 1991;15:315–321.

19. Piehler JM, Crichlow RW. Primary Carcinoma of the gallbladder. *Surg Gynecol Obstet* 1978;147:929–942.

20. Olken SM, Bledsoe R, Nemark H 3rd. The ultrasonic diagnosis of primary carcinoma of the gallbladder. *Radiology.* 1978;129:481–482.

21. Ozmen MM, Patankar RV, Hengirmen S, et al. Epidemiology of gallbladder polyps. *Scan J Gastroenterol* 1994;29:480.

22. Koga A, Watanabe K, Fukuyma T, et al. Diagnosis and operative indications for polypoid lesions of the gallbladder. *Br J Surg* 1985;72:728–730.

23. Damore LJ 2nd, Cook CH, Fernandez KL, et al. Ultrasonography incorrectly diagnoses gallbladder polyps. *Surg Laparosc Endosc Percutan Tech* 2001;11:88–91.

24. Csendes A, Burgos AM, Csendes P, et al. Late follow-up of polypoid lesions of the gallbladder smaller than 10 mm. *Ann Surg* 2001;234:657–660.

25. Terzi C, Sökmen S, Seçkin S, et al. Polypoid lesions of the gallbladder: report of 100 cases with special reference to operative indications. *Surgery* 2000;127:622–627.

26. Chattopadhyay D, Lochan R, Balupuri S, et al. Outcome of gallbladder polypoid lesions detected by transabdominal ultrasound scanning: a nine year experience. *World J Gastroenterol* 2005;11:2171–2173.

27. Grand D, Horton KM, Fishman EK. CT of the gallbladder: spectrum of disease. *AJR* 2004;183:163–170.

28. Yoshimitsu K, Honda H, Shinozaki K, et al. Helical CT of the local spread of carcinoma of the gallbladder: evaluation according to the TNM system in patients who underwent resection. *AJR* 2002;179:423–428.

29. Schwartz LH, Black J, Fong Y, et al. Gallbladder carcinoma: findings at MR imaging with MR cholangiography. *J Comput Assist Tomogr.* 2002;26:405–410.

30. Meara RS, Jhala D, Eloubeidi MA, et al. Endoscopic ultrasound-guided FNA biopsy of bile duct and gallbladder: analysis of 53 cases. *Cytopathology* 2006;17:42–49.

31. Sadomoto Y, Kubo H, Harada N, et al. Preoperative diagnosis and staging of gallbladder carcinoma by EUS. *Gastrointest Endosc* 2003;58:536–541.

32. Jacobson BC, Pitman MB, Brugge WR. EUS-guided FNA for the diagnosis of gallbladder masses. *Gastrointest Endosc* 2003;57:251–254.

33. Donahue JH. Present status of the diagnosis and treatment of gallbladder carcinoma. *J Hepatobiliary Pancreat Surg* 2001;8:530–534.

34. Weber S, DeMatteo RP, Fong Y, et al. Staging laparoscopy in patients with extrahepatic biliary carcinoma: analysis of 100 patients. *Ann Surg* 2002;235:392–399.

35. Rodriguez-Fernandez A, Gomez-Rio M, Llamas-Elvira JM, et al. Positron-emission tomography with fluorine-18-fluoro-2-deoxy-D-glucose for gallbladder cancer diagnosis. *Am J Surg* 2004;188:171–175.

36. Anderson CD, Rice MH, Pinson CW, et al. Fluorodeoxyglucose PET imaging in the evaluation of gallbladder carcinoma and cholangiocarcinoma. *J Gastroint Surg* 2004;8:90–97.

37. Nevin JE, Moran TJ, Kay S, et al. Carcinoma of the gallbladder: staging, treatment, and prognosis. *Cancer* 1976;37:141–148.

38. Donahue JH, Nagorney DM, Grant CS, et al. Carcinoma of the gallbladder: does radical resection improve outcome? *Arch Surg* 1990;125:237–241.

39. Fong Y, Jarnagin W, Blumgart LH. Gallbladder cancer: comparison of patient presenting initially for definitive operation with those presenting after prior noncurative intervention. *Ann Surg.* 2000;232:557–569.

40. Hawkins WG, DeMatteo RP, Jernigan WR, et al. Jaundice predicts advanced disease and early mortality in patients with gallbladder cancer. *Ann Surg Oncol* 2004;11:310–315.

41. Suzuki K, Kimura T, Ogawa H. Long-term prognosis of gallbladder cancer diagnosed after laparoscopic cholecystectomy. *Surg Endosc* 2000;14:712–716.

42. Contini S, Dalla Valle R, Zinicola R. Unexpected gallbladder cancer after laparoscopic cholecystectomy: an emerging problem? Reflections on four cases. *Surg Endosc* 1999;13:264–267.

43. Taner CB, Nagorney DM, Donahue JH. Surgical treatment of gallbladder cancer. *J Gastrointest Surg* 2004;8:83–89.

44. Shimizu Y, Ohtsuka M, Ito H, et al. Should the extrahepatic bile duct be resected for locally advanced gallbladder cancer? *Surgery* 2004;136:1012–1017.

45. Shirai Y, Yoshida K, Tsukada K, et al. Radical Surgery for gallbladder carcinoma. *Ann Surg* 1992;216:565–568.

46. Bartlett DL, Fong Y, Fortner JG, et al. Long-term results after resection for gallbladder cancer: implications for staging and management. *Ann Surg* 1996;224:639–646.

47. Matsumoto Y, Fujii H, Aoyama H, et al. Surgical treatment of primary carcinoma of the gallbladder based on the histologic analysis of 48 surgical specimens. *Am J Surg* 1992;163:239–245.

48. Yamaguchi K, Tsuneyoshi M. Subclinical gallbladder carcinoma. *Am J Surg* 1992;163:382–386.

49. Oertli D, Herzog U, Tondelli P. Primary carcinoma of the gallbladder: operative experience during a 16-year period. *Eur J Surg.* 1993;159:415–420.

50. de Arextabala X, Roa IS, Burgos LA, et al. Curative resection in potentially resectable tumours of the gallbladder. *Eur J Surg* 1997;163:419–426.

51. Boerma EJ. Towards an oncological resection of gall bladder cancer. *Eur J Surg Oncol* 1994;20:537–544.

52. Shinkai H, Kimura W, Sata N, et al. A case of gallbladder cancer with para-aortic lymph node metastasis who has survived more than seven years after the primary extended radical operation. *Hepatogastroenterology* 1996;43:1370–1376.

53. Shimada H, Endo I, Togo S, et al. The role of lymph node dissection in the treatment of gallbladder carcinoma. *Cancer* 1997;80:61–667.

54. Nimura Y, Hayakawa N, Kamiya J, et al. Hepatopancreatoduodenectomy for advanced carcinoma of the biliary tract. *Hepatogastroenterology* 1991;38:170–175.

55. Nakamura S, Nishiyama R, Yokoi Y, et al. Hepatopancreatoduodenectomy for advanced gallbladder carcinoma. *Arch Surg* 1994;129:625–629.

56. Shirai Y, Yoshida K, Tsukada K, et al. Identification of the regional lymphatic system of the gallbladder by vital staining. *Br J Surg* 1992;79:659–662.

57. Yamamoto M, Onoyama H, Ajiki T, et al. Surgical results of operation for carcinoma of the gallbladder. *Hepatogastroenterology* 1999;46:1552–1556.

58. Sasaki R, Hidenori I, Fujita, et al. Significance of extensive surgery including resection of the pancreas head for the treatment of gallbladder cancer–from the perspective of the mode of lymph node involvement and surgical outcome. *World J Surg* 2006;30:36–42.

59. Sun CD, Zhang BY, Wu LQ, et al. Laparoscopic cholecystectomy for treatment of unexpected early-stage gallbladder cancer. *J Surg Oncol.* 2005;91:253–257.

60. Steinert R, Nestler G Sagynaliev E, et al. Laparoscopic cholecystectomy and gallbladder cancer. *J Surg Oncol* 2006;93:682–689.

61. Ouchi K, Mikuni J, Kakugawa Y; Organizing Committee, the 30th Annual Congress of the Japanese Society of Biliary Surgery. *J Hepatobiliary Pancreat Surg* 2002;9:256–260.

62. Misra MC, Guleria S. Management of cancer gallbladder found as a surprise on a resected specimen. *J Surg Oncol* 2006;93:690–698.

63. National Comprehensive Cancer Network Practice Guidelines in Oncology v. 1.2006. http://www.nccn.org/professionals/physician_gls/PDF/hepatobiliary.pdf accessed July 29, 2006.

64. Fong Y, Heffernan N, Blumgart LH. Gallbladder carcinoma during laparoscopic cholecystectomy; aggressive reresection is beneficial. *Cancer* 1998;83:423–427.

65. Pack GT, Miller TR, Brasfield RD. Total right hepatic lobectomy for cancer of the gallbladder. *Ann Surg* 1955;142:6–16.

66. Kresl JJ, Schild SE, Henning GT, et al. Adjuvant external beam radiation therapy with concurrent chemotherapy in the management of gallbladder carcinoma. *Int J Radiation Oncol Biol Phys* 2002;52:167–175.

67. Czito BG, Hurwitz HI. Clough RW. Adjuvant external-beam radiotherapy with concurrent chemotherapy after resection of primary gallbladder carcinoma: a 23 year experience. *Int J Radiation Oncol Biol Phys* 2005;62:1030–1034.

68. Todoroki T. Chemotherapy for gallbladder carcinoma—a surgeon's perspective. *Hepatogastroenterology* 2000;47:948–955.

69. Hadjis NS, Collier NA, Blumgart LH. Malignant masquerade at the hilum of the liver. *Br J Surg.* 1985;72:659–661.

70. Corvera CU, Blumgart LH, Darvishian F, et al. Clinical and pathologic features of proximal biliary strictures masquerading as hilar cholangiocarcinoma. *J Am Coll Surg* 2005;201:862–869.

71. Shaib Y, El-Serag HB. The epidemiology of cholangiocarcinoma. *Semin Liv Dis* 2004;24:115–125.

72. Vauthey JN, Blumgart LH. Recent advances in the management of cholangiocarcinoma. *Semin Liv Dis* 1994;14:109–114.

73. Welzel TM, McGlynn KA, Hsing AW, et al. Impact of classification of hilar cholangiocarcinomas (Klatskin tumors) on the Incidence of intra- and extrahepatic cholangiocarcinoma in the United States. *J Natl Cancer Inst* 2006;98:873–875.

74. Carriaga MT, Henson DE. Liver, gallbladder, extrahepatic bile ducts, and pancreas. *Cancer* 1995;75(Suppl 1):171–190.

75. Patel T. Cholangiocarcinoma. *Nat Clin Pract Gastroenterol Hepatol* 2006;3:3–42.

76. Broome U, Olsson R, Loof L, et al. Natural history and prognostic factors in 305 Swedish patients with primary sclerosing cholangitis. *Gut* 1996;38:610–615.

77. Bergquist A, Glaumann H, Persson B, et al. Risk factors and clinical presentation of hepatobiliary carcinoma in patients with primary sclerosing cholangitis: a case control study. *Hepatology* 1998;27:311–316.

78. Chalasani N, Baluyut A, Ismail A, et al. Cholangiocarcinoma in patients with primary sclerosing cholangitis: a multicenter case-control study. *Hepatology* 200;31:7–11.

79. Burak K, Angulo P, Pasha TM, et al. Incidence and risk factors for cholangiocarcinoma in primary sclerosing cholangitis. *Am J Gastroenterol.* 2004;99:523–526.

80. Watanapa P. Watanapa WB. Liver fluke-associated cholangiocarcinoma. *Br J Surg* 2002;89:962–970.

81. Honjo S, Srivatanakul P, Sriplung H, et al. Genetic and environmental determinants of risk for cholangiocarcinoma via Opisthorchis viverrini in a densely infested area in Nakhon Phanom, northeast Thailand. *Int J Cancer* 2005;117:854–860.

82. Sher L, Iwatsuki S, Lebearu G, et al. Hilar cholangiocarcinoma associated with clonorchiasis. *Dig Dis Sci* 1989;34:1121–1123.

83. Ona FV, Dytoc JN. Clonorchiasis-associated cholangiocarcinoma: a report of two cases with unusual manifestations. *Gastroenterology* 1991;101:831–839.

84. Chung CS, Lee SK. An epidemiologic study of primary liver carcinomas in Pusan area with special reference to clonorchiasis. *Korean J Pathol* 1976;10:33–64.

85. Shin HR, Lee CU, Park HJ, et al. Hepatitis B and C virus, Clonorchis sinensis for the risk of liver cancer a case-control study in Pusan, Korea. *Int J Epidemiol* 1996;25:933–940.

86. Metcalfe MS, Wemyss-Holden SA, Maddern GJ. Management dilemmas with choledochal cysts. *Arch Surg* 2003;138:333–339.

87. Song HK, Kim MH, Myung SJ, et al. Choledochal cyst associated the with anomalous union of pancreaticobiliary duct (AUPBD) has a more grave clinical course than choledochal cyst alone. *K Intern Med* 1999;14:1–8.

88. Liu CL, Fan ST, Lo CM, et al. Choledochal cysts in adults. *Arch Surg* 2002;137:465–468.

89. Stain SC, Guthrie CR, Yellin AE, et al. Choledochal cyst in the adult. *Ann Surg.* 1995;222:128–133.

90. Kato O, Hattori K, Suzuki T, et al. Clinical significance of anomalous pancreaticobiliary union. *Gastrointest Endosc* 1983;29:94–98.

91. Olnes MJ, Erlich R. A review and update on cholangiocarcinoma. *Oncology* 2004;66:167–179.

92. Isa T, Tomita S, Nakachi A, et al. Analysis of microsatellite instability, K-ras mutation and p53 protein overexpression in intrahepatic cholangiocarcinoma. *Hepatogastroenterology* 2002;49:604–608.

93. Rashid A, Ueki T, Gao YT, et al. K-ras mutation, p53 overexpression, and microsatellite instability in biliary tract cancers: a population based study in China. *Clin Cancer Res* 2002:8:3156–3163.

94. Diamantis I, Karamitopoulou E, Perentes E, et al. p53 immunoreactivity in extrahepatic bile duct and gallbladder cancer: correlation with tumor grade and survival. *Hepatology* 1995;22:774–779.

95. Wu T. Cyclooxygenase-2 and prostaglandin signaling in cholangiocarcinoma. *Biochem Biophys Acta* 2005;1755:135–150.

96. Renshaw K. Malignant neoplasms of the extrahepatic biliary ducts. *Ann Surg* 1922;76:205–221.

97. Altemeier WA, Gall EA, Zinninger MM, et al. Sclerosing carcinoma of the major intrahepatic bile ducts. *AMA Arch Surg* 1957;75:450–461.

98. Klatskin G. Adenocarcinoma of the hepatic duct at its bifurcation within the porta hepatis: an unusual tumor with distinctive clinical and pathological features. *Am J Med* 1965;38:241–256.

99. Huang Z, Zhou NX, Wang DD, et al. Changing trends of surgical treatment of hilar bile duct cancer: clinical and experimental perspectives. *World J Gastroenterol.* 2000;6:777–782.

100. Starzl TE, Francavilla A, Halgrimson CG, et al. The origin, hormonal nature, and action of hepatotrophic substances in portal venous blood. *Surg Gynecol Obstet* 1973;137:173–199.

101. Hadjis NS, Carr D, Blenkharn I, et al. Expectant management of patients with unilateral stricture and atrophy. *Gut* 1986;27:1223–1227.

102. Jarnagin WR, Fong Y, DeMatteo RP, et al. Staging, resectability, and outcome in 225 patients with hilar cholangiocarcinoma. *Ann Surg* 2001:234;507–519.

103. Chamberlain RS, Blumgart LH. Hilar cholangiocarcinoma: a review and commentary. *Ann Surg Oncol* 2000;7:55–66.

104. Hochwald SN, Burke EC, Jarnagin WR, et al. Association of preoperative biliary stenting with increased postoperative infectious complications in proximal cholangiocarcinoma. *Arch Surg* 1999;134:261–266.

105. Lillemoe K, Cameron JL. Surgery for hilar cholangiocarcinoma: the Johns Hopkins approach. *J Hepatobiliary Pancreat Surg* 2000;7: 115–121.

106. Hemming AW, Reed AI, Fujita S, et al. Surgical management of hilar cholangiocarcinoma. *Ann Surg* 2005;241:693–702.

107. Hanninen EL, Pech M, Jonas S, et al. Magnetic resonance imaging including magnetic resonance cholangiopancreatography for tumor localization and therapy planning in malignant hilar obstructions. *Acta Radiol* 2005;46:462–470.

108. Manfredi R, Barbaro B, Masselli G, et al. Magnetic resonance imaging of cholangiocarcinoma. *Semin Liver Dis.* 2004;24:155–164.

109. Hann LE, Fong Y, Shriver CD, et al. Malignant hepatic hilar tumors: can ultrasonography be used as an alternative to angiography with CT arterial portography for determination of resectability? *J Ultrasound Med* 1996;15:37–45.

110. Singh P, Patel T. Advances in the diagnosis and management of cholangiocarcinoma. *Curr Opin Gastroenterol* 2006;22:294–299.

111. Reinhardt MJ, Strunk H, Gerhardt T, et al. Detection of Klatskin's tumor in extrahepatic bile duct strictures using delayed 18F-FDG PET/CT: preliminary results for 22 patient studies. *J Nucl Med* 2005;46:1158–1163.

112. Wakabayashi H, Akamoto S, Yachida S, et al. Significance of fluorodeoxyglucose PET imaging in the diagnosis of malignancies in patients with biliary stricture. *Eur J Surg Oncol* 2005;31:1175–1179.

113. Eloubeidi MA, Chen VK, Jhala NC, et al. Endoscopic ultrasound-guided fine needle aspiration biopsy of suspected cholangiocarcinoma. *Clin Gastroenterol Hepatol* 2004;2:209–213.

114. Fritscher-Ravens A, Broering DC, Knoefel WT, et al. EUS-guided fine-needle aspiration of suspected cholangiocarcinoma in potentially operable patients with negative brush cytology. *Am J Gastroenterol* 2004;99:45–51.

115. Bismuth H, Corlette MB. Intrahepatic cholangioenteric anastomosis in carcinoma of the hilus of the liver. *Surg Gynecol Obstet.* 1975; 140(2):170–178.

116. Greene FL, Page DL, Fleming ID, et al., eds, for the American Joint Committee on Cancer. *AJCC Cancer Staging Manual*, 6th ed. New York, NY: Springer-Verlag; 2002.

117. Nishio H, Nagino M, Oda K, et al. TNM classification for perihilar cholangiocarcinoma: comparison between 5ᵗʰ and 6ᵗʰ editions of the AJCC/UICC staging systems. *Langenbecks Arch Surg* 2005;390:319–327.

118. Nakeeb A, Pitt HA, Sohn TA. Cholangiocarcinoma: a spectrum of intrahepatic, perihilar, and distal tumors. *Ann Surg* 1996;224:463–475.

119. Robles R, Figueras J, Turrion VS, et al. Spanish experience in liver transplantation for hilar and peripheral cholangiocarcinoma. *Ann Surg* 2004;239:265–271.

120. Alessiani M. Tzakis A. Todo S, et al. Assessment of 5-year experience with abdominal organ transplantation. *J Am Coll Surg* 1995; 180:1–9.

121. Goldstein RM, Stone M, Tillery GW, et al. Is liver transplantation indicated for cholangiocarcinoma: *Am J Surg* 1993;166:768–771.

122. Pichlmayr R, Weimann A, Klempnauer J, et al. Surgical treatment in proximal bile duct cancer. A single-center experience. *Ann Surg* 1996;224:628–638.

123. Sudan D, DeRoover A, Chinnakotla S, et al. Radiotherapy and transplantation allow long-term survival for nonresectable hilar cholangiocarcinoma. *Am J Transplantation* 2002;2:774–779.

124. Rea DJ, Heimbach JK, Rosen CB, et al. Liver transplantation with neoadjuvant chemoradiation is more effective than resection for hilar cholangiocarcinoma. *Ann Surg* 2005;242:451–461.

125. Callery M. Transplantation for cholangiocarcinoma: advance or supply-demand dilemma? *Gastroenterology* 2006;130:2242–2244.

126. Rea DJ, Munoz-Juarez M, Farnell MB, et al. Major hepatic resection for hilar cholangiocarcinoma: analysis of 46 patients. *Arch Surg.* 2004;139:514–525.

127. Gerhards MF, van Gulik TM, González DG, et al. Results of postoperative radiotherapy for resectable hilar cholangiocarcinoma. *World J Surg* 2003;27:173–179.

128. Nakeeb A, Tran KQ, Black MJ, et al. Improved survival in resected biliary malignancies. *Surgery* 2002;132:555–564.

129. Sagawa N, Kondo S, Morikawa T, et al. Effectiveness of radiation therapy after surgery for hilar cholangiocarcinoma. *Surg Today* 2005;35:548–552.

130. Pitt HA, Nakeeb A, Abrams RA. Perihilar cholangiocarcinoma: postoperative radiotherapy does not improve survival. *Ann Surg* 1995;221:788–798.

131. Berr F, Wiedmann M, Tannapfel A, et al. Photodynamic therapy for advanced bile duct cancer: evidence for improved palliation and extended survival. *Hepatology* 2000;31:291–298.

132. Witzigman H, Berr F, Ringel U, et al. Surgical and palliative management and outcome in 184 patients with hilar cholangiocarcinoma: palliative photodynamic therapy plus stenting is comparable to R1/R2 resection. *Ann Surg* 2006;244:230–239.

COMMENTARY
Leslie H. Blumgart and Michael D'Angelica

TUMORS OF THE GALLBLADDER

As the authors of Chapter 57 clearly point out, gallbladder cancer is quite rare. The incidence, however, has remarkable ethnic and geographic variation. Although not well studied, surgeons in endemic areas often perform prophylactic cholecystectomy in patients with asymptomatic stones, whereas in North America, the low incidence of this cancer does not justify such an approach to prevent the development of cancer. Some studies have correlated size and/or volume of stones with a higher risk of cancer but these studies must be interpreted cautiously (1,2). The main issue is that these studies are not population-based but rather based on resected specimens and, therefore, the true denominator is not well defined. There may be a case for cancer prevention by prophylactic cholecystectomy in a young patient in a high incidence area with a large stone or multiple stones, but such an approach is not justified in low incidence areas such as North America.

The association of molecular and genetic changes with gallbladder cancer still requires much work, but unfortunately the rarity of this tumor will make such studies difficult. Other associated risk factors are discussed, including adenomatous changes, squamous metaplasia, and porcelain gallbladder. Although it is likely to be a very uncommon predecessor of gallbladder cancer, adenomatous polyps can progress to malignancy. Studies have demonstrated an increased risk in patients with single polyps >1cm in size. We and others advocate cholecystectomy for these patients, who should be carefully counseled about the possibility of finding cancer and the operations to treat such a cancer should it be found at operation. For patients with polyps less than 1 cm, observation is appropriate. Although porcelain gallbladder was once believed to be associated with a very high risk of cancer, the chapter appropriately stresses that more modern studies, which likely have more accurate denominators, show this risk to be quite low and probably well under 5% (3).

The pathology of gallbladder cancer is relatively straightforward as the great majority of cases are adenocarcinomas and are usually of the more invasive nodular type. Well-differentiated or papillary tumors are less often invasive and represent a distinct minority of cases. It should be stressed that although there is a long list of histologic possibilities in gallbladder tumors, the great majority will be the invasive nodular type, which is overwhelmingly responsible for the clinical data on the presentation, treatment, and outcome of gallbladder cancer.

The imaging for gallbladder cancer is composed of ultrasound to evaluate the primary tumor and cross-sectional imaging (computed tomography or magnetic resonance imaging) to evaluate the rest of the abdominal cavity for evidence of regional or distant metastases. Although the authors review the use of direct cholangiography for the jaundiced patient with gallbladder cancer, we believe that magnetic resonance cholangiopancreatography has largely replaced this modality for diagnostic purposes (4). Of course, direct cholangiography may be necessary for therapeutic stenting options. It is worth mentioning that differentiating gallbladder cancer with diffuse biliary involvement from hilar cholangiocarcinoma can often be quite difficult. Gallbladder cancer involving the bile duct has a typical radiographic appearance of a midbile duct stricture correlating with the insertion of the cystic duct into the common hepatic duct. Lastly, gallbladder cancer presenting with jaundice is a sign of advanced disease. In our experience, <10% of jaundiced patients are resectable and no patient has survived >3 years from the date of diagnosis, regardless of resection (5). There are, however, uncommon situations in which jaundice in association with gallbladder cancer is not such an ominous sign. Such situations include stones causing jaundice or a primary tumor of the cystic duct/infundibulum of the gallbladder with limited involvement of the bile duct. Unfortunately, the great majority of cases of gallbladder cancer patients presenting with jaundice are due to diffuse biliary involvement or extensive invasive nodal metastases, which portend a very poor prognosis.

Inevitably, any discussion of the diagnostic workup of gallbladder cancer leads to a discussion about biopsy, and the authors mention the use of endoscopic ultrasonography and biopsy "in patients considered for resection." We do not believe that biopsy has a role in the evaluation of suspicious gallbladder lesions that are radiologically resectable; the "biopsy" for this situation should be the definitive resection. However, these patients with a clinical diagnosis of gallbladder cancer not confirmed by preoperative biopsy should be advised of the small possibility of finding benign disease on the final pathologic examination. Unfortunately, despite great improvements in cross-sectional imaging, a large number of patients with gallbladder cancer are found to be unresectable at operation. We believe that diagnostic laparoscopy should be employed routinely before a planned open exploration and resection inasmuch as about half of the patients with unresectable disease can be identified by this method. These patients are spared laparotomy with the

additional benefits of shorter hospital stay, reduced morbidity, and earlier initiation of nonsurgical therapy (6). In addition, we even perform laparoscopy selectively in patients who have had a recent laparoscopic cholecystectomy in whom an occult malignancy was found on complete pathologic examination.

The appropriate operation for gallbladder cancer is based on a complete resection with a reasonable margin of normal tissue and a regional lymph node dissection. Outcome after complete resection is largely dictated by T and N stage. In our experience, N stage is the most important factor because long-term survival with node-positive disease is uncommon. Since our original reports on gallbladder cancer, we have now documented a small number of long-term survivors with node-positive disease and continue to resect patients with nodal metastases limited to the porta hepatis. It is important to recognize that a subset of patients with advanced T-stage disease are node-negative and potentially curable with an operation. We agree that lymph node metastases beyond the porta hepatis (mostly celiac and retropancreatic) represent systemic disease and are incurable with an operation. These nodal basins should be explored at operation before proceeding with a definitive resection.

We generally believe that the appropriate operation for gallbladder cancer is based on the anatomic location of the tumor and what structures are involved. The basic operation would be a cholecystectomy with an en bloc resection of liver segments IVb and five along with a portal lymph node dissection. A major hepatic resection (hemihepatectomy or greater) should be performed only when the tumor location involves inflow structures such that there is no other way to resect the tumor with negative margins. Although we used to routinely resect the bile duct to enhance the nodal dissection, we have become more selective about this and generally preserve the bile duct. Indications to remove the bile duct would be a positive cystic duct margin or tumor involving the duct, mandating such a resection for oncologic adequacy.

We agree that T1a tumors (invasion extends to the laminas propria) are cured with a simple cholecystectomy but a negative cystic duct margin must be ensured, and in rare cases an excision of the bile duct may be necessary. Treatment of T1b tumors (invasion extends to the muscle layer) is more controversial, and there are very limited data to base the appropriate extent of resection. It has been suggested that there is a significant failure rate after laparoscopic cholecystectomy for T1b tumors and these are mostly accounted for by locoregional failure (7). Acknowledging limited proof, we advocate selectively re-resecting patients with T1b tumors, especially in the young healthy patient. We agree with the authors that re-resection of port sites is a diagnostic, not therapeutic, procedure as patients with tumor in these specimens almost always develop rapid progression in the peritoneal cavity. We do not believe that re-excision of port sites is a mandatory part of a reoperation for gallbladder cancer.

The evidence for re-resection after a simple cholecystectomy for a T2 or greater gallbladder tumor is retrospective and fraught with selection bias but convincing nonetheless. Retrospective comparisons of survival comparing simple cholecystectomy with extended cholecystectomy (en bloc liver resection and portal lymphadenectomy) have shown a consistent survival advantage associated with an extended cholecystectomy. Data from our institution and others have also demonstrated that when comparing patients undergoing re-resection after simple cholecystectomy with those undergoing a cancer operation initially, there are no differences in resectability, survival, or recurrence patterns (8). Of course, this must be interpreted in the context of our selection. These data are based on the patients who are referred to a hepatobiliary surgeon after a laparoscopic cholecystectomy and omitting from analysis those patients who progress rapidly. Furthermore, a higher percentage of tumors diagnosed at laparoscopic cholecystectomy are in an early stage compared with those diagnosed preoperatively.

The management of a patient who presents with a diagnosis of gallbladder cancer after a noncurative cholecystectomy is difficult. In general, the workup should include consultation with the surgeon who performed the cholecystectomy to review operative findings; a review of the precholecystectomy imaging to try to retrospectively identify the location of the tumor; a re-review of the pathology report to accurately stage the tumor and assess margins, and finally, repeat imaging to rule out early metastatic disease. Despite such a complete evaluation, the operation is still somewhat "blind," and differentiating scar from tumor is often difficult if not impossible. Patients should be warned that sometimes major operations are performed and final pathologic examination will reveal no tumor.

Generally speaking, there is no effective adjuvant therapy for completely resected gallbladder cancer. Systemic chemotherapy for advanced disease is not effective and the rarity of the disease has precluded adequate randomized trials of adjuvant approaches. There is one trial from Japan that reported a modest benefit to adjuvant chemotherapy with mitomycin and 5-fluorouracil. Unfortunately, the details of the final pathology and surgical findings are not presented, thus making the interpretation of the data difficult (9). There is no standard adjuvant therapy; hopefully, multi-institutional studies can eventually address this problem. It is important to understand recurrence patterns when considering the adjuvant treatment. We have published that 85% of recurrences involve distant sites, highlighting the importance of systemic therapy in any potential adjuvant strategy (10).

TUMORS OF THE BILE DUCT

Cholangiocarcinoma can develop from biliary epithelium anywhere along the biliary tract from the distal intrapancreatic bile duct to small intrahepatic ducts. Chapter 57 primarily deals with extrahepatic hilar and midbile duct tumors. The authors review the incidence of benign obstructive lesions masquerading as malignancy with an incidence of approximately 10% in resected specimens. It should be stressed that although benign lesions can masquerade as malignant biliary obstruction, differentiating the two is often impossible and negative biopsies do not ensure a benign diagnosis. Therefore, all mass lesions obstructing the biliary tree must be assumed to be malignant and treated as such. When preparing patients for resection of a biliary tumor that has not been histologically proven a malignancy, it is important to document and explain to the patient that the resection may ultimately reveal benign disease.

Hilar cholangiocarcinoma is a relatively rare disease, and changes in incidence are likely related to better imaging and

awareness of the diagnosis. The risk factors for hilar cholangiocarcinoma are nicely reviewed by the authors and generally relate to chronic inflammatory conditions of the biliary tree such as parasitic infections, choledochal cysts with anomalous pancreatobiliary junction, and sclerosing cholangitis. The relative rarity of hilar cholangiocarcinoma makes epidemiologic associations difficult to study and prove.

The majority of extrahepatic cholangiocarcinomas are nodular and/or sclerosing tumors that are notorious for both longitudinal and radial spread beyond the palpable tumor. Local invasion of the hepatic artery and/or portal vein is common, making resection particularly challenging. In our experience, papillary tumors are found both in the hilar location as well as in the distal bile duct, but overall account for the minority of tumors. Papillary tumors are less invasive, more easily resected, and associated with a better prognosis (11). It is interesting that in the early reports on hilar cholangiocarcinoma, it was emphasized that the tumors tend to cause problems mainly from prolonged biliary obstruction rather than metastases (12). Although these tumors can certainly metastasize, in our experience the biggest problem in managing patients with hilar cholangiocarcinoma is managing the biliary obstruction and resultant cholangitis and liver disease, which are often responsible for patients' demise. The authors appropriately stress that cholangiocarcinoma usually presents with jaundice but there is typically a period before the onset of jaundice, when the obstruction is incomplete or unilobar. During this period the patient is typically asymptomatic and the only abnormality may be a raised alkaline phosphatase level. We have always emphasized that an incidentally found rise in alkaline phosphatase without obvious other causes should prompt an investigation of the biliary tree.

Because a margin-negative resection is the only chance of long-term survival, preoperative assessment of resectability is critical. Based on cross-sectional imaging and an ultrasound, we have devised a T-staging system that is simple and correlates very well with resectability (Table 57C.1) (13). In our analysis the resectability of T1, 2, and 3 tumors was 59%, 31%, and 0%, respectively. This T-staging system also correlates well with the risk of finding metastatic disease during an open exploration or at diagnostic laparoscopy and, therefore, can serve as a good method of selecting patients for staging laparoscopy. The yield of laparoscopy in identifying unresectable disease was 9% for T1, whereas the yield for T2 or T3 tumors was 36% (14). Consequently, we advocate diagnostic laparoscopy in advanced T-stage tumors to avoid unnecessary laparotomy.

The radiologic workup for hilar cholangiocarcinoma is variable depending on institutional biases and expertise. Direct cholangiography is frequently used and advocated by many, including the authors. Although the majority of our patients come to us having had a direct cholangiography, we do not have a policy of deliberate intubation of the bile ducts for relief of jaundice or for diagnostic purposes. We advocate ultrasound and magnetic resonance cholangiography, which in our experience provides excellent preoperative imaging and avoids invasive procedures, which may increase the risk of perioperative infectious complications (4,15,16). The role of endoscopic ultrasonography and fine-needle aspiration is discussed by the authors. This approach has been only minimally studied, and we do not favor

Table 57C.1

Proposed Preoperative T Stages for Patients with Hilar Cholangiocarcinoma

Stage	Description
T1	Tumor involving the biliary confluence with or without unilateral extension to second-order biliary radicles
T2	Tumor involving the biliary confluence with or without unilateral extension to second-order biliary radicles **and** *ipsilateral* portal vein involvement with or without *ipsilateral* hepatic lobe atrophy
T3	Tumor involving the biliary confluence with bilateral extension to second-order biliary radicles; **or** unilateral extension to second-order biliary radicles with *contralateral* hepatic lobar atrophy; **or** main or bilateral portal venous involvement.

From Jarnagin WR, Fong Y, DeMatteo RP, et al. Staging, resectability, and outcome in 225 patients with hilar cholangiocarcinoma. *Ann Surg.* 2001;234:507–519.

preoperative biopsy in a patient who is potentially resectable because a negative result does not rule out a malignancy.

Staging hilar cholangiocarcinoma in a clinically relevant manner is difficult. The American Joint Committee on Cancer TNM system presented by the authors is limited it in its clinical utility. Because series on resected hilar cholangiocarcinoma are relatively small, prognostic factors are not that well documented. For example, nodal metastases are not uniformly predictive of outcome but are a major part of the American Joint Committee on Cancer staging system. We use the T-staging system proposed here to help predict resectability and outcome. Although not specifically addressed in any staging system, almost all series report that a margin-negative resection and concomitant hepatic resection are the two most important factors that determine outcome. Because the biliary confluence is intimately associated with the liver, it is mandatory to perform a liver resection to obtain a negative margin in nearly all cases, and this is well documented in the literature. Therefore, the most important issues in predicting outcome in hilar cholangiocarcinoma are ruling out distant metastases and obtaining a margin-negative resection, which almost universally requires a partial hepatectomy.

The authors review the principles of resection. Although a discussion of local resection of the bile duct is common in most publications on this subject, this is rarely possible except for the small midbile duct tumor that does not involve any liver parenchyma. As previously discussed, a resection for a true hilar cholangiocarcinoma mandates a liver resection on the involved side in almost all cases. This dramatically increases the margin negativity rate and therefore improves outcome. An en bloc resection of the caudate lobe is generally advocated for central hilar tumors and tumors involving the left hepatic duct because small branches from these areas of the bile duct drain directly from the caudate lobe, and complete resection is less likely without a caudate resection.

Orthotopic liver transplantation has been advocated as an 'ideal' treatment for hilar cholangiocarcinoma, and the authors review recent results from the Mayo Clinic (17). At initial glance, transplantation is an appealing treatment modality but its use is severely limited by a number of issues. The results from the Mayo Clinic represent extreme selection bias as patients require a laparotomy to rule out nodal metastases and then must survive without metastases the waiting time for a transplant. The true denominator of patients is not well known and these results must be interpreted cautiously. Of course, there is a severe shortage of organs, which significantly hampers the use of transplant for this disease. Lastly, many centers have reported significant rates of morbidity and mortality that are higher than other indications for transplant (18). Nonetheless, the use of transplantation should continue to be studied on well-designed research protocols.

Most patients with hilar cholangiocarcinoma are unresectable, and the biggest clinical challenge with these patients is managing their obstructive jaundice. The problem in managing biliary obstruction in patients with unresectable disease is that the obstruction often extends to segmental branches, and therefore one or two stents often will not adequately drain the liver. Unfortunately, any intubation of the biliary tree contaminates the whole biliary system, and contamination in an undrained segment of the liver can result in segmental cholangitis, which can be life-threatening and miserable for a patient with an incurable malignancy. These patients should be managed by experienced hepatobiliary surgeons and interventional radiologists. The goals of drainage should be clearly outlined and a careful review of good cross-sectional imaging should be performed. Goals of drainage include relief of infection, relief of itching, or to decrease serum bilirubin such that chemotherapy can be administered. These goals are extremely important because itching can be relieved with incomplete drainage, whereas complete relief of jaundice or improvement in quality of life may not occur (19).

Overall, hilar cholangiocarcinoma is an extremely challenging disease to manage, but great strides have been made. Imaging has improved our ability to better categorize patients. Interventional radiologic procedures have enhanced our ability to treat complex biliary obstruction. Improved surgical techniques have increased the number of patients who can undergo a margin-negative, potentially curative resection. Despite these improvements, we have a long way to go in developing more effective adjuvant regimens and providing better palliative therapies.

REFERENCES

1. Zatonski WA, Lowenfels AB, Boyle P, et al. Epidemiologic aspects of gallbladder cancer: a case control study of the SEARCH Program of the International Agency for Research on Cancer. *J Natl Cancer Inst.* 1997;89:1132–1138.
2. Lowenfelds AB, Walker AM, Althaus DP, et al. Gallstone growth, size, and risk of gallbladder cancer: an interracial study. *Int J Epidemiol.* 1989;18:50–54.
3. Stephen AE, Berger DL. Carcinoma in the porcelain gallbladder: a relationship revisited. *Surgery.* 2001;129:699–703.

4. Schwartz LH, Coakley FV, Sun Y, et al. Neoplastic pancreatico-biliary duct obstruction: evaluation with breath-hold MR Cholangiopancreatography. *AJR Am J Roentgenol.* 1998;170:1491–1495.

5. Hawkins WG, DeMatteo RP, Jarnagin WR, et al. Jaundice predicts advanced disease and early mortality in patients with gallbladder cancer. *Ann Surg Oncol.* 2004;11:310–315.

6. D'Angelica M, Fong Y, Weber S, et al. The role of staging laparoscopy in hepatobiliary malignancy: prospective analysis of 401 cases. *Ann Surg Oncol.* 2003;10:183–189.

7. Wagholikar GD, Behari A, Krishnani N, et al. Early gallbladder cancer. *J Am Coll Surg.* 2002;194:137–141.

8. Shoup M, Fong Y. Surgical indications and extent of resection in gallbladder cancer. *Surg Oncol Clin North Am.* 2002;11:985–994.

9. Takada T, Amano H, Yasuda H, et al. Study Group of Surgical Adjuvant Therapy for Carcinomas of the Pancreas and Biliary Tract. Is postoperative adjuvant chemotherapy useful for gallbladder carcinoma? A phase III multicenter prospective randomized controlled trial in patients with resected pancreaticobiliary carcinoma. *Cancer.* 2002;95(8):1685–1695.

10. Jarnagin WR, Ruo L, Little SA, et al. Patterns of initial disease recurrence after resection of gallbladder carcinoma and hilar cholangiocarcinoma: implications for adjuvant therapeutic strategies. *Cancer.* 2003;98(8):1689–1700.

11. Jarnagin WR, Bowne W, Klimstra DS, et al. Papillary phenotype confers improved survival after resection of hilar cholangiocarcinoma. *Ann Surg.* 2005;241:703–714.

12. Klatskin G. Adenocarcinoma of the hepatic duct at its bifurcation within the porta hepatis. An unusual tumor with distinctive clinical and pathological features. *Am J Med.* 1965;38:241–256.

13. Jarnagin WR, Fong Y, DeMatteo RP, et al. Staging, resectability, and outcome in 225 patients with hilar cholangiocarcinoma. *Ann Surg.* 2001;234:507–519.

14. Weber SM, DeMatteo RP, Fong Y, et al. Staging laparoscopy in patients with extrahepatic biliary carcinoma. Analysis of 100 patients. *Ann Surg.* 2002;235:392–399.

15. Hochwald SN, Burke EC, Jarnagin WR, et al. Association of preoperative biliary stenting with increased postoperative infectious complications in proximal cholangiocarcinoma. *Arch Surg.* 1999;134:261–266.

16. Hann LE, Fong Y, Shriver CD, et al. Malignant hepatic hilar tumors: can ultrasonography be used as an alternative to angiography with CT arterial portography for determination of resectability? *J Ultrasound Med.* 1996;15:37–45.

17. Rea DJ, Heimbach JK, Rosen CB, et al. Liver transplantation with neoadjuvant chemoradiation is more effective than resection for hilar cholangiocarcinoma. *Ann Surg.* 2005;242:451–461.

18. Nagorney DM, Kendrick ML. Hepatic resection in the treatment of hilar cholangiocarcinoma. *Adv Surg.* 2006;40:159–171.

19. Robson PM, Heffernan N, Holmes R, et al. Effect of Percutaneous biliary drainage (PBD) for malignant biliary obstruction (MBO) on quality of life (QOL). In: Proceedings from the American Society of Clinical Oncology; June 1–5, 2007; Chicago, IL. Abstract 9029.

58

Radiologic Intervention in Malignant Biliary Obstruction

Marc L. Friedman

Malignant biliary obstruction accounts for approximately 90% of biliary strictures seen at the time of percutaneous transhepatic cholangiography (1). The most common cause is pancreatic carcinoma, which is the fourth leading cause of cancer death in the United States. Cholangiocarcinoma, gallbladder carcinoma, ampullary carcinoma, lymphoma, hepatoma, and metastases can produce malignant biliary obstruction. It is generally an unfavorable prognostic sign when jaundice appears in patients with malignancy. The pruritus that accompanies the jaundice is miserable for the patient. Surgical intervention for the construction of a biliary-enteric bypass imposes a significant recuperative period on an individual whose life expectancy may be already limited. This chapter will focus on numerous percutaneous techniques that enable the radiologist to not only image, but to biopsy and treat patients with malignant biliary obstruction.

Although the technique of transhepatic cholangiography was originally described by Burckhardt and Muller (2) in 1921, it was not until several decades later that percutaneous biliary intervention gained momentum. The Seldinger arteriographic technique (3) was modified for use in the biliary tract. In 1964, Weichel (4) published his work with biliary catheters that were inserted by a percutaneous transhepatic approach. Decompression of obstructed bile ducts by transhepatically placed catheters was first reported by Molnar and Stockum (5) in 1974. This coincided with the demonstration that modified angiographic catheters could be manipulated through the biliary tree and across obstructing lesions (6). Early reports suggested that preoperative biliary drainage improved hepatic function while diminishing surgical morbidity and mortality (7,8). This has never been substantiated. Furthermore, cancer patient survival is not affected by surgical or nonsurgical biliary drainage (9). Preoperative biliary decompression is currently being performed only in selected patients. Most commonly, this occurs in patients with cholangitis who require medical management prior to elective surgery. Preoperative biliary stenting has recently been described as a prequel to pancreatic resection in selected patients with profound comorbidities associated with jaundice (10). Some surgeons prefer a catheter in the bile duct as a landmark to guide anatomic identification in the porta hepatis, which can be difficult when extensive scarring from previous surgery is present. Following choledochoenterostomy, the transhepatic catheter can be used to stent the anastomosis and allow for postoperative cholangiography. Today, the overwhelming majority of percutaneous biliary drainage procedures are performed for palliative treatment of malignant biliary obstruction. Many investigators have published their work using a variety of catheters and stents, and accompanying techniques for placing them into the biliary tree (11–21). Although percutaneous transhepatic cholangiography and biliary drainage are technically demanding procedures, the low risk/benefit ratio is extremely desirable for the quality of life and sense of well-being of the jaundiced cancer patient.

PREPROCEDURE EVALUATION

Malignant biliary obstruction classically presents with painless jaundice. This can be associated with weight loss, anorexia, acholic stools, dark urine, abnormal liver function tests, and pruritus. The diagnosis is usually suspected before the interventionalist is consulted. Prior to intervention, it is incumbent on the radiologist to review all imaging studies as these may provide anatomic information that might alter the percutaneous approach, convey the potential need for multiple drainage catheters, or even contraindicate the procedure. Demonstration of dilated intrahepatic ducts by cross-sectional imaging techniques including ultrasound, computed tomography, and magnetic resonance imaging confirms bile duct obstruction. These studies often demonstrate the level of the obstruction as evidenced by an abrupt change in duct caliber. In addition, the presence of a mass at the level of obstruction, or ascites in the planned percutaneous access route, is easily delineated.

A large amount of perihepatic ascites is a relative contraindication to percutaneous biliary drainage. Catheters and guidewires tend to buckle in the easily compressible, fluid-filled space between the abdominal wall and liver. This can result in dislodgement during stent placement, especially when catheter advancement across a tight obstruction is attempted. If dislodgement occurs, percutaneous access to a decompressed system can become difficult or impossible. The risk of intraprocedural catheter dislodgement can be lessened by several factors. Preprocedure paracentesis can significantly decrease the size of the perihepatic fluid-filled space. Subxiphoid left hepatic duct approach may be preferred, as there tends to be much less peritoneal fluid collection anterior to the liver.

Puncturing an intrahepatic duct that ultimately limits the degree of tortuosity of the transhepatic catheter course is crucial. In addition, maximum stiffness of the working guidewire and presence of a safety guidewire are recommended. Perihepatic ascites also tends to leak around a transhepatic catheter and can present an annoying clinical problem for the patient as the skin becomes irritated and prone to infection.

Review of the cross-sectional imaging studies is also important for evaluation of hepatic parenchymal disease. The presence of liver masses can alter the planned access route. For example, the risk of secondary infection of liver cysts by a transhepatic catheter and anaphylaxis from puncture of hydatid cysts must be avoided (22). In patients with extensive hepatic metastases, percutaneous biliary drainage may not significantly lower the level of jaundice. In addition, multifocal obstruction with isolation of hepatic segments often requires multiple procedures to place several drainage catheters. This may not be advantageous for a patient with limited life expectancy. Incomplete drainage of the biliary tree can reduce jaundice; however, there is a significant risk of cholangitis in the undrained segments.

Preprocedure laboratory evaluation is essential prior to percutaneous biliary intervention. This includes a complete blood count, coagulation profile, and blood chemistries. Baseline hematocrit allows evaluation of any subsequent bleeding complication.

Although a bleeding diathesis is the only absolute contraindication to percutaneous biliary drainage, coagulation disorders can usually be corrected by the administration of various blood products. If the platelet count is <50,000, platelet transfusions are performed. If the coagulation profile is abnormal, administration of vitamin K, fresh-frozen plasma, or specific blood coagulation products will usually allow the procedure to be performed. Postprocedure metabolic abnormalities can occur, especially when external biliary drainage is fashioned, and therefore baseline electrolyte evaluation is essential. Patients receive intravascular contrast media during needle interrogation of the liver through various hepatic venous and portal venous radicals, especially patients with minimally dilated intrahepatic ducts. Therefore, baseline serum urea nitrogen and creatinine should be documented. Lastly, preprocedure liver function tests provide a reference for chemical monitoring of the postprocedure effects of biliary drainage.

Antibiotic prophylaxis is mandatory during percutaneous transhepatic biliary drainage. There is a relatively high risk of infectious complications from manipulation in the biliary tree secondary to the likelihood of bacterial pathogens in an obstructed system (23). Antibiotics should be initiated <2 hours before the start of the procedure. Most commonly, they are administered by the nurse when the patient arrives in the interventional suite. Various agents have been recommended. Ampicillin/sulbactam (Unasyn) has greater activity against enterococcus and has been described as the most appropriate choice in the setting of biliary obstruction (24).

Third-generation cephalosporins (e.g., ceftriaxone) may be more effective than second-generation cephalosporins because they have enhanced biliary excretion and thus reach higher concentrations in the bile. If a patient is already receiving antibiotics, the timing of the last dose as well as its spectrum of coverage should be assessed. Patients with a documented history of anaphylactic reaction to penicillin should receive vancomycin (Gram-positive prophylaxis) and/or a monobactam such as aztreonam (Gram-negative prophylaxis). Single-dose

therapy is usually sufficient assuming that successful drainage is accomplished.

The patient is carefully informed of the methods and expectations from percutaneous biliary drainage. The risks, benefits, and therapeutic alternatives are discussed. The principle risks include bleeding, infection (e.g., peritonitis and septicemia), possible need for emergency surgery or intervention (e.g., transcatheter embolotherapy for significant hemobilia), and possible loss of life (22). The patient must understand the potential need for multiple procedures and possible requirement for an externally draining catheter. This is associated with transhepatic catheter-related pain, which often requires intravenous or intramuscular analgesia following the procedure. If drainage is not internalized, transhepatic catheter-related pain diminishes daily and usually resolves within 7 to 10 days.

Intravenous sedation and analgesia are important factors in accomplishing successful percutaneous biliary drainage as percutaneous access, tract dilation, and manipulation within the biliary system can be extremely painful for the patient. It is not possible for the interventional radiologist to administer medication and monitor conscious sedation while concurrently performing percutaneous transhepatic biliary drainage. Therefore, it is essential that an anesthesiologist or trained interventional nurse specialist be present. The vital signs, electrocardiogram, and pulse oximetry are routinely monitored. We usually administer a benzodiazepine and an opiate derivative. Midazolam produces amnesia, anxiolysis, and sedation. Fentanyl provides analgesia while blunting the autonomic response to painful stimulation. If an anesthesiologist is present, the patient is usually administered a continuous infusion of propofol. This short-acting sedative/hypnotic demonstrates modest respiratory effects if doses are kept low. It has a much shorter recovery time than benzodiazepines or barbiturates and has a low incidence of postprocedure nausea and vomiting. Thoracic paravertebral block (25), celiac plexus block (26), and pleural block (27) have been used to accomplish analgesia for deep visceral pain sensation transmitted from the liver. Ultimately, the choice depends on the condition of the patient and the experience of the interventionalist.

TECHNIQUE

Percutaneous transhepatic biliary drainage is initiated by opacifying the intrahepatic ducts using a fine needle (21 gauge). The interventionalist must decide whether a right-sided or left-sided approach to the biliary tree is appropriate. When the obstruction involves the extrahepatic duct, a branch of the right hepatic duct is usually chosen as the entry site (Figure 58.1). If the obstruction is in the porta hepatis, as with cholangiocarcinoma involving the junction of right and left hepatic ducts or metastatic disease to the liver hilum, multiple duct stenoses are more likely to occur on the right (28). Consequently, left hepatic duct drainage is preferred as one catheter is more likely to drain a larger percentage of the biliary tree. The left lobe must not be atrophic or in a high position under the costal margin, which can make duct puncture from a subxiphoid approach technically difficult. Ultrasound guidance allows puncture of the segment II or III duct (Figure 58.2), which is preferred because of the extrahepatic position

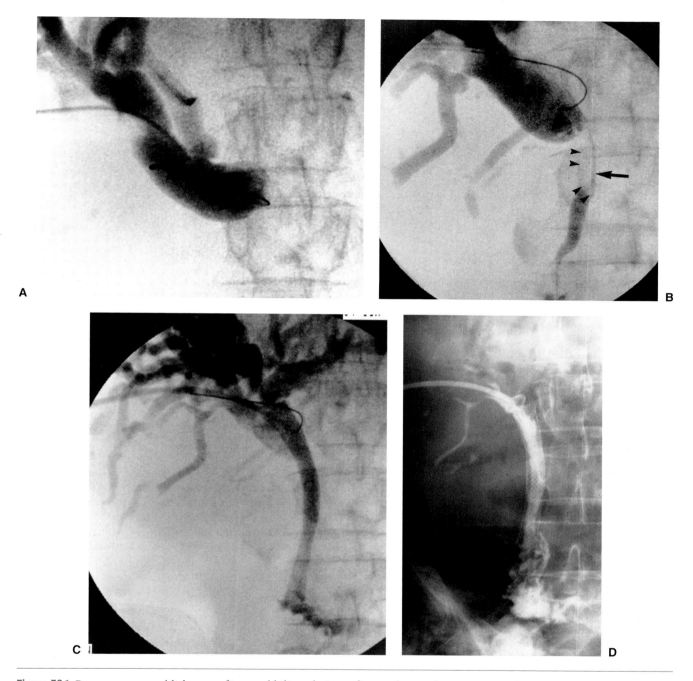

Figure 58.1 Percutaneous establishment of internal biliary drainage from right transhepatic approach. (**A**) Malignant-appearing obstruction of common bile duct (CBD). (**B**) Catheter (*arrow*) opacifies normal distal CBD beyond intraluminal mass (*arrowheads*). (**C**) Metallic endoprosthesis extends from proximal common hepatic duct into duodenum. (**D**) Follow-up cholangiogram confirms patent endoprosthesis with decompressed intrahepatic bile ducts. External drain was removed.

of the left hepatic duct medial to the falciform ligament. Extrahepatic duct puncture increases the risk of bile leakage (29). The segment III duct is positioned more anteriorly and inferiorly than the segment II duct and is usually more approachable with ultrasound guidance from the subxiphoid approach. In addition, ultrasound guidance will help avoid inadvertent puncture of the lung, stomach, and transverse colon. The subcostal location of an anterior left hepatic duct catheter is often better tolerated by

the patient than the intercostal position of a lateral right hepatic duct catheter. The left-sided approach can be more technically demanding because of the tendency of the fluoroscopic field to include the hands of the interventionalist.

The right-sided approach is more commonly used. The puncture site is selected at an intercostal space caudal to the costophrenic angle but cephalad to the colon. Although a more cephalic entry point is desirable as this typically allows a less

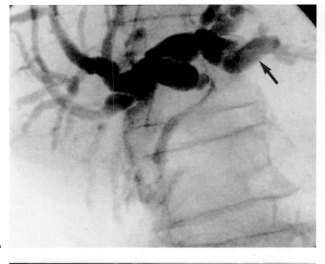

A

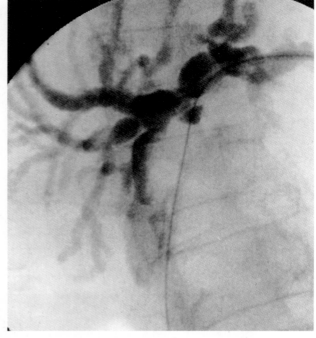

B

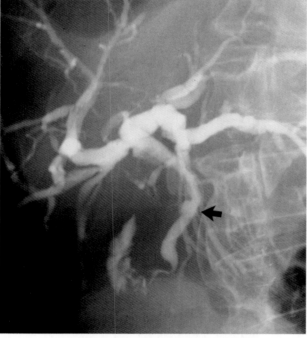

C

Figure 58.2 Percutaneous establishment of internal biliary drainage from left transhepatic approach. Computed tomography scan suggested proximal common hepatic duct obstruction. (**A**) Needle puncture of segment III duct (*long arrow*). Note the incomplete obstruction and marked deviation of common bile duct course by metastatic gastric cancer. (**B**) Stiff guidewire advanced across obstruction and into duodenum. (**C**) Metallic endoprosthesis is positioned in common duct so that distal end (*short arrow*) is just below the level of obstruction. Sphincter function is preserved.

angled path to the extrahepatic duct, the risk of pleural transgression increases with a more cephalic entry. A midaxillary or slightly anterior to midaxillary entry point typically in the tenth intercostal space tends to avoid the posteriorly deepening pleural space. Under fluoroscopic guidance, the needle is generally aimed toward the upper 12th vertebral body along a coronal plane that is typically parallel to the table top. Needle excursion stops approximately 2 cm from the lateral spinal margin. The needle is then slowly withdrawn while small dilute contrast pulses are administered under fluoroscopy. Entry into a bile duct is recognized by slow flow away from the needle tip within a tubular structure. Hepatic vein and portal vein opacification is recognized by faster tubular flow with washout directed toward the right atrium and liver periphery respectively. Periportal lymphatic opacification appears as a delicate network of tubular channels extending toward the porta hepatis. Once a bile duct

is entered, opacification of the biliary tree is accomplished and multiple spot films are obtained. A tilting table is advantageous in this regard as it allows dependent maneuvering of the contrast material to define the level of obstruction. Attempts are made to limit the amount of ductal distention with contrast material. This lessens the risk of septicemia caused by manipulation within the infected biliary tree.

The suitability of the initially punctured duct for establishment of percutaneous drainage depends on several factors. A peripheral rather than central duct entry is preferred as this reduces the risk of venous or arterial injury and subsequent hemobilia. Peripheral puncture also provides more room for drainage catheter side holes above an obstruction. Maximizing a straight line course from the skin to the level of obstruction facilitates subsequent manipulation, including crossing the obstruction and placing a stent. If the entered bile duct is suboptimal,

C-arm fluoroscopic guidance is used to directly puncture a suitable duct using a second 21-gauge needle.

Once a suitable duct has been entered, a 0.018-inch guidewire with a steerable radio-opaque tip is advanced through the fine needle into the biliary tree. A coaxially tapered dilator/stiffening cannula/sheath assembly is then directed over the guidewire into the biliary tree. The dilator/stiffening cannula is removed, leaving a working sheath and 0.018-inch safety guidewire. Following advancement of a standard 0.035-inch working guidewire into the bile duct, the tract is dilated and one of several options is pursued.

If the patient is unstable or there is evidence of grossly purulent bile or clinical septicemia, simple external drainage is established by leaving a catheter positioned proximal to the obstruction and connecting the external hub to a bile drainage bag. A Cope loop-design (30) anchoring mechanism is recommended to prevent catheter withdrawal, which may occur as a result of normal respiratory motion. The external portion of the drainage catheter is fixed to the skin by an adhesive device or suture. Further percutaneous manipulation is delayed until the patient's condition stabilizes.

In most patients with an apparently complete obstruction, a torquing guidewire and catheter can usually be negotiated through the narrowed ductal lumen into the distal common bile duct and duodenum. If the narrowed lumen cannot be traversed initially, a repeat attempt after 2 or 3 days of biliary drainage is almost always successful as the edema that is associated with high-grade obstruction resolves.

TRANSCATHETER BILIARY BIOPSY

Although the cholangiographic appearance of a malignant biliary obstruction is characteristic (e.g., abruptly tapered, shouldered, irregular, rounded), morphologic distinction between malignant and benign disease is not entirely reliable. If a malignant etiology has not been established, several transcatheter biopsy methods are available once a stable guidewire has been advanced into duodenum. Simple bile aspiration has a low sensitivity (34%) (31). Brush biopsy can be performed by advancing a 9F peel-away sheath just beyond the obstruction (Figure 58.3). The sheath dilator is removed and a cytologic biopsy brush is then advanced to the level of the obstruction. The tip of the sheath is withdrawn so that the brush is uncovered at the level of obstruction and brush biopsy is performed by moving the brush across the stricture multiple times. The brush is then removed from the sheath and cut from the remainder of the instrument. It is placed in saline and sent for cytologic examination. Cytologic brush biopsy is a useful method to establish a diagnosis of malignant biliary stenosis with 75% sensitivity, but the negative predictive value is not satisfied (32). The procedure is typically repeated 3 times as it has been shown that the probability of having bile duct carcinoma after three sequential negative cytologic brushings is <6% (33).

Scrape biopsy has also been described in which the biopsy instrument is a dilator into which 4 to 6 flaps are fashioned with an 11-scalpel blade. This is positioned through a sheath in collapsed form at the level of the obstruction. The sheath is withdrawn to expose the flaps and a back-and-forth motion collects the specimen. A sensitivity of 60% and a false-negative rate of 13% have been demonstrated with this technique (34).

Transcatheter needle biopsy can also be performed through a guiding sheath with the needle tip positioned using C-arm fluoroscopy (35). This technique is limited by the rigid nature of the needle and the often tortuous course of the transhepatic tract. However, this technique can produce histologic core specimens using a variety of automated biopsy devices (36). Transcatheter tissue biopsy specimens can also be obtained with an atherectomy device (37) and a flexible biopsy forceps (38).

RADIOTHERAPEUTIC APPLICATIONS

Once unresectable malignant bile duct obstruction has been confirmed and transhepatic internal/external drainage has been established, palliative internal radiotherapy using iridium-192 or another source can be instituted (39–44). The iridium wire is placed into the transhepatic catheter using a modified angiographic guidewire.

The length of active iridium wire is positioned directly at the level of the tumor under fluoroscopic control and fixed at the catheter hub. A high radiotherapeutic dose can be delivered directly to the tumor bed while limiting radiation damage to surrounding organs. Intraluminal high-dose rate brachytherapy with metallic stenting leads to an improved quality of life in patients with obstructive jaundice from extrahepatic bile duct carcinoma (44). Depending on the isodose distribution, the radionuclide source may be used as the only source of radiation or may be supplemented by external-beam therapy.

BILIARY ENDOPROSTHESIS PLACEMENT

Endoprosthesis placement for biliary drainage was introduced by Pereiras et al. (45) in 1978 when they described a method to place a completely detached internal tube. Over the years, several different designs or plastic and metallic stents have been developed that are intended to ensure antegrade bile flow without the disadvantages of external drainage. These include the need for regular catheter flushing and dressing, possible bile and peritoneal fluid leakage, infection and pain at the catheter entry site, and the psychological problems associated with an external drainage tube. The patient's emotional attachment to the catheter and the catheter's significance as a reminder of impending death tend to diminish the patient's quality of life. Occlusion or migration of an indwelling endoprosthesis is its major disadvantage because a repeat percutaneous and/or endoscopic procedure to re-establish drainage is required.

Biliary endoprostheses were initially constructed of plastic. These stents were prone to migration and premature occlusion (46). Plastic tubes typically occlude with debris, which may be triggered by bacterial adherence to the tube surface. This is followed by the deposition of glycoproteins, deconjugation of bilirubin, and deposition of calcium bilirubinate crystals.

Attempts to prolong plastic stent patency with chronic antibiotic therapy, ursodeoxycholic acid, change in type of polymer used, or coating the inner lining used with a variety of agents to preclude bacterial colonization have proven unsuccessful. As a result, the development of metallic biliary stents gained

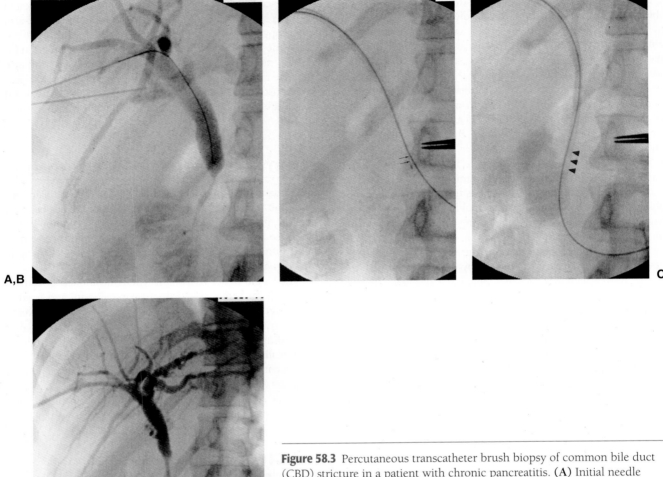

Figure 58.3 Percutaneous transcatheter brush biopsy of common bile duct (CBD) stricture in a patient with chronic pancreatitis. **(A)** Initial needle puncture of caudal branch of right hepatic duct is suboptimal for transhepatic drainage. A more suitable duct entry is accomplished. Distal CBD stricture is demonstrated. **(B)** Following placement of a stiff guidewire into duodenum, a 9F sheath (*arrowheads*) is situated across the stricture. **(C)** Once the brush (*arrows*) is in position, the sheath is withdrawn and brush biopsy is completed. Three specimens demonstrated no malignant cells. **(D)** Internal/external drainage is established. Subsequent biliary-enteric bypass was performed. No tumor was found.

momentum and metallic biliary endoprostheses became widely available in the late 1980s. These self-expandable or balloon expandable stents are delivered through small-caliber sheaths (6F to 7F) and attain internal diameters up to 12 mm. The small introducer allows placement of the endoprostheses during the initial percutaneous intervention. Typically, an external biliary drainage catheter is left in place overnight. On the following day, if cholangiography confirms satisfactory stent position, distal antegrade flow and absence of significant clot or debris above the endoprosthesis, the external catheter is removed (Figures 58.1 and 58.2). Unfortunately, metallic endoprostheses tend to develop ingrowth or marginal overgrowth of tumor and or granulation tissue, which ultimately lead to occlusion.

Although it is difficult to determine long-term patency rates in patients with median survival of 6 months (47), the small number of randomized, prospective, comparative studies have

confirmed that metallic stents are associated with fewer complications and probably have a lower rate of occlusion than their plastic counterparts 48–52). Although metallic stents are significantly more expensive, cost-effectiveness analyses have shown that the cost of treatment of each patient was lower when Wallstents were used because of the lower rate of reintervention (49,50). Covered metallic stents (Schneider Stent, a division of Pfizer, Inc., Minneapolis, MN) represent an evolution of noncovered types, and are intended to prevent obstruction caused by tumor ingrowth within the stent lumen (53). The use of covered biliary stents is becoming common clinical practice in the management of malignant biliary obstruction in some centers. The use of partially or fully polyurethane-covered Wallstents, polyurethane-covered nitinol stents, and expanded polytetrafluoroethylene/fluorinated ethylene propylene-covered nitinol stents have been described in several series (54), but

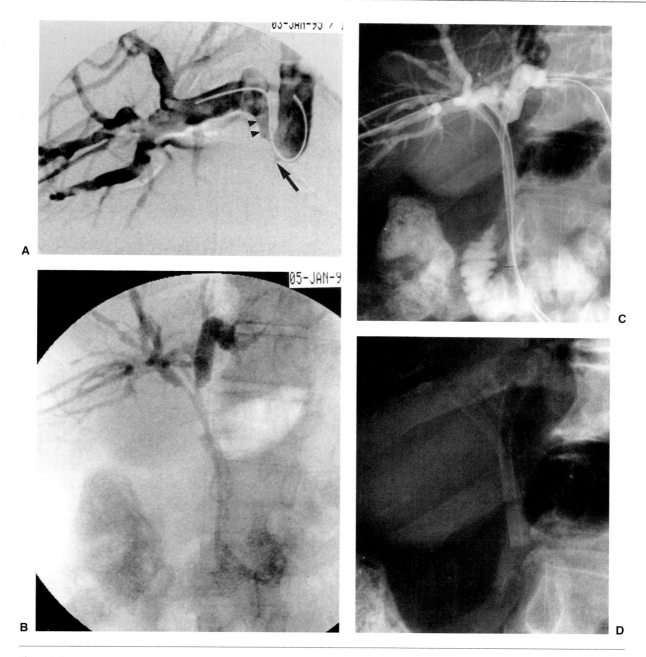

Figure 58.4 Percutaneous internal biliary drainage in a patient with hilar cholangiocarcinoma. (A) Initial transhepatic cholangiogram demonstrates malignant obstruction at confluence of left hepatic duct (*arrow*) and posterior sector right hepatic duct (*arrowheads*). Anterior sector right hepatic duct is not opacified. (B) Following needle puncture of isolated anterior sector duct, complete internal/external drainage is established with two catheters. However, left hepatic duct obstruction appears imminent. (C) Left hepatic direct drainage is accomplished from subxiphoid approach. Three metallic endoprostheses are placed and appear widely patent. (D) Plain-film appearance of endoprostheses. The patient died 8 months later with no evidence of recurrent biliary obstruction.

no randomized prospective comparison evaluating patency and complications of covered stents versus bare stents in malignant biliary obstruction is available.

Endoscopic placement of an endoprosthesis remains a compelling alternative to percutaneous biliary drainage in many patients. Advantages include direct visualization of the periampullary region, controlled sphincterotomy, and biopsy of dis-

tal lesions. These procedures tend to be well tolerated by the patient and require only a brief period of recuperation. Patients with ascites are also better suited for endoscopic placement because of the tendency for peritoneal fluid to leak externally around the transhepatic catheter.

Endoscopic stenting of hilar lesions is less successful as it is often difficult for the endoscopist to direct the endoprosthesis

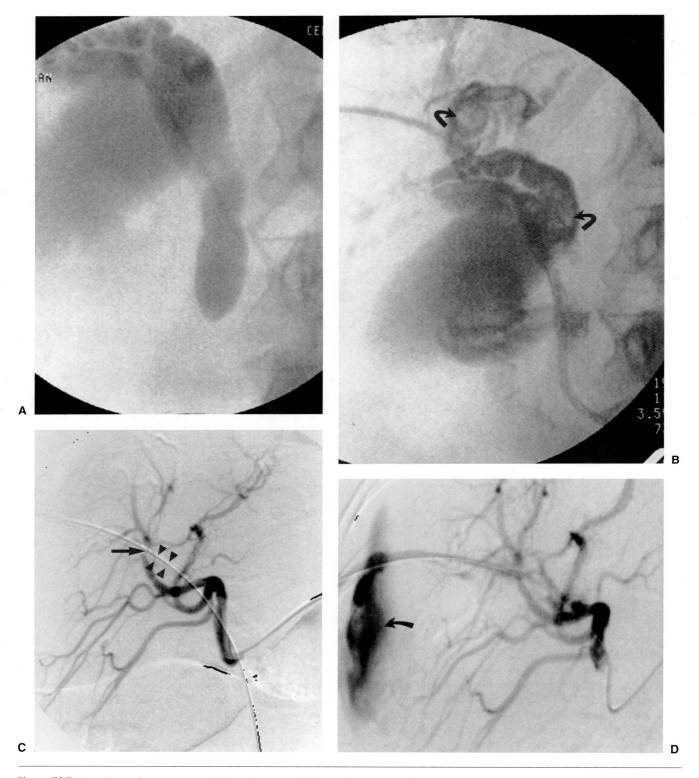

Figure 58.5 Complicated percutaneous biliary drainage. (**A**) Distal common bile duct (CBD) obstruction secondary to pancreatic cancer. (**B**) Thrombus caste (*hooked arrows*) seen in CBD and intrahepatic ducts. Brisk pulsatile bleeding was noted from the tract during catheter exchanges. (**C**) Right hepatic arteriogram demonstrates focal narrowing of artery (*closed arrow*) at the crossing of transhepatic catheter tract. The introducer sheath (*arrowheads*) tamponades the bleeding. (**D**) Repeat arteriogram following sheath removal confirms arterial-biliary fistula with blood collecting on patient's skin (*curved arrow*). (*continued*)

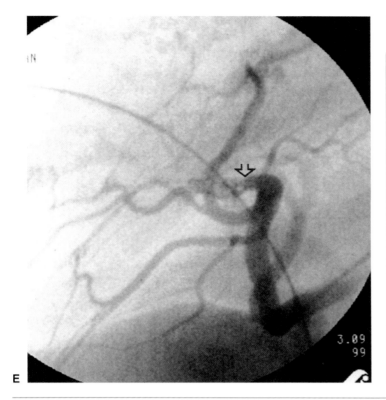
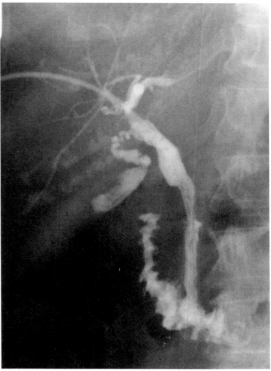

Figure 58.5 *(continued)* **(E)** Successful embolic occlusion *(open arrow)* of right hepatic artery branch with no further extravasation seen. **(F)** Follow-up cholangiogram demonstrates widely patent endoprosthesis and decompressed ducts. External drain was removed uneventfully.

into a particular hepatic lobe or segment. Therefore, hilar lesions are best managed by the interventional radiologist who can use one or more access routes to gain maximum drainage of the biliary tree (Figure 58.4). In addition, patients who have had prior gastroenteric reconstruction are better suited for percutaneous manipulation because of altered retrograde access to the chole-dochoenteric junction. The advantages of percutaneous and endoscopic approaches can be combined in a rendezvous procedure in which a long guidewire is manipulated transhepatically through a 3F catheter well into the Roux limb of the hepaticoje-junostomy. The wire is then snared by the endoscopist and used to guide retrograde cannulation and stenting of the bile duct. Once drainage is accomplished, the small-caliber transhepatic catheter can be removed. The decision on which drainage technique to use ultimately may be determined by the availability of the physician with the appropriate skills.

COMPLICATIONS

Major complications of percutaneous biliary drainage include hemorrhage, septic shock, and death. Literature review indicates the incidence of major complications is 4.6% to 25%, and the incidence of procedure-related deaths is 0% to 5.6% (55). With careful technique, major complications are infrequent but unavoidable, especially when considering the often debilitated condition of the patient with malignant biliary obstruction. Fever and chills may occur in 5% to 26% of patients undergoing bil-

iary drainage. If frank septicemia is apparent (e.g., fever spike, chills, tachycardia), fluid administration and antibiotic therapy are initiated. Simple establishment of external biliary drainage is expedited and further manipulation is avoided.

Hemobilia occurs in 2.6% to 9.6% of cases (55). Bleeding is the most common cause of serious morbidity but it is rarely a cause of death. Venous bleeding into the bile ducts occurs frequently during the procedure but is of no consequence if clotting function is adequate. On follow-up cholangiography, clotted blood usually clears completely within 24 to 48 hours. It is important to make sure that catheter side holes have not migrated into the intraparenchymal tract where they can communicate with hepatic or portal veins. Advancement of the catheter side holes into the biliary tree should resolve the hemobilia. Occasionally, upsizing the catheter to tamponade the bleeding is necessary. With biliary-cutaneous tract maturation, venous bleeding typically resolves.

Arterial bleeding is much more serious. A thrombus caste of the biliary tree associated with poor drainage of sanguinous bile is usually noted at the initial procedure. If pulsatile, bright red blood emanates from the transhepatic tract especially during catheter exchanges, arterial injury should be suspected. This typically occurs from a traumatic hepatic artery pseudoaneurysm with an arterial biliary fistula (Figure 58.5). This can be successfully treated with arterial embolization techniques (51). A hepatic arteriogram performed while the transhepatic biliary drainage catheter has been withdrawn over a guidewire will usually delineate the bleeding source. The hepatic artery branch is then embolized with gel foam (Upjohn, Kalamazoo, MI) or embolic coils. The incidence of arterial trauma can be minimized by avoiding central duct puncture. Patients with cirrhosis, who have an increased arterial blood flow, are at increased risk for arterial injury.

Significant bile leakage occurs rarely. In the case of a transhepatic catheter, this usually occurs because a side hole is positioned within the biliary-cutaneous tract. Bile can accumulate in the subcapsular space, intraperitoneal cavity, or at the skin entrance site. Biliary ascites can occur following acute occlusion or migration of a percutaneously-placed endoprosthesis. Repeat cholangiography should identify the cause of leakage and enable tube repositioning or appropriate placement of a drainage catheter.

Late complications are related to occlusion and migration of the transhepatic catheter or endoprosthesis. Stent occlusion is inevitable; however, its occurrence depends on the length of patient survival. Recurrent obstruction typically presents with cholangitis (e.g., fever, chills), right upper quadrant pain, jaundice, or bile leak around an external drainage tube. If a transhepatic biliary drainage tube occludes, it is easily and safely replaced over a guidewire in the outpatient setting. Recurrent biliary obstruction in a patient with an indwelling endoprosthesis requires a new interventional procedure. If the endoprosthesis protrudes into the duodenum, endoscopic replacement is recommended as this procedure is better tolerated by the patient. Occluded plastic stents are typically removed and replaced with a new endoprosthesis. If a metallic stent has occluded, a second endoprosthesis is placed that overlaps the first and restores antegrade bile flow into the duodenum. If the occluded endoprosthesis does not extend into the duodenum, or if the site of obstruction is at the level of the liver hilum, repeat percutaneous intervention is recommended.

CONCLUSION

Percutaneous biliary drainage remains an important method of nonsurgical palliation in malignant biliary obstruction. The technique allows relief of cholestasis and its clinical sequela, with low risk for the patient.

REFERENCES

1. Soulen MC. Treatment of biliary strictures. In: LaBerge JM, Venbrux AC, eds. *Biliary Interventions*. Fairfax, VA: SCVIR; 1995;221–232.
2. Burckhardt H, Muller W. Versuche uber die Punktion der Gallenblase und ihre Rontgendarstellung. *Deutsche Zeitschrift fur Chirurgie*. 1921;162:168–197.
3. Seldinger SI. Catheter replacement of needle in percutaneous arteriography: New technique. *Acta Radiol (Stockh)*. 1953;39:368–376.
4. Weichel KL. Percutaneous transhepatic cholangiography: technique and application with studies of hepatic venous and biliary duct pressures, the chemical blood and bile and clinical results in a series of jaundiced patients. *Acta Chir Scand*. 1964, vol 130, suppl 300, 1–99.
5. Molnar W, Stockum AE. Relief of obstructive jaundice through percutaneous transhepatic catheter: a new therapeutic method. *Am J Roentgenol Radium Ther Nucl Med*. 1974;122:356–367.
6. Ring EJ, Oleaga JA, Freiman DB, et al. Therapeutic applications of catheter cholangiography. *Radiology*. 1978;128:333–338.
7. Denning DA, Ellison EG, Carey BC. Preoperative percutaneous transhepatic biliary decompression lowers morbidity in patients with obstructive jaundice. *Am J Surg*. 1981;14:61–65.
8. Gobien RP, Stanley JM, Soucek CD, et al. Routine preoperative biliary drainage: Effect on management of obstructive jaundice. *Radiology*. 1984;152:353–356.
9. Bonnell D, Ferucci JT, Mueller PR, et al. Surgical and radiological decompression in malignant biliary obstruction: a retrospective study using multivariated risk factor analysis. *Radiology*. 1984;152:347–351.
10. Anderson F, Clarke DL, Thomson SR. Pre-operative biliary stenting: a prequel to pancreatic resection selected patients. *S Afr J Surg*. 2004;42:128–130.
11. Ishikawa Y, Oishi I, Miyai M, et al. Percutaneous transhepatic drainage; experience in 100 cases. *J Clin Gastrenterol*. 1980;2:305–314.
12. Berquist TH, May GR, Johnson CM, et al. Percutaneous biliary decompression: internal and external drainage in 50 patients. *AJR Am J Roentgenol*. 1981;136:901–906.
13. Mueller PR, vanSonnenberg E, Ferrucci JT, Percutaneous biliary drainage: technical and catheter related problems in 200 procedures. *AJR Am J Roentgenol*. 1982;138:17–23.
14. Carrasco CH, Zounoza J, Bechtel WJ. Malignant biliary obstruction; complications of percutaneous biliary drainage. *Radiology*. 1984;152:343–346.
15. Hamlin JA, Friedman M, Stein MG, et al. Percutaneous biliary drainage: complications of 118 consecutive catheterizations. *Radiology*. 1986;158:199–202.
16. Lammer J, Neumayer K. Biliary drainage endoprostheses: experience with 201 placements. *Radiology*. 1986;159:625–629.
17. Dick BW, Gordon RL, La Berge JM. Percutaneous transhepatic placement of biliary endoprostheses: results in 100 consecutive patients. *J Vasc Interv Radiol*. 1990;1:97–100.
18. Gordon RL, Ring EJ, La Berge JM. Malignant biliary obstruction: treatment with expandable metallic stents-follow-up of 50 consecutive patients. *Radiology*. 1992;182:697–701.
19. Lameris JS, Stoker J, Nijs HGT. Malignant biliary obstruction: percutaneous use of self-expandable stents. *Radiology*. 1991;179:702–707.
20. Becker CD, Giatti A, Malbach R. Percutaneous palliative of malignant obstructive jaundice with the Wallstent endoprostheses: follow-up and re-intervention in patients with hilar and non-hilar obstructions. *J Vasc Interv Radiol*. 1993;4:597–604.
21. Rossi P, Bezzi M, Soni M. Metallic stents in malignant biliary obstruction: results of a multicenter European study of 240 patients. *J Vasc Interv Radiol*. 1994;5:279–285.
22. Venbrux AC, Osterman FC. Percutaneous transhepatic cholangiography and percutaneous biliary drainage: step by step. In: LaBerge JM, Venbrux AC, eds. *Biliary Interventions*. Fairfax, VA: Society of Cardiovascular and Interventional Radiology; 1995;129–150.
23. Yee AC, Ho C-S. Complications of percutaneous drainage: benign versus malignant diseases. *AJR Am J Roentgenol*. 1987;148:1207–1209.
24. Ryan JM, Ryan BM, Smith TP. Antibiotic prophylaxis in interventional radiology. *J Vasc Interv Radiol*. 2004;15:547–556.
25. Culp WC Jr., Culp WC. Thoracic paravertebral block for percutaneous transhepatic biliary drainage. *J Vasc Interv Radiol*. 2005;16:1397–1400.
26. Savader SJ, Bourke DL, Venbrux AC, et al. Randomized double-blinded clinical trial of celiac plexus block for percutaneous biliary drainage. *J Vasc Interv Radiol*. 1993;4:539–542.

27. Rosenblatt M. Robalino J, Bergman A, et al. Pleural block: technique for regional anesthesia during percutaneous hepatobiliary drainage. *Radiology.* 1989;172:279–280.

28. Mueller PR, Ferrucci JT, van Sonnenberg E, et al. Obstruction of the left hepatic duct: diagnosis and treatment by selective fine-needle cholangiography and percutaneous biliary drainage. *Radiology.* 1982;145:297–302.

29. Russell E, Yrizzary JM, Montalvo BM, et al. Left hepatic duct anatomy: implications. *Radiology.* 1990;174:353–356.

30. Cope C. Improved anchoring of nephrostomy catheters: loop technique. *AJR Am J Roentgenol.* 1980;135–402.

31. Muro A, Mueller PR, Ferrucci JT, et al. Bile cytology: a routine addition to percutaneous biliary drainage. *Radiology.* 1983;149:846–847.

32. Xing GD, Geng JC, Han XW. Endobiliary brush cytology during percutaneous transhepatic cholangiodrainage in patients with obstructive jaundice. *Hepatobiliary Pancreat Dis Int.* 2005;4:98–103.

33. Rabinovitz M, Zajko AB, Hassanein T, et al. Diagnostic value of brush cytology in the diagnosis of bile duct carcinoma: a study in 60 patients with bile duct strictures. *Hepatology.* 1990;12:747–752.

34. Yip CKY, Leung JWC, Chang MKM, et al. Scrape biopsy of malignant biliary structure through percutaneous transhepatic biliary drainage tracts. *AJR Am J Roentgenol.* 1989;152:529–530.

35. Cope C, Marinelli DL, Weinstein JK. Transcatheter biopsy of lesions obstructing the bile ducts. *Radiology.* 1988;169:555–556.

36. Mladinich CR, Ackerman N, Berry CR, et al. Evaluation and comparison of automatic biopsy devices. *Radiology.* 1992;184:845–847.

37. Kim D, Porter DH, Siegel JB, et al. Common bile duct biopsy with the Simpson atherectomy catheter. AJR 1990;154:1213–1215.

38. Terasaki K, Wittich GR, Lycke E. Percutaneous transluminal biopsy of biliary strictures with a bioptome. *AJR Am J Roentgenol.* 1991;156:77–78.

39. Herskovic A, Heaton D, Engler MJ, et al. Irradiation of biliary carcinoma. *Radiology.* 1981;139:219–222.

40. Conroy RM, Shahbazian AA, Edwards KC, et al. A new method for treating carcinomatous biliary obstruction with intracatheter radium. *Cancer.* 1982;49:1312–1327.

41. Karani J, Fletcher M, Brinkley D, et al. Internal biliary drainage and local radiotherapy with iridium-192 wire in treatment of hilar cholangiocarcinoma. *Clin Radiol.* 1985;36:603–606.

42. Haffty BG, Mate TP, Greenwood LH, et al. Malignant biliary obstruction: intracavitary treatment with a high-dose rate remote after loading device. *Radiology.* 1987;164:574–576.

43. Hayes JK, Sapozink MD, Miller FJ. Definitive radiation therapy in bile duct carcinoma. *Int J Rad Oncol Biol Phys.* 1988;15:734–744.

44. Kocak Z, Ozkan H, Adli M. Intraluminal brachytherapy with metallic stenting in the palliative treatment of malignant obstruction of the bile duct. *Radiat Med.* 2005;23:200–207.

45. Pereiras RV, Owen JR, Hutson D, et al. Relief of malignant obstructive jaundice by percutaneous insertion of a permanent prosthesis in the biliary tree. *Ann Intern Med.* 1978;89:489–593.

46. Mueller PR, Ferrucci JR Jr, Teplick SK, et al. Biliary stent endoprosthesis: analysis of complications in 113 patients. *Radiology.* 1985;156:637–639.

47. Lichtenstein DR, Carr-Locke DL. Endoscopic palliation for unresectable pancreatic carcinoma. *Surg Clin North Am.* 1995;75:969–987.

48. Adam AN, Biliary stent placement for malignancy. In: SCVIR 1995 Program. Fairfax, Va. SCVIR, 1995;89–90.

49. Davids PHP, Groen AK, Ruacos EAJ, et al. Randomized trial of self-expanding metal stents versus polyethylene stents for distal malignant biliary obstruction. *Lancet.* 1992;340:1488–1492.

50. Kaassis M, Boyer J, Dumas R, et al. Plastic or metal stents for malignant strictures of the common bile duct? Results of a randomized prospective study. *Gastrointest Endosc.* 2003;57:178–182.

51. Wagner HJ, Knyrim K, Vakil N, Klose KJ. Plastic endoprostheses versus metal stents in the palliative treatment of malihnant hilar biliary obstruction. A prospective and randomized trial. *Endoscopy.* 1993;25(3):213–218.

52. Lammer J, Hausegger KA, Flueckiger F, et al. Common bile duct obstruction due to malignancy: treatment with plastic versus metal stents. *Radiology.* 1996;201:167–172.

53. Bezzi M, Zolovkins A, Cantisani V. New ePTFE/FEP: covered stent in the palliative treatment of malignant biliary obstructions. *J Vasc Interv Radiol.* 2002;13:581–598.

54. Han Y, Gong-Yong J, Seung-Ok L. Flared polyurethane-covered self-expandable nitinol stent for malignant biliary obstructions. *J Vasc Interv Radiol.* 2003;14:1291–1301.

55. Savader SJ, Trerotola SO, Merine DS, et al. Hemobilia after percutaneous transhepatic biliary drainage: treatment with transcatheter embolotherapy. *J Vasc Interv Radiol.* 1992;3:345–352.

COMMENTARY
LeAnn S. Stokes and Steven G. Meranze

As endoscopic equipment and techniques have improved, the role of interventional radiology (IR) in the management of malignant biliary obstruction has changed. Percutaneous biliary drainage has been replaced as a primary means of nonoperative biliary decompression, and the focus for IR has shifted to minimally invasive management of postoperative complications in patients who have undergone resection and to treatment of patients with unresectable disease who have failed endoscopy. The following discussion will expand on some of the key technical points mentioned in the previous chapter and will describe a few potential advances in the percutaneous management of malignant biliary obstruction.

MANAGEMENT OF POSTOPERATIVE COMPLICATIONS

For the 30% of patients with pancreatobiliary malignancy who are candidates for resection, the incidence of postoperative complications after pancreatoduodenectomy may be as high as 30%; however, the overall length of postoperative stay has decreased over the past decade. This decreased length of stay has been attributed to an improvement in the management of complications, specifically the increasing use of minimally invasive, image-guided techniques rather than repeat surgical intervention (1).

In a retrospective review of just over 1,000 patients who underwent pancreatoduodenectomy at a single institution between 1995 and 2000, 12% of patients had a percutaneous procedure for treatment of a surgical complication. These complications included intra-abdominal abscess or biloma in 8%; bile leak, undrained biliary segment or T-tube dislodgement in 4%; and hemobilia or gastrointestinal bleeding requiring angiography in

2%. In 85% of these patients, the IR procedure prevented reoperation and resulted in a shorter recovery time. Of note, routine preoperative drainage was the indication for percutaneous biliary drainage in the other 88% of patients in this study (1). Preoperative drainage is now rarely performed because it has been not been shown to improve outcome and may actually be associated with an increased risk of overall postoperative complications (2,3).

In patients with a suspected postoperative complication, cross-sectional imaging is essential for diagnosis and for determining whether the problem can be managed nonoperatively. Computed tomography provides postsurgical anatomic details and readily identifies fluid collections, abscesses, or bilomas that may be amenable to percutaneous drainage. If a biliary anastomotic leak is suspected, the degree of biliary ductal dilatation can be assessed. If biliary drainage is indicated and a jejunal access loop is present, the site of fixation and the course of the loop to the biliary-enteric anastomosis can be visualized.

Jejunal Access Loop

The routine creation of a jejunal access loop has been recommended in all biliary-enteric anastomoses and should be the first choice for access in patients who have a surgically affixed loop. Several advantages have been described for transjejunal over transhepatic access. The transjejunal approach avoids the discomfort of the transhepatic approach, has a lower complication rate, and allows access to all parts of the biliary tree from a single percutaneous puncture, which can be particularly helpful in patients with multiple strictures, isolated segments, or multifocal carcinoma. If biliary access is easily gained via the jejunal loop, there is no need to leave a catheter in place in anticipation of repeat procedures, as is often the case with transhepatic access.

If a loop has been created, it has hopefully been done in a way that will optimize access to the loop and to the biliary tree. The site of subcutaneous fixation should be well marked, and the efferent limb should be straight and relatively short. The longer and more tortuous the access limb, the more difficult it is to navigate a catheter into the biliary tree. In a retrospective review of 43 patients who underwent 196 attempts at percutaneous transjejunal biliary intervention, primary access of the biliary tree was successful in 92% with a complication rate of 4% (4).

Biliary Anastomotic Leak

The reported incidence of a fistula or anastomotic leak following hepatopancreatobiliary surgery is 3% to 10%, most of which heal spontaneously. If the leak does not close, percutaneous biliary drainage should be attempted even if the biliary tree is not dilated. In a retrospective review that included 17 patients with postoperative leaks and nondilated systems, a technical success rate of 100% was reported for access and stenting of the biliary tree, with an 88% rate of healing. The mean time to closure was 31 days, and there was no difference in outcome with external verses internal-external drainage. The authors of this study concluded that percutaneous biliary drainage is safe and reliable even in postoperative patients in poor general condition who have a postoperative anastomotic leak and a nondilated biliary tree (5).

Healing of a postoperative anastomotic leak can be facilitated by a combination of internal-external biliary drainage and percutaneous drainage of any associated fluid collections or bilomas. A leak that persists despite optimal drainage may be a good indication for use of a retrievable stent graft, such as the Viabil stent graft that is described in detail later. In fact, a case report has recently been published of successful treatment of a refractory biliary anastomotic leak with placement of a stent graft that was removed 15 days after placement (6).

MANAGEMENT OF UNRESECTABLE DISEASE

Approximately 70% of patients with pancreatobiliary carcinoma are not candidates for curative resection at presentation, and the patients who do undergo resection are at risk for benign or recurrent malignant biliary strictures. The cause of death in these patients is commonly related to biliary obstruction, making effective biliary drainage and control of local disease the goals of palliative therapy. When percutaneous biliary intervention is considered, the indications for the procedure should be discussed with the clinical team caring for the patient, and plans for the procedure should take into account the need for tissue sampling, the life expectancy of the patient, and any therapeutic options that may be available to the patient.

Selecting an Approach for Drainage

Preprocedural imaging is indispensable in planning the percutaneous approach for biliary drainage. In patients with malignant biliary obstruction, computed tomography can demonstrate the level or levels of obstruction, the presence of hepatic lobar atrophy, intrahepatic lesions that should be avoided, and other anatomic considerations such as the location of the lung, stomach, and colon relative to the liver.

Because only 25% to 30% of the liver must be drained to relieve obstructive jaundice, a single well-positioned percutaneous catheter can often achieve this goal. Biliary drainage via a left lateral segmental duct is preferable to right-sided drainage unless the left lobe is atrophied or cannot be accessed from a subxiphoid approach. The left intrahepatic ducts are less likely to become isolated than the right and are often easier to access, especially with sonographic guidance. A left subcostal drain is usually better tolerated than a right intercostal drain and has a lower risk of pleural complications and intercostal vessel injury.

Placement of bilateral percutaneous biliary drains or stents means multiple passes through the liver and is typically avoided if possible. Unilateral drainage is cheaper, simpler, and has a lower complication rate than bilateral drainage. Bilateral or multiple drains may be necessary, however, in patients with sepsis from undrained, infected ducts, and care should be taken to avoid contamination of poorly drained or isolated ducts during drain placement.

Tissue Sampling

The etiology of a biliary stricture can be difficult to diagnose, and the sensitivity for bile aspiration and/or brush biopsy is low. If a definitive diagnosis is necessary and routine cytology has been indeterminant, the use of advanced cytologic testing or cholangioscopic guidance for biopsy should be considered. Digital image analysis (DIA) and fluorescence in situ hybridization (FISH) are advanced cytologic techniques for detecting aneuploidy that have become available. In a recent study, tissue samples from 233 consecutive patients who underwent endoscopic retrograde cholangiopancreatography for pancreatobiliary strictures were analyzed using routine cytology, DIA, and FISH, with the conclusion that FISH and DIA increase the sensitivity for diagnosis of malignant strictures over that obtained by routine cytology alone while maintaining an acceptable specificity (7).

The other technique that may aid in making a definitive diagnosis is the use of cholangioscopic guidance. In patients with abnormal findings on imaging studies, cholangioscopy can improve assessment of the extent of disease and enable directed biopsy. Visual inspection may reveal unsuspected areas of friability that warrant biopsy, and increased sensitivity and specificity for cholangioscopically guided biopsy have been reported (8). In order to perform percutaneous cholangioscopy with a 5.2-mm scope, the hepatic parenchymal tract must be dilated to 16Fr or 18Fr and then allowed to mature for several days. Despite the larger tract size, the main risks of percutaneous cholangioscopy appear to be related to the initial placement of the biliary drainage catheter, and the complications described with cholangioscopy, including bile duct injury, cholangitis and bacteremia, are more common with therapeutic than diagnostic procedures (9).

Externalized Drains

Percutaneous biliary drainage is often accomplished initially with placement of an 8F or 10F drain that may allow for external drainage only or for both internal and external drainage. External drainage is less secure, can result in electrolyte abnormalities, and is only indicated when the biliary obstruction cannot be traversed. Internal-external biliary drains maintain access to the biliary tree, can be capped for internal drainage but are easily returned to external drainage during episodes of cholangitis, are relatively well tolerated, and are easy to exchange as needed. Long-term relief of biliary obstruction can be accomplished with an internal-external biliary drain, but most patients prefer internalized stents.

Internalized Stents

Self-expandable metal stents (SEMS) are preferred over plastic stents in patients who have a life expectancy >3 to 6 months because they have higher 6-month patency rates, decreasing the need for reintervention and making them more cost-effective. Reintervention rates with uncovered SEMS range from 11% to 40%, usually for occlusion due to tumor ingrowth or overgrowth, bile sludge, or stones. Although overgrowth can be addressed by overstenting, covered stents that could potentially prevent ingrowth and resist the deleterious effects of bile and other secretions have not been as effective as hoped (10).

Several studies of a newer generation covered biliary endoprosthesis, the Viabil stent graft (W.L. Gore & Associates, Flagstaff, AZ), have now been published. The Viabil consists of an inner lining of ultra thin, low-porosity expanded polytetrafluoroethylene and fluorinated ethylene propylene (ePTFE/FEP)

supported by a helically wound nitinol wire. Several sections of the wire are elevated to anchor the stent graft and prevent migration. The device is available in 8- or 10-mm diameters and 4-, 6-, and 8-cm lengths, all of which are placed via a 10F sheath. The two longer stents come with or without drainage holes cut in the proximal 1.5 cm of the lining. The extremely low porosity lining of the Viabil should prevent ingrowth to a greater degree than the materials used in older covered stents, theoretically resulting in improved patency rates for the Viabil.

An early prospective, nonrandomized multicenter study of 42 patients with inoperable malignant biliary obstruction of the common bile or hepatic ducts treated with the Viabil stent graft found primary patency rates of 90%, 76%, and 76% at 3, 6, and 12 months, respectively, with no instances of migration. This study documented a device-related complication rate of 10%, including one case of mild pancreatitis and three cases of acute cholecystitis related to covering the pancreatic or cystic ducts, and a procedural complication rate of 5%. Although the patency rate of the Viabil at 12 months was slightly better than for uncovered stents, 78% versus 51% to 68%, the risk of pancreatitis and cholecystitis was also higher than expected (11).

In a more recent report of Viabil stent grafts placed in 37 patients with malignant biliary obstruction, primary patency rates of 100%, 55.5%, and 25% were shown at 3, 6, and 12 months, respectively, while secondary patency was 100% at 12 months. Unlike the earlier study, Viabil stents with side holes were placed when necessary to avoid branch duct obstruction. The patency rates were consistently higher for the fully covered Viabil, 75% at 6 months compared with 40% for the Viabil with side holes. None of the patients in this study developed cholecystitis or pancreatitis but at the cost of a significantly lower patency rate (10).

One promising attribute of the Viabil endoprosthesis is that it has proven to be retrievable but has not been found to migrate. The option of retrieval gives the interventional radiologist greater latitude in determining when and in which patients to place a stent, which may be particularly beneficial when the underlying lesion is not well characterized. In a small series of five patients, one with a malignant cause of biliary obstruction, seven Viabil stent grafts were placed and removal of six stent grafts was attempted. Removal was 100% successful after a mean implantation time of 38 days, and no complications related to retrieval were described. The authors of this study suggested that the subset of patients who have malignant obstruction but a relatively long life expectancy might particularly benefit from a covered stent that could be changed periodically (12).

Local Control of Disease

Because patients with biliary drains often die within 6 to 12 months after placement from liver failure or cholangitis secondary to chronic or recurrent obstruction, local control of disease is a key issue in palliative treatment. Brachytherapy with iridium-192, photodynamic therapy (PDT) and high-intensity ultrasound are potential options for local disease control. The use of an iridium-192 wire allows direct delivery of high-dose radiation to the tumor bed while limiting the dose to surrounding tissues. The goal of PDT is to selectively destroy tumor cells by direct illumination after photosensitization, and high-intensity ultrasound is aimed at focal tissue destruction.

Intraluminal brachytherapy has been evaluated in several retrospective studies with different protocols and mixed results. In one of the most encouraging studies, Eschelman et al. (13) described 22 patients with inoperable malignant biliary obstruction who were treated with percutaneous biliary drainage followed by intraluminal iridium-192. In this study, brachytherapy was combined with external-beam radiation therapy plus systemic chemotherapy as a radiosensitizer, and a SEMS was placed 1 to 3 days after completion of brachytherapy. Brachytherapy was shown to prolong patient survival and improve stent patency in patients with cholangiocarcinoma but not in patients with other malignancies. The mean survival in patients with cholangiocarcinoma was 22.6 months, and the mean stent patency without intervention was 19.5 months (13).

PDT involves the intravenous administration of a photosensitizer that preferentially accumulates in neoplastic tissue and is then activated by exposure to a light source with a specific wavelength. The depth of tissue necrosis varies from <2 to 4 mm. PDT appears to be well tolerated, and several small studies have shown favorable results, including stable or improved quality of life, in patients with unresectable cholangiocarcinoma. One prospective randomized study of biliary stenting with or without PDT in patients with inoperable cholangiocarcinoma demonstrated a significantly longer median survival and significantly improved physical function and quality of life in the group of patients who received PDT (14).

Although most studies with PDT are encouraging, a 2007 study of 13 patients treated with a second-generation photosensitizer for recurrent obstructive jaundice following initial metal or plastic stent placement reported a significant complication rate, including two procedure-related deaths. The increased risk of complications in this study was attributed to the treatment protocol, underscoring the need for further investigation regarding the optimal light dose for the photosensitizer and the safest interval for repeat treatment (15).

One other potential local therapy is intraductal high-intensity ultrasound, and the results of a feasibility study using this technology were reported by Prat et al. (16) in 2002. In this study, high-intensity ultrasound was delivered across both intra- and extrahepatic malignant strictures via an 8-mm flexible transducer from an endoscopic approach. A total of ten patients were treated and two later underwent surgical resection. Treatment response was present in the two surgical specimens, complete response allowing stent removal was seen in one patient, and a partial response was noted in four patients.

CONCLUSION

The management of pancreatobiliary malignancy is complex and is best provided by a multidisciplinary team that ideally includes an oncologic surgeon, medical oncologist, radiation oncologist, endoscopist, and interventional radiologist. Because of the advanced stage of disease at presentation in the majority of patients with malignant biliary obstruction, the interventional radiologist may be the only specialist who can actually access and decompress the biliary tree; however, decisions regarding the timing, site, and type of drainage are best made when all specialties are involved. Although the overall prognosis for patients with pancreatobiliary malignancies remains poor, interventional radiologists may be able to perform minimally invasive procedures that can improve quality of life and survival both in patients who have undergone surgical resection and those who have not.

REFERENCES

1. Sohn TA, Yeo CJ, Cameron JL, et al. Pancreaticoduodenectomy: role of interventional radiologists in managing patients and complications. *J Gastrointest Surg.* 2003;7:209–219.
2. Povoski SP, Karpeh MS Jr, Conlon KC, et al. Association of preoperative biliary drainage with postoperative outcome following pancreaticoduodenectomy. *Ann Surg.* 1999;230:131–142.
3. Hochwald SN, Burke EC, Jarnagin WR, et al. Association of preoperative biliary stenting with increased postoperative infectious complications in proximal cholangiocarcinoma. *Arch Surg.* 1999;134:261–266.
4. McPherson SJ, Gibson RN, Collier NA, et al. Percutaneous transjejunal biliary intervention: 10-year experience with access via Roux-en-Y loops. *Radiology.* 1998;206:665–672.
5. Cozzi G, Severini A, Civelli E, et al. Percutaneous transhepatic biliary drainage in the management of postsurgical biliary leaks in patients with nondilated intrahepatic bile ducts. *Cardiovasc Intervent Radiol.* 2006;29:380–388.
6. Gwon DI, Shim JC, Lee YK, et al. Retrievable biliary stent-graft management of refractory postoperative bile leakage. *J Vasc Interv Radiol.* 2007;18:1036–1041.
7. Moreno Luna LE, Kipp B, Halling KC, et al. Advanced cytologic techniques for the detection of malignant pancreatobiliary strictures [published online ahead of print August 16, 2006]. *Gastroenterology.* 2006;131:1064–1072.
8. Simon T, Fink AS, Zuckerman AM. Experience with percutaneous transhepatic cholangioscopy (PTCS) in the management of biliary tract disease. *Surg Endosc.* 1999;13:1199–1202.
9. Oh HC, Lee SK, Lee TY, et al. Analysis of percutaneous transhepatic cholangioscopy-related complications and the risk factors for those complications. *Endoscopy.* 2007;39:731–736.
10. Hatzidakis A, Krokidis M, Kalbakis K, et al. ePTFE/FEP-Covered metallic stents for palliation of malignant biliary disease: can tumor ingrowth be prevented? [published online ahead of print May 17, 2007.] *Cardiovasc Intervent Radiol.* 2007;30:950–958.
11. Schoder M, Rossi P, Uflacker R, et al. Malignant biliary obstruction: treatment with ePTFE-FEP-covered endoprostheses initial technical and clinical experiences in a multicenter trial. *Radiology.* 2002;225:35–42.
12. Kuo MD, Lopresti DC, Gover DD, et al. Intentional retrieval of viabil stent-grafts from the biliary system. *J Vasc Interv Radiol.* 2006;17:389–397.
13. Eschelman DJ, Shapiro MJ, Bonn J, et al. Malignant biliary duct obstruction: long-term experience with Gianturco stents and combined-modality radiation therapy. *Radiology.* 1996;200:717–724.
14. Ortner ME, Caca K, Berr F, et al. Successful photodynamic therapy for nonresectable cholangiocarcinoma: a randomized prospective study. *Gastroenterology.* 2003;125:1355–1363.
15. Pereira SP, Ayaru L, Rogowska A, et al. Photodynamic therapy of malignant biliary strictures using meso-tetrahydroxyphenylchlorin. *Eur J Gastroenterol Hepatol.* 2007;19:479–485.
16. Prat F, Lafon C, De Lima DM, et al. Endoscopic treatment of cholangiocarcinoma and carcinoma of the duodenal papilla by intraductal high-intensity US: results of a pilot study. *Gastrointest Endosc.* 2002;56:909–915.

59

Management of Pain in Cancer and Cancer Treatment

Howard L. Rosner

Pain is one of the most feared effects of cancer and cancer treatment among cancer sufferers. The lack of successful management of cancer-related pain, or merely the fear of potential pain, can interfere with the overall treatment of patients with cancer. There are more than 4 million people worldwide with some form of cancer. The prevalence of chronic pain among cancer patients who are being actively treated ranges from 30% to 50% and rises to more than 80% of patients with advanced disease (1), yet up to 90% of patients could attain adequate pain control with simple drug-management techniques. Inadequate management of pain is a complex issue with multiple sources that include fear of government regulators, underutilization of medications by clinicians with insufficient knowledge of pain assessment and therapy, inappropriate concerns about medication side effects and opiate addiction, a tendency to give lower priority to symptom control than to cancer treatment, patient fear and misunderstanding of medication and fear of diverting treatment away from the active disease, noncompliance and underreporting of symptoms, and health care delivery system impediments and costs. Pain in cancer pain remains undertreated and neglected and a significant public health problem (2). Pain is more prevalent in some types of cancer than others. Table 59.1 reflects the locations of cancers and the percentage of patients who suffer pain as a result (3).

An understanding of the pathophysiology, etiologies, and management strategies of various aspects of cancer-related pain is essential to treatment of patients with cancer. The clinical management of all pain begins with an attempt to identify—and then treat—the underlying cause of the pain. Regardless of cause, the objective of pain treatment is threefold: to reduce discomfort, decrease anxiety, and return the patient to his or her previous level of function. There are no easy formulas for achieving these objectives. The treatment of pain must always be individualized, because individuals exhibit a remarkably wide range of pain tolerance and an equally wide range of responsiveness to therapy. In an attempt to formulate sensible management plans, numerous classification schemas have been promoted. In past years, the most common description of pain was either as acute (the normal painful response to trauma or disease) or chronic (any pain syndrome of longer than some set duration of time, usually more than 6 months). However, this became problematic as evidence grew that the acute pain model of tissue damage could be applied to many disease states that, by their nature, affected the patient for far longer than 6 months. Table 59.2 presents pain as classified by both duration of symptoms and underlying diagnosis (4).

DIAGNOSING PAIN

Most pain complaints among hospitalized patients arise from the first two categories of pain listed in Table 59.2: acute and subacute pain. Here the underlying pain generator is tissue injury resulting from a single event (e.g., surgery). The incidence of moderate postoperative pain can be as high as 29% and 10.9% for severe pain; poor pain relief, 3.5%; and fair-to-poor pain relief, 19.4% (5). Pain that is not adequately controlled can lead to numerous known complications such as atelectasis, pneumonia, and prolonged hospitalization. Additionally, inadequately controlled pain can lead to changes in the central nervous system, which include central sensitization and the development of chronic pain and psychopathology. Ongoing acute and recurrent acute pain occurs as a result of continuing tissue injury from disease, malignant or nonmalignant, respectively. In these states, the acute pain model can be applied for management. Yet, adequate pain management in cancer remains elusive for many patients.

There are significant long-term problems associated with undertreated acute pain. Both the biological and psychological foundations for long-term persistent pain begin within hours of acute injury (6). The pain associated with acute injury usually lasts for <1 month; however, in some cases, it can persist >6 months from the time of injury (7). Nerve remodeling and sensitization begins within 20 minutes of injury and may rapidly evolve into a chronic pain syndrome. In the neonate, simple lancing of the heel can result in weeks of hypersensitivity to touch (8). Conversely, good postoperative pain control in adults lowers analgesic requirement and improves functional status (9).

Another means of classifying pain is by the type of injury the patient suffers, which further delineates the direction of management. In this model, pain is subdivided into pain arising from stimulation of pain receptors (nociceptors) and is described as *nociceptive pain*, or pain arising from damage to either the peripheral or central nervous system, or *neuropathic pain*. Table 59.3 categorizes the differences between nociceptive and neuropathic pain.

Because pain is inherently subjective, a patient's self-report is vital. Important considerations in a pain assessment include temporal features (onset, daily variation), location (pain sites, radiation patterns), severity (some form of consistent and reproducible scale; e.g., mild, moderate, or severe, or a 0–10 numeric scale), quality (e.g., aching, throbbing, stabbing, shooting, burning, tingling), and finally, alleviating and exacerbating factors. This history, coupled to a physical examination and evaluation

Table 59.1

Cancer Type and Its Association With Pain

Type/Location of Cancer	% With Pain
Bone	85
Oral cavity	80
Genitourinary (men/women)	75/78
Breast	52
Lung	45
Gastrointestinal	40
Lymphoma	20
Leukemia	5

Adapted from Warfield CA, ed. *Manual of Pain Management*. Philadelphia: J.B. Lippincott Co; 1991.

Table 59.2

Pain Classification by Duration of Symptoms

1. **Acute**
   Duration: 0–7 days
   Degree of pain: Mild to severe
   Cause: Known or unknown, but usually a single event (e.g., surgery)
   Drug treatment: Narcotic and nonnarcotic
   Emotional state: Mild psychological symptoms

2. **Subacute**
   Duration: 7 days to 6 months
   Degree of pain: Mild to severe
   Cause: Same as in acute pain
   Drug treatment: Narcotic and nonnarcotic
   Emotional state: Mild psychological symptoms

3. **Ongoing acute**
   Duration: Any length of time
   Degree of pain: Usually severe
   Cause: Due to ongoing tissue damage from neoplasms
   Drug treatment: Narcotic and nonnarcotic
   Emotional state: Depression and anxiety common

4. **Recurrent acute**
   Duration: Any length of time
   Degree of pain: Mild to severe
   Cause: Due to chronic organic process
   Drug treatment: Nonnarcotic and coanalgesics; narcotics sometimes indicated
   Emotional state: Depression and anxiety common

5. **Chronic intractable benign pain syndrome**
   Duration: Greater than 6 months
   Degree of pain: Mild to severe
   Cause: Unknown
   Drug treatment: Nonnarcotic and coanalgesics are primary medications; usually no need for narcotics
   Emotional state: Psychological factors very important, psychotherapy indicated

Adapted from Rosner HL: The pharmacologic management of postoperative pain. In: Lefkowitz M, Lebovits A, Wlody D, et al., eds. *A Practical Approach to Pain Management*. Boston: Little Brown and Co.; 1996.

of laboratory and imaging studies, helps define the pain generator, and therefore can more clearly direct the clinician in the direction of pain management.

It is essential to perform a comprehensive pain assessment in order to properly manage pain. By international definition, pain is primarily subjective; therefore, the patient's self-report is the primary means used for assessment. Many different pain assessment tools are routinely used and many different standardized approaches exist. As long as there is uniformity in the particular tools used, most assessment tools achieve the same ends. Patient complaints are viewed in terms of their underlying disease state, as well as a separate diagnosis for the pain. Pain is then assessed in terms of its severity (e.g., 10-point scale, visual analogue scale), location (primary sites and radiating patterns), characteristics (neuropathic vs. nociceptive), temporal relationships (onset, diurnal variation, and progression), exacerbating and alleviating factors, the impact of the pain on quality of life, and other comorbidities. The assessment, coupled with the remainder of the history, physical examination, and review of diagnostic studies, provides the basis for the pain diagnosis in addition to understanding the underlying disease process.

The remainder of this chapter is devoted to consideration of many of the pain syndromes seen in patients with cancer; pain secondary to the cancer itself, as well as pain related to its treatment. Certainly, patients with cancers develop or experience exacerbations of benign problems such as herniated discs, which often require pain management. These topics are beyond the scope of this chapter.

Opioids and other conventional analgesics play an important role in the management of cancer-related acute, subacute, and ongoing acute pain. However, of the various pain-management problems confronted by clinicians, neuropathic pain, which sometimes can respond to conventional analgesics, represents the largest number of severe cancer pain patients who do not respond well to traditional painkillers (10).

CANCER PAIN SYNDROMES

Pain in patients with cancer occurs from both cancer and non-cancer sources. Most patients, up to 75%, suffer their pain as a direct result of the tumor; the others as a result of treatment or other disease states (11).

Direct involvement by tumor into bone, muscle, joint, or connective tissue leads to significant somatic pain. The spine is the most common site of bony metastases; many patients with cancer have back pain, although the factors that convert a painless lesion into a painful one are unknown. Only a small proportion of bony metastases become painful, and the mechanisms by which a lesion becomes painful is unclear. Spinal involvement by tumor has the added risk of potential damage to the spinal cord and/or spinal nerve roots. This can produce not only severe neuropathic pain, but also neurologic deficits including numbness, weakness, and incontinence. Back pain from vertebral metastasis must be vigorously examined to prevent compressive lesions

Table 59.3

Nociceptive and Neuropathic Pain

Nociceptive Pain	Neuropathic Pain
Etiology: 　Mediated by nociceptor stimulation 　Classified as thermo-, mechano- or chemoreceptors 　Systemic distribution: cutaneous and connective tissue, 　　bone, muscle, viscera 　Somatic or visceral Pain characteristics: 　Normal expected responses to stimulus 　Described as "sharp, dull, aching, throbbing" Usually opiate monotherapy-sensitive Pain elicited by (nonneural) tissue injury 　Traumatic pain 　Postoperative pain 　Cancer pain 　　Tumor-induced 　　Treatment-induced 　Bone pain 　Pressure pain	Etiology: 　Damage to peripheral or central nervous system Pain characteristics: 　Hyperesthesia, hyperalgesia, hyperpathia, allodynia 　Hypersensitivity, exaggerated response to stimuli 　Described as "burning, tingling, shooting" Usually opiate monotherapy-resistant Examples 　Neuralgias and neuropathies 　Mono- and polyneuropathies, postherpetic neuralgia, 　　diabetic neuropathy, drug-induced neuropathy 　Deafferentation neuropathy 　Nerve transection or compression injury 　"Failed back" with radicular pain 　Plexopathies 　Complex regional pain syndrome 　Causalgia and reflex sympathetic dystrophy 　HIV-related neuropathies 　Cancer-induced neuropathic pain 　　Tumor-induced 　　Treatment-induced

HIV, human immunodeficiency virus.

and cauda equina syndrome. With early diagnosis and treatment of the tumor, the impending neurologic disorder can be circumvented. Tumor involvement in long bones can lead to both bony pain and pathologic fractures, all painful sequelae. Tumor involvement into nervous tissue, either centrally or peripherally, can lead to significant neuropathic pain and neurologic deficits. The emergence of Horner syndrome can be an early sign of a brachial plexopathy prior to the onset of upper extremity pain.

Treatment of the underlying cancer can also cause significant acute and chronic pain. Physicians sometimes forget that even the simplest of diagnostic studies can be tremendously painful for those who are chronically ill. Even venipuncture for a patient who has undergone several rounds of chemotherapy or multiple blood draws can be difficult. There are many chronic pain syndromes associated with the treatment of cancer, including chemotherapy-induced neuropathies and mucous membrane syndromes, radiation, and surgically induced neuropathies. Even the acute postsurgical pain in a patient with chronic cancer can be challenging, particularly in those patients who are already being treated for some chronic pain issues. Finally, patients with chronic illness and pain are at greater risk to develop psychological problems, which make the overall management more difficult. Table 59.4 lists many of the tumor-related and diagnostic/therapeutic pain syndromes in cancer (12).

For the majority of patients with cancer pain, the mainstay of therapy has become the use of systemic opioids. Once considered dangerous and open for misuse, proper opioid management has improved the lives of generations of cancer pain sufferers.

Over the past 20 years, with the development of many commercially available sustained-release preparations of opioids from morphine to oxycodone to hydromorphone to fentanyl, opioid management has become easier to deliver and safer to maintain.

Severe episodic worsening of pain over a baseline of chronic moderate pain has been described as "breakthrough pain" (13) or episodic pain (14). Unlike constant pain, which is best managed with a long-acting or sustained-release opiate, breakthrough or episodic pain is better treated with an immediate-acting, short-duration medication.

Neuropathic problems are far more difficult to manage. Empirical evidence suggests that the symptomatic therapy of severe pain should start with an opioid, irrespective of its mechanism (15). There is tremendous variability in opioid pharmacokinetics and dynamics from patient to patient; therefore, analgesia should be reached through the gradual upward titration of opioids dose until satisfactory pain control is achieved or side effects become unmanageable. Some patients have been reported to require very high doses of systemic opioids to control pain (16). Many authors believe the absolute dose is immaterial as long as the side effects, inconvenience, discomfort, or costs are not excessive (15). Over time, some patients require escalations of their opioids doses; others do not (17). Most, however, are able to attain an analgesic dose that remains constant for an extended period.

Increasing pain can occur from progression of disease, tolerance, hyperalgesia, or unrelated pain issues. Hyperalgesia, a phenomenon associated with the development of opioid tolerance, may explain why certain patients have increasing pain as

Table 59.4	
Cancer-Related Pain	
Pain due to Tumor	**Pain due to Diagnostics or Treatment**
Nociceptive pain syndromes	Diagnostic studies
Bone, joint, or soft-tissue metastases or invasion	Venipuncture
Pathologic long bone fractures.	Lumbar puncture
Hypertrophic osteoarthropathy	Postdural-puncture headache
Vertebral syndromes	Bone marrow biopsy
Pathologic compression fractures.	Angiography
Bone marrow expansion	Therapeutic procedures
Paraneoplastic pain syndromes	Medication infusion
Visceral pain	Paracentesis
Intestinal obstruction	Thoracentesis
Visceral carcinomatosis	Pleurodesis
Hepatic distension	Embolization
Lymphedema	Nephrostomy
Neuropathic pain syndromes	Treatment-induced pain
Plexopathies	Thrombophlebitis
Cervical	Mucositis
Brachial	Proctitis
Lumbosacral	Radiation neuritis/neuropathy/plexopathy/myelopathy
Sacral	Acute postoperative pain
Radiculopathy	Postsurgical neuropathic pain syndromes
Epidural spinal cord compression	Postmastectomy syndrome
Central or peripheral neuropathies	Postthoracotomy syndrome
	Postradical neck dissection syndrome
	Postnephrectomy syndrome
	Stump pain and phantom pain
	Chemotherapy-induced pain
	Headache
	Bone
	Muscle
	Joint
	Peripheral neuropathies

Adapted from Portenoy RK, Lesage P. Management of cancer pain. *Lancet.* 1999;353:1695–1700.

their doses of opiates are raised. It has been postulated that neural plasticity associated with the development of opioid tolerance may activate a pronociceptive mechanism that could counteract the analgesic effects of opioids, thus, part of the mechanisms leading to the reduced opioid analgesic efficacy in chronic opioid therapy (18). One way that has been suggested to decrease the need for dose escalation is to change opioid medications periodically (19). By rotating different medications, slightly different receptor affinities of the various opioids can provide similar analgesia at equipotent doses.

PHARMACOLOGIC APPROACHES

Opioid Therapy

There is no drug class with greater efficacy or safety than opioids. This class of medication is the mainstay of pain management with moderate-to-severe cancer pain. The "analgesic ladder" approach of the World Health Organization was created to provide basic guidance for an approach to cancer pain (2,20). Many routes of administration for opioids have been developed, although the oral route remains preferable. Transdermal and transbuccal administration can be effective for lipophilic drugs such as fentanyl, but less effective for hydrophilic medications such as morphine or hydromorphone. Additionally, subcutaneous or intravenous delivery systems can be used, particularly for patients whose dosing requirements are high.

Opioid doses are often based on their equianalgesic potency. All pure opioids act at the opiate receptors with similar effect. The dose required to obtain that effect differs from drug to drug. The equianalgesic dose of opioids, therefore, is the dose needed of that particular drug to achieve the same analgesic effect as another opioid. For the most part, all opioids are equianalgesic, at their equipotent doses. Table 59.5 lists the more commonly used opioid medications and their equipotency to 10 mg of parenteral morphine (21,22).

Most patients with chronic cancer pain will be treated with some combination of long-acting medication to manage their

Table 59.5

Opioid Analgesics for Management of Severe Pain

| Medication | Equianalgesic Dose to 10 mg of Parenteral Morphine[b] | | | | |
	IM/IV/SC	Oral	$T_{1/2}$ (h)	Duration (h)	Comments
Fentanyl	0.25	—	2–3	2–4	Lipophilicity can lead to accumulation over time (100 mcg/h infusion approximates morphine 4 mg/h)
Fentanyl transmucosal	—	800 mcg transmucosal	2–3	2–4	200 mcg lozenge approximates 5 mg PO oxycodone or 6.5 mg PO morphine
Fentanyl transdermal	—	—	2–3	16–24	25 mcg patch approximates 15 mg/day parenteral morphine
Hydromorphone	1.5–2	5–7.5	2–3	2–4	Range of potency may reach 3:1 with chronic use
Methadone	10	20	3–190	4–12	Accumulation of methadone leads to increased duration of action and half-life
Levorphanol	1.5–2	4	4–24	4–12	Can accumulate with repeated dosing
Morphine	**10**	**30**	**2–3**	**2–4**	**Standard of comparison**
Morphine CR	10	30	2–3	8–12	
Morphine SR	10	30	2–3	24	
Oxycodone	—	20	2–3	3–4	
Oxycodone CR	—	20	2–3	8–12	
Oxymorphone	1	10	2–3	2–4	Oral oxymorphone has been newly released to the U.S. market in both an immediate and controlled-release preparation
Oxymorphone CR	1	10	2–3	8–12	Oral oxymorphone has been newly released to the U.S. market in both an immediate and controlled-release preparation

IV, intravenously; IM, intramuscularly; SC, subcutaneously; PO, orally; CR, controlled release; SR, sustained-release.
[a]Equianalgesic studies are based on IM morphine; IV/SC routes are usually equivalent.
Adapted from Brunton L, Lazo J, Parker K. *Goodman & Gilman's The Pharmacological Basis of Therapeutics*, 11th ed. New York: McGraw-Hill Medical Publishing, 2005; and Derby S, Chin J, Portenoy RK. Systemic opioid therapy for chronic cancer pain: practical guidelines for converting drugs and routes of administration. *CNS Drugs*. 1998;9:99–109.

baseline, constant pain, plus an immediate-acting preparation to manage painful episodic or breakthrough pain. There are no set formulae for the "correct" combination of baseline sustained-release and breakthrough medications. Once baseline analgesia is established, the size of the rescue dose usually ranges from 5% to 15% of the total daily dose. The dosing interval is based on the onset and duration of the breakthrough medication employed and should be long enough to observe the full effect of each dose. With oral dosing, the minimum interval is usually 2 hours, whereas with intravenous administration it can be as short as 8 to 10 minutes, although most authorities agree that if a patient requires more than four to six doses of breakthrough medication per day, consideration should be made to increase the dose of the baseline medication (23).

Less than ideal opioid analgesia can be due to multiple factors including tolerance, progression of disease, misunderstand-

ing, or improper prescribing. Additionally, dose-limiting side effects can diminish the effectiveness of opioids by preventing the patient from achieving a therapeutic dose. Ideally, a patient should be titrated to analgesia, side effects increasing with dose. When patients become analgesic but have significant side effects, a subsequent reduction in the dose of the opioid usually results in a reduction of the dose-related side effects while preserving analgesia (24). However, if the dose of opioid cannot be reduced without the loss of analgesia, a more synergistic, multimodal polypharmaceutical approach must be taken. This includes the addition of nonopioid coanalgesics (e.g., acetaminophen or nonsteroidal anti-inflammatory drugs [NSAIDs]), analgesic adjuvants (e.g., antidepressants or antiepileptic medications), and/or the employment of an anesthetic or surgical neuroablative or neuroaugmentative procedure (e.g., celiac plexus chemoneurolysis or spinal opiate infusions).

Table 59.6	
Adjuvant Analgesics	
Adjuvant	Indication
Acetaminophen	Generalized pain Minimal anti-inflammatory effects
Alpha-2-adrenergic agonists (e.g., clonidine, tizanidine)	Neuropathic pain
Antidepressants (tricyclics and SNRIs) (e.g., amitriptyline, nortriptyline) (e.g., venlafaxine, duloxetine)	Neuropathic pain
Antiepileptic drugs (e.g., pregabalin, gabapentin, valproate, carbamazepine, lamotrigine)	Neuropathic pain
Benzodiazepines (e.g., diazepam, lorazepam, clonazepam)	Anxiety
Bisphosphonates (e.g., pamidronate, zoledronate)	Bone pain
Calcitonin	Bone pain
Corticosteroids (e.g., dexamethasone, hydrocortisone)	Nerve compression, bone pain, visceral pain
Hydroxyzine	Nausea, anxiety
Local anesthetics (IV: e.g., lidocaine) (PO: e.g., mexiletine, tocainide)	Neuropathic pain
NSAIDs (e.g., ibuprofen, naproxen, diclofenac,) (celecoxib)	Bone pain, inflammatory pain
NMDA receptor antagonists (e.g., ketamine, dextromethorphan, Memantine)	Neuropathic pain
Phenothiazines (e.g., chlorpromazine, trifluoperazine)	Neuropathic pain, anxiety, delirium, nausea
Stimulants (e.g., methylphenidate, pemoline) (Modafinil[a])	Sedation

SNRI, serotonin-norepinephrine reuptake inhibitor; NSAID, nonsteroidal anti-inflammatory drug; NMDA,
   N-methyl-D-aspartate acid; PO, by mouth.
[a] Not a stimulant but useful in managing sedation.

Nonopioid Adjuvant Therapy

The nonopioid analgesics include acetaminophen and the NSAIDs. Adjuvant analgesics are medications whose primary use is in conditions other than pain, but possess analgesic properties that are independent of opioids. Acetaminophen and NSAIDs are considered safe for most patients, routinely employed, and produce dose-dependent analgesic effects. Unlike opioids, these classes of medications have both a minimum effective dose and a ceiling dose for analgesia. NSAIDs can be useful and should be considered for coadministration with the opioids. Although all NSAIDs possess similar pharmacokinetics and should act in a similar fashion, there remains variability among patients with respect to maximum efficacy and side effects. Most NSAIDs posses some degree of gastrointestinal toxicity, most are platelet aggregation inhibitors, and all are renally toxic to some degree. The newer class of cyclo-oxygenase II inhibitors possesses less gastrointestinal toxicity, but still has the same degree of cardiovascular risk and renal toxicity as their older siblings.

Analgesic adjuvants are composed of medications from multiple classes. Included in this group are medications as diverse as corticosteroids and antiepileptic medications. Table 59.6 briefly summarizes many of the analgesic adjuvants, and in which pain syndromes they are useful. These medications are usually started after opioid analgesics have been employed and optimized; however, in cases of primary neuropathic pain, an appropriate adjuvant coanalgesic, including antidepressants, anticonvulsants, and oral local anesthetics, may be started at the same time as an opioid (25). Steroids are used for a variety of purposes including plexopathies, inflammatory, and bone pain, and are used commonly in patients with advanced disease to improve anorexia, nausea, and malaise. Other adjuvant analgesics are used to manage opioid-refractory malignant bone pain including bisphosphonates, radiopharmaceutical drugs (e.g., strontium), and calcitonin (26,27).

NEUROAUGMENTIVE AND NEUROABLATIVE PROCEDURES

Neuroaugmentation is the term given to the application of therapies directly to the central nervous system to modify painful input from the periphery. This includes the infusion of opiates and/or other medications directly into the cerebrospinal fluid or epidural space, or the application of electricity to the spinal cord or brain to modify or interfere with the painful signal. Often in patients with cancer, electrical stimulation of any sort is contraindicated. However, intraspinal approaches (epidural or intrathecal) can be invaluable among selected patients who for one reason or another are unable to benefit from systemic therapy (28). Opioid delivery to the sites of action in the spinal cord may decrease central opiate receptor-mediated side effects (29). The intrathecal route delivers more consistent and higher-grade pain control with lower doses, particularly if the implant is to be used for an extended period. The epidural route is preferred if higher concentrations of local anesthetic are needed, if a full intrathecal implant is not possible, or if the cost factors of the implant are not warranted by patient longevity (30).

The selection of an opioid, or a mixture of medications, is influenced by multiple factors. The type of pain experienced (nociceptive, neuropathic, or mixed) is one point on the decision tree. Other important points are the location of the pain in proximity to the portal of drug delivery, the degree of tolerance to opioids experienced by the patient, and the types of comorbidities with which the patient suffers. Hydrophilic drugs, such as morphine and hydromorphone, have a prolonged presence in cerebrospinal fluid and significant cephalad distribution. These drugs are therefore very useful for widespread pain problems or those problems in which the spinal site of action is distant from the tip of the implanted catheter. Lipophilic opioids, such as fentanyl and sufentanil, have minimal redistribution, remaining in cord tissue in proximity to the tip of the infusion catheter, and therefore may be preferable for segmental analgesia at the level of spinal infusion.

Spinal administration of medications allows for multimodal polypharmacy as well. Very common is the addition of a low concentration of a local anesthetic, such as 0.125% to 0.25% bupivacaine (31), which has been demonstrated to increase analgesic effect without increasing toxicity. Other medications that can be highly efficacious in spinal administration, particularly for neuropathic pain syndromes, include the α_2-adrenergic agonist clonidine (32), the γ-aminobutyric acid (GABA)B receptor agonist baclofen (33), and the N-calcium channel blocker ziconotide (34).

Neuroablative Therapy

Destruction of parts of the pain conduction pathways limits the ability for a painful signal to reach the brain. Table 59.7 describes the invasive techniques used for pain control according to the site of pain. Over the years, these types of interventions have been more infrequently performed as analgesic management and neuromodulatory procedures have improved.

However, there remains a place in our treatment armamentarium for guided injections of neurolytic substances such as alcohol, phenol, glycerol, or hypertonic saline (chemoneurolysis), which chemically denervate part or parts of the nervous system (35). Chemical denervation can be performed on sensory nerves only. Mixed nerves, which are far more commonly involved, cannot be undergo neurolysis unless the functional loss is anticipated, understood by all parties, and will not increase the suffering experienced by the patient (36).

MANAGEMENT OF ACUTE POSTOPERATIVE PAIN

In the acute period following surgery or injury, or when a patient experiences a rapid increase in pain and requires hospitalization, systemic opiate administration effectively manages acute pain by raising serum opiate concentration into the therapeutic range. This therapeutic range is different for every patient and is affected by factors such as (a) severity of pain, (b) patient age, (c) pre-existing tolerance to medications, or (d) ratio of nociceptive to neuropathic components of a mixed pain syndrome. Certainly we expect that postoperative pain is primarily nociceptive and would be responsive to conventional opiate therapy. To attain the desired increase in serum concentration of opiates, parenteral administration (intramuscular, subcutaneous, or intravenous) is more rapid than enteral administration. Once a patient is titrated to an analgesic therapeutic range, analgesia can be maintained by the use of a patient-controlled analgesia (PCA) device or periodic dosing through nurse-administered parenteral administration. PCA units are programmed based on the (a) medication selected, (b) basal rate (continuous infusion rate), (c) patient demand dose, (d) lockout interval (how often a patient can get the demand dose), and (e) contingencies if the original parameters are inadequate.

The advantage of PCA includes the ability to administer a small, low-dose infusion, small preprogrammed doses of opiate on patient demand and need, larger boluses by prescription, and rapid changes of dosing if needed, and for patients who understand how to use one, it provides smoother and more consistent blood levels than nurse-administered on-demand dosing (4). When dosing opiates, it is important to understand the concept of equipotency; the dose required of each agent needed to achieve similar analgesic effect. Table 59.8 is a list of opiate analgesics commonly used for management of acute and postoperative pain.

Patients who are deemed opiate-tolerant prior to surgery have much higher opiate requirements in the postoperative period. Patients who have been maintained on opiates in the preoperative period are at risk of having inadequate analgesia following surgery, even in the best of hands. Opiate hyperalgesia plays an important role in this phenomenon and cannot be discounted (37). Inadequate pain control can lead to a host of postoperative complications. Therefore, there must be preoperative planning for postoperative analgesia to be ideal. The preoperative dose of opiate must be replaced fully in the postoperative period. However, this dose of opioid will be inadequate to achieve analgesia for most surgical procedures. Therefore, aggressive titration of opiate above and beyond the patient's usual daily dose must be performed. Often, because of their hyperalgesia, patients will

Table 59.7	
Invasive Techniques According to the Site of Pain	
Site	Procedure
Face (unilateral)	Gasserian gangliolysis Trigeminal neurolysis Intraventricular opioid
Pharyngeal	Glossopharyngeal neurolysis Intraventricular opioid
Arm/brachial plexus	Spinal opioid ± local anesthetic Chemical or surgical rhizotomy
Chest wall spinal opioid ± local anesthetic	Intercostal neurolysis Paravertebral neurolysis Chemical rhizotomy Surgical rhizotomy
Abdominal wall (somatic)	Spinal opioid ± local anesthetic Chemical rhizotomy Surgical rhizotomy Cordotomy (unilateral pain)
Abdomen (visceral)	Celiac plexus neurolysis Bilateral splanchnic neurolysis
Low abdomen (visceral)	Celiac plexus neurolysis Bilateral splanchnic neurolysis
Pelvic structures and perineum	Spinal opioid ± local anesthetic Hypogastric neurolysis Ganglion impar neurolysis Chemical rhizotomy Surgical rhizotomy Transsacral nerve root neurolysis Caudal neurolysis
Pelvis + lower limb	Spinal opioid ± local anesthetic Chemical rhizotomy Surgical rhizotomy
Unilateral lower quadrant	Cordotomy
Multifocal or generalized pain with upper body or head pain or severe diffuse pain	Pituitary ablation Cingulotomy

Adapted from Cherney NI. The management of cancer pain. *CA Cancer J Clin.* 2000;50:70–116.

require up to twice their preoperative opiate dose in the immediate postoperative period to achieve analgesia. In those situations in which analgesia cannot be achieved with opiates alone, the addition of ketamine, a potent NMDA (N-methyl-D-aspartate acid) receptor blocker, in subanesthetic doses can be very helpful (38). Ketamine could, in addition to having an opioid-sparing effect, conceivably reduce the development of chronic postoperative pain through NMDA receptor blockade and reduction of wind-up and central sensitization (39).

Postoperative Epidural Analgesia

The application of opiates in the epidural space to provide analgesia began in the late 1970s and early 1980s. Early observations indicated this to be a well-tolerated means of pain control, requiring doses far lower than parenteral administration (40,41). However, shortly thereafter, side effects were described including nausea, vomiting, itching, and respiratory depression (42–44). Morphine, because of its hydrophilicity, was demonstrated to circulate quickly in the cerebrospinal fluid, reaching the brainstem in as little as 15 to 20 minutes after epidural injection (45).

Over the past 20 years, epidural opiate analgesia has been added to the commonly used techniques for postoperative analgesia. In the early days, morphine was administered by bolus injection in the epidural catheter, either once or twice daily. The more contemporary practice is to use infusion pumps to provide a steady-state, thus avoiding some of the side effects that large boluses can cause. With patient-controlled epidural analgesia, patient demand features on newer infusion pumps add another level of improvement, allowing patients to bolus themselves with a preset dose if they feel pain, much like an intravenous PCA (46). With infusions comes the ability to mix a local anesthetic or other medications with the opioid, enhancing the overall level of analgesia by modulating pain signals at more than one location (47). In lower extremity surgical procedures, epidural analgesia has been employed frequently with superior benefits (48), and in abdominal surgery, epidural analgesia has been demonstrated superior to intravenous opioid in the postoperative setting (49,50).

The longer a spinally administered drug remains in the cerebrospinal fluid, the greater the chance of developing a central side effect. Rostral spread with the resultant side effects of itching, nausea, vomiting, and respiratory depression is more common with the use of hydrophilic opioids such as morphine, which can remain in the aqueous phase of the cerebrospinal fluid for up to 24 hours (51). To avoid these phenomena, many clinicians use lipophilic opioids such as fentanyl or sufentanil mixed with a local anesthetic such as bupivacaine (52). These combinations are more frequently administered by infusion or patient-controlled epidural analgesia than by intermittent bolus.

CONCLUSIONS

Pain in cancer occurs in a broad array of settings that include pain from the disease itself, pain secondary to diagnostic studies, and pain due to therapeutic interventions. There are no clear-cut formulae for managing all pain; we must work at length to identify the source of pain and use the appropriate treatment protocols to achieve analgesia. In some settings, such as the postoperative period, the source of pain and its management are clear. In others, the source can be more elusive, and optimal management may depend on our ability to isolate the generator. We must be prepared to take the patient's psychological state into account and realize that what we are treating is beyond the pain itself. Overall impairments including the physical, psychological, social, spiritual, and existential may be reported as pain. These taken together comprise "suffering" or "total pain" (53–55) and which together must be addressed if the outcome is to be favorable. Open communication between all parties, comprehensive

Table 59.8

Parenteral Opioid Analgesics for Acute Postoperative Pain, Common Starting Doses (Patient-Controlled Analgesia [PCA]) in Opiate-Naïve Patients

Generic Name	Demand Dose (PCA Dose)	Basal Rate (Continuous Infusion)	Equipotency to 1 mg of Parenteral Morphine	Comments
Fentanyl	10–25 mcg q3–5 min	25–50 mcg/h	25 mcg	Lipophilicity may lead to accumulation; 100 mcg/h infusion approximates morphine 4 mg/h
Hydromorphone	0.1–0.2 mg q6–10 min	0.1–0.2 mg/h	0.15–0.2 mg	Minimal histamine release compared to morphine, no active metabolites
Meperidine	5–10 mg q6–10 min	5–10 mg/h	10 mg	Not commonly used; anticholinergic side effects; normeperidine accumulation can lead to CNS excitation and seizures
Morphine	0.5–1 mg q6–8 min	0.5–1 mg/h	1 mg	Morphine-6-glucuronide can accumulate in renal insufficiency leading to overdose
Methadone	0.5–1 mg q6–10 min	0.5–1 mg/h	1 mg	Protein binding and lipophilicity may lead to accumulation, dose reductions may be appropriate after loading period
Oxymorphone	50–100 mcg q6–10 min	50–100 mcg/h	0.1 mg	Recently offered on the market as immediate release and sustained oral preparations.

assessment, and an understanding of the pathophysiology and pharmacology of pain forms the foundation of the management of cancer pain.

REFERENCES

1. Bruera E, Lawlor P. Cancer pain management. *Acta Anaesthesiol Scand.* 1997;41:146–153.
2. Jacox A, Carr DB, Payne R, et al. *Management of Cancer Pain: Clinical Practice Guideline no. 9.* Rockville, MD: US Department of Health and Human Services, Public Health Service; 1994. AHCPR publication. 94-O592.
3. Warfield CA, ed. *Manual of Pain Management.* Philadelphia: Lippincott; 1991.
4. Rosner HL: The pharmacologic management of postoperative pain. In: Lefkowitz M, Lebovits A, Wlody D, et al., eds. *A Practical Approach to Pain Management.* Boston: Little Brown and Co.; 1996.
5. Dolin SJ, Cashman JN, Bland JM. Effectiveness of acute postoperative pain management: I. Evidence from published data. *Br J Anaesth.* 2002;89:409–423.
6. Niv D, Devor M. Transition from acute to chronic pain. In: Aronoff GM, ed. *Evaluation and Treatment of Chronic Pain,* 3rd ed. Baltimore: Williams & Wilkins, 1998.
7. Merskey H, Bogduk N, eds. Classification of chronic pain: descriptions of chronic pain syndromes and definition of pain terms. *Report by the International Association for the Study of Pain Task Force on Taxonomy.* 2nd ed. Seattle: IASP Press, 1994.
8. Fitzgerald M, Millard C, McIntosh N. Cutaneous hypersensitivity following peripheral tissue damage in newborn infants and its reversal with topical anesthesia. *Pain.* 1989;39:31–36.
9. Carr DB. Preempting the memory of pain. *JAMA.* 1998;279:1114–1115.
10. Portenoy RK, Foley KM, Inturrisi CE. The nature of opioid responsiveness and its implications for neuropathic pain: new hypotheses derived from studies of opioid infusions. *Pain.* 1990;43:273–286.
11. Cherny NI, Portenoy RK. Cancer pain: principles of assessment and syndromes. In: Wall PD, Melzack R, eds. *Textbook of Pain,* 5th ed. Edinburgh: Churchill Livingstone, 2005.
12. Portenoy RK. Lesage P. Management of cancer pain. *Lancet.* 1999; 353:1695–1700.
13. Portenoy RK, Hagen NA. Breakthrough pain: definition, prevalence and characteristics. *Pain.* 1990;41:273–281.
14. Mercadante S, Radbruch L, Caraceni A et al. Episodic (breakthrough) pain: consensus conference of an expert working group of the European Association for Palliative Care. *Cancer.* 2002;94:832–839.
15. Cherny NI. How to deal with difficult pain problems. *Ann Oncol.* 2005;16(Suppl 2):ii79–ii87.
16. Bercovitch M, Adunsky A. Patterns of high-dose morphine use in a home-care hospice service: should we be afraid of it? *Cancer.* 2004; 101:1473–1477.
17. Schug SA, Zech D, Grond S et al. A long-term survey of morphine in cancer pain patients. *J Pain Symptom Manage.* 1992;7:259–266.
18. Mao J. Opioid-induced abnormal pain sensitivity. *Curr Pain Headache Rep.* 2006;10:67–70.
19. Indelicato RA, Portenoy RK. Opioid rotation in the management of refractory cancer pain. *J Clin Oncol.* 2002;20:348–352.
20. American Pain Society. *Principles of Analgesic Use in the Treatment of Acute Pain and Cancer Pain.* Skokie, IL: American Pain Society; 1992.

21. Brunton L, Lazo J, Parker K. *Goodman & Gilman's The Pharmacological Basis of Therapeutics,* 11th ed. New York: McGraw-Hill Medical Publishing; 2005.

22. Derby S, Chin J, Portenoy RK. Systemic opioid therapy for chronic cancer pain: practical guidelines for converting drugs and routes of administration. *CNS Drugs.* 1998;9:99–109.

23. Bruera E. Kim HN. Cancer pain. *JAMA.* 2003;290:2476–2479.

24. Cherny N, Ripamonti C, Pereira J, et al. Strategies to manage the adverse effects of oral morphine: an evidence-based report. *J Clin Oncol.* 2001;19:2542–2554.

25. Breitbart W. Psychotropic adjuvant analgesics for pain in cancer and AIDS. *PsychoOncol.* 1998;7:333–345.

26. Portenoy RK. Adjuvant analgesics in pain management. In: Doyle D, Hanks GW, MacDonald N, eds. *Oxford Textbook of Palliative Medicine.* New York: Oxford University Press; 1998:361–390.

27. Dafermou A, Colamussi P, Giganti M, et al. A multicentre observational study of radionuclide therapy in patients with painful bone metastases of prostate cancer. *Eur J Nucl Med.* 2001;28:788–798.

28. Waldman SD, Leak DW, Kennedy LD, et al. Intraspinal opioid therapy. In: Patt RB, ed. *Cancer Pain.* Philadelphia: JB Lippincott; 1993: 285–38.

29. Smith TJ, Staats PS, Deer T, et al. Randomized clinical trial of an implantable drug delivery system compared with comprehensive medical management for refractory cancer pain: impact on pain, drug-related toxicity, and survival. *J Clin Oncol.* 2002;20:4040–4049.

30. Muir A, Molloy AR. Neuraxial implants for pain control. *Int Anesthesiol Clin.* 1997;35:171–196.

31. Deer TR, Caraway DL, Kim CK, et al. Clinical experience with intrathecal bupivacaine in combination with opioid for the treatment of chronic pain related to failed back surgery syndrome and metastatic cancer pain of the spine. *Spine J.* 2002;2:274–278.

32. Obata H, Li X, Eisenach JC. Spinal adenosine receptor activation reduces hypersensitivity after surgery by a different mechanism than after nerve injury. *Anesthesiology.* 2004;100:1258–1262.

33. Middleton JW, Siddall PJ, Walker S, et al. Intrathecal clonidine and baclofen in the management of spasticity and neuropathic pain following spinal cord injury: a case study. *Arch Phys Med Rehabil.* 1996; 77:824–826.

34. Wermeling DP. Ziconotide, an intrathecally administered N-type calcium channel antagonist for the treatment of chronic pain. *Pharmacotherapy.* 2005;25:1084–1094.

35. Miguel R. Interventional treatment of cancer pain: the fourth step in the World Health Organization analgesic ladder? *Cancer Control.* 2000;7:149–156.

36. Cherney NI. The management of cancer pain. *CA Cancer J Clin.* 2000;50:70–116.

37. Li X, Angst MS, Clark JD. Opioid-induced hyperalgesia and incisional pain. *Anesth Analg.* 2001;93:204–209.

38. Hayes C, Armstrong-Brown A, Burstal R. Perioperative intravenous ketamine infusion for the prevention of persistent postamputation pain: a randomized, controlled trial. *Anaesth Intensive Care.* 2004;32:330–338.

39. Bell RF, Dahl JB, Moore RA, et al. Perioperative ketamine for acute postoperative pain. *Cochrane Database Syst Rev.* 2006;(1): CD004603.

40. Behar M, Magora F, Olshwang D, et al. Epidural morphine in treatment of pain. *Lancet.* 1979;i:527–529.

41. Magora F, Olshwang D, Eimrei D, et al. Observations on extradural morphine analgesia in various pain conditions. *Br J Anaesth.* 1980; 52:247–252.

42. Bromage PR, Camporesi EM, Durant PA, et al. Nonrespiratory side effects of epidural morphine. *Anesth Analg.* 1982;61:490–495.

43. Camporesi EM, Nielsen CH, Bromage PR, et al. Ventilatory CO_2 sensitivity after intravenous and epidural morphine in volunteers. *Anesth Analg.* 1983;62:633–640.

44. Gourlay GK, Cherry DA, Cousins MJ. Cephalad migration of morphine in CSF following lumbar epidural administration in patients with cancer pain. *Pain.* 1985;23:317–326.

45. Bromage PR, Camporesi EM, Durant PA, et al. Rostral spread of epidural morphine. *Anesthesiology.* 1982;56:431–436.

46. Lubenow TR, Tanck EN, Hopkins EM, et al. Comparison of patient-assisted epidural analgesia for postoperative patients. *Reg Anesth.* 1994;19:206–211.

47. Sveticic G. Gentilini A, Eichenberger U, et al. Combinations of bupivacaine, fentanyl, and clonidine for lumbar epidural postoperative analgesia: a novel optimization procedure. *Anesthesiology.* 2004;101:1381–1393.

48. Weinbroum AA. Superiority of postoperative epidural over intravenous patient-controlled analgesia in orthopedic oncologic patients. *Surgery.* 2005;138:869–876.

49. Blake DW, Stainsby GV, Bjorksten AR. Patient-controlled epidural versus intravenous pethidine to supplement epidural bupivacaine after abdominal aortic surgery. *Anaesth Intensive Care.* 1998;26:630–635.

50. Niiyama Y, Kawamata T, Shimizu H, et al. The addition of epidural morphine to ropivacaine improves epidural analgesia after lower abdominal surgery. *Can J Anaesth.* 2005;52:181–185.

51. Nordberg G. Pharmacokinetic aspects of spinal morphine analgesia. *Acta Anaesthesiol Scand Suppl.* 1984;79:1–38.

52. Gourlay GK, Murphy TM, Plummer JL, et al. Pharmacokinetics of fentanyl in lumbar and cervical CSF following lumbar epidural and intravenous administration. *Pain.* 1989;38:253–259.

53. Saunders C. The philosophy of terminal care. In: Saunders C, ed. *The Management of Terminal Malignant Disease.* London: Edward Arnold; 1984:232–241.

54. Cassell EJ. The nature of suffering and the goals of medicine. *N Engl J Med.* 1982;306:639–645.

55. Cherny NI, Coyle N, Foley KM. Suffering in the advanced cancer patient: a definition and taxonomy. *J Palliat Care.* 1994;10:57–70.

COMMENTARY
Karen S. Sibert

Whether or not we agree with the currently popular concept of pain as "the fifth vital sign" to be assessed quantitatively along with blood pressure, temperature, pulse, and respiratory rates, there is no question that control of pain receives much public attention today and is considered a right rather than a privilege for patients. The state of California recently instituted a requirement for all physicians to complete 12 hours of continuing medical education in pain management and end-of-life care as a condition for license renewal. As Dr. Rosner has discussed, poorly managed postoperative pain causes patients emotional and physiologic stress, and increases the risk for development of chronic pain syndromes. The focus of this commentary will be on the anesthesiologist's role in perioperative pain management, and specifically on the management of intraspinal (both epidural and intrathecal) techniques in major oncologic surgeries.

PATIENT SELECTION

At Cedars-Sinai Medical Center, the option of epidural analgesia as an adjunct to general anesthesia is offered routinely to many patients undergoing major upper abdominal and open thoracic operations. A number of studies have documented improved respiratory function as measured by spirometry, improved ability to cough and clear secretions, and earlier mobilization when epidural analgesia is working well to control pain (1–4). At Cedars-Sinai Medical Center, we sometimes use epidural analgesia for lower abdominal procedures such as colectomy, but the benefits are less clear-cut as postoperative respiratory function is less impaired. There appears to be little reason to provide epidural analgesia for laparoscopy-assisted cases because the analgesic requirements of these patients are reduced, or for thoracoscopic cases unless bilateral thoracoscopy is required. The rest of this discussion therefore should be assumed to apply to open cases in which upper midline, chevron, or thoracotomy incisions are planned.

There are some absolute contraindications to epidural analgesia, and a few relative contraindications. Coagulopathy or thrombocytopenia could result in the development of epidural hematoma; if recognized promptly, a hematoma can be surgically evacuated, but otherwise could lead to permanent neurologic damage, including paraplegia. Infection near the planned insertion site or systemic sepsis could lead to epidural abscess formation. Prior history of neurologic disease such as spinal stenosis, disk disease, diabetic polyneuropathy, or other peripheral neuropathy is not an absolute contraindication but increases the risk for neurologic complications (5). Previous spinal surgery may distort or obliterate the epidural space and cause difficulty with catheter insertion; even if a catheter is placed, epidural medications may not spread evenly, and the analgesia may be suboptimal. Patient refusal or reluctance must be taken seriously, and the patient must be informed of the risks of epidural catheter insertion including failure, headache, back pain, and potential damage to nerve roots or spinal cord. It is vitally important that the patient be able to communicate well with caregivers if epidural analgesia is contemplated, as continuous assessment of neurologic function as well as pain control is critical in the postoperative period. For this reason, impaired cognitive function is a contraindication, and language barrier also may be an issue unless fluent interpreters are immediately available.

TIMING OF CATHETER INSERTION

Surgeons occasionally are reluctant to request epidural analgesia because of the extra time needed to place a catheter before surgery begins. We have found that to be a minor issue. With advance planning, the surgical team is aware of the plan for epidural analgesia but does not need to be present for catheter placement, and can make rounds or attend to other duties during the 15 to 20 minutes needed by an experienced anesthesiologist. Although some anesthesiologists are comfortable inserting an epidural catheter in an anesthetized adult patient at the end of the case, there are strong arguments to be made against this practice (6,7). The most devastating complication of epidural catheter insertion—direct injury to the spinal cord or a major

nerve root—may be heralded by localized or radiating pain, or by a marked paresthesia, in an awake patient. The needle then may be redirected or the procedure abandoned altogether, avoiding a catastrophic event such as direct intracordal injection of local anesthetic. We typically provide sedation with midazolam and small increments of fentanyl to achieve a state wherein the patient is very relaxed but able to cooperate with positioning and able to respond to questions about pain or paresthesia during both needle and catheter insertion. If a patient is anxious or uncooperative enough to make this impractical, perhaps another form of postoperative analgesia should be recommended.

Another reason to place the epidural catheter prior to surgery is that it is not uncommon for a dilutional coagulopathy to develop during lengthy operations such as a Whipple procedure or hepatic resection. As long as the patient has normal coagulation parameters prior to the start of the procedure, we do not consider this risk to contraindicate epidural catheter placement. Even in vascular procedures in which complete heparinization is necessary, epidural anesthesia is accepted practice as long as there is an adequate interval (an hour is usually recommended) between insertion of the catheter and anticoagulation. In our patients, epidural catheters are left in place postoperatively for up to 72 hours, which allows ample time for correction of any coagulation abnormalities with appropriate blood products before the catheter is removed. If insertion of the epidural catheter is deferred to the end of the case, a number of patients would be ineligible for epidural analgesia because of abnormal coagulation parameters and thus would be deprived of the benefits.

THROMBOTIC RISK IN ONCOLOGY PATIENTS

Trousseau first described the association between thromboembolic events and visceral cancers in 1861, and it is well acknowledged that patients with pancreatic, pelvic, and other malignant tumors are at increased risk of deep venous thrombosis (DVT) and pulmonary embolism in the perioperative period. For this reason, many surgeons prescribe injections of subcutaneous heparin, or more recently low-molecular-weight heparins (LMWHs), for these patients. Several questions arise in relation to epidural analgesia. If a patient is already receiving subcutaneous heparin or LWMH, should an epidural catheter be inserted at all, and if so, how much time needs to elapse between the last dose and catheter insertion? Is it necessary or safe to administer subcutaneous heparin or LMWH while an epidural catheter is in place? How long a time interval should elapse between removing an epidural catheter and instituting therapy with heparin or LWMH?

Some of these questions have been addressed in the context of orthopaedic joint-replacement surgery, in which there is a known risk of thromboembolism but a decreased incidence if the surgery is performed under regional anesthesia (spinal or epidural) as opposed to general anesthesia (8). After a number of case reports described the development of epidural or spinal hematomas in orthopaedic patients who received regional anesthesia and LWMH, the American Society of Regional Anesthesia developed a consensus statement to guide practitioners (9). The group's recommendations may be summarized briefly:

- Subcutaneous prophylaxis with unfractionated heparin presents no contraindication to regional anesthesia. Heparin should be withheld for 1 hour after needle placement, and an indwelling epidural catheter should be removed 2 to 4 hours after the last heparin dose.
- Prophylaxis with LMWH is not an absolute contraindication to regional anesthetic techniques, but greater caution is necessary. Needle placement should take place not less than 12 hours after low-dose prophylaxis, or 24 hours after a higher dose with confirmation of normal coagulation studies. Epidural catheter removal should occur 10 to 12 hours after the last dose. Subsequent dosing of LWMH should be deferred until 2 hours after catheter removal.

In our practice, we have chosen to avoid the use of preoperative use of unfractionated heparin or LWMH when epidural anesthesia is planned for our major oncology cases. Rigorous attention is paid to the application of sequential compression devices before the induction of general anesthesia and their continuation in the postoperative period. It has been our observation that epidural analgesia increases the likelihood of immediate postoperative extubation in these patients, so that they need no sedation and are able to move their extremities on the day of surgery. The majority are able to be up in a chair or ambulating on the first postoperative day. If a patient is not moving well, subcutaneous unfractionated heparin is started after the epidural catheter is removed, usually on the second or third postoperative day. We have not seen any patient in our large series develop DVT or pulmonary embolism using this approach. If a patient has a pre-existing condition requiring anticoagulation or antiplatelet therapy (previous DVT or pulmonary embolism, chronic atrial fibrillation, anticardiolipin antibody, drug-eluting coronary stent), then epidural analgesia is not used and the patient's usual therapy is resumed as soon as possible after surgery.

THORACIC VERSUS LUMBAR EPIDURAL ANALGESIA

Anesthesiologists learn the technique of epidural catheter insertion at the lumbar level, which is used for obstetric anesthesia and for surgery of the lower extremities or lower abdomen. The technique is very safe because the needle is inserted caudad to the spinal cord, which terminates at the level of vertebrae L1 or L2 in 95% of adult patients. However, the lumbar approach is suboptimal for analgesia in upper abdominal or thoracic cases. Superior analgesia is obtained by insertion of the epidural catheter at the lower thoracic level for upper abdominal incisions or at the midthoracic level for thoracotomy. This allows infusion of local anesthetic solutions directly at the level of the source of pain, producing a segmental block, which is highly effective. Thoracic epidural analgesia with low-concentration local anesthetic solutions does not block the lumbar sympathetic nerves, thus avoiding vasodilation of the lower extremities and the hypotension that can result.

Lastly, the use of thoracic epidural analgesia permits the patient to ambulate with the catheter in place, which encourages early mobilization, improves pulmonary function, and reduces the risk of thromboembolic complications. Because a thoracic epidural catheter by definition is inserted cephalad to the termination of the spinal cord, it is inherently a higher risk technique, and its use should be restricted to anesthesiologists with substantial experience.

INTRAOPERATIVE AND POSTOPERATIVE MANAGEMENT

Major oncologic surgeries may be prolonged and often are associated with blood loss and fluid shifts. Our practice for upper abdominal and thoracic cases is to place the thoracic epidural catheter first and then induce general anesthesia. Arterial, central venous, and/or pulmonary artery catheters are inserted once the patient is asleep. With a functioning epidural catheter in place, it is always tempting to make use of it by injecting local anesthetic solutions as part of the anesthesia during the case: the "combined epidural-general" technique. However, if local anesthetics such as bupivacaine or lidocaine are used in a high enough concentration to provide surgical anesthesia, they inevitably will block the sympathetic chain as well and can lead to hemodynamic instability. The sudden onset of surgical bleeding, which may happen even in the most careful hands, will be more difficult to manage and can result in profound hypotension. In elderly patients, particularly those with atherosclerotic disease, permanent neurologic injury from anterior spinal artery syndrome (10) or spinal cord infarction (11) has been described.

Our preference, therefore, is to test the epidural catheter after insertion but not activate it fully until the operation is concluding, when the tumor has been removed and any major blood loss has ended. The only medication usually given via the epidural catheter early in the case is preservative-free morphine. Epidural morphine is the most hydrophilic of the narcotics, which makes it take longer to be absorbed into the cerebrospinal fluid (CSF) but allows it to remain sequestered in the CSF for longer than other narcotics. The onset of action of epidural morphine is approximately 1 hour and the duration of action varies from 10 to 24 hours. Giving epidural morphine early during the surgery helps minimize the amount of parenteral narcotics needed during the general anesthetic, and contributes to the patient waking up in less pain and more alert. The usual dose is 2.5 to 4 mg, with the lower dose recommended for older and more fragile patients. Epidural morphine alone does not significantly affect systemic vascular resistance or blood pressure.

As surgical wound closure is beginning, the concentration of anesthetic gas breathed by the patient is reduced, and we begin to titrate in a loading dose of 0.125% bupivacaine in combination with fentanyl. The dose range again is adjusted to the patient's age and size, but usually consists of 5 to 10 mL of 0.125% bupivacaine with 50 to 100 mcg of fentanyl. At the conclusion of the case, muscle relaxation is reversed and the patient is extubated if respiratory effort and oxygen saturation are satisfactory. If the patient complains of pain, additional bupivacaine and fentanyl may be administered. On arrival in the postanesthesia recovery area, a continuous epidural infusion of bupivacaine and fentanyl is started promptly. The usual solution is bupivacaine 0.05% to 0.0625% with fentanyl 5 mcg/mL, at a rate of 4 to 8 mL/h. When the patient is alert enough, he or she is instructed in the use of patient-controlled epidural analgesia, which allows the patient to self-administer an additional dose of 2 to 4 mL when needed to supplement the continuous infusion. The advantage of fentanyl, which is a very lipid-soluble narcotic, is that the onset of action is fast and a constant plasma level of drug is reached. This works in concert with the segmental block provided by the bupivacaine. Thus, a patient with a xiphoid-to-pubis midline incision, or an Ivor-Lewis esophagectomy, can still be maintained in relative comfort as the narcotic helps to relieve pain in the lower portion of the incision that is not covered by the local anesthetic in the thoracic epidural space.

With appropriate education of nursing staff, we do not find it necessary to send patients to the intensive care unit just because of a thoracic epidural infusion. Vital signs are monitored per routine. The nursing staff understands that no motor block of the lower extremities is expected with a thoracic epidural infusion, and that the new onset of any motor block should be reported immediately to a physician. Severe hypotension is rarely a problem, but a relative decrease in blood pressure usually reflects a need for additional volume infusion. The Department of Anesthesiology at Cedars-Sinai Medical Center always has an anesthesiologist specializing in pain management on call to cover acute pain issues, and during the day both an anesthesiologist and a pain service nurse make rounds on all patients with epidural infusions. Side effects such as nausea and pruritus are seldom severe, and respond to treatment with antiemetics and diphenhydramine.

INTRATHECAL NARCOTICS

One useful tool that should not be overlooked is the administration of intraspinal narcotics as an alternative to epidural analgesia. Preservative-free morphine in combination with fentanyl or sufentanil may be injected directly into the CSF at the lumbar level as a one-time dose. Technically, intrathecal injections are easier than epidural catheter placement, with an easily identifiable goal of aspirating CSF. This technique can be very helpful for the patient who has had previous spinal surgery with probable obliteration of the epidural space. We have also used it to good effect when a thoracoscopic case has turned unexpectedly into an open thoracotomy, and I often use it at the end of abdominal aortic aneurysm repair after all coagulation parameters are normalized. Although we avoid placing a thoracic epidural catheter in an already anesthetized patient, the injec-

tion of spinal narcotics at the lumbar level has a long record of safe use (12) and can be performed easily at the end of surgery by turning the patient to the lateral position before emergence from anesthesia. The combination of fentanyl (25 to 50 mcg) and preservative-free morphine (0.5 to 0.8 mg) provides onset of analgesia within 15 minutes and duration of action from 12 to 24 hours.

REFERENCES

1. Bromage PR. Spirometry in assessment of analgesia after abdominal surgery. *Br J Anaesth.* 1955;2:539–542.
2. Craig DB. Post-operative recovery of pulmonary function. *Anesth Analg.* 1981;60:46–52.
3. Simpson BP, Parkhouse J, Marshall R, et al. Extradural analgesia and the prevention of post-operative respiratory complications. *Br J Anaesth.* 1961;33:623–641.
4. Yeager MP, Glass DD, Nett RF, et al. Epidural anesthesia and analgesia in high-risk surgical patients. *Anesthesiology.* 1987;66:729–736.
5. Hebl JR, Kopp SL, Schroeder DR, et al. Neurologic complications after neuraxial anesthesia or analgesia in patients with preexisting peripheral sensorimotor neuropathy or diabetic polyneuropathy. *Anesth Analg.* 2006;103:1294–1299.
6. Kao MC, Tsai SK, Tsou MY, et al. Paraplegia after delayed detection of inadvertent spinal cord injury during thoracic epidural catheterization in an anesthetized elderly patient. *Anesth Analg.* 2004;99:580–583.
7. Rosenquist RW, Birnback DJ. Epidural insertion in anesthetized adults: will your patients thank you? *Anesth Analg.* 2003;96:1545–1546.
8. Modig J, Borg T, Karlstrom G, et al. Thromboembolism after total hip replacement: role of epidural and general anesthesia. *Anesth Analg.* 1983;62:174–180.
9. American Society of Regional Anesthesia and Pain Medicine. Second Consensus Conference on Neuraxial Anesthesia and Anticoagulation. *Reg Anesth Pain Med.* 2003;28:172–197.
10. Hong DK, Lawrence HM. Anterior spinal artery syndrome following total hip arthroplasty under epidural anesthesia. *Anaesth Intensive Care.* 2001;29:62–66.
11. Weinbert L, Harvey WR, Marshall RJ. Post-operative paraplegia following spinal cord infarction. *Acta Anaesthesiol Scand.* 2002;46:469–472.
12. Gwirtz KH. Intraspinal narcotics in the management of postoperative pain: the Acute Pain Service at Indiana University Hospital. *Anesthesiol Rev.* 1990;17:16–28.

Index

Page numbers followed by *f* indicate figures; page numbers followed by *t* indicate tables.

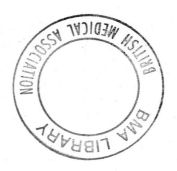